Universal Precautions

Human immunodeficiency virus (HIV), the virus that causes acquired immunodeficiency syndrome (AIDS), is transmitted during sexual contact, through the sharing of intravenous drug needles and syringes while "shooting" drugs, through exposure to infected blood or blood components, and perinatally from mother to neonate. Currently there is neither a cure for nor an immunization to prevent AIDS. The increasing prevalence of HIV increases the risk that health care workers will be exposed to blood from patients infected with HIV.

The Centers for Disease Control in Atlanta has developed "Universal Precautions" (formerly called "Universal Blood and Body Fluid Precautions") as recommendations to all health care workers. Under universal precautions, blood and certain body fluids of **all** patients are considered potentially infectious for HIV, hepatitis B virus (HBV), and other bloodborne pathogens. Universal Precautions are intended to prevent parenteral, mucous membrane, and nonintact skin exposures of health care workers to bloodborne pathogens. In addition, immunization with HBV vaccine is recommended as an important adjunct to universal precautions for health care workers who have been exposed to blood. (The implementation of control measures for HIV and HBV does not obviate the need for continued adherence to general infection-control principles and general hygiene measures.) The following is a summary of the CDC's recommendations.

BODY FLUIDS TO WHICH UNIVERSAL PRECAUTIONS APPLY

Universal precautions apply to blood and other body fluids containing visible blood. **Blood is the single most important source of HIV, HBV, and other bloodborne pathogens in the health care facility.** Infection control efforts for HIV, HBV, and other bloodborne pathogens must focus on both preventing exposures to blood and delivering HBV immunization. Universal precautions also apply to semen and vaginal secretions, tissues, and the following fluids: cerebrospinal, synovial, pleural, peritoneal, pericardial, and amniotic.

BODY FLUIDS TO WHICH UNIVERSAL PRECAUTIONS DO NOT APPLY

Universal precautions *do not* apply to feces, nasal secretions, sputum, sweat, tears, urine, and vomitus unless they contain visible blood. The risk of transmission of HIV or HBV from these fluids is extremely low or nonexistent.

GENERAL PRECAUTIONS

- Use universal precautions for **all** patients.
- Use appropriate barrier precautions routinely when contact with blood or other body fluids of any patient is anticipated.

    Wear gloves when touching blood and body fluids, mucous membranes, or nonintact skin; when handling items or surfaces soiled with blood or body fluids; and when performing venipuncture and other vascular access procedures.

    Change gloves after each contact with patients.

    Wear masks and protective eyewear or face shields during procedures that are likely to generate drops of blood or other body fluids to prevent exposure of mucous membranes of mouth, nose, and eyes.

    Wear gowns or aprons during procedures that are likely to generate splashes of blood or other body fluids.

- Wash hands and other skin surfaces immediately and thoroughly if contaminated with blood or other body fluids.
- Wash hands immediately after gloves are removed.
- Take precautions to prevent injuries caused by needles, scalpels, and other sharp instruments or devices during procedures; when cleaning used instruments; during disposal of used needles; and when handling sharp instruments after procedures.

    Discard needle units uncapped and unbroken after use.

    Place disposable syringes and needles, scalpel blades, and other sharp items in puncture-resistant containers.

    Place puncture-resistant containers as near as practical to the area of use.

- Although saliva has not been implicated, to minimize the need for emergency mouth-to-mouth resuscitation, make mouthpieces, resuscitation bags, or other ventilation devices available for use in areas where the need for resuscitation is predictable.
- If you have exudative lesions or weeping dermatitis refrain from all direct patient care and from handling patient care equipment until the condition resolves.

PRECAUTIONS FOR INVASIVE PROCEDURES

- If you participate in invasive procedures, use appropriate barrier methods: gloves, surgical masks, protective eyewear, face shields, gowns, and aprons.
- If you perform or assist in vaginal or cesarean deliveries, wear gloves and gowns when handling the placenta or the infant until blood and amniotic fluid have been removed from the infant's skin and during postdelivery care of the umbilical cord.
- If a glove is torn or a needlestick or other injury occurs, remove the gloves and use a new glove as promptly as patient safety permits; remove the needle or instrument used in the incident from the sterile field.

ENVIRONMENTAL CONSIDERATIONS

- Standard sterilization and disinfection procedures currently recommended for use in health care settings are adequate.
- Sterilize instruments or devices that enter sterile tissue or the vascular system before reuse.
- Clean and remove soiled surfaces on walls, floors, and other surfaces routinely; extraordinary attempts to disinfect or sterilize are not necessary.
- Use chemical germicides approved as hospital disinfectants (and tuberculocidals) to decontaminate spills of blood and other body fluids.

PRECAUTIONS WITH SOILED LINEN

- Observe hygienic and common-sense storage and processing of clean and soiled linens.
- Handle soiled linen as little as possible and with minimum agitation.
- Bag all soiled linen at the location where it is used.
- Place and transport linen soiled with blood or body fluids in bags that prevent leakage.

INFECTIVE WASTE

- It is practical to identify those wastes with the potential for causing infection during handling and disposal and for which some special precautions seem prudent (e.g., microbiology laboratory waste, pathology waste, and blood specimens or blood products).
- Incinerate or autoclave infective waste before disposal in a sanitary landfill.
- Carefully pour bulk blood, suctioned fluids, excretions, and secretions down a drain connected to a sanitary sewer.

From Guidelines for Prevention of Transmission of Human Immunodeficiency Virus and Hepatitis B Virus to Health-Care and Public-Safety Workers. U.S. Department of Health and Human Services, Centers for Disease Control, Atlanta, GA, February 1989; Update: Universal Precautions for Prevention of Transmission of Human Immunodeficiency Virus, Hepatitis B Virus, and Other Bloodborne Pathogens in Health-Care Settings. Morbidity and Mortality Weekly Report, 1988; Recommendations for Prevention of HIV Transmission in Health-Care Settings. Morbidity and Mortality Weekly Report, 1987.

Fundamentals of
NURSING

Ruth F. Craven, EdD, RN
Assistant Dean, Continuing Nursing Education
Associate Professor
School of Nursing
University of Washington
Seattle, WA

Constance J. Hirnle, MN, RN
Lecturer, School of Nursing
University of Washington
Seattle, WA

Fundamentals of
NURSING

Human Health and Function

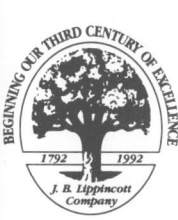

J.B. LIPPINCOTT COMPANY
Philadelphia

New York   London   Hagerstown

Dedication

To Bob, Scott, John, and Sarah Hirnle
Bill, Brent, Judy, and Kyle Craven
for their love, support, sacrifice, and encouragement that allowed us to make this book a reality.

Sponsoring Editor: Donna L. Hilton, BSN, RN
Developmental Editor: Eleanor Faven
Editorial Assistant: Susan Perry
Project Editor: Mary Rose Muccie
Indexer: Alexandra Nickerson
Designer: Holly Reid McLaughlin
Design Coordinator: Susan Hermansen
Production Manager: Helen Ewan
Compositor: Circle Graphics
Printer/Binder: Courier Westford

1 3 5 6 4 2

Library of Congress Cataloging-in-Publication Data
Craven, Ruth F.
    Fundamentals of nursing : human health and function /
Ruth F. Craven, Constance J. Hirnle.
        p.   cm.
    Includes bibliographical references and index.
    ISBN 0-397-54669-6
    1. Nursing.   I. Hirnle, Constance J.   II. Title.
    [DNLM: 1. Health Promotion—nurses' instruction.
    2. Nursing.   3. Nursing Process.   WY 100 C898f]
RT41.C86   1992
610.73—dc20
DNLM/DLC
for Library of Congress   91-29838
                                              CIP

Any procedure or practice described in this book should be applied by the health-care practitioner under appropriate supervision in accordance with professional standards of care used with regard to the unique circumstances that apply in each practice situation. Care has been taken to confirm the accuracy of information presented and to describe generally accepted practices. However, the authors, editors, and publisher cannot accept any responsibility for errors or omissions or for any consequences from application of the information in this book and make no warranty, express or implied, with respect to the contents of the book.

Every effort has been made to ensure drug selections and dosages are in accordance with current recommendations and practice. Because of ongoing research, changes in government regulations and the constant flow of information on drug therapy, reactions and interactions, the reader is cautioned to check the package insert for each drug for indications, dosages, warnings and precautions, particularly if the drug is new or infrequently used.

Contributors

Joan M. Baker, MS, RN, CS
Clinical Nurse Specialist
Psychiatric Service
University of Washington Medical Center
Seattle, WA

Chapter 41:   Sensory Perception

Debra A. Beauchaine, MN, RN
Former Lecturer
School of Nursing
University of Washington
Seattle, WA

Chapter 37:   Urinary Elimination*
Chapter 38:   Bowel Elimination

Diane Britt, MN, RN
Medical-Surgical Clinical Nurse Specialist
University of Washington Medical Center
Seattle, WA

Chapter 42:   Cognitive Processes

Margaret Bruya, DNSc, RN, C
Associate Professor
Intercollegiate Center for Nursing Education
Spokane, WA

Chapter 5:   Nursing Research

Karen K. Carlson, MN, RN, CCRN
Critical Care Clinical Nurse Specialist
Group Health Cooperative of Puget Sound
Seattle, WA

Chapter 19:   Vital Sign Assessment*

Dona Marie Carpenter, EdD, RN
Assistant Professor of Nursing
Department of Nursing
University of Scranton
Scranton, PA

Chapter 1:   The Profession of Nursing: Theory, Education,
*   and Practice*

Ann Tyler Chadwick, MN, RN, CRRN
Clinical Instructor
School of Nursing
University of Washington
Seattle, WA

Chapter 25:   Safety

B. Jane Cornman, PhD, RN
Assistant Professor
Department of Parent-Child Nursing
University of Washington
Seattle, WA

Chapter 11:   Health and Wellness

Ruth F. Craven, EdD, RN
Assistant Dean
Continuing Nursing Education
and
Associate Professor
School of Nursing
University of Washington
Seattle, WA

Chapter 29: Body Mechanics and Mobility*

Teresa A. Delarose, MN, RN, CNOR
Lecturer
School of Nursing
Perioperative Staff Nurse
University of Washington Medical Center
University of Washington
and
Doctoral Candidate
Seattle University
Seattle, WA

Chapter 23:   Perioperative Nursing
Chapter 33:   Nutrition

Alice S. Demi, DNSc, FAAN
Professor
Georgia State University
Atlanta, GA

Chapter 46:   Loss and Grieving

*Chapter cowritten with another contributor.

Linda Dunn, MN, RN (deceased)
Former Nurse Educator
Providence Medical Center
Seattle, WA
and
Clinical Faculty
School of Nursing
University of Washington
Seattle, WA

Chapter 18:   Health Assessment of Human Function

Mary P. Farley, MN, RN, CCRN
Nursing Supervisor
Evergreen Hospital Medical Center
Kirkland, WA

Chapter 22:   Asepsis
Chapter 35:   The Body's Defenses Against Infection

Polly E. Gardner, MN, RN
Critical Care Clinical Nurse Specialist
Evergreen Hospital Medical Center
Kirkland, WA
and
Clinical Instructor
School of Nursing
University of Washington
Seattle, WA

*Chapter 24:   Medication Administration**

Laina M. Gerace, PhD, RN
Assistant Professor of Psychiatric Nursing
University of Illinois at Chicago
Chicago, IL

*Chapter 17:   Communication: The Nurse–Patient
   Relationship*

Mikell Goe, MN, RN, CCRN
Medical-Surgical Clinical Nurse Specialist
Evergreen Hospital Medical Center
Kirkland, WA
and
Clinical Instructor
School of Nursing
University of Washington
Seattle, WA

*Chapter 20:   Diagnostic Tests and Procedures**
*Chapter 31:   Oxygenation: Cardiac Function and Tissue
   Perfusion*

Joanne Woodhull Goepfert, MN, RN, PHC
Doctoral Candidate
Oregon Health Sciences University
Portland, OR

Chapter 28:   Self-Care and Hygiene

Mary Sue Gorski, MN, RNC
Assistant Professor
Lewis-Clark State College
Lewiston, ID

*Chapter 10:   Communication of the Nursing Process:
   Recording and Reporting*

Celia L. Hartley, MN, RN
Director of Nursing Education and Professor of Nursing
Shoreline Community College
Seattle, WA

Chapter 2:   The Health-Care Delivery System

Judy A. Hartmann, MSN, RN
Vice President for Nursing
Sacred Heart Rehabilitation Hospital
Milwaukee, WI

Chapter 44:   Communication: Social Interaction

Kathryn Van Dykes Hayes, MSN, RN, C
Doctoral Candidate
The Catholic University of America
Washington, DC

*Chapter 9:   Nursing Management: Planning,
   Implementation, and Evaluation*

Constance J. Hirnle, MN, RN
Lecturer
School of Nursing
University of Washington
Seattle, WA

*Chapter 29:   Body Mechanics and Mobility**

Emily Wurster Hitchins, EdD, RN
Associate Professor of Nursing
Seattle Pacific University
Seattle, WA

Chapter 16:   Values
Chapter 49:   Spiritual Health

L. Michele Issel, PhD, RN
Program Evaluator
Robert Wood Johnson/Pew Charitable Trusts
Providence Medical Center
Portland, OR

Chapter 27:   Home Maintenance Management

Don Johnson, PhD, RN
Associate Professor
University of Texas
Health Science Center
San Antonio, TX

Chapter 32:   Fluid, Electrolyte, and Acid-Base Balance

Ann E. Kelly, MSN, RNCS
Clinical Nurse Specialist
San Diego Veterans Affairs Medical Center
San Diego, CA

Chapter 43:   Self-Concept

Joy Miller Knopp, MN, RN, OCN
Oncology Clinical Nurse Specialist
Overlake Hospital Medical Center
Bellevue, WA

*Chapter 40:   Pain Perception and Comfort**

*Chapter cowritten with another contributor.

Kathleen Kovarik, MN, RN
Instructor
Intercollegiate Center for Nursing Education
Spokane, WA

Chapter 34: Skin Integrity and Wound Healing*

Claudia Kroll, MSEd, MSN, ARNP
Nursing Instructor
Spokane Community College
Spokane, WA

Chapter 34: Skin Integrity and Wound Healing*

Valerie G. Larson, MN, ARNP, CS
Project Coordinator, Fitness and Aging
University of Washington
Seattle, WA

Chapter 20: Diagnostic Tests and Procedures*

Alice Lind, BSN, RN
HIV/AIDS Consultant
Department of Health
Olympia, WA

Chapter 3: Ethical and Legal Concerns

Mary McGregor, MN, RN, CDE
Acute Care Clinical Nurse Specialist
General Hospital Medical Center
Everett, WA

Chapter 24: Medication Administration*

Beverly S. McKenna, MN, RN
Manager, Clinical Systems
Overlake Hospital Medical Center
Bellevue, WA

Chapter 40: Pain Perception and Comfort*

Kristine Iwersen Moore, MN, RN, CDE
Clinical Nurse Specialist
Group Health Cooperative of Puget Sound
Seattle, WA

Chapter 21: Patient Teaching

Marjorie A. Muecke, PhD, RN
Professor of Nursing
Adjunct Professor of Anthropology
and
Adjunct Professor of Health Services
University of Washington
Seattle, WA

Chapter 15: Culture and Ethnicity

Georgia R. Narsavage, PhD, RN
Assistant Professor
and
Director of RN Program
Department of Nursing
University of Scranton
Scranton, PA

Chapter 45: Families and Their Relationships

Ellen F. Olshansky, DNSc, RNC
Associate Professor
Department of Parent-Child Nursing
University of Washington
Seattle, WA

Chapter 48: Human Sexuality

Jane W. Peterson, PhD, RN
Professor
School of Nursing
Seattle University
Seattle, WA

Chapter 14: Individual, Family, and Community

Cheryl M. Prandoni, MSN, RNC
Director of Learning Resources
and
Adjunct Assistant Professor
School of Nursing
The Catholic University of America
Washington, DC

Chapter 12: Human Needs

Marlene Reimer, MN, RN
Assistant Professor of Nursing
The University of Calgary
Calgary, Alberta, Canada

Chapter 39: Sleep and Rest

Barbara J. Ruff, MN, RN
Case Manager, Adult Outpatient Service
Community Psychiatric Clinic
Seattle, WA

Chapter 47: Stress, Coping, and Adaptation

Jennifer M. Schaller-Ayres, MNSc, RN, C
Doctoral Student
Oregon Health Sciences University
Portland, OR

Chapter 26: Health Maintenance

Margaret L. Snyder, MN, RN, CCRN
Critical Care Clinical Nurse Specialist
Northwest Hospital
Seattle, WA

Chapter 19: Vital Sign Assessment*

Sheila M. Sparks, DNSc, RN, CS
Assistant Professor
Georgetown University
Washington, DC

Chapter 6: The Nursing Process in Human Health and Function
Chapter 7: Nursing Assessment
Chapter 8: Nursing Diagnosis

Karen A. Thomas, PhD, RN
Assistant Professor
Department of Parent-Child Nursing
University of Washington
Seattle, WA

Chapter 13: Lifespan Development

*Chapter cowritten with another contributor.

Wendy L. Walker, MN, RN
Lecturer
School of Nursing
University of Washington
Seattle, WA

*Chapter 37:   Urinary Elimination**

Lorraine A. Watson, PhD, RN
Assistant Professor
Faculty of Nursing
The University of Calgary
Calgary, Alberta, Canada

Chapter 36:   Thermoregulation

Karen S. Wulff, EdD, RN
Executive Staff Specialist
Swedish Hospital Medical Center
Seattle, WA

Chapter 4:   Leadership and Management

Special Contributions

Terry F. Cicero, MN, RN, CCRN
Lecturer
School of Nursing
University of Washington
Seattle, WA

Procedures

Joan M. Jenks, MSN
Assistant Professor
College of Allied Health Sciences
Department of Nursing
Thomas Jefferson University
Philadelphia, PA

Consultant

*Chapter cowritten with another contributor.

Reviewers

Donna Adams, DNSc, RN
Assistant Professor
Arizona State University
College of Nursing
Tempe, AZ

Janet S. Anderson, MSN, RN
Assistant Professor
Director of the Teaching and Learning Center
University of Rochester
School of Nursing
Rochester, NY

Mary Ann Anglim, ME, BSN, RN
Assistant Professor
University of Minnesota
School of Nursing
Minneapolis, MN

Shirley Bell, EdD, MSN, BSN, RN
Assistant Professor
Arizona State University
College of Nursing
Tempe, AZ

Barbara Boland, MSN, RN
Clinical Specialist, Educational Coordinator
Rehabilitation Center
Good Samaritan Hospital
Baltimore, MD

Penny S. Brooke, JD, MSN, RN
Associate Professor
University of Utah
College of Nursing
Salt Lake City, UT

Bonita M. Cavanaugh, PhD, RN
Assistant Professor
University of Colorado
School of Nursing
Denver, CO

Mary F. Crowley, MSN, BA, RN
Nursing Instructor
New England Baptist Hospital
School of Nursing
Boston, MA

Judy Davy, MHS, RN
Professor of Nursing
Humboldt State University
Arcata, CA

Susan Dudek, RD
Former Nutrition and Diet Therapy Instructor
Sisters Hospital School of Nursing
Buffalo, NY

Marjorie L. Garrity, MS, RN
Assistant Professor
Arizona State University
College of Nursing
Tempe, AZ

Judith A. Halstead, RNC, MSN
Lecturer in Nursing
Indiana University
School of Nursing
Indianapolis, IN

Phyllis G. Hummel, MSN, RN
Executive Director
Roger Maris Cancer Center
Fargo, ND

Mary Sue Jack, PhD, RN
Assistant Professor
University of Rochester
School of Nursing
Rochester, NY

Judy Johnson, PhD, MSN, RN
Assistant Professor
Indiana State University
School of Nursing
Terre Haute, IN

Margaret Ann Kerr, MSN, BS, RN, ANP
Medical University of South Carolina
College of Nursing
Charleston, SC

Mary L. Killeen, PhD, RN
Assistant Professor
Arizona State University
College of Nursing
Tempe, AZ

Kathryn Lackey, MSN, BSN, RN
Former Assistant Professor
Angelo State University
Department of Nursing
San Angelo, TX

Peggy Tracy Leapley, PhD, RN
Associate Professor
California State University
Bakersfield, CA

Ruth Lindquist, PhD, RN
Assistant Professor
University of Minnesota
School of Nursing
Minneapolis, MN

Judith Maroni, DNSc, RN, CS
Assistant Professor
Catholic University of America
School of Nursing
Washington, DC

Edwina A. McConnell, PhD, RN
Independent Nurse Consultant
Madison, WI

Faye Medley, MSN, RN
Assistant Professor
University of Florida
College of Nursing
Gainesville, FL

Sandra Millon-Underwood, PhD, RN
Assistant Professor
University of Wisconsin
School of Nursing
Milwaukee, WI

Suzanne M. Philip, MA, BEd, BScNEd, RN
Humber College
Health Sciences Division
Rexdale, Ontario, Canada

Mildred M. Russin, MSN, RN
Education Director
Division of Surgical Nursing
Shands Hospital at the University of Florida
Gainesville, FL

Mariah Snyder, PhD, RN, FAAN
Professor
University of Minnesota
School of Nursing
Minneapolis, MN

Barbara Thomas, EdD, RN
Associate Professor
University of Windsor
School of Nursing
Windsor, Ontario, Canada

Darla Ura, MN, RN
Instructor
Emory University
Nell Hodgson Woodruff School of Nursing
Atlanta, GA

Judith A. Vessey, PhD, RN, C
Associate Professor and Research Facilitator
University of Arkansas for Medical Sciences, and
    Arkansas Children's Hospital
Little Rock, AR

Nancy Wells, DNSc, RN
Clinical Nurse Researcher
Strong Memorial Hospital
and
Behavior Therapist
Pain Treatment Center
University of Rochester Medical Center
Rochester, NY

Ann Windsor, DNS, RN
Clinical Associate Professor
University of Wisconsin–Madison
School of Nursing
Madison, WI

Preface

"I use the word nursing for want of a better. It has been limited to signify little more than the administration of medicines and the application of polices. It ought to signify the proper use of fresh air, light, warmth, cleanliness, quiet and the proper selection and administration of diet—all at the least expense of vital power to the patient.

The same laws of health or of nursing, for they are in reality the same, obtain among the well as among the sick (Florence Nightingale (1859). Notes on Nursing: What It Is and What It Is Not. Reprint, J.B. Lippincott, 1946)."

Although more than a century has passed since Florence Nightingale wrote these words, her description of nursing is remarkably current. Nursing today includes attributes similar to those advocated by Florence Nightingale in 1860—the maintenance of health, the management of the environment and other factors, and care of the ill. Two basic premises of *Fundamentals of Nursing: Human Health and Function* relate to Florence Nightingale's beliefs.

The first is that the art and science of professional nursing practice focuses on the health, function, and wellness of the person with the goals of maintaining, supporting, and restoring health and function. Achieving these goals requires that the nurse promptly identify potential altered function and recognize manifestations of altered function and their impact on activities of daily living. The second premise is that contemporary nursing practice is based on the appropriate selection and use of nursing interventions. In nursing practice these activities involve the "diagnosis and treatment of human responses to potential or actual health problems" (ANA (1980). Nursing: A Social Policy Statement, Kansas City, MO, ANA).

Through the incorporation of both of these premises, we have attempted to create an innovative text that helps nursing faculty prepare beginning students for the challenging and dynamic nursing practice of today and tomorrow. The intent is to provide the beginning student with the knowledge base to assess a patient's ability to function independently, evaluate the patient's ability to cope with altered function, and intervene to maximize function. These nursing responsibilities are critical as health care delivery moves away from acute-care facilities and focuses on promoting the patient's self-responsibility. Both nurses and patients find themselves in a changing health care environment with evolving health care delivery patterns.

In this text, the person who seeks and receives health care services is referred to as a "patient." The authors have struggled with the use of the terms "client" and "patient" and are aware of the different meanings nurses attach to each term. We believe that "patient" conveys the vulnerability and health-sustaining needs of the person seeking health care. The use of "patient" is intended to imply both a high degree of compassion for the person and competence on the part of the nurse. This distinction seems particularly important in today's changing health care environment, in which a patient may be assigned a number and a physician, as in an HMO or PPO.

ORGANIZATION

The text is organized in two main sections, **Section I, Conceptual Foundations of Nursing,** and **Section II, Human Function and Clinical Nursing Therapeutics.**

Section I presents the professional and clinical concepts essential to nursing today. This section contains five units.

Unit I, Concepts Essential for Professional Nursing introduces the student to the profession of nursing. *Chapter 1, The Profession of Nursing: Theory, Education, and Practice* provides the foundation. A discussion of the nursing role within the health care delivery system follows in Chapter 2. The remaining chapters discuss topics that underscore nursing's vital role within that system: ethical and legal concerns, leadership and management, and nursing research.

Unit II, The Nursing Process: Framework for Clinical Nursing Therapeutics, introduces the beginning student to the nursing process and explores each component in detail. This unit discusses the skills and activities needed to assess a patient's health status, analyze and cluster data to formulate a nursing diagnosis, formulate a plan of care and select nursing interventions based on patient goals, and evaluate the effectiveness of those interventions using outcome criteria. The final chapter discusses all forms of recording and reporting, the communication aspect of the nursing process. This unit provides the framework for the application of the nursing process throughout the text.

Unit III, Concepts Essential for Human Function and Nursing Management, provides foundational concepts and knowledge about patients essential for providing safe, effective nursing care. This unit begins with a discussion of the concepts of health and wellness, illness, and human needs. *Chapter 13, Lifespan Development,* presents the concepts of human growth and development. The information in this chapter sets the stage for the "Lifespan Considerations" section in each nursing care chapter in Section II. Other chapters explore the individual as part of a family and a community, culture, ethnicity, and values. *Chapter 17, Communication: The Nurse–Patient Relationship* focuses on the skills needed to establish an effective nurse–patient relationship. This chapter has been coordinated with *Chapter 44, Communication: Social Interaction,* to focus strongly on communication and its importance in all human relationships.

Unit IV, Essential Assessment Components, explores the fundamental skills in each component of health assessment. *Chapter 18, Health Assessment of Human Function,* details an overall health assessment. The next chapter describes vital sign assessment. The final chapter in this unit discusses the role of the nurse in assisting with diagnostic tests and procedures and how the data from these tests factor into overall health assessment.

Unit V, Selected Clinical Nursing Therapeutics, focuses on nursing responsibilities associated with common clinical situations that provide the basis for many aspects of nursing care, including patient teaching, asepsis, caring for the patient before and after surgery, and medication administration.

Section II, Human Function and Clinical Nursing Therapeutics, is organized by areas of human function and uses a consistent nursing process format to present the concepts and nursing responsibilities for helping patients meet patient needs in each area of function. Each clinical nursing care chapter in the 11 units in this section focuses on assessment and diagnosis of altered function and human responses, followed by implementation of appropriate nursing care strategies and evaluation of those interventions. Normal function is discussed first, to allow the student to fully understand normal or expected function before proceeding to altered function. Both normal and altered function set the framework for assessment of subjective and objective data and for the nursing interventions. Each chapter in this section emphasizes North American Nursing Diagnosis Association (NANDA) nursing diagnoses, patient goals, and possible outcome criteria. Additionally, each clinical chapter in Section II includes step-by-step, highly illustrated procedures that cover purpose, assessment, equipment, and procedure steps with rationale. "Lifespan Considerations" and "Home Care Modifications" assist the student in modifying a procedure or making adjustments while caring for all types of patients regardless of the environment.

SPECIAL CHAPTERS

Special chapters in **Section II, Human Function and Clinical Nursing Therapeutics,** focus on the future, discussing timely nursing care topics. These chapters provide the student with an expanded knowledge base and put a current focus on information presented in traditional fundamentals texts. *Chapter 26, Health Maintenance,* discusses how people perceive their own health, what they do to improve or maintain it, and how a nurse can assist in this endeavor. The nursing diagnoses of Altered Health Maintenance and Health Seeking Behaviors are featured. *Chapter 27, Home Maintenance Management,* explores how patients can maintain their own environment and what types of support might be needed to provide assistance, and essential information for appropriate discharge planning.

In *Chapter 31,* the clinical topic of *Oxygenation: Cardiac Function and Tissue Perfusion* explores the essential role of circulation in fulfilling the body's need for oxygenation, particularly relevant topics as cardiovascular disease continues to be the leading cause of death in the United States. *Chapter 36, Thermoregulation,* and *Chapter 42, Cognitive Processes,* focus on two areas of particular concern in the elderly population. Finally, *Chapter 44, Communication: Social Interaction,* and *Chapter 45, Families and Their Relationships,* emphasize the impact these areas of psychosocial function have on human health and wellness.

NURSING PROCESS

Fundamentals of Nursing: Human Health and Function provides students with a solid grounding in the nursing process and nursing diagnosis. Each clinical nursing care chapter in Section II employs a nursing process format in which each component is examined in relation to an area of human function. The assessment portion of each chapter presents both subjective and objective data collection. Each chapter then explores the definition, defining characteristics, and related factors of appropriate nursing diagnoses as defined by NANDA. This provides the beginning student with a firm foundation in the knowledge and application of nursing diagnoses. A section on related diagnoses demonstrates the interrelationship among diagnoses in the spectrum of human responses. Patient goals and possible outcome criteria are presented in a consistent format throughout the text to help students understand the relationship between the nursing diagnosis and the patient goal. This awareness helps students plan effective care.

Each chapter presents nursing interventions in three categories to illustrate the scope of nursing care for patient needs in each area of function. The first category, "Nursing Interventions to Promote Health and Function," focuses on nursing activities that promote wellness, maximize patient strengths, and maintain health and function. "Nursing Interventions for Altered Function," the second section, covers those basic nursing interventions that address the nursing care needs for common problems associated with dysfunction. The last category, "Discharge Planning and Home Care," emphasizes those nursing activities that promote continuity of care and help the patient move from one level of care to another. Finally, Nursing Management Plans in each chapter teach students how to use nursing diagnoses and provide examples of appropriate nursing care along with scientific rationale.

KEY FEATURES

Fundamentals of Nursing: Human Health and Function presents the essential concepts, processes, and skills that help students build a solid foundation for professional nursing practice. To achieve this goal, the text incorporates the following key features.

- **Emphasizes human health, function, and wellness.** Building on the foundational sciences helps students fully understand normal function, which provides a solid foundation for understanding the scientific rationale for basic nursing care.

- **Emphasizes how normal function and dysfunction vary throughout the life cycle.** This emphasis encourages students to view people and their differing needs within the context of their developmental stage.

- **Discusses the impact of dysfunction on activities of daily living.** Understanding how a person's daily life is affected by dysfunction enables students to better assist patients to maintain optimal function.

- **Reinforces nursing responsibility for promoting optimal function in wellness and illness.** This thread runs throughout the text and helps students understand the

impact of health and illness on human response and implement nursing care strategies for people throughout the health–illness continuum.

- **Emphasizes holistic care across the life cycle.** This emphasis helps students to see people as having equally important physiologic, psychosocial, and spiritual needs.

- **Provides a strong nursing process and nursing diagnosis framework.** The nursing process is fundamental to nursing care. This organizing structure creates a strong theoretical underpinning and assists student understanding of how to use nursing process and nursing diagnosis in clinical practice.

- **Emphasizes patient goals and outcome criteria.** Nursing interventions relate to outcome, and measurable patient behaviors help students evaluate the effectiveness of the interventions carried out.

- **Includes discharge planning and home care.** Both components assist students with understanding the importance of continuity of care.

- **Features a family focus.** This perspective encourages students to view patients in light of their families and to view families as critical for patient support.

- **Emphasizes communication.** A thorough understanding of communication as an essential component of all human relationships enables students to become effective listeners, competent caregivers, and reliable health care team members.

- **Emphasizes nursing research.** By introducing research early, beginning students learn to be discriminating consumers of nursing research, understand its relevance to clinical practice, and value the importance of research in the advancement of professional nursing.

PEDAGOGICAL FEATURES

To reinforce and enhance learning and involve the student in the learning process, numerous pedagogical aids summarize or highlight text information.

- **Learning Objectives, Key Terms, and Chapter Outlines** alert students as to what to expect in the chapter and help them focus on chapter content.

- **Key Concepts** highlight essential chapter concepts and information.

- **Separate References and Bibliographies** provide students with current nursing research and a broad base of authoritative resources.

- **Boxed displays, tables, and charts** emphasize essential material. Special boxed displays recur throughout the text—"Nursing Research," "Safety Alert," "Patient Teaching," and "Selected Nursing Interventions for

Common Problems"—as do the Nursing Management Plans.

- **Abundant illustrations and photographs** clarify the text and enhance understanding.

TEACHING–LEARNING PACKAGE

Fundamentals of Nursing: Human Health and Function has an extensive ancillary package to ensure a smooth transition to this new text. The ancillary package was designed with both the student and instructor in mind.

The *Instructor's Manual with Transparency Masters and Syllabus Conversion Charts (Teaching–Learning Plans)* enhances the use of the text and provides a template for an instructor-designed syllabus. *Procedure Checklists* provide guidelines for student practice and evaluation tools for faculty. A student *Study Guide* augments the text and provides a means of student self-evaluation. Finally, a *Computerized Testing Program* in Apple and IBM versions facilitates instructor-designed queries and examinations.

Ruth F. Craven, EdD, RN
Constance J. Hirnle, MN, RN

Acknowledgments

Sincere appreciation and warmest thanks are extended to the many people who contributed to the production of this book

- The contributors, who worked diligently to provide content in their areas of expertise and were patient with revision.

- Our students, for their contributions to the completion of the manuscript. They were consulted throughout the project for their opinions regarding organization and level of content, and their ideas regarding what would facilitate learning. In particular we would like to single out
  - Kristi Prinos
  - Rosemarie Taylor
  - Anne Millman
  - Holly Tomashek

- Diana Itenzo, Publisher; Donna Hilton, Senior Editor; and Eleanor Faven, Developmental Editor, for encouragement, patience, competence, and faith that "it would work!"

- Mary Rose Muccie, Project Editor, for her patience, reliability, and good-natured support while completing the book.

- Susan Hermansen, Art Director, and Helen Ewan, Production Manager, for seeing the production process through with patience and professionalism.

- Joan Jenks, RN, MSN, who consulted with the authors, reviewed the organization of the book, provided suggestions on each chapter, and offered many valuable points on functional health.

- Sandy Nettina, RN, MSN, ANP, who assisted in formatting content in selected chapters.

- Charlene Clark, RN, MEd; Neysa Dobson, RN; Gail Pilant; and the Intercollegiate Center for Nursing Education, Spokane, for their contribution to the photographs used in this book.

- Beverly Ernst and Willow Wolfe, whose accurate and competent typing assisted in manuscript preparation.

- University of Washington School of Nursing, University of Washington Medical Center, Seattle Pacific University, Seattle University, Shoreline Community College, Overlake Hospital Medical Center, friends, colleagues, and all others who contributed photos for use in this text.

Finally, but most important, we acknowledge with love and gratitude the constant support and encouragement of family, friends, and colleagues throughout this project.

Contents

Expanded Contents   xix
Nursing Procedures and Skills   xxxv
Nursing Diagnoses   xl
Nursing Management Plans   xli
Summary of Recurring Displays   xlii

section one
Conceptual Foundations of Nursing   1

UNIT I: Concepts Essential for
           Professional Nursing   2

1   The Profession of Nursing: Theory,
    Education, and Practice   4
2   The Health-Care Delivery System   26
3   Ethical and Legal Concerns   40
4   Leadership and Management   58
5   Nursing Research   70

UNIT II: The Nursing Process:
           Framework for Clinical
           Nursing Therapeutics   80

6   The Nursing Process in Human
    Health and Function   82
7   Nursing Assessment   94
8   Nursing Diagnosis   110
9   Nursing Management: Planning,
    Implementation, and Evaluation   126
10 Communication of the Nursing
    Process: Recording and Reporting   148

UNIT III: Concepts Essential for
           Human Function
           and Nursing
           Management   170

11 Health and Wellness   172
12 Human Needs   184

13 Lifespan Development   196
14 Individual, Family, and Community   222
15 Culture and Ethnicity   236
16 Values   254
17 Communication: The Nurse–Patient
    Relationship   272

UNIT IV: Essential Assessment
           Components   292

18 Health Assessment of Human
    Function   294
19 Vital Sign Assessment   348
20 Diagnostic Tests and Procedures   378

UNIT V: Selected Clinical
           Nursing Therapeutics   406

21 Patient Teaching   408
22 Asepsis   426
23 Perioperative Nursing   464
24 Medication Administration   498

section two
**Human Function and Clinical Nursing
Therapeutics**   559

UNIT VI: Health Perception and
           Health Management   560

25 Safety   562
26 Health Maintenance   592
27 Home Maintenance Management   612

UNIT VII: Activity and Exercise   638

28 Self-Care and Hygiene   640
29 Body Mechanics and Mobility   692
30 Oxygenation: Respiratory Function   746

31   Oxygenation: Cardiac Function and
Tissue Perfusion   **800**

UNIT **VIII:**   Nutrition and
Metabolism   **842**

32   Fluid, Electrolyte, and Acid–Base
Balance   **844**

33   Nutrition   **890**

34   Skin Integrity and Wound Healing   **934**

35   The Body's Defenses Against
Infection   **980**

36   Thermoregulation   **1016**

UNIT **IX:**   Elimination   **1038**

37   Urinary Elimination   **1040**

38   Bowel Elimination   **1088**

UNIT **X:**   Sleep and Rest   **1134**

39   Sleep and Rest   **1136**

UNIT **XI:**   Cognition and
Perception   **1158**

40   Pain Perception and Comfort   **1160**

41   Sensory Perception   **1190**

42   Cognitive Processes   **1210**

UNIT **XII:**   Self-Perception and
Self-Concept   **1238**

43   Self-Concept   **1240**

UNIT **XIII:**   Roles and
Relationships   **1262**

44   Communication: Social Interaction   **1264**

45   Families and Their Relationships   **1286**

46   Loss and Grieving   **1308**

UNIT **XIV:**   Coping and Stress
Management   **1332**

47   Stress, Coping, and Adaptation   **1334**

UNIT **XV:**   Sexuality and
Reproduction   **1358**

48   Human Sexuality   **1360**

UNIT **XVI:**   Values and Beliefs   **1388**

49   Spiritual Health   **1390**

Appendices
A.   Equivalents   1413
B.   Laboratory Values   1415
C.   Medical Terminology: Prefixes, Roots, and
Suffixes   1438
D.   Recommended Dietary Allowances, USA   1445
E.   Nutrition Recommendations for
Canadians   1448

Glossary   1449

Index   1467

Expanded Contents

Nursing Procedures and Skills   xxxv
Nursing Diagnoses   xl
Nursing Management Plans   xli
Summary of Recurring Displays   xlii

section one
Conceptual Foundations of Nursing   1

UNIT I: Concepts Essential for
          Professional Nursing   2
1   The Profession of Nursing: Theory,
    Education, and Practice   4
The Profession of Nursing   5
Historic Evolution of Modern Nursing   6
Socialization to Professional Nursing   10
Nursing and Professionalism Defined   11
Conceptual Frameworks and Theories of Nursing   11
Four Major Concepts   12
Concerns About Nursing Theory   12
Educational Preparation and Career Opportunities   13
Nursing Education   13
Nursing Practice Settings   16
Nursing Roles and Responsibilities   17
Career Development and Expanded Nursing
    Roles   19
Professional Nursing Practice   20
Standards of Practice   20
Nurse Practice Acts   20
Nursing Organizations   20
Current and Future Trends in Nursing Practice   23
Key Concepts   23

2   The Health-Care Delivery
    System   26
Defining the Health-Care Delivery System   27
**Factors Affecting the Delivery of Health-Care
    Services**   28
Health Care as a Right   28
Increasing Longevity of Americans   28
Technologic Advances and Ethical Dilemmas   28
Rising Consumerism   29
Changing Health Services   29
Increasing Legislative Activity   29

The Health-Care Delivery Setting   29
Types of Services   30
Agencies Providing Inpatient Services   30
Agencies Providing Outpatient Services   32
Community-Based Agencies   32
Funding of Health-Care Services   33
Private Health Insurance   33
Government Involvement in Health-Care Funding   33
Charitable Funding of Health Care   35
Colleagues in the Health-Care System   35
Physicians   35
Focused Care Providers   35
Technicians and Technologists   35
Therapists   35
Others Providing Necessary Services   36
Challenges to the Health-Care Delivery System   36
Quality of Care   36
Fragmentation of Service   37
Limited Medical and Financial Resources   37
Access to Health Care   37
Ethical and Bioethical Decisions   38
Key Concepts   38

3   Ethical and Legal Concerns   40
Legal and Ethical Dilemmas   41
Ethical Issues in Nursing   42
What Is Ethics?   42
Professional Codes of Ethics   42

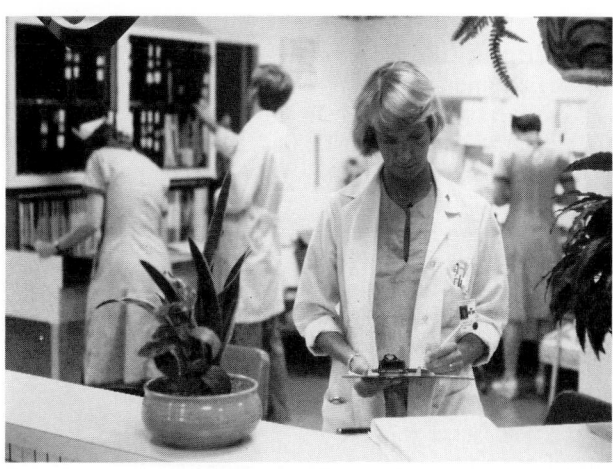

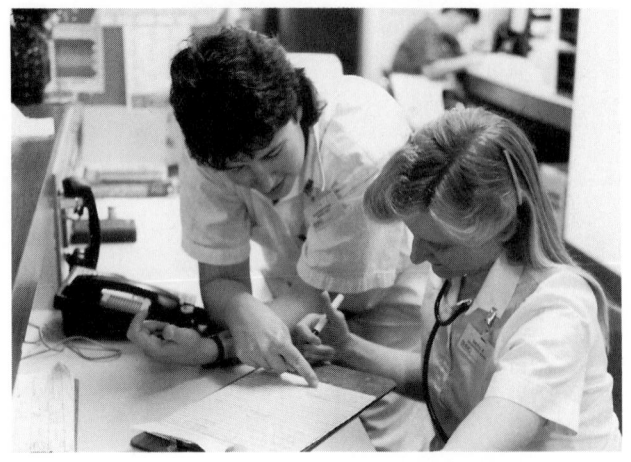

Examples of Ethical Philosophy   42
Moral Development   44
Analysis of an Ethical Dilemma   45
Role Conflict   45
Legal Issues In Nursing   **45**
Sources of Laws   47
Licensure   47
Standards of Care   48
Torts and Crimes   48
Controlled Substances   52
Death and Dying   52
Protecting Yourself   54
Key Concepts   **56**

4   Leadership and Management   **58**
Leadership   **59**
Styles of Leadership   59
Management   **60**
Functions of Managers   60
Skills for Effective Management   62
**Applying Leadership and Management
to Nursing Roles**   **63**
Clinical Practice Roles   63
Nursing Management Roles   66
Teaching Roles   67
Key Concepts   **68**

5   Nursing Research   **70**
Research and Nursing   **71**
Evolution of Nursing Research   72
Characteristics of Nursing Research   73
Scientific Process and Nursing Research   73
The Research Process   **73**
Research Design   73
Where Does One Start?   74
Legal and Ethical Issues   **76**
Institutional Review Boards   76
Subject Rights   76
Research and the Professional Nurse   **77**
Roles of Nursing Personnel at Different Levels 77
Clinical Nursing Practice   77
Key Concepts   **79**

**UNIT II: The Nursing Process:
Framework for Clinical
Nursing Therapeutics**   **80**

**6   The Nursing Process in Human
Health and Function**   **82**
Historical Development of the Nursing Process   **83**
Components of the Nursing Process   **84**
Definition   84
Phases   84
Interactive Nature of Each Phase   87
**Theoretical Foundations for the Use of the
Nursing Process**   **87**
Systems Theory   87
Problem-Solving Theory   87
Decision-Making Process   88
Information-Processing Theory   88
Diagnostic Reasoning Process   89
**Requirements for Effective Use of the Nursing
Process**   **89**
Professional Relevance of the Nursing Process   **90**
**Functional Health Approach to the Nursing
Process**   **90**
Future Nursing Process Trends   **90**
Key Concepts   **92**

7   Nursing Assessment   **94**
Preparing for Assessment   **96**
Types of Assessment   96
Setting and Environment   97
Assessment Skills   **97**
Observation   98
Interviewing   99
Physical Examination Techniques   100
Intuition   101
Assessment Activities   **101**
Collect Data   102
Validate Data   103
Organize Data   105
Key Concepts   **107**

8   Nursing Diagnosis   **110**
Historical Development   **111**
Nursing Diagnosis Taxonomy   **112**
What is a Taxonomy?   112
Nursing Diagnosis Taxonomy Development   113
**Nursing Diagnosis and Other Health-Care
Problems**   **116**
Components of a Nursing Diagnosis   **117**
Diagnostic Label   118
Qualifiers   118
Definition   118
Defining Characteristics   118
Risk Factors   118
Related Factors   118
Diagnosis Activities   **118**
Identify Pattern   118
Validate Diagnosis   120
Formulate the Diagnostic Statement   121
Significance of Nursing Diagnosis   **122**
**Nursing Diagnoses Organized by Functional
Health Patterns**   **124**
Key Concepts   **125**

9   Nursing Management: Planning, Implementation, and Evaluation   **126**
Planning   **127**
  Planning Activities   128
  Planning Organized by Functional Health   134
Implementation   **134**
  Implementation Skills   135
  Implementation Activities   135
  Implementation Using a Functional Health Approach   139
Evaluation   **139**
  Evaluation Skills   140
  Types of Evaluation   141
  Evaluation Activities   142
  Quality Assurance Monitors   144
  Evaluation Using the Functional Health Approach   146
Key Concepts   **146**

10   Communication of the Nursing Process: Recording and Reporting   **148**
Written Communication: The Patient Record   **149**
  Purpose   150
  Principles of Charting   150
  Types of Documentation   154
  Nursing Entries on the Patient Record   155
Oral Communication: Reporting   **165**
  Change-of-Shift Reports   165
  Nursing Rounds   167
  Telephone Reports   167
  Patient Transfers   167
  Report to Physician   167
  Reports from Other Departments   168
  Care Plan Conferences   168
  Confidentiality   168
Key Concepts   **169**

UNIT III: Concepts Essential for Human Function and Nursing Management   170

11   Health and Wellness   **172**
Health and Wellness   **173**
  Clinical Model   174
  Host–Agent–Environment Model   174
  Health Belief Model   174
  High-Level Wellness Model   175
  Holistic Health Model   175
Wellness and Holistic Health Care   **176**
  Holistic Practice   177
  Meaning of Disease, Illness, and Dysfunction   178
  Effect of Stress   179
Nursing in Wellness and Holistic Health Care   **179**
  Promoting Health and Preventing Illness   179
  Nursing as a Therapeutic Partnership   180
  Nursing Diagnoses for Wellness   180
  Examples of Holistic Health Care Modalities   180
Key Concepts   **182**

12   Human Needs   **184**
Maslow's Hierarchy of Needs   **185**
  Physiologic Needs   185
  Safety Needs   187

  Love Needs   188
  Esteem Needs   188
  Self-Actualization Needs   188
Lifespan Considerations   **188**
Nursing Theorists' Perceptions of Human Needs   **189**
  Florence Nightingale   189
  Virginia Henderson   189
  Ida Jean Orlando   190
  Dorothea Orem   190
  Yura and Walsh   190
  Imogene M. King   190
  Sister Callista Roy   190
  Martha E. Rogers   190
  Faye Glenn Abdellah   190
  Lydia E. Hall   190
  Jean Watson   191
Functional Health Patterns and Assessing Human Needs   **192**
Key Concepts   **193**

13   Lifespan Development   **196**
Genetics and Environment   **198**
Concepts of Development   **199**
  Principles of Growth and Development   199
  Growth and Development Theory   199
Growth and Development Through the Lifespan   **201**
  Intrauterine Development   201
  Neonate (Birth to 1 Month)   204
  Infant (1 Month to 1 Year)   204
  Toddler (1 to 3 Years)   205
  Preschooler (3 to 6 Years)   206
  School-Age Child (6 to 11 Years)   206
  Adolescent (11 to 21 Years)   207
  Young Adult (21 to 40 Years)   207
  Middle Adult (40 to 50 Years)   208
  Older Adult (60 Years and Older)   208
Functional Health and Lifespan Development Related to Health Problems and Anticipatory Guidance   **209**
  Health Perception and Health Management   209
  Nutrition and Metabolism   211
  Elimination   212
  Activity and Exercise   212
  Cognition and Perception   213

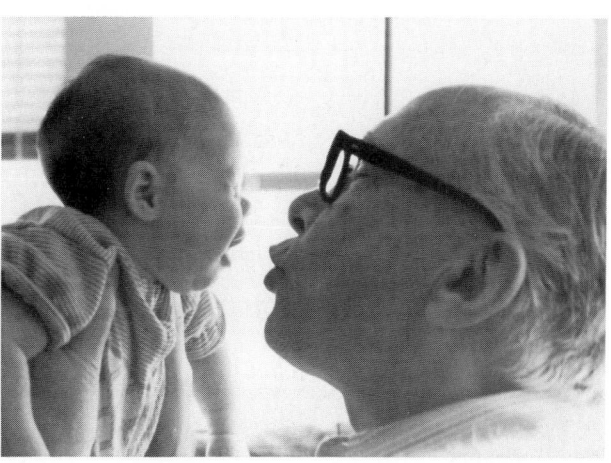

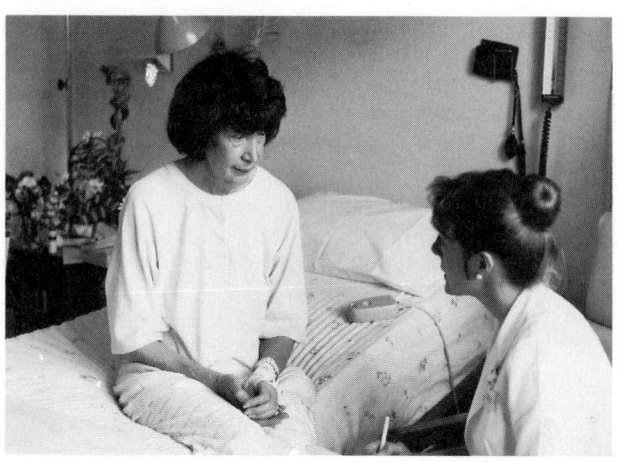

Sleep and Rest   214
Self-Perception and Self-Concept   215
Roles and Relationships   215
Sexuality and Reproduction   216
Coping and Stress Tolerance   217
Values and Beliefs   218
Key Concepts   **219**

**14 Individual, Family,
    and Community**   **222**
The Individual   **223**
The Family   **224**
Family Conceptual Frameworks   225
Family Assessment   228
Family Responsibility for Functional Health   229
The Community   **229**
Definition of Community   229
Community Assessment   233
Community Responsibility for Functional Health   233
Advanced Community Concepts   233
Key Concepts   **233**

15 Culture and Ethnicity   **236**
What is Culture?   **237**
Characteristics of Culture   238
Concepts Related to Culture   **241**
Ethnicity or Ethnic Identity   241
Minority   242
Race   242
Racism   242
Subculture   242
Stereotype   243
**Implications of the Concept of Culture
for Nursing**   **243**
Need for Culturally Sensitive Nursing Care   243
Taking Account of Biocultural Variation   246
Grounding Nursing Assessments in the Patient's
Perspective   247
When the Patient Does Not Speak the Nurse's
Language   248
Increased Effectiveness of Patient Education   250
Key Concepts   **250**

16 Values   **254**
Value and Belief Patterns   **256**
Major Categories of Values   256
Professional Values in Nursing   256
Values Clarification   257
Values Inquiry   258
Applied Ethics   258
Sources of Values   **259**
Community   259
Peer Culture   259
Role Models   259
Interaction with People of Differing Values and
Viewpoints   260
Experiences that Challenge One's Way of
Thinking   260
Decision-Making   260
Manifestations of Values   **260**
Effect of Values on Functional Health   261
Manifestations of Nurses' Values   265
Lifespan Considerations   **266**
Hall's Value Development Theory   267
Value Conflicts   **267**
Patient and Family Conflicts   267
Patient and Health-Care Conflicts   268
Resolving Value Conflicts in the Health-Care
System   268
Values Assessment   **269**
Level of Values Development   269
View of Hospitalization and Illness   269
Activities of Daily Living   269
Discharge Planning   270
Key Concepts   **270**

**17 Communication: The Nurse–Patient
    Relationship**   **272**
The Communication Process   **274**
Types of Communication   274
Elements of the Communication Process   275
Importance of Language and Experience   275
**The Nurse–Patient Relationship: A Helping
Relationship**   **277**
Phases   277
Contract-Setting   277
Advocacy   278
Circle of Confidentiality   279
Ingredients of Therapeutic Communication   **279**
Empathy   280
Positive Regard   280
Comfortable Sense of Self   281
Communication and Nursing Process   **281**
Assessment   281
Intervention   283
Key Concepts   **291**

**UNIT IV: Essential Assessment
              Components**   **292**

**18 Health Assessment of Human
    Function**   **294**
Purpose and Preparation   **296**
Purpose of the Assessment   296
Preparation of the Patient and Environment   296

Organization and Documentation 297
Types of Data Collection 297
  Obtaining Subjective Data: The Interview 297
  Obtaining Objective Data: The Physical
    Examination 303
Assessment of Individual Aspects of Functional
  Health 307
Assessment of Health Perception and Health
  Management 307
Assessment of Activity and Exercise 308
  Mobility and Self-Care Assessment 308
  Respiratory Assessment 310
  Cardiovascular Assessment 316
Assessment of Nutrition and Metabolism 321
Assessment of Elimination 327
  Urinary Elimination 327
  Bowel Elimination 328
Assessment of Sleep and Rest 328
Assessment of Cognition and Perception 328
  Cognitive Function 329
  Sensory Function 333
  Pain Assessment 336
Assessment of Self-Perception and Self-Concept 337
Assessment of Roles and Relationships 339
Assessment of Coping and Stress Tolerance 340
Assessment of Sexuality and Reproduction 341
Assessment of Values and Beliefs 343
Concluding the Assessment 343
Lifespan Considerations 344
Key Concepts 346
Procedure 18-1 Auscultating Breath Sounds 315
Procedure 18-2 Auscultating Heart Sounds 319
Procedure 18-3 Measuring Weight 323
              Weight with Chair Scale 323
              Weight with Standing Scale 323
              Weight with Bed Scale 323
Procedure 18-4 Auscultating Bowel Sounds 324
Procedure 18-5 Assessing the Neurologic
              System 330

19 Vital Sign Assessment 348
Body Temperature 349
  Factors Affecting Body Temperature 350
  Factors Affecting Body Temperature
    Measurement 351
  Assessing Temperature 351
Pulse 354
  Characteristics 354
  Factors Affecting Pulse Rate 354
  Assessing the Pulse 357
Respirations 361
  Factors Affecting Respirations 361
  Assessing Respirations 362
Blood Pressure 364
  Physiologic Factors Determining Blood Pressure 364
  Factors Affecting Blood Pressure 365
  Assessing Blood Pressure 366
Lifespan Considerations 373
Documenting Vital Signs 376
Key Concepts 376
Procedure 19-1 Assessing Body Temperature 355
              Assessing Oral Temperature 355

              Assessing Axillary Temperature 355
              Assessing Rectal Temperature 356
Procedure 19-2 Obtaining a Pulse 359
              Radial Pulse 359
              Apical Pulse 359
Procedure 19-3 Assessing Pulse Deficits 362
Procedure 19-4 Assessing Respirations 365
Procedure 19-5 Obtaining Blood Pressure 367
Procedure 19-6 Assessing for Orthostatic
              Hypotension 373

20 Diagnostic Tests and Procedures 378
The Nurse as a Facilitator for Diagnostic Testing 380
  Patient Preparation 380
  Responsibilities During Testing 383
  Responsibilities After Testing 384
  Using Data to Individualize Care 385
Laboratory Tests 385
  Blood Specimen Collection 385
  Hematologic Tests 388
  Urine Testing 392
  Culture and Sensitivity Testing 392
Diagnostic Tests 393
  Noninvasive Viewing Techniques 393
  Invasive Viewing Techniques 397
  Aspiration Diagnostic Procedures 399
  Diagnostic Procedures That Evaluate Electrical
    Conduction 402
Lifespan Considerations 403
Key Concepts 404
Procedure 20-1 Preparing the Patient for
              Diagnostic Procedures 381
Procedure 20-2 Measuring Blood Glucose by
              Skin Puncture 389

UNIT **V:**   **Selected Clinical
             Nursing Therapeutics** 406

21 Patient Teaching 408
Teaching–Learning Process 410
  Sequence of Events in Learning 410
  Domains of Knowledge 410
  Learning Styles 411

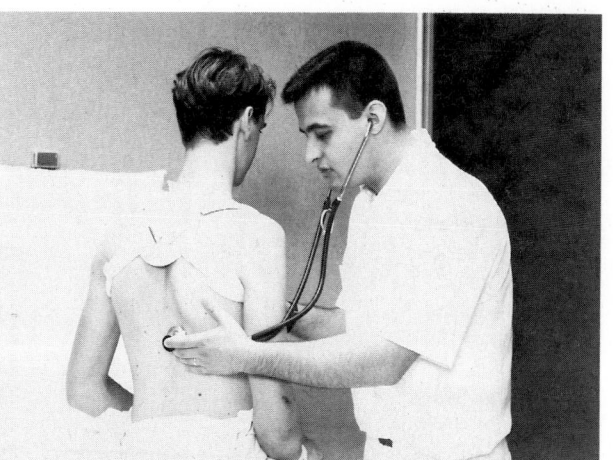

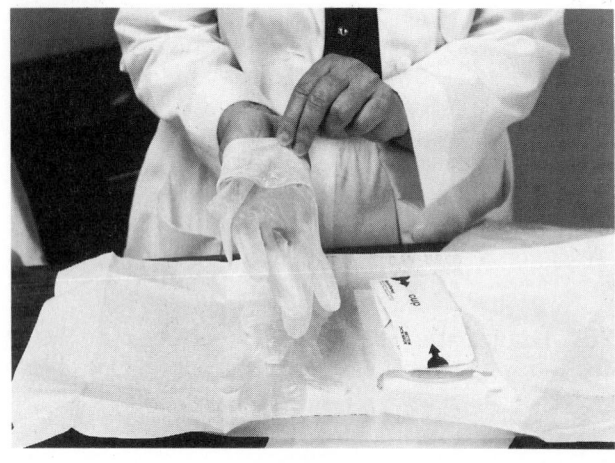

Patient Teaching to Promote Health and Function 412
Preventive Health Education 412
Patient Teaching for Acute Problems 412
Patient Teaching for Chronic Problems 413
Assessment for Learning 413
Assessing Learning Needs 413
Assessing Learning Readiness 414
Nursing Diagnoses and Patient Goals 415
Planning for Learning 415
Appropriate Family and Friend Involvement 415
Implementation of Patient Teaching 416
Sensitivity 416
Environment Control 417
Structured Teaching Sessions 417
Audiovisual Aids 417
Communication 417
Repetition 418
Teaching Methods 418
Teaching Strategies 419
Evaluation of Learning 420
Documentation of Patient Teaching 420
Lifespan Considerations 421
Key Concepts 423

22 Asepsis 426
Role of Microorganisms in Infection 428
Agents Causing Infection 428
Chain of Infection 428
Progress of an Infection 430
Nosocomial Infections 432
Infection Hazards in Nonacute Care Setting 433
Infection Control 434
Recognition of Factors 434
Regulatory Agencies 434
Employee Health 435
Waste Disposal 438
Aseptic Practices 438
Categories of Asepsis 439
Handwashing 440
Cleaning, Disinfection, and Sterilization 443
Use of Barriers 445
Isolation Systems 448
Surgical Asepsis 453
Lifespan Considerations 457

Key Concepts 461
Procedure 22-1 Handwashing 441
Procedure 22-2 Donning and Removing a Mask
      and Gown 446
      Donning Mask 446
      Donning Clean Gown 446
      Removing Contaminated Gown 447
Procedure 22-3 Practicing Strict Isolation
      Technique 452
Procedure 22-4 Applying and Removing Sterile
      Gloves 459
      Applying Gloves 459
      Removing Gloves 460

23 Perioperative Nursing 464
Surgical Intervention 466
Classification of Surgery 466
Surgical Facilities 466
Phases of Perioperative Nursing 466
Impact of Surgery on Functional Health 468
Lifespan Considerations 473
Preoperative Nursing 474
Nursing Assessment 474
Nursing Diagnoses and Patient Goals 474
Nursing Interventions 474
Evaluation 483
Intraoperative Nursing 484
Nursing Assessment 484
Nursing Diagnoses and Patient Goals 484
Nursing Interventions 485
Evaluation 490
Postoperative Nursing 490
Nursing Assessment 490
Nursing Diagnoses and Patient Goals 491
Nursing Interventions 491
Evaluation 495
Key Concepts 496

24 Medication Administration 498
Drugs and Medications 500
Names of Drugs 500
Types and Forms of Drugs 500
Sources of Information About Medications 500
Medication Standards 502
Systems of Medication Distribution 503
Nonprescription and Prescription Medications 504
Components of a Drug Order 504
Types of Orders 504
Systems of Drug Measurement 505
Legal Aspects of Medication Administration 507
Laws Affecting Drugs and Medications 507
Drug Enforcement Agencies 508
The Nurse's Role 508
The Patient's Rights 510
Substance Abuse 511
Principles of Drug Action 511
Pharmacokinetics 511
Pharmacodynamics 512
Factors Affecting Drug Action 514
Medication Assessment 515
Information Collected on Admission 515
Assessment Before Medication Administration 516
Assessment of Knowledge and Compliance 518

Nursing Diagnoses | **518**
Diagnostic Statement: Noncompliance | 518
Diagnostic Statement: Knowledge Deficit | 518
Related Nursing Diagnoses | 519
Medication Administration | **519**
Process to Ensure Safety | 519
Oral Medications | 523
Topical Medications | 528
Inhaled Medications | 530
Parenteral Medications | 530
Discharge Planning and Home Care | 553
Evaluation | **554**
Lifespan Considerations | **554**
Key Concepts | **556**
Procedure 24-1 **Administering Oral Medications** | **524**
Procedure 24-2 **Drawing up Two Medications in a Syringe** | **535**
Modification for Insulin | **536**
Procedure 24-3 **Administering Subcutaneous Injections** | **538**
Variations for Administering Heparin | **540**
Procedure 24-4 **Administering Intramuscular Injections** | **543**
Variations for Air Lock Injection Technique | **545**
Variations for Z-track Injections | **545**
Procedure 24-5 **Administering IV Medications Using Intermittent Infusion Technique** | **551**
Using a Heparin Lock | **552**

---

section two
Human Function and Clinical Nursing Therapeutics

559

UNIT **VI:**   **Health Perception and Health Management**

560
25   Safety | **562**
Normal Safety Function | **564**
Characteristics of Safety | 564
Normal Functional Pattern | 564
Factors Affecting Safety | 565
Lifespan Considerations | 567
Altered Safety Function | **569**
Potential for Altered Safety | 569
Manifestations of Altered Safety | 572
Impact of Safety Dysfunction on Activities of Daily Living | 575
Assessment | **576**
Subjective Data | 576
Objective Data | 577
Nursing Diagnoses and Patient Goals | **578**
Diagnostic Statement: High Risk for Injury | 578
Related Nursing Diagnoses | 578
Patient Goals | 578
Implementation | **579**
Nursing Interventions to Promote Health and Safety Function | 579

Nursing Interventions for Altered Safety Function | 586
Discharge Planning and Home Care | 587
Evaluation | **589**
Key Concepts | **590**
26   Health Maintenance | **592**
Normal Health Maintenance | **593**
Characteristics of Normal Health Maintenance | 594
Normal Functional Health Maintenance | 595
Factors Affecting Health Maintenance | 596
Lifespan Considerations | 598
Altered Health Maintenance Function | **599**
Potential for Altered Function | 599
Manifestations of Altered Function | 600
Impact of Dysfunction on Activities of Daily Living | 601
Assessment | **601**
Subjective Data | 601
Objective Data | 602
Nursing Diagnoses and Patient Goals | **604**
Diagnostic Statement: Altered Health Maintenance | 604
Diagnostic Statement: Health-Seeking Behaviors | 604
Related Nursing Diagnoses | 605
Patient Goals | 605
Implementation | **605**
Nursing Interventions to Promote Health and Function | 605
Nursing Interventions for Altered Function | 607
Discharge Planning and Home Care | 608
Evaluation | **608**
Key Concepts | **609**
27   Home Maintenance Management | **612**
Normal Home Maintenance Management | **614**
Environment | 614
Characteristics of Normal Home Maintenance Management | 614
Normal Home Maintenance Functional Pattern | 615
Factors Affecting Home Maintenance Management | 615
Lifespan Considerations | 617
Altered Home Maintenance Management | **618**
Potential for Altered Home Maintenance Management | 618

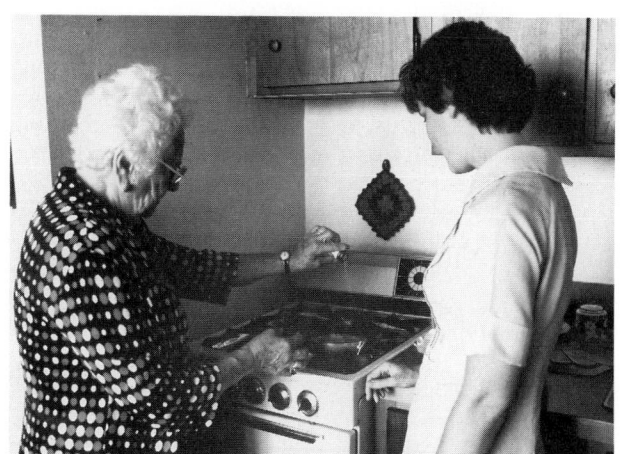

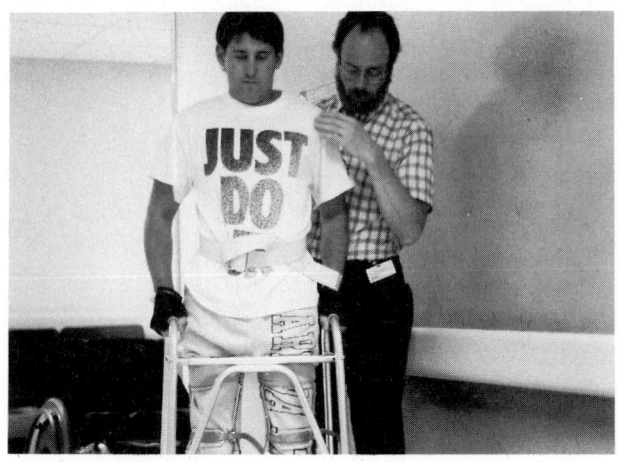

Manifestations of Altered Home Maintenance
  Management   619
Assessment   **620**
  Subjective Data   620
  Objective Data   621
Nursing Diagnoses and Patient Goals   **623**
  Diagnostic Statement: Impaired Home
    Maintenance Management   623
  Related Nursing Diagnoses   624
  Patient Goals   624
Implementation   **625**
  Nursing Interventions to Promote Health
    and Function   625
  Nursing Interventions for Altered Home
    Maintenance Management   626
Evaluation   **633**
Key Concepts   **635**

UNIT VII: Activity and Exercise   **638**
28 Self-Care and Hygiene   **640**
Normal Self-Care Function   **642**
  Characteristics of Normal Self-Care   642
  Normal Self-Care Functional Patterns   644
  Factors Affecting Normal Self-Care   644
  Lifespan Considerations   645
Altered Self-Care Function   **646**
  Potential for Altered Self-Care   647
  Manifestations of Altered Self-Care   648
Assessment   **648**
  Subjective Data   648
  Objective Data   650
Nursing Diagnoses and Patient Goals   **651**
  Self-Care Deficit, Bathing/Hygiene   651
  Self-Care Deficit, Dressing/Grooming   652
  Self-Care Deficit, Toileting   652
  Self-Care Deficit, Feeding   653
  Related Nursing Diagnoses   653
  Patient Goals   653
Implementation   **653**
  Nursing Interventions to Promote Health
    and Self-Care   653
  Nursing Interventions for Altered Self-Care   653
  Discharge Planning and Home Care   682

Evaluation   689
Key Concepts   691

Procedure 28-1 **Bathing a Patient in Bed**   **657**
Procedure 28-2 **Assisting with the Bath
                    or Shower**   **661**
Procedure 28-3 **Massaging the Back**   **664**
Procedure 28-4 **Performing Foot and Nail Care**   **666**
Procedure 28-5 **Shampooing Hair of a
                    Bedridden Patient**   **668**
Procedure 28-6 **Providing Oral Care**   **670**
                  **Variation for the
                    Unconscious Patient**   **671**
Procedure 28-7 **Using a Bedpan**   **679**
                  Placing the Bedpan   **679**
                  Removing the Bedpan   **680**
Procedure 28-8 **Making an Unoccupied Bed**   **683**
Procedure 28-9 **Making an Occupied Bed**   **686**

29 Body Mechanics and Mobility   **692**
Normal Mobility   **694**
  Anatomy of the Musculoskeletal System   694
  Normal Physiologic Function   695
  Characteristics of Normal Movement   701
  Factors Affecting Normal Mobility   702
  Lifespan Considerations   704
Altered Mobility   **705**
  Potential for Altered Mobility   705
  Manifestations of Altered Mobility   706
  Impact of Immobility on Functional Health   707
  Impact of Altered Mobility on Activities of Daily
    Living   714
Assessment   **714**
  Subjective Data   715
  Objective Data   715
Nursing Diagnoses and Patient Goals   **717**
  Impaired Physical Mobility   717
  Activity Intolerance   717
  High Risk for Disuse Syndrome   718
  Related Nursing Diagnoses   718
  Patient Goals   718
Implementation   **718**
  Nursing Interventions to Promote Health
    and Function   718
  Nursing Interventions for Altered Mobility   718
  Discharge Planning and Home Care   735
Evaluation   **742**
Key Concepts   **743**
Procedure 29-1 **Using Proper Body Mechanics**   **698**
Procedure 29-2 **Positioning a Patient in Bed**   **723**
                  **Moving a Patient up in Bed
                    (One Nurse)**   **723**
                  **Moving Helpless Patient up
                    in Bed (Two Nurses)**   **723**
                  **Positioning Patient in
                    Side-Lying Position**   **724**
                  Logrolling   **725**
Procedure 29-3 **Providing Range-of-Motion
                    Exercises**   **728**
Procedure 29-4 **Assisting with Ambulation**   **730**
                  One Nurse   **730**
                  Two Nurses   **731**
                  Using a Walker   **731**

Procedure 29-5   **Helping Patients with Crutch**
                   Walking   733
                   Four-Point Gait   733
                   Three-Point Gait   734
                   Two-Point Gait   734
                   Swinging-to Gait   735
                   Swinging-through Gait   735
                   Climbing Stairs   735
                   Descending Stairs   735
Procedure 29-6   **Transferring a Patient to**
                   a Stretcher   736
Procedure 29-7   **Transferring a Patient to**
                   a Wheelchair   737

30   Oxygenation: Respiratory Function   746
Normal Respiratory Function   748
Normal Anatomy of the Respiratory System   748
Normal Function of the Respiratory System   748
Normal Breathing Pattern   751
Factors Affecting Normal Respiratory Function   751
Lifespan Considerations   752
Altered Respiratory Function   753
Potential for Altered Function   753
Manifestations of Altered Respiratory Function   755
Impact of Respiratory Dysfunction on Activities
of Daily Living   758
Assessment   759
Subjective Data   759
Objective Data   761
Nursing Diagnoses and Patient Goals   764
Diagnostic Statement: Ineffective Breathing
Pattern   764
Diagnostic Statement: Ineffective Airway
Clearance   764
Diagnostic Statement: Impaired Gas Exchange   764
Related Nursing Diagnoses   765
Patient Goals   765
Implementation   765
Nursing Interventions to Promote Health
and Respiratory Function   765
Nursing Interventions for Altered Respiratory
Function   772
Discharge Planning and Home Care   788
Evaluation   795
Key Concepts   797
Procedure 30-1   **Teaching Coughing and Deep**
                   Breathing Exercises   768
                   Deep Breathing   768
                   Controlled Coughing   768
Procedure 30-2   **Promoting Breathing with the**
                   Incentive Spirometer   771
Procedure 30-3   **Administering Oxygen by Nasal**
                   Cannula or Mask   776
Procedure 30-4   **Suctioning Oropharyngeal and**
                   Nasopharyngeal Areas   782
Procedure 30-5   **Suctioning Nasotracheal**
                   Secretions   786
Procedure 30-6   **Providing Tracheostomy Care**   789
Procedure 30-7   **Managing an Obstructed Airway**
                   (Heimlich Maneuver)   793
                   Conscious Adult
                   (Heimlich Maneuver)   793

                   Unconscious Patient
                   (Heimlich Maneuver,
                   Abdominal Thrust)   794
                   Infants Under 1 Year
                   of Age (Back Blows
                   and Chest Thrusts)   794
                   Children Over 1 Year
                   of Age   794
                   Pregnant Women or Very
                   Obese Adults (Chest Thrusts)   794

31   Oxygenation: Cardiac Function and
Tissue Perfusion   800
Normal Cardiovascular Function   802
Anatomy of the Cardiovascular System   802
Normal Function of the Heart and Blood Vessels   803
Normal Cardiovascular Functional Pattern   806
Factors Affecting Normal Cardiovascular Function   807
Lifespan Considerations   808
Altered Cardiovascular Function   809
Potential for Altered Cardiovascular Function   809
Manifestations of Altered Cardiovascular Function   813
Impact of Cardiovascular Dysfunction
on Activities of Daily Living   817
Assessment   817
Subjective Data   817
Objective Data   819
Nursing Diagnoses and Patient Goals   822
Diagnostic Statement: Altered Tissue Perfusion
(Renal, Cerebral, Cardiopulmonary,
Gastrointestinal, Peripheral)   823
Diagnostic Statement: Decreased Cardiac Output   823
Diagnostic Statement: Activity Intolerance   823
Related Nursing Diagnoses   823
Patient Goals   823
Implementation   824
Nursing Interventions to Promote Health
and Function   825
Nursing Interventions for Altered Cardiovascular
Function   825
Evaluation   837
Key Concepts   839
Procedure 31-1   **Applying Antiembolic Stockings**   828

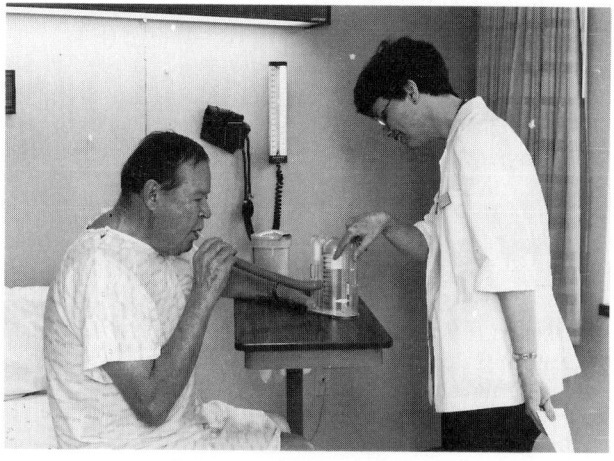

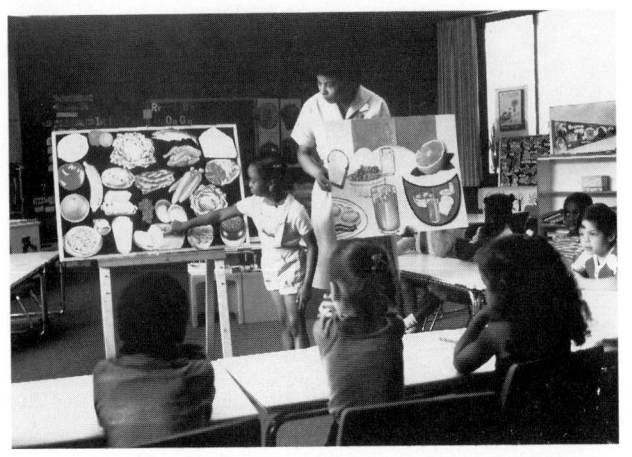

Procedure 31-2 **Administering Cardiopulmonary**
        Resuscitation (CPR)   **833**
        One Rescuer—Adult Patient   **833**
        Two Rescuers—Adult Patient   **835**
        One Rescuer—Infant
        and Child   **835**

UNIT **VIII:**   Nutrition and
            Metabolism   **842**

32 Fluid, Electrolyte, and Acid–Base
    Balance   **844**
Normal Fluid and Electrolyte Balance   **846**
  Fluid Compartments   846
  Total Body Water   846
  Electrolytes   846
  Fluid and Electrolyte Distribution   848
  Factors Affecting Fluid and Electrolyte Balance   850
  Lifespan Considerations   852
Normal Acid–Base Balance   **853**
  Acids, Bases, and pH   853
  Acids and Bases in the Blood   854
  Factors Affecting Acid–Base Balance   854
Altered Fluid, Electrolyte, and Acid–Base
  Balance   **855**
  Altered States of Fluid, Electrolyte, or Acid–Base
    Balance   855
  Potential for Altered Fluid, Electrolyte, and
    Acid–Base Balance   858
  Manifestations of Fluid, Electrolyte, or Acid–Base
    Imbalances   860
  Impact of Fluid, Electrolyte, or Acid–Base
    Imbalance on Activities of Daily Living   861
Assessment   **861**
  Subjective Data   861
  Objective Data   862
Nursing Diagnoses and Patient Goals   **866**
  Diagnostic Statement: Fluid Volume Deficit   866
  Diagnostic Statement: Fluid Volume Excess   866
  Related Nursing Diagnoses   867
  Patient Goals   867
Implementation   **867**
  Nursing Interventions to Promote Health
    and Function   867

  Nursing Interventions for Altered Fluid
    and Electrolyte Status   868
  Discharge Planning and Home Care   884
Evaluation   **886**
Key Concepts   **887**
Procedure 32-1 **Monitoring an Intravenous**
        Infusion   **873**
Procedure 32-2 **Changing Intravenous Solution**
        and Tubing   **877**
        Changing Solution Container   **877**
        Changing Solution and Tubing   **878**
Procedure 32-3 **Administering a Blood**
        Transfusion   **883**

33 Nutrition   **890**
Normal Nutritional Function   **892**
  Anatomy of the Digestive System   892
  Normal Physiologic Function of Nutrients   893
  Normal Physiologic Function of the Digestive
    System   900
  Characteristics of Normal Nutrition   901
  Normal Nutritional Functional Pattern   902
  Factors Affecting Normal Nutrition   905
  Lifespan Considerations   907
Altered Nutritional Function   **909**
  Potential for Altered Nutritional Function   909
  Manifestations of Altered Nutrition   911
Assessment   **912**
  Subjective Data   912
  Objective Data   913
Nursing Diagnoses and Patient Goals   **915**
  Altered Nutrition: Less than Body Requirements   915
  Altered Nutrition: More than Body Requirements   915
  Altered Nutrition: High Risk for More than Body
    Requirements   915
  Impaired Swallowing   915
  Related Nursing Diagnoses   916
  Patient Goals   916
Implementation   **916**
  Nursing Interventions to Promote Health
    and Function   916
  Nursing Interventions for Altered Function   917
  Discharge Planning and Home Care   929
Evaluation   **930**
Key Concepts   **932**
Procedure 33-1 **Assisting an Adult with Feeding**   **918**
Procedure 33-2 **Administering Nutrition via**
        Nasogastric or Gastrostomy
        Tube   **924**
        Bolus or Intermittent Feeding   **925**
        Continuous Feeding   **925**
Procedure 33-3 **Administering Total Parenteral**
        Nutrition (TPN)   **926**
        Monitoring TPN Therapy   **926**
        Changing TPN Tubing
        and Dressing   **927**
        Administering Intralipids   **927**

34 Skin Integrity and Wound Healing   **934**
Normal Integumentary Function   **936**
  Anatomy   936
  Normal Physiologic Function   937
  Characteristics of Normal Skin   937

Normal Integumentary Functional Pattern 938
Factors Affecting Normal Integumentary Function 938
Lifespan Considerations 938
Altered Integumentary Function **939**
Potential for Altered Integumentary Function 939
Manifestations of Altered Integumentary Function 944
Wound Healing in Altered Integumentary Function 945
Impact of Integumentary Dysfunction on Activities
of Daily Living 950
Assessment **951**
Subjective Data 951
Objective Data 952
Nursing Diagnoses and Patient Goals **954**
Diagnostic Statement: Impaired Skin Integrity 954
Diagnostic Statement: Impaired Tissue Integrity 954
Related Nursing Diagnoses 954
Patient Goals 954
Implementation **954**
Nursing Interventions to Promote Health
and Integumentary Function 955
Nursing Interventions for Altered Integumentary
Function 957
Discharge Planning and Home Care 976
Evaluation **976**
Key Concepts **978**
Procedure 34-1 **Changing a Dry Sterile**
Dressing 961
Procedure 34-2 **Applying Wet-to-Dry Dressings** 964
Procedure 34-3 **Maintaining a Portable**
(Hemovac) Wound Suction 968
Procedure 34-4 **Irrigating a Wound** 970
Procedure 34-5 **Applying a Cold Pack** 973
Procedure 34-6 **Applying Aquathermia Pads** 975

35   The Body's Defenses
Against Infection **980**
Normal Resistance to Infection **982**
Characteristics of Normal Resistance to Infection 982
Factors Affecting Normal Resistance to Infection 985
Lifespan Considerations 986
Altered Resistance to Infection **992**
Potential for Infection 992
Manifestations of Infection 998
Impact of Infection on Activities of Daily Living 1000
Assessment **1000**
Subjective Data 1001
Objective Data 1001
Nursing Diagnoses and Patient Goals **1005**
Diagnostic Statement: High Risk for Infection 1005
Related Nursing Diagnoses 1005
Patient Goals 1006
Implementation **1006**
Nursing Interventions to Promote Health
and Function 1006
Nursing Interventions for Altered Function 1009
Discharge Planning and Home Care 1012
Evaluation **1014**
Key Concepts **1014**

36   Thermoregulation **1016**
Normal Thermoregulation **1018**
Heat Production 1018
Heat Loss 1020

Normal Pattern of Body Temperature 1021
Factors Affecting Normal Body Temperature 1022
Lifespan Considerations 1023
Altered Thermoregulation **1024**
Potential for Altered Thermoregulation 1024
Manifestations of Altered Thermoregulation 1026
Impact of Altered Temperature on Activities
of Daily Living 1028
Assessment **1028**
Subjective Data 1028
Objective Data 1029
Nursing Diagnoses and Patient Goals **1030**
Diagnostic Statement: High Risk for Altered
Body Temperature 1030
Diagnostic Statement: Hypothermia 1030
Diagnostic Statement: Hyperthermia 1030
Diagnostic Statement: Ineffective
Thermoregulation 1030
Related Nursing Diagnoses 1030
Patient Goals 1031
Implementation **1031**
Nursing Interventions to Promote Health 1031
Nursing Interventions for Altered
Thermoregulation 1032
Discharge Planning and Home Care 1034
Evaluation **1035**
Key Concepts **1036**

UNIT **IX:**   Elimination 1038
37   Urinary Elimination **1040**
Normal Urinary Function **1042**
Anatomy of the Urinary Tract 1042
Normal Function of the Urinary System 1043
Characteristics of Normal Urine 1045
Normal Pattern of Urinary Elimination 1046
Factors Affecting Normal Urinary Elimination 1046
Lifespan Considerations 1047
Altered Urinary Function **1048**
Potential for Altered Urinary Function 1048
Manifestations of Altered Urinary Function 1051
Impact of Urinary Dysfunction on Activities
of Daily Living 1054

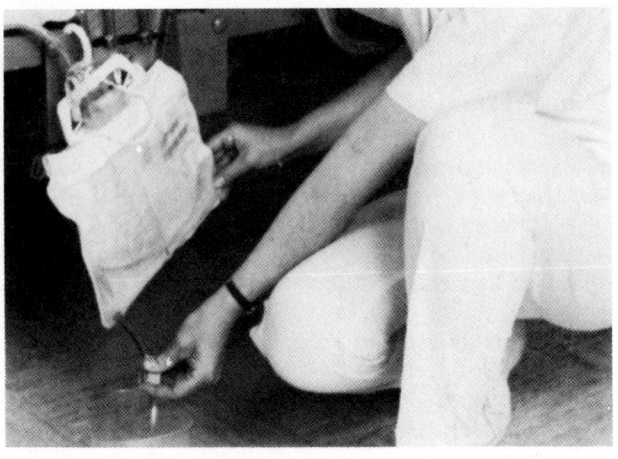

Characteristics of Normal Feces   1093
Normal Functional Bowel Pattern   1093
Factors Affecting Normal Bowel Elimination   1094
Lifespan Considerations   1095
Altered Bowel Function   **1096**
Potential for Altered Bowel Function   1096
Manifestations of Altered Bowel Function   1098
Impact of Bowel Dysfunction on Activities
   of Daily Living   1101
Assessment   **1102**
Subjective Data   1102
Objective Data   1103
Nursing Diagnoses and Patient Goals   **1108**
Diagnostic Statement: Colonic Constipation   1108
Diagnostic Statement: Perceived Constipation   1109
Diagnostic Statement: Diarrhea   1109
Diagnostic Statement: Bowel Incontinence   1109
Related Nursing Diagnoses   1110
Patient Goals   1110
Implementation   **1110**
Nursing Interventions to Promote Health
   and Function   1110
Nursing Interventions for Altered Bowel Function   1111
Discharge Planning and Home Care   1125
Evaluation   **1129**
Key Concepts   **1131**
Procedure 38-1   **Assessing Stool for Occult
        Blood**   **1107**
Procedure 38-2   **Administering an Enema**   **1115**
        Large-Volume Enema   **1115**
        Small-Volume Enema   **1116**
Procedure 38-3   **Inserting a Nasogastric Tube**   **1121**
Procedure 38-4   **Applying a Fecal Ostomy Pouch**   **1126**
Procedure 38-5   **Irrigating a Colostomy**   **1127**

UNIT **X:**   Sleep and Rest   1134

39   Sleep and Rest   **1136**
Normal Sleep/Rest Function   **1137**
Normal Physiologic Function   1138
Characteristics of Normal Sleep/Rest Function   1142
Normal Functional Sleep/Rest Pattern   1142
Factors Affecting Sleep and Rest   1143
Lifespan Considerations   1144
Altered Sleep/Rest Function   **1145**
Potential for Altered Sleep Function   1145
Manifestations of Altered Sleep Function   1148
Impact of Sleep Dysfunction on Activities
   of Daily Living   1150
Assessment   **1150**
Subjective Data   1150
Objective Data   1151
Nursing Diagnosis and Patient Goals   **1151**
Diagnostic Statement: Sleep Pattern Disturbance   1151
Related Nursing Diagnoses   1151
Patient Goals   1151
Implementation   **1151**
Nursing Interventions to Promote Health
   and Sleep/Rest Function   1151
Nursing Interventions for Altered Function   1153
Discharge Planning and Home Care   1154
Evaluation   **1154**
Key Concepts   **1155**

Assessment   **1054**
Subjective Data   1054
Objective Data   1055
Nursing Diagnoses and Patient Goals   **1064**
Diagnostic Statement: Stress Incontinence   1064
Diagnostic Statement: Urge Incontinence   1064
Diagnostic Statement: Reflex Incontinence   1064
Diagnostic Statement: Functional Incontinence   1065
Diagnostic Statement: Total Incontinence   1065
Diagnostic Statement: Urinary Retention   1065
Related Nursing Diagnoses   1065
Patient Goals   1065
Implementation   **1066**
Nursing Interventions to Promote Health and
   Urinary Function   1066
Nursing Interventions for Altered Function   1068
Discharge Planning and Home Care   1083
Evaluation   **1085**
Key Concepts   **1086**
Procedure 37-1   **Collecting Urine Specimens**   **1057**
        **Collecting Sterile Specimen
        from an Indwelling Catheter**   **1057**
        **Collecting Midstream Urine
        Specimen for a Female**   **1057**
        **Collecting Midstream Urine
        Specimen for a Male**   **1058**
        **Collecting a Specimen
        from a Child Without
        Urinary Control**   **1058**
Procedure 37-2   **Testing Specific Gravity
        of Urine**   **1061**
Procedure 37-3   **Applying a Condom Catheter**   **1070**
Procedure 37-4   **Inserting a Straight or
        Indwelling Urinary Catheter**   **1073**
        **Inserting Catheter for
        a Woman**   **1073**
        Inserting Catheter for a Man   **1075**
        **Removing an Indwelling
        Catheter**   **1077**
Procedure 37-5   **Performing Continuous Bladder
        Irrigation**   **1080**

38   Bowel Elimination   **1088**
Normal Bowel Function   **1090**
Anatomy of the Gastrointestinal Tract   1090
Normal Function of the Intestine   1092

UNIT XI: Cognition and Perception   1158

40   Pain Perception and Comfort   1160
Normal Function of Pain   **1162**
Anatomy   1162
Normal Physiology of Pain   1163
Characteristics of Pain   1165
Normal Function of Pain Perception   1166
Factors Affecting Normal Pain Function   1166
Lifespan Considerations   1167
Altered Function Resulting in Pain   **1168**
Potential Causes of Pain   1168
Manifestations of Pain   1168
Impact of Pain on Activities of Daily Living   1170
Assessment   **1170**
Subjective Data   1170
Objective Data   1172
Nursing Diagnoses and Patient Goals   **1174**
Diagnostic Statement: Pain   1174
Diagnostic Statement: Chronic Pain   1175
Related Nursing Diagnoses   1175
Patient Goals   1175
Implementation   **1175**
Nursing Interventions to Promote Health and Function   1175
Nursing Interventions for Altered Comfort   1176
Discharge Planning and Home Care   1185
Evaluation   **1186**
Key Concepts   **1186**

41   Sensory Perception   1190
Normal Sensory Perception Function   **1191**
Normal Function of Sensory Perception   1191
Characteristics of Normal Sensory Perception   1192
Normal Functional Sensory Pattern   1192
Factors Affecting Normal Sensory Perception   1192
Lifespan Considerations   1193
Altered Sensory Function   **1193**
Potential for Altered Sensory Function   1193
Manifestations of Altered Sensory Function   1196
Impact of Dysfunction on Activities of Daily Living   1196
Assessment   **1197**
Subjective Data   1197
Objective Data   1198
Nursing Diagnosis and Patient Goals   **1199**
Diagnostic Statement: Sensory/Perceptual Alterations   1199
Related Nursing Diagnoses   1199
Patient Goals   1200
Implementation   **1200**
Nursing Interventions to Promote Sensory Health and Function   1200
Nursing Interventions for Altered Sensory Function   1201
Discharge Planning and Home Care   1203
Evaluation   **1206**
Key Concepts   **1207**

42   Cognitive Processes   1210
Normal Cognitive Function   **1212**
Anatomy   1212
Normal Physiologic Function   1213
Characteristics of Normal Cognition   1214
Normal Cognitive Functional Pattern   1215

Factors Affecting Normal Cognitive Function   1216
Lifespan Considerations   1217
Altered Cognitive Function   **1219**
Potential for Altered Cognition   1219
Manifestations of Altered Function   1221
Impact of Dysfunction on Activities of Daily Living   1223
Assessment   **1223**
Subjective Data   1223
Objective Data   1226
Nursing Diagnosis and Patient Goals   **1229**
Diagnostic Statement: Altered Thought Processes   1229
Related Nursing Diagnoses   1229
Patient Goals   1229
Implementation   **1229**
Nursing Interventions to Promote Cognitive Health and Function   1229
Nursing Interventions for Altered Cognitive Function   1231
Discharge Planning and Home Care   1234
Evaluation   **1235**
Key Concepts   **1236**

UNIT XII: Self-Perception and Self-Concept   1238

43   Self-Concept   1240
Normal Function of Self   **1242**
Characteristics of Normal Self-Concept   1242
Normal Functional Self-Concept Patterns   1243
Factors Affecting Normal Self-Concept   1244
Lifespan Considerations   1245
Potential for Altered Self-Concept   1249
Manifestations of Altered Function   1250
Impact of Dysfunction on Activities of Daily Living   1252
Assessment   **1252**
Subjective Data   1252
Objective Data   1253
Nursing Diagnoses and Patient Goals   **1253**
Diagnostic Statement: Body Image Disturbance   1253
Diagnostic Statement: Self-Esteem Disturbance   1253
Diagnostic Statement: Personal Identity Disturbance   1253
Diagnostic Statement: Altered Role Performance   1254
Related Nursing Diagnoses   1254
Patient Goals   1254

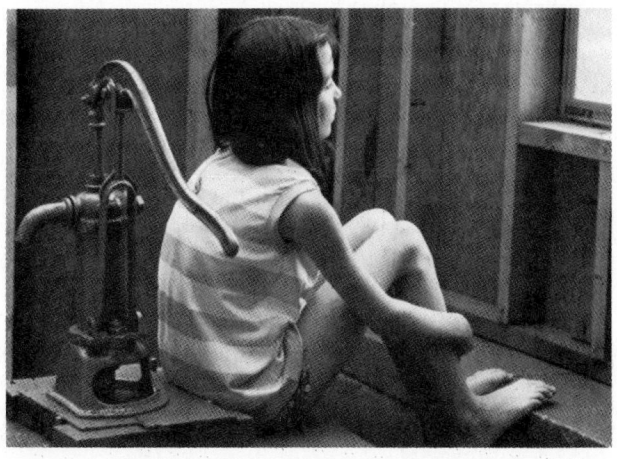

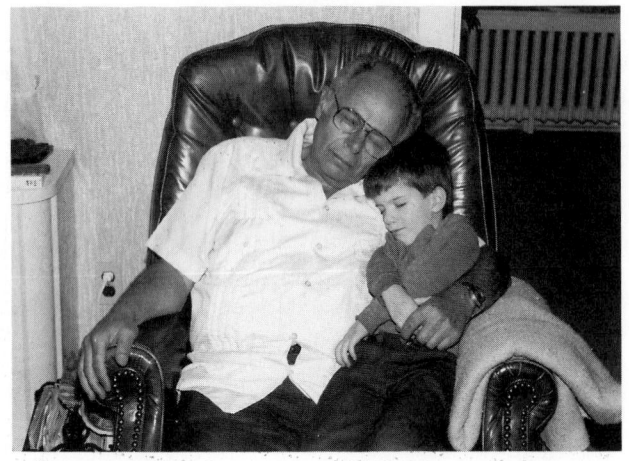

Implementation   **1254**
Nursing Interventions to Promote Health
   and Function   1254
Nursing Interventions for Altered Self-Concept   1256
Discharge Planning and Home Care   1257
Evaluation   **1258**
Key Concepts   **1259**

UNIT **XIII:**   Roles and
               Relationships   **1262**

44   **Communication: Social Interaction**   **1264**
Normal Communication   **1265**
Anatomy of Communication Centers   1266
Normal Function of Communication   1267
Characteristics of Normal Communication   1267
Factors Affecting Normal Communication   1268
Lifespan Considerations   1269
Altered Communication   **1270**
Potential for Altered Communication   1270
Manifestations of Altered Communication   1271
Impact on Activities of Daily Living   1273
Assessment   **1273**
Subjective Data   1274
Objective Data   1275
Nursing Diagnosis and Patient Goals   **1276**
Diagnostic Statement: Impaired Verbal
   Communication   1276
Related Nursing Diagnoses   1276
Patient Goals   1276
Implementation   **1277**
Nursing Interventions to Promote Health
   and Function   1277
Nursing Interventions for Altered Communication
   Function   1277
Discharge Planning and Home Care   1280
Evaluation   **1281**
Key Concepts   **1283**

45   **Families and Their Relationships**   **1286**
Normal Family Function   **1287**
Characteristics of a Normal Family   1288
Normal Functional Family Pattern   1290
Factors Affecting Normal Family Function   1290
Lifespan Considerations   1291

Altered Family Function   **1292**
Potential for Altered Function   1292
Manifestations of Altered Family Function   1294
Impact of Family Dysfunction on Activities
   of Daily Living   1295
Assessment   **1296**
Subjective Assessment   1296
Objective Data   1298
Nursing Diagnoses and Patient Goals   **1298**
Diagnostic Statement: Altered Family Processes   1298
Diagnostic Statement: Ineffective Family Coping:
   Disabling   1298
Diagnostic Statement: Ineffective Family Coping:
   Compromised   1299
Diagnostic Statement: Altered Parenting   1300
Related Nursing Diagnoses   1300
Patient Goals   1300
Implementation   **1300**
Nursing Interventions to Promote Family Health
   and Function   1300
Nursing Interventions for Altered Family Function   1302
Discharge Planning and Home Care   1303
Evaluation   **1304**
Key Concepts   **1304**

46   **Loss and Grieving**   **1308**
Normal Grief Function   **1309**
Characteristics of Normal Grief and Loss   1309
Normal Functional Grief Pattern   1315
Factors Affecting Normal Function   1315
Lifespan Considerations   1316
Altered Grieving Function   **1318**
Potential for Altered Grieving Function   1318
Manifestations of Altered Grieving Function   1318
Assessment   **1319**
Subjective Data   1319
Objective Data   1321
Nursing Diagnoses and Patient Goals   **1321**
Diagnostic Statement: Anticipatory Grieving   1321
Diagnostic Statement: Dysfunctional Grieving   1321
Related Nursing Diagnoses   1322
Patient Goals   1322
Implementation   **1322**
Nursing Interventions to Promote Health
   and Grieving Function   1322
Nursing Interventions for Altered Grieving
   Function   1325
Discharge Planning and Home Care   1325
Evaluation   **1325**
Key Concepts   **1330**

UNIT **XIV:**   Coping and Stress
              Management   **1332**

47   **Stress, Coping, and Adaptation**   **1334**
Normal Coping and Adaptation to Stress   **1335**
Normal Function of Stress and Coping   1336
Characteristics of Normal Coping and Adaptation   1337
Normal Pattern of Coping and Adaptation   1340
Factors Affecting Normal Coping and Adaptation   1341
Lifespan Considerations   1342
Altered Coping and Adaptation to Stress   **1343**
Potential for Altered Coping   1343

Manifestations of Altered Coping 1344
Impact of Coping Dysfunction on Activities
of Daily Living 1345
Assessment **1345**
Subjective Data 1346
Objective Data 1347
Nursing Diagnosis and Patient Goals **1348**
Diagnostic Statement: Ineffective Individual
Coping 1348
Related Nursing Diagnoses 1349
Patient Goals 1349
Implementation **1349**
Nursing Interventions to Promote Health
and Function 1349
Nursing Interventions for Altered Coping Function 1353
Discharge Planning and Home Care 1354
Evaluation **1354**
Key Concepts **1356**

UNIT XV: Sexuality and
Reproduction **1358**

48   Human Sexuality **1360**
Normal Human Sexuality **1362**
Anatomy 1362
Normal Function of Male and Female
Reproductive Systems 1362
Characteristics of Normal Sexuality 1366
Normal Sexual Functional Pattern 1368
Factors Affecting Sexuality 1368
Lifespan Considerations 1369
Altered Sexual Function **1371**
Potential for Altered Sexuality 1371
Manifestations of Altered Sexuality 1372
Impact of Sexual Dysfunction on Activities
of Daily Living 1373
Assessment **1374**
Subjective Data 1374
Objective Data 1376
Nursing Diagnoses and Patient Goals **1377**
Diagnostic Statement: Sexual Dysfunction 1377
Diagnostic Statement: Altered Sexuality Patterns 1378
Related Nursing Diagnoses 1378
Patient Goals 1378
Implementation **1378**
Nursing Interventions to Promote Health
and Function 1378
Nursing Interventions for Altered Function 1383
Discharge Planning and Home Care 1383
Evaluation **1384**
Key Concepts **1385**

UNIT XVI: Values and Beliefs **1388**

49   Spiritual Health **1390**
Normal Spiritual Function **1391**
Characteristics of Normal Spirituality 1392
Normal Spiritual Functional Pattern 1393

Factors Affecting Normal Spiritual Expression 1394
Lifespan Considerations 1394
Altered Spiritual Function **1396**
Potential for Altered Spiritual Function 1396
Manifestations of Altered Spiritual Function 1397
Impact of Spiritual Dysfunction on Activities
of Daily Living 1397
Assessment **1399**
Subjective Data 1399
Objective Data 1401
Nursing Diagnoses and Patient Goals **1401**
Diagnostic Statement: Spiritual Distress
(Distress of the Human Spirit) 1401
Related Nursing Diagnoses 1402
Patient Goals 1402
Implementation **1402**
Nursing Interventions to Promote Spiritual Health
and Function 1402
Nursing Intervention for Altered Spiritual Function 1404
Discharge Planning and Home Care 1408
Evaluation **1409**
Key Concepts **1410**

Appendices
A. **Equivalents** **1413**
B. **Laboratory Values** **1415**
C. **Medical Terminology: Prefixes, Roots,**
and Suffixes **1438**
D. **Recommended Dietary Allowances, USA** **1445**
E. **Nutrition Recommendations for Canadians** **1448**

Glossary **1449**

Index **1467**

Nursing Procedures and Skills

CHAPTER 7: Nursing Assessment
Nursing Skill Collecting Data 102
Nursing Skill Validating Data 103
Nursing Skill Organizing Data 105

CHAPTER 8: Nursing Diagnosis
Nursing Skill Identifying Patterns 118
Nursing Skill Validating Diagnoses 120
Nursing Skill Formulating the Diagnostic
               Statement 121

CHAPTER 9: Nursing Management:
           Planning, Implementation,
           and Evaluation
Nursing Skill Establishing Priorities 128
Nursing Skill Establishing Patient Goals and
               Outcome Criteria 128
Nursing Skill Planning Nursing Interventions 129
Nursing Skill Writing the Nursing Care Plan 130
Nursing Skill Reassessing 135
Nursing Skill Setting Implementation Priorities 135
Nursing Skill Performing Nursing Interventions 136
Nursing Skill Recording Actions 139
Nursing Skill Reviewing Patient Goals and
               Outcome Criteria 142
Nursing Skill Collecting Data for Evaluation 142
Nursing Skill Measuring Goal Attainment 143
Nursing Skill Recording Judgment and
               Measurement of Goal Attainment 144
Nursing Skill Revising and Modifying the
               Nursing Care Plan 144

CHAPTER 10: Communication of the
            Nursing Process:
            Recording and Reporting
Nursing Skill Recording 149
Nursing Skill Reporting 165

CHAPTER 14: Individual, Family, and
            Community
Nursing Skill Assessing the Family 228
Nursing Skill Assessing the Community 233

CHAPTER 15: Culture and Ethnicity
Nursing Skill Assessing the Patient Using
               Cultural Sensitivity 247

CHAPTER 16: Values
Nursing Skill Assessing Values 269

CHAPTER 18: Health Assessment of
            Human Function
Nursing Skill Preparing the Patient and
               Environment for Assessment 296
Nursing Skill Positioning and Draping for
               Assessment 297
Nursing Skill Obtaining Subjective Data: The
               Interview 297
Nursing Skill Obtaining Objective Data: The
               Physical Examination 303
Nursing Skill Assessing Health Perception and
               Health Management 307
Nursing Skill Assessing Activity and Exercise 308
Procedure 18-1 Auscultating Breath Sounds 315
Procedure 18-2 Auscultating Heart Sounds 319
Nursing Skill Assessing Nutrition and
               Metabolism 320
Procedure 18-3 Measuring Weight 323
                Weight with Chair Scale 323
                Weight with Standing Scale 323
                Weight with Bed Scale 323
Procedure 18-4 Auscultating Bowel Sounds 324
Nursing Skill Assessing Elimination 327
Nursing Skill Assessing Sleep and Rest 328
Nursing Skill Assessing Cognition and
               Perception 328
Procedure 18-5 Assessing the Neurologic
                System 330
Nursing Skill Assessing Self-Perception and
               Self-Concept 337
Nursing Skill Assessing Roles and
               Relationships 339
Nursing Skill Assessing Coping and Stress
               Tolerance 340
Nursing Skill Assessing Sexuality and
               Reproduction 341
Nursing Skill Assessing Values and Beliefs 343

CHAPTER 19:   Vital Sign Assessment

Procedure 19-1	*Assessing Body Temperature*	355
	Assessing Oral Temperature	355
	Assessing Axillary Temperature	355
	Assessing Rectal Temperature	356
Procedure 19-2	*Obtaining a Pulse*	359
	Radial Pulse	359
	Apical Pulse	359
Procedure 19-3	*Assessing Pulse Deficits*	362
Procedure 19-4	*Assessing Respirations*	365
Procedure 19-5	*Obtaining Blood Pressure*	367
Procedure 19-6	*Assessing for Orthostatic Hypotension*	373

CHAPTER 20:   Diagnostic Tests and Procedures

Nursing Skill	Preparing the Patient for Diagnostic Tests	380
Procedure 20-1	*Preparing the Patient for Diagnostic Procedures*	381
Nursing Skill	Nursing Responsibilities During Testing	383
Nursing Skill	Nursing Responsibilities After Testing	384
Procedure 20-2	*Measuring Blood Glucose by Skin Puncture*	389

CHAPTER 21:   Patient Teaching

Nursing Skill	Assessing Learning Needs	413
Nursing Skill	Assessing Learning Readiness	414

CHAPTER 22:   Asepsis

Procedure 22-1	*Handwashing*	441
Nursing Skill	Cleaning, Disinfecting, and Sterilizing	443
Nursing Skill	Creating and Maintaining a Sterile Field	445
Procedure 22-2	*Donning and Removing a Mask and Gown*	446
	Donning Mask	446
	Donning Clean Gown	446
	Removing Contaminated Gown	447
Procedure 22-3	*Practicing a Strict Isolation Technique*	452
Nursing Skill	Using Sterile Technique	453
Nursing Skill	Preparing Skin for Surgery	454
Nursing Skill	Handwashing for Surgery	456
Procedure 22-4	*Applying and Removing Sterile Gloves*	458
	Applying Gloves	458
	Removing Gloves	460

CHAPTER 23:   Perioperative Nursing

Nursing Skill	Assessing the Preoperative Patient	474
Nursing Skill	Preparing the Patient for Surgery	480
Nursing Skill	Assessing the Intraoperative Patient	484
Nursing Skill	Assessing the Patient in the Recovery Room	490
Nursing Skill	Assessing the Postoperative Patient	491

CHAPTER 24:   Medication Administration

Nursing Skill	Assessing Before Medication Administration	516
Nursing Skill	Calculating Medication Dosages	519
Nursing Skill	Calculating Pediatric Medication Dosages	521
Nursing Skill	Dispensing Medications According to the Five Rights	521
Procedure 24-1	*Administering Oral Medications*	524
Nursing Skill	Administering Medications Through Tubes	527
Nursing Skill	Administering Medications by Sublingual Route	528
Nursing Skill	Administering Buccal Medications	528
Nursing Skill	Administering Irrigating Solutions	528
Nursing Skill	Administering Creams and Lotions	528
Nursing Skill	Administering Transdermal Medications	529
Nursing Skill	Administering Ophthalmic Medications	529
Nursing Skill	Administering Otic Medications	529
Nursing Skill	Administering Nasal Medications	529
Nursing Skill	Administering Rectal Medications	529
Nursing Skill	Administering Vaginal Medications	530
Nursing Skill	Administering Inhaled Medications	530
Procedure 24-2	*Drawing up Two Medications in a Syringe*	535
	Modification for Insulin	536
Procedure 24-3	*Administering Subcutaneous Injections*	538
	Variations for Administering Heparin	540
Nursing Skill	Giving IM Injections at the Deltoid Site	542
Nursing Skill	Giving IM Injections at the Rectus Femoris and Vastus Lateralis Sites	542
Procedure 24-4	*Administering Intramuscular Injections*	543
	Variations for Air Lock Injection Technique	545
	Variations for Z-track Injections	545
Nursing Skill	Giving IM Injections at the Ventrogluteal Site	545
Nursing Skill	Giving IM Injections at the Dorsogluteal Site	546
Nursing Skill	Giving Medications by IV Push	547
Procedure 24-5	*Administering IV Medications*	
	Using Intermittent Infusion Technique	551
	Using a Heparin Lock	552
Nursing Skill	Giving Medications by Continuous Infusion	552
Nursing Skill	Planning for Medications After Discharge	553

CHAPTER 25:   Safety

Nursing Skill	Assessing for Safety	576
Nursing Skill	Planning for Discharge Related to Safety	587

CHAPTER 26:   **Health Maintenance**

Nursing Skill   Assessing for Health Maintenance   601
Nursing Skill   Teaching About Common Illnesses   605
Nursing Skill   Teaching Self-Examination Techniques   607
Nursing Skill   Providing Routine Health Care   607
Nursing Skill   Planning for Discharge Related to Health Maintenance   608

CHAPTER 27:   **Home Maintenance Management**

Nursing Skill   Assessing for Home Maintenance Management   620
Nursing Skill   Assessing the Home for Home Maintenance   622
Nursing Skill   Assessing the Community for Support   622
Nursing Skill   Contracting with the Patient for Home Maintenance Management   628
Nursing Skill   Planning for Discharge in Impaired Home Maintenance Management   629

CHAPTER 28:   **Self-Care and Hygiene**

Nursing Skill   Assessing for Self-Care and Hygiene   648
Procedure 28-1   *Bathing a Patient in Bed*   657
Procedure 28-2   *Assisting with the Bath or Shower*   661
Nursing Skill   Providing Perineal Care   662
Nursing Skill   Brushing and Combing the Patient's Hair   663
Procedure 28-3   *Massaging the Back*   664
Nursing Skill   Shaving the Patient   665
Procedure 28-4   *Performing Foot and Nail Care*   666
Procedure 28-5   *Shampooing Hair of a Bedridden Patient*   668
Procedure 28-6   *Providing Oral Care*   670
    Variation for the Unconscious Patient   671
Nursing Skill   Caring for Dentures   672
Nursing Skill   Providing Eye Care   673
Nursing Skill   Caring for Eyeglasses   673
Nursing Skill   Caring for Contact Lenses   673
Nursing Skill   Caring for the Patient with an Artificial Eye   676
Nursing Skill   Caring for the Eyes of a Comatose Patient   676
Nursing Skill   Providing Ear Care   676
Nursing Skill   Caring for Hearing Aids   676
Nursing Skill   Feeding Patients   677
Nursing Skill   Providing a Urinal   678
Nursing Skill   Helping the Patient Dress   678
Procedure 28-7   *Using a Bedpan*   679
    Placing the Bedpan   679
    Removing the Bedpan   680
Nursing Skill   Planning for Discharge Related to Self-Care Hygiene   682
Procedure 28-8   *Making an Unoccupied Bed*   683
Procedure 28-9   *Making an Occupied Bed*   686

CHAPTER 29:   **Body Mechanics and Mobility**

Procedure 29-1   *Using Proper Body Mechanics*   698
Nursing Skill   Assessing Mobility   714
Nursing Skill   Assessing Alignment   716
Nursing Skill   Assessing Balance   716
Nursing Skill   Assessing Coordination   716
Nursing Skill   Assessing Gait   716
Nursing Skill   Assessing Joint Structure and Function   716
Nursing Skill   Assessing Muscle Mass and Strength   716
Nursing Skill   Assessing the Risk for Falls   716
Nursing Skill   Assessing Activity Tolerance   717
Procedure 29-2   *Positioning a Patient in Bed*   723
    Moving a Patient up in Bed (One Nurse)   723
    Moving Helpless Patient up in Bed (Two Nurses)   723
    Positioning Patient in Side Lying Position   724
    Logrolling   725
Procedure 29-3   *Providing Range-of-Motion Exercises*   728
Procedure 29-4   *Assisting with Ambulation*   730
    One Nurse   730
    Two Nurses   731
    Using a Walker   731
Procedure 29-5   *Helping Patients with Crutch Walking*   733
    Four-Point Gait   733
    Three-Point Gait   734
    Two-Point Gait   734
    Swinging-to Gait   735
    Swinging-through Gait   735
    Climbing Stairs   735
    Descending Stairs   735
Nursing Skill   Using a Hydraulic Lift for Transfer   735
Nursing Skill   Planning for Discharge Related to Mobility   735
Procedure 29-6   *Transferring a Patient to a Stretcher*   736
Procedure 29-7   *Transferring a Patient to a Wheelchair*   737

CHAPTER 30:   **Oxygenation: Respiratory Function**

Nursing Skill   Assessing for Respiratory Function   759
Nursing Skill   Teaching Pursed-Lip Breathing   767
Procedure 30-1   *Teaching Coughing and Deep-Breathing Exercises*   768
    Deep Breathing   768
    Controlled Coughing   768
Nursing Skill   Assisting with IPPB Treatment   769
Nursing Skill   Promoting Deep Coughing   770
Nursing Skill   Promoting Stacked Coughing   770
Nursing Skill   Promoting Low-Flow (Huff) Coughing   770
Nursing Skill   Promoting Quad Coughing   770
Nursing Skill   Using Handheld Nebulizers   771

Procedure 30-2   *Promoting Breathing with the Incentive Spirometer*   771

Procedure 30-3   *Administering Oxygen by Nasal Cannula or Mask*   776

Nursing Skill   Managing Hyperventilation   780

Nursing Skill   Managing Hypoventilation   780

Nursing Skill   Providing Chest Physiotherapy   780

Procedure 30-4   *Suctioning Oropharyngeal and Nasopharyngeal Areas*   782

Procedure 30-5   *Suctioning Nasotracheal Secretions*   786

Nursing Skill   Planning for Discharge Related to Respiratory Function   788

Procedure 30-6   *Providing Tracheostomy Care*   789

Procedure 30-7   *Managing an Obstructed Airway (Heimlich Maneuver) Conscious Adult (Heimlich Maneuver)*   793

   Unconscious Patient (Heimlich Maneuver, Abdominal Thrust)   794

   Infants Under 1 Year of Age (Back Blows and Chest Thrusts)   794

   Children Over 1 Year of Age   794

   Pregnant Women or Very Obese Adults (Chest Thrusts)   794

CHAPTER 31:   **Oxygenation: Cardiac Function and Tissue Perfusion**

Nursing Skill   Assessing Cardiac Function and Tissue Perfusion   817

Procedure 31-1   *Applying Antiembolic Stockings*   828

Nursing Skill   Elevating Limbs   829

Nursing Skill   Positioning for Cardiovascular Dysfunction   829

Nursing Skill   Managing Chest Pain   830

Nursing Skill   Using Energy Conservation   830

Nursing Skill   Helping the Cardiovascular Patient Rehabilitate   831

Procedure 31-2   *Administering Cardiopulmonary Resuscitation (CPR)*   833

   One Rescuer—Adult Patient   833

   Two Rescuers—Adult Patient   835

   One Rescuer CPR—Infant and Child   835

CHAPTER 32:   **Fluid, Electrolyte, and Acid–Base Balance**

Nursing Skill   Assessing Fluid, Electrolyte, and Acid–Base Balance   861

Nursing Skill   Monitoring Intake and Output   862

Nursing Skill   Monitoring Body Weight   864

Nursing Skill   Assessing Integumentary Function   864

Nursing Skill   Assessing Veins   864

Nursing Skill   Increasing Oral Fluids   868

Nursing Skill   Restricting Oral Fluids   868

Nursing Skill   Replacing Electrolytes   869

Nursing Skill   Doing a Venipuncture   871

Procedure 32-1   *Monitoring an Intravenous Infusion*   873

Procedure 32-2   *Changing Intravenous Solution and Tubing*   877

   Changing Solution Container   877

   Changing Solution and Tubing   877

Nursing Skill   Discontinuing an Intravenous Infusion   880

Nursing Skill   Selecting Blood Donors   881

Procedure 32-3   *Administering a Blood Transfusion*   883

Nursing Skill   Planning for Discharge Related to Fluid, Electrolyte, and Acid–Base Balance   884

CHAPTER 33:   **Nutrition**

Nursing Skill   Assessing Nutritional Status   912

Nursing Skill   Evaluating Swallowing   914

Procedure 33-1   *Assisting an Adult with Feeding*   919

Procedure 33-2   *Administering Nutrition via Nasogastric or Gastrostomy Tube*   924

   Bolus or Intermittent Feeding   925

   Continuous Feeding   925

Procedure 33-3   *Administering Total Parenteral Nutrition (TPN)*   926

   Monitoring TPN Therapy   926

   Changing TPN Tubing and Dressing   927

   Administering Intralipids   927

Nursing Skill   Planning for Discharge Related to Nutrition   929

CHAPTER 34:   **Skin Integrity and Wound Healing**

Nursing Skill   Assessing Skin Integrity and Wound Healing   951

Nursing Skill   Inspecting the Skin   952

Nursing Skill   Inspecting the Wound   952

Nursing Skill   Inspecting for Infection   953

Nursing Skill   Preventing Pressure Sores   956

Nursing Skill   Providing Pruritus Relief   957

Nursing Skill   Providing First Aid for Minor Wounds   957

Nursing Skill   Providing First Aid for Minor Burns   958

Nursing Skill   Caring for Sutures, Staples, and Clips   960

Procedure 34-1   *Changing a Dry Sterile Dressing*   961

Nursing Skill   Applying Bandages   963

Procedure 34-2   *Applying Wet-to-Dry Dressings*   964

Nursing Skill   Applying Binders   965

Nursing Skill   Managing Wound Drainage   966

Nursing Skill   Advancing and Removing Drains   967

Procedure 34-3   *Maintaining a Portable (Hemovac) Wound Suction*   968

Nursing Skill   Packing Wounds   969

Procedure 34-4   *Irrigating a Wound*   970

Nursing Skill   Applying Cold Compresses   972

Nursing Skill   Applying Warm Compresses   972

Procedure 34-5   *Applying a Cold Pack*   973

Nursing Skill   Providing a Sitz Bath   974

Nursing Skill   Applying Hot Packs   974

Nursing Skill   Using Heating Pads   974

Nursing Skill   Using Heat Lamps   974

Nursing Skill Using Heat Cradles 974
Procedure 34-6 *Applying Aquathermia Pads* 975
Nursing Skill Planning for Discharge Related to Skin Integrity and Wound Healing 976

CHAPTER 35: **The Body's Defenses Against Infection**

Nursing Skill Assessing Body Defenses and Signs of Infection 1000
Nursing Skill Enhancing Host Defenses 1009
Nursing Skill Preventing Spread of Infection 1011
Nursing Skill Instituting Isolation 1011
Nursing Skill Disposing of Secretions 1012
Nursing Skill Planning for Discharge Related to Infection Control 1012

CHAPTER 36: **Thermoregulation**

Nursing Skill Assessing Thermoregulation 1028
Nursing Skill Managing a Fever 1032
Nursing Skill Managing Hyperthermia 1034
Nursing Skill Managing Hypothermia 1034
Nursing Skill Planning for Discharge Related to Thermoregulation 1034

CHAPTER 37: **Urinary Elimination**

Nursing Skill Assessing Urinary Elimination 1054
Procedure 37-1 *Collecting Urine Specimens* 1057
  Collecting Sterile Specimen from an Indwelling Catheter 1057
  Collecting Midstream Urine Specimen for a Woman 1057
  Collecting Midstream Urine Specimen for a Man 1058
  Collecting a Specimen from a Child Without Urinary Control 1058
Procedure 37-2 *Testing Specific Gravity of Urine* 1061
Nursing Skill Promoting Fluid Intake 1066
Nursing Skill Preventing Urinary Tract Infection 1066
Nursing Skill Promoting Perineal Muscle Tone 1066
Nursing Skill Providing Bladder Training 1069
Procedure 37-3 *Applying a Condom Catheter* 1070
Procedure 37-4 *Inserting a Straight or Indwelling Urinary Catheter* 1073
  Inserting Catheter for a Woman 1073
  Inserting Catheter for a Man 1075
  Removing an Indwelling Catheter 1076
Procedure 37-5 *Performing Continuous Bladder Irrigation* 1080
Nursing Skill Using Bladder Credé 1081
Nursing Skill Caring for the Patient Undergoing Peritoneal Dialysis 1082
Nursing Skill Caring for the Patient Undergoing Hemodialysis 1083
Nursing Skill Planning for Discharge Related to Urinary Function 1083

CHAPTER 38: **Bowel Elimination**

Nursing Skill Assessing for Bowel Function 1102
Nursing Skill Measuring Abdominal Girth 1105
Nursing Skill Examining the Perirectal Area 1105

Nursing Skill Collecting Stool Specimens 1105
Procedure 38-1 *Assessing Stool for Occult Blood* 1107
Nursing Skill Teaching Regarding Healthy Bowel Function 1110
Procedure 38-2 *Administering an Enema* 1115
  Large-Volume Enema 1115
  Small-Volume Enema 1116
Nursing Skill Using a Rectal Tube 1117
Nursing Skill Caring for the Patient with Nasogastric Intubation 1120
Procedure 38-3 *Inserting a Nasogastric Tube* 1121
Nursing Skill Removing Fecal Impaction 1122
Nursing Skill Using a Bowel Training Program 1123
Nursing Skill Planning for Discharge Related to Bowel Function 1125
Procedure 38-4 *Applying a Fecal Ostomy Pouch* 1126
Procedure 38-5 *Irrigating a Colostomy* 1127

CHAPTER 39: **Sleep and Rest**

Nursing Skill Assessing for Sleep and Rest 1150
Nursing Skill Using Hypnotics 1153
Nursing Skill Planning for the Discharged Patient's Sleep and Rest 1154

CHAPTER 40: **Pain Perception and Comfort**

Nursing Skill Assessing for Pain 1170
Nursing Skill Positioning and Providing Hygiene for Patients in Pain 1176
Nursing Skill Providing Distraction for Pain Relief 1177
Nursing Skill Massaging for Pain Relief 1178
Nursing Skill Applying Heat and Cold for Pain Relief 1178
Nursing Skill Using Meditation for Pain Relief 1179
Nursing Skill Using Guided Imagery for Pain Relief 1179
Nursing Skill Planning for Pain Management After Discharge 1185

CHAPTER 41: **Sensory Perception**

Nursing Skill Assessing Sensory Function 1197
Nursing Skill Teaching Regarding Sensory Function 1200
Nursing Skill Preparing the Patient for Procedures 1200
Nursing Skill Providing Stimulation 1201
Nursing Skill Reducing Stimulation 1202
Nursing Skill Using Sensory Aids 1203
Nursing Skill Providing Safety for the Patient with Sensory Dysfunction 1203
Nursing Skill Planning for Discharge Related to Sensory Function 1203

CHAPTER 42: **Cognitive Processes**

Nursing Skill Assessing for Cognitive Function 1223
Nursing Skill Promoting Healthy Lifestyle for Cognitive Function 1229
Nursing Skill Helping the Patient Maintain Learning Skills 1231

Nursing Skill	Providing Safety for the Patient with Cognitive Dysfunction	1232
Nursing Skill	Using Reality Orientation	1233
Nursing Skill	Using Socialization Therapies	1234
Nursing Skill	Planning for Discharge Related to Cognitive Function	1234

CHAPTER 43:   Self-Concept

Nursing Skill	Assessing for Self-Concept	1252
Nursing Skill	Helping Patient Identify Strengths	1254
Nursing Skill	Helping the Patient Evaluate Self	1256
Nursing Skill	Helping the Patient Make Behavior Changes	1257
Nursing Skill	Planning for Discharge Related to Self-Concept	1257

CHAPTER 44:   Communication: Social Interaction

Nursing Skill	Assessing for Social Communication	1273
Nursing Skill	Teaching for Functional Communication	1277
Nursing Skill	Orienting the Patient to Surroundings	1278
Nursing Skill	Using Alternative Communication Skills	1278
Nursing Skill	Setting Environmental Restrictions	1280
Nursing Skill	Assisting with Coping Measures	1280
Nursing Skill	Planning for Discharge Related to Communication Dysfunction	1280

CHAPTER 45:   Families and Their Relationships

Nursing Skill	Assessing for Family Relationships	1296
Nursing Skill	Reinforcing Family Strengths	1301
Nursing Skill	Helping Families Problem Solve	1302
Nursing Skill	Planning for Discharge Related to Family Dysfunction	1303

CHAPTER 46:   Loss and Grieving

Nursing Skill	Assessing for Grieving	1319
Nursing Skill	Teaching Regarding Grieving and Loss	1323

Nursing Skill	Helping the Patient Work Through Grief Stages	1323
Nursing Skill	Caring for the Body of the Deceased	1324
Nursing Skill	Planning for Discharge of the Grieving Patient	1325

CHAPTER 47:   Stress, Coping, and Adaptation

Nursing Skill	Assessing for Stress and Coping	1345
Nursing Skill	Managing Stress in Nursing	1349
Nursing Skill	Reducing Stressors	1350
Nursing Skill	Addressing Perfection	1350
Nursing Skill	Changing Internal Messages	1350
Nursing Skill	Promoting Lifestyle Changes	1351
Nursing Skill	Assisting with Relaxation Techniques	1352
Nursing Skill	Reducing Environmental Stressors in the Health Care Facility	1354
Nursing Skill	Planning for Discharge Related to Stress Adaptation	1354

CHAPTER 48:   Human Sexuality

Nursing Skill	Assessing Sexual Function and Sexuality	1374
Nursing Skill	Teaching Regarding Sexuality	1378
Nursing Skill	Teaching Kegel Exercises	1381
Nursing Skill	Providing Sex Education	1381
Nursing Skill	Teaching Responsible Sex	1381
Nursing Skill	Providing Information about Contraceptives	1381
Nursing Skill	Counseling Regarding Sexual Dysfunction	1383
Nursing Skill	Planning for Discharge Related to Sexual Dysfunction	1383

CHAPTER 49:   Spiritual Health

Nursing Skill	Assessing for Spiritual Health	1399
Nursing Skill	Supporting Spiritual Practices	1403
Nursing Skill	Listening and Supporting Spiritual Needs	1404
Nursing Skill	Planning for Discharge Related to Spiritual Needs	1408

Nursing Diagnoses

CHAPTER 24	Noncompliance	518
	Knowledge Deficit	518
CHAPTER 25	High Risk for Injury	578
CHAPTER 26	Altered Health Maintenance	604
	Health-Seeking Behaviors	604
CHAPTER 27	Impaired Home Maintenance Management	623

CHAPTER 28	Self-Care Deficit: Bathing, Hygiene	651
	Self-Care Deficit: Dressing, Grooming	652
	Self-Care Deficit: Toileting	652
	Self-Care Deficit: Feeding	653
CHAPTER 29	Impaired Physical Mobility	717
	Activity Intolerance	717
	High Risk for Disuse Syndrome	718

CHAPTER 30	Ineffective Breathing Pattern	764
	Ineffective Airway Clearance	764
	Impaired Gas Exchange	764
CHAPTER 31	Altered Tissue Perfusion	823
	Decreased Cardiac Output	823
	Activity Intolerance	823
CHAPTER 32	Fluid Volume Deficit	866
	Fluid Volume Excess	866
CHAPTER 33	Altered Nutrition: Less Than Body Requirements	915
	Altered Nutrition: More Than Body Requirements	915
	Altered Nutrition: High Risk for More Than Body Requirements	915
	Impaired Swallowing	915
CHAPTER 34	Impaired Skin Integrity	954
	Impaired Tissue Integrity	954
CHAPTER 35	High Risk for Infection	1005
CHAPTER 36	High Risk for Altered Body Temperature	1030
	Hypothermia	1030
	Hyperthermia	1030
	Ineffective Thermoregulation	1030
CHAPTER 37	Stress Incontinence	1064
	Urge Incontinence	1064
	Reflex Incontinence	1064
	Functional Incontinence	1065
	Total Incontinence	1065
	Urinary Retention	1065

CHAPTER 38	Colonic Constipation	1108
	Perceived Constipation	1109
	Diarrhea	1109
	Bowel Incontinence	1109
CHAPTER 39	Sleep Pattern Disturbance	1151
CHAPTER 40	Pain	1174
	Chronic Pain	1175
CHAPTER 41	Sensory/Perception Alterations	1199
CHAPTER 42	Altered Thought Processes	1229
CHAPTER 43	Body Image Disturbance	1253
	Self-Esteem Disturbance	1253
	Personal Identity Disturbance	1253
	Altered Role Performance	1254
CHAPTER 44	Impaired Verbal Communication	1276
CHAPTER 45	Altered Family Processes	1298
	Ineffective Family Coping: Disabling	1298
	Ineffective Family Coping: Compromised	1299
	Altered Parenting	1300
CHAPTER 46	Anticipatory Grieving	1321
	Dysfunctional Grieving	1321
CHAPTER 47	Ineffective Individual Coping	1348
CHAPTER 48	Sexual Dysfunction	1377
	Altered Sexuality Patterns	1378
CHAPTER 49	Spiritual Distress	1401

Nursing Management Plans

CHAPTER 25	The Patient at Risk for Injury	589
CHAPTER 26	The Patient with Health-Seeking Behavior	609
CHAPTER 27	The Patient with Impaired Home Maintenance Management	634
CHAPTER 28	The Patient with Self-Care Deficit	690
CHAPTER 29	The Patient with Impaired Physical Mobility	741
CHAPTER 30	The Patient with Ineffective Airway Clearance	796
CHAPTER 31	The Patient with Activity Intolerance	838
CHAPTER 32	The Patient with Fluid Volume Deficit	885

CHAPTER 33	The Patient with Altered Nutrition	931
CHAPTER 34	The Patient with Impaired Skin Integrity	977
CHAPTER 35	The Patient at Risk for Infection	1013
CHAPTER 36	The Patient with Ineffective Thermoregulation	1035
CHAPTER 37	The Patient with Urge Incontinence	1084
CHAPTER 38	The Patient with Constipation	1130
CHAPTER 39	The Patient with Sleep Pattern Disturbance	1156
CHAPTER 40	The Patient Experiencing Pain	1187
CHAPTER 41	The Patient with Sensory/Perceptual Alterations	1205

CHAPTER 42   The Patient with Altered Thought
Processes   1236

CHAPTER 43   The Patient with Body Image
Disturbance   1259

CHAPTER 44   The Patient with Impaired Verbal
Communication   1282

CHAPTER 45   The Infant and Family with Altered
Parenting   1305

CHAPTER 46   The Patient Who Is Grieving   1326

CHAPTER 47   The Patient with Ineffective
Individual Coping   1355

CHAPTER 48   The Patient with Sexual Dysfunction 1385

CHAPTER 49   The Patient with Spiritual Distress 1409

Summary of Recurring Displays

CHAPTER 1: The Profession of Nursing:
Theory, Education, and
Practice

CHAPTER 2: The Health-Care Delivery
System
Nursing Research   36

CHAPTER 3: Ethical and Legal Concerns
Nursing Research   43
Safety Alert   56
Patient Teaching   56

CHAPTER 4: Leadership and
Management
Nursing Research   68

CHAPTER 5: Nursing Research

CHAPTER 6: The Nursing Process in
Human Health and
Function
Nursing Research   91

CHAPTER 7: Nursing Assessment
Nursing Research   107

CHAPTER 8: Nursing Diagnosis
Nursing Research   122

CHAPTER 9: Nursing Management:
Planning, Implementation,
and Evaluation
Nursing Research   130

CHAPTER 10: Communication of the
Nursing Process: Recording
and Reporting
Nursing Research   155
Safety Alert   168

CHAPTER 11: Health and Wellness
Nursing Research   181

CHAPTER 12: Human Needs

CHAPTER 13: Lifespan Development
Nursing Research   218

CHAPTER 14: Individual, Family, and
Community
Nursing Research: Family   225
Nursing Research: Community 229

CHAPTER 15: Culture and Ethnicity
Nursing Research   247

CHAPTER 16: Values
Nursing Research   269

CHAPTER 17: Communication:
The Nurse–Patient
Relationship
Nursing Research   290

CHAPTER 18: Health Assessment of
Human Function
Patient Teaching   303
Nursing Research   344
Safety Alert   345

CHAPTER 19: Vital Sign Assessment
Safety Alert   351
Nursing Research   372
Patient Teaching   374

CHAPTER 20: Diagnostic Tests and
Procedures
Patient Teaching   380
Safety Alert   383
Nursing Research   403

CHAPTER 21: **Patient Teaching**
Nursing Research   418

CHAPTER 22: **Asepsis**
Safety Alert   433
Nursing Research   456
Patient Teaching   460

CHAPTER 23: **Perioperative Nursing**
Nursing Research   468
Patient Teaching   478
Safety Alert   485

CHAPTER 24: **Medication Administration**
Safety Alert   510
Nursing Research   512
Patient Teaching   553

CHAPTER 25: **Safety**
Nursing Research   576
Selected Nursing Interventions for Common Problems   579
Patient Teaching: Childproofing the Home   583
Patient Teaching: Preventing Childhood Poisoning   585

CHAPTER 26: **Health Maintenance**
Nursing Research   599
Selected Nursing Interventions for Common Problems   605
Patient Teaching   606
Safety Alert   608

CHAPTER 27: **Home Maintenance Management**
Selected Nursing Interventions for Common Impaired HMM Problems   627
Patient Teaching   630
Nursing Research   631

CHAPTER 28: **Self-Care and Hygiene**
Nursing Research   652
Selected Nursing Interventions for Common Self-Care Problems   654
Safety Alert   655
Safety Alert: Bathing   656
Patient Teaching: Self-Care and Hygiene   689

CHAPTER 29: **Body Mechanics and Mobility**
Nursing Research   714
Selected Nursing Interventions for Common Altered Mobility Problems   719
Safety Alert   727
Patient Teaching   740

CHAPTER 30: **Oxygenation: Respiratory Function**
Nursing Research   756
Selected Nursing Interventions for Selected Respiratory Dysfunctions   765
Patient Teaching   766
Safety Alert   772

CHAPTER 31: **Oxygenation: Cardiac Function and Tissue Perfusion**
Nursing Research   814
Selected Nursing Interventions for Common Cardiac Problems   825
Patient Teaching   824
Safety Alert   830

CHAPTER 32: **Fluid, Electrolyte, and Acid–Base Balance**
Nursing Research   857
Patient Teaching   868
Safety Alert   881
Selected Nursing Interventions for Common Fluid and Electrolyte Problems   882

CHAPTER 33: **Nutrition**
Patient Teaching   917
Selected Nursing Interventions for Common Nutritional Problems   920
Safety Alert   921
Nursing Research   930

CHAPTER 34: **Skin Integrity and Wound Healing**
Nursing Research   942
Patient Teaching   955
Selected Nursing Interventions for Common Skin Integrity Problems   957
Safety Alert   969

CHAPTER 35: **The Body's Defenses**
Against Infection
Nursing Research   1007
Patient Teaching   1009
Safety Alert   1012

CHAPTER 36: **Thermoregulation**
Nursing Research   1026
Selected Nursing
Interventions for
Alterations in
Thermoregulation   1031
Patient Teaching:
Thermoregulation   1031
Safety Alert   1034

CHAPTER 37: **Urinary Elimination**
Selected Nursing
Interventions for
Common Urinary
Problems   1068
Safety Alert   1076
Patient Teaching   1081
Nursing Research   1082

CHAPTER 38: **Bowel Elimination**
Nursing Research   1099
Patient Teaching   1110
Selected Nursing
Interventions for
Common Bowel
Problems   1112
Safety Alert   1123

CHAPTER 39: **Sleep and Rest**
Patient Teaching   1152
Safety Alert   1152
Nursing Research   1153
Selected Nursing
Interventions for
Common Sleep
Problems   1154

CHAPTER 40: **Pain Perception and**
Comfort
Nursing Research   1174
Selected Nursing
Interventions for
Common Pain
Problems   1176
Safety Alert   1177
Patient Teaching   1186

CHAPTER 41: **Sensory Perception**
Patient Teaching   1200
Nursing Research   1201
Selected Nursing
Interventions for
Common Sensory
Problems   1203
Safety Alert   1204

CHAPTER 42: **Cognitive Processes**
Nursing Research   1231
Selected Nursing
Interventions for
Common Problems
of Confusion   1232
Safety Alert   1232

CHAPTER 43: **Self-Concept**
Safety Alert   1254
Selected Nursing
Interventions for
Common Body-Image
Problems   1257
Patient Teaching   1257
Nursing Research   1258

CHAPTER 44: **Communication: Social**
Interaction
Patient Teaching   1277
Selected Nursing
Interventions for
Common Communication
Problems   1278
Selected Nursing
Interventions for
Communicating with
Patients with
Comprehension Deficits   1279
Safety Alert   1279
Nursing Research   1280
Family Teaching: Patients
with Expression Deficits   1281

CHAPTER 45: **Families and Their**
Relationships
Nursing Research   1299
Patient Teaching   1301
Selected Nursing
Interventions for
Common Family
Problems   1302
Safety Alert   1303

CHAPTER 46: **Loss and Grieving**
Nursing Research   1322
Patient Teaching   1323
Selected Nursing
Interventions to
Help the Patient Move
Through Grief Stages   1324

CHAPTER 47: **Stress, Coping, and**
Adaptation
Nursing Research   1343
Safety Alert   1349
Patient Teaching   1351
Selected Nursing
Interventions for
Common Stress
Problems   1354

CHAPTER 48: **Human Sexuality**
Nursing Research 1368
Safety Alert 1377
Selected Nursing
Interventions for
Common Sexuality
Problems 1378
Patient Teaching 1379, 1380

CHAPTER 49: **Spiritual Health**
Nursing Research 1401
Safety Alert 1402
Patient Teaching 1403
Selected Nursing
Interventions for
Common Spirituality
Problems 1404

Conceptual Foundations of Nursing

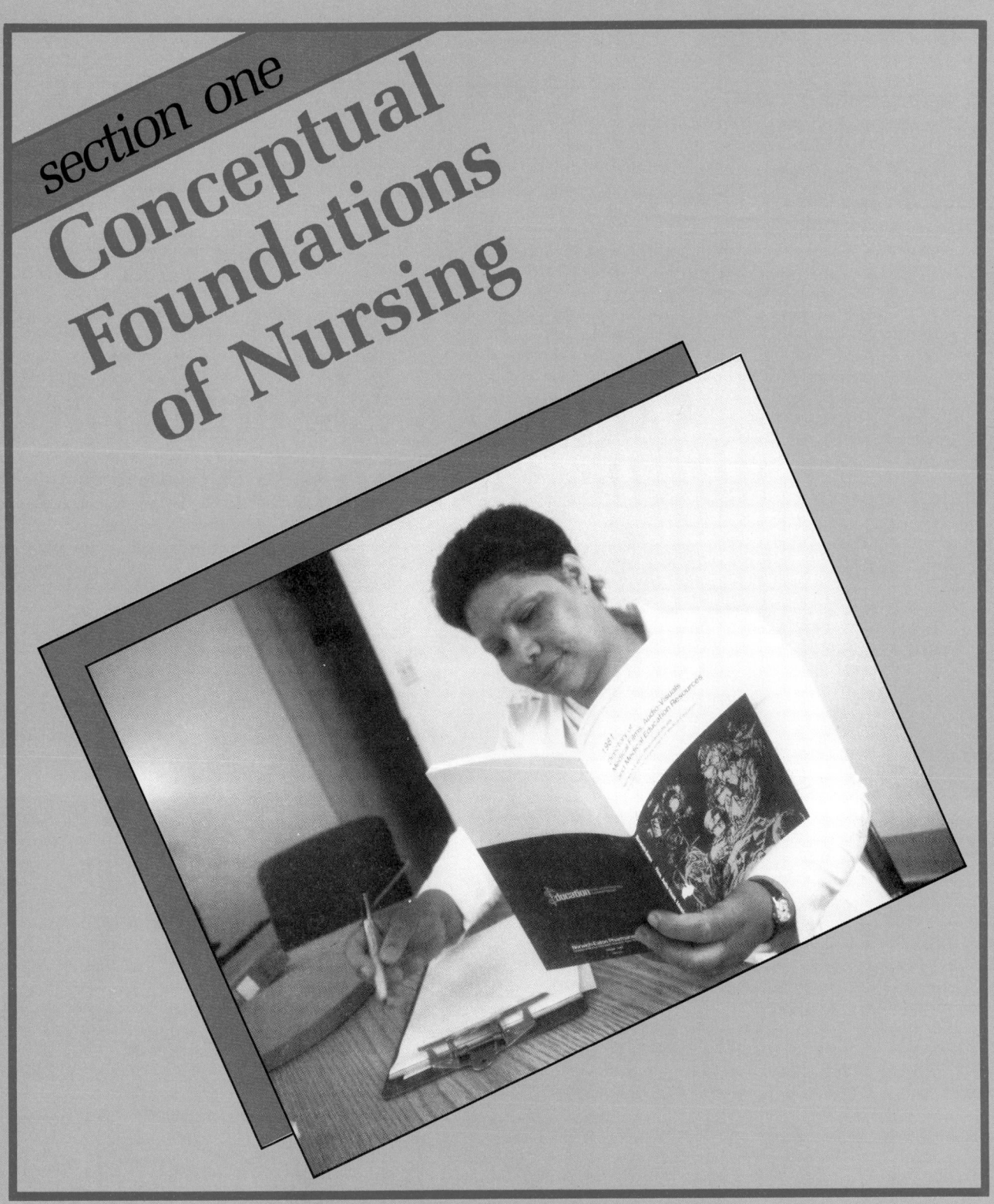

UNIT I
Concepts Essential for Professional Nursing

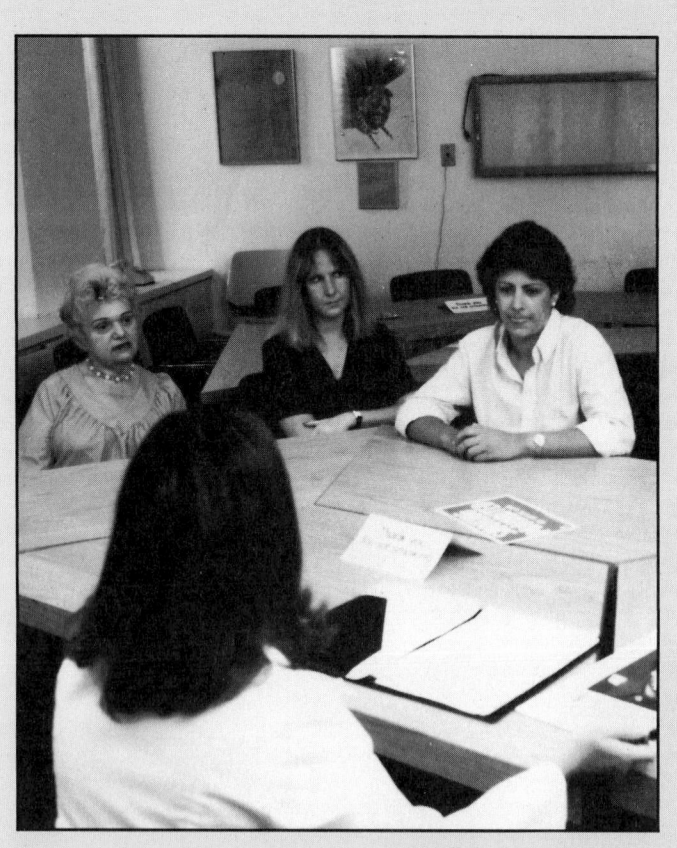

CHAPTERS

1 The Profession of Nursing: Theory, Education, and Practice

2 The Health-Care Delivery System

3 Ethical and Legal Concerns

4 Leadership and Management

5 Nursing Research

Professional nursing has a strong history and a solid foundation in theory and education. The practice of nursing today is dynamic and challenging and builds on historical and theoretical foundations. Unit I introduces the profession of nursing and explores the principles and concepts that underlie its theory, education, and practice.

The first chapter provides the knowledge base for understanding professional nursing and explores its history, practice guidelines, education, and organizations. Additionally, the work of various nursing theorists is presented in a way that promotes a beginning understanding and appreciation of this important basis for professional nursing. The next chapter discusses today's complex health care delivery system and the vital role of nursing within it. Chapter 3 considers the ethical and legal principles and concepts that underlie professional nursing practice and relationships. Chapter 4 provides a beginning discussion of leadership and management, skills and knowledge essential for practice in today's demanding and diverse health care environment. The final chapter in this unit introduces nursing research, which allows beginning practitioners to appreciate its relevance to clinical practice, to learn to be discriminating consumers of nursing research, and to value its importance in the advancement of professional nursing.

Unit I provides a strong foundation for understanding the many facets of the profession of nursing.

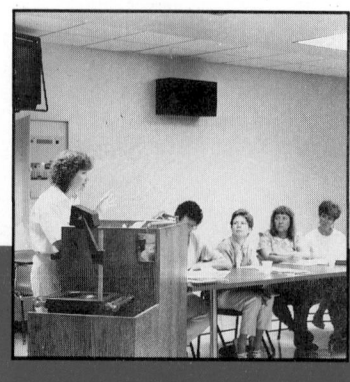

The Profession of Nursing: Theory, Education, and Practice

LEARNING OBJECTIVES

Upon completion of this chapter, the student will be able to do the following:

- Describe the evolution of professional nursing.
- Recognize major nursing theories and their relevance to nursing practice.
- Explain types of educational programs.
- Identify roles and responsibilities of professional nursing within the health-care delivery system.
- Describe career development opportunities and expanded nursing roles.
- Describe the purpose and function of professional nursing organizations.
- Discuss the impact of current and future social trends on professional nursing practice.

KEY TERMS

American Nurses Association
Clinical nurse specialist
In-service education
International Council of Nurses

Licensed practical nurse
National League for Nursing
Nurse administrator
Nurse anesthetist

Nurse educator
Nurse midwife
Nurse practice acts
Nurse practitioner
Nurse researcher

1

The Profession of Nursing
 Historic Evolution of Modern Nursing
  Pre-Christian Era
  Early Christian Era
  Contributions of the Greeks
  The Middle Ages
  The Renaissance
  The Reformation
  Nursing in the 18th Century
  Nursing in the 19th Century
  20th-Century Nursing
 Socialization to Professional Nursing
 Nursing and Professionalism Defined
Conceptual Frameworks and Theories of Nursing
 Four Major Concepts
 Concerns About Nursing Theory
  Does Nursing Have a Theory?
  Should Nursing Use a Single-Theory Approach
   or Multiple-Theory Approach?
  What Is the Relationship of Nursing Theory
   to Nursing Practice?

Educational Preparation and Career Opportunities
 Nursing Education
  Types of Educational Programs
  Advanced Nursing Education Opportunities
 Nursing Practice Settings
 Nursing Roles and Responsibilities
 Career Development and Expanded Nursing Roles
Professional Nursing Practice
 Standards of Practice
 Nurse Practice Acts
 Nursing Organizations
  American Nurses Association
  Canadian Nurses Association
  National League for Nursing
  National Student Nurses' Association
  International Council of Nurses
Current and Future Trends in Nursing Practice
Key Concepts

Nursing is a word that brings to mind a multitude of ideas and images. For some these images include white uniforms, nursing caps, needles, and bedpans; for others they include kindness, skill, compassion, and intelligence. Many factors have influenced the way nursing is perceived by the public, by nursing professionals, and by those beginning their nursing careers. Socialization of women, the portrayal of nursing in the media, and our history have had a considerable impact on the image of nursing today.

Nursing is caring, commitment, and dedication to meeting the functional health needs (physiologic, psychological, and sociologic) of all people. Nurses are people committed to identifying and meeting the health-care needs of individuals, families, and communities. As technology increases and society's health-care needs change, the need for well-educated nurses who are devoted to maintaining expertise in practice becomes critical.

Nursing is no longer isolated in hospital settings. Nursing means caring for communities and the homeless, addressing issues such as human rights and AIDS. Nursing means being socially responsible, involved, and committed to the health of all people.

As society's health-care needs continue to change, nursing continues to grow and change in response to these needs. Nursing offers a multitude of challenging, exciting career opportunities. As a profession, nursing continues to promote excellence in health care by attracting the brightest and most dedicated people. Students embarking on a professional nursing career accept responsibility for the health-care needs of society, as well as for the advancement of nursing as a profession.

This chapter provides a starting point for understanding where nursing has been, where it is now, and where it is headed as we move into the 21st century.

THE PROFESSION OF NURSING

The practice of professional nursing has evolved over many years. Contemporary nursing practice is different from that of the past, but issues affecting the profession today are connected to our history. Developing a sense of nursing's evolution provides the background necessary to understand current nursing practice. Figure 1-1 illustrates a training program in the early 20th century. Table 1-1 highlights events in nursing's history and shows how the past affects current nursing issues.

Historic Evolution of Modern Nursing

Although nursing in some form has probably existed throughout human history, documentation of the history of nursing goes back only 150 years. Nursing probably began as women intuitively identified and provided for their families' health-care needs. As individuals emerged with the desire and ability to nurture and provide care, the profession of nursing began to evolve.

Pre-Christian Era

Pre-Christian history makes few references to nursing; any discussions of nursing or medical roles were blurred. During the ancient cultures of the Babylonians, Egyptians, and Sumerians, the role of the nurse emerged. Then wealthy families were the primary recipients of

nursing care. If and when nursing care was made available outside wealthy homes, the nurse was primarily a servant. Subservient roles for women and nurses were rooted in the sexual discrimination and overall devaluation of human life reflective of this era. Cultural attitudes toward the sick, combined with the low status of women, provided major obstacles to nursing (Dolan, Fitzpatrick, & Herrmann, 1983).

Early Christian Era

Evidence of nursing roles became apparent in the early Christian era. Women performed roles that reflected components of today's nursing practice: dietitian, physical therapist, pharmacist, and counselor. Providing hygiene and comfort measures was the central focus of nursing (Dolan, et al., 1983).

The influence of Christianity raised nursing's social position by placing more value on human life and individuality. Compassion, charity, and willingness to serve were qualities associated with nurses. Deacons and deaconesses (individuals working for the church ministry) were designated to perform services for the sick because women's roles primarily involved marriage and childbearing (Kelly, 1985).

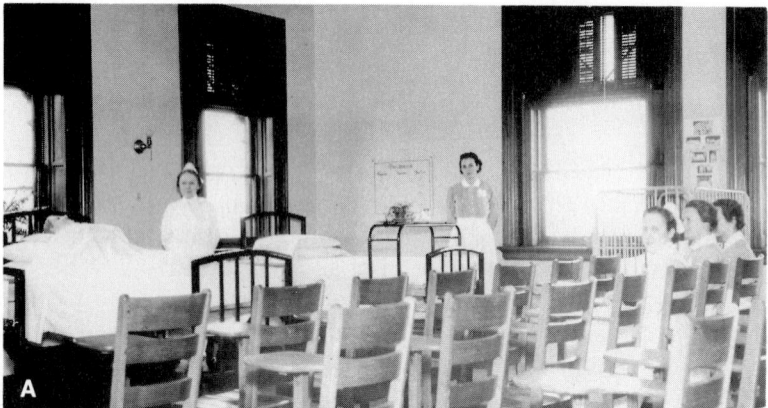

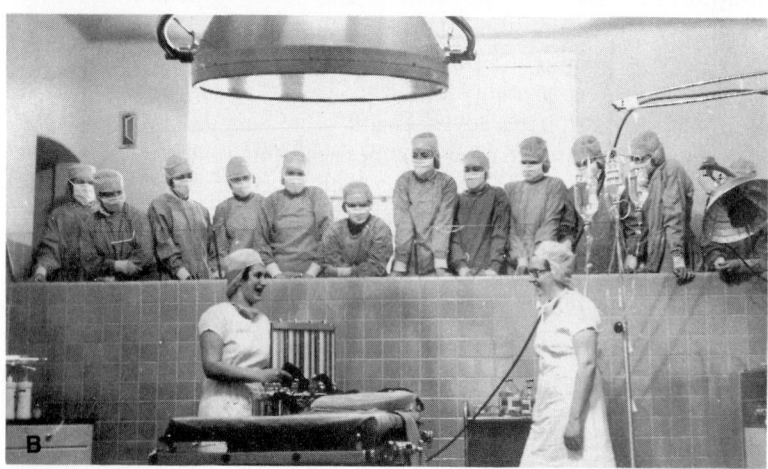

Figure 1–1.   Nurses' training in the early 20th century.   **A:** Classroom in an early training program.   **B:** Operating amphitheater for training students. (Courtesy of Moses Taylor Hospital, Scranton, PA)

TABLE 1–1

Significant Events in the History of Nursing

Date	Then	Now
1–500 (approximately)	Nursing care primarily involved meeting hygiene and comfort needs of individuals and families. Care was provided by Christians working in close association with an organized church.	Nursing care today involves a high degree of technology and includes responsibilities above and beyond hygiene and comfort measures, although these components of care continue to be very important. Today's nurse must be highly skilled and have knowledge in the sciences and humanities. Responsibilities are multiple and require an ability to think critically and to function safely. Nursing is no longer tied to the church, and nurses are educated in colleges and universities.
1836	Theodor Fleidner opened a small hospital and training school in Kaiserswerth, Germany, where Florence Nightingale, "The Founder of Modern Nursing" received her training.	Hospital-based schools of nursing continue to exist today, but numbers are declining as nursing maintains control of practice and our scientific knowledge base is expanded.
1854–1860	Florence Nightingale made major contributions to modern nursing, was named superintendent of nursing, cared for soldiers in the Crimean War, opened a training school at St. Thomas Hospital in London, and published "Notes on Nursing."	Nightingale's many contributions to nursing continue to affect the profession. The components of her theory are applicable even today, and nurses around the world recognize the courage, hard work, and dedication exemplified by this early nursing leader.
1861–1865	Dorothea Dix established the Nurse Corps of the U.S.A. Dix was not a nurse, but an advocate for the mentally ill.	Nurses continue to be offered the opportunity for exciting and rewarding careers in the armed services.
1872	America's first trained nurse, Linda Richards, graduated from the New England Hospital for Women in Boston.	Nursing continues to prepare educated, competent individuals to provide nursing care in institutions of higher education.
1873	Three nursing schools patterned after the Nightingale plan developed in the United States. Bellevue Training School, Connecticut Training School, Boston Training School.	New nursing programs continue to develop. Nursing now offers several routes to a career in nursing, including diploma, associate degree, baccalaureate degree, and the generic master's and doctoral degrees.
1882	American National Red Cross was organized by Clara Barton.	The Red Cross continues to exist today, offering care to victims of disasters and maintaining the nation's blood supply.
1893	Lillian Wald and Mary Brewster founded the Henry Street Settlement, the first home visiting nurse organization in the United States. The Henry Street Settlement can still be visited in New York City.	Visiting nurse associations have grown and become essential health-care components in society.
1897	Nurses' Associated Alumnae of United States and Canada organized. Renamed the American Nurses Association in 1911.	The American Nurses Association continues to function as American nursing's professional organization.
1899	International Council of Nurses (ICN) established.	ICN continues to represent and speak to international nursing concerns.
1900	American Journal of Nursing, the first nursing journal to be owned, operated, and published by nurses, was developed.	American Journal of Nursing continues to be a major reference for clinical nursing practice.
1923	Goldmark Report of the Rockefeller Foundation published, advocating financial support of university-based schools of nursing.	There is currently a decline in available financial support to incoming students of nursing. However, nursing organizations and leaders are working to improve financial assistance to students.
1940	World War II resulted in another nursing shortage. Esther Lucille Brown completed the Brown Report on nursing education, which said nursing education belonged in colleges and universities, not in hospitals.	Although hospital-based schools of nursing continue to exist, they are declining and students are more frequently choosing college educations.

(continued)

TABLE 1–1
(continued)

Date	Then	Now
1953	National Student Nurses' Association founded.	NSNA continues today to encourage nursing students to become involved in professional issues.
1965	ANA issued its first position paper on nursing education, calling for all nursing education to take place in institutions of higher education and stipulating the baccalaureate as the minimum preparation for professional nursing, the associate degree for technical nursing practice.	The entry-level debate continues into the 1990s, although baccalaureate and associate degree programs increase and hospital-based nursing programs decrease.
1990		Nursing is moving forward. Key issues are image, recruitment, solutions to the nursing shortage, and the ever-changing health-care delivery system.

Contributions of the Greeks

The Greeks made significant contributions to the care of the sick and, to a certain extent, to the profession of nursing. Hippocrates, known as "the father of medicine," made a major advance in medicine by rejecting the belief that diseases had supernatural causes. He is also credited with developing assessment standards for patients, establishing overall medical standards, and recognizing a need for nurses (Kelly, 1985).

The Middle Ages

Poverty was a critical problem during the Middle Ages, but nursing continued to shape the purpose and direction of health care and provide leadership in the field. These advancements were enhanced by the continuing spread of Christianity, which had positive effects on cultural values and institutions. The influence of Christianity also improved the status of nursing by attracting intelligent individuals from respected families (Dolan, et al., 1983). The Crusades resulted in the establishment of military nursing orders and the recruitment of men into nursing. Hospitals and religious orders were formed to meet specific health-care needs.

The Renaissance

During the Renaissance (1400 to 1600) recognition of the need for sound educational preparation in nursing contributed to further advancement of the profession. Unfortunately, the continued lack of effective sanitation as well as increasing poverty resulted in serious health-care problems. The immediate need for health-care providers, due to a significant increase in medical problems, further delayed the move toward improving nursing education (Dolan, et al., 1983).

The Reformation

Nursing encountered a severe setback during the Reformation. The dispersion of religious orders, which had been the primary source of health care, resulted in a serious deterioration in hospital conditions and nursing care. Attempts to improve nursing education and the image of nurses were destroyed (Dolan, et al., 1983).

Nursing in the 18th Century

Revolutions and epidemics resulted in further expansion of nursing roles. The prevention of illness became a primary objective of the nursing profession. Continuing problems with poor sanitation and low standards of living increased the need for what we know today as public-health nursing (Dolan, et al., 1983).

By the end of the 18th century there was evidence of nursing in hospitals, but nurses' working conditions were poor, resulting in a loss of social status for the profession. As nursing's social status deteriorated, fewer qualified individuals chose to enter the profession. Nursing was considered a last-resort occupation.

Society's attitudes about nursing during this time were reflected in Charles Dickens' *Martin Chuzzlewit* (1884), in which nursing care was provided by criminals and women of low moral standards. One of the book's characters, Sarah Gamp, was a nurse who abused alcohol and was cruel to her patients. This negative portrayal of nursing seriously damaged the profession's image, and fragments of such images can still be found in media portrayals of nursing today (Dolan, et al., 1983).

Nursing in the 19th Century

New problems and social changes affected the profession and the role of the nurse. The 19th century brought the

Industrial Revolution and was characterized by political, economic, and social expansion. Poverty, long work days for women and children, and the prevalence of disease increased the need for community health nurses. Continued emphasis was placed on the need for proper preparation of nurses. Nursing was once again influenced by religion: the caring image of the nurse was believed to be based on a spiritual calling to the profession. Poverty, innocence, and submissiveness were qualities associated with potential nursing candidates (Dolan, et al., 1983).

Florence Nightingale. Florence Nightingale has been called "the founder of modern nursing." Unyielding and stubborn, Nightingale improved health laws, reformed hospitals, reorganized military medical services, and established nursing as a profession with two missions: sick nursing and health nursing. Nightingale saw "sick nursing" as helping patients to use their own reparative processes to get well, and "health nursing" as the prevention of illness (Dolan, et al., 1983; Kelly, 1985).

Nightingale was born May 12, 1820, in Florence, Italy, to a wealthy English family and was educated in languages, philosophy, and the liberal arts. Much to her family's dismay, she entered nurses' training when she was 31 in the hope of replacing the "Sarah Gamp" image with that of well-educated, intelligent, kind nurses (Dolan, et al., 1983).

Nightingale's contributions to nursing were many. She was the superintendent of nurses at King's College Hospital until she left to care for soldiers during the Crimean War. Her efforts during this war were credited with halving the mortality rate, and she soon became known as "the lady with the lamp" as she made midnight rounds to the soldiers. In 1859 Nightingale published *Notes on Nursing* and in 1860 started the Nightingale Training School for Nurses. Nightingale was gracious and hardworking, and her contributions continue to influence the profession today (Dolan, et al., 1983).

Nursing During the American Civil War. During the Civil War (1861 to 1865), there was a need for more hospitals, as well as more and better prepared nurses. Although she was not a nurse, Dorothea Dix established the Nurse Corps of the U.S. Army, further expanding nursing's role. Another early nursing leader, Clara Barton, practiced nursing on Civil War battlefields. Barton founded the American Red Cross, an organization that continues to make significant contributions to society and health care today (Dolan, et al., 1983).

Nursing Education in the 19th Century. In 1869 the American Medical Association developed the Committee on the Training of Nurses, and as a result of this committee's recommendations hospital-based schools of nursing under medical supervision emerged. In 1874, Linda Richards, America's first trained nurse, gradu-

ated from the Bellevue Hospital Training School in New York City.

The central focus of nursing during this time was caring for the sick. Despite improvements in nursing education, major problems remained. Nursing students were expected to perform such nonnursing duties as scrubbing floors and doing laundry. They also were used as free labor in hospitals as they gained clinical experience (Dolan, et al., 1983).

As the 19th century came to a close, the profession saw the emergence of public-health nursing. Two early nursing leaders, Lillian Wald and Mary Brewster, established the first public-health nursing service for the sick and poor, the Henry Street Settlement on New York City's Lower East Side. The Henry Street Settlement is now a famous center of public-health nursing (Dolan, et al., 1983).

20th-Century Nursing

In the early 20th century, professional organizations such as the American Nurses Association (ANA), the Canadian Nurses Association (CNA), the International Council of Nurses (ICN), and the National League for Nursing (NLN) emerged. Nursing journals were developed and research was conducted into the need for higher education in nursing. The American Journal of Nursing (AJN), first published in 1900, was the first nursing journal to be owned, operated, and published by nurses. AJN continues to be a significant nursing publication (Dolan, et al., 1983).

A noteworthy milestone in the history of nursing education occurred in 1923 with the publication of the Goldmark Report, which advocated financial support for university-based schools of nursing. This report's findings eased the transition from hospital-based schools of nursing to university settings, marking a major advance in nursing education (Dolan, et al., 1983).

The casualties of World War II brought a critical nursing shortage, prompting quick solutions to increase the number of nurses and providing a setback for the move toward university-based nursing education. Nonetheless, Esther Lucille Brown, in her report on nursing education published at that time, wrote that nursing education belonged in colleges and universities, not in hospitals. This report provided further documentation of the need for university-based nursing education programs (Dolan, et al., 1983).

In 1965, a report by the National Commission on Nursing and Nursing Education addressed several nursing issues, including supply and demand for nurses, clarification of nursing roles and functions, nursing education, and available career opportunities for nurses. The report, called the Lysaught Report in honor of the study's director, helped clarify the role of professional nursing practice (Dolan, et al., 1983).

The latter part of the 20th century has been marked by rapid scientific advances and increasingly complex technology. Longer lifespans, increased incidence of chronic illness, and new family structures have had a dramatic impact on where and how nurses practice. Despite these changes, nursing continues to focus on the delivery of care that is safe, comprehensive, and effective.

Nursing's historic antecedents affect the profession today. Education, practice settings, and roles have all been influenced by the profession's history. Likewise, when, how, and why the profession evolves will be directly related to the contributions made by present and future nursing professionals. Social forces can be expected to influence future definitions of nursing, just as these forces have affected nursing practice to date.

Socialization to Professional Nursing

Socialization is a process that involves learning theory and skills and internalizing an identity appropriate to a specific role. Internalizing a specific role allows one to participate as a member of a group.

Students often enter nursing with the perception that their professional identity will center on providing service to individuals who are ill or who require care in regaining health. Although this initial perception may be true, it is only a small part of the professional identity that students must internalize when they join the profession. Socialization to nursing involves changes that ultimately affect a student's knowledge base, attitudes, and values regarding professional nursing practice. This socialization is a lifelong process that occurs as the individual grows personally and professionally. As the student becomes socialized to nursing, an understanding of the nursing profession develops and is internalized.

Professions generally have a specific body of knowledge, a specific set of values, and specific skills that differentiate them from one another. Professional nursing curriculums teach foundations of the discipline of nursing. Theoretical and clinical instruction facilitate the development of a professional identity and prepare students to function as beginning professional nurses. Beyond this initial socialization to nursing, continuing socialization occurs as the nurse gains experience in the workplace and perhaps pursues advanced education.

Patricia Benner, in *From Novice to Expert* (1984), discusses socialization and skill acquisition in nursing using the Dreyfuss model (Table 1-2). According to this model, a student passes through five levels of proficiency in acquiring and developing a skill: novice, advanced beginner, competent, proficient, and expert. Differences in each level reflect changes in three areas of skill performance. In the first level, the student moves from relying on abstract principles to using past concrete experiences. The second level involves a change from seeing situations in parts to seeing them more conceptually, or as a whole. Finally, in the third level, the student is no longer outside the situation observing, but is involved directly in the situation.

TABLE 1-2
Dreyfuss Model of Skill Acquisition Applied to Nursing

Novice	A beginning nursing student, or any nurse entering a situation where he or she has had no previous experience. Behavior is governed by established rules and is limited and inflexible.
Advanced beginner	The advanced beginner can demonstrate marginally acceptable performance. He or she has had enough experience in actual situations to identify meaningful aspects or global characteristics that can be identified only through prior experience.
Competent	Competence is reflected by the nurse who has been on the same job for 2 or 3 years and who consciously and deliberately plans nursing care in terms of long-range goals.
Proficient	The proficient nurse perceives situations as wholes rather than in terms of aspects and manages nursing care rather than performing tasks.
Expert	The expert nurse no longer relies on rules or guidelines to connect understanding of a situation to an appropriate action. The expert nurse, with an enormous background of experience, has an intuitive grasp of the situation and zeroes in on the problem immediately.

The five levels of proficiency listed in the left column were developed by Stuart Dreyfuss and Hubert Dreyfuss. The second column reflects the author's summary of a discussion by Patricia Benner in *From Novice to Expert: Excellence and Power in Clinical Nursing Practice*. (San Francisco: Addison-Wesley, 1984).

Nursing and Professionalism Defined

Because definitions of nursing reflect the values and influences of society, there are times when the profession is subject to misinterpretation. One common misconception is that nurses are handmaidens to physicians; other misconceptions can readily be seen on television and in films and novels. Beginning nursing professionals must form a clear, accurate understanding of professional nursing practice if precise interpretations of the role of the nurse are to be shared by other members of the health-care team and the public.

Nursing is a multifaceted profession and, as such, has been defined in a variety of ways. Florence Nightingale defined nursing as "the act of utilizing the environment of the patient to assist him in his recovery" (Nightingale, 1860/1969). The ANA defined nursing as "the diagnosis and treatment of human responses to actual or potential health problems" (ANA Social Policy Statement). The CNA published this definition (CNA, 1980):

> "Nursing" or "the practice of nursing" means the identification and treatment of human responses to actual or potential health problems and includes the practice of and supervision of functions and services that directly or indirectly, in collaboration with a client or providers of health care other than nurses, have as their objectives the promotion of health, prevention of illness, alleviation of suffering, restoration of health, and optimum development of health potential and includes all aspects of the nursing process."

Despite the multitude of definitions, common themes emerge. Holism, caring, teaching, supporting, promoting, maintaining, and restoring health are all components of nursing practice. Nursing care involves creativity, sensitivity, and care based on scientific rationale. All of these components are part of the practice, but nurses should not limit themselves to these themes alone.

The question of whether nursing is a profession has been a topic of ongoing debate. To answer this question, it is first helpful to examine the established criteria for a profession. Several criteria to evaluate nursing's professional status have been proposed, including the need for higher education, a specific body of knowledge, public interest and responsibility, and internal organization. Table 1-3 compares the patterns identified in developing professions with characteristics specific to nursing.

From Table 1-3, one can see that nursing is a profession that is evolving and growing. The growth of professionalism in nursing has been influenced by higher and more specialized education, as well as by increased autonomy in practice. As more nurses obtain master's and doctoral degrees, the profession's specific body of knowledge becomes clearer and more accurately defined. Furthermore, increased levels of research activity, accountability, and responsibility have contributed to enhance nursing's status as a profession.

CONCEPTUAL FRAMEWORKS AND THEORIES OF NURSING

The science and practice of nursing have been identified as nursing's two major dimensions. Without nursing science, nursing practice could not exist (Rogers, 1970). The science of nursing incorporates the study of relation-

---

TABLE 1–3
Professional Development Patterns Compared to Nursing

Patterns of Developing Professions	Nursing Profession
Professions require critical thinking ability and higher education.	Nurses are educated in institutions of higher learning and provide responsible and accountable nursing care to patients and families.
Professions are based on a specific body of knowledge.	Nursing has identified and continues to develop its own specific body of knowledge from which nursing practice emerges. Application of theory derived from research provides rationale for action.
Professions characteristically are accompanied by acceptance of responsibility and are fueled by public interest.	Nursing professionals accept a great deal of responsibility in providing for the health-care needs of people. The profession evolved in response to needs identified by society and is guided by an ethical code.

ships among nurses, patients, and their environments within the context of health. From nursing science, nursing theories evolve. As the nursing profession continues to develop its own body of knowledge, we can expect that concepts and theories will continue to develop to support the practice component of nursing.

Conceptual frameworks and theories of nursing are essential to understanding as nursing continues to define its body of knowledge. What nurses do and the way they provide care must be described to promote a clearer understanding of the profession. A *conceptual framework* can be viewed simply as a group of related concepts. A *theory* goes one step beyond this: a theory is a way to relate concepts by using definitions that state significant relationships between concepts. Conceptual frameworks and nursing theories can help describe and clarify approaches to nursing practice and can help describe the relationships between the concepts of person, environment, health, and nursing (Nursing Theories Conference Group, 1980).

Nursing theory provides the foundation for nursing knowledge and gives direction for nursing practice. It also facilitates development of future nursing research (Webster & Jacox, 1985). Although nursing theory development is crucial, a comprehensive discussion of the process is beyond the scope of this chapter. Therefore, only an overview of nursing theory follows.

Four Major Concepts

Nursing theories address the concepts of person, environment, health, and nursing by specifying relationships among the four concepts. Definitions of these four concepts vary.

The concept of *person*, in a broad sense, refers to all humans, but in many nursing theories the concept of person has evolved into the view of all people as biologic, psychological, and social beings. (Nursing theorists take this broad view and then articulate the definition of person in a manner specific to their theory.) Given this broad interpretation, nurses can be seen as caring for the biologic, psychological, and social aspects of all people.

The second major concept is *environment*, which usually includes all factors that affect people internally and externally. Individuals may experience different responses to internal and external environmental stimuli. The concept of environment also includes the individual's intellectual, psychological, and interpersonal aspects that may influence environmental responses. (Again, each theorist specifies the relationship of environment within the particular nursing theory to the concepts of person, health, and nursing.)

Health, the third major concept, can be seen as dynamic and in a constant state of change. Health is related to how the individual adapts to internal and external stressors. Through adaptation, people move toward living their lives to the fullest by achieving their maximum potential. Because nursing theorists believe that many factors influence health, definitions of health are less consistent than the definitions of the other three concepts.

Nursing, the fourth concept, is central to all nursing theories. Definitions of nursing describe what nursing is, what nurses do, and what the role of the nurse is in his or her interaction with patients. Some of the actions for which nurses are responsible are providing emotional support, implementing comfort measures, assisting patients with physical care, and helping patients with basic hygiene measures. Nurses also teach and promote healthy lifestyles and illness prevention activities.

In summary, nursing theories, as varied as they may be, have in common four central concepts: person, environment, health, and nursing. Table 1-4 lists major nursing theorists, the central purpose of each theory, and each theorist's definitions of the four major concepts.

Concerns About Nursing Theory

Many questions have been raised about the applicability and need for nursing theory. A discussion of some of these questions follows.

Does Nursing Have a Theory?

Some argue that nursing theory does not exist. Arguments against nursing theory include the belief that theories are not congruent with practice and cannot be validated unless they are linked to the practice component of the discipline. Others argue that nursing theories have not been sufficiently developed to define a body of nursing knowledge, and that nursing has not achieved the status of science. Others believe that theory is the substance of the field, and that poorly defined phenomena must be given definition (Webster & Jacox, 1985). Although opinions vary, continued theory development and refinement is imperative for nursing science.

Should Nursing Use a Single-Theory Approach or Multiple-Theory Approach?

The profession's multifaceted nature has resulted in the development of nursing theories with components of theories from other disciplines. The question remains: should we attempt to narrow our focus to such an extent as to have only one theory, when we probably need theories from basic sciences and social sciences? Cohesive arguments can be made in support of one theory or multidisciplinary theories (Stevens, 1985). Differences in opinion and beliefs regarding single-theory approaches or multiple-theory approaches stem from differing philosophies about what constitutes nursing science and practice.

What Is the Relationship of Nursing Theory to Nursing Practice?

One of the most critical arguments related to theory development is the fact that there is not enough evidence that nursing theories are grounded in practice. Those arguing this view believe that theories look good on paper but cannot be applied in practice. Those who believe that theory offers guidelines for practice hold that nursing theory arises out of practice, is verified in practice, and returns to explain or direct practice (Firlit, 1985). Research in the application of nursing theory to practice settings would provide valuable data for the resolution of this argument.

Studies and discussions on theory development in nursing have proliferated since the publication of *Theory Development: What? Why? How?* by the NLN in 1975, and will continue as the nursing profession further develops a scientific base for practice. No definitive answer to the questions asked about nursing theory exists, but all nursing theories challenge the reader to approach the world of nursing in different and increasingly complex ways (Moccia, 1986).

EDUCATIONAL PREPARATION AND CAREER OPPORTUNITIES

Educational preparation in nursing has long been a topic of debate among members of the profession. Three distinct pathways exist for entrance into professional nursing practice, and new approaches are continually emerging. Basic preparation and selected examples of newer approaches will be presented in this section.

Directly related to the issue of educational preparation is the topic of career opportunities in nursing. Depending on the individual's educational preparation and area of clinical expertise, a wide variety of career opportunities exists in professional nursing.

Nursing Education

The issue of educational preparation for entry into practice has been debated since the 1930s and 1940s, when the Brown and Goldmark reports recommended two levels of nursing preparation. In 1965, the ANA adopted a resolution proposing that minimum preparation for beginning professional practice should be a baccalaureate degree in nursing, and the minimum preparation for technical practice should be an associate degree in nursing. The ANA's 1965 resolution also prompted the 1985 ANA statement adopting the titles of *associate nurse,* a nurse prepared in an associate degree program, and *professional nurse,* a nurse possessing the baccalaureate degree in nursing, for these two levels of educational preparation.

Many critical issues in professional nursing practice continue to be affected by the debate over entry-level preparation. Included in this debate are the competencies of new nursing graduates, the public view of nursing roles, the need for professional status within the health-care community, the organization of nursing education, and the supply and demand for nursing professionals. Finally, the variety of programs available for entry into nursing practice is confusing to students, employers, and the public. Professional nursing must resolve the problems of entry-level requirements.

Nursing continues to have three major routes leading to the *registered nurse* licensure. Educational preparation may be the diploma, associate, or baccalaureate degree. Now emerging are programs that have the master's degree and nursing doctorate degree as entry-level preparation.

All nursing programs require, at a minimum, state approval. In addition to state approval, the NLN provides accreditation standards for all types of nursing programs. Accreditation from the NLN signifies excellence in nursing education.

Types of Educational Programs

Would-be nurses may enter licensed practical nursing programs or may pursue diploma, associate, baccalaureate, master's, or doctoral degrees. Students may choose the educational route that best suits their personal needs and goals.

Practical Nursing Program. People interested in a practical nursing career attend 1-year programs that prepare them to perform technical skills under the supervision of a registered nurse. Students successfully completing the program requirements may sit for the licensure examination given by the state board of nursing to become a **licensed practical nurse** (LPN) or licensed vocational nurse (LVN). LPNs are employed in hospitals, long-term care facilities, and rehabilitation centers and by health-care providers such as physicians. LPNs differ from registered nurses in two areas: educational preparation and scope of practice.

Diploma Nursing Program. Diploma nursing schools were the first type of educational preparation available for registered nurses. Diploma programs usually require 3 years of study. Students earn some college credit, but college credit is not awarded for nursing courses. Clinical experience is extensive, and this is seen as an advantage of this route.

Students successfully completing diploma programs take the state board of nursing examination for registered nurse licensure. Graduates of diploma programs work as beginning practitioners in acute, intermediate, long-term, and ambulatory health-care facilities. Graduates must demonstrate competency in the assessment,

(Text continues on page 16)

TABLE 1–4

Summary of Major Nursing Theorists

Theorist	Purpose	Person
Florence Nightingale (1860) "Notes on Nursing"	To help individuals responsible for caring for the sick to "think how to nurse." The theory addresses fundamental needs of the sick and basic principles of good health care.	An individual with vital reparative processes to deal with disease.
Hildegard E. Peplau (1952) "Interpersonal Relations in Nursing"	To develop an interpersonal interaction between the patient and the nurse.	An organism striving to reduce tension generated by needs.
Lydia E. Hall (1959) "Nursing: What Is It?"	To provide professional nursing care to persons past the acute stage of illness. Founded the philosophy care at the Loeb Center at Montefiore Hospital, Bronx, N.Y.	Unique individual, past the acute stage of long-term illness, capable of learning and growing.
Faye Glenn Abdellah (1960) "Patient-Centered Approaches to Nursing"	To deliver nursing care for the whole individual.	The recipient of nursing care.
Ida Orlando (1961) "The Dynamic Nurse-Patient Relationship"	To offer the professional nursing student a theory of effective nursing practice.	A unique individual.
Virginia Henderson (1966) "The Nature of Nursing"	To assist the patient in gaining independence as rapidly as possible.	Individual composed of biological, psychological, and spiritual components.
Martha E. Rogers (1970) The science of unitary man	To help the patient achieve a maximum level of wellness.	Unitary man, a four-dimensional energy field.
Imogene M. King (1971) Open systems model	To use communication to help the patient reestablish a positive adaptation to his or her environment.	Biopsychosocial being.
Dorothea E. Orem (1971) "Nursing: Concepts of Practice"	To provide care and to assist the patient in self-care.	Biopsychosocial being capable of self-care. Includes physical, psychological, interpersonal, and social aspects of human functioning.
Myra Estrin Levine (1973) Conservation model	To use conservation activities aimed at optimal use of patient's resources.	A holistic being.
Sister Callista Roy (1976 & 1984) Adaptation model	To identify the types of demands placed on a patient and the patient's adaptation to the demands.	A biopsychosocial being and the recipient of nursing care.
Dorothy E. Johnson (1980) "The Behavioral System Model for Nursing"	To reduce stress so the patient can recover as quickly as possible.	Person is viewed as having two major systems: biological and behavioral.
Betty Neuman (1982) "The Neuman Systems Model"	To address the effects of stress and reactions to stress on the development and maintenance of health.	A composite of physiologic, psychological, sociocultural, and developmental variables.
Jean Watson (1988) "Nursing: Human Science and Human Care"	To focus on carative factors derived from a humanistic perspective and scientific knowledge.	A valued person in and of him or herself to be cared for, respected, nurtured, understood, and assisted. A fully functional, integrated self.

TABLE 1–4

(continued)

Environment	Health	Nursing
External conditions that affect life and the development of the individual. Focus is on ventilation, warmth, odors, and light.	The focus is on the reparative process of getting well.	The goal of nursing is to place the individual in the best condition for nature to act by manipulating the environment.
Environment is not directly addressed. The psychodynamic milieu is given attention, with some emphasis on the patient's culture and mores.	Ongoing human process in the direction of creative, constructive, productive, personal, and community living.	Interpersonal therapeutic process. "A human relationship between an individual who is sick, or in need of health services, and a nurse especially educated to recognize and to respond to the need for help."
Environment should facilitate the achievement of the patient's personal goals.	Development of a mature self-identity that assists in the conscious selection of actions that facilitate growth.	Caring is the primary function of the nurse. The nurse assists other members of the health-care team in the curing of illness.
No definition. Includes society in "planning for optimum health on local, state, national, and international levels."	The purpose of nursing is achieving health. Health may be viewed as a dynamic pattern of functioning, with continuous interaction between internal and external stimuli.	Broadly grouped into "21 Nursing Problems" that center around needs for hygiene, comfort, activity, rest, safety, oxygen, nutrition, elimination, hydration, physical and emotional health promotion, interpersonal relationships, and development of self-awareness.
Interactions occurring between nurse and patient.	Not specified. Primarily addressed illness.	Central focus of theory. Unique, independent consideration of a patient's immediate needs.
Physical, biological, social, and cultural surroundings.	Independent functioning within 14 components: breathing, eating and drinking, comfort, sleep and rest, clothing, body temperature, safety, communication, worship, work, recreation, and continued development.	Assists and supports the individual in life activities and the attainment of independence.
Encompassing all that is outside any given human field. Person exchanging matter and energy.	Not specifically addressed, but emerges out of interaction with the human and the environment, is forward moving, maximizes human potential.	A learned profession that is both a science and an art.
Internal and external environment continually interacting to assist in the adjustment to change.	A dynamic life experience with continued goal attainment and adjustment to stressors.	Perceiving, thinking, relating, judging, and acting with an individual who comes to a nursing situation.
Internal and external stimuli. Requisites for self-care have their origins in human beings and the environment.	State of wholeness or integrity of human beings, including physical, mental, and social well-being.	A creative effort of one human being to help another human being. Consists of three nursing systems, wholly compensatory, partially compensatory, supportive-educative.
A person interacting with physical and psychosocial surroundings. Viewed broadly and includes all experiences of the individual.	The maintenance of unity and integrity of the patient.	A discipline rooted in the organic dependency of the individual human on his or her relationships with other humans.
All conditions, circumstances, and influences surrounding and affecting the development of an organism or group of organisms.	The person encounters adaptation problems in changing environments.	A theoretical system of knowledge that prescribes a process of analysis and action related to the care of the ill or potentially ill person.
All forces that impinge on the person and to which the person adjusts.	Equilibrium with eight subsystems of the person. "Purposeful adaptive response, physically, mentally, emotionally, and socially, to internal and external stimuli.	Promotion of behavioral system balance and stability.
The internal and external forces surrounding humans at any time. Constant environmental interaction.	Health or wellness exists when all parts and subparts are in harmony with the whole person. Not specified. Primarily addressed illness.	A unique profession concerned with all the variables affecting an individual's response to stressors.
Social environment, caring, and the culture of caring effect on health.	Physical, mental, and social well-being.	"A human science of persons and human health/illness experiences that are mediated by professional, personal, scientific, esthetic, and ethical human care transactions."

planning, implementation, and evaluation phases of the nursing process (National League for Nursing, 1978b).

The number of diploma programs is declining as nursing education moves into institutions of higher learning. This decline is related to nursing's efforts to achieve professional status and control over practice.

Associate Degree Nursing Program. Associate degree nursing, a concept introduced by Mildred Montag, developed in response to a nursing shortage and continues to exist successfully today. The student pursuing this degree attends a junior college for 2 years, receiving college credit for all courses and clinical experience in nursing. The goal of this program is to prepare a technical nurse to function under the supervision of a professional nurse. The student successfully completing the requirements of an associate degree program also takes the state board of nursing examination for registered nurse licensure.

As a provider of nursing care, the associate degree nurse uses the nursing process to formulate and maintain individualized nursing care plans. The associate degree nurse also teaches clients who need information or support to maintain health. As a manager, the associate degree nurse provides care for a group of clients with common, well-defined health problems in structured settings (National League for Nursing, 1978c).

Baccalaureate Degree Nursing Program. The baccalaureate degree in nursing offers the student a full college education with a background in liberal arts. The programs are rigorous and provide the student with college credit for nursing courses and clinical experience in all areas of nursing practice. There is an added emphasis in baccalaureate degree programs on community health nursing, research, leadership, and management. Baccalaureate programs in nursing are offered in college or university settings.

Students successfully completing the baccalaureate degree in nursing take the state board of nursing examination for registered nurse licensure. Nurses are prepared as generalists at the baccalaureate level and provide comprehensive service that assesses, promotes, and maintains the health of individuals and groups (National League for Nursing, 1978a).

Advanced Nursing Education Opportunities

Master's Degree Nursing Program. Several colleges offer a generic master of science degree in nursing in preparation for professional nursing practice. Usually students begin the programs with a baccalaureate degree in a field of study other than nursing. Candidates also take the state board of nursing registered nurse licensure examination. Students completing generic master's programs have advanced research capabilities and some opportunity for clinical concentration in a nursing specialty area.

Nurse Doctorate Program. The newest nursing program to emerge for entrance into professional nursing practice is the nurse doctorate program. Case Western Reserve University began the first program in 1985, and the University of Colorado has recently begun a program. The candidate takes the state board of nursing examination for licensure as a registered nurse before completing the program. Advanced preparation in research is a major component of the program.

Graduate Degree Programs. Nurses interested in attaining advanced education in a specialty area may complete graduate programs in their area of interest. Graduate education prepares the nurse for advanced, independent practice with continued emphasis on research. Graduate education requires independent critical thinking, and nurses pursuing graduate education must have a high degree of scholastic ability.

Doctoral Degree Programs. Students interested in careers as nurse researchers or nurse educators usually must obtain doctoral degrees. Doctoral education has become more available to nurses, and the number of nurses earning doctoral degrees continues to increase. Doctoral education in nursing may be obtained after completing a generic program, or students may enter doctoral nursing programs directly from high school.

In-Service Education. In-service education is provided by hospital employees to newly hired nurses or other health-care providers to ensure quality care. In-service education helps nurses provide the most accurate and up-to-date care to patients. For example, in-service educators may provide information on a new piece of equipment or on fire safety. A primary goal of in-service educators is to upgrade employees' knowledge and skills.

Nursing Practice Settings

With the changing health-care needs of society and the rising cost of health care, the settings for nursing practice have also changed. In addition to hospitals, nurses are now found in community health nursing, private-duty nursing, health promotion activities, long-term care facilities, rehabilitation centers, and nursing centers.

Hospital. Nurses have always been and probably always will be at the bedside caring for patients and helping to meet their health-care needs. Hospital nursing involves caring for patients with medical and surgical needs and may include specialty areas such as orthopedics, obstetrics and gynecology, outpatient chemotherapy, emergency room nursing, operating room nursing (Fig. 1-2), cardiac rehabilitation, and pediatrics. Opportunities are diversified and challenging in the hospital setting, as nurses continually meet their patients' complex health-care needs.

Community. Community health nurses are responsible for teaching health and providing for their patients' health-care needs as they recover or are treated in home-care situations. With the increasing cost of hospitalization, the need for community health nurses will grow as more people have their health-care needs met in the home and community situation.

Private-Duty. Private-duty nursing, which involves caring for one patient for the duration of his or her illness, may take place in the hospital or at home. The request for a private-duty nurse is usually made by the patient or family. Private-duty nurses help meet the health-care needs of patients with complex problems that require individualized, continuous attention.

Health Promotion Centers. Nurses are becoming increasingly involved in health promotion activities. In this setting, nurses serve in a teaching and supportive role, helping patients to achieve goals such as losing weight, quitting smoking, and establishing exercise programs. Prevention and health promotion provide the major focus of health care today, and nursing plays a significant role in this setting. Nurses working in health promotion centers may be employed by a hospital sponsoring such programs, or they may work independently.

Long-Term Facilities Long-term care facilities provide nursing care to elderly patients or those who require long-term assistance in meeting their health-care needs.

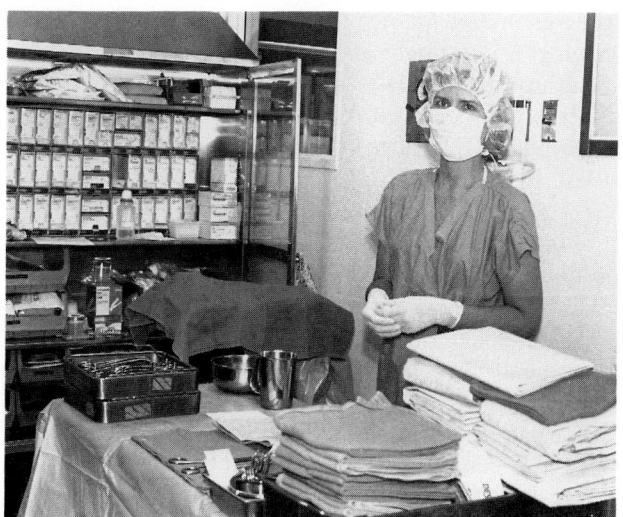

Figure 1–2. Hospital nursing may involve a specialty area such as the operating room.

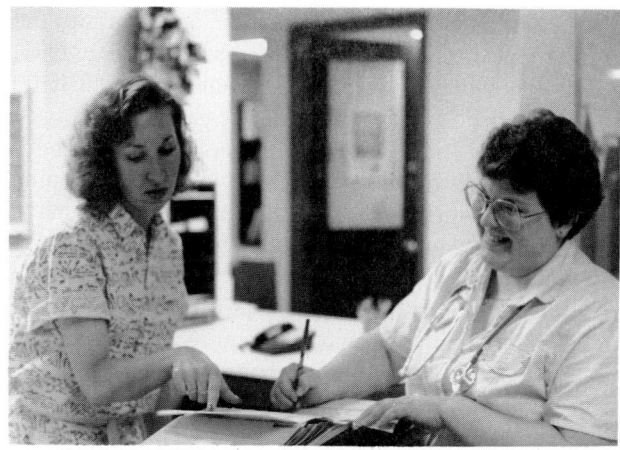

Figure 1–3. Nursing centers are new health-care facilities that address basic needs of individuals and communities.

Patients in a long-term care facility have complex needs and require intensive nursing care. As our elderly population increases and technology helps individuals to live longer lives, the special health-care needs of the elderly will continue to grow.

Rehabilitation Centers. Patients needing help in regaining their abilities to perform activities of daily living are cared for by nurses in rehabilitation centers. Nurses in these centers work with patients who may have experienced traumatic injury such as a car accident or a stroke and need long-term assistance and therapy to regain maximum independence.

Nursing Centers. Nursing centers are one of the newest arenas for the practice of nursing (Fig. 1-3). Colleges and universities have been among the first to develop nursing centers to meet their students' health-care needs and also to provide settings for nursing practice. Nursing centers help to meet the community's health-care needs by providing such services as physical examinations, basic diagnostic studies, and physician referrals when indicated.

Nursing Roles and Responsibilities

Historically, the sole duty of a nurse was to provide care and comfort to the sick, but as technology, knowledge, health promotion, and prevention have expanded, so have the roles and functions of the nurse.

Nursing functions include activities that the nurse performs dependently, interdependently, or independently. *Dependent* functions include skills that require a physician's order to be implemented. For example, one nursing function is giving medication to patients. Although the physician must prescribe the medication, the nurse must have a thorough understanding of the medication, observe for side effects, and teach the patient about the medication. Therefore, this particular nursing function requires nursing judgment. Nurses also perform *independent* functions, those nursing measures that do not require a physician's order to be implemented. Examples include providing comfort measures, repositioning patients, providing back and mouth care, and having patients cough and deep-breathe. *Interdependent* nursing functions are those activities that are collaborative in nature and are completed with or without a physician's order. Interdependent functions require mutual recognition of separate spheres of responsibility.

In addition to these roles, the profession has many other requirements, including assertiveness; a sound knowledge base in the sciences, humanities, and arts; the ability to make safe judgments; the ability to communicate, in written and oral forms, the health-care needs of patients; and a spirit of collegiality with other members of the health-care team. The professional nurse is an autonomous individual, functioning in both independent and interdependent ways and assuming the responsibilities of provider of care, decision-maker, patient advocate, manager and coordinator of health-care needs, educator, and communicator.

Caregiver. As a provider of care, the nurse assumes responsibility for helping the patient in promoting, restoring, and maintaining health and wellness (Fig. 1-4). The patient is seen as a unique human being, and the entire person is considered in the caring process. Patients' physiologic concerns are addressed as well as their spiritual, emotional, and social needs. Nurses must set priorities for care and assist patients in meeting all their needs in the most timely and cost-effective manner possible while ensuring excellence in patient care.

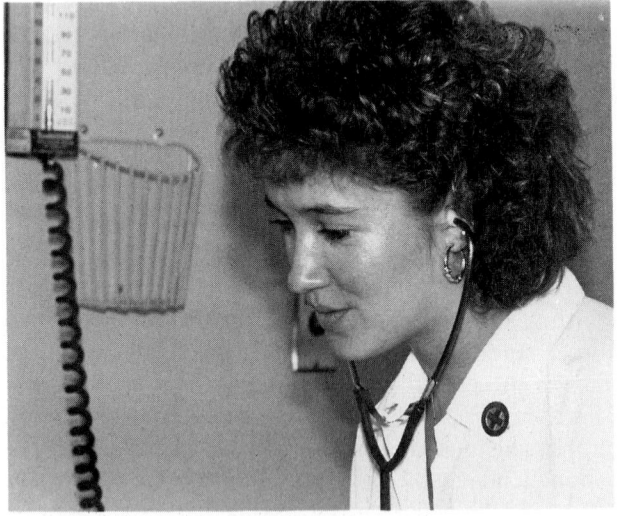

Figure 1–4. The nurse, as caregiver, views the patient as unique, and uses a holistic approach to assist the patient in promotion, restoration, and maintenance of health and wellness.

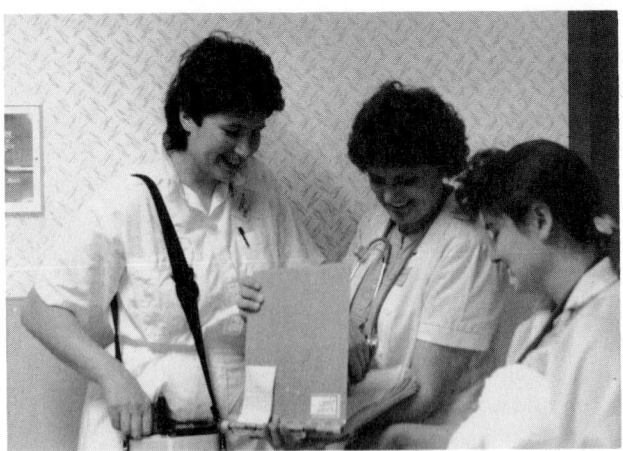

Figure 1–5. The nurse is responsible for involving other members of the health-care team in decision-making.

Decision-Maker. Nurses are continually identifying obstacles or difficulties in the promotion, restoration, and maintenance of health. Problem resolution requires the ability to make sound judgments and decisions. Nurses must make choices about the best approach to patient care, help patients to participate in this decision-making process, and use safe and effective judgments in providing patient care. The nurse also is responsible for involving other members of the health-care team and the patient's family in the decision-making process to ensure that sound, well-thought-out choices are made (Fig. 1-5).

Patient Advocate. One of the most important functions of the nurse is to protect the patient. Nurses act as patient advocates in many situations; examples include communicating the patient's needs and concerns and ensuring that patients understand their treatment. Nurses must promote a safe environment that facilitates the restoration of health. Nurses are responsible for having a thorough understanding of their patients' health problems, past history, and potential problems. Nurses consistently take responsibility for protecting their patients' legal rights and helping patients to assert these rights.

Manager and Coordinator. Promoting, restoring, and maintaining health involves coordinating the services offered by a variety of health-care professionals. In addition to managing his or her own time, the nurse must also coordinate all activities or treatments that involve the patient. The goal of the manager/coordinator role is to have patient care completed effectively and efficiently and in a manner that benefits the patient.

Communicator. Central to all other roles is the role of communicator. Because the nurse is the person who spends the most time with the patient, he or she has the greatest opportunity for observing, communicating, and identifying problems or improvements in the care plan. The nurse is responsible for communicating findings to the health-care team, in oral and written form. The quality of communication is a critical factor in meeting patients' health-care needs: the nurse must be knowledgeable, articulate, and capable of effective written and verbal expression.

Educator. Health promotion and illness prevention have become a growing concern and focus of the health-care delivery system. Educating patients about the disease process, how to prevent disease, nutritional factors, and healthy behaviors is essential. The nurse must explain treatments and procedures for which he or she is responsible, answer any questions the patient has, and evaluate the patient's progress toward health. Education is involved in all nursing activities.

Career Development and Expanded Nursing Roles

There are many additional opportunities for career development and advancement in nursing. These opportunities, some requiring advanced education, lead to new and varied roles and challenging and exciting responsibilities and opportunities. Some of these expanded nursing roles include nurse practitioner, clinical nurse specialist, nurse midwife, nurse anesthetist, nurse researcher, nurse administrator, and nurse educator.

Nurse Practitioner. **Nurse practitioners** have advanced education, often a master's degree in nursing, and are graduates of a nurse practitioner program. Nurse practitioners function with more independence and autonomy and are highly skilled at making nursing assessments, performing physical examinations, counseling, teaching, and treating minor health problems. Nurse practitioners may be generalists or may have a specialty, such as obstetrics or pediatrics.

Clinical Nurse Specialist. **Clinical nurse specialists** hold a master's degree in nursing and may have advanced experience and expertise in a specialized area of practice (e.g., gerontology, pediatrics, critical care, oncology, endocrinology, or cardiovascular or pulmonary disease). They work in a variety of settings, depending on their specialty (Fig. 1-6). Their roles include clinician, educator, manager, consultant, and researcher.

Nurse Midwife. A **nurse midwife** is educated in nursing and midwifery and is certified by the American College of Nurse Midwives. The nurse midwife provides independent care for women during normal pregnancy, labor, and delivery. The nurse midwife practices in conjunction with a specific health-care agency where medical services are available should the patient develop complications. The nurse midwife may also do routine Pap smears, breast examinations, and family planning.

Nurse Anesthetist. **Nurse anesthetists** provide general anesthesia for patients undergoing surgery under the supervision of a physician prepared in anesthesiology. The nurse anesthetist is a registered nurse with advanced education in anesthesiology. He or she works in a hospital.

Nurse Researcher. **Nurse researchers** are responsible for the continued development and refinement of nursing knowledge and practice through the investigation of nursing problems. Nurse researchers have advanced education, usually at the doctoral level. They work in large teaching hospitals and research centers such as the Na-

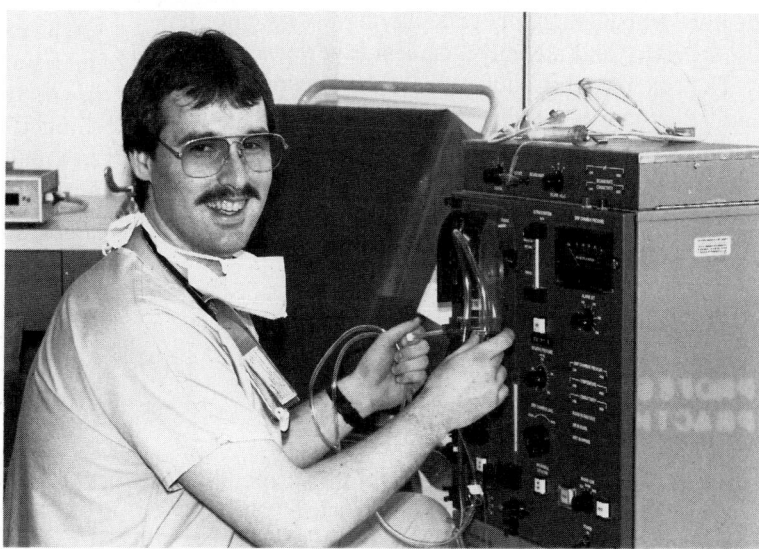

Figure 1–6.   Nurses in the renal dialysis unit specialize in helping patients with specific health problems.

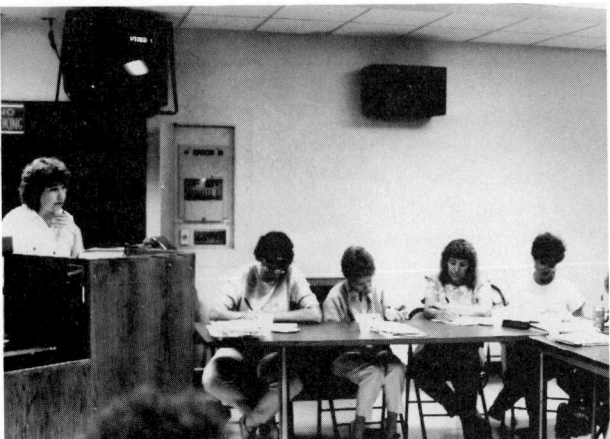

Figure 1–7.   Nurse educators bring a variety of abilities and responsibilities to the classroom.

tional Institute for Nursing Research in Bethesda, Maryland.

All nurses have a responsibility to do research to improve nursing care. Even nurses without advanced preparation in research can work with individuals who have such training.

Nurse Administrator. Nurse administrators manage and control patient care. They are responsible for specific nursing units and also serve as liaisons between the staff and the director of nursing. Educational preparation for the role of nurse administrator requires at least a baccalaureate degree in nursing and in some cases a master's or doctoral degree.

Nurse Educator. The **nurse educator** role can be developed in a variety of settings, in schools of nursing or hospital staff development departments, for example. Advanced education is required, usually a master's degree in nursing. Teaching at the baccalaureate, master's, or doctoral level in nursing usually requires a doctoral degree. Nurse educators generally have a specific clinical specialty and advanced clinical experience.

The role of nurse educator is a challenging one. The individual in this career role must continue to maintain expertise in the practice setting, develop expert knowledge of theory, perfect classroom presentation style, and have in-depth knowledge of curriculum development and higher education (Fig. 1-7).

PROFESSIONAL NURSING PRACTICE

As the nursing profession became more independent, it began to set its own standards of practice.

Standards of Practice

Standards of practice are essential because they serve as guidelines for providing and evaluating nursing care. Standards of practice ensure high-quality care and serve as criteria in legal questions of whether adequate care was provided.

The ANA's standards of practice designate the responsibilities of professional nursing as data collection, nursing diagnosis, planning, implementation, and evaluation. These responsibilities are inherent in the nursing process and are discussed later in the text.

The CNA has set similar standards of practice. The CNA's four central standards of nursing practice are the use of a conceptual model for nursing, effective use of the nursing process, initiation of helping relationships between the patient and nurse, and the fulfillment of professional responsibilities.

Nurse Practice Acts

Each state's **nurse practice act** defines the practice of nursing within that state. Requirements for licensure are set by the state licensing board in conjunction with the board of nursing. New graduates must take and pass the nursing licensure examination to qualify for a nursing license. With the emergence of more autonomous and expanded roles for nurses, many states have begun to revise their nurse practice acts to reflect those changes.

Nursing Organizations

As the nursing profession has developed and advanced, the organizations that have become an integral part of the profession have also increased. The number of associations continues to grow at local, state, and national levels. Nursing organizations may be related to a specialty or they may encompass all areas of nursing.

The organizations that involve most nurses or student nurses are the ANA, the CNA, the NLN, and the National Student Nurses' Association. The International Council of Nurses includes nurses throughout the world and addresses international health-care concerns in nursing. See the display for a list of nursing specialty organizations.

American Nurses Association

The **American Nurses Association** is American nursing's professional organization. Membership in state constituents of the ANA is open only to registered professional nurses. The ANA is important because it makes decisions about the functions, activities, and goals of the nursing profession. The ANA serves as a voice for nurses

Standards of Practice

American Nurses Association Standards of Practice*

1. The collection of data about the health status of the client is systematic and continuous. The data are accessible, communicated, and recorded.
2. Nursing diagnoses are derived from health status data.
3. The plan of nursing care includes goals derived from the nursing diagnoses.
4. The plan of nursing care includes priorities and the prescribed nursing approaches or measures to achieve the goals derived from the nursing diagnoses.
5. Nursing actions provide for client participation in health promotion, maintenance, and restoration.
6. The nursing actions assist the client to maximize his health capabilities.
7. The client's progress or lack of progress toward goal achievements is determined by the client and the nurse.
8. The client's progress or lack of progress toward goal achievement directs reassessment, reordering of priorities, new goal-setting, and revision of the plan of care.

Canadian Nurses Association Standards of Nursing Practice†

STANDARD I. Nursing practice requires that a conceptual model(s) for nursing be the basis for that practice.
Nurses are required (in any practice setting) to have a clear idea, or conception of the:

1. *Distinct goal of nursing*
2. *Client*
3. Their *role* in response to the health needs of society
4. *Source of client difficulty*
5. *Focus and modes of nursing intervention*
6. Expected *consequences* of nursing activities.

STANDARD II. Nursing practice requires the effective use of the nursing process. Nurses are required (in any practice setting) to:

1. *Collect data* in accordance with their conception of the client
2. *Analyze data* collected in accordance with their conception of the goal of nursing, their role, and the source of client difficulty
3. *Plan* their nursing actions on the identified actual and potential client problems, in accordance with their conception of the focus and modes of intervention
4. Perform nursing actions that *implement* the plan
5. *Evaluate* all steps of the nursing process in accordance with their conceptual model for nursing.

STANDARD III. Nursing practice requires that the helping relationship be the nature of the client-nurse interaction.
Nurses are required (in any practice setting) to:

1. *Initiate interaction* in a way that increases the likelihood that the client will perceive the health-service experience as understandable, manageable, and meaningful at the outset
2. Set *mutually agreed-upon expectations* as a means of increasing the likelihood that the client will perceive the health-service experience as understandable, manageable, and meaningful
3. Ensure a *successful termination* of the helping relationship.

STANDARD IV. Nursing practice requires nurses to fulfill professional responsibilities.
Nurses are required to:

1. Respect *statutes and policies* relevant to the profession and the practice setting
2. Comply with the *code of ethics* of their profession
3. Function as members of a *health team.*

* (From American Nurses Association. (1973). *Standards of practice.* Kansas City, MO: ANA.)
† From Canadian Nurses Association. (1980). *A definition of nursing practice: Standards for nursing practice.* Ottawa: CNA.

Selected Nursing Specialty Organizations

American Association of Critical Care Nurses
American Association of Occupational Health Nurses
American Nephrology Nurses Association
American Association of Neurosurgical Nurses
American Association of Nurse Anesthetists
American College of Nurse Midwives
Association of Operating Room Nurses
Emergency Department Nurses Association
National Association of School Nurses
Nurses Association of the American College of Obstetricians and Gynecologists
Public Health Nursing Section, American Public Health Association
American Organization of Nurse Executives
American Society of Ophthalmic Registered Nurses
American Society of Plastic and Reconstructive Surgical Nurses
American Society of Post-Anesthesia Nurses
Association of Practitioners in Infection Control
Association of Rehabilitation Nurses

International Association for Enterostomal Therapy
National Association of Pediatric Nurse Associates and Practitioners
National Intravenous Therapy Association
National Nurses Society on Alcoholism
Nurse Consultant Association
Oncology Nursing Society
Alpha Tau Delta, Nursing Fraternity
American Assembly for Men in Nursing
American Association of Colleges of Nursing
American Association for the History of Nursing
American Association of Neuroscience Nurses
American Association of Nurse Attorneys
American Association of Pediatric Oncology Nurses
American Holistic Nurses Association
American Indian/Alaskan Native Nurses' Association
National Black Nurses Association
Nurses' Environmental Health Watch
Nurses' Alliance for the Prevention of Nuclear War
Mid-Atlantic Regional Nursing Association

---

because it acts on issues and wishes expressed by the membership (Kelly, 1985).

The ANA's functions and activities have been adapted or expanded in accordance with the changing needs of the profession and the public. Its goals, as stated in the current bylaws, are to work for the improvement of health standards and the availability of health-care services for all, to foster high standards of nursing, and to stimulate and promote the professional development of nurses and advance their economic and general welfare (Kelly, 1985).

Canadian Nurses Association

The *Canadian Nurses Association,* Canada's professional nursing organization, promotes high standards of practice and professional development for Canadian nursing. It functions in a similar fashion to the ANA.

National League for Nursing

The main purpose of the **National League for Nursing** is to ensure that the public need for nursing will be met. The NLN's members include nurses and other members of the health team, laypeople, and agencies concerned with nursing education and service. The NLN works within the community and in association with individuals and groups outside of nursing. The NLN is the accrediting body through which nursing education programs seek accreditation, signifying excellence in nursing education (Kelly, 1985).

National Student Nurses' Association

The National Student Nurses' Association (NSNA), established in 1953, is the national organization for nursing students in the United States. Its goals are to assume responsibility for contributing to nursing education to provide for the highest-quality health care; to provide programs representative of fundamental and current professional interests and concerns; and to aid in the development of the whole person, his or her professional role, and his or her responsibility for the health care of people in all walks of life. The NSNA is autonomous, student-financed, and student-run. It serves as the voice of nursing students, speaking out on issues of concern to nursing students and nursing (Kelly, 1985).

International Council of Nurses

The oldest international association of any professional women is the **International Council of Nurses.** This non-political group brings together people from many countries who have a common interest in nursing and the common purpose of developing nursing throughout the world (Kelly, 1985).

CURRENT AND FUTURE TRENDS IN NURSING PRACTICE

Professional nursing is changing to reflect the values of society. Examples of issues and trends that affect the profession include health-care cost containment, scientific and technologic advances, and the women's movement.

Given the limits on resources, cost containment has become imperative. Patients enter the health-care system acutely ill and leave much sooner than they did in the past, increasing the demand on nurses to ensure high-quality, comprehensive care before discharge. The health-care system must shift its focus: emphasis is increasingly placed on such areas as illness prevention, nutrition, and healthy lifestyles.

Nursing practice must change in response to current social transitions and directions. Current trends in nursing practice include the development of nursing centers, wellness promotion programs, care of the elderly, birthing centers, and home and community health care. As nursing practice changes, so too must the preparation of its practitioners.

Science and technology also continue to affect the nursing profession. In the past nurses relied on their experience, observation, and intuition. Today nursing has defined a body of knowledge specific to the profession and continues to develop this knowledge through research and practice. Nurses today work in a more technical and more controversial health-care delivery system that demands a high degree of skill. New ethical dilemmas and questions continue to arise in the process of providing health care.

The women's movement has also affected nursing practice. The movement has brought attention to the need for equality and the recognition of universal human rights; as a result, nurses are becoming more assertive as professionals and are demanding more autonomy in patient care. Some believe, however, that the movement has hurt nursing by encouraging women to enter non-traditional careers, thus diminishing the pool of capable women from which nursing has traditionally drawn.

Social issues and concerns are intimately linked to the provision of health care. Just as social issues of the past have affected today's nursing practice, the issues of today will influence what happens in the future. The profession must remain dynamic in its attempts to meet the health-care needs of society.

Key Concepts

- The nursing profession has evolved over hundreds of years and continues to grow in response to the needs of society.
- The history of nursing has affected the modern profession's educational requirements, roles, and practice settings.
- Conceptual frameworks and nursing theories are major components in the establishment of a scientific knowledge base for nursing.
- Nursing theories attempt to clarify the practice of nursing, provide guidelines for nursing education, and promote nursing research.
- Many nursing theorists have attempted to clarify nursing, and theories continue to emerge that help nurses clarify their practice.
- Educational preparation and career opportunities in nursing are numerous.
- Diploma, associate, baccalaureate, master's, and doctoral degrees are available to those seeking a career in nursing.
- Nursing roles have expanded as nursing has developed more autonomy and gained status as a profession.
- Nurses function as caregivers, decision-makers, patient advocates, managers, communicators, and educators.
- The practice of nursing is governed by individual state nurse practice acts that define the scope of nursing practice within each state.
- The American Nurses Association's standards of practice guide and direct the practice of nursing, designating nursing responsibilities to include collecting data, making nursing diagnoses, planning and implementing care, and evaluating outcomes of patient care.
- Nursing organizations have emerged to represent nurses in general and nurses involved in specialties. The American Nurses Association is the professional organization for American nurses.
- Trends in nursing practice develop in response to changes in society. Trends affecting modern nursing practice include advances in technology, shorter hospital stays for patients, and the women's movement.

References

Abdellah, F. G. (1960). *Patient-centered approaches to nursing.* New York: Macmillan.

American Nurses Association. (1973). *Standards of practice.* Kansas City, MO: ANA.

American Nurses Association. (1980). *Nursing: A social policy statement.* Kansas City, MO: ANA.

Benner, P. (1984). *From novice to expert: Excellence and power in clinical nursing practice.* Menlo Park, California: Addison-Wesley.

Canadian Nurses Association. (1980). *A definition of nursing practice: Standards for nursing practice.* Ottawa: CNA.

Dolan, A. J., Fitzpatrick, M. L., & Herrmann, E. K. (1983). *Nursing in society: A historical perspective* (15th ed.). Philadelphia: W. B. Saunders.

Firlit, S. L. (1985). Nursing theory and nursing practice: Separate or linked? In J. C. McCloskey & H. K. Grace (Eds.), *Current issues in nursing* (2nd ed.). St. Louis. MO: Blackwell Mosby Book Distributors.

Hall, L. (1959). Nursing: What is it? *Publication of the Virginia State Nurses Association,* Winter, p. 1

Henderson, V. (1966). *The nature of nursing.* New York: Macmillan.

Johnson, D. E. (1980). The behavioral system model for nursing. In J. P. Riehl & C. Roy (Eds.), *Conceptual models for nursing practice* (2nd ed.). New York: Appleton-Century-Crofts.

Kelly, L. Y. (1985). *Dimensions of professional nursing,* 5th ed. New York: Macmillan.

King, I. M. (1981). *A theory for nursing: Systems, concepts, process.* New York: Wiley.

Levine, M. E. (1973). *Introduction to clinical nursing* (2nd ed.). Philadelphia: F. A. Davis.

Moccia, P. (Ed.). (1986). *New approaches to theory development.* New York: National League for Nursing.

National League for Nursing. (1978a). *Characteristics of baccalaureate education in nursing,* Pub. No. 15-1758. New York: Author.

National League for Nursing. (1978b). *Roles and competencies of graduate of diploma programs in nursing,* Pub. No. 16-1735. New York: Author.

National League for Nursing. (1978c). *Roles and competencies of the associate degree nurse on entry into practice,* Pub. No. 23-17211. New York: Author.

Neuman, B. (1982). *The Neuman systems model: Application to nursing education and practice.* New York: Appleton-Century-Crofts.

Nightingale, F. (1969). *Notes on nursing.* New York: Dover. (Original work published 1860)

Nursing Theories Conference Group. (1980). *Nursing theories: The base for professional nursing practice.* Englewood Cliffs, NJ: Prentice-Hall.

Orem, D. E. (1985). *Nursing: Concepts of practice* (3rd ed.). New York: McGraw-Hill.

Orlando, I. J. (1961) *The dynamic nurse–patient relationship: Function, process, and principles.* New York: G. P. Putnam.

Peplau, H. E. (1952). *Interpersonal relations in nursing.* New York: G. P. Putnam.

Rogers, M. E. (1970). *An introduction to the theoretical basis of nursing.* Philadelphia: F. A. Davis.

Roy, C. (1984). *Introduction to nursing: An adaptation model* (2nd ed.). Englewood Cliffs, NJ: Prentice-Hall.

Stevens, B. J. (1985). Nursing theories: One or many? In J. C. McCloskey & H. K. Grace (Eds.), *Current issues in nursing,* 2nd ed. St Louis, MO: Blackwell Mosby Book Distributors.

Watson, J. (1985). *Nursing: Human science and human care, a theory of nursing.* Norwalk, CT: Appleton-Century-Crofts.

Webster, G. & Jacox, A.K. (1985). The liberation of nursing theory. In J. C. McCloskey & H. K. Grace (Eds.), *Current issues in nursing,* 2nd ed. St Louis, MO: Blackwell Mosby Book Distributors.

Bibliography

Ashley, J. (1976). *Hospitals, paternalism, and the role of the nurse.* New York: Teachers College Press.

Buhler-Wilkerson, K., et al. (1987). Missing data: Nurses with their patients. *Nursing Research, 36*(1), 38–41.

King, J. E. (1986). A comparative study of adult developmental patterns of R.N. and generic students in a baccalaureate nursing program. *Journal of Nursing Education, 25*(9), 366–371.

Lawler, T. G., et al. (1987). Professionalization : A comparison among generic, baccalaureate, associate degree and R.N./B.S.N. nurses. *Nurse Educator, 12*(3), 19–22.

McDaniel, C. (1987). Qualitative study of nursing adult learners. *Nurse Educator, 12*(4), 4–5.

O'Brian, P. A. (1987). All a woman's life can bring: The domestic roots of nursing in Philadelphia, 1830–1885. *Nursing Research, 36*(1), 12–17.

Reverby, S. (1987). A caring dilemma: Womanhood and nursing in historical perspective. *Nursing Research, 36*(10), 5–11.

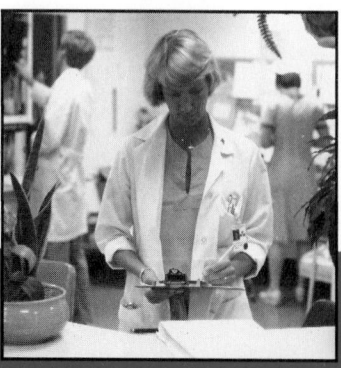

The Health-Care Delivery System

LEARNING OBJECTIVES

Upon completion of this chapter, the student will be able to do the following:

- Discuss the factors that affect the delivery of health-care services.
- Identify the services provided by the health-care delivery system.
- Describe the services offered by inpatient and outpatient services and services provided by the community.
- Identify several methods of funding health care.
- Outline the role and educational preparation of at least 10 colleagues in the health-care delivery system.
- Explain how quality assurance can be assessed, and why it is important.
- Discuss concerns related to fragmentation of care, limited resources, and access to health care.
- Identify some ethical and bioethical concerns.

KEY TERMS

Ambulatory care centers
Consumerism
Health-care delivery system
Health insurance
Health maintenance organizations
Hospices
Long-term care
Medicaid
Medicare
Prospective payment
Quality assurance
Urgent care centers

2

Defining the Health-Care Delivery System
Factors Affecting the Delivery of Health-Care Services
  Health Care as a Right
  Increasing Longevity of Americans
  Technologic Advances and Ethical Dilemmas
  Rising Consumerism
  Changing Health Services
  Increasing Legislative Activity
The Health-Care Delivery Setting
  Types of Services
    Health Promotion and Illness Prevention
    Diagnosis and Treatment
    Rehabilitation
  Agencies Providing Inpatient Services
    Acute-Care Hospitals
    Long-Term Care Facilities
    Retirement Communities
    Health Maintenance Organizations
    Preferred Provider Organizations
    Specialized Inpatient Services
  Agencies Providing Outpatient Services
    Physicians' Offices
    Ambulatory Care Centers and Clinics
    Urgent Care Centers
    Day-Care Centers

  Community-Based Agencies
    Mental Health Centers
    Rural Health Centers
    Home-Health Agencies
    Hospices
Funding of Health-Care Services
  Private Health Insurance
  Government Involvement in Health-Care Funding
    Medicare and Medicaid
    Prospective Payment
  Charitable Funding of Health Care
Colleagues in the Health-Care System
  Physicians
  Focused Care Providers
  Technicians and Technologists
  Therapists
  Others Providing Necessary Services
Challenges to the Health-Care Delivery System
  Quality of Care
  Fragmentation of Service
  Limited Medical and Financial Resources
  Access to Health Care
  Ethical and Bioethical Decisions
Key Concepts

The health-care delivery system may be the largest industry in the United States: it employs an estimated 8 million people (Jonas, 1986), many of whom work in one of the almost 7,000 hospitals in the country. A tremendous variety of products are consumed by the system (for instance, drugs, hospital supplies and equipment). Each year the health-care delivery system becomes larger and more complex, offering more challenges and demanding more changes.

DEFINING THE HEALTH-CARE DELIVERY SYSTEM

The term **health-care delivery system** refers to the complex system of services intended to help people lead healthier lives. These services are preventive, therapeutic, and rehabilitative. They are provided in hospitals, nursing homes, government agencies, and voluntary agencies in the form of inpatient care, outpatient care, ambulatory care, home care, hospice care, and urgent care. The care is provided by a long list of health professionals, including physicians, nurses, dentists, psychologists, pharmacists, osteopaths, chiropractors, and technicians and technologists. The care is paid for by patients, private insurance companies, and government agencies.

It is appropriate to call health-care delivery a system, because a system is a set of things that are connected to form a whole. For instance, a physician and a hospital are mutually dependent: the physician cannot do surgery or carry out certain treatments without the hospital's facili-

Commonly Used Abbreviations in Health-Care Delivery	
AHA	American Hospital Association
AMA	American Medical Association
ANA	American Nurses Association
APHA	American Public Health Association
APhA	American Pharmaceutical Association
CAHEA	Committee on Allied Health Education and Accreditation
CDC	Centers for Disease Control
CHAMPUS	Civilian Health and Medical Program of the Uniformed Services
CNA	Canadian Nurses Association
DHHS	Department of Health and Human Services (formerly the Department of Health, Education and Welfare)
DRG(s)	Diagnosis-related group(s)
EPA	Environmental Protection Agency
FDA	Food and Drug Administration
GNP	Gross national product
HCFA	Health-Care Financing Administration
HMO	Health maintenance organization
HSA	Health Service Administration
ICF	Intermediate-care facility
ICN	International Council of Nurses
JCAHO	Joint Commission on Accreditation of Healthcare Organizations
MCH	Maternal–child health
NCHS	National Center for Health Statistics
NCNR	National Center for Nursing Research
NIH	National Institutes of Health
NHI	National Health Insurance
NIA	National Institute on Aging
NFSNO	National Federation for Specialty Nursing Organizations
NLN	National League for Nursing
OSHA	Occupational Safety and Health Administration
PHS	Public Health Service
PPO	Preferred provider organization
RFP	Request for proposal
SMI	Supplementary Medical Insurance
SNF	Skilled nursing facility
UR	Utilization review
VA	Veterans Affairs (or Administration)
VNA	Visiting Nurses Association
WHO	World Health Organization

ties, and the hospital relies on the physician to admit patients, thus generating the revenues that guarantee continued operation. Other pieces of the system include other health-care workers and health-care services, the pharmaceutical industry, manufacturers, suppliers, insurers, and researchers.

As the health-care delivery system has grown in size and complexity, it has also become more expensive. In 1987, $500 billion was spent on health care, a figure double that of 1977. United States citizens spent 11.1% of the gross national product on health care in 1987, or $1987 per person (Jecker & Pearlman, 1989). The *gross national product* is the value of all the goods and services produced within the country. This annual spending on health care is higher than that of any other nation. The increasing cost of health care is a growing concern and the focus of much debate.

FACTORS AFFECTING THE DELIVERY OF HEALTH-CARE SERVICES

Several factors have contributed to the growth and complexity of our health-care delivery system.

Health Care as a Right

At one time in the United States, access to health care was the privilege of the rich. The poor either went without or had to be satisfied with lesser quality care. But values have changed, and today equal access to health care is viewed as everyone's right, rich or poor.

Increasing Longevity of Americans

Americans born in 1987 can expect to live an average of 75 years (men 71.5, women 78.4), compared to 47.3 years for those born in 1900 (U.S. Department of Health and Human Services, 1990). The fastest-growing age group is that of people 85 and older. Because the heaviest users of health services are the elderly, more emphasis is being placed on their needs, and gerontology has become a significant branch of medicine and nursing (Fig. 2-1). Topics such as living wills and powers of attorney are becoming more widely discussed as people become concerned about the ability to maintain life and the quality of that life.

Technologic Advances and Ethical Dilemmas

The advances made in technology have drastically changed health care. Ever more powerful and costly

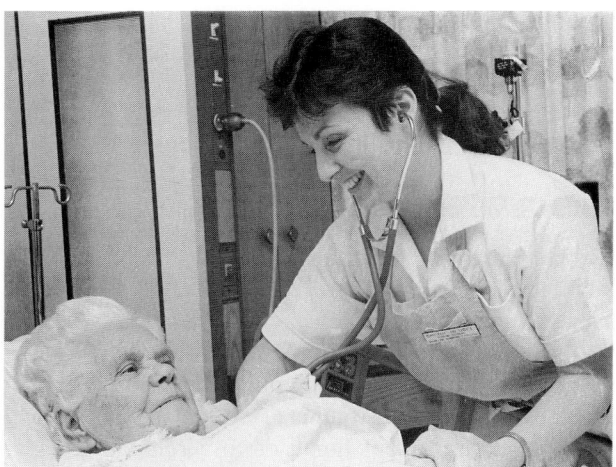

Figure 2–1   As the population ages, there will be a need for more retirement homes and nursing homes and a need for nurses to staff these health-care facilities. (Photo courtesy of Shoreline Community College.)

antibiotics ward off deadly diseases. Better diagnostic tools assist in recognizing conditions while they are treatable. Heart, lung, and liver transplants, unheard of two decades ago, are becoming commonplace. Life can be maintained mechanically long after biologic systems have ceased to support life.

Changing technology alters the profile of the hospitalized patient. For example, after insulin was developed in the 1920s, people with diabetes could manage their disease at home instead of in the hospital. The polio vaccine eliminated the need for patients to undergo hospital treatment with the iron lung.

But these advances have given rise to questions. Should elderly people be placed on respirators? Should a person be required to donate bone marrow if that person is the only acceptable match? Should major health-insurance plans cover expensive transplants? Medical ethicists wrestle with these and other implications of technology.

Rising Consumerism

Consumerism is the public's expectation that it will have a voice in determining the type, quality, and cost of health care. Americans are better informed than ever before and are asserting their rights in the delivery of health care. Previously the health-care system operated on the assumption that physicians knew what was best for patients and should make decisions for them; now, patients expect—and demand—to be involved in health-care decisions, and a new relationship has developed between the consumer and the health-care provider.

The consumer movement was fostered in part by the advent of health maintenance organizations, which promote the prevention as well as the treatment of illness. It

was also encouraged by legislation that required the patient to give informed consent before receiving certain treatments.

Changing Health Services

Health services in the 1980s and 1990s have been marked by a holistic approach. Today, health promotion and disease prevention receive as much emphasis as the diagnosis and treatment of disease. As people realize the importance of exercise, specialties such as sports medicine have emerged. More emphasis is being placed on nutrition, and wellness and health-promotion programs abound.

Increasing Legislative Activity

Nothing has affected the health-care delivery system more than federal legislation. For example, the Hill-Burton Act of 1946 drastically affected the health-care delivery system by providing funds for the construction of many small rural hospitals. In 1965, the Social Security Act was amended to incorporate Medicare and Medicaid; until that time, no branch of the government had been responsible for providing aid to nonindigent people when they were ill. **Medicare** provides health insurance to people who are either over age 65 or disabled. **Medicaid** provides health benefits to the poor. These two programs will be discussed later in the chapter.

In 1984, hospital funding based on diagnosis-related groups (DRGs) was established; it was determined that most hospital patients could be classified into one of 467 DRGs. Historically, hospitals had been paid on a retrospective cost or near-cost basis. This legislation shifted to a **prospective payment** system in which a fixed schedule of payment was established based on diagnosis.

THE HEALTH-CARE DELIVERY SETTING

A person seeking health care today faces a tremendous array of settings in which care is provided. Some suggest that this maze is so complex that the average person needs an advocate to help him or her move through it. Services may vary: some concentrate on health promotion and illness prevention, while others focus on diagnosis and treatment, rehabilitation, or custodial care.

Because of the recent increases in the number and variety of agencies that provide health care, any attempt at categorization would be incomplete. We will divide these agencies into inpatient and outpatient ones, however, although some facilities could fall into either category.

Types of Services

Health Promotion and Illness Prevention

Health promotion and illness prevention services have grown in popularity in the last decade as Americans have taken more responsibility for their health (Fig. 2-2). Health clubs may offer classes on nutrition and healthy eating, and other programs are available that emphasize weight control, stress reduction, smoking cessation, and moderation in the use of alcohol.

Diagnosis and Treatment

Treatment of illness may take many forms and may occur in various settings depending of the seriousness of the diagnosis and the equipment and facilities required to correct the condition. Traditionally, diagnosis and treatment has been the major service offered by the health-care delivery system. This care is generally provided in a physician's office; if needed, the patient may be admitted to a hospital. More recently, some diagnostic services, such as mammograms, have been offered in clinics or walk-in emergent care facilities. Some tests, such as screening for blood cholesterol levels, are even being done in shopping malls.

Rehabilitation

The goal of rehabilitation is to help the patient with an injury or disabling illness to achieve maximum function and independence. Rehabilitation services may be offered at a large medical complex or a free-standing agency. Often the rehabilitation program involves a vari-

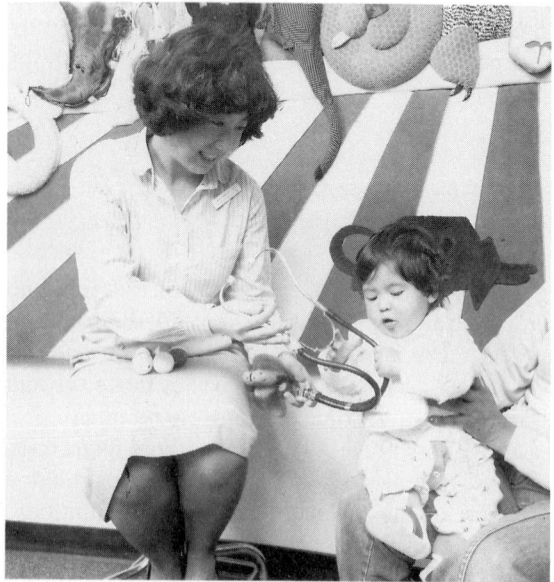

Figure 2–2 Nurse practitioners actively participate in health-promotion activities. (Photo courtesy of University of Washington School of Nursing.)

ety of health professionals, including physicians, nurses, physical therapists, and social workers.

Agencies Providing Inpatient Services

Acute-Care Hospitals

Hospitals provide a wide range of services, including surgical treatment, diagnostic procedures, care of mothers and babies, rehabilitation, emergency services, and more recently outpatient care. They are seen as acute-care facilities; that is, they provide care during the acute phase of an illness, surgery, or trauma. As soon as recovery begins, patients are sent home or to a rehabilitation or extended-care facility. Many hospitals have added substance-abuse treatment units, oncology units, health-promotion programs, and home health services.

Hospitals can be classified as those owned by the federal, state, or local government or by a private organization.

The federal government owns the hospitals that are run by the Department of Veterans Affairs, the Department of Defense, the Department of Health and Human Services (DHHS), the Alcohol, Drug Abuse and Mental Health Administration, which functions under DHHS, and the Department of Transportation. Also included in this category are hospitals in federal prisons.

States own the hospitals at state-run medical schools and prisons. They also often own hospitals that offer long-term care, such as psychiatric facilities.

On the local government level are hospitals organized by a district, county, or city. These hospitals are usually funded by local bonds and often have an elected board of directors or commissioners.

Privately owned hospitals are further classified as being voluntary (not for profit) and proprietary (for profit). Voluntary hospitals are operated by religious or charitable groups; they may also be independent or represent health maintenance organizations or cooperatives. Proprietary hospitals have individual owners or are owned by a partnership or corporation. The last decade has seen an increase in investor-owned hospital corporations; the stock of these corporations is traded on the stock exchange (Wilson & Neuhauser, 1987).

The size of a hospital is generally reported as the number of available beds; the average size in the United States is about 200 beds.

Long-Term Care Facilities

Long-term care can be defined as "a set of health, personal care, and social services delivered over a sustained period of time to people who have lost or never acquired some degree of functional capacity" (Kane & Kane, 1987, p. 4). Long-term care is most often provided to the elderly, but some people need long-term care from birth; others need long-term care after spinal cord injuries or a debilitating disease such as multiple sclerosis. Long-term care focuses on maintaining as much function as possible and emphasizes activities of daily living (basic needs such as eating, dressing, toileting, bathing, and ambulating).

The term long-term care is used because patients spend much longer in one of these facilities than in an acute-care facility; often, patients spend their last days at a long-term care center (Fig. 2-3). Because of this, patients may see the facility as their home. Greater accommodation must be made for visits from family and friends and for outings. Because patients have varying degrees of functional ability, the staff must be flexible and tailor their care to each patient's needs.

Most long-term care is provided by nursing homes. An estimated 5% of the population over 65 lives in nursing homes, and one in every four Americans will spend some time in a nursing home (U.S. Senate Special Committee Report on Aging, 1987). Nursing homes may also be certified as skilled nursing facilities, intermediate-care facilities, or both. As with acute-care facilities, the ownership of nursing homes may be voluntary, proprietary, or governmental; in 1985, almost 75% of the homes were proprietary, with an average bed capacity of 85 (Kane & Kane, 1987, p. 56).

Retirement Communities

In the last 20 years, the number of retirement communities has increased significantly. These communities can take many forms: self-contained towns, retirement villages, retirement subdivisions, retirement residences, and continuing-care communities (Matteson & McConnell, 1988). Although the services provided vary from one community to another, continuing-care communities usually provide a number of levels of care. In an arrangement known as assisted living, older people can live independently in condominiums or apartments while still having care nearby when they need it. A convalescent center may be associated with the facility, and services such as physical and occupational therapy may be provided. Other health-care services such as dental care may also be available.

Residents are guaranteed access to various health-care services, and the financial responsibilities are spread over the entire community. Some of the fees are prepaid. As might be anticipated, entry fees may be substantial, often $60,000 or more. Monthly maintenance fees are also high, thus limiting access to these facilities to more affluent retirees (Matteson & McConnell, 1988).

Health Maintenance Organizations

Health maintenance organizations (HMOs) are prepaid health plans that offer complete health-care services to their members for an established fee, thus combining traditional insurance and health-care delivery in one organization. HMOs provide a wide range of services, including inpatient and outpatient hospital care, infertility and mental health services, therapeutic radiologic treatment, alcohol and drug addiction treatment, and physical therapy. HMOs were first established in 1973 under a federal program. Enrollment is voluntary; members have the option to select another plan.

Because the fee paid by members is fixed, the organization tries to minimize its costs. To do this, HMOs place greater emphasis on health promotion and disease prevention. Physicians who work for HMOs may receive a monthly salary regardless of the number of patients they see, and such costs as malpractice insurance are paid by the organization.

Preferred Provider Organizations

In a preferred provider arrangement, patients select their care provider from a list of people, groups, or institutions that have contracted to offer services at a certain price. Generally, the cost of care is somewhat lower because these arrangements place a greater emphasis on health maintenance and limit expensive procedures. If a consumer chooses to seek services from a provider who has not contracted with the plan, a substantial deductible fee is assessed, or the service is not covered at all.

Specialized Inpatient Services

Some facilities, such as psychiatric hospitals, offer only specialized services. Another example is a respite care facility, which provides short-term inpatient services to patients who usually are cared for at home. The purpose of respite care is to offer relief to the primary caregiver, usually a family member.

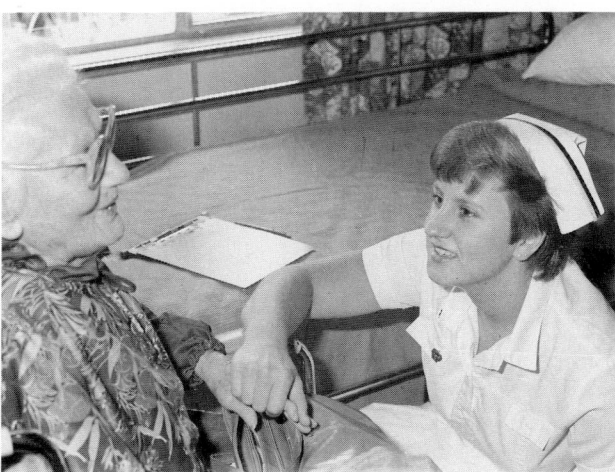

Figure 2–3   A warm, loving environment is important in the remaining years of the patient's life in a nursing home. (Photo courtesy of Shoreline Community College.)

Rehabilitation centers might also be considered specialized inpatient facilities, although outpatient services may also be available. Rehabilitation centers focus on helping patients to return to normal functioning or to achieve the highest possible level of functioning after an illness or injury.

Agencies Providing Outpatient Services

Because of rising hospital costs, more procedures and treatments are being done on an outpatient basis. Patients come to an outpatient facility for care and do not stay there for any period of time. A hallmark of good outpatient care is thorough family and patient education. The role of nurses in an outpatient center may vary considerably, depending on their education and the management of the center.

Physicians' Offices

In the physician's office, the traditional center for outpatient care, patients are treated for minor injuries and illnesses and may have diagnostic work-ups such as electrocardiograms, radiographs, and ultrasonograms. Laboratory diagnostic services, such as analysis of blood and urine specimens, may be available. Other services may also be offered depending on the physician's specialty.

Ambulatory Care Centers and Clinics

Patients can also receive care for conditions not requiring hospitalization at **ambulatory care centers.** Many ambulatory care centers and clinics are affiliated with a hospital, but others operate independently, often in major shopping areas. Traditional "walk-in" clinics have existed for many years and are often used by people of lower economic status in lieu of a family physician. Centers may operate on an appointment or drop-in basis. Some clinics are specialized, such as family-planning clinics or those offering women's health care only.

Urgent Care Centers

Urgent care centers, which operate in a manner similar to drop-in clinics, are often located in major shopping areas or malls and are open during regular business hours. Patient who need services at other hours of the day must seek care elsewhere, such as at a hospital emergency department. Urgent care centers offer a variety of services, from treatment of minor illnesses and injuries to routine physical examinations.

Day-Care Centers

Day-care centers target a particular patient population; for instance, many day-care centers serve elderly pa-

tients who cannot be left alone for long periods of time but who can carry out activities of daily living. Other day-care centers serve patients who are physically or mentally challenged, such as those with cerebral palsy or Down's syndrome, or people with chemical dependencies. These centers care for patients when family members are working and offer such services as meals, rehabilitation, and occupational therapy.

Community-Based Agencies

Community health-care agencies offer care to a given neighborhood or community. Many of the care facilities discussed earlier, such as day-care centers, may also be community-based. Many have come into existence as a result of federal legislation.

Mental Health Centers

Mental health centers offer a wide range of mental health services within a given "catchment" area. They may be a network of coordinated services rather than a single entity, and may provide short-term and crisis intervention approaches to treatment (Wilson & Neuhauser, 1987). Centers may be associated with a hospital or may operate as independent nonprofit entities.

Rural Health Centers

Also developed as a result of federal financing, rural health centers were established to provide care in rural, impoverished areas that have few physicians (Fig. 2-4). Much of the care is provided by nurse practitioners or physician's assistants.

Home-Health Agencies

As the impact of prospective payment has forced pa-

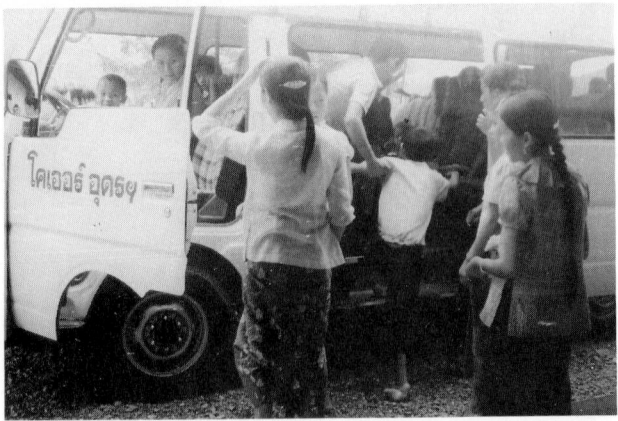

Figure 2–4 Transportation is often necessary to help immigrants in rural areas gain access to health care. (Photo courtesy of Marjorie A. Muecke.)

tients to be discharged from the hospital earlier, home health care has become an essential part of the health-care delivery system. Much of the care is given by registered nurses skilled in assessment, but practical nurses and aides also are employed. Agencies receiving reimbursement under the Medicare program must be certified and must meet conditions and standards established by federal legislation. These services may be provided by a visiting nurse association, the local health department, or proprietary or voluntary agencies established for this purpose.

In addition to skilled nursing care, home health care may include therapeutic services as such physical, occupational, or speech therapy. Home care in a broader sense may include homemaker services, in-home services to the elderly, and home-delivered meals.

Hospices

Hospices, run by public or private agencies, help terminally ill patients and their families by providing supportive, palliative services. Many patients receiving these services are suffering from cancer, although conditions such as AIDS, multiple sclerosis, congestive heart failure, or end-stage renal disease may also require hospice care. The first hospice in the United States was established in 1974 in New Haven, Conn., and was modeled after St. Christopher's Hospice in London (Wilson & Neuhauser, 1987).

Although nurses play a major role in hospice care, a team approach involving physicians, therapists, trained volunteers, and members of the clergy is often used. Nursing activities focus on managing pain, treating symptoms, and preparing the patient and family for death and bereavement. Hospice care was initially provided in the home, but more recently hospital and community-based units have been developed.

FUNDING OF HEALTH-CARE SERVICES

Who should pay for the ever-increasing costs of health care and hospitalization? The astronomical cost of some forms of treatment has made it impossible for the average patient to personally pay for all medical and nursing services. Bills well above $10,000 are no longer the exception. **Health insurance** provides protection against the cost of medical care and hospitalization arising from illness or injury.

There has been much debate about whether the United States should adopt a national health insurance plan. Under a national plan, taxpayers would foot the bill, much as insurance companies collect funds from subscribers. It is worth remembering that no health insurance plan, national or private, is free.

Private Health Insurance

Many people have private health insurance plans, which are offered as a benefit by employers or purchased on an individual basis. Because the insurance company pays the medical bill, this system is known as *third-party reimbursement.* One of the earliest health insurance programs in the United States was started at Baylor University Hospital in Texas in 1929. Teachers prepaid half a dollar a month to ensure up to 21 days of semiprivate hospitalization annually (McCarthy & Thorpe, 1986). From this evolved the Blue Cross program.

Today a wide variety of organizations provide private health insurance programs. Health insurance benefits have become a major negotiable item in labor contracts. The available programs vary tremendously: some cover all medical costs, others have sizable deductibles and force subscribers to shoulder some of the cost. Whether policies should cover extremely expensive procedures such as transplants is a subject of debate.

The term *catastrophic health insurance* generally refers to plans that protect the insured (particularly the elderly) and their families from bankruptcy due to major or long-term illness. A workable plan for catastrophic health coverage has yet to be developed.

Private and group insurance policies can provide significant assistance to people struggling to meet rising health-care costs, but provide no assistance to people who are unemployed or those who do not receive health insurance benefits. Who pays for health-care services for the growing segment of the population ineligible for health insurance?

Government Involvement in Health-Care Funding

The federal government helps to cover health-care costs for some citizens. The Department of Health and Human Services (DHHS) is the second-largest department of the federal government; only the Department of Defense is larger. Some of the services offered by the federal government have been mentioned earlier, such as services provided in government hospitals. Care is also provided under the Medicare and Medicaid programs, started in 1965.

Medicare and Medicaid

Medicare provides medical and hospital insurance to people age 65 or older and to disabled people. Hospital insurance, provided under Part A of the plan, covers inpatient care, care in a skilled nursing facility, and home health care. It is financed by Social Security taxes. Part B of Medicare, which provides supplemental medical insurance (SMI), is optional. People choosing to enroll in this plan in addition to Part A must pay for the services, and the cost is deducted from their Social Security check. Part B covers physicians' charges, outpatient or emergency room services, unlimited home health visits, and other services such as speech and physical therapy, x-rays, and wheelchairs and similar supplies. The Health Care Financing Administration (HCFA) oversees the Medicare program. Medicare expenditures are increasing each year, raising concerns for the program and the public it serves.

Medicaid is a federally funded program administered through the states to provide services to two groups of people:

The *categorically needy* are blind, disabled, or aged people and those receiving public assistance from Aid to Families with Dependent Children.
The *medically needy* are those who meet other low-

income standards as defined by the state in which they live.

Medicaid's benefit structure varies from state to state. Some states pay for dental care, eyeglasses, or prescription drugs, but other states do not. Like Medicare, the cost of this program has grown and is a matter of public concern.

Prospective Payment

Two acts passed by Congress have significantly affected the methods by which hospitals are reimbursed for care. The Tax Equity and Fiscal Responsibility Act of 1982 (TEFRA) established a cost-per-case basis for hospital payment. Of even greater significance were the 1983

Health-Care Delivery in Canada

Similar forces have affected health-care delivery in Canada, but they have been dealt with in a substantially different manner because of intrinsic differences in the health-care delivery systems. Health care in Canada is based on five fundamental principles (Canada Health Act, 1984):

- Universality–the entitlement of all citizens to insured health services
- Accessibility–the availability of health services on uniform terms and conditions without extra charges and user fees
- Comprehensiveness–the insurance of essentially all health services provided by hospitals and physicians and, where legislated in the provinces, similar or additional services provided by other health-care practitioners
- Portability–the continuation of health insurance coverage when residents are temporarily absent or move between provinces
- Public administration–the administration and operation of provincial health-care insurance plans on a nonprofit basis by an appointed or designated public authority.

In other words, comprehensive health-care insurance is provided to all Canadians through government sources. Constitutionally, health care is a provincial responsibility, but it is financed largely through transfer payments from the federal government.

The early 1960s saw increasing erosion of the previously mentioned principles. Hospital costs were escalating. Many physicians were augmenting the fees for service set by various provincial plans by direct extra billing to patients. Through the 1984 Canada Health Act, the federal government used its control over funding to reverse the extra billing trend and to increase health promotion, community and home care program incentives (Canada Health Act, 1984).

The Canadian Nurses Association (CNA) has played a major role in the lobbying for health-care reform. It was a major breakthrough to have included in the Canada Health Act the provisions for access to the health-care system through physicians *and* other practitioners. Unlike the United States, where other health-care providers such as nurse practitioners have been an access point for health care, physicians have been essentially the sole entry point for insured services in Canada. The CNA continues to press for reallocation of resources to further emphasize health promotion, illness prevention, and community involvement in decision-making. This position is in keeping with the move toward primary health care. As defined by the World Health Organization (1978), primary health care is "essential health care made universally accessible to individuals and families in the community by means acceptable to them, through their full participation and at a cost that the community and country can afford."

The section on health-care delivery in Canada was written by Marlene Reimer, RN, MN, Assistant Professor, University of Calgary, Calgary, Alberta, Canada.

DIAGNOSIS RELATED GROUP

amendments to the Social Security Act, which established a method of paying for inpatient care to Medicare patients based on DRGs. In an attempt to control rising costs, a predetermined (prospective) and fixed rate was established for reimbursing for the care for each of 467 diagnoses or procedures. Hospitals receive no more than this figure, regardless of the cost they may have incurred in delivering the care. Costs above the established amount must be absorbed by the hospital, but if the care is delivered for less than the established amount, the hospital keeps the difference and makes a profit. Different rates were set for urban and rural hospitals, and rates are adjusted each year to reflect the increasing costs of goods and services. Many states have adopted DRGs as the basis for reimbursement of care provided to patients other than those covered by Medicare.

Charitable Funding of Health Care

The largest percentage of charitable care is offered through hospitals to the uninsured. Some charitable funding is directed toward special populations, such as children suffering from muscular dystrophy or cancer.

COLLEAGUES IN THE HEALTH-CARE SYSTEM

Nurses are the single largest group of health-care professionals, but as health care has become more complex, the number and variety of people involved in providing services has increased proportionately. Raffel and Raffel (1989) identified 24 allied health training occupations accredited through the Committee on Allied Health Education and Accreditation, and many other jobs are accredited by other groups. Collaboration with these other professionals is critical to providing quality care.

Physicians

Physicians make up the second-largest group of health-care professionals. They diagnose and treat patients in an attempt to cure or improve the condition. Nurses follow physicians' orders for medications and develop nursing care plans that are compatible with the medical regimen. Because they generally are responsible for the patient's entry into the health-care system, physicians are considered primary health-care providers; however, nurses working in extended roles may also serve in this capacity.

Physicians attend 4 years of college and 4 years of medical school, then train as residents. The practice of medicine has become highly specialized, either around a body part (e.g., cardiology, gynecology) or around conditions and their treatment (oncology, rheumatology). Physicians may be allopathic (MDs) or osteopathic (DOs).

Focused Care Providers

Within the health-care delivery system, certain groups of professionals provide *focused care services* (those limited to or concentrated on a particular aspect of healthy living). Examples are clinical psychologists, dentists, podiatrists, and optometrists. (Optometrists are often confused with ophthalmologists. Ophthalmologists are medical specialists; optometrists are trained and licensed to examine eyes for vision problems and to prescribe and fit eyeglasses, but do not diagnose or treat eye diseases or injuries.)

These professionals are licensed, although standards vary from state to state. They are usually addressed as "doctor." Their prescriptive authority also varies from state to state. In some areas they may have hospital privileges (that is, they can admit and treat patients in a hospital setting).

Technicians and Technologists

Many people who provide ancillary health-care services are called technicians or technologists; examples include the medical laboratory technician or medical technologist, the medical record technician, the radiologic technician, and the dietary technician. At one time, the term *technologist* was used for people with a bachelor's degree and the term *technician* for those with a 2-year degree. In recent years the terms have been applied indiscriminately, however, so no conclusions can be drawn from the titles.

Technicians or technologists provide a service that contributes to patient care. For example, the medical laboratory technician works in the hospital's clinical laboratory, testing body fluids and tissues to help diagnose a patient's condition.

Therapists

Still other professionals are called therapists; examples are respiratory, occupational, physical, and speech therapists. Each is educated and licensed to provide a specific service. For example, the respiratory therapist helps patients with pulmonary function and oxygenation, and the speech therapist helps the patient to speak more clearly or correct speech disturbances.

Others Providing Necessary Services

Pharmacists are specialists in the science of drugs and can make recommendations about drug therapy. Most programs preparing pharmacists are five years long and include an internship. Pharmacists make up the third-largest group of health-care providers.

Social workers are assuming increasingly important roles in today's health-care delivery system. These professionals counsel patients and families, often directing them to various health-care resources. Social workers are also involved in discharge planning. Social workers have bachelor's degrees, although a master's degree is often preferred for employment in health care.

Chaplains try to meet the spiritual and emotional needs of patients and families. Chaplains usually are nondenominational and may contact a member of the clergy of the patient's faith.

The *physician's assistant* (PA) is a relative newcomer to the health-care delivery system; the first training program for PAs was started at Duke University in 1966 (Raffel and Raffel, 1989, p. 113). Because PAs assume many of the responsibilities of physicians, they can substitute for physicians in areas where a shortage exists. The training program, typically two years long, focuses on medical science and clinical skills. PAs work under the supervision of physicians, who are responsible for their performance.

CHALLENGES TO THE HEALTH-CARE DELIVERY SYSTEM

As the delivery of health-care services has become more complex and sophisticated, it has become a challenge to maintain the quality of care. Five major areas of concern are discussed here.

Quality of Care

Quality assurance, one of the most discussed topics in health care today, means the techniques or methods used to measure the quality of medical care delivered by people or institutions (Jonas & Rosenberg, 1986). Licensing, accreditation, and certification are examples of attempts to guarantee that people and places are prepared to do what the public expects.

Both people and institutions may be licensed. Mechanisms, often tests, are established to recognize minimal competence in a profession. Practicing without a license is a criminal offense. Institutions are licensed based on their ability to meet established criteria. Typical factors considered are physical structure, administration, qualification of personnel, and standards for provision of services. Hospitals, nursing homes, and pharmacies are licensed in all states; licensing of other facilities and nonhospital services varies from state to state.

Accreditation, a popular approach to quality measurement, is a voluntary system used in institutions. Groups with mutual interests establish standards of quality and proceed to inspect themselves according to these standards. Although not a legal requirement, strong incentives exist to attain and maintain accreditation. In many instances, accreditation is a requisite for securing federal funding. For hospitals, an important accrediting organization is the Joint Commission on Accreditation of Healthcare Organizations (JCAHO). Nursing programs can seek accreditation from the National League for Nursing.

Nursing Research

Selected Nursing Research Studies

Baggs, J. C., & Schmitt, M. H. (1988). Collaboration between nurses and physicians. *Image, 20*(3), 145–149.

Berne, A. S., Dato, D., Mason, D. J., et al. (1990). A nursing model for addressing the health needs of homeless families. *Image, 22*(1), 8–13.

Hays, J. C. (1986). Hospice policy and patterns of care. *Image, 18*(3), 92–97.

McCullock, McInyk, K. A. (1990). Barriers to care: Operationalizing the variable. *Nursing Research, 39*(2), 108–112.

Reinardy, J. R., & Quam, J. (1989). Providing health services to elderly in public housing: A case for clinical experience. *Journal of Nursing Education, 28*(3), 127–132.

Weitzel, M. H. (1989). A test of the health promotion model with blue-collar workers. *Nursing Research, 38*(2), 99–103.

Possible Topics for Nursing Inquiry

- If nurses were to do all charting at the patient's bedside, would the amount of overtime paid to nurses be reduced, thus lowering hospital operating expenses?
- When nurses are added to hospital ethics committees, are the decisions more patient-centered?
- Do patients express more satisfaction with the care provided by a nurse practitioner or a physician's assistant?
- Are graduates of nurse practitioner programs today seeking more positions outside the acute-care setting than did 5 years ago?

Certification, the third approach to quality control, combines features of licensing and accreditation. Standards for education, experience, and performance on examinations are used to determine a person's competence. Although certification is usually voluntary, there are incentives for people to become certified. Certification is often used to designate a person's professional specialty.

More recently, quality assurance methods have been used to evaluate the care of patients or groups of patients. Often these methods of evaluating care compare the care given to actual patients with an established standard. This type of assessment requires that some type of peer review, either retrospective or concurrent, be built into the system.

A popular method of evaluating care is to review patient care outcomes. In this system, medical charts are reviewed and patients are reexamined and interviewed, then compared with established standards that are usually based on indicators of health status. Quality assurance checks are also done by third-party payers, who review a hospital's charts and records to determine the quality and appropriateness of the care provided.

Quality assurance is a critical element of the health-care delivery system, but it is time-consuming and therefore costly. Standards for assessment must be developed and refined, a process requiring time and constant updates.

Fragmentation of Service

The explosive growth in medical information has led to specialization throughout the health-care system. The traditional family physician who treated cuts and fractures, delivered babies, performed minor surgery, and treated medical emergencies with equal poise and confidence is seldom found today. Likewise, the nurse who could work on any hospital unit has become a rarity. The sophisticated technology throughout today's hospital requires more than a generalist's knowledge and skill.

The price we pay for these technologic advances is fragmented care. For example, a surgical patient who suffers from diabetes receives care from a surgeon and an endocrinologist or internist. If that same patient has heart problems during surgery, a cardiologist is called in. The patient may spend time in surgery, the recovery room, the intensive or coronary care unit, a step-down unit, or a medical or surgical unit; in fact, the same patient may spend some time in all these areas! After discharge, this fragmentation may continue as different specialists prescribe different medications and require follow-up visits. This can confuse and upset the patient and family.

The nurse can help ensure that the health-care delivery system always puts the patient's needs first, and can help minimize fragmented care. As a coordinator of care

and patient advocate, the nurse can advise patients and reduce confusion (Fig. 2-5).

Limited Medical and Financial Resources

As discussed above, health-care costs in the United States are increasing steadily. Some of the reasons are the growing elderly population, increasing technology, increasing specialization in services, and changing values. In an effort to offset some of the rising costs, several measures have been adopted. For example, health-care delivery through HMOs has been encouraged, and the government has established prospective payment for Medicare.

Such attempts at cost containment have led to earlier discharges and the rebirth of home health nursing. Nurses are increasingly filling the gaps in service and assuming greater roles in patient care. Nursing as a profession must begin to put a dollar value on its services, inside and outside of hospitals. Including the costs of nurse-delivered care in expenses covered by third-party payers is critical.

Access to Health Care

Although more people are involved in the health-care system than ever before, some areas of the United States still lack adequate health-care resources. Often rural areas cannot afford to establish and maintain sound health-care delivery. Nurses can often provide many of these services; in some small communities, a nurse practitioner is the only health-care professional. Nurse midwives, community health nurses, and nurses specializing

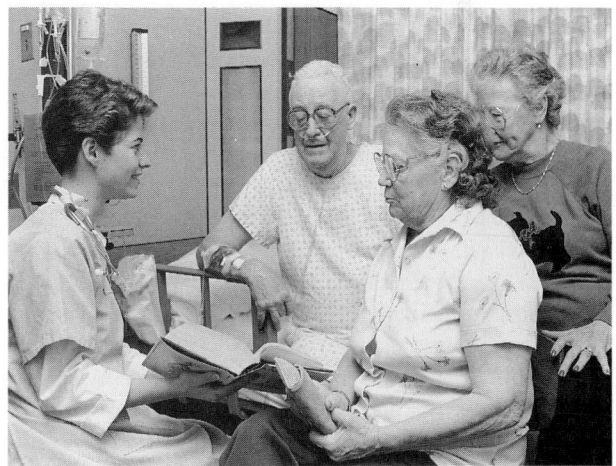

Figure 2–5   The nurse is responsible for providing quality care, and one way to do this is by coordinating health care. She works with the patient and family members to plan for discharge and home care. (Photo courtesy of Shoreline Community College.)

in areas such as gerontology, pediatrics, and family health can make a considerable contribution.

Ethical and Bioethical Decisions

As technology makes available more options of care, ethical and bioethical decision-making becomes critical. Many hospitals have formed ethics committees that make decisions and establish policies on such controversial issues as allocation of scarce medical and financial resources and development of appropriate treatment protocols. Nurses play a critical role in making decisions on bioethical issues and often serve on these ethics committees. Because they have the most contact with the patient, nurses are in a unique position to know the patient's and family's wishes and to be advocates on the patient's behalf. See Chap. 3 for more discussion on ethical concerns in nursing.

Key Concepts

- The U.S. health-care delivery system has experienced phenomenal growth, and this pattern will continue.
- Health care is becoming increasingly expensive.
- Nurses are assuming increasingly significant roles in the delivery of care. They serve as primary caregivers, develop collaborative roles, and respond to the increasing specialization in health care.
- Americans have come to view health care as a right rather than a privilege and are demanding a greater voice in determining the type and quality of care.
- Two other factors affecting the health-care system are that Americans are living longer and that technology is increasing.
- The federal government continues to assume a large role in the health-care system.
- Several types of health services are available in the United States: health promotion and illness prevention, diagnosis and treatment, and rehabilitation.
- Agencies providing inpatient services include acute-care hospitals, long-term care facilities, health maintenance organizations, preferred provider organizations, and organizations providing specialized services.
- Outpatient services are offered in a variety of settings, including physicians' offices, ambulatory care centers and clinics, urgent care centers, and day-care centers.
- Community-based agencies include mental health centers, rural health centers, home-health agencies, and hospices.
- Health-care benefits are available to consumers through private health insurance, programs initiated by the federal government (such as Medicare and Medicaid), and charitable funding.

- The introduction of prospective payment has greatly affected the structure of care delivery.
- To provide quality care, a collaborative approach is needed between nurses and other health-care professionals.
- Significant challenges face nurses and other health-care professionals, such as ensuring the quality of care, minimizing the fragmentation of service, managing limited medical and financial resources, providing access to health care, and making ethical and bioethical decisions.

References

Government of Canada. (1984). *Canada Health Act*. Ottawa: Author.
Jecker, N. S., & Pearlman, R. A. (1989). Ethical constraints on rationing medical care by age. *Journal of American Geriatrics Society, 37*, 1067–1075.
Jonas, S. (1986). *Health care delivery in the United States* (3rd ed). New York: Springhouse.
Jonas, S., & Rosenberg, S. N. (1986). Ambulatory health care. In S. Jonas (Ed.), *Health care delivery in the United States* (3rd ed.). New York: Springhouse, pp. 125–165.
Kane, R. A., & Kane, R. L. (1987). *Long-term care: Principles, programs and policies*. New York: Springer.
Matteson, M. A., & McConnell, E. S. (1988). *Gerontological nursing: Concepts and practice*. Philadelphia: Harcourt-Brace-Jovanovich.
McCarthy, C. M., & Thorpe, K. E. (1986). Financing of health care. In S. Jonas (Ed.), *Health care delivery in the United States* (3rd ed.). New York: Springhouse, pp. 303–331..
Raffel, M. W. & Raffel, N. K. (1989). *The U.S. health system: Origins and functions* (3rd ed.). New York: John Wiley & Sons.
Thompson, F. J. (1983). *Health policy and the bureaucracy: Politics and implementation*. Cambridge, MA: MIT Press.
Thorpe, K. E., Thorpe, J. L., & Barhydt-Wezenaar, N. (1986). Health Maintenance Organizations. In S. Jonas (Ed.), *Health care delivery in the United States* (3rd ed.). New York: Springhouse, pp. 166–182.
U.S. Department of Health and Human Services. (1990). *Vital statistics for the United States: 1987 life tables* (Vol. 2, Sec. 6). Pub. #PHS 90-1104. Hyattsville, MD: U.S. Government Printing Office.
U.S. Senate Special Committee Report on Aging. (1987). *Aging America: Trends and projections, 1985–1986*. Washington, DC: Public Health Service, Department of Health and Human Services.
Wilson, F. A., & Neuhauser, D. (1987). *Health services in the United States* (2nd ed.). Cambridge, MA: Ballinger.
World Health Organization. (1978). *Report of the International Conference on Primary Health Care*. Geneva: Author.

Bibliography

Abrahamson, L. (1990). *Healing our health-care system*. New York: Grove Weidenfeld.
Cahill, C. W. (1990). Health-care rationing through inconvenience. *New England Journal of Medicine, 322*, 1816.
Callahan, D. (1990). *What kind of life: The limits of medical progress*. New York: Simon & Schuster.
Callahan, D. (1990). Rationing medical progress: The way to affordable health care. *New England Journal of Medicine, 322*, 1810–1813.
Colby, W. H. (1990). Missouri stands alone. *Hastings Center Report, 20*(5), 5–6.
Cranford, R. E. (1990). A hostage to technology. *Hastings Center Report, 20*(5), 9–10.

Del Bueno, D. (1988). The promise and the reality of certification. *Image, 20,* 208–211.

Fagin, C. M. (1990) Nursing's value proves itself. *American Journal of Nursing, 90*(10), 17–18.

Garland, M. J., & Hasnain, R. (1990). Health care in common: Setting priorities in Oregon. *Hastings Center Report, 20*(5), 16–18.

Ginsburg, J. A., & Prout, D. M. (1990). Access to health care. *Annals of Internal Medicine, 112,* 641–661.

Grace, H. (1990). Can health-care costs be contained? *Nursing & Health Care, 11*(3), 125–130.

Grumet, G. W. (1989). Health-care rationing through inconvenience: The third party's secret weapon. *New England Journal of Medicine, 321,* 607–611.

Johnson, P. A. (1990) A national health insurance program: A nursing perspective. *Nursing & Health Care, 11,* 416–418.

Lohr, K. N. (Ed.). (1990). *Medicare: A strategy for quality assurance,* Vol. I. Washington, DC: National Academy Press.

Lynn, J., & Glover, J. (1990). Cruzan and caring for others. *Hastings Center Report, 20*(5), 10–11.

Reinhardt, U. W. (1987). Health insurance for the nation's poor. *Health Affairs, 6*(1), 101–112.

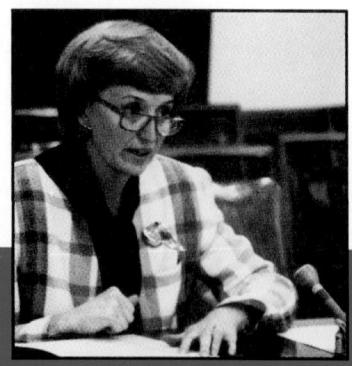

Ethical and Legal Concerns

LEARNING OBJECTIVES

After completion of this chapter, the student will be able to do the following:

- Define ethics.
- Differentiate morals from values.
- Describe the ethical principles inherent in the American Nurses Association code.
- Explain ethical philosophy.
- Give theories of moral development.
- Describe a systematic approach to resolve ethical dilemmas.
- Analyze an ethical dilemma, citing ethical principles.
- Explain licensure.
- Describe standard of care.
- Explain and give examples of crimes and torts.
- Define four elements of negligence.
- Describe legal protections for nurses and cite measures to be taken.

KEY TERMS

Assault	Laws	Plaintiff
Battery	Liability	Respondeat
Crime	Malpractice	superior
Defendant	Morals	Teleology
Deontology	Negligence	Tort
Ethics		

3

Legal and Ethical Dilemmas
Ethical Issues in Nursing
What is Ethics?
Professional Codes of Ethics
Ethical Principles
Codes of Ethics for the Nursing Profession
Examples of Ethical Philosophy
Teleologic Approach
Deontologic Approach
Moral Development
Lawrence Kohlberg
Carol Gilligan
Analysis of an Ethical Dilemma
Analytic Skills
Role Conflict
Legal Issues in Nursing

Sources of Laws
Licensure
Standards of Care
Patient's Bill of Rights
Informed Consent
Torts and Crimes
Intentional Torts
Unintentional Torts
Liability
Crimes
Controlled Substances
Death and Dying
Protecting Yourself
Good Samaritan Law
Key Concepts

Nurses taking courses on legal and ethical issues in health care are enthusiastic participants. They want to discuss what is "good." They want a wise teacher to tell them what is legally right and wrong. They want guidance for acting on their moral convictions.

In this era of technologic advances and cost-containment problems, legal and ethical dilemmas in nursing are becoming more difficult. Nurses have an obligation to their patients to help them attain their goals, but nurses also have an obligation to the institutions for which they work, and the society of which they are a part.

Advocacy in this environment means that nurses must act as interpreters. They must explain to lawmakers what it means to be a patient in today's health-care setting. They also must translate to patients how cost constraints will limit their choices. The legal and moral rights of patients must be balanced against the obligations incumbent on all health professionals.

Nurses bring unique values of holism and humanism to health care. They nurture their patients in a way that empowers the patients (that is, they promote independence rather than fostering a dependent role).

LEGAL AND ETHICAL DILEMMAS

Mr. North was an 86-year-old who had prostate surgery. His surgery went well, but afterwards he developed problems with his breathing. After being on a ventilator for several days, the doctors took a gamble and extubated him, and he did well. That is, as far as the doctors saw, he looked well. We were keeping his lungs clear by nasotracheally suctioning him every 4 hours, tying down his hands and feet so he wouldn't kick and hit us during the procedure. He hated it. It got to the point that whenever a nurse came into his room, he became agitated. We had to give him huge amounts of sedatives just to take his blood pressure. The family supported this; they wanted to see their father get better. But every time Mr. North looked at me with that fear and anger in his eyes, I felt less like a nurse and more like a prison guard.

This nurse faced both an ethical and a legal dilemma. Her ethical dilemma was that she wanted to promote Mr.

North's health by keeping his lungs clear, but she also wanted to promote his independence and dignity. Her legal dilemma was that the patient could charge her with battery for intentionally touching his body without his permission, whereas the family could sue her if her failure to suction him caused his death by pneumonia.

Some nurses may believe that they know what is right to do in such a situation. Unless they study the ethical and legal principles of nursing, however, they are acting largely on their hunches or intuition. They may make decisions in this way for years—many nurses do. But there will probably come a difficult time when they are unsure of the consequences of their actions.

If nurses want to take actions that are at odds with medical orders or the accepted practices of their institution, they must understand the *legal principles* of their action, which will help them understand the risks to which they are subject, and the *ethical principles* of their action, which will provide them with a rationale for their moral choice. Substantiating a decision with a reference to state case law or a quote from the American Nurses Association *Code for Nurses* goes a long way toward reducing personal risk.

No book or teacher can give all the answers to the ethical and legal problems nurses encounter, but this chapter provides some guidelines.

ETHICAL ISSUES IN NURSING

What Is Ethics?

Ethics is a branch of philosophy. It is the systematic intellectual pursuit of standards of behavior; it asks the major questions about right and wrong. When we ask a theoretical question such as "How do we know what is good?" we are doing metaethics. When we ask a practical question such as "Am I doing the right thing in this situation?" we are doing normative ethics. Most questions about medicine, nursing, and patient care are examples of normative ethics, and that is what this section of the chapter explores.

The word **morals** generally refers to a more informal, personal commitment to a set of values (Jameton, 1984). *Values* are standards for decision-making that endure over a significant period of time (Hall, 1982). As we think about our values, we learn what we are willing to fight for, what we are willing to speak out in favor of, what we are silently committed to, and what we prefer but may be willing to surrender. Values are discussed further in Chapter 16.

Nurses must examine their personal values to understand how they fit into professional codes of ethics. Nursing codes of ethics are important because they advise both the nurse and the general public of expected conduct of professional nurses. The goals established in the codes also provide standards on which members may be disciplined.

Professional Codes of Ethics

Ethical Principles

Ethical principles are introduced in the American Nurses Association's *Code for Nurses* (1985), which states:

> When making clinical judgments, nurses base their decisions on universal moral principles which both prescribe and justify moral actions. The most fundamental of these is respect for persons. Other important principles which stem from this basic one are: autonomy, beneficence, nonmaleficence, veracity, confidentiality, fidelity, and justice.

These moral principles are useful in looking at individual cases, but it is important to remember that there is no absolute hierarchy of principles. In many ethical dilemmas, two or more principles may come into conflict and may point in different directions. When this occurs, it is helpful to reflect on the ethical philosophies from which such principles arise. To understand the principles introduced in the American Nurses Association code, consider how they are used to reflect on the ethical issue of informed consent (which is discussed later in the chapter).

Beneficence and Nonmaleficence. In the past, physicians guided treatment decisions by the principles of beneficence and nonmaleficence (*beneficence,* to promote good; *nonmaleficence,* to avoid harm). The patient was the passive recipient of the physician's good intention to cure the illness. Consent was uninformed: Hippocrates admonished physicians to "do no harm" but also to reveal "nothing of the patient's future or present condition" (President's Commission for the study of Ethical Problems in Medicine and Biomedical and Behavioral Research, 1982).

Beneficence and nonmaleficence are still guiding principles when the patient does not participate in decision-making. That may be the patient's choice: "I'll go along with whatever the doctors and nurses say I should do." Or the patient may be unable to voice his or her wishes, and no one may be available to speak for him or her. In such a case, health-care providers seek the patient's best interests.

Autonomy. *Autonomy,* the principle of self-determination, is the foundation for informed consent decisions. The President's Commission for the Study of Ethical Problems in Medicine described its findings on the issue of informed consent in *Making Health Care Decisions.* In the report, Gerald Dworkin defined autonomy as "an individual's exercise of the capacity to form, revise, and pursue personal plans for life." The report goes on to describe autonomy as both a shield and a sword: the shield protects the patient from interference, whereas the sword is "creative self-agency." Thus, the principle of autonomy allows a patient to make health-care decisions based on individual goals and values.

Veracity. The American Nurses Association code links autonomy to the other principles in its statement on respect for human dignity. Since each patient has the moral right of self-determination, the principle of **veracity,** or truth-telling, becomes a moral obligation for nurses. Patients have the right "to be given accurate information necessary for making informed judgments" (President's Commission, 1982).

Fidelity. The American Nurses Association code charges nurses with the responsibility of supporting patients who are making treatment decisions and helping them to weigh the risks and benefits. This role comes from the principle of *fidelity,* or faithfulness. Patients trust nurses to help them, and nurses abide by their commitments to patient care.

Nursing Research

Selected Nursing Research Studies

Cassidy, V. R., et al. (1988). Professional autonomy and ethical decision-making among graduate and undergraduate nursing majors. *Journal of Nursing Education.*

Davis, A. J. (1989). Clinical nurses' ethical decision-making in situations of informed consent. *Advances in Nursing Science, 11*(3), 63–69.

Holly, C. (1989). Critical care nurses' participation in ethical decision-making. *Journal of the New York State Nurses Association, 20*(4),

Janson, L., et al. (1989). Ethical reasoning concerning the feeding of terminally ill cancer patients: Interviews with registered nurses experienced in the care of cancer patients. *Cancer Nursing, 12,* 352–358.

Possible Topics for Nursing Inquiry

- What are the ethical dilemmas encountered by nurses in long-term care who work with ill and frail elderly patients?
- How do nurses in critical care balance ethics and the life-sustaining need of critically ill patients?
- What are the most useful methods for teaching ethics to nursing students?
- What are the most common documentation errors by nurses in cases that are brought to litigation?

Confidentiality. Nurses promise to keep patients' disclosures confidential. Whether patients accept or refuse treatment, and regardless of the basis for their decision, the principle of confidentiality dictates that nurses respect patients' rights to privacy.

Justice. Autonomy is meaningless without the principles of veracity, fidelity, and confidentiality to support it. But as essential as autonomy is to health-care decisions, it is limited by the principle of *justice.* Justice can be seen as fairness in allocating health-care resources.

Health-care resources are becoming increasingly limited in many ways. Limitations are seen in the scarcity of some resources (for example, beds in extended-care facilities and organs for transplantation). Our society has not arrived at a fair method of allocating these goods. It is too tempting to give the bed to the patient with the wealthiest family, and to give the liver to the child with the most media coverage.

Nurses, who are committed to the principle of justice, are leading the fight for fair access to health care. These decisions are best made on the basis of policies developed at the institutional, state, and federal level.

Codes of Ethics for the Nursing Profession

The American Nurses Association and Canadian Nurses Association have developed codes of ethics, and an international code of ethics also exists. Although they differ in presentation, the principles remain the same in all three. Nursing students should study them carefully, and nurses should attempt to follow these codes of ethics in their professional life.

Examples of Ethical Philosophy

As stated before, normative ethics considers questions about how to act in a given situation. Someone making an ethical decision must amass and analyze data that help to answer those questions. Philosophers have developed ethical theories that require the decision-maker to consider different sets of data, analyze them in different ways, and ask different questions. The various approaches may lead to the same or different answers (Davis and Aroskar, 1983). Two examples follow.

Teleologic Approach

Teleologic approaches examine the results of actions in question. The word **teleology** is from the Greek "telos" (the end). These philosophies look at the consequences of actions to judge right and wrong.

Utilitarianism. The most familiar such philosophy is *utilitarianism,* espoused by British philosopher John Stuart Mill. In an 1863 essay, he wrote:

The creed which accepts as the foundation of morals, Utility, or the Greatest Happiness Principle, holds that actions are right in proportion as they tend to promote happiness, wrong as they tend to produce the reverse of happiness. By happiness is intended pleasure, and the absence of pain; by unhappiness, pain, and the privation of pleasure."(Gorovitz, 1971)

Mill did not want to defend an "egoist" position (that is, that whatever makes *me* happy is the right thing to do). Instead, he insisted that the happiness we ought to seek is the good of the whole, "the greatest amount of happiness altogether"(Gorovitz, 1971).

One way utilitarianism relates to moral decisions in health care is in the consideration of limited resources. For example, if there are only 10 beds in intensive care and 12 critically ill patients, the team must decide who will benefit most by intensive care. What is the greatest good?

This philosophy can be difficult to practice, since nurses recognize the individual patient as the most important consideration. Generally, even if five family members would be made "unhappy" by the outcome of a certain decision, but the patient would be made "happy," we do what the patient prefers.

Another problem with all teleologic theories lies in attempting to predict the consequences of a particular decision. Consider this case from an acute-care hospital.

> *A patient was admitted to the intensive care unit with an aortic aneurysm. Shortly after his arrival, the aneurysm began to dissect, and the patient suffered a cardiac arrest. Resuscitation was initiated promptly and continued with little success for 30 minutes. The attending physician arrived and consulted the family about their wishes: should the team continue its efforts? The patient's wife answered that if the patient would be left paralyzed, he would not want to live. So the attending physician returned to the patient's room and asked the resuscitation team, "Has anyone seen the patient's legs move?" No one had. Neurologic tests on the patient's extremities were negative. Resuscitation was ceased. Moments later, the patient's toes wiggled. The attending physician, seeing this, ordered resuscitation resumed. It continued another 30 minutes, but the team was unsuccessful, and the patient died.*

Deontologic Approach

How would this situation have been different if the basis of the ethical decision had not been on the ends or consequences of the action? Formalist philosophies look to the action itself to judge its rightness. **Deontology** is an example of a formalist theory. "Deon" is the Greek word for duty; deontologic philosophy examines our duty to moral law or moral principles.

Immanuel Kant. Immanuel Kant, an 18th-century German philosopher, formulated his theory of deontology in a series of maxims, or rules. The most important rule, the "categorical imperative," states that we ought to act "according to the maxim which can at the same time make itself a universal law" (Kant, 1785). In other words, we should look at the underlying principle of our action. Is it a principle we would like everyone to follow? Kant's example is the false promise. He stated that we should never lie to another person, no matter what the consequences may be, for if that principle were universal, there could be "no promises made at all" (Kant, 1785). Similarly, he stated that we must always act so as to treat any person as an end in him or herself, never as a means only.

Deontology, in its infinite respect for the person, seems most akin to nursing philosophy; however, in practice it is difficult to ignore the consequences of a moral action and focus on the principle alone. Take Kant's example of the lying promise: as nurses, we promise our patients that we will keep them comfortable after surgery, but when a patient wakes up from surgery with a dangerously low blood pressure, administering pain medicine may be life-threatening. Should we ignore the consequences to keep our promise?

We must strive for a balance that recognizes both the means and the ends, the principle that underlies the action as well as the consequences of that action. When two colleagues express differing moral views, their arguments may be based on such opposite approaches to the problem.

Moral Development

The ability to integrate ethical principles into one's personal moral decisions has been recognized as the highest stage of moral development. Two theories of moral development follow, which contrast the more traditional approach with what new research describes as the norm for women.

Lawrence Kohlberg

Lawrence Kohlberg, a developmental psychologist, described three levels of moral development. At the first level, *preconventional* judgment, good and bad are interpreted as reward and punishment; the focus progresses from obedience to a recognition of the exchange of favors producing good. Level two is the *conventional* level, in which one learns to conform to the rules and expectations of society. Here one progresses from seeking approval for being "nice" to a "law-and-order" orientation. At the third level, one begins to define *personal* values and moral principles. There are two stages: a utilitarian view of social policies, and the "universal ethical-principle orientation." At this final stage, one uses abstract, universal principles of justice to make moral decisions (Turner, 1987).

One problem with this well-defined sequence of moral development is that Kohlberg based his longitudinal study on a group of 84 boys; therefore women judged against this scale appear to be morally deficient.

Carol Gilligan

In her 1982 book *In A Different Voice,* Carol Gilligan described a distinct pattern of moral development for women. She found that for women, moral development centered around the issues of caring and selfishness. In the first stage, one focuses on caring for the self, with survival as the goal. In the second stage, that view is seen as selfish, and the woman/girl progresses to caring for others based on responsibility. Finally, there is an evolution to a new understanding of the interconnectedness of the self and others: "Care becomes the self-chosen principle of a judgment that remains psychological in its concern with relationships and response but becomes universal in its condemnation of exploitation and hurt" (Gilligan, 1982).

Analysis of an Ethical Dilemma

These different perspectives help us to weigh and sort out moral problems when they occur. Moral dilemmas typically involve a choice between conflicting values or moral principles. They are often complex problems, because we are faced with alternatives that have both good and bad aspects.

Many texts in bioethics offer methods for analyzing moral problems (Davis & Aroskar, 1983; Francoeur, 1983; Jameton, 1984). What follows is a structural approach to analyzing moral dilemmas, with examples.

Analytic Skills

When examining patient problems, it is helpful to ask yourself what other information you need to make a decision.

1. Gather data about the problem. Use as many different sources as possible, including family, friends, and other members of the health-care team. Ask for the patient's perspective in a sensitive and caring way. Ask yourself, what would I do if I were the patient in this situation, or if this patient were my parent? Who is acting as the patient's advocate, and what is his or her opinion?

2. Identify the nature of the problem. Is it really an ethical problem (that is, are there ethical principles in conflict)? Or is it a problem of communication between patient and family, patient and physician, or nurse and physician?

3. Clarify the decision that needs to be made. Has a definitive decision been made, or is it still open to discussion? How much of an impact can you have on the decision? Who is making the decision, and for whom?

4. Apply principles of ethical reasoning to the decision. Which ethical principles are involved? Is the focus on the action or on the end result? Are the rights of the patient being honored?

5. Participate in the decision-making process. Be sure to communicate your values as a nurse. If no one is speaking for the patient's values, bring those forth as well. Encourage the decision to be made in an open forum, not in a covert way. Ensure that these questions are answered: Is the decision final or revocable? When is the action to take place? Who needs to know the results of this process? How will the process be documented?

6. Evaluate your reaction to the process and the resulting action. Based on your analysis, was the decision right or wrong? If you are morally opposed to the decision, how will you act on that stance? From whom can you obtain support for your feelings or your action? How will you act on similar problems in the future?

Role Conflict

Although nurses assume responsibility for their patients, they concomitantly become accountable to the families, physician, and other health-care professionals. If a nurse disagrees with a physician's orders or another nurse's treatment of a patient, must he or she carry out the orders or overlook the incident? To whom is the nurse primarily accountable?

These interdependent relationships incite ethical dilemmas. Despite the role conflict, the analytic approach taken is exactly the same.

Consider your responses to the examples in the display using information you have on ethical considerations of nursing dilemmas. Then, reconsider your response after reading the section on legal issues. How does an understanding of the law applied to nursing issues change your response?

LEGAL ISSUES IN NURSING

Creighton (1986) defined **laws** as "those standards of human conduct established and enforced by the authority of an organized society through its government."

Professional Codes of Ethics for Nurses

American Nurses Association Code for Nurses*

1. The nurse provides services with respect for human dignity and the uniqueness of the client unrestricted by considerations of social or economic status, personal attributes, or the nature of health problems.
2. The nurse safeguards the client's right to privacy by judiciously protecting information of a confidential nature.
3. The nurse acts to safeguard the client and the public when health care and safety are affected by the incompetent, unethical, or illegal practice of any person.
4. The nurse assumes responsibility and accountability for individual nursing judgments and actions.
5. The nurse maintains competence in nursing.
6. The nurse exercises informed judgment and uses individual competence and qualifications as criteria in seeking consultation, accepting responsibilities, and delegating nursing activities to others.
7. The nurse participates in activities that contribute to the ongoing development of the profession's body of knowledge.
8. The nurse participates in the profession's efforts to implement and improve standards of nursing.
9. The nurse participates in the profession's efforts to establish and maintain conditions of employment conducive to high-quality nursing care.
10. The nurse participates in the profession's effort to protect the public from misinformation and misrepresentation and to maintain the integrity of nursing.
11. The nurse collaborates with members of the health professions and other citizens in promoting community and national efforts to meet the health needs of the public.

Canadian Nurses Association Code of Ethics for Nursing†

Clients

1. A nurse is obliged to treat clients with respect for their individual needs and values.
2. Based upon respect for clients and regard for their right to control their own care, nursing care should reflect respect for the right of choice held by clients.
3. The nurse is obliged to hold confidential all information regarding a client learned in the health-care setting.
4. The nurse has an obligation to be guided by consideration for the dignity of clients.
5. The nurse is obligated to provide competent care to clients.
6. The nurse is obliged to represent the ethics of nursing before colleagues and others.
7. The nurse is obligated to advocate the client's interest.
8. In all professional settings, including education, research, and administration, the nurse retains a commitment to the welfare of clients. The nurse bears an obligation to act in such a fashion as will maintain trust in nurses and nursing.

Health team

9. Client care should represent a cooperative effort, drawing upon the expertise of nursing and other health professions. Acknowledging personal or professional limitations, the nurse recognizes the perspective and expertise of colleagues from other disciplines.
10. The nurse, as a member of the health-care team, is obliged to take steps to ensure that the client receives competent and ethical care.

The social context of nursing

11. Conditions of employment should contribute to client care and to the professional satisfaction of nurses. Nurses are obliged to work towards securing and maintaining conditions of employment that satisfy these connected goals.

Responsibilities of the profession

12. Professional nurses' organizations recognize a responsibility to clarify, secure, and sustain ethical nursing conduct. The fulfillment of these tasks requires that professional organizations remain responsive to the rights, needs, and legitimate interests of clients and nurses.

International Council of Nurses Code for Nurses‡

The fundamental responsibility of the nurse is four fold: to promote health, to prevent illness, to restore health, and to alleviate suffering.

(continued)

Professional Codes of Ethics for Nurses *(continued)*

The need for nursing is universal. Inherent in nursing is respect for life, dignity, and rights of man. It is unrestricted by considerations of nationality, race, creed, color, age, sex, politics, or social status.

Nurses render health services to the individual, the family, and the community and coordinate their services with those of related groups.

Nurses and people

The nurse's primary responsibility is to those people who require nursing care.

The nurse, in providing care, promotes an environment in which the values, customs, and spiritual beliefs of the individual are respected.

The nurse holds in confidence personal information and uses judgment in sharing this information.

Nurses and practice

The nurse carries personal responsibility for nursing practice and for maintaining competence by continual learning. The nurse maintains the highest standards of nursing care possible within the reality of a specific situation.

The nurse uses judgment in relation to individual competence when accepting and delegating responsibilities.

The nurse when acting in a professional capacity should at all times maintain standards of personal conduct that reflect credit upon the profession.

Nurses and society

The nurse shares with other citizens the responsibility for initiating and supporting action to meet the health and social needs of the public.

Nurses and coworkers

The nurse sustains a cooperative relationship with coworkers in nursing and other fields. The nurse takes appropriate action to safeguard the individual whose care is endangered by a coworker or any other person.

Nurses and the profession

The nurse plays the major role in determining and implementing desirable standards of nursing practice and nursing education.

The nurse is active in developing a core of professional knowledge.

The nurse, acting through the professional organization, participates in establishing and maintaining equitable social and economic working conditions in nursing.

* From American Nurses Association. (1985). *Code for nurses.* Kansas City, MO: Author.

† This represents only one element of the code—*values. Standards,* which provide more specific directions for conduct than values, and *limitations,* which describe exceptional circumstances in which a value or standard cannot receive its usual application, are provided with each value in the publication. From Canadian Nurses Association (1985). *Code of Ethics for Nursing.* Ottawa: Author.

‡ From International Council of Nurses. (1973). *ICN Code for Nurses: Ethical concepts applied to nursing.* Geneva: Imprimeries Populaires.

Laws are established to protect the rights of society in general. As a society changes its moral standards, the laws generally evolve to correspond with those standards.

In health care and other areas of society where technology has a major impact, moral and legal standards lag behind technologic advances. Thus, even a thorough knowledge of the law may not provide the answers to difficult health-care dilemmas. Nurses have a responsibility to understand the existing legal guidelines as well as to attempt to modify the laws to meet the changing needs of society.

Sources of Laws

English law served as the model for the American system of law that was established when this country was founded. Laws derive from two major sources: *common,* or court-made, law from the judgments in court cases, and *civil* law, which is created by legislative bodies (Creighton, 1986). Civil law encompasses constitutional law, which defines the framework of government; statutes, which define rules for behavior in society; and administrative law, which specifies how those laws are to be interpreted (Fiesta, 1988).

Licensure

One type of law that directly affects nursing practice is the nurse practice act. The purpose of these acts is to carefully circumscribe current nursing practice: to delineate what does and does not constitute nursing. These acts are designed to protect the profession from encroachment by other groups, and to protect the public

---

Analytical Skills: Information Needed in Making a Decision

- Gather data about the problem.
- Identify the nature of the problem.
- Clarify the decisions that need to be made.
- Apply principles of ethical reasoning to the decision.
- Participate in the decision-making process.
- Evaluate your reaction to the process and the resulting action.

---

from those who would practice nursing without a license. Roles and competencies of graduates of diploma, associate degree, and baccalaureate programs are highlighted in Chapter 1.

Licensure is mandatory (that is, to practice nursing one must be licensed as a nurse). In all states there are exceptions for those who provide nursing care to ill friends or family members (Creighton, 1986).

Two of the current challenges to state boards of nursing are increasing the scope of practice to include the expanding role of the nurse in clinical specialist, nurse practitioner, or other entrepreneurial positions; and establishing the baccalaureate degree as the educational requirement for registered nursing. The North Dakota Board of Nursing in 1986 was the first to tackle the latter challenge, and was supported in this change by the North Dakota Supreme Court in 1987 (McCarty, 1987). Other issues being defined state by state are third-party reimbursement for nursing services, prescriptive authority for nurse practitioners, and ensuring liability insurance for nurses in expanded practice (Trandel-Korenchuk, 1980).

Standards of Care

Each state's nurse practice act provides one set of guidelines for the standard that nursing care should meet. The standard of care is also defined on the national level by the American Nurses Association and other specialty organizations. The Joint Commisssion on Accreditation of Healthcare Organizations (JCAHO) accredits hospitals and sets Nursing Standards for things such as documentation. Locally, each institution should have policies and procedures defining the minimum standard for nursing care. Standardized nursing care plans may also reflect the care expected for a specific patient group (Guarriello, 1984). The care provided by each nurse is also measured against the expected behavior of a nurse with a similar level of expertise and experience.

Patient's Bill of Rights

In 1973 the American Hospital Association published *A Patient's Bill of Rights,* which delineates the responsibilities of the hospital and its staff toward the patient and family. Promoting 12 specific rights, the Bill offers guidance and protection for the patient. Although not a legally binding document, it does affirm the patient's right to know his or her diagnosis, treatment, and prognosis in terms that he or she understands.

Informed Consent

As discussed earlier, nurses have a moral obligation to ensure that patients give informed consent for their care. Health care providers are also *legally* required to involve patients in health care decisions. The law has evolved from first demanding that physicians simply obtain permission for experimental treatment and surgery to the modern concept of giving patients full information regarding all therapeutic and diagnostic procedures. These elements must be covered for consent to be "informed:"

- The patient's current medical status and the general course of the illness;
- The proposed treatment and its rationale;
- Risks and benefits of the proposed treatment;
- Risks of not consenting to the treatment;
- Alternatives to the proposed treatment and their associated risks and benefits.

The health care provider who performs a procedure is charged with obtaining informed consent; however, it is generally the nurse's responsibility to obtain the patient's signature verifying that he or she was informed about a proposed treatment. The Joint Commission on Accreditation of Healthcare Organizations stipulates that hospitals specify in their policies which procedures require signed consent. Once a consent form is signed, the burden of proof falls to the plaintiff in a legal action against the hospital or employee. A sample informed consent form is shown in Chapter 23.

In some states, informed consent is addressed in statutory language. These statutes may strengthen the case for informed consent by addressing the need for legal competency of the patient, and stipulating who is authorized to give consent for an incompetent patient. The law grants hospital permission to administer emergency treatment without consent if it is impossible to obtain.

Torts and Crimes

Torts and **crimes** are legal wrongs committed against a person or property. A tort is subject to action in a civil

---

Examples of Ethical Dilemmas

Mrs. Miller has been a patient in the intensive care unit for 3 weeks following major abdominal surgery for metastatic cancer. She has been on a ventilator, receiving multiple drugs to support her blood pressure, and intravenous hydration and nutrition. During this time she has been unconscious and steadily deteriorating; the primary nurse has been planning a family conference with the physicians to discuss future treatment plans.

Today the primary nurse is off, and you are caring for Mrs. Miller. When you start the shift, you notice new orders on the chart discontinuing the IV fluids and medications, and lowering the oxygen on the ventilator to 21%. In addition, there is an order not to resuscitate Mrs. Miller in the event of a cardiac arrest. On the progress notes, the attending physician has written, "The family has been informed of the patient's poor prognosis, and agrees to withdraw life support at this time." The patient's daughter then comes out of her room and says, "The doctor told us she doesn't need the oxygen and the IVs anymore. Isn't that great?"

• What do you tell the daughter?

• What do you do when the heart rate starts to drop?
• What if you can't reach the physician?

Mr. Jones has a longstanding history of circulatory disease. He was admitted to the hospital because of a painful, cold foot. After several days of medical treatment, the circulation has not improved, and the physicians are considering surgery for a below-the-knee amputation. On their physical work-up, they find enlarged nodes in both the axillary and liver regions. They suspect cancer, but do not communicate their suspicions to the patient. The wife is told, and she agrees that her husband should not be informed. However, she does want him to make the final decision regarding the amputation. After she leaves the hospital for the evening, Mr. Jones asks you, "How do you think I'll do after the surgery? Do you think I should have it?"

• What do you tell him?
• What if he specifically asks you, "Do you think the doctors are telling me the whole story?" How do you answer?

---

court; a crime is a violation punishable by the state (Table 3-1).

The purpose of a tort action is to keep the peace, and the goal is to compensate for damages. Torts are usually settled by fines but rarely by imprisonment. Torts may be intentional (assault and battery, invasion of privacy, false imprisonment, defamation of character) or unintentional (negligence, malpractice).

A crime, which is prosecuted in the criminal-justice system, is any wrong punishable by the state. Two elements are necessary: evil intent and a criminal act; however, crimes may exist in which a matter of intent is not spelled out. A person may claim ignorance of the law or be negligent in a gross manner (Creighton, 1986). Crimes are classified as felonies (e.g., murder) or misdemeanors (lesser offenses punishable by a fine of less than $1000 or imprisonment of less than 1 year).

Intentional Torts

Assault and Battery. The most common suit brought against nurses is assault and battery. **Assault** is the threat of touching another person without his or her consent. **Battery** is the actual carrying out of such a threat (that is, the unlawful touching of a person's body). A nurse can be sued for battery any time he or she fails to get consent for a procedure. For example, if an alert, competent patient refuses an injection, it is unlawful for a nurse to apply restraints to carry out the procedure.

Defamation of Character. *Defamation of character* includes false communication or communication resulting in injury to a person's reputation by means of print (libel) or spoken word (slander). The nurse is permitted to make statements about patients *only* as part of his or her nursing practice and *only* to other health-care professionals.

Fraud. *Fraud* is the willful, purposeful misrepresentation of self or an act that may cause harm to a person or property. A nurse who misrepresents the outcome of a procedure is committing a fraud.

Invasion of Privacy. The fourth amendment of the U.S. Constitution protects every citizen's right to privacy. The nurse is bound to limit discussion of the patient to appropriate parties. Disclosing confidential information to an inappropriate third party subjects the nurse to a possible slander charge or liability. The nurse should discuss the patient with others only when the discussion is directly related to treatment and care.

False Imprisonment. Prevention of movement or unjustified retention of a person without consent may be

TABLE 3–1
Differences Between Crimes and Torts

Crime

Results in prison term or fine and/or short jail sentence to punish offender.

Felony

Intentional (1st-degree murder)
Unintentional (2nd-degree murder; manslaughter)

Misdemeanor

An offense punishable by imprisonment of less than 1 year or a fine of less than $1,000. Does not amount to a felony.

Tort

Results in civil trial to assess compensation for plaintiff.

Intentional

Assault and battery
Defamation of character
Fraud
Invasion of privacy
False imprisonment

Unintentional

Negligence (e.g., error in sponge counts, causing a burn, failure to use aseptic technique, falls, medical errors, misadministration of blood)
Malpractice

false imprisonment. Nurses must use restraints carefully and under the approval of a physician. A patient cannot be forced to remain in the hospital against his or her will (assuming that the patient is mentally alert and oriented and capable of participating in care decisions). If the patient refuses to remain in the hospital, the agency will have him or her sign a release stating that he or she left without medical approval. Those with mental impairments may be committed involuntarily if they are dangerous to themselves or others.

Unintentional Torts

Negligence. **Negligence** may be an act of omission or commission (neglecting to do something that a reasonably prudent person would do, or doing something that a reasonably prudent person would not do). **Malpractice** is the act of negligence on the part of a professional. Professional negligence is the lowest level of culpability for malpractice, and as such is considered inadvertent risk-creation for the patient. The person committing an act of negligence is unaware that a risk is being created for another (Kadish, 1983).

To prove nursing negligence, a lawyer must prove that there has been a deviation from the standard of care. In a malpractice case, negligence may be proven or disproven by expert testimony. Another nurse who is a known expert (an expert witness) or has experience in a given field of nursing will be called to testify as to the standard of practice as it relates to the particular case. This is one way in which nurses can define the standard of care in their community; thus, it is dangerous when courts allow others (e.g., physicians) to give expert testimony on nursing.

To prove negligence, four conditions must be met:

There must be a duty to provide care according to the standard described above.
There must be a failure to meet that standard, or a breach of duty.
Causation must be proven (that is, that the breach of duty led to the injury).
Damages must be proven; an actual injury to the patient must exist.

These elements will now be described in greater detail, with examples.

Duty. *Duty* describes the relationship between the **plaintiff** (the person bringing suit) and the **defendant** (the person being sued). Hospitals have a legal duty to treat patients who come to their emergency rooms; nurses as hospital employees have a duty to treat patients admitted by the hospital.

In a few recent cases, patients were denied emergency treatment because they could not pay hospital fees. A nurse who thus refuses care to a patient can be held liable for injuries resulting from such refusal. "The only non-statutory right to medical care U.S. citizens have is the right to be treated in an emergency room for an emergency condition" (Annas, 1985).

Breach of Duty. *Breach of duty* is the failure to conform to the standard of practice, thus creating a risk for another that a reasonable person would have foreseen. Breach of duty may be charged when a patient falls in a hospital; indeed, falls are common causes for malpractice suits against nurses. Although there is currently controversy regarding the use of restraints, the courts have held that the appropriate use of siderails and restraints is a nursing judgment (O'Reilly-Yob, 1988). Nurses can best assess their patients' needs for safety measures, following their facility's policies and procedures regarding restraints. The nurse has a duty to protect patients who are confused, elderly, have recently returned from surgery, sedated, or are in any way less than alert and competent (Greenlaw, 1982).

A patient suffering from pneumonitis was admitted to the hospital acutely ill, feverish, lacking in coordination and with blurred vision. He was placed in a private room that had a small balcony with a railing 2 or 3 feet high. Not long before the subsequent accident, he was seen on the balcony calling for a ladder from construction workers, who notified hospital personnel. The nurse returned the disoriented patient to his room, placed a Posey belt and cloth wristlets on him and notified his physician, who told the nurse to keep an eye on him. The nurse then called the patient's wife at her place of work to come and sit with him, since none of the hospital staff was free to do so. The wife told the nurse she would call her mother and ask her to go to the hospital immediately, and asked the nurse to have someone watch him until her mother arrived. The patient fell from the balcony just before his mother-in-law arrived. The New York appellate court affirmed a judgment for the plaintiff, finding the hospital negligent in failing to supervise the patient until the arrival of his mother-in-law (Creighton, 1986).

Proximate Cause. Causation must be proven for the courts to find negligence. A nurse's carelessness might not result in injury, or injury may occur without the nurse's carelessness as its proximate cause. This was true in the case of one patient who suffered a cardiovascular accident. The court found that the nurse failed to meet the standard of care because she failed to take vital signs as frequently as ordered. The patient's paralysis was not directly caused by the nurse's failure to take the patient's blood pressure, however (Fiesta, 1988).

Courts frequently use foreseeability as a criterion for determining whether a cause is considered proximate (Prosser, 1971). The question becomes whether a reasonable person should have foreseen that injury would result from a failure to conform to the standard of care.

It is difficult to prove proximate cause with hospital-acquired infections, but in one case a hospital was found liable for a patient's infection when he testified that the nurses did not wash their hands after caring for his roommate, who had a staph infection (Fiesta, 1988). The nurse should have foreseen that failure to wash her hands after caring for the roommate could spread infection to the plaintiff.

When it is obvious that the patient's injury was the result of someone's negligence, but it is impossible to prove who was at fault, the doctrine of *res ipsa loquitur* ("the thing speaks for itself") may be invoked. Three elements must be proven (Fiesta, 1988):

The injury could not have occurred if negligence were not present.
The defendant (e.g., nurse, doctor, or hospital) was in complete control of the instrument causing the injury.
The plaintiff (patient) did not voluntarily act to create the injury.

Damages. For a court to find liability, the plaintiff must have suffered actual damages. The purpose of delineating these damages is to compensate for them. *General* damages are those resulting from the injury itself, and may include pain and suffering, disfigurement, and disability. *Special* damages are for the losses and expenses related to injury. In addition, the court may find

emotional damages. *Punitive* damages are found when there is evidence of especially malicious behavior on the part of the defendant, and generally result in a larger judgment (Fiesta, 1988).

Malpractice. In the past, nurses were generally not sued for malpractice because it was considered better to sue the person or institution with the most money or insurance, and it was usually the physician or hospital who had the deepest pockets. Nurses are increasingly subject to malpractice litigation, however, both because of higher salaries and because of their increasing autonomy.

A 10-year study of malpractice suits against nurses found a significant increase, from 177 cases in the first 5-year period to 213 cases in the second (Campazi, 1980). Most negligence cases were related to the administration of treatments, followed by communication, supervision of patients, administration of medications, foreign objects left in patients, and postoperative injuries and infections. In almost 20% of the cases, communication was faulty; examples included informed consent decisions, errors or omissions in charting, the failure to report a patient's worsening condition, and conflicts in communications with physicians.

If the ANA Standards of Nursing Practice (see Chap. 1) are followed, the nurse may avoid being named in a malpractice lawsuit.

Liability

When the four elements of negligence are proven (that is, when the nurse's breach of a duty owed to the patient was the proximate cause of injury to the patient), then the nurse can be found liable for the patient's injury. The hospital may be held responsible for a nurse's negligence under the doctrine of *respondeat superior* ("let the master answer").

This notion of vicarious **liability** can be applied whenever the nurse is acting within the scope of employment. The hospital may attempt to prove that the nurse was not acting within the scope of employment when the negligent act occurred; this is one reason why all nurses should have liability insurance. Defining scope of employment has been a difficult legal question, but nurses are generally covered by vicarious liability when they are acting under the control of their employer.

Crimes

Criminal proceedings may be distinguished from civil tort proceedings in that the state brings charges against the defendant who has violated a criminal statute (e.g., robbery, rape, or manslaughter). The state seeks punishment for that wrongdoing. Negligence that leads to the death of a patient may be tried as a civil tort, which may be a lawsuit filed by the patient's family, or may be tried as a criminal action, filed by the state. In a criminal procedure, the prosecution must prove guilt beyond a reasonable doubt; in a civil case, the plaintiff need only prove a preponderance of evidence in his or her favor (Creighton, 1986).

In some states, a nurse can be criminally prosecuted if there is evidence of criminal action and intent (that is, the nurse must have been aware that the action was unlawful when committing it). This is a case of gross negligence or recklessness, such as one in which the nurse failed to report eclampsia developing in a postpartum patient. The nurse failed to notify the physician, and the patient subsequently died (Creighton, 1986).

Assault and battery (described above as torts) may also be criminally tried. Other examples of crimes nurses have been tried for include robbery, narcotics laws violations, and murder. In one notorious case, a nurse who wanted to prove the need for a pediatric intensive care unit administered succinylcholine to several children in a pediatrician's office. The first five children experienced respiratory arrest and survived. When the sixth one died, she was tried and convicted for murder (Tammelleo, 1986).

Another case resulted in criminal charges when a nurse forcefully searched a patient whom she suspected of stealing money from another patient. When the patient objected to being searched, a guard held the patient's arms so the nurse could search the pockets. Finding no money, they left the patient, who subsequently suffered a cardiac arrest and died. Criminal intent was shown because she should have been aware that her search was illegal (Tammelleo, 1985).

Controlled Substances

In 1970 the Comprehensive Drug Abuse Prevention and Control Act was passed in the United States. In most states nurses may administer controlled substances (narcotics, depressants, stimulants, and hallucinogens) only under the direction of a licensed physician. Misuse can lead to criminal penalties. In institutions, most controlled substances must be kept secure and monitored closely.

Death and Dying

It is the nurse's duty to recognize legal death to document all events that occur while caring for the patient. In some states, the nurse may pronounce death at the bedside; however, in most states the physician has the legal responsibility of pronouncing the person dead.

Death occurs when there is an absence of brain function, despite the function of other body organs. Clinical signs of impending death are:

- Failure to swallow.
- Pitting edema.
- Decreased gastrointestinal and urinary tract activity.
- Incontinence.
- Fever with cold or clammy skin.
- Dysfunctional motion and reflexes.
- Cyanosis.
- Hypotension.
- Noisy or irregular respiration.
- Cheyne-Stokes respirations.

Physician- or nurse-assisted death (active euthanasia) is a controversial issue. Many health care providers believe that actively causing death of a patient would violate their professional ethics. In the United States it is illegal to assist a terminally ill patient to die, although it is rarely prosecuted. Despite most practitioners' reluctance to participate in active euthanasia, there is growing support for its legalization. The proposed laws generally require that the patient be mentally competent; declared terminally ill by more than one physician; and theat the patient make a repeated, written request for help ending his or her life.

Living Wills. The nurse must become familiar with statutes that authorize a *living will,* a person's signed request to be allowed to die when life can be only supported by mechanical or heroic measures. These statutes list specific procedures to follow while granting civil and criminal immunity to those following guidelines. Living wills do not generally allow the removal of life support once it has already been initiated, but allow the withholding of support measures. In some states with a Natural Death Act, however, an adult person may execute a directive to withhold or withdraw life-sustaining procedures in a terminal condition. The living will should be prepared when the person is healthy, rather than waiting until he or she becomes suddenly incapacitated.

Codes. The nurse must know the code status of her patients. A *no code* status requires no effort to resuscitate the patient; it may be written as DNR (do not resuscitate) or "no heroics." In some institutions, policies allow the use of mechanical or chemical support only in a resuscitation order. The nurse verifies the code on the patient's order sheet and follows agency policy regarding codes. The physician periodically reviews the order in case a patient's condition necessitates a change of order.

Death Certificate. Laws are specific in the United States and Canada regarding a death certificate. Each patient requires a separate death certificate. It is the physician's responsibility to sign a death certificate.

Care of the Body. After the death pronouncement by the physician, the nurse is responsible for preparing the

A Patient's Bill of Rights

1. The patient has the right to considerate and respectful care.
2. The patient has the right to obtain from his physician complete current information concerning his diagnosis, treatment, and prognosis in terms the patient can be reasonably expected to understand. When it is not medically advisable to give such information to the patient, the information should be made available to an appropriate person in his behalf. He has the right to know by name the physician responsible for coordinating his care.
3. The patient has the right to receive from his physician information necessary to give informed consent prior to the start of any procedure and/or treatment. Except in emergencies, such information for informed consent should include but not necessarily be limited to the specific procedure and/or treatment, the medically significant risks involved, and the probable duration of incapacitation. Where medically significant alternatives for care or treatment exist, or when the patient requests information concerning medical alternatives, the patient has the right to such information. The patient also has the right to know the name of the person responsible for the procedures and/or treatment.
4. The patient has the right to refuse treatment to the extent permitted by law, and to be informed of the medical consequences of his action.
5. The patient has the right to every consideration of his privacy concerning his own medical care program. Case discussion, consultation, examination, and treatment are confidential and should be conducted discreetly. Those not directly involved in his care must have the permission of the patient to be present.
6. The patient has the right to expect that all communications and records pertaining to his care should be treated as confidential.
7. The patient has the right to expect that within its capacity, a hospital must make reasonable response to the request of a patient for services. The hospital must provide evaluation, service, and/or referral as indicated by the urgency of the case. When medically permis-

sible, a patient may be transferred to another facility only after he has received complete information and explanation concerning the needs for and alternatives to such a transfer. The institution to which the patient is to be transferred must first have accepted the patient for transfer.
8. The patient has the right to obtain information as to any relationship of his hospital to other health-care and educational institutions insofar as his care is concerned. The patient has the right to obtain information as to the existence of any professional relationships among individuals, by name, who are treating him.
9. The patient has the right to be advised if the hospital proposes to engage in or perform human experimentation affecting his care or treatment. The patient has the right to refuse to participate in such research projects.
10. The patient has the right to expect reasonable continuity of care. He has the right to know in advance what appointment times and physicians are available and where. The patient has the right to expect that the hospital will provide a mechanism whereby he is informed by his physician or a delegate of the physician of the patient's continuing health-care requirements following discharge.
11. The patient has the right to examine and receive an explanation of his bill, regardless of source of payment.
12. The patient has the right to know what hospital rules and regulations apply to his conduct as a patient.

No catalogue of rights can guarantee for the patient the kind of treatment he has a right to expect. A hospital has many functions to perform, including the prevention and treatment of disease, the education of both health professionals and patients, and the conduct of clinical research. All these activities must be conducted with an overriding concern for the patient and, above all, the recognition of his dignity as a human being. Success in achieving this recognition assures success in the defense of the rights of the patient.

(Reprinted with permission of the American Hospital Association, copyright 1972.)

body for the morgue or mortuary. The nurse must be familiar with the hospital's instructions for care, including the religious beliefs of the deceased and family. The body should be treated with dignity. Identification tags are placed on the ankle of the body, any of the patient's belongings (e.g., dentures, eyeglasses), and the shroud or body bag.

Organ Donation. The nurse must check to see if the deceased wished to donate organs to a transplant program. If the death was accidental and no donor card is available, the nurse may discuss with the family the possibility of donating the organs of the deceased. Figure 3-1 shows a sample organ donor card. A section of the living will, discussed earlier in this chapter, also provides this information. If functional organs are to be donated, the hospital should have specific care instructions for the body.

Autopsy. An *autopsy* is a postmortem examination of the organs and tissues of the body to determine the cause of death or pathological conditions contributing to the death. Consent for an autopsy is a legal requirement. It is the physician's responsibility to request an autopsy, but the nurse may be asked for clarification by family members. Consent may be given by the deceased before death or by a close family member. Because of religious beliefs, some families may not consent to an autopsy, but the consent law is overruled if the death was by murder or suicide or was of suspicious origin.

Signed by the donor and the following two witnesses in the presence of each other:

Sophie Cyzewski — Signature of Donor
5/10/66 — Date of Birth of Donor
12/6/91 — Date Signed
Pittsburgh, PA — City and State
Dave Jarrett — Witness
Debbie Smith — Witness

This is a legal document under the Uniform Anatomical Gift Act or similar laws in all 50 states

Delaware Valley TRANSPLANT PROGRAM

For further information call
800 KIDNEY-1
2401 Walnut St., Suite 404
Philadelphia, PA 19103

UNIFORM DONOR CARD

Sophie Cyzewski
Print or type name of donor

In the hope that I may help others, I hereby make this anatomical gift, if medically acceptable, to take effect upon my death. The words and marks below indicate my desires.
I give: a) ✓ any needed organs or parts
b) ____ only the following organs or parts

Specify the organ(s) or part(s)

for the purpose of transplantation, therapy, medical research or education:
c) No my body for anatomical study if needed

Limitations or special wishes, if any

Figure 3–1. Organ donor card.

Wills. The nurse may be asked to witness a *will,* a declaration by a person regarding how his or her property is to be handled after death. Many institutions have policies that prohibit nurses from witnessing legal documents. If a nurse does witness a will, the nurse makes a note on the patient's chart about the patient's mental and physical condition at the time of the signing and of the nurse's role in the procedures. A nurse cannot be a beneficiary to any will he or she witnesses.

Protecting Yourself

The best way to guard against lawsuits is to use sound judgment and to maintain good relationships with your patients.

Be aware of the standards that apply to nurses. Know the standards of care for your hospital, your specialty area, and your state. Keep current with changes in the profession by attending continuing education courses and by reading journals. Apply that knowledge to the care you give your patients. Follow legislative changes that affect your practice, and the case law that applies to nursing.

Document thoroughly and carefully (Fig. 3-2). It will be difficult to prove what you have done if it is not recorded in written form. Notes can be admitted into evidence in a court case and may show a nurse's attention or lack of attention to patient care. Gaps in documentation may lead to a conclusion of nursing negligence (Cushing, 1982). Charting should include all pertinent facts. Notes should be written legibly and should include direct quotations whenever possible. Avoid making judgments of character or conclusions about a patient's motivations; simply state facts and observations. Errors should be indicated by making one straight line through the words, and initialing and dating the correction above; a nurse can be charged with fraud for otherwise altering a patient's record.

Be sure that you have personal liability insurance (Reinert & Buck, 1989). As stated previously, the doctrine of **respondeat superior** merely gives the plaintiff an additional avenue for recourse; it does not protect the individual nurse from suit. Your employer's insurance may cover you, but it might not provide you with your own counsel. For a reasonable cost, insurance can be obtained through a professional association that will cover the damages awarded against you within the limits of the policy, the costs of the attorneys hired to defend you, and the bond that may be required if the case goes to an appeals court (Mancini, 1984).

Suggested Format For a Uniform Living Will/Durable Power of Attorney/Organ Donation Document

by Belding H. Scribner, M.D.

I, _Doris M. Montex_ being of sound mind hereby express my wishes regarding life-support treatment.

A. Conditions which must prevail in order for this document to become activated.
1. I must have an incurable illness or injury.
2. That illness or injury must render me incapable of communicating my wishes regarding treatment, as judged by my physician in consultation with another physician.

B. Designation of surrogate(s) (persons who will make the decisions regarding termination of life-support treatment).
Choose one:
1. (X) My physician in consultation with my family.
2. ( ) I appoint _____ as my surrogate. If for any reason he/she is unable to serve then choice #1 will become operative. Note: If choice #2 is made, a separate power of attorney document must be executed and attached to this document.

C. Specific instructions
( ) I want all forms of life-support treatment.

WANT	DO NOT WANT	DEFER TO MY SURROGATE	
( )	( )	(X)	IV fluids
( )	(X)	( )	Feeding by a tube in my stomach
(X)	( )	( )	Antibiotics
( )	(X)	( )	Artificial kidney treatment
( )	(X)	( )	Support by respirator
( )	(X)	( )	Cardiopulmonary resuscitation
( )	( )	( )	Other _____

D. Time of decision to terminate the life-support treatment as designated in Part C. Choose one:
1. ( ) When I am in a terminal condition and the moment of my death is being postponed by artificial means.
2. ( ) When I am not in a terminal condition, but my survival depends on life-support treatment. My qualify of life as determined by my surrogates has irreversibly deteriorated to the point where I would have refused further treatment had I been able to do so.

E. ORGAN DONATION
1. (X) I wish to donate my corneas.
2. (X) I wish to donate other organs (kidney, heart, etc.).
3. ( ) I wish to donate my body for scientific study.
(Note: If any of these items are checked, carry an organ donor card.)

F. Verification: Date _1/22/92_
1. Print your name _Doris M. Montex_
2. Signature _Doris M. Montex_
3. Witnesses (must not be family members, physicians, etc.)
   a) Signature _John Martin_
   b) Signature _Joyce Martin_

To register this document and carry a numbered registration card in your wallet, contact Concern for Dying, 250 West 57th Street, New York, NY 10107.

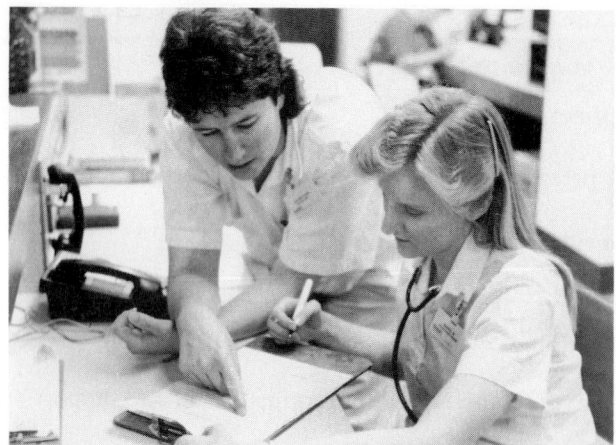

Figure 3–2. Careful documentation and reporting are nursing responsibilities and also maintain legal records.

If a specific incident such as a fall or medication error occurs, follow these principles:

Maintain rapport with the patient. Don't avoid communication with the patient who is experiencing stress and uncertainty. Offer simple explanations if you can do so honestly, calmly, and without blaming anyone.

Document the incident in both the progress notes and the appropriate forms used by your institution. Incident reports are useful to remind you of the events surrounding the incident (Doll, 1980), and they are also useful in bringing about needed changes in the institution (Communique, 1988).

Nursing students must perform *only* those duties that are in the scope of their professional training to date. These acts are performed with the same degree of competence an RN would exhibit. Under the auspices of a clinical supervisor, they may carry out assignments. Nursing students assume liability for their negligent or wrong acts.

Good Samaritan Law

The "Good Samaritan Law" offers legal immunity for health-care professionals who assist in an emergency and render the best care possible under such circumstances. Although most states do not require nurses or citizens to aid the distressed, such assistance becomes an ethical rather than a legal duty. Although this law limits liability for the nurse, he or she is required to follow the ANA code.

Patient Teaching

Instruct the patient as follows:

- Ask questions about all procedures and treatments so that you can be fully informed.
- Prepare a living will or make your wishes known to your family and health-care providers.
- Patient advocacy should be a priority of care. If you do not feel you are supported by your health-care providers (nurse, physician, others), seek other health-care providers.

Safety Alert

- Use responsible professional judgment in performing all procedures; you are legally accountable for your actions.
- Carry out physicians' orders. Question orders you feel are detrimental or in error; you are held accountable independent of the physician.
- Take responsibility only for assignments for which you have been prepared; ask for supervision for tasks in which you have less skill.
- Know the limits of the nurse practice act in your state; you are accountable for practice within the limits of that act.

Key Concepts

- Morals are an informal, personal commitment to a set of values.
- Nurses as professionals must examine their values.
- The ANA code is the nurses' value statement to the public.
- Universal moral principles include autonomy, beneficence, nonmaleficence, veracity, confidentiality, fidelity, and justice.
- In developing morally, one integrates ethical principles into one's personal moral decisions.
- A moral dilemma involves choosing between conflicting values or moral principles and basing the solution on a structured analysis.
- Each state's nurse practice act lists the guidelines for standard nursing care.
- Nurses are subject to review when a tort or crime is committed.
- The Patient Bill of Rights gives a code of ethics for nurses to follow.
- The four elements of negligence are duty, breach of duty, proximate cause, and damage.

- Although the Good Samaritan Law provides immunity for professionals under specific circumstances, nurses should carry personal liability insurance.
- One way to avoid malpractice litigation is to follow the ANA code, documenting all events and treatments involving patients.
- The nurse has legal responsibilities regarding the dying patient and the deceased (e.g., living wills, codes, the death certificate, care of the body, organ donations, the autopsy, and wills).

References

American Nurses Association. (1985). *Code for nurses.* Kansas City, MO: Author, p. 1.

Annas, G. J. (1985). Adam Smith in the emergency room. *Hastings Center Report, 15,* 4.

Campazi, B. C. (1980). Nurses, nursing and malpractice litigation: 1967–1977. *Nursing Administration Quarterly, 5,* 1–18.

Communique, Q. A. (1988). Development of an incident reporting system. *Quarterly Review Bulletin, 14,* 245–250.

Creighton, H. (1986). *Law every nurse should know* (5th ed.). Philadelphia: W. B. Saunders, pp. 2, 148, 227, 233.

Cushing, M. (1982). Gaps in documentation. *American Journal of Nursing, 82,* 1899–1900.

Davis, A. J., & Aroskar, M. A. (1983). *Ethical dilemmas and nursing practice* (2nd ed.). Norwalk, CN: Appleton-Century-Crofts.

Doll, A. (1980). What to do after an incident. *Nursing '80, 10,* 73–79.

Fiesta, J. (1988) *The law and liability: A guide for nurses* (2nd ed.). St. Paul, MN: John Wiley & Sons.

Francoeur, R. T. (1983). *Biomedical ethics.* New York: John Wiley & Sons.

Gilligan, C. (1982). *In a different voice.* Cambridge, MA: Harvard University Press, p. 74.

Gorovitz, S. (Ed.). (1971). *Utilitarianism with critical essays.* New York: Bobbs-Merrill, pp. 18, 21.

Greenlaw, J. (1982). When leaving siderails down can bring you up on charges. *RN, 45,* 75–78.

Guarrielo, D. L. (1984). Legal booby-traps in nursing standards. *RN, 47,* 19–21.

Hall, B., Kalven, J., Rosen, L., & Taylor, B. (1982). *Readings in value development.* Ramsey, NJ: Paulist Press.

Jameton, A. (1984). *Nursing practice: The ethical issues.* Englewood Cliffs, NJ: Prentice-Hall, p. 5.

Kadish, S., Schulhofer, S., & Paulsen, M. (1983). *Criminal law and its processes* (4th ed.). Boston: Little, Brown, p. 274.

Kant, I. (1785). *Groundwork of the metaphysics of morals.* New York: Bobbs-Merrill, p. 22, 63.

Kaufmann, W. (1970). Prologue. In M Buber, *I and Thou* (p. 20). New York: Charles Scribner's Sons.

Mancini, M. (1984). What you should know about malpractice insurance. *American Journal of Nursing, 84,* 985–986.

McCarty, M. (Ed.). (1987). Legislature upholds North Dakota Board of Nursing's power. *The American Nurse, 19,* 3.

O'Reilly-Yob, M. (1988). Use of restraints: Too much or not enough? *Focus of Critical Care, 15,* 32–33.

President's Commission for the Study of Ethical Problems in Medicine and Biomedical and Behavioral Research. (1982). *Making health care decisions* (Vol. 1). Washington, DC: U.S. Government Printing Office, pp. 2, 32, 44, 46.

Prosser, W. L. (1971). *Handbook of the law of torts* (4th ed.). St. Paul, MN: West, p. 267.

Reinert, B. R., & Buck, E. A. (1989). Issues in liability insurance and the nursing consultant. *Clinical Nurse Specialist, 3,* 42–45.

Tammelleo, A. D. (Ed.). (1985). Chaos in the O.R. *The Regan Report on Nursing Law, 26,* 4.

Tammelleo, A. D. (Ed.). (1986). Nurse murders pediatric patient. *The Regan Report on Nursing Law, 27,* 6.

Tammelleo, A. D. (Ed.). (1986). R.N. searches patient—death results. *The Regan Report on Nursing Law, 27,* 2.

Trandel-Korenchuk, D. M., & Trandel-Korenchuk, K. M. (1980). Current legal issues facing nursing practice. *Nursing Administration Quarterly, 5,* 37–45.

Turner, J. S., & Helms, D. B. (1987). *Lifespan development.* New York: Holt, Rinehart & Winston.

Bibliography

Andrews, J. (1989). Whose right is it, anyway? When treatment should cease. *Nursing Times, 85*(47), 24.

Aroskar, M. A. (1989). Community health nurses: Their most significant ethical decision-making problems. *Nursing Clinics of North America, 14,* 967–975.

Botter, M. L., et al. (1989). Allocation of resources: Nurses, the key decision-makers. *Holistic Nursing Practice, 4,* 44–45.

Cassidy, V. R., et al. (1988). Professional autonomy and ethical decision-making among graduate and undergraduate nursing majors. *Journal of Nursing Education, 27,* 405–410.

Davis, A. J. (1989). Clinical nurses' ethical decision-making in situations of informed consent. *Advances in Nursing Science, 11,* 63–69.

Fowler, M. D. M. (1989). Ethical decision-making in clinical practice. *Nursing Clinics of North America, 14,* 955–965.

How each state stands on legislative issues affecting advanced nursing practice. (1990, January). *Nurse Practitioner, 15,* 11–18.

Janson, L., et al. (1989). Ethical reasoning concerning the feeding of terminally ill cancer patients: Interviews with registered nurses experienced in the care of cancer patients. *Cancer Nursing, 12,* 352–358.

Killian, W. H. (1990). Nurses face increasing liability. *American Nurse 22,* 43.

Murphy, E. K. (1990). Legal concerns of the next decade. *Association of Operating Room Nurses, 51,* 258, 260–261.

Patient Identifying Confidentiality Act of 1989. (1989). *Journal of the American Medical Records Association, 60,* 17–18.

Penticuff, J. H. (1990). Ethical issues in redefining death. *Journal of Neuroscience Nurses, , 22,* 48–49.

Pierce, S. F. (1989). The critical care nurse: An ethicist by trade. *Critical Care Nursing Quarterly, 12,* 75–78.

Rogers, B. (1989). AIDS and ethics in the workplace. *Nursing Outlook, 37,* 254–255, 290.

Sawyer, L. M. (1989). Nursing code of ethics: An international comparison. *International Nursing Review, 36,* 145–148.

Selekman, J. (1989). When the nurse knows and the patient does not: Waiting for a diagnosis. *Holistic Nursing Practice, 4,* 1–7.

St. Amant, J. L. S. (1989). The nurse as a witness in a medical malpractice case. *Veterans Administration Nurse, 57,* 44–46.

Varga, K. (1989–1990). How to protect yourself against malpractice. *Imprint, 37,* 33–37.

Wilkinson, J. M. (1989). Moral distress: A labor and delivery nurses's experience. *Journal of Obstetrical, Gynecological, and Neonatal Nursing, 18,* 513–519.

Willis, C., et al. (1989). Medical records and legal implications for the nurse. *Dimensions of Oncology Nursing, 3,* 9–10.

Wolf, Z. R. (1989). Medication errors and nursing responsibility. *Holistic Nursing Practice, 4,* 8–17.

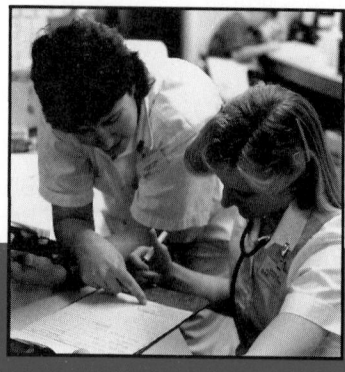

Leadership and Management

LEARNING OBJECTIVES

Upon completion of this chapter, the student will be able to do the following:

- Define the differences between leadership and management.
- Describe the four components of the management process.
- Identify three skills required for effective management.
- List interventions that can control perceptions and reactions to change.

- Describe common clinical practice, management, and education roles in nursing.
- Characterize leadership and management functions of common nursing roles.
- Identify and describe the three most popular models of nursing-care delivery.
- Explain why problem-solving, management, and nursing processes are similar.

KEY TERMS

Charge nurse
Clinical nurse
  specialist
Controlling
Directing
Directive
  leadership
Leadership

Managed care
Management
Nurse anesthetist
Nurse executive
Nurse midwife
Nurse practitioner
Organizing

Participative
  leadership
Planning
Primary nursing
Problem-solving
Team leader
Team nursing

Leadership
  Styles of Leadership
Management
  Functions of Managers
    Planning
    Organizing
    Directing
    Controlling
  Skills for Effective Management
    Problem-Solving

Communication
Managing Change
**Applying Leadership and Management to Nursing
  Roles**
  Clinical Practice Roles
    Staff Nurse
    Advanced Clinical Practice Roles
  Nursing Management Roles
  Teaching Roles
Key Concepts

As professionals, nurses have a responsibility to provide a defined service that meets the needs of society. The American Nurses Association's social policy statement (1980) defines that service as "the diagnosis and treatment of human responses to actual or potential health problems." The profession needs internal organization and leadership so that it can provide that service. At the institutional level, leadership abilities and management skills are required to provide the circumstances in which nurses can practice. At the individual nurse–patient level, leadership and good management skills are required to determine the plan of nursing care and to integrate that plan of care effectively with other health-care professionals.

We cannot discuss all the specific leadership roles in the nursing profession because of the diverse specialties, the variety of work settings in which nurses practice, and the vast number of roles. Nurses may decide to specialize in medical, surgical, parent–child, psychiatric, or home health fields, or any subcomponent of these specialties, such as cardiac, oncology, or gerontology nursing. Nurses may also choose to care for patients with either acute or chronic illnesses. Although most nurses work in hospitals, others work in community nursing, clinics, physicians' offices, nursing homes, schools, industry, the military, or in missionary work. Nurses may choose among clinical practice roles, teaching roles, or management roles. Although most nurses are clinicians, education and management roles exist in most organizations where nurses practice to provide the education, management, communication, and representation required for nurses to practice nursing.

Many options are available to new nursing graduates.

Throughout their nursing careers, they may choose different work settings and roles in nursing. This chapter will discuss leadership, the management process, management skills, and leadership and management aspects of some of the common roles in nursing.

LEADERSHIP

Leadership is the ability to influence others to strive for a goal or to change. Leadership results from the effective practice of behaviors that are selected to meet the needs of the situation. These behaviors can be learned.

There is no one best way (or one best set of behaviors) for effective leadership. Research on leaders and leadership has shown that different leaders have different inherent traits and abilities (Hitt, 1988; Yukl, 1989). Although certain personality traits are more common in leaders than in followers, no single set of traits is always found in leaders. Although many leaders are assertive, decisive, logical, thorough, and innovative, not all leaders are; indeed, some followers have these traits. According to more recent leadership research, a leader's effectiveness depends not only on his or her traits, skills, and behaviors, but also on characteristics of the followers and factors in the situation (Hitt, 1988; Tannenbaum & Schmidt, 1973; Vroom & Jago, 1988; Yukl, 1989).

Styles of Leadership

Effective leadership occurs when a person with the right combination of personality traits and abilities uses behaviors appropriate for the circumstances. A leader who is effective in one situation may not be effective in another. Leaders are often described by the style of leadership they predominantly use. Leadership style describes how the leader interacts with followers or subordinates. That style reflects the traits, values, abilities, and behaviors used by the leader.

In a classic article that has been the basis for many subsequent leadership theories, Tannenbaum and Schmidt (1973) described leadership styles along a continuum from directive to participative (Fig. 4-1).

Directive leadership describes a leader who makes all the decisions and tells followers what to do. The leader is in complete control. The directive leader does not involve followers in problem-solving, discussion, or decision-making. This type of leadership is also called authoritarian or autocratic. It was formerly used in hospitals: physicians told nurses what to do, and nurses told patients what to do. But as the roles of nurses and patients changed, leadership style changed. A participative or democratic leadership is usually preferred. In an emergency, however, leadership may require one person to make decisions and instruct others what to do.

Participative leadership, also referred to as democratic, is at the opposite end of the continuum. The participative leader involves followers in goal-setting, problem-solving, and decision-making. This involvement promotes followers' sense of importance to the overall goal or organization and promotes a sense of control over the situation. To be effective, a participative leader must also provide overall direction to the group process.

Under most circumstances, some degree of participation is appropriate to promote job satisfaction and commitment. But in a crisis or emergency, when there is no time for group discussion and decision, directive leadership is most appropriate. A more directive style may also be appropriate when the leader is sharing new skills or knowledge with immature, insecure, or unskilled followers. The effective leader learns how to vary his or her style to match the circumstances.

MANAGEMENT

The management process is a systematic process similar to the problem-solving process and the nursing process (see Chap. 6). All are similar because they are based on the scientific or research process.

Functions of Managers

Management is getting a job done or accomplishing a goal by planning, organizing, directing, and controlling (Fig. 4-2). In any setting, these four management functions provide a way to organize people, things, and activities and to direct them toward overall objectives. These management functions provide the glue that holds the organization together. In health-care organizations, managers must organize the health-care professionals and support staff, the building space, supplies, and equipment, and the patient care and support activities.

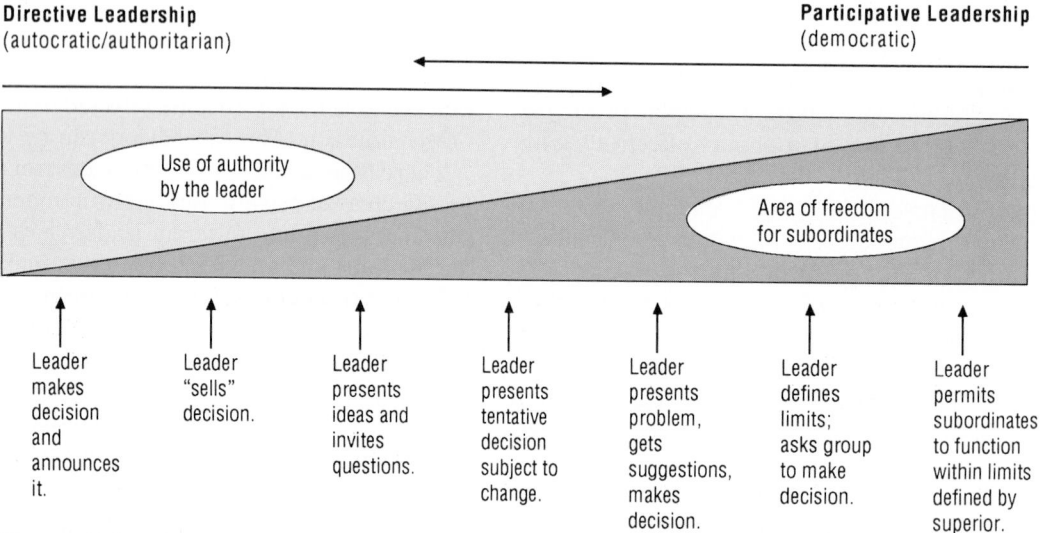

Figure 4–1.   Leadership style is often described along a continuum from directive to participative. Directive leadership is sometimes called autocratic, authoritative, or boss-centered. The opposite end of the continuum is participative leadership, also called democratic or subordinate-centered leadership. (Adapted by permission of *Harvard Business Review.* An exhibit from "How to choose a leadership pattern" by R. Tannenbaum & W. H. Schmidt (May/June 1973). Copyright © 1973 by the Presidents and Fellows of Harvard College; all rights reserved.)

The four management functions help to accomplish the overall objective of providing quality patient care.

All managers perform these functions, although the scope, specific details, and the amount of time devoted to each varies at different organizational levels (Callahan & Fleenor, 1988; Hersey & Duldt, 1989; Hitt, 1988; Sheridan, Bronstein, & Walker, 1984; Sullivan & Decker, 1988).

Planning

Planning is deciding what to do, when, where, how, by whom, and with what resources. Planning is an ongoing process that involves assessing, setting goals, establishing priorities, developing action plans, and evaluating whether the actions are meeting the objectives. Planning provides direction for the people involved, meaning for the work activities, and a scheme for efficient use of the people, space, and equipment.

In a nursing department, the top-level manager, the **nurse executive,** devotes a great deal of time to planning. The nurse executive plans the department's goals and services and determines the numbers and types of nurses and other personnel required to provide those services.

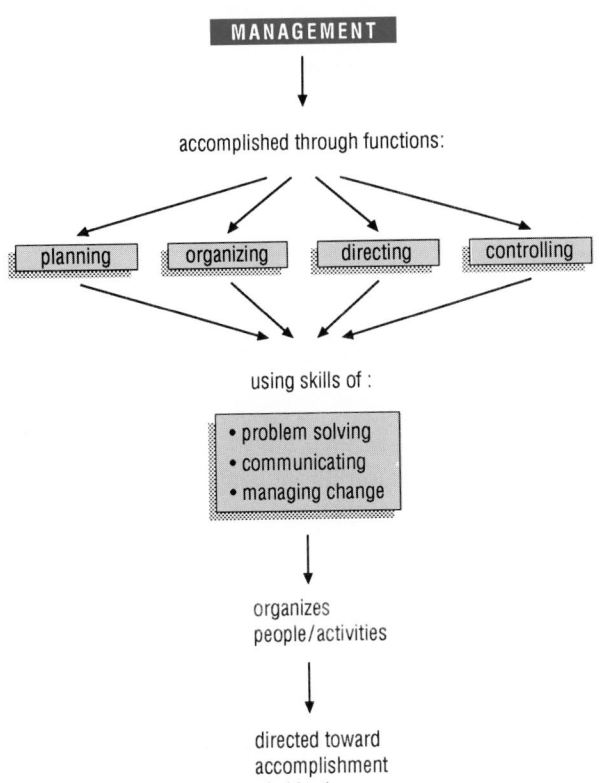

Figure 4–2. The management process includes the functions of planning, organizing, directing, and controlling. To perform each of these functions effectively, managers must be skilled in problem-solving, communicating, and managing change.

In contrast, the department's lowest-level manager, the staff nurse, devotes less time to planning. The staff nurse assesses each patient and determines needs, sets priorities, and develops a plan for his or her nursing care. The care plan answers the questions of what to do, when, where, and how.

Organizing

Organizing is arranging the work to be done in small units so that it can be accomplished. Organizing involves setting expectations, determining responsibilities, and establishing lines of communication and reporting relationships. The nurse executive ensures that the department has objectives that establish the priorities, job descriptions that assign responsibilities and reporting relationships, and standards and procedures that describe the expectations.

The nurse executive delegates to others the responsibility and accountability for much of the work. For example, the responsibility for direct nursing care is delegated to staff nurses. The nurse executive typically spends less time on organizing than on planning and controlling (Callahan & Fleenor, 1988).

The staff nurse organizes patient care by establishing the goals, interventions (things to be done), and expected outcomes of the care. The care plan and nursing shift report are used to communicate priorities to other nurses who are delegated responsibility for delivering some of the nursing care.

Directing

Directing involves supervision and ongoing decision-making to carry out the plans. Directing includes assigning responsibilities for the work to be done, providing instructions, communicating expectations, and guiding others as needed to reach the overall objectives. The nurse executive directs much of the change for the department of nursing by supervising the next-level managers; he or she devotes much less time to directing than to planning and controlling.

The **charge nurse** directs the work of the shift by assigning patients, scheduling meal and break times, and determining who will admit and care for patients admitted during the shift. The staff nurse directs the care for patients by ordering nursing care, communicating the care on the written care plan and in shift reports, and supervising the care delivered by others.

Controlling

Controlling is checking that plans are being carried out as planned and evaluating the outcomes of the actions. Controlling also includes evaluating staff. Some steps in the control process are measuring results against pre-established standards or expectations and taking action to positively reinforce effective actions and to change ineffective ones.

The nurse executive monitors the results of recruitment, staff turnover, and budget performance against expectations. He or she uses the performance appraisal process to acknowledge positive performance and to promote further growth in subordinates.

The staff nurse reassesses the patient to determine whether the prescribed nursing interventions are resulting in patient improvement, whether interventions need to be changed, and whether other interventions should be added.

Skills for Effective Management

Because managers deal with people, ideas, and things, the effective manager must be skilled in problem-solving, communicating, and managing change.

Problem-Solving

Problem-solving is a systematic process (see Chap. 6) that involves the following steps:

1. Identifying and analyzing the problem.
2. Determining possible solutions.
3. Considering the consequences of each possible solution, and choosing a solution.
4. Implementing the solution.
5. Evaluating the results.

Identifying and analyzing the problem involves collecting information about the issue to clarify the problem and its circumstances. Gathering information helps to clarify the problem and also offers clues to possible solutions and their consequences. After speculating on the possible consequences of each proposed solution, the manager chooses the solution that is expected to result in the most positive outcome. After the solution is implemented, another assessment is done to determine whether the desired results were obtained.

Managers use problem-solving in each step of the management process (planning, organizing, directing, and controlling). Staff nurses use problem-solving in each step of the nursing process to manage patient care.

Communication

Research shows that managers spend 75% to 90% of their time communicating in one form or another with others (Glueck, 1980). Staff nurses spend a large amount of their time communicating with patients, families, other nurses, physicians, and other health-care professionals and support staff.

Effective communication involves the transfer of the meaning of information between two or more people (see Chap. 17). To successfully implement the manage-

ment process, managers must have effective communication skills in writing, speaking, and listening. For effective communication, the sender must be able to send a clear message, and the receiver must be able to receive and objectively interpret that message. The interpretation of the message can be influenced by factors such as differences in the sender's and receiver's skills, background experiences, education, values, semantics, and emotional states. The status difference between the leader and followers may also affect communication effectiveness.

The nonverbal cues accompanying the message are essential aspects of verbal communication. If the sender's tone, speed, or inflection of voice, facial expression, or other nonverbal behaviors are consistent with the verbal message, communication will be enhanced. But if any of these are inconsistent with the verbal mes-

---

Skills for Effective Management

Problem-Solving

- Identify and analyze the problem
- Determine possible solutions
- Consider consequences and choose solution
- Implement the solution
- Evaluate results

Communicating

- Ability to send a clear message
- Ability to receive and objectively interpret the message
- Verbal: writing and speaking
- Listening:
  - Pay full attention to speaker
  - Listen to both facts and feelings
  - Avoid prematurely judging meaning
  - Avoid premature formulation of response
  - Use questions to clarify
- Nonverbal: body language

Managing Change

- Assess current needs
- Anticipate future needs
- Determine if change is needed
- Implement change cooperatively with others
- Address resistance to change

(Adapted by permission of *Harvard Business Review*. An exhibit from "How to choose a leadership pattern" by R. Tannenbaum & W. H. Schmidt (May/June 1973). Copyright © 1973 by the Presidents and Fellows of Harvard College; all rights reserved.)

sage, the receiver will believe the nonverbal message instead of the verbal one.

Listening is an important part of effective verbal communication. Listening can be hampered by the listener's lack of interest in the topic, premature interpretation of the message, or preoccupation with preparing a response. Good listening is a choice of actions that can be improved with practice. To be more effective, the listener should:

Give full attention to what the speaker is saying.
Listen to both the facts and feelings.
Avoid formulating a response or judging the meaning until the speaker has finished.
Use questions to clarify meanings.

Communication skills are necessary for successful implementation of the management process. Managers depend on communication to keep informed, to assist with planning and decision-making, and to convey decisions to others. Staff nurses rely on communication to care for patients and families, to relate to coworkers, and to function as an effective interdisciplinary team member.

Managing Change

This age of technology is bringing rapid change. To be effective, managers must be masters of the change process. They need to be able to assess the current situation and anticipate future needs, to determine when change is needed, and to implement the needed change. Managers also must be able to manage change that is imposed by others.

Managers need to know how to overcome resistance to change in themselves, their followers, and in the overall organization (Fig. 4-3). Lack of knowledge, inaccurate information, fear of the unknown, threats to status or position, and threats to economic benefits can cause resistance to change. Education and enhanced communication are the best ways to reduce resistance caused by a lack of information or inaccurate information. Participation and involvement are effective approaches when the initiators of the change do not have all the information they need to design the change and when others have the power to resist the change. When people are resisting the change because of emotional adjustment problems, the best interventions are facilitation and support. Negotiation and agreement may be appropriate approaches when the change adversely affects the person's position or economic status.

People can control their perceptions and reactions to change by being aware of emotional reactions associated with change and by actively seeking information, increasing communication, and getting involved in the change process. Those who perceive change as an opportunity for learning and personal growth see change as positive and offer less resistance to the change.

To effectively implement change, managers must as-sess the implications of any change for themselves and their followers, and must intervene by providing needed communication, information, support, and involvement. For instance, illness represents a change for patients and their family members. The nurse increases communication, teaches, involves the patient and family in care, and offers support to ease patient and family adjustment to illness.

APPLYING LEADERSHIP AND MANAGEMENT TO NURSING ROLES

There is a subtle difference between leadership and management. Leadership focuses on people and inspiring them to perform or change. Management focuses on getting the job done by planning, organizing, directing, and controlling people and activities. The use of leadership and management in nursing care is discussed in the following section.

Clinical Practice Roles

Nursing delivers its service to society through clinical practice roles. The teaching and administrative roles within the profession exist to support and represent the clinical practice roles.

Staff Nurse

The core role of nursing is the staff nurse role. Most nurses are staff nurses, and they deliver most of the nursing care directly to patients. The staff nurse fulfills many functions in the delivery of patient care: provider of care, decision-maker, patient advocate, team member, communicator, and educator. Whether working in a hospital, clinic or office setting, or in the community, the staff nurse initiates the nursing process. He or she assesses the patient and family, determines nursing diagnoses, establishes a plan of care (nursing orders), and evaluates the outcome of the care. In addition, the staff nurse consults with other health-care professionals, reports the most current patient status, and coordinates the care by those professionals with the nursing care. Thus, the staff nurse uses management skills to integrate the nursing care plan with the therapy plans of the other health-care professionals, and to coordinate the care for the patient.

In hospitals today, the most popular models of care delivery are team nursing, primary nursing, and managed care.

Team Nursing. In **team nursing,** a team cares for a group of patients, with team members assigned specific care functions or procedures to perform for all the patients. Members of the team usually include nurses, licensed practical nurses, and nursing assistants. The

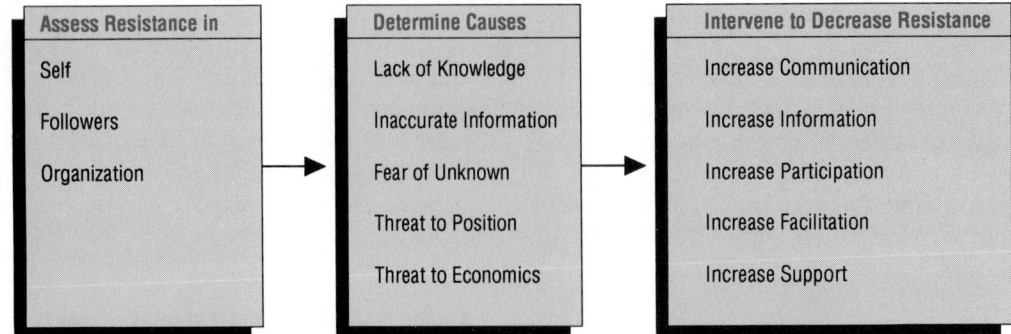

Assess Resistance in	Determine Causes	Intervene to Decrease Resistance
Self	Lack of Knowledge	Increase Communication
Followers	Inaccurate Information	Increase Information
Organization	Fear of Unknown	Increase Participation
	Threat to Position	Increase Facilitation
	Threat to Economics	Increase Support

Figure 4–3.   To be effective, managers must be masters of the change process. They need to know how to intervene to overcome resistance to change in themselves, their followers, and the overall organization.

team leader is the nurse who manages the team by using the management process (planning, organizing, directing, and controlling).

Some of the advantages of team nursing include the natural group discussion and decision-making about the plan of care for each patient. Team nursing also provides an easy mechanism for more experienced nurses to supervise and teach less experienced nurses.

One disadvantage is that more staff members deliver care to each patient. This fragmentation may result in decreased accountability for the overall plan and delivery of care, and can result in decreased quality of patient outcomes. The patient and family are also less likely to develop rapport with the nursing staff and are less likely to receive consistent care.

Primary Nursing. In **primary nursing,** a professional nurse assumes responsibility for developing a 24-hour nursing care plan and for integrating that plan with the therapy plan of the other health-care professionals. The primary nurse accepts total responsibility for the quality of the nursing care for a patient. He or she uses good management skills in planning and coordinating patient care. The primary nurse also uses leadership abilities in ensuring that the prescribed plan is implemented and that the nursing care is integrated with the care delivered by others.

Difference Between Leadership and Management

- **Leadership** is focused on personnel and inspiring them to perform or change.
- **Management** is focused on getting the job done by planning, organizing, directing, and controlling people and activities.

Primary nursing results in increased continuity of care, improved interdisciplinary communication, and enhanced coordination of the total therapy plan. Primary nursing provides improved quality and consistency of nursing care for patients. The primary nursing model can also result in increased job satisfaction for nurses because it provides increased autonomy in practice, a close working relationship with patients and families, enhanced collaboration with other health-care professionals, and increased focus of the nurse's role on planning and delivering patient care.

Primary nursing requires the hospital to have enough registered nurses so that all patients have a nurse responsible for their plan of care, while allowing a reasonable caseload for each registered nurse. A staff of all registered nurses may be impossible because of availability and costs. The professional nurse must have enough direct contact with the patient to make critical judgments about the patient's diagnoses, required care, and response to therapy and the ongoing disease process.

Other potential disadvantages of the primary nursing model are lack of a built-in system for experienced nurses to supervise and teach less experienced nurses, and the lack of a natural nurse-to-nurse consultation. The busy routine in the work setting detracts from nurse-to-nurse consultation and joint decision-making.

Managed Care. In some institutions, primary nursing has evolved into a **managed care** delivery model. In the managed care model, the primary nurse uses a predetermined critical pathway to establish and monitor the extent and timing of care within an anticipated length of hospital stay. For commonly treated cases, nurses and physicians jointly develop a standard plan of care that includes a time frame. Some of the key elements that are slotted at specific times in the plan include diagnostic tests, consultations, treatments, activities, procedures, and discharge planning and teaching.

Within the first day after admission, the primary nurse reviews the standard critical pathway with the patient's

Applying Roles of Leadership and Management to Nursing in Clinical Practice

Staff Nurses

- Function as providers of care, decision-makers, patient advocates, team members, communicators, educators
- Initiate the nursing process
- Consult with other health professionals
- Report current patient status
- Integrate the nursing care plan with therapy plans of other professionals
- Coordinate patient care.

Team Nursing

A team cares for a group of patients; different team members are assigned specific care functions for all patients. Team leader is a nurse and manages the team.
- Organizes group discussion and decision-making on the plan of care for each patient
- Provides a mechanism for more experienced nurses to supervise and teach less experienced nurses.

Primary Nursing

- Assumes responsibility for developing a 24-hour nursing care plan
- Integrates that plan with the therapy plan of the other health-care professionals
- Accepts total responsibility for quality of care
- Has autonomy and professional accountability.

Managed Care

- Works jointly with a physician to develop and individualize a standard plan of care, which includes a time frame

- Evaluates daily the patient's progress with the physician and plans corrections and changes.

Advanced Clinical Practice Roles

Clinical Nurse Specialists
(Registered nurses with a master's degree and advanced preparation in a specialty area)

- Give direct patient care
- Consult with staff nurses
- Provide advanced education for nurses in specialty areas
- Evaluate nursing care outcomes
- Develop new nursing practice to support new therapy or new technology.

Nurse Practitioners
(Registered nurses with advanced degrees in a specialty area and either certification or advanced licensing)

- Practice independently in a specialty area (usually practice in community clinics or offices as independent practitioners or as members of a group practice)
- Use good management techniques in planning and implementing patient care, consultation efforts, and educational programs
- Deliver advanced care
- Consult on complex care issues
- Develop new nursing practice
- Participate in nursing research and publication.

physician. They jointly individualize the plan to reflect unique patient circumstances that are expected to alter the timing or the type of care required. They evaluate the patient's progress daily against the critical pathway and deal with variances. If the variance is due to a hospital system or the actions or inaction of caregivers, corrections are made. If the variance is due to an unanticipated reaction of the patient, changes in care are considered and added to the plan as needed. The primary nurse manages and closely controls patient care, using the critical pathways to evaluate patient progress and to determine the need for corrective action (Zander, 1989).

Circumstances such as the availability of nurses, changing patient populations, changes in technology, hospital system variations, and altered financial conditions lead to the development of new models of care delivery or variations in current models. Nurses use their knowledge of systems, the current circumstances, and the priorities of care to adjust the current model of care delivery or to create a new one.

Advanced Clinical Practice Roles

Advanced nurses provide direct patient care and consultation to staff nurses. Some provide direct nursing care through group or independent practice.

Clinical Nurse Specialists. Clinical nurse specialists are registered nurses who have a master's degree and advanced preparation in a specialty area of nursing (e.g., cardiovascular, neuroscience, critical care, psychosocial, or rehabilitation). Clinical nurse specialists usually practice in hospitals, hospital clinics, community home health agencies, or private practice. They provide direct patient care, consultation to staff nurses, advanced education for nurses in specialty areas, evaluation of nursing care outcomes, and development of new nursing practices to support new therapy or new technology.

Nurse Practitioners. Nurse practitioners are registered nurses with advanced degrees and preparation in health assessment in a specialty area such as pediatrics, geriatrics, women's health, or adult health. These nurses also hold either certification or advanced licensing to allow them to practice independently in a specialty area. They usually work in community clinics or offices as independent practitioners or as a member of a group practice.

Other advanced specialty roles within the nursing profession include nurse midwives and nurse anesthetists. A **nurse midwife** is a registered nurse with advanced education and certification in the care of women during uncomplicated pregnancy and delivery. The **nurse anesthetist** is a registered nurse with additional education in anesthesiology. The nurse anesthetist administers anesthesia to surgical patients under the supervision of an anesthesiologist.

To be effective, these advanced practitioners must use good management techniques in planning and implementing patient care, consultation efforts, and educational programs. Others in the nursing profession also expect these advanced practitioners to be leaders in the profession through delivery of advanced care, consultation on complex care issues, development of new nursing practices, and participation in nursing research and publication. Often through their pioneering efforts, nursing is clarified, refined, and in some instances redefined.

Nursing Management Roles

Beginning Managers. Through experience, staff nurses gain increasing abilities to manage care for a group of patients, to assist team members, and to serve as a resource for new nurses. These enhanced abilities are an indication to supervisors that staff nurses are ready to assume beginning management functions. Two such beginning management roles are team leader and charge nurse.

In hospitals or community nursing, where team leading is the model of nursing care delivery, the team leader manages a team of nurses, licensed practical nurses, and nursing assistants to provide nursing care for a group of patients. The team leader is responsible for the performance of team members and the quality of nursing care delivered.

The charge nurse is responsible for the functioning of a nursing unit for a particular work shift. The charge nurse makes management decisions and supervises the unit's staff as needed to provide quality patient care on that shift. The charge nurse serves as a resource person for other staff members and may be pulled into issues that require interdepartmental or interdisciplinary problem-solving. During the shift, the charge nurse determines staff work assignments and evaluates whether the numbers and skills of the staff on the next shift are adequate to safely meet the current patient needs.

Although the staff supervision and decision-making functions of the team leader and the charge nurse are similar, the scope of responsibility is different. The charge nurse has responsibility for the entire unit, which may have more than one team. The charge nurse supervises the team leaders (or if primary, managed, or other model of care delivery is used, supervises the total unit staff) and facilitates communication and work between the teams (or staff).

Unit Managers. Permanent management roles at the hospital unit level are *head nurse* and *assistant head nurse*. The head nurse role is a pivotal one within the hospital. In many hospitals, the head nurse is recognized as a department head and is held accountable for 24-hour operations of the nursing unit. Operations include such functions as staff scheduling and supervision, budget management, staff education, and quality patient care. The head nurse provides a vital communication link between patients, direct caregivers, and the administration. The head nurse alerts the administration to changing patient needs and care preferences and changing staff characteristics. The head nurse also represents the administration to the staff and patients by communicating changes in the organization that may affect them.

The assistant head nurse helps the head nurse with overall management of the nursing unit by performing functions delegated by the head nurse (e.g., hiring, evaluating, and counseling staff; preparing work schedules; preparing and monitoring the unit budget). In addition to performing delegated management functions, the assistant head nurse often serves as a unit-based clinical resource and educator.

In community home health agencies, staff nurses are similarly organized into teams by geographic or specialty areas. A supervisor, coordinator, or director manages each team and is the pivotal person and communication link between the patients, staff, and agency administration.

Middle Managers. Depending on the size and complexity of the hospital or agency, there may be several levels of middle management (Fig. 4-4). Between the head nurse or coordinator and the nurse executive may be managers with titles of supervisor, assistant director, associate director, or assistant administrator. These middle managers are usually responsible for the activities of several departments and programs. They spend more of their time in strategic planning and interdepartmental or interdisciplinary problem-solving than the head nurse, but spend less of their time dealing with day-to-day patient care management than the head nurse does.

Nurse Executives. The nurse executive has a variety of titles and duties, depending on the type and complexity of the institution (Fig. 4-5). Some of the titles currently in use are vice president, associate administrator, assistant administrator, or director of nursing. The nurse executive is an administrator and a leader of professionals. Because he or she is involved in strategic planning and decision-making for the institution, the nurse

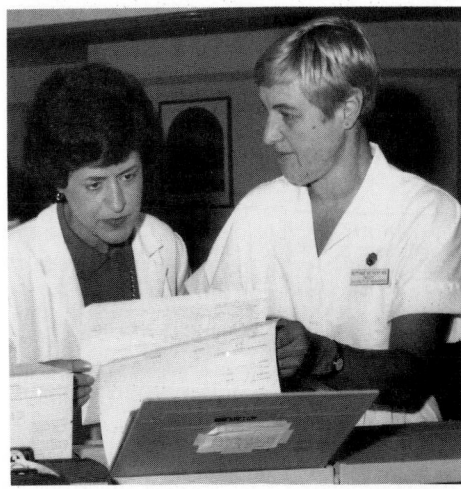

Figure 4–5.   The Dean of the School of Nursing and a faculty member confer on courses and credits. The dean, as an executive manager, needs strong management techniques and effective leadership skills. (Courtesy of University of Washington School of Nursing)

executive must effectively negotiate with non-clinical administrators and the medical director (the other top-level clinical administrator). The nurse executive must also be able to lead, influence, and represent nursing professionals.

To be effective in all of these management roles, people must be skilled in the techniques of planning, organizing, directing, and controlling. The proportion of time spent doing each of these activities varies with each role. The beginning managers, the head nurse, and assistant head nurses primarily focus on current operations and patient care management. The nurse executive primarily focuses on strategic planning and on issues within the agency that affect nursing practice or issues with the community or other agencies.

A manager's success depends on strong management techniques and effective leadership practices. The higher the level of the manager, the more essential it is for him or her to be an effective leader. Nurse executives are expected to be leaders within their agency, as well as leaders in the nursing profession itself. Effective nurse executives establish circumstances that allow nurses to function as professionals in providing quality patient care.

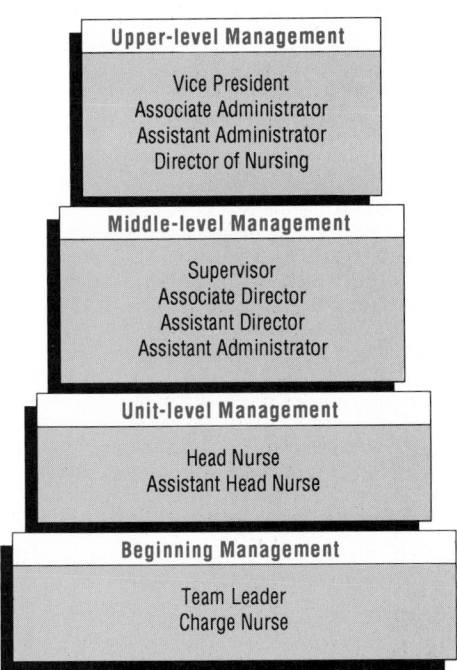

Figure 4–4.   Depending on the size and complexity of the hospital or agency, there may be several levels and roles in management. These management roles exist to support and represent the clinical practice roles in nursing.

Teaching Roles

Formal or informal teaching is an inherent part of all roles in nursing. The staff nurse teaches the patient and family about health, disease, and self-care. The experienced nurse teaches the less experienced nurse. The head nurse coaches staff nurses, team leaders, and

Nursing Research

Selected Nursing Research Studies

Rogers, M. A. (1989). Dimensions of leadership of assistant/associate deans in collegiate schools of nursing. *Journal of Nursing Education, 28,* 415–421.

Bradham, C. U., Dalme, F. C., & Thompson, P. J. (1990). Personality traits valued by practicing nurses and measured in nursing students. *Journal of Nursing Education, 29,* 225–232.

Pooyan, A., Eberhardt, B. J., & Szigeti, E. (1990). Work-related variables and turnover among registered nurses. *Nursing and Health Care, 11,* 255–258.

Mitchell, P., Armstrong, T. F., & Lentz, M. (1989). American Association of Critical-Care Nurses demonstration project: Profile of excellence in critical care nursing. *Heart & Lung, 18,* 219–237.

Potect, G. W. (1989). Nursing administrators and delegation. *Nursing Administration Quarterly, 13,* 23–32.

Possible Topics for Nursing Inquiry

- What are the leadership behaviors of staff nurses who are identified as experts by their peers?
- What are the relative priorities of various management skills of staff nurses at different career stages?
- What is the impact of varying leadership styles of head nurses on staff nurse job satisfaction and retention?
- What is the impact of varying leadership styles and management skills of nurse executives on nurse recruitment and retention?

charge nurses. The nurse executive coaches middle managers. In addition, most agencies have an educator who is responsible for orientation and continuing education programs. Effective teachers influence others through leadership skills and role-modeling.

Key Concepts

- Nurses are professionals responsible for providing a service to society through effective leadership behaviors and management skills.

- Leadership is the ability to influence others to strive for a goal or to change. Management is getting the job done or the goal accomplished through planning, organizing, directing, and controlling.
- The management process is similar to both the problem-solving process and the nursing process because all are based on the scientific or research process.
- As managers, nurses need to be skilled in problem-solving, communicating, and managing change.
- The five steps of the problem-solving process are identifying and analyzing the problem; determining possible solutions; considering the consequences of each possible solution and choosing a solution; implementing the solution; and evaluating the results.
- Effective communication involves the transfer of the meaning of information between people, using good verbal communication and effective listening.
- Change is inevitable, and people can influence their own perceptions and reactions to change by being aware of the emotions associated with change and by actively seeking information, increasing communication, and getting involved in the change process.
- New nursing graduates have many options available in work settings and roles within nursing.
- Effective leadership behaviors and management skills contribute to the success of nurses in the many clinical, management, and teaching roles.

References

American Nurses Association. (1980). *Nursing: A social policy statement.* Kansas City, MO.
Callahan, R. E., & Fleenor, C. P. (1988). *Managing human relations.* Columbus: Merrill Publishing, p. 95.
Glueck, W. G. (1980). *Management.* Hinsdale, IL: Dryden Press, pp. 564–565.
Hersey, P., & Duldt, B. W. (1989). *Situational leadership in nursing.* Norwalk, CT: Appleton & Lange, p. 137.
Hitt, W. D. (1988). *The leader-manager.* Columbus, OH: Battelle Press, pp. 4, 105.
Sheridan, D. R., Bronstein, J. E., & Walker, D. D. (1984). *The new nurse manager.* Rockville, MD: Aspen, p. 128.
Sullivan, E. J., & Decker, P. J. (1988). *Effective management in nursing* (2nd ed.). Menlo Park: Addison-Wesley, p. 43.
Tannenbaum, R., & Schmidt, W. H. (1973). How to choose a leadership pattern. *Harvard Business Review, 51,* 164–173.
Vroom, V. H., & Jago, A. G. (1988). *The new leadership.* Englewood Cliffs, NJ: Prentice-Hall, pp. 49, 50.
Yukl, G. A. (1989). *Leadership in organizations* (2nd ed.). Englewood Cliffs, NJ: Prentice-Hall, pp. 9, 174, 273, 274.
Zander, K. (1989). Second-generation critical paths. *Definition, 4,* 1.

Bibliography

Baillie, V. K., Trygstad, L., & Cordoni, T. I. (1989). *Effective nursing leadership.* Rockville, MD: Aspen.
Bernhard, L. A., & Walsh, M. (1990). *Leadership: The key to the professionalization of nursing* (2nd ed.). St. Louis: C. V. Mosby.
Blanchett, S. S. (Ed.). (1988). *Classics from JONA.* Philadelphia: J. B. Lippincott.
Clark, C. C. (1987). *The nurse as group leader.* New York: Springer.

Douglass, L. M. (1988). *The effective nurse leader and manager* (3rd ed.). St. Louis: C. V. Mosby.

Dunham, J., & Klafehn, K. A. (1990). Transformational leadership and the nurse executive. *Journal of Nursing Administration, 20*(4), 28–34.

Fiedler, F. E., & Garcia, J. E. (1987). *New approaches to effective leadership.* New York: John Wiley & Sons.

Hein, E. C., & Nicholson, M. J. (Eds.). (1986). *Contemporary leadership behavior: Selected readings.* Boston: Little, Brown & Co.

Hersey, P., & Blanchard, K. H. (1988). *Management of organizational behavior* (5th ed.). Englewood Cliffs, NJ: Prentice-Hall.

Holle, M. L., & Blatchley, M. E. (1987). *Introduction to leadership and management in nursing* (2nd ed.). Boston: Jones & Bartlett.

Innes, B. S. (1989). *Common characteristics of nurse change agents.* Unpublished doctoral dissertation, Seattle University.

Keane, C. B. (1987). *Management essentials in nursing.* Philadelphia: J. B. Lippincott.

Kouzes, J. M., & Posner, B. Z. (1987). *The leadership challenge.* San Francisco: Jossey-Bass.

Kron, T., & Gray, A. (1987). *The management of patient care* (6th ed.). Philadelphia: W. B. Saunders.

Loveridge, C. E., Cummings, S. H., & O'Malley, J. (1988). Developing case management in a primary nursing system. *Journal of Nursing Administration, 18*(10), 36–39.

Marriner-Torrey, A. (1988). *Guide to nursing management* (3rd ed.). St. Louis: C. V. Mosby.

Marriner-Torrey, A. (1990). *Case studies in nursing management: Practice, theory, and research.* St. Louis: C. V. Mosby.

Moore, K., Biordi, D., Holm, K., & McElmurry, B. (1988). Nurse executive effectiveness. *Journal of Nursing Administration, 18*(12), 23–27.

Morford, J. A. (1987). Effective leadership: Research and theory. *Journal of Correctional Education, 38*(2), 42–46.

O'Leary, J. G., Wendelgass, S. T., & Zimmerman, H. E. (1986). *Winning strategies for nursing managers.* Philadelphia: J. B. Lippincott.

Peterson, M. E., & Allen, D. G. (1986). Shared governance: A strategy for transforming organizations, part 2. *Journal of Nursing Administration, 16*(2), 11–16.

Pinkerton, S. E., & Schroeder, P. (1988). *Commitment to nursing excellence: Developing a professional nursing staff.* Rockville, MD: Aspen.

Porter-O'Grady, T. (1986). *Creative nursing administration.* Rockville, MD: Aspen.

Sullivan, E. J., & Decker, P. J. (1988). *Effective management in nursing* (2nd ed.). Menlo Park: Addison-Wesley.

Vestel, K. W. (1987). *Management concepts for the new nurse.* Philadelphia: J. B. Lippincott.

Young, L. C., & Hayne, A. N. (1987). *Nursing administration from concept to practice.* Philadelphia: W. B. Saunders.

Zander, K. (1985). Second-generation primary nursing. *Journal of Nursing Administration, 15*(3), 18–24.

Zander, K. (1990). Mindset transitions for 1990. *Definition, 5*(1), 1–2.

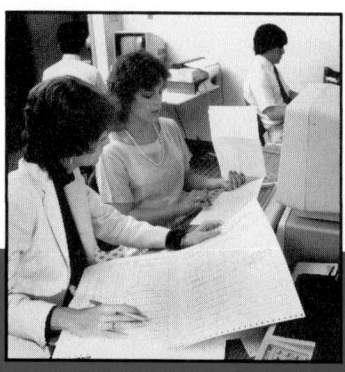

Nursing Research

LEARNING OBJECTIVES

Upon completion of this chapter, the student will be able to do the following:

- Explain the contributions that research has made to nursing.
- Discuss the role of research in nursing.
- Review the research process for the beginning professional student in nursing.

KEY TERMS

Anonymity
Conceptual
  framework
Confidentiality
Dependent variable

Hypothesis
Independent
  variable
Literature review
Method

Nursing research
Problem statement
Research design
Theory

5

Research and Nursing
  Evolution of Nursing Research
  Characteristics of Nursing Research
  Scientific Process and Nursing Research
The Research Process
  Research Design
  Where Does One Start?
    Literature Review
    Theoretical Framework
    Problem Statement
    Research in Practice

    Dissemination
Legal and Ethical Issues
  Institutional Review Boards
  Subject Rights
Research and the Professional Nurse
  Roles of Nursing Personnel at Different Levels
  Clinical Nursing Practice
    Clinical Research
    Applying Research to Practice
Key Concepts

One of the many responsibilities that nurses have is providing safe patient care. Nursing students learn that to provide this safe care, nursing practice requires a sound scientific base. The clinical practice of nursing is enhanced when the nurse decides to use a method of treatment that has a research base over another, untested treatment. Research-based nursing practice should lead to improved care.

Biomedical and sociologic research have resulted in monumental advances in modern health care. Research into the human immune system has led to the ability to transplant body organs and has provided essential information about the care and treatment of individuals with AIDS. Nursing research also has had a major impact on the provision of safe, quality care.

Nursing is a science that draws heavily on other sciences to substantiate and prescribe nursing therapies. Because nursing draws so heavily on other professionals' work, particularly in the biopsychosocial fields, a nurse must be able to discriminate "good" research from "poor" research. Therefore, the nurse must have a working knowledge of research and a beginning ability to critique research.

Displays on nursing research are provided throughout this textbook. The displays are divided into two sections: Selected Nursing Research Studies and Possible Topics for Nursing Inquiry. The first section lists recent research articles; the second section may lead to class discussion or future study.

RESEARCH AND NURSING

For the purposes of this chapter, *research* is defined as a formalized process of systematic investigation designed to test a research question or **hypothesis** and draw conclusions from the data collected. Many similarities exist between the formalized research process and the nursing process format that is an integral part of nursing education. When using the formalized research process, the nurse contributes to the body of professional nursing knowledge.

Nursing research is defined as a "systematic inquiry into the problems encountered in nursing practice and into the modalities of patient care, such as support and comfort, prevention of trauma, promotion of recovery, health education, health appraisal and coordination of health care" (Gortner, 1975).

Nursing research is similar to that of any other discipline in which practitioners are interested in seeking the truth. Nurses interested in discovering the truth about nursing practice attempt to describe events and phenomena, define and describe the relationships among the phenomena, and eventually control and predict the phenomena studied.

Nurse researchers hope to affect the clinical practice of nurses in their speciality, particularly in relation to the goals of nursing (Fig. 5-1). Nursing research "develops knowledge about health and the promotion of health over the full life span, care of persons with health prob-

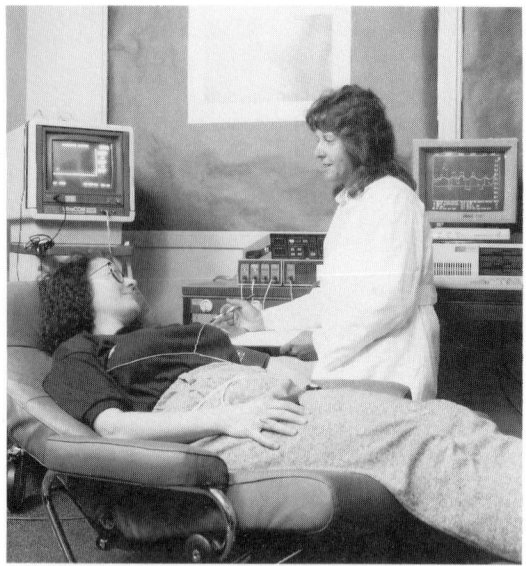

Figure 5–1. Clinical research defines nursing practice and raises the standards of nursing care.

lems and disabilities, and nursing actions to enhance the ability of individuals to respond to actual or potential health problems" (American Nurses Association, 1981).

Although many problems nurses encounter in their clinical practice affect people of all ages, such as nursing actions to facilitate optimum wound healing, some problems are age- or person-specific. One nurse may be interested in the health benefits of aerobic exercise in a healthy geriatric population; another nurse may be interested in the effect of positioning on the oxygen saturation of postoperative coronary artery bypass surgery patients. Each researcher contributes to the body of nursing knowledge in a specific way, and all nurses should contribute in some fashion to the expansion of nursing knowledge.

A major reason for conducting research is to expand a profession's knowledge base. The focus of nursing research must be on generating fundamental knowledge to guide nursing practice (Barnard, 1980). Making progress in nursing service, nursing practice, or the administration of nursing requires systematic analyses of research (Fig. 5-2).

Evolution of Nursing Research

Appreciation of the place of research in nursing has grown significantly over the last 30 years, but nursing research has been an integral part of the profession since Florence Nightingale documented the care of soldiers in the Crimean War (Sarkis & Conners, 1986). Her carefully kept statistical records are a model for nurses and social scientists alike (Cohen, 1984).

According to Polit and Hungler (1987), several events led to the recent developments in nursing research. From 1900 to 1940, research centered around nursing education, methods of teaching, and methods of evaluating how nurses learned. During World War II, interest turned to the supply and demand of nurses because of the increased need for nurses.

During the 1950s, more master's programs in nursing were developed, and most of these courses included courses on research methods. Federal funding enabled more nurses to continue their studies at the master's level, and publications of nursing research became more commonplace. The journal *Nursing Research* began publishing the results of studies by individuals and schools of nursing. At about the same time, a 5-year research project sponsored by the American Nurses Association (ANA) focused on nurses' activities and functions.

Federal funding for graduate study and research continued in the 1960s. The profession of nursing was strengthened with the development of conceptual frameworks, an early stage of theory development wherein interrelated concepts help shape the proposed research, and the use of scientific method in nursing practice. Nursing organizations established priorities for research investigations. Such research led to improvements in the quality of nursing care.

Rapid growth in nursing research continued in the 1970s and 1980s. Three more journals of nursing research were born in the 1970s: *Advances in Nursing Science*, *Research in Nursing and Health*, and *Western Journal of Nursing Research*.

The ANA Commission on Nursing Research in 1980 recommended further research in areas of health pro-

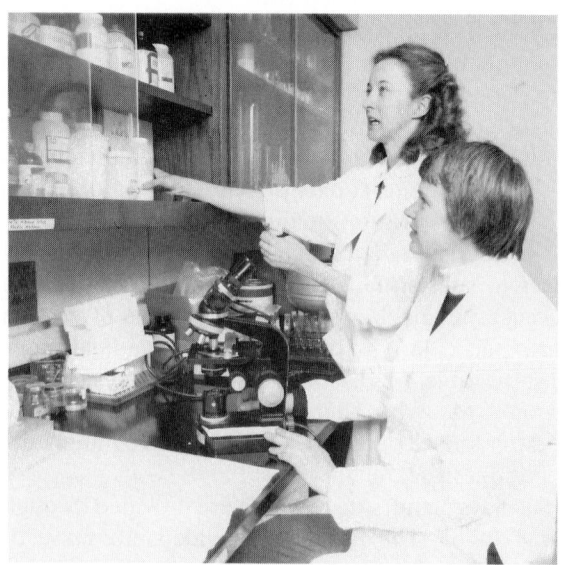

Figure 5–2. Some nurses are involved in laboratory research.

motion, illness prevention, cost-effective health care, and nursing care for high-risk patients. Researchers examined the **conceptual frameworks** that arose in the 1960s and 1970s.

The Institute of Medicine, in a 1983 study, urged the federal government to increase the level of funding for nursing. As a result, the National Center for Nursing Research was established under the National Institutes of Health. The purpose of the center was to place nursing securely in the sphere of scientific investigation and to support research and training into patient care, health promotion, disease prevention, and the mitigation of effects of acute and chronic disabilities (Merritt, 1986).

Characteristics of Nursing Research

Nursing has traditionally been concerned with the whole person, not the individual parts. Likewise, nursing research also encompasses the whole person. Nursing research differs from biomedical research in that it has a *holistic* perspective. When nurses do research, they focus on the physiologic, psychological, sociologic, cultural, and economic factors that affect that person.

Diers (1979) listed three properties of nursing research that maintain the holistic perspective:

The focus of nursing research must be on a difference that matters for improving patient care.

Nursing research has the potential for contributing to theory development and the body of scientific nursing knowledge.

A research problem is a nursing research problem when nurses have access to and control over phenomena being studied.

Scientific Process and Nursing Research

Research is a broad term that generally means the search for a valid answer to a question. How the question is raised and by whom often is the key to solving the problem. Techniques that use a method of research are the scientific method, the problem-solving method, and the nursing process (see Chap. 6).

Ways of seeking and finding answers and acquiring knowledge in any field include classes, clinical experience, discussions with classmates, scientific problem-solving, continuing education, and research studies relevant to the area of interest. These methods of seeking knowledge have the following in common:

1. Identifying what one needs to know.
2. Deciding how to approach the goal of answering the problem.
3. Devising a plan to do so.

4. Implementing the plan.
5. Assessing the results.

The similarities between the research process and the nursing process are discussed in Unit II. Similarities between clinical practice and nursing research are listed in Table 5-1.

The first step for the practicing nurse is to assess a problem, and for the researcher the first step is to recognize the general problem area. The next step for the practicing nurse is to make a nursing diagnosis, whereas defining the specific problem is the second step in the research process. The clinical nurse then proceeds with planning and intervention, whereas the nurse researcher proposes hypotheses and manages data. In the final step, the clinician evaluates outcomes, whereas the researcher analyzes results and disseminates his or her findings.

Beginning nurses can use the nursing process framework to begin to formulate and answer questions. The outcome will be improved patient care and services and the advancement of nursing as a profession.

THE RESEARCH PROCESS

An understanding of the step-by-step process used by nurse researchers is essential for the beginning practitioner and user of nursing research. Knowing the process helps the nurse judge the appropriateness of the research presented and allows him or her to apply the findings to the clinical situation.

Research Design

Research design is the overall plan for the collection and analysis of the data. The design of a study is crucial. If the design can limit the number of research problems before the study, the outcome may be more useful. If an instrument is to be used in a study or a new instrument needs to be developed, a consultant in methods (methodologist) can alleviate some problems with reliability and validity by helping the novice researcher select or develop an instrument.

TABLE 5–1

Similarities Between the Practicing Nurse and the Nurse Researcher

Practicing Nurse	Nurse Researcher
Assessment	Problem area identification
Nursing diagnosis	Definition of specific problem
Planning	Proposed hypotheses
Intervention	Data management
Evaluation	Analysis of results and dissemination of findings

Since most nursing research is done outside a laboratory setting, the policies, parameters, and constraints of the institution must be taken into account. The researcher must consider the costs of the facilities, equipment, and personnel time (Fig. 5-3). Sometimes a study cannot be conducted because the costs outweigh the benefits.

Where Does One Start?

Practical experience, scientific literature, and untested theories influence the development of a research idea. For the practicing nurse, clinical practice can provide daily opportunities to piece together observations that may lead to a researchable problem. For example, nurses working in the recovery room observe that temperatures taken with an aural (in-the-ear) device appear to be quicker but just as accurate as more traditional methods. The nurses note the differences in methods, speculate about other factors that might contribute to these differences, and agree to study the problem.

The scientific literature may be a valuable source for research ideas. For example, articles on how a family adapts to a child's head injury (Baker, 1990) or how prepared childbirth classes affect obstetric outcome (Hetherington, 1990) may be valuable for your clinical practice area.

Untested theories serve as good starts for nursing research. For example, Haase (1987) studied critically ill adolescents using a "courage" theory. The study gave insight into this special population and also served to further develop a knowledge base surrounding adolescent care.

Literature Review

Literature review is the process of selecting published materials (both research-based and anecdotal) that contribute to and substantiate a summary of the concepts to be studied.

Critical appraisal of the scientific literature may lead a nurse to speculate about a problem area, particularly if the literature is in conflict or inconsistent with his or her practice. For example, a nurse working in coronary care may read two articles on pain management in percutaneous transluminal coronary angioplasty patients that suggest two different protocols. The nurse may wonder which protocol is the most valid. Because of the conflict in the literature, an evaluation of the area may give the answer.

The literature review must be systematic and exhaustive. The researcher must take a critical, almost suspicious, approach to the material. Because the critical appraisal of the literature is the basis for the current study, such review is essential. All research builds on previous work; hence, an extensive literature review, properly executed, allows the researcher to place current ideas in the context of previous work.

A complete review also helps develop the conceptual frame of reference for the study. It gives clues on how to study the problem (the **methods**) and suggests instruments that might help.

The search for nursing literature can seem overwhelming to a beginner. An indispensable skill is the ability to identify and locate pertinent documentation on a particular topic. To do so, the student must know which library sources to use. Books and indexes of journals, reports, and abstracts are a few places to start.

Books provide an overview of a topic or deal with a specific, detailed topic. Bibliographies in books are valuable resources because they provide information about past references.

Indexes are the gateway to the enormous volume of literature in the health sciences. Indexes such as the *International Nursing Index, Index Medicus, Nursing Studies Index, Grateful Med*, and *Nursing Research Index* are invaluable to the nursing researcher. They are available in print and on computer databases; consult a librarian for details.

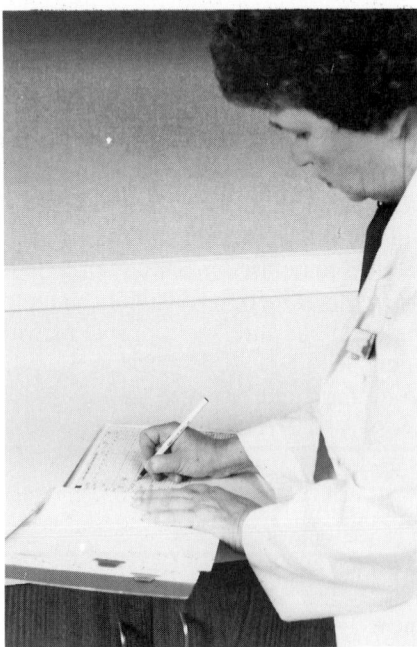

Figure 5–3. Nursing research requires careful note-taking and accurate records. The process can be time-consuming for personnel, and the value of research must be weighed against the cost.

Theoretical Framework

Nursing science and theory development are in the early stages of refinement. A **theory** is a set of interrelated constructs or propositions that attempt to present or explain, systematically, some phenomenon. Several nursing theorists have developed models and theories that remain incompletely tested. This incomplete testing and the evolving nature of models and theories give the researcher a wonderful opportunity to use the work of a nursing theorist to test concepts from that theory for practice application. An example might be a nurse who wants to study Orem's self-care model for patients undergoing outpatient surgical procedures. The nurse might design a study to investigate factors influencing self-care abilities of the adult surgical patient before and after surgery.

The nursing model or theory should be used as a guide to systematically identify and study the logical relationships between variables. Each nursing model depends on the individual researcher's philosophy of human behavior, and how that philosophical behavior meshes with other ways of looking at science.

Often a theoretical framework is likened to an architectural blueprint. These renderings, although not exact models of the real item, help the user get from one place to another. They provide a way for the nurse to construct theories that deal with the phenomena of concern to nursing and help distinguish nursing from other disciplines.

Problem Statement

One of the key steps in the research process is the ability to formulate the problem statement. The **problem statement** identifies the direction that a research project will eventually take. As a beginning consumer of research literature, the nursing student will be in a position to evaluate whether the study is a logical extension of that problem. Sometimes the problem area is not clearly stated, and the reader is unsure of the direction of the study. The problem statement should be clear and unambiguous, should express a relationship between two or more variables, should identify the population to be studied, and should encourage empirical testing. The problem statement is introduced early in the research and should reflect a well-defined, specific focus.

Stating the problem requires specifying the population to be studied. In the problem statement, the researcher states who will be the focus. For instance, the problem statement "Is there a relationship between fathers who have been abused as children and their school-aged sons' emergency-room records for suspicious injury?" suggests that the populations to be studied are fathers and sons.

The researcher must consider what significance the problem has for nursing. Research should be applicable to nursing practice, education, or administration. It should have the potential for altering nursing practice or protocol and benefiting patients, other nurses, or students. It should be theoretically relevant.

Questions about judgments, ethics, morals, or values are not amenable to the scientific research process. For example, the question, "Is it better to tell patients about their diagnosis of terminal cancer or to let them discover it themselves?" is impossible to answer. What is meant by "better"? Whose value system is being considered? The study of values has no right answer. If the question were framed differently, it would be researchable through clinical inquiry. For instance, a nurse interested in determining how often each method for letting the patient know was used could investigate attitudes toward each method.

Variables. In the problem statement, the relationship is expressed between two or more variables, or operationalized concepts. *Variables,* or properties that vary from each other, are the focus of the study. For example, a researcher studying postoperative patients might be interested in preoperative preparation in relation to the outcome of respiratory function.

Variables can be dependent or independent, given the role they play in a particular study. An **independent variable** has the presumed effect on the dependent variable. It may be manipulated if the researcher is doing an experimental study; in a nonexperimental study it is assumed to have occurred naturally before or during the study. The **dependent variable** is the consequence or presumed effect that varies as changes occur in the independent variable. The dependent variable is the one that the researcher is interested in understanding and explaining.

For example, a nurse may study the problem that cardiac output measurement (the dependent variable) will vary with the temperature of the injectate solution (the independent variable). In this case, the researcher would try to explain the effects of temperature on the measurements.

Testability. The final consideration in evaluating a research problem is that of testability. The problem must be measurable by qualitative or quantitative methods. If the question is posed in such a way that there is a relationship between an independent and a dependent variable, and that relationship can be measured, it is probably a researchable question.

Research in Practice

When a research report has been critically evaluated and is being considered for use in the clinical practice area, preparation for change is made. Bringing together those professionals who are affected is essential if the change is to be made smoothly. For example, nurses in one unit may read a study concluding that selective decontamination of the digestive tract of mechanically ventilated patients may reduce the incidence of nosocomial infections (Meijer, Van Saene, & Hill, 1990) and decide they want to implement the findings. Making such a change would involve a number of health professionals. Nurses would collaborate with physicians, hospital microbiologists, pharmacists, and respiratory therapists to consider how this change would influence patient care. During the period of evaluation, everyone involved in patient care must be aware that each patient in the study should be treated according to the standards of care in the unit. Research subjects need to be given the same treatment in order to be compared to each other on outcome variables.

Dissemination

Increasing the body of nursing theory and knowledge is a primary goal of nursing research. Therefore, once the results of a study are determined, the findings must be disseminated so that clinical application or research replication by other nurses can occur. Conclusions are strengthened and validated by similar findings in more than one research study. Findings can be disseminated by oral and poster presentations at research meetings or in print through research and clinical journals.

Presenting and publishing study results allows other nurses interested in improving nursing practice to act on the findings. Nurses may adopt the finding for clinical practice. Another nurse may choose to do the same study, but with a different group of study subjects or subjects in another clinical area, to see how useful the findings would be in this other group. Others may extend the same study, or stop using a clinical procedure or therapy that has shown little or no merit. A bonus of presenting at meetings or publishing the results of studies may be that the researcher will meet other nurses with similar interests.

LEGAL AND ETHICAL ISSUES

Institutional Review Boards

In 1974 the National Research Act was passed, requiring any agency applying for funding for any project involving biomedical or behavioral research on humans to submit assurances that it had an institutional review board to review the research and protect the rights of human subjects. At agencies where no federal money has been awarded, there is usually a review mechanism similar to the institutional review board.

Why are institutional review boards necessary? After World War II, the Nuremberg military tribunal was charged with prosecuting Nazis who had done biomedical research on concentration camp prisoners. Because the tribunal had no measures against which to test the defendants, a set of basic principles of ethical, moral, and legal concepts for the conduct of acceptable experiments had to be written. The Articles of the Nuremberg Tribunal are listed in the display.

Subject Rights

The first tenet of the Nuremberg code, developed in 1949, addressed the rights of research subjects. Paramount are voluntary consent; the right to withdraw from investigations; protection from physical and mental suffering; injury, disability, and death; and a balance between benefits and risks (Levine, 1981). Nursing researchers must provide the following information to human subjects (Commission on Nursing Research, 1981):

- Explanation of the study.
- Procedures to be followed and their purposes.
- Clear description of physical and mental discomforts, any invasion of privacy, and any threat to dignity.

Articles of the Nuremberg Tribunal

- The voluntary consent of the human subject is absolutely essential.
- The experiment should be such as to yield fruitful results for the good of society, unprocurable by other means of study, and not random and unnecessary in nature.
- The experiment should be so designed and based on the results of animal experimentation and knowledge of the natural history of the disease or other problems under study that the anticipated results will justify the performance of the experiment.
- The experiment should be conducted to avoid all unnecessary physical and mental suffering and injury.
- No experiment should be conducted where there is a prior reason to believe that death or disabling injury will occur.
- The degree of risk to be taken should never exceed that determined by the humanitarian importance of the problem to be solved by the experiment.
- Proper preparations should be made and adequate facilities provided to protect the subject against . . . injury, disability, or death.
- The experiment should be conducted only by scientifically qualified persons.
- The human subject should be at liberty to bring the experiment to an end.
- During the experiment the scientist . . . if he has probable cause to believe that a continuation of the experiment is likely to result in injury, disability, or death due to the experiment subject . . . will bring it to a close.

(From Katz, J. (1972). *Experimentation with human beings.* New York: Russell Sage Foundation, pp. 289–290.)

• Methods used to protect the anonymity and ensure confidentiality.

These may seem obvious, but before 1974 several human research studies were conducted in the United States that probably would not be allowed today. Subjects in these studies underwent unethical experimental procedures including sterilization, euthanasia, injection with live cancer cells, and the withholding of treatment for syphilis (Diers, 1979; Faulder, 1985; LoBiondo-Wood & Haber, 1986; Tetting, 1990).

Patients involved in research assume that their privacy is being protected. **Anonymity** is the protection of the subject so that not even the researcher can link the subject with the information provided. **Confidentiality** ensures that the subjects' identities will not be linked with the information they provided and will not be publicly divulged.

Although a student may have few opportunities to seek or obtain informed consent from individuals selected as potential subjects for research, a student may have a role in data collection or may provide medications or treatments in a research study. The role that a nurse or student is to play in a research study must be clarified with the involved faculty member.

RESEARCH AND THE PROFESSIONAL NURSE

Roles of Nursing Personnel at Different Levels

Some nurses may think that they have little to contribute to research, but this is not so. Nurses actually have a great deal to contribute by observing patient responses to treatments and techniques. A nurse with several years of clinical experience in a particular unit may generate many unanswered questions. He or she would be in a position to initiate research with a skilled researcher, or would heartily value someone else's research project, assisting with patient management or data collection.

The education of nurses who are clinical specialists often emphasizes clinically relevant research. In the practice arena they can do their own research, act as consultants to novice researchers, and collaborate with other health-care professionals on more complex patient situations. For example, a clinical specialist in oncology may collaborate with a clinical psychologist to study stressors of hospitalization.

The American Nurses Association's Commission on Nursing Education has developed guidelines for the investigative function of nurses. These standards give information about how different educational levels may enhance the research contributions that nurses can make.

Clinical Nursing Practice

Clinical Research

Whitney and Roncoli (1986) describe the relationship between the daily practice of nursing and researchable problems. They emphasize how the problem-solving methods used by nurses can help practicing nurses translate clinical problems into research projects.

Nurses in clinical areas regularly raise questions that could be considered researchable. Because of daily interactions with patients, nurses have the opportunity to problem-solve, but in the strict sense do not research nursing questions.

A nurse interested in research, especially in the clinical area, uses the resources at hand: patients. Patient care allows the nurse to define and seek solutions to a variety of problems. Using observation skills, discussions with colleagues, and personal clinical experience, the nurse can learn to organize priorities and proceed to offer the patient the most efficient and timely care.

Nurse researchers use techniques similar to those they developed first as a student and then refined as a skilled clinician. The nurse researcher broadens the area of study and tries to discover the variety of conditions (variables) that affect the situation.

For example, a nurse in the neonatal unit might be concerned with the temperature balance of neonates receiving phototherapy for physiologic jaundice. The researcher recognizes that to study this problem, the related fields of physical thermodynamics and developmental physiology have to be investigated. The researcher also needs to investigate the placement of temperature probes, site selection, nurse technique, and the soundness of previous research.

The nurse researcher recognizes that other experts need to be consulted and other organizational patterns must be considered. Recruitment of those skilled in particular areas ensures that the results will be more useful and gives the design and statistical analysis more merit. Often the skills of a statistician, for example, are needed.

Applying Research to Practice

The student nurse and the beginning practicing nurse are not usually involved in direct research, except in the role of data collection or administering medications and treatments as a protocol in a research project. But even with limited direct participation in research, the beginning nurse should be a consumer of research. He or she can read research literature applicable to the practice setting and attempt to evaluate it. For the beginning nurse, the ability to read articles carefully and critically is important. Critiquing does not necessarily mean finding flaws and faults. Rather, it is the conscious decision

---

Guidelines for the Investigative Function of Nurses

Associate Degree in Nursing

- Demonstrates awareness of the value or relevance of research in nursing.
- Assists in identifying problem areas in nursing practice.
- Assists in collection of data within an established, structured format.

Baccalaureate in Nursing

- Reads, interprets, and evaluates research for applicability to nursing practice.
- Identifies nursing problems that need to be investigated and participates in implementation of scientific studies.
- Uses nursing practice as a means of gathering data for refining and extending practice.
- Applies established findings of nursing and other health-related research to nursing practice.
- Shares research findings with colleagues.

Master's Degree in Nursing

- Analyzes and reformulates nursing practice problems so that scientific knowledge and scientific methods can be used to find solutions.
- Enhances the quality and clinical relevance of nursing research by providing expertise in clinical problems and by providing knowledge about the way in which these clinical services are delivered.
- Facilitates investigation of problems in clinical settings through such activities as contributing to a climate supportive of investigative activities, collaborating with others in investigations, and enhancing nursing's access to clients and data.
- Conducts investigations for the purpose of monitoring the quality of the practice of nursing in a clinical setting.
- Assists others to apply scientific knowledge in nursing practice.

Doctoral Degree in Nursing or Related Discipline

Graduate of a practice-oriented doctoral program
- Provides leadership for the integration of scientific knowledge with other sources of knowledge for the advancement of practice.
- Conducts investigations to evaluate the contribution of nursing activities to the well-being of clients.
- Develops methods to monitor the quality of the practice of nursing in a clinical setting and to evaluate contributions of nursing activities to the well-being of clients.

Graduate of a research-oriented doctoral program
- Develops theoretical explanations of phenomena relevant to nursing by empirical research and analytical processes.
- Uses analytic and empirical methods to discover ways to modify or extend existing scientific knowledge so that it is relevant to nursing.
- Develops methods for scientific inquiry of phenomena relevant to nursing.

This language was developed as part of the work of the ANA Commission on Nursing Education and was included in the report of that commission to the 1980 ANA House of Delegates. From Commission on Nursing Research. (1981). *Guidelines for the investigative function of nurses*. Kansas City, MO: Author.

---

to undertake an objective and careful evaluation of the research project in light of how the practicing nurse, working directly with a patient or patient population, would be able to use this knowledge.

After a study or research project has been evaluated, the findings might be used in clinical practice. The nurse should not jump to the conclusion that just because something has been published, it is appropriate for clinical practice, however. On the contrary, because something is published, the contents should be viewed with some degree of skepticism.

Applying research findings to clinical practice has some urgency as the explosion of health-care knowledge continues. Nurses need to narrow the gap between research and application by selecting useful studies to put into place. While research is emerging, a planned program of evaluation and implementation will help nurses find appropriate approaches to patient-care situations. The journal *Focus on Critical Care* has a column, "Research Review," that helps critical-care nurses to "apply relevant research to their practice." Other journals provide similar information.

Tetting, D. W. (1990). Preparing for human subjects review. *Critical Care Nursing Quarterly, 12*(4), 10–16.
Whitney, P. W., & Roncoli, M. (1986). Turning clinical problems into research. *Heart & Lung, 15*(1), 57–59.

Key Concepts

- Expanding the knowledge base of nursing is an important goal of nursing research.
- Nursing research is the systematic inquiry into clinical practice problems and modes of patient care.
- The scientific method of research and the nursing process are similar.
- Research is a step-by-step process of defining ideas, reviewing the literature, developing a theoretical framework, formulating a problem statement, proceeding with the study, and disseminating findings.
- Nursing research must be disseminated so that the profession can evaluate and apply the findings.
- Ethical consideration of the rights of human subjects, anonymity, and confidentiality are central to any research study.
- Practicing nurses encounter many questions that may be a basis for a research study.

References

American Nurses Association. (1981). *Research priorities for the 1980s: Generating a scientific base for nursing practice.* Publication No. D-68. Kansas City, MO: Author.
Baker, J. L. (1990). Family adaptation when one member has a head injury. *Journal of Neuroscience Nursing, 22,* 232–237.
Barnard, K. E. (1980). Knowledge for practice: Directions for the future. *Nursing Research, 29,* 208–212.
Cohen, I. B. (1984). Florence Nightingale. *Scientific American, 250*(3), 128–137.
Commission on Nursing Research. (1981). *Guidelines for the investigative function of nurses.* Kansas City, MO: Author.
Diers, D. (1979). *Research in nursing practice.* Philadelphia: J. B. Lippincott.
Faulder, C. (1985). *Whose body is it?* London: Virago.
Fonteyn, M. E. (1990). The need for nurse involvement in critical care research. *Critical Care Quarterly, 12*(4), 1–4.
Gortner, S. (1975). Research for a practice profession. *Nursing Research, 24*(6), 193–197.
Haase, J. E. (1987). Components of courage in critically ill adolescents: A phenomenological study. *Advances in Nursing Science, 19*(2), 64–80.
Hetherington, S. L. (1990). A controlled study of the effects of prepared childbirth classes on obstetric outcome. *Birth, 17*(2), 86–89.
Levine, R. J. (1981). *Ethics and regulation of clinical research.* Baltimore: Urban & Schwarzenberg.
LoBiondo-Wood, G., & Haber, J. (1986). *Nursing research: Critical appraisal and utilization.* St. Louis: C. V. Mosby.
Meijer, K., Van Saene, R., & Hill, J. (1990). Infection control in patients undergoing mechanical ventilation: Traditional approach versus a new development—Selective decontamination of the digestive tract. *Heart & Lung, 19*(10), 11–20.
Merritt, D. H. (1986). The National Center for Nursing Research, *Image: Journal of Nursing Scholarship, 18*(2):84.
Polit, D. F., & Hungler, B. P. (1987). *Nursing research: Principles and methods* (3rd ed.). Philadelphia: J. B. Lippincott.
Sarkis, J. M., & Conners, V. L. (1986). Nursing research: Historical background and teaching information strategies. *Nursing Research, 14*(2), 121–125.

Bibliography

American Nurses Association. (1976). *Research in nursing: Toward a science of health care.* Publication No. D-525M. Kansas City, MO: Author.
Bostrom, A. C., et al. (1989). Staff nurses' attitudes toward nursing research: A descriptive survey. *Journal of Advanced Nursing, 14,* 915–923.
Brent, N. J. (1990). Legal issues in research: Informed consent. *Journal of Neuroscience Nursing, 22*(3), 189–191.
Briones, T., and Bruya, M. A. (1990). The professional imperative: Research utilization in the search for scientifically based nursing practice. *Focus on Critical Care, 17*(1), 78–81.
Burns, N. (1989). The research process and the nursing process: Distinctly different. *Nursing Science Quarterly, 2*(4), 162–171.
Chicuye, P. S. (1989). Nursing in action: Nurses' influence in research and health policy development. *Journal of Professional Nursing, 5,* 326–329.
Clayton, G. M., (1989). Instruments for use in nursing education research. *Council on Social Research in Nursing Education* NLN Publication #15-2248, 1–70.
Heaney, R. P., & Barger-Lux, M. J. (1986). Priming students to read research critically. *Nursing and Health Care, 7,* 421–424.
Hinshaw, A. S. (1989). Nursing science: The challenge to develop knowledge. *Nursing Science Quarterly, 2*(4), 162–171.
Jackre, M. (1989). Presenting research to nurses in clinical practice. *Applied Nursing Research, 2*(4), 191–193.
Jones, J. A. (1989). The verbal protocol: A research technique for nursing. *Journal of Advanced Nursing, 14,* 1062–1070.
Kingry, M. J., Tiedje, L. B., and Friedman, L. L. (1990). Focus groups: A research technique for nursing. *Nursing Research, 39*(2), 124–125.
Leininger, M. (1990). Ethnomethods: The philosophic and epistemic bases to explicate transcultural nursing knowledge. *Journal of Transcultural Nursing, 1*(2), 40–51.
Lindeman, C. A. (1989). Using nursing research. Research in nursing practice. NLN Publication #15-2232, 1–17. (pamphlet)
Maerker, M., Lisper, H., and Rickberg, S. (1990). Role-playing as a method in nursing research. *Journal of Advanced Nursing, 15*(2), 180–186.
Marchette, L. (1986). Professional survival tips: Basing your practice decisions on research. *Perioperative Nursing Quarterly, 2*(2), 68–70.
Moody, L. E. (1986). Generating researchable problems. *Nurse Educator, 11*(5), 8–9.
Neidich, B. (1990). A method to facilitate student interest in research: Chart review. *Nurse Educator, 29*(3), 139–140.
O'Brien, D., and Heyman, B. (1989). Changes in nurse education and the facilitation of nursing research: an exploratory study. *Nurse Education Today, 9*(6), 392–396.
Oddi, L. F., and Cassidy, V. R. (1989). Nursing research in the United States: The protection of human subjects. *International Journal of Nursing Studies, 27*(1), 21–33.
Rempusheski, V. F. (1990). Ask an expert: Formulating research questions. *Applied Nursing Research, 3*(1), 44–46.
Selby, M. L., Tornquist, E. M., and Finerty, E. J. (1989). How to present your research: The ABCs of creating and using visual aids to enhance your research presentation, part 2. *Nursing Outlook, 37,* 236–238.
Stark, J. L. (1989). A multiple-strategy leased research program for staff nurse involvement. *Journal of Nursing Administration, 19*(9), 7–8.
Thiele, J. E. (1989). Guidelines for collaborative research. *Applied Nursing Research, 2*(4), 150–153.

UNIT II
The Nursing Process: Framework for Clinical Nursing Therapeutics

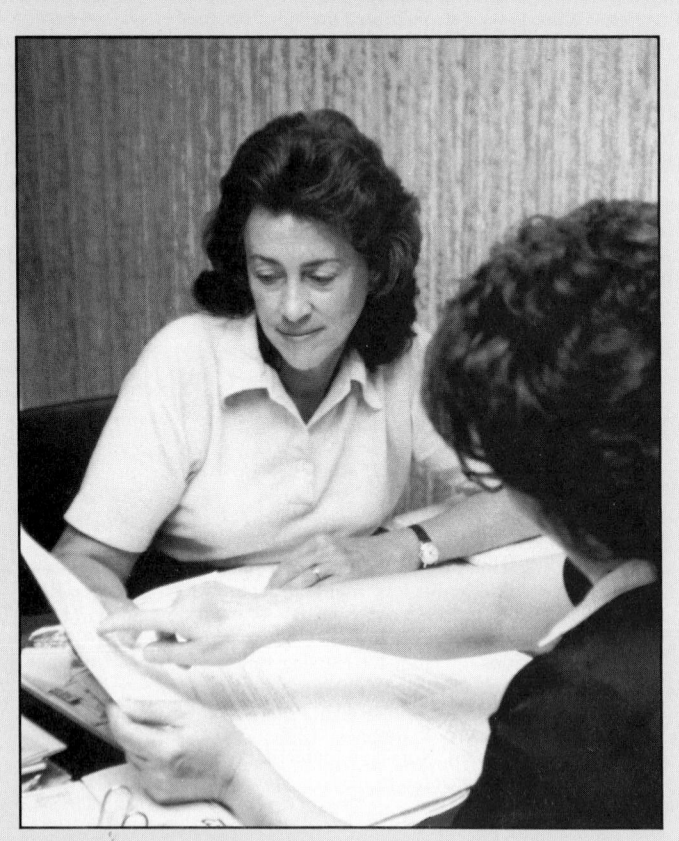

CHAPTERS

6 The Nursing Process in Human Health and Function

7 Nursing Assessment

8 Nursing Diagnosis

9 Nursing Management: Planning, Implementation, and Evaluation

10 Communication of the Nursing Process: Recording and Reporting

The nursing process is a systematic method of providing holistic, individualized nursing care that is goal directed and client centered. The five chapters in Unit II discuss the five steps of the nursing process in detail: assessment, diagnosis, planning, implementation, and evaluation. This discussion provides a solid grounding in the essential concepts.

Chapter 6 "The Nursing Process in Human Health and Function," provides an overview of the nursing process, describing the components and their relationships. The nursing process takes a cyclical rather than linear approach, allowing the nurse to use knowledge, experience, and skills to help patients maintain, support, and restore health and function. The other chapters in this unit explore the skills and activities needed to assess a patient's health status, to analyze and cluster data to formulate a nursing diagnosis, to prepare a plan of care and select nursing interventions based on mutually decided patient goals, and to evaluate the effectiveness of those interventions using outcome criteria. A final chapter discusses all forms of recording and reporting, the communication aspects of the nursing process.

The nursing process underlies nursing actions. This unit provides the framework for the application of the nursing process throughout the clinical nursing care chapters of the text.

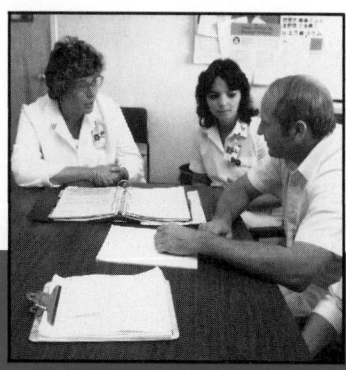

The Nursing Process in Human Health and Function

LEARNING OBJECTIVES

Upon completion of this chapter, the student will be able to do the following:

- Identify the components of the nursing process.
- Recognize significant historical developments in the evolution of the nursing process.
- Discuss the requirements for effective use of the nursing process.
- Explain the major theoretical foundations on which the nursing process is based.
- Describe the functional health approach to the nursing process.
- Appraise future trends that influence the nursing process.

KEY TERMS

Decision-making
Diagnostic reasoning process

Functional health pattern
Information-processing theory

Nursing process
Problem-solving process
Systems theory

6

Historical Development of the Nursing Process
Components of the Nursing Process
  Definition
  Phases
    Assessment
    Diagnosis
    Planning
    Implementation
    Evaluation
  Interactive Nature of Each Phase
Theoretical Foundations for Use of the Nursing
      Process

Systems Theory
Problem-Solving Process
Decision-Making Process
Information-Processing Theory
Diagnostic Reasoning Process
Requirements for Effective Use of the Nursing Process
Professional Relevance of the Nursing Process
Functional Health Approach to the Nursing Process
Future Nursing Process Trends
Key Concepts

Nursing process is the foundation of nursing practice. This method of practicing nursing is composed of five phases: assessment, diagnosis, planning, implementation, and evaluation. The phases are interrelated and form a framework for providing nursing care to patients, families, and communities. Skill in using the nursing process is necessary for the clinical application of knowledge and theory in nursing practice.

This chapter contains an overview of each phase of the nursing process, discusses its historical development, and gives a brief review of the theoretical foundations of the nursing process. The chapter also describes the requirements for the effective use and professional relevance of the nursing process. The chapter concludes with a discussion of the functional health patterns approach to the nursing process, and future nursing process trends.

HISTORICAL DEVELOPMENT OF THE NURSING PROCESS

The term **nursing process** is synonymous with the problem-solving approach for discovering the health care and nursing care needs of patients and their families. Before the widespread use of the term nursing process in the late 1960s, nurses cared for patients using a loosely structured framework based on the medical model. Since then, several nursing leaders have been instrumental in developing today's nursing process (Table 6-1). Many models of the nursing process have been developed.

Lydia Hall is credited with originally introducing the term "nursing process" in 1955 (George, 1985), but it was not used extensively in nursing publications until the 1960s. A few years later, a three-step nursing process was described by Dorothy Johnson (1959), Ida Jean Orlando (1961), and Ernestine Wiedenbach (1963). In 1967 Lois Knowles published a five-step nursing process using "the five Ds": discover, delve, decide, do, and discriminate. The *discover* and *delve* steps are synonymous with the assessment phase; *decide* is the planning stage; *do* is the implementation phase; and *discriminate* is the evaluation of patient responses to nursing interventions.

In 1967, several publications defined the nursing process and delineated the steps. The Western Interstate Commission on Higher Education (WICHE) and the faculty at the Catholic University of America were instrumental in moving the nursing process forward. WICHE (1967) published this definition: "The nursing process is that which goes on between a patient and a nurse in a given setting; it records the behaviors of patient and nurse and the resulting interaction. The steps of the process are perception, communication, interpretation, and evaluation." Although this definition was never widely accepted, it was an impetus to the further development of the nursing process.

Helen Yura and Mary Walsh, along with the nursing faculty at the Catholic University of America, identified the steps of the nursing process as assessing, planning, implementing, and evaluating. Since 1967, Yura and

TABLE 6–1

Contributions of Selected Individuals and Organizations to the Development and Evolution of the Nursing Process

Decade	Individual/Organization	Contribution
1950s	L. Hall (1955)	Originally used the term "nursing process."
		Identified three aspects of nursing care as care, cure, and core.
		Three steps of nursing process: note observations, ministration of care, validation.
	D. Johnson (1959)	Nursing seen as fostering the behavioral functioning of the patient.
		Three steps of nursing process: assessment, decision, nursing action.
1960s	I. J. Orlando (1961)	Nursing process set into motion by patient behavior.
		Three steps of nursing process: patient behavior, nurse reaction, nurse's actions.
	Western Interstate Commission of Higher Education (1967)	Nursing defined as an interactive process between patient and nurse.
		Four steps of nursing process: perception, communication, interpretation, evaluation.
	H. Yura & M. Walsh (1967)	Four components of nursing process: assessing, planning, implementing, evaluating.
	Knowles (1967)	Described nursing practice as: discover, delve, decide, do, discriminate.
1970s	American Nurses Association (1973)	Published *Standards of Nursing Practice.*
		Diagnosis distinguished as separate step of nursing process.
1980s	American Nurses Association (1980)	Published *Nursing: A Social Policy Statement.*
		Diagnosis of actual and potential health problems delineated as integral part of nursing practice.

Walsh have continued to develop and refine the nursing process concept.

In 1973, the American Nurses Association (ANA) distinguished diagnosis as a separate step of the nursing process in their *Standards of Nursing Practice.* The standards were arranged according to the five steps of the nursing process (see Chap. 1). Thus, the use of the five-step nursing process model by nursing educators and practitioners began around this time.

In the 1980s, further support was gained for making diagnosis a distinct nursing function and a separate step of the nursing process. In *Nursing: A Social Policy Statement,* the ANA (1980) again identified diagnosis of actual and potential health problems as an integral part of nursing practice. Table 6-1 summarizes selected contributions of people and organizations to the development and evolution of the nursing process.

COMPONENTS OF THE NURSING PROCESS

Definition

The generally accepted definition of **nursing process** is a systematic problem-solving approach of giving individualized nursing care, but others have defined the term differently. The nursing process is used in all settings with patients of all ages to identify and treat human responses to potential or actual health problems. By incorporating the unique aspects of each patient, the nursing process facilitates the development of individualized care.

The nursing process complements the current role of consumers in health care; that is, patients play an active role in decisions affecting their health. Patients no longer passively accept the decisions made by health-care professionals.

The nursing process has been defined in various ways by a number of nursing authors. A few definitions are included in the display for your consideration. Note the similarities between the definitions.

The nursing process serves as a guide for professional nursing practice. It has the following characteristics:

- It is a framework for providing nursing care to patient, family, and community.
- It is orderly and systematic.
- It is cyclical.
- It is interrelated.
- It provides individual care.
- It is patient-centered (uses patient's strengths).
- It is practical for use over the lifespan.
- It can be used in all settings.

Some of these features are shown in Fig. 6-1.

Phases

Assessment

Assessment commonly refers to evaluation or appraisal. In nursing, assessment is the systematic collection of subjective and objective data with the goal of making a clinical nursing judgment about a patient or family. During assessment, the nurse appraises the patient's total situation by considering the physical, psychological,

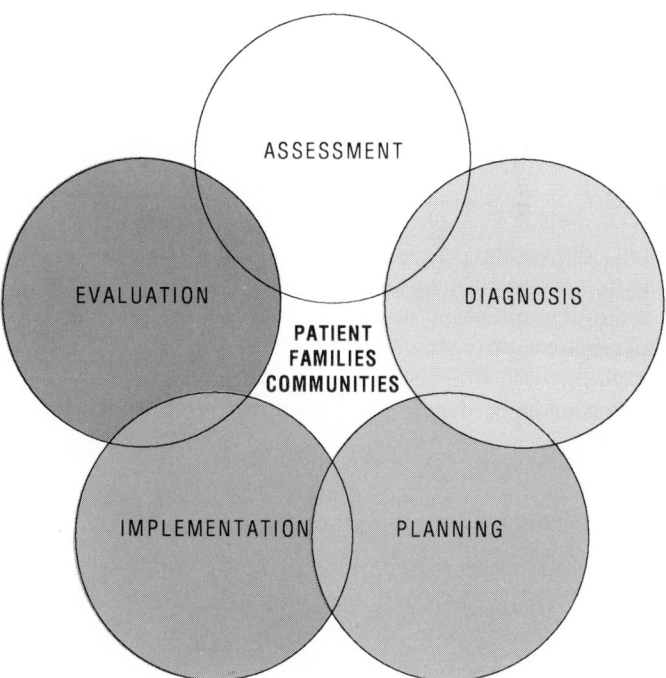

Figure 6-1. Five phases of the nursing process.

emotional, sociocultural, and spiritual factors that may affect his or her health status.

All relevant information about the patient's present and past problems must be gathered to develop a complete database. Data collection takes place during every nurse–patient interaction and from every available source (Gordon, 1987). The patient is the primary source of information for assessment. Secondary sources include family members, significant others, other health-care professionals, health records, and literature review.

Assessment data are gathered by observing, interviewing, and examining the patient, and interpreting laboratory data. Observation begins with the first encounter with the patient and is an ongoing process. The nursing interview allows for the systematic assessment of functional health patterns, including the patient's perception and interpretation of problems (Gordon, 1982; 1987). During the physical examination, the nurse uses the techniques of inspection, percussion, palpation, and auscultation to obtain data. Objective information from health records, including laboratory, diagnostic, and radiologic data, completes the database.

An in-depth nursing history and physical assessment are usually required at admission. This initial database becomes the reference point for all further nursing assessments. Thorough assessment data provide the foundation for nursing diagnoses (Yura & Walsh, 1988).

Diagnosis

Diagnosing human responses to actual or potential health problems is the second phase of the nursing proc-

ess. Diagnosis is both the clinical act of diagnosing and the term given to the patient's problem. To diagnose means to analyze assessment information and derive meaning from this analysis.

Registered nurses are educated and licensed to make nursing diagnoses. They are responsible for identifying nursing diagnoses for their patients and have a duty to identify and plan patient management based on nursing diagnoses.

The North American Nursing Diagnosis Association (1990) defines nursing diagnosis as "a clinical judgment about an individual, family, or community responses to actual or potential health problems/life processes. Nursing diagnoses provide the selection of nursing interventions to achieve outcomes for which the nurse is accountable" (NANDA, 1990). The registered nurse is responsible for identifying nursing diagnoses for those patients under his or her care.

The clinical skills used to make nursing diagnoses are the nursing diagnostic process and the nursing diagnosis statement. The nursing diagnostic process uses cue clustering, cluster interpretation, and diagnostic validation to ensure accuracy in the selection of the correct diagnoses. Formulating the diagnostic statement requires knowledge of the differences among actual, high risk, and possible nursing diagnoses.

Planning

Once nursing diagnoses have been determined, priorities are established and the planning phase begins, in which nursing strategies to resolve or reduce patient problems are established. The planning phase involves preparing a nursing care plan, which directs the activities of the nursing staff in the provision of patient care.

The nursing care plan is a written summary of the care to be given a patient. The Joint Commission on Accreditation of Healthcare Organizations (1990) requires a written plan of care for each patient. Although many institutions have developed standardized plans of care, all care plans must be individualized. Nursing care plans are further discussed in Chapter 9. The skills involved in planning include establishing patient goals and outcome criteria and determining nursing interventions.

Writing the care plan on the medical record formally recognizes what the nurse planned and carried out to assist the patient. Since the care plan remains a permanent part of the record, the beginning practitioner is sometimes intimidated to write information that may be criticized or changed by another nurse. As skill develops in writing care plans and nurses begin to recognize their responsibility to carry out other nurses' plans of care, this fear should be reduced. Once the care plan is written it must be implemented on behalf of the patient.

Implementation

Implementation is the action phase of the nursing process. It is the actual initiation of the plan, evaluation of response to the plan, and recording of nursing actions and patient response to these actions. To implement means to carry out, to perform, to do something. Bloch (1979) defined implementation as the "administration, execution, and provision" of nursing care. Nursing actions are goal directed and should assist the patient to reach maximum functional health. Standards for nursing practice stipulate that nursing actions should include patient participation and "assist the client/patient to maximize his health capabilities" (ANA, 1973).

Since nursing care is provided to assist in meeting patient goals, it is imperative that nurses focus on their actions. The nurse should make sure that each action undertaken is necessary and required.

The components of implementation are reassessment, initiation of the plan, evaluation of the response, and recording actions taken. Nursing actions focus on resolving, dissolving, or diminishing a patient's functional health status problems.

Implementation requires the use of intellectual, interpersonal, and technical skills. Developing expertise in each of these skills is required for professional nursing practice. Once the care has been provided, it is evaluated.

Evaluation

Evaluation commonly refers to rating, grading, and judging. In the evaluation phase, the nurse discovers why the nursing care plan was a success or failure (Alfaro, 1990). The nurse determines the patient's reaction to nursing interventions and judges whether the goals of the care plan have been achieved (the management plan provides the basis for evaluation). Reassessing the patient provides new information for changing or eliminating nursing diagnoses, goals, or interventions. Determining goal achievement is a joint decision between the patient and the nurse (Yura & Walsh, 1988).

There are five components of evaluation:

- Reviewing pre-established goals and outcome criteria
- Collecting data
- Measuring goal achievement
- Recording the judgment or measurement of goal attainment
- Revising or modifying the nursing management plan.

Evaluation focuses on both individual patients and groups of patients. Quality assurance monitors provide input for development and refinement of standards of care for groups of similar patients.

Although evaluation is a separate and distinct phase, it is also an ongoing and continuous process performed throughout all phases of the nursing process. Judgments in previous phases of the nursing process result in prompt reassessment, rediagnosing, and replanning. The evaluation phase involves a detailed reassessment of the entire nursing management plan. An in-depth, comprehensive judgment about patient goal attainment and fulfillment of outcome criteria takes place in this phase (Yura & Walsh, 1988).

The process of evaluation requires a variety of skills for judging the nursing management plan. These include knowledge of standards of care, knowledge of normal patient responses, knowledge of conceptual models of nursing, ability to monitor the effectiveness of nursing interventions, and awareness of clinical research.

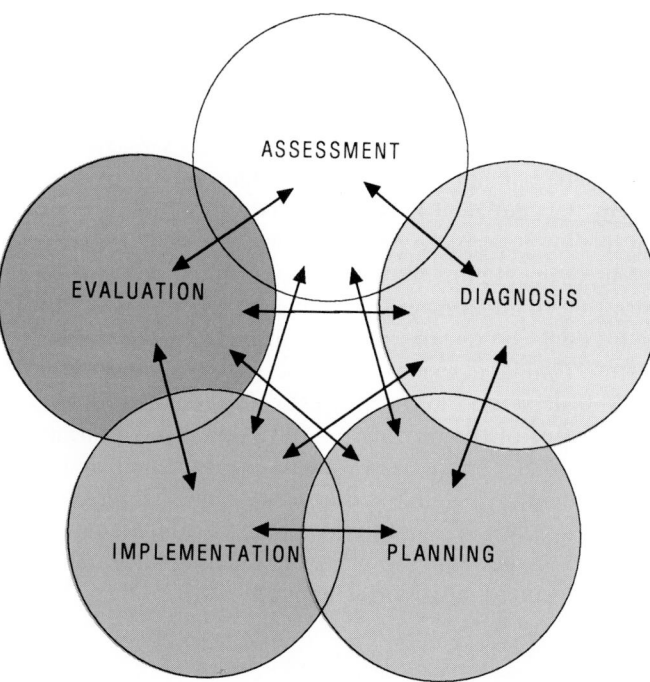

Figure 6–2.   Interactive nature of the nursing process.

Interactive Nature of Each Phase

Each phase of the nursing process interacts with and is influenced by the other phases (Fig. 6-2). For example, a nurse collecting assessment information may implement some aspects of care at the same time. In a similar manner, as the nurse evaluates nursing care, new plans are made and implemented. During an emergency, all phases of the nursing process may be carried out with no apparent division among them.

As the patient's condition changes, new data are gathered and incorporated into the plan of care. When care is provided, evaluation of the patient's response may indicate a need for immediate revision of the plan or for the identification of new nursing diagnoses.

THEORETICAL FOUNDATIONS FOR THE USE OF THE NURSING PROCESS

An understanding of the theoretical foundations of the nursing process is necessary for effectively applying it. Systems theory, problem-solving process, decision-making process, diagnostic reasoning process, and information processing theory are the basic structural units of the nursing process.

Systems Theory

Systems theory is the basis on which the nursing process is built. Systems theory illustrates how the steps of the nursing process interact with each other, forming a

unique blend that is greater than the sum of its parts (Fig. 6-3). Systems terminology provides a common language for the members of the health-care team (Fawcett, 1989; George, 1985).

All systems have cyclical patterns, and the nursing process is no exception. The steps of the nursing process overlap and influence subsequent steps. A system is composed of a set of subsystems, and each higher level is made up of systems of the lower levels. The nursing process has five subsystems: assessment, diagnosis, planning, implementation, and evaluation.

Input, the information that enters a system, is the data collected during the assessment step (the nursing interview and physical examination). Input includes assessment data about the patient and his immediate environment. *Throughput* is the process by which a system transforms, creates, and organizes input, resulting in a reorganization of the input. After the nurse identifies nursing diagnoses and plans and implements nursing care, throughput takes place. *Output,* the end-product of a system, is the patient's health status (that is, whether the patient's health has been maintained or improved). Evaluation of the attainment of goals and the need for modification provides *feedback* for revising the plan, thereby completing the cycle. See Figure 6-3 for a comparison of systems theory to the nursing process.

Problem-Solving Process

Nurses encounter problems that require solutions, ranging from a simple question to a complex clinical situation. Nurses confront problems with patients, family

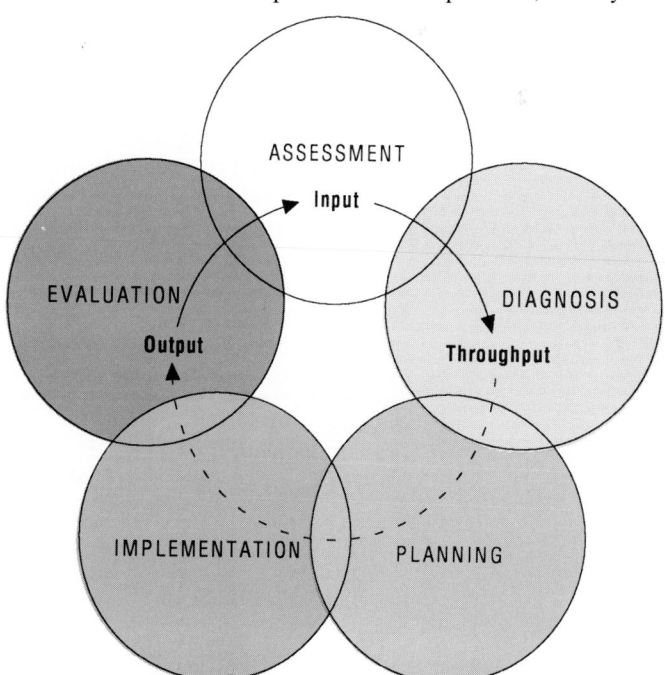

Figure 6–3.   Systems theory in comparison to the nursing process.

members, other health-team members, or equipment. Approaches to problem-solving vary depending on the complexity of the problem, the problem-solver's intellect, experience, and ability, and the method chosen to solve the problem (Francis, 1967).

Problem-solving is the basis for the nursing process. The **problem-solving process** is a modified version of the scientific problem-solving method, which focuses on one problem, is carried out in a laboratory, has an extended time element, and controls as many variables or factors as possible. In contrast, the problem-solving process takes place in a clinical setting and involves patients with multiple problems. It occurs under shorter time constraints, and unforeseeable factors and events frequently intervene. The problem-solving process allows for the flexibility needed in the "real world" of clinical nursing practice.

Problem-solving does not occur in isolation. The nurse solves problems by interacting and working with patients, family members, and other health-team members. It is an interpersonal approach that may involve two or more people (Sinnott, 1989). The patient, whenever possible, is involved in the solution of problems.

The problem-solving process is composed of six steps. The phases of the nursing process are similar to the steps of the problem-solving process. Table 6-2 illustrates the similarities of the scientific problem-solving method, the problem-solving process, and the nursing process.

Decision-Making Process

Making decisions about patient care is the essence of nursing practice. Decision-making is integral to every step of the nursing process. In its simplest form, **decision-making** consists of three phases: identifying the problem, determining the alternatives, and selecting the most appropriate alternative. People make decisions constantly, such as what to wear, what to eat, and when to study. All of the decisions we make are influenced by past experiences and exposure to different life events.

In a clinical situation, the nurse must decide which patient should receive care first, when care may be delegated to other health-team members, and which patient-care activity will be done. Each decision is carried out or changed depending on the immediate circumstances. Some days proceed smoothly, and decisions made early in the day present no problems. But given the constant changes in patients, the usual scenario is one of changing priorities in meeting emergent needs. The nurse usually must deal with uncertainty and must be adept at making astute clinical decisions.

The steps used in this process can be compared with the phases of the nursing process. Gathering information is analogous to assessment, identification of the problem area is similar to diagnosing, considering alternative courses of action and selecting a course may be likened to the planning phase. Evaluating information and the course of action is implied in this process.

Information-Processing Theory

After the interview is completed, the chart reviewed, and the patient examined, the nurse must synthesize the data. This is a complex task (Benner & Tanner, 1987): the processing of information requires the cognitive skills of logical and inductive/deductive thinking as well as the decision-making and diagnostic processes.

Information-processing theory (Fig. 6-4) can be used to help cluster data to arrive at a diagnosis (Newell & Simon, 1972; Simon, 1979). Since the brain can process only five to seven pieces of information at once, data need to be organized in a framework or outline (the model used in this textbook is the functional health approach; see below). In this way, the nurse can see where each piece fits into the whole. Studies have shown that experienced nurses need fewer cues to make accurate diagnoses (Benner, 1984).

Gathering and processing information can proceed inductively or deductively. Both approaches are used by

---

TABLE 6–2

Similarities and Differences Among the Scientific Problem-Solving Method, the Problem-Solving Process, and the Nursing Process

Scientic Problem-Solving Method	Problem-Solving Process	Nursing Process
Define problem	Recognize existence of problem	Assessment
Collect data	Collect data	Assessment
Formulate a hypothesis	Analyze data; specify problem	Diagnosis
Select method to test hypothesis	Determine ways to achieve solution to problem	Planning
Test hypothesis	Execute the planned actions	Implementation
Formulate conclusion; evaluate hypothesis	Judge the effectiveness of selected actions	Evaluation

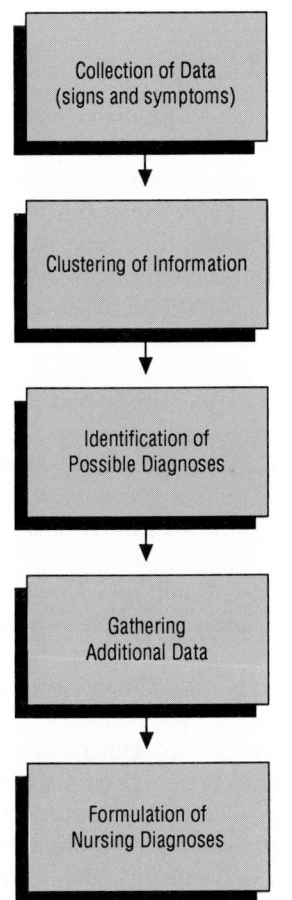

Figure 6–4.   Information processing model.

nurses to identify and resolve problems. *Induction* is a reasoning process that proceeds from the specific to the general. For example:

A rose has petals.
A daisy has petals.
A petunia has petals.
Therefore, all flowers have petals.

Deduction proceeds from the general to the specific. For example:

All flowers have petals.
A rose has petals.
Therefore, a rose is a flower.

Diagnostic Reasoning Process

The **diagnostic reasoning process** is used to make accurate clinical diagnoses about patient problems. It is a complex process composed of several interrelated steps and affected by variables such as the background of both the diagnostician and the patient. Although the steps are discussed sequentially, in practice there is much overlap

until the diagnosis is made and confirmed (Woods, 1984). The steps include:

- Background of both the diagnostician and the patient
- Initiation of the process
- Gathering individual cues
- Development of cue clusters
- Identification of possible diagnoses
- Collection of specific data
- Confirmation/refutation of the diagnosis.

REQUIREMENTS FOR EFFECTIVE USE OF THE NURSING PROCESS

To use the nursing process successfully, the nurse must have a general understanding of the basic sciences and humanities. Nursing uses this scientific knowledge during assessment, planning, implementing, and evaluating patient care. For example, several factors may influence the patient with chronic obstructive pulmonary disease that produce changes in the physiology of his or her lungs. He or she must adapt based on culture and ethnic background. Also, the course of the disease may have been influenced by exposure to pollutants acquired at work. Drawing all the pieces together to plan care requires a broad knowledge base.

Nurses add to their basic knowledge formally and informally by attending continuing-education programs, reading professional journals, learning about related fields, and having discussions with peers and others. Incorporating new research findings into practice is necessary to achieve better patient outcomes, develop new standards for practice, and provide cost-effective care.

Writing skills are needed to communicate information on the patient's health record and other institutional forms. Writing enables others to develop a picture of the patient at one point in time. Records are often the only way to discover historical information about the progression of a disease and the patient's response to it. Skillful writing requires the ability to summarize information while remaining comprehensive and accurate. Succinct descriptive terms are useful in providing an accurate, detailed written report.

A key way to obtain information for written reports is by listening. Active listening implies that the nurse is responsive to the cues the patient is sending. If patients are anxious or preoccupied, they may respond to questions with short or inappropriate answers. The astute nurse listens to what the patient says and does not say to follow up on misconceptions and misunderstandings, or to correct misinformation.

Being an active listener is hard work. It involves paying attention to nonverbal cues as well as the spoken response. Patients may hesitate to give certain information. Although it is important to respect the patient and not to pry, the nurse needs to gather data essential for good patient care. As interviewing skills develop, the nurse learns how to phrase certain questions and how to approach personal matters. Often the way a question is asked can make the difference between a complete or a superficial response.

PROFESSIONAL RELEVANCE OF THE NURSING PROCESS

The nursing process is a systematic, organized way of providing nursing care for any patient in any situation. Its adaptability and practicality contribute to high-quality nursing care. Because a concise nursing care plan is written, continuity of care is facilitated and communication among nurses is enhanced.

The nursing process focuses on the patient's unique problems. The patient or family members are involved in developing goals, setting priorities, and selecting nursing interventions, and thereby play an important role in decisions that directly affect patient care. The patient's responses to nursing interventions are continually assessed and evaluated, which fosters individualized nursing care.

Legally, the nursing process is recognized as the standard for nursing practice. The nurse is held accountable to practice according to legal statutes and the nurse practice act of the state. Most states use the term nursing process in describing the act of nursing.

Professionally, the nursing process is generally recognized as the method of practicing nursing. It is the model on which professional nursing standards are based. Although sometimes criticized for not being adaptable to the changing health-care environment, the nursing process remains the almost universally accepted method for providing nursing care.

FUNCTIONAL HEALTH APPROACH TO THE NURSING PROCESS

Gordon (1982; 1987) developed a method for organizing nursing assessment data that involves the appraisal of 11 **functional health patterns.** These functional health patterns provide a framework for the collection of assessment data.

Gordon originally developed the functional health pattern typology (a systematic classification) in 1974 while teaching nursing assessment and diagnosis content to nursing students at Boston College. The incorporation of comments from nurse scholars, nurse educators, clinical nurse specialists, and students who used the categories in their practice resulted in some modification of the original health pattern categories.

Functional health patterns help the nurse ascertain the patient's strengths and any dysfunctional or potentially dysfunctional pattern that exists. All 11 patterns are considered a composite of the patient–environment situation and are examined collectively. The typology of

---

Typology of 11 Functional Health Patterns

Health perception–health management: Describes patient's perceived pattern of health and well-being and how health is managed

Nutritional–metabolic: Describes pattern of food and fluid consumption relative to metabolic need and pattern indicators of local nutrient supply

Elimination: Describes patterns of excretory function (bowel, bladder, skin)

Activity–exercise: Describes pattern of exercise, activity, leisure, and recreation

Cognitive–perceptual: Describes sensory-perceptual and cognitive pattern

Sleep–rest: Describes patterns of sleep, rest, and relaxation

Self-perception–self-concept: Describes self-concept pattern and perceptions of self (e.g., body comfort, body image, feeling state)

Role–relationship: Describes pattern of role-engagements and relationships

Sexuality–reproductive: Describes patient's patterns of satisfaction and dissatisfaction with sexuality pattern; describes reproductive patterns

Coping–stress tolerance: Describes general coping pattern and effectiveness of the pattern in terms of stress tolerance

Value–belief: Describes patterns of values, beliefs (including spiritual), or goals that guide choices or decisions

(From Gordon, M. (1987). *Nursing diagnosis: Process and application* (2nd ed). New York: McGraw-Hill.)

---

the 11 patterns is given in the display. The patterns are built on the data collected during the interview and physical examination and are relevant for the individual, family, or community (Gordon, 1982; 1987).

Functional health patterns act as the blueprint for the rest of the nursing process. In this way, the functional health approach permeates every phase of the nursing process. Although functional health patterns guide the collection of assessment data, they also serve as a guide for the identification of nursing diagnoses, development of the nursing management plan, implementation of the plan, and the organization of evaluative data for revision of the plan. Figure 6-5 diagrams the relationships between functional health and the nursing process.

FUTURE NURSING PROCESS TRENDS

Although the steps of the nursing process are likely to remain the same, the way the nursing process is used will

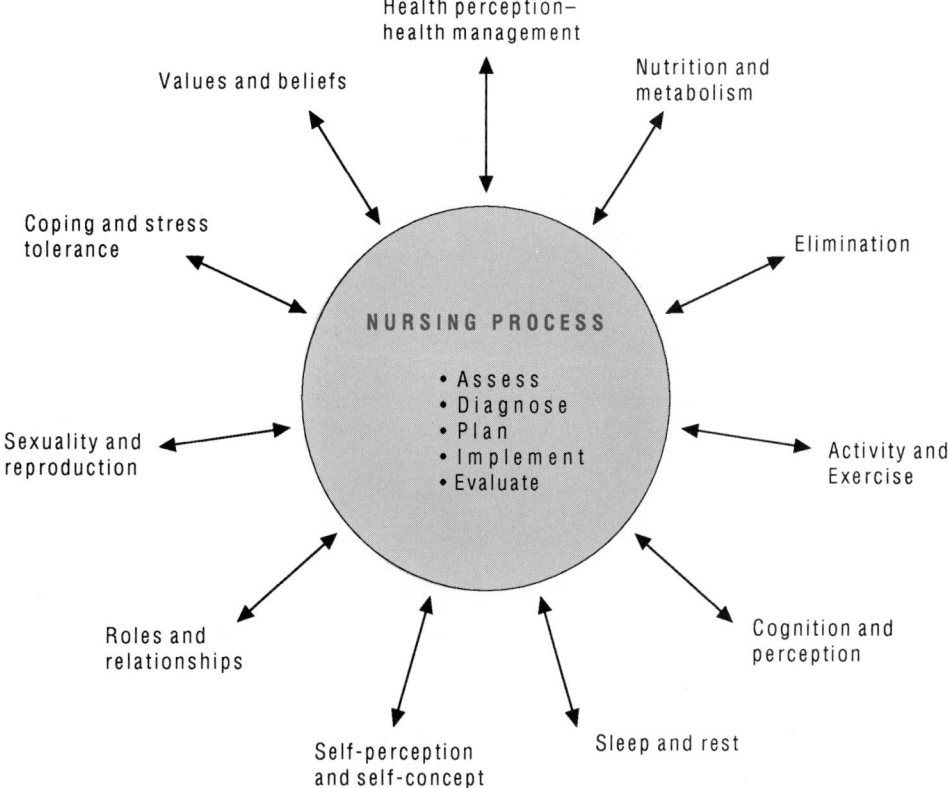

Figure 6–5.   Functional health permeates every phase of the nursing process.

change. Many institutions have computerized their data-collection methods and nursing management plans. Written documentation is often minimal; instead, the nurse systematically enters data into a computer terminal, often at the patient's bedside, providing easy access to all types of information necessary for quality patient care. For example, a patient's laboratory test results may be available for rapid interpretation and possible changes in the nursing management plan.

Computerization should not be equated with a lack of personalized care that fails to consider the uniqueness of the patient. Computerization aims to provide a larger, more comprehensive data base for the provision of improved patient care and outcomes. Frequently patients require complex medical treatment and nursing care. Often the treatment involves the use of sophisticated technologic devices. In this technologic environment, it is important not to lose sight of the patient's need for human touch. Technology can "never replace the caring touch and voice of the nurse" (Selby, 1987, p. 1).

As nursing diagnoses are researched and the taxonomy is scientifically validated, standardized approaches to nursing care delivery can be taken. Use of national health databases will assist in evaluating and modifying nursing care. Nursing efforts are focusing on the development of a nursing intervention taxonomy and a patient outcome taxonomy (Lang & Marek, 1990; McCloskey, et al., 1990). There may be a need to develop a nursing assessment taxonomy as well.

Nursing Research

Harvey, R.M. (1991). Nursing diagnosis by neural networks: A new aid for nursing practice. In R.M. Carroll-Johnson (ed.), *Classification of nursing diagnoses: Proceedings of the ninth conference.* Philadelphia: J.B. Lippincott.

This pilot study was done to test the ability of neural networks (ART-2), a computer technology, to make clinical decisions about nursing diagnoses. An assessment tool based on Gordon's functional health pattern, elimination, was designed that produced diagnostic "patterns" and was taught to the ART-2. The diagnoses made by the ART-2 agreed with those made by the researcher. The advantage of this approach is that it can incorporate new material; a disadvantage is that a case example must be available to teach the neural network.

Key Concepts

- The nursing process is the systematic, problem-solving approach to providing nursing care to patients, families, and communities.
- The nursing process has evolved over the last 35 years to consist of five phases: assessment, diagnosis, planning, implementation, and evaluation.
- The nursing process is used in all settings with patients of all ages to identify actual and potential health problems and design strategies to resolve them.
- Systems theory, the problem-solving process, decision-making process, information processing theory, and diagnostic reasoning process serve as the theoretical foundations for the nursing process.

References

Alfaro, R. (1990). *Applying Nursing Diagnosis and Nursing Process: A step-by-step guide* (2nd ed.). Philadelphia: J. B. Lippincott.

American Nurses Association. (1973). *Standards of nursing practice.* Kansas City, MO: Author.

American Nurses Association (1980). *Nursing: A social policy statement.* Kansas City, MO: Author.

Benner, P. (1984). *From novice to expert.* Menlo Park, CA: Addison-Wesley.

Benner, P., & Tanner, C. (1987). Clinical judgment: How expert nurses use intuition. *American Journal of Nursing, 87,* 23–31.

Carpenito, L. J. (1989). *Nursing diagnosis: Application to clinical practice* (3rd ed.). Philadelphia: J. B. Lippincott.

Fawcett, J. (1989). *Analysis and evaluation of conceptual models of nursing* (2nd ed.). Philadelphia: F. A. Davis.

Francis, G. (1967). This thing called problem-solving. *Journal of Nursing Education, 6*(4), 27–33.

George, J. B. (1985). *Nursing theories: The base for professional nursing practice* (2nd ed.). Englewood Cliffs, NJ: Prentice-Hall.

Gordon, M. (1982). *Nursing diagnosis: Process and application.* New York: McGraw-Hill.

Gordon, M. (1987). *Nursing diagnosis: Process and application* (2nd ed). New York: McGraw-Hill.

Harvey, R. M. (1991). Nursing diagnosis by neural networks: A new aid for nursing practice. In R. M. Carroll-Johnson (Ed.), *Classification of nursing diagnoses: Proceedings of the ninth conference.* Philadelphia: J. B. Lippincott.

Johnson, D. (1959). A philosophy of nursing. *Nursing Outlook, 7,* 198–200.

Joint Commission on Accreditation of Healthcare Organizations. (1990). *Accreditation manual for hospitals.* Chicago: Author.

Knowles, L. (1967). *Decision-making in nursing: A necessity for doing.* New York: Appleton-Century-Crofts.

Lang, N. M., & Marek, K. D. (1990). The classification of patient outcomes. *Journal of Professional Nursing, 6*(3), 158–163.

McCloskey, J. C., Bulechek, G. M., Cohen, M. Z., et al. (1990). Classification of nursing interventions. *Journal of Professional Nursing, 6*(3), 151–157.

Newell, A., & Simon, H. A. (1972). *Human problem-solving.* Englewood Cliffs, NJ: Prentice-Hall.

North American Nursing Diagnosis Association. (1990). *NANDA taxonomy I* (rev.). St. Louis: Author.

North American Nursing Diagnosis Association. (1990). *Guidelines for submission.* St. Louis: Author.

Orlando, I. J. (1961). *The dynamic nurse–patient relationship.* New York: G. P. Putnam.

Selby, T. L. (1987). Nurses add human touch to technology. *The American Nurse, 19*(4), p. 1.

Simon, H. A. (1979). *Models of thought.* New Haven: Yale University Press.

Sinnott, J. D. (1989). *Everyday problem-solving.* New York: Praeger.

Western Interstate Commission on Higher Education. (1967). *Defining clinical content, graduate nursing programs, medical and surgical nursing.* Boulder, CO: Author.

Wiedenbach, E. (1963). The helping art of nursing. *American Journal of Nursing, 63*(11), 54–57.

Woods, N. F. (1984). Methods for studying diagnostic reasoning in nursing. In D. L. Carnevali, P. H. Mitchell, N. F. Woods, et al. (Eds.), *Diagnostic reasoning in nursing.* Philadelphia: J. B. Lippincott.

Yura, H., & Walsh, M.B. (1973). *The nursing process: Assessing, planning, implementing, evaluating.* Norwalk, CT: Appleton-Century-Crofts.

Yura, H., & Walsh, M. B. (1988). *The nursing process: Assessing, planning, implementing, evaluating* (5th ed.). Norwalk, CT: Appleton & Lange.

Bibliography

Coyle, L. A., & Sokop, A. G. (1990). Innovation adoption behavior among nurses. *Nursing Research, 39,* 176–180.

Fry, V. (1953). The creative approach to nursing. *American Journal of Nursing, 53,* 301–302.

Solomon, J. (1990). Physical assessment skills in undergraduate curricula. *Nursing Outlook, 38,* 194–195.

Tanner, C. A. (1987). Theoretical perspectives for research on clinical judgment. In K. J. Hannah, M. Reimer, W. C. Mills, et al. (Eds.), *Clinical judgment and decision-making: The future with nursing diagnosis.* New York: John Wiley & Sons.

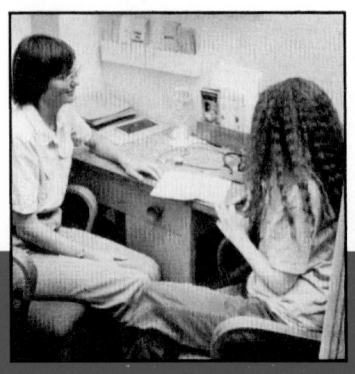

Nursing Assessment

LEARNING OBJECTIVES

Upon completion of this chapter, the student will be able to do the following:

- Define the assessment phase of the nursing process.
- Discuss the purpose of assessment in nursing practice.
- Identify the skills required for nursing assessment.
- Differentiate the three major activities involved in nursing assessment.
- Describe the process of data collection.
- Explain the rationale for data validation.
- Discuss the frameworks used to organize assessment data.
- Perform a nursing assessment based on functional health patterns.

KEY TERMS

Assessment	Intuition	Physical
Auscultation	Objective data	examination
Cue	Observation	Subjective data
Inspection	Palpation	Validation
Interviewing	Percussion	

7

Preparing for Assessment
  Types of Assessment
    Initial Assessment
    Focus Assessment
    Time-Lapsed Reassessment
    Emergency Assessment
  Setting and Environment
Assessment Skills
  Observation
    Vision
    Smell
    Hearing
    Touch
  Interviewing
    Preparatory Phase
    Introductory Phase
    Maintenance Phase

    Concluding Phase
  Physical Examination Techniques
    Inspection
    Palpation
    Percussion
    Auscultation
  Intuition
Assessment Activities
  Collect Data
    Types of Data
    Sources of Data
    Recording Data
  Validate Data
  Organize Data
    Body Systems Model
    Functional Health Patterns
Key Concepts

The first phase of the nursing process is called **assessment.** Assessment is the collection of data for nursing purposes. The nurse uses many skills to collect the information; including observation, interviewing, physical examination, and intuition. Data or information are collected from many sources, including patients, their family members or significant others, health records, other health team members, and literature review. Data are grouped, collected, and organized during assessment. Figure 7-1 shows the assessment phase in relation to the other phases in the nursing process. Interpretation or analysis of the data takes place in the diagnosis phase of the nursing process. Many frameworks have been developed to organize assessment data; they are discussed at the end of the chapter.

Assessment is the first phase of the nursing process during which data are gathered for the purpose of identifying actual or potential health problems. Accurate assessment information is essential for the provision of quality nursing care.

Although there may be overlap in the collection of some data by other members of the health-care team, the specific way in which the data are used differs from one profession to another. Nursing assessment focuses on the gathering of data about a patient's state of wellness, functional ability, physical status, strengths, and responses to actual and potential health problems (Gordon, 1987).

The purpose of nursing assessment is to gather data about the patient that can be used in diagnosing, planning, and implementing care. Assessment is done to:

- Establish baseline information on the patient
- Determine the patient's normal function
- Determine the presence or absence of dysfunction
- Determine the patient's strengths
- Provide data for the diagnosis phase.

The activities that make up the assessment phase are data collection, validation, and organization; these are discussed later in this chapter. Many frameworks have been developed to organize assessment data, and these also are discussed later in the chapter.

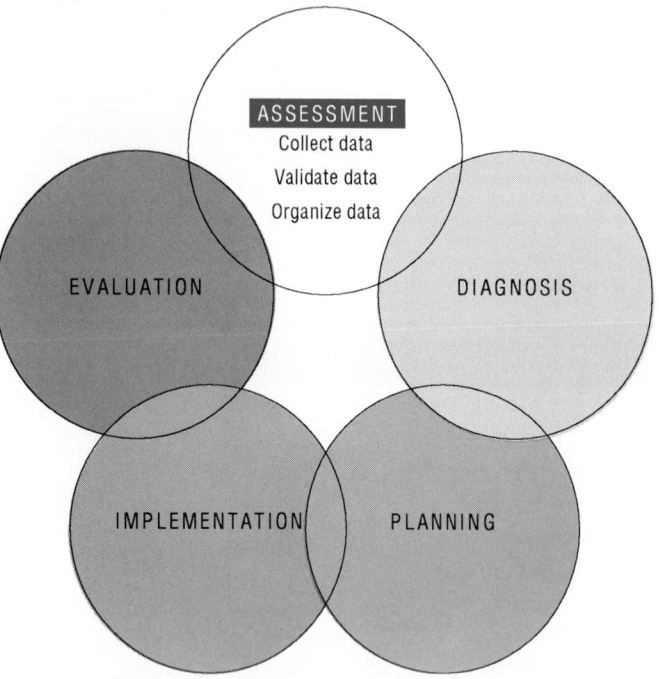

Figure 7–1. The relationship of assessment to the entire nursing process.

PREPARING FOR ASSESSMENT

Types of Assessment

Assessment takes many forms depending on the clinical situation, patient status, time available, and purpose of data collection. The types of assessment are the initial assessment, focus assessment, time-lapsed reassessment, and emergency assessment (Table 7-1).

Initial Assessment

An initial assessment, also called an admission assessment, is performed at the time the patient enters the health-care facility. The purposes are to evaluate the patient's health status, to identify functional health patterns that are problematic, and to provide an in-depth, comprehensive database, which is critical for evaluating changes in the patient's health status in subsequent assessments (Gordon, 1982; 1987).

This type of assessment is usually performed by a professional registered nurse. If a thorough assessment cannot be completed because of the patient's health status or urgency of specific health problems, it is finished at a later time. Frequently, parts of the admission assessment are delegated to nonprofessional staff members. Even if parts of the assessment are delegated to others, however, the professional registered nurse is ultimately responsible for the completeness and accuracy of the information. The Joint Commission on the Accreditation of Healthcare Organizations (1990) mandates that each patient have a documented nursing admission assessment that follows institutional policies.

Focus Assessment

The goal of the focus assessment is to collect data about a problem already identified. This type of assessment has a narrower scope and a shorter timeframe than the initial assessment. The nurse determines if the problem still exists and whether the status of the problem has changed (e.g., improved, worsened, or resolved). This assessment also includes the appraisal of any new, overlooked, or misdiagnosed problems. In the intensive care unit, the

TABLE 7–1

Types, Aims, and Timeframe for Assessment

Type	Aim	Timeframe
Initial assessment	Initial identification of normal function, functional status, and collection of data concerning actual or potential dysfunction. Provide baseline for reference and future comparison	Within the specified timeframe after admission to a hospital, nursing home, ambulatory health-care center, or home health-care setting
Focus assessment	Determine status of a specific problem identified during previous assessment	Ongoing process; integrated with nursing care; a few minutes to a few hours between assessments
Time-lapsed assessment	Comparison of patient's current status to baseline obtained previously; detection of changes in all functional health patterns after an extended period of time has passed	Several months (3, 6, or 9 months or more) between assessments
Emergency assessment	Identification of life-threatening situation	Anytime a physiologic, psychological, or emotional crisis occurs

nurse may perform focus assessments every few minutes for a critically ill patient; for example, a severely burned patient requires frequent monitoring of fluid requirements due to fluid volume deficits caused by the excessive fluid losses that result from the burn injury.

Often, the nurse assesses the patient for a specific problem and provides nursing care at the same time. For example, while bathing a patient with weakness in the lower extremities, the nurse can assess the patient's muscular strength and ability to perform self-care activities (Gordon, 1982; 1987).

Time-Lapsed Reassessment

Time-lapsed reassessment is another type of assessment that takes place after the initial assessment is performed. The aim of the time-lapsed reassessment is to evaluate any changes in the patient's functional health. It is performed when substantial periods of time have elapsed between assessments. Like the focus assessment, it determines the status of problems already identified. Due to the varying time interval between reassessments (e.g, 3 to 12 months), a complete review of all functional health patterns is carried out. For example, several weeks or months may lapse between reassessments of a patient in an outpatient setting. Time-lapsed reassessment is usually less comprehensive than the initial assessment (Gordon, 1987).

Emergency Assessment

Emergency assessment takes place in life-threatening situations where the preservation of life is the top priority. Time is of the essence for rapid identification of and intervention for the patient's health problems. Often the patient's difficulties involve airway, breathing, and circulatory problems (the ABCs). Abrupt changes in self-concept (suicidal thoughts) or roles or relationships (social conflict leading to violent acts) can also initiate an emergency (Gordon, 1987). Emergency assessment focuses on a few essential health patterns and is not comprehensive.

Setting and Environment

Assessment can take place in any setting where nurses care for patients and their family members: in the patient's home, at a clinic, in a hospital room, at a health fair, or at the patient's workplace. The patient's physical comfort helps facilitate data collection, so the assessment should be scheduled at an appropriate time of day so that the patient is not tired, hungry, or in pain.

The nurse must be aware of environmental factors conducive to the collection of accurate and complete assessment data. An assessment is best performed in a quiet, private setting that lends itself to the discussion of sensitive, personal, and confidential information. The setting must be restricted or secluded to prevent the patient's undue embarrassment during the interview and physical examination. The nurse may ask visitors and family members to leave the room temporarily (Brunner & Suddarth, 1988). Distractions should be minimized (e.g., television or radio, announcements over the intercom, a too-hot or too-cold room). The nurse may need to close the door, pull the curtains, turn down the heat, or move the patient to another place if the environment cannot be modified.

ASSESSMENT SKILLS

Nurses use a variety of skills as they assess patients and their family members. Assessment skills are important in obtaining comprehensive data. One can read about various skills, but it is through actual clinical experience and use of these skills that proficiency in nursing assessment is developed. Assessment involves recognizing and collecting **cues,** pieces of information about a patient's health status. Cues may be overt (objective) or covert (subjective). Examples of overt cues are a description of an incision site ("reddened, swollen") or a blood-pressure measurement (180/110); an example of a covert clue is the patient's statement, "I have a sharp pain in my shoulder." In the diagnosis phase, these cues are interpreted, clustered, and analyzed. Subjective and objective data are further defined under Assessment Activities in this chapter.

The clinical skills of observation, interviewing, physical examination, and intuition are used to assess patients across the lifespan in a variety of settings. The nurse uses these skills simultaneously when assessing patients. For example, during the patient interview, the nurse asks questions, observes the patient, listens to the patient's answers, and mentally stores information for further exploration during the physical examination. The clinical skills used in assessment are summarized in Table 7-2.

TABLE 7–2

Clinical Skills Used in Assessment

Type	Definition
Observation	The act of noticing patient cues
Interviewing	Interaction and communication process for gathering data by questioning and information exchange
Physical examination	Analysis of bodily functioning using the techniques of inspection, palpation, percussion, and auscultation
Intuition	Use of one's insights, instincts, or clinical experience to make judgments about patient care

Nurses come in contact with patients of all ages. Assessment techniques are modified according to the age and developmental stage of the patient. Assessing a child often involves parental assistance; the parent may hold the child on his or her lap to facilitate examination. Distraction techniques, such as flashing a light or moving an object, are helpful to divert an infant's attention during assessment (e.g., when examining the ear) (Bates, 1987). When assessing an obese patient, a larger blood-pressure cuff may be needed. The nurse may need to speak more slowly and distinctly when examining an elderly patient with degenerative hearing loss. An elderly patient with joint problems or muscular weakness may require additional time to change positions during the physical examination.

Observation

Observation lays the groundwork for collecting other kinds of assessment data. As assessment proceeds, the nurse anticipates the type of information that will be necessary or appropriate to obtain for a particular patient. **Observation** is more than the nurse's ability to "see" the patient; the nurse uses the senses of vision, smell, hearing, and touch (the sense of taste is rarely used) (Gordon, 1987; Yura & Walsh 1988).

Observation begins the moment the nurse meets the patient. As the patient walks into the room, gets out of the wheelchair, or is assisted into bed, the nurse is constantly observing, via sensory modalities. Observation includes looking, watching, examining, scrutinizing, surveying, scanning, or appraising. Using his or her knowledge of nursing care, physical assessment, basic sciences, social sciences, and pathophysiology, nurses observe patients in a sophisticated manner. Intellectual skills also come into play as the nurse makes decisions about what data are needed to complete the assessment.

Vision

The sense of vision is used in a specialized manner. The nurse's ability to survey how the patient "looks" is key. Does the patient show signs of distress or discomfort, such as grimacing, scowling, or frowning, and guarding or holding a body part? Is the patient sitting upright in a chair with arms resting comfortably at the sides, or curled up in bed? What is the patient's body size and nutritional status: overweight, obese, normal weight, or undernourished and emaciated? What is the patient's preferred posture? Can he or she walk? Are there abnormal movements?

How is the patient groomed and dressed? Is the patient's clothing clean, excessively worn, or inappropriate for the season or weather? If a patient's appearance and clothing are disheveled, further information is needed to determine if the patient is homeless or has a physical or mental condition contributing to self-neglect. The nurse must compare the patient's appearance to the probable norm for the patient, taking into account the patient's lifestyle, occupation, age, and socioeconomic group (Bates, 1987; Yura & Walsh, 1988).

Smell

A keen sense of smell is used when observing the patient. The nurse notes any body or breath odors that may indicate an underlying physical condition. For example, foul-smelling breath may signify an oral or pulmonary infection. A fruity breath odor may indicate a metabolic disorder such as ketosis in diabetes mellitus. Alcohol on the patient's breath does not always mean that alcohol intake is the exclusive explanation for mental and physical findings (Bates, 1987). Body odors indicate sweat and sebaceous gland function and the patient's overall cleanliness. A homeless person may have body odors related to lifestyle circumstances and the inability to bathe.

Hearing

Observation includes the nurse's ability to listen to and hear what the patient says. The patient's level of consciousness and awareness of the surroundings is noted. The patient's ability to state his or her name, location, and date accurately is determined as the nurse asks questions and observes how the patient answers. The ability to initiate conversation or to respond only when spoken to gives clues about the patient's mental and physical condition. If the patient is confused, the nurse should question the validity of the information obtained; family members or significant others, if available, can provide information for the confused or incapacitated patient.

Nonverbal behavior is noted during every interaction with the patient. The patient's nonverbal demeanor yields information about feelings toward the nurse, staff, and family (Sundeen, et al., 1989). Does the patient show any signs of anger, suspiciousness, anxiety, or hostility? For example, the patient may deny any anxiety or apprehension about health problems, but may have an anxious facial expression or tear-filled eyes. The patient may be argumentative and hostile with family members but cooperative and friendly with staff.

Touch

General observations continue through the use of touch. Touch is used to greet the patient (a handshake), to provide nonverbal communication and reassurance, and to perform a preliminary appraisal of skin temperature and moisture. The nurse observes the presence of perspiration, warmth or coldness, and strength of the patient's handshake. A gentle touch on the arm or hand may reassure the patient and at the same time reveal dry, scaly skin indicative of dehydration or thyroid problems. A specialized kind of touching called palpation is performed during the physical examination.

The nurse must consider the patient's sociocultural background when using touch. In some cultures, the use of touch must be modified to minimize the patient's sense that privacy has been invaded. Patients of some cultures may interpret touching as a hostile action. A specialized kind of touching called palpation is performed during physical examination. Detailed examination of the skin is performed during the nutritional–metabolic health pattern assessment (Gordon, 1987).

Interviewing

The nurse must be an effective communicator to conduct a successful interview. Among the factors affecting the quality and comprehensiveness of the interview are the nurse's skill and experience and the patient's willingness to share information.

There are several techniques that facilitate communication between the nurse and the patient. These techniques establish rapport, help the nurse elicit the patient's thoughts and feelings, encourage conversation, and ensure mutual understanding (Stuart & Cash, 1985; Sundeen, et al., 1989). Barriers that hinder interaction have the opposite effect on communication (Carpenito, 1989; Sundeen, et al., 1989). Table 7-3 summarizes the facilitators and barriers to effective communication. Communication techniques are further discussed in Chapter 17.

Interviewing is an essential skill for obtaining information for the nursing history, which consists of questions designed to elicit subjective data from the patient or family members. The nursing history focuses on the patient's account of the impact of actual or potential health problems on his or her functional health status. The nursing history helps to:

- Clarify and verify the patient's perception of his or her functional health status.
- Compare the patient's present and past functional health status, lifestyle behaviors, and coping abilities.
- Identify actual and potential nursing diagnoses.
- Develop the nursing management plan.
- Implement nursing interventions supportive of the patient's adaptive responses.

Health-care institutions usually have a form for the systematic collection and documentation of the nursing history. Such documentation improves communication between nursing staff and other health-team members.

A nursing history can take 30 to 60 minutes to perform. Although usually completed in one session, it may be obtained over several sessions. If the patient's condition (e.g., severe pain, breathing difficulties) or setting (e.g. excessive noise, lack of privacy) makes data collection difficult, the nurse can collect information about urgent problems and defer other questions until a more suitable time.

An interview can be divided into four phases: preparatory, introductory, maintenance, and concluding.

Preparatory Phase

The preparatory or preinteraction phase occurs before the nurse meets the patient. Actions taken in this phase help ensure that the interview will be as productive as possible. The nurse's attention is directed toward preparing for the first nurse–patient interaction. During this phase, the nurse does the following (Sundeen, et al., 1989):

- Reviews as much information as possible about the patient.
- Decides what data are needed and what type of data collection form will be used.
- Reviews the literature pertinent to the patient's devel-

TABLE 7–3

Techniques that Facilitate and Block Communication During an Interview

Facilitators of Communication	Barriers to Communication
Use broad opening statements	Make stereotyped comments
Give general leads	Give advice or state your opinion
Listen	Agree with the patient
Acknowledge the patient's feelings	Defend
Use silence	Give approval
Give information	Use reassuring clichés
Reflect or repeat the patient's words	Request an explanation
Share observations	Express disapproval
Clarify	Belittle the patient's feelings
Summarize	Change the subject
Validate	Disagree with the patient
Verbalize implied thoughts or feelings	

opmental age, psychosocial aspects, and pathophysiologic considerations, if needed.

- Assesses his or her feelings or reactions to previous patients that may interfere with the nurse–patient relationship.
- Seeks assistance from more experienced nurses, mentors, or supervisors if concerned about how to carry out the interview.
- Plans for a private, quiet setting for the interview, schedules a mutually convenient time of day, and determines the length of time needed for data collection.
- Modifies the environment to facilitate the interview.

Introductory Phase

The second phase of an interview is called the introductory phase. Also known as the orientation phase, the introductory phase begins when the nurse and patient meet. The nurse's actions in this phase assist in establishing rapport, clarifying roles, and alleviating anxiety. The nurse and patient are actively involved in asking questions, getting acquainted, and exchanging their expectations for the interview and health assessment. During this phase, the nurse does the following (Sundeen, et al., 1989):

- Introduces himself or herself and states his or her position and the purpose and content of the interview.
- Begins to establish rapport with the patient by conveying a caring, interested attitude. Rapport is essential for a trusting, helpful nurse–patient relationship.
- Observes the patient's behavior and listens attentively to determine the patient's self-perceptions and the way the patient sees his or her health problems; validates the patient's perceptions as the interview progresses.
- Lets the patient know how long the nurse–patient relationship is expected to last (e.g., until discharge).
- Informs the patient how the information collected will be used.
- Starts with nonthreatening specific questions and proceeds to open-ended questions.
- Establishes a verbal contract with the patient, incorporating the goals of the interview.

Maintenance Phase

The maintenance phase is the third phase of an interview. In the maintenance or working phase, the nurse and patient work toward achieving the specific task or goal agreed on in the introductory phase. Both participants maintain the interaction for the purpose of getting the "work" done, but it is the nurse's responsibility to ensure that the goals are met. The goals may be mutually revised by the patient and nurse. In this phase, the nurse does the following (Sundeen, et al., 1989):

- Keeps focused on the tasks or goals to ensure that needed data is obtained and goals are achieved.

- Encourages the patient to express his or her feelings, concerns, and questions.
- Uses techniques that facilitate communication between the nurse and patient (e.g., silence, using general leads, validating).
- Observes the nonverbal behavior that accompanies verbal responses (e.g., a patient may say she is not nervous, worried, or anxious, but she bites her fingernails, moves constantly, and smokes throughout the interview).
- Assesses the patient's ability to continue the interview (e.g., grimace of pain, shortness of breath, fatigue).
- Facilitates goal attainment by moving to the next topic of discussion after needed data are collected.

Concluding Phase

In the concluding or termination phase, the nurse–patient relationship is completed. Actions taken in this phase can help ensure that the termination will be a positive experience for both participants. The nurse focuses on reviewing goals or tasks attained and expressing concerns related to this phase. In this phase, the nurse does the following (Sundeen, et al., 1989):

- Reviews goal or task attainment. Such a review can foster a sense of achievement in the patient and nurse.
- Summarizes the highlights of the interview and its meaning to the nurse and the patient.
- Encourages the patient to express and share his or her feelings regarding the termination of the nurse–patient relationship.
- Uses language congruous with the patient's cultural background and local custom (e.g., "good-bye" may mean a final farewell in some cultures; promises to contact the patient in the future may be taken literally).

Physical Examination Techniques

The **physical examination** is a systematic data collection method that uses the senses of sight, hearing, smell, and touch to detect health problems. It is divided into four techniques: inspection, palpation, percussion, and auscultation. Usually, the nursing interview is completed before the physical examination is performed. The physical examination is used to verify and expand the data gathered during the nursing interview (Gordon, 1982; 1987). More details on physical examination techniques can be found in Chapter 18.

Inspection

Inspection is a visual examination of the patient done in a methodical and deliberate manner so that important data are not omitted. It begins with the nurse's first contact with the patient and is conducted intentionally and continuously so that important data are not omitted. Inspection is not haphazard or passive. It is an important first step in the physical examination process. As the nurse inspects the patient, the underlying anatomic structures are considered and any abnormalities that may be present are identified. Factors such as color, shape, symmetry, movement, pulsations, and texture of the involved body part are noted (Bates, 1987; Fuller & Schaller-Ayers, 1990).

Inspection is carried out during the interview and subsequent physical examination. For example, an enlarged thyroid or growth in the neck may be visible while interviewing a patient. Detailed inspection of the neck would take place after the interview.

Palpation

Palpation is the specialized use of touch for the collection of data that augments the inspection process. By using the fingertips and palms of the hand, the nurse can determine the size, shape, and configuration of underlying body structures. The pulsations of blood vessels; the outline of organs such as the thyroid, spleen, or liver; the size, shape, and mobility of masses; the temperature of the skin; vibration or movement of blood in a blood vessel; and tenderness or sensitivity of a body part are detected.

Percussion

Percussion is a technique in which one or both hands are used to strike the body surface to produce a sound called a percussion note. Underlying body structures have characteristic percussion notes that indicate their denseness or hollowness. Percussion is used to discover the location and level of organs (liver, heart, diaphragm), the consistency of body structures (fluid-filled, air-filled, or solid), the presence of tenderness (over the kidneys or near the spine), and the identification of masses or tumors.

Auscultation

Auscultation is the technique of listening to body sounds with a stethoscope. It yields information about the movement of air or fluid in the body. The stethoscope is placed on the body surface to amplify normal and abnormal sounds. Mastery of auscultation lies in the interpretation of the findings. This is accomplished by consulting those nurses who are more experienced and proficient in identification of auscultation sounds. Various body systems, including the respiratory, cardiovascular, and gastrointestinal systems are auscultated for characteristic sounds. Bowel sounds, breath sounds, heart sounds, and the sound of blood moving through a narrowed or twisted blood vessel (known as a bruit) are heard through auscultation.

Intuition

Intuition has only recently been acknowledged as a legitimate part of nursing practice. It is defined as the use of insight, instinct, and clinical experience to make clinical judgments about the patient. "Although not validated or valued in traditional ways, intuitive knowledge appears to be used by nurses, particularly expert nurses, in many aspects of clinical practice" (Beckett, 1990, p. 2).

Intuition plays a role in the nurse's ability to rapidly analyze cues, make clinical decisions, and implement nursing actions even though assessment data may be incomplete or ambiguous (Rew, 1988). In the past, the concept of intuition appeared infrequently in nursing literature, but nurse researchers and scholars are beginning to examine its role in the various phases of the nursing process. Each phase of the nursing process is sequential and builds on the activities of the previous phase. Assessment data are systematically collected until the information compiled for every health pattern is complete. Each subsequent phase of the nursing process is built on the initial data base. Research results imply that the nursing process addresses only part of the problem-solving process used by nurses (Rew & Barrow, 1989). Rew (1988) found that most experienced nurses used intuition in the assessment and implementation phases of the nursing process.

Intuition comes into play when assessment data are incomplete, sketchy, or vague, or when the patient looks alright on the surface but the nurse senses that something is not quite right. For example, before obtaining complete assessment data, a nurse may enter a patient's room and get a strong "feel" about the patient's condition without performing a physical examination or reading the chart. Or a nurse may sense that a patient with normal vital signs, skin color, and neurologic status is going to have a cardiac or respiratory arrest (Rew, 1988). In the two situations described, the nurse uses intuitive knowledge to analyze cues, make clinical decisions, and implement nursing interventions on behalf of the patient. Intuition results in decisions that might not have been made had the nurse used the nursing process alone.

ASSESSMENT ACTIVITIES

During the assessment phase, the nurse collects, validates, and organizes data. Because these activities are so closely related, the nurse often shifts from one to another, perhaps collecting and organizing data at the same time. The nurse may choose to validate information as it is collected rather than at the completion of data collection. As data are organized, the nurse may discover an ambiguous cue that requires further clarification and validation with the patient.

Collect Data

The process of compiling information about the patient is called data collection. Data collection begins with the first contact with the patient and is done by observation, interviewing, and physical examination. Usually, data are collected using a systematic format that ensures comprehensive, accurate information.

Types of Data

Objective and subjective data, both integral parts of assessment, are obtained during data collection. Table 7-4 shows the differences in the methods of obtaining subjective and objective data, and provides examples of each type.

Subjective data, also known as symptoms or covert cues, include the patient's feelings and statements about his or her health problems. Subjective data are supplied by the patient, and it is not always feasible to validate, confirm, or substantiate through other sources. Often the nurse tries to validate subjective data through objective data collection. Subjective data are obtained through the interview and are best recorded as a direct quote from the patient:

"I haven't felt good for the last couple of months."
"I get a sharp pain in my stomach after I eat."
"Every time I move, I feel nauseated."

Objective data, also known as signs or overt cues, are observable, perceptible, and measurable. They can be validated or verified by others. Examples include bowel sounds, temperature reading, peripheral pulses, distended neck vessels, and skin rashes. Objective data may be obtained by the senses (e.g., vision, touch, smell) or by measuring devices or equipment (e.g., thermometer, sphygmomanometer), laboratory studies (e.g., complete blood count), radiologic tests (e.g., x-rays, barium enema), or diagnostic procedures (e.g., colonoscopy).

Sources of Data

Two major sources of data exist for the collection of information about the patient. The patient is considered the primary source of data, since only he or she can give a first-hand description of the health problem and its effects on his or her lifestyle. All other sources, such as family members, significant others, other members of the health-care team, laboratory tests, and literature review are considered secondary sources.

Primary Sources. The patient is the primary source of data. Information collected from the patient is considered to be the most reliable. Skills used for obtaining information from the patient include observation, interview, and physical examination. Assessment data is elicited from the patient unless circumstances such as altered level of consciousness, severe pain, impending surgery, acute illness, or age make data collection impossible. The patient is deemed unreliable if he or she is confused or suffering from physical or mental conditions that alter thinking, judgment, or memory. In situations where the patient is unreliable, secondary sources help provide the necessary assessment information.

Secondary Sources. There are several secondary sources of data. Secondary sources provide data that supplement, clarify, and validate information obtained from the patient. These include family members or significant others, the health record, laboratory tests and

---

TABLE 7–4
Comparison of Subjective and Objective Data

Type	Subjective Data (Covert Cues)	Objective Data (Overt Cues)
Method of Obtaining Data	Interview	Techniques of inspection, palpation, percussion, and auscultation Measurement devices Health record Laboratory studies, radiologic tests, diagnostic procedures
Examples	Symptoms Values Perceptions Feelings Attitudes Sensations Beliefs	Physical examination findings: heart sounds, palpable tumor, discolored skin Blood pressure, temperature, intracranial pressure Written reports of other health team members on health record Complete blood count results, chest x-ray results

diagnostic procedures, health team members, and literature review.

Family members or significant others supplement and verify information obtained from the patient. They can provide information that the patient forgets to mention or is unwilling to reveal. They may be the only source of data for children or for confused, unresponsive, or severely ill patients. Data provided by family members and significant others include a description of how the patient reacts to illness, the patient's perceptions of changes in functional health, the patient's ability to cope with life stressors, and information about the patient's home situation.

Usually the patient's permission is obtained *before* seeking information from family members or significant others. All people involved must understand the confidential nature of the information they provide. The patient's permission must also be obtained to divulge any information (e.g., diagnosis of cancer, AIDS, pregnancy) to family members or significant others.

Past and current health records—items such as consultation reports, medical and nursing histories, and physical examination findings—contain a wealth of information about the patient and are helpful in completing assessment data. Facts about the patient's previous illnesses, hospitalizations, and functional and dysfunctional health patterns are obtained. The health record may also reveal data not expressed by the patient or picked up by the nurse. Reviewing health records can also reduce the number of times a patient is asked the same questions by various health-team members.

Laboratory tests and diagnostic procedures are another secondary source of data for the completion of the data base. They clarify, supplement, and verify findings from the interview and physical examination. Laboratory tests are always interpreted in relationship to the patient's underlying health problems and treatment modalities. These results can also identify actual or potential health problems not disclosed by the patient or explored by the nurse. Sometimes laboratory tests and diagnostic procedures are used to judge the effectiveness of nursing interventions.

Written and verbal reports from other health-team members are another source of assessment data. The nurse can take advantage of the expertise of other colleagues caring for the patient: all of them are valuable sources of information about the patient's current and past health status. By consulting other health-team members, the nurse verifies and supplements the assessment data. Health-team members include professional staff such as nurses, social workers, physical therapists, physicians, clergy, and respiratory therapists, and nonprofessional personnel such as nursing assistants.

Reviewing the literature helps complete the patient's database. Pertinent literature includes textbooks, journals, dissertation abstracts, and unpublished monographs presented at professional meetings. The patient's health patterns must be viewed in relation to current knowledge and theory. A thorough review of the literature provides information on recent developments in nursing and medical practice.

Recording Data

Using a framework or outline, assessment data are systematically recorded and become a permanent part of the medical record. Institutions usually have a specific form for recording data and facilitating its use by other nurses caring for the patient. Baseline assessment data are referred to periodically to reaffirm assessment findings and to compare the patient's current status to his or her initial condition. Two methods can be used: the traditional written assessment record and the computerized assessment record.

Traditional Written Assessment Record. Traditionally, while assessment data are collected, the nurse takes notes throughout the nursing interview and physical examination. After the health assessment, an in-depth recording of findings is made. The nurse follows institutional policy and records the data by hand on the appropriate forms. Depending on the examiner's skill and the number of health problems the patient has, recording assessment data can be time-consuming. The more experienced nurse can take notes on the appropriate forms as the interview proceeds and summarize comments quickly and efficiently.

Computerized Assessment Record. Computerization of health records has led to a new format for recording assessment data: the computerized nursing assessment record. In many institutions, assessment data can be entered into a computer at the patient's bedside. Instead of writing the data on the medical record forms, data are entered into the computer by typing on the keyboard. The time required to enter the data depends on the nurse's familiarity with computers and typing proficiency. Some computerized systems incorporate other types of data, such as laboratory test data and diagnostic study results. This facilitates the retrieval of these data for nursing purposes. For example, a laboratory blood test result can be obtained by computer, rather than waiting for the report to arrive on the patient care unit or calling the laboratory personnel for a verbal report. The nurse can immediately incorporate these data into the patient's functional health assessment.

Validate Data

Validation is the process of confirming the accuracy of assessment data collected. It is commonly referred to as double-checking the information at hand. As the nurse collects data, multiple cues are identified. Inferences are made about the cues; that is, a meaning or interpretation is attached to the cue. One or more inferences can be made about a particular cue or group of cues (Alfaro, 1990). See the accompanying examples.

The nurse must make sure that the cues and inferences are correct. Validation assists in the verification and clarification of cues and inferences and increases the likelihood that cues and inferences are accurate, free from bias, and interpreted correctly (Alfaro, 1990). Incorrect cues and inferences lead to the development of inappropriate nursing diagnoses and nursing management plans. Figure 7-2 illustrates the connection between cues and inferences and methods for the validation of data.

Identification of relevant cues and correct inferences depends on the nurse's clinical nursing knowledge, assessment skills, personal values, and past experience (Alfaro, 1990). Inferences must be validated before the clustering and analysis of cues and identification of nursing diagnoses.

Methods of validating data include (Alfaro, 1990; Phipps, Long, & Woods, 1983):

- Comparing cues to normal function. For example, Mr.

Jones is a professional athlete and has a resting pulse of 50 beats per minute; the nurse knows that physiologic heart changes in physically fit people can result in a slower pulse rate (bradycardia).
- Referring to textbooks, journals, and research reports. For example, the nurse may consider brown macules or "liver spots" on the hands and forearms of an elderly patient as abnormal. After checking a textbook on physical changes that occur with aging, the nurse learns that they are common in the elderly.
- Checking consistency of cues. Data can be checked, for example, by retaking the patient's temperature or blood pressure or by using another piece of equipment. Subjective and objective data can be compared. For example, the patient may state, "I feel hot," but his or her temperature is 98.6°F., or the patient may state, "I can't get my breath," but respirations are 20 and lung sounds are clear.
- Clarifying the patient's statements. Ask specific, closed-ended questions, share observations with the patient and family members, clarify ambiguous or vague statements, and verify inferences.
- Seeking consensus with colleagues about inferences. This is usually done after the data have been validated

---

Examples of Cues and Inferences

Example 1

Group of Cues

Patient has
- Blurry vision or visual defects
- Headache
- Tingling and numbness in extremities
- Dizziness

Possible Inferences
1. Patient has a brain tumor.
2. Patient is having warning signals of a stroke.
3. Patient may be diabetic.
4. Patient is anxious.

Example 2

Cue
Mr. Spencer has dry, flaky skin.

Possible Inferences
1. Mr. Spencer may be dehydrated.
2. Mr. Spencer has hypothyroidism.
3. Mr. Spencer has some type of dermatitis.

Example 3

Cue
Patient has frequency and burning on urination.

Inference
Patient has a urinary tract infection.

Example 4

Cue
Mrs. Smith's blood sugar is 55 mg/dL.

Inference
Mrs. Smith is suffering from a hypoglycemic reaction.

Example 5

Cue
Patient states, "I just can't seem to shake this pain in my joints."

Inference
Patient has inadequate pain management.

DATA VALIDATION

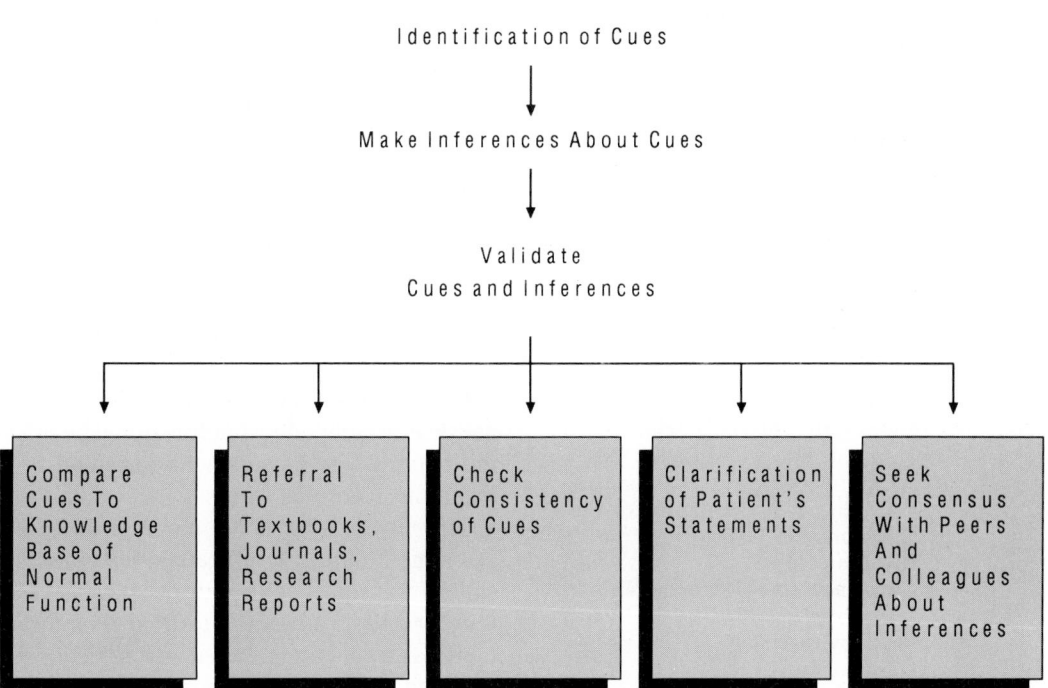

Figure 7–2.   Methods for the validation of cues and inferences.

using the above methods, as peers and colleagues may have made their own inferences that may be incorrect.

Organize Data

There are a variety of frameworks for the orderly collection and recording of assessment data. The framework serves as a guide during the nursing interview and physical examination, helps prevent the omission of pertinent information, and fosters data analysis in the diagnosis phase. The framework may be modified based on the patient's physical status and on the nurse's personal preference (Fuller & Schaller-Ayers, 1990).

TABLE 7–5

Selected Nursing Theorists and Their Nursing Conceptual Models

Theorist	Conceptual Model
Orem	Self-care model
Roy	Adaptation model
Neuman	Health-care system model
Johnson	Behavioral system model
Rogers	Life process model
King	Open systems model
Levine	Conservation model
Parse	Man-living-health model
Paterson & Zderad	Humanistic nursing model
Yura & Walsh	Human needs model

Nursing conceptual models provide one such framework. Institutions, nursing schools, and individual nurses use one or more of these frameworks to guide their nursing practice. Each conceptual framework has a frame of reference for carrying out nursing care. Some examples are Orem's self-care model, Roy's adaptation model, Neuman's systems model, and Johnson's behavioral model (Fawcett, 1989). The reader who uses one of these frameworks should refer to specific texts that describe these models in detail. Table 7-5 summarizes selected nursing theorists and their nursing conceptual models.

Body Systems Model

The body systems model (also called the medical model, review of systems, or head-to-toe approach) focuses on the patient's major anatomic systems. This framework is used to collect data about the past and present condition of each organ or body system and to thoroughly examine all body systems for actual and potential problems. This review often reveals information that the patient did not consider important or neglected to mention. It starts with an assessment of the patient's general state of health, followed by the assesssment of the skin. The examiner uses a top-to-bottom approach to cover all body systems. Table 7-6 indicates the order of the physical assessment as performed by the staff nurse using a body systems framework.

TABLE 7–6
Physical Assessment Using the Body Systems Model

Body System	Criteria
Sensory-perceptual	Mental status
	Vision and appearance of eyes
	Hearing
	Touch
	Taste and smell
Skin	Condition (color, turgor, character)
	Lesions
	Edema
	Hair distribution
	Breast
Respiratory	Rate, character
	Breath sounds
	Cough
Cardiovascular	Pulses (rate, quality, rhythm)
	Apical Radial
	Carotid Dorsalis pedis
	Brachial Posterior tibial
	Femoral
	Blood pressure
	Circulation (mucous membranes, nailbeds)
Neurologic	Pupillary reactions
	Orientation
	Level of consciousness
	Grasp strength
Gastrointestinal	Mouth, gums, teeth, and tongue (color and condition)
	Gag reflex
	Bowel sounds
	Presence of distention, impaction, hemorrhoids (external)
Genitourinary	Presence of retention
	Discharge (vaginal, urethral)
	Uterine response (pregnancy, postpartum)
	External genitalia
Musculoskeletal	Muscle tone, strength
	Gait, stability
	Range of motion

From Carpenito, L. J. (1989). *Nursing diagnosis: Application to clinical practice* (3rd ed.). Philadelphia: J. B. Lippincott, p. 50.

Functional Health Patterns

The patient's strengths, talents, and functional health patterns (see Chap. 6) are an integral part of the assessment data. Sometimes, this information is obscured or forgotten in some assessment frameworks. An assessment of functional health focuses not only on the patient's normal function but also on his or her altered function or risk for altered function. Because the information gathered using the 11 functional health patterns is basic to nursing, it is applicable to all conceptual models of nursing practice (Gordon, 1982; 1987). Functional health assessment can be used for patients of all ages and in all specialty areas and is relevant for the assessment of the person, family, or community (Beyea & Matzo, 1989; Tompkins, 1989).

The use of functional health patterns for the assessment and documentation of nursing care is predicted to rise from a reported 34% in 1989 to 48% in 1992 (Wake, 1990). This increase may be due to the advantages of a functional health framework:

- Patient strengths or assets—not merely deficits, problems, or limitations—can be identified.
- The focus is on nursing diagnoses, not medical diagnoses.
- Clustering is easier to do because of the simple categories and concise typology.
- It may contribute to the delineation of basic assessment areas relevant for all patients.

Components of Functional Health Assessment. There are several components of functional health assessment: the pattern label, assessment parameters for each pattern, and recording of assessment data.

The *pattern label* is the name given to a category of assessment data. Eleven categories of assessment data, called functional health patterns, have been identified by Gordon (1982; 1987). Pattern labels indicate if the patient has a functional (asset, strength) or dysfunctional (nursing diagnosis) health pattern.

Assessment parameters help the nurse gather specific information about each functional health pattern. Assessment parameters have been identified for each functional health pattern. Specific interview questions, physical examination techniques, and other information such as laboratory data or health records help the nurse identify health problems in each pattern.

There are various forms for *recording assessment parameters* and identifying the patient's functional or dysfunctional health patterns (Beyea & Matzo, 1989; Gordon, 1987). The nurse uses the approved institutional form at the place of employment or school of nursing. Data may be recorded by handwriting the information on a form or by entering the information into a computer.

Description of Functional Health Patterns. The 11 functional health patterns identified by Gordon (1982; 1987) are described below. For in-depth information about the assessment parameters for each functional health pattern, see Chapter 18.

Health perception and health management focuses on the patient's perception of his or her state of health and well-being and general management of health. Assessment parameters include a general survey of the patient's health status and usual health behaviors.

Nutrition and metabolism focuses on the patient's dietary pattern and food and fluid consumption in relationship to metabolic need. The patient's skin integrity and wound-healing status are also considered. Assessment parameters include eating habits, appraisal of appetite, weight loss or gain, and changes in skin, hair, or nails.

Nursing Research

Selected Nursing Research Studies

Davis, M. J., & Nomura, L. A. (1990). Vital signs of class I surgical patients. *Western Journal of Nursing Research, 12*(1), 28–41.

Itano, J. K. (1989). A comparison of the clinical judgment process in experienced registered nurses and student nurses. *Journal of Nursing Education, 28,* 120–126.

Mulhearn, S. (1989). The nursing process: Improving psychiatric admission assessment. *Journal of Advanced Nursing, 14,* 808–814.

Rew, L. (1988). Intuition in decision-making. *Image, 20,* 150–154.

Possible Topics for Nursing Inquiry

- Do graduate nurses and experienced nurses differ in the way they view functional health pattern assessment?
- What is the effect of the documentation of functional health pattern assessment on nurses' participation in patient-care decisions?
- Does functional health pattern assessment facilitate the development of new nursing diagnoses?
- What is the relationship between intuitive nursing knowledge and the diagnostic process in nurses with 10 years of experience?

Self-perception and self-concept focuses on the patient's feelings of self-worth and body image. Assessment parameters include the patient's descriptions of himself or herself, physical appearance, effects of illness, and major life accomplishments.

Role and relationships focuses on the patient's satisfaction and dissatisfaction with family and social roles and relationships. Assessment parameters include the patient's perceptions of key relationships and observations of interactions with others.

Sexuality and reproduction focuses on the patient's sexual expression in relationship to his or her developmental stage, perceptions of satisfaction and dissatisfaction, and reproductive patterns. Assessment parameters include the patient's appraisal of his or her sexual role and sexual health. Physical examination, if appropriate, is carried out if problems are identified from subjective data.

Coping and stress tolerance focuses on the patient's perception of stressors and coping patterns and their effectiveness in terms of stress tolerance. Assessment parameters concentrate on the patient's evaluation of current stress level, coping ability, and ability to endure life stressors. Physiologic responses to stress are also assessed (e.g., blood pressure, heart rate).

Values and beliefs focuses on the patient's beliefs or goals that guide decision-making and preferences in life, including spiritual beliefs. Assessment parameters include the patient's identification of valued people and possessions, sources of support, and religious practices.

Elimination centers on excretory function (bowel, bladder, and skin). Routines, laxatives, or devices used to control excretion are examined. Assessment parameters include the patient's usual bowel and bladder elimination habits as well as the excretory function of the skin (e.g., excessive perspiration).

Activity and exercise focuses on the patient's pattern of energy expenditure in exercise, activity, leisure, and recreation. Assessment parameters include the patient's mobility status, exercise routine, and leisure activities.

Cognition and perception focuses on cognitive functions such as memory, language, reasoning, and problem-solving, and sensory/perceptual abilities such as vision, hearing, and sensory overload and deprivation. Assessment parameters include changes in cognitive function; ability to hear, see, and speak; and the presence of pain, numbness, or other sensations.

Sleep and rest focuses on the patient's perception of sleep, rest, and relaxation patterns. Assessment parameters include the patient's regular sleep habits and routine.

Key Concepts

- Assessment is the collection of subjective and objective data from the patient and other sources for the purpose of describing health problems.
- Types of assessment vary depending on the clinical situation, the patient's health status, the time available, and the purpose of data collection.
- An in-depth, comprehensive appraisal of a patient's functional health patterns at the time of entry to a health-care facility is called an admission assessment.
- Environmental factors can facilitate or hinder collection of assessment data.
- Observation helps the nurse anticipate appropriate data to be collected during the nursing interview and physical examination.
- Proficient interviewing skills are necessary for obtaining comprehensive assessment data.
- The physical examination is a systematic analysis using inspection, palpation, percussion, and auscultation.

■ Intuition, a legitimate aspect of nursing practice, involves the nurse's use of insight, instinct, and clinical experience.

■ The patient, family and significant others, health-team members, and health records are sources of assessment data.

■ Assessment data are recorded and become a permanent part of the health record.

■ The functional health pattern assessment provides a framework for the collection and organization of patient data and provides a foundation for the development of nursing diagnoses.

References

Alfaro, R. (1990). *Applying nursing diagnosis and nursing process: A step-by-step guide* (2nd ed.). Philadelphia: J. B. Lippincott.

Bates, B. (1987). *A guide to physical examination* (4th ed.). Philadelphia: J. B. Lippincott.

Beckett, J. E. (1990). Intuition in clinical nursing. *Research review: Studies in nursing practice, 6*(3), 2.

Beyea, S., & Matzo, M. (1989). Assessing elders using the functional health pattern assessment model. *Nurse Educator, 14*(5), 32–37.

Brunner, L. S., & Suddarth, D. S. (1988). *Textbook of medical-surgical nursing* (6th ed.). Philadelphia: J. B. Lippincott.

Carpenito, L. J. (1989). *Nursing diagnosis: Application to clinical practice* (3rd ed.). Philadelphia: J. B. Lippincott.

Fuller, J., & Schaller-Ayers, J. (1990). *Health assessment: A nursing approach*. Philadelphia: J. B. Lippincott.

Gordon, M. (1982). *Nursing diagnosis: Process and application*. New York: McGraw-Hill.

Gordon, M. (1987). *Nursing diagnosis: Process and application* (2nd ed.). New York: McGraw-Hill.

Joint Commission on Accreditation of Healthcare Organizations. (1990). *Accreditation manual for hospitals*. Chicago: Author.

Phipps, W. J., Long, B. C., & Woods, N. F. (1983). *Medical-surgical nursing: Concepts and clinical practice* (2nd ed.). St. Louis, MO: Mosby-Year.

Rew, L. (1988). Intuition in decision-making. *Image, 20,* 150–154.

Rew, L., & Barrow, E. M. (1987). Intuition: A neglected hallmark of nursing knowledge. *Advances in Nursing Science, 10*(1), 49–62.

Rew, L., & Barrow, E. M. (1989). Nurses' intuition: Can it coexist with the nursing process? *AORN Journal, 50,* 353–358.

Stuart, C. J., & Cash, W. B. (1985). *Interviewing principles and practices* (4th ed.). Dubuque, IA: William C. Brown.

Sundeen, S. J., Stuart, G. W., Rankin, E. D., et al. (1989). *Nurse–client interaction: Implementing the nursing process* (4th ed.). St. Louis, MO: C. V. Mosby.

Tompkins, E. S. (1989). In support of the discipline of nursing: A nursing assessment. *Nursingconnections, 2*(3), 21–29.

Wake, M. M. (1990). Nursing care delivery systems: Status and vision. *Journal of Nursing Administration, 20*(5), 47–51.

Yura, H., & Walsh, M. B. (1988). *The nursing process: Assessing, planning, implementing, evaluating* (5th ed.). Norwalk, CT: Appleton and Lange.

Bibliography

Davis, M. J., & Nomura, L. A. (1990). Vital signs of class I surgical patients. *Western Journal of Nursing Research, 12*(1), 28–41.

Fawcett, J. (1989). *Analysis and evaluation of conceptual models of nursing* (2nd ed.). Philadelphia: F. A. Davis.

Itano, J. K. (1989). A comparison of the clinical judgment process in experienced registered nurses and student nurses. *Journal of Nursing Education, 28,* 120–126.

Mulhearn, S. (1989). The nursing process: Improving psychiatric admission assessment. *Journal of Advanced Nursing, 14,* 808–814.

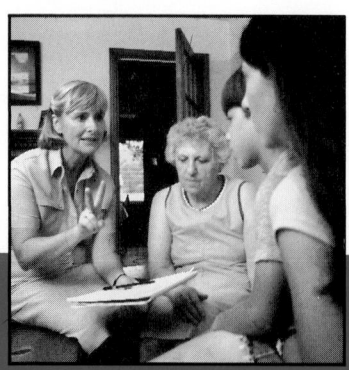

Nursing Diagnosis

LEARNING OBJECTIVES

Upon completion of this chapter, the student will be able to do the following:

- Define diagnosis in relation to the nursing process.
- State the meaning of nursing diagnosis.
- Describe the components of a nursing diagnosis.
- Discuss the significance of nursing diagnosis for nursing practice.
- Differentiate between a nursing diagnosis and other health-care problems.
- Identify the clinical skills needed to make nursing diagnoses.
- Formulate nursing diagnoses given a patient situation.
- Discuss the categorization of nursing diagnoses by functional health patterns.

KEY TERMS

Actual nursing diagnosis
Cluster
Collaborative health problem
Cue
High risk nursing diagnosis
Medical diagnosis
Nursing diagnosis
Possible nursing diagnosis
Taxonomy
Validation

8

Historical Development
Nursing Diagnosis Taxonomy
  What is a Taxonomy?
  Nursing Diagnosis Taxonomy Development
   Human Response Patterns
Nursing Diagnoses and Other Health-Care Problems
Components of a Nursing Diagnosis
  Diagnostic Label
  Qualifiers
  Definition
  Defining Characteristics
  Risk Factors
  Related Factors

Diagnosis Activities
  Identify Pattern
   Cue Clustering
   Cluster Interpretation
  Validate Diagnosis
  Formulate the Diagnostic Statement
   Actual Nursing Diagnoses
   High-Risk Nursing Diagnoses
   Possible Nursing Diagnoses
Significance of Nursing Diagnosis
Nursing Diagnoses Organized by Functional Health Patterns
Key Concepts

Diagnosing human responses to actual or potential health problems is the second phase of the nursing process. After the nurse collects relevant patient information, the data needs to be analyzed and interpreted. The result of this interpretation is the nursing diagnosis. This term serves as both the label and the action of describing a patient's functional health problems. Registered nurses are the health care professionals educated and licensed to make nursing diagnoses. As such, nurses have a duty to identify and plan patient management based on nursing diagnoses.

The North American Nursing Diagnosis Association (NANDA) defines a **nursing diagnosis** as

> . . . a clinical judgment about individual, family, or community responses to actual or potential health problems/life processes. Nursing diagnoses provide the basis for selection of nursing interventions to achieve outcomes for which the nurse is accountable (NANDA, 1990).

The term, nursing diagnosis, serves as both the label and the action of describing a patient's functional health problems. The purpose of a nursing diagnosis is to identify problems and synthesize the information gathered during the nursing assessment. Reasons for doing this are to:

- Analyze collected data
- Identify the patient's strengths
- Identify the patient's normal functional level and indicators of actual or potential dysfunction
- Formulate a diagnostic statement in relation to this synthesis.

In the diagnosis phase, the nurse does the following:

- Identifies patterns
- Validates the diagnosis
- Formulates the nursing diagnosis statement.

Figure 8-1 shows the diagnosis phase in relation to the other phases of the nursing process.

HISTORICAL DEVELOPMENT*

As early as 1926, Harmer suggested that nurses should include problem statements when documenting patient care. In 1947, Lesnich and Anderson argued that diagnosis was within the scope of nursing practice. Fry (1953)

*Acknowledgment is made to Margaret Lunney (1990) for the outline for this section.

111

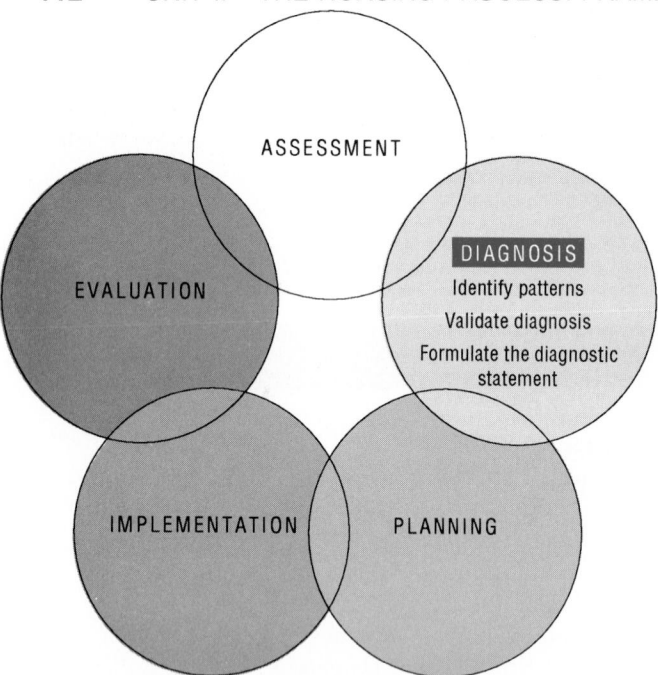

Figure 8–1. The relationship of nursing diagnosis to the entire nursing process.

is generally credited with the first use of the term nursing diagnosis in the nursing literature. During the 1960s, a series of research studies focused on the nurse's ability to make clinical judgments using patient cues (Hammond, 1966). These studies revealed that knowledge and interpretation varied widely and that the terms used to describe patient problems were not standardized.

In 1972, Gordon completed her dissertation on diagnostic reasoning in nursing. The formal development of the identification and classification of nursing diagnoses began with the 1st National Conference on the Classification of Nursing Diagnoses convened by Gebbie and Lavin in 1973.

Although implied in the assessment phase of the nursing process (Yura & Walsh, 1973, 1988), nursing diagnosis emerged as a separate phase in the early 1970s. Recognition of the act of diagnosing was made explicit by the American Nurses Association (ANA) in *Standards of Nursing Practice* (1973). It gained further support when the ANA included diagnosis as a separate activity in *Nursing: A Social Policy Statement* (1980). Since that time, most state nurse practice acts have included diagnosis as part of the domain of nursing practice for which the nurse is held accountable. Standards developed by the Joint Commission on the Accreditation of Healthcare Organizations (JCAHO) mandate that "each patient's nursing care is based on identified nursing diagnoses and/or patient care needs" (JCAHO, 1990, p. 132).

Nurses continue to develop new nursing diagnoses, refine existing diagnoses, and organize them into a classification system useful to practicing nurses. NANDA has been the leader in nursing diagnosis classification

and has been endorsed by the ANA as having the responsibility to do so. To date, nine conferences have been held to refine the classification system for nursing diagnoses.

NURSING DIAGNOSIS TAXONOMY

Professions require a sound scientific base; the nursing process is nursing's scientific base. To achieve this scientific foundation, nursing requires a **taxonomy,** or classification system, to provide a structure for nursing practice. According to Kritek, "the generation and classification of nursing diagnoses is an embryonic theory with significant potential for the nursing profession" (1979, p. 122). Developing a classification system for nursing diagnoses involves a knowledge of nursing practice, theoretical frameworks, and the characteristics of taxonomies. The North American Nursing Diagnosis Association (NANDA) has been acknowledged by the nursing profession as the leader in nursing diagnosis classification. To date, nine conferences have been held to suggest a classification system for nursing diagnoses. In order to understand the complexity of this task, a discussion of types of taxonomies and the selection of a nursing taxonomy is presented below.

What is a Taxonomy?

A taxonomy is a method for ordering complex information. Each classification system is based on a single principle or set of principles (criteria). These principles establish the ground rules for the selection and placement of individual elements in the system. A simple example of an ordering system is an outline:

I.
   A.
   B.
   C.
      1.
      2.
         a.
         b.

The set (in this case, I, II, III) is a well-defined collection. The subset is a smaller unit or category of the set (A, B, C). These elements, or subsets, can be further subdivided into smaller units (1 or 2, a or b). The further down the classification, the more concrete the unit becomes. It may name a real thing or may be observable and measurable.

An example of a simple classification system is the dictionary: words are grouped under each letter of the alphabet, which simplifies finding them. (Imagine searching for a word in the dictionary arranged with no organizing principle; it would be mind-boggling.) Mathematics also uses a precise hierarchical arrangement with definitions for each category and mutually exclusive and exhaustive classes.

The goal of a taxonomy is to produce a workable classification system. If the system is too complex, it confuses its users. But if the system is too simple, the categories may be vague and there may be duplication. "In every system the component classes must have something different. Without the sameness there is no identifiable class; without the differences there are no discrete entities to group" (Gebbie & Lavin, 1975, p. 34).

The classification of diseases has been evolving since the 1770's. Today, the most widely accepted classification system of diseases is the International Classification of Diseases-9-CM (ICD-9-CM). It is constantly undergoing revision, and NANDA and the ANA are working to incorporate nursing diagnoses into this system. The ICD-9-CM codes diseases by cause or manifestation. Other classification systems include SNO MED, the Systemized Nomenclature of Medicine, published by the College of American Pathologists, and CPT, or Current Procedural Terminology, published by the American Medical Association. In psychiatry, the Diagnostic and Statistical Manual of Mental Disorders, or DSM-III-R, is used to classify mental health disorders. All of these systems respond to changes in epidemiology, as well as changing practice, to maintain accuracy.

The development of a nursing diagnosis taxonomy has bee the goal of the North American Nursing Diagnosis Association.

Nursing Diagnosis Taxonomy Development

NANDA's goal has been to develop a nursing diagnosis taxonomy. At the first conference in 1973, 86 nursing diagnoses were listed alphabetically and published for use and development by all registered nurses (Gebbie & Lavin, 1975). There was no claim as to the validity of the diagnoses, nor was the list considered a final one. No classification system was selected.

Through the first six conferences, the listing of nursing diagnoses remained an alphabetical one, but attention was being given to the selection of a classification system. Nursing theorists were involved with the classification from the outset, and in 1977 were formally asked to participate in the development of the classification system.

As of 1990, 99 nursing diagnoses had been accepted by NANDA for clinical use and testing.

A summary of the activities of each conference is presented in Table 8-1. To illustrate the development of the taxonomy, one nursing diagnosis, *Grieving,* has been selected to highlight changes made throughout the nine conferences. The numbers indicate its placement in the classification system.

Human Response Patterns

The complete NANDA Taxonomy I (Rev.) is presented in the display. The nursing diagnoses are organized according to human response patterns: exchanging, communicating, relating, valuing, choosing, moving, perceiving, knowing, and feeling. Human response patterns characterize the essence of nursing practice. Each pattern describes an abstract concept; taken together, the patterns describe the alterations of human responses that nurses are prepared and educated to treat.

As abstract labels, the titles of each pattern are intended to be inclusive of all the nursing diagnoses that fit that particular pattern. The more detailed the taxonomy, the more concrete (real) and clinically useful the entity becomes. This specificity enables the nurse to plan and deliver care that is tailored to resolve specific patient problems. (Consider the nursing care needs of a patient unable to feed himself compared to a patient who cannot dress himself.) The ability and knowledge to assist patients in resolving clearly identified problems enables the nurse to demonstrate what *nursing* does in providing health-care services.

Not all nursing diagnoses are at the same level. Some are broadly stated concepts that must be individualized before they can become clinically useful. In practice nurses continue to identify new nursing diagnoses and refine existing ones.

Each human response pattern is presented below, with a definition and description of the nursing diagnoses included in each. This overview illustrates where there are gaps in nursing knowledge, suggests directions for nursing research, and provides guidance for implementing specific interventions and evaluating patient outcomes.

Pattern 1. Exchanging. This pattern involves mutual giving and receiving; to give, relinquish, or lose: giving up something while receiving something in return. The nursing diagnoses are mostly physiologic. The major concepts are nutrition, physical regulation, elimination, circulation, oxygenation, and physical integrity.

Pattern 2. Communicating. This pattern involves sending messages; to convey, impart, confer, or transmit thoughts, feelings, or information, either verbally or nonverbally. The only nursing diagnosis in this pattern is Impaired Verbal Communication, but alterations in nonverbal communication probably exist. Other communication problems, as yet undefined, may be described in the future.

Pattern 3. Relating. This pattern involves establishing bonds; to connect, to establish a link between, to stand in some association to another thing, person, or place. The major concepts in this pattern are socialization, parenting, and sexuality. There is recognition of the individual as well as the family unit.

TABLE 8–1

Summary of the Classification of Nursing Diagnosis Conferences

Year/#	Accomplishments	Chronological Development of the Nursing Diagnosis: Grieving
1973 1st National Conference	86 nursing diagnoses identified, listed alphabetically Establishment of clearinghouse for nursing diagnoses	11.73 Grieving 11.74 Normal Grieving 11.75 Normal Grieving, Potential 11.76 11.77 Arrested Grieving 11.78 Arrested Grieving, Potential 11.79 Delayed Onset of Grieving 11.80 Delayed Onset of Grieving, Potential
1975 2nd National Conference	Further identification of nursing diagnoses, listed alphabetically	11.73 Grieving, Acute 11.76 Grieving, Anticipatory 11.77 Grieving, Delayed
1978 3rd National Conference	Diagnoses listed alphabetically "Unitary Man"schema introduced as classification	11.73 Grieving
1980 4th National Conference	Patterns of nursing diagnoses discussed, no definite recommendations Diagnoses listed alphabetically	11.73 Grieving, Dysfunctional 11.74 Delete 11.75 Delete 11.76 Grieving, Anticipatory 11.77 Delete 11.78 Delete 11.79 Delete 11.80 Delete
1982 5th National Conference	Patterns of Unitary Man described Diagnoses listed alphabetically Vote to become NANDA	Grieving, Anticipatory Grieving, Dysfunctional
1984 6th Conference	First conference open to nursing public Further refinement to patterns of unitary man Diagnoses listed alphabetically	Grieving, Anticipatory Grieving, Dysfunctional
1986 7th Conference	Endorsement of NANDA Taxonomy I Human response patterns replaced patterns of unitary man Development of rules for submission of new diagnoses	9.2.2 Grieving 9.2.2.1 Dysfunctional 9.2.2.2 Anticipatory 9.2.2.3
1988 8th Conference	Endorsement of NANDA Taxonomy I (rev.)	9.2.1.1 Dysfunctional Grieving 9.2.1.2 Anticipatory Grieving
1990 9th Conference	NANDA Taxonomy II proposed Definition of nursing diagnosis approved	9.2.1.1 Dysfunctional Grieving 9.2.1.2 Anticipatory Grieving

Pattern 4. Valuing. This pattern involves the assigning of relative worth; to be concerned about, to care, to equate in importance. The only nursing diagnosis in this pattern is Spiritual Distress, but again there is a presumed lack of completeness and need for further development in this area.

Pattern 5. Choosing. This pattern involves the selection of alternatives; to determine in favor of a course; to decide in accordance with inclinations. The nursing diagnoses range from Coping to Noncompliance. Two distinct concepts, coping and participation, are evident. The individual and family are recognized by accepted diagnoses; the community is a discrete entity yet to be described.

Pattern 6. Moving. This pattern involves activity; to change the place or position; to put or keep in motion. There are several nursing diagnoses in this category. The main concepts are activity, rest, recreation, and activities of daily living.

Pattern 7. Perceiving. This pattern involves the reception of information; to apprehend what is not open or present to observation. The nursing diagnoses include Disturbance in Body Image, Self-Esteem, or Personal Identity; Visual, Sensory-Perceptual Alterations; Hopelessness; and Powerlessness. The major concepts are self-concept, sensory responses, and meaningfulness.

Pattern 8. Knowing. This pattern involves the mean-

Approved Nursing Diagnoses NANDA, 1990, Organized by Human Response Patterns

PATTERN 1: EXCHANGING
  Altered Nutrition: More Than Body Requirements
  Altered Nutrition: Less Than Body Requirements
  Altered Nutrition: Potential for More than Body Requirements
  High Risk for Infection*
  High Risk for Altered Body Temperature*
  Hypothermia
  Hyperthermia
  Ineffective Thermoregulation
  Dysreflexia
  Constipation
  Perceived Constipation
  Colonic Constipation
  Diarrhea
  Bowel Incontinence
  Altered Urinary Elimination
  Stress Incontinence
  Reflex Incontinence
  Urge Incontinence
  Functional Incontinence
  Total Incontinence
  Urinary Retention
  Altered (specify type) Tissue Perfusion (renal, cerebral, cardiopulmonary, gastrointestinal, peripheral)
  Fluid Volume Excess
  Fluid Volume Deficit
  High Risk for Fluid Volume Deficit*
  Decreased Cardiac Output
  Impaired Gas Exchange
  Ineffective Airway Clearance
  Ineffective Breathing Pattern
  High Risk for Injury*
  High Risk for Suffocation*
  High Risk for Poisoning*
  High Risk for Trauma*
  High Risk for Aspiration*
  High Risk for Disuse Syndrome*
  Altered Protection
  Impaired Tissue Integrity
  Altered Oral Mucous Membrane
  Impaired Skin Integrity
  High Risk for Impaired Skin Integrity*
PATTERN 2: COMMUNICATING
  Impaired Verbal Communication
PATTERN 3: RELATING
  Impaired Social Interaction
  Social Isolation

  Altered Role Performance
  Altered Parenting
  High Risk for Altered Parenting*
  Sexual Dysfunction
  Altered Family Processes
  Parental Role Conflict
  Altered Sexuality Patterns
PATTERN 4: VALUING
  Spiritual Distress (distress of the human spirit)
PATTERN 5: CHOOSING
  Ineffective Individual Coping
  Impaired Adjustment
  Defensive Coping
  Ineffective Denial
  Ineffective Family Coping: Disabling
  Ineffective Family Coping: Compromised
  Family Coping: Potential for Growth
  Noncompliance (specify)
  Decisional Conflict (specify)
  Health-Seeking Behaviors (specify)
PATTERN 6: MOVING
  Impaired Physical Mobility
  Activity Intolerance
  Fatigue
  High Risk for Activity Intolerance*
  Sleep Pattern Disturbance
  Diversional Activity Deficit
  Impaired Home Maintenance Management
  Altered Health Maintenance
  Feeding Self-Care Deficit
  Impaired Swallowing
  Ineffective Breastfeeding
  Effective Breastfeeding
  Bathing/Hygiene Self-Care Deficit
  Dressing/Grooming Self-Care Deficit
  Toileting Self-Care Deficit
  Altered Growth and Development
PATTERN 7: PERCEIVING
  Body Image Disturbance
  Self-Esteem Disturbance
  Chronic Low Self-Esteem
  Situational Low Self-Esteem
  Personal Identity Disturbance
  Sensory/Perceptual Alterations (specify) (visual, auditory, kinesthetic, gustatory, tactile, olfactory)
  Unilateral Neglect
  Hopelessness
  Powerlessness
PATTERN 8: KNOWING
  Knowledge Deficit (specify)
  Altered Thought Processes

(continued)

Approved Nursing Diagnoses NANDA, 1990, Organized by Human Response Patterns (continued)

PATTERN 9: FEELING
  Pain
  Chronic Pain
  Dysfunctional Grieving
  Anticipatory Grieving
  High Risk for Violence: Self-Directed or
    Directed at Others*

Post-Trauma Response
Rape-Trauma Syndrome
Rape-Trauma Syndrome: Compound Reaction
Rape-Trauma Syndrome: Silent Reaction
Anxiety
Fear

* These diagnoses were formerly lableled "Potential for."

ing associated with information; to be cognizant of something through observation, inquiry, or information. The nursing diagnoses include Knowledge Deficit and Altered Thought Processes. The main concepts are knowledge, learning, and thinking. This pattern clearly indicates a need to be able to describe more clearly the subsets of knowing.

Pattern 9. Feeling. This pattern involves the subjective awareness of information; to be consciously or emotionally affected by a fact, event, or state. The nursing diagnoses in this pattern include Pain, Grieving, Post-Trauma Response, Rape-Trauma Syndrome, Violence, Anxiety, and Fear. The major concepts are loss, aggression, and mental or physical distress.

NURSING DIAGNOSES AND OTHER HEALTH-CARE PROBLEMS

Nursing diagnoses must be distinguished from medical diagnoses. A **medical diagnosis** describes a disease or pathology for which treatment focuses on correcting or preventing specific pathology of specific organs or body systems. Medical diagnoses convey information about the signs and symptoms of disease processes and provide a convenient means of communicating treatment requirements. The physician focuses on treating the underlying pathology.

In contrast, a nursing diagnosis describes an actual or high-risk human response to a health problem that

TABLE 8–2

Comparison of Nursing Diagnoses with Collaborative Problems and Medical Diagnoses

	Nursing Diagnoses	**Collaborative Problems and Medical Diagnoses**
Focus of assessment activities	Main focus is on monitoring human responses to actual and potential health problems.	Main focus is on monitoring for pathophysiologic response of body organs or systems.
Problem identification	Nurse identifies and validates that problem exists independently.	Nurse may identify problem but is required to refer to physician for validation that problem exists (may require additional diagnostic studies to label the problem). Nurse may not be qualified to diagnose exact nature of problem, but refers abnormal data to physician.
Treatment	Nurse initiates interventions for treatment independently.	Nurse collaborates with physician to initiate interventions for treatment. Nurse may have standing orders from physician or institution (delegated authority) to initiate diagnostic studies or treatment interventions for the problem without physician's orders.

From Alfaro, R. (1990). *Applying nursing diagnosis and nursing process: A step-by-step guide* (2nd ed.). Philadelphia: J. B. Lippincott, p. 67.

nurses are responsible for treating independently. Nursing diagnoses describe the patient's response to the disease process, developmental stage, or life change and provide a convenient way to communicate nursing therapies or interventions.

Nursing diagnoses carry legal ramifications. Only those health-care problems within the scope of nursing practice can be identified as nursing diagnoses. The nurse cannot diagnose a medical disease and is not licensed to treat such problems. Care must be taken to identify patient problems within the scope, practice abilities, and education of the registered nurse.

When identifying problems from assessment data, the nurse determines if the problem is one that can be addressed legally and independently by nurses; if so, it is a nursing diagnosis. If the problem requires both medical treatment and nursing treatment, however, it is a **collaborative health problem.** A collaborative problem refers to actual or potential physiologic complications that can result from disease, trauma, treatment, or diagnostic studies for which nurses intervene in collaboration with other disciplines (Carpenito, 1992, p. 38).

Table 8-2 compares nursing diagnoses with collaborative and medical diagnoses, and Figure 8-2 shows how a nurse makes these determinations.

Procedures, medical terminology, symptoms, patient needs, and treatments are often confused with nursing diagnoses. For example, if the nurse writes "Foley catheter," this is a treatment, not the response the patient may have to the treatment. Other examples include "need for oxygen" or "dyspnea," terms that describe symptoms and do not provide enough information to validate the presence of a nursing diagnosis. Another common mistake is to write "lack of adequate nutrition" as the nursing diagnosis. This phrase describes a patient need, but it is not a nursing diagnosis. The nursing diagnosis, in this case, would be Altered Nutrition: Less Than Body Requirements.

The following list shows the proper use of a variety of terms for a patient with a specific breathing problem. These terms are often confused.

- Medical diagnosis: Pneumonia
- Nursing diagnosis: Ineffective Airway Clearance Related to Tracheobronchial Secretions
- Patient need: Oxygenation
- Procedure: Bronchoscopy
- Treatment: Oxygen therapy.

Formulating an accurate nursing diagnosis is a clinical judgment, but nursing diagnoses should not be written in judgmental terms. For example, it is incorrect to write "failure to carry out medical regimen related to drug use." The reasons for the patient's noncompliance with the regimen should be explored and analyzed to avoid labeling or stereotyping a patient's behavior based on insufficient evidence.

COMPONENTS OF A NURSING DIAGNOSIS

The parts of a nursing diagnosis are the diagnostic label, definition, defining characteristics (major and minor), risk factors, related factors, and qualifiers. All of the

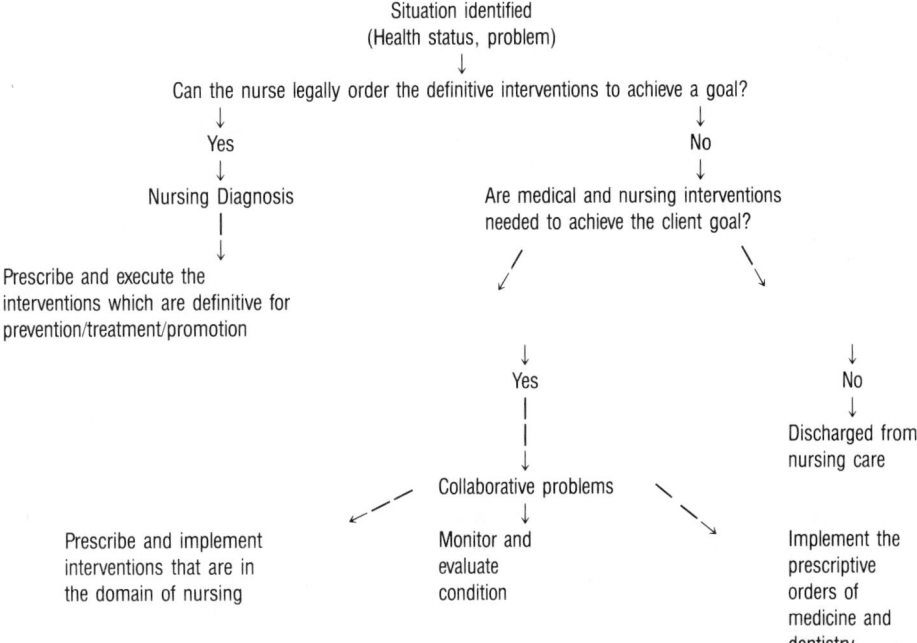

Figure 8–2. Differentiating a nursing diagnosis from other client problems. (From Carpenito, L. (1992). *Nursing diagnosis: Approach to Clinical Practice* (4th ed.). Philadelphia: J. B. Lippincott, p. 40.)

diagnoses discussed in Section II describe each of these points.

Diagnostic Label

The diagnostic label is the name of the nursing diagnosis, as listed in the taxonomy display. It describes the essence of the problem using as few words as possible. Some examples are Stress Incontinence, Anxiety, and Self-Care Deficit. Each nursing diagnosis represents a pattern of related patient cues.

Qualifiers

Qualifiers are words used to give additional meaning to the nursing diagnosis. They describe changes in condition, state of the patient, or some quantification of the specific nursing diagnosis. They accompany the label in the Taxonomy display. Examples used by NANDA include:

- Altered: a change from baseline
- Impaired: made worse, weakened, damaged, reduced, deteriorated
- Depleted: emptied wholly or partially exhausted of
- Deficient: inadequate in amount, quality, or degree; defective, not sufficient, incomplete
- Excessive: greater than necessary, desirable, or useful
- Dysfunctional: abnormal or incomplete
- Disturbed: agitated, interrupted, or interfered with
- Ineffective: not producing the desired effect
- Decreased: smaller in size, amount, or degree
- Increased: greater in size, amount, or degree
- Acute: severe or of short duration
- Chronic: lasting a long time, recurring, or constant
- Intermittent: stopping and starting again at intervals.

Definition

Each nursing diagnosis approved by NANDA for clinical use and testing has a definition that describes the characteristics of the human response under consideration. For example, the definition of the diagnostic label Hypothermia is "the state in which an individual's body temperature is reduced below normal range" (NANDA, 1990, p. 15).

Defining Characteristics

Defining characteristics are the major and minor clinical cues that validate the presence of and *actual nursing diagnosis*. Each piece of patient information is considered a clinical cue; a set of clinical cues forms a cluster that is present if the diagnosis is accurate.

Major defining characteristics are present 80% to 100% of the time in researched nursing diagnoses and 100% of the time in nonresearched ones. Minor defining characteristics are present 50% to 79% of the time in researched nursing diagnoses and less than 100% of the time in nonresearched ones (NANDA, 1990).

Risk Factors

The term *risk factors* is used to described clinical cues in *high risk nursing diagnoses*. They are identifiable intrinsic (inside, somatic) and extrinsic (outside, environmental) characteristics of the patient. The presence of specific risk factors indicate that the individual, family, or community is vulnerable to or at risk for a particular problem. Examples of risk factors for the nursing diagnosis High Risk for Fluid Volume Deficit include extremes of age, physical immobility, and excessive losses. If the risk factors are not addressed, a potential problem may well become an actual problem.

Related Factors

Related factors describe the etiology or likely cause of the problem. Although there is usually not a direct causal relationship between the nursing diagnosis and the cause, some relationship can be described. Terms that can be used are "associated with," "related to," or "contributing to." Identifying related factors helps the nurse to develop specific interventions to resolve the health problem. For example, different nursing interventions would be used in caring for a patient with Stress Incontinence related to high intra-abdominal pressure than for a patient with Stress Incontinence related to overdistention between voidings.

DIAGNOSIS ACTIVITIES

Identify Pattern

After the nurse completes the patient assessment, the data obtained are analyzed to identify specific patient problems. The data, both subjective symptoms and objective signs, form **cues.** All data are examined but not all will be clustered to identify problems. Significant cues to be clustered are subjective and objective data that deviate from standards or from what is considered normal. Several cues form a **cluster,** which is then interpreted and validated. The end result is a nursing diagnostic label that accurately reflects the specific patient problem. Because the clustering, interpretation, and validation of these patient cues is integral to nursing practice, each step will be described separately. It should be noted, however, that this process is cyclical; that is, as new information is obtained, new cue patterns may emerge and cue clusters may change. As nurses develop skill in diagnosing patient problems, they may intuitively cluster information correctly rather than going through each step consciously (Benner & Tanner, 1987).

Cue Clustering

A cue is any piece of information, subjective or objective, that is collected during the nursing assessment. As cues are collected, some organizing of data has already taken place. Usually, the nurse uses a standardized assessment form (see Chap. 18) that automatically puts information into categories. Clustering goes beyond systems. Cue clustering brings together cues that, if viewed in separate systems, would not convey the same meaning. It is the purpose of cue clustering to take individual cues and group them to derive meaning from them.

Cue clustering can be compared with piecing together a puzzle. All the puzzle pieces form one picture (the patient problem); each piece is a cue. Figure 8-3 illustrates the puzzle concept. The puzzle shows a sky with a cloud. All the pieces of the puzzle with the cloud form a cluster. Placing the white cloud pieces into a cluster helps identify the pattern of the puzzle (the diagnosis). A separate and distinct cue cluster forms each nursing diagnosis. Taken together, all the cue clusters form one patient.

During cue clustering, the nurse uses critical thinking to analyze and synthesize the cues. Each cue is analyzed for its fit into a particular problem. The cues are then put together to form meaningful clusters that describe specific patient problems.

To see how this process works in a patient situation, use the following case study. Read the clinical example and then see which cues belong together in describing a particular problem.

> *Mr. J. M., a 42-year-old white carpenter, is admitted for surgical repair of a 10 × 20-cm sacral pressure ulcer. He has been a wheelchair-dependent quadriplegic for 6 months after a construction accident. He is not working, considers himself to be the provider for his family (wife and two children), and displays anger that his wife is paying the bills, working, and disciplining the children.*

Although the first tendency is to identify Impaired Skin Integrity as a nursing diagnosis—and it is present—the nurse should also look at other cues the patient has given. For the purpose of illustration, one nursing diagnosis has been selected, but the reader is encouraged to select other cues and describe additional nursing diagnoses that may be present. The relevant cues are:

- Not currently working
- Recent change from active, mobile individual to wheelchair-dependent quadriplegic person
- Considers self to be provider
- Anger at wife for carrying out role of breadwinner.

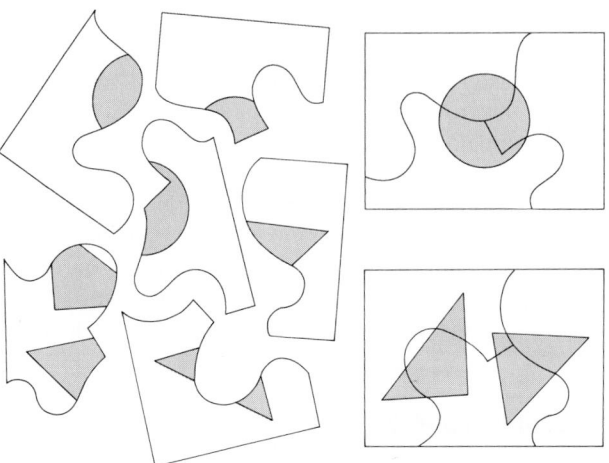

Figure 8–3. Collecting the puzzle pieces is assessment. Pieces that are similar form a cluster. Identifying the pattern and putting the puzzle together is nursing diagnosis. Other parts of the puzzle (a tree, for instance) would form another diagnosis. All the clusters form one patient.

Taken together, these cues fit the defining characteristics of a specific nursing diagnosis. The knowledgeable nurse will recognize this cue cluster and proceed with the next step, cluster interpretation. But before doing that, some of the problems that can occur in cue clustering must be described.

Problems in Cue Clustering. The major problems in cue clustering are insufficient cues, inaccurate cues, and inconsistent cues. Skill in cue clustering comes with experience and practice. The beginning practitioner should expect to use a variety of reference materials to develop these skills.

Having insufficient cues is a problem: the nurse cannot plan effective care because the problem cannot be determined with confidence. Using the clinical example, the nurse might select the cue 10 × 20 sacral pressure ulcer, and write this nursing diagnosis: Impaired Skin Integrity related to immobilization. But not enough information has been presented in the case to lead to this conclusion. This lack of adequate cues can also be called premature closure, selecting a diagnosis before analyzing pertinent information. Additional cues that would be needed in this example are the characteristics of the pressure ulcer (size, depth, color, exudate), patient knowledge about skin care regimens, patient's perception of why the problem occurred, medical treatment planned, nutritional status, self-care abilities, and frequency of pressure-relieving activities.

Not accurately clustering the cues is a problem because the nurse may cluster unrelated information and make judgments based on incorrect clusters. Inaccuracy in clustering occurs when the nurse is unfamiliar with the diagnosis, or when the cues for different diagnoses overlap. If, for example, the cues wheelchair-dependent quadriplegic, not working, and anger are clustered and the nursing diagnosis of Impaired Mobility related to dependency is made, nursing interventions will be geared toward resolving the dependency, not the problem of impaired mobility.

Inconsistent cues are a problem because the meaning attached to one cue may be altered based on another cue. For example, one patient may say that she cannot eat a regular diet, but is later seen eating a steak and potatoes. Because the cues do not match, further information is needed to validate the problem and the cues.

Cluster Interpretation

Cluster interpretation means synthesizing the cue clusters. It is an intellectual activity that requires the nurse to see the whole picture and to attach meaning to the cluster, looking at the pattern the cluster suggests. It is the ability to derive the meaning and implications of the human response for a patient. In the clinical example used above, the cue cluster was presented. Please review it now and think of possible nursing diagnoses.

Clinical Examples. The following nursing diagnoses are listed as possible choices from the situation presented above:

Ineffective Individual Coping related to dependency. Cues: anger, wheelchair-dependent quadriplegic.
Impaired Adjustment related to disability requiring change in lifestyle. Cues: wheelchair-dependent quadriplegic for 6 months, not working.
Altered Role Performance related to recent change. Cues: not working, anger at wife for carrying out breadwinner role, perceives self as provider, recent change from active, mobile person to wheelchair-dependent quadriplegic.

Analyzing these suggested nursing diagnostic statements would involve reviewing each definition and associated defining characteristics.

The first two cannot be supported by clinical cues. Ineffective Individual Coping relies on two cues that are not defining characteristics of this diagnosis. This diagnosis requires evidence of a patient's verbalization of the inability to cope or ask for help or the inability to solve problems. More information is needed to support the use of this diagnosis. The diagnosis of Impaired Adjustment may or may not describe this patient. The nurse has assumed that by becoming a wheelchair-dependent quadriplegic, this patient has not made a satisfactory adjustment to his new lifestyle. The presence of additional defining characteristics would be needed to evaluate the presence of this problem.

In the third diagnosis, Altered Role Performance, all the cues supporting the defining characteristics for this diagnosis are present. The patient had a change in the perception of his role, change in his physical capacity to resume a previous role, and change in his usual patterns of responsibility, and there is evidence of conflict, as shown by his anger toward his wife. The nurse can make this diagnosis with confidence and plan nursing interventions to assist the patient in resolving this problem.

Problems in Cluster Interpretation. The analysis of cue clusters can be impeded by incorrect clustering of data and misinterpretation of cue clusters. "Making a clinical inference from several pieces of data requires theoretical knowledge, experience, and the use of cognition" (Fredette, 1988, p. 33).

If the cues are not clustered correctly, the nurse cannot make accurate clinical judgments. For example, if the cues malnourished, feeds self, and dependent in mobility are clustered, the nurse may arrive at the erroneous diagnosis of Self-Care Deficit related to inadequate intake. There is no information here about the daily intake of food. The fact that the patient feeds himself does not explain the cue of dependent in mobility. Does the patient use assistive devices? What is the state of malnourishment? Are supplemental feedings being given? By forming this particular cue cluster, the nurse has neglected other important areas for analysis. In this example, these include defining characteristics for the nursing diagnoses of Altered Nutrition: Less Than Body Requirements and Impaired Physical Mobility.

Misinterpretation of cue clusters occurs when the nurse fails to recognize the correct pattern. This can happen if the nurse is unfamiliar with the nursing diagnosis or is inexperienced in relating these particular cues. If the defining characteristics for the diagnosis under consideration are complex and require extensive analysis for correct interpretation, it would be prudent to ask an experienced clinician to assist in interpreting the cues.

Validate Diagnosis

After a nursing diagnosis is selected (Altered Role Performance, in the clinical example), it should be validated with the patient (Fig. 8-4). **Validation** legitimizes the diagnosis and helps to discover its significance for the patient. The patient may deny that there is a problem, may not want to deal with it, or may acknowledge it but want to deal with it later. These are acceptable reasons for not dealing with an identified diagnosis, but the presence of the problem and its status should be documented. For most problems, the patient will agree that there is a dysfunctional health pattern problem that can be resolved with nursing assistance.

Diagnostic validation occurs in two stages. In the first stage, the cue clusters that have been interpreted are compared to norms for the patient and for patients in general. In the second stage, the specific nursing diag-

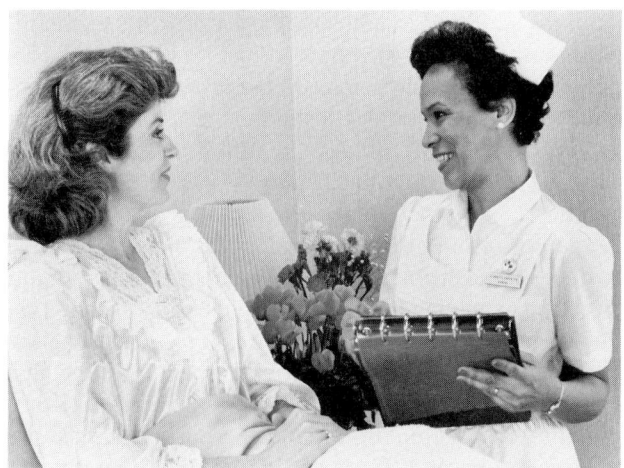

Figure 8–4. The nurse and patient work together to establish a nursing diagnosis and make plans for further care.

nosis is evaluated for its nursing research base. This research base is different for each nursing diagnosis.

In the clinical example, these diagnoses may be made if additional collection identifies cues to support them:

- Ineffective Individual Coping
- Impaired Adjustment
- Impaired Skin Integrity

For each of these diagnoses, the nurse should talk with the patient about the significance of the problem, determine the patient's perception of the reason for the problem, and ask the patient if help is desired to resolve or diminish the problem. Some patients are not ready or motivated to seek help even when a problem clearly exists.

Problems in Diagnostic Validation. Problems can occur in diagnostic validation because of limited experience of the nurse, lack of a knowledge base about the nursing diagnosis, or insufficient research to support the defining characteristics of a diagnosis.

If the nurse has limited clinical experience, exposure to a variety of patients under the guidance of an instructor, mentor, or expert practitioner can provide an opportunity to practice these skills. Each nursing diagnosis and defining characteristics should be discussed and errors corrected. This requires a nonthreatening environment and patience and understanding from both parties. It is helpful to trace the steps taken to arrive at a particular problem; errors in logic or missing steps in the process can sometimes be identified and suggestions made for avoiding them.

The nurse who is not knowledgeable about a specific nursing diagnosis should refer to articles, books, or other materials that discuss the identification of the problem and its management. For example, the proceedings of the NANDA conferences on the classification of

nursing diagnoses and *Nursing Diagnosis: Applications to Clinical Practice* (Carpenito, 1990) can be used to learn about individual nursing diagnoses.

The problem of insufficient research about specific nursing diagnoses can be corrected by participating in clinical research studies sponsored by institutions, organizations, and individual researchers. The registered nurse has an obligation to contribute to the scientific development of the profession. Current research on nursing diagnoses can be found in nursing journals and the previously mentioned proceedings of the NANDA conferences. The term "nursing diagnosis" is listed as a subject heading in the *Cumulative Index for Nursing and Allied Health,* enabling the nurse to find nursing diagnosis information quickly.

Formulate the Diagnostic Statement

Formulating the nursing diagnostic statement involves writing the label of the actual, high-risk, or possible nursing diagnosis(es) that have been made through the nursing diagnostic process. The correct way of stating these diagnoses is presented in the following sections.

Actual Nursing Diagnoses

Actual nursing diagnoses describe a human response to a health problem that is currently being manifested. They are written as three-part statements: the diagnostic label, the related factors, and defining characteristics. The patient cues supporting the existence of the problem can be found in the documentation of the assessment data. In the nursing diagnosis statement, they are identified by "as manifested by."

Problems sometimes occur when the nurse inverts the label and the "related to" phrase. This problem can be avoided by determining the main focus of this problem (the diagnostic label), and the factor that is contributing to the patient's inability to resolve it (related factor).

Clinical Examples. Examples of accurate and inaccurate diagnostic statements for actual nursing diagnoses are presented below.

Accurate. Ineffective Airway Clearance related to increased secretions

Inaccurate. Airway Clearance, Ineffective: related to presence of yellow, purulent, thick secretions. (The nurse has reversed the label phrase and included cues in the "related to" section instead of summarizing this information into a succinct statement.)

Accurate. Impaired Physical Mobility related to pain

Inaccurate. Ineffective Movement related to surgical incision, which causes pain when moving. (The nurse has selected an incorrect qualifier, has not used an approved diagnostic label, has repeated the problem in the "related to" phrase, and has used a cue incorrectly.)

Nursing Research

Selected Nursing Research Studies

Aden, C. (1991). A validation study of NANDA's Taxonomy I. In R. M. Carroll-Johnson, *Classification of nursing diagnoses: Proceedings of the ninth conference.* Philadelphia: J. B. Lippincott.

Brutwitzki, G., Holmgren, C., & Maibusch, R. (1991). Validation of the defining characteristics of the nursing diagnosis: Ineffective Airway Clearance. In R. M. Carroll-Johnson, *Classification of nursing diagnoses: Proceedings of the ninth conference.* Philadelphia: J. B. Lippincott.

Del Bueno, D. J. (1990). Experience, education, and nurses' ability to make clinical judgments. *Nursing & Health Care, 11*(6), 290–294.

Henning, M. (1991). Comparison of nursing diagnostic statements using a functional health pattern and a health history/body systems format. In R. M. Carroll-Johnson, *Classification of nursing diagnoses: Proceedings of the ninth conference.* Philadelphia: J. B. Lippincott.

Possible Topics for Nursing Inquiry

- What is the relationship between years of nursing practice and the ability to recognize a cue cluster for a selected nursing diagnosis?
- Given a simulated patient database, what is the relationship between the number and accuracy of nursing diagnoses made by nurses educated about nursing diagnoses using two teaching methods?
- Are there nursing diagnoses that occur together in specific patient situations?
- Is the classification system used to organize nursing diagnoses valid and reliable?
- What is the cost-effectiveness of a reimbursement system using nursing diagnoses as the organizing framework?
- What is the minimum number of cues necessary to make a specific nursing diagnosis?

High Risk Nursing Diagnoses

NANDA has replaced the term "potential" with the term "high risk" because it is believed that this term is more descriptive of some patients' particular vulnerability to health problems. For example, all patients who are admitted to a hospital are at risk for infection. Some are at higher risk than others, however, such as a person with a compromised immune system, for instance. This terminology also could assist in third-part reimbursement for nursing care and is the term used in the ICD-10 list of nursing diagnoses. A **high risk nursing diagnosis,** as defined by NANDA, is a clinical judgment that a person, family, or community is more vulnerable to develop the problem than others in the same or similar situation. The diagnosis is supported by risk factors that guide nursing interventions to reduce or prevent the occurrence of the problem. Problems in identifying high risk nursing diagnoses include lack of knowledge of a patient's risk factor profile and the particular risks involved in care and treatment of the underlying health problem.

Clinical Examples. Examples of high risk nursing diagnosis statements are:

Accurate. High Risk for Activity Intolerance related to prolonged bedrest

Inaccurate. Activity Intolerance, High Risk for. (The nurse has reversed the phrases.)

Accurate. High Risk for Aspiration related to reduced level of consciousness

Inaccurate. High Risk for Secretions entering the airway from impaired swallowing. (The nurse has listed part of the definition and one of the risk factors in the label.)

Possible Nursing Diagnoses

A **possible nursing diagnosis** is made when there is not enough evidence to support the presence of the problem, but the nurse thinks that it is highly probable and wants to collect more information. The statement is phrased in the same way as an actual problem, except the "related to" phrase is "unknown cause."

An example of a possible nursing diagnosis statement is:

Accurate: Possible Impaired Adjustment related to unknown etiology. (One of the first interventions will be to collect additional assessment data.)

Inaccurate: Adjustment Impaired, Possibly due to recent car accident that resulted in quadriplegia. (The nurse has reversed the diagnostic label and included cues in the "related to" phrase.)

SIGNIFICANCE OF NURSING DIAGNOSIS

Nursing diagnoses provide a means of communicating the nursing requirements for patient care to other nurses, the health-care team, and the public. "Nursing

Nursing Diagnoses Organized by Functional Health Patterns

**Health Perception
and Health Management Pattern**

High Risk for Disuse Syndrome
Dysreflexia
Altered Health Maintenance
Health-Seeking Behaviors
High Risk for Infection
High Risk for Injury
Noncompliance
High Risk for Poisoning
Altered Protection
High Risk for Suffocation

Nutritional and Metabolic Pattern

High Risk for Altered Body Temperature
Effective Breastfeeding
Ineffective Breastfeeding
Fluid Volume Excess
Fluid Volume Deficit
High Risk for Fluid Volume Deficit
Hyperthermia
Hypothermia
Altered Nutrition: Less than Body Requirements
Altered Nutrition: More than Body Requirements
Altered Oral Mucous Membrane
Impaired Skin Integrity
High Risk for Impaired Skin Integrity
Impaired Swallowing
Ineffective Thermoregulation
Impaired Tissue Integrity

Elimination Pattern

Constipation
Diarrhea
Bowel Incontinence
Functional Incontinence
Reflex Incontinence
Stress Incontinence
Total Incontinence
Urge Incontinence
Altered Urinary Elimination
Urinary Retention

Sleep and Rest Pattern

Fatigue
Sleep Pattern Disturbance

Cognitive and Perceptual Pattern

Knowledge Deficit
Pain
Chronic Pain
Sensory/Perceptual Alterations
Altered Thought Process

Self-Perception or Self-Concept Pattern

Impaired Adjustment
Anxiety
Fear
Anticipatory Grieving
Hopelessness
Powerlessness
Personal Identity Disturbance
Chronic Low Self-Esteem
Self-Esteem Disturbance
Situational Low Self-Esteem
High Risk for Violence

Role or Relationship Pattern

Anticipatory Grieving
Dysfunctional Grieving
Altered Family Processes
Parental Role Conflict
Altered Parenting: Actual or High Risk for
Impaired Social Interaction
Social Isolation
Impaired Verbal Communication
High Risk for Violence

Sexuality and Reproductive Pattern

Rape-Trauma Syndrome
Sexual Dysfunction
Altered Sexuality Patterns

(continued)

Nursing Diagnoses Organized by Functional Health Patterns *(continued)*

Activity or Exercise Pattern

Activity Intolerance
Ineffective Airway Clearance
High Risk for Aspiration
Ineffective Breathing Pattern
Decreased Cardiac Output
Diversional Activity Deficit
Impaired Gas Exchange
Impaired Home Maintenance Management
Impaired Mobility
Unilateral Neglect
Self-Care Deficit
Altered Tissue Perfusion

Coping and Stress-Tolerance Pattern

Defensive Coping
Ineffective Denial
Family Coping
Ineffective Family Coping
Ineffective Individual Coping
Decisional Conflict
Dysfunctional Grieving

Value and Belief Pattern

Spiritual Distress

---

diagnoses facilitate the development of nursing autonomy and accountability by focusing the attention of nurses on the phenomena that are uniquely nursing and by providing a common language for communication of the phenomena" (Maas, 1986, p. 39). The nursing diagnostic labels can serve as shorthand for specific patient problems.

Although many nursing diagnoses need further research to be clinically useful, all of them have suggested lists of defining characteristics or risk factors that validate the existence of the problem. Making accurate nursing diagnoses helps to ensure that patients receive quality nursing care.

By focusing attention on the actual or potential health needs of patients, nursing diagnoses increase the specificity of nursing interventions for each patient. This specificity can be measured and monitored to make sure that effective interventions are acknowledged for their contribution to resolving the health care problem. Coding of nursing diagnoses in computerized systems allows direct reimbursement of nurses. This acknowledgment of nursing's specific contribution in resolving health problems advances the development of professional nursing practice.

Studies of specific nursing diagnoses improve our understanding of the nursing diagnostic process and contribute to examination of the nurse's role in health care. As nursing diagnoses become supported by research, a clear description of the scope of nursing practice will emerge. The development and publication of a taxonomy of nursing diagnoses should have a significant impact on practice, education, research, legislation, and nursing as a profession. A nursing diagnosis taxonomy will help to bridge the gap between knowledge and practice and will articulate the scope of nursing practice. This is essential to developing nursing's professional role in health care.

Each nurse will decide the usefulness of the nursing diagnosis taxonomy. As the profession develops, it is expected that the taxonomy will be critically reviewed, revised, and tested. For today's practitioner the taxonomy meets the need for organization of nursing diagnoses.

The limitations of NANDA Taxonomy I (Rev.) do not mean that it cannot or should not be used in clinical practice. In fact, all nurses have the opportunity and responsibility to use the taxonomy in practice. The challenge for each practitioner is to learn the concepts and skills required to assist clients by accurately diagnosing, planning, and implementing nursing care.

NURSING DIAGNOSES ORGANIZED BY FUNCTIONAL HEALTH PATTERNS

The nursing process and nursing diagnosis taxonomy continue to evolve. New nursing diagnoses are added and existing diagnoses are reworded. The human response pattern evolved from the Unitary Man classification. Gordon (1987) suggested a framework for the organization of nursing diagnoses based on her functional health patterns.

Functional health patterns offer a convenient way to cluster similar diagnoses. Since this book has a functional health focus and data collected during the assessment phase is discussed and organized in this fashion, it is useful to organize nursing diagnoses in the same manner. See the complete list of nursing diagnoses organized by functional health patterns in the display.

Reviewing the functional health patterns and possible nursing diagnoses for each pattern ensures that the nurse has given consideration to all actual, possible, or high-risk nursing diagnoses. In this manner, the nurse can ensure that physiologic problems do not overshadow the patient's emotional, social, or spiritual needs.

Key Concepts

- There is a direct link between the collection of assessment data and the identification of nursing diagnoses.
- Registered nurses are the health-care professionals educated and licensed to make nursing diagnoses.
- A nursing diagnosis is a clinical judgment about individual, family, or community responses to actual or potential health problems/life processes.
- Activities of nursing diagnoses are pattern identification, diagnostic validation, and formulation of the nursing diagnosis statement.
- NANDA-accepted nursing diagnoses currently are organized according to the human response pattern.
- A nursing diagnosis must address a problem within the scope and education of the registered nurse in which the nurse can intervene independently.
- The nurse is responsible and accountable to identify and treat collaborative problems, which focus on pathophysiologic responses, in collaboration with the physician.
- The parts of a nursing diagnosis are the diagnostic label, definition, defining characteristics (major and minor), risk factors, related factors, and qualifiers.
- A cue is a piece of information, subjective or objective, collected during the nursing assessment.
- Cluster interpretation is synthesis of the cue clusters. It is an intellectual activity requiring the ability to see the whole picture, attach meaning to the cluster, and discern the pattern the cluster suggests.
- Diagnostic validation occurs in two stages: comparing the clusters to norms, and evaluating the specific nursing diagnosis for its particular nursing research base.
- Formulating the nursing diagnostic statement involves writing the actual, high-risk, or possible nursing diagnosis(es).

References

Aden, C. (1992). A validation study of NANDA's Taxonomy I. In R. M. Carroll-Johnson, *Classification of nursing diagnoses: Proceedings of the ninth conference.* Philadelphia: J.B. Lippincott.

Alfaro, R. (1990). *Applying nursing diagnosis and nursing process: A step-by-step guide* (2nd ed.). Philadelphia: J. B. Lippincott.

American Nurses Association. (1973). *Standards of nursing practice.* Kansas City, MO: Author.

American Nurses Association. (1980). *Nursing: A social policy statement.* Kansas City, MO: Author.

Benner, P., & Tanner, C. (1987). Clinical judgment: How expert nurses use intuition. *American Journal of Nursing, 87,* 23–31.

Brutwitzki, G., Holmgren, C., & Maibusch, R. (1991). Validation of the defining characteristics of the nursing diagnosis: Ineffective Airway Clearance. In R. M. Carroll-Johnson, *Classification of nursing diagnoses: Proceedings of the ninth conference.* Philadelphia: J.B. Lippincott.

Carpenito, L. J. (1992). *Nursing diagnosis: Application to clinical practice* (4th ed.). Philadelphia: J. B. Lippincott.

Carroll-Johnson, R. M. (Ed.). (1989). *Classification of nursing diagnoses: Proceedings of the eighth conference.* Philadelphia: J. B. Lippincott.

Carroll-Johnson, R. M. (Ed.). (1992). *Classification of nursing diagnoses:* Proceedings of the ninth conference. Philadelphia: J. B. Lippincott.

Del Bueno, D. J. (1990). Experience, education, and nurses' ability to make clinical judgments. *Nursing & Health Care, 11*(6), 290–294.

Fredette, S. L. (1988). Common diagnostic errors. *Nurse Educator, 13*(3), 31–35.

Fry, V. (1953). The creative approach to nursing. *American Journal of Nursing, 53,* 301–302.

Gebbie, K., & Lavin, M. (1975). *Classification of nursing diagnoses: Proceedings from the first national conference.* St. Louis: C. V. Mosby.

Gordon, M. (1987). *Nursing diagnosis: Process and application* (2nd ed.). New York: McGraw-Hill.

Hammond, K. R. (1966). Clinical inference in nursing: A psychologist's viewpoint. *Nursing Research, 15,* 27–38.

Henning, M. (1991). Comparison of nursing diagnostic statements using a functional health pattern and a health history/body systems format. In R. M. Carroll-Johnson, *Classification of nursing diagnoses: Proceedings of the ninth conference.* Philadelphia: J. B. Lippincott.

Joint Commission on Accreditation of Healthcare Organizations. (1990). *Accreditation manual for hospitals.* Chicago: Author.

Kritek, P. (1979). The struggle to classify our diagnoses. *American Journal of Nursing, 79*(6), 122.

Lunney, M. (1990). *Concept of nursing diagnosis: History.* Prepared for NANDA. New York: Author.

Maas, M. L. (1986). Nursing diagnoses in a professional model of nursing: Keystones for effective nursing administration. *Journal of Nursing Administration, 16*(12), 39–42.

North American Nursing Diagnosis Association. (1990). *NANDA taxonomy I* (rev.). St. Louis: Author.

North American Nursing Diagnosis Association. (1990). *NANDA guidelines for submission.* St. Louis: Author.

Yura, H., & Walsh, M. B. (1973). *The nursing process.* Norwalk, CT: Appleton-Century-Crofts.

Yura, H., & Walsh, M. B. (1988). *The nursing process* (5th ed.). Norwalk, CT: Appleton & Lange.

Bibliography

Avant, K. C. (1990). The art and science in nursing diagnosis development. *Nursing Diagnosis, 1*(2), 51–55.

Aydelotte, M. (1987). Keynote address. In A. McLane, *Classification of nursing diagnoses: Proceedings of the seventh conference.* St. Louis: C. V. Mosby.

Fitzpatrick, J., Kerr, M., Saba, V., et al. (1989). Translating nursing diagnosis into ICD code. *American Journal of Nursing, 89*(4), 493–495.

Hurley, M. E. (Ed.). (1986). *Classification of nursing diagnoses: Proceedings of the sixth conference.* St. Louis: C. V. Mosby.

Kim, M. J., McFarland, G. K., & McLane, A. M. (Eds.) (1984). *Classification of nursing diagnoses: Proceedings of the fifth national conference.* St. Louis: C. V. Mosby.

Kim, M. J., & Moritz, D..A. (Eds.) (1982). *Classification of nursing diagnoses: Proceedings of the third and fourth national conferences.* New York: McGraw-Hill.

McLane, A. (1987). *Classification of nursing diagnoses: Proceedings of the seventh conference.* St. Louis: C.V. Mosby.

Radwin, L. E. (1990). Research on diagnostic reasoning in nursing. *Nursing Diagnosis, 1*(2), 70–77.

Simon, H. A. (1979). *Models of thought.* New Haven: Yale University Press.

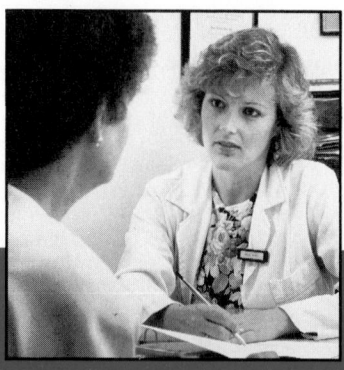

Nursing Management: Planning, Implementation, and Evaluation

LEARNING OBJECTIVES

Upon completion of this chapter, the student will be able to do the following:

- Define planning, implementation, and evaluation.
- Discuss the purposes of planning, implementation, and evaluation.
- Formulate a nursing care plan for a patient given a nursing assessment database.
- Describe the components of the nursing care plan.
- Describe the clinical skills needed to implement the nursing care plan.
- Describe methods for revising or modifying the nursing care plan.
- Describe the activities the nurse carries out during the evaluation step of the nursing process.
- Discuss quality assurance monitors used in nursing settings.
- Use a functional health pattern approach to plan, implement, and evaluate patient care.

KEY TERMS

Goal	Outcome criteria	Quality assurance
Implementation	Peer review	monitors
Nursing	Planning phase	Scientific rationale
interventions	Priority	Standards
Nursing monitors		

9

Planning
  Planning Activities
    Establish Priorities
    Establish Patient Goals and Outcome Criteria
    Plan Nursing Interventions
    Write a Nursing Care Plan
  Planning Organized by Functional Health
Implementation
  Implementation Skills
    Intellectual Skills
    Interpersonal Skills
    Technical Skills
  Implementation Activities
    Reassess
    Set Priorities
    Perform Nursing Interventions
    Record Actions
  Implementation Using a Functional Health
    Approach
Evaluation
  Evaluation Skills
    Knowledge of Standards of Care
    Knowledge of Normal Patient Responses

    Knowledge of Conceptual Models of Nursing
    Ability to Monitor the Effectiveness of Nursing
      Interventions
    Awareness of Clinical Research
  Types of Evaluation
    Structure Evaluation
    Process Evaluation
    Outcome Evaluation
  Evaluation Activities
    Review Patient Goals and Outcome Criteria
    Collect Data
    Measure Goal Attainment
    Record Judgment or Measurement of Goal
      Attainment
    Revise and Modify the Nursing Care Plan
  Quality Assurance Monitors
    American Nurses Association
    The Joint Commission on Accreditation of
      Healthcare Organizations
    Peer Review
  Evaluation Using the Functional Health Pattern
    Approach
Key Concepts

Once assessment data have been collected and analyzed and nursing diagnoses have been identified and validated, the nurse moves to the remaining phases of the nursing process: planning, implementing, and evaluating patient care. Skill in planning, implementing, and evaluating patient care is necessary for professional nursing practice. As nursing is a practice discipline, its practitioners must be experts at applying theoretical knowledge to actual patient situations.

In the third phase of the nursing process, *planning,* a nursing care plan is developed to direct nursing care activities for an individual patient. The purposes of the plan also include promoting continuity of care, directing documentation of care, and specifying nursing actions.

Implementation refers to the activity of providing care. Purposes include support, teaching, counseling, supervision, and carrying out technical and therapeutic nursing interventions to achieve an optimal level of health.

Evaluation, the fifth phase of the nursing process, consists of measuring the patient's status in response to the nursing care provided. The purpose of evaluation is to judge the effectiveness of the nursing care given.

PLANNING

The **planning phase** refers to the design of nursing strategies designed to resolve patient problems. The written nursing care plan directs the activities of the nursing staff in the provision of patient care. There are two kinds of nursing care plans; 1) students write instructional nursing care plans, and 2) nurses in practice write clinical nursing care plans. The reasons for planning are to:

- Direct patient care activities
- Promote continuity of care
- Focus charting requirements
- Allow for the delegation of specific activities.

Formats for plans can be individual, generic, or computer-generated. To meet the standards of the Joint Commission for Accreditation of Healthcare Organizations (JCAHO, 1990), the plan must be developed by a registered nurse, must be documented in the patient's health record, and must reflect the standards of care established by the institution and the profession.

Planning requires skill in writing behavioral objectives and patient goals, prioritizing needs, and determining nursing interventions to resolve patient problems. The planning phase of the nursing process in relation to the other phases is shown in Figure 9-1.

Activities of the planning phase are:

- Establish priorities.
- Establish patient goals and outcome criteria.
- Plan nursing interventions.
- Write the nursing care plan.

Planning Activities

Establish Priorities

Nursing priorities are based on the identified nursing diagnoses and patient needs. This skill requires clinical expertise and practice. If the patient has life-threatening problems, for instance, maintaining an airway and hemodynamic monitoring take precedence. But if the patient is being discharged the next day, the focus is on determining what further teaching is needed and ensuring that referrals and supplies are ready.

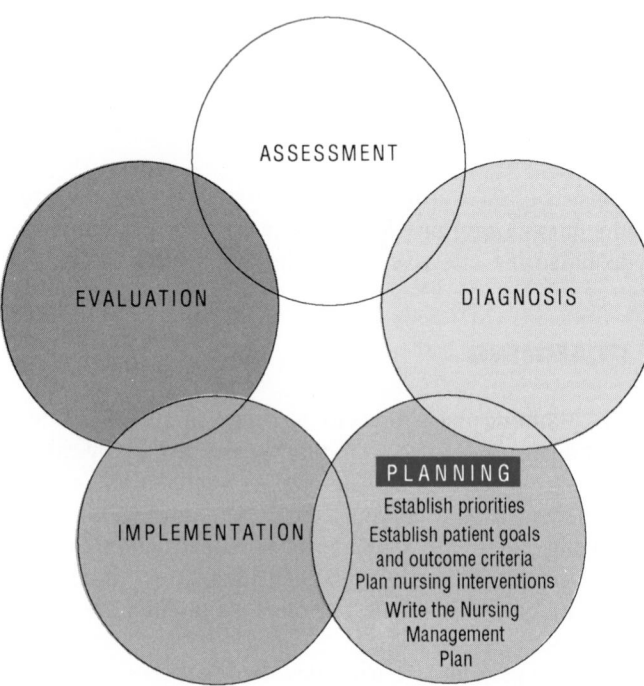

Figure 9–1.   The relationship of planning to the entire nursing process.

Because each patient is different, the sequence of nursing interventions must be individualized. One patient may be ready to discuss home-care needs after colostomy surgery; another may need a visit from a colostomy patient before this topic can be broached. The ability to alter routine plans is the hallmark of an expert nurse.

Establish Patient Goals and Outcome Criteria

Often the terms goals, objectives, and outcomes are used interchangeably; they are statements of expectations. The nurse in a health-care facility must know how terms are used in the clinical setting. In this textbook, a distinction is made, and the term patient goals and patient outcomes are not used interchangeably.

A patient **goal** is an educated guess, made as a broad statement, about the state of the patient after the nursing interventions are carried out. It addresses directly the problem stated in the nursing diagnosis.

Using clinical knowledge and experience, the nurse writes a goal that he or she believes can be achieved. Human beings are unpredictable; the disease may progress faster that usual, a complication may occur, or the family may stop visiting. Any number of things can happen to invalidate the goal. When this happens, the goal needs to be revised. For example, the nurse may set the goal of ''ambulates with a quad cane'' for a stroke patient. But if this patient suffers an extension of the stroke (unpredictable, unexpected, and not within your control), the goal may need to be changed to ''transfers to chair with two-person assist.'' Changes in the patient's condition require revision of goals.

Behavioral goals are written to indicate a desired state. They contain an action verb and a qualifier that indicates the level of performance needed to achieve it. Some commonly used behavioral verbs are presented in the display. The qualifier is a description of the parameters for achieving the goal. For example, ''walks'' would not be a sufficient patient goal. An appropriate goal may be ''ambulates 30 feet using a quad cane.'' This is easily understood and can be measured. If the nurse caring for the patient observes that dyspnea occurs after 15 feet, this would be noted in the record and the goal would be revised. In this way, goals are measured against actual performance.

Goals may be short-term or long-term. A short-term goal can be met in a relatively short time (within 24 hours, by the end of the week). A long-term goal requires more time to achieve, perhaps several weeks or months. A long-term goal may also indicate an ongoing activity. Long-term goals are usually stated by using ''every day'' or ''will maintain'' (Alfaro, 1990).

Outcome criteria are specific, measurable, realistic statements of goal attainment. They may restate the goal, but they also present information that will guide the evaluation phase of the nursing process. When shifts

Behavioral Verbs Used in Care Plans	
Calculate	List
Classify	Maintain
Communicate	Name
Compare	Participate
Construct	Perform
Contrast	Practice
Define	Recall
Demonstrate	Recite
Describe	Record
Discuss	Stand
Distinguish	State
Draw	Use
Explain	Verbalize
Express	Walk
Identify	

change, the outcome criteria help other nurses know specifically what the patient and nurse are striving to accomplish (Fig. 9-2).

To be specific and measurable, certain requirements must be met in writing outcome criteria. Outcome criteria answer the questions who, what actions, under what circumstances, how well, and when (Alfaro, 1990). For the stroke patient whose goal is ambulation with a quad cane, the outcome criteria would be: The patient (*who*) ambulates (*what action*) with a quad cane (*under what circumstances*) 30 feet (*how well*) before shift change (*when*).

Patient goals and outcome criteria are used throughout Section II of this text. They appear in the text after nursing diagnoses and in the Evaluation section of each chapter. The same patient goals and outcome criteria are used in the nursing care plan at the end of the chapter.

Plan Nursing Interventions

Selecting appropriate nursing interventions is the next activity in the planning phase and directs activities to be carried out in the implementation phase. **Nursing interventions** are "any direct care treatment that a nurse performs on behalf of a client, which includes nurse-initiated treatments, physician-initiated treatments, and performance of daily essential functions" (Bulechek & McCloskey, 1990, p. 26). Interventions are usually considered to be broad conceptual labels and are written as specific activities on the nursing care plan.

Determining which nursing interventions are appropriate for a specific patient requires clinical knowledge and practice. Generally, interventions can be grouped to describe the activity being suggested, but work in this area of classification is just beginning (McCloskey, et al., 1990). Types of interventions include:

- Psychomotor (positioning, inserting, applying)
- Psychosocial (supporting, exploring, encouraging)
- Educative (demonstrating, teaching, observing return demonstrations)
- Maintenance (skin care, hygiene)
- Surveillance (detecting changes)
- Supervisory (other health-care providers)
- Sociocultural (spending time, incorporating cultural differences into care regimen).

Clinical examples of accurate and inaccurate nursing intervention statements are listed below.

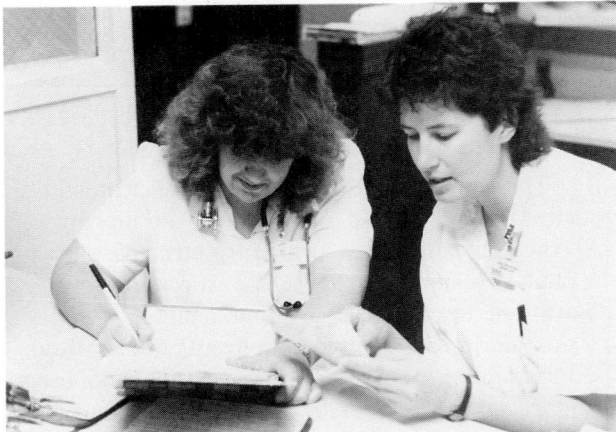

Figure 9–2. Outcome criteria clarify what is expected of the patient as a result of nursing care. Such criteria, as part of the nursing care plan, are useful when shifts change and for evaluation of the patient and care provided.

Requirements for Writing Outcome Criteria
Subject: *Who* is the person expected to achieve the goal?
Verb: *What actions* must the person do to achieve the goal?
Condition: *Under what circumstances* is the person to perform the actions?
Criteria: *How well* is the person to perform the action?
Specific time: *When* is the person expected to perform the action?

From Alfaro, R. (1990). *Applying nursing diagnosis and nursing process: A step-by-step guide* (2nd ed.). Philadelphia: J. B. Lippincott, p. 100.

Clinical Examples

Accurate. Position the patient in correct body alignment and change position every 2 hours.

Inaccurate. Position patient on left side. (The nurse in this case could leave the patient in one position and it could be incorrect alignment.)

Accurate. Demonstrate skin-care regimen (use standard protocol) to patient and family.

Inaccurate. Demonstrate skin care program. (The nurse in this case has not specified which regimen to use and has not indicated who is to be shown the care.)

Accurate. Supervise patient's self-administration of insulin on 8/8/92.

Inaccurate. Supervise medication administration. (The nurse in this case has not indicated who is to be supervised or for what medication.)

Write a Nursing Care Plan

The problem-solving process is documented in the nursing care plan.* The ability to create the nursing care plan has become a standard expected of every nurse. The care plan is a critical element in focusing nursing activity. This documentation and communication of the problem solving process used by the nurse also serves as evaluation criteria for the Joint Commission for Accreditation of Healthcare Organizations (JCAHO). Medicare and Medicaid standards are require nursing care plans for each patient.

Students should remember two important guidelines when learning to write nursing care plans:

- The care plan is *nursing*-centered.
- The care plan is a step-by-step process.

Keeping the care plan *nursing*-centered is essential to identify the scope and depth of nursing practice. By focusing on the treatment of human responses to actual or potential health problems, the nurse remains in the nursing practice domain. The second guideline is that the nursing care plan follows a step-by-step process (Fig. 9-3). There must be enough data collected to substantiate the nursing diagnosis. There must be at least one goal specified for each nursing diagnosis. The nursing interventions must be specifically designed to meet the identified goal. Each intervention should be supported by scientific rationale. Finally, the evaluation must address whether each goal was achieved or not. Care plans can be developed using a variety of approaches.

Types of Nursing Care Plans. The nursing care plan can be written in a variety of ways. Institutions may use a

---

* Nursing care plans are called nursing management plans in this text because they describe how the nurse manages the care of patients with specific dysfunctional problems. Nursing Care Plans and Nursing Management Plans are used interchangably in this chapter.

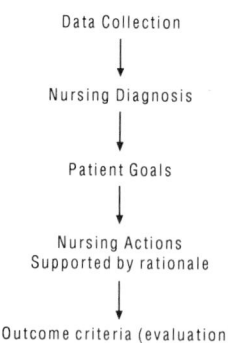

Figure 9–3. Step-by-step process for developing a care plan.

portable metal card file format, a notebook, or a computerized care plan design. (These are discussed further in Chap. 10.) Despite these design differences, the care plans usually contain three key elements. These are the nursing diagnosis (patient problem), patient goals, and nursing interventions (nursing orders, nursing actions). In addition, the care plan can be written for the individual patient, be standardized for a patient population, be generic for a specific problem, or be computer-generated from assessment data. Students learning to write care plans use the instructional nursing care plan format. In practice settings nurses use the clinical nursing care plan format. Each of these plans is discussed in the next section.

Instructional Nursing Care Plans. The type of care plan used to learn the nursing process is comprehensive, in-depth, and sometimes requires the student to speculate on likely consequences. These "instructional nursing care plans" allow the student to learn about a variety of patient problems and the processes nurses use to solve them. Scientific rationales from nursing literature are

---

Nursing Research

Henderson, P., & Southern, D. (1990). Making caring plans. *Nursing Times, 80*(4), 33–35.

This study looked at the influence of an individualized care plan on the attitudes of the nurse. When the patient was included as an active participant in planning care, there was a more positive attitude toward teaching and dealing with the problem than when the patient was not involved. Interventions were more imaginative and used more professional skills. The authors conclude, "Warning: Care plans can seriously affect your attitude and the actions you take toward your patient."

given as references for the information and to illustrate the nurse's decision-making process. Specific recommendations for completing this type of care plan will be given using each step of the nursing process. These guidelines will also be applicable to writing a clinical nursing care plan as a practicing nurse and will be refined further in Section II of this text.

Clinical Nursing Care Plans. The clinical care plan used in the practice setting to plan nursing care is different from the required instructional care plan done by students. The nursing process is used, but the plan is organized in a practical, concise format for daily use. There is less specific detail and rationales are not documented. The focus is to individualize the care plan for each patient using findings from the nursing assessment and identified nursing diagnoses.

Individual care plans are written for each patient by a registered nurse. The nursing diagnoses are listed, along with specific goals and interventions to resolve the problem. Ideally, this method provided individualized care for all patients, but it is time-consuming.

Standardized care plans are written by a group of nurses who are experts in a given area of practice, e.g., obstetrics, rehabilitation, or orthopedics. The plan is written for a patient population with a specific medical diagnosis, i.e., total hip repalcement, vaginal delivery, or coronary artery bypass surgery. These experts identify the most common nursing diagnoses for this patient population and write the goals and interventions usually necessary to resolve the problem. Each time a standardized care plan is used, it must be individualized for a specific patient. This method assures the nurse that the plan is correct for most patients. The danger lies in the fact that standardized care plans may not fit a specific patient. Nurses must make judgments as to the degree standardized care plans should be modified, or if they should not be used in individual cases.

Generic care plans are usually written for a specific nursing diagnosis. They contain the goals and interventions most commonly seen when that particular nursing diagnosis is identified. Again, the generic care plan must be individualized for a specific patient. Because generic care plans are written by experts in a particular diagnostic area, they may serve as a learning tool for the inexperienced nurse who is unfamiliar with the content.

Computerized care plans are generated from assessment data entered into a computer about a specific patient. The plan is written by experts in the area and the content is similar to that of the standardized or generic care plan. Once the plan is on the computer screen the nurse has an opportunity to customize it for the patient. Since these care plans are linked to assesment data, it is critical that all pertinent information be collected and entered into the system. The generated care plan is only as good as the data on which it is based.

With the increased emphasis on computerized nursing systems, the "speed, quality, comprehensiveness, and effectiveness of creating patient-specific care plans" (Walters, 1986, p. 33) can be enhanced.

Preparing the Instructional Nursing Care Plans. Students learning to write care plans use the instructional nursing care plan format; in practice settings, nurses use the clinical nursing care plan format. Each of these plans is described in the following sections.

Student nurses usually are required to complete some form of an instructional nursing care plan. The purpose is to demonstrate in a written format an understanding of the problem-solving process used in assisting patients to regain a higher level of functional health. Once assessment data have been collected, organized, and synthesized, one or more nursing diagnoses are identified (see Chaps. 7 and 8). Each nursing diagnosis is used to develop a part of the care plan.

Nursing Management Plan Format Used in This Text

Nursing Diagnosis: _____

Patient Goal: _____

Patient Outcome Criteria

- _____
- _____
- _____

Nursing Intervention	**Scientific Rationale**
1. _____	1. _____
2. _____	2. _____

Components of instructional nursing care plans usually are nursing diagnosis, patient goals or patient outcome criteria, nursing interventions, scientific rationale, and evaluation.

The format used in Section II of this text consists of one nursing diagnosis, one or more patient goals, several patient outcome criteria, nursing interventions, and scientific rationales. The goals and outcome criteria reflect patient goals and outcome criteria discussed in the specific chapter. The Nursing Management Plans are designed in the sample format given here; they appear at the end of Chapters 25 through 49. To help the student understand what to include in each section of the Plan, a second copy of the format with instructions for completion is also included here.

Nursing Diagnosis. The nursing diagnostic statement is recorded in the space labeled "nursing diagnosis." It is composed of the diagnostic label (using NANDA terminology, if possible), "related to" (the related factor), and "manifested by" (the supporting defining characteristics). For high-risk diagnoses (formerly called potential nursing diagnoses), there is no related factor listed. Using the functional health pattern approach helps the nurse focus on real or potential functional health problems rather than on disease pathology. All of the identified nursing diagnoses for a particular patient should be listed in order of priority for patient care.

Clinical Examples

Accurate. Feeding Self-Care Deficit (level 3) related to right-sided weakness, manifested by inability to pick up spoon, lack of attention to food on tray, and inability to open containers.

Inaccurate. Self-Care Deficit, Feeding: due to left cerebrovascular accident, manifested by not eating. (The nurse in this case has inverted the diagnostic phrase, used a medical diagnosis as a direct causative agent for the problem, and not shown clinical indicators in the form of defining characteristics for the validation of the diagnosis.)

Patient Goal. One or more patient goals are established for each nursing diagnosis. The goal is a broadly stated objective that indicates an overall picture of the state of the patient if the problem is resolved. Each goal must be measurable, realistic, or observable. Some examples of goal statements include: maintains present weight, no evidence of infection, and administers insulin correctly. The goal describes a patient outcome in broad terms. The patient goal must reflect resolution or correction of the identified problem (diagnostic label).

Clinical Examples

Accurate. Patient demonstrates correct skin care regimen.

Inaccurate. Patient's skin is free of eczema. (The nurse in this case has set a goal that is not achievable through nursing interventions. Furthermore, it may not be realistic to expect this goal to be accomplished even with medications and other therapy.)

Patient Outcome Criteria. Patient outcome criteria are specific, measurable, realistic statements that can be evaluated to judge goal attainment. They should include a time reference. Outcome criteria are stated in terms of behavioral objectives. They include a verb that denotes the action and a short phrase that describes the specific measure to be accomplished. Examples include:

Information to Be Placed in Nursing Management Plan

Nursing Diagnosis: (Use the NANDA-accepted list of nursing diagnoses. List in priority order. Use the diagnostic label and "related to" [related factor], followed by "manifested by" [supporting defining characteristics].)

Patient Goal: (One or more patient goals established from nursing diagnosis. A broadly stated objective that indicates an overall picture of the state of the patient if the problem is resolved.)

Patient Outcome Criteria: (Specific, measurable, realistic statements that can be evaluated to judge goal attainment. Stated as behavioral objectives, they include a verb, a short phrase describing the specific measure to be accomplished, and a time reference.)

Nursing Intervention	Scientific Rationale
(Write interventions [nursing orders] that are specific and relate to the goal. The "related to" phrase of the nursing diagnostic statement directs choice of nursing interventions. Interventions include who, what, when, and how the order is to be carried out.)	(Gives justification for carrying out the intervention. Demonstrates synthesis of physiologic and pathophysiologic concepts.)

- Draws up correct dosage of insulin at next administration.
- Demonstrates accurate deep-breathing and coughing exercises at afternoon teaching session.
- Verbalizes a basic understanding of the relationship between excessive stimuli and feelings of loss of control to nurse during evening shift.

Clinical Examples

Accurate. Ambulates 30 feet using walker this afternoon.

Inaccurate. Walks in hall. (The nurse in this case has failed to be specific and to include necessary qualifiers for the outcome.)

Nursing Interventions. Sometimes called nursing orders, nursing interventions are written in specific terms that relate to the goals. The "related to" phrase of the nursing diagnostic statement directs the choice of nursing interventions. Each nursing intervention must specify who, what, when, and how the order is to be carried out. The statements should be comprehensive but brief; the nurse may be referred to procedures, protocols, or standing policies for further information. In some cases, nursing interventions include specific measures needed to carry out the medical regimen (Table 9-1).

Clinical Examples

Accurate. Staff will give passive range of motion exercises to the right upper extremity during morning care, once on evenings, and once during the night.

Inaccurate. Range of motion three times a day. (The nurse in this case has not specified who is to carry out the order, whether or not it is to be active or passive range of motion, and the time frame.)

Scientific Rationale. The **scientific rationale** is the justification or reason for carrying out the intervention. It should synthesize psychological and pathophysiologic concepts. The rationale—the "why" of the intervention—describes a research-based reason for the significance of the intervention. Usually student nurses are required to supply scientific rationales to show they understand the basic reasons for carrying out specific nursing interventions. In clinical practice settings, the nurse may use rationales to illustrate new research findings or to support a controversial approach to a problem.

Whether the rationale is stated or not, the nurse should be able to state the reason for the intervention. A reference for each scientific rationale must be given, citing the author, year, title, and page of the article or book used. Sometimes nurses think that interventions are based on common sense, but this is not so: many nursing interventions previously thought to be sensible have turned out to be unsafe, impractical, or unnecessary. Asking why certain nursing interventions are performed aids in the scientific development of nursing practice.

Clinical Examples

Accurate. Small shifts of body weight promote circulation and help to prevent skin breakdown (Seiler & Stahelein, 1985, p. 223).

Inaccurate. Change position every 2 hours. (The nurse in this case has neither given a reason for the position change nor referenced it.)

Evaluation. The evaluation of a nursing intervention is a written statement that determines the patient's status in relation to the outcome criteria at a particular point in time. The evaluation stage answers the question: was the goal achieved? It provides the necessary feedback to guide revision of the care plan or resolution of the problem. Changes may be needed in the time frame for goal achievement, progression or regression of the patient, or to facilitate new skill development in the patient. In some cases, the student will state what *would* have been evaluated if nursing care had been provided during additional clinical experiences. Case studies using hypothetical patient situations can also be effective supplements to clinical learning. The procedure for evaluation of care can be just as effective using this method.

Evaluation of care is usually recorded in the narrative nursing note and includes the patient's response to the intervention as well as the objective clinical findings. Each intervention is evaluated for effectiveness, modified if needed, and deleted if not necessary.

Clinical Examples

Accurate. Unable to complete passive range of motion to right upper extremity after morning care because of report of pain when arm elevated above level of shoul-

---

TABLE 9–1

Examples of Nursing Interventions to Include the Medical Regimen

Medical Order	Nursing Intervention
Weigh qd, report loss > 5#	Bedscale weight every day at 6 AM; report weight <(specify #) to team leader and physician.
Increase caloric intake	Provide between-meal snack at 10 AM, 2 PM, and 10 PM. Request consultation with dietitian (done 10/19). Transfer patient to chair for each meal and snack.

der. Physician notified, patient instructed to rest arm until further evaluation is made.

Inaccurate. Range of motion discontinued due to pain. (In this case the nurse has failed to evaluate the patient's response and what was done to follow up on the problem.)

Preparing the Clinical Nursing Care Plans. The clinical care plan differs from the plan used by students. The differentiation between clinical and instructional care plans assists the student in his or her transition into the professional role. It is vital that nurses continue to refine the process of writing care plans, as well as actively using them in implementing daily nursing care. The nursing process is used, but the plan is organized in a practical, concise format for daily use. There is less specific detail, and rationales are not documented. The goal is to individualize the plan for each patient using findings from the nursing assessment and identified nursing diagnoses. A well-written, continually updated nursing care plan is an invaluable tool. The following section will focus on the application of the instructional care plan previously described, to the clinical care plan. The examples given will assist the student in moving from the type of comprehensive care plan required for learning to a workable plan for nursing care used by practicing nurses. Mayers differentiates the two "tools" as follows:

> The primary purpose of an educational tool [instructional nursing care plan] is to provide a medium for learning about patients' health problems and the rationales for solving them. The primary purpose of a care delivery tool [clinical care plan] is to communicate relevant data rapidly and efficiently to other team members regarding the required strategies for care which contribute to the overall patient objectives (Mayers, 1978, p. 9).

The specific differences seen in a clinical care plan will be discussed further as they relate to each step of the nursing process. The steps of a clinical care plan are as follows:

Assessment/Data Collection. The collection of data and patient assessment are completed on an ongoing basis by the nurse. The admission history and physical assessment serve as guidelines for the initial care plan. Data are gathered in each subsequent meeting with the patient to revise the plan.

Nursing Diagnosis. The nursing diagnosis in a working care plan is written using the guidelines in Chapter 8. The instructional care plan includes all possible patient problems; the clinical care plan focuses on individual patient needs and priority nursing problems.

Patient Goals. Patient goals and outcome criteria are often seen in the same statement. The goals are specific to meeting the patient problems identified in the nursing diagnoses.

Interventions. Nursing actions are documented in essentially the same way as on the clinical care plan. This phase is also made more specific to each patient's needs. An important step in this phase is to identify the health-care worker responsible for performing the nursing action. The action may be most appropriately completed by the rehabilitation nurse aide, or the registered nurse. This leads to better communication and use of plans for daily assignments, and is particularly important in practice.

Rationale. Although rationale is not a step in the nursing process, selecting a scientific rationale for interventions is an important step in the instructional plan, and although it is not documented in the clinical plan it is no less important. The nurse must know the rationale behind the nursing actions, or must question and review the rationale before performing the action. This is a professional responsibility and is expected of every practicing nurse.

Evaluation. The process of evaluation is ongoing. It begins with initial care planning and ends when the diagnoses identified are solved. The evaluation in the clinical plan is based on the specific observations made of patient progress toward the outcome criteria as outlined in the plan. The plan is updated and changed—minute by minute in critical and acute care, weekly or monthly in long-term care.

Planning Organized by Functional Health

In today's health-care environment, the nurse must meet high standards to satisfy professional mandates, including legal, social, and institutional expectations of professional practice. Using a functional health patterns approach facilitates professional nursing practice.

Because functional health patterns are useful in organizing assessment data and identifying nursing diagnoses, they are also useful in focusing the plan of care. Some patients will be functional in many areas, but may require nursing care for dysfunctional problems. Understanding the concepts of function and dysfunction allows the nurse to see what strengths and limitations the patient has; functional areas may be used to address dysfunctional ones. The functional health approach provides a strong focus for planning nursing interventions.

IMPLEMENTATION

Whether or not computer-generated care plans are used, the nurse is responsible for implementing nursing care. Most of Section II of this text focuses on specific activities performed to meet patient needs for nursing care.

Implementation refers to the action phase of the nursing process in which nursing care is provided. It is defined as the actual initiation of the plan, evaluation of response to the plan, and recording of nursing actions. The purpose of implementation is to provide the nursing care required to meet patient needs. Competence in intellectual, interpersonal, and technical skills is required to carry out the implementation phase of the nursing process. Parts of the care plan can be delegated to other members of the health-care team, but the registered nurse maintains accountability for the supervision and evaluation of these people. The activities of implementation are illustrated in Figure 9-4 and include:

- Reassess
- Set priorities
- Perform nursing interventions
- Record actions

Implementation Skills

The implementation phase demands competence in intellectual, interpersonal, and technical skills. Developing expertise in each of these is required for professional nursing practice.

Intellectual Skills

The intellectual skills used in implementation include problem-solving, decision-making, and teaching. To solve problems, the nurse asks the patient pertinent questions, discusses alternatives, and is open to new ideas. To enrich the patient's decision-making ability, the nurse gives him or her opportunities to help choose which treatments are performed, when, and in what sequence. Teaching patients requires a knowledge base of teaching–learning principles and the information to be conveyed.

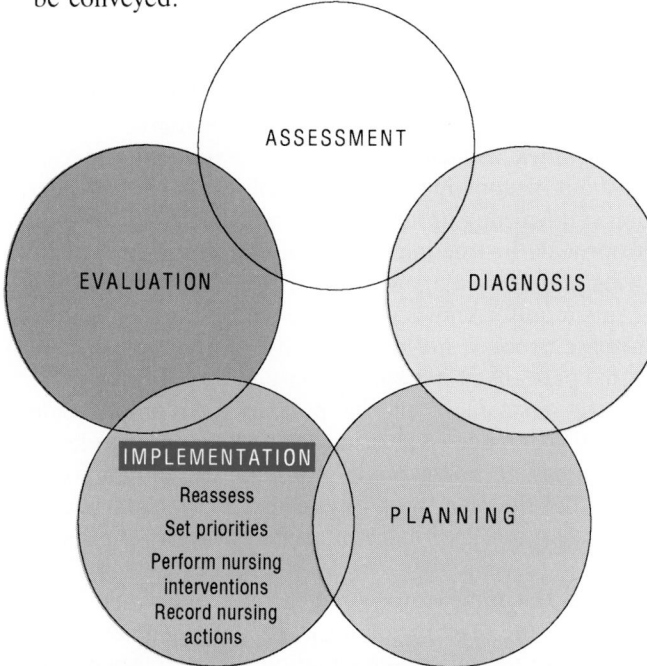

Figure 9–4.   The relationship of implementation to the entire nursing process.

Interpersonal Skills

The ability to work with others to accomplish a goal is critical to nursing. The nurse uses communication skills to carry out planned nursing interventions. Skill at both verbal and nonverbal communication is refined through practice. More details on communication are given in Chapter 17.

Technical Skills

Technical skills are used to carry out treatments and procedures. The specific skills are learned through clinical practice. Technical competence means learning how to use equipment, machines, and supplies in a particular specialty. For example, the nurse working in the delivery room must be familiar with fetal monitoring, positioning on the delivery-room table, and infant resuscitation devices. On the other hand, the nurse working on a medical unit may need technical competence in using the hypothermia blanket, therapeutic beds, or feeding pumps. The clinical skills necessary for practice are discussed in Section II of this text.

Implementation Activities

The activities of the implementation of the nursing process, illustrated in Figure 9-4, are:

- Reassess
- Set priorities
- Perform nursing interventions
- Record actions

Reassess

During each patient encounter, the nurse assesses the patient's functional health. This ensures that prompt attention is paid to emerging problems. Since the condition of the patient can change quickly and dramatically, the astute nurse remains alert to subtle cues and inferences that the patient gives. For example, the patient experiencing pain may become quiet and withdraw from external stimuli. Recognizing this change, the nurse can intervene, validate, and assist the patient to become more comfortable. A patient who is demanding and irritable may be masking anxiety about a surgical procedure or fear about the results of a diagnostic test. As the nursing care plan is initiated, care must be taken to make sure that the planned interventions are still relevant.

Set Priorities

Priorities are based on the information collected during reassessment. A **priority** is a nursing problem that takes on a position of prominence. When setting priorities, the nurse ranks nursing problems in order of importance based on several factors (Fig. 9-5), including:

- The patient's condition
- New information from reassessment
- Time and resources available for nursing interventions
- Feedback from the patient, family, and health-care staff
- The nurse's experience in assessing situations and setting priorities.

A nursing intervention for a priority problem would be done before another intervention, but setting priorities does not entail skipping any interventions. Setting priorities affects only the order in which nursing interventions are carried out.

Priorities can be set every few minutes, hourly, daily, weekly, or for longer periods of time. For example, in the critical care unit, priorities may need to be set every few minutes for an unstable multiple trauma patient on several life-support systems. Usually maintaining a patent airway, breathing, and circulation (the ABCs) are top priorities in these cases. Nursing interventions for the nursing diagnosis of High Risk for Disuse Syndrome would be done after the patient was stabilized. In the long-term care unit, however, priorities may be set for

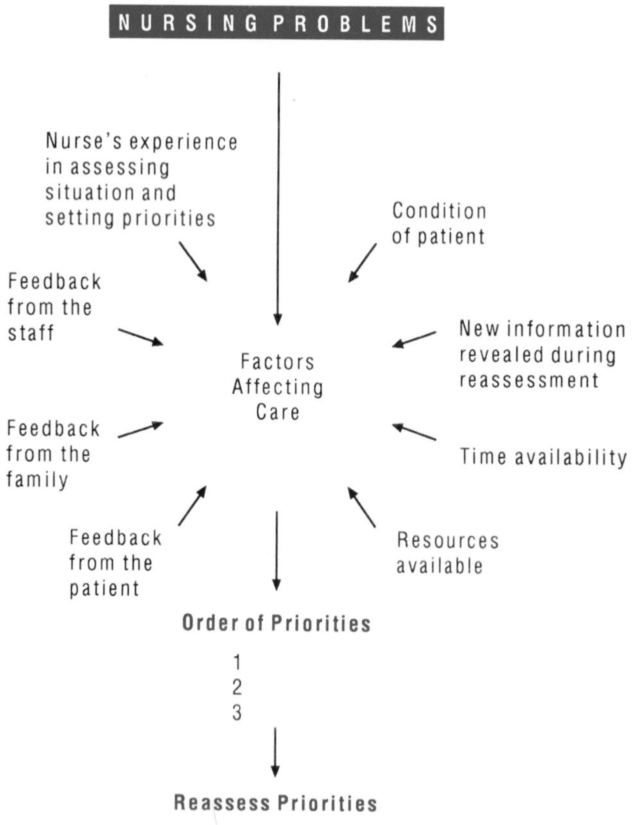

Figure 9–5.   Priorities (position of prominence) are set by considering factors affecting care.

much longer periods of time. For example, a priority for a stroke patient for a specific period of time may be fostering independent transferring from bed to chair.

Perform Nursing Interventions

To initiate the plan, the nurse (or designee) carries out the nursing interventions listed on the nursing care plan. If the nurse is caring for several patients, a schedule for carrying out the interventions is developed. The actual procedures or protocols to be used are discussed in the appropriate chapters of this book. For example, if the intervention is to provide range of motion exercises, the nurse is referred to that chapter in this text.

Interventions for Collaborative Problems.   Collaborative problems (see Chap. 8) are those for which "nurses are responsible and accountable to identify and treat *in collaboration with the physician*" (Alfaro, 1990). Nursing diagnoses are determined, in part, when the nurse asks, "Is this a problem that a nurse can legally treat without an order from a physician?" Interventions based on such diagnoses are *independent* actions. When the nurse follows a physician-prescribed order, the action is *dependent*. Both types of interventions involve nursing judgment because both require legal mandates. When the nurse uses both independent and dependent interventions to give nursing care to the patient, the problem is a *collaborative problem.* (Carpenito, 1989)

Types of Nursing Interventions.   Nursing interventions fall within three major categories: those using cognitive skills, those using interpersonal skills, and those using technical skills (Table 9-2). Selection of the type of nursing intervention to be used in patient situations depends on the patient's functional health requirements and dysfunctional health pattern. Each type of nursing intervention is discussed in the next section.

Cognitive. Educative nursing interventions are carried out by applying general principles about the teaching and learning process. Teaching plans are developed to provide instruction about specific health-care problems and their management. The ability to teach patients requires knowledge of the pathophysiology of the disease process, normal anatomy and physiology, and usual patterns of patient response to health changes. A careful assessment of the patient yields information about his or her level of motivation, knowledge level, willingness to follow the health regimen, and ability to carry out the plan, both physically and psychologically. See Chapter 21 for more information on patient teaching.

Once the nurse is aware of how ready the patient is for learning, the teaching plan can be implemented. Goals specific to the individual situation are established, and instruction is given in a way that optimizes a successful outcome.

TABLE 9–2

Types of Interventions

Cognitive	Interpersonal	Technical
Teach/educate	Coordinate activities	Provide basic hygiene, skin care
Relate knowledge to ADLs	Provide caregiving	Perform routine nursing activities
Provide feedback	Use therapeutic communication	Detect change from baseline data
Create strategies for patients with dysfunctional communication	Provide a personal presence	Recognize abnormal responses
Supervise nursing team	Set limits	Provide independent and dependent treatment
Supervise patient in performance	Provide opportunity to examine values and attitudes	Assist with ADLs
Supervise family in performance	Explore and legitimize feelings	Provide appropriate sensory stimulation
Alter the environment as needed	Provide spiritual support	Mobilize equipment
	Use humor	Maintain supplies
	Provide individual therapy	Use special abilities or talents
	Provide group therapy	
	Become patient's advocate	
	Support patient and family plans	
	Make referrals for followup	
	Serve as a role model	

Clinical Example

Accurate. During administration of medications on 10/23, review purpose and schedule of antihypertensive drugs.

Inaccurate. Give patient antihypertensive drug handout. (The nurse in this case has failed to involve the patient in discussion, specify by whom and when the intervention is to be carried out, and has not individualized the teaching for the patient.)

Supervisory nursing interventions include ensuring that other members of the nursing team carry out specified aspects of the management plan, and those involved with the patient or family return demonstration of skills. To supervise nursing team members requires an in-depth knowledge of the job descriptions and capabilities of each person on the team. Nurses may delegate specific aspects of care to nonprofessional staff, but the registered nurse is held accountable for the selection of appropriate nursing care measures that can be performed by these personnel. The nurse also maintains the responsibility to ensure that these nursing care measures have been carried out correctly and that important information about the patient's response to the care is communicated verbally and in written form to the nurse responsible for the patient.

Supervising the patient or family in skill performance is essential to provide encouragement, to provide feedback about correct and incorrect performance, or to facilitate introduction of new skills to be learned. Patients and their families are often unfamiliar with nursing care regimens, equipment, and supplies. They should be given ample opportunity to carry out the intervention before discharge. Given today's shortened hospital stay, this requires immediate attention and inclusion of the patient and family in planning and implementing care from the time of admission. The nurse

familiar with usual routines for managing of specific health care problems can introduce the patient or family responsibility for care during the admission interview. Each nurse taking care of the patient subsequently should be informed about the capabilities of the patient and family to carry out the intervention. Skills are built with practice; doing an activity once usually is not sufficient for proficiency. The astute nurse ensures that patients and their families can practice interventions several times before discharge.

Clinical Example

Accurate. Using a long-handled mirror, patient carries out skin inspection on 10/24 without being reminded by the nurse.

Inaccurate. Patient does skin inspection. (The nurse in this case has failed to specify the equipment needed and the conditions under which the patient is to carry out the intervention.)

Interpersonal. *Coordinating* patient activities serves many purposes. The nurse carries out the coordination function by acting as a patient advocate, making referrals for followup care, communicating with other health-team members, and ensuring that the patient's schedule is therapeutic.

For some patients, the nurse fulfills the advocate role by speaking for the patient or encouraging the patient to ask questions. For example, a patient may need help in refusing a suggested treatment or requesting a second opinion about surgery. In the advocacy role, the nurse presents the patient's point of view and suggests ways in which the patient's requests can be met.

The nurse is in a position to know what type of nursing follow-up the patient needs after discharge. Referrals should be made to home health agencies, visiting nurse associations, or other health-care providers to facilitate return of optimal functional health. A variety of self-help groups and community services are available to provide assistance to patients with health related problems; creativity in matching patients with these services can help ensure that the patient's health status will be monitored and that relapses may be minimized.

Clinical Example

Accurate. Refer to Home Health agency for dressing changes after discharge.

Inaccurate. Needs dressing changes at home. (The nurse in this case has identified a patient need but has not specified by whom or how this intervention will be carried out.)

Supportive nursing interventions emphasize use of communication skills, relief of spiritual distress, and caring behaviors. A combination of good communication and caring provides comfort and promotes a healthy response to dysfunctional health problems. Being supportive means recognizing the need for encouragement, unconditional acceptance of behaviors, and the positive effects of "being there" for a patient during stress or crisis. The nurse may sit with a patient who is anxious, listen to a grieving patient's experience with the loss of a loved one, or touch the forehead of a patient with a spinal-cord injury. This is called "therapeutic use of self."

Spiritual support can be provided by giving the patient time to carry out religious practices, meditation, or reading. Respecting the patient's privacy during these times conveys acceptance and understanding. If the patient wants to talk, the nurse should listen to assess spiritual distress without being judgmental. If the patient asks for a spiritual support person, the patient's minister, rabbi, or priest or the hospital chaplain can be contacted.

Clinical Example

Accurate. Encourage patient to express feelings and concerns about terminal illness; spend time in the room each shift sitting at the bedside.

Inaccurate. Talk to patient about terminal illness. (The nurse in this case is not giving the patient a chance to open and guide the discussion. By forcing information on the patient, too much or too little material may be conveyed. The patient is the best judge of when and how much information he or she can digest.)

Psychosocial nursing interventions focus on resolving emotional, psychological, or social problems. Humor, individual or group therapy, role-modeling social skills, and exploring feelings are all ways of carrying out psychosocial nursing interventions.

Some patients and families respond to stress by joking, teasing, or laughing about it. The nurse, too, can use humor as a way to relieve stress and to give the patient examples of difficult situations and ways to resolve them. Humor must always be used judiciously, however. The nurse must recognize underlying themes or deeper problems and respond appropriately. A patient may jokingly

say to the nurse, "Gee, my arm must be target practice for everyone learning how to draw blood." The nurse should pick up on this cue and find out how many times the patient has been "stuck," determine why there was such a problem, and instruct the patient to speak up and request special consideration for future blood-drawing attempts.

Providing individual and group therapy is part of the nursing practice domain for nurses in a variety of settings. Individual therapy, used as a means of resolving psychological problems, usually requires additional training or certification. Group therapy is often used to provide support and guidance for patients and their support persons with similar needs or problems. Recognizing the need for individual or group therapy, the nurse makes referrals to healthcare providers with the required expertise. On some units, nurses hold group meetings with spouses of Alzheimer's patients, families of children with cancer, or patients who have had a stroke. Most group therapy sessions have a stated purpose and schedule of activities. Group members rely on their own experiences and gain new ways of dealing with problems from others who have experienced the same problems. The nurse therapist serves as the group facilitator and assists group members to share feelings, advice, and helpful hints with one another.

Sometimes a group member can offer a suggestion that would not be acceptable to the person if made by a health-care professional. For example, in a group for spouses of Alzheimer's patients, one wife reported that her husband continued to drive even though he admitted that he often got lost and couldn't remember the way home. Another group member simply said, "Take the keys away! I don't want to be on the street with him." The wife accepted this blunt advice and followed it. She had previously refused this advice from the therapist because she said driving was his only pleasure; she did not want to rob him of this last piece of independence.

If the nurse recognizes the need for individual or group therapy, he or she makes referrals to health-care providers with the required expertise.

Role-modeling social skills need to be taught to patients who have not acquired them, either due to lack of exposure or lengthy hospitalizations. In some long-term care settings, patients have grown to depend on the staff to make all their decisions. In other cases, patients have never practiced acceptable social behaviors. By treating the patient with respect and using appropriate language and social behaviors (saying "please" and "thank you" and not interrupting, for instance), the nurse can help the patient to become socially adept. Some psychiatric patients need to learn how to regulate their behavior; for example, if they become agitated in a crowd, they can go to a quiet place. Helping the patient recognize and act on these cues is important for decreasing readmissions and improving the patient's feelings of self-worth.

Exploring feelings is another way of providing psychosocial nursing interventions. Many patients with chronic or life-threatening illnesses need an opportunity to explore their feelings in a nonjudgmental setting. The nurse is in a prime position to help.

Clinical Example

Accurate. Encourage attendance at Stroke Club meeting, Thursday evening at 7 PM in the conference room.

Inaccurate. Refer to Stroke Club. (The nurse in this case has not assumed responsibility for providing support in terms of encouragement and has not indicated when the meeting is to take place.)

Technical. The goal of *maintenance* nursing interventions is to keep the patient in a certain state of health. Maintenance activities prevent deterioration of physical or psychological functioning and preserve independence. Maintenance interventions include basic hygiene, skin care, and other routine nursing activities.

Maintenance nursing interventions are sometimes undervalued or considered insignificant, but they allow the patient to preserve function and reduce the chance of developing complications. Nurses should take proper credit for maintaining healthy states and should receive acknowledgement for these activities in their job evaluations and recognition awards for excellence in practice.

Clinical Example

Accurate. Give complete bath, inspect skin surfaces every shift (report any redness or signs of breakdown), massage bony prominences with each position change.

Inaccurate. Total patient care. (The nurse in this case has failed to specify the level of care and reportable conditions.)

Surveillance nursing interventions include detecting changes from baseline data and recognition of abnormal responses. This activity can also be categorized as observation, inspection, or vigilance. The nurse relies on use of the senses to detect changes. Hearing, vision, touch, and smell are routinely used; taste is rarely involved. The nurse observes through vision the appearance and characteristics of the patient. Nurses hear by auscultation, pitch, and tone. Odors are detected and compared with past experience and knowledge of specific problems. Using touch, the nurse assesses body temperature, skin condition, clamminess, or diaphoresis. All of these surveillance activities are used to determine the patient's current status and changes from previous states. Subtle changes in a patient's condition are often detected by the nurse and communicated to the physician to minimize problems. Expert nurse clinicians develop skill in detection and prevention of complications and usually receive positive feedback for their accurate and timely interventions based on this "sense" of something being wrong.

Clinical Example

Accurate. Monitor respiratory status every 2 hours; report rate above 24, rales, dyspnea, or restlessness.

Inaccurate. Vital signs every 2 hours. (The nurse in this case has failed to specify the parameters of reportable findings and has not stated which vital signs are of concern.)

Psychomotor nursing interventions—those requiring technical expertise—include inserting, removing, changing, applying, administering, cleansing, or any other activity that requires a psychomotor action. The management and care of equipment, supplies, treatments, and procedures also falls into this category of nursing interventions. The nurse gains technical competence by practice.

Clinical Example

Accurate. Irrigate gastrointestinal tube every 8 hours, check patency, and measure output (record characteristics of the drainage).

Inaccurate. Give gastrointestinal tube care. (The nurse in this case has failed to specify the frequency of the intervention and the additional requirements for carrying out this intervention.)

Record Actions

After nursing interventions have been carried out, they are recorded in the patient's health record. Each institution determines the specific requirements for documentation and should prepare written guidelines for the use of all forms. With today's emphasis on efficiency, new charting methods are being developed. It is anticipated that in 1992, focus charting will be the method of choice in 35% of hospitals, and charting by exception will be used in 27% of hospitals (Wake, 1990). The recording of information is discussed more fully in Chapter 10.

Implementation Using a Functional Health Approach

When thinking about implementation, the nurse should consider the overall perspective of nursing. In a functional health approach, nursing tries to maximize a patient's functional status. To achieve this goal, the focus is resolving dysfunctional health. With each patient encounter, the nurse reassesses functional status, revises care when needed, and evaluates the patient's response. By focusing on areas of strength or healthy functioning (as discussed in the Planning section of this chapter), the nurse can optimize interventions to help the patient reach his or her healthiest state.

EVALUATION

Evaluation is the fifth phase of the nursing process. It follows implementation of the nursing management plan. Evaluation is defined as the judgment of the effectiveness of nursing care to meet patient goals; it is the phase in which the nurse compares the patient's behavioral responses with predetermined patient goals and outcome criteria. This phase involves a thorough, systematic review of the effectiveness of nursing interventions and determination of whether or not patient goals have been met and outcome criteria achieved. The nurse uses a variety of skills to judge the effectiveness of nursing care. These skills include knowledge of standards of care, knowledge of normal patient responses, knowledge of conceptual models of nursing, ability to monitor the effectiveness of nursing interventions, and awareness of clinical research. Critical appraisal of goal attainment is determined jointly by the nurse and patient.

Although evaluation is a separate and distinct phase, it is also an ongoing process performed throughout the nursing process (Alfaro, 1990). Judgments made in previous steps usually result in prompt reassessment, rediagnosis and replanning (Yura & Walsh, 1988). The nurse continually assesses the patient's response to a particular nursing intervention, establishes different priorities for nursing diagnoses, and alters the nursing care plan. An in-depth, comprehensive judgment about goal attainment and fulfillment of outcome criteria is performed only during the evaluation phase of the nursing process (Yura & Walsh, 1988).

The nursing care plan serves as the foundation for evaluation. The identified nursing diagnoses, patient goals, outcome criteria, and nursing interventions serve as the guide for evaluation. Through the evaluation process, the appropriateness, accuracy, and relevance of these nursing care components can be determined. Evaluation also helps the nurse discover any errors that may have occurred in previous steps of the nursing process. The nurse always considers evaluation in light of how the patient responded or reacted to the planned course of action (Yura & Walsh, 1983; 1988). Figure 9-6 illustrates the relationship of the activities of the evaluation phase to the other steps of the nursing process.

There are several purposes for carrying out the evaluation step of the nursing process. They include the collection of subjective and objective data to make judgments about the nursing care delivered, examination of the patient's behavioral responses to nursing interventions, and comparison of the patient's behavioral responses to predetermined outcome criteria. In addition, evaluation provides an appraisal of the extent to which patient goals were attained or problems resolved, and evidence of involvement and collaboration of the patient, family members, nurses, and other health-term members in health-care decisions and revision of the nursing care plan. Finally, evaluation identifies changes needed in nursing diagnoses, patient goals, outcome criteria, and nursing strategies, and monitors the quality of nursing care and its effect on the patient's health status (Alfaro, 1990; Brunner & Suddarth, 1988; Carpenito, 1989; Yura & Walsh, 1988).

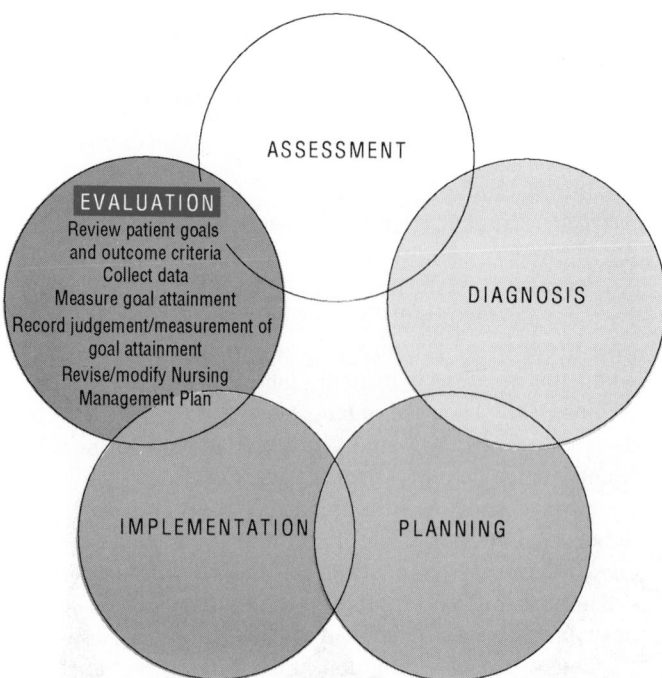

Figure 9–6. The relationship of evaluation to the entire nursing process.

The evaluation phase consists of a number of specific activities. These activities include

- Review patient goals and outcome criteria
- Collect data
- Measure goal attainment
- Record judgment/measurement of goal attainment
- Revise/modify the nursing care plan

These activities will be discussed later in this chapter.

Evaluation Skills

A variety of intellectual, interpersonal, and technical skills are required to evaluate the nursing care plan. These skills include knowledge of standards of care, knowledge of normal patient responses, knowledge of conceptual models of nursing, ability to monitor the effectivenss of nursing interventions, and awareness of clinical research.

Knowledge of Standards of Care

The nurse must know about the current standards of care proposed by nursing organizations (e.g., the American Nurses Association [ANA]), external review boards (e.g., the Joint Commission on the Accreditation of Healthcare Organizations [JCAHO]), and his or her own institution (e.g., policies and procedures) to evaluate nursing care. See the section on quality assurance monitors for discussion on the above standards.

Knowledge of Normal Patient Responses

To evaluate normal patient responses, the nurse's knowledge of many subjects, such as physiology, pathophysiology, biochemistry, psychology, sociology, and pharmacology, comes into play. A tremendous amount of knowledge about patient responses is obtained during the basic nursing educational program. Additional knowledge and updating of information is acquired through formal and informal continuing education. Obtaining college credits in nursing is an example of formal continuing education. Attendance at nursing conferences and seminars is an example of informal continuing education. The nurse also sharpens skills and updates knowledge about patient responses through clinical experience, through guidance and assistance from mentors, and by reading textbooks and journal articles.

Knowledge of Conceptual Models of Nursing

Conceptual models of nursing provide information that facilitates evaluation of the nursing care plan. Every conceptual model sets out specified goals of action and consequences of those actions that enhance the objective nature of evaluation. Because the conceptual model guides development of patient goals and outcome criteria, the goal of action or desired result of a particular conceptual model is revealed in these components of the plan (Ziegler, Vaughan-Wrobel, & Erlen, 1986). If a patient's behavioral responses match the patient goal statements and patient outcome criteria, the conceptual model's goal has been reached. For example, the goal of the Roy (1981) Adaptation Model of Nursing is the adaptation of the patient in four adaptive modes. The consequences of nursing actions lead to effective coping mechanisms, maximal level of functioning, and adaptive responses.

Ability to Monitor the Effectiveness of Nursing Interventions

Many intellectual and technical skills are required to monitor the effectiveness of nursing interventions. Interviewing techniques and physical assessment skills are needed to obtain subjective and objective data from the patient and family members. Knowledge of interviewing techniques such as types of questions, interview phases, and the appropriate environment for interviewing facilitates the collection of subjective data for evaluation of the nursing care plan. For further information about interviewing see Chapter 7. Physical assessment skills are necessary to monitor the effectiveness of nursing interventions (see Chap. 18). The ability to inspect, palpate, percuss, and auscultate proficiently provides objective data about the effectiveness of nursing interventions. For example, if a patient has a gas exchange impairment related to altered oxygen supply, ausculta-

tion of breath sounds yields information about the effectiveness of nursing interventions.

Knowledge and skill in the use of measurement devices yields further information about the effectiveness of nursing interventions. Many technologic advances in medicine and nursing make it mandatory for nurses to have knowledge and skill in the use of multiple measurement devices. Nurses use devices such as blood pressure cuffs, thermometers, arterial lines, intracranial pressure monitors, and central venous pressure lines frequently depending on the practice setting. Measurement devices provide information for the evaluation of nursing strategies. The nurse also requires knowledge and skill in interpreting laboratory data. Laboratory studies such as complete blood counts, arterial blood gases, and routine urinalysis tests produce data for evaluation of nursing interventions. For example, in the same patient with gas exchange impairment related to altered oxygen supply, arterial blood gas measurements help the nurse determine oxygenation, ventilation, metabolic status, and whether endotracheal intubation is needed.

Awareness of Clinical Research

Current research findings are used to develop innovative methods to sharpen assessment and diagnostic skills; establish future standards for developing patient goals, patient outcomes, and nursing interventions in the planning step; and provide the latest, up-to-date knowledge to enhance nursing practice. Nurses can use current research findings in several ways. (Moloney, 1986; Ziegler, Vaughan-Wrobel, & Erlen, 1986).

Types of Evaluation

Evaluation can center on one of three areas: structure, process, or outcome.

Structure Evaluation

Structure evaluation focuses on the attributes of the setting or surroundings where the health care is provided (Donabedian, 1966). It deals with the environmental aspects that directly or indirectly influence the quality of care provided. Availability of equipment, layout of physical facilities, nurse–patient ratios, administrative support, and maintenance of nursing staff competence are some areas of concern for structure evaluation (Miller, 1989; Ziegler, Vaughan-Wrobel, & Erlen, 1986).

Process Evaluation

Process evaluation focuses on the performance of the nurse and whether the nursing care provided was appropriate and competent (Ziegler, Vaughan-Wrobel, & Erlen, 1986). The steps of the nursing process are used

Nursing Research

Pasquarello, M. A. (1990). Measuring the impact of an acute stroke program on patient outcomes. *Journal of Neuroscience Nursing, 22,* 76–82.

This study examined the impact of a nurse-managed stroke program in an acute-care facility on several patient outcome criteria. Some of the outcome criteria included length of stay, type of facility where patient was placed after hospitalization, complications, and compliance with followup appointments and medication regimen. The stroke program had an inpatient, followup, and research component. Family members were an integral part of all aspects. Study findings showed a decrease in length of stay, an increase in patients discharged to home after hospitalization, a decrease in complications, and an increase in keeping followup appointments and medication compliance. The nurse-managed stroke program made a significant impact on patient outcomes in this particular group of patients. The authors suggest that a collaborative approach among nurse practitioners, researchers, and educators would facilitate the development of nursing strategies for stroke patients based on patient outcomes.

as the framework for the evaluation of nursing care (Yura & Walsh, 1988). Areas of concern for this type of evaluation include the type of information obtained by interview and physical assessment, the validity of the nursing diagnostic statements, and the technical competence of the nurse (Donabedian, 1966; 1976).

Outcome Evaluation

Outcome evaluation, which focuses on the patient and the patient's functional health status, is currently receiving a great deal of emphasis. Outcome evaluation determines the extent to which the patient's behavioral response to nursing intervention reflects the desired patient goal and outcome criteria (Ziegler, Vaughan-Wrobel, & Erlen, 1986). Outcome evaluation can take place only after standards have been developed. An example of an outcome evaluation would be to establish standards of care for a specific diagnosis and then to compare actual patient outcomes with that standard.

Evaluation Activities

The evaluation phase of the nursing process includes these activities: review patient goals and outcome crite-

ria; collect data; measure goal attainment; record judgment of goal attainment; and revise the nursing care plan and record judgments made about goal attainment.

Review Patient Goals and Outcome Criteria

The nurse begins measuring goal attainment by reviewing the patient goals and outcome criteria developed for each nursing diagnosis. Outcome criteria, written in measurable terms in the planning phase, are used to judge goal attainment. Review of the expected patient behaviors includes examining the time-frames and methods for measurement of goal fulfillment. This review helps the nurse focus on data needed to assess the accuracy and realistic nature of the goals and outcome criteria (Alfaro, 1990).

Collect Data

Systematic data collection is required to determine if goals have been attained and if patient outcome criteria have been fulfilled. Subjective and objective data are collected to judge the patient's behavioral responses to nursing interventions. Objective data is collected from many sources, including the patient, family members or significant others, nursing staff, and other health-team members. Information from observation (e.g., posture, skin color, behavior), health records (e.g., laboratory results, reports from other health-team members), physical assessment (e.g., breath sounds, strength of extrem-

Nursing Research

Morgan, S. P. (1990). A comparison of three methods of managing fever in the neurologic patient. *Journal of Neuroscience Nursing, 22,* 19–24.

This study measured the effect of three methods of reducing fever in adult neurologic patients and the effect of these methods on patient shivering. Twenty-one patients with elevated temperatures were randomly assigned to one of the three temperature reduction groups. Study results indicated no significant difference among the three methods in the rate of decreasing body temperature. Statistical analysis revealed a significant relationship between the frequency of shivering and the use of a hypothermia (cooling) blanket. The authors recommended replication of this study using a larger sample. In addition, research is needed on nursing strategies to reduce the harmful effects of shivering when a hypothermia blanket is used.

ities), and measurement devices (e.g., blood pressure, temperature) are examples of objective data.

Subjective data is also used to evaluate the effectiveness of nursing care provided. For example, a patient with a nursing diagnosis of Pain related to a recent surgical procedure may have as a goal, "Patient will state that his pain is relieved within 30 minutes after he is repositioned." The patient's subjective statement would be needed to judge whether this goal had been achieved. More information on subjective and objective data can be found in Chapter 18.

Measure Goal Attainment

After collecting data, the nurse forms a comprehensive picture of the patient's behavioral responses to nursing interventions. The next step is to make a judgment about goal attainment. The evaluative data are used to compare the patient's actual behavioral responses to the predicted responses or predetermined outcome criteria developed in the planning phase. When possible, the patient is involved in the judgment of goal attainment.

The four possible judgments that may be made are (Alfaro, 1990):

- The goal was completely met.
- The goal was partially met.
- The goal was completely unmet.
- New problems or nursing diagnoses have developed (this can exist simultaneously with any of the first three).

The fourth judgment can exist simultaneously with any of the first three. Figure 9-7 displays some examples of a completely met goal, a partially met goal, and a completely unmet goal. Once the judgment about the attainment or lack of attainment of the outcome criteria is made, revision of the nursing management plan takes place. See the section on revision and modification of the nursing care plan.

Assess for Facilitators of Goal Attainment. Patients, family members, significant others, and other health-team members are invaluable in facilitating or helping with goal attainment. Occasionally, only those closest to the patient can identify the subtle or elusive factors that helped (or hindered) goal achievement. Examples of facilitators include audiovisual materials, written handouts, repetition of material, and easily accessible and interested nursing staff.

Assess for Barriers to Goal Attainment. Several barriers to goal attainment have been identified including the patient, family members, significant others, nurse, and other health-team members. Examples of how goal attainment may be blocked include providing incorrect information, withholding information, having an unexpected reaction to treatment (e.g., allergic response to

Goal Completely Met

Nursing Diagnosis: Impaired swallowing related to neuromuscular impairment
↓
Patient Goal: Patient will demonstrate correct eating techniques to maximize swallowing
↓
Subjective Data: Patient states, "I sit up in a chair for a half hour after I eat."
↓
Objective Data: Wears dentures when eating; performs return demonstration of facial exercises; bends head forward when eating; checks mouth for any remaining food particles; remains in Fowler's position for at least 30 minutes after eating; lies on side while lying in bed.

Goal Partially Met

Nursing Diagnosis: Chronic low self-esteem
↓
Patient Goal: Patient interacts verbally in group therapy session.
↓
Subjective Data: Patient states, "I feel uncomfortable when speaking in front of others."
↓
Objective Data: Patient observed sitting in group session, looking at floor, and not participating in discussion.

Goal Completely Unmet

Nursing Diagnosis: Impaired mobility related to neuromuscular impairment.
↓
Patient Goal: Patient will carry out prescribed mobility regimen.
↓
Subjective Data: Patient states, "I can't do anything by myself. I need a lot of help with everything."
↓
Objective Data: Unable to perform active range of motion exercises independently; unable to transfer from bed to wheelchair; unable to dress and groom independently.

Figure 9–7. Clinical examples of evaluation of patient goals: goals completely met, partially met, and completely unmet.

therapy), inadequate coping ability, and worsening of underlying pathologic condition (Yura & Walsh, 1988).

Family members are also barriers to goal attainment. Family members or significant others may hinder goal achievement in multiple ways. For example, their lack of understanding of the plan of care, their lack of interest in the patients, or their failure to realize the patient actually has a problem can impede movement toward goal achievement. The cultural heritage, moral values, and religious influences of a family can also be barriers to goal attainment (Yura & Walsh 1988).

The nurse may unwittingly block goal achievement, for instance, by neglecting to collect pertinent assessment data, assigning an inappropriate priority rating to nursing diagnoses, and delegating nursing care to inappropriate nursing staff members. The nurse may fail to include the patient in the planning step, fail to incorporate facets of the medical regimen when developing the nursing management plan, and neglect to share critical information with other members of the health team (Yura & Walsh, 1988).

Other health-team members may be the source of barriers to goal attainment. They may have a lack of communication among themselves, inability to work together as a team, and failure to coordinate the activities of all health-team members (Yura & Walsh, 1988). When health-team members do not share information among themselves, continuity in the planning and implementation of care is hampered. The evaluation phase identifies the barriers that interfere with the patient's advancement toward goal achievement.

Record Judgment or Measurement of Goal Attainment

Written documentation of the subjective and objective data gathered and the judgment made about goal attainment is required on the patient's health record. Judgments about goal attainment are written clearly and concisely. Avoid ambiguous terms such as "inadequate," "good," or "extremely well," which can be interpreted differently by different people (Ziegler, Vaughan-Wrobel, & Erlen, 1986).

Revise and Modify Nursing Management Plan

Revision and modification of the nursing management plan is part of the evaluation phase. It provides a feedback mechanism that starts the entire chain of events again. Figure 9-8 illustrates the feedback mechanism, which starts with a complete reassessment of the patient, and the cyclic nature of the nursing process.

Nursing diagnoses that were resolved require no further nursing intervention. Resolved nursing diagnoses may be deleted from the nursing care plan. To maintain the patient's "problem-free status," a nursing care plan is developed that incorporates potential nursing diagnoses and gears nursing actions toward maximal functional health (Yura & Walsh, 1988). The nurse periodically reassesses the level of functioning and health status changes to determine if new problems or nursing diagnoses have developed.

Some patient goals will be partially met or completely unmet. Modification begins with a complete reassessment of the patient. Changes in patient goals, patient outcome criteria, and nursing interventions are required. If new problems have arisen, new nursing diagnoses must be identified and a nursing care plan written. Figure 9-9 illustrates the steps taken after judgment of goal attainment and needed revisions of the nursing care plan.

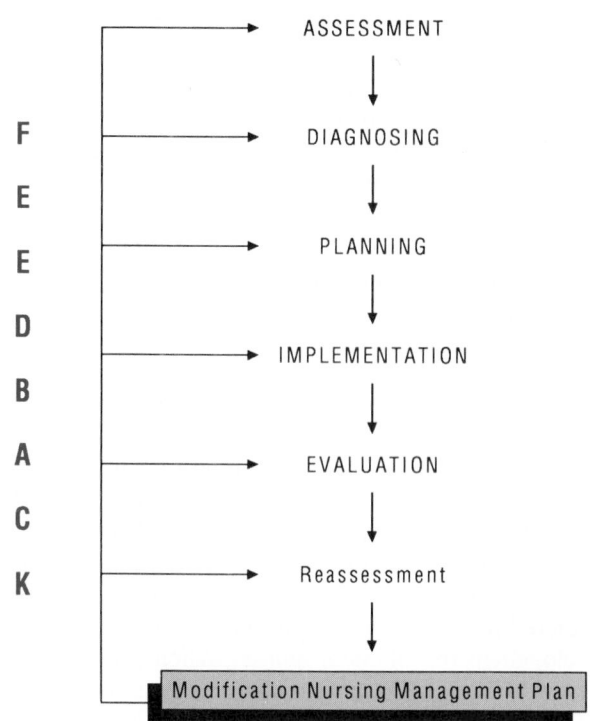

Figure 9–8. Feedback mechanism and cyclic nature of nursing process.

Quality Assurance Monitors

Up to this point, the discussion has centered on the evaluation of the individual patient. The patient's nursing care plan, with unique nursing diagnoses, patient goals, outcome criteria, and nursing interventions has been the center of attention. Evaluation has focused on the attainment of patient's goals and outcome criteria for a single patient. The evaluation of the quality of nursing care provided to groups of patients with similar problems or nursing diagnoses is also conducted. **Quality assurance monitors** provide input for the development and refinement of standards of care for groups of similar patients. Peer review is another method of evaluating the quality of patient care.

Quality assurance monitors are mechanisms that ensure quality patient care is provided and standards are upheld. Standards provide the basis for quality assurance monitors "because they are statements of accountability and define requirements for quality nursing care" (Moriconi, 1989, p. 176). Quality assurance involves measuring "the extent to which there is deviation from the standard or the extent to which the standard is met" (Yura & Walsh, 1988, p. 174). Focus on quality assurance monitors is the combined result of the consumer's demand for high-caliber health services and soaring healthcare costs. Also, governmental agencies, accreditation groups, and regulatory bodies have pressured the

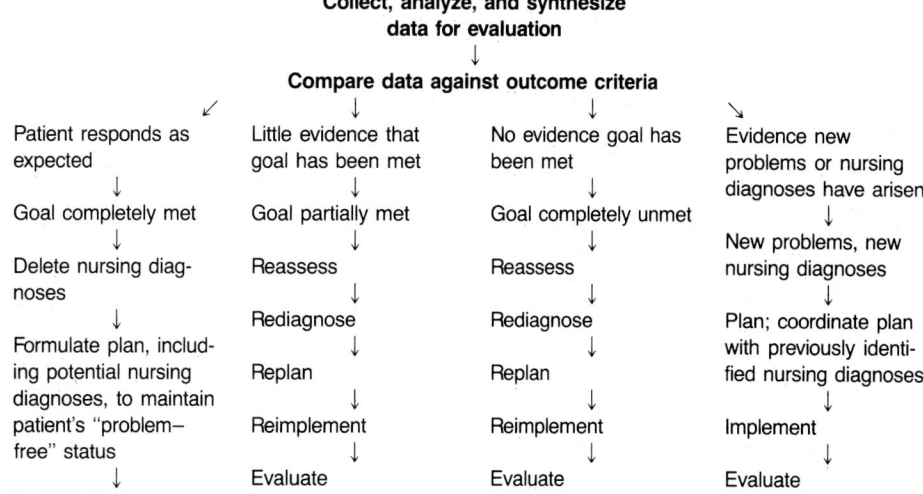

Figure 9–9. Flowchart to identify actions taken after judgment of goal achievement.

Collect, analyze, and synthesize
data for evaluation
↓
Compare data against outcome criteria

Patient responds as expected	Little evidence that goal has been met	No evidence goal has been met	Evidence new problems or nursing diagnoses have arisen
↓	↓	↓	↓
Goal completely met	Goal partially met	Goal completely unmet	New problems, new nursing diagnoses
↓	↓	↓	↓
Delete nursing diagnoses	Reassess	Reassess	Plan; coordinate plan with previously identified nursing diagnoses
↓	↓	↓	↓
Formulate plan, including potential nursing diagnoses, to maintain patient's "problem–free" status	Rediagnose	Rediagnose	Implement
	↓	↓	↓
	Replan	Replan	Evaluate
	↓	↓	
	Reimplement	Reimplement	
↓	↓	↓	
Periodically reassess	Evaluate	Evaluate	

nursing profession to respond to quality assurance issues. Standards of care have been proposed by the American Nurses Association (ANA), the JCAHO, specialty nursing organizations (e.g, the American Association of Neuroscience Nurses), and by individual health-care institutions.

American Nurses Association

The American Nurses Association established the *Standards of Nursing Practice* in 1973 (see Chapter 1). Based on a nursing process framework, these standards consist of eight nursing goals to be attained by every patient. They are broad, general standards used to measure the quality of nursing care. Standards 7 and 8 specify the nurse's role in the evaluation process. Stadard 7 requires that the nurse measure the patient's progression or lack of progression toward goal attainment. Standard 8 states that the progression or lack of progression toward goal attainment directs the nurse to reassess, reorder priorities, set new goals, and revise the nursing care plan.

In conjunction with the ANA, some specialty nursing groups have developed processes and outcome criteria for a number of nursing diagnoses. For example, the Association of Rehabilitation Nurses and the American Association of Neuroscience Nurses have set standards based on nursing diagnoses.

The Joint Commission on Accreditation of Healthcare Organizations

The JCAHO is an external review board that establishes standards for institutions. These standards help to ensure that the institution functions within specified guidelines (Miller, 1989). The hospital standards for nursing

care are applicable to all patients in every setting where nursing care is provided. Recent changes in the JCAHO guidelines require the continuous monitoring and evaluation of the quality of nursing care provided by the department of nursing. The guidelines are general and each institution develops a specific quality assurance program suited to its organizational structure (Miller 1989).

Peer Review

Peer review is the evaluation and judgment of performance by other nurses. It is another mechanism for evaluating and monitoring nursing care provided. There are two types of peer review—nursing monitors and individual peer review.

Nursing Monitors. Nursing monitors, previously called nursing audits, are "a review, by a nurse, of the client's care or records to determine the extent to which that care or records meet established standards" (Yura & Walsh, 1988, p. 177). Nursing monitoring committees usually established the "standards against which their observations will be measured" (Yura & Walsh, 1988, p. 178). Although nursing departments develop their own standards for particular nursing care settings, the ANA *Standards of Nursing Practice* is often used as a source of generating unique standards for a particular setting or institution. Members of the monitoring committee may review a nurses' documentation of care in the health record, or may determine the patient's health status through observation. Observing the nurse actually providing nursing care is the focus of individual peer review.

Individual Peer Review. The second type of peer review is individual peer review, which focuses on the

---

Possible Topics for Nursing Inquiry

- Given a simulated functional health pattern assessment data base, what patient goals and nursing interventions are written by experienced and novice nurses?
- Which nursing interventions are effective in resolving a specific nursing diagnosis?
- Do certain conceptual nursing models facilitate comprehensive evaluation more than others?
- What is the effect of functional health pattern assessment on the evaluation phase of the nursing process?
- What is the relationship between a nursing conceptual model, personal practice ethics, and the evaluation process in new graduate nurses?

---

nurse. An individual nurse's performance is evaluated and judged by other nurses with similar education and experience. This type of review is also based on pre-established standards (Yura & Walsh, 1988). Individual peer review adds to nursing monitoring data.

Evaluation Using the Functional Health Approach

Evaluation using the functional health approach requires a specific perspective. Instead of measuring attainment of patient goals and patient outcomes, the patient's functional status for each of the 11 health patterns is established. The patient's functional status is ascertained after the nursing care plan is implemented and is based on data from the evaluation phase. Subjective and objective data are used to determine the patient's movement toward functionality or dysfunctionality in each health pattern. Evaluation using the functional health approach provides a framework for organization and evaluation of data for revision or modification of the nursing care plan.

Key Concepts

- The nursing care plan is designed to direct patient care activities, promote continuity of care, focus charting requirements, and specify who is to carry out the nursing actions.
- The key elements of the nursing care plan are the nursing diagnosis, patient goals and outcome criteria, and nursing interventions.

- Patient goals are stated as behavioral objectives and indicate the desired state of the patient if the problem has been resolved.
- Nursing interventions are dependent, independent, and interdependent activities that nurses carry out to provide patient care.
- Implementing the nursing care plan requires intellectual, interpersonal, and technical skills.
- Evaluation is a judgmental process for determining the effectiveness of nursing interventions to meet patient goals.
- Evaluation occurs throughout all steps of the nursing process but is also a distinct, separate step.
- An in-depth, comprehensive judgment about patient goal attainment and fulfillment of patient outcome criteria is performed during the evaluation step of the nursing process.
- The nursing care plan forms the foundation for evaluation.
- The nurse and patient determine goal attainment.
- The nurse, patient, family members, significant others, and other health-team members may help or hinder goal attainment.
- Quality assurance involves the monitoring and evaluating of nursing care against standards of nursing practice.
- Revising the nursing care plan involves reassessment, rediagnosis, and replanning.
- Evaluation determines the reasons why the nursing care plan was a success or failure.

References

Alfaro, R. (1990). *Applying nursing diagnosis and nursing process: A step-by-step guide* (2nd ed.). Philadelphia: J. B. Lippincott.

American Nurses Association (1973). *Standards of nursing practice.* Kansas City, MO: author.

Brunner, L. S., & Suddarth, D. S. (1988). *Textbook of medical-surgical nursing* (6th ed.). Philadelphia: J. B. Lippincott.

Bulechek, G. M., & McCloskey, J. C. (1990). Nursing intervention taxonomy development. In J. C. McCloskey & H. K. Grace (Eds.), *Current issues in nursing* (3rd ed.). St. Louis: C. V. Mosby, pp. 23–28.

Carpenito, L. J. (1989). *Nursing diagnosis: Application to clinical practice* (3rd ed.). Philadelphia: J. B. Lippincott.

Donabedian, A. (1966). Evaluating the quality of medical care. *Milbank Memorial Fund Quarterly, 44*(3), 166–203 (part 2).

Donabedian, A. (1976). Some basic issues in evaluating the quality of health care. In American Nurses Association, *Issues in evaluation research: An invitational conference* (pp. 3–28). Kansas City, MO: American Nurses Association.

Henderson, P., & Southern, D. (1990). Making caring plans. *Nursing Times, 80*(4), 33–35.

Joint Commission on the Accreditation of Healthcare Organizations. (1990). *Accreditation manual for hospitals.* Chicago: Author.

Mayers, M. G. (1978). *A systematic approach to the nursing care plan* (pp. 8–9). New York: Appleton-Century-Crofts.

McCloskey, J. C., Bulechek, G. M., Cohen, M. Z., et al. (1990). Classification of nursing interventions. *Journal of Professional Nursing, 6*(3), 151–157.

Miller, E. (1989). *How to make nursing diagnosis work: Administrative and clinical strategies.* Norwalk, CT: Appleton & Lange.

Moloney, M. M. (1986). *Professionalization of nursing: Current issues and trends.* Philadelphia: J. B. Lippincott.

Morgan, S. P. (1990). A comparison of three methods of managing fever in the neurologic patient. *Journal of Neuroscience Nursing, 22,* 19–24.

Moriconi, D. (1989). Quality assurance in diagnosis-based nursing practice. In E. Miller (Ed.), *How to make nursing diagnosis work: Administrative and clinical strategies.* Norwalk, CT: Appleton & Lange.

Pasquarello, M. A. (1990). Measuring the impact of an acute stroke program on patient outcomes. *Journal of Neuroscience Nursing, 22,* 76–82.

Roy, C., & Roberts, S. L. (1981). *Theory construction in nursing: An adaptation model.* Englewood Cliffs, NJ: Prentice-Hall.

Seiler, W., & Stahelin, H. (1985). Decubitus ulcers: Treatment through five therapeutic principles. *Geriatrics, 40*(90), 30–42.

Walters, S. (1986). Computerized care plans help nurses achieve quality patient care. *Journal of Nursing Administration, 16*(11), 33–39.

Yura, H., & Walsh, M. B. (1983). *The nursing process: Assessing, planning, implementing, evaluating* (4th ed.). Norwalk, CT: Appleton-Century-Crofts.

Yura, H., & Walsh, M. B. (1988). *The nursing process: Assessing, planning, implementing, evaluating* (5th ed.). Norwalk, CT: Appleton & Lange.

Ziegler, S. M., Vaughan-Wrobel, B. C., & Erlen, J. A. (1986). *Nursing process, nursing diagnosis, nursing knowledge: Avenues to autonomy.* Norwalk, CT: Appleton-Century-Crofts.

Bibliography

Kirchhoff, K. (Ed.). (1990). Computer voice documentation system. *Research review: Studies for nursing practice, 6*(5), 3.

Lang, N. M., & Marek, K. D. (1990). The classification of patient outcomes. *Journal of Professional Nursing, 6*(3), 158–163.

Masson, V. (1990). Nursing the charts. *Nursing Outlook, 38*(4), 196.

Ohs, C. A. (1990). Dictated patient assessments. *Journal of Nursing Administration, 20*(4), 4–5.

Wake, M. M. (1990). Nursing care delivery systems: Status and vision. *Journal of Nursing Administration, 20*(5), 47–51.

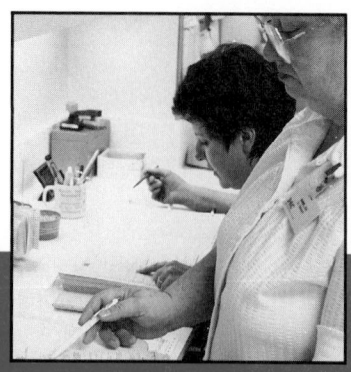

Communication of the Nursing Process: Recording and Reporting

LEARNING OBJECTIVES

Upon completion of this chapter, the student will be able to do the following:

- Describe the purposes of the patient record.
- List principles of charting.
- Differentiate formats of source-oriented recording and problem-oriented recording.
- Understand how to use a nursing Kardex.
- Properly record nursing progress notes by SOAP or narrative format.

- Identify flowsheets used in the patient record.
- Fill out a nursing history admission sheet and a nursing discharge summary.
- Identify important data for the change-of-shift report.
- Describe the procedure for telephone reporting.
- Discuss the importance of confidentiality.

KEY TERMS

Audit
Care plan conferences
Change-of-shift report
Flowsheets

Incident
Kardex
Nursing care plan
Problem-oriented medical record

Recording
Reporting
SOAP note
Source-oriented record

10

Written Communication: The Patient Record
 Purpose
  Communication
  Assessment
  Care Planning
  Education
  Research
  Auditing
  Legal Documentation
 Principles of Charting
  Conciseness
  Accuracy
  Completeness
  Organization
  Legibility
  Timeliness
  Confidentiality
 Types of Documentation
  Source-Oriented Record
  Problem-Oriented Medical Record

  Computer Documentation
 Nursing Entries on the Patient Record
  Nursing Care Plan
  Kardex
  Nursing Progress Notes
  Flowsheets
  Admission Entries
  Nursing Discharge Summary
  Medication Records
  Incident Report
Oral Communication: Reporting
 Change-of-Shift Reports
 Nursing Rounds
 Telephone Reports
 Patient Transfers
 Report to Physician
 Reports from Other Departments
 Care Plan Conferences
 Confidentiality
Key Concepts

The nursing process is communicated both verbally and in writing. Effective communication enhances patient care by ensuring comprehensive, coordinated care by a variety of providers. All members of the health-care team share information through recording and reporting.

Written communication, or **recording,** serves as a permanent document of patient information and care. The patient record or chart provides information during the present visit or admission and may also be consulted in the future to review the patient's history and for educational, research, and legal purposes.

Reporting takes place when two or more people share information about patient care, either face to face (as in a nursing report from one shift to the next), by audiotape, or by telephone (as in laboratory reports given to the nursing unit).

Nurses are responsible for accurate, complete, and timely recording and reporting. As an instrument of continuous patient care and as a legal document, the patient record should contain all pertinent assessments, planning, interventions, and evaluations for that patient.

WRITTEN COMMUNICATION: THE PATIENT RECORD

The patient record is essential for the communication of goals, overall plan of care, and progress for each patient. It is prepared in written or computerized form and is accessible to members of the health-care team caring for the patient. If a patient record is misplaced on a nursing unit, a vital line of communication is blocked.

Nurses should become familiar with the type of recording done in their hospital. Nurses' entries on the patient record are important because they show that medical orders were carried out and independent assessments and interventions were performed, and the exact dates and times of care and progress are documented.

Purposes of Patient Records

- Communication
- Assessment
- Care planning
- Education
- Research
- Auditing
- Legal documentation

Purpose

The patient record is kept for the following reasons: communication, assessment, care planning, education, research, auditing, and legal documentation.

Communication

Clearly documented information on the patient record communicates the care plan and the patient's progress to all members of the health-care team. Team members who interact with the patient at different times and in different ways get a clear picture of what took place in their absence. This communication ensures continuity of care.

Assessment

Nurses and other team members can gather assessment data from the patient record. By reading about the patient's history and initial assessment and comparing additional subjective and objective information that has been documented, the nurse can assess current health status and progress toward goals. Progressive assessments of a wound, for example, might alert the nurse to a developing infection or tell him or her the wound is healing properly.

Care Planning

Formulating a care plan should flow from assessment when working with the patient record. All data on the patient record should be considered when developing nursing diagnoses, goals, interventions, and evaluation criteria for that patient. An individualized nursing care plan is essential for each patient and may become part of the permanent patient record.

Education

Members of the health-care team, including students of nursing, medicine, and other disciplines, often use the patient record as an educational tool. It contains valu-

able information about signs and symptoms of disease, diagnostic tests, treatment modalities, and patient responses to the disease and treatment. A nursing student, for example, may read the record of a stroke patient to learn what signs and symptoms the patient initially experienced, what a CAT scan might show, what medications are used to minimize brain injury, and what type of physical therapy is helpful.

Research

Nursing and medical research is often carried out by studying patient records. Data may be gathered from groups of records to determine significant similarities in disease presentation, to identify contributing factors, or to determine the effectiveness of therapies. For example, a nurse researcher may review the records of patients who have had appendectomies to determine how long they needed pain medication postoperatively. This information, then, might be used in preoperative teaching.

Auditing

An **audit** is a review of records. Audits of patient records serve a dual purpose: quality assurance and reimbursement.

Auditing is done for quality assurance by randomly selecting records to see if certain standards of care have been met and documented. The Joint Commission on Accreditation of Healthcare Organizations (JCAHO) audits patient records yearly and encourages hospitals to set up ongoing quality assurance programs. Any identified deficiencies can be remedied by educating the staff.

Auditing may also take place for the purpose of reimbursement. Insurance coverage may not be provided unless an audit of the patient record justifies the care for which the company is being billed. The patient record is key in a prospective payment system based on diagnosis-related groups (DRGs).

Legal Documentation

The patient record serves as a legal document of the patient's health status and the care given. It may be used in court to prove or disprove injuries to a patient incurred in an accident, or to implicate or absolve a health-care professional for improper care. Since nurses and other health-care team members cannot remember specific assessments or interventions about a patient years after the fact, accurate and complete documentation is essential. The care may have been excellent, but documentation must prove it.

Principles of Charting

Principles of good charting are easier to accept and adopt if the purposes of the record are kept in mind. Remem-

TABLE 10–1

Abbreviations Commonly Used in Documentation

Abbreviation	Meaning	Abbreviation	Meaning
ā	before	NG	nasogastric
abd	abdomen	noc	night
ac	before meals	NPO	nothing by mouth
ADLs	activities of daily living	os	mouth
ad lib	as needed	OOB	out of bed
adm.	admitted, admission	oz	ounce
amp.	ampule	p̄	after
ant.	anterior	p.c.	after meals
AP	anterior–posterior	post	posterior
ax.	axillary	prep	preparation
b.i.d.	twice a day	prn	when necessary
BP	blood pressure	q̄, q	every
BR	bed rest	q̄ 2 (3, 4, etc.) h	every 2 (3, 4, etc.) hours.
BRP	bathroom privileges	qd	every day
C	Centigrade	qh	every hour
c̄	with	q.i.d.	four times a day
caps	capsule	q.o.d.	every other day
C.C.	chief complaint	q.s.	quantity sufficient
cc	cubic centimeter (1 cc = 1 mL)	R/O	rule out
CVP	central venous pressure	ROM	range of motion
c/o	complains of	s̄	without
D/C	discontinue	SBA	stand by assistance
disch; DC	discharge	SC	subcutaneous
drsg	dressing	SL	sublingual
dr	dram	SOB	shortness of breath
elix	elixir	sol, soln	solution
ext	extract or external	spec	specimen
F	Fahrenheit	S/P	status post
fx.	fracture, fractional	sp. gr.	specific gravity
gm	gram	S.S.E.	soapsuds enema
gr	grain	ss	one-half
gtt	drop	stat	immediately
"H," SC, or sub q	hypodermic or subcutaneous	tab	tablet
h	hour	t.i.d.	three times a day
HOB	head of bed	tinct or tr.	tincture
h.s.	bedtime (hour of sleep)	TKO	to keep open
hx	history	TPN	total parenteral nutrition, hyper-alimentation
I & O	intake & output		
IM	intramuscular	TPR	temperature, pulse, respiration
IV	intravenous	tsp	teaspoon
kg	kilogram	TO	telephone order
KVO	keep vein open	TWE	tap water enema
L	left; liter	VO	verbal order
lat	lateral	VS	vital signs
MAE	moves all extremities	VSS	vital signs stable
mg	milligram	W/C	wheelchair
ml, mL	milliliter (1 mL = 1 cc)	WNL	within normal limits
NAD	no apparent distress		

Selected Abbreviations Used for Specific Descriptions

Abbreviation	Meaning	Abbreviation	Meaning
AKA	above-knee amputation	Nsy.	nursery
ASCVD	arteriosclerotic cardiovascular disease	NWB	non-weight-bearing
		O.D.	right eye
ASHD	arteriosclerotic heart disease	O.S.	left eye
BKA	below-knee amputation	O.U.	each eye
ca	cancer	OPD	outpatient department
chest clear to A & P	chest clear to auscultation & percussion	ORIF	open reduction internal fixation
		Ortho	orthopedics
CMS	circulation movement sensation	OT	occupational therapy
CNS	central nervous system	PE	physical examination

(continued)

TABLE 10–1

(continued)

Abbreviation	Meaning	Abbreviation	Meaning
DJD	degenerative joint disease	PERRLA	pupils equal, round, & react to light and accommodation
DOE	dyspnea on exertion		
DT's	delerium tremens	PID	pelvic inflammatory disease
D₅W	5% dextrose in water	PI	present illness
FUO	fever of unknown origin	PM & R	physical medicine & rehabilitation
GB	gall bladder	Psych	psychology; psychiatric
GI	gastrointestinal	PT	physical therapy
GYN	gynecology	RL (or LR)	Ringer's lactate; lactated Ringer's
H₂O₂	hydrogen peroxide	RLE	right lower extremity
HA	hyperalimentation; headache	RLQ	right lower quadrant
HCVD	hypertensive cardiovascular disease	RR, PAR	recovery room, post-anesthesia room
HEENT	head, ear, eye, nose, throat	RUE	right upper extremity
HVD	hypertensive vascular disease	RUQ	right upper quadrant
ICU	intensive care unit	Rx	prescription
I & D	incision and drainage	STSG	split-thickness skin graft
LLE	left lower extremity	Surg	surgery, surgical
LLQ	left lower quadrant	T & A	tonsillectomy & adenoidectomy
LOC	level of consciousness; laxatives of choice	THR; TJR	total hip replacement; total joint replacement
LMP	last menstrual period	URI	upper respiratory infection
LUE	left upper extremity	UTI	urinary tract infection
LUQ	left upper quadrant	vag	vaginal
MI	myocardial infarction	VD	venereal disease
Neuro	neurology; neurosurgery	WNWD	well-nourished, well-developed
NS	normal saline		

Selected Abbreviations Related to Common Diagnostic Tests

Abbreviation	Meaning	Abbreviation	Meaning
BE	barium enema	hct	hematocrit
B.M.R.	basal metabolism rate	Hgb	hemoglobin
Ca⁺⁺	calcium	IVP	intravenous pyelogram
CAT	computed axial tomography	K⁺	potassium
CBC	complete blood count	LP	lumbar puncture
Cl⁻	chloride	MRI	magnetic resonance imaging
C & S	culture & sensitivity	Na⁺	sodium
Dx	diagnosis	RBC	red blood cell
ECG, EKG	electrocardiogram	UGI	upper gastrointestinal x-ray
EEG	electroencephalogram	UA	urinalysis
FBS	fasting blood sugar	WBC	white blood cell

Commonly Used Symbols

Symbol	Meaning	Symbol	Meaning
$>$	greater than	@	at
$<$	less than	+	positive
$=$	equal to	−	negative
$\approx$	approximately equal to	$\pm$	positive or negative
$\leq$	equal to or less than	F_1	first filial generation
$\geq$	equal to or greater than	F_2	second filial generation
$\uparrow$	increased	$P\,O_2$	partial pressure of oxygen
$\downarrow$	decreased	$P\,CO_2$	partial pressure of carbon dioxide
♀	female	:	ratio
♂	male	$\therefore$	therefore
°	degree	%	percent
#	number or pound	2°	secondary to
$\times$	times	Δ	change

ber that any entry made in the nursing notes can serve not only as communication, but may also be scrutinized carefully by students, lawyers, and researchers. Principles of good charting include conciseness, accuracy, completeness, organization, legibility, timeliness, and confidentiality.

Conciseness

Good charting is concise and brief. Use partial sentences and phrases; drop the patient's name and terms referring to the patient. Use abbreviations, but only those that are commonly accepted (Table 10-1). Unnecessary elabora-

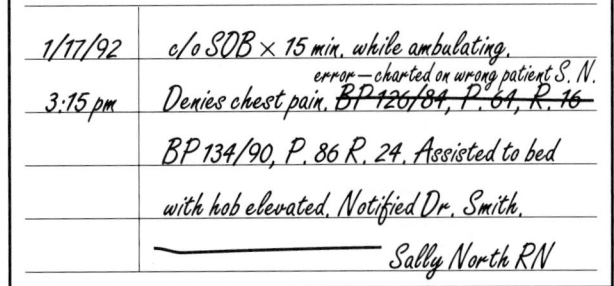

Principles of Charting

- Conciseness
- Accuracy
- Completeness
- Organization
- Legibility
- Timeliness
- Confidentiality

All entries must be made in ink; no erasures or White Out.

Figure 10–1.   Sample correction of an error in recording.

tion confuses important issues. Being concise is also helpful in time management: the nurse will spend less time at the desk and more time with patients.

Accuracy

Entries must be accurate. The nurse must write only observations that he or she has seen, heard, smelled, or felt; an observation made by another health professional must be clearly discriminated from the nurse's personal assumptions. Charting that a patient "states he is upset that surgery has been postponed" is more accurate than charting "patient mad at doctor." Precise measurements and times should be used when possible. For example, a wound should be described as "3 cm by 0.5 cm" rather than "small." To avoid confusion, make sure that the names of physicians or other professionals are correct. Correct spelling and correct use of medical terms are important.

When an error occurs, no erasure is permissible, so a notation about the error must be made (Fig. 10-1). A single line should be drawn through the error and the word "error" and the nurse's initials should be written above it. Some hospitals require an explanation of the error, such as "charted for wrong patient."

Completeness

Obviously, not every observation and intervention is recorded, but information about the nursing process must be complete. Other team members may consider that an action not recorded may not have been done. For example, if a patient's temperature of 100.8°F at 2 PM was not recorded, the nurse coming on at 4 PM might not take the patient's temperature; it may be significantly higher, the patient will be uncomfortable, and infection may be flourishing. Complete, pertinent assessment data, such as other vital signs, wound drainage, and patient complaints, as well as who was notified and what interventions were carried out, give the night-shift nurse a complete picture, so that he or she can make objective evaluations and revise the care plan as needed.

The following information is essential in charting:

- Signs and symptoms
- Patient behavior
- Nursing interventions
- Medications given
- Physician's orders carried out
- Patient teaching
- Patient responses.

Most significant is any new or changed information.

Organization

Each entry must clearly show a logical and systematic grouping of important information. Information is grouped by problem or occurrence and flows in a logical format. For example, assessment is recorded with subjective and objective data, followed by a physician's order, the nursing interventions, and the patient's response. Information about a routine laboratory test is recorded elsewhere if it does not pertain to this problem.

There must be a chronologic flow of information about patient care according to time and procedures completed, with patient reaction documented. Recording as the events of the day unfold can prevent out-of-sequence or fragmented entries that can cause confusion.

Legibility

The nurse's writing must be clear and easily read by others. Legibility is especially important when recording numbers and medical terms. For example, a pulse rate of 164 may look similar to 104, but has more serious implications. The term *dysphasia* (difficulty speaking) may be mistaken for *dysphagia* (difficulty swallowing).

Timeliness

Timely recording is especially important when a patient's condition is changing frequently. For example, suppose a nurse gives a postoperative patient an injection of meperidine (Demerol) 75 mg, but does not record the injection. She then enters an isolation room to care for another patient. Another nurse discovers that the postoperative patient's blood pressure has dropped. She notifies the surgeon, who takes steps to determine if the patient has internal bleeding. In fact, the patient was having an adverse reaction to meperidine, but because the injection was not charted, other team members were unaware of it. Nurses should not leave the unit for breaks or other long periods until important information is recorded.

Timeliness is also important in recording so nurses do not forget important information. Waiting until the end of the shift to record the day's events on several patients may cause the nurse to omit important data or enter inaccurate information.

Confidentiality

All patient care should be confidential. This is a basic nursing responsibility. Nurses should treat the patient record as a confidential document entrusted to the health-care team. It should never be left in public areas or where a patient or family member can read it without a physician's order and explanation of medical terms.

Types of Documentation

Documentation may be of three types:

- Source-oriented record
- Problem-oriented medical record (POMR)
- Computer documentation.

Nurses should become familiar with the type used in their hospital. All team members should use the same type of documentation.

Source-Oriented Record

In the **source-oriented record,** documentation is organized according to who is making the entry (Table 10-2). Each type of health-care provider documents separately. For example, nurses record only in the area designated for nursing, and physical therapists document separately in their area. This may cause fragmentation and replication of documentation and may hinder coordination between team members. Other components of this type of record that nurses do not record include the physician's history and physical assessment, physician's progress notes, discharge summary, and respiratory therapy notes. Table 10-2 explains components of the source-oriented record.

Source-oriented documentation makes recording easier, but it makes it more difficult to review a particular event or to follow the overall progress of a patient. For example, if an elderly patient falls getting out of bed, the nurse records the event in the nurses' notes. The physician charts his or her assessment on the physician's progress notes and makes orders on the physician's order sheet. A physical therapist who teaches the patient how to use a cane records in physical therapy notes. The x-ray report appears in its section. Reviewing the entire incident would require flipping back and forth and scanning much information.

Some nurses think that source-oriented recording

TABLE 10–2

The Source-Oriented Record and Its Components

Component	Information Included
Admission sheet	Patient's name, address, age, sex, Social Security number, occupation, employer, religion, attending physician, admitting diagnosis, health insurance
Physician's order sheet	Specific orders for medications, treatment, diagnostic tests
Graph/flowsheets	Temperature, pulse, respirations, blood pressure, daily weights, intake and output measurements, urine sugar and acetone, daily activity, routine treatments performed
Nursing admission assessment	Nursing history and functional assessment on admission
Nurses' notes	Chronological documentation of the nursing process (ongoing assessment, nursing diagnosis, planning, intervention, and evaluation of patient care)
Medication sheet	Name, dosage, route, and time of medication given with initials and signature of nurse who gave it
Physician's history and physical examination	Medical history, physical examination, diagnosis, and tentative plan of care
Physician's progress notes	Chronological assessment and interpretation of patient's progress with revisions in plan of care
Discharge summary	Physician's summary of patient's course of illness, response to treatment, prognosis, status at discharge, and plan for rehabilitation or followup
Nurse's discharge sheet	Patient's vital signs and health status at discharge, as well as followup and other instructions
Miscellaneous forms	Laboratory reports, x-ray reports, consultations, respiratory therapy notes, physical therapy notes, dietary notes, social services notes

makes it easier to evaluate nursing care, because it can be done simply by reviewing the nurses' notes. In the source-oriented record traditional narrative nurses' notes are preferred to newer formats for recording nursing care.

Problem-Oriented Medical Record

Weed (1971) introduced a new method of organizing the medical record by using a patient problem approach or **problem-oriented medical record** (POMR). The POMR includes a database, problem list, plans, and progress notes; the focus is the patient's problem list. Because the same problem list and progress notes are used by all team members, the care plan is coordinated. Two examples of POMRs are given in Figures 10-2 and 10-3.

The *database* consists of all information known about the patient, including physician and nursing histories, physical assessment data, and diagnostic test results. Any team member may provide information for the database.

The *problem list* is made up of problems identified by different team members as they occur or are discovered. Problems include medical diagnoses, nursing diagnoses, signs and symptoms, abnormal diagnostic tests, behavioral problems, or risk factors. These problems are numbered, but not necessarily in order of importance. Problems are dated as to when they happened and when they were resolved.

Following the database and problem list is the *initial care plan*. Initial medical and nursing care plans may be listed after each problem. Physician's orders also appear in this section. The nursing care plan is located here, rather than in a separate file (or Kardex).

Next come *progress notes*. The POMR system uses a SOAP format of progress recording (S, subjective; O, objective; A, assessment; P, plan). SOAP is discussed later in the chapter.

Computer Documentation

Computer documentation is becoming increasingly popular. The computer can save time in both storage and retrieval of information. The use of the Hospital Information System for improving documentation of nursing practice started as early as the 1960s (Saba & McCormick, 1986, p. 265). The functions of the computer in a hospital include ordering supplies and services for a patient; storing admission assessment data; developing and revising nursing care plans; documenting progress notes; listing treatments, procedures, and medications; and storing diagnostic test results.

Computer programs used on nursing units are patient centered. Data for a particular patient can be entered or retrieved easily (Fig. 10-4). This eliminates phone calls to other departments to order supplies, reading through a whole patient record to evaluate progress, or sorting through stacks of reports to determine a patient's test result. Patient information is permanently recorded, and caregivers in various departments can communicate with one another.

Basic computer skills are usually taught through in-service education. Each nursing unit or each bed has a computer screen to display information, a keyboard to enter data, and possibly a printer to produce printed copy. The entire patient record or just parts of it (such as the medication record or laboratory tests) may be computerized.

Nursing Entries on the Patient Record

Nurses make entries on a variety of components in the patient record, including the nursing care plan, the Kardex, nursing progress notes, flowsheets, admission record, discharge instruction sheet, and medication record. Hospitals vary in their use of these components and the format for recording.

Nursing Care Plan

A **nursing care plan** also called a nursing management plan, should be generated at admission and revised to reflect changes in the patient's condition. The nursing care plan must contain nursing diagnoses, goals, outcome criteria, nursing interventions, and evaluation. Standardized care plans designed for patients with certain medical diagnoses may be used, but must be individualized. Nursing care plans are often part of the permanent patient record. See Chapter 9 for information on writing nursing care plans.

(Text continues on page 158)

Nursing Research

Selected Nursing Research Studies

Edelstein, J. (1990). A study in nursing documentation. *Nursing Management, 21*(11), 40–46.
Lucatorto, M., Petras, D. M., Drew, L. A., et al. (1991) Documentation: A focus of cost saving. *Journal of Nursing Administration, 21*(3), 32–36.

Possible Topics for Nursing Inquiry

- What are barriers to documenting nursing care?
- What nursing activities can be documented on flowsheets as compared to progress notes?
- What is the relationship between daily nursing documentation and effective discharge planning?

PATIENT CARE NEEDS
NURSING ASSESSMENT

(Date and initial column for significant problems)

PROBLEMS

NEURO
(Date/Initials)
_____ Altered thought processes
_____ Ineffective thermoregulation
_____ Altered tissue perfusion (cerebral)

SENSORY – PERCEPTUAL ALTERATION
_____ Thermoregulation:
hypothermia/hyperthermia
_____ Sensory/Perceptual alterations
_____ (specify)
(visual, auditory, kinesthetic,
gustatory, tactile, olfactory)
_____ Impaired verbal communication
_____ Impaired auditory
_____ Input excess/deficit
_____ Impaired swallowing
_____ Powerlessness

MUSCULO-SKELETAL
_____ Impaired physical mobility
_____ Activity intolerance
_____ Fatigue
_____ Altered health maintenance
_____ Potential for injury

CARDIOVASCULAR
_____ Decreased cardiac output
1. (3-14 SS) Impaired gas exchange
_____ Altered tissue perfusion
_____ (specify) (renal,
cardiopulmonary, GI, peripheral)

PULMONARY
_____ Impaired gas exchange
2. /3-14 SS Ineffective airway clearance
_____ Ineffective breathing pattern
_____ Impaired verbal communication

URINARY ELIMINATION
_____ Retention
_____ Incontinence
_____ Altered patterns

BOWEL ELIMINATION
_____ Constipation
_____ Diarrhea

NUTRITION: ALTERED
_____ More than body requirements
_____ Less than body requirements
_____ Breastfeeding: effective/ineffective

FLUID VOLUME: ALTERED
_____ Excess
_____ Deficit
                                    PG\CA2361

PROBLEMS

SKIN INTEGRITY
(Date/Initials)
_____ Impaired _____
(specify area on body)
_____ Potential for impairment _____
_____ High risk for infection
_____ Altered protection

ALTERATION IN COMFORT
3. (3-16 SS) Pain *chest muscles* (specify)
_____ Fear
_____ Sleep pattern disturbance
_____ Other _____

PSYCH – SOCIAL: ALTERED
_____ Anxiety
_____ Body image disturbance
(dysfunctional or anticipatory)
_____ Ineffective individual coping
_____ Ineffective family coping
_____ Altered family processes
_____ Parental role conflict
_____ Grieving:
anticipatory/dysfunctional
_____ Potential for self harm
_____ Diversional activity deficit
_____ Impaired home maintenance
management
_____ Other _____

KNOWLEDGE DEFICIT
_____ Specify _____
(cognitive impairment, lack of
exposure, lack of motivation)

HEALTH PERCEPTION
_____ Altered growth and development
_____ Noncompliance
_____ Spiritual distress

SELF-CARE DEFICIT
_____ Specify _____
(feeding, bathing and hygiene,
dressing and grooming, toileting)

OTHER (Refer to nursing diagnoses checklist)
_____ Specify _____
_____ Specify _____

_____
| PATIENT STAMP:
|
| James, John
| Age 52
| K. Subramanian, MD

Figure 10–2. Sample problem list. (Courtesy of Evergreen Hospital Medical
Center, Seattle, WA.)

LONG TERM GOAL The patient will maintain optimal gas exchange and a patent airway.

DATE AND HOUR	PROB. NO.	PROBLEMS/NEEDS/ CONCERNS	PATIENT OUTCOMES	INTERVENTIONS/TEACHING AND DISCHARGE PLANS	INITIAL & DATE RESOLVED
1-4	1	Impaired gas exchange related to inflammatory process in lungs.	no dyspnea on exertion; decreased restlessness; arterial blood gases within normal limits	Assess and document respiratory rate, depth, and sounds q 4 hours Administer O_2 2L per nasal cannula Elevate head of bed or have patient up in a chair to maximize air exchange	
1-4	2	Ineffective airway clearance related to pulmonary inflammation.	experiences effective coughing; has adequate fluid intake	Encourage deep breathing and coughing q 2 hours while awake. Offer fluids frequently (1000cc / shift) Change position q 2 hours	

PT. NO. James, John

Age 52

NAME

K. Subramanian, M.D.

D.O.B.

PRIMARY NURSE J. Sidney, RN

UNIVERSITY OF WASHINGTON HOSPITALS
HARBORVIEW MEDICAL CENTER
UNIVERSITY HOSPITAL
SEATTLE, WASHINGTON

PATIENT CARE PLAN

UH 0570 REV SEP 78 1-78-2059

Figure 10–3. Combined problem list and care plan.

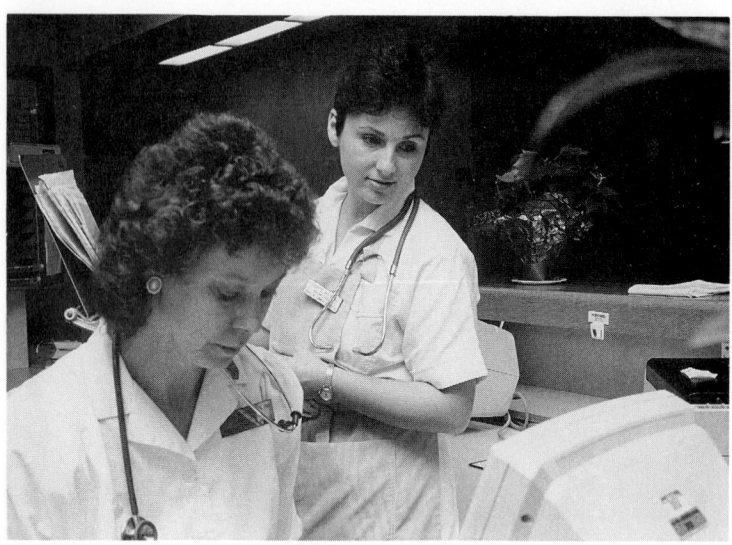

Figure 10–4. The computer in the nursing unit is a time-saver for both storage and retrieval of information in the patient record.

Kardex

The **Kardex** is a series of flip cards kept in a portable file (Fig. 10-5). Information entered on the Kardex includes the following:

- Pertinent data such as name, age, occupation, religion, physician, admission date, diagnosis, surgery, and emergency contact
- Basic needs such as diet, activity, hygiene, how bowel and urinary elimination is accomplished, assistive devices, and safety precautions
- Allergies
- Diagnostic tests
- Intravenous therapy
- Daily nursing procedures such as dressing changes, vital signs, and irrigations
- Medications
- Respiratory therapy such as use of oxygen, mechanical ventilation, or suctioning.

The Kardex serves as a way to ensure continuity of care from one shift to another, as well as from one day to the next. The Kardex is commonly used for the change-of-shift report, discussed later in this chapter. This most current record of a patient's health care is updated at least once every 8 hours or more frequently as the patient's condition changes.

Kardex entries are often in pencil so that they can be changed as the patient's condition changes. This means that the Kardex is for planning and communication purposes *only*; nursing care and patient progress must still be documented in the progress notes and appropriate flowsheets. If the Kardex is to become part of the permanent patient record, it should be written in ink. In either case, nurses are responsible for initiating and updating the Kardex and ensuring that data has been transcribed correctly from the patient record.

Nursing Progress Notes

Nursing progress notes are recorded for all patients, but vary in format. Narrative notes are often used in the source-oriented system, SOAP notes in the POMR system. Figure 10-6 gives examples of narrative and SOAP nursing progress notes.

Narrative Notes. This type of documentation serves as a method for recording all the patient's relevant behavior and activities throughout a shift. The note includes the date and time of the entry and specific activities accomplished. Typical notes include the type of morning care given (for example, bath or shower) and the patient's response. The meals given are included in the narrative, with the time given and how much the patient ate. Nursing procedures such as dressing changes and intravenous care are documented as they are completed throughout the day. Nursing assessment data is recorded as it is gathered.

Since recording in this method describes nursing actions and procedures, specific nursing identification of patient problems is not required. These activities should support information recorded on the nursing care plan and the nursing Kardex, however.

A disadvantage of narrative notes is that much reading is required to learn about a specific problem. The use of abbreviations and concise language decreases space and time used in recording. Many hospitals combine the use of flowsheets and narrative notes to shorten recording time and reduce redundancy. This is called charting by exception. Routine assessments (such as vital signs) or routine activities (such as intravenous care and bowel elimination) are recorded on flowsheets. Charting by exception can be used effectively only when the criteria are clear and all nurses in the facility consistently use these criteria.

EVERGREEN HOSPITAL MEDICAL CENTER

LEVEL OF CARE

DIET: *3-12 2gm Na diet* **ALLERGIES:**	**DAILY ORDER:** *3-12 weigh daily*
	SPECIAL EQUIPMENT
	PULMONARY: *3-12 O₂ 2L per nasal cannula* *Turn, cough, deep breathe q 2h while awake*
HYGIENE: BATH: *Assist c̄ bath* SKIN: *Observe for pressure* ORAL: *Assist*	**CARDIAC:**
	VASCULAR: *3-12 D5 ½ NS TKO*
ACTIVITY: *Up as tolerated* *Bathroom or bedside* *commode, as tolerated*	
ELIMINATION I and O: *record q shift* FOLEY: ✗	**GASTRIC:**
	OTHER:
LAST BM: *3-12*	

LAB	X-RAY	PROCEDURE OR CONSULTS	TREATMENTS
3-12 CBC, electrolytes, chemistry profile	*3-12 Chest X-ray PA & lateral*	*3-12 Respiratory Therapy*	*3-12 Antiembolic stockings*

ADMIT *3-12* **ROOM** *230* NUR-191 8603854 (3/89)	**NAME PLATE** *Bradley, Scott* *Age 91* *Brant Kyle, MD*	**CARE CLASSIFICATION** **DIAGNOSIS** *Congestive Heart Failure*	

Figure 10–5.   Example of a nursing Kardex.

SOAP Notes Examples

Correct

Problem #3	2/18/92 0900	"S" "My head hurts right in the back of my eyes." Pt describes pain worse bending over, like sinus headaches in past. "O" Eyes closed, lights dim, hesitant to move head when questioned. HR 80 R 20 BP 140/90 T 98.6 "A" HA probable 2° sinus pressure. "P" 1. Decongestant prn as ordered 2. Warm wash cloth to eyes 3. Monitor temp q 4° 4. Assess pain after med and contact physician as indicated. ———————— MS Gorski RN

Incorrect

#3	2/18/92 0900	"S" Pt states "My head hurts." "O" History of constipation, ate well at breakfast, took shower without assist, lungs clear. "I hurt all over now." "A" Headache "P" Contact physician for futher orders. ———————— MS Gorski RN

Narrative Note Example

Correct

2/18/92	0730 Patient awake, alert, denies complaints, sitting up in bed watching TV, VS taken, IV infusing s̄ difficulty, IV site (R) hand s̄ redness, (L) hip drsg dry and intact. 0830 Full liq BF take 100% 0900 Partial bath at bedside during linen △, pt tolerated sitting in chair × 30 min s̄ fatigue. 0930 △ Drsg to (L) hip approx 50cc pink drng, sutures intact, Ø redness or edema at incision line, pt tol s̄ pain 1015 1000cc D51/2 NS added to present IV to run at 125cc/hr, pt resting. 1100 To x-ray via stretcher. 1145 Returned from x-ray, back to bed for rest. 1200 Reg lunch taken 100% ———————— MS Gorski RN

Incorrect

2/18/92	0730 Pt fine, states "I like the TV program." 0830 Took a good breakfast s̄ problems. 0900 Linen changed with pt up in chair, used own toothpaste and hairbrush, doesn't like our brand. 0930 Changed drsg, incision site looks good, new dressing applied with cloth tape. 1015 New bag hung. 1145 Returned to room, tol procedure well. 1200 Eating lunch. ———————— MS Gorski RN

Figure 10–6. Nursing progress notes may be done in the form of SOAP notes (above) or NARRATIVE notes (below).

SOAP Notes. The **SOAP note** is a progress note that relates to only one health problem. All health-care team members use the same format. The left-hand column of the SOAP note refers to the number of the problem being addressed from the master problem list. Using this method, the patient's progress on that particular problem can be assessed without sorting through the whole chart. The team member need only read down the left-hand column of the interdisciplinary progress notes and read the notes of all disciplines that relate to that numbered problem. However, some nurses think that the SOAP format focuses too narrowly on the identified problem list and does not highlight routine nursing care as well as traditional narrative notes do.

After documenting the problem to be addressed, the next step is organizing the information in the SOAP note format. The "S" stands for *subjective* and refers to data or symptoms the patient expresses. Quotation marks are often used to document the patient's specific statements; quoting the patient allows for different interpretations than the nurse's. If the patient cannot give information or gave none relevant to this problem, the "S" may be omitted or followed by "none."

"O" refers to *objective* findings and includes data collected by the nurse relevant to the problem. Objective data include what the nurse can see, feel, smell, or hear, as well as relevant laboratory data, diagnostic tests, and vital signs.

"A" stands for *assessment,* which represents a diagnosis, an impression, or a condition change. This assessment is made after analyzing the data from the subjective and objective portions and must be supported by those data. If assessment cannot be made from the data gathered, write "further data-gathering necessary" or "abdominal pain, unknown etiology" under the "A" portion of the SOAP note.

"P" stands for *plan.* This portion deals with nursing interventions specifically related to the identified problem. The plan section may simply state "continue present regimen" when the assessment is made that the patient is progressing adequately using the plan already outlined. The plan can also specify revisions of the present nursing interventions as the need is assessed.

Some hospitals use the SOAPIER format of recording (I, intervention; E, evaluation; R, revision). This allows the team member to record interventions that were done, the patient's response to the plan, and any revisions needed to the plan. The nurse must remember that all information recorded under the SOAP or SOAPIER headings must pertain to the same problem.

In some circumstances, a full SOAP note may be unnecessary. Routine care may be documented on a flowsheet. Routine nursing assessments need not be written as a SOAP note if they are not specifically related to a problem (for example, routine temperature and blood pressure on a patient who has had no problem with fever and has stable blood pressure).

Flowsheets

Flowsheets are designed to document routine nursing procedures and to free the nurse from writing out procedures done repeatedly. One example is a sheet for vital signs that gives a graphic representation of pulse, blood pressure, respirations, and temperature so that trends can be evaluated. It also serves as a documentation for frequent vital signs monitoring, as shown in Figure 10-7. The intake and output sheet is used to maintain an ongoing record of all fluid intake and output. A sample chart is given in Chapter 32. On another common flowsheet, the nurse documents all routine care, such as activity, dressing changes, meals taken, and breath sounds (Fig. 10-8). Critical care flowsheets are used in the intensive care unit to document frequently changing data, specific nursing interventions, patient responses, and multiple medications and intravenous fluids administered.

Admission Entries

When a patient is admitted, a nursing history is completed. The data gathered include most or all of the functional health patterns as described by Gordon (1987). The nutrition, activity, sleep, and coping patterns are assessed and documented, as well as pertinent medical history and history relating to the reason for admission. A complete physical assessment is performed and fully documented. See Chapter 7 for a full description of nursing admission history and physical assessment. A sample admission assessment form is shown in Figure 18-1.

In addition to recording the nursing history and physical assessment on admission, the nurse must document the admission procedure. This information may be entered on the nursing admission history and physical assessment sheet, on another standardized form, or in nursing progress notes. The admission procedure includes identifying the patient by identification bracelet, introducing the nurse and the patient's roommate, unit orientation, measuring vital signs, helping the patient to undress and get into bed, and explaining the disposition of personal items and valuables. During orientation, the nurse should try to allay anxiety and make the patient feel secure. The nurse describes the use of the call system, adjustable bed controls, telephone, television, radio, lights, location of the bathroom, visiting hours, meal times, and any other pertinent unit activities. Any special equipment, such as oxygen or an intravenous infusion, should be explained and documented on the progress notes or other appropriate form.

Nursing Discharge Summary

A nursing discharge summary should be started at admission and completed at discharge (Fig. 10-9). It should

(Text continues on page 165)

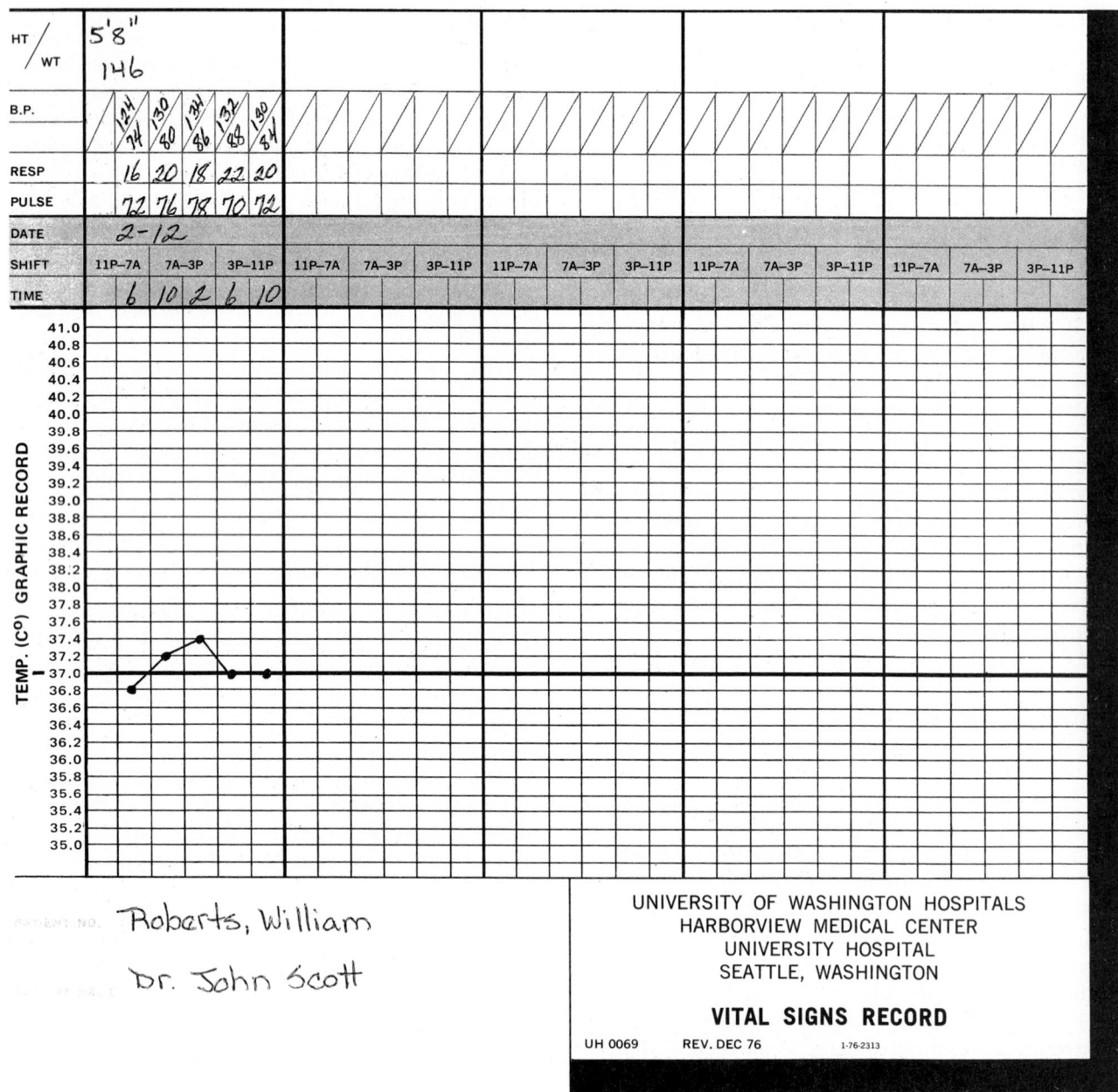

HT / WT	5'8" 146															
B.P.	124/74 130/90 134/86 132/88 130/84															
RESP	16 20 18 22 20															
PULSE	72 76 78 70 72															
DATE	2-12															
SHIFT	11P–7A	7A–3P	3P–11P	11P–7A	7A–3P	3P–11P	11P–7A	7A–3P	3P–11P	11P–7A	7A–3P	3P–11P	11P–7A	7A–3P	3P–11P
TIME	6	10 2	6 10												

TEMP. (C°) GRAPHIC RECORD

41.0 40.8 40.6 40.4 40.2 40.0 39.8 39.6 39.4 39.2 39.0 38.8 38.6 38.4 38.2 38.0 37.8 37.6 37.4 37.2 37.0 36.8 36.6 36.4 36.2 36.0 35.8 35.6 35.4 35.2 35.0

Roberts, William

Dr. John Scott

UNIVERSITY OF WASHINGTON HOSPITALS
HARBORVIEW MEDICAL CENTER
UNIVERSITY HOSPITAL
SEATTLE, WASHINGTON

VITAL SIGNS RECORD

UH 0069   REV. DEC 76   1-76-2313

Figure 10–7. Vital signs record.

EVERGREEN HOSPITAL MEDICAL CENTER
KIRKLAND, WASHINGTON
DAILY NURSING SUMMARY

NUR-010 (REV. 1/90)   DATE: 2-14

		0700	0800	0900	1000	1100	1200	1300	1400	1500	1600	1700	1800
VITAL SIGNS	TEMPERATURE	36^2				36^6				37^2			
	PULSE	92				88				86			
	RESPIRATIONS	20				22				22			
	BLOOD PRESSURE	110/82				116/92				120/88			
CNS	MENTATION	alert oriented		A/O						A/O			
	RESPONSE / MOTOR VERBAL	appropriate											
SAFETY	SIDERAILS / CALL LIGHT FALL PRECAUTIONS	2↑				2↑				2↑			
	RESTRAINTS												
ACTIVITIES OF DAILY LIVING	REST/ACTIVITY / TYPE TOL	Up in room		Up walking				Up chair					
	PERSONAL HYGIENE			Bath/linen change									
	NUTRITION / TYPE % TAKEN	ice chips			ice chips			ice chips		ice chips			
	FLUID INTAKE												
PHYSICAL CHANGES	FLUID OUTPUT / FOLEY CARE	500				250							
	EMESIS/NG / AMT APPEARANCE												
	BOWEL / GUAIAC APPEARANCE	passing flatus				+ Bowel sounds				flatus			
	LUNGS BS, TCDB / O₂ AMOUNT												
	SKIN	warm dry					warm dry						
	IV CHECK / SOLUTION RATE IV SITE	patent no redness			ice parlour			ice parlour		patent			
	DRAINS / CHEST TUBES	J-P = 20 cc. recompressed						J-P = 30cc recompressed					
PAIN	TYPE, LOCATION	Abd.											
	INTERVENTION/RESPONSE												
WOUND	HEALING/APPEARANCE	incision intact											
	DRESSING ✓/CHANGE	minimal drainage											
OTHER	PHYSICIAN			Dr. Stuart in									
	NURSES INITIALS	JS	JS	JS	JS	JS	JS	JS	JS	JS			

Identify Initials with Signature on Back

INTAKE	TYPE	DAYS	EVES.	NOCS	24 HR. TOTAL
	oral	150	150	100	400
	IV	1000	950	1000	2950
	TOTAL	1150	1100	1100	3350

TODAY'S MEASURED WEIGHT 146

YESTERDAY'S MEASURED WEIGHT 145

OUTPUT	TYPE	DAYS	EVES.	NOCS	24 HR. TOTAL
	urine	750	1250	800	2800
	J-P	50	40	20	110
	TOTAL	800	1290	820	2910

▼ STAMP HERE ▼

Harvey, Judith
Age 54
K. Stuart, MD

Figure 10-8.   Nursing assessment flowsheet.

Diagnosis	SELF CARE STATUS LEVEL (Check ✓ either I—Independent, A—Assistance, U—Unable)		I	A	U
Congestive Heart Failure					
	DRESSES SELF				✓
Procedures/Surgeries: (Include Dates)	SHAVES SELF				✓
	TRANSFERS SELF				✓
	AMBULATES				✓
How Patient Discharged	FEEDS SELF		✓		
☐ Ambulatory ✓ Wheelchair ☐ Ambulance ☐ Cabulance	BATHES SELF ☐ TUB ✓ SHOWER				✓
Who Patient Discharged With:	ORAL HYGIENE				✓
☐ Alone ✓ M. Hazelet (daughter)	● BLADDER				
Name and Relationship to Patient					
Discharged To:	● BOWEL				
☐ Nursing Home (Name)					
☐ Own Home or Apt. ✓ Other (Name) Daughter's home					
Family/Support System (Name, Relationship, Phone)	● WOUNDS/DRESSINGS/TUBES				
May Hazelet (daughter) 698-8650	(Type and Location) none				
Sensory Needs ✓ Hard of Hearing					
Hearing ☐ w/in Normal Limits ☐ Aids Ø					
Vision ☐ w/in Normal Limits ✓ Aids glasses	(Supplies/Amt. Provided)				
Speech ☐ w/in Normal Limits ☐ Aphasic					
☐ Aids					
Languages Spoken:	● SPECIAL EQUIPMENT/APPLIANCES SENT HOME WITH PATIENT				
English					
Allergies: ✗ None	(if Rental, Obtained From)				
☐ Specify					

YOUR MEDICATIONS

NAME	DOSAGE	WHEN TO TAKE	SPECIAL INSTRUCTIONS	LAST DOSE GIVEN AT
Digoxin	0.125 mg	1 tablet ē other day in morning		0900 3-21
Lasix	40 mg	1 tablet every morning		0900 3-21
Potassium	40 mEq	every morning		0900 3-21

PATIENT TEACHING	RETURN DEMONSTRATION	NEEDS PRACTICE	NEEDS MORE INSTRUCTION	SATISFACTORY	REFERRAL AT DISCHARGE
Skills/Topics					Agency Name

FOLLOW-UP CARE

SPECIAL INSTRUCTIONS	CLINIC NAME/PHYSICIAN	DATE	TIME	
Diet 2 Gm Na Activity Up ad lib	Lake Beach Clinic Dr. B. Kyle	3-29-92	9⁰⁰ am	Address
Lab work				Phone # Date Phoned
				Referral For:
				☐ NURSING CARE
				☐ P.T. ☐ O.T.
				☐ MEAL SERVICE
Other				☐ CHORE WORKER
				☐ COMPANION
	PHONE NUMBER WHERE YOU CAN BE REACHED			☐ OTHER
	AT UWMC CALL (206-548-4333) TO MAKE APPOINTMENT(S)			3-21-92 11:30
	AT HMC CALL_____TO MAKE APPOINTMENT(S)			Discharge Date/Time

I have been informed and I understand my home discharge instructions.

Patient Signature or Care Giver	Primary Nurse Signature	R.N.	Discharge Unit/Phone Number
X Scott Bradley	X J. Sidney RN		689-5342

Date 3-21-92   Ord. Sta. No.

Pt. No. 029345

Name Bradley, Scott

D.O.B.

UNIVERSITY OF WASHINGTON MEDICAL CENTERS
HARBORVIEW MEDICAL CENTER
UNIVERSITY OF WASHINGTON MEDICAL CENTER
SEATTLE, WASHINGTON

PATIENT DISCHARGE STATUS REPORT
DIVISION OF NURSING

WHITE—CHART COPY
CANARY—PATIENT COPY
(BELOW PERFORATION)
PINK—REFERRAL COPY
GOLDENROD—CLINIC COPY

UH 0021   REV JUL 89

Figure 10–9. Patient discharge summary.

list the discharge planning and patient teaching that took place since admission. (Discharge planning is discussed in Chapter 27 and in each chapter in Section II of this text.) The discharge summary notes the patient's condition at discharge and provides specific information about care after discharge. A copy of the discharge summary is given to the patient or sent to a home health nurse or extended-care facility.

Nursing discharge summary forms are usually standardized and contain space to write specific instructions. Information includes medications, diet, activity, follow-up care, and special instructions such as dressing changes, heat applications, and circumstances requiring notification of the physician. Most nursing discharge summary forms also contain space for vital signs, condition at discharge, method of discharge, time, and to whom and where the patient was discharged.

Any pertinent discharge information should be documented on the nursing progress notes if it is not on the nursing discharge summary, such as assessment of the patient's home environment, support system, and self-care abilities. The patient's response to patient teaching should be recorded throughout the hospital stay. Any written information or teaching plans given to the patient should be documented. A note to the home health provider should mention any further health-education needs.

Medication Records

The medication record and intravenous flowsheets are important parts of documentation. Nurses should record administration of medications promptly to avoid confusion about missed doses and to prevent inadvertent double-dosing.

The medication record distinguishes between routine medications and prn ("as needed") medications (Fig. 10-10). On the form are routine times for medication administration such as 8 AM, 12 PM, 4 PM, with a space for the initials of the nurse giving the drug. When giving a prn drug, the nurse records the time given and the effectiveness of the drug. When a patient refuses or does not receive a drug for any reason, the nurse's initials must be circled, and the reason the patient did not receive the drug is noted. Intravenous flow records ensure continuity by recording the total intake over 8 hours and the volume remaining.

Incident Report

An **incident** is any unusual happening in the hospital, such as a patient fall, a medication error, or a malfunction in equipment. Each hospital has a standardized form on which the witnessing nurse can record patient or visitor incidents. The form includes the date and time of the incident, the events leading up to it, the patient's response, and a full nursing assessment. Do not be judg-

mental or accusatory in documenting the incident. There should be a place on the form for physician notification, which is usually advisable, and an area for additional medical orders and assessment.

Some hospitals use incident reports related to nursing procedures as a way to evaluate the quality of care; these are called quality assurance memos. These reports are used to assess patterns of errors and the need to change the procedures involved. For example, a monthly review of incident reports reveals three identical errors by three different nurses. The same medication was involved in each instance. Discussion with each nurse may reveal that a simple change in the medication's packaging may prevent further incidents. It is important to remember this use of incident reports. It is difficult to admit that a mistake was made, but it is important to document the error for the patient's sake, as well as for the prevention of future errors.

ORAL COMMUNICATION: REPORTING

Oral communication is used to communicate the nursing process to other health-care personnel. Reporting is done face to face, on the telephone, or by taped messages. Reporting enhances patient care and serves to educate caregivers. It should be organized, concise, complete, and professional.

Change-of-Shift Reports

In the **change-of-shift report,** one nurse reports to another about patient status and care plans. This report is a way of ensuring continuity in patient care from one shift to the next. It may be taped or given face to face; audiotaping saves time but does not allow for clarification of details.

A change-of-shift report in an acute-care hospital includes the following information:

- Name, age, and room number
- Medical diagnosis(es), surgery (date)
- Significant nursing diagnoses and progress toward goals
- Significant assessment findings, including diagnostic test results
- Specific treatments (i.e., dressing changes, respiratory therapy)
- Intravenous rate and amount remaining.

Information about changes in status should be reported comprehensively and should include assessment data, nursing diagnoses pertaining to the change, planning, interventions, and evaluation. The patient's emotional response and behavior should be reported as well.

ROUTINE MEDICATIONS

DATE			MEDICATION STRENGTH—DOSAGE—ROUTE		DATE	DATE	DATE	DATE
US	RN	RPh			TIME & INITIAL	TIME & INITIAL	TIME & INITIAL	TIME & INITIAL
3-6	⨂		Digoxin 0.125 mg p.o. qd TIME 0800	2400-0800				
				0800-1600	0800/JS	0800/JS		
				1600-2400				
3-6	⨂		Procardia 10 mg p.o. bid TIME 0800 2000	2400-0800				
				0800-1600	0800/JS	0800/JS		
				1600-2400	2000/JS	2000/JS		
3-6	⨂		Atarax 50 mg p.o. qid TIME 0600 1200 1800 2400	2400-0800	0600/JS	0600/JS		
				0800-1600	1200/JS	1200/JS		
				1600-2400	1800/JS 2400/JS	1800/JS 2400/JS		
3-6	⨂		Amitriptyline 50 mg qhs TIME 2200	2400-0800				
				0800-1600				
				1600-2400	2200/JS	2200/JS		
			TIME	2400-0800				
				0800-1600				
				1600-2400				
			TIME	2400-0800				
				0800-1600				
				1600-2400				
			TIME	2400-0800				
				0800-1600				
				1600-2400				
			TIME	2400-0800				
				0800-1600				
				1600-2400				
			TIME	2400-0800				
				0800-1600				
				1600-2400				

	DATE	I.V. DRIP MEDICATION	US	RN	RPh	DATE	I.V. DRIP MEDICATION	US	RN	RPh
I.V. DRIP MEDICATION										

SIGNATURE INITIAL			SIGNATURE INITIAL		ALLERGY: NKA
	1. J.S. *Sidney RN*			6.	
	2. J.J. *James RN*			7.	DIAGNOSIS: CHF
	3.			8.	
	4.			9.	▼ PATIENT STAMP ▼
	5.			10.	

EVERGREEN HOSPITAL MEDICAL CENTER
KIRKLAND, WASHINGTON
MEDICATION RECORD

Herbert, Howard
Age 58
N. Dean, MD

A - RIGHT ARM	F - LEFT THIGH
B - LEFT ARM	G - RIGHT VENTROGLUTEAL
C - RIGHT BUTTOCK	H - LEFT VENTROGLUTEAL
D - LEFT BUTTOCK	I - RIGHT ABDOMEN
E - RIGHT THIGH	J - LEFT ABDOMEN

RX-229A

Figure 10–10. Medication record.

Exact times, dosages, and measurements should be given.

Both oral and taped reports use the nursing Kardex and nursing care plan as a basis for the information to be included. The listener also uses the Kardex as a guide to clarify information given by the previous nurse and to fill in the details of routine care.

Variations in shift reports occur according to the specialty nursing area. For example, the report in a critical-care setting may include an in-depth evaluation of each patient's body systems (i.e., respiratory status by assessment and ventilator readings, cardiovascular status by rhythm strips and blood pressure measurements). The report in a long-term care setting might include only those patients with significant status changes and might not mention those with no change in condition.

Nursing Rounds

Another method of reporting is nursing rounds (also called walking rounds). Rounds may be used for change-of-shift reports or for care planning. Two or more nurses visit a group of patients, and the nurse assigned to each patient summarizes the patient's current status and care plan.

The advantage of nursing rounds is that there is optimal communication between nurses, and patient status is confirmed by direct observation. For instance, it may be easier to describe various intravenous lines and dressing changes when the oncoming nurse is at the patient's bedside. Two disadvantages are that rounds are time-consuming because other topics may be discussed, and that the patient may feel excluded or alienated by the medical terms being used. Using understandable language and encouraging the patient to participate can help.

Telephone Reports

Telephone reports can be used when transferring a patient to another facility or to another unit within the hospital. Telephone reports are also used extensively to update physicians about patient status and to communicate between hospital departments. Since telephone reports do not rely on written verification or direct observation, accuracy is vital. Clarification should be made if any question exists. The sender should state the message clearly and concisely, and the receiver should repeat pertinent data for verification.

Patient Transfers

When transferring a patient to a different facility (such as from the hospital to an extended-care facility), a form must be completed to provide necessary information for the patient's continued care. Forms vary, but the basic information includes physician orders, nursing orders, specific patient needs, patient limitations, and other pertinent data for planning care. The telephone report includes the patient's status at the time of transfer and a verbal reiteration of information included on the form. The receiving nurse needs to know what to expect, and the telephone report enables the nurse to prepare for the patient before his or her arrival. It also allows the receiving nurse to clarify any information.

When transferring a patient to a different unit, the patient record is transferred with the patient, but the receiving nurse needs to have the most current information on patient status as well as a summary of the patient's progress and general care. Information to be included in the transfer report is:

- Patient name and age
- Current diagnosis and medical history
- Reason for transfer
- Most current assessment, particularly abnormalities
- Equipment to be transferred with patient (i.e., oxygen, intravenous infusion, wheelchair)
- Time and method of expected transport.

Report to Physician

A telephone report to a physician usually involves a change in the patient's condition. The most important preparation for this type of communication is completion of a focused nursing assessment. The assessment may be focused on the system involved, but all pertinent data should be gathered and communicated as appropriate. It may help to outline on paper the information that needs to be communicated to the physician. Have the patient's chart handy for reference. Important information to give a physician for status reports or possible medical intervention is:

- Patient name and diagnosis
- Stated symptoms
- Changes in nursing assessment
- Vital signs (compared to normal)
- Laboratory tests (compared to normal)
- Nursing treatment initiated and patient response.

The following is an example of a nurse–physician telephone call:

Mr. Jones, who is here for knee surgery, has a history of unstable angina. He now complains of epigastric pain; he states it's like "gas pain." The pain does not get worse with ambulation. His vital signs remain normal and he has no abdominal tenderness or distention. Mylanta 30 mL prn as ordered relieves pain within 15 minutes. I wanted to let you know of this change because of his cardiac history.

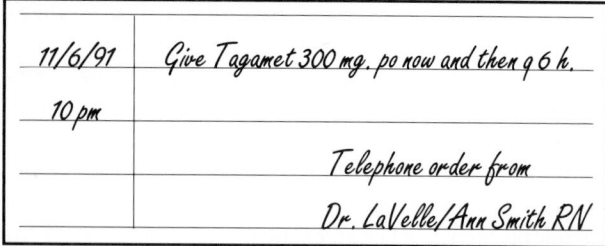

11/6/91	Give Tagamet 300 mg. po now and then q 6 h.
10 pm	
	Telephone order from
	Dr. LaVelle/Ann Smith RN

Figure 10–11. Documentation of a telephone order from a physician by a nurse.

A telephone report to a physician is often followed by telephone orders that must be documented in the patient record and carried out by the nurse. For example, the physician may order a medication for Mr. Jones that should be started before the physician can visit the patient. The nurse writes the order in the patient record on the physician's order sheet and labels it as a telephone or verbal order. The nurse is responsible for correctly identifying the medication, dose, time, route, and the physician who ordered it. To ensure accuracy, the nurse should repeat the information and ask the physician to spell the medication or his or her name as necessary. Figure 10-11 is an example of a correctly transcribed telephone order.

Reports from Other Departments

Nurses often receive telephone reports from other departments, such as radiology or the laboratory. Information is exchanged that is crucial to patient care, and numbers for laboratory values and complex terminology for diagnostic procedures may easily be misunderstood.

When requesting information from another department, the nurse should be courteous. The nurse should identify herself or himself and identify the patient, room number, and identification number, if necessary. When a report is given, the nurse should repeat the information and speak clearly to verify numbers.

Likewise, nurses often give reports to other departments. Usually information such as name, room number, age, and diagnosis is reported. This takes place when a nurse reports a new patient to the dietary department or requests a consultation from physical therapy.

Care Plan Conferences

Care plan conferences are discussions about patient care, involving either several departments or just the nursing staff on the unit.

Interdisciplinary conferences help to coordinate services so that the patient care plan can be developed and implemented in the most efficient way. Nurses usually initiate these conferences and invite members of the

---

Safety Alert

- Familiarize yourself with the type of recording done in your institution.
- Include all potential assessments, planning, interventions, and evaluations in the patient record.
- Be concise and brief on the patient record; use precise measurements and times.
- Use commonly accepted abbreviations and symbols on the patient record.
- Write only observations seen, heard, smelled, or felt in nursing notes. Clearly distinguish between observation and assumption.
- Note any errors on the record. Do not erase.
- Be complete in your notes.
- Be logical and systematic in your information.
- Write legibly so others can read your notes.
- Record information immediately or as soon as possible for proper care. This is vital in medication administration.
- Keep all patient care confidential. Do not leave patient information in public areas or where the patient or family can read it.
- Initiate discharge planning at admission and complete the summary at discharge.
- Document all incidents, including everything leading up to the occurrence, response, and full nursing assessment. Do not be judgmental or accusatory.
- Be accurate in giving and taking telephone reports. Clarify anything not understood.
- Organize or outline your notes in preparation for a telephone report to the physician.

---

health-care team from other departments, such as physical therapy, social services, and dietary. Patients who most benefit from such conferences are those with multiple, complex problems.

A conference with other nurses may be held to "brainstorm" ideas about a particular patient's care. These conferences are initiated by the nurses caring for the patient in hopes of enhancing the quality and continuity of care.

Confidentiality

The patient record is the property of the hospital, clinic, or physician's office. Its contents are not to be discussed or shared with anyone not directly involved in the patient's care. This includes the patient's minister, family members, and physicians or nurses who are friends of the family. The patient's right to confidentiality must be actively guarded, and nurses often serve as "gate-keepers" for charts.

Patients have the right to see their records, but permission must be obtained from the owner of the record (the hospital or physician). When a patient sees the record, a physician is usually present to explain medical terms.

When using computers in documentation, access codes must be issued and kept secret. When making a telephone report or engaging in other verbal communication, nurses must make sure they are speaking in a private place and that they are speaking to authorized people. Communication should remain professional.

brief. They should highlight changes in the past 24 hours.

■ In telephone reporting, the sender of the message should speak clearly and the receiver should repeat the message to avoid errors.

References

Gordon, M. (1987). *Nursing diagnosis: Process and application* (2nd ed.). New York: McGraw-Hill.

Saba, V. K., & McCormick, K. A. (1986). *Essentials of computers for nurses.* Philadelphia: J. B. Lippincott.

Weed, L. L. (1969). *Medical records, medical education, and patient care.* Chicago: Year Book.

Key Concepts

■ The purposes of the patient record are communication, assessment, care planning, education, research, auditing, and legal documentation.

■ Principles of recording are conciseness, accuracy, completeness, organization, legibility, timeliness, and confidentiality.

■ A source-oriented record is divided into sections according to the type of caregiver (i.e., nurses, physicians, respiratory therapists).

■ A problem-oriented medical record is divided into sections by problem. All caregivers record on the same set of progress notes.

■ Computers are becoming increasingly common in documentation. Either the entire patient record or just parts of it, such as nursing care plans, can be computerized.

■ The nursing Kardex is a series of cards containing background information, routine care information, and specific treatments for each patient. It is used in giving care and for change-of-shift reporting.

■ The SOAP format organizes information into subjective, objective, assessment, and plan categories. Chronologic narrative nursing progress notes may be difficult to follow when checking the progress of the patient on a specific problem.

■ Flowsheets for vital signs, intake and output, and routine nursing assessment and care make recording quicker and less redundant.

■ A nursing discharge summary reports the patient's status at discharge and gives instructions for diet, activity, home care, and followup.

■ Change-of-shift reports should be comprehensive but

Bibliography

Afferbach, D. (1986). A flow sheet that saves time and trouble. *RN, 49*(1), 42–44.

Bailey-Allen, A. M. (1986). Avoid legal pitfalls in charting. *Orthopedic Nursing, 5*(1), 21–23.

Bailey-Allen, A. M. (1988). More about charting with a jury in mind. *Nursing '88, 18*(4), 50–54.

Brunt, B. A. (1990). The documentation maze: Finding the right path. *Journal of Nursing Staff Development, 6*(1), 21–24.

Edelstein, J. (1990). A study in nursing documentation. *Nursing Management, 21*(11), 40–46.

Gruber, M., & Gruber, J. M. (1990). Nursing malpractice: The importance of documentation, or saved by the pen! *Gastroenterological Nursing, 12,* 255–259.

Lucatorto, M., Petras, D. M., Drew, L. A., et al. (1991). Documentation: A focus of cost saving. *Journal of Nursing Administration, 21*(3), 32–36.

McKiel, R. E., & Rogers, C. A. (1986). The chart critique: A learning activity for nursing students. *Nurse Educator, 11*(2), 23–24.

Miller, P., & Pastorino, C. (1990). Daily nursing documentation can be quick and thorough. *Nursing Management, 21*(11), 47–49.

Murphy, J., & Burkem, L. J. (1990). Charting by exception: A more efficient way to document. *Nursing '90, 20*(5), 65–69.

Philpott, M. (1986). Twenty rules for good charting. *Nursing '86, 10*(8), 63.

Rauen, K. K. (1990). Documentation of the nursing process in the outpatient clinic. *Journal of Nursing Quality Assurance, 4*(4), 55–62.

Reiley, P. J., & Stengrevics, S. S. (1989). Change of shift report: Put it in writing! *Nursing Management, 20*(9), 47–51.

Rich, P. L. (1985). With this flowsheet, less is more. *Nursing '85, 15*(7), 25–29.

Schmidt, D., Gathers, B., Stewart, M., et al. (1990). Charting for accountability. *Nursing Management, 21*(11), 50–55.

Sklar, C. L. (1984). The patient's record, an invaluable communication tool. *Canadian Nurse, 80*(5), 50–52.

Wakefield, B., Miller, P., Farzad, R., et al. (1990). Documentation of the nursing process in the operating room. *Journal of Nursing Quality Assurance, 4*(4), 45–54.

Weed, L. L. (1971). *Medical records, medical education, and patient care: The problem-oriented record as a basic tool.* Cleveland: Case Western Reserve University Press.

Woolery, L. K. (1990). Professional standards and ethical dilemmas in nursing information systems. *Journal of Nursing Administration, 20*(10), 50–53.

UNIT III
Concepts Essential for Human Function and Nursing Management

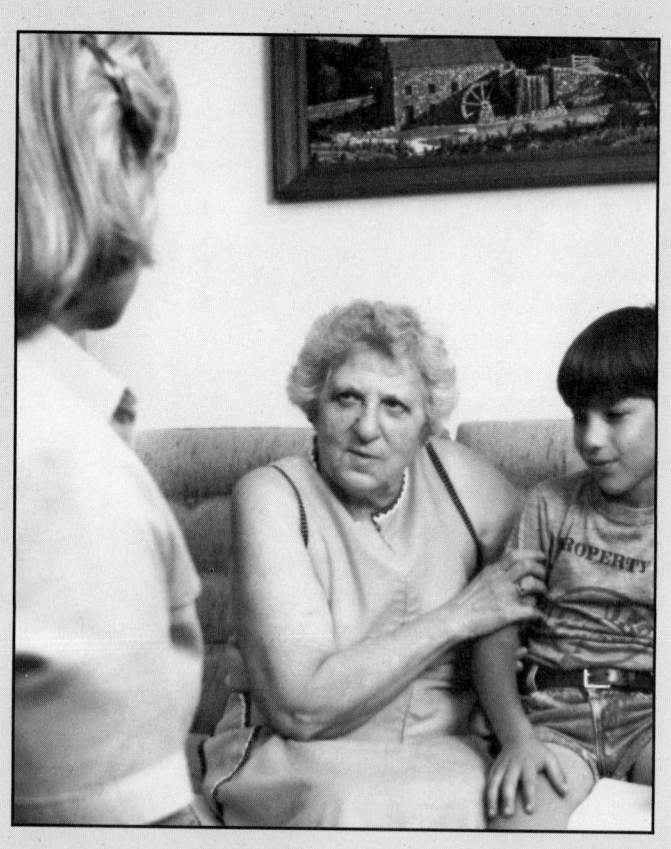

CHAPTERS

11 Health and Wellness

12 Human Needs

13 Lifespan Development

14 Individual, Family, and Community

15 Culture and Ethnicity

16 Values

17 Communication: The Nurse–Patient Relationship

The chapters in Unit III explore the foundational concepts essential for the nurse to provide safe, effective, holistic nursing care. The first chapter considers the concepts of health, wellness, and illness with an emphasis on maintaining health and wellness. An awareness of basic human needs, detailed in Chapter 12, enables the nurse to plan and prioritize nursing care that meets patient needs.

Chapter 13 discusses human growth and development throughout the lifespan. This chapter sets the stage for "Lifespan Considerations" in each clinical chapter, an integrated approach that enables the nurse to see how these concepts are applied clinically. The next chapter considers the patient as an individual, part of a family, and part of a larger community. This chapter begins a family focus carried throughout the text.

Culture, ethnicity, and values are considered in the next two chapters. These issues affect a patient's attitudes and feelings about health practices and underlie his or her decisions about health care. The final chapter in this unit focuses on the knowledge and skills needed to establish an effective nurse–patient relationship. This chapter is coordinated with Chapter 44 to focus on communication and its importance in all human relationships.

The chapters in this Unit provide a strong foundation for understanding less tangible patient needs and planning individualized, holistic nursing care.

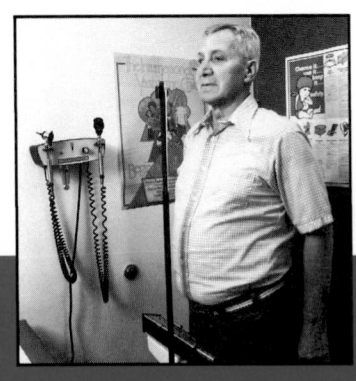

Health and Wellness

LEARNING OBJECTIVES

Upon completion of this chapter, the student will be able to do the following:

- Define wellness, holism, and holistic care.
- Compare and contrast the different methods of health care.
- Identify the connection between mind, body, and spirit and symptoms.
- Explain the role of the holistic nurse as a colleague to the patient.
- Give examples of holistic health care modalities.

KEY TERMS

Disease	Holism	Meditation
Dysfunction	Homeostasis	Self-awareness
Health	Illness	Therapeutic Touch
High-level wellness	Imagery	Wellness

Health and Wellness
  Clinical Model
  Host–Agent–Environment Model
  Health Belief Model
  High-Level Wellness Model
  Holistic Health Model
Wellness and Holistic Health Care
  Holistic Practice
    Self-Responsibility
    Informed Choices
    Self-Worth
  Meaning of Disease, Illness, and Dysfunction
  Effect of Stress

Nursing in Wellness and Holistic Health Care
  Promoting Health and Preventing Illness
    Preventive Activities
    Nurturative Activities
    Generative Activities
  Nursing as a Therapeutic Partnership
  Nursing Diagnoses for Wellness
  Examples of Holistic Health Care Modalities
    Lifestyle Modification
    Meditation
    Imagery
    Therapeutic Touch
Key Concepts

Emma Rose lay in her hospital bed, considering her situation. Here she was, 25 years old, an independent woman, who had had unexpected surgery for appendicitis just yesterday. She had never been in a hospital before. She overheard the physician on rounds refer to her as "the appendectomy in Room 304." Between being in a hospital bed and overhearing this comment, she felt like a piece of furniture one minute and a child the next. No one seemed interested in how this relatively simple operation had affected her. She had always taken her health for granted. Now she felt sick and disabled.

The nurse on the morning shift said she practiced holistic nursing. What would be different about that? she wondered. Would it be better just to avoid all these "health" people?

Health-care professionals are changing the way they think about health. Kuhn (1962) wrote that scientific models are replaced when the "watershed point" is reached: an increasing body of information cannot be fitted into the old model, which has reached its limit of creativity. It becomes more profitable to seek a new model than to patch up the old one. The concepts of health and holism must be examined to understand this new health-care model.

HEALTH AND WELLNESS

The World Health Organization (WHO, 1947) defined **health** as "a state of complete physical, mental, and social well-being, not merely the absence of disease or infirmity." This was a dramatic departure from the traditional view, which considered a person healthy if he or she were merely symptom-free.

This definition of health is a useful starting point. It considers the total person (functioning physically, psychologically, and socially) as essential to the state of health and wellness. According to Allen (1986), the WHO's definition was designed to prevent health from being defined in a Western "disease" orientation. He suggested that when trying to define health, we should consider historical meanings and implications and understand whose interests were served; this enables us to recognize what is necessary for present and future social change.

Each person has a personal definition of health. Some people describe their state of health as "good," even though they may actually have one or more diagnosed illnesses. That is because each person defines health in relation to personal expectations and values.

The concept of health must allow for this individual variability. Health is a dynamic state in which the person is constantly adapting to changes in the internal and external environments. For example, a person may see himself or herself as healthy while experiencing a respiratory infection. Someone who has a temporary disability related to mobility may consider himself or herself "not healthy," but a person with a permanent disability may consider that a "normal" state and will define health differently.

The concept of wellness also allows for individual variability. **Wellness** can be thought of as a balance of the physical, psychological, social, and spiritual aspects of a person's life. This is a dynamic state. As with health, each person would also define wellness in relation to personal expectations. Wellness behaviors are those that promote healthy functioning and help prevent illness. These include, for example, stress management, nutritional awareness, and physical fitness.

There are various models of the concept of health. Some models are based narrowly on the presence or absence of definable illness. Others are based more conceptually on health beliefs, wellness, and holism.

Clinical Model

In the clinical model, health is interpreted narrowly as the absence of signs and symptoms of disease or injury; thus, the opposite of health is disease. Dunn (1961) defined health in this model as "a relatively passive state of freedom from illness . . . a condition of relative homeostasis." Illness, therefore, is something that happens to a person. Many health-care providers focus on the relief of signs and symptoms of disease and conclude that when these are no longer present, the person is healthy.

This model may not take into consideration the person's health beliefs or the lifestyle factors that may continue to place him or her at high risk for disease. Relieving obvious signs and symptoms may not address larger issues in the person's life that may affect his or her health. For example, the person who persists in smoking cigarettes and living a sedentary life will eventually develop signs and symptoms that relate to these lifestyle patterns.

Host–Agent–Environment Model

The host–agent–environment model was developed to help identify the cause of an illness (Leavell, 1965). In this model, the following definitions apply:

Host: the person (or group) who may be at risk for or susceptible to an illness.
Agent: any factor (internal or external) that can lead to illness by its presence or absence.
Environment: those factors (physical, social, economic, emotional, spiritual) that may create the likelihood or the predisposition for the person to develop disease.

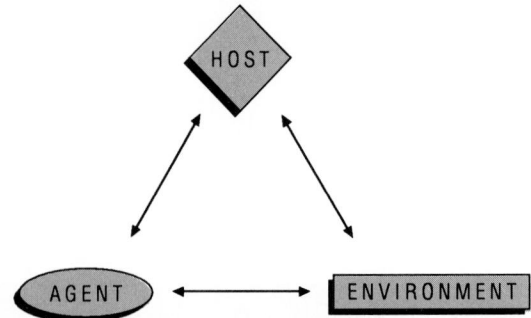

Figure 11–1.   Host–agent–environment model.

In this model, health and illness depend on the interaction of these three factors (Fig. 11-1). For example, a person (host) may be exposed to the virus for the common cold (agent), but whether or not a cold develops depends on a variety of conditions (environment). Poor nutrition, inadequate sleep, and unusual stress before the exposure would predispose the host to develop a cold. Conversely, a person who was well nourished and physically fit and who felt in control of the stresses of life would be less likely to develop symptoms.

Health Belief Model

In the health belief model (Rosenstock, 1974), there is a relation between a person's beliefs and actions (Fig. 11-2). The factors that influence those beliefs include the following:

• Personal expectations in relation to health and illness.
• Earlier experiences with illness and health.
• Sociocultural context.
• Age and developmental state.

Someone who expects to have a cold at the same time every year may find that those expectations come true. Conversely, positive, health-oriented expectations might keep the person from developing an illness. Previous experience with an illness has a major influence on how the person reacts to subsequent challenges: previous pain experiences, for example, shape future experiences with pain.

Peer influence, personality characteristics, ethnicity, and socioeconomic factors may all affect a person's response to illness. Someone who gets sick, but whose experience is similar to that of his or her peers or socioeconomic group, may not consider that he or she is in "poor health." Group values influence the health beliefs of each person.

Age and developmental stage are important considerations in the health belief model. For example, an elderly person may be more tolerant of a particular illness or disability than a younger person, because of perceived greater susceptibility to "poor health." In-

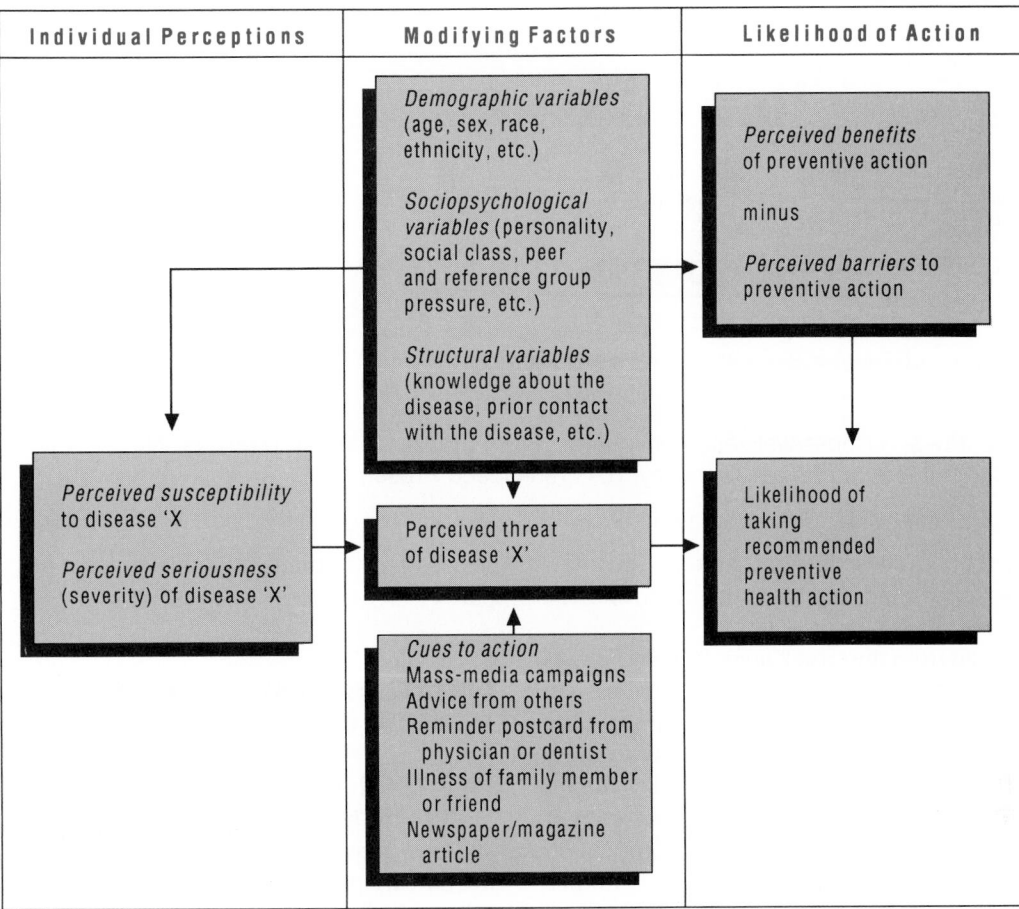

| Individual Perceptions | Modifying Factors | Likelihood of Action |

Demographic variables (age, sex, race, ethnicity, etc.)

Sociopsychological variables (personality, social class, peer and reference group pressure, etc.)

Structural variables (knowledge about the disease, prior contact with the disease, etc.)

Perceived benefits of preventive action

minus

Perceived barriers to preventive action

Perceived susceptibility to disease 'X

Perceived seriousness (severity) of disease 'X'

Perceived threat of disease 'X'

Likelihood of taking recommended preventive health action

Cues to action
Mass-media campaigns
Advice from others
Reminder postcard from physician or dentist
Illness of family member or friend
Newspaper/magazine article

Figure 11–2.   Health belief model.

fants and very young children do not differentiate illness from health because they have not developed a conscious memory of one state compared with another.

The health belief model provides insight into the connection between the way a person sees his or her state of health and his or her response to health, illness, and treatment.

High-Level Wellness Model

Dunn (1961) introduced the term **high-level wellness** and recognized health as an ongoing process toward the person's highest potential of functioning. This process involves the person, the family, and the community. Dunn described high-level wellness as "the experience of a person alive with the glow of good health, alive to the tips of their fingers with energy to burn, tingling with vitality—at times like this the world is a glorious place."

The wellness–illness continuum (Travis & Ryan, 1988) is a visual comparison of high-level wellness and traditional medicine's view of wellness (Fig. 11-3). At the neutral point, there are no signs or symptoms of disease. A person moving toward the left experiences a

worsening state of health. Someone with wellness-oriented goals wants to move beyond the neutral point (mere absence of disease) to the right (toward high-level wellness). This person evaluates the current conduct of his or her life, learns about the available options, and grows toward self-actualization by trying out these options in the search for high-level wellness.

High-level wellness, according to Ardell (1977), is "a lifestyle-focused approach which you design for the purpose of pursuing the highest-level health within your capability." A person's lifestyle is a dynamic process that involves beliefs, needs, and values. Choices in life become opportunities to move toward wellness, using methods such as self-responsibility, nutritional awareness, stress management, physical fitness, spiritual growth, and environmental sensitivity.

Holistic Health Model

Holism is seen as a "new" model of health, but actually it is not new at all. Holism has been a major theme in the humanities, Western political tradition, and major religions throughout history. Holism is a different approach

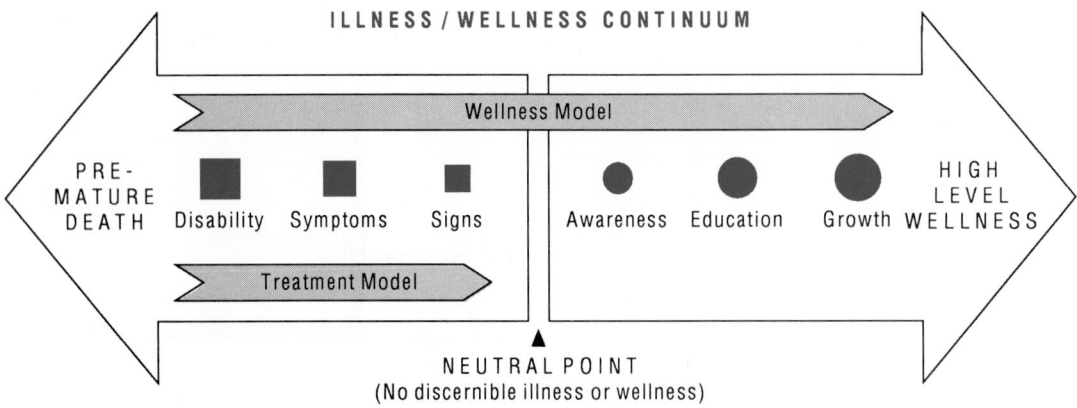

Figure 11–3.   Illness/wellness continuum. (From Travis, J. W., & Ryan, R. S. (1988). *Wellness workbook.* Berkeley, CA: Ten-Speed Press.)

to health care that acknowledges and respects the interaction of a person's mind, body, and spirit within the environment (Fig. 11-4).

Holism, derived from the Greek *holos* ("whole"), was first used by South African philosopher Jan Christian Smuts (1926) in *Holism and Evolution.* Smuts saw holism as an antidote to the atomistic approach of contemporary science. An atomistic approach takes things apart, examining the person piece by piece in an attempt to understand the larger picture by examining the smallest molecule or atom. In Emma Rose's case, this atomistic approach concentrated on her appendix and ignored the rest of her life.

Holism is based on the belief that people (or even their parts) cannot be fully understood if examined solely in pieces apart from their environment. People are seen as ever-changing systems of energy. As Figure 11-4 illustrates, the organism and the system in which it lives are

seen as greater than and different from the sum of their parts.

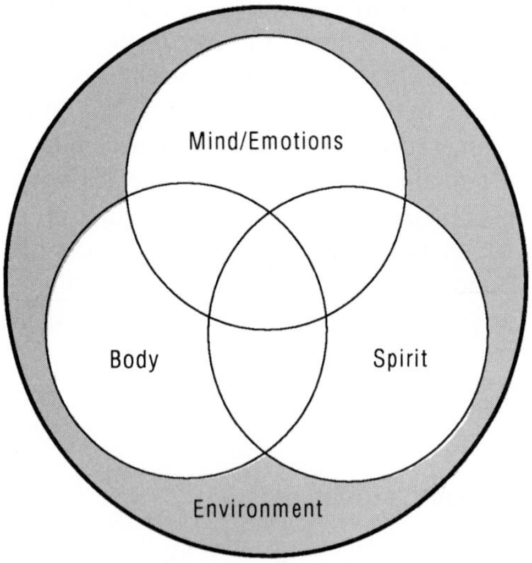

WELLNESS AND HOLISTIC HEALTH CARE

Holistic health care is different from traditional Western health care because it emphasizes humanism, choices, self-care activities, and a peer relationship between the health-care provider and the client. These interventions focus on the interrelated needs of body, mind, emotions, and spirit.

For years, the health-care community thought of body and mind as distinct entities. An illness labeled psychosomatic (*psyche,* mind, and *soma,* body) was considered a mental-health problem, and often the client was referred to a mental-health practitioner. But holistic practitioners see the psychosomatic process differently. They use the term psychosomatic to mean not simply that the mind or emotions cause illness, but that the mind and body are so interrelated that they act on each other in an intimate, direct, inseparable way. Therefore, holistic health practitioners acknowledge the interactive process of the mind, body, and spirit.

Emma Rose decided to talk to the nurse, Barbara, to discuss ideas related to holistic care. Barbara gave her some questionnaires to fill out to gather information about her current lifestyle, including questions on nutrition, exercise, stress reduction, spirituality, expression of feelings, even environmental awareness. Just answering the questions made her think about lifestyle choices and their role in her desire for wellness. For instance, the questionnaire about nutrition made her realize that she usually had a doughnut for breakfast but found herself hungry by mid-morning. Her morning coffee really seemed to increase her jitters.

Figure 11–4.   Schematic representation of holism. The system is greater than and different from the sum of the parts.

Holistic Practice

Holistic health practitioners do not want to abandon the established successes of traditional health care. Instead, they try to combine the best of both worlds: the proven success of Western modern medicine and a wide range of alternatives. This balance is illustrated by the T'ai-chi T'u symbol (Fig. 11-5). This symbol shows the symmetry of *yin* and *yang*, or the feminine and masculine principles of Chinese thought. The diagram depicts the equality of power and mutual interdependence of two major forces. This is the intent of holistic care: to acknowledge and use the best elements of both systems of health care.

Holistic practitioners recognize the incredible strides that traditional medicine has made toward wellness (e.g., antibiotics and surgery). But they are especially mindful of the risk of *iatrogenic* illness, illness that results from treatment and may be traced to the overuse and abuse of prescription medications. Holistic practitioners strive to reduce unnecessary, invasive care. For example, using stress reduction or relaxation techniques with a hypertensive client can reduce or eliminate the need for medication and its accompanying risk of side effects.

Emma Rose was in pain when Barbara, the staff nurse, stopped by her room. She had asked for pain medication and had been told it was not time and she would have to wait another 30 minutes. Emma Rose felt uncomfortable and anxious. Barbara suggested that using imagery might help her to relax and be more comfortable. Barbara suggested that Emma Rose picture herself on a warm, soft stretch of sand, looking out over a calm, blue-green body of water under a clear blue sky. Before long, Emma Rose realized she was no longer counting the minutes until her pain medication. She did feel calmer.

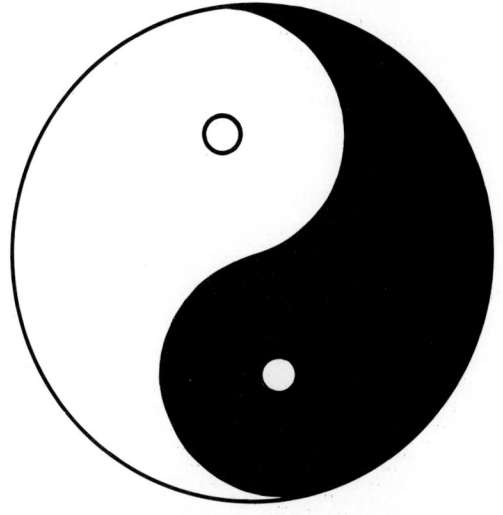

Figure 11-5. T'ai-chi T'u (yin-yang) symbol.

Emma Rose realized that working with a holistic health practitioner meant that she would be a partner, an active participant in her own care. Later in the day she again used the imagery to feel calmer, and she liked feeling that she was in charge.

Self-Responsibility

The first dimension of a wellness lifestyle is *self-responsibility,* a personal sense of accountability for one's own well-being. To make informed choices, the client must first be aware of himself or herself. **Self-awareness** means knowing and caring for oneself, recognizing one's strengths and limitations. Holistic health practices add to self-knowledge. This knowledge of self on all levels (physical, psychological, social, and spiritual) enables the person to identify his or her status of being and decide the priorities of knowledge and service required. Self-knowing may be the first step toward self-caring.

Informed Choices

Making informed choices, being an active participant rather than a passive pawn, can benefit one's self-concept. This altered self-concept may facilitate a fundamental change in the person's belief system. The holistic health practitioner can use this decision to change by encouraging the person to examine his or her lifestyle and consider moving toward high-level wellness.

For example, people learning to use biofeedback to reduce tension headaches must first gather data on their own tension signals and triggers. To initiate relaxation techniques at an early stage, they become aware of the bodily symptoms or signals that warn of a tension buildup. By becoming aware of the situations that trigger a stress response, they can learn ways to change those situations, or change their view of the situation to prevent the stress response before it occurs.

Self-Worth

Psychologist Yetta Bernhard (1975) proposed that self-respect and self-worth are developed in the process of caring for oneself.

After having been taught by the holistic nurse what to watch for, Emma Rose began to monitor her own wound healing. Looking at her scar on the 3rd day, she recognized the red puffy tissue without drainage as a healthy sign. She felt a sense of control that was not present when the physician made rounds and briefly glanced at her scar without commenting or explaining how the incision should look at various stages of healing.

Participating in self-care gives the client a greater feeling of independence and control. The altered concept of self as an active agent can help the person move toward high-level wellness. The concept of self as an active health agent extends across the wellness–illness continuum and applies to people at all developmental levels.

Meaning of Disease, Illness, and Dysfunction

Disease. Since health is a state of harmony, **disease** is a state of disharmony of mind, body, emotions, and spirit. Pelletier, in *Holistic Medicine* (1979), discussed the holistic view of disease as an opportunity to discover meaning. Traditional medicine often equates disease with failure, either of medicine or of the person. Even language such as "chief complaint" conveys a negative message. When going to see the school nurse, a child is often asked, "What's wrong?"

According to the holistic view, the manifestation and course of a disease depend on how the client integrates the experience into his or her life. The school nurse can ask the child, "How are things going for you today?" Disease can be transformed into a positive experience of personal value and growth.

Illness. **Illness** is a product of the disharmonious interaction (disease) between mind, body, emotions, and spirit. Claude Bernard, a 17th-century French physiologist, developed the concept of **homeostasis,** the organism's attempt to restore balance. With self-regulatory mechanisms, our bodies respond to constant challenges from the external environment in an effort to maintain equilibrium or health. Illness is our body's way of signaling that we have exceeded our natural ability to mediate between our internal and external environment. Illness can be an opportunity to discover meaning in life and to heal ourselves. We can identify areas of disharmony or "dis-ease" and determine how to best move toward a natural state of harmony.

Illness is a product of a complementary interaction between mind and body. Meek (1977) observed that if the client's mind is fed a daily diet of anger, remorse, revenge, hate, jealousy, suspicion, and envy, the very cells of the client's body reflect this environment. Increased vulnerability to specific diseases seems to correlate with problems expressing certain emotions. For instance, people who deny anxiety seem more prone to cardiac disease. Psychologist Lawrence LeShan (1961) found that cancer patients had a higher-than-normal incidence of feelings of helplessness and hopelessness before their diagnosis. Cancer also seems to correlate with difficulty expressing feelings such as anger and depression (Eysenck, 1988).

Feelings do not cause disease, but they do interfere with the immune system and may create an atmosphere in which disease can develop. One study of cancer patients and their families found a powerful relationship between negative images surrounding cancer and treatment outcomes (Simonton, Matthews-Simonton, & Creighton, 1978). The authors counseled patients and their support systems about psychological awareness and self-care to achieve the best treatment outcome.

Illness can be a signal that important needs are not being met. It can be an invitation from within to look at the balance between activity and rest or self- and other-oriented care. Do we really prefer to ignore this balance until we become ill (and are forced to curtail our activities)? Or should we openly acknowledge or even anticipate these signals and provide ourselves with an opportunity to prevent illness and enjoy ourselves in the process?

Getting Well Again (Simonton, Matthews-Simonton, & Creighton, 1978) suggests a simple exercise to identify the needs being met through illness and ways to find other avenues:

> List the five most important benefits you received from an illness in your life. Consider the needs that were met by your illness: relief from stress, love and attention, opportunity to renew energy, etc. Identify the rules or beliefs that limit you from meeting each of these needs when you are well.

Emma Rose used this exercise to examine her hospitalization. Up to this point she had focused only on the negative aspects. She realized that the surgery allowed her to take a break from a project she didn't enjoy at work. She loved the caring messages from her friends when they sent cards or flowers. She decided to ask her boss to assign her to a project she enjoyed more. She also reorganized her calendar so that she could have more contact with the friends who had responded to her in such caring ways.

Dysfunction. **Dysfunction** is an action (abnormal, inadequate, or impaired) that does not meet expected norms. The action "generates therapeutic concern on the part of the client, family, or friends, and the nurse" (Gordon, 1987).

Emma Rose felt pain when she moved in bed or stood to walk. She also wondered if she would continue her usual pattern of daily bowel movements. She voiced her concerns to Barbara. Barbara told her that she would have altered mobility and altered bowel elimination for several days as a result of pain and trauma to her internal organs. In the meantime, Barbara taught Emma Rose how to sit up in bed from a side position while swinging her feet to the bed stool. Barbara said that she should take short walks and then rest, and told her it was normal to feel tired after surgery. Barbara advised her not to push herself beyond endurance but to move within the limitations of discomfort. Barbara also told her to drink plenty of liquids and eat as her appetite dictated. "Normal function will return in a few days," Barbara said.

Therapeutic interventions for dysfunctional problems are directed at contributing factors. Interventions for potential dysfunction are directed at prevention by reducing risk factors (Gordon, 1987). "An outgrowth of the disease orientation is a disability orientation; an outgrowth of the health orientation is an ability orientation" (Hopkins & Smith, 1988). Therefore, the person with altered function is not necessarily disabled, but should be able to adapt strengths toward being abled. This transformation is evident in the lives of famous role models such as Helen Keller and President Franklin D. Roosevelt.

Effect of Stress

Holistic practitioners recognize that life stresses affect how and when an illness will be manifested. Any change, even a positive one, results in a certain amount of stress. Psychosocial stress, such as the death of a spouse or being diagnosed with a progressively deteriorating illness, can lead to depression, anger, and despair, all of which harm the immune system. A cluster of events that require life adjustment is associated with illness onset. Underlying both cardiovascular disease and cancer, the two leading causes of disability and death, is a prolonged state of sympathetic nervous system activity mediated through the hormonal pathways. This is the body's response to prolonged stress reactivity.

Holistic practitioners recognize the impact of stress on health and teach skills to notice and decrease it, when possible. See Chapter 47 for more information on stress.

NURSING IN WELLNESS AND HOLISTIC HEALTH CARE

Holistic professionals are committed to participating and cooperating with clients. The holistic nurse acts as a "caring colleague" of the client (Blattner, 1981). Holistic nurses help their clients toward high-level wellness while acknowledging that each has the right to choose his or her own path. Holistic nurses also recognize a duty to provide the healthiest environment for themselves and generations to come.

According to Martha Rogers, the primary purpose of nursing is to help people achieve their maximum health potential. The first line of defense is promotion of health and prevention of illness. By promoting high-level wellness and preventing illness whenever possible, the holis-

tic nurse uses an approach that minimizes risk and empowers the client.

Promoting Health and Preventing Illness

"The goal of holistic nursing is to use preventive, nurturative, and generative activities to assist clients towards achieving their own high-level wellness" (Blattner, 1981). A major goal is to prevent unnecessary disruptions in the clients' lives.

Preventive Activities

The prevention aspect of holistic nursing has three levels:

Primary prevention, preventing disease before it occurs, might involve enforcing environmental controls (e.g., prohibiting excessive noise in the workplace to prevent hearing loss).

Secondary prevention involves screening or education to promote early diagnosis and treatment (e.g., a program identifying hypertensive clients to teach stress-reduction techniques).

Tertiary prevention applies to rehabilitation situations, where the goal is to minimize residual dysfunction. A good example would be a program for a myocardial infarction patient that includes lifestyle changes such as dietary and exercise habits, as well as attitude changes or modified responses to stress.

Prevention is discussed further in Chapter 26.

Nurturative Activities

The nurturative activities of the holistic nurse involve caring, supporting, and sustaining clients. These activities may range from giving antibiotics to giving a massage.

Emma Rose felt a personal connection with the holistic nurse. When Emma Rose began to ambulate, Barbara stopped by her room. Emma Rose said she felt so uprooted surrounded by unfamiliar objects and wearing a patient gown. Barbara suggested she have a friend bring in her own pajamas from home and a few things, such as a photograph or cassette tapes, that would make the environment more comfortable. "If you can't be home you can bring some home here," said Barbara.

Generative Activities

Generative activities are those that encourage self-care. Examples are teaching relaxation techniques to children with cancer to help them cope during traumatic procedures, or researching alternate healing methods to provide an objective database for future decision-making.

Nursing as a Therapeutic Partnership

The holistic practitioner sees the nurse–client relationship as a therapeutic partnership rather than a dependent relationship. Some nurses believe the word *patient* connotes a passive, helpless person rather than a person seeking wellness, which at times includes the support of a health-care provider; as an alternative, many nurses use the term *client*. The nurse is no longer the "pill fairy" in a culture that has become accustomed to a quick fix. Instead, the nurse is an agent for change, helping clients to take responsibility and to take charge of their lives and health.

True helping can occur only when the client wants and needs it. Some helpers become rescuers by entering into what Steiner (1971) calls the victim, rescuer, and persecutor triangle (Fig. 11-6). In the triangle, the client can be seen as a victim, acting as if he or she wants help. The health-care provider, as a rescuer, decides to help. But the rescuer neglects to determine if the help being offered is needed or wanted. The rescuer usually ends up as a victim of the same person he or she was trying to rescue, since the help is ineffective and the efforts are wasted. The rescuer then may feel persecuted by the client and experience resentment ("After all I've done for you!").

People in these roles go around and around the triangle. Rescuing leads to burnout on the part of the health-care provider, since the energy expended does not result in the desired outcome. Table 11-1 lists characteristics of helpers and rescuers (Travis & Ryan, 1988).

A health-care provider cannot change or help others unless they want to be changed or helped. Clients cannot be made well unless they want to be well more than they want to be ill (Meek, 1977). Once healed, they will not stay well unless they want to stay well. Clients may be unaware that they want to be well or ill. In these cases, practitioners may help clients clarify and explore their desires in terms of wellness. Is the payoff for becoming well greater than the gains of remaining ill?

Nursing Diagnoses for Wellness

Nursing diagnoses are used to provide organization and clarity when communicating with the health-care team. Nursing diagnoses for wellness serve several purposes. They encourage the nurse and client to examine positive, life-affirming behaviors that contribute to healthy functioning. When written as part of the client's health-care

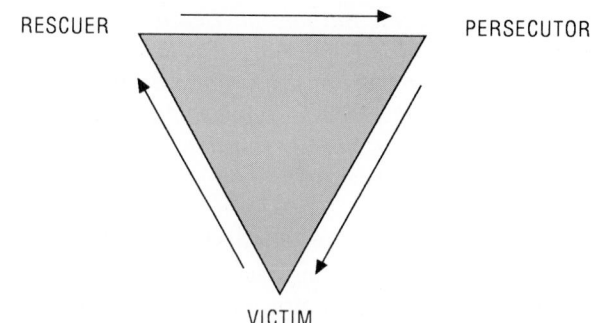

Figure 11–6.   Victim–rescuer–persecutor triangle.

record, the diagnoses can be used to reinforce continued health promotion. "Assessment of strengths and health-promoting behaviors, shared and supported in collaboration with the recipient of nursing care, encourages the continued use of positive strategies in similar circumstances" (Houldin, Saltstein, & Ganley, 1987). There are currently four wellness diagnoses on the North American Nursing Diagnostic Association (NANDA) accepted list. They are: Effective Breastfeeding; Health Seeking Behaviors; Family Coping, Potential for Growth; and Anticipatory Grieving.

Nurses in all settings can use these and other wellness diagnoses to focus on promoting health. Each person should be seen as a whole person with the physical, psychological, and spiritual potential for optimal functioning across the lifespan.

Examples of Holistic Health Care Modalities

Lifestyle Modification

Holistic practitioners advocate the use of lifestyle modification skills, such as meditation, exercise, or relaxation, that alleviate stress and promote a state less susceptible to disease. These skills increase energy flow rather than reduce awareness of tension.

Norman Cousins (1976), in his courageous fight against a serious connective tissue disorder, called the placebo effect "the doctor who resides within." He recognized the importance of how he thought about his illness, how much control he perceived himself as having in his life, and how much he was enjoying his life.

Cousins took the bold step of accepting responsibility for his disorder. He decided to check out of the hospital where his condition was termed hopeless and made his relationship with his physician into a partnership. He started a self-care regimen that included watching comedies by the Three Stooges and the Marx Brothers because he had noticed that laughter eased his symptoms. Rather than focusing on the negative connotations of his disease, he became an active agent to change his outlook in a more positive direction. After months of recuperation, he resumed his work and his mobility improved.

TABLE 11–1

Characteristics of Helpers and Rescuers

Helper	Rescuer
Listens for request	Gives when not asked
Presents offer	Neglects to find if offer is welcome
Gives only what is needed	Gives more help and for longer time than needed
Checks periodically with patient	Omits feedback
Checks results that patient	Does not check results and feels good when accepted, bad when turned down by client
Functions better	
Meets goals	
Solves problems independently	
Uses suggestions successfully	

From Travis, J., & Ryan R. S. (1988). *Wellness workbook*. Berkeley, CA: Ten-Speed Press.

Meditation

Meditation, deep personal thought and reflection, may be one of the most basic and powerful self-care activities that we can incorporate into our lives. It stills the chattering mind and sharpens our understanding of internal and external worlds. Meditation is a way to tune and train the mind that leads to greater efficiency in everyday life. It helps to decrease anxiety and helps us handle stress with less negative impact. Meditators withstand more life changes with less illness.

Although meditation seems like simple tool, it can have powerful results. It is not a strange and complicated technique requiring great effort and skill: it is merely a way of switching our concentration from the external world to the internal world. Many types of meditation are clearly described in Joel Levey's *The Fine Arts of Relaxation, Concentration and Meditation* (1987).

Imagery

Imagery is the "internal experience of a perceptual event in the absence of the actual external stimuli" (Achterberg & Lawlis, 1980). In the Simontons' (1978) work with cancer patients, they teach their patients to use daily relaxation and mental imagery to enhance their immune system response. The patients are taught to picture cancer cells being destroyed by the current treatment and by their body's white blood cells. The imagery process includes seeing themselves as whole, well, and full of energy. Using these methods, the Simontons report encouraging results: surviving patients in one study lived on the average twice as long as those patients who received medical treatment alone, and even those patients who died lived 1.5 times longer than the control group.

Therapeutic Touch

Therapeutic Touch, a technique derived from the ancient "laying on of hands," incorporates many aspects of holism and holistic health care. Dora Kunz and Dolores Krieger developed this approach, which has been taught to nurses worldwide.

According to their philosophy, the client's state of health is reflected in the vital energy field that surrounds him or her. The Therapeutic Touch practitioner learns to

---

Nursing Research

Selected Nursing Research Studies

Laffrey, S. C. (1982). Health behavior choice as related to self-actualization, body weight, and healthy conception. *Dissertation Abstracts International, 43,* 3536B. (University Microfilms No. 83-06904)

English-Lueck, J. A. (1990). Health in the New Age: A study in California holistic practices. Albuquerque: University of New Mexico Press.

Kunz, D. & Peper, E. (1982, December). Fields and their clinical implications. *American Theosophist,* p. 215.

Possible Topics for Nursing Inquiry

- How does a person's value of health affect his or her health-promoting behaviors and resulting wellness?
- What are effective noninvasive holistic treatments to reduce unnecessary usage of medications and surgery in treating disease?
- How can nurses support the patient's health-care choices while evaluating the efficacy of these choices objectively?

attune to this energy field by first centering, or achieving a sense of peace and wholeness within himself or herself. Krieger described **Therapeutic Touch** as a healing meditation, since the centered state is maintained throughout the process. The practitioner assesses and treats the client's energy field with the goal of restoring harmony. If the flow of energy is perceived as obstructed, disordered, or depleted, the practitioner attempts to direct energy to the client to release congestion and balance the areas where flow may be disordered.

Therapeutic Touch relaxes the client, who experiences slower, deeper breathing, decreased muscle tension, and warmer hands and feet. This method has been reported to alleviate discomfort and to speed healing (MacCrae, 1988). Therapeutic Touch is a noninvasive process that may decrease patients' need for medication and may enable them to tap into their natural healing potential. It is said to be a healing experience for both practitioner and client.

Therapeutic Touch is only one healing method in the expanding field of holistic nursing. It represents a powerful shift in medicine that has influenced health-care practitioners and clients alike.

Key Concepts

- Health, as defined by the World Health Organization, is a state of complete physical, mental, and social well-being.
- Wellness is a dynamic state that allows for different personal beliefs about health.
- In the clinical model, health is seen as the absence of indications of illness.
- The host–agent–environment model of health seeks a source or cause of illness.
- The health belief model is characterized by the relationship between a person's beliefs and actions.
- In the high-level wellness model, health is an ongoing process toward the person's highest potential.
- The holistic health model recognizes the unique interaction of a person's mind, body, and spirit within the environment.
- Holistic health care combines the proven success of modern medicine, participation of the client, and additional activities to complement medical protocol.
- The nursing diagnoses relating to health and wellness are important for initiating and reinforcing health promotion.
- Holistic health care interventions include lifestyle modification, exercise, meditation, and imagery.

References

Achterberg, J. A., & Lawlis, G. F. (1980). *Bridges of the bodymind.* Champaign, IL: Institute for Personality and Ability Testing, p. 27.

Allen, D. G. (1986). Using philosophical and historical methodologies to understand the concept of health. In P. Chinn (Ed.), *Nursing research methodology* (pp. 157–168). Rockville, MD: Aspen.

Ardell, D. B. (1977). *High-level wellness.* Emmaus, PA: Rodale, p. 65.

Bernhard, Y. (1975). *Self-care.* Millbrae, CA: Celestial Arts.

Blattner, B. (1981). *Holistic nursing.* Englewood Cliffs, NJ: Prentice-Hall.

Coddington, R. D. (1972). The significance of life events as etiologic factors in the diseases of children. *Journal of Psychosomatic Research, 16,* 7–18.

Cousins, N. (1976). Anatomy of an illness. *New England Journal of Medicine, 12,* 4–51.

Davis, B. (1978). *The magical child within you.* Millbrae, CA: Celestial Arts.

Dunn, H. L. (1961). *High-level wellness.* Arlington, VA: R. W. Beatty.

Eysenck, H. J. (1988). Personality, stress and cancer prediction and prophylaxis. *British Journal of Medical Psychology, 61,* 57–75.

Ferguson, M. (1980). *The Aquarian conspiracy: Personal and social transformation in the 1980s.* Los Angeles: J. P. Tarcher.

Fuerst, M. L. (1983, July 25). Holistic medicine: Just what is it anyway? *Medical World News,* pp. 34–53.

Goleman, D. (1976, February). Meditation helps break the stress spiral. *Psychology Today,* p. 2.

Gordon, M. G. (1987). *Nursing diagnosis: Process and application* (2nd ed.). New York: McGraw-Hill, p. 135.

Harman, W. (1977). The coming transformation. *The Futurist, 4,* 106–112.

Hopkins, H. L., & Smith, H. D. (1988). *Willard and Spackman's occupational therapy* (7th ed.). Philadelphia: J. B. Lippincott, p. 435.

Houldin, A., Saltstein, S., & Ganley, K. (1987). *Nursing diagnosis for wellness.* Philadelphia: J.B. Lippincott.

Jacoban, L. (1982, February). Nursing amidst the Aquarian conspiracy. *The Washington Nurse,* pp. 3–6.

Kuhn, T. S. (1962). *The structure of scientific revolutions.* Chicago: University of Chicago Press.

Leavell, H. R., et al. (1965). *Preventive medicine for the doctor in his community* (3rd ed.). New York: McGraw-Hill.

LeShan, L. (1961). A basic psychological orientation apparently associated with malignant disease. *Psychiatric Quarterly, 35,* 314.

LeShan, L. (1974). *How to meditate.* New York: Bantam.

Levey, J. (1987). *The fine arts of relaxation, concentration and meditation: Ancient skills for modern minds.* London: Wisdom Publications.

MacCrae, J. (1988). *Therapeutic Touch: A practical guide.* New York: Alfred A. Knopf.

Mayeroff, M. (1971). *On caring.* New York: Harper & Row.

Meek, G. W. (1977). *Healers and the healing process.* Wheaton, IL: Theosophical Publishing House.

Pelletier, K. (1979). *Holistic medicine.* New York: Delacorte.

Pender, N. (1987). *Health promotion in nursing practice* (2nd ed.). Los Altos, CA: Appleton & Lange.

Rahe, R. H., Meyer, M., Smith, M., Kjaer, G., & Holmes, T. H. (1964). Social stress and illness onset. *Journal of Psychosomatic Research, 8,* 35–44.

Rosenstock, I. (1974). Historical origin of the health belief model. *Health Education Monographs, 2,* 334.

Rogers, M. (1990). *An introduction to the theoretical basis of nursing.* Philadelphia: F. A. Davis.

Selye, H. (1974). *Stress without distress.* New York: Dutton.

Simonton, O. C., Matthews-Simonton, S., & Creighton, J. L. (1978). *Getting well again.* New York: Bantam.

Smuts, J. C. (1926). *Holism and evolution.* New York: Macmillan.

Steiner, C. (1971). *Transactional analysis made simple.* San Francisco: Transactional Publications.

Travis, J. W., & Ryan, R. S. (1988). *Wellness workbook.* Berkeley, CA: Ten-Speed Press.

World Health Organization. (1947). Constitution of the World Health Organization. *Chronicles of WHO, 1,* 1–2.

Bibliography

Allen, C. J. (1989). Incorporating a wellness perspective for nursing diagnosis in practice. *Classifications of Nursing Diagnoses Proceedings Eighth Conference,* 37–42.

Bar, B. (1990). Patients teach holistic nursing care. *Advances in Clinical Care, 5,* 18.

Benson, E. R., McDevitt, J. Q. (1989). Home care and the older adult: Illness care vs. wellness care. *Holistic Nursing Practice, 3*(2), 30–38.

Buchanan, M., et al. (1989). *Nursing centers: Meeting the demand for quality health care.* National League of Nursing: Publication #21-2311, pp. 111–116.

Butterfield, P. G. (1990). Thinking upstream: Nurturing a conceptual understanding of the societal context of health behavior. *ANS, 12*(2), 1–8.

De Leeuw, E. (1989). Concepts in health promotion: The notion of relativism. *Soc Sci Med, 29,* 1281–1288.

Gorton, D. (1988). Holistic health techniques to increase individual coping and wellness. *J Holistic Nurs, 6,* 25–30.

Keiley, M. (1989). Holistic health care: The roles of the self and the nurse. *Dimens Health Serv, 66*(4), 17–19.

Loreno, P., and Drick, C. (1990). Self-care identity formation: A nursing education perspective. *Holistic Nurs Pract, 4*(2), 79–86.

Nagai-Jacobson, M. G., and Burkhardt, M.A. (1989). Spirituality: Cornerstone of holistic nursing practice. *Holistic Nurs Pract, 3*(3), 18–26.

Nemcek, M. A. (1990). Health beliefs and preventive behavior: A review of research literature. *AAOHN J, 38*(3), 127–138.

Sherman, J. B., Clark, L., and McEwen, M. M. (1989). Evaluation of worksite wellness program: Impact on exercise, weight, smoking, and stress. *Public Health Nurs, 6*(3), 114–119.

Smith, J. M., and Sorrel, V. (1989). Developing wellness centers: A nurse-managed "stay well center" for senior citizens. *Clin Nurs Spec, 3*(4), 198–202.

Smith, M. J. (1988). Perspectives of wholeness: The lens makes a difference. *Nursing Science Quarterly, 1*(3), 94–95.

Spencer, E. A. (1989). Toward a balance of work and play: Promotion of health and wellness. *Occup Ther Health Care, 5*(4), 87–99.

Utz, S. W. (1990). Motivating self-care: A nursing approach. *Holistic Nurs Pract, 4*(2), 13–21.

Volden, C. et al. (1990). The relationship of age, gender, and exercise practices to measures of health, life-style, and self-esteem. *Appl Nurs Res, 3*(1), 20–26.

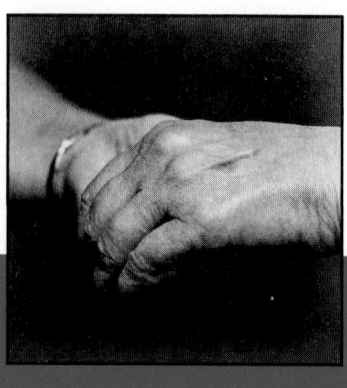

Human Needs

12

Maslow's Hierarchy of Needs
  Physiologic Needs
  Safety Needs
  Love Needs
  Esteem Needs
  Self-Actualization Needs
Lifespan Considerations
  Newborn and Infant
  Toddler and Preschooler
  Child and Adolescent
  Adult and Older Adult
Nursing Theorists' Perceptions of Human Needs
  Florence Nightingale

Virginia Henderson
Ida Jean Orlando
Dorothea Orem
Yura and Walsh
Imogene M. King
Sister Callista Roy
Martha E. Rogers
Faye Glenn Abdellah
Lydia E. Hall
Jean Watson
Functional Health Patterns and Assessing Human Needs
Key Concepts

The "territory of nursing" has been described as "the preservation of, the maintenance of, and the facilitation of the integrity of all human needs" (Yura & Walsh, 1988, p. 70). A **human need** is any physiologic or psychological factor necessary for a healthy existence. No matter where we live, all of us have the same basic needs.

Human needs are said to be motivational forces (Yura & Walsh, 1988). The motivational strength and manner of expression of these needs is influenced by culture, socioeconomic factors, personal values, and health status. All people develop behaviors that help them meet their needs. They can learn to delay meeting needs and modify the specific behaviors that satisfy a need, depending on the need's motivational strength. If a need goes unmet, physical illness, psychological disequilibrium, or death can occur. This chapter will examine human needs theory, nursing and human needs, and how the concept of functional health patterns relates to human needs theory.

MASLOW'S HIERARCHY OF NEEDS

The most prominent theorist to focus on human needs has been Abraham Maslow (1970); others have included

Lederer (1980), McHale and McHale (1978), Montague (1970), and Murray (1938). Maslow believed that all humans are born with instinctive needs. These needs can be grouped into five categories, and they can be arranged in order of importance from those essential for physical survival to those necessary to develop our fullest human potential. His hierarchy of human needs provides an ideal framework for understanding the characteristics and motivational force behind each human need (Fig. 12-1).

The pyramid is helpful in understanding Maslow's theory of human needs. Just as a pyramid must be constructed from its base to its apex, people must meet lower-level needs to some degree before they can address higher-level needs. A person is not motivated by all five categories of human needs at the same time; only the category most relevant to the person's circumstances at a particular time is the primary motivation (Yura & Walsh, 1988). Meeting needs is a dynamic process. It involves the continual resolution of, progression beyond, and return to any given category of needs.

Physiologic Needs

Physiologic needs are the fundamental motivating force in human existence and thus provide the base for Mas-

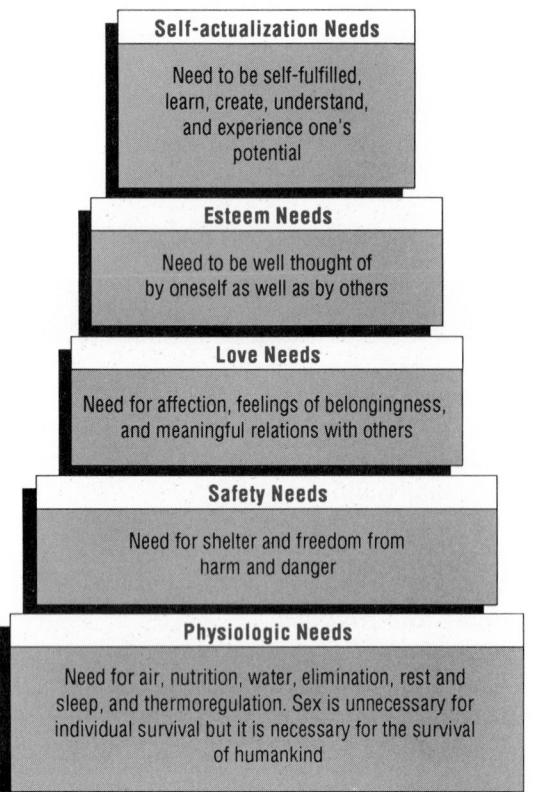

Figure 12–1. A pyramid represents Maslow's hierarchy of human needs. According to Maslow, basic physiologic needs, such as nutrition and water, must be met before the person can move on to higher-level needs. Nursing helps people to meet needs they cannot meet by themselves.

low's pyramid. Existence requires air, food, water, elimination, sleep and rest, temperature maintenance, and sex. If any one of these needs goes unmet, the existence of the person or species is threatened (Montague, 1970). Nurses assess the patient's ability to meet his or her physiologic needs, and identify the nature and degree of nursing interventions necessary to enable the person to satisfy them.

Air. Oxygen is essential for the body's metabolic processes. Satisfying this need requires a properly functioning respiratory and cardiovascular system. Poor oxygenation of body tissues leads to tissue ischemia and eventual death. Although a person's respiratory status may be sufficient for proper oxygenation, air quality can affect his or her ability to meet this need. Pollution from automobiles, industry, and cigarette smoke have prompted clean-air legislation so that this human need can be met.

The nurse helps the patient to meet this need based on a thorough physical assessment, including respiratory rate, breath sounds, muscles used in breathing, activity tolerance, past medical history, and supporting laboratory data. Environmental factors, such as living or working in a polluted area, must also be assessed.

If the nurse determines that this need is not being met, interventions might include teaching the patient about good nutrition and proper exercise, and advising him or her not to smoke and to wear masks in polluted areas. Patients in both acute-care and home settings may require external mechanical assistance for proper oxygenation. Nursing interventions in this situation involve maintaining a patent airway in the patient and monitoring equipment to ensure that it functions properly.

Nutrition. Proper nutrition is essential for energy production and the body's metabolic processes. Satisfying this need requires adequate food and a properly functioning gastrointestinal tract and metabolism. If this need goes unmet, hunger, destruction of vital tissues, and ultimately death will occur. Throughout history, humans have recognized this critical need. The need for food is documented in the drawings of early cave-dwellers and is reflected in contemporary efforts to address hunger in the world.

Assessing the patient's ability to meet this need involves examining his or her weight, diet, and eating patterns, and reviewing available laboratory data. Appropriate nursing interventions depend on the particular barrier to adequate nutrition. Lack of knowledge about a balanced diet requires nutritional counseling. Insufficient financial resources could be addressed by a referral for financial assistance or supplemental food. Psychological disorders such as anorexia or bulimia require referrals for mental health and medical treatment.

Mechanical interventions for meeting this need include gastrostomy tubes, nasogastric tubes, or hyperalimentation. The patient and family members may require teaching if these interventions are carried out at home.

Water. Fluids are necessary for metabolic processes of the body, and proper fluid balance is critical for life. A depletion or excess of fluid can be life-threatening; the very young, the old, and the critically ill are especially at risk (Mountcastle, 1980).

Assessment can range from the basic steps of weighing the patient and measuring fluid intake and output to the complex measurements conducted in the intensive care unit. Nursing interventions include having patients weigh themselves daily and measure their fluid intake and output. Judging whether this need has been met is critical when a patient's urinary or cardiovascular system becomes compromised.

Elimination. Elimination, a crucial part of the metabolic process, enables the body to dispose of waste products and to maintain fluid and electrolyte balance. The gastrointestinal and renal systems and certain metabolic processes must be working for successful elimination to occur. Satisfying this need also requires a nutritionally balanced diet and proper fluid intake. Failure to meet this need leads to a buildup of waste products, eventually endangering health and life. Kidney failure or bowel obstructions from feces or a tumor are examples of life-threatening conditions that can develop if this need goes unmet. Medical and nursing interventions are critical to sustain life and reestablish healthy physiologic functioning in these circumstances.

The nurse should assess how the patient's needs for food and water are being met and should review the patient's bowel and urine elimination patterns. Improper diet, inappropriate use of laxatives, and insufficient fluid intake are all problems that require nursing intervention.

Sleep and Rest. Sleep and rest are necessary for the body to revitalize itself. People vary considerably in the total amount, frequency, and duration of sleep and rest periods they need to feel refreshed. Requirements for sleep and rest also vary throughout the lifespan. But regardless of the particular pattern of sleep and rest, failure to meet this need leads to fatigue, irritability, behavioral changes, difficulty concentrating, and eventual exhaustion. Major obstacles to meeting this need are failure to allocate sufficient time for rest and sleep and the inability either to fall asleep or to remain asleep. Insomnia typically is caused by a combination of physiologic, psychological, and environmental factors.

Nursing assessment requires a detailed history of sleep habits and patterns and activity level. It should also include an evaluation of the patient's current health status and the sources of stress in his or her life. Interventions, which are developed from information obtained during the assessment, may include helping to modify the patient's lifestyle, developing an exercise program, or teaching stress-reduction techniques.

Thermoregulation. Temperature maintenance is necessary for life. Extremes in either direction can lead to death. The body monitors and maintains its temperature through sensors in the skin, the hypothalamus, and the effector system (Vander, Sherman, & Luciano, 1985). Any alteration in these structures can affect temperature regulation. The body can adapt to environmental temperatures within broad limits, but age and health status greatly affect this capacity. The very young, very old, and chronically ill patients do not have optimal adaptive capabilities and are at risk when temperature alterations are severe.

Nursing assessment involves a careful evaluation of the patient's living situation and daily activities. The nurse must assess for signs of hypo- or hyperthermia. Nursing interventions are based on the person's health status, lifestyle, and economic resources.

Sex. Sex is not essential for the person's survival, but it is necessary for the continuation of the human race.

The importance of this need varies widely among people, and meeting this need can affect how the person deals with higher-order needs such as love, belonging, and self-esteem. The role that sex plays in the patient's life depends on a complex set of cultural, religious, social, and psychological variables.

Assessing this need requires considerable skill and sensitivity. Some patients readily discuss sexual issues; others see such questions as intrusive. The nurse must be attentive to cues from the patient and must respect his or her wishes. Recognizing individual differences and variations that can occur across the lifespan should serve as a framework for evaluation. An adequate assessment must consider the patient's past and current sexual behavior, the patient's satisfaction with this behavior, and the effect of the patient's health status on sexual activity.

Nursing interventions may involve helping the patient develop alternate strategies for satisfying this need when his or her health status is compromised, or referring the patient for counseling if a sexual dysfunction is identified.

Safety Needs

Once basic physiologic needs are met, the person must address **safety needs.** Humans need to be physically safe and free from the fear and anxiety that can result from a lack of security and protection. If this need goes unmet, the person may experience or fear pain, injury, or death. This need begins at birth. Infants and children depend on adult caretakers to meet this need, and the degree to which safety and security needs are met in early life can have a profound effect on the person's physical and psychological health and ability to focus on higher-order needs.

Safety can often be a dominant motivating need. For example, in a war-torn country, safety becomes a primary motivating force among the inhabitants as long as their physiologic needs are met at a minimal level. The same is true during natural disasters such as floods or tornadoes. Such events cause major disruptions in personal, family, and societal routines and can lead to chaos. According to Maslow (1970), an essential aspect of safety is the need for predictability and routine.

Illness can represent a major threat to the safety needs of both the patient and family. The severe stress that arises from illness and hospitalization can threaten safety and security because the patient's normal routine is typically disrupted, independence is threatened, and there may be uncertainty about what is wrong and what to expect. Patients' reactions vary greatly and can include anger, withdrawal, and depression.

The nursing assessment of safety and security needs must evaluate health status, social supports, and the environment. The specific issues to be considered in each of these areas vary depending on the patient's age.

Nursing interventions should address the patient's needs while in the hospital and after discharge.

Love Needs

The need for love and belonging (**love needs**) is the next tier on the pyramid. Once we achieve a sense of safety, we need to feel as if we belong and are loved to avoid loneliness and isolation. People seek caring, friendship, love, and intimacy in diverse ways, either by developing relationships with people in general or with a specific person. This can be done by joining groups or clubs that share common values, interests, and beliefs, or by establishing personal relationships such as friendships or marriage. To meet this need, the person must both give and receive love. Maslow (1970) wrote that this group of needs is becoming increasingly difficult to fulfill in our mobile society.

Illness and hospitalization can alter the patient's ability to satisfy this need. The nurse must assess how illness affects the patient's typical way of meeting this need, and must also determine how the significant people in the patient's life respond to the illness. Nursing interventions typically consist of helping the patient and significant others to deal with the illness. The patient and significant others should be included in planning and participating in care. Interventions may also involve referrals to appropriate support groups.

Esteem Needs

We must develop and maintain a sense of our own value if we are to meet our **esteem needs.** According to Maslow (1970), there are two types of esteem needs: esteem derived from others and self-esteem. People need esteem from others: we need to know that others think well of us, admire and respect us. We also need self-esteem, an internal sense of our own adequacy and worth. In Maslow's view, esteem from others is primary and is critical if a person is to develop an internal sense of worth. It is difficult to feel worthwhile if others do not value us and provide us with positive feedback. In contrast, self-esteem develops from within. To be genuine, it must be firmly grounded in a realistic appraisal of who we are and what our strengths and weaknesses are. If esteem needs go unmet, the person is doomed to a life characterized by self-doubt and feelings of helplessness and worthlessness.

What others value in us and what we value in ourselves varies greatly and is influenced by cultural, social, and psychological variables. During assessment, the nurse must recognize this and try to understand the patient's frame of reference rather than impose his or her own values on the patient. Nursing assessment should focus on the patient's usual ways of achieving self-esteem and how alterations in health status affect them. Nursing interventions should help the patient explore the feelings associated with a change in health status and should help the patient develop new ways of satisfying esteem needs.

Self-Actualization Needs

Once we satisfy lower-order needs, we strive for self-actualization. According to Maslow (1970), the need for **self-actualization** is the innate need to fully realize all our abilities and qualities: we try to develop our maximum potential. Maslow sees this as a never-ending process. Although it is affected by early life experiences, we have the capacity to change and reach a stage of optimal psychological health as we strive for self-actualization.

The nurse must assess the effect that illness has on the patient's self-actualization. Does the loss of health alter the patient's ability to function in a previous role, making him or her dependent on others for many basic needs? This dependency affects self-image, problem-solving and control issues, and stress management, and behavioral changes occur.

The goal of nursing intervention is to give the patient some control over decisions pertaining to treatment. The nurse encourages hobbies that may relax the patient, giving the patient private time and a sense of accomplishment. The patient begins to work toward his or her potential. Self-confidence increases as he or she again experiences success and control in the environment.

LIFESPAN CONSIDERATIONS

No matter what their age, all humans have the same basic needs. Differences in how they meet their needs or have their needs met are a result of the stage of their psychophysiologic development. The human organism is in a constant state of flux as a result of both developmental processes and external and internal events (Turner & Helm, 1987). Consequently, there is a continuous emergency, resolution, and reemergency of each of Maslow's five categories of human needs throughout life.

Newborn and Infant

During the first stages of human development, physiologic and safety needs predominate. The infant depends on others for the satisfaction of most human needs. The infant must rely completely on others for food and safety needs; both are crucial for the rapid physiologic and psychological development that occurs at this time. The infant can meet his or her needs for air, sleep, and elimination, but does depend on others for help with elimination. A key characteristic of need satisfaction during this period is that the infant cannot delay or modify gratification of physiologic needs.

Toddler and Preschooler

During this period, the child begins to develop considerable autonomy in meeting lower-level needs, but still depends heavily on adults for a facilitating environment. The child can satisfy basic physiologic needs and begins to learn how to meet safety needs. During this stage, the foundation is laid for the person's ability to meet love, belonging, and esteem needs, through interactions with the significant adults in his or her life (Turner, 1987).

Child and Adolescent

Basic physiologic and safety needs continue to be motivating factors. Parental guidance in how best to meet these needs is still warranted (although not always welcome). Provided these lower-level needs are adequately met, the need for love, belonging, and esteem is increasingly prominent during this period. The child looks to peers and adults to meet these needs. The child's and adolescent's experiences with others and their ability to meet these higher-level needs have a profound effect on their self-concept.

Adult and Older Adult

Healthy, fully functioning adults have mastered the developmental tasks of earlier life stages, giving them the freedom to move successfully through the hierarchy of human needs and strive for self-actualization. Such people can use their physical and psychological resources and experiences to respond to the vicissitudes of life.

As the adult ages, physical and mental abilities decline, and lower-order needs may again predominate. The person's health status, social and family supports, and financial resources all play a significant role in determining the dominant needs of the aging adult. Meeting basic physiologic needs such as food, water, and elimination may become an increasing focus in the older adult's life and may require intervention from a family member or outside resource. Safety and security needs may also return to prominence, especially if the older adult suffers a stroke or chronic degenerative disease that compromises physical or psychological functioning.

Aging and changes in health status can result in the loss of previous ways for satisfying needs for love and belonging. The loss of belonging is difficult because it occurs at a time when many people are least able to develop new strategies to meet this need.

NURSING THEORISTS' PERCEPTIONS OF HUMAN NEEDS

Nursing theories through the years have incorporated ideas from human needs theory. Typically, nurses identify a patient's needs and base the care they deliver on this information. Human needs theory has led to the development of nursing models and frameworks for holistic nursing.

Florence Nightingale

In *Notes on Nursing* (1860/1946), Nightingale wrote that nurses should create an environment in which healing could take place; the need for a positive environment, free from filth and vermin, was seen as paramount to the patient's recovery. She was also concerned with the patient's response to illness.

Virginia Henderson

More than a century later, Henderson (1966) set out 14 principles of nursing (see the display). The first eight focus on physiologic needs; the rest address social, psychological, and spiritual needs. The ninth principle deals with the environment in much the same way as Florence Nightingale did. Henderson's principles address the patient's basic human needs and delineate the nurse's responsibilities. They also expand on Henderson's definition of nursing, which is to assist:

> the individual, sick or well, in the performance of those activities contributing to health or its recovery (or to a peaceful death) that he could perform unaided if he had the necessary strength or knowledge; and to do this in such a way as to help him gain independence as rapidly as possible.

Each of Henderson's needs can vary in importance depending on the situation. The nursing assessment identifies the relative importance of each need for a particular patient and assists in developing a systematic nursing care plan.

Henderson's Principles of Nursing

- Breathe normally.
- Eat and drink adequately.
- Eliminate body wastes.
- Move and maintain posture.
- Provide for sleep and rest.
- Wear suitable clothing.
- Maintain body temperature.
- Keep body clean and well-groomed.
- Avoid dangers in environment.
- Communicate.
- Worship according to one's faith.
- Feel good about work accomplishment.
- Participate in recreation.
- Learn, discover, or satisfy curiosity.

Ida Jean Orlando

Orlando (1961) defined a need as a "requirement of the patient which, if supplied, relieves or diminishes his immediate distress or improves his immediate sense of adequacy or well-being." The concept of need is central to her theory, which focuses on patients and their unmet needs. Orlando believed that the purpose of nursing was "to supply the help patients require in order for their needs to be met." Her model identified three categories of needs, which may also be seen as problem areas requiring nursing interventions:

Physical limitations (age, illness, or disability).
Adverse reactions to a setting.
Experiences that prevent communication of needs.

Dorothea Orem

Orem (1985), noted for her theory of self-care in nursing, placed human needs into three categories:

Universal self-care requisites: air, food, water, elimination, and safety. She also included self-concept, rest and activity, and social interaction time in this group.
Developmental self-care requisites, which address human needs through the lifespan.
Health deviation: needs that develop as a result of illness.

Yura and Walsh

According to Yura and Walsh (1988), the nurse's primary role is to meet human needs by using the nursing process. They divided human needs into two groups (Table 12-1). The first group addresses the person's needs, the second the needs of the family and community. By considering both the patient and his or her social context, this holistic approach incorporates human needs into nursing theory. Nursing care is delivered after considering the biopsychosocial and spiritual aspects of the patient and family, situation, and community.

Imogene M. King

King (1981) saw nursing as a "process of action, reaction, interaction and transaction." The nurse operates on the belief that each person is an open system who interacts with interpersonal and societal systems. The patient and nurse establish a relationship to cope with or improve a health state. Both identify the patient's needs: "Each perceives the other and the situation, and through communication they set goals, explore means, and agree on means to achieve goals."

Sister Callista Roy

The goal of nursing, according to Sister Callista Roy, is to promote "adaptive responses in relation to four adap-tive modes" (George, 1990, p. 238). Her adaptation model identified five essential elements: person, goal of nursing, nursing activities, health, and environment. Each person, as a complete entity, constantly interacts with the environment, and central to her theory is the need for a person to adapt to that environment. Four modes of adaptation are:

- Physiologic needs (adaptation to satisfy basic needs).
- Self-concept (adaptation to maintain psychological integrity).
- Role function (adaptation to society's roles and duties).
- Interdependence (adaptation to enable need fulfillment; support system).

Each person adapts according to his or her individual coping mechanisms. Output behaviors are either adaptive (which promote integrity, meeting of goals, survival) or ineffective (which do not promote growth). Using the nursing process, the nurse assesses how effectively the patient is adapting; diagnosis, goal-setting, intervention, and evaluation follow.

Martha E. Rogers

Rogers (1970) described nursing as a humanistic science dedicated to compassionate concern for maintaining and promoting health. Preventing illness and rehabilitating the sick and disabled are also primary goals. Nursing promotes a symphonic interaction between humans and their environment. Central to nursing's purpose is serving humanity; intellectual judgment, abstract knowledge, and compassion are foundations for professional practice.

Faye Glenn Abdellah

Abdellah described nursing as a service to people, families, and society. The nurse helps people, sick or well, to cope with their health needs. In Abdellah's model, nursing care means providing information to the patient or doing something to the patient with the goal of meeting needs or alleviating an impairment (Marriner-Tomey, 1989). For example, Number 18 of her 21 Nursing Problems (George, 1990) is to facilitate awareness of self as a person with varying physical, emotional, and developmental needs. The nurse helps the patient to identify and resolve a problem. If each problem is resolved, the patient can return to a healthy state.

Lydia E. Hall

Hall saw nursing as having different functions in three interlocking circles:

- Care circle (patient's body).
- Cure circle (disease).

TABLE 12–1

Basic Human Needs Amenable to Nursing Intervention

Human Needs For the Person Who Is the Patient	Human Needs and Their Categories For the Family and the Community As Patients*
Acceptance of self and others, by others	Survival needs:
Activity	Activity
Adaptation, to manage stress	Adaptation, to manage stress
Air	Air
Appreciation, attention	Elimination
Autonomy, choice	Fluids
Beauty and esthetic experiences	Interchange of gases
Belonging	Nutrition
Challenge	Protection from excessive fear, anxiety, and chaos
Conceptualization, rationality, problem-solving	Effective percentage of reality
Confidence	Rest and leisure
Elimination	Safety
Fluids (intake)	Sensory integrity
Freedom from pain	Sleep
Humor	Skin integrity
Interchange of gases	Structure, law, and limits
Nutrition (intake)	Closeness needs:
Effective perception of reality	Acceptance of self and others
Personal recognition, esteem, respect	Appreciation, attention
Protection from excessive fear, anxiety, and chaos	Belonging
Rest and leisure	Confidence
Safety	Humor
Self-control, self-determination, responsibility	Personal recognition, esteem, respect
Self-fulfillment, to be, to become	Sexual integrity
Sensory integrity	Tenderness
Sexual integrity	To love and be loved
Skin integrity	Wholesome body image
Sleep	Freedom needs:
Spiritual integrity	Autonomy, choice
Structure, law, and limits	Beauty and esthetic experiences
Tenderness	Challenge
Territoriality	Conceptualization, rationality, problem-solving
To love and be loved	Freedom from pain
Wholesome body image	Self-control, self-determination, responsibility
Value system	Self-fulfillment, to be, to become
	Spiritual experience
	Territoriality
	Value system

From Yura, H., & Walsh, M. (1983). *The nursing process: Assessing, planning, implementing and evaluating* (4th ed.). Norwalk, CT: Appleton-Century-Crofts, pp. 136–137.

* Category labels for survival needs, closeness needs, and freedom needs adapted from Gahung, J. (1980). The basic needs approach. In K. Lederer (Ed.). *Human needs*. Cambridge, MA.: Oelgeschlager, Gunn, & Horn, p. 59.

• Core circle (patient's inner feelings and motivations).

The therapeutic use of self is evident in the core circle (George, 1990). Using reflection, the nurse helps the patient become aware of his or her needs, feelings, and motivations. It then becomes the patient's task to set goals and priorities. This learning process encourages maximum growth. The patient freely expresses ideas regarding the disease process and his or her own needs, and through this expression the patient gains self-identity and moves toward self-actualization.

Jean Watson

Watson believed that nursing's focus is on 10 carative factors that combine a humanistic perspective with scientific knowledge. These carative factors result in satisfaction of certain needs. The nurse recognizes the biophysical, psychosocial, psychophysical, and interpersonal needs of her patient (George, 1990). Caring is central to nursing, because a caring environment allows the patient to grow and to choose the best action for himself or herself. By establishing rapport and caring, the nurse develops a helping, trusting relationship with the patient.

Watson's hierarchy is similar to Maslow's: patients must satisfy lower-order needs before attaining higher ones. Her carative factor Number 9 (assistance with gratification of human needs) includes the lower needs of survival (food, fluid, etc.) and function (activity, sexuality) and the higher needs of integration (achievement, affiliation) and growth-seeking (self-actualization).

According to Watson, each person must be seen in the context of the whole. Each need is viewed in relation to all others, and all are valued in the promotion of health and nursing care.

FUNCTIONAL HEALTH PATTERNS AND ASSESSING HUMAN NEEDS

The ideal approach to nursing should be a holistic one, because the body cannot be separated from the rest of the person. The nurse must deal with the entire person, including the physical, psychological, interpersonal, and spiritual aspects of his or her life. The patient's family and community must be considered in making a comprehensive nursing assessment; this is becoming increasingly important because the community has become a major location for the delivery of health care.

One way to ensure a holistic approach to nursing is by using Marjorie Gordon's **functional health patterns** (1987), as listed in Chapter 6. These patterns delineate the human needs of the person, family, and community. These patterns, which focus on behaviors that occur over a period of time, present a total picture of the patient rather than just a small part of his or her life. Functional health patterns represent basic health needs, and they develop as people strive to meet their needs. These patterns are unique because they are interrelated: one pattern often provides answers to another. No pattern can be studied as a separate category.

Gordon's patterns are consistent with the human needs philosophy and can be considered along with Maslow's hierarchy to provide a framework for holistic nursing assessment. Gordon provides a comprehensive discussion of patient needs; Maslow's hierarchy offers a rationale for determining the order in which needs should be addressed. A closer look at functions helps provide a better understanding of the relationship between human needs theory, functional health patterns, and the delivery of nursing care (Fig. 12-2).

Health perception–health management is the umbrella for the other 10. It focuses on health values and beliefs and the resources in the community available to meet health needs. This pattern is based on the awareness that although nursing promotes health as one of its primary functions, it is actually the patient who manages his or her own health. Success in meeting human needs by the person, family, and community in this pattern relies heavily on culture, societal beliefs, personal expectations, and one's own health. The patient's family may play an important part in this function because a family member other than the patient may be the one who makes major health decisions for family members.

An assessment of how the community meets the needs of this pattern would reveal how it thinks about health needs and how it provides health services and allocates funds. Differences in geographic location could also be assessed using this pattern. If there are no resources within a community to meet identified health management requirements, then the community must obtain outside assistance. Just because a community has resources does not mean that it uses them to the fullest extent to meet human needs, however; the failure to do so is itself a pattern.

Nutrition and metabolism are the second functions. Life cannot be sustained without meeting human needs in this category. A careful assessment reveals the patient's ability to address these needs. People establish patterns for meeting these needs early in life, and many of these behaviors are learned in the family setting. It is not simply a matter of eating: it is a complex pattern of food knowledge, food preparation, financial limits, and cultural ideas. The community is also important because of the resources it can offer (e.g., nutrition programs).

The third function, *elimination*, is closely related to nutrition and metabolism, and often these areas can be assessed simultaneously. Both are crucial to understanding the patient's needs.

Energy must be expended to meet human needs; this is examined in *activity and exercise*. Patients must be evaluated for their ability to engage in self-care activities to meet basic physiologic needs. Another aspect involves determining how much energy they have to ensure the safety of their environment. For example, the requirements for an elderly person living alone are vastly different from those of a young adult living in an intact family. Assessment reveals the patient's attitudes toward activity and exercise and his or her usual activity level. The relationship to health perception–health management is evident here because the nurse must learn how important the person, family, or community thinks this category of needs is. The community may not have adequate transportation for its members to engage in such activities. Problems meeting needs in this category may affect other needs, such as human companionship and food.

Assessment of *cognition and perception* examines the extent of the patient's awareness of human needs, which ties in with the first pattern. Lifespan considerations are also important in evaluating this pattern.

The sixth function, *sleep and rest,* is a primary human need. Patterns begin to develop at birth and change

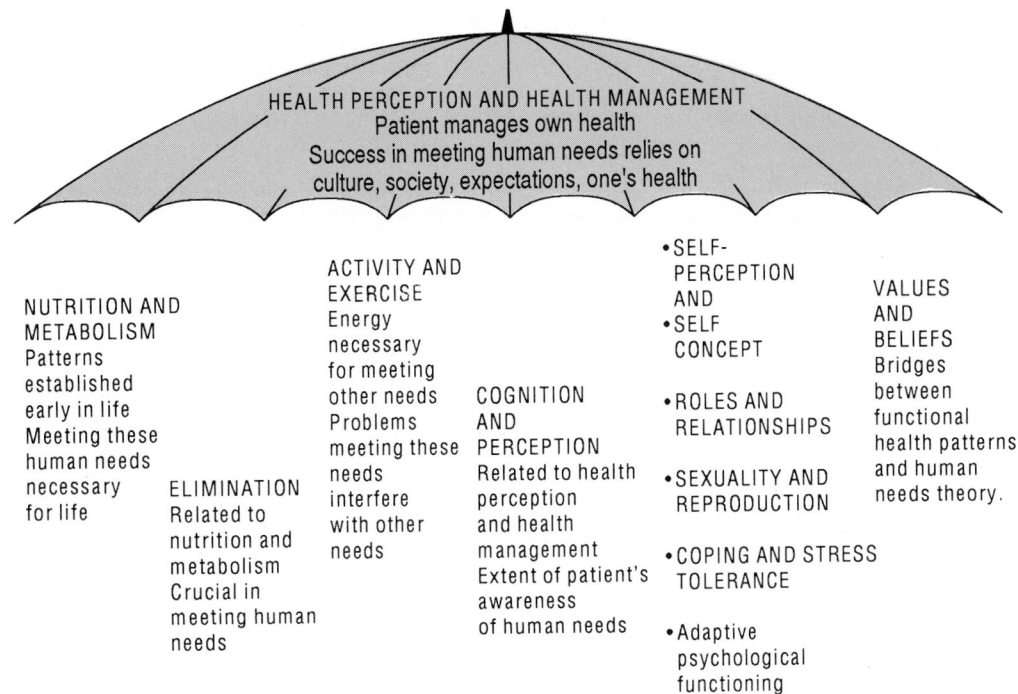

HEALTH PERCEPTION AND HEALTH MANAGEMENT
Patient manages own health
Success in meeting human needs relies on
culture, society, expectations, one's health

NUTRITION AND
METABOLISM
Patterns
established
early in life
Meeting these
human needs
necessary
for life

ELIMINATION
Related to
nutrition and
metabolism
Crucial in
meeting human
needs

ACTIVITY AND
EXERCISE
Energy
necessary
for meeting
other needs
Problems
meeting these
needs
interfere
with other
needs

COGNITION
AND
PERCEPTION
Related to health
perception
and health
management
Extent of patient's
awareness
of human needs

•SELF-
PERCEPTION
AND
•SELF
CONCEPT

•ROLES AND
RELATIONSHIPS

•SEXUALITY AND
REPRODUCTION

•COPING AND STRESS
TOLERANCE

•Adaptive
psychological
functioning

VALUES
AND
BELIEFS
Bridges
between
functional
health patterns
and human
needs theory.

Figure 12–2.   Relationship of functional health patterns, human needs theory, and delivery of nursing care. The first function, health perception and health management, forms an umbrella for the remaining 10.

throughout life. Infants, for example, spend a great deal of time sleeping; parents can reveal the amount of time and how the infant sleeps, thus showing a pattern. The person's environment may prove a help or hindrance with this category of needs. Assessment focuses on the role of the person, the family, and the environment.

The last six functions, *self-perception, self-concept, roles and relationship, sexuality, coping and stress tolerance,* and *values and beliefs,* involve a complex group of needs that are intimately related to the person's level of adaptive psychological functioning. Adequate examination of these patterns requires assessment of the patient's intrapsychic and interpersonal functioning, which means looking at the patient in relationship to himself or herself, the family, significant others, and the community.

Values and beliefs provide the bridge between functional health patterns and human needs theory. Understanding the patient's value and belief system is crucial: this information tells the nurse how important each human need is as a motivating factor in the patient's life, the life of his or her family, and the patient's life as a community member.

Key Concepts

■ A human need is any physiologic or psychological factor in life necessary for a healthy existence.
■ Human needs are a motivational force influenced by

culture, socioeconomic factors, personal values, and health status.
■ Maslow's theory of human needs presents a hierarchical ordering of human needs.
■ Physiologic needs include air, food, water, elimination, sleep and rest, temperature maintenance, and sex.
■ Safety needs include the freedom from fear and anxiety as well as from injury, pain, and death.
■ "Belongingness" and love needs involve developing attachments or relationships with others and seeking caring, friendship, love, and intimacy.
■ Esteem needs are of two types: esteem derived from others and self-esteem.
■ Self-actualization needs are met when the person attempts to develop his or her maximum potential.
■ Although all humans have the same basic needs, age and stage of development influence the priority of other needs.
■ Using functional health patterns is a holistic approach to nursing. Patterns delineate the human needs of the patient, family, and community.
■ Functional health patterns provide a comprehensive discussion of patient needs, while Maslow's hierarchy offers a rationale for determining the order in which a patient's needs could be addressed.

References

George, J. B. (Ed.). (1990). *Nursing theories: The base for professional nursing practice* (3rd ed.). Norwalk, CT: Appleton & Lange.

Gordon, M. (1987). *Nursing diagnosis, process and application* (2nd ed.). New York: McGraw-Hill.

Henderson, V. (1966). *The nature of nursing.* New York: Harper & Row.

King, Imogene M. (1981). *A theory of nursing.* New York: John Wiley & Sons.

Lederer, K. (Ed.). (1980). *Human needs.* Cambridge, MA: Oegleschlager, Gunn, & Horn.

Marriner-Tomey, A. (1989). *Nursing theorists and their work* (2nd ed.). Philadelphia: C. V. Mosby.

Maslow, A. H. (1970). *Motivation and personality* (2nd ed.). New York: Harper & Row.

McHale, J., & McHale, M. (1978). *Basic human needs: A framework for action.* New Brunswick, NJ: Transaction Books.

Montague, A. (1970). *The direction of human development.* New York: Hawthorn.

Mountcastle, V. B. (Ed.). (1980). *Medical physiology* (14th ed.). Vol. 2. St. Louis: C. V. Mosby.

Murray, H. A. (1938). *Explorations in personality.* New York: Oxford University Press.

Nightingale, F. (1946). *Notes on nursing.* Philadelphia: J. B. Lippincott. (Original work published 1860)

Orem, D. E. (1985). *Nursing: concepts of practice* (3rd ed.). New York: McGraw-Hill.

Orlando, I. J. (1961). *The dynamic nurse-patient relationship: Function, process and principles.* New York: Putnam.

Rogers, M. E. (1970). *An introduction to theoretical basis of nursing.* Philadelphia: Davis.

Turner, J. S., & Helm, D. B. (1987). *Lifespan development* (3rd ed.). San Francisco: Holt, Rinehart & Winston.

Vander, A. J., Sherman, J. H., & Luciano, D. S. (1985). *Human physiology: The mechanisms of body function.* San Francisco: McGraw-Hill.

Yura, H., & Walsh, M. (1988). *The nursing process: Assessing, planning, implementing and evaluating* (5th ed.). Norwalk, CT: Appleton & Lange.

Lifespan Development

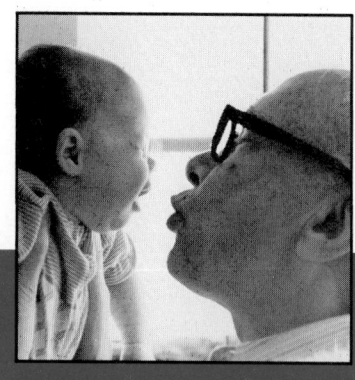

Lifespan Development

LEARNING OBJECTIVES

Upon completion of this chapter, the student will be able to do the following:

- Relate theories of development to health patterns exhibited across the lifespan.
- Identify the major health needs of specific developmental age groups.
- Describe the influence of development on health.
- Describe the influence of health status on development.

KEY TERMS

Development	Environment	Maturation
Developmental tasks	Fetus	Neonatal period
Embryo	Genetics	Perception
	Growth	Puberty

13

Genetics and Environment

Concepts of Development

  Principles of Growth and Development

  Growth and Development Theory

    Psychodynamic Theories

    Cognitive Development Theory

    Developmental Task Theory

    Human Needs Theory

    Moral Development Theory

Growth and Development Through the Lifespan

  Intrauterine Development

    Physical Development

    Cognitive Development

    Psychosocial Development

  Neonate (Birth to 1 Month)

    Physical Development

    Cognitive Development

    Psychosocial Development

  Infant (1 Month to 1 Year)

    Physical Development

    Cognitive Development

    Psychosocial Development

  Toddler (1 to 3 Years)

    Physical Development

    Cognitive Development

    Psychosocial Development

  Preschooler (3 to 6 Years)

    Physical Development

    Cognitive Development

    Psychosocial Development

  School-Age Child (6 to 11 Years)

    Physical Development

    Cognitive Development

    Psychosocial Development

  Adolescent (11 to 21 Years)

    Physical Development

    Cognitive Development

    Psychosocial Development

  Young Adult (21 to 40 Years)

    Physical Development

    Cognitive Development

    Psychosocial Development

  Middle Adult (40 to 60 Years)

    Physical Development

    Cognitive Development

    Psychosocial Development

  Older Adult (60 Years and Older)

    Physical Development

    Cognitive Development

    Psychosocial Development

Functional Health and Lifespan Development Related to Health Problems and Anticipatory Guidance

  Health Perception and Health Management

  Nutrition and Metabolism

  Elimination

  Activity and Exercise

  Cognition and Perception

  Sleep and Rest

  Self-Perception and Self-Concept

  Roles and Relationships

  Sexuality and Reproduction

  Coping and Stress Tolerance

  Values and Beliefs

Key Concepts

D evelopment is the process of ongoing change, reorganization, and integration occurring throughout life. This process includes changes in body structure and function as well as changes in psychosocial behaviors and cognition. As a result of development, a person's competence and capabilities increase so he or she can participate more fully in life.

Traditionally, development was seen as a characteristic of infancy and childhood with little attention given to development beyond the teen years, yet there is mounting evidence that predictable patterns of change occur throughout life. Researchers (Gilligan, 1982; Levinson, 1978) have delineated phases of adult development. In attempting to understand human behavior as it relates to health, lifespan development is a central and critical issue. When the word development is used in this chapter, "lifespan" is always an assumed qualifier.

GENETICS AND ENVIRONMENT

Two primary factors drive development—genetics and environment. **Genetics** involves the potential for human function determined by the inheritance of 46 single chromosomes carrying genetic information from each birth parent. The code contained in the chromosomes provides complete information governing the growth, differentiation, and function of all body cells. Our knowledge of the inheritance of physical characteristics, such as eye color, is substantial; less well understood is behavioral genetics or the extent to which behavior is also inherited. Because of the enormous numbers of possible combinations of inherited characteristics, each person possesses a unique genetic makeup, contributing to the wide variety of observed individual differences.

Environment defines the context in which the person exists, including both animate and inanimate surroundings (Bronfenbrenner, 1979). The animate environment comprises specific people (parents, siblings, spouses, partners, extended family, friends, classmates, workmates, and colleagues) and, more broadly, social and cultural groups. The inanimate environment describes all aspects of the physical surroundings. Sensory components of the physical environment include sound and light as well as motion. The inanimate environment at a broader level includes housing, transportation, resources, economics, and other ecologic factors. Although genetic makeup is stable over generations, surroundings change. Two important factors influencing individual development are history and cohort; that is, environment is decidedly different based on the year of birth and the experiences of the cohort or counterparts of people born at that time. In 1961, school children across the United States gathered in classrooms and gymnasiums to watch television coverage of Alan Shepherd, the first American astronaut to fly in space—quite a different experience from children in 1927 who learned from the newspaper or radio of Charles Lindbergh's flight to Europe.

Although the environment can be arbitrarily divided into components, the environment is experienced as a whole. **Perception,** a highly individual process, is the neurosensory process that allows the environment to be experienced by each person. Even when environments may appear to be similar, individual perceptions are different. Thus, two siblings who share the same family, home, school, and community have differing perceptions of their environments.

Development is the expression of genetic inheritance as it is modified by the environment. Genetic inheritance is fixed; that is, you can be only as good as the genes you

inherited. Although genetics may set the ceiling for human function, the environment serves to promote maximum potential or hinder development. For example, there has been long and continued debate regarding the inheritance of intelligence. Although evidence does support some basis for children's intelligence being related to parental intelligence, the environment of rearing is critical. An infant who is nurtured, talked with, responded to contingently, provided appropriate sensory stimuli, and assisted in regulating sleep and feeding patterns evidences higher intelligence than an infant who does not receive such early experiences.

Although people are different, the changes in body structure and function, psychosocial behaviors, and cognition show similar characteristics when described in similar age groups. Development occurs as a pattern, that is, certain predictable processes follow a time course (e.g., puberty occurs in the early teenage years). Patterns provide a way of describing the commonalities of development while preserving the consideration of individual differences. By understanding patterns of development with change, reorganization, and integration, we can better understand individual behavior at a point in the lifespan.

Change. Development starts with conception and continues through death. Development, although ongoing, is not consistent across time nor is it a simple linear process. The school-age child's ability to determine that a set volume of liquid is the same, regardless of the shape of the container does not demonstrate a gradual change. Neither does development peak at 18 years of age and plateau until old age. Development includes periods of both relative stability and change. Infancy and adolescence are short in duration but are known for rapid changes in a multitude of functions including growth, coordination, and cognitive skills.

Although all aspects of the human function change with development, not all changes occur on the same time schedule. Body development and social development are not entirely synchronized. The social behaviors of the adolescent may indicate an increasing interest in sexuality, although there may be little change in endocrine activity or physical evidence of puberty. A 3-month-old infant may focus intently on a toy and attempt to reach the toy using a batting motion of the arms. The desire to handle the toy is spurred by cognitive development; however, the infant's motor development has not progressed to the level of obtaining the toy.

Reorganization and Integration. Development is not only a process of continual change, but also one of reorganization and integration with behavior becoming more complex and sophisticated. For example, the problem-solving abilities of the adult and child are different. The adult brings to the problem-solving situation an appreciation of cause–effect relationships, the ability to determine consequences of actions, the ability to see the problem from multiple perspectives, and past experiences. The child's problem-solving abilities are determined by cognitive development and, therefore, the child's perception of how the world operates.

CONCEPTS OF DEVELOPMENT

Principles of Growth and Development

Growth and development knowledge is drawn from biologic and psychosocial sciences and involves certain principles that generally affect all people. These principles, as listed in the display, express commonalities of the process of growth and development.

Growth and Development Theory

Theories of development describe why development occurs as it does and what factors shape developmental outcomes.

Theories tend to fall into groupings based on the theoretical perspectives of the theory development.

Psychodynamic theories are based on the perspective that humans are essentially emotional, responding to instinctive drives without rationality. By studying childhood events, psychodynamic theorists attempt to explain human behavior throughout the lifespan. Freud and Erikson are two well-known psychodynamic theorists, although Freud's perspectives are currently controversial.

Piaget has conducted considerable research on *cognitive development theory,* which deals with perception and thinking, focusing on intellectual processes at each stage of development. Intellectual growth involves changes in the mental operations of the person at various ages. Children at the various ages respond to cognitive tasks in comparable ways according to this theory.

Other theories include the *developmental task theory* (Havighurst), *human needs theory* (Maslow), and *moral development theory* (Kohlberg). These theorists propose that there are specified tasks, needs, or stages of moral development that the child or person must meet or complete to continue to develop and mature.

Principles of Growth and Development

Principle 1: The process of growth and development is continuous and systematic following a purposeful sequence. The development of a child is orderly with maturational milestones occurring at predictable points in time. The sequence of growth and development tends to be from head to toe (cephalocaudal), proximal to distal, and symmetric.

Principle 2: The process of growth and development is ongoing and complex. The most active time for growth and development is during the childhood and adolescent years, but they continue through the lifespan. Intellectual development and physical changes occur throughout life.

Principle 3: The process of growth and development is distinctive and predetermined and occurs at a discrete rate for each person. Every person has a unique genetic program inherited from biologic parents. That genetic program determines the growth and developmpent process for that person and the rate at which it occurs.

Principle 4: The process of growth and development has both quantitative and qualitative aspects. While the person is increasing in size and general motor ability (quantitative), he or she is also increasing in skills in expression and in personality (qualitative).

Principle 5: The process of growth and development requires experience and practice as well as energy. Learning each developmental skill or task demands repetition and practice and that, in turn, requires energy.

Principle 6: The process of growth and development occurs through adaptation to the conflict of equilibrium versus disequilibrium. The whole process of maturing is an adaptation to stages of disequilibrium balanced by stages of equilibrium. Change occurs in response to conflict, and the conflict of different stages of development is the initiating force in maturation.

Principle 7: The process of growth and development produces individuality from interaction of genetic heredity and environment. One's inherited genetic program is influenced by the catalyst of environment that helps shape development and maturation. The influences of culture, family, friends, religion, and community shape values, morals, mores, and behavior.

Principle 8: The outcome of growth and development is the attainment of personal potential. The goal of maturation is the achievement of a person's greatest potential, or self-realization. A positive outcome of the developmental process indicates that the person has achieved personal integrity or self-actualization.

Selected developmental theories are summarized in Table 13-1.

Psychodynamic Theories

Freud. The work of Freud characterizes psychosexual development across the lifespan, encompassing the oral, anal, phallic, latency, and genital phases. Freud's view of the mind included the *id* (concerned with self-gratification), the *ego* (the mediator between the id and reality), and the *superego* (the conscience). Freud theorized that all people pass through the five phases, confronting and resolving conflicts of the id–ego–superego in the process. If the person does not resolve these conflicts, movement through succeeding stages may not be successful.

Erikson. Although based on Freud's theory, Erikson's theory of development encompassed social and cultural influences as well. He was the first theorist who recognized that development is a lifelong process. The eight stages of his theory progress from birth to death and are presented as developmental crises (e.g., trust versus mistrust), which must be mastered before proceeding to the next stage.

TABLE 13–1

Overview of Selected Developmental Theories

Theorist	Stages/Tasks	Characteristics
Sigmund Freud	Oral—birth to 1 year	Seeking pleasure through oral gratification
	Anal—2 to 3 years	Delayed gratification through controlling anal sphincter
	Phallic—4 to 5 years	Curiosity regarding genitals and gender differences
	Latent—6 to 12 years	Transition; peer relationships and identification with parent of same sex
	Genital—13 to death	Sexual interest and maturation
Erik Erikson	Trust vs. mistrust—Birth to 1 year	Development of trust (or mistrust) in parents
	Autonomy vs. shame—2 to 4 years	Gaining independence through parents' encouraging
	Initiative vs. guilt—4 to 6 years	Developing confidence in abilities
	Indusry vs. inferiority—8 to 12 years	Pleasure from accomplishments
	Identity vs. role confusion—13 to 20 years	Achieving stable sense of identity
	Intimacy vs. isolation—20 to 30 years	Developing close personal relationships
	Generativity vs. stagnation—30 to 60 years	Creativity, productivity in work
	Integrity vs. despair—> 60 years	Attainment of purpose, fulfillment
Jean Piaget	Sensorimotor—Birth to 2 years, 6 substages	Development of senses, motor activity
	Preoperational—2 to 7 years, 2 subtages	Beginning intellectual ability
	Concrete operations—7 to 11 years	Reasoning, organizing, relationships
	Formal operations—11 to death	Abstract thinking, deductive reasoning
Robert Havighurst	Infancy, early childhood	Learning neuromuscular control
	Middle childhood	Developing physical, intellectual, emotional skills
	Adolescence	Achieving gender roles, independence
	Early adulthood	Marriage, family, career
	Middle age	Assisting grown children, parents; social, civic responsibility
	Later maturity	Retirement, declining physical ability, loss of relationships
Abraham Maslow	Physiologic	Hierarchic human needs; lower order needs must be fulfilled to achieve higher order needs
	Safety	
	Love and belongingness	
	Esteem	
	Self-actualization	
Lawrence Kohlberg	Premoral (perconventional)	Development of moral reasoning: governed by egocentricity
	Obedience, punishment	
	Hedonistic	
	Conventional morality	Concrete thinking; follows orders and requests for approval
	Approval seeking	
	Respect for authority	
	Postconventional morality	Autonomous decision-making regarding moral issues
	Democratic contractual morality	
	Principles of conscience morality	

Cognitive Development Theory

Piaget. Piaget's theory of cognitive development is based on the assumption that human nature is essentially rational and that the person's basic goal is to learn to master the environment. The resulting satisfaction received from learning prompts the person's curiosity, problem-solving, imitation, practice, and play activities (Piaget, 1952). Two functions that assist the person in learning and intellectual growth are organization and adaptation. *Organization* involves the rearranging and structuring of one's knowledge and thoughts. *Adaptation* relates to the process of assimilating and accommodating new information. To integrate new learning with old and adapt it to expanding environments, the infant uses the complementary processes of assimilation and accommodation. *Assimilation* is the ongoing process of organizing new information into existing knowledge. *Accommodation* is the process of resolving the disequilibrium resulting from the modifications needed in thought processes to incorporate new data. The four cognitive development stages identified by Piaget include sensorimotor, preoperational, concrete operations, and formal operations.

Developmental Task Theory

Havighurst. Havighurst's theory of development is based on learning and learned behaviors, called **developmental tasks,** that emanate from biologic, psychological, and social origins during the lifespan. Specific developmental tasks are assigned to the various stages of life. Failure to complete the tasks assigned to each stage may lead to failure in tasks in subsequent stages. According to this theory, success in achieving the developmental tasks leads to success with tasks in later stages of life (Havighurst, 1972).

Human Needs Theory

Maslow. Abraham Maslow is one of the better known humanistic theorists. Humanistic theories (also called phenomenologic theories) propose that people are basically good when born and attempt to become all they are capable of becoming throughout their lives. People vary in their experiences, and have a free will and ability to grow and become what they self-determine. As a consequence, people should not be categorized into stages or levels of development.

Maslow organized human needs into a hierarchic framework with a base of physiologic needs and an apex of self-actualization (see Table 13-1). To reach the apex of the hierarchy, a person must have each of the preceding levels of needs met beginning with physiologic needs and moving up toward self-actualization. Because of its positive approach, Maslow's theory is a basis of holistic health through illness prevention and individual responsibility for health (Freiberg, 1987).

Moral Development Theory

Kohlberg. Lawrence Kohlberg amplified the work of Piaget by studying the development of moral judgment and reasoning. Moral development has been described as occurring in three phases (Kohlberg, 1976). Themes in moral development include external versus internal controls; the role of authority and relationship with authority figures; the influence of punishment and rewards; and the sense of right and wrong. Moral development is not strictly age-based; differences in development reflect the rationale for behavior rather than the behavior itself. Moral development moves from the egocentric approach to right and wrong of infancy to autonomous social consciousness regarding moral issues. Kohlberg's stages of development parallel those of Piaget's theory.

GROWTH AND DEVELOPMENT THROUGH THE LIFESPAN

Normal growth and development are orderly, predictable processes in the human experience (Table 13-2), yet each person progresses and develops at an individual pace. For example, in the child, there is a time range during which developmental phases are expected to occur (e.g., walking, talking). If a child progresses through a stage outside of the usual time range, there may be no significant effect on overall development, or it may affect the ability to move on to or complete subsequent phases of development.

Intrauterine Development

Life begins and growth and development are initiated at the moment of conception. During the 9 months of the intrauterine stage, development moves from the single cell of the fertilized ovum to a complete human being at the time of birth. Cognitive and psychosocial development begins during intrauterine development, setting the stage for further development after birth.

Physical Development

The period of intrauterine gestation is divided into three stages or trimesters. The first trimester begins with the fertilization of the ovum by the sperm and unites the two sets of chromosomes, creating the genetic program of the new organism. From this program, the genetically produced characteristics, such as eye and hair color are passed on to the child. During each of the trimesters, the fetus experiences different types of development.

First Trimester. The first trimester, the developmental period, produces all the organ systems, and the **embryo** (the stage of development between the 2nd and 8th weeks) continues to develop rapidly. By the 8th week,

(*Text continues on page 204*)

TABLE 13–2

Physical and Psychosocial Development through the Lifespan

Stage	Physical	Psychosocial
Neonate (birth to 1 month)	Reflexive physical functioning	Parents and infants develop deep attachment normally.
	Major organ systems are stabilizing.	Interactions during routine care enhance or detract from attachment process.
	Heart rate decreases from 130–160 to 120–140.	Infant's waking hours include feedings and short play periods.
	Systole and diastole shorten in length.	Attachment may be altered if either parent or child experiences health problems after birth.
	Respiratory movements are primarily abdominal (30–50/min).	
	Fontanelle is palpable between unfused skull bones.	
	Behavior—crying, sucking, sleeping, and activity	
	Sporadic, symmetric movements in all four extremities	
	Smiles reflexively	
	Responds to sensory stimuli (particularly caregiver's voice, face and touch)	
	Reflex—blinks in response to light, and startles to loud sudden noise, Babinski's, Landau, Moro, palmar grasp, placing, rooting, neck righting	
Infant (1 month to 1 year)	Doubles birthweight by 6 months and triples it at 12 months	Differentiates self from others (external world)
	Grows 10 to 12 in	Smiles responsively.
	Walks on hands and feet like a bear	Deals with environment through emergence of trust
	Walks—one hand held	Sensory and cognitive abilities improve; recognizes differences in people
	Reaches for objects	Establishes close attachment with caregiver
	Sucks/mouths objects	Plays simple social games (peek-a-boo)
	Progresses from holding head up to sitting alone, crawling, pulling to stand, cruising	More meaningful interaction with environment
	Throws objects to floor	
	Patterns of body function stabilize—predictable sleep, elimination, and feeding routines	
	Fine motor prehension (cortically controlled individual movements of fingers and thumbs); also uses both hands simultaneously	
Toddler (1–3 years)	Rate of increase in height and weight slows (smaller food intake)	Child develops autonomy. Explores immediate environment.
	Heart rate slows to 110 beats, respiration to 24 beats/min	Needs emotional support and encouragement from parents
	Cardiopulmonary system stabilizes—110/60 blood pressure	Parent is most significant person in toddler's life.
	Walks upright with broad gait	Parallel plays with others
	Gross motor skills advance—walking up and down stairs, kicks a ball, jumps and stands on one foot, rides a tricycle, runs	Learns to control one's possessions and oneself
	Fine motor—scribbles spontaneously; draws circles, crosses, stick people; stacks a tower of small blocks	Extremely active and unable to set limits on own behavior. Parents must set limits.
	Handedness appears around 19 months.	Parents must create safe environment for exploratory behavior (automobile safety, poisoning).
	Toilet training—develops sphincter control	
	Able to undress	
Preschool (3–6 years)	Heart (90 beats/min) and respiratory rates (24 beats/min) continue to stabilize.	Relies heavily on parents/primary caregivers for security
	Weight increases 5 lb/year. Average (by age 5) is 45 lb.	Ventures out to seek contact with children and adults
	Height increases 2 in/year. Average (by age 5) is 42 in.	Asks questions

(continued)

TABLE 13-2

(continued)

Stage	Physical	Psychosocial
	Large and fine muscle coordination improves. Runs well, climbs stairs with ease, hops, skips, jumps, throws and catches a ball Fine motor—copies circles, squares, and triangles; begins printing letters and numbers	Is less afraid of strangers
School age (6–11 years)	Height increases 1–2 in/year. Variable weight increases (averages 3–6 lb/year). Cardiovascular functioning refines: heart rate = 65–90 beats/min, blood pressure = 110/70 mm Hg, and respiratory rate = 16–18 beats/min. Until age 9, boys are 1–2 in taller and 2 lb heavier than girls. Girls begin rapid growth period (9–12 years). At age 12, girls are 2 lb heavier and 1 in taller than boys. Prepubertal physical changes and growth spurts can occur between the ages of 9 and 14 for girls, 12 and 16 for boys. Steady skeletal growth in trunk and extremities. Minimal secondary sex characteristics are present. Strength doubles Majority of permanent teeth have erupted. Refined neuromuscular functioning—good body balance, rides bicycle, engages in team sports, climbs trees; eye–hand coordination improves (punts, writes in script, paints, detailed drawing, plays computer games)	Develops a sense of achievement Psychosocial development is influenced by physical and cognitive skil development. Is independent in ADLs Possesses need to maintain control Develops strong preferences (food, clothes) Engages in group-oriented play Prefers same sex peers Regards rules as necessary Considers motivation and behavior when making judgments
Adolescence (11–21 years)	Sexual maturation with development of primary and secondary characteristics Increased growth rate of skeleton, muscle, and viscera	Establishes independence from family; close peer relationships Makes major decisions about life and vocation Refines adult cognitive skills Establishes moral code Establishes own identity Adjusts to own sexuality Establishes unique identity (personal and group) Develops moral judgment
Young and middle adulthood (21–65 years)	Physical structure stabilizes and few changes are noted (except for pregnancy). Young adults—quite active, experience less severe illnesses and tend to ignore physical symptoms when ill Health concerns and risk factors center around lifestyle, family history, and community. Middle adults—the aging process varies for all individuals; decreases appear in hormone levels, basal metabolic rate, respiratory, cardiovascular and circulatory functioning.	Emotional health is related to one's ability to resolve personal and social tasks (family, job stresses). 23 to 28 years—refines self-perception and intimacy 29 to 34 years—energy is put toward achievement in world 35 to 43 years—examines life goals and relationships Decides between singlehood and marriage Decides on family, parenthood Develops sense of generativity Makes lasting contributions though involvement with others
Late adult (65–77 years)	All systems are affected by the aging process: reproductive, urinary, neurologic, musculoskeletal, respiratory, head and neck, breasts, skin, and nails. Effects vary with the person's lifestyle, genetic predisposition, and freedom from disease.	Puts life in order Recognizes sense of integrity and wisdom Learns to accept life accomplishments, retirement, death

the embryo possesses a face, legs, arms, brain, heartbeat, and a productive digestive system and liver (red blood cell production). When the first bone cells appear in the upper arms, the embryo becomes a **fetus** (child in utero from 3rd month of gestation to birth). The fetus is approximately 3 inches long and weighs 1 oz. The critical development of organ systems during this trimester renders the embryo susceptible to developmental or environmental influences that may cause malformations.

Second Trimester. Fetal movement is felt by the mother during the second trimester. During this growth period lanugo (downy hair) develops on the fetus' arms, legs, and back. Head hair, eyelashes, eyebrows, fingernails, and toenails appear. Skeletal ossification continues. The skin is red and wrinkled. The fetus is nonviable at this point and cannot survive out of the uterine environment. Toward the 20th week, fetal growth slows and the lower limbs are fully formed. The fetus is 11 to 14 inches long and weighs 1 lb, 4 oz.

Third Trimester. During the last trimester, fetal features are refined. The hair on the head grows, fingernails grow, and lanugo almost disappears. Teeth buds for permanent teeth appear behind milk teeth buds. The fetus responds to bright lights and internal and external sounds. As the fetus increases in growth, his or her activity may diminish because space becomes less available. Arms and legs increase in flexion during the third trimester; early in the third trimester the fetus is extended. The head remains large in comparison to the body. Arms and legs are in flexed position. The lungs mature. Chances for survival improve with the advent of the delivery date. The baby receives short-term immunity from the mother; antibodies pass through the placenta.

Cognitive Development

During the last trimester, the fetus responds to internal and external sounds. Fetal activity represents a form of mother–baby communication fostering bonding. At birth the neonate is capable of differentiating the voice of the mother. Is this caused by maternal familiarity? Mothers report infants appear to prefer music heard while previously in utero. Maternal stress and neonatal stressors are known to affect development adversely. A mother's emotional state influences fetal motility and hyperactivity later in the neonatal period. Research shows that periods of diminished oxygen and severe, long-term malnutrition prenatally adversely affect later cognitive functioning (Schuster & Ashburn, 1986).

Psychosocial Development

It has not yet been determined if events occurring during intrauterine life affect the psychosocial development of the fetus. The current methods rule out objective study of psychological interactions between fetus and mother. It appears that prebirth events do help to mold cognitive, language, or affective development (Schuster & Ashburn, 1986). A fetus' activity ranges from constant movement to alternating periods of calm and peak activity to quiet. Because the mother's emotional state influences the fetus' biochemical environment, any stressor plays a significant role in the psychosocial development in utero.

Neonate (Birth to 1 Month)

Physical Development

During the **neonatal period** (from birth to 6 weeks), the baby depends on others to have all his or her physiologic and emotional needs met. The baby's day and family life must be recorded. The baby must learn new ways of intaking food, oxygen, and also of elimination. All arm, leg, and hand movements are reflexive. The baby thrusts extremities in play. Although he cannot support his head while lying on his abdomen, he is able to lift his head briefly. When pulled to a sitting position, he may hold his head in line with his back. The baby is capable of rolling part way to side from back. The month-old baby generally keeps his or her hands fisted or slightly open. If fingers are pried, the baby is able to grasp the handle of a spoon or rattle briefly. He stares at objects, coordinating his eyes; however, he does not reach for objects.

Cognitive Development

Piaget's first period of cognitive development, the sensorimotor stage, begins with the coordination of such activities as grasping objects and basic reflexes. Although historically neonates were thought to exhibit reflexive behavior only, current knowledge reveals that, even at birth, neonates are capable of a wide range of behaviors, particularly the ability to provide cues to parents and caregivers regarding interactional needs. The cerebral cortex has not fully developed.

Psychosocial Development

The infant responds positively to comfort and satisfaction and negatively to pain. The baby smiles back at a face or voice. The mother or primary caregiver is often able to comfort the baby when making direct eye contact. Attachment or bonding develops at this time (Fig. 13-1).

Infant (1 Month to 1 Year)

Physical Development

The infant progresses physically in a sequential pattern. There may be slight discrepancies with each baby. Voluntary motor skills begin to replace reflexive behavior

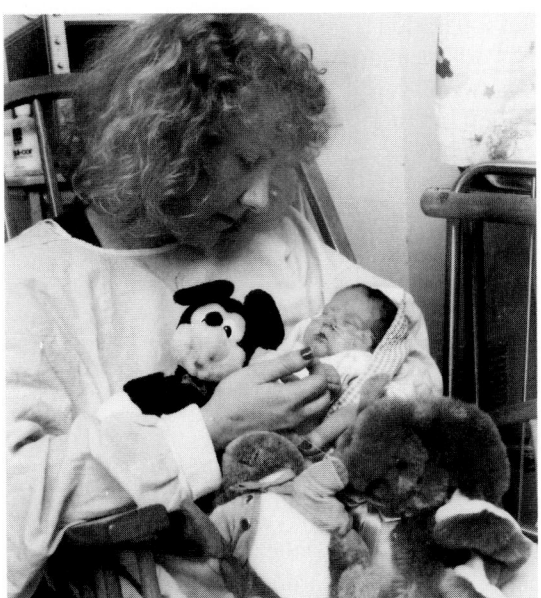

Figure 13–1. Attachment formation between mother and child is an important task in early infancy. (Photo courtesy of the University of Washington School of Nursing.)

(Schuster & Ashburn, 1986). Weight and height increase at rates faster than during any other period. Visual acuity also develops, rapidly facilitating eye–hand coordination (Brazelton, 1979). The infant begins by holding his head up for brief periods of time and advances to supported sitting, independent sitting, creeping, standing with support, and walking while holding on to objects. A pincer grasp (picking up objects) replaces the whole-hand carry. The infant gains increasing efficiency in energy expenditure while increasing the speed and accuracy of movement.

Cognitive Development

He engages in systematic imitative behavior. He also babbles as actions become goal-oriented. The infant is able to solve simple problems by using previously mastered activities or actions. He attaches meanings to words. He utters a few words. When an infant discovers a pleasurable activity, he repeats this behavior. Through manipulation of objects and motor activities, the infant differentiates self and environment. Infants are fascinated with their own extremities. The infant achieves personal satisfaction from the ability to direct or control objects. Play remains an important component in self-concept development. Sensory impressions and motor activities provide the groundwork for the infant's knowledge of the world. He is capable of coordinating one action with another. The "power of association" (Turner & Helms, 1987) assists the infant in understanding a cause–effect relationship. The concept of object permanence develops.

Psychosocial Development

The infant's primary gratification is in sucking and having needs met by the caregiver. Social responsiveness is evident later on as he or she smiles in response to a familiar face. Laughing indicates pleasure as the infant shows preferential treatment or response to caregiver. The infant shows fear of strangers or separation from his parent (Freiberg, 1987). Many theorists consider attachment to be a lifelong process. The infant begins to explore the environment while separating briefly from parents. He or she is capable of making simple needs known by gestures or holophases. The infant enjoys simple games, toys, water and sand play, books and nursery rhymes.

Toddler (1 to 3 Years)

Physical Development

The anterior fontanelle closes between 12 and 18 months of age. The toddler possesses a large head, a long trunk, and short stubby legs. Weak abdominal muscles account for a "pot-bellied" look. Baby fat is present. During the second year, the growth of legs and arms increases. In comparison to the first 12 months of life, the toddler's growth is less accelerated. Height and weight slow down. The toddler gains 5 lb per year and grows 3 to 5 inches. Nutritional needs are met by solid foods. Central nervous system, musculoskeletal, cardiopulmonary, and gastrointestinal systems continue to develop. Gross motor skills rapidly develop; he kicks a ball, jumps, walks stairs, rides a tricycle, and runs. Fine motor abilities progress from stacking a tower of blocks to drawing stick people.

Cognitive Development

The toddler has definite ideas about how his world should operate, often expressing individual preferences. At the age of one and a half years, the toddler responds negatively to requests. "No" is a favorite reply. Self-identity and competency are reflected in common phrases such as "mine" and "I do it." The egocentricity characteristic of this age contributes to sense of self. The child sees the world from his perspective. He becomes aware of the approval or disapproval of others. Fear, an emotional response to threat of self, is expressed (Dixon & Stein, 1987). The toddler develops a perception of who he is. The toddler learns to use upper muscles of the arms and legs before finger or toe muscles. He progresses to manipulate objects and explore his environment. Piaget's sensorimotor period extends from birth to approximately 2 years. Concepts mastered include object permanence, causality, spatial relationships, and the use of instruments (Hill & Humphrey, 1982). At 2 years, the toddler is impulsive, rigid, domineering, demanding, and energetic. The older toddler becomes more cooperative. He advances to the preoperational stage (2 to 6 years) in which the child assigns meaning or identity to an object governed by his own perceptions. Internal and external reality are one. The toddler's speech progresses from simple words, short sentences, to talking continually by 3 years. The toddler questions everything and is capable of following simple commands.

Psychosocial Development

The role of the toddler expands to include peers or playmates. In becoming autonomous, he sees himself as distinct, although emotionally attached to parents. Toddlers' play is often parallel (side by side). The toddler begins to learn socially responsible behaviors. He learns basic social skills, which contribute to these interactions. Sensory capabilities are the focal point for interaction.

Preschooler (3 to 6 Years)

Physical Development

Physical changes occur at a slow, even, and continuous pace. Development proceeds from cephalocaudal (head to toe) and proximal-distal direction. The 5-year-old child's head circumference is 50 cm (90% of adult size), whereas leg circumference is 22.5 cm (only 45% of adult size). By age 5, the child weighs 39 lb and is 40 inches tall. Arms and legs grow faster; trunk growth follows later. By the age of 5, the pot-bellied appearance of the toddler is that of a miniature adult. Neuromuscular skills refine. He dresses himself, washes his face and hands, brushes his teeth, and takes care of his own toilet needs.

Cognitive Development

Piaget's preoperational stage allows the preschooler to use mental symbols; thinking can include past or future events or events happening elsewhere in the present. Preconceptual thinking (based on concrete perceptions) progresses to intuitive (internally representing events). Questions from the preschooler begin; ''why'' progresses to ''where'' and ''how.'' He asks meaning of words, talks constantly, counts, identifies coins, knows the day of the week, follows three-step direction in order, and memorizes his address. Magical thinking occurs in which the preschooler believes his thinking influences the outside world.

Psychosocial Development

Play is critical for early development (Bellack & Fleming, 1985). The play style of preschoolers is termed associative. Children play together, demonstrating preferences for friends, and sharing materials or objects. There is little organization or goal-oriented behavior. The securely attached preschool child easily tolerates limited separation from parents while enjoying the company of other children. This is a period of rapid fluctuations between dependence and independence, competence and ineptitude, maturity and infantilism, and growing affection and antisocial destructiveness. As the child strives for individuality, he questions and explores his own abilities (Turner & Helms, 1987). His increasing language, motor, and cognitive skills facilitate this process. He learns to express emotions acceptably along with developing a conscience for moral development and control of his actions.

School-Age Child (6 to 11 Years)

Physical Development

The school-age child is taller and thinner than the preschooler. Steady growth occurs; height increases 2 to 3 inches per year, and weight increases 3 to 6 lb. Baby fat decreases and muscle mass increases. The child's body is forming new bony tissue constantly as bones lengthen and harden. Proportions continue to be more adultlike. Lordosis of early childhood has disappeared. Facial proportions change (forehead broadens, nose grows larger, lips get fuller, jaw juts out). They engage in large muscle activities—walking, running, skating, swimming, riding skateboards and horses, and team sports. Small muscle activities include sewing, printing and script writing, painting, clay modeling, and model building.

Cognitive Development

During middle childhood, tremendous growth in the ability to use words occurs. Vocabulary increases, and the school-age child uses rules of grammar and syntax. The cognitive operation of concrete thinking is mastered. These children use more logic in their thinking (Piaget, 1952). However, logic is limited to the here and now. Comprehension of cause–effect relationships increases, and the concept of time is better understood. Becoming less egocentric, the school-age child begins to appreciate another's perspective. He or she recognizes that physical properties of objects remain the same despite changes in shape. The school-age child demonstrates a public and private self.

Psychosocial Development

The family and the school are major socializers affecting the school-age child's developing personality and self-image. He enjoys brief separation from family (overnight). Play is cooperative; he plays in groups with fixed rules and goals. Friendships are an important part of social contacts, usually with children of the same sex. Rivalry for friends is often evident. Friends are chosen largely by similarity. Although relationships are quickly formed and dissolved, they may be intense. The school-aged child observes and imitates the attitudes, values, and behaviors of those significant people in his environment. In this age of industry (Erikson, 1963), the child is determined to master tasks, becoming a competent member of his culture. Cooperative work is valued.

Adolescent (11 to 21 Years)

Physical Development

The early years of adolescence are ones of rapid growth. This period begins with **puberty,** a maturation of the sex organs and reproductive functions along with the appearance of secondary sex characteristics. Girls begin adolescence at approximately 10 to 11 years of age, whereas boys enter at 11 to 12 years (Hill & Humphrey, 1982). The end of adolescence varies. Skeletal growth, dependent on the secretion of growth hormones regulated by the pituitary and thyroid glands, occurs through a combination of lengthening of the bones and changes in the ossification centers. Girls (11 to 13 years) achieve a growth spurt 2 years earlier than boys and plateau in height by 17 years of age. Although girls are initially taller than boys, boys grow rapidly between the ages of 14 to 21. They then surpass girls in height. Weight gain follows a similar pattern for both sexes. One's body image and concept of self depend on these physiologic changes. Chronologic age does not always coincide with these changes. One may see a 4-year spread in sexual development among adolescents. These variations become a developmental crisis for some young people. Concern over body normalcy, sports competition, and social and peer relationships can create major hurdles. Late adolescence (18 to 22 or 25 years) is often categorized as a period of transition to adulthood.

Cognitive Development

Formal thinking begins to emerge around 12 years of age (Piaget). This level is characterized by ability to think abstractly. Ideas can be expressed conceptually. The thinking of this age group reflects formal logic. Formal thinking allows seeing a situation from multiple perspectives. It is not entirely related to chronologic age, and its acquisition may vary with the person. Adolescents engage in introspection, self-examination, and personal critique. The changing body of the adolescent challenges the sense of identity as physical maturation and sexuality are integrated into self-image. The adolescent tries to establish a personal identity. This process occurs within the context of peers.

Psychosocial Development

The psychosocial development of the adolescent is characterized by an identity search and self-discovery. Piaget refers to this stage as adolescent egocentrism, in which adolescents do not distinguish between their own conceptualizations and those of the rest of society (Frieberg, 1987). Instability and emotional upheaval characterize early adolescence (11 to 13 years). Increasing independence from parents and family is coupled with increasing time spent with members of peer group, creating changes that may cause tension between the adolescent and family. He or she develops a personal value system. Peer contacts and being a part of a group are important. Roles and relationships take on abstract meaning cognitively. Initial experience with dating and early intimate relationships occur in adolescence. First forays into the working world are often attempted. The adolescent develop a more mature morality based on his or her own judgment. Late adolescents (17 to 20 years) develop a smoother relationship with their parents. Physical growth slows, allowing the person to adapt to a new body image. He or she refines interpersonal skills and gains mastery over drives and emotions as he prepares to enter the world of the adult. Drug abuse, alcoholism, and cigarette smoking present challenges the adolescent must conquer.

Young Adult (21 to 40 years)

Physical Development

The young adult's physical structure stabilizes. Maturational development is complete at this time with most systems operating at peak efficiency. However, weight and muscle mass may change due to the environmental influence of diet and exercise. Dental maturity is evident in the mid 20s. Hearing and vision, in the absence of deficits for other reasons, are generally normal and functionally acute. Sexuality is fully mature, and function is at a peak. Physiologic changes related to reproduction are considered normal physiologic development for the procreation of the children.

Cognitive Development

During the 20s, cognitive functioning reaches a peak. In some groups the need to achieve intellectually is strong. The young adult is creative, has effective problem-solving abilities, is realistic, and is less egocentric. Formal educational opportunities along with apprenticeship-type education are common.

Psychosocial Development

Young adulthood (from 18 to 22 or 25 years) is a period of transition from childhood to adulthood. The careers of adulthood emerge: work, intimacy, and parenting. An adult assumes a multitude of roles: citizen, taxpayer, homeowner. Social support is important because role conflict often arises. One must juggle the many hats of parent, grandparent, husband, wife, brother, sister, daughter, friend, and worker while prioritizing to achieve success and happiness.

Middle Adult (40 to 60 years)

Physical Development

The middle adult years are a time of transition from the active, building years of young adulthood and the later years of older adulthood. Physiologically, adults in their middle years begin to slow down. Body tissue tends to redistribute with increased thickening noticed around the middle portion of the trunk. The earliest signs of aging begin to show. Hair starts to gray, wrinkles begin to show, men may begin to lose hair, and visual acuity for near vision begins to diminish (presbyopia). Decreased function in other body systems is evidenced as beginning loss of muscle strength and agility, decreased cardiac output, decreasing hormone production, and increased fatigue.

The physical changes of the middle years occur gradually and insidiously and do not interfere with the person's vitality or function in life. In the absence of disease or disabilities, the ability to function physically is unaffected. A lifestyle emphasizing adequate diet, regular exercise, control of stress, and limiting or eliminating unhealthful habits (e.g., no smoking, moderate alcohol intake) contributes to successful life in the middle years.

Cognitive Development

Adults in their middle years continue to be interested in learning and show no decrease in ability to learn. Education is particularly motivating if the knowledge is relevant and personally applicable. Although the ability to perform may remain unchanged, a reduction in speed of problem-solving or motor skills may interfere with some aspects of functioning (e.g., eye–hand coordination is not as keen as before, leading to a slower reaction time).

Psychosocial Development

During the middle years, changes in roles occur. Children may be grown and have left home, although in recent years many parents have delayed having children until they are well into their thirties or forties. If married, the marriage may be stressed or strengthened by these changes. At this time of life, people may be faced with providing support to children who may not be totally independent, and at the same time have elderly parents who may require care. Women in particular may feel the burden of both responsibilities. Illness or death of parents often brings grief and lifestyle disruption.

The middle-aged person often views himself or herself more favorably with more time for social and leisure activities. A greater commitment to enjoying relationships may exist. Interpersonal impoverishment or stagnation may develop if the mature adult does not develop generativity (Erikson, 1963). One accomplishes this by possessing a genuine concern for oneself, one's children, community, peers, and society. Inability to accept the physical changes and psychosocial challenges of this time may foster depression and low self-esteem.

Older Adult (60 Years and Older)

Physical Development

Growth and maturation occur during late life with the physical changes accompanying old age appearing at different times and manifesting themselves in different ways. All physiologic systems decline in overall function and efficiency. Chronologic age alone is not a predictor of physical decline, however. Genetic influence, lifestyle factors, and self-concept combine in determining aging.

Stamina and strength may decrease. Basal metabolic rate decreases, and the gastrointestinal system has decreased digestive juices, less tone, and slower peristalsis. The older person often finds it difficult to adapt to changing temperatures because there is a decrease in subcutaneous fat, diminished circulation to the skin, and a decrease in core body temperature. Age-related changes in the function of the heart, circulatory, and respiratory systems contribute to diminished output of left ventricle, less anaerobic support to muscles, less efficient ventilatory ability, and increased time for recuperation and healing.

Neurologic changes in aging include increased time required for impulses to travel over multisynaptic pathways, less efficient sleep, and decline in senses of balance. Special senses that began to decline in middle age continue to show decreased function. Vision and hearing changes (presbyopia and presbycusis) become more prominent in the older adult. Urinary function diminishes with age because the plasma flow to the kidney may decrease as much as 50% from age 30 to age 80, leading to a comparable decrease in glomerular filtration rate. Decreased urinary bladder tone can contribute to incomplete emptying of the bladder, urinary frequency, and bladder infections in the older adult. Degenerative changes in connective tissue and cartilage, along with demineralization of the bone, can lead to age-related problems with posture, mobility, and injury as a result of accidents (e.g., falls).

Although the older adult experiences many physical changes with aging, these changes occur gradually and to varying extents. As a result, the older person has been adapting and accommodating to these changes over a period of years and, in the absence of illness or specific debilities, can function adequately in the later years of life.

Cognitive Development

Although the stereotype of the aging person is one of memory loss and reduced cognitive skills, the actual cognitive changes seen in the latter part of the lifespan do not fit the description. With aging, there is a reduction in visual and auditory acuity, potentially affecting function. Changes in cognition are more often a difference in speed rather than ability (i.e., learning a new task takes longer and performance time is longer). An older adult is more concerned about accuracy than speed of performance than younger adults. Along with age comes increasing experiential knowledge (Clayton, 1975).

Intellectual loss in later life may reflect interrelated physiologic decrements caused by disease (e.g., atherosclerosis causes blood vessels to narrow). Perfusion to the brain is diminished. Malignancies may metastasize to the brain and other body parts. Cardiovascular disease, emphysema, high blood pressure, poor nutrition, or effects of surgery may temporarily reduce blood supply to the brain, limiting or altering performance. Cognitive dysfunctions that may result from dementia, delirium, chronic brain disorders, or Alzheimer's disease are not synonymous with old age. Most older adults do not experience cognitive impairments. Physical fitness and intellectual stimulation help maintain intellectual functioning in old age.

Psychosocial Development

Older adults must make the transition from working to retirement. Retirement entails the loss of the work role and relationships at work and substantial changes in one's lifestyle. Some people welcome retirement with the opportunity for more time for activities such as church, community, and leisure projects. Other people find that retirement makes them feel useless and as though they are waiting to die. Losses are common for elderly people who experience the death of spouses, friends, and possibly children. Social contacts and role performance may be limited by physical changes associated with aging. Preretirement planning and a prior devotion to hobbies make the transition easier (Freiberg, 1987).

If an older adult successfully accomplishes "ego" integrity (Erikson, 1963), he or she still participates in life and does not fear death. Family support, friends, and coworkers influence the retiree. Although marriage and divorce occur in later life, marital satisfaction before retirement greatly affects marital satisfaction in retirement. Women outlive men by an average of 7 years.

Although many older people maintain their own houses or apartments, a minority live in retirement homes for the aged or nursing homes.

FUNCTIONAL HEALTH AND LIFESPAN DEVELOPMENT RELATED TO HEALTH PROBLEMS AND ANTICIPATORY GUIDANCE

Knowledge of lifespan development and an understanding of how humans operate physiologically as well as behaviorally are basic components of nursing. A key to appreciating human function is knowledge of how development produces qualitative and quantitative differences in function across the lifespan and how these differences relate to health. Development and health are intricately related—health has an impact on development and development has an impact on health.

The focus of discussion in this section is how functional health varies with age, the way in which health needs are modified by age, and the way in which anticipatory guidance can assist with maximizing function and minimizing health problems. Functional health and health problems are highly interrelated, change over the lifespan, and are responsive to anticipatory guidance.

Health Perception and Health Management

Fetal, Newborn, and Infant. The earliest effects of health behaviors are seen during the period of fetal development. The intrauterine environment and its effects on the growing fetus produce a lifelong impact on health and shape functional health throughout the remainder of the lifespan. Maternal factors, including drug and alcohol use, smoking, exposure to toxins, diet, stress, rest, and exercise, are important determinants of fetal outcome. The fetus and the newborn infant may experience dysfunction (e.g., problems affecting the cardiac, musculoskeletal, or nervous systems) related to intrauterine environment.

Getting neonates off to the best possible start is an important means of influencing lifelong health. For this reason, women's health management during the prenatal period is of paramount importance in anticipatory guidance. Pregnant women need to be encouraged to seek prenatal care early in pregnancy.

After birth, an infant depends on the parents' health behaviors. Parents should be encouraged to seek well-child care with regular health monitoring, immunizations, and preventive teaching (Fig. 13-2). Facilitating the transition to the parent role may help prevent future health and relationship problems.

Neonates and young infants are particularly prone to infection because of immaturity of the immune system.

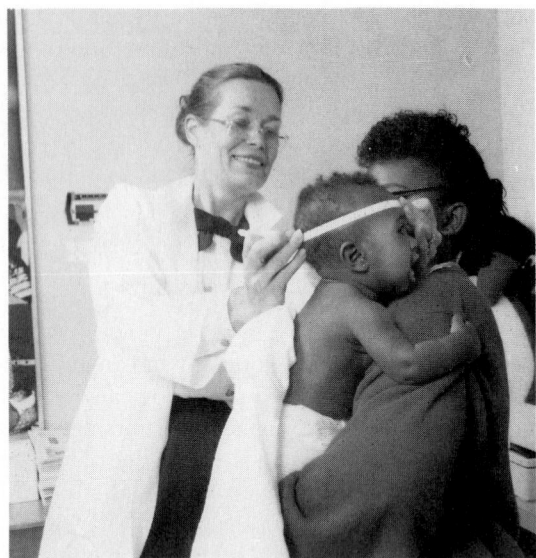

Figure 13–2. Well-child care includes assessing cranial circumference and fontanelle size. (Photo courtesy of the University of Washington School of Nursing.)

Certain behaviors of infants and toddlers, such as mouthing objects, increase the occurrence of infection. Since day-care situations provide more opportunity for exposure it is not surprising that infants in day care have more infections, especially upper respiratory infections. The effect of economics and living conditions on infant health are evidenced by a greater incidence of infections in infants of lower-class families.

Infants are totally dependent on caregivers for all safety concerns. Chief health concerns for infants include safe sleeping conditions and prevention of falls. The increasing mobility involved in rolling over, creeping, crawling, and walking requires modifications in the home to prevent falls and other hazards. In older infants, hand-to-mouth behavior could cause choking or ingestion of harmful substances.

Toddler and Preschooler. The toddler and preschooler continue to be prone to infections and minor illnesses. Although rubella, mumps, and rubeola can be prevented through immunization, chickenpox remains as a common communicable disease, often experienced in early childhood. Immunization (discussed in Chap. 35) is a means of reducing the incidence of certain infections and is a component of normal well-child health care.

The toddler's advancing motor and cognitive skills promote exploration, and high levels of energy and activity are often the basis for injury. Injuries can range from falls and minor injuries that occur as a part of play, to life-threatening accidents such as drownings, burns, poisoning, or motor vehicle accidents.

Anticipatory guidance for parents of toddlers and preschoolers includes providing a safe environment that encourages exploration, such as storing chemicals, household cleaning products, and medications in safe and protected places. Use of seatbelts in motor vehicles, life vests when around water, and close supervision wherever there is a potentially dangerous situation (e.g., in bathtubs, by swimming pools, at playgrounds) is essential.

The toddler and preschooler's normal level of curiosity makes them prone to participate in dangerous activities. Parents need to view the world from the level of their child and protect the child from danger at that level (e.g., wall outlets, stove burners and knobs, stairs, space heaters).

School Age and Adolescent. Accidents and minor illnesses continue to be the most common health problems of the school-age child. Exposure to larger numbers of children in school and play environments adds to the kinds and types of infections to which the child may be susceptible. Advances in motor skills throughout childhood are associated with the use of bicycles, tricycles, skateboards, and other riding toys and, consequently, their related safety concerns. Independent excursions away from home make traffic accidents a concern as well as precautions about strangers. Daring exploits, imagination, and industry of school-age children determine safety needs.

Adolescence is a time of trying on different identities and testing limits, coupled with the perception of invulnerability. Some of these actions involve health risks, such as smoking, drug use, alcohol consumption, fast driving, or drinking and driving. In adolescence, the risk of sexually transmitted disease (STD) is increased with sexual activity and is added to the usual infectious possibilities of being a young person. AIDS becomes an additional risk, particularly if experimentation with intravenous drugs or homosexuality occurs. Suicide and gang activity are on the rise among adolescents and create significant concern.

Although the adolescent may have a working knowledge of how the body functions, there may be limited ability to appreciate a cause-and-effect relationship between health behaviors and outcomes. Additionally, intense privacy needs may impede adequate health care.

Anticipatory guidance involves teaching and counseling by the nurse in regard to safety concerns, sex education, appropriate nutrition, and hygiene. Supporting and encouraging positive family relationships is particularly important during these transitional years.

Adult and Older Adult. Young adulthood is characterized by separation from family of origin, career development, and family establishment. Occupation may determine specialized safety concerns. Health behaviors begun in adolescence may continue into adulthood, such as smoking, drinking, or sexuality behaviors. As the person proceeds in adulthood, the physical effects of health behaviors may become apparent. For example, cigarette smoking results in progressive decline in pulmonary function. Health problems common to the middle adult group include hypertension, adult-onset diabetes, elevated cholesterol, or serious illness (e.g., cancer or cardiac disease).

The older adult may find that the ability to manage health independently may be impaired by changes associated with aging. Alterations in hearing, vision, and mobility affect health management practices such as hygiene, diet, and exercise. Changes in sensory and motor abilities intensify safety needs and make falls a major source of injury in the elderly. Because the immune response is decreased, the elderly have increased risk of infection at a time when poor nutrition and other factors may further impede natural defenses (Fig. 13-3).

Acute and chronic illnesses related to lifestyle patterns are manifested late in life. The cumulative effects of smoking, poor nutrition, inadequate exercise, and other health risks are demonstrated in aging. The common health problems include chronic pulmonary conditions, cardiovascular problems, and joint degeneration.

Anticipatory guidance for adults includes health teaching for health behavior modifications, such as a regular program of exercise, lifestyle management, stress reduction, and appropriate diet. Adults need to be encouraged to have regular physical examinations and to seek referrals as may be warranted for physical or mental health as well as for relational challenges. For more information, see Chapter 26.

Nutrition and Metabolism

Newborn and Infant. Infancy is a period of high metabolic rate and nutritional need. Nutrient intake is partic-

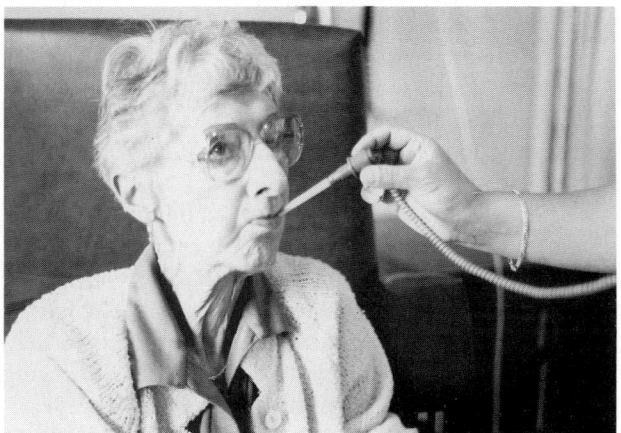

Figure 13–3. Monitoring the older adult for the risk of infections involves assessing body temperature as well as other health factors. Because of the thermoregulatory changes that accompany aging, temperature may not be an effective assessment of infection.

ularly important during infancy because brain growth occupies a large share of the body's metabolic rate. The infant's complex nutritional needs can be met by breast milk or formula during the first 6 months of life. Health problems related to nutrition focus mainly on the infant receiving adequate amounts of mild and properly prepared formula. With the eruption of teeth and the introduction of solid foods, nutrient intake is expanded to many types of foods, and breast milk or formula becomes less essential in the diet.

Increased metabolic rate and immature renal function lead to high fluid requirements in infancy. Resulting inherent health problems include reduced ability to remove drugs or other substances from the body, greater potential for fluid loss, and difficulty concentrating or diluting urine.

Anticipatory guidance encompasses teaching parents regarding infant nutrition, proper preparation of formula, and monitoring of the infant's weight. Helping parents understand when and how to introduce new foods is supportive.

Toddler and Preschooler. Appetite during toddlerhood and preschool years is extremely variable, and changes are usually a normal consequence of slowing of growth and change in body composition. Toddlers and preschoolers often prefer simple foods served separately, rather than mixed. The primary health problem relates to intake of adequate nutrition because the parent is beginning to have less control. At this age, there is also a potential for children to chew food incompletely and possibly choke on pieces of food.

Anticipatory guidance for the parents should include encouragement to present the child with an adequate quantity and variety of food. From this, the child generally selects enough for sufficient nutrition.

School Age and Adolescent. As the child moves beyond the home environment, social influences on food consumption become increasingly important. The food choices of school-age children and teenagers are highly related to peer influences and media advertisements. Adolescence is a period of rapid growth and high nutritional requirements. For some teens, the conflict between eating and the desire to be thin is expressed in the health problems of fad dieting, bulimia, or anorexia. For other teens, the response to stress may be overeating, leading to obesity. These types of health problems may set lifelong patterns.

Anticipatory guidance depends on teaching and attempting to influence peer groups in a positive way to encourage good nutrition. Working with teens in groups tends to be more effective in changing behavior.

Adult and Older Adult. Metabolic activity decreases in adults, but not the need for adequate nutrients. Bone growth, which is accelerated during adolescence, continues in young adulthood. During childbearing years, nutrition is particularly important to women and to the outcome of the pregnancy. Health problems can be avoided by an optimal nutritional intake during the active young adult years. Obesity, bulimia, or anorexia may begin or continue to be problems in young adults. Metabolic disorders, such as diabetes, may be manifested in childhood, adolescence, or young adult years.

Through the middle and older adult years, there is increased concern about health problems related to nutrition. Cardiovascular changes make blood cholesterol levels and fat in the diet a concern. The sodium content of food is important for people with disorders of the kidney or with high blood pressure. People with diabetes need to regulate total dietary intake. Meeting nutritional needs using fewer calories is a challenge, and many people must be concerned about excess weight.

Aging changes in the kidney may limit adaptability to fluid changes. Decreased glomerular filtration rate can lead to fluid retention and inability to remove drugs or their metabolites.

Anticipatory guidance in the adult years includes providing the patient with access to reliable information about nutrition so that fact and myth can be identified. Referral to dietitians, nutrition classes, and support groups may be beneficial. For more information, see Chapter 33.

Elimination

Newborn and Infant. The infant is too immature to have control over either bowel or bladder elimination. Health problems relate primarily to skin disorders resulting from the need to wear diapers. Monilial infections and diaper rash are common problems. Anticipatory guidance by the nurse is directed toward teaching proper diapering, disposal of stool and diapers, and care of the skin. Parents will want to learn about skin hygiene, frequency of diaper changes, and differences in skin rashes and their treatment.

Toddler and Preschooler. Between 2 and 3 years of age, toddlers have begun to develop control over elimination functions. Health problems relate to skin care during this development period as well as to delay in progressing toward continence. Continence, once achieved, is not guaranteed, and "accidents" are not uncommon during the preschool years.

Anticipatory guidance can help parents understand that the attitudes conveyed during this time of achieving continence and reactions to incidences of incontinence influence not only feelings about body function, but also about personal mastery and competency. Patience and allowing the child to progress at his or her own pace are the hallmarks of this stage of development.

School Age and Adolescent. Older children occasionally have difficulty with nocturnal enuresis or "bed-wetting" after preschool and young school-age years. This problem is often related to maturation of both urinary control mechanisms and sleep, but may have emotional or structural causes. Nocturnal enuresis after the age of 6 years is a matter of concern. It is not uncommon to identify a familial pattern of enuresis. The main health problem is related to embarrassment and self-consciousness of the child who may limit social activities as a result of the enuresis.

Anticipatory guidance is directed toward helping parents and child understand nocturnal enuresis, encouraging a thorough evaluation, and realizing that, in most cases, the child eventually matures and becomes continent. Although a physical assessment is essential, psychosocial support is imperative.

Adult and Older Adult. Continence may be disrupted by "normal" life events, such as pregnancy or childbirth, which result in changes of the pelvic musculature. Decreasing estrogen levels that occur during menopause affect sphincter control, resulting in an increased occurrence of stress incontinence (Henderson & Taylor, 1987). Illnesses, such as a cerebral vascular accident, or procedures, such as prostatic surgery, ureterostomy placement, or a colostomy alter normal elimination patterns and threaten the sense of mastery and personal control at any age. In the elderly, alterations in innervation and changes in muscle tone may produce incontinence or nocturia (excessive urination at night).

The nurse shapes patient teaching to the specific problem related to elimination, either teaching how to manage the alterations or therapies the patient can use to regain continence. For more information, see Chapters 37 and 38.

Activity and Exercise

Newborn and Infant. Newborns and infants are prone to respiratory difficulties as a result of the relative immaturity of the lungs. Premature infants can be at risk for respiratory distress syndrome, and babies born by cesarean section may have excessive mucus in their lungs. These situations lead to potential health problems related to adequate ventilation.

The developing motor activity of an infant can lead to potential health problems related to safety. As infants learn to reach and grasp objects and to roll over, they are placing themselves at risk for injury. In anticipatory guidance, the nurse can work with the parents to help them understand how rapidly their infant is changing and what factors may constitute danger. Close supervision of motor activities and, if needed, of respiratory function are central elements in teaching.

Toddler and Preschooler. Energy production of the heart and lungs in the toddler and preschooler is adequate. The occurrence of respiratory infections and the management of congenital problems with the heart or lungs are the leading health problems of this age group.

As their motor control increases, the desire to explore and curiosity of toddlers and preschoolers cause them to be adventurous and to take risks. Safety and accident prevention are the focus of health problems.

Anticipatory guidance is centered on prevention of respiratory infections, when possible, and early treatment when they occur. Parents of children with congenital problems need support and individual teaching to manage their child's difficulty. Awareness of safety needs remains paramount. (See the section entitled "Health Perception and Health Management" above.)

School Age and Adolescent. The school-age child without congenital abnormalities or chronic problems has few health problems. Respiratory infections continue to occur as a result of contact with classmates. As motor control develops, children become more active, but their bones are not mature and are susceptible to some types of fracture, but since they are not completely ossified, they are somewhat more resistant to fractures. Because the rib cage is not yet rigid, the school-age child is vulnerable to injury to the heart and lungs from blows to the chest.

The adolescent's health problems are related to lifestyle factors and risk-taking behaviors. Smoking and the use of smokeless tobacco predispose the adolescent to changes in the mucosa of the mouth and the respiratory tract with the potential of malignant changes in the tissues and in vital capacity changes in ventilation. Increased physical activity in sports, motor vehicle driving, and, possibly, gang activity place the adolescent at risk for serious injuries.

In anticipatory guidance, the nurse needs to be a teacher, counselor, and confidant when working with and advising school-age children and adolescents. Helping parents and their children understand ways they can minimize health problems and prevent injury is the nursing focus.

Adult and Older Adult. With progression through the adult years and into aging, the effects of smoking or other pollution sources become apparent. When combined with the decline in function that normally occurs with age, the resulting health concerns include decreased vital capacity of the lungs, reduced stroke volume and force of contraction of the heart, and ischemia of tissues that are not adequately perfused. Additionally, the vascular system shows accumulation of atherosclerotic plaque and reduced resilience of vessel walls with age.

In adulthood, changes in motor abilities are noticeable. Throughout life, the motor system operates under the "use it or lose it" principle (i.e., activity is essential for maintenance of muscle and atrophy results from decreased use). Exercise is increasingly important in the maintenance of muscle function. During aging, mobility is affected not only by muscular changes, but also by skeletal changes such as arthritis or loss of bone mineral. Visual and motor changes associated with aging impair use of means of transportation.

Anticipatory guidance includes encouragement to participate in a regular program of exercise; maintain a low-fat, high-fiber diet; and to develop pleasurable leisure activities. The adult is capable of making modifications in lifestyle to extend wellness late into life. For more information, see Chapter 26.

Cognition and Perception

Newborn and Infant. Special senses are important components of cognitive-perceptual development in infancy. Sensory stimulation is a basic human need (Fig. 13-4). Studies of sensory deprivation indicate that sensory stimulation is an important requirement for central nervous system function. Sensory stimulation is critical during the early years of life and essential for normal development. Work by Spitz (1945) first showed that infants raised in foundling homes who received little sensory stimulation and handling had retarded growth and reduced mental performance compared to infants raised in normal home environments.

Although sensory stimulation during early development is extremely important, it is also important to identify that the notion "if a little is good, a lot is better" is not applicable. The central nervous system of the neonate and infant is easily overwhelmed by excess stimulation. Infants provide caregivers with behavioral cues indicating the appropriateness of stimulation for particular infant's neurobehavioral development (Als, Lester, & Brazelton, 1979).

Health problems that interfere with the accuracy of sensory input, such as hearing, affect cognitive-perceptual development. In connection with immature anat-

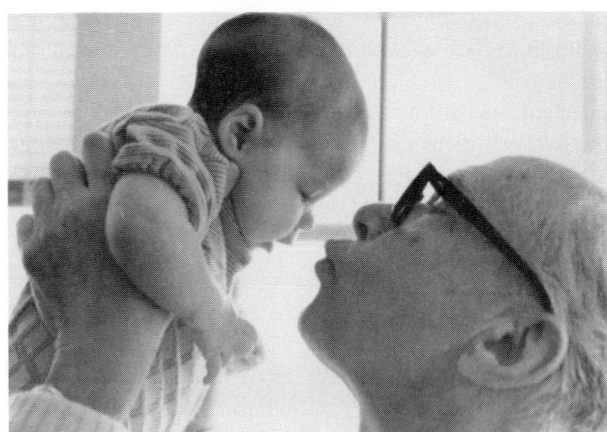

Figure 13-4. Sensory stimulation involves the senses and movement. A grandfather instills trust while providing stimulation to his grandchild. (Photo courtesy of the University of Washington School of Nursing.)

omy and immune response, the infant is prone to the development of middle ear infections, which, if they become chronic and recurring, may interfere with hearing perception. Infants express pain through pulling on or rubbing the ear, disturbances in sleep or eating, or crying or fussiness.

Observation of the infant's responses to sounds and expressions of pain is an important form of anticipatory guidance for parents. Helping parents understand the need for physical contact and sensory stimulation for adequate cognitive-perceptual development is an important nursing function. Holding and cuddling provide physical sensory stimulation, whereas colorful mobiles, pictures, sounds, and toys in the environment stimulate the special senses.

Toddler and Preschooler. At this age, children are developing cognitive skills, such as language, and are more verbal about indicating the presence of pain. Hearing and vision problems can impede progress and may relate to misperceptions by the child. It takes careful and informed observation to identify the subtle pain behaviors in children of this age. Although one might expect to see reduction in activity, children often continue to participate in play despite being in pain. Regression and withdrawal are also common pain behaviors of children.

Anticipatory guidance includes encouraging regular hearing and vision examinations as a part of well-child care, as well as additional assessment if the child's hearing or vision seems to be questionable. Assisting parents in becoming observant of subtle behaviors that may be linked to pain and an underlying health problem is part of patient teaching.

School Age and Adolescent. Health problems for school-age children and adolescents may be related to previous problems of sensory input. Additionally, physiologic, emotional, and environmental factors may have influence on cognitive-perceptual function (see Chap. 42). Use of drugs and alcohol alters cognition. Mental health problems become more prominent at these ages than at earlier ages, and suicide is a major health concern.

The nurse can provide anticipatory guidance at regular well-child exams at which vision and hearing are examined. The nurse should encourage parents to be aware of indications of substance use or mental health problems, such as poor academic performance, withdrawal, or change in personality, and to seek appropriate care.

Adult and Older Adult. In the absence of chronic conditions, the young and middle adult years have few health problems related to cognition and perception. With aging, the decline in sensory function can contribute to cognitive misperceptions. Pain perception in the older adult may vary from the typical pattern seen in younger people and needs careful evaluation. Chapter 42 presents a complete discussion of the various factors that affect the older adult's cognition. Reversible confusion and dementia are two major health problems for older adults.

The nurse can provide anticipatory guidance for older adults by prompting them to seek evaluation of pain, sensory deficits, and cognitive changes. Abnormalities should not be accepted as a "normal" part of aging.

Sleep and Rest

Newborn and Infant. Infants are in the process of organizing sleep and rest. As the infant matures, sleep periods consolidate and become longer. Sleep moves from being free running to becoming linked to nighttime (Coons, 1987; Hoppenbrouwers, 1987). Health problems of sleep in the infant are usually related to problems in the maturation of neurologic integration. Anticipatory guidance for parents should include counseling that the infant normally organizes sleep in an orderly fashion. Uncommon deviations from orderly progression should be assessed by a health-care provider.

Toddler and Preschooler. Toddlers and preschoolers have organized sleep patterns; the majority of sleep occurs at night with one or two naps during the day. During the second year of life, nightmares often emerge as cognitive development increases memory and the ability to represent experiences mentally, including fearful situations (Terr, 1987). In anticipatory guidance, the nurse can remind the parents to reassure the anxious child in an unhurried manner and talk in a quiet voice.

School Age and Adolescent. Nightmares continue to occur in early school-age children, producing nighttime awakenings. Nighttime bedwetting, a common problem in young children, may disrupt sleep (Nino-Murcia & Keenan, 1987). Anticipatory guidance by the nurse includes support for the parents in reassuring their children regarding nightmares. Nighttime bedwetting needs to handled by not drawing excessive attention to the behavior, once it has been determined not to have a pathophysiologic base. As a rule, the child outgrows the problem, and scolding and punishment are ineffective.

The adolescent actually has increased sleep needs as a result of the rapid growth and endocrine changes. Sleep deprivation may, in reality, be a health problem for adolescents who are pressured by school, jobs, and multiple activities (Carskadon & Dement, 1987). The nurse can provide anticipatory guidance to the adolescent by counseling regarding time management and balance of activities, so that the adolescent can be active and, yet, get enough sleep.

Adult and Older Adult. Sleep problems in adults are often related to stress and schedules that lead to sleep deprivation. Older adults often experience changes in sleep pattern that are within the range of normal. Environmental situations, such as nighttime problems of children in the family, pregnancy, or late-night exercising or eating, may interfere with sleep as well. In anticipatory guidance, the nurse needs to counsel the adult with respect to activities before bedtime that foster sleep. Insomnia and sleep apnea are frequent sleep disorders for adults. Insomnia, a disorder of initiating or maintaining sleep, may become a health problem for which the adult may choose to seek evaluation. Sleep apnea is the absence of breathing for 10 seconds or longer five times during an hour and may require thorough assessment and intervention. For more information, see Chapter 39.

Self-Perception and Self-Concept

Newborn and Infant. The infant's perception of self begins with the parent–child relationship in which the infant learns a sense of worthiness. The infant's successful use of cues in conveying and satisfying needs is early evidence of competency. Health problems arise when the infant is unable to respond to the usual parent–child interactions. The nurse can provide anticipatory guidance in supporting parents in interactions that engender trust.

Toddler and Preschooler. Toddlers and preschoolers are egocentric in their relationships with peers. Expressions of anger, jealousy, and even regression are not uncommon. Health problems exist for the child who is at either extreme from this: lack of egocentric response or exaggerated responses. Excessive fears of injury or altered body image may give indication of problems with self-concept. The nurse can help parents understand the range of normal behaviors and can provide anticipatory guidance about behaviors outside of that range that require further evaluation.

School Age and Adolescent. At these ages, children's self-concept is tied closely to peers and peer relationships. One's self-concept may be challenged by the response and acceptance given by peers. Use of drugs and exposure to STDs and AIDS may be indications of the need for peer acceptance to have a positive self-concept. The nurse can provide anticipatory guidance to the child and family by encouraging open communication, interactions with groups that promote development of positive self-concept (church, Scouts, sports), and health education regarding the consequences of drug use and sexual activity.

Adult and Older Adult. Throughout the lifespan, self-concept and self-perception are reinforced or altered as a consequence of life events and interpersonal relationships. In adulthood, this pattern is extremely individual and less predictable, although certain commonalities exist. The older adult may have depression regarding life events or for no definable reason. Evidences of disturbed self-concept that interfere with the ability to carry out activities of daily living require referral for evaluation and treatment. In providing anticipatory guidance, the nurse needs to be supportive to the patient and family during periods when self-concept may be altered. Referral to support groups, counselors, or psychiatrists may be the appropriate guidance.

Roles and Relationships

Newborn and Infant. The infant's primary relationship is with the parents (Ainsworth, Blehar, Waters, & Wall, 1978). Attachment is not a magical or mystic occurrence, but rather a process in which the ongoing interaction between the infant and parent produces a special bond, offering the infant a safe base from which to launch into the world. The sensitive parent learns to "read" the infant's cues and provides for the infant's needs. The infant in turn responds by cessation of crying, by smiling, or by sleeping. Problems in either party can alter the interaction and interfere with attachment. The change in the relationship produces a sense of loss, which leads to altered ability to form relationships. In anticipatory guidance, the nurse can encourage the parent and infant in their mutual bonding through providing opportunities for positive interaction and teach the parent the importance of reciprocal interactions with the infant.

Toddler and Preschooler. As the child begins to perceive self as separate from parents, separation is equated with loss. In late infancy and toddlerhood, the child expresses the sense of loss of changes in relationships through separation anxiety and protest. The degree of anxiety and protest, however, are not necessarily direct evidence of attachment. The nurse can provide anticipatory guidance by assisting the parents in understanding the response of the child and recognizing when it exceeds normal bounds.

School Age and Adolescent. Peer relationships are increasingly important in the school-age years. The two key influences during adolescence are sexual development and peer group. Time spent with friends is increased, whereas time spent with parents and family is decreased. Changing relationships with family and forming new relationships are normal during these years. The child who has difficulty relating to peers, leaving home and family, or managing sexuality appropriately may be exhibiting problems in roles and relationships. In anticipatory guidance, the nurse can be a safe confidant and counselor for the child, a support and encouragement for parents, and an appraiser and evaluator of the need for further intervention.

Adult and Older Adult. Adults assume many roles including career, intimacy, marriage, and parenthood. Although these categories help structure our thinking, the patterns of resultant roles and relationships are not as clear-cut. Patterns of intimacy and parenting are not predictable or set. Although physical intimacy is required for the bearing of biologic offspring, intimacy is not always linked with parenting. There are differing patterns of parenting as well. Parenting may be deferred in favor of establishing a career, parenting may be inhibited due to infertility or lack of a mate, or the person may make a choice to not parent. Parenting may occur as a result of the conscious choice to conceive or by chance, or may also involve adoption of children or formation of a blended family. Parenting styles can be categorized as authoritative, authoritarian, or permissive (Baumrind, 1968). These roles are increasingly complex and the number of roles far exceeds those of childhood. Because of this, the demands of disparate roles may lead to role conflict.

For middle and older adults, the loss of relationships through relocation, divorce, death, or illness is equally challenging. Altered role relationships that disturb daily living may occur. The middle-aged person may have elderly parents who require care, and death of parents often occurs in middle age. Middle age is also a time of evaluation and reflection, which may lead to some role conflicts and altered relationships. Older adults experience loss of the work role, reduced mobility and activity which may limit social contacts, and changes in family roles and relationships.

Nurses can be helpful in counseling adults who are experiencing altered roles and relationships by knowing community resources for referral and for support for the specific problems. Parents of young children can be counseled regarding parenting skills and sources for improving and reinforcing them. Middle-aged adults can be reassured that midlife review is a normal developmental process and that there are resources available to assist them in sorting through feelings and conflicts that arise. Preparing for retirement years through developing new interests and activities helps to minimize the adjustment to the various role losses and changed relationships that most older adults experience (Fig. 13-5). This is discussed further in Chapter 45.

Sexuality and Reproduction

Newborn and Infant. Gender is determined at the time of fertilization. In the first weeks of embryologic life, sexual differentiation is determined by exposure to hormones. At the time of birth, the gender of the infant is established based on the physical sexual appearance.

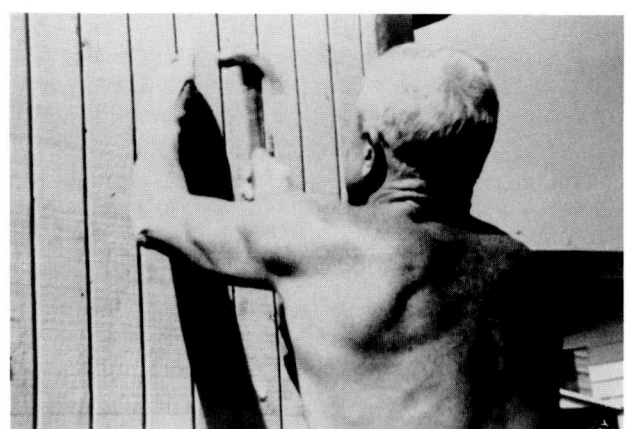

Figure 13–5. Developing hobbies and leisure activities promotes successful retirement. (Photo courtesy of the University of Washington School of Nursing.)

Health problems arise if gender identification based on the appearance of the genitalia is not clear or if there are structural anomalies. The nurse can provide anticipatory guidance by encouraging parents to provide love, comfort, intimacy, and nurturance, the basis for later sexuality.

Toddler and Preschooler. The explorative behavior of toddlers includes exploration of the body, and preschoolers recognize physical differences between the sexes identifying gender based on body parts and appearances. This age group often has exhibitionistic-type behaviors of removing clothing and discussing sexual organs, their own and others. Anticipatory guidance includes reminding parents that exploratory behavior and interest in sexuality is to be expected. The nurse can also communicate to parents the importance of affection and acceptance of the child as a basis for future sexuality and positive self-concept.

School Age and Adolescent. The school-age child has increasing curiosity about sexual function, although peer relationships and friendships are almost exclusively with children of the same gender. Sexual behavior becomes a problem only when the child seems to be turning to masturbation as a primary source of comfort.

Health problems for adolescents are associated with lifestyle activities of the adolescent and peer group. STDs and AIDS are significant potential problems for the sexually active adolescent, with drug use as a contributory factor. Use of birth control methods is inconsistent with the attitude of invulnerability characteristic of adolescents. Although the causes of homosexuality are poorly understood, this lifestyle demonstrates alternate patterns of sexual development that have not been clearly explicated (Bidwell, 1988).

Children of any age are the potential victims of sexual abuse. Children who are preschool age may demonstrate indications of anxiety, fear, sleep disturbances, and holding on to parents. School-age children have similar clues as younger children plus phobias and interference with school performance. Adolescents may exhibit socially unacceptable behavior, sexual promiscuity, running away from home, and failing academic performance. In anticipatory guidance, the nurse needs to participate in teaching children of all ages to tell someone (friend, pastor, teacher) when they have been approached or touched in a way that makes them uncomfortable. Encouraging parents to listen to their children carefully and not discount what the parents might term as "imaginative" is important.

Adult and Older Adult. Reproduction is a prime concern of early adult years with the major related health problems being infertility, STDs, and specific sexual dysfunction. During the middle years, menopause occurs in women and may present health problems related to decreased estrogen production (e.g., hot flashes, osteoporosis). STDs and AIDS remain as potential problems throughout adulthood.

Body structure and function, sexual expression, and intimacy are primary aspects of human function in the older adult. Sexuality, which is more than the act of intercourse, is still important. In normal aging, decreased mobility and energy production may limit sexual activity. Health problems are related to interference with sexual expression that may be the result of illness (e.g., stroke), death of a spouse, or environment (e.g., nursing homes).

In anticipatory guidance, the nurse who works with couples experiencing infertility needs to be sensitive to their feelings and support their efforts to identify therapies to correct the problem. Encouraging couples to maintain their personal intimacy as well as sexual intimacy is essential to promote the integrity of the couple. Preventing STDs and AIDS is a continuing problem with which the nurse is concerned. Nurses can also help older adults to understand that age alone is not a barrier to sexual function and can counsel (or refer to counselors) elderly people on alternate forms of sexual expression if intercourse is not possible. Sensitivity by nurses in anticipating privacy needs for older adults in health-care settings is a valuable nursing function. For further information, see Chapter 48.

Coping and Stress Tolerance

Newborn and Infant. Infants are not immune to stress. Thomas and Chess (1977) have used the concepts of adaptability and rhythmicity to describe infant behaviors and have classified infant temperament styles as easy, slow-to-warm-up, and difficult.

Sources of stress in infancy involve satisfaction of basic needs within the context of the caregiving or parental relationship. The major stressor of infancy and childhood is separation, indicating the impact of attachment (Garmezy, 1983). A limited understanding of time and the absence of the parent or caregiver during this period of trust development are the reasons for this anxiety. Expressions of anxiety that exceed usual expectations of separation anxiety may indicate a problem.

Nurses can provide anticipatory guidance in counseling with parents and caregivers regarding the reason for separation anxiety and the range of normal for this response. Within the context of the early parent–infant interaction, coping behaviors are established. Infants employ self-regulating and soothing behaviors, such as sucking, crying, motor activity, or withdrawal. The responsiveness of the caregiver is an important determinant in how the infant learns to cope.

Toddler and Preschooler. The stressors of toddlerhood include separation and loss as well as dealing with increasing autonomy. Death, divorce, and illness of a family member can affect toddlers (Rutter, 1983). Additionally, birth of a sibling is a common stressor, not only during the toddler years, but throughout childhood. With the birth of a sibling, the toddler loses their role as "the baby in the family." Hospitalization is an especially stressful occurrence for toddlers and preschoolers.

Cognitive development includes changes in memory. The role of memory in coping is twofold. First, the child can relate to previous stressful events, learning from such experiences; this learning can be positive or negative depending on the coping behaviors used and the outcome. Second, memory sensitizes the child to stressors. A child who is bitten by a dog may become afraid not only of dogs, but all furry animals. Fears and fantasy are also characteristic of preschoolers and cause related stress. Motor development increases the possibilities for coping behaviors. Mobility can be used to avoid or exit a stressful situation, to change the situation directly, or for aggression.

Nurses can assist parents in recognizing the stressor that their toddlers or preschoolers are encountering and learning to nurture their children by teaching them coping skills for managing these stressors. This anticipatory guidance allows the child to learn from the experience how to manage similar situations in the future.

School Age and Adolescent. Performance expectations, academic pressures, and widening interpersonal contacts are characteristic sources of stress in the school-age child. Although performance is the primary stressor at this age, many of the stressors that were problematic as a preschooler may continue to some degree in the school-age child. The nurse can provide anticipatory guidance to the child and the parents by being supportive of coping abilities and helping them understand the pressures that are being encountered.

Academic demands, conflicts over issues of independence, threats to identity, and peer pressures dominate the stresses of adolescents. Substance use and abuse become more common means of coping. The increased suicide rate among adolescents reflects the seriousness of the effects of stress on this age group. Anticipatory guidance to parents regarding observing for signs of excessive stress and dysfunctional coping mechanisms in their adolescent is particularly crucial for nurses. Adolescents need to feel supported and accepted regarding their stress experiences, and nurses are often in the best position to participate in this.

Adult and Older Adult. The various roles of adulthood involve specific kinds of stressors. Balancing these roles is a further form of stress. The underlying features in stressful events are change and loss. Coping is a function of both the stressors or demands posed by the environment as well as the person's or family's capabilities and vulnerabilities (Rose, 1984, 1987). Health problems related to stress include cardiac, nutrition, sleep, and substance use disorders. Chapter 47 presents a complete discussion of stress, coping, and adjustment. The nurse can provide anticipatory guidance by encouraging the person to learn a variety of methods for managing stress, such as exercise, relaxation, imagery, and biofeedback.

Values and Beliefs

Newborn and Infant. Infants have a limited understanding of right and wrong and do not appreciate the cause–effect relationship between their actions and punishment or reward. The nurse can support the parents in understanding that, because the infant is not deliberately defying them, punishment is not appropriate.

Toddler and Preschooler. At this age, egocentricity results in a self-centered approach to right and wrong—whatever the child wants is deemed right. Punishment and reward guide behavior, and authority figures, external to the child, determine and dispense rewards and punishment. Toddlers and preschoolers learn religious practices through family activities and imitation, although without understanding. The nurse's role is to help parents use this stage to enhance positive behavior through rewarding desired behavior. Encouraging parents to include their child in their religious practices fosters spiritual beliefs and development (Fowler, 1974; Shelly, 1982).

School Age and Adolescent. The school-age child tends to follow orders and requests to gain the approval of others. Because of the desire for conformity and wanting to fit in, the will to do right guides behavior and there is less emphasis on punishment and rewards. Religious beliefs reflect a beginning appreciation of the existence of a "god" or deity. Because doing right is associated

---

Nursing Research

Selected Nursing Research Studies

Eyler, F. E., Edens, M. J., Nelson, Resnick, M. B. Courtway-Meyers, C., Hellrung, D. J., & Eitzman, D. V. (1989). Effects of developmental intervention on heart rate and transcutaneous oxygen levels in low-birthweight infants. *Neonatal Network, 8,* 17–23.

Free, T., Russell, F., Mills, B., & Hathaway, D. (1990). A descriptive study of infants and toddlers exposed prenatally to substance abuse. *Maternal–Child Nursing, 15,* 245–249.

Gillis, A. J. (1990, April). Nurses' knowledge of growth and development principles in meeting psychosocial needs of hospitalized children. *Journal of Pediatric Nursing, 5*(2), 78–87.

Saucier, B. L. (1989, January–February). The effects of play therapy on developmental achievement levels of abused children. *Pediatric Nursing, 15*(1), 27–30.

Storm, D. S., Metzger, B. L., Therrien, B. (1989). Effects of age on autonomic cardiovascular responsiveness in healthy men and women. *Nursing Research, 38,* 326–330.

Possible Topics for Nursing Inquiry

- What are cultural indicators affecting cognitive development among school-age children?
- What specific stressors affect the accomplishment of developmental tasks of older adults?
- What cultural factors affect parents of infants seeking access to well-child care?

---

with reward, the school-age child may engage in making "deals" with the deity figure. Parents can be influenced, through anticipatory guidance, to reinforce desired behavior in their child. Being aware of the child's spiritual development enhances the parents' ability to further development.

Adolescents learn to make moral judgments that are situation-specific, to transfer moral judgments across situations, and finally to make autonomous decisions regarding moral issues. Problems occur when the adolescent tries out various activities and behaviors, such as substance use and promiscuous sexual behavior. At this time, faith and religious beliefs are questioned and challenged as the adolescent develops a personal identity and expands independence from the family. The nurse can assist the adolescent and parents in awareness of the developmental aspects of this stage.

Adult and Older Adult. Values and moral development are at the level of autonomous decisions, applying principles to differing situations. Moral reasoning is less bound by rules, and actions are guided to a greater extent by personal values. Spiritual beliefs evolve and are applicable across a variety of situations. Health problems occur when disharmony occurs between spiritual beliefs and events in the adult's life. Chapter 49 has a complete discussion of spirituality and alterations in spirituality.

Key Concepts

■ Growth and development occur throughout the lifespan.

■ Development is the process of ongoing change, reorganization, and integration occurring throughout the life of a person, including body structure and function, psychosocial behaviors, and cognition.

■ Genetics and environment are the two primary factors driving development.

■ Principles of growth and development are drawn from biologic and psychosocial sciences and express commonalities in the process.

■ Theorists have attempted to explain growth and development within various contexts, such as psychodynamics, cognitive development, human needs, developmental tasks, and moral development.

■ There are progressive, sequenced aspects of development for various stages of life on which future development expands.

■ The nurse's primary role in growth and development is understanding the person's position in the process, being aware of expectations in terms of functional health, and recognizing functional health problems related to development.

References

Ainsworth, M. D. S., Blehar, M. C., Waters, E., & Wall, S. (1978). *Patterns of attachment.* Hinsdale, N. J.: Lawrence Erlbaum Associates.

Als, H., Lester, B. M., & Brazelton, T. B. (1979). Dynamics of the behavioral organization of the premature infant: A theoretical perspective. In T. M. Field, A. M. Sostek, S. Goldberg, & H. H. Shuman (Eds.), *Infants born at risk: Behavior and development* (pp. 173–192). New York: Spectrum Publications.

Baumrind, D. (1968). Authoritarian versus authoritative parental control. *Adolescence, 3,* 255–272.

Bellack, J. P., & Heming, J. W. (1985). Theoretical and practical aspects of play: a universal need. In C. Fore & E. C. Poster (eds.) *Meeting psychosocial needs of children and families in health care.* Washington D.C.: Child Health Care Association.

Bidwell, R. J. (1988). The gay and lesbian teen: A case of denied adolescence. *Journal of Pediatric Health Care, 2,* 3–8.

Brazelton, T. (1979). Behavioral competence in the newborn infant. *Seminars in Perinatology, 3,* 35–44.

Bronfenbrenner, U. (1979). *The ecology of human development.* Cambridge, MA: Harvard University Press.

Carskadon, M. A., & Dement, W. C. (1987). Sleepiness in the normal adolescent. In C. Guilleminault (Ed.), *Sleep disorders in children* (pp. 53–66). New York: Raven Press.

Clayton, V. (1975). Erikson's theory of human development as it applies to the aged: Wisdom as contradictive cognition. *Human Development, 18,* 119–128.

Coons, S. (1987). Development of sleep and wakefulness during the first 6 months of life. In C. Guilleminault (Ed.), *Sleep and its disorders in children* (pp. 17–28). New York: Raven Press.

Dixon, S., & Stein, M. (1987). *Encounters with children. Pediatric behavior and development.* Chicago: Year Book Medical Publishers.

Erikson, E. (1963). *Childhood and society* (2nd ed.). New York: Norton.

Fowler, J. W. (1974). Toward a developmental perspective on faith. *Religious Education, 69,* 207–219.

Freiberg, K. L. (1987). *Human development—A life-span approach.* Boston: Jones & Bartlett.

Garmezy, N. (1983). Stressors of childhood. In N. Garmezy & M. Rutter (Eds.), *Stress, coping, and development in children* (pp. 43–84). New York: McGraw-Hill.

Gilligan, C. (1982). *In a different voice.* Cambridge, MA: Harvard University Press.

Havighurst, R. J. (1972). *Developmental tasks and education* (3rd ed.). New York: David McKay.

Henderson, J. S., & Taylor, K. H. (1987). Age as a variable in an exercise program for the treatment of simple urinary stress incontinence. *Journal of Obstetric, Gynecologic, and Neonatal Nursing, 16*(4), 266–272.

Hill, P. M., & Humphrey, P. (1982). *Human growth and development through life: A nursing perspective.* New York: John Wiley & Sons.

Hoppenbrouwers, T. (1987). Sleep in infants. In C. Guilleminault (Ed.), *Sleep and its disorders in children* (pp. 1–16). New York: Raven Press.

Kohlberg, L. (1976). Moral stages and moralization: The cognitive-developmental approach. In T. Lickkona (Ed.), *Moral development and behavior.* New York: Holt, Rinehart, & Winston.

Levinson, D. J. (1978). *The seasons of a man's life.* New York: Knopf.

Nino-Murcia, G., & Keenan, S. (1987). Enuresis and sleep. In C. Guilleminault (Ed.), *Sleep and its disorders in children* (pp. 1–16). New York: Raven Press.

Piaget, J. (1952). *The origins of intelligence in children.* New York: International Universities Press.

Rose, M. H. (1984). The concepts of coping and vulnerability as applied to children with chronic conditions. *Issues in Comprehensive Pediatric Nursing, 7,* 177–186.

Rose, M. H. (1987). Individual adaptations of children with chronic conditions. In M. H. Rose & R. B. Thomas (Eds.), *Children with chronic conditions: Nursing in a family and community context* (pp. 13–28). Orlando, FL: Grune & Stratton.

Rutter, M. (1983). Stress, coping, and development: Some issues and some questions. In N. Garmezy & M. Rutter (Eds.), *Stress, coping, and development in children* (pp. 1–42). New York: McGraw-Hill.

Schuster, C. S., & Ashburn, S. S. (1992). *The process of human development* (3rd ed.). Philadelphia: J. B. Lippincott.

Shelly, J. A. (1982). *The spiritual needs of children: A guide for nurses, parents and teachers.* Downers Grove, IL: InterVarsity Press.

Spitz, R. A. (1945). Hospitalism: An inquiry into the genesis of psychiatric conditions in early childhood. *Psychoanalytic Study of the Child, 2,* 113–117.

Terr, L. C. (1987). Nightmares in children. In C. Guilleminault (Ed.), *Sleep and its disorders in children* (pp. 231–242). New York: Raven Press.

Thomas, A., & Chess, S. (1977). *Temperament and development.* New York: Brunner/Mazel.

Turner, J., & Helms, D. (1987). *Lifespan development* (3rd ed.). San Francisco: Holt, Rinehart & Winston.

Bibliography

Dorbusch, S. M. (1987, October). The relation of parenting style to adolescent school performance. *Child Development, 58*(5), 1244–1257.

Hopkins, B. (1983, January). The development of early non-verbal communication: An evaluation of its meaning. *Journal of Child Psychology and Psychiatry and Allied Discipline, 24*(1), 131–144.

Lesser, H. (1985, February). The socialization of authoritarianism in children. *The High School Journal, 68*(4), 162–166.

Pardeck, J. T., & Pardeck, J. A. (1988, October). The influence of the family system on the development of adolescent autonomy. *Child Psychiatry Quarterly, 21*(4), 179–189.

Shapiro, T., & Sherman, M. (1983, June). Long term follow up of children with psychiatric disorders. *Hospital and Community Psychiatry, 34*(6), 522–527.

Stringer, S. A., Starrett, A. L., & Parker, L. R. (1986). Perceptions of neonatal behaviors by different caretakers. *Infant Mental Health Journal, 7*(3), 189–199.

Wadsworth, M. E. (1986, September). Effect of parenting style and preschool experience in children's verbal attainment. *Early Childhood Research Quarterly, 1*(3), 237–248.

Woodson, R. H. (1983, January). Newborn behavior and the transition of extrauterine life. *Infant Behavior and Development, 6*(1), 139–144.

Yogman, M. W. (1982–83). Assessing effects of serotonin precursors on newborn behavior. *Journal of Psychiatric Research, 17*(2), 123–133.

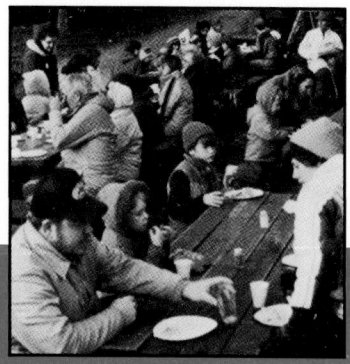

Individual, Family, and Community

LEARNING OBJECTIVES

Upon completion of this chapter, the student will be able to do the following:

- State the interaction between individual, family, and community based on Maslow's hierarchy of basic needs.
- State the key concepts of two different conceptual frameworks used to study the family.
- Describe three methods a nurse can use to assess a family.
- Discuss family responsibilities for functional health.

- Describe the components that could be included in a definition of community.
- Define family and community.
- Differentiate among the various types of community.
- Discuss the implications of different types of communities for nursing care.
- Discuss community responsibilities for functional health and the nurse's participation in community.

KEY TERMS

Community	Family	Systems theory
Developmental stages	Feedback loop	

The Individual
The Family
   Family Conceptual Frameworks
     Developmental Framework
     Systems Framework
   Family Assessment
   Family Responsibility for Functional Health

The Community
   Definition of Community
     Types of Communities
   Community Assessment
   Community Responsibility for Functional Health
   Advanced Community Concepts
Key Concepts

Mrs. Nellie Benoli is a 78-year-old Italian American. She was born in Italy and came to the United States at the age of 19. She and her husband have three grown children, six grandchildren, and two great-grandchildren. The Benoli family is devoutly Catholic. A hard worker all her life, Mrs. Benoli enjoys gardening and sewing. She retired at the mandatory age despite her desire to continue working as a seamstress in a small dress shop. She continues to go to the dress shop daily to gossip with her friends.

Mrs. Benoli states that she has lived in the same neighborhood since her arrival in the United States. The area is bordered by a high school, the Catholic church, a main boulevard, and a power plant. She has never had a reason to leave the neighborhood except to visit relatives in Italy. Mrs. Benoli never finished high school; she married her high school sweetheart, who brought her to the United States once he was established in a small grocery store.

Mrs. Benoli suffered a cerebrovascular accident and was hospitalized. Now that she has passed the acute phase of her illness, members of the health care team, along with Mrs. Benoli and her family, are planning for her discharge from the hospital. A primary concern is family and community support. Mr. Benoli is frail and spends most of his time on the porch chatting with friends. He never participated in any domestic chores.

The nurses are most concerned about Mrs. Benoli's ability and attitude in the following areas. She expresses no motivation to walk. She prefers to skip meals to avoid the embarrassment of "eating as babies do." Her speech is slurred, so she would prefer not to talk. At present she cannot continue her hobbies; she refuses to develop other hobbies. Her one interest is to continue to go to church on Sundays and Holy Days of Obligation, if at all possible.

In summary, Mrs. Benoli believes that if she goes home she would be least burdensome to her husband if she stayed quietly in bed all day and ate only when necessary.

Until recently the health care professions have focused on the patient as the recipient of care; however, care of the patient is enhanced when the nurse understands the patient as an individual in the context of what that individual brings to the nurse–patient relationship. The beliefs and values individuals hold and the support they receive come in large measure from the family and are reinforced by the community. Understanding family dynamics and the community context assists the nurse in planning care that, because it is compatible with the patient's everyday life, has the greatest chance of success.

THE INDIVIDUAL

Nurses have traditionally cared for the individual, ill, potentially ill, or well. Individuals are not isolates, however; they influence and are influenced by other people, beliefs, values, and the environment. The other chapters in this unit address other issues related to the individual: issues of lifespan, culture and ethnicity, values, and communication.

In Maslow's hierarchy of basic human needs (Maslow 1968), described in Chapter 12, there are five categories of needs: physiologic needs, safety, love, esteem, and self-actualization. A person can meet some of the basic needs independently, wheras some require interaction with family and community, and others may require the interventions of a nurse to be met (Fig. 14-1). Nursing care can be organized around the unmet basic needs in Maslow's hierarchy. These are prioritized and one must be able to satisfactorily meet the lower-level need to meet the next-level need fully.

The case of Mrs. Benoli can be used to illustrate basic needs of the individual according to Maslow. The nurse needs to note, however, that an individual's needs are sometimes best met in the family or in the community.

Physiologic Needs. Mrs. Benoli can no longer independently meet her need for adequate nutrition. The nurse will assist Mrs. Benoli in food preparation and feeding. Mr. Benoli has agreed to buy the groceries and Mrs. Benoli's friends from the dress shop plan to rotate cooking duties and assist in feeding her.

Safety Needs. Mrs. Benoli is emotionally insecure. She is fearful that her husband is too frail to assist her. The nurse will teach Mrs. Benoli to set realistic expectations for her husband so that she can trust in his ability to carry them out. The Benolis' oldest son will install grab

bars in the bathroom to facilitate her independence in toileting. The local Easter Seal Society has agreed to build a ramp with hand rails to the front door so Mrs. Benoli will not have to climb stairs getting in and out of her house.

Love Needs. Mrs. Benoli feels a strong sense of belonging within her family, in the community, and in her ties to Italy. Mrs. Benoli does not need the nurse to help her fulfill basic needs in this area.

Esteem Needs. Mrs. Benoli sees herself as "burdensome" to her husband because she is losing her independence. The nurse will assist Mrs. Benoli in building feelings of self-worth based on those things that she can do. Her family, under her direction, will take care of her garden and encourage her to participate as she is able. The Community Garden Club plans to honor her for a hybrid rose that she grew just before becoming ill.

Needs for Self-Actualization. Mrs. Benoli has not accepted her present state of health; she is focused on herself and views events subjectively. The nurse will refocus Mrs. Benoli on her likes, abilities, and accomplishments, and help her draw on her spirituality as a source of strength for her daily life.

THE FAMILY

The renewed interest in the role of the nurse in family and community emerged in the 1970s and was reflected in the American Nurses Association's description of nursing practice as "a direct service, goal oriented and adaptable to the needs of the individual, the family and the community during health and illness" (American Nurses Association, 1973, p. 2).

The family traditionally has been considered the basic unit of human society, and has played a central role in the organization of social relations. Although there is debate among social scientists about the universality of the functions of the family, the consensus among anthropologists provides a useful perspective on this issue. Most agree that the family provides for the following needs: sexual, reproductive, economic, nurturing, educational, caring, status, and political. Several if not all functions seem to be necessary to designate a group as a family. This is not to say that these functions cannot be carried out by other individuals or institutions, but that over time the family has proven to be a successful social institution in fulfilling these functions. Family functions are discussed more fully in Chapter 45.

For the purposes of this chapter's discussion of the **family,** the following general definition is offered:

> The family is a social group whose members share common values, occupy specific positions, and interact with each other over time. Adults bear and rear children, engage in economic and political cooperation, and care for the elders.

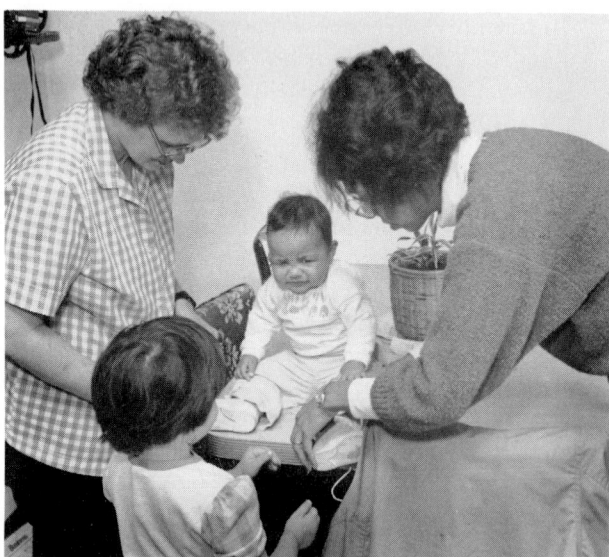

Figure 14-1. The nurse assesses individual family members and the function of the family in relation to each individual. Different developmental levels need different types and amounts of care from the family and nurse. (Courtesy of Seattle University)

Nursing Research: Family

Selected Nursing Research Studies

Frey, M. A. (1989). Social support and health: A theoretical formulation derived from King's conceptual framework. *Nursing Science Quarterly, 2,* 130–148.

Glanz, D., Ganong, L., & Coleman, M. (1989). Client, gender, diagnosis, and family structure. *Western Journal of Nursing Research, 11,* 726–735.

Phillips, L. R., Rempusheski, V. F., & Morrison, E. (1989). Developing and testing the beliefs about caregiving scale. *Research in Nursing and Health, 12,* 207–220.

Quayhagen, M. P., & Roth, P. A. (1989). From models to measurers in assessment of mature families. *Journal of Professional Nursing, 5*(3), 144–151.

Stanley, S. R. (1989). Disclosure of sexual abuse: The secret is out—what now? *Journal of Child and Adolescent Psychiatric Mental Health Nursing, 2,* 154–160.

Stewart, M. J. (1989). Social support instruments created by nurse investigators. *Nursing Research, 38*(5), 268–275.

von Windeguth, B. J. (1989). Cocaine-abusing mothers and their infants: A new morbidity brings challenges for nursing care. *Journal of Community Health Nursing, 6*(3), 147–153.

Possible Topics for Nursing Inquiry

- What is the relationship of a family's perception of an illness and an individual's collaboration with nursing interventions?
- What kinds of support will family members accept during a relative's terminal illness?
- Does viewing a problem from a systems perspective versus an individual perspective increase the probability of resolution of the problem?
- Do nurses who use a theoretical framework to collect family assessment data provide more individualized nursing care than nurses who do not?

Family Conceptual Frameworks

Conceptual frameworks provide useful guidelines for organizing family information. Each framework analyzes the family from a different perspective. No one framework is inherently right or wrong, but each requires the nurse to obtain somewhat different information. There are many frameworks, and it is not the intent here to acquaint the nurse with all of these but rather to show briefly the implications of their use.

By comparing two frameworks the nurse can see how each guides nursing care. The two frameworks chosen for this chapter are a developmental framework and a systems framework.

Developmental Framework

The developmental framework is popular in the study of families. In the early 1950s Duvall (1962) directed a group that studied the concept of family developmental tasks. This research focused on developmental tasks and role expectations of parents and children throughout a life cycle. The framework was meant to allow for biological and cultural differences as well as differences in values.

Duvall's framework, essentially based on the individual life cycle, demonstrated that families move through a series of eight **developmental stages.** These stages are based on the developmental stage of the oldest child in the family, and address marriage, childbearing, preschool years, school years, adolescent years, young adulthood, middle-aged parents whose children have left home, and aging parents. The critical family developmental tasks for these stages include learning to be a marital partner, adjusting to parenthood, stimulating the curiosity of preschool children, adapting to other school-age families, assisting adolescents to balance independence and autonomy, launching young adults into the work world, redefining the marital dyad without children, and coping with loss (Duvall, 1977). Tasks not completed at any one developmental stage produce chronic difficulties as the family struggles to master tasks at the next stage. Carter and McGoldrick (1980) refined this framework to reflect the changing times and make it applicable to divorced families.

In 1959 anthropologist Meyer Fortes noted in the introduction to *The Developmental Cycle in Domestic Groups* (1971) that the family life cycle consisted of three phases: expansion, dispersion or fusion, and replacement. The papers in that collection point out the universality of the family developmental cycle, describing families in Southeast Asia, Africa, and the Western Pacific.

The developmental cycle of the family, combining the

TABLE 14–1

Developmental Cycle of the Family and Task Accomplishment

Family Developmental Stage	Developmental Task
Pre-expansion	
Unattached adult	Stabilize image
	Develop independence
Expansion	
Unit formation	Develop mutual satisfaction
	Develop independence
Having children (by birth or adoption)	Adjust to child expectation
	Adjust to birth/adoption of child
	Establish a home for the family
Raising children	
Newborn through preschool	Nurture growth and development
School-age child	Adjust to less privacy
	Encourage education of children
	Develop community socialization
Adolescent	Balance freedom and responsibility
	Promote adolescent's independence
Dispersion	
Assist children to move on	Release children with appropriate assistance
Readjust unit	and stable home base
	Reestablish own interests and careers
	Readjust the relationships
Replacement	
	Maintain connection with other generations
Aging	Cope with loss of job, significant other,
Death	friends, home
Children become adults	Adjust to altered living space

work of Duvall, Fortes, and Carter and McGoldrick, is shown in Table 14-1. At each stage Duvall and Carter and McGoldrick identified specific tasks for the family to accomplish.

Systems Framework

First described in the social science context by the biologist von Bertalanffy (1968), systems theory has become popular because it takes a holistic approach and tries to encompass all data collected at all levels of abstraction. **Systems theory** looks at the interaction of the parts that make up the whole. There is input to the system, throughput (input from one member in the system to another), and output from the system. When the system is under stress, it tries to regulate itself by use of **feedback loops,** in which some of the output is rerouted back to the system as input, which in turn affects subsequent output. This response restores the system's balance, or homeostasis.

Because there are many feedback loops, some of which overlap, systems theory describes a circular process, not a deterministic one. When feedback to the system causes the system to move away from homeostasis, it is called positive feedback; when the feedback causes the system to maintain homeostasis, it is called negative

feedback. Systems are also considered to be either open or closed. These terms refer to the amount of exchange that takes place between a system and its environment. In a closed system no exchange occurs, whereas in an open system exchange occurs readily.

Families are basically open systems; however, the degree to which they are willing to exchange resources with other systems varies greatly. Healthy, functioning families exchange to a greater degree than dysfunctional families (Fig. 14-2).

Within the systems perspective there are many different schools of thought. Systems theorists include Virginia Satir (1988), Murray Bowen (1978), Salvador Minuchin (1974), Salvador Minuchin and H. Charles Fishman (1981), and Jay Haley (1971).

Several concepts are important for the nurse to understand when viewing a family as a system. These concepts are wholeness, circular interaction, lack of an identified patient, and holistic thinking, and are defined as follows:

Wholeness means that the whole is greater than the sum of its parts. Wholeness includes family values, beliefs, themes, and the rules by which the themes are carried out.

Circular interaction means that all parts of the system are acting, reacting, and interacting at the same time.

There is no identified patient in systems thinking.

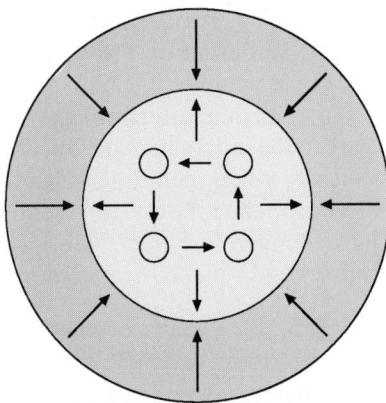 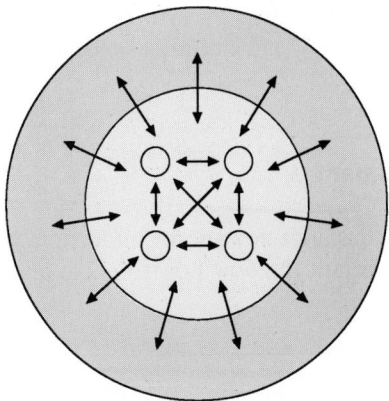

Figure 14–2.   In a simple systems framework, the family and its members are in the center, and feedback loops interlap. The outer circle is the environment, or, in this chapter, the community: ethnic group, school, church, places of employment, institutions. According to systems theory, the whole is greater than the sums of the parts. In other words, there is no identified person at the center but all are equal and interrelated. All systems are acting, reacting, and interacting at the same time. Holistically, *everything* counts. The functional family (*left*) has interaction among all systems. The boundary between family and community is a broken circle, allowing for input and output between family and community. The dysfunctional family (*right*) has limited interaction that goes in only one direction with a boundary between family and community that does not allow for input and output between those two systems.

TABLE 14–2

Family Assessment Based on Four Specific Frameworks

Areas to Assess	Developmental Stage	Wholeness	Communication	Support
Observe	Family behavior is consistent with their developmental stage.	Family themes and rule are explicit and implicit.	Family interaction and patterns of communication between members are recognized.	Types of support (such as emotional or financial) family members give each other.
Compare	Family behavior is similar to that of other families at the same stage of development.	Family rules derive from themes and fit a community standard.	Differences and similarities of interaction and communication patterns are noted among different families.	Family members are able to give and receive the amount of support needed for self and each other.
Interview	Tasks and stage of development the family is working on are clear and understood by members.	Members can articulate what is important in their family and what happens if a member breaks a rule.	Members can state functional and dysfunctional communication patterns within the family.	Members can state if they are receiving sufficient support from others in the family.
References	Duvall (1962, 1977).	Smoyak (1982) uses pictures of the family structure called genograms to display information graphically. This allows the nurse to see patterns of themes and rules repeated over generations.	Satir (1988) describes four dysfunctional patterns. Holman (1983) and Hartman (1978) describe how to depict graphically communication patterns among family members using an ecomap. Minuchin (1974) and Minuchin and Fishman (1981) describe techniques to establish family and communication boundaries.	Attneave (1975, 1976) and LaFargue (1984) use family network maps to assess family support.

From a holistic perspective everything—the biologic, psychological, social, and cultural aspects of the family's life—counts.

Family Assessment

Once the nurse has a framework for understanding the family, it is important to know how to make an assess-

ment of the family. For each framework the nurse will collect slightly different data and organize the data according to the focus and principles of the selected framework. Many nursing interventions related to family process are independent nursing functions. In some situations, such as when medication is indicated or admittance to a hospital necessary, interventions are dependent. There is much interdependent collaborative work among nurses and between nurses and other members of

---

Functional Health: Suggestions to Elicit Information Related to Functional Health in the Family

Health Perception and Health Management

- What is your perception of your family's state of health?
- Are you able to cope with family health problems?
- Name one thing you do to promote healthy living for yourself, and for each member of the family.

Nutrition and Metabolism

- Describe your family's eating patterns.
- What are typical meals and when are they served?
- Do you have any special way of preparing family meals?
- Who is the best cook in the house? Why?

Elimination

- Is garbage disposal a problem for your family?
- How is waste and specifically human excrement disposed of in this family?
- What hygiene practices are followed by members of this family after using the toilet?

Activity and Exercise

- How would you characterize the activity level in this family?
- What types of activities does the family engage in as a group? How often does this occur?
- What are the favorite leisure time activities of this family?

Sleep and Rest

- What is the general sleep pattern in this family?
- What happens when this pattern is disturbed?

Cognition and Perception

- How are decisions made in this family?
- Are your decisions more concerete or more abstract, related more to the past, present, or future?

Self-Perception and Self-Concept

- What does each member like and dislike about being part of this family?
- How would each member describe the family?

Roles and Relationships

- Do you consider the relationship among and between family members to be healthy and supportive? Please explain.

Sexuality and Reproduction

- Is it acceptable to discuss issues of sexuality openly in this family?
- When, how, and what are children told about sexuality? Are you satisfied with your expression of sexuality within the family?
- Have there been any reproductive problems in the family? Please explain.

Coping and Stress Tolerance

- Name a stressful event in the family. What was each member's perception of the event? How did each member cope with it?

Values and Beliefs

- What are important beliefs this family holds? How does each member carry out such beliefs?
- How valued are the activities in which members of the family are engaged?

the health team related to family process interventions, however.

It is beyond the scope of this chapter to discuss the various assessment tools in detail. The reader is referred to the references for additional information. At the beginning level, a basic family assessment can be done by observation, comparison, and interview. The areas to be assessed depend on the framework the nurse chooses. Basic areas the nurse might assess are developmental stage, wholeness, communication, and support. These areas can be assessed by observation of behavior in the family, comparison of family behavior to the literature and to other families in similar circumstances, and interview (Table 14-2).

Nursing process in relation to the family is discussed further in Chapter 45.

Family Responsibility for Functional Health

Interaction between the individual and family is all-involving and ongoing. The nurse cannot plan nursing care for the one without assessing the other. Gordon (1982), in her typology of functional health patterns, discusses both of these levels. (Gordon's functional health patterns are discussed in detail in Chapter 6.)

Family members share responsibility with each other for the functional health of all the members. For example, a functional family should discuss health issues and how to lead more healthy lives—issues of prevention. The family can walk or bike together or plan vacations that include activities such as hiking or swimming. Does the person who shops, plans, and cooks meals buy nutritious food, plan healthful meals, and cook without frying?

The accompanying display suggests questions the nurse can ask to elicit information on the interaction of the individual and family as it relates to functional health.

THE COMMUNITY

Nurses in every setting must be aware of their patients' interactions with and within the community. For beginning nursing students, the focus is on resources for the patient and family that exist within the community. The student is encouraged to see patients as individuals within a family in the context of a community. This means that nursing care incorporates the interaction of patients with family members and with other institutions such as employer, religious institution, school, or other social group.

As the student progresses through the nursing curriculum, this foundation will be built on so that the nurse can focus appropriate nursing care on any level of need

---

| Nursing Research: Community |

Selected Nursing Research Studies

Badger, F., Cameron, E., & Evers, H. (1989). The nursing auxiliary service and care of the elderly patients. *Journal of Advanced Nursing, 14,* 471–477.

Christiano, A., & Susser, I. (1989). Knowledge and perceptions of HIV infection among homeless pregnant women. *Journal of Nurse Midwifery, 34,* 318–322.

Crocker, K. S., & Coker, M. H. (1990). Initiation of a home hemotherapy program using a primary nursing model. *Journal of Intravenous Nursing, 13*(1), 13–19.

Melnyk, K. A. M. (1990). Barriers to care: Operationalizing the variable. *Nursing Research, 39,* 108–112.

Stewart, M. J. (1989). Social support intervention studies: A review and prospectus of nursing contributions. *International Journal of Nursing Studies, 26,* 93–114.

Stewart, M. J. (1989). Target populations of nursing research on social support. *International Journal of Nursing Studies, 26,* 115–129.

Possible Topics for Nursing Inquiry

- Does a person's definition of community make a difference in his/her recovery from an illness?
- Do nurses who assess community data write more individualized Visiting Nurse Service referrals than nurses who do not assess community data?
- Is early discharge of hospitalized patients related to resources within their community?
- Are active community participants as likely to become ill as those who are passive?

(individual, family, or community) while not losing sight of the relationships between all three levels (Fig. 14-3).

Definition of Community

A definition of community and knowledge of types of communities form the foundation for understanding more advanced concepts of community. Much has been written about community, but there is no agreement on a single definition. Each attempt at a definition has had a

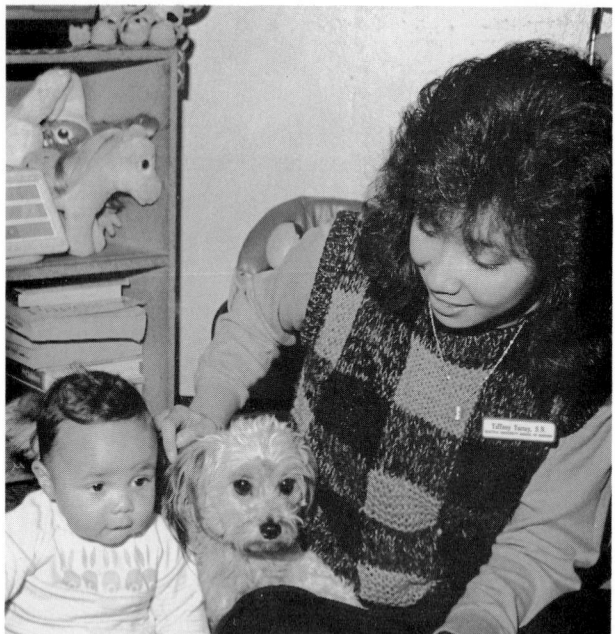

Figure 14–3. The nursing student learns about the individual, family, and community during a family home health-care visit. (Courtesy of Seattle University)

perspective on community as the integration of linkages between individuals. They place these characteristics on a continuum. Along this continuum eight forms of community emerge. At one end is the "highly affective" or traditional community, such as a rural village, and at the opposite end is the "strictly interest group" or community of interest, such as the American Nurses Association.

Higgs and Gustafson (1985) believe that communities are social units and like individuals have a hierarchy of needs. They developed a community typology analogous to Maslow's hierarchy of individual needs. Because they view the community as the client they do not discuss types of communities, but rather enumerate functions of a community (1985, p. 12):

- Use of space
- Means of livelihood
- Production, distribution, and consumption of goods and services
- Protection of its members
- Education
- Participation
- Linkage with other systems

particular focus, the one most appropriate to the community in question. A brief overview of how the definition of community has been summarized gives the nurse a sense of this variety.

Archer (1985) describes three general types of communities: emotional, structural, and functional communities. These community types are similar to Tucker's view of community "as a spatial unit, as an ethnic group with a common culture, and as an aggregate of people with shared values, interests and goals" (Tucker, 1983, p. 173).

Rubin and Rubin (1986) summarize the sociologists'

For the purposes of this chapter, **community** is defined as a social group whose members may or may not share common geographic boundaries, yet who interact because of common interests or shared values to meet their needs within a larger society.

Types of Communities

A list of the types of communities with examples gives the nurse an awareness of the scope of communities. The purpose in doing this is to make the nurse aware of resources that can be used for patients.

TABLE 14–3

Types of Communities: Their Focus and Selected Examples

Type	Focus	Example
Space	Geographic boundaries	Town; hospital; unit of a hospital
People	Characteristics of people	Cajun population in New Orleans; group of adolescent diabetic campers
Institution and Shared Values	Common beliefs and values of a group and their behavior based on those values	American Jesuit Universities; support groups for the caretakers of Alzheimer victims
Interaction of People	Usually centered around interest	Parent–teacher association of a specific school; local nurses association
Distribution of Power	When influence is exerted over others so that, despite resistance, a favorable outcome is obtained	Grey Panther party; American Medical Association
Social System	Interaction between systems	Family–school–hospital–church system
Emotional Security	Emotional ties between people and emphasis on ascribed characteristics	Prenatal classes; ethnic neighbors

TABLE 14–4
Implications for Specific Nursing Interventions for Mrs. Benoli by Types of Communities

Types of Communities	Nursing Needs				
	Mobility	*Nutrition*	*Communication*	*Interests*	*Spirituality*
Space Neighborhood	Set walking criteria within neighborhood boundaries	Eat frequent small meals alone or with one trusted friend	Start with face-to-face communication and a one-to-one interaction with a trusted friend	Engage in gross motor activities around light gardening	Allow priest to come to home while planning how to get to church
People Friends in dress shop	Walk to dress shop to meet with friends	Eat with friends; allow them to assist periodically	Communicate first face-to-face, then in writing, and eventually by phone	Accept suggestions from friends to start new hobbies with them	Allow friends to take to church
Values Do for self	Walk short distances alone versus longer ones with assistance	Use assistive feeding devices	Use electric typewriter or computer where no assistance is needed and message is clear	Remain with known hobbies and learn to readjust to limitations	Go to church rather than have priest come to home
Interaction Stroke support group	Do what others in same circumstances suggest	Do as suggested by leader of the stroke support group	Read and keep abreast of what is new for members of stroke group; try various methods of communication as encouraged within the group	Consider hobbies other members of the stroke support group can do successfully	Use resources of group to get to and from church
Power Italian female elders in the neighborhood	Sees very little need to walk as others will come to her; must walk to maintain independence	Eat with family to maintain public image of being in control	Speak within small sphere of other elderly women	Select a hobby which reflects status and can be mastered	Be physically present at church to act as a role model for the younger generation
Social System Interaction between family–dress shop–neighborhood–church–hospital–elders	Walk outdoors daily to carry out necessary chores	Eat a balanced diet daily with family	Contact two people daily; this can be done either face-to-face, in writing, or by phone	Select one hobby that can be done either alone or in a group	Set aside one hour a day for spiritual reflection; allow neighbors to take to church
Emotional Security Place of birth: Caravaggio, Italy; ethnic group: Italian	Walk as much as possible; would like to visit Caravaggio once again	Eat the foods her grandmother fixed, which she felt had a therapeutic value	Speak Italian and English; make contact with relatives in Italy	Select a hobby which centers around "the old days," and "the old country"	Pray, which takes a large part of the day; going to church is not as meaningful as it once was

Health Perception and Health Management

- Is your community a safe community in which to live? Why?
- What are the major health problems in your community?
- What health problems are on the decline/increase in this community? Why has this decline/increase happened?
- Review morbidity and mortality statistics for the community.

Nutrition and Metabolism

- Do residents seem well nourished in your community?
- Are there any specific nutritional programs in your community?
- Observe specific groups in the community such as children, pregnant women, and the elderly. What does their nutritional status appear to be?

Elimination

- How is hazardous waste disposed of in your community?
- Does your community have a recycling plan? How does it work?
- How is household waste disposed of in your community?
- What infectious diseases in your community can be traced to improper waste disposal?

Activity and Exercise

- How efficient is the public transportation system in your community?
- What are the recreational activities in your community? Who plans them?
- Are there parks, bike, and hike paths?
- What are the cultural activities in your community?

Sleep and Rest

- What is the noise level like in your community at night?
- Do noises in the community interfere with your sleep and rest?

Cognition and Perception

- Are the schools providing a good education?
- How are decisions made in this community? Who participates in decisions that affect all community members?
- Observe the process used by any one group to make their voice heard in the community.

Self-Perception and Self-Concept

- Is there a sense that the community "cares for" its residents?
- Are residents proud of their community? Are they fearful?

Roles and Relationships

- Do community institutions collaborate with each other?
- Can individuals access agencies easily in terms of health-related issues?

Sexuality and Reproduction

- What is the attitude towards sex education in your community? Who should be teaching this material? Are they?
- Review the marriage and birth statistics for the community. Note birth rate, age of mother at pregnancy, abortions, and adoptions.

Coping and Stress Tolerance

- What are the issues causing stress in your community? (Examples drawn from other communities are racial tension, child molestation, AIDS, and noise pollution.)

Values and Beliefs

- How effective are the local media (newspaper, radio, television)? Who makes decisions on programming?
- Do people feel strongly about local government? Do they vote?
- What health-related issues would your community spend money on? What issues would they not?
- How would you complete this sentence related to health issues in your community? We believe that health _____

_____.

The early work of Warren (1963) still provides a useful approach to ways of examining types of communities. His six types of communities (space, people, institution, interaction, distribution, and social system) are discrete and provide useful guidelines for nursing care. Definitions previously discussed combine several of the types described by Warren. Archer's emotional community and Rubin and Rubin's affective community are not addressed in Warren's list, however. These can be combined into a seventh category: emotional security. Table 14-3 summarizes seven types of communities.

Community Assessment

When the nurse is able to understand a patient's community, nursing care and discharge planning are enhanced by using appropriate community resources. The case of Mrs. Benoli illustrates this point.

The nurse might ask Mrs. Benoli to describe her community. Such assessment focuses discharge planning on two points: a method the client finds acceptable, and a method using community resources to a maximum. The implications for Mrs. Benoli's nursing care, based on the type of community, are summarized in Table 14-4. This matrix shows possible goals on which the nurse and client could agree. The table is by no means exhaustive, but is meant to show the nursing student a preliminary way to think of resources based on client needs and types of communities.

Community Responsibility for Functional Health

The community environment affects the well-being of the individual and the family. Government, educational, recreational, and health care services affect all phases of functional health. One community may have suitable grocery stores with fresh produce and meats at a reasonable price whereas another neighborhood may sell questionable products at a higher price. One community may provide free smoke detectors and teach people how to check batteries whereas another community ignores the issue of fires and safety. Conversely, some communities may be more prone to fires, such as run-down, crowded, inner-city areas with boarded-up houses and litter-strewn fire hazards.

Systems theory suggests that the community has responsibilities toward the family, but the family also is responsible for taking part in community activities and promoting good services. In the same vein, the community is responsible to the health-care system for providing adequate facilities and resources. Health-care workers participate in a feedback loop by volunteering in community activities, acting as resources, and assessing community needs and services.

The display covering family health in the community lists questions to be asked of individuals, community representatives, and nurses. The questions apply to the community at large or, on a smaller scale, to institutions such as hospitals, schools, and factories.

Advanced Community Concepts

Organizing and intervening at a community level are advanced concepts that are beyond the level of the beginning nursing student. These concepts require the nurse to conceptualize community as the unit receiving care. There are several approaches to studying community in this way. Higgs and Gustafson (1985), for example, discuss community assessment and diagnosis from four perspectives: epidemiologic, descriptive, systems, and adaptive.

The concept of "at risk" is also a useful concept, since it targets the group most likely to encounter health-related problems. In so doing, preventive measures can be taken to stop those problems either before they occur or in the early stages. Research and health programs in the community target "at risk" communities.

Key Concepts

- People need to be understood in terms of their priority needs based on Maslow's hierarchy of basic needs.
- Nursing care for the individual is best developed in the context of the patient's family and community.
- An individual can meet some basic needs independently but often needs the family and community for help in meeting needs.
- Gordon's functional health patterns are useful at the individual, family, and community levels.
- Conceptual frameworks provide useful guidelines for organizing family information.
- Developmental frameworks focus on developmental tasks and role expectations of parents and children throughout the life cycle.
- Family systems frameworks look at the interaction of the parts, such as individual members, that make up the whole, the family.
- Methods for assessing family functioning are observation, comparison, and interviewing.
- Different types of communities offer different types of resources to their residents.
- Nurses need to use community resources for their patients.
- Nurses should find a means of participating in the community.

References

American Nurses Association. (1973). *Standards: Nursing practice.* Kansas City, MO: Author.

Archer, S. E. (1985). Selected concepts and process for client-centered community health nursing. In S. E. Archer & R. P. Fleshman (Eds.), *Community health nursing* (3rd ed.) (pp. 96–130). Monterey, CA: Wadsworth Health Sciences.

Attneave, C. L. (1975). *Family network map.* Available from The Boston Family Institute, 315 Dartmouth Street, Boston, MA 02116.

Attneave, C. L. (1976). Social network as the unit of intervention. In P. Guerin (Ed.), *Family therapy: Theory and practice* (pp. 220–231). New York: Gardner Press.

Bowen, M. (1978). *Family therapy in clinical practice.* New York: Janson Arson.

Carter, E. A., & McGoldrick, M. (Eds.). (1980). *The family life cycle: A framework for family therapy.* New York: Gardner Press.

Duvall, E. M. (1962). *Development* (2nd ed.). Philadelphia: J. B. Lippincott.

Duvall, E. M. (1977). *Marriage and family development* (5th ed.). Philadelphia: J. B. Lippincott.

Fortes, M. (1971). Introduction. In J. Goody (Ed.), *The developmental cycle in domestic groups* (reprint) (pp. 1–14). Cambridge: The University Press.

Gordon, M. (1982). *Nursing diagnosis: Process and application.* New York: McGraw-Hill.

Haley, J. (1971). Approaches to family therapy. In J. Haley (Ed.), *Changing families, a family therapy reader* (pp. 227–236). New York: Grune & Stratton.

Higgs, Z. R., & Gustafson, D. D. (1985). *Community as a client: Assessment and diagnosis.* Philadelphia: F. A. Davis.

Hartman, A. M. (1978). A diagrammatic assessment of family relationships. *Social Casework, 59,* 465–476.

Holman, A. M. (1983). *Family assessment tools for understanding and intervention.* Beverly Hills: Sage Publications.

LaFargue, J. P. (1984). Application of cultural concepts to nursing care: Working with family networks. In J. Uhl (Ed.), *Proceedings of the Ninth Annual Transcultural Nursing Conference* (pp. 14–26). Salt Lake City: The Transcultural Nursing Society.

Maslow, A. H. (1968). *Toward a philosophy of being* (2nd ed.). New York: Van Nostrand Reinhold.

Minuchin, S. (1974). *Families and family therapy.* Cambridge: Harvard University Press.

Minuchin, S., & Fishman, H. C. (1981). *Family therapy techniques.* Cambridge: Harvard University Press.

Rubin, H. J., & Rubin, I. (1986). *Community organizing and development.* Columbus, OH: Merrill.

Satir, V. (1988). *The new peoplemaking.* Mountain View, CA: Science and Behavior Books.

Smoyak, S. (1982). Family systems: Use of genograms as an assessment tool. In I. W. Clements & D. M. Buchanan (Eds.), *Family therapy: A nursing perspective* (pp. 245–250). New York: John Wiley & Sons.

Tucker, W. H. (1983). The nature of a community. In M. J. Fromer (Ed.), *Community health care and the nursing process* (2nd ed.) (pp. 173–198). St. Louis: C. V. Mosby.

von Bertalanffy, L. (1968). *General system theory: Foundations, development, applications.* New York: George Braziller.

Warren, R. L. (1963). *The community in America.* Chicago: Rand McNally.

Bibliography

Thompson, M. K. (1984). Family development theory. *Nurse Practitioner, 9*(6), 54–58.

Uphols, C. R., & Strickland, O. L. (1989). Issues related to the unit of analysis in family nursing research. *Western Journal of Nursing, 11,* 405–417.

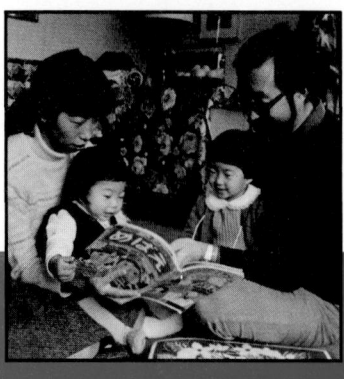

Culture and Ethnicity

LEARNING OBJECTIVES

Upon completion of this chapter, the student will be able to do the following:

- Discuss characteristics of culture.
- Define concepts related to culture.
- View human responses in a cultural context from which to build an understanding of people.
- Identify patterns of behavior that reflect cultural and ethnic influences.
- Communicate effectively with people of diverse orientations.
- Increase awareness of personal culturation and its influence on nursing practice.
- Recognize and discuss cultures and ethnic groups represented in the community.

KEY TERMS

Belief
Cultural relativity
Cultural sensitivity
Culture
Culture shock

Ethnicity or ethnic
  identity
Ethnocentrism
Key informant
Minority

Race
Racism
Stereotype
Subculture

15

What is Culture?
  Characteristics of Culture
Concepts Related to Culture
  Ethnicity or Ethnic Identity
  Minority
  Race
  Racism
  Subculture
  Stereotype

Implications of the Concept of Culture for Nursing
  Need for Culturally Sensitive Nursing Care
  Taking Account of Biocultural Variation
  Grounding Nursing Assessments in the Patient's
    Perspective
  When the Patient Does Not Speak the Nurse's
    Language
  Increased Effectiveness of Patient Education
Key Concepts

Nursing is concerned with human responses to actual or potential health problems (American Nurses' Association, 1980). In this chapter, the student is encouraged to think about how those responses might be affected by the patient's and the nurse's cultural backgrounds. The learner is invited to recast such common patient descriptors as "noncompliant," "uncooperative," "resistant," "malingering," or "uncommunicative" into cultural assessments of the patient or family and of the health-care system that labels them. To arrive at a more accurate and empathic understanding of patients (MacGregor, 1976). Cultural assessments identify patterns of behavior over time from the same person and from people of similar background. They are fundamental ways to "locate" culture in carrying out the nursing process.

This chapter will help students take account of culture—their own, their patients', and nursing's—in their nursing care. Understanding culture and ethnicity helps improve the quality of nursing care in several ways: by increasing the diversity of people with whom nurses communicate effectively; by enabling nurses to attend more accurately to the integrity of the patient as a socially and culturally connected person; and by preventing nurses from imposing, however unintentionally, their own culturally shaped presuppositions on patients and peers.

In the first part of the chapter, theoretical interpretations of culture and related concepts are examined. Related concepts include ethnicity or ethnic identity, minority, race, racism, subculture, and stereotype. In the second part of the chapter, implications of culture and ethnicity for nursing are discussed. Particular emphasis is placed on nursing assessment and intervention.

WHAT IS CULTURE?

Nursing derives the concept of culture and methods for studying it from anthropology. The anthropologic concept of culture is relatively new; it was first defined in print only in 1871 (Tylor, 1871). Since then, various schools of thought about culture have waxed and waned, but most anthropologists would agree that "culture controls behavior in deep and persisting ways, many of which are outside of awareness and therefore beyond conscious control of the individual" (Hall, 1959). In this chapter, the following definition of culture is explained:

> **Culture** is a belief system that the culture members hold, consciously or unconsciously, as absolute truth. That belief system guides everyday behavior and makes it routine; it provides answers to the unanswerable questions of life, sickness and death; and it makes the world make sense. Culture thus enables a person to behave reasonably in contexts that s/he shares with members of the same culture.

There are many other definitions of culture. *Culture* can imply qualitative enrichment: the intellectual and aesthetic content of civilizations is called *culture,* and people become *cultured* by engaging in the fine arts; bees, fish, and oysters are *cultured* to increase their supply. Culture is also thought to make humans qualitatively distinct, distinguishing *Homo sapiens* from other orders of being. Both psychological and sociologic characteristics have been found in plants (Goetschs, 1937; Rhoades, 1985; Tompkins & Bird, 1972) and animals (Darling, 1937; Goodall, 1986), but neither is thought to have and create culture. This is because other animals and phylogenetically lower forms of life are believed not to have the capacity that humans do to communicate in symbols. Construction and use of symbols as effective and powerful vehicles of human communication reflects the human capacity for culture (Douglas, 1973).

Almost anything can carry symbolic meaning. Colors, for example, tend to do so universally, but their meaning varies across cultures and by context (Berlin & Kay, 1969). Black signifies death and mourning among Westerners, but white does the same for Chinese. Westerners color-code sex (pink and blue) and movement (red and green), but not time or social status. The Thai color-code time and social status, but not sex or movement: they designate a specific color as auspicious for each day of the week and reserve blue for royalty and yellow-gold for monks and the king. Christians clothe their priests in black and white; Mahayana Buddhists clothe their monks in gray; Mien* clothe their shamans in red. The traditional white of hospital nurses' uniforms symbolizes the cleanliness and purity of nursing. Physicians, in contrast, wear white jackets or coats that convey the same symbolic meaning, but with dark pants or skirts, the dark color signifying authority.

Nurse anthropologists generally concur that "whatever a person believes to be true or right about any aspect of his [sic] life stems from his culture" (Brink, 1976). Culture patterns ways of perceiving, interpreting and evaluating, and responding to life and the world (Boyle & Andrews, 1989a). It provides a blueprint for reacting, feeling, behaving, and interacting socially. People who grow up or live together in the same thought and communication community share a culture. Their experiences are carved by a shared cultural heritage. That heritage shapes their behavior just as grammar shapes a language: it provides rules that are so well-known to a native that they are followed automatically.

In Western society, for example, spitting in public is considered dirty and aggressive, but exposing the nude body for physical examination by nurses or physicians is generally accepted protocol. In Moslem societies, in contrast, spitting during ritual ablutions is understood as a religious act of cleansing, and exposure of the bare body, particularly to people of the opposite sex, is highly embarrassing and offensive because it violates strong cultural mores associated with intimacy. Such different interpretations of the same behaviors indicate that culture is learned and taught within a society. Culture is the

---

*The Mein are a people who live a seminomadic lifestyle of agricultural self-subsistence in the hills of Laos. Some of them fought with the CIA against the communists in the 1960s and 1970s in the Vietnam War. With the 1975 takeover of the Laotian government by the communists, many Mien fled as refugees, and some have resettled in the United States.

accumulated "common sense" shared and generated among members of a group. It provides solutions to common problems of living that have been handed down through generations (Leininger, 1970b).

In Western society, spitting was not disparaged for centuries. Spitting became an unattractive behavior in the West only when public health science changed the understanding of the world by showing that bacteria cause disease and that sputum carries bacteria. What triggered the reversal of Westerners' attitude toward spitting was the association of spitting with tuberculosis, which in the late 19th century was highly prevalent and feared. This example shows that culture is created by people, often unconsciously, when their old common sense doesn't work, as when they attempt to deal with new knowledge, situations, challenges, or threats.

It is *vital* for nurses to understand how culture affects behavior and what functions it serves, for two reasons. First, nurses are accountable for observing and assessing patients' responses; second, culture influences all learned human responses. *Culture is, consequently, an integral component of the knowledge base of nursing.* Culture makes communication highly efficient among people who share the same culture, but it can seriously distort and squelch communication among people who don't understand each other's cultures. Culture enables people of similar cultural heritage to understand the meanings of each other's words as part of the particular context in which they are expressed, to "read" each other's nonverbal behavior fairly accurately (often so well that they are barely aware they are doing so; Hall, 1969), and to communicate through symbols.

It has been estimated that at least *two thirds of the meaning of a social interaction is communicated nonverbally,* that is, in gestures, vocalizations (sighs, throat clearing, laughter, grunts, whistling, and so forth), and use of space and distance (Birdwhistell, 1970). This means that even when a nurse cares for a patient who speaks English, if the nurse and the patient don't understand each other's cultures, they are likely to misconstrue at least two thirds of each other's messages or information.

Characteristics of Culture

Characteristics of culture are summarized in the accompanying display.

Culture Is Learned. By sustained contact between groups and by repeated observations of and participation in a group, culture is learned. It takes time to learn a culture. Some of the learning is purposeful, and some is absorbed without awareness. When the culture one has learned is different from the culture learned by the people in one's environment, one can become radically disoriented and stressed. The acute experience of not com-

---

Characteristics of Culture

Culture Is

Learned, not innate
Learned from other people
Shared by people who communicate with each other over time
Shared unequally by its members: some learn and use more of it than others, and some have and use more access to it than others
Always changing, at variable rates
Reasonable from the perspective of the members of the culture
Implicit, not easily described by its own members
Habituated assumptions
Ethnocentric
Relative
Pervasive and holistic
Recognizable in patterns at many levels

Culture Is Not

Predictable at the level of the individual
Necessarily logical or reasonable to the outside observer
A set of traits

Culture Functions To

Guide behavior by providing a "blueprint" for action
Interpret or give meaning to experience
Explain what otherwise is unknowable: why we are born; why we are born into the families we are; why we suffer our afflictions, dream our dreams, die our deaths, and have experiences different from others

---

Culture Is Unequally Shared. Because culture is unequally shared by its members, not all members of the same culture act and think alike. Knowing a cultural norm does *not* enable one to predict a person's response. It is particularly inappropriate to generalize about cultural norms in contemporary urban societies because people belong to more than one subcultural group and are influenced uniquely by multiple diverse reference groups. There are always exceptions to cultural norms. For example, Americans pride themselves on being generous and altruistic and admire others who are the same. Yet millions of people and families with children are homeless on U.S. streets, or do not get basic health care because they cannot afford it. Much of American international aid is actually disposal of surplus or obsolete material that otherwise would not be used. Americans also think of themselves as friendly, yet people from other cultures may view this friendliness as insensitively intrusive or aggressive; and patients waiting in public hospital and clinic waiting rooms are not likely to find the atmosphere there friendly.

People who know certain aspects of their culture better than others are called **key informants.** Usually, key informants not only have an especially rich base of cultural knowledge, they also are reflective, like to talk, and have consciously considered their culture so that they can discuss it. Nurses, for example, often make excellent key informants on hospital culture (Anderson, 1979; Germain, 1979).

Culture Changes. Culture changes as people come into contact with new beliefs and ideas. Culture change is much more rapid in the 20th century than ever before because of the vast reduction in distances between different peoples that the communication and transportation industries have achieved (Fig. 15-1). Immigrants and refugees from developing countries who resettle in North America change their cultures quickly—consciously or not, they revise their culture by blending

prehending the culture in which one is situated is called **culture shock** (Oberg, 1954). Culture shock is a stress syndrome that normally progresses through a series of recognizable stages (honeymoon, disenchantment, beginning resolution, and effective function) to its resolution (Brink & Saunders, 1976). Patients from other cultures or countries where health-care systems are not as technologically complex as in North America are at risk for culture shock if they are suddenly hospitalized here. Resolution of culture shock requires time, opportunity to observe and participate in the new setting, and careful anticipatory guidance that introduces people, behaviors, and events of the new environment as they affect daily routine.

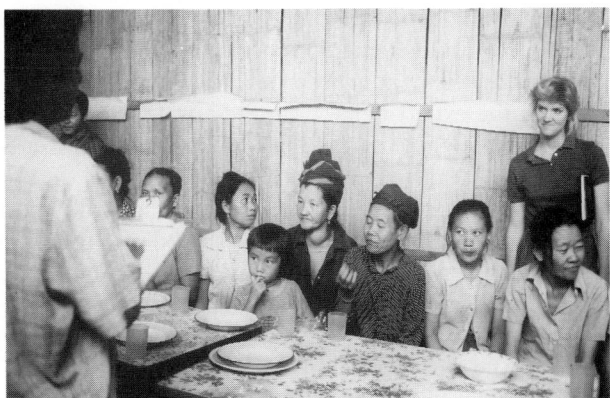

Figure 15–1. A nurse-facilitated support group in a refugee camp, Chiang Kham, Thailand. (Photo courtesy of Marjorie A. Muecke.)

those things from their original culture that seem to work in their new surroundings with new behaviors, attitudes, or beliefs that they find, often by trial and error, work and make life easier for them. Simultaneously, North American society is changed by the introduction of cultural ideas from refugees, immigrants, foreign business, and media from abroad. For example, there has been a rise in demand for and use of (Chinese) acupuncture in medicine and a surge in popularity of "ethnic" food and restaurants, clothes, and music.

Culture Is Reasonable from the Perspective of Its Members. Members of the culture in question find their culture reasonable, even though it might seem illogical, counterproductive, or insensitive to an outsider. People such as spouses in cross-cultural marriages, resettling refugees, patients who come from abroad for specialized health care, or those who for whatever reasons move quickly from one culture to another tend to act according to the rules of their culture of origin. When those rules do not make a reasonable fit with cultural rules in their new setting, they are culturally stressed, at risk for culture shock. Ways in which the culturally informed nurse can minimize this stress are addressed in the section of this chapter entitled "Grounding Nursing Assessment in the Patient's Perspective."

Culture Is Not Easily Described by Its Own Members. Much of culture is implicit, a combination of habit and habituated assumptions about the world. Habits are enacted without reflection in the daily course of living. Thus, asking patients directly "What do you believe about (for example) prenatal care?" may be a less productive a approach than reading about a cultural group or talking with a key informant about it.

Culture Is Habituated Assumptions. Culture is habituated assumptions that people learn through socialization as they grow up and become deeply involved in different subcultures. Cultural habituation is advantageous in that it reduces the extent to which we have to take environmental cues into account—it allows us to respond to routine situations almost without thinking. This is a key element in expertise. Benner (1984) differentiates the expert nurse from the novice nurse on the basis of being able to take in a large number of cues rapidly; to scan, assess, and prioritize them; and to respond appropriately and effectively in unusually short order. To the extent that culture is shared with others in our community, cultural habituation makes our world familiar and predictable. Having a predictable environment, being able to perceive the world as coherent, is essential for our functioning. Without it, we suffer extreme mental stress (Antonovsky, 1980), a mild form of which is culture shock.

Culture Is Ethnocentric. Because culture is generally learned from authority figures (parents, priests, peers,

and so forth), one tends to hold cultural beliefs as truth. The use of one's own culture as the only correct standard by which to view people of other cultures is **ethnocentrism.** It reflects a fear of difference from one's belief system, and consequent derision or disqualification of people and practices that do not conform to one's own view. Because cultural habituation makes us unaware of many of our cultural assumptions, we are not always aware of our cultural biases. This is why, for example, some whites have difficulty accepting the charge of white supremacy that may be leveled against them by blacks, or why some men have trouble understanding charges of their being male chauvinists by women.

Culture Is Relative. The example of variation in the meanings of colors across cultures given above demonstrates the principle of cultural relativity. Another example is the handshake. Westerners attribute trust and agreement to the handshake, and view it as a positive social act. Asians may avoid handshaking because it involves touching a stranger or touching hands that may be dirty. A cultural interpretation of the difference is that the handshake by itself is meaningless; when carried out by Westerners it is invested with one meaning and when enacted by Asians it has another. At its extreme, the principle of cultural relativity would assume that there is no absolute, that nothing has meaning by itself, that the meaning or significance of any act or symbol is created and assigned by human groups. It has been argued that such an extreme position is untenable because it is amoral. Most nurses accept the principle of cultural relativity only up to a certain (but variable) degree.

Culture Is Pervasive. A culture is a systematic way of interpreting people, behaviors, and events holistically. The holistic nature of culture is congenial with nurses' concern that nursing care be holistic, individualized, and safe. Both the cultural and nursing approaches regard people in their entire humanity, and both direct attention to the total context of a person or group (Leininger, 1970a). Culture links a wide variety of disparate behaviors and events in unique ways. For example, for Western nurses, autopsy is culturally linked to medical beliefs (that cause of death can be discovered or validated by examination of the internal organs and tissues; and that by learning organic causes of death, death can be postponed or prevented); to the Cartesian belief in the separation of the body and soul; and to the Judeo-Christian belief that the body ultimately decomposes into "dust" or generic organic matter. Peoples of other cultural heritages may link autopsy with other belief systems and practices. For example, Hmong† who have not converted to Christianity tend to link autopsy to their recent experience of genocide in Laos and to their beliefs in

---

† Like the Mien, the Hmong have resettled in Western countries as refugees from the Vietnam War.

reincarnation, multiple souls, and the inseparability of body and spirit. They tend to interpret autopsy as preventing the continuation of their society by preventing the union of a person's souls with its body after death, thereby making it impossible to be reborn.

Culture Is Recognizable at Many Levels. The easiest level of culture to recognize is *material*—in artwork, drama, tools, clothes, food, buildings, rituals. Generally, we think of rituals as events such as Thanksgiving dinner, weddings, funerals, and parades; however, there are also nursing rituals—report, handwashing, gowning, nursing rounds, annual professional meetings, and so forth. Harder to recognize are *values and beliefs.* Sometimes they can be accessed by asking about items of material culture. For example, interested, nonjudgmental inquiry about a tattoo on a patient's arm could lead to explanations about the person's religious background (from a Coptic Christian), belief in magic (from a Thai), or occupational history (from an American sailor). Sometimes understanding a people's values and beliefs requires long-term contact with careful observation and inquiry about patterns in behavior. Although this is the approach of anthropologists, it takes too long for most nurses. Its results are available to nurses in books, journals, documentary movies/videos, lectures, and coursework.

CONCEPTS RELATED TO CULTURE

A number of concepts are so closely related to the concept of culture that each may sometimes be used synonymously with culture, but each also carries some specific connotation. The concepts to be discussed are ethnicity or ethnic identity, minority, race, racism, subculture, and stereotype. In North American society, blacks, Chinese, Hmong, Mexican-Americans, whites, and similar categories of peoples may be legitimately referred to as ethnic groups, minorities, or subcultures, depending on context, and each group may be stereotyped. The accompanying display illustrates that there may be statistically definable differences among groups differentiated by such cultural labels.

Ethnicity or Ethnic Identity

Ever since Erik Erikson published his "Reflections on the American Identity" in *Childhood and Society* (Erikson, 1950), ethnicity has implied a culturally informed identity (Petersen, Novak, & Gleason, 1980). **Ethnicity or ethnic identity** refers to a *self-conscious past-oriented* form of identity that is based on a notion of shared cultural and perhaps ancestral heritage, and current position in larger society. Whites in North America, for example, have an ethnic identity that is grounded in a sense of common European heritage and the associated migration to the land where they were free to develop

---

> **Cultural Variation in Health: Birthweight and Infant Mortality**
>
> People of the same cultural background share some learned standards of behavior that may be reflected in characteristic morbidity, mortality and fertility patterns. For example, in the United States, the proportion of low-birthweight (<2500 g) infants among total births is lower among Chinese (4.9%) than among other groups for whom figures are available: Whites (5.6%), Mexican-Americans (5.7%), Hmong (9.9%), and blacks (12.4%). Similarly, infant mortality rates (per 1000 live births) are lowest among Chinese (5.9), almost twice as high among whites (11.4), and over three higher among blacks (21.8).
>
> From Hahn, R. A., & Muecke, M. A. (1987). The anthropology of birth in five populations: Implications for obstetrical practice. *Curr Probl Obstet Gynecol Fertil, 10*(4), 133–171.

---

frontiers. The ethnicity of blacks in North America is linked to a belief in common descent from African peoples and a history of having been brought from there against their wills as slaves to white supremacists.

What distinguishes ethnic identity from culture is that ethnic identity is self-conscious, specifically about select symbolic elements that are taken as the cynosure or emblem of social identity. In one context, an ethnic group might use native language as its cynosure, as Hmong or Mien do to distinguish themselves from other groups in North America. In another context, the group might draw on other ethnic indicators, such as style of dress (as when Hmong of one tribe encounter Hmong of another tribe) or religion (as when animist Hmong exclude Christian Hmong from the ranks of "true" Hmong).

Ethnicity involves the selection of certain shared cultural characteristics as symbols of a common group origin, history, or descent. That selection may be made by the ethnic group or by the larger society to which it is subordinate. Margaret Mead (1982, p. 175) has documented a history of change in North Americans' images of Native Americans:

> The early explorers in the south painted the portraits of the southeast Indians as royalty and nobles, placing on their impressive physiognomy the mark of European aristocracy and dressing them in the clothing of the courts. Faced with a need to come to terms with those who possessed the land and knew how to live on it, the settlers elevated them to petty princes before whom it was no shame to ask for help or to admit failure, in the disease-ridden, inexpertly managed colonies of the southeast.

And, after centuries of subjection, ruthless pillage, and exile into remote reservations, the ethnic emblems of Native Americans remained ambiguous status symbols:

> Thus, in the 1930s the Indians of Oklahoma who were oil rich used to go to New York and buy theatric Indian costumes for the poorer members of other tribes to wear in local rodeos. In Florida the remnants of different tribes gathered into an artificial synthesis, costumed in European materials, and set themselves up in tourist-oriented Seminole villages.

Ethnic emblems preserve and create a sense of special social identity (e.g., the valuable Indian Head nickel), but even such romanticized images as those described by Mead deny regard for ethnically badged groups as human beings.

Minority

Several parameters define the term **minority**: social power, size of the population, and ethnicity. Generally, the term refers to a disadvantaged or less powerful group rather than to a numeric minority (Wirth, 1945). A minority does not have the preeminent authority over the society's value system and the allocation of its resources that the dominant segment does (Schermerhorn, 1978a). People in ethnic groups are usually considered minorities because more ethnic groups are in subordinate than dominant positions in society. Thus, the term emphasizes the political dimension of cultural identity in a pluralistic society such as the United States or Canada, each of which has numerous ethnic groups.

Race

Although the terms *race* and *ethnic group* sometimes refer to the same people, **race** takes biologic characteristics as the markers of separate social status, and ethnic group takes them as markers of cultural identity. The biologic features used to differentiate racial groups are easily identifiable only in the extreme or at the level of large population groups such as Asians, blacks, or whites. They include blood type, bone length, and the size, shape, and number of teeth. There are *no* true or readily identifiable physiologic boundaries between races, however, because interracial marriages have made countless people part of more than one racial heritage. Because criteria for identifying race are so loose, the U.S. Census Bureau no longer uses standardized criteria to identify racial heritage; rather, it asks each person to identify his or her own race or racial mix without regard for the criteria for doing so. This practice equates race with ethnic identity.

Racism

Since the Renaissance, European expansion occurred at the expense of peoples whose skin was of darker hue. As a result, skin color has become the symbol of both social status or power and cultural difference. **Racism** takes skin color as the only indicator of social value. In Western society, racism reserves legitimate dominance only for those with white skin. This form of racism defines peoples with darker skin as inferior because of accidents of history that denied them resources and privileges of the elite, rather than because of innate difference. In its maximal form, racism defines people as inferior on the basis of skin color as part of a natural order of existence. Extreme racism is an ideology of the elite who use it to legitimate and perpetuate their dominance and their oppression and exploitation of peoples of different skin color (Schermerhorn, 1978b).

Subculture

A **subculture** is a holistic belief system that is marginal and subordinate to the belief system of a culture, and that is held most expertly by a recognizable portion of the larger population. The beliefs and standards of a subculture are active only when a person or group acts in a particular social capacity, such as an occupational group or an ethnic group (Harwood, 1981b).

Nursing is a middle class subculture of Western society, particularly of Western medicine. It epitomizes the valued role of nurturers and caregivers. Nurses reflect many values of the dominant group: they generally adhere to the work ethic whereby work is seen as a reward, independent of other compensation; they spend much talent and time on planning for the future; they are keenly sensitive to use of time. Nurses are recognizable as a subgroup in numerous ways: by their authoritative stance vis-a-vis patients and the general public; by their dress; by their language ("nursese" includes a large vocabulary of acronyms specific to health-care professions). Nurses must be aware of their own subcultural values and behaviors so that they can modify them when working with patients for whom they are unfamiliar or uncomfortable.

Subcultural identity, like ethnic identity, can be a source of social support or it can be a target for stigma and exploitation (Fig. 15-2). For example, in the 1960s, Oscar Lewis' work (Lewis, 1966) spread the notion that poverty is a subculture. Poverty was held to be the vehicle for personal and family disorganization, and for fatalism (Harrington, 1962). The theory that culture accounts for poverty blames the poor for being poor: it implies that if people weren't fatalistic and if they pulled themselves up by their bootstraps, they would not be poor. Critics of the culture of poverty school have disproven the theory by demonstrating that societal mecha-

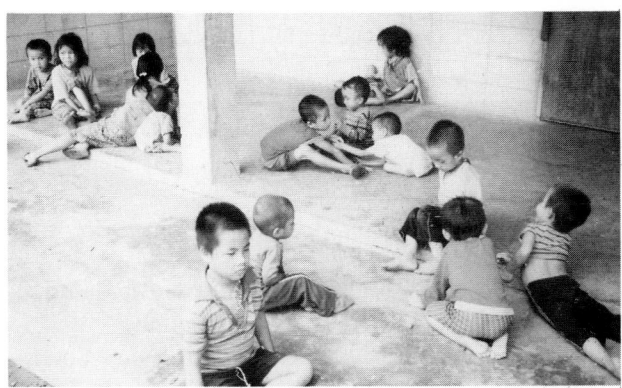

Figure 15–2. Day care for physically disabled children in a refugee camp, Baan Vinai, Thailand. (Children with obvious disabilities would otherwise be kept at home and not sent to school.) (Photo courtesy of Marjorie A. Muecke.)

nisms such as the welfare system and the lack of adequate day care for children are structural and value characteristics of the larger society that maintain people in poverty. They have noted that many of the features said to be characteristic of the culture of poverty, such as unemployment and low wages, are characteristic of poverty, not of culture (Stack, 1974; Valentine, 1968). Informed professionals no longer adhere to the notion of a subculture of poverty.

Stereotype

Assigning people to specific categories because of their culture, race, or ethnic emblems is stereotypic thinking. **Stereotypes** are preconceived and untested beliefs about people. They are exaggerated descriptors of character or behavior that are commonly reiterated in the mass media, idiomatic expressions, and folklore. They may be denigrating ("people on welfare are lazy, just living off handouts"; "the rich are greedy and selfish") or idealizing ("Vietnamese are the valedictorians"; "nurses are patient people"; "physicians are gods on feet"). Either way, they mislead the hearer and deny the individuality of the person.

Use of stereotypes in nursing results in wrong assessments and, consequently, inappropriate and potentially harmful and unethical interventions or nonaction. For example, acting on the stereotype that "Orientals are stoic" could result in the nurse's failure to assess pain and to undertake nursing measures to alleviate pain in a patient who looks "Oriental."

IMPLICATIONS OF THE CONCEPT OF CULTURE FOR NURSING

Culture shapes all learned human responses. Patients and clients have the right to receive care that is culturally

acceptable to them. Because nursing focuses on human responses to actual or threatened health problems, nurses increase the quality and safety of their care insofar as they take account of cultural influences on a patient's, family's, or community's responses to illness. Culture is an integral component of the knowledge base of nursing.

Need for Culturally Sensitive Nursing Care

The culturally sensitive nurse is alert to the possibility of cultural influences on behavior as part of routine assessments of patients, families, and communities. Common cues to subcultural or ethnic identity that should be assessed include religion, native language or language spoken at home, strong food preferences, characteristic body adornments (including tattoos, amulets, head coverings, and jewelry), and communication style (including decision-making, relationship to authority figures, and relationships to the same and opposite sexes). Once identified, the culturally sensitive nurse arranges to adapt nursing *and* medical care to respect the patient's subcultural characteristics to the extent that puts the patient at greatest ease while ensuring medical safety. The nurse should expect to find cultural variation in patient responses to pain, hygiene practices and exposure of the body, food preferences and eating styles, gestures (eye contact, touch), the sex and age of the health-care provider, isolation and quiet, and visitors, among other areas.

The cultural assessment should identify not only cultural characteristics of the patient to take into account for nursing care, but also areas of discrepancy between the patient's culture and the culture of the nurse and health-care setting. Areas of discrepancy indicate the need for providing anticipatory guidance and for clarifying nursing and medical expectations for the patient. This clarification might require the assistance of a trained interpreter. Culturally informed case management prevents or minimizes culture shock for the patient who is embedded in the subculture of a hospital or health-care agency. It also reinforces the patient's sense of competency, thereby promoting learning for self-care.

It is becoming increasingly important for nurses to exercise cultural sensitivity. Demographic trends, such as the rise in average age of the population and the increasing ethnic heterogeneity of the population, expand the proportion of patients for whom primary prevention, health education, and long-term care are fundamental intervention strategies. If these interventions are to result in effective outcomes, the nurse must understand the patient's lifestyle, living environment, and values and beliefs.

Other major but more recent changes in society—the emergence of the AIDS pandemic, the practice of early

Health/Illness Considerations Among Five Major Ethnic Groups in North America

Asian American

Health/Wellness Concept

Spiritual and physical harmony among body, mind, spirit, and nature. Equilibrium among natural forces (*yin* and *yang* for Chinese; humoral elements of earth, fire, air, and water for Southeast Asian). Body is a gift from parents, ancestors, or gods, and should be cared for.

Illness Concept

Imbalance between *yin* and *yang,* or among humoral elements may cause illness, either immediately or years later (as in the case of postpartal imbalances). Eating the wrong food, breaking obligations to parents or ancestors, or dishonoring religious principles are also seen as possible causes of illness.

Treatment Concept

Strong self-care component: Chinese or herbal domestic medicine, massage, skin rubbing or pinching (Southeast Asians), dietary modifications, and over-the-counter medications for symptom abatement. Prefer physicians of own ethic group, and health-care providers of same sex as patient. Some groups (e.g., Japanese, Vietnamese) seek intrusive care, others (e.g., Hmong) strongly avoid it. Adults are responsible for the care of their children and of their aged parents.

Examples of Significant Health Problems

Lactose intolerance, hemoglobinopathies, hepatitis B.

Urban Black

Health/Wellness Concept

Good health is the responsibility of the individual adult, and of the wife/mother for children. It is maintained by cleanliness, adequate rest and nutrition, and observing the dictates of religion (usually Protestant, also Muslim).

Illness Concept

Divine punishment, stress, worry, or sorcery can cause illness. Widespread use of ethnic illness labels such as *low blood* (anemia?), *high blood* ("swimming in the head"), *bruised blood* (hematoma?), *sugar* (diabetes mellitus), *falling out* (brief state of semiconsciousness). Emotional or mental illness is stigmatizing.

Treatment Concept

Self-care with home medications mostly by mother or oldest daughter. Consult friends, relatives, folk healers, religious leaders. Use prayer, song. Seek medical care for sexually transmitted diseases, problems with pregnancy, wounds; treat for symptom abatement. Tend *not* to seek medical care when believe they are seriously ill. Some religious groups avoid medical care (e.g., Jehovah's Witnesses eschew blood transfusion).

Examples of Significant Health Problems

Hypertension, sickle cell anemia, smoking-related cancers, diabetes, male homicide, high infant and maternal mortalities, high cancer mortalities.

Native American

Health/Wellness Concept

Maintain health through harmonious relationships with people, nature, and the supernaturals. Avoid taboos to avoid illness. Both education and religious affiliation affect the nature of concepts of health.

Illness Concept

Illness may develop from a variety of causes: "soul loss," breach of taboo (e.g., incest, contact with a "dangerous" object), witchcraft or sorcery, evil spirits or good spirits angered by improper human behavior, natural phenomena (lightning), animals, ceremonials. Pain, or anxiety-provoking dreams, rather than symptoms, tend to be regarded as indicators of illness.

Treatment Concept

Diagnosis is *not* made on the basis of symptoms. The healing system is sacred; healing rituals are performed to remove the *cause* of illness rather than to alleviate symptoms. Adults are responsible for the care of their children and of the aged parents. Home treatment centers on the use of plant medicines and sweat baths.

Examples of Significant Health Problems

Prevalence patterns strongly reflect poverty conditions and other barriers to care. Accidents, suicide,

(continued)

Health/Illness Considerations Among Five Major Ethnic Groups in North America (continued)

alcoholism, depression, diabetes, homicide, tuberculosis, nutritional deficiencies in children, high infant and maternal mortalities (maternal mortality due to toxemia of pregnancy and anemia-related hemorrhage).

Hispanic

Health/Wellness Concept

Eating well, keeping warm, and staying clean give one the signs of good health: functioning well with strength, color, plumpness, and absence of pain.

Illness Concept

The hot–cold (humoral) theory of illness is prevasive; the notions of "hot" and "cold" are ethnic and do not signify thermal temperature. Situational factors (worry, too many problems), viruses, "allergy," germs, parasites, and spirits may also cause disease, as can soul loss. Illness is recognized in a plethora of symptoms, both somatic and psychological.

Treatment Concept

Treatment is symptom-focused. Treat sickness classified as "cold" with "hot" foods and medications, and "hot" states with "cool" substances. Self-care in the home, at the pharmacy or herb shop, or at a folk healer's dispensary. Self-care medications include herbal and over-the-counter drugs; cathartics are used liberally for a variety of "infections." Women are the primary diagnosticians and caregivers. Healers (*curanderos/curanderas*) treat with botanicals and massages; care may also be sought from spiritists and faith healers. Primary contact with the biomedical system is through the emergency room.

Examples of Significant Health Problems

Prevalence patterns strongly reflect poverty conditions and other barriers to care. Respiratory disease (infants and children). Accidents and drugs (urbanites), diabetes mellitus, cirrhosis of the liver, tuberculosis, uterine cancer. High suicide, some stomach cancer (men). *Ataques* (sudden partial loss of consciousness, sometimes with seizures: Puerto Rican Syndrome), *mal de ojo* (sudden onset of any, minor or severe, sickness condition in a child: evil eye); *susto* (trauma-induced soul loss: fright). Some lactose intolerance.

White

Health/Wellness Concept

Ability to carry out normal roles and functions; absence of symptoms and known diseases. Physical and emotional well-being.

Illness Concept

Inability to carry out normal activities and functions; presence of symptoms and biomedically relevant signs of disease. Physical illness more acceptable than emotional or mental instability.

Treatment Concept

Self-care with over-the-counter medications, home remedies made of soft foods and topical applications, variety of folk treatments. Seek care from a physician or other health-care professional; appreciate high-tech diagnostic equipment and treatments. Strong orientation to the maxim "doctor knows best."

Examples of Significant Health Problems

Lifestyle-related problems leading to cancer, heart disease, hypertension, diabetes, accidents, and sexually transmitted diseases.

discharge from hospital—also demand that the nurse take account of the patient's cultural orientations. The stigma and emotional responses attached to AIDS require that nurses be skilled in eliciting the meanings of the illness from their patients and their support persons, and from the public at large *before* undertaking health education about AIDS prevention and control. The shift in site of nursing care away from hospitals to patient's natural environments (homes, workplaces, schools, ambulatory care settings; Aiken & Gortner, 1982) changes the nurse : patient power balance in favor of the patient. In the hospital, the patient was the guest/visitor at the nurse's domain; outside the hospital, the nurse is the guest of the patient. When caring for patients outside the hospital, the nurse needs to learn more from their patients.

Taking Account of Biocultural Variation

People's adaptation to different econiches over the years, group in-marriage, and the transmission of cultural traditions across generations together probably account for much of the genetic variation that occurs among different ethnic and racial groups. Nurses need to take account of the variation in assessing patients. The discussion here is limited to noting variations in growth and development, nutritional tolerance, body odor, and skin color.

Growth and Development. Populations differ in their average adult size, their tempo of growth, and their shape because of complicated interactions of genetic and environmental factors (Fig. 15-3). There is some racial difference in size, with Asian children distinctly smaller than African or European children, even when all children compared are raised in well-off environments. This difference in standing height should be taken into account when evaluating growth curves of children, whether in well-child screening or for pediatric assessment of response to treatment. Asian and African children also have a faster tempo of growth than Europeans (e.g., on average, girls reach menarche at a younger age), but African children are more advanced in skeletal maturity and motor development than Europeans from birth on to adolescence (Tanner, 1978a). Nutritional status has a strong influence on growth. However, even though disease may cause some growth retardation among children with inadequate diets, the growth usually catches up after the disease is cured. Socioeconomic status also affects growth, most likely because it is associated with type of diet available to the child. In every society studied, children in the upper socioeconomic sector are larger and grow more rapidly (Tanner, 1978b).

Nutritional Tolerance. Dietary tolerance is associated with both cultural food preferences and biologic variation. White people, for example, have inherited the ability to continue digesting milk sugar after weaning through adulthood, but most of the rest of the world's population become lactose-intolerant after the age of 5 years. Symptoms of lactose intolerance are dose-dependent; they include bloating, cramps, flatulence, and sometimes diarrhea after the ingestion of milk. Because of the associated poor absorption, milk should be withheld. However, it is hard to obtain adequate calcium unless milk and milk products are used or unless the diet is high in other calcium-rich foods (nuts, peanut butter, canned fish, cracked roast meat bones in soups, dark green leafy vegetables, and so forth).

There is also a racial difference in reaction to the ingestion of alcohol and alcoholic beverages. Enzymatic differences (alcohol dehydrogenase [ADH] and acetaldehyde dehydrogenase [ALDH]) account for the finding that most Asians and American Indians experience a rapid onset followed by a slow decrease of blood acetaldehyde levels when alcoholic beverages are consumed. This leaves them with a long period of exposure to the substance that is thought to cause many of the symptoms of alcohol intoxication (facial flushing and other vasomotor symptoms) that are found much less often among blacks and whites (Overfield, 1985).

Body Odor. Both body odor and the ways people respond to it vary among populations. Body odor results from deterioration of apocrine sweat, particularly in the axillary area. Populations that have fewer apocrine glands have less body odor; they include Asians and American Indians (Boyle & Andrews, 1989b). In other populations, cultural patterns determine the extent to which the body odor is disguised, ignored, or enhanced.

Skin Color. Skin color darkens with greater amounts of melanin. Melanin protects the skin from the sun's ultraviolet rays; its presence accounts for the low prevalence of skin cancers found among blacks and American Indians. *Mongolian spots* are clusters of melanocytes that commonly appear (80% to 90% prevalence) among American Indian, Asian, and black newborns as poorly circumscribed macular blue-black areas of pigmentation, particularly on the lower back around the buttocks. The pigmentation usually disappears by early childhood. Assessment of oxygenation of the tissues by examination of people with darkly pigmented skin requires practice. Color changes, as in anemic pallor, cyanosis, and jaundice, are most easily observable in the areas that are least densely pigmented: the sclera, conjunctiva, nailbeds, buccal mucosa, tongue, palms and soles. It is normal for

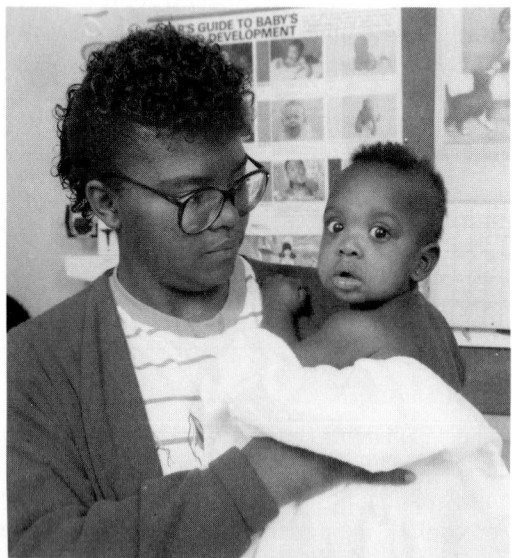

Figure 15–3. Fostering the parent's understanding of growth and development contributes to family health. (Photo courtesy of the University of Washington School of Nursing.)

some blacks to have bluish pigmentation of the gums and deposits of brown melanin in the sclera.

Grounding Nursing Assessments in the Patient's Perspective

Accurate nursing assessments require that the nurse minimize ethnocentric tendencies and maximize cultural sensitivity.

Subjective data represent the patient's/family's view of themselves, their health, their patterns of daily living, demands that are made on them, their usable and unusable resources, and their values and goals. In the subjective data realm the interviewee is *the expert*. It is his [sic] life, his experi-

---

Nursing Research

Selected Nursing Research Studies

Anderson, J. M. (1985). Perspectives on the health of immigrant women: A feminist analysis. *Advances in Nursing Science, 8*(1), 61–76.

Flaskerud, J. H. (1988). Is the Likert Scale format culturally biased? *Nursing Research, 37*(3), 185–186.

Johnson, M. N., et al. (1987). Psychological stress and blood pressure levels in black women. *Journal of the National Black Nurses' Association, 12,* 41.

Kulig, J. C. (1990). Childbearing beliefs among Cambodian refugee women. *Western Journal of Nursing Research, 12*(1), 108–118.

Reizian, A., & Meleis, A. L. (1986). Arab-Americans' perceptions of and responses to pain. *Critical Care Nurse, 6*(6), 30–37.

Possible Topics for Nursing Inquiry

- What are cultural variations in use of immunizations among parents for their school-age children?
- How does the health–wellness concept of a specific ethnic group affect adherence to treatment programs?
- How does use of prenatal care services relate to cultural identity?
- What cultural factors in a specific ethnic group have a relationship with access to health care?
- How does cultural background influence response to pain?

---

ence, his responses, his resources, and his world as he sees it. In the domain of nursing, gathering and recording subjective data without adulterating it is critical (Carnevali, 1983).

There are several ways to obtain an understanding of the patient's perspective. Usually combining several of the methods yields more complete and accurate results than relying on any single one. The most effective methods are open-ended interviewing, a variant of which is the ethnographic interview; the use of key informants; and observation over time.

Open-Ended Interviewing. A variety of techniques are used in open-ended interviewing to elicit responses from the interviewee that are as free from influence by the interviewer's comments as possible. Open-ended questions require that the respondent use his or her own words to answer. Silent pauses are sometimes useful because they give the respondent time to think about more things to say. Prompts, such as "Could you tell me more about _____?," encourage the patient to elaborate on a point of interest to the nurse.

The Ethnographic Interview. The ethnographic interview is a structured way to elicit the respondent's concepts and understandings (Spradley, 1979). The nurse-interviewer asks questions, the patient answers; the nurse-interviewer asks for repeated clarification of the patient's response. Highly skilled nurse-interviewers conduct ethnographic interviews that sound so much like a friendly conversation that the respondent does not feel he or she is being interviewed. In effect, the nurse-interviewer guides the patient to teach about the subject at hand. The nurse does this by expressing interest in the topic, incorporating the patient's own words, and using hypothetical examples. Asking the patient to clarify words reveals their individual meaning. Most important is the sense of mutual effort to gain understanding of the patient's perspective that the nurse conveys.

There are three parts to an ethnographic interview.

1. It begins with an open-ended, general question such as "How have you been feeling since I saw you yesterday?" or "I'm wondering about your family. . . ."
2. From the patient's response, the nurse selects some *key terms* and asks for clarification. For example, "You felt 'hot in your throat'? I'm not sure what you mean, would you tell me more?" or "You said your 'absent father'—what did you mean by that?" Note the nurse repeats exactly the words and phrases that the patient used. The terms are clues to what is important to the patient, so the nurse asks the patient to talk more about them.
3. The last part of the ethnographic interview is documentation. Information on the patient's view of himself or herself or of the issue discussed should be

recorded as soon as possible after the interview to retain it as accurately and completely as possible.

Key Informant Technique. The key informant technique is a method in which the interviewer looks for, locates, and interviews people who have expert or a native's knowledge about a culture the interviewer needs to know. They must be willing to discuss it with the interviewer, and there must be rapport. The optimal key informant about a patient is the individual patient, but medically or culturally compromised patients might not be able to fill the role. Nurses' direct, regular, and ubiquitous (in hospital, clinic, home, school, or workplace) contact with their patients enables nurses to observe and assess patient behaviors, social support system, and environmental constraints and resources. But without an understanding of the cultural meaning of what is observed, the nurse's observations have little value.

For most patients with limited English-speaking ability, the most useful key informants in the hospital or clinic situation are bilingual, bicultural, *trained* interpreters (Berkanovic, 1980; Diaz-Duque, 1982; Putsch, 1985; U.S. Department of Health and Human Services, 1985). Unfortunately, only a small proportion of healthcare agencies have hired such experts. Others who might make useful key informants for nurses include the ethnic herbalist or druggist, and the religious official (particularly on matters relating to preparation for death, emotional disturbances and social crises, and for explanations of illness; Muecke, 1987). The role of the religious official in health is often overlooked. It is important, however, because people usually interpret life–death and health–illness issues in terms of their cultural heritage of religious beliefs.

The following examples indicate the diversity of religious practitioners who might serve as key informants for different ethnic groups in the USA. For *blacks*, ministers and church mothers can be excellent informants because the church plays a strong central role in black communities (Jacques, 1976). Church mothers are particularly well informed about pregnancy, childbirthing, and women's health in general. For *Haitian Americans,* a voodoo priest is the expert in the mythology of spirits and the use of plants for home remedies (Laguerre, 1981). For *Mexican Americans* who are Roman Catholic, the priest as well as the *curandera* (secular folk healer; Kiev, 1968) may be useful informants on people's self-diagnoses and self-care practices. Many Mexicans are Protestant; a minister of the patient's particular sect should be sought because there is a vast difference between the nonpossessional sects (those that do not believe in spirit possession, such as Baptist, Methodist, Seventh-Day Adventist) and the possessional sects (Pentecostals believe in spirit possession and the healing power of prayer, and oppose the use of medicines and biomedical services; Clark, 1970; Kay, 1977; Rubel, 1966; Schreiber & Homiak, 1981). For *Native Ameri-*

cans, candidates for key informants vary by tribe. *Navajo* practice a wide diversity of religious practices: on the reservation, a peyote leader would be an important informant on health-related problems and behavior; other informants would be ministers of evangelical groups (Baptist, Nazarene, Pentecostals; Kunitz & Levy, 1981). The *Apache* and *Pueblo* of the Southwest rely heavily on medicine men (Joe, Gallerito, & Pino, 1976). For *Puerto Ricans,* both spiritist healers (people who are said to lend their bodies to spirits who communicate through them) and Pentecostal ministers may be helpful informants for conditions not recognized or curable by biomedicine, such as emotional disturbances, incurable chronic or terminal illness, intractable somatic symptoms, and life crisis adjustments (Garrison, 1977; Harwood, 1981a).

When the Patient Does Not Speak the Nurse's Language

A deliberate search for the meaning behind patient responses enables the nurse to plan and provide safe and individualized patient care. Language differences between the nurse and patient compound cultural differences between them, however, and can keep the nurse from getting at the patient's point of view. When the patient does not speak the same language or does so only to a limited extent, the nurse may decide to act in the patient's best interests—without actually knowing what the patient thinks those interests are. For example, when a patient from an ethnic minority is alert but nontalkative or responds with only affirmatives, health-care providers might conclude that the patient does not understand English. If there is no interpreter at hand, they might do what they think is best or necessary for the patient even if they do not have the subjective data normally required to guide clinical decision-making. The result can be tragic in terms of patient welfare and in terms of loss of trust with a subcultural community (Fink & Doua Yang, 1983).

For example:

> An international patient of limited English-speaking ability underwent major surgery and recuperated without complications in the intensive care unit (ICU) of a tertiary care hospital. The staff liked him very much. After he was transferred to a regular care unit, his behavior changed dramatically: he exhibited anxious and paranoid behavior. When a psychiatric consultant and interpreter were brought in to handle the problem, they became the first health-care providers to attempt to access the patient's point of view. They found that the transfer from the ICU to a regular unit did not signify recuperation to the patient at all. In fact, he interpreted it as meaning the hospital had given up on him because

they thought he was so sick that he was no longer worth caring for. In his view, he had been moved from an environment of expert care and the best of technologic assistance into an old part of the hospital that was practically devoid of technologic props and wanting in staff to tend to him. The health-care team's belief that the transfer was a self-explanatory demonstration of recuperation is a classic example of medical/nursing ethnocentrism because they neglected to assess the patient's perspective.

The patient's confusion, fear, and isolation were all preventable: they could be considered iatrogenic, that is, caused by hospitalization. Cases such as this could be defined as negligent in today's health-care system because an interpreter should have been obtained to explain to the patient what the plans for him were before transferring him to another unit. *Hospitals are obliged to provide trained language interpreters for "the patient who does not speak or understand the predominant language of the community" (Joint Commission on Accreditation of Hospitals, 1985)."* Furthermore, hospitals that receive Medicare or Medicaid reimbursement are subject to Title VI of the Civil Rights Act. This Act prohibits recipients of federal funds from discriminating or denying benefits on the basis of race, color, or national origin: hospitals that fail to provide trained interpreters for non- or limited-English speaking people, or for deaf people who use sign language, are in violation of the law (U.S. Department of Health and Human Services). The nurse who is frustrated in efforts to communicate with a patient due to language differences or impaired hearing or speech, and unable to provide the quality of care deemed appropriate has legal recourse *to encourage a hospital to provide a trained interpreter to resolve the difficulty* (U.S. Department of Health and Human Services, 1985).

It is important to secure trained interpreters rather than bilingual members of the patient's family or friends, however well-intentioned the latter might be. Much of the vocabulary of the medical world is difficult to translate into some languages. For example, the phrase "the lab tech dialed the wrong number" could not be translated into a language of a culture that did not have telephones or scientific laboratories (Werner & Campbell, 1973). Furthermore, the emotional burden of responsibility should the patient's condition deteriorate could be overwhelming on someone close to the patient. For example:

A Vietnamese woman was hospitalized with cancer; her 20-year-old daughter was in a nursing home with leukemia. The husband-father spoke little English. The hospital staff relied on the 12-year-old daughter-sister to interpret for them. First the sister died, then the mother. The twelve-

year-old, suffering from a sense of complicity in their deaths because of her closeness to them in the last days in her role as translator, had an acute psychotic episode for which she had to be institutionalized.

A person's need for an interpreter should be established at first contact with the health-care agency. An interpreter should be provided whenever requested, and definitely at any time when plans for the patient are being made or change in procedure inaugurated: during admission, for consent for treatment, during treatments, for discharge planning, for patient education, and so forth. Tips for communicating through an interpreter are given in the display.

Tips for Communicating Through an Interpreter

- Speak *to the patient* rather than to the interpreter: this enables the patient to "read" your nonverbal language.
- Watch the verbal and nonverbal interactions between the interpreter and patient: "read" their nonverbal language.
- Speak slowly.
- Use simple sentences.
- Avoid using metaphors: they are too hard to translate (e.g., "Have you been feeling blue?", "Once in a blue moon," "Does it feel like pins and needles?").
- Rephrase a question in different words or ask it indirectly if the answer you received is inappropriate or inconsistent with other indications.
- Expect that it might take an interpreter much longer to say or explain something in another language than in English: this is particularly true when the concept is a medical one for which there is no equivalent in the other language or culture, or when the topic is considered taboo or embarrassing in the other culture. The best culturally sensitive interpreters do not always translate verbatim, word for word; they couch your words in phrasings that are culturally appropriate in the patient's language.
- When unsure how to bring up a delicate subject, ask the interpreter for advice; use the interpreter as a key informant on the culture of the patient.
- Try to work consistently with the same interpreter; with practice you both can learn to communicate better with each other.
- Relate to the interpreter as a professional colleague; your nursing care depends on the interpreter's skill.

Increased Effectiveness of Patient Education

The culturally sensitive nurse looks for patterns in the occurrence of unusual behavior in a patient from a sub-culture or ethnic group other than his or her own. The nurse who understands the principle of cultural relativity expects that there is an underlying explanation for behavior, particularly for behavior that is repeated by different people of the same culture or ethnic group (Fig. 15-4). When refugees from rural and mountainous areas of Southeast Asia first arrived in the United States, health-care and social-service providers had many stories of the "funny" and "bad" things they did. Analysis of these stories identified clusterings of similar tales, each cluster representing unfamiliarity with Western ways. The nurses interpreted the unfamiliarity as areas of poor previous communication and, therefore, as the starting points for health education. Some of the frequent problems were:

When women who were taking birth control pills forgot to take a pill, they either took two pills the next day, or gave the extra pill to their husbands to take.

A large number of newborns in families of non-English speaking refugees were brought into the emergency room with dehydration.

Many refugee households with newborns put the heat on in their apartments even during the hot summer, and they swaddled infants and toddlers who had fevers in layers of clothing.

By using the ethnographic interview, observing in patient's homes, and consulting key informants, the nurses discovered the following rationales for the refugee behaviors:

The women who forgot to take a birth control pill were trying to compensate for its omission. Because they did not know the principles on which the pills work, they made legitimate guesses about how to overcome their oversight. Also, their cultural heritage had taught them not to ask questions of authority figures lest they be considered rude and offensive.

The mothers of dehydrated babies had followed infant feeding instructions that they had been given in the postpartum unit. A hospital nurse who researched the problem discovered that the mothers had learned their lesson well. The problem was that the method they were taught was correct only for the ready-to-use formula for which the hospital gave out free samples. Once those samples were used up, the women began using formula from the Women, Infants, and Children (WIC) Program. The WIC milk was dry powder. Because the women could not read the English language directions on the labels, they guessed how to mix the dry formula. Many guessed wrong, resulting in dehydrated babies.

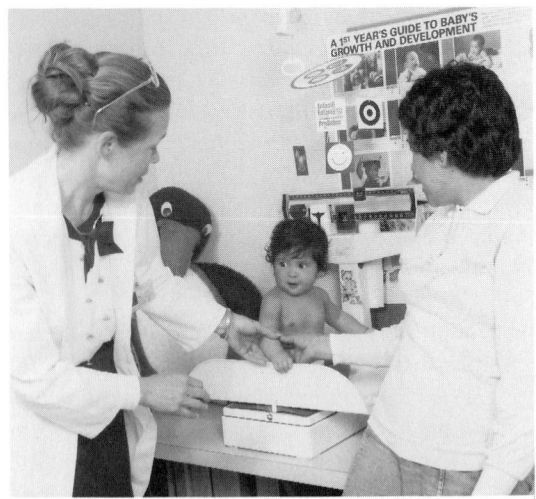

Figure 15–4. The nurse and the parent of an Hispanic child evaluate the child's health. (Photo courtesy of the University of Washington School of Nursing.)

The households that turned the heat up and overdressed children with fevers were exercising their belief in the humoral theory of physiology that is prevalent in Southeast Asia (Muecke, 1976). According to this theory, blood is "hot." Because women lose blood during delivery, they lose heat; to keep them from getting sick, their bodies must be kept so warm that they regain the "heat" they have lost. Similarly, children, who tend to have higher fevers than adults, are thought to lose "heat" when they have a fever; dressing them warmly is thought to prevent "heat" from leaving their bodies.

The culturally sensitive nursing assessments that revealed the above rationales for untoward self-care practices provided a highly valid basis for nursing diagnoses and related patient education. The health education that resulted from these assessments increased the patients' and their ethnic communities' trust of nurses and of health-care agencies.

Key Concepts

■ Culture is defined as a belief system that the culture members hold, consciously or unconsciously, as absolute truth.

■ This belief system guides everyday behavior and makes it routine; provides answers to the unanswerable questions of life, sickness, and death; and makes the world make sense.

■ Culture enables a person to behave reasonably in contexts that the person shares with members of the same culture.

■ Culture is an integral component of the knowledge base of nursing.

■ Accurate nursing assessments require that the nurse minimize ethnocentric tendencies and maximize cultural sensitivity.

■ Physical assessment skills require knowledge of biocultural variation in such areas as growth, nutritional tolerance, skin color, and body odor.

■ Patient assessments that take account of the patient's perspective are most likely to yield diagnoses and interventions appropriate to the patient.

■ Methods to gain the patient's perspective include open-ended interviewing, a variant of which is the ethnographic interview; the use of key informants; observation over time; and use of the patient's language.

References

Aiken, L. H., & Gortner, S. R. (Eds.). (1982). *Nursing in the 1980s: Crises, opportunities, challenges* (p. 57). Philadelphia: J. B. Lippincott.

American Nurses Association. (1980). *Nursing: A social policy statement* (p. 9). Kansas City: Author.

Anderson, P. (1979). *Nurse.* New York: Berkley.

Antonovsky, A. (1980). *Health, stress and coping.* San Francisco: Jossey-Bass.

Benner, P. (1984). *From novice to expert: Excellence and power in clinical nursing practice.* Menlo Park, CA: Addison-Wesley.

Berkanovic, E. (1980). The effect of inadequate language translation on Hispanic's responses to health surveys. *American Journal of Public Health, 70*(12), 1273–1276.

Berlin, B., & Kay, P. (1969). *Basic color terms: Their universality and evolution.* Berkeley: University of California Press.

Birdwhistell, R. L. (1970). *Kinesics and context: Essays on body motion communication.* Philadelphia: University of Pennsylvania Press.

Boyle, J. S., & Andrews, M. M. (1989a). *Transcultural concepts in nursing care* (p. 12). Boston: Scott, Foresman.

Boyle, J. S., & Andrews, M. M. (1989b). *Transcultural concepts in nursing care* (p. 79). Boston: Scott, Foresman.

Brink, P. J. (Ed.). (1976). *Transcultural nursing: A book of readings* (p. 3). Englewood Cliffs, NJ: Prentice-Hall.

Brink, P. J., & Saunders, J. M. (1976). Culture shock: Theoretical and applied. In P. J. Brink (Ed.), *Transcultural nursing: A book of readings* (pp. 126–138). Englewood Cliffs, NJ: Prentice-Hall.

Carnevali, D. L. (1983). *Nursing care planning: Diagnosis and management* (3rd ed.; p. 93). Philadelphia: J. B. Lippincott.

Clark, M. (1970). *Health in the Mexican-American culture* (2nd ed.). Berkeley: University of California Press.

Darling, F. F. (1937). *A herd of red deer.* London: Oxford University Press.

Diaz-Duque, O. F. (1982). Advice from an interpreter. *American Journal of Nursing, 82,* 1376–1379.

Douglas, M. (1973). *Natural symbols.* Middlesex, England: Penguin Books.

Erikson, E. H. (1950). *Childhood and society.* New York: W. W. Norton.

Fink, J., & Doua Yang. (1983). *Peace has not been made: A case history of a Hmong family's encounter with a hospital* (video). Rhode Island Office of Refugee Resettlement.

Garrison, V. (1977). Doctor, *espiritista* or psychiatrist: Health-seeking behavior in a Puerto Rican neighborhood of New York City. *Medical Anthropology, 1*(2), 54–180.

Germain, C. (1979). *The cancer unit: An ethnography.* Wakefield, MA: Nursing Resources.

Goetschs, W. (1937). *The ants.* Ann Arbor: University of Michigan Press.

Goodall, J. (1986). *The chimpanzees of Gombe: Patterns of behavior.* Cambridge, MA: Belknap Press.

Hall, E. T. (1959). *The silent language* (p. 35). Greenwich, CT: Fawcett Premier.

Hall, E. T. (1969). *The hidden dimension.* Garden City, NY: Anchor Press/Doubleday.

Harrington, M. (1962). *The other America.* New York: Macmillan.

Harwood, A. (1981a). Mainland Puerto Ricans. In A. J. Harwood (Ed.), *Ethnicity and medical care* (pp. 397–481). Cambridge, MA: Harvard University Press.

Harwood, A. (Ed.). (1981b). *Ethnicity and medical care* (p. 27). Cambridge, MA: Harvard University Press.

Jacques, G. (1976). Cultural health traditions: A black perspective. In M. F. Branch & P. P. Paxton (Eds.) *Providing safe nursing care for ethnic people of color* (pp. 115–134). New York: Appleton-Century-Crofts.

Joe, J., Gallerito, C., & Pino, J. (1976). Cultural health traditions: American Indian perspectives. In M. F. Branch & P. P. Paxton (Eds.), *Providing safe nursing care for ethnic people of color* (pp. 81–98). New York: Appleton-Century-Crofts.

Joint Commission on Accreditation of Hospitals. (1985). Rights and responsibilities of patients. In *AMH-85 Accreditation manual for hospitals* (p. xi).

Kay, M. A. (1977). Health and illness in a Mexican-American barrio. In E. Spicer (Ed.), *Ethnic medicine in the Southwest.* Tucson: University of Arizona Press.

Kiev, A. (1968). *Curanderismo.* New York: The Free Press.

Kunitz, S. J., & Levy, J. E. (1981). Navajos. In A. J. Harwood (Ed.), *Ethnicity and medical care* (pp. 337–396). Cambridge, MA: Harvard University Press.

Laguerre, M. S. (1981). Haitian Americans. In A. J. Harwood (Ed.), *Ethnicity and medical care* (pp. 172–210). Cambridge, MA: Harvard University Press.

Leininger, M. M. (1970a). *Nursing and anthropology: Two worlds to blend* (pp. 21–22). New York: John Wiley & Sons.

Leininger, M. M. (1970b). *Nursing and anthropology: Two worlds to blend* (p. 49). New York: John Wiley & Sons.

Lewis, O. (1966). The culture of poverty. *Scientific American 215*(4), 19–25.

MacGregor, F. C. (1967). Uncooperative patients: Some cultural interpretations. *American Journal of Nursing 67*(1), 88–91 (Reprinted in Brink, P. J. (Ed.). (1976). *Transcultural nursing: A book of readings* (pp. 36–43). Englewood Cliffs, NJ: Prentice-Hall.

Mead, M. (1982). Ethnicity and anthropology in America. In G. De Vos & L. Romanucci-Ross (Eds.). *Ethnic identity: Cultural continuities and change* (pp. 175–177). Chicago: University of Chicago Press.

Muecke, M. A. (1976). Health care systems as socializing agents: Childbearing the North Thai and Western ways. *Social Science and Medicine, 10*(8–9), 377–383.

Muecke, M. A. (1987). Resettled refugees' reconstruction of identity: Lao in Seattle. *Urban Anthropology 16*(1), 273–290.

Oberg, K. (1954). *Culture shock.* Indianapolis: Bobbs-Merrill.

Overfield, T. (1985). *Biologic variation in health and illness: Race, age, and sex differences* (pp. 80–81). Menlo Park, CA: Addison-Wesley.

Petersen, W., Novak, M., & Gleason, P. (1980). *Concepts of ethnicity* (pp. 56, 116). Littleton, MA: Harvard University Press.

Putsch, R. W., III. (1985). The special case of interpreters in health care. *Journal of the American Medical Association, 254*(23), 3344–3348.

Rhoades, D. F. (1985). Pheromonal communication between plants. In G. A. Cooper-Driver, T. Swain, & E. E. Conn (Eds.), *Chemically mediated interactions between plants and other organisms* (pp. 195–218). New York: Plenum.

Rubel, A. J. (1966). *Across the tracks: Mexican Americans in a Texas city.* Austin: University of Texas Press.

Schermerhorn, R. A. (1978a). *Comparative ethnic relations: A framework for theory and research* (pp. 12–14). Chicago: University of Chicago Press.

Schermerhorn, R. A. (1978b). *Comparative ethnic relations: A framework for theory and research* (pp. 73–77). Chicago: University of Chicago Press.

Schreiber, J. M., & Homiak, J. P. (1981). Mexican Americans. In A. J. Harwood (Ed.), *Ethnicity and medical care* (pp. 264–336). Cambridge, MA: Harvard University Press.

Spradley, J. P. (1979). *The ethnographic interview.* New York: Holt, Rinehart & Winston.

Stack, C. (1974). *All our kin: Strategies for survival in a black community.* New York: Harper & Row.

Tanner, J. M. (1978a). *Foetus into man: Physical growth from conception to maturity* (pp. 137–141). Cambridge, MA: Harvard University Press.

Tanner, J. M. (1978b). *Foetus into man: Physical growth from conception to maturity* (pp. 141–153). Cambridge, MA: Harvard University Press.

Tompkins, P., & Bird, C. (1972). *The secret life of plants.* New York: Avon Books.

Tylor, E. B. (1871). *Primitive culture.* London: Murray.

U.S. Department of Health and Human Services. *Your rights under Title VI of the Civil Rights Act of 1964 in Health and Human Service Programs, HHS 391.* Washington, D.C.: US DHHS.

U.S. Department of Health and Human Services, Office for Civil Rights. (1985, February). *How to establish effective communication procedures for people with limited English proficiency and for people with impaired hearing, vision, or speech.* Region X, Seattle, WA.

Valentine, C. A. (1968). *Culture and poverty: Critique and counterproposals.* Chicago: University of Chicago Press.

Werner, O., & Campbell, D. T. (1973). Translating, working through interpreters and the problem of decentering. In R. Naroll & R. Cohen (Eds.), *A handbook of method in cultural anthropology* (pp. 398–420). Irvington-on-Hudson, NY: Columbia University Press.

Wirth, L. (1945). The problem of minority groups. In R. Linton (Ed.), *The science of man in the world crisis.* New York: Columbia University Press.

Bibliography

Abu-Saad, H. (1984). Cultural group indicators of pain in children. *Maternal Child Nursing Journal 13,* 187–196.

Hahn, R.A., & Muecke, M. A. (1987). The anthropology of birth in five U.S. ethnic populations: Implications for obstetrical practice. *Current Problems in Obstetrics, Gynecology and Fertility, 10*(4), 133–171.

LaFargue, J. P. (1972). Role of prejudice in rejection of health care. *Nursing Research 2,* 53–58.

Lipson, J. G., Reizian, A. E., & Meleis, A. I. (1987). Arab-American patients: A medical record review. *Social Science and Medicine, 24*(2), 101–107.

Powers, B. A. (1982). The use of orthodox and black American folk medicine. *Advances in Nursing Science, 4,* 35–47.

Tripp-Reimer, T. (1982). Barriers to health care: Variations in interpretation of Appalachian client behavior by Appalachian and non-Appalachian health professionals. *Western Journal of Nursing Research, 4,* 179–191.

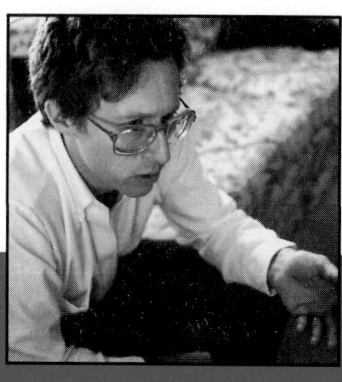

Values

LEARNING OBJECTIVES

Upon completion of this chapter, the student will be able to do the following:

- Define values.
- Identify sources of professional nursing values.
- Apply developmental and cultural perspectives when identifying values.
- Relate values with functional health patterns.
- Examine values conflict and resolution in nursing care situations.
- Integrate values assessment into nursing care.
- Appreciate the impact of values in situations such as the initial nursing assessment and discharge planning.

KEY TERMS

Attitudes
Action values
Behaviors
Beliefs
Choice values
Cultural value orientation

Hierarchy of skills
Imaginal skills
Instrumental skills
Interpersonal skills
Moral values
Operative (means) values

Systems skills
Terminal (ends) values
Values
Value conflict
Value system
Vision values

Value and Belief Patterns
  Major Categories of Values
  Professional Values in Nursing
    Socialization
    Classroom Study
    Clinical Study
  Values Clarification
  Values Inquiry
  Applied Ethics
Sources of Values
  Community
  Peer Culture
  Role Models
  Interaction with People of Differing Values and
    Viewpoints
  Experiences that Challenge One's Way of
    Thinking
  Decision-Making
Manifestations of Values
  Effect of Values on Functional Health
    Health Perception and Health Management
    Nutrition and Metabolism
    Elimination
    Activity and Exercise

    Sleep and Rest
    Cognition and Perception
    Self-Perception and Self-Concept
    Roles and Relationships
    Sexuality and Reproduction
    Coping and Stress Management
    Values and Beliefs
  Manifestations of Nurses' Values
Lifespan Considerations
    Infant, Toddler, and Preschooler
    Child and Adolescent
    Adult and Older Adult
  Hall's Value Development Theory
Value Conflicts
    Patient and Family Conflicts
    Patient and Health-Care Conflicts
  Resolving Value Conflicts in the Health-Care
    System
Values Assessment
  Level of Values Development
  View of Hospitalization and Illness
  Activities of Daily Living
  Discharge Planning
Key Concepts

What is really important in your life? How do you decide what actions to take? On what do you base your decisions? The answers to these questions are found when you examine your attitudes, beliefs, and values. People who do not take time to reflect on these issues often are unclear in their purpose in life; they may find that decision-making is difficult because they cannot effectively articulate or defend their position. They lack an awareness of their inner self or being.

As beginning students of nursing you have decided that you want to work with people and help them in some way improve their health. If you examine the thoughts and feelings connected with this decision, you will also find that you have a positive attitude toward people, that you like to be with people. You also probably like the study of the biologic and social sciences. There may have

been a variety of other influences on your choice to become a nurse, such as other family members who are health-care professionals. Perhaps you understood the critical need for nurses and saw the opportunity for job security. Thus, your decision to become a professional nurse is a deep one, reflecting your core attitudes, beliefs, and values. Ultimately, these values, beliefs, and attitudes will emerge in the way you care for patients and their families.

Just as you have core attitudes, beliefs, and values, so do the patients, their families, and the health-care organizations within which you will be working. Patients and families will demonstrate their values by their behaviors, whereas health-care organizations demonstrate values in mission statements and policies.

Usually, the conflicts that nurses observe or deal with

have a value base. These value conflicts represent a variety of preferences and levels of development, and they can lead to ethical dilemmas for both nurses and patients. Whatever the conflict, it is important for nurses to understand their own attitudes, beliefs, and values and be sensitive to others' value systems to be effective health caregivers.

VALUE AND BELIEF PATTERNS

Values are standards for decision-making that endure over a significant period of time in one's life (Hall, et al., 1982). As such, values have four parts: thinking, choosing, feeling, and behaving (King, 1984). The first aspect of a value is that it is an abstract idea, for example "truth." The word "truth" means little until one makes a choice about being honest and consequently behaves in a truthful manner. Unless a person has thought about the concepts of truth and honesty, these values remain unchosen ones and would not be easily articulated unless behaviors or choices were questioned or explored.

A **value system** is an enduring set of principles and rules organized into a hierarchy (Rokeach, 1973). As one is choosing between alternative actions and making decisions, one must weigh which value is the most important. To use the example of truth and honesty again, suppose a nurse believes in truth and honesty and a patient asks what the medical diagnosis is. The nurse might not want to give an answer immediately, especially if the diagnosis were unusual, complicated, or a disease that usually causes death. Other values with which the nurse might balance with truth could include caring, harmony, duty, or responsibility. The situation might be further complicated if the nurse knew that the family or other health-care team members had different preferences. This scenario represents an internal, personal values conflict as well as a conflict within the family and health-care team.

Attitudes, beliefs, and behaviors are often linked with values, but are not the same as values (Hall, et al., 1982). An **attitude** is one's disposition toward an object or a situation; it can be a mental or emotional mind-set and it may be positive or negative. Attitudes can be seen in one's behavior or the opinions one expresses. **Beliefs** are ideas that are accepted as true; they may be expressed by such things as decisions, opinions, or creeds. **Behaviors** are observable actions. To continue with the example of truth-telling and the medical diagnosis, a nurse's attitudes and beliefs about the medical diagnosis would influence the valuing process. The ultimate behavior, however, would demonstrate the value that held priority. Attitudes, beliefs, and behaviors are value indicators, and if the nurse is encouraged to take time to reflect on them, his or her values cand value system will be realized and articulated.

Major Categories of Values

There are several ways of categorizing values. For the purpose of this discussion, three categories are considered: operative (or means), terminal (or ends), and moral values. **Operative values** are those that are indicated by a specific behavior, which may be a response or a preference (Hall, et al., 1982). For example, honestly sharing one's observations indicates that honesty is valuable to that person. **Terminal values** are values that are regarded as good in themselves; they transcend immediate needs and shape long-term goals (Rokeach, 1973). Truth is in this category as an ends value, while honesty is a means value. **Moral values** are those values involving correct behavior, such as having some sense of right and wrong or "oughtness." (Rokeach, 1973) They deal with such issues as how to treat life and people; truth and honesty are also moral values. Nonmoral values are those that serve a personal preference or purpose, or make a contribution. They do not involve right and wrong behavior. For example, the value of a healthy lifestyle is seen as good, but if people choose not to take care of their health, it is not considered immoral unless, of course, their habits and decisions affect others, as would be the case in driving while intoxicated.

Professional Values in Nursing

Professional nursing values can be traced in the history and traditions of nursing. Beginning with the Nightingale Pledge in 1893 (see the display) through to the current American Nurses Association's Code for Nurses (see Chap. 3), nurses have endeavored to identify and define standards of practice. These standards are based on universal moral principles or values, the central one being respect for people or human dignity. Other values

---

Nightingale Pledge

"I solemnly pledge myself before God and in the presence of this assembly to pass my life in purity and to practice my profession faithfully. I will abstain from whatever is deleterious and mischievous, and will not take or knowingly administer any harmful drug. I will do all in my power to maintain and elevate the standard of my profession, and will hold in confidence all personal matters committed to my keeping and all family affairs coming to my knowledge in the practice of my calling. With loyalty will I endeavor to aid the physician in his work, and devote myself to the welfare of those committed to my care."

based on human dignity include self-determination, doing good, avoiding harm, truth-telling, respecting privileged information, keeping promises, and treating people fairly. When one enters nursing, however, one also "inherits a measure of both the responsibility and the trust that have accrued to nursing over the years . . . ," thus, one becomes a part of the nursing tradition of service.

A second statement of values, advanced by the American Association of Colleges of Nursing (AACN) in *Essentials of College and University Education for Professional Nursing* (AACN, 1986), identifies seven core values for nurses: altruism, equality, esthetics, freedom, human dignity, justice, and truth. The AACN stresses that it is especially important for nurses to adopt these essential values to have a sense of commitment and social responsibility, a sensitivity and responsiveness to the needs of others, and responsibility for themselves and their actions.

Although the American Nurses Association (ANA) and the AACN both have statements on the importance of values (Table 16-1), how do nursing students develop these values? There are at least three ways in which values are developed in nursing: socialization, classroom study, and clinical study.

Socialization

Based on some beginning nursing research, it appears that pre-nursing students already have values similar to those of nursing faculty (Thurston, et al., 1989). For example, the top four means values selected by both faculty and students were to be responsible, honest, loving, and forgiving. One explanation for this is that our society already has some accurate perceptions about values basic to nursing, despite the distortions of the television image. Thus, the process of socialization to nursing begins long before one is in a nursing education program.

TABLE 16–1
Values in Professional Nursing

ANA Code of Ethics (Ethical Values)	AACN Essentials (Professional Values)
Human dignity	Altruism
Autonomy	Equality
Doing good	Esthetics
Avoiding harm	Freedom
Truth-telling	Human dignity
Confidentiality	Justice
Keeping promises	Truth
Justice	

From American Nurses' Association (1985). *Code for nurses with interpretive statements.* Kansas City, MO: Author; American Association of Colleges of Nursing (1986). *Essentials of colleges and university education for professional nursing.* Washington, DC: Author.

Classroom Study

Several different approaches to values education have been adopted by nurse educators: values clarification, values inquiry, and applied ethics (King, 1984). Requisite to any study of values is an understanding of growth and development and, in particular, moral development. Since children and adults view the world differently, they make different moral choices when deciding on what is right and wrong behavior toward other human beings. Children and adults also have different needs or motivators that influence their value choices.

Clinical Study

The major learning experience in clinical study is patient care. After the nurse becomes proficient in giving basic patient care, he or she often begins to examine such questions as was the care effective, what made it effective, or was it acceptable to the patient. In answering these questions, what is important to both the patient and the nurse becomes apparent. In fact, the whole care-planning process is a value-laden situation: the questions that are asked during the nursing assessment, the prioritizing of nursing diagnoses, and the establishment of patient goals all reflect values.

If the care-planning process is mutual and the patient's values are taken into account, then the nursing care will support the patient's unique qualities, for "if a person's values are ignored or replaced with the values of others, the person ceases to exist as a singular human being" (Curtin & Flaherty, 1982, p. 90). Therefore, if the patient's values are affirmed during the caring process, the patient is also affirmed as a worthwhile person. Thus, the study of patient care includes a consciousness of the patient's values and the nurse's values and how these interact in the caregiving process.

Values Clarification

Values clarification is "a method of self-discovery by which people identify their personal values and their value rankings" (King, 1984, p. 25). This process does not evaluate the values as such, but rather helps people identify their own values. According to Raths, Harmin, and Simon (1966), there are three phases to this process (choosing, prizing, and acting) and seven steps (as listed in the display).

This process can be used in several ways:

- To examine past situations and decisions.
- To conduct a general case study.
- To explore how time is spent by listing activities in a typical 24-hour period.

Whatever the vehicle for examination of values, there are certain assumptions underlying the process. First,

Phases and Steps in Values Clarification

Choosing Ones's Beliefs and Behaviors

1. Choosing freely
2. Choosing from among alternative
3. Choosing after consideration of the consequences

Prizing One's Beliefs and Behaviors

4. Prizing and cherishing
5. Affirming

Acting on One's Beliefs

6. Acting upon choices
7. Repeating

Adapted from Raths, L. E., Harmin, M., & Simon, S. B. (1966). *Values and teaching* (2nd ed.). Columbus, OH: Charles E. Merrill.

1. What are the facts?
2. What can be inferred from the facts?
3. What can be inferred from the person's value system?
4. What evidence supports these inferences?

Another set of questions useful in assisting with values inquiry is based on problem-solving:

1. What is the problem?
2. What other alternatives were options?
3. What are the possible consequences of each alternative?
4. What was the evidence that these consequences might occur?
5. What are the advantages and disadvantages of each consequence? Why?
6. What would you do if you were in this situation? Why?

Unlike values clarification, which can be either an individual or a group experience, values inquiry lends itself more exclusively to group discussion (Fig. 16-2). The process increases understanding and enhances empathy within a broader social context, as well as increasing communication skills and the ability to verbalize one's position.

Applied Ethics

Nurses must acknowledge and be aware of their personal and professional values when they confront ethical di-

for people freely to choose beliefs and behaviors, they must have a sense of who they are, or a sense of self (King, 1984) (Fig. 16-1). This generally begins to occur in late childhood, and individuation is well developed by young adulthood. If individuation has not occurred to some degree, the chosen values will reflect others' values and be externalized rather than internalized. Second, people need to have basic self-esteem to be confident in relying on their feelings, beliefs, and behaviors as guides for decisions (King, 1984).

The prizing and cherishing of one's beliefs and behaviors tend to affirm self-worth and contribute to a sense of inner harmony, purpose, and meaning (King, 1984). These feelings are rewarding in themselves and enable one to act more easily on the indicated choices. As the beliefs are acted on repeatedly and consistently in a variety of situations, they become values, and a mature, self-conscious, personal value system begins to emerge.

Values Inquiry

Whereas values clarification is a method of self-discovery of personal values, values inquiry (King, 1984) is a method of examining social issues and the values that motivate human choice. Case studies and issue-laden incidents provide ways to facilitate the inquiry process. A predetermined series of questions aids in discussing the issues. One set of questions is:

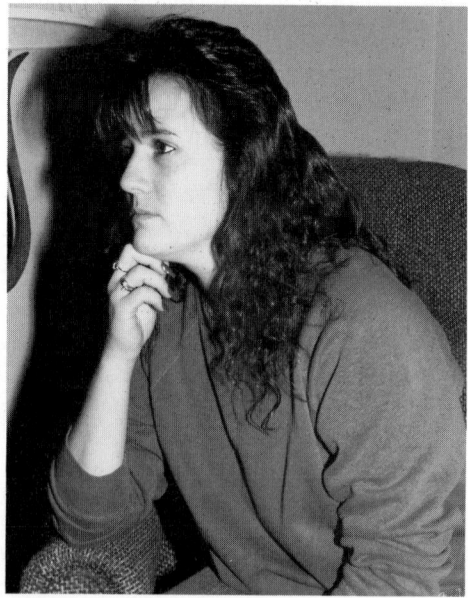

Figure 16–1.   Values clarification helps people identify their own values and gives them a sense of who they are.

lemmas. Of particular importance here are moral values, or those that deal with right and wrong behavior toward other human beings. Analyzing and critiquing case studies assists in applying certain ethical principles, or values, such as respect for persons, honesty, and justice. Consideration of case studies also aids in developing moral reasoning skills, and, if done in a group discussion, develops communication skills (King, 1984).

SOURCES OF VALUES

Values come from many sources. Some authors, such as Fromm and Maslow, believe that values are rooted in the very conditions of human existence, intrinsic in the structure of human nature, both genetically and culturally (Fromm, 1959). Others believe that values are learned from the culture and society in which one grows up, particularly in the social institutions of family, school, and religion.

There are several ways in which children learn values: parents reward and punish behavior, language colors thinking and perception, significant others model behavior, the media floods us with a variety of images, and unspoken expectations direct behavior (Hall et al., 1982). As one enters adolescence and young adulthood one is more likely to encounter a variety of values, and become more aware of value differences. The process of value refinement continues throughout life. It may be a result of a planned self-conscious discovery process or it may be a matter of living and dealing with life situations as they are encountered. Lifespan considerations are discussed later in this chapter.

Two more phenomena that make it possible to become more conscious of different values manifest themselves in adolescence: social perspective-taking and formal rea-

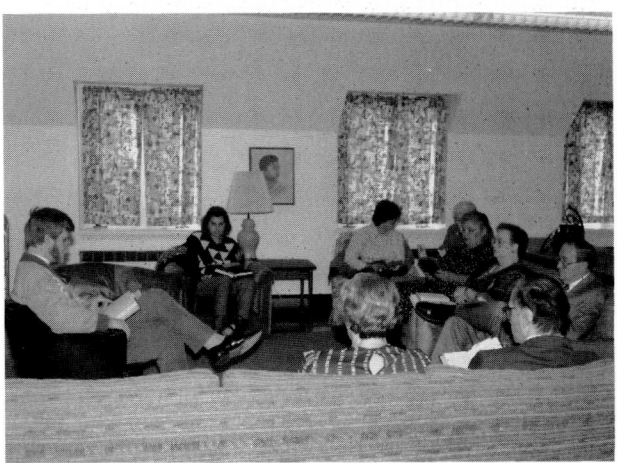

Figure 16–2. Values inquiry uses group discussion to examine social issues and values that motivate human choice.

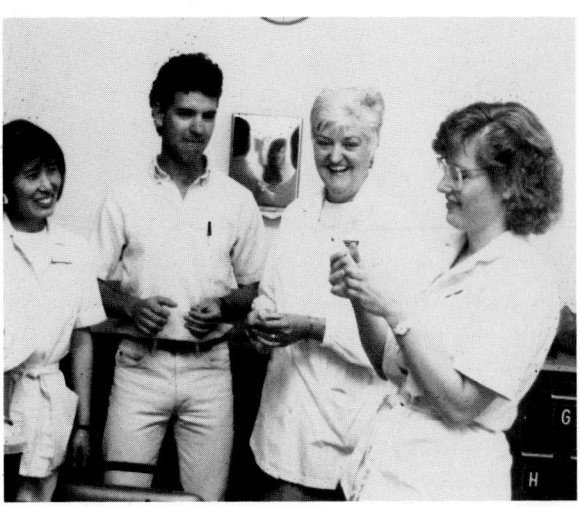

Figure 16–3. A community experience supports stated values and goals.

soning. Both of these abilities enable a person to understand and have empathy for another's thoughts, feelings, and point of view. In addition to these abilities, several other critical factors enhance values development; various social institutions, particularly colleges, plan their programs in view of these factors: community, peer culture, role models, interactions with people of differing values and viewpoints, experiences that challenge one's way of thinking, and decision-making (Dalton, 1985).

Community

A sense of community is formed in an institution, e.g., colleges, by fostering values and goals that are consistently integrated into the various classroom and extracurricular activities. It is further enhanced when people are treated with consideration, according to the stated values. The experience of community also provides a supportive environment in which one can experiment more freely with different attitudes, beliefs, and behaviors (Dalton, 1985) (Fig. 16-3).

Peer Culture

Although a sense of community has a strong influence on value development, the attitudes, beliefs, and behaviors that grow out of peer group relationships are powerful. Peer groups define themselves by common interests, needs, and problems. Out of these similar interests and bonds, values are clarified (Dalton, 1985).

Role Models

Effective role models are conscious of their values as they seek to demonstrate those in which they believe and prize. Affirming values in this manner has a more powerful impact than "preaching." Young adults, quick to recognize incongruities between talking and doing, respond to more mature adults who make an effort to live the difference. Unfortunately, there are many role models who fail to reflect on their own values, and thus model conflict and confusion (Dalton, 1985).

Interaction with People of Differing Values and Viewpoints

Values development is also promoted when one interacts with others of differing values and viewpoints (Fig. 16-4). "Such experiences tend to encourage and even demand reflectiveness and re-examination of what one may know or believe" (Dalton, 1985, pp. 55–56). In addition to being challenged by different values, which often stem from lifestyle, ethnicity, age, religion, or rural or urban living, one is also challenged to become more reasoned and articulate in defending one's own values. In dealing with people from different backgrounds, one also becomes more aware of larger social issues and values. Finally, one learns to disagree with others without necessarily rejecting them (Dalton, 1985).

Experiences that Challenge One's Way of Thinking

As one emerges from adolescence into young adulthood, often one's environment changes from home to college, the armed forces, or an independent living situation.

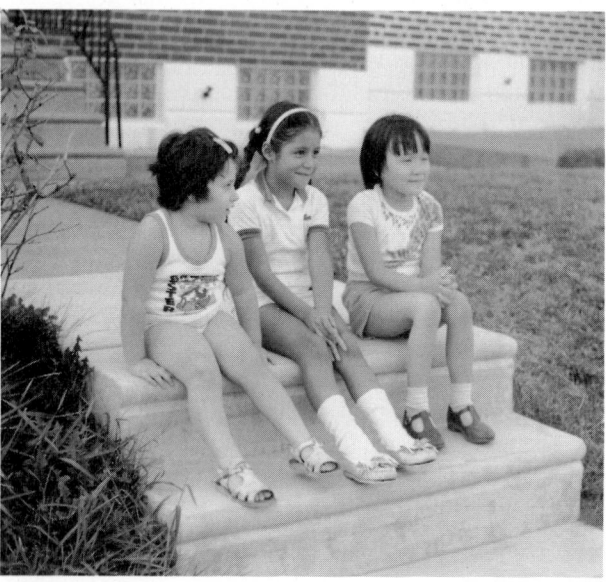

Figure 16–4. Interaction with peers from other cultures enriches one's values and viewpoints. The children are enriched by sharing their heritages: Italian, Hispanic, and Chinese.

This [new] environment often imposes new patterns of daily living and a variety of new relationships and social interactions. These changes in the individual's environment often force new adaptations and adjustments in one's values . . . (Dalton, 1985).

These environmental changes are so potent that some institutions plan them to create a sense of disorganization in their new members, and then provide a climate for reintegration, thus promoting more mature and consistent values.

Decision-Making

Choosing one of several alternative behaviors, either real or hypothetical, makes one more aware of one's personal values. The awareness can be heightened if this is done in a discussion where various individual decisions can be compared and contrasted (Dalton, 1985). This process shares aspects with the values clarification and values inquiry processes.

MANIFESTATIONS OF VALUES

As discussed earlier, values are reflected through attitudes, beliefs, and behaviors. It is behavior, however, that really demonstrates whether or not a person truly holds and lives out a value. A researcher in the area of values, Brian Hall (1980), identified three levels of valuing: action, choice, and vision (Fig. 16-5).

In this schema, there are two kinds of behavior that indicate a held value. One kind is habitual; the person does not have to think about it. For example, such health practices as brushing and flossing teeth can become a routine part of morning care; this habit would indicate an **action value**. Another type of behavior relies on choice; this behavior is done only when the person sets it as a goal. To continue with the dental care example, let us say that the dentist recommends that one also use a water-spray oral hygiene device. To add this procedure to one's morning routine, one would need to purchase the equipment and allow additional time to use it. It might also entail setting the alarm to get up earlier. Until these additional behaviors become habits, the extra dental care would remain a **choice value.** If the person only thought about buying a water-spray device, however, telling the dentist that he or she thought it was a good idea, the value of additional dental care would remain a **vision value**; this is a value projected into the future that will not become "real" until the person acts. The dentist might demonstrate the water-pic or show before-and-after pictures of gum tissue improvement with its use, but until the person actually carried out the procedure, it would remain a vision value, not an action value. Vision

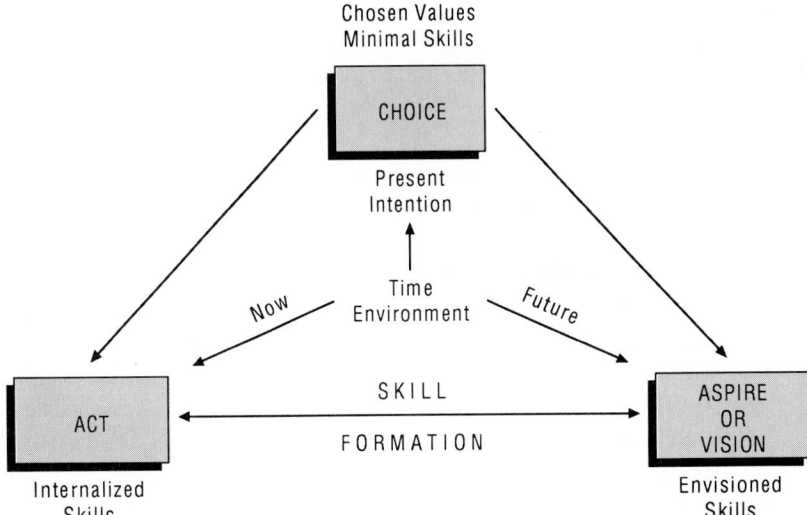

Figure 16–5.   Three levels of valuing: choice, act, and vision. (From Hall, B. (1980). *The personal discernment inventory* (p. 36). New York: Paulist Press.)

values are those we ultimately would like to hold, but for which we lack, momentarily, the knowledge or skills necessary to integrate them into our lives.

Effect of Values on Functional Health

In assessing values related to functional health, there are three levels of information of which the nurse needs to be aware: general human needs, social and culture-specific needs, and individual or personal needs. These needs are discussed in detail in Chapters 12, 14, and 15. These three levels of need determine patient behaviors and, thus, indicate the values that influence health status.

The nursing profession has identified 11 functional health patterns that represent general, basic human needs. For example, the preceding discussion about values and dental care comes under the second pattern, Nutritional and Metabolic Patterns.

> All human beings have in common certain functional patterns that contribute to their health, quality of life, and achievement of human potential. These patterns are the focus of nursing assessment. Description and evaluation of health patterns permits the nurse to identify functional patterns (client strengths) and dysfunctional patterns (nursing diagnoses) (Gordon, 1987).

The culture or social group also defines how the patient views health. The culture may promote specific beliefs about health, the body, and the cause and cure of illness, which dictate certain behaviors and indicate values. For example, in a Southeast Asian culture, the top of a person's head is sacred; if something should cover this area, the person's spirit is harmed. Thus, certain diagnostic procedures, medical treatments, or surgeries are very frightening, causing conflicts between values of spiritual well-being and medical care.

Finally, each patient is a unique person, expressing personal preferences and values. For example, there are individual preferences regarding sensory modes; some patients like touch whereas others do not, depending on their personal history.

Thus, in understanding and being sensitive toward patient values and their interactions with functional health patterns, the nurse should move from the perspective of general human needs, to cultural or social needs, and finally to unique individual needs. The following briefly reviews the 11 health patterns, relating values issues to each. The values identified with each pattern are taken from the list of 120 values (as shown in the accompanying display) identified by Hall (1980).

Health Perception and Health Management

Personal health is a value. The basis of this value resides in people's value to themselves, usually expressed as self-esteem or self-acceptance. Health values also reflect beliefs about the nature of health and health practices; most of these beliefs and practices are culturally or socially defined. For example, good health may be seen as an indicator of balance in life or of being a good person. To maintain health as a value, additional values are necessary to carry out health practices; these might include discipline, planning, responsibility, education, and cooperation. In working with specific persons, nurses need to assess how the patients experience health and what they do to maintain health, all within their cultural and social environment. Their level of self-esteem, which is also a value, will reflect their ability to incorporate new health behaviors into their lifestyle.

Nutrition and Metabolism

The essential value represented by the nutrition and metabolism pattern is survival; however, the various atti-

Hall's Value List with Skills

Values	Skills	Values	Skills
1. Accountability/Mutual Responsibility	IS	47. Evaluation/Self System	IP
		48. Expressiveness/Freedom	IM
2. Achievement/Success	I_2	49. Faith/Risk	IP
3. Adaptability/Flexibility	IP	50. Family/Belonging	IP
4. Administration/Control	I_2	51. Fantasy/Play	IM
5. Affection/Physical	IP	52. Food/Warmth/Shelter	I_2
6. Art/Beauty/As Pure Value	IM	53. Friendship/Belonging	IP
7. (Self) Assertion	IP	54. Function	I_2
8. Being Liked	IP	55. Generosity/Service	IP
9. Being Self	IS	56. Growth/Expansion	IS
10. Care/Nurture	IP	57. Harmony/System	IS
11. (Self) Centeredness	IP	58. Health/Personal	IS
12. Communications	I_2	59. Hierarchy/Property/Order	IS
13. Community/Personalist	IS	60. Honor	IS
14. Community/Supportive	IS	61. Human Dignity	IS
15. Competition	I_2	62. Independence	IP
16. (Self) Competence/Confidence	I_2	63. Instrumentality	I_2
17. Congruence	IP	64. Integration/Wholeness	IP
18. Construction/New Order	IS	65. Interdependence	IS
19. Contemplation/Asceticism	I_2	66. Intimacy	IP
20. (Self) Control	IP	67. Intimacy and Solitude as Unitive	IP
21. Control/Order/Discipline	I_2	68. Justice	IS
22. Convivial Tool/Intermediate Technology	IS	69. Knowledge/Discovery/Insight	I_2
		70. Law/Guide	IS
23. Cooperation	IS	71. Law/Rule	I_2
24. Corporation/Construction/ New Order	IS	72. Life/Self-Actualization	IP
		73. Limitation/Celebration	IP
25. Courtesy/Respect	IP	74. Loyalty/Respect	IP
26. Creativity/Ideation	IM	75. Macro Economics	IS
27. Criteria/Rationality	I_2	76. Management	I_2
28. (Self) Delight	IM	77. Membership	I_2
29. Detachment/Solitude	IS	78. Mission/Goals	IS
30. Decision/Initiation	IP	79. Obedience/Duty	IP
31. Design/Pattern/Order	I_2	80. Obedience/Mutual Accountability	IS
32. (Self) Directedness	IP	81. Objectivity	I_2
33. Discovery/Delight	IM	82. Ownership	IP
34. Discernment/Communal	IS	83. Patriotism/Esteem	IP
35. Duty/Obligation	IP	84. Pioneerism/Innovation/Progress	IS
36. Economics/Profit	I_2	85. Play/Leisure	IP
37. Economics/Success	I_2	86. Poverty/Simplicity	IS
38. Ecority/Beauty/Aesthetics	IM	87. Pluriformity	IS
39. Education/Certification	I_2	88. Power Authority/Honesty	IP
40. Education/Knowledge/Insight	I_2	89. Presence/Dwelling	IP
41. Efficiency/Planning	I_2	90. (Self) Preservation	IP
42. Empathy	IP	91. Prestige/Image	IP
43. Equilibrium	IS	92. Productivity	I_2
44. Equality/Liberation	IP	93. Property/Control	I_2
45. Equity/Rights	IP	94. Recreation/Freesence	IM
46. Ethics/Accountability/Values	I_2	95. Relaxation	IS

(continued)

Hall's Value List with Skills *(continued)*

Values	Skills	Values	Skills
96. Research/Originality/Knowledge	IM	109. Synergy	IS
97. Responsibility	IP	110. Tradition	IS
98. Ritual/Meaning	IS	111. Transcendence/Global Confluence	IS
99. Rule/Accountability	I_2	112. Truth/Wisdom/Intuitive Insight	IM
100. Safety/Survival	I_2	113. Unity/Solidarity	IP
101. Search/Meaning	IM	114. Wonder/Awe/Fate	IM
102. Security	IP	115. Wonder/Curiosity	IM
103. Sensory Pleasure/Sex	IP	116. Word	IS
104. Service/Vocation	IS	117. Work/Labor	I_2
105. Sharing/Listening/Trust	IP	118. Workmanship/Craft	I_2
106. Simplicity/Play	I_2	119. Worship/Duty/Creed	I_2
107. Social Affirmation	IS	120. (Self) Worth	IP
108. Support Peer	IP		

I_2, instrumental skills; IP, interpersonal skills; IM, imaginal skills; IS, systems skills.
Adapted from Hall, B. (1980). *The personal discernment inventory.* New York: Paulist Press.

tudes and beliefs about nutrition represent cultural and personal preferences. The presentation of food may also reflect esthetic values, such as art and beauty, and socialization values, such as family, work, service, or ritual. For example, some cultures consider color, texture, and design as part of food preparation; others may emphasize the social interaction at meal time.

Elimination

Values associated with excretory functions of the bowel, bladder, and skin may include sensory pleasure, control, discipline, and self-competence. Practices associated with these functions are learned within cultural and family frameworks. For example, adolescent Americans learn to be self-conscious regarding body odor and body hair, whereas those from other parts of the world may not.

Activity and Exercise

The activity and exercise pattern deals with an person's energy level. Persons who have a sensory orientation to the world tend to be more physically active. Values associated with this pattern might include sensory pleasure, competition, image, play, leisure, relaxation, and recreation. For example, in American society, where values of knowledge and research are a priority, physical fitness—especially through aerobic exercise—has been shown to reduce risks of heart disease. Not all people at risk exercise, however; they might give priority to other values or they might not have the time management

skills to incorporate an exercise program into their schedule.

Sleep and Rest

Survival is the value basic to the sleep and rest pattern, but culture and family also support practices related to sleep and rest; siestas and coffee breaks are examples. Also, the manner of sleeping varies across cultures and families; family members might sleep in separate beds and bedrooms or in a large family room on mats on the floor. Generally, all people need 6 to 8 hours of sleep per day, but much variability occurs with age, occupation, and individual needs.

Cognition and Perception

The cognition and perception pattern involves the five senses, language, memory, and decision-making. Values associated with this area include sensory pleasure, expressiveness, communication, rationality, evaluation, and intuition. Language is probably the most important of these aspects, because it reflects cultural patterns of thinking in such areas as time, space, and world-view. Within that culture a person's sentence structure indicates the thinking process, reality orientation, and sensory preference.

Further delineation of the world-view concept is other concepts in understanding **cultural value orientations.** These are human–nature orientation, time orientation, activity orientation, and relational orientation (Brink,

1984). A combination of Brink's cultural value orientations and Hall's value list (Table 16-2) is another way to study cultural value.

For example, if one believes that humans are masters of nature, then one values problem-solving and intervention. If one believes in harmony with nature, however, then one values balance. The subjugation-to-nature view values wonder, awe, or fate, focusing more on safety and survival. Time orientation refers to past, present, and future. If one has a future orientation, one values goals and planning, whereas a person with a past orientation values order, ritual, and tradition. Present orientation values include sensory pleasure, wonder, play, flexibility, and sharing. Activity orientation expresses the type of involvement one has with life. For example, a person whose orientation is toward "doing" values productivity as a measure of success or happiness, whereas a "being" person values self-acceptance, and a "being-in-becoming" person values self-development or self-actualization.

The three relational orientations or styles are individual, collateral, and lineal. The main distinctions between these styles revolve around the value of individual versus group well-being or goals. Collateral relationships emphasize such values as duty, mutual accountability, responsibility, and membership, and focus on the group rather than the individual. Lineal relationships value hierarchical group relationships based on authority, order, discipline, and tradition. These four value orientations, discussed earlier, have numerous implications for nurses and patient care; they affect the understanding of the illness process, intervention in the process, the deci-sion as to which people are to be involved in the process, and acceptable treatment activities.

One interesting way to understand this pattern is to read Tony Hillerman's detective novels, set in the Navajo culture of the southwestern United States (Hillerman, 1990). He successfully captures the value orientations of "present," harmony with nature, collateral or tribal relationships, and "doing" as the investigation unfolds. Since there is usually a murder involved, one should pay particular attention to the understanding of the body and the spirit.

Self-Perception and Self-Concept

Values underlying this pattern are self-preservation, self-delight, self-worth, self-competency, self-assertion, self-actualization, integration, and being one's self. Initially, the family and the larger society prescribe how one should think and feel about one's self. In American culture, where individuality and independence are valued, the emphasis is on one's unique sense of self apart from the group.

Roles and Relationships

How we relate to others is often defined by our function or role. Some of the values associated with the many possible role relationships include belonging, social affiliation, support, work, duty, ownership, membership, education, service, power, authority, cooperation, and intimacy. The major roles in our society are family roles, student or work roles, and social roles (Fig. 16-6).

TABLE 16–2

Cultural Value Orientations with Associated Values from Hall

Orientations	Associated Values		
Man–Nature	**Mastery**	**Subjugation**	**Harmony**
	Control	Fate	Equilibrium
	Order	Awe	Balance
	Planning	Survival	Integration
Time	**Future**	**Present**	**Past**
	Management	Wonder	Tradition
	Achievement	Flexibility	Ritual
	Research	Sensory pleasure	Obligation
Relational	**Individual**	**Collateral**	**Lineal**
	Independence	Mutual accountability	Authority
	Competition	Belonging	Discipline
	Success		Heirarchy
Activity	**Doing**	**Being**	**Being-in-Becoming**
	Productivity	Being self	Self-actualization
	Efficiency	Expressiveness	Wholeness
	Profits	Celebration	Search/meaning

From Brink, P. J. (1984). Values orientation as an assessment tool in cultural diversity. *Nursing Research, 33,* 198–203; Hall, B. (1980). *The personal discernment inventory.* New York: Paulist Press.

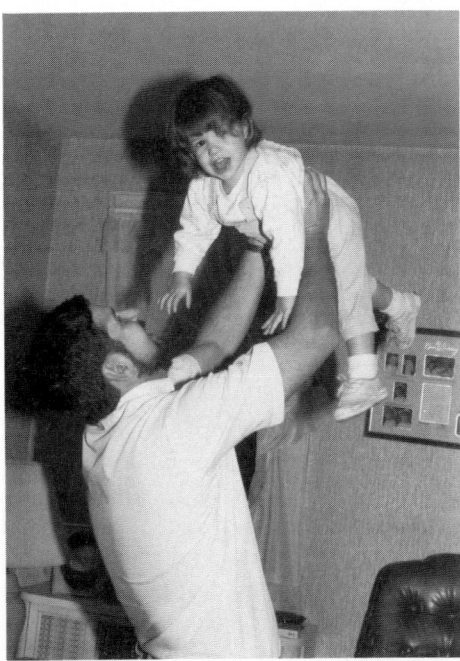

Figure 16–6. Values are displayed through roles and relationships in the family. The child learns values through time spent with the parents.

Sexuality and Reproduction

The pattern of sexuality and reproduction is closely associated with self-concept and role relationships. Self-delight, self-control, belonging, sharing, wholeness, being one's self, and intimacy are values associated with this pattern. Participation and levels of satisfaction are usually defined within the society and culture. For example, the focus of sexuality may be primarily on reproduction, or it may be on intimacy and pleasure.

Coping and Stress Management

Though people respond to stress in many ways, the basic values underlying this pattern are self-preservation, safety, and survival. Other values related to this pattern reflect various coping styles; some of these values include support, competition, equilibrium, control, planning, management, flexibility, assertion, relaxation, sharing, listening, education, creativity, detachment, cooperation, and insight.

Values and Beliefs

The values and beliefs pattern reflects a person's overall attitude or feeling about life, and is associated with hope, meaning, and purpose. It may also involve spiritual and religious issues that support the person's worldview, his or her attitudes about the importance of life and the meaning of death. Values typical of this pattern include wonder, duty, loyalty, tradition, worship, de-

sign, law, unity, service, search, human dignity, intimacy, justice, mission, faith, truth, and transcendence.

Manifestations of Nurses' Values

Nurses demonstrate their values in their attitudes and behaviors. For example, a nurse may say that he or she values family and belonging. Observation of the nurse's interaction with families—supporting them, sharing information with them, and consulting them for discharge planning—might indicate a discrepancy between what the nurse says and does. The nurse's value of family and belonging might be questioned. In this case, where a nurse claims to value family and belonging but does not demonstrate this when caring for patients, the nurse might be deficient in communication skills or not understand family dynamics. Thus, this value would be a vision value or an ideal, not yet committed to behavior.

In Hall's schema, values can also be organized in a **hierarchy of skills** (Hall, 1980). These skills are instrumental, interpersonal, imaginal, and systems. **Instrumental skills** comprise the first level of skills and are associated with basic physical and intellectual competencies that enable one to shape both ideas and the external environment. An example in nursing of instrumental skills would be the knowledge and clinical application necessary in providing basic patient care (i.e., skin care, wound care, range of motion, vital signs). **Interpersonal skills** determine the ability to relate happily and productively with others. Communication skills such as listening and sharing, problem-solving skills, teaching, and counseling are some of the interpersonal skills necessary in nursing. **Imaginal skills** bring imagination and creativity into play, enabling the nurse to envision a plan for adapting and personalizing patient care. The values that support imaginal skills are esthetic; esthetics is also an essential value of nursing, as identified by the American Association of Colleges of Nursing (1986). **Systems skills** are those that aid one in seeing the whole picture and how various parts relate. As nurses initiate changes in one aspect of patient care, they need to be aware of how this may affect other departments in the hospital such as housekeeping, pharmacy, physical therapy, and x-ray or laboratory services.

Returning to the example of the nurse whose vision value is family and belonging, we can define knowledge of family dynamics and communication as instrumental skills. Understanding the process of the nurse–patient relationship and being able to form relationships built on trust are interpersonal skills. For the value of family and belonging to become a behavioral reality, the nurse sets goals to use family dynamics knowledge and to practice communication. That is, this value is a choice value until the nurse "does" the behaviors automatically.

One of the essential values of the nursing profession discussed earlier was human dignity. Both knowledge of family dynamics and communication are values that will ultimately support the higher value of human dignity. In Hall's schema, human dignity is a systems skill, the most complex of all the skills. It requires incorporation not only of instrumental and interpersonal skills, but also imaginal skills. When these skills are integrated, the nurse can move beyond a particular family and begin to think of family health programs in the larger health care system. It is at this level that human dignity for all families becomes an action value.

This hierarchy of instrumental, interpersonal, imaginal, and systems value-skills, as well as other concepts in Hall's theory, has implications for growth and development.

LIFESPAN CONSIDERATIONS

Values can also reflect the person's age and stage of development. Although not everyone automatically develops all values, most people's values change or are refined by various life experiences. Table 16-3 illustrates key values during different stages of life, combining Erikson's (1982) and Hall's theories of development.

Infant, Toddler, and Preschooler

At the most basic level, an infant begins value development with the evolution of trust and autonomy. Moral development and cognitive ability are closely related. As the child progresses to toddlerhood, moral and values development begin with the child identifying which behaviors elicit reward or punishment. Kohlberg (1964) refers to this as the first-level preconventional stage, where the child learns to distinguish right from wrong and understand the choice between obedience and punishment.

The preschool-aged child learns that rules are unchanging and are imposed by parents and adults. In this later stage of development the child recognizes and accepts fairness and cooperation, although these are limited by the child's self-interest and self-will. Children are concerned when the situation seems "unfair" to them, yet do not have enough maturity to project that same sense of fairness to their peers.

Child and Adolescent

The school-aged child is industrious, recognizing the need for moral codes and social rules. The younger child

---

TABLE 16-3
Stage of Human Development: Parallels

Eras	Erikson's Eight Stages	Hall's Four Phases of Consciousness
Infancy	Trust (Hope)	Phase I
		Security
	Autonomy	Survival
		Pleasure
Early Childhood	(Will)	Wonder
	Initiative (Purpose)	
Childhood	Industry (Competence)	Phase II
		Belonging
		Work
Adolescence	Identify (Fidelity)	Self-competence
		Self-worth
Young Adulthood	Intimacy (Love)	Phase III
		Independence
Adulthood	Generativity (Care)	Service/vocation
		Creation
		Being self
Maturity	Integrity (Wisdom)	Phase IV
		Harmony
		Interdependence
		Intimacy
		Esthetics

maintains a strict understanding and application of the rules, seeing things in clearly dichotomous ways (i.e., right or wrong). As the child grows into preadolescence, he or she becomes more flexible. The threat of discipline becomes less important than social expectations. Kohlberg (1964) refers to this as the second-level or conventional stage, characterized by conformity to expectations and behaviors of others.

For the adolescent, the influence of peer identification reaches its greatest persuasiveness. Although this period of development is often characterized by rebellion, the adolescent has a high level of moral judgment with a law-and-order orientation. The adolescent understands that morality is derived from principles of conscience and that rules are cooperative agreements that can be modified. As the person reaches late adolescence, he or she begins to move away from the strong peer influence based on individual principles, and peer group values decrease in importance.

Adult and Older Adult

The adult focuses on generativity and intimacy as careers and families are formed. The primary moral concerns are now directed to meeting the expectations of employer, family, and adult social group. Values that were taught and caught in childhood generally develop into what the adult will accept as guiding principles for life.

The older adult's attention is on personal integrity and the wisdom that has been accumulated over a lifetime. Values are firmly ingrained in the adult, yet the older adult is often more accepting of values of others that may be different from his or her own.

Hall's Value Development Theory

Hall's theory of values and value development is complex and draws on many sources, two of which are Freire's work on "Conscientization" and Maslow's hierarchy of needs (Hall, 1986). Building on these sources, Hall outlines a potential natural growth process for a values hierarchy. In this framework, needs are the basis of values that flow from different stages of life.

Table 16-3 identifies Hall's four phases of consciousness or world-views (Hall, 1980, 1986; Hall, et al., 1982). The perspective in Phase I is that of the infant or child where the self is center, focusing on physical existence; the world is a mystery over which the self has no control. The basic needs or values are food, shelter, and pleasure. The era of adolescence through young adulthood deals with the world as problem of Phase II, seeing the world as a problem to be solved. The self copes by doing and learning, as well as by belonging to a social or peer group. The basic values are social acceptance, affirma-

tion, approval, and achievement. At the Phase III level of consciousness, the self, similar in nature to Maslow's self-actualizer, views the world as a project and invention. The basic values include personal authority, freedom, dignity, and integrity. The self seeks to satisfy the personal need of independence. In Phase IV the worldview is one of mystery, but unlike the child, the self reaches out to care. This caring is in the global sense, beyond one's own immediate environment. The values are truth, community, harmony, and interdependence. This stage is possible from adult mid-life through old age; however, not everyone is able to reach this level of function.

These phases of consciousness or levels of development are significantly different from other developmental theories in that they are not necessarily related to age, but to experience and self-reflection (Hall, 1986). For example, in the first few years of life, a child experiences the world as a mystery over which he or she has no control, but also perceives it with wonder, awe, curiosity, and self-delight. If the child's survival needs are not met, however, then as an adult, the experience of the world will continue in Phase I as the self struggles to survive in an environment perceived as hostile, alien, oppressive, and capricious. In this example, the adult continues to struggle with basic needs or values. If the environment is supportive, however, the young adult emerges secure and competent. Then, as a mid-life adult, the person is able to move toward self-actualization.

The nurse can apply these phases of consciousness and values in the initial assessment; however, the patient's life experience and reflection on this experience determines the actual level of values development.

VALUE CONFLICTS

Wherever there is human interaction there is likely to be **value conflicts.** These conflicts can be worked out if the nurse is aware of his or her own values and the patient's values. Working out these conflicts may entail a clarification of values and an appreciation and acceptance of value differences. Since value conflicts may also affect compliance with nursing care, appreciation and acceptance of value differences by the nurse can be the basis of negotiation and compromise leading to acceptable care for the patient.

Patient and Family Conflicts

Value conflicts between family members arise from developmental differences, experience differences, and personal preference differences. One fairly common example is when one spouse refuses to take the time to have a health check-up. Depending on how the healthcare system was experienced in early life or interpreted by the culture, the person refusing care may have values of tradition, self-control, competition, self-directedness, independence, fate, and risk that may appear to counter values of regular preventive health care. These values may reflect an underlying struggle with other values such as security, self-competence, or self-worth. The nurse's role might lie in helping the spouses explore their personal health history and needs rather than continuing the argument about the health check-up. Ideally, the nurse could assist each spouse in setting some attainable personal health goals, helping them realize the values of sharing, listening, trust, accountability, and responsibility.

Patient and Health-Care Conflicts

Areas of conflict between patient and health-care caregivers can evolve around values related to knowledge, cultural differences, and developmental differences, as well as personal preference.

For example, in the case of an American family where the grandmother has died, the parents may prefer that the children not go to the funeral, stating that the children do not understand death and it might be difficult for them. The nurse, who values communication, support, and the research findings on children and death, might disagree with the parents. Realizing that death is a traumatic event for the survivors, and that the parents' protection of the children is really a protection of their own feelings, the nurse might explore other ways in which the children's grief and loss needs could be met and that the family could more readily accept. Depending on the ages of the children, these might include stories, drawing, or playing with a doll house family that includes a grandmother (Cook & Oltjenbruns, 1989).

Resolving Value Conflicts in the Health-Care System

Three main issues that arise in thinking about the resolution of value conflicts are the perception of conflict, the meaning of resolution, and the values underlying the resolution process.

When nurses face value conflicts it is important for them to examine their own values regarding conflict. If the nurse views conflict as negative, he or she might feel threatened; his or her own values of self-competence, duty, success, authority, and esteem are questioned. If the nurse views conflict as positive, however, the values of respect, communication, care, equilibrium, harmony, service, and creativity are enhanced. These two views of conflict are based on the nurse's life experience and level of values development. For example, if a nurse was raised in a dysfunctional family, conflict is very threatening and to be avoided; the core value is security. For the nurse who has experienced more functional patterns of family interaction, the core value might be interdependence or innovation.

There are several definitions of the word "resolution" that help in thinking about resolving value conflicts. One definition of resolution is that it is a clarifying or explanatory process. For example, as discussed earlier, many people have not reflected on their values, and so when conflicts occur they are not able to articulate their position. Therefore, one of the first goals for the nurse is to assist the patient in exploring and defining the relevant issues, attitudes, and beliefs. This clarification or explanation may be the resolution, or it may be the first step in a resolution process.

A second definition of resolution is that it takes place through the answering of questions. Patients have many questions related to their care. What nurses take for granted as routine care may be strange to the patient. Encouraging questions by saying something like, "I have asked you a lot of questions, now do you have some that you would like to ask?" can be helpful. For example, an adolescent woman is admitted for a suicide gesture; she cut her wrist. After a lengthy assessment, the nurse asks her if she has any questions. Her question is, "How is the food here?" Although a suicide attempt indicates that the patient is dealing with survival issues, this question also is a concrete demonstration that the patient is in the Phase I value development mode or basic survival mode, focusing on food and shelter. She is not able to focus on setting goals related to communication skills, assertiveness, or dealing with loss and grief, although the nurse has mentioned that these are some areas she might consider working on during her hospitalization. The first nursing intervention is getting the patient something to eat. Had the nurse insisted on focusing on the counseling goals of communication or assertiveness in the ensuing 24 hours, there would have been a values conflict. The patient is not ready to deal with feelings on a verbal level.

Another kind of resolution lies in coming to a decision or a determination for future action. For example, there may be several treatment options from which a patient can choose. Even after examining all the facts and getting a second opinion, a patient decides to take a course of action that the nurse does not like. If the nurse were to impose his or her decision on the patient at this point, it is highly likely that a value conflict would arise and the patient might not comply with any treatment.

A fourth definition of resolution involves breaking up the issue or problem into its elements. Perhaps there are some elements of the situation on which the nurse and patient can agree, thus facilitating care. This is especially important with patients from different sociocultural backgrounds. The patient often has a different belief system regarding the cause of illness, resulting in different values regarding prevention and cure. For example, a male refugee from Africa becomes psychotic because of major losses and culture shock. He is hospitalized for several months, discharged, and then rehospitalized because he did not take the prescribed psychotropic medications. In exploring the patient's belief system, it is found that he believes that his problems are due to displeasing his family and being a coward. Mental illness is viewed as a punishment. Rather than focusing on the scientific explanation supported by Western values of knowledge, the nurse assists the patient in learning about the community by taking him to various activities and facilities. The patient likes this approach, finding that a prayer meeting held at a church of his ethnic group was especially helpful.

In summary, it is useful to view conflict and its resolution as part of an ongoing process in human relationships. Value conflict resolution, based on respect, involves a process that includes understanding one's perception of conflict, values clarification, answering or encouraging questions, making decisions, and finding elements for agreement or negotiation and compromise.

VALUES ASSESSMENT

The nursing history is one place where values assessment takes place, but any interaction with a patient may give the nurse value indicators. The following discussion identifies how the nurse can assess a patient's values.

Level of Values Development

The age and experiences of a patient may indicate the primary values associated with the four phases of consciousness. For example, young adult values are concerned with family and belonging, self-worth, and self-competence, whereas adult values at midlife may be more concerned with life/self-actualization, and service and vocation. Asking the patient to share a major turning point in his or her life or a life-changing experience may clarify the phases. If the patient has had some traumatic experiences, or currently faces a life-threatening illness, he or she may temporarily focus on values of self-preservation and security typical of the Phase I level of consciousness.

View of Hospitalization and Illness

Useful initial openings for a nursing assessment are "Tell me what brought you in for the hospitalization?" (if the person has been in several times), and "What is your understanding of your condition (illness)?" These questions clarify the patient's perception of health and illness, and elicit information on the patient's world-view, defined earlier as mastery over nature or problem-solv-

---

| Nursing Research |

Possible Topics for Nursing Inquiry

- What changes in values occur during the nursing education process?
- What are the value differences at various levels of nursing education? nursing service?
- Define nursing values assessment.
- Test values as they relate to functional health.

Selected Nursing Research Studies

Bloomquist, B. L. et al. (1980). Values of basic nursing students in secular and religious schools. *Nursing Research, 29,* 379–383.

Furham, A. (1988). Values and vocational choice. *Social Science Medicine, 2,* 613–618.

Garvin, B., & Kuznik, K. (1985). Values of entering nursing students: Changes over 10 years. *Research in Nursing and Health, 3,* 235–241.

Thurston, H. I., et al. (1989). Values held by nursing faculty and students in a university setting. *Journal of Professional Nursing, 5,* 199–207.

Ulrich, B. (1987). Value differences between practicing nurse executive and graduate nurse educators. *Nurse Educator, 6,* 287–291.

---

ing, acceptance of natural forces or fate, and harmony with nature or balance (Brink, 1984). These views indicate the patient's probable acceptance of therapy; for example, a patient who saw the illness as a problem to be solved might be more open to the problem-solving process and goal-setting than the patient who saw the illness as fate.

Activities of Daily Living

When the nurse asks patients questions about how they spend their time, that is, how a typical day or week in their life is, he or she is gathering information related to operative or action values. The behaviors patients describe indicate their value commitments. Many of these action values can be identified as functional health is assessed. These include nutrition and metabolism, elimination, activity and exercise, sleep and rest, roles and relationships, sexuality and reproduction, and coping and stress management. "How" the patients describe their day would indicate the patterns of health-perception and health-management, self-perception, and values and beliefs.

Discharge Planning

Final discharge planning, coming near the end of a hospitalization, is a busy time for the nurse, the patient, and the patient's family. By this time, the patient and the nurse should have been involved in a mutual goal-setting process of which discharge planning is an extension. In clarifying follow-up care, teaching self-care skills, evaluating living arrangements, and meeting with the family, the nurse will continue to identify patient values. Three value orientations are particularly useful in assessment at this time: role relationships, activity modes, and time orientation (Brink, 1984).

In terms of role relationships, it is important for the nurse to assess the patient's view of him- or herself and his or her relationships to family and friends. If the patient comes from the general American culture, he or she is more likely to have a smaller nuclear family and value individualism and will want to have more say about his or her own follow-up care unless, of course, the patient is a dependent child or elderly. If the patient comes from a larger extended family, the group opinion is more valued. If the extended family is hierarchical in nature, the senior group members may have more decision-making power. Thus, it is important to understand these role relationships and how they may effect the discharge planning process.

The goal-setting process will be influenced by the activity values orientation. For example, those patients who like to "do" things might be more involved in a physical rehabilitation program, because it is concrete and measurable. By contrast, those who have a "being" orientation might be less planned or more sporadic in their program. In working with the being-oriented person, the nurse might assist the patient and family to find a variety of ways to meet the physical rehabilitation needs, thus allowing for more spontaneity.

The goal-setting process is also influenced by the patient's time orientation values. Patients who are future-oriented can think more easily of goals than ones who have past or present orientations. For patients who have tradition as a value, the nurse may explore ways to relate some of these rituals to new health-care regimens. Present value orientation patients may need activities that are fun, stimulating, calming, and so forth, which give immediate feedback or sensation.

Discharge planning may also be a time when patients discuss the need for behavior change, which brings into play their choice or vision values. To help accomplish these changes, the nurse could assist patients in assessing additional skills and values they need. For example, a newly diagnosed diabetic patient who values independence might be concerned about the impact of the illness on his or her family. To maintain independence, he or she might become involved in the instrumental skills of learning how to manipulate a glucose-monitoring machine, self-administering insulin, and managing his or her diet, but the patient might avoid talking about feelings or concerns with his or her family. The nurse, assessing this lack, could assist the patient in exploring his or her feelings about the diagnosis. The nurse then could discuss the values of sharing, listening, and trust as they relate to the well-being of the family. In this example, the vision values would be interdependence, expressiveness, and intimacy.

In summary, values are an integral part of all human interactions. An understanding of values and their influence on the nurse–patient–family interaction is vital if there is to be acceptance of health care, as well as an integration of the value of personal health into the lives of patients and families (Uustal, 1987).

Key Concepts

- All human interactions are value-based.
- Nurses must clarify and respect the values of others, as well as examine their own values.
- Sources of values for professional nursing are parents, family, and significant others; they are absorbed through observation and experience, throughout a lifetime.
- Values are enhanced and refined by experiences that cultivate values development, such as interactions with persons of differing values and viewpoints and experiences that challenge one's way of thinking.
- The *Code for Nurses* by the American Nurses Association is a set of standards based on universal moral principles or values.
- The American Association of Colleges of Nursing identifies seven core values for nurses.
- Values in nursing are developed through socialization, classroom study, and clinical study.
- Values clarification is a method of self-discovery by which people identify their personal values without evaluating the values as such.
- Hall's developmental theory of values can be related to functional health patterns, to how patients and nurses manifest their values, to values conflict and resolution, and to values assessment.
- An understanding of values and their influence on the nurse–patient–family interaction is vital for acceptance of health care and the integration of the value of personal health into the lives of the patient and family.

References

American Association of Colleges of Nursing. (1986). *Essentials of colleges and university education for professional nursing.* Washington, DC: Author.

American Nurses Association. (1985). *Code for nurses with interpretive statements.* Kansas City, MO: Author.

Brink, P. J. (1984). Values orientations as an assessment tool in cultural diversity. *Nursing Research, 33,* 198–203.

Cook, A. S., & Oltjenbruns, K. A. (1989). *Dying and grieving: Lifespan and family perspectives.* New York: Holt, Rinehart and Winston.

Curtin, L., & Flaherty, M. J. (1982). *Nursing ethics: Theories and pragmatics.* Bowie, MD: Robert J. Brody.

Dalton, J. C. (1985). Promoting values development in college students. *NASPA Monograph Series, 4,* 47–59.

Erikson, E. (1982). *The life cycle completed.* New York: W. W. Morton & Co.

Fromm, E. (1959). Values, psychology and human existence. In A. Maslow (Ed.), *New knowledge in human values.* New York: Harper and Row.

Gordon, M. (1987). *Nursing diagnosis process and application* (2nd ed.). New York: McGraw-Hill.

Hall, B. (1980). *The personal discernment inventory.* New York: Paulist Press.

Hall, B. (1986). *The genesis effect.* New York: Paulist Press.

Hall, B., Kalven, J. Rosen, L. and Taylor, B. (1982). *Readings in value development.* Ramsey, NJ: Paulist Press.

Hillerman, T. (1990). *The coyote waits.* New York: Harper & Row.

King, E. C. (1984). *Affective education in nursing.* Rockville, MD: An Aspen Publication.

Kohlberg, L. (1964). Development of moral character and moral ideology. In M. L. Hoffman & L. N. W. Hoffman (Eds.), *Review of child development research, Vol. 1.* New York: Russell Bage Foundation.

Raths, L. E., Harmin, M., & Simon, S. B. (1966). *Values and teaching.* Columbus, OH: Charles E. Merrill.

Rokeach, M. (1973). *The nature of human values.* New York: The Free Press.

Thurston, H. I. (1989). Values held by nursing faculty and students in a university setting. *Journal of Professional Nursing, 5,* 199–207.

Uustal, D. B. (1987). Values: The cornerstone of nursing's moral art. In M. D. M. Fowler & J. Levine-Ariff (Eds.), *Ethics at the bedside.* Philadelphia: J. B. Lippincott.

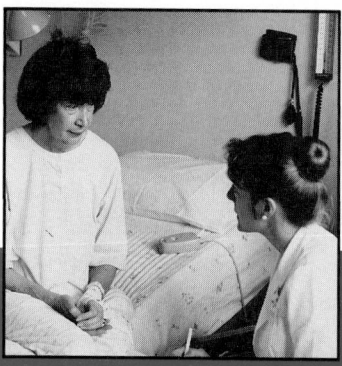

Communication: The Nurse–Patient Relationship

LEARNING OBJECTIVES

Upon completion of this chapter, the student will be able to do the following:

- Define various types of communication.
- Discuss elements of the communication process and their relevance to nursing.
- Discuss the relationship of language and experience to the communication process.
- Explain the nature of the nurse–patient relationship.
- Distinguish between a professional and a social relationship.
- Name the elements of an informal nurse–patient contract.
- Discuss four key aspects of therapeutic communication.
- Give examples of areas of assessment applied to nurse–patient communication.
- Define and give examples of a variety of therapeutic communication techniques.
- Name key nontherapeutic responses and explain how these interfere with therapeutic communication.
- Describe some special situations that affect communication.

KEY TERMS

Advocacy
Circle of
  confidentiality
Communication
  channel

Decode
Empathy
Encoding
Metacommuni-
  cation

Nonverbal
  communication
Therapeutic
  communication

17

The Communication Process
  Types of Communication
    Relationship of Types
  Elements of the Communication Process
  Importance of Language and Experience
The Nurse–Patient Relationship: A Helping
     Relationship
  Phases
  Contract-Setting
  Advocacy
  Circle of Confidentiality
Ingredients of Therapeutic Communication
  Empathy

Positive Regard
Comfortable Sense of Self
Communication and Nursing Process
  Assessment
  Intervention
    Helping the Patient Get Started
    Active Listening
    Exploring
    Developing Communication Skills
    Nontherapeutic Responses
    Special Situations
Key Concepts

Effective communication within the nurse–patient relationship is not so much a natural process as it is a learned skill. It is a way of being helpful to patients that differs from the way a clerk in a grocery store is helpful, or the way friends are helpful to each other. For example, when the grocery clerk gives a courteous answer to a question about a product, the result is a satisfied customer. In a conversation between two friends who are sharing their problems, each friend feels cared for and understood. Although nurse–patient communication may include some of the elements in these examples, it differs considerably.

The main subject of communication in the nurse–patient relationship is the *patient* and his or her experiences and problems. The results are directed toward improving coping skills related to the patient's health status and well-being. Thus, **therapeutic communication** is a way of being helpful by facilitating interactions that are focused on the patient and the patient's concerns. The purpose of therapeutic communication is to help the patient express and work through feelings and problems related to his or her condition, treatments, and nursing care (Fig. 17-1).

What kind of a process is therapeutic communication and how does it fit into the context of nursing practice? Because nursing is a practice based on the sciences, nurses master many scientific principles and technical skills. Nursing is also an interpersonal process, however. Interaction between the nurse and the patient has a great deal to do with the outcomes of care. The following happens during the communication process:

The nurse and patient work together to solve problems centered around the patient's health-care needs.
The patient feels cared for and understood.
The family is included in the care.
Health teaching is conducted.
Preventive care is delivered.

Peplau, a psychiatric nurse and nurse theorist, considered nursing to be a "significant therapeutic interpersonal process" and defined nursing as a "human relationship between an individual who is sick or in need of health services and a nurse especially educated to recognize and respond to the need for help" (Peplau, 1952). In short, communication is at the heart of all nursing care.

To understand therapeutic communication, we must first understand the communication process and the importance of language and experience. Specific ingredients and techniques of communication, knowledge about the nurse–patient relationship, contract-setting, advocacy, and confidentiality, and developmental issues

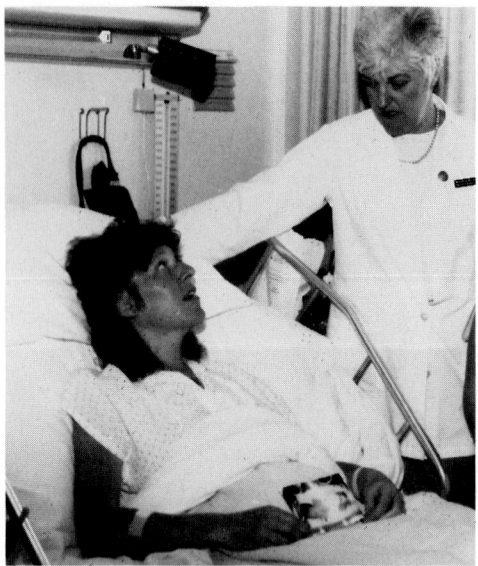

Figure 17–1. Listening and investigating are ways to address patient concerns. This occurs in all aspects of care and is the purpose of therapeutic communication.

related to communication are important as well. This chapter gives an overview of these and other concepts related to therapeutic communication.

THE COMMUNICATION PROCESS

There are many definitions of communication. To communicate means to impart information, to exchange ideas, to express ourselves in such a way that we are understood. Communication can be defined as a system of sending and receiving messages that forms a connection between the sender and the receiver (Fig. 17-2). It is a process for giving and receiving information, a form of interaction or transaction.

Communication is a continuous function of human life, much like breathing or cardiac functioning. The process goes on all the time. In many ways, the saying, "You cannot NOT communicate," is true. For example,

when a person decides not to share information, or one person stops talking to another person because of hurt or anger, communication has still taken place.

Communication is basic and essential to being human. Through communication, people relate to their environment and to each other. Without it, we would be unable to learn, to direct our lives, and to work together cooperatively in families, organizations, and communities. Communication is basic to human feeling and intellect; without it, we could not survive (Berlo, 1960; Thayer, 1968).

Types of Communication

People communicate in a variety of ways. *Verbal communication* involves the spoken or written word. It is an exchange using the elements of language (see Chap. 44). Equally important is **nonverbal communication.** A person communicates by gestures, facial expressions, posture, body movement, voice tone, rate of speech, and even dress. Silence is a form of nonverbal communication.

Another kind of communication, **metacommunication,** is a message *about* a message. It looks beyond the literal level of communication (that is, beyond just the words of the message). It includes anything that is taken into account when interpreting what is happening, such as the role of the communicator, the nonverbal messages sent, and the context of the communication taking place.

Relationship of Types

The relationship of these kinds of communication (verbal, nonverbal, and metacommunication) is important. The way they fit or do not fit together reflects just how complex communication is. The following two examples illustrate this.

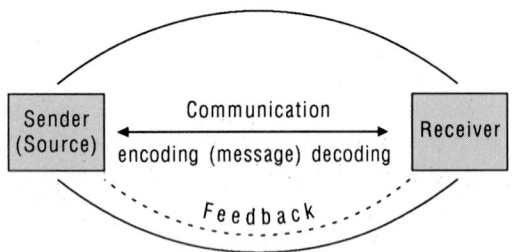

Figure 17–2. Communication is a process in which information is sent and received. It is a form of interaction that is continuous and ever-changing.

Examples of Types of Communication

Verbal	Nonverbal
Written	Touch
Spoken	Eye contact
Television and radio	Facial expression
Movies	Body posture
Magazines	Gestures
Books	Physical appearance
Computers	Voice tone
Posters	Rate of speech
Brochures	Neatness
	Movement

Incongruence. A patient and a nurse have been working together on diabetic teaching. After the teaching session is completed, the patient says to the nurse, "Yes, I understand my diabetic diet and how to take my insulin." On the surface, this seems to be a straightforward communication indicating that the patient understands the components of care needed to successfully deal with diabetes. If, however, the words of the message were said with an irritated facial expression and a harsh tone of voice, the nonverbal and metacommunication aspects of the message do not "fit" with the verbal message; they are incongruent. The metacommunication in this example may be conveying, "I am tired of being told how to run my life. I am angry about having a chronic illness." Furthermore, if the patient is later seen sneaking a candy bar, this nonverbal communication may convey the message that the patient has not yet accepted the illness. Thus, incongruence between kinds of communication gives the nurse clues about the patient's experience.

Congruence. A nurse makes rounds on his or her assigned primary patients at the beginning of the shift. He or she explains his or her role to each patient, confers with them about their nursing care needs, and schedules with them the care tasks to be done on that shift. The nurse is dressed in a professional manner and wears a name tag and hospital identification badge. He or she speaks in a well-modulated voice and listens carefully to what each patient says.

In this example, each kind of communication conveys messages that are congruent. The messages say, "I am your professional nurse. We will work together to meet your nursing care needs. I respect you." There is a "good fit" between verbal, nonverbal, and metacommunication.

Elements of the Communication Process

As shown in Figure 17-2, communication is a continuous operation, dynamic, ongoing, and ever-changing. Although it is somewhat artificial to break down communication into components, doing so can be useful. Knowing the individual elements of a process can be helpful in identifying where in the process a problem is occurring. The elements of the model presented here are based on the work of Berlo (1960), a communication theorist.

All communication has a *source* (a person or group with a purpose for the communication). The source's purpose must be translated into a code. This is done with language or nonverbal signals such as gestures, facial expressions, or body cues. The process of getting the purpose translated into the code is called **encoding.** Encoding results in a *message*. The fourth element in the communication process is the **communication channel,** the medium or carrier of the message. Television is a channel. The voice or written word are channels. Touch can be a channel.

If the communication process were to stop at the fourth element, no communication has taken place because there must be someone at the other end of the channel: the *receiver*. The receiver is the target of the communication. The receiver must be able to understand or **decode** the message. Once messages are decoded and received, *feedback* occurs. Feedback means that the source and the receiver use the reaction of the other to produce further messages.

Knowledge about the elements of the communication process can be useful to the nurse because sometimes specific difficulties in communication can be traced to one or more of the elements identified. A basic example is the patient who speaks a different language. In this case the nurse needs to attend to the communication channel. An interpreter may be needed to help the patient decode the nurse's messages. Pictures may also be used to convey messages.

Problems in the encoding process may occur as well. These problems can occur in patients with thought disorders or certain forms of brain damage. The patient has an intent to communicate but impairment in encoding results in a garbled message. A frightened patient whose thoughts are disturbed may say, "The F.B.I. is after me," when he really means, "I am very frightened and out of control." In the case of a patient suffering from a stroke, the patient may understand communication directed at him, but cannot encode a returning message because of brain damage.

Importance of Language and Experience

The importance of language and experience to the process of communication cannot be overestimated. Language distinguishes humans from other animals. It is used not only to communicate, but also to develop the person's view of life and the world. Thus, language and experiences are closely related. This idea was explained by Brandler and Grinder (1975) and the following discussion is based on their work.

A person's view of the world is developed through several kinds of filters. One such filter consists of the neurologic receptor systems: sight, hearing, touch, taste, and smell. Stimuli processed through these receptor systems enable the person to experience the outside world, and through language such experiences can be compared with others' experiences. Alterations in sensory perceptions can change the person's view of the world. A person with poor hearing or vision, for example, experiences the world differently than someone with perfect hearing and vision.

Another filter through which a person experiences the world is the particular language system into which the person is socialized. Words and sentences give meaning to things and events. Language allows us to conceptualize the world. If a language has only three words for all the color distinctions possible to see, for example, then a person would conceptualize colors differently than someone whose language offered more choices. Someone with a limited vocabulary has more difficulty describing experiences than does someone with a rich, diverse vocabulary. In fact, limitations in language skills may actually limit the person's choices in life.

A third filter through which a person experiences the world is his or her unique personal history. Every human has a set of experiences that are unique. Cultural background enters into personal history, as do family relationships, the person's place in the sibling ranking, the type of parenting received, the genetic makeup of the person, and other factors.

Both nurse and patient bring language and personal experiences into the communication that occurs between them. Some aspects of each person's language and experience are shared; in other words, they are similar in nature. Other aspects are unique to each person. An example is the word "mother." A mother has been a key person in almost everyone's life. Based on past experiences with one's mother, the feelings evoked by the word "mother" may vary from warmth and unconditional love to feelings of conflict to feelings of intense deprivation and longing. These feelings can be brought into the health-care situation as the nurse cares for the patient. Depending on past experiences with his or her mother, the patient may trust or not trust the nurse, manifest hostility to the nurse, or work collaboratively with the nurse. Similarly, the nurse brings his or her own feelings to the situation.

The interaction of the nurse and patient is productive when a method of communication is at work that identifies and uses common meanings (Peplau, 1952). Developing a common understanding is the underlying aim of communication, especially therapeutic communication. To communicate therapeutically, the nurse must first understand and appreciate the language and experiences that he or she brings to the situation. After that, the nurse must understand and appreciate the viewpoint of the patient, even if it differs from his or her own.

In the clinical setting, the extent to which patients and nurses successfully exchange information is affected by the degree to which their realities are mutually compatible. The medical system in which most nurses work produces barriers to communication. For example, technical language, such as medical jargon, can be a barrier to communication. Studies have shown that the inability of working-class patients to understand technical language intimidates them and prevents them from asking questions on their own behalf. Other barriers include talking about the patient in front of him or her, withholding information from the patient, and being too busy to spend time with the patient (Matthews, 1983).

Peplau (1952) identified two overriding principles that guide communication: clarity and continuity. Table 17-1 illustrates the concepts of clarity and continuity.

Clarity refers to words and sentences used that clarify events when they occur within the frame of reference and common experience of both nurse and patient. Meaning is established or made understandable as a result of the joint and sustained effort of everyone involved in the communication. Clarity is facilitated when the patient's perceptions are expressed and discussed.

Continuity in communication occurs when language is used as a tool for the promotion of coherence or connections of ideas expressed. Continuity is promoted when the nurse picks up threads or cues of conversation offered by the patient. A conversational thread or cue is a vaguely expressed word, phrase, or idea that hints at a problem or concern. The nurse helps the patient focus on and elaborate on these cues. By doing so, the patient is helped to express underlying problems or concerns.

TABLE 17–1

Examples of Clarity and Continuity

Clarity	Continuity
Patient: I am having pain. ("Pain" can mean many things.)	Patient: This place is crazy. Things are confusing here. ("Crazy" and "confusing" are conversational cues.)
Nurse: Where is the pain?	Nurse: Confusing?
Patient: In my stomach.	Patient: Yes, I can't tell what is going on. ("Going on" is a cue.)
Nurse: What kind of pain is it? Can you describe to me?	Nurse: "Going on" in what sense?
(Patient describes exact nature and place of pain.)	Patient: About my condition. No one is explaining it to me.
Outcome: Nurse and patient come to a common understanding about the patient's experience.	Outcome: Patient is helped to focus on the real problem because the nurse helped him elaborate on conversational cues.

TABLE 17–2

Comparison of Professional with Social Relationship

	Nurse-Patient	**Social**
Key Focus	Patient	Both participants
Goals	Meeting patient's needs. Help patient identify feelings and concerns; problem-solve, cope, and adapt in relation to health-care situation.	Meeting own needs. Mutual companionship, enjoyment, and interaction. May lead to intimacy and commitment.
Parameters	Limited primarily to the needs incurred by the health-care situation. Nurse self-discloses only what is appropriate for the patient's benefit. Relationship is terminated when goals are met and service no longer needed.	Sharing of life's events, activities, or other aspects of self. May stay superficial or lead to long-term relationship. Relationship may be terminated when own needs are no longer met.
Self-assessment	Nurse assesses own role, communication skills, values, etc. and how these affect the professional relationship.	Each person assesses how own needs for enjoyment, affection, and sharing, or love and intimacy, are met in the relationship.

THE NURSE–PATIENT RELATIONSHIP: A HELPING RELATIONSHIP

Within the nurse–patient relationship, the nurse assumes the role of a professional, a helper. The patient is the one seeking help. This kind of relationship differs from a social or intimate relationship. The nurse–patient relationship is focused on the patient, is goal-directed, and has defined parameters. Another important way that the nurse–patient relationship differs from a social one concerns the nurse's self-assessment. In the professional relationship, the nurse learns to assess his or her own role, communication skills, personal history, and values in terms of how these may be affecting the nurse–patient relationship and interactions. Table 17-2 compares the nurse–patient relationship with a social relationship.

Phases

The nurse–patient relationship can be thought of in terms of three phases: orientation, working, and termination. The *orientation* phase consists of introductions and an agreement between nurse and patient about their mutual roles and responsibilities. The nurse and patient get to know each other and trust is developed.

The *working* phase is when the nurse and patient participate together in nursing care activities. During this period the patient "uses" the nurse's expertise and abilities on his or her behalf. The nurse functions as the patient's advocate, caring for his or her physical and emotional health-care needs.

Termination is the closure of the relationship. The nurse reviews with the patient aspects of care and how they have dealt with physical and emotional responses. Discharge planning is a key component in the termination process. Termination can take various forms. For example, the nurse–patient relationship can end when the patient is discharged or the nurse is reassigned.

In psychiatric nursing, the nurse–patient relationship tends to be more formal, with the nurse functioning as a therapeutic counselor, but in the more general nursing setting, the nurse–patient relationship tends to be less formal. Other nurses and professionals often share in the care of the patient. The nurse's days off interrupt the continuity of the relationship. Even though the professional relationship may lack some continuity, however, it is still important that the relationship retain some structure. Attention needs to be given to the appropriate roles and functions within each phase of the relationship.

Contract-Setting

The professional relationship can take various forms. Generally, the nurse–patient relationship is based on an informal contractual model. In the contractual relationship, patients are seen as having control over the significant decisions affecting their lives (Aroskar, 1980; Smith, 1986). Aspects of care, goals of treatment, and necessary adaptations are discussed with the patient, and the nurse takes no major action without consulting the patient or a family member representing the patient. The basic attitude in the contractual relationship is one of collaboration. The nurse discusses his or her role with the patient, as well as the patient's condition, treatment, and nursing care. Decisions about nursing and health care are made collaboratively.

The contractual relationship between nurse and patient is an informal one, which means that contracting is done verbally and is an assumed attitude toward the relationship. In the area of psychiatric nursing practice, contracts tend to be more formal, sometimes even written, and tend to be used as a therapeutic tool to help a patient develop more insight and control over his own behavior (Loomis, 1985).

The elements of an informal contract between nurse and patient are summarized in the display. The usual way for a nurse to establish an informal contract with a patient is to make a verbal agreement as to how they are to work together. A nurse might approach a patient as follows: "I'm your primary nurse while you are a patient here. This means I'm responsible for planning your care. I'll be here every day this week but will be off on the weekend, when an associate primary nurse will take over your care. On the evening and night shifts, other nurses will care for you according to the plan we decide on together. This afternoon we'll review your care plan together and decide how we can best meet your nursing care needs. How does that sound to you?"

An important advantage to the informal contractual relationship has to do with values and rights. The nurse maintains his or her own rights while respecting those of the patient. For instance, what if a nurse disagrees with abortion, but the patient under her care is considering having one? She can contract with the patient to provide the information, but she need not participate in the procedure. The nurse must respect the patient's rights. Because abortion is a legal procedure, she cannot re-

strain the patient from having one. Indeed, she is obligated to provide the patient with information so that the patient can make a decision based on such information. The nurse, however, has every right to participate in organized protests against legalized abortion. She may also decide not to work for an institution that performs abortions.

Advocacy

Nurses are the most constant professional in the patient's environment. The ideologic orientation that nursing as a profession holds toward communication is one of **advocacy,** or taking the patient's side. Advocacy holds that patients have a right to information so that they can make their own decisions about treatment options and nursing care. Patients need information about their health status and the course of illness so that they can make the necessary adjustments in their lives. Nursing believes that sharing information reduces anxiety and is an integral part of being therapeutic (Matthews, 1983).

Being an advocate for the patient means that nurses must avoid taking a *maternalistic* approach (Taylor, 1985). Maternalism is the female counterpart of paternalism, but either men or women can be paternalistic or maternalistic in their relationships. The paternalistic approach is taken by professionals in authority, such as physicians. This approach assumes that the professional will make the decisions for the patient ("father knows best"). The maternalistic approach takes the attitude of wanting what is best for the person by laying out consequences, not alternatives. The patient is led to choose between "hurting" and "caring" or "being selfish" and "being responsible."

An example of a maternalistic approach is telling a child, "I cooked this dinner especially for you and now you aren't going to eat it." The underlying message is "because you did not eat the dinner, mother is hurt and you are selfish." When used in child-rearing situations, maternalistic approaches are often appropriate because the child learns how his or her behavior affects another. But in the nurse–patient relationship, the maternalistic approach is inappropriate and manipulative. Table 17-3 compares paternalistic and maternalistic approaches with the advocacy approach.

Open communication between the nurse and patient sometimes conflicts with the physician's viewpoint (Barry, 1984; Matthews, 1983). Physicians tend to see the physician–patient relationship as primary and exclusive and tend to see themselves as in control of information. The best approach to this problem is for the nurse to develop a working relationship with the physician so that open communication and information-sharing can occur between physician and nurse. The nurse can also help the patient become more assertive with the physician.

Elements of an Informal Nurse–Patient Contract

Nurse and patient know each others' names
Roles and responsibilities are clarified
Parameters of the professional relationship are clear
Mutual expectations are agreed on
Circle of confidentiality is respected

TABLE 17–3

Comparison of Paternalistic, Maternalistic, and Advocacy Approaches

Clinical example: Surgery has been recommended but the patient is reluctant to have the operation.

	Paternalistic	**Maternalistic**	**Advocacy**
Approach	No choice	Choice based on consequences of actions	Choice based on information and examination of alternatives
Response	"The surgery has been scheduled. You need this operation."	"If you don't have the surgery, you may not live to see your grandchildren. Your family needs you."	"Whether or not you have the surgery is your choice. It is your body. What is your understanding of the situation?"
Underlying message	The professional knows best and should make the decisions for you.	If you don't do what the professional recommends, you and others will get hurt.	The professional is here to help you make informed choices about your health and well-being.

For instance, a patient may confide in the nurse that she believes she is not receiving enough information about her condition. The patient complains that the physician does not spend enough time with her and she feels left out of the decisions made about treatment. If the nurse provides the information to the patient without conferring with the physician, he or she has intruded into the physician–patient relationship; after all, the patient's perception is that they needs more information from the physician.

In this instance, the nurse can do several things. He or she can discuss the problem with the patient and help the patient assert herself through such means as writing a list of questions to ask the physician. With the patient's permission, the nurse can seek out the physician and share the patient's perceptions with him or her. By handling the situation in this manner, the nurse has not interfered in the physician–patient relationship but has acted on the patient's behalf. This action is true to the role of advocacy.

Circle of Confidentiality

Every patient has a right to privacy, but it is important for patient information to be shared with all the professionals involved in his or her care. The people with whom patient information can be shared can be thought of as a **circle of confidentiality.** This circle includes all the people in a nursing unit who have responsibility for the patient. It usually includes the family, unless the patient objects.

The nurse should clarify with the patient that he or she is part of a team. For instance, a nurse has been caring for a patient with a serious prognosis. The patient says to the nurse, "If I tell you something, will you promise to keep it in the strictest confidence? Don't tell anyone else, not even my family." The nurse agrees. Then the patient says that he plans to kill himself after he is discharged, stating that he has a loaded gun at home.

The nurse in this example failed to adhere to the concept of the circle of confidentiality. The proper response to the above conversation would be to tell the patient that the nurse is part of the health-care team, and important information is shared with the team if the nurse believes that to be in the patient's best interest. This protects both nurse and patient.

Transmitting information beyond the nursing unit, however, needs to be carefully considered. It is best to obtain written permission from the patient before information is given out. The patient's right to privacy is important. A patient may not want others to know about his or her hospitalization, for example, or may not want anyone to know the nature of his or her illness. This is especially true in psychiatric illness. Within the therapeutic relationship, patients may reveal information of an intimate nature, and it is up to the nurse to protect confidentiality. Nurses need to consider this in such mundane situations as talking about patients at lunch or at home.

INGREDIENTS OF THERAPEUTIC COMMUNICATION

Up to this point, we have presented theory related to the communication process and the nurse–patient relationship. Now we move on to therapeutic communication. What makes communication therapeutic? How is therapeutic communication different from other forms of communication? For this discussion, we turn to the work of Carl Rogers (1961), who studied the process of therapeutic communication.

Rogers believed that a person cannot be separated from the techniques of communication he or she uses. Based on his research, the characteristics of a therapeutic, "helpful" person were identified. Empathy, positive regard, and a comfortable sense of self were among the key ingredients.

Empathy

Empathy is the ability to enter into another person's experience to accurately perceive it and to understand how the situation is viewed from the patient's perspective (Kalisch, 1973). Empathy includes the ability to receptively respond to the other person's experience while still maintaining objectivity. It also implies the ability to communicate to the person that they are understood. This is done through the process of reflective or "active" listening, which is explained in the intervention section of this chapter.

Empathy is a complex process. The nurse must:

1. Have enough knowledge and experience to accurately perceive the patient's perspective.
2. Feel secure enough not to be intimidated if the patient experiences a situation differently.
3. Feel comfortable enough with himself or herself to be able to imagine what a situation might be like for someone else, while remaining outside that situation to maintain objectivity.
4. Know how to let the patient know that the nurse perceives the patient's feelings, thoughts, and experiences accurately.

Empathy can be communicated to the patient both verbally and nonverbally (Fig. 17-3). In two studies (Hardin & Gerace, 1983; Hardin & Halaris, 1983), researchers videotaped nurse–patient interactions. The patients in the study and objective raters were asked to rate how empathic they thought the nurses were. Raters were then asked to identify behaviors they thought were

TABLE 17-4

Emphatic and Nonemphatic Behaviors

Emphatic	Nonemphatic
Verbal	
Focus on feelings	Ignore feelings
Reflect feelings	Closed (yes-no) questions
Open-ended questions	Judgmental attitude
Nonjudgmental atittude	Flat vocal tone
Warm vocal tone	
Nonverbal	
Eye contact	Looking away
Head nods	Nods too much
Some smiling	Picking at clothing on body
Smooth gestures	Too few smiles; inexpressive
Open arms	
Leaning towards	Laughs too much
Looking comfortable	Stabbing gestures
Movement synchronized	Crossed arms
	Leaning away
	Looking uncomfortable
	Movements not synchronized with patient

From Hardin, S. & Gerace, L. (1983). Verbal and nonverbal counterparts in nurses' emphatic communication. Paper presented at Midwest Nursing Research Society, University of Iowa.

empathic or nonempathic. After this, the researchers analyzed the identified behaviors by looking systematically at the behaviors on the videotapes. The results are summarized in Table 17-4.

It can be seen that focusing on feelings and being warm and nonjudgmental play an important role in empathic communication. Body orchestration, in terms of looking comfortable, is important as well. Moderate amounts of movement, such as tilting the head toward the patient, smiling, leaning forward, and keeping the arms open, seem to communicate empathy. But looking away, stabbing gestures, closed or leaning-away body posture, sitting too still, or moving too much were experienced as nonempathic.

Positive Regard

Positive regard means warmth, caring, interest, and respect for the person. It is a way of seeing the person unconditionally or nonjudgmentally. Respect for the person does not depend on the person's behavior; instead, the person is regarded as worthwhile simply for being human.

How can this work? What if, for example, the nurse cares for a person who has been convicted of a serious crime? Does that mean that the nurse condones the things this person has done?

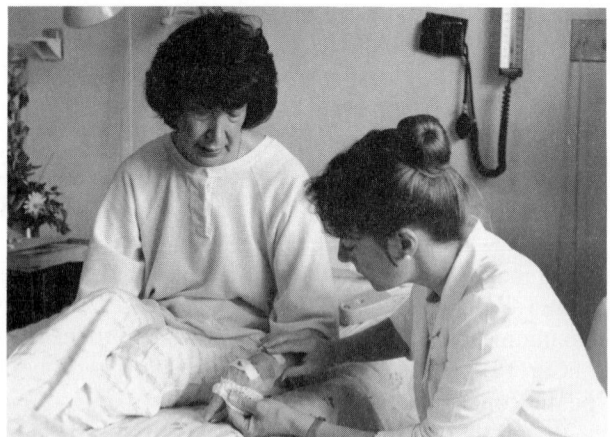

Figure 17–3.   The nurse communicates empathy verbally and nonverbally.

Positive regard does *not* mean that the nurse accepts all aspects of a person's behavior. The nurse does not condone or encourage behavior that is socially inappropriate or abusive. However, the nurse must separate that behavior from the person. The assumption is that the person is worthwhile and has value and dignity.

Positive regard also means that the professional avoids unnecessarily labeling patients. The focus of health-care professionals on disease tends to label the patient as an object (for example, a diabetic, an amputee, or an alcoholic). As a result, the patient is seen as someone who is defective. There is an undeniable tendency to see patients not as if they *have* a disease, but rather that they *are* the disease (Remen, 1980). This attitude can interfere with seeing the person behind the label, and tends to come through in the communication process. When the person is ignored, it becomes more difficult to know and understand his or her response to health and illness and to use his or her strengths and potential.

Comfortable Sense of Self

Before a nurse can communicate therapeutically, it is important for him or her to have a comfortable sense of self. The nurse should be aware of his or her own personality, values, cultural background and style of communication. Rogers (1961) used the term "becoming a person" to mean dropping the false fronts we sometimes assume in our professional roles and becoming the people we are inside.

A person with a comfortable sense of self is open to experiences and is aware of his or her feelings and attitudes. Doing so allows the person to take a more flexible view of life. For example, the nurse may notice that not all patients respond the same way to a similar surgical procedure, and that not all people in a given culture fit those cultural stereotypes. The differences between the nurse and patient can be seen as interesting or challenging, not as threatening or "bad."

A person's sense of self is made up of a collection of characteristics. For example, a nurse may be a professional, a parent, and a sibling, and may be overweight, tall, athletic, or a host of other characteristics. How the nurse experiences these characteristics influences how he or she sees others.

The nurse with a comfortable sense of self can evaluate his or her strengths and weaknesses. For example, one nurse may say, "I work well with postoperative patients, but I have less aptitude for working with rehabilitation patients because I like things to happen more quickly." Another nurse might enjoy working with psychiatric patients so that he can learn more about himself.

Self-evaluation also means taking responsibility for our actions as professionals. For example, a nurse might think, "I could have said something more supportive," or, "I should have included the family in the planning phase." Through this process, the nurse grows in professional competency.

The professional with a comfortable sense of self feels separate from others. This is an important aspect of being therapeutic, because it is easy for a nurse to overidentify with patients. A nurse who becomes too involved in the suffering he or she sees soon burns out, and lacks the objectivity it takes to be therapeutic. A comfortable sense of separation from others also means that the nurse does not need patients to depend on him or her. The nurse gives appropriate support and care, but leaves patients the freedom to make choices about their health and lives.

Having a comfortable sense of self is in part accomplished by having a well-rounded life. Nursing is demanding work and can be emotionally draining and physically tiring. To maintain professional enthusiasm and job satisfaction, nurses must attend to their needs as people. They should get enough rest and exercise and should eat a balanced diet. They must take care of themselves emotionally by having supportive relationships, interesting activities, and time to relax and enjoy themselves. Being therapeutic with ourselves is necessary before we can be therapeutic with others.

COMMUNICATION AND NURSING PROCESS

The nurse–patient relationship and therapeutic communication are instruments used to implement the nursing process. The nursing process can also be applied to the communication that takes place between nurse and patient, as well as the professional relationship. There are specific things to assess about the patient's communication, and specific therapeutic communication techniques are part of nursing intervention. Also, developmental considerations affect communication with different age groups.

Assessment

Because therapeutic communication takes place within the nurse–patient relationship, the first area of assessment concerns the goals of the relationship. Goals vary depending on the patient's needs, the area of nursing practice, and the specific role of the nurse in each particular clinical situation.

For example, a nurse works on a postpartum unit where the average length of stay is only 2 days. Each nurse cares for an average of eight patients per shift. The nurse's role is primarily to care for the mother's physical needs, facilitate mother–infant bonding, and assess and conduct whatever teaching is necessary to help the family care for and adjust to the new baby. In this situation,

---

Communication Assessment Tool

Name _____   Age _____   Sex _____   Diagnosis _____

I. Sender or receiver impairments
   Structural deficit _____
   Same deficits: hearing, sight, smell,
   touch, taste _____
   Loss of functions _____
   Disease _____
   Drugs _____
   Other _____

II. Message variables
   Nonverbal communication
      1. Facial expression _____
      2. Gestures _____
      3. Body movements _____
      4. Affect _____
      5. Tone of voice _____
      6. Posture _____
      7. Eye contact _____
      8. Voice volume, quality, pitch _____
      9. Other _____
   Verbal communication
      1. Content of message _____
      2. Themes _____
      3. Emotions _____
   Communication Patterns
      1. Blocking _____
      2. Slow _____
      3. Rapid _____
      4. Quiet _____
      5. Halting _____
      6. Aphasic _____
      7. Continuity _____
      8. Excessive _____
      9. Detailed _____
     10. Stammering _____
     11. Circumstantial _____
     12. Tangential _____
     13. Long silences _____
     14. Other _____

III. Communication skills
   Openness, spontaneity _____
   Use of clarification _____
   Request for feedback _____
   Tolerance of silence _____
   Acceptance of confrontation _____
   Other _____

IV. Feedback
   Precise _____
   Pertinent _____
   Goal-directed _____
   Informative _____
   Solicited _____
   Positive _____
   Negative _____
   Clarified _____
   Opportune _____

V.   Environment
   External influences
      1. Temperature _____
      2. Physical arrangement _____
      3. Personal space _____
      4. Lighting _____
      5. Noise level _____
      6. Privacy _____
   Internal influences
      1. Beliefs _____
      2. Experiences _____
      3. Thoughts _____
      4. Attitudes _____
   Cultural influences
      1. Health practice _____
      2. Religious implications _____
      3. Language barriers _____
      4. Food preferences _____
      5. Other _____

Adapted from Johnson, B. S. (1989). *Psychiatric/mental health nursing: Adaptation and growth*, (2nd ed.). Philadelphia: J. B. Lippincott

---

the nurse–patient relationship is short-term and focused. The nurse renders little direct physical care, working instead as an adviser and health teacher. The nurse and patient move through each phase of the nurse–patient relationship quickly.

In contrast, another nurse works for a hospice program and gives care in the homes of terminally ill patients. The nurse spends 2 hours three times a week with the patient and family. Her role is to give direct physical care, to support the patient and family, and to teach the family how to care for the patient. This relationship is intense and demanding. During the orientation phase, the nurse needs to establish a working relationship with the family and the patient. She talks with the patient and family about how they will communicate and work together, thus establishing a verbal contract. In this situation the nurse works as a direct caregiver, teacher, and therapeutic counselor.

After the nurse has established appropriate goals for the nurse–patient relationship, the nurse introduces herself and calls the patient by name. The nurse then clarifies the nature of their relationship and the purpose of the interactions to take place. An agreement is made that includes the frequency, length, and goals of nurse-patient contacts.

During this initial phase of the relationship, the nurse assesses the patient's communication, using the theoretical base presented earlier in this chapter. Some key areas of communication assessment are summarized in the display. Are verbal and nonverbal communications congruent? What are the feelings and themes conveyed by the patient? What emotions are expressed? What are the patient's communication patterns? Does he or she speak slowly or rapidly? Does he or she get caught up in minute details? Are there long silences? Can the patient express himself or herself openly and ask the questions he or she needs to ask? When messages are sent by the nurse, does the patient return feedback that is precise, pertinent, and directed toward the goals of the nurse–patient relationship?

Assessing the environment in which communication takes place is also important. The external environment must be conducive to communication. How are the nurse and patient positioned in relation to each other? How far apart are they? Noise is another important consideration. Telephones, televisions, radios, and machines such as ventilators, cardiac monitors, and suctioning machines can be distracting. Privacy is another important factor. The presence of other patients and employees can interfere with comfortable communication.

The patient's internal environment is made up of his or her cultural background, beliefs, and experiences. Assessing how these affect nurse–patient communication is important. For example, do the patient's religious beliefs pervade all aspects of his life and decision-making? If so, this will affect communication, especially if the nurse has a different belief system. Language and cultural practices should also be assessed.

Many of the same factors assessed in the patient pertain to the nurse as well. The nurse needs to consider his or her voice tone, quality, and pitch, body language, facial expressions, and verbal fluency, and should know how anxiety may affect them. The nurse must constantly assess his or her communication and feedback skills, and must also examine how his or her cultural beliefs and personal history affect his or her perception of the patient.

General Principles for Facilitating Communication

- Speak in a normal tone.
- Do not raise your voice or shout unless the patient is deaf.
- Realize that speaking louder does not increase comprehension.
- Speak to the patient on an adult level.
- Remember that impaired communication does not indicate impaired intelligence.
- Avoid carrying on more than one conversation at a time.
- Ask simple questions that require simple answers.
- Keep the atmosphere quiet and relaxed.
- Reduce or eliminate environmental noises.
- Make sure you have the patient's attention before you speak.
- Maintain eye contact with the patient throughout the conversation.
- Assume patients can understand you. Do not discuss their cases or other inappropriate topics in front of them.
- Do not rush the patient. Give him or her adequate time to respond.
- Do not correct mistakes.
- If you do not understand, ask the patient to repeat what he or she said.
- Praise patients for their attempts at speech.

Intervention

Once communication has been assessed, how does the nurse use communication as a therapeutic intervention? Specific techniques to facilitate therapeutic communication are summarized in Table 17-5. The therapeutic communication skills highlighted in this section are considered basic to any therapeutic relationship. More advanced skills are usually studied in psychiatric nursing, especially at the clinical specialist level.

Helping the Patient Get Started

General nurses are usually involved in informal therapeutic relationships, which can be important to the patient (Barry, 1984). In the hospital, the nurse often combines physical care with a discussion about the patient's concerns. One of the most important things a nurse can do to encourage a patient to express concerns is to sit down. Patients do not feel like expressing themselves to someone who is always in a hurry or seems too

TABLE 17-5

Therapeutic Communication Techniques

Technique	Definition
Offering self	Making self available to listen to the patient
Open-ended questions	Neutral questions that encourage the patient to express concerns
Opening remarks	General statements based on observations and assessments about the patient
Restatement	Repeating to the patient the main content of his or her communciation
Reflection	Identifying the main feeling themes contained in a communication and directing these back to the patient
Focusing	Asking goal-directed questions to help the patient focus on key concerns
Encouraging elaboration	Helping the patient to describe more fully the concerns or problems under discussion
Seeking clarification	Helping the patient put into words unclear thoughts or ideas
Giving information	Sharing with the patient relevant information for his or her health care and well-being
Looking at alternatives	Helping the patient see options and participate in the decision-making process related to his or her health care and well-being
Silence	A pause in communication that allows nurse and patient time to think about what has taken place
Summarizing	Highlighting the important points of a conversation by condensing what was said

busy. It helps to draw the curtain between beds, and to see that the patient faces away from any roommates and toward the nurse.

The nurse should call the patient by name, asking if the patient prefers to be called by the first or last name. Many older people find being called by their first name intrusive or rude. The nurse should convey interest and readiness to listen. By leaning toward the patient, making eye contact, and assuming a relaxed, open posture, the nurse offers himself or herself to the patient.

Open-Ended Questions. An *open-ended question* is one that elicits more than a "yes" or "no" answer. Such questions ask how, what, where, and when. Examples of appropriate questions are, "How are things going for you at this point?" or "What have your experiences been like?"

Opening Remarks. Other ways to help a patient get started include *opening remarks* based on observations and assessment about the patient. Having assessed the communication and behavior of the patient, the nurse can make statements such as, "You've been having a pretty rough time," "I notice you're going through some important changes," or "You seem to be feeling better."

These questions and statements must be neutral and tentative, not probing or interrogating. "Why" questions are generally not considered therapeutic because they are too intrusive; newspaper reporters and school-

teachers ask "why" questions. For example, asking a patient why they are upset is more threatening than just noting that they seems upset.

Active Listening

Listening is an active process that takes a great deal of skill (Fig. 17-4). The nurse must be able to focus on the patient and what the patient's messages are about. Listening actively means that the nurse conveys back to the patient an accurate picture of what the patient is expressing.

Listening actively means that the listener must constantly decode the messages sent. The nurse listens for both content and feeling. The content part of the message includes thoughts, words, opinions, and ideas; the feeling part refers to the patient's emotions. Emotions may be described verbally, but usually are manifested more accurately through nonverbal means such as facial expression, body posture, laughter, or crying. Noting congruence or incongruence between these messages helps the nurse understand how patients are experiencing the things they are discussing.

The nurse must also observe what is behind the message sent by the patient. For example, is the patient conveying an attitude of helplessness, rejection, or aggression toward the nurse?

As the nurse decodes the conversation, he or she listens actively by using two important techniques: re-

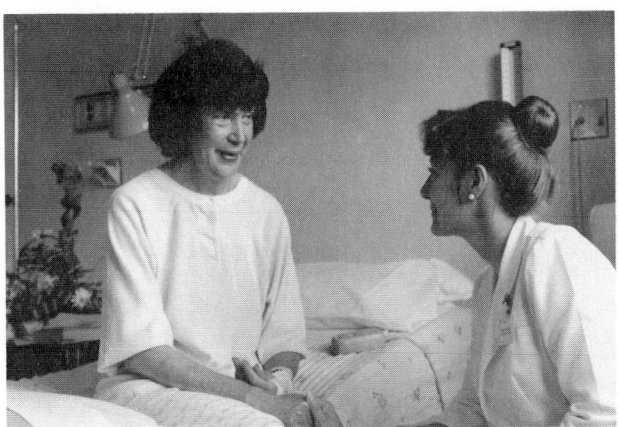

Figure 17–4. Listening is an active process. Listening intently and with interest sends a message to the receiver.

statement and reflection. These key techniques are used to help a patient feel listened to and understood.

Restatement refers mainly to the content portion of the communication. The nurse listens carefully to the patient and restates the content of the communication back to the patient, to verify the nurse's understanding with the patient. By restating the content back to the patient, he or she has the opportunity to hear himself or herself, and to gain understanding of his or her own communication.

Reflection means identifying the main feeling themes contained in a communication and directing them back to the patient. The nurse listens for the underlying feeling that a patient is conveying, then states his or her understanding of that feeling in a neutral, open manner. The purpose is to verify the feelings that are being heard and to check what is being heard with the patient. As a result, the patient gains a clearer understanding of the feelings being experienced.

The following example shows how these might be used in an informal therapeutic relationship:

Patient: I can't sleep. It's too hot in here and the noise is bothering me.
Nurse: You can't sleep because it's uncomfortable in here. (Restatement.)
Patient: That's right. All I can think about is having that operation in the morning. (Sounds irritable, looks anxious.)
Nurse: You seem upset about having the surgery. (Reflection.)
Patient: I am. (Starts to cry.)

In this situation, the nurse listened carefully and found that it was not really the environment but the anxiety about having surgery that was keeping the patient awake. By communicating back to the patient in a careful way the things she was hearing, the nurse opened up an opportunity for the patient to discuss her fears about the impending surgery.

Exploring

Exploring is a way of communicating therapeutically without giving direct advice. Instead, the nurse helps patients express their concerns and solve their own problems by exploring the situation, how the patient feels about it, and what some alternatives might be.

Focusing. Focusing means asking goal-directed questions that help the patient stay on the topic and talk more about it. The questions should still be open-ended, but are directed toward the key concerns. An example of focusing is, "You were talking about your fears about how people will respond to your mastectomy. Can you say more about that?"

Asking focused questions helps the patient to discuss the main issues of concern. It keeps the conversation on target by not changing the subject or becoming too generalized. By staying on the subject, the nurse is conveying that he or she will stay with the patient and help explore his or her concerns.

Sometimes helping a patient express things of importance can be frightening. The nurse encounters a variety of suffering when working with ill and dying patients. To be therapeutic, a nurse must develop maturity and a sense of perspective about life. This takes time and experience. It helps to remember that just helping patients focus on their concerns is helpful. The patients feel less alone and may better understand their situations.

Encouraging Elaboration. Encouraging elaboration is a technique used to help the patient describe more fully the concerns or problems under discussion. By nodding one's head, using an attentive demeanor, and making comments such as "go on" or "I see," the nurse encourages the patient to keep talking and to express himself or herself more thoroughly. This helps the nurse to learn about the patient's emotional state and his or her coping abilities and view of the situation.

Seeking Clarification. Seeking clarification means helping the patient put into words unclear thoughts or ideas. It can also be used to clarify events by putting them in a time sequence. Examples are, "I'm not sure I understand what you mean," "What else happened?" and "What happened then?" Such questions help the patient to order his or her thoughts, put events into context, and place things in a more manageable perspective. By clarifying the problem or event being discussed, the patient gains new insight into his or her situation.

Giving Information. Giving information means sharing information about the patient's health and well-being. This must be done in a timely manner and should be based on what is currently known about the patient's condition. Giving information can mean sharing what is known about a patient's illness, treatment, and recovery. It can also mean correcting misperceptions.

For example, a young woman is brought to the emergency room after she was raped. After medical care is completed, police reports filled out, and her family notified, the nurse sits with her for a few minutes while she waits for a family member to come. The patient says, "I should have been more careful. I was wearing a short skirt. Maybe that caused the rape."

Based on what the nurse knows about rape victims' perceptions, a timely intervention might be for the nurse to say, "When people are raped, it is usual for them to look for the cause within themselves. But the rape is not your fault. You're a victim in this situation." This information is based on research showing that rape victims commonly assume that they provoked the rape. In addition to giving this information, the nurse might also refer the patient to a rape counseling center in the community.

Giving information is a skill used by nurses in health teaching and is often done while the nurse is giving physical care. Information must be distinguished from suggestions or advice. A typical way to give advice is to start by saying, "Why don't you?" or "You should." Such advice-giving reinforces the patient's dependency on the nurse. A more useful strategy is to give the information the patient needs so he or she can make a decision. If the patient has difficulty making a decision, the nurse might explore why. The nurse might also give information about how other patients have dealt with a similar situation.

Looking at Alternatives. Looking at alternatives means presenting options for the patient's consideration. This increases the patient's perceived choices (Fig. 17-5). The nurse does not always need to present the alternatives; the patient can be asked for them instead. Examples of questions to use are as follows:

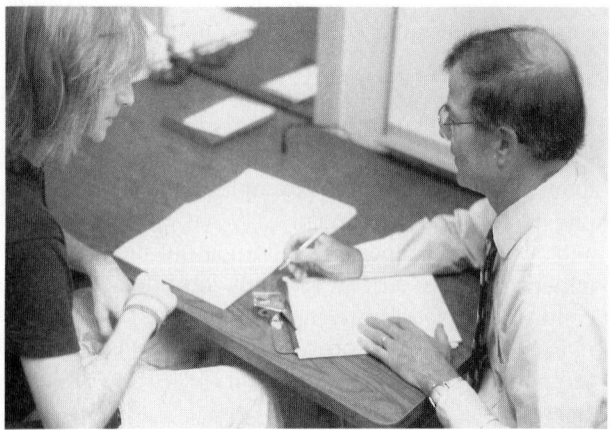

Figure 17–5. Examining alternatives increases the patient's perceived choices.

What are some of your ideas about how to handle this?
Have you thought about (alternate courses of action)?
What else could you do?
If you met someone in the same situation as you, what would you advise him or her to do?
What are some advantages (disadvantages) of (alternates)?

Discussing alternatives should not be done too early or before the patient has a clear understanding of the current situation. Sometimes the patient must first express feelings such as grief or anger before he or she can explore how to deal with the situation.

Silence. Another useful therapeutic technique is using silence, a pause in communication that allows the nurse and patient to reflect on what has taken place. By waiting quietly and attentively, the nurse encourages the patient to initiate and maintain conversation.

Summarizing. Summarizing means highlighting the important points of a conversation by condensing what was said. This is useful toward the end of a therapeutic conversation. Summarizing helps both nurse and patient review the main themes of the conversation and gives a sense of closure. It also enables the nurse and patient to think about what else needs to be thought or talked about in the future. It emphasizes the progress made towards self-understanding and problem-solving. Examples of summarizing include, "Today it seems that you've thought about . . . " and "Let's review what we've talked about today."

Developing Communication Skills

These and other therapeutic techniques are helpful in maintaining the boundaries of the nurse–patient relationship. Communication between nurse and patient in the clinical setting is based on patient needs, not on personal or social interests. By maintaining a professional approach and being patient-centered, the nurse maintains a focus on the patient's health and well-being.

It takes time and experience for the nurse to become skilled at using therapeutic communication. One way to develop this skill is to study one's interactions either by tape-recording a therapeutic conversation (after obtaining the patient's permission) or by recreating the conversation from memory. Once a transcript of the conversation is made, the nurse can then analyze his or her skill. The nurse should look at what techniques were used, their timing and appropriateness, and how the patient responded to the nurse. The nurse's own thoughts and feelings should also be noted, because these affect how he or she responds to the patient. An example of a process recording is shown in Table 17-6.

TABLE 17–6

Sample Process Recording

Situation: The patient is a 35-year-old man who sustained burns on his face and upper body due to a car accident. He was transferred from the burn unit to the rehabilitation unit 2 days ago.

Verbal and Nonverbal Interaction	Analysis
Nurse: When I left you yesterday things weren't going very well for you.	Opening remark establishes that nurse remembers events from previous day. Indicates working phase of relationship.
How are you doing today? (Nurse sits down, facing patient.)	Open-ended question to help patient get started. Nurse offers self.
Patient: It has been a rough 2 days.	Patient makes a general statement.
Nurse: . . . rough 2 days . . .	Restatement.
SILENCE	Nurse allows silence so that patient can collect his thoughts.
Patient: I've come to the realization that I'm not going to look the same as I did . . .	Patient begins to clarify what he means.
Nurse: . . . and . . .? (Remains attentive.)	Encouraging elaboration.
Patient: It's hard. (Beomes tearful.)	Patient showing feelings nonverbally.
Nurse: (Gently) It is upsetting to deal with the after-effects of your burns.	Reflection. The nurse reflects the patient's feelings so he can own them.
Patient: I shouldn't cry. (Appears embarrassed.)	Nurse assesses that patient's past experiences and personal history have led him to the conclusion that men should not cry.
Nurse: You think men shouldn't cry when they have a really difficult adjustment to make?	Reflection of metacommunciation (embarrassment about crying). The nurse shows the patient what he feels about his feelings.
Patient: (Laughs slightly.) I guess it's okay for me to cry. My situation isn't easy to deal with.	The patient gained understanding of his feelings and his metacommunication.
SILENCE	
Patient: (Looks sad. Remains thoughtful.)	
Nurse: Some of what you are experiencing is a natural grieving process that people in your situation go through. You have lost part of your former self, and that is a painful experience.	Giving information. The nurse is experienced and well-read in the rehabilitation of burn patients. She shares this information in a timely manner. The nurse realizes that there is no easy solution for this patient's problem. She provides support.

Table developed by Laina Gerace, Ph.D., R.N., Assistant Professor, University of Illinois at Chicago, College of Nursing.

Nontherapeutic Responses

Nontherapeutic responses are those that interfere with or block therapeutic communication. Often such responses are the more natural ones that might be made in social situations. Nontherapeutic responses may prevent the nurse from functioning as a professional and a therapeutic agent in the patient's care.

The nurse's own needs must be met outside the therapeutic context. A nurse might, for example, become overly involved with patients because he has not developed his social life in a way that meets his needs. Another nurse might be uncomfortable with patients who express feelings because she has never been allowed to express her own. The nurse must engage in self-evaluation to determine his or her own strengths and weaknesses.

Inexperienced health-care workers may believe that serious problems can be easily solved. After all, on television, dire problems are solved in half an hour. But in real life this is not always the case, and presenting quick solutions and unwarranted cheerfulness blocks the therapeutic process. Some people have incurable illnesses. Others must adapt to situations for which there are no quick or simple answers. Through experience, nurses learn that they cannot always provide solutions. It is more important for them to maintain a supportive presence while the patient struggles through a difficult situation. Nurses can help by listening carefully and exploring the patient's main concerns. They can give health-care information and provide the best technical bedside care available.

A variety of nontherapeutic responses block the therapeutic communication process.

Rescue Feelings. A nurse has rescue feelings when he or she feels essential to the patient's welfare. The nurse thinks that he or she has exceptional abilities to help the patient, and his or her expectations for the patient will be high.

Some rescue feelings may be useful, because having confidence in one's abilities to be helpful is part of being therapeutic. Strong rescue feelings impede the therapeutic process, however. The nurse may believe that only he or she can meet the patient's needs, alienating himself or herself from the health-care team. The nurse may also raise the patient's expectations too high; when these expectations are not met, the patient is disappointed.

False Reassurance. False reassurance means giving reassurance that is not based on fact. It is a way of minimizing the patient's situation. For example, saying, "Don't worry, everything will be fine," minimizes the patient's concerns. Other forms of false reassurance include telling a patient not to dwell on his or her problems or saying that an injection will not hurt. Although the intention of such comments is to reassure the patient, they actually serve to diminish trust in the professional.

Real reassurance must be based on fact. For example, telling a patient that there will be postoperative pain and how it will be controlled is much more reassuring than saying, "There's nothing to this operation. We do it all the time." An operation may seem routine to the nurse, but to the patient it is a major event. The patient will feel much more supported if he or she is allowed to express anxiety about it.

The nurse who gives false reassurance violates the patient's trust. If the nurse tells a patient not to worry when the patient actually is worried, or that something doesn't hurt when it does hurt, how can the patient have confidence in the nurse? It is much better to first let the patient express his or her concern. After this, the nurse can supply any needed information and give reassurances based on facts.

Giving Advice. Giving advice is another common nontherapeutic response. Giving advice focuses on the nurse and his or her experiences and opinions. Examples of giving advice include statements that begin, "I think you should," "Why don't you," and "The same thing happened to me and I." The problem with advice-giving is that it diminishes the patient's responsibilities and choices and tends to be controlling. Patients may feel that they must do what the nurse says, even though the advice might not work well for them.

Giving advice is different from giving a suggestion, an alternative idea for the patient's consideration. If carefully done, a suggestion increases the patient's perceived options. Usually, however, it is better if the patient comes up with his or her own ideas. A helpful way to give a suggestion is to frame it tentatively, such as, "I wonder if you have thought about (an alternate course of action)?"

Changing the Subject. Changing the subject is a nontherapeutic response that usually indicates anxiety on the nurse's part. It is a way of resisting hearing about a patient's distress, sadness, and difficulties. The nurse might change the subject in an attempt to cheer the patient up or to distract the patient from painful thoughts; however, changing the subject can be a way to avoid listening to what the patient has to say.

Being Moralistic. Being moralistic means seeing a situation in terms of goodness or badness, or right or wrong. It is a judgmental approach. The nurse must become aware of how he or she uses the word "should." Talking to patients in terms of "shoulds" means the nurse has a preconceived idea about the "right" thing to do. For instance, a nurse would be moralistic by saying to an unwed mother, "I think you should keep the baby." Many factors go into making a decision of this magnitude. What might work for one person may not work for another.

Another way of being moralistic is to give approval or disapproval by judging the patient's actions as good or bad. Everyone has moral attitudes, and being moral is part of being human. Nurses have a right to their own values, but in the clinical situation they must transcend them and view their patients in more objective terms.

Nonprofessional Involvement. Nonprofessional involvement means being overly friendly or trying to be the patient's friend or buddy (Burgess, 1985). Although it is sometimes appropriate, too much social chit-chat points to a nonprofessional relationship. Nurses who talk too much with patients about themselves and their own goals and problems are nonprofessional. Sometimes the nurse may chat with the patient about the weather or a major news event. After all, nurses and patients share many hours together and sometimes the experiences they share are intense. But if most of a nurse's relationships with patients are social or overly friendly, this is a red flag that the nurse's involvements are nontherapeutic.

It is nonprofessional to call patients after discharge, to be seductive with patients, or to date or otherwise socially engage patients. Of course, sometimes there are unit parties when long-term patients are discharged, or there are reunions of discharged premature infants, and occasionally a nurse may develop a romantic relationship with a patient she has cared for.

Being nontherapeutically involved has pitfalls for both nurse and patient. The patient is receiving nursing care because he or she needs professional services. The nurse must maintain a professional attitude to remain objective in clinical decision-making. The patient wants to feel confident that a professional is in charge of nursing care. If the nurse becomes a friend to the patient, he or she has abdicated their professional role.

Special Situations

Several situations call for particular communication techniques. Communication with the person with sensory dysfunctions is discussed in Chapter 41. Communication techniques and skills for the unconscious patient and special lifespan considerations are presented in Chapter 44.

Children and Adolescents. Children and adolescents present unique challenges to effective communication. These age groups are undergoing many changes that make clear communication more difficult.

Children are responsive to nonverbal communication, such as body movements, voice tone, and eye contact. The nurse should talk to a child at the child's eye level in an effort to minimize intimidation. Speaking gently and calmly and using quiet body movement engenders greater trust.

When children first learn words, it is sometimes difficult to understand what they mean. The way words are combined does not always convey the exact meaning intended. The nurse should clarify meanings with the child until the message can be understood, using restatement and clarification.

Child: "Baby socks."
Nurse: "You have little socks?"
Child: No response.
Nurse: "You have socks?"
Child: Shakes head to indicate "no."
Nurse: "You want your socks?"
Child: Smiles and nods head to indicate "yes."

Young children are more attentive to simplified speech. The nurse should use language the child can understand. When speaking to a child who does not respond, the nurse should rephrase the communication. For example:

Nurse: "It's time for your dinner now."
Child: No response.
Nurse: "Time to eat now."
Child: Takes nurse's hand to go to dining area.

The nurse can use play to help children deal with the stress of hospitalization. For example, having children play with dolls representing physicians and nurses can help them enact their fears. By observing play, the nurse can identify a child's concerns. By participating in such play, children can develop feelings of mastery over the situation. Many hospitals caring for young children provide structured play to help patients deal with their illnesses and treatments.

Hospitalization for physical problems in this age group can produce anxiety. Children and adolescents often feel embarrassed about their bodies, and they feel vulnerable to the control of adults. Therefore, it is important that the nurse be considerate of the child or adolescent's personal space. The nurse should not be too intrusive. Touch should be judicious, and the patient's modesty should be maintained. Adolescents are particularly conscious of the need for privacy and modesty in communication situations with health professionals.

Information about procedures and treatments should be given in a straightforward manner, and it is especially important not to give false reassurance. For example, if a procedure might be painful, it is best to share this matter-of-factly.

To work effectively with children and adolescents, the nurse needs a sense of give-and-take. The nurse might be a little less formal than with an adult but must maintain some professional distance. Limit-setting is a key factor in working effectively with children and adolescents, and to set limits the nurse must be seen as authoritative. Being *authoritative* means being in charge but permitting freedom within reasonable limits (Hetherington and Parke, 1986). This is different from being *authoritarian,* which means exerting power over another person. Being authoritative means the nurse clearly communicates the limits of behavior and elicits participation in their reinforcement.

Adults and Older Adults. It is difficult to specify communication strategies for any phase of development, especially for adulthood. Adulthood is an ongoing developmental period, not the end of growth and development. As people grow and age, they must constantly adapt to many changes, and less is known about adulthood than any other phase of development.

Hospitalization can create a period of transition in which adults question the progress of their lives, their goals, and even life's meaning. Their responsibilities are interrupted by the illness, and feelings of vulnerability may overwhelm them. It can be difficult for an active, achieving adult to be dependent on the nurse, and the adult may sometimes behave in ways that are difficult for the nurse to manage.

The nurse also may experience a range of feelings in relation to various adult patients. For example, an elderly male patient may remind a nurse of her grandfather. She may relate to him as she does to her grandfather, or may treat him as if he is helpless and cannot make any decisions. If the patient is a physician or a wealthy or well-known person, the nurse may feel intimidated. Numerous complex situations come into play when communicating therapeutically with adults. Nurses must recognize their feelings and share them with fellow professionals, because these feelings affect the way in which communication takes place.

Communication strategies with adults draw on all the concepts discussed in this chapter. The contractual approach provides an opportunity to work out with the patient how communication will take place. For example, whether to call an adult by their first or last name can be discussed at the outset. It helps to remember that all human beings, no matter what their job, social status, or wealth, at some point in their lives are vulnerable and suffer anxiety and worry. The therapeutic communication skills presented in this chapter will facilitate expression and problem-solving with any adult.

The Person Who Speaks a Foreign Language. The nurse should learn what non-English-speaking groups live in the community and should become familiar with common phrases related to nursing care (e.g., identity, bathing, eating, eliminating, walking). A dictionary of common conversational phrases in the other language is helpful.

The nurse should remember that the non-English-speaking patient has a language barrier, not a hearing problem (unless one exists). The nurse should speak clearly and distinctly in a normal tone of voice, using hand motions and demonstrations when appropriate. But even with the most careful efforts, misunderstandings may occur, and in health care it is particularly important to avoid them. Therefore, an interpreter should be used whenever possible. The interpreter can also provide insight into cultural meanings and nuances of the language and the related culture that may have a bearing on the patient's health-care needs.

The Person in the ICU. The intensive care unit (ICU) is an environment designed to help maintain the lives of seriously ill patients. It is characterized by unfamiliar sounds and noises, artificial lighting, and undefined colors (Williams, 1989). Being admitted to the ICU is a stressful event: the patient fears the diagnosis and the extent of the injury and may be unable to communicate. Communication is hindered if the patient does not know or understand the severity of the illness, feels a lack of control over what is being done, does not know the reason for therapies, receives care from several different providers, and loses contact with the outside world, including a sense of day and time (Chyun, 1989).

It is easy for the nurse to get caught up in the complexities and technology of the unit and as a result to have

---

Nursing Research

Selected Nursing Research Studies

Chyun, D. (1989). Patients' perceptions of stressors in intensive care and coronary care units. *Focus on Critical Care, 16,* 206–211.

Williams, M. A. (1989). Physical environment of the intensive care unit and elderly patients. *Crit Care Nurs Quarterly, 12,* 52–60.

Hardin, S. & Halaris, A. (1983). Nonverbal communication of patients and high- and low-empathy nurses. *Journal of Psychosocial Nurs Mental Helath Services, 21,* 14–20.

Possible Topics for Nursing Inquiry

- What are nonverbal communication cues in the intensive care unit patient?
- What are nonverbal confirmations of verbal communication in the patient in pain?
- What nurse responses promote communication with the preschool child?

---

minimal communication with the patient. The nurse must be constantly aware that the patient in this life-threatening situation is a person for whom communication is more important than ever. Even when the patient cannot answer (because of decreased level of consciousness, intubation, or other reasons), the nurse should assume that the patient can hear. The nurse should talk to the patient about what is being done as he or she would with any other patient. Nonverbal communication, such as touch and facial expressions, is especially meaningful for ICU patients.

To give cues about day and time, the nurse can provide clocks and calendars where the patient can see them. For patients who can use their hands but cannot speak, note pads or magic slates aid in communication. Call bells within easy reach help the patient to communicate his or her needs.

Once the patient has been stabilized, the nurse can help the patient understand the illness and the reason for various therapies. Explanations must be clear, direct, and simply stated. Because of the patient's state, the nurse should expect to repeat them. When the patient is able, discussing his or her perceptions and understanding enhances the patient's sense of control and decreases stress. Nurses in the ICU have an valuable opportunity to facilitate communication between the patient and the health-care system.

Key Concepts

- Effective communication within the nurse–patient relationship focuses on the patient and the patient's experiences and results in improved health status and well-being.
- Communication is a system of sending and receiving messages that forms a connection between the sender and the receiver.
- Verbal communication involves language; nonverbal communication includes gestures, facial expressions, body posture, body movement, voice tone, rate of speech, and dress.
- The elements of communication are the source, the message, and the receiver with the processes of encoding, decoding, and feedback.
- The nurse–patient relationship is focused on the patient, is goal-directed, and has defined parameters.
- The three phases in the nurse–patient relationship are orientation, working, and termination.
- Empathy, positive regard, and a comfortable sense of self are among the key ingredients of the nurse–patient relationship.
- The nurse–patient relationship and therapeutic communication are instruments used to implement the nursing process.
- Skillful use of therapeutic responses is essential to accurate assessment and interventions.
- Ineffective communication can be avoided if the nurse is aware of nontherapeutic responses.
- Patients in special situations need modified communication techniques.

References

Aroskar, M. A. (1980). Ethics of nurse-patient relationship. *Nurse Educator,* March–April, 18–20.

Barry, P. D. (1984). *Psychosocial nursing assessment and intervention.* Philadelphia: J. B. Lippincott.

Berlo, D. K. (1960). *The process of communication: An introduction to therapy and practice.* New York: Holt, Rinehart & Winston.

Brandler, R., & Grinder, J. (1975). *The structure of magic: A book about language and therapy.* Palo Alto, CA: Science & Behavior Books.

Burgess, A. W. (1985). *Psychiatric nursing in the hospital and the community.* Englewood Cliffs, NJ: Prentice-Hall.

Chyun, D. (1989). Patients' perceptions of stressors in intensive care units. *Focus on Critical Care, 16*(3), 206–211.

Hardin, S., & Gerace, L. (1983). Verbal and nonverbal counterparts in nurses' empathic communication. Paper presented at the Midwest Nursing Research Society, University of Iowa.

Hardin, S., & Halaris, A. (1983). Nonverbal communication of patients and high- and low-empathy nurses. *Journal of Psychosocial Nursing & Mental Health Services, 21,* 14–20.

Hetherington, E. M., & Parke, R. D. (1986). *Child psychology: A contemporary viewpoint.* New York: McGraw-Hill.

Johnson, B. S. (1989). *Psychiatric/mental health nursing: Adaptation and growth.* Philadelphia: J. B. Lippincott.

Kalisch, B. (1973). What is empathy? *American Journal of Nursing, 73,* 1548.

Loomis, M. (1985). Levels of contracting. *Journal of Psychosocial Nursing & Mental Health Services, 23*(3), 9–14.

Matthews, J. J. (1983). The communication process in clinical settings. *Social Science Medicine, 17,* 1371–1378.

Peplau, H. E. (1952). *Interpersonal relations in nursing.* New York: G. P. Putnam's Sons.

Remen, N. (1980). *The human patient.* New York: Doubleday.

Rogers, C. (1961). *On becoming a person.* Boston: Houghton-Mifflin.

Smith, L. (1986). Talking it out. *Nursing Times,* March 26, 38–39.

Taylor, S. (1985). Rights and responsibilities: Nurse–patient relationship. *Image, 17*(1), 9–13.

Thayer, L. (1968). *Communication and communication systems in organization, management and interpersonal relations.* Homewood, IL: Richard D. Irwin.

Williams, M. A. (1989). Physical environment of the intensive care unit and elderly patients. *Critical Care Nursing Quarterly, 12*(1), 52–60.

Bibliography

Clark, R. (1978). Some even simpler ways to learn to talk. In N. Waterson & C. Snow (Eds.), *The development of communication.* London: Wiley.

Emde, R. N., Gaensbauer, T. J., & Marmon, R. J. (1976). Emotional expression in infancy: A biobehavioral study. *Psychological Issues, 10*(37). New York: International.

Field, T. M., Cohen, D., Garcia, R., & Greenberg, R. (1984). Mother-stranger face discrimination by the newborn. *Infant Behavior and Development, 7,* 19–25.

Garvey, C. (1984). *Children's talk.* Cambridge, MA: Harvard University Press.

U N I T IV
Essential Assessment Components

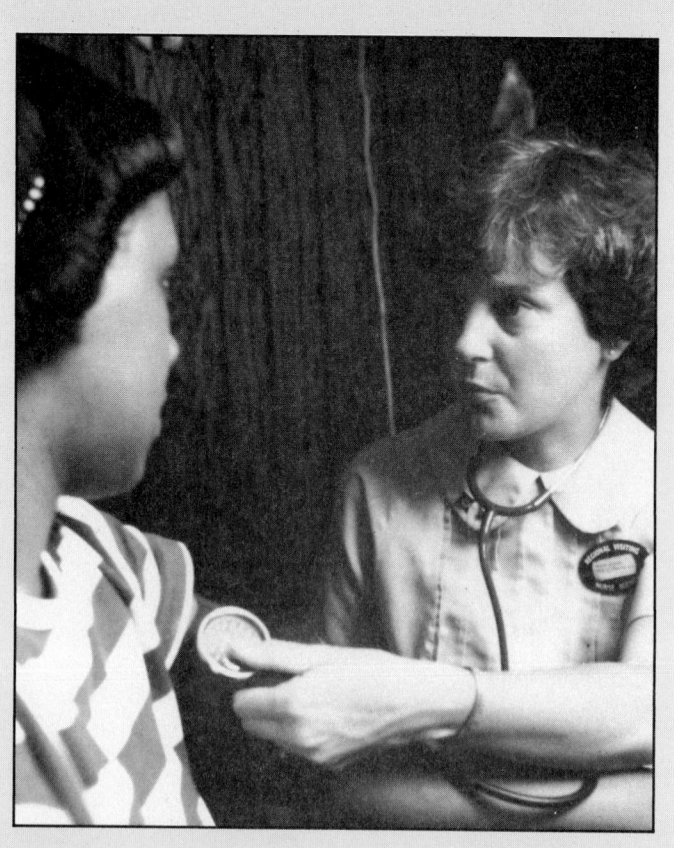

CHAPTERS

18 Health Assessment of Human Function

19 Vital Sign Assessment

20 Diagnostic Tests and Procedures

The chapters in Unit IV detail the fundamental skills and knowledge needed to carry out each component of health assessment. The information gathered during health assessment and vital sign assessment, combined with information from diagnostic tests and procedures, forms a data base from which many nursing care decisions are made.

The chapter on health assessment and human function describes the systematic and continuous gathering of subjective and objective data, beginning with a health history and physical examination. Along with discussing normal or acceptable findings, this chapter provides a knowledge base that is basic to identifying patient strengths and responses to health problems.

The next chapter presents the knowledge and skills required for accurate and timely vital sign measurement along with a discussion of normal parameters and variations. An awareness of both are essential components of nursing practice.

The final chapter in this unit discusses the role of the nurse in assisting with or performing diagnostic tests and procedures and describes how the data from these tests factor into the patient's overall health assessment.

Unit IV focuses on gathering data from and about a patient. These chapters provide a composite picture of essential assessment components, providing a strong foundation for the first step of the nursing process.

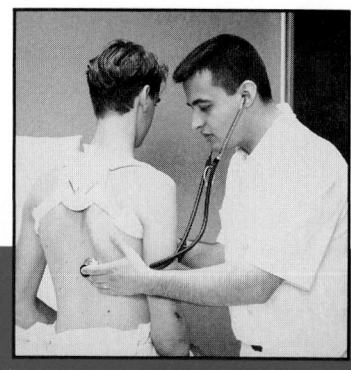

Health Assessment of Human Function

LEARNING OBJECTIVES

Upon completion of this chapter, the student will be able to do the following:

- Organize a nursing assessment using functional health patterns as a framework for data collection.
- Discuss preparation of the patient and the environment to foster data collection during assessment.
- Differentiate between objective and subjective data.
- Discuss methods to obtain subjective information using the patient interview.
- Describe the techniques of inspection, palpation, percussion, and auscultation.
- Describe the appropriate use of the stethoscope's bell and diaphragm during auscultation.
- Select a few appropriate interview questions to assess each of the functional patterns for a patient.
- Individualize functional nursing assessment based on lifespan considerations.

KEY TERMS

Auscultation	Palpation	Resonance
Bruit	Percussion	Stethoscope
Frequency	Pleximeter	Symmetry
Inspection	Plexor	Tangential lighting
Intensity		

18

Purpose and Preparation
  Purpose of the Assessment
  Preparation of the Patient and Environment
    Introduction
    Environment
    Positioning and Draping
Organization and Documentation
Types of Data Collection
  Obtaining Subjective Data: The Interview
  Obtaining Objective Data: The Physical
    Examination
    Inspection
    Palpation
    Percussion
    Auscultation
    Odors
Assessment of Individual Aspects of Functional Health
Assessment of Health Perception and Health
    Management
    Subjective Data
    Objective Data
Assessment of Activity and Exercise
  Mobility and Self-Care Assessment
    Subjective Data
    Objective Data
  Respiratory Assessment
    Subjective Data
    Objective Data
  Cardiovascular Assessment
    Subjective Data
    Objective Data
Assessment of Nutrition and Metabolism
    Subjective Data
    Objective Data
Assessment of Elimination
  Urinary Elimination
    Subjective Data
    Objective Data

Bowel Elimination
  Subjective Data
  Objective Data
Assessment of Sleep and Rest
  Subjective Data
  Objective Data
Assessment of Cognition and Perception
  Cognitive Function
  Subjective Data
  Objective Data
  Sensory Function
  Subjective Data
  Objective Data
  Pain Assessment
  Subjective Data
  Objective Data
Assessment of Self-Perception and Self-Concept
  Subjective Data
  Objective Data
Assessment of Roles and Relationships
  Subjective Data
  Objective Data
Assessment of Coping and Stress Tolerance
  Subjective Data
  Objective Data
Assessment of Sexuality and Reproduction
  Subjective Data
  Objective Data
Assessment of Values and Beliefs
  Subjective Data
  Objective Data
Concluding the Assessment
Lifespan Considerations
  Newborn and Infant
  Toddler and Preschooler
  School Age and Adolescent
  Adult and Older Adult
Key Concepts

A functional health assessment is an evaluation of mind, body, and environment and their effect on a person's ability to perform the tasks of daily living. A nurse conducts a functional health assessment by gathering and analyzing data. From these data, conclusions are formulated about the patient's functional abilities, about risk factors that can contribute to dysfunction, and about actual functional deficits. A clear description of health status and identification of health-related problems are the desired outcomes of a functional health assessment.

A comprehensive health assessment encompasses the physical, psychological, social, and spiritual dimensions of living. Physical health includes basic functions such as breathing, eating, and walking, as well as complex functions such as learning, reproducing, and sensing. Psychological health involves intellect, self-concept, emotions, and behavior. The social dimensions of health encompass relationships and interactions among family, friends, and coworkers. Spiritual health is influenced by belief in a higher being, personal interpretation of the meaning of life, and attitudes toward moral decisions and personal conduct. In performing a comprehensive health assessment, the nurse considers all of these dimensions.

This chapter discusses how the nurse can perform assessments using a functional health framework as a structure for data collection. Much information is provided concerning data collection for each health pattern. The nurse must select the most important interviewing questions or assessment techniques to use. Selection often depends on time constraints and the patient's current status.

A comprehensive functional health assessment may be performed routinely as a patient enters a health-care facility. Usually such an assessment includes collecting subjective data by interviewing the patient and obtaining objective data by physically examining the patient. A comprehensive functional health assessment should take approximately 30 minutes but can vary in length depending on the specific patient. Although a comprehensive assessment is ideal, it may not always be practical or feasible.

Most health-care facilities develop standards of care related to patient assessment, which emphasize the most common needs of the patient in specific situations. Agencies require a comprehensive health assessment when a patient enters a health-care facility, and subsequent focused assessments thereafter, depending on the patient's situation. Different types of nursing assessment are discussed in more detail in Chapter 7.

PURPOSE AND PREPARATION

Purpose of the Assessment

The purpose of a functional health assessment is to establish a database for the patient concerning normal functional patterns, risk factors that can contribute to dysfunction, and actual alterations in normal function. From this information, the nurse and the patient together can plan strategies to encourage continuation of healthy patterns, prevent potential health problems, and alleviate or manage existing health problems. Assessment data are used to individualize patient care in promoting optimum health for the patient. A detailed initial database has long-term usefulness in measuring a patient's progress toward health-related goals.

Preparation of the Patient and Environment

Thoughtful preparation of the patient and the environment before beginning a health assessment is advantageous for both the patient and the nurse. Understanding the process and knowing what to expect ensures the patient's physical and emotional comfort. The nurse who is well organized and competent is efficient and reassuring to the patient.

Most patients undergoing a health examination are anxious. Pain, fear, and embarrassment may all contribute to a patient's distress. By thoughtfully preparing the patient and environment before the assessment, some of the controllable sources of anxiety for the patient can be eliminated.

Introduction

To begin, the nurse should introduce himself or herself to the patient and explain the nature and purpose of the health assessment. Assessment can be described as a series of questions about the patient's past and present state of health, followed by a physical examination. The nurse should explain that information obtained in the assessment will be used to understand the patient's current state of health and illness, to monitor progress, and to determine ways to make treatment more effective and comfortable. During this introductory phase, the nurse should tell the patient approximately how long the assessment will take. The patient should also be assured that information obtained during the assessment process is confidential and will be shared only with other health-care professionals participating in provision of care.

Environment

The environment should be comfortable for both nurse and patient. A warm, quiet, well-lit room is ideal. All necessary equipment should be accessible and fully functional. Leaving the patient to find equipment is distracting and time-consuming.

Privacy and confidentiality are important concerns for the patient who is about to share personal information and submit to a physical examination. The patient should feel confident that he or she will not be viewed or overheard by others during the interview or physical examination. This can be a challenge in the hospital if the patient shares a room with another patient. Planning the interview for a time when the roommate is out of the room, asking the roommate to step out for a short period of time, or using an examining room on the nursing unit may help to ensure privacy. Family members and visitors should be asked to leave, unless the patient requests otherwise.

The patient should be as physically comfortable as possible during the assessment. A relaxed patient is more attentive and can provide more accurate and complete information. Ask the patient to void before beginning the assessment, especially if an abdominal assessment is anticipated. The nurse may be unable to provide relief to the patient in acute pain or distress until an assessment of the patient's condition has been accomplished. When this occurs, the nurse should acknowledge the distress and promptly begin the assessment, focusing immediately on the patient's primary problem. Physical examination usually takes priority over obtaining a detailed patient history when a patient is acutely ill.

Positioning and Draping

One way to provide privacy is to draw the curtain around the bed or close the door of the examining room. Draping is a second concern. During the examination, the nurse covers the patient's body parts not included in the specific examination taking place, exposing only the part of the body being examined. As the nurse examines another part of the body, the patient is redraped. Draping also keeps the patient warm during examination. Draping materials include paper sheets, special cloths, or bed linens.

The patient may need to assume various positions for the physical examination. Positions are discussed and illustrated in Chapter 20 (see Fig. 20-1). Patients may need assistance with positioning and, if in pain, should not remain in any position for an extended length of time. Organization and planning of the assessment should take positioning and the patient's present status into consideration.

ORGANIZATION AND DOCUMENTATION

The major portion of the patient interview is usually conducted before the physical examination is performed, but dialogue with the patient is continued throughout the assessment as more information is gathered and new questions are formulated.

During most health assessments, a preprinted form is used to record information. An example of a completed health assessment is found in Figure 18-1. Health assessment forms vary in title and format, depending on the institution, the patient population, and the purpose of the assessment. Some common titles for health assessment forms include Nursing History, Nursing Admission Form, Patient Database, and Nursing Assessment Form. The format may be structured, using specific questions and lists of required data, or the format may be unstructured, defining broad areas of health. Following a printed form is useful, particularly when the nurse is learning to perform health assessment, because it provides a structure for moving logically from one health area to another. It also helps to prevent the omission of any pertinent information.

TYPES OF DATA COLLECTION

The information (or data) obtained during the assessment falls into two categories: subjective and objective. Subjective data are the information only the patient can provide. They relate to the patient's own feelings and experiences, and cannot be verified by an outsider. Subjective data include the patient's descriptions of bodily sensations (such as pain, dizziness, fatigue) and emotional states, and the feelings about past and current health status. Interviewing is the technique used to obtain subjective data. This process is the basis for taking a nursing history. The nursing history is discussed in Chapter 7 as part of the nursing process.

The second category of data obtained during the assessment is objective. Objective data are the tangible, observable facts about the patient. They include observations (such as an unsteady gait, limp, or excessive perspiration) and measurements such as blood pressure, cholesterol level, and pupil size). Objective data are obtained by physical examination and diagnostic testing. Diagnostic testing includes an array of laboratory, x-ray, and special procedures (see Chap. 20).

Obtaining Subjective Data: The Interview

The health history, or interview, is a goal-directed conversation between nurse and patient. Goals may include the following:

* Obtain a description of the patient's health and related problems.
* Identify factors that either positively or negatively influence health.
* Describe how aspects of life are influenced by health status.
* Identify patient's strengths.
* Identify patient's deficits.

The interview component of a health assessment is often the patient's first encounter with the nurse and, therefore, the first step toward establishing a trusting and therapeutic nurse–patient relationship. (Phases of interviewing are discussed in Chap. 7.) The nurse should be professional, concerned, and attentive throughout the interview. When the patient responds to a question, it is important to convey interest by maintaining eye contact, occasionally nodding, or verbally responding to remarks made. Nonverbal behavior, particularly the nurse's body language, can convey a strong message during an interview. The nurse who sits at eye level with the patient, appears unhurried and alert, and takes notes, conveys to the patient that the information being shared is important and deserves attention (see Fig. 17-4). In contrast, the nurse who stands over a patient

(Text continues on page 303)

Inspiratory
capacity
(IC)

BRONSON METHODIST HOSPITAL
Kalamazoo, Michigan

Medical/Surgical-Critical Care Admission Assessment

A. Name: *Jane Smith*

Prefers to be called: *Jane*   Age: *62*

Date: *1/19/91*   Time of arrival to unit: *1700*

Mode of admission: *Amb*

I.D. bracelet on and coincides with addressograph: ☒ Yes ☐ No Information given by: _____

If unable to reach next of kin/legal guardian, contact: *Bill Wright*   Phone: *(206) 186-2964*

Valuables (list and state disposition): *∅*

Admitted from: ☒ Home ☐ Nursing Home ☐ Assisted Living ☐ Foster Care ☐ Senior Citizens' Apartments ☐ Other

Facility Name: _____   Adm. Medical Diagnosis: _____

(DEMOGRAPHIC DATA)

B. Ht *5'4"*   Wt: *134*   Kg

Temp: *98*   ☒ Oral ☐ Ax. ☐ Rectal

Pulse: *82*   ☒ Reg. ☐ Irreg.

Resp: *16*   ☒ Reg. ☐ Irreg.

BP: Left: *142/86*

   ☐ Lying ☒ Sitting ☐ Standing

Right: _____

   ☐ Lying ☐ Sitting ☐ Standing

(VITAL SIGNS)

C. (The following have been explained):

Call system/bed–bathroom	☒ Yes ☐ N/A	Floor restrictions	☒ Yes ☐ N/A
Bed operation/siderails	☒ Yes ☐ N/A	Visitation Policy	☒ Yes ☐ N/A
Bathroom/bedpan–urinal	☒ Yes ☐ N/A	Lounge	☒ Yes ☐ N/A
TV/CH2/telephone	☒ Yes ☐ N/A	Newspaper/mail	☒ Yes ☐ N/A
Meal/cafeteria hours	☒ Yes ☐ N/A	Siderails policy	☒ Yes ☐ N/A
Smoking policy	☒ Yes ☐ N/A	Chaplain services	☒ Yes ☐ N/A

Signature: *Jane Smith*

(ORIENTATION TO UNIT)

D. **Health Patterns Assessment:** Complete information, **including patient's words.** Indicate N/A if non-applicable. Circle, code, or check all other findings as appropriate.

1. Reason for hospitalization/chief complaint: *To have my gall bladder removed*

Recent illness/exposure to communicable disease: *Cold 3 weeks ago*

Previous hospitalizations/surgeries: *Hysterectomy 1982, Appendectomy 1957*

What other health problems have you had? *∅*

Things done to manage health: *See my doctor regularly*

Statement of patient's general appearance (include condition of hair, skin, nails): *Well groomed white female with no observable skin lesions*

Tobacco use: ☐ Yes ☐ No ☒ Used to smoke: _____

EtOH use: *Socially*

Allergies: ☒ Yes (list with reaction experienced)   ☐ No

Food: *Shellfish — hives*

Medications/anesthetics: *∅*

Other (e.g., wool, tape, pollens): *∅*

(HEALTH PERCEPTION/HEALTH MANAGEMENT)

FORM 102 (Revised 10/84) — Page 1

Figure 18–1. Database assessment form organized according to functional health patterns. (Reprinted with permission from the Bronson Methodist Hospital, Kalamazoo, Michigan.)

Patient's Name: _____ Hospital No.: _____ Date: _____

Medications: (e.g., prescript., non-prescript.) ☐ Yes ☐ No Did you bring? ☐ Yes ☐ No Taken home? ☐ Yes ☐ No ☐ N/A

NAME	DOSE	SCHEDULE	REASON	PRESCRIBING PHYSICIAN

Have you been taking your medication(s) as prescribed? _____
_____

OTHER PERTINENT DATA: _____

| | initials |

2. Special diet? _Ø_____ Supplements: _Ø_____

Pattern of daily food/fluid intake: _3 Regular meals with snacks_
___Avoid fatty foods — cause pain___

Appetite: _good_____ Wt. loss/gain: _____

Nausea/Vomiting: _Occasionally_____

GI pain: _3 episodes of severe pain   MD says it's gall bladder__

Condition of oral mucous membranes: _good_____

Dental condition: _Good including gums_____ Dentures: ☐ Upper ☐ Lower ☐ Partial ☒ N/A

Skin: ☒ Warm ☒ Dry ☐ Cool ☐ Moist ☐ Other: _No breaks___

Turgor: ☒ Supple ☒ Firm ☐ Fragile ☐ Dehydrated ☐ Other: _____

Color: ☒ Pink ☐ Pale ☐ Dusky ☐ Cyanotic ☐ Jaundiced ☐ Mottled ☐ Other: _____

Edema: _Ø_____

Wounds/drains/dressings: _Ø_____

Skin problems (description and location): _____

I.V.'s: _____ ☐ N/A

OTHER PERTINENT DATA _____

(left margin, vertical: NUTRITION / METABOLIC)

| | _CJH_ | initials |

3. Abd. tenderness/guarding/distention: _Previous episodes of abd pain_

Bowel sounds: _____ Stoma (type): _____

Any problems with hemorrhoids/involuntary stool? _____

Usual bowel pattern (frequency, character, consistency, etc.) _QD — mornings_
_____ Date of last BM _Yesterday_

If problem, describe _____

Use of anything to manage bowels (e.g., laxatives, enemas, suppositories, "home remedies", anti-diarrheals): _____
Occasionally MOM if constipated

Usual urinary pattern (frequency, character, amount, incontinence, nocturia, etc.): _____
4—5 times per day
_____ Last void (time) _1 hr ago_

If problem, describe: _Ø pain or UTI_____

Perspiration/nocturnal sweats: _____

OTHER PERTINENT DATA: _____

(left margin, vertical: ELIMINATION)

| | _CJH_ | initials |

Figure 18–1   *(Continued)*

4.

CARDIO-VASCULAR STATUS

Peripheral pulses: *Pedal palpable equal Bilaterally*

_____ ☐ N/A

Neurovascular check (e.g., capillary refill): *WNL*

_____

Chest pain/radiation: _Ø_____

_____

Jugular vein distention: ☐ Yes ☒ No

Hx of murmur: ☐ Yes ☒ No

Pacemaker: ☐ Yes ☒ No

Presence of A-V Shunt: _____ ☒ No

Arterio-venous bruit: _____ ☒ N/A

Monitor/rhythm: _____ ☐ N/A

Hemodynamic monitoring: _____ ☐ N/A

ACTIVITY / EXERCISE

RESPIRATORY STATUS

Respiratory pattern: ☒ No problem ☐ Dyspnea ☐ Nocturnal Dyspnea ☐ S.O.B. at rest

☐ S.O.B. on exertion: _____ ☐ Other: _____

Lung sounds: *Clear* _____ Use of accessory muscles? ☐ Yes ☒ No

Cough/production: _Ø_____ O₂ supplement: _____ ☒ N/A

Resp. tubes (e.g., ET, trach, chest/describe secretions/drainage): _____
_____ ☐ N/A

Ventilatory assistance: _____ ☐ N/A

ACTIVITIES OF DAILY LIVING/MOBILITY STATUS

Use the **Activity Level Code** below to assess admission statuses:

	ADL Status		**Mobility Status**
0–total independence	Feeding _0_	Meal Preparation _0_	Bed mobility _0_
1–assist with device	Bathing _0_	Cleaning _0_	Cart transfer _0_
2–assist with person	Dressing _0_	Shopping _0_	Chair/toilet transfer _0_
3–assist with device & person	Grooming _0_	Laundry _0_	Ambulation _0_
4–total dependence	Toileting _0_	Other ____	R.O.M. _0_

Handedness: ☒ Right ☐ Left

Able to use? ☒ Yes ☐ No

Reasons for ADL/Mobility limitations: _____
_____ ☒ N/A

Devices used for assist: _____ ☒ N/A

Do you need assistance with transportation? ☐ Yes ☒ No If "Yes", specify _____

Where do you plan to be discharged? _Home_____ Will you need assistance? ☐ Yes ☒ No

If "Yes", describe: _____

OTHER PERTINENT DATA _____
_____ | *CJH* | initials |

5.

COGNITIVE / PERCEPTUAL

Level of consciousness _Alert_____ Oriented to: ☒ Person ☒ Place ☒ Time

Behaviors (describe): _____

Hx of epilepsy/seizures/Parkinson's, etc.: _No_____

REFLEXES

Reflexes: ☒ No problem ☐ Problem (If "No problem", do not complete this section.)

Eyes: Pupil size: r_____ l_____ Equal? ☐ Yes ☐ No Reaction to light: r_____ l_____

Accommodation: r_____ l_____ Deviation: _____

Handgrasp: r_____ l_____ Gag: _____ Swallow: _____

Movement of extremities: _____

SENSORIUM

Eyes/sight:	☐ No problem ☒ Deficit	_____	Aid: *Bifocals*
Ears/hearing:	☒ No problem ☐ Deficit	_____	Aid: _____
Nose/smell:	☒ No problem ☐ Deficit	_____	
Tongue/taste:	☒ No problem ☐ Deficit	_____	
Skin/touch:	☒ No problem ☐ Deficit	_____	
Numbness/tingling:	☒ No problem ☐ Deficit	_____	
Dizziness:	☒ No problem ☐ Deficit	_____	

FORM 102 (Revised 10/84) — Page 3

Figure 18–1 *(Continued)*

Patient's Name _Jane Smith_   Hospital No. _____   Date: _1/19/91_

COGNITIVE / PERCEPTUAL

PAIN

Pain: ☐ No problem ☒ Problem (If "No problem", do not complete this section.)

If "Problem", describe location, type, intensity, onset, duration: _3 Episodes of sudden acute colicy pain_
following dinner
Currently in no apparent distress

Methods of pain management: _Nonprescription pain med last episode to ER_

COGNITION

Primary language: _English_ _____ Speech deficit: _____ Aid: _Ø_
Any learning difficulties? _Ø_
OTHER PERTINENT DATA: _High school education_

| | CJH | initials |

SLEEP / REST

6.   Usual sleep/rest pattern: _8 hours at night, no naps_
Adequate? ☒ Yes ☐ No   Factors affecting sleep/rest: _pain_
Methods to promote sleep: _warm milk, soft music_
Hx of sleep disturbances: _Ø_
OTHER PERTINENT DATA: _____

| | CJH | initials |

SELF-PERCEPTION SELF-CONCEPT

7.   Are there any ways you feel differently about yourself since you've been ill/hospitalized? _____
Am not able to take care of my husband & my home

Description of non-verbal behaviors: _Appears calm_
OTHER PERTINENT DATA: _____

| | CJH | initials |

ROLE / RELATIONSHIP

8.   Marital status: _Married_ _____ Children: _3_
Do you live? ☐ Alone ☒ With family ☐ Other: _____
Family feelings regarding hospitalization: _Worried, but want the pain to stop_
Who are the people that will help you most at this time? _Husband_
Are you presently employed? ☐ Yes ☒ No   Occupation: _Housewife_   ☐ N/A
Are you presently in school? ☐ Yes ☒ No   Will illness/hospitalization interfere? _____   ☐ N/A
Upon discharge, if necessary, will you be able to afford?
              Medications: ☒ Yes ☐ No   Supplies: ☒ Yes ☐ No   Medical Care: ☒ Yes ☐ No
OTHER PERTINENT DATA: _____

| | CJH | initials |

SEXUALITY / REPRODUCTIVE

9.   Female: ☐ N/A   Menopausal: ☒ Yes ☐ No   Menstrual pattern: _____   ☐ N/A
     Problems/changes: _____
     Date of L.N.M.P. _1978_ _____   ☒ N/A   Possibly pregnant? ☐ Yes ☐ No ☐ N/A
     Pregnancy history: _____
     Use of birth control measure ☐ Yes ☐ No ☒ N/A   Type: _____
     Any problems with use? _____
     Monthly self-breast exam? ☐ Yes ☒ No ☐ N/A
     Vaginal discharge/bleeding/lesions _____
     Receiving medical attention? ☐ Yes ☒ No ☐ N/A
     OTHER PERTINENT DATA: _____

| | CJH | initials |

Male: ☒ N/A   Prostate problems? _____
Monthly self-testicular exam? ☐ Yes ☐ No ☐ N/A
Penile discharge/bleeding/lesions _____
Receiving medical attention? ☐ Yes ☐ No ☐ N/A
OTHER PERTINENT DATA: _____

| | CJH | initials |

FORM 102 (Revised 10/84) — Page 4

Figure 18–1   *(Continued)*

COPING/STRESS

10. Have you experienced any recent stressful situations in addition to your illness/hospitalization? ☐ Yes ☒ No

If "Yes", please describe briefly: _____

_____

_____

_____

Are there any ways we can be of assistance? _____

How do you usually manage stresses? *Talk with family & friends*

_____

What do you do for relaxation? *Read, watch TV*

Support groups/counselling resources used: _____

Were they helpful? _____ ☒ N/A

OTHER PERTINENT DATA: _____

_____ | *CJH* | initials |

VALUE/BELIEF

11. Will illness/hospitalization interfere with any of the following?

Spiritual or religious practices? ☒ Yes ☐ No

Cultural beliefs or practices? ☐ Yes ☒ No

Familial traditions? ☐ Yes ☒ No

If "Yes", to any of the above, please describe briefly: *Active in my church*

_____

_____

_____

_____

Would you like your clergy or hospital chaplain to be contacted? ☒ Yes ☐ No ☐ N/A

OTHER PERTINENT DATA: _____

_____ | *CJH* | initials |

IMPRESSIONS

E. Include: a. Possible nursing diagnostic concept labels to consider for care planning.
b. Possible referral resources to consider for discharge planning needs.
c. Other pertinent information

Potential for acute pain related to gall bladder dysfunction and surgical intervention

Knowledge deificit regarding pre & postoperative management related to lack of instruction

Potential altered breathing patterns related to surgical intervention & history or recent cold

_____

_____

_____

_____

_____ | initials |

DATE	TIME	INITIALS	SIGNATURES	
1/19/91	*1700*	*CJH*	*Constance J Hirnle*	(1st Adm. R.N.)
				(2nd Adm. R.N.)
				(3rd Adm. R.N.)
				(4th Adm. R.N.)

Figure 18–1 *(Continued)*

during an interview communicates that the nurse's stay will be brief, and the patient may feel powerless or conclude that the nurse is in a hurry or has more important tasks to do. Throughout the interview, the nurse should be aware of his or her verbal and nonverbal messages. These messages can either promote or discourage the patient's trust and confidence.

Questioning patients about their health is a skill that requires study and practice to achieve competence. Before the first assessment and interview, the nurse should prepare a few questions in each functional health area. Open-ended questions are preferable to questions that can be answered yes, no, or in one word. For example, the statement, "Describe what you eat on a normal day" will yield more valuable information than "How is your appetite?" Follow-up or probing questions should be asked when a problem area is discovered or suggested. Further detail can be solicited by statements such as, "Tell me more about that" or "That seems to concern you." After the planned interview questions have been covered, it is important to ask the patient, "Is there anything you would like to discuss that I have not yet mentioned?" This question invites the patient to add information that was overlooked or was not anticipated by the nurse.

Special techniques may be necessary to control the interview if a patient is overly talkative, particularly in relation to unrelated information. Many patients have difficulty staying on a topic or limiting their answers to significant points. A sensitive yet effective method for directing the patient might be, "Because our time is limited, we won't be able to discuss that in detail now. I would like to hear more about. . . ." The ability to skillfully, yet sensitively control the interview is essential for obtaining pertinent information in a timely manner. Later in the chapter discussion concerning each functional health area guides the nurse in the skill of communication.

Chief Complaint. The first subject usually discussed in a patient interview is the patient's specific reason for seeking medical attention. This subject is often called the patient's "chief complaint" or "chief concern." The nurse should listen carefully to the patient's description of the primary problem and document it, quoting the patient's exact words. In-depth questioning and discussion of this problem should follow. After the patient's chief complaint has been addressed, the nurse should proceed with a systematic survey of each functional health pattern.

Approaches. In most circumstances, the patient interview precedes the physical examination. Some nurses prefer to interview the patient regarding all of the functional patterns before physical examination. Other nurses prefer to address functional health patterns one at a time, collecting subjective and objective information

for each area. Either approach is acceptable. Subjective data collection should always precede physical examination of the related area, however. Information obtained during the interview alerts the nurse to areas of pain or probable abnormality so that the examination of the affected areas can be more careful, thoughtful, and thorough.

Obtaining Objective Data: The Physical Examination

Physical examination involves the use of one's senses (seeing, hearing, touching, smelling, as described in Chap. 7) to obtain information about the structure and function of an area being observed or manipulated. The four basic techniques of physical examination are inspection, palpation, percussion, and auscultation. With few exceptions, they should be performed in that order because each technique reinforces and refines what was discovered in the previous step. It is often suggested that beginning students practice newly learned physical assessment skills on fellow students or willing friends. This helps to acquire some skill, confidence, and organization before approaching a patient. Expertise in the techniques of physical examination can only be learned through practice.

Inspection

Inspection uses the sense of sight, or looking at a patient, to make specific observations of physical features and behavior. Inspection is the natural beginning to physical examination because it starts immediately upon meeting the patient.

The general inspection, or survey of a patient, includes easily observable features. These initial observa-

Patient Teaching

Instruct the patient as follows:

- Understand what the nurse is planning to do and how you can assist him or her.
- All information collected will be used to help plan and individualize your nursing care and will be kept confidential.
- Alert the nurse if you are becoming fatigued or uncomfortable during the assessment.
- Slowly exhale during palpation. This prevents tensing muscles, which can make palpation difficult and cause you discomfort.
- Perform self-assessment (such as breast self-exam) following the technique used by the nurse during assessment.

tions provide an overall impression of the patient's present state of health. General inspection of a patient focuses on the following areas:

- Overall appearance of health or illness (Does the patient appear weak, frail, or chronically ill?)
- Signs of distress (Is the patient grimacing, as if in pain? Is breathing labored?)
- Body size (Does the patient appear thin and malnourished or overweight?)
- Grooming and personal hygiene (Are the patient and his or her clothing clean and neat?)
- Unusual odors (Is there a smell of alcohol, acetone, or urine?)
- Facial expression and mood (Does the patient appear anxious, depressed, angry, or uninterested?).

In addition to the role of inspection in the general survey of a patient, inspection is the first method used in physical examination of a specific area. The chest and abdomen, for example, are inspected before palpation, percussion, or auscultation are performed.

The optimal conditions for effective inspection are full exposure of the area and adequate lighting. Removal of clothing and bed linen is necessary; however, in respect for the patient's modesty and comfort, only the specific area being examined should be exposed. A well-lit room is essential for good visualization. Special instruments are used to provide intense and more focused light, such as an otoscope, for inspecting the ears, and an ophthalmoscope, for inspecting the eyes. **Tangential lighting** is provided by indirectly shining light with a lamp or flashlight so that a shadow is created over the area being examined. The shadow brings out subtle differences in contour and movement. Tangential lighting is often used for inspecting the blood vessels of the neck and the area of the chest that lies over the heart.

The inspection phase of physical examination consists of the general survey as well as focused inspection of specific areas. The physical examination is organized so that each step builds on information obtained in the previous step. Inspection, therefore, builds on data from the patient interview. Subjective patient data should be considered and applied during inspection of the patient because looking "for" something generally yields more information than simply looking "at" something.

Palpation

Palpation uses the tactile sense and is a special form of touching. Palpation usually follows inspection because it defines what was seen and reveals what cannot be seen. Palpation is used to discriminate texture, dimension, temperature, and consistency of different areas of the body. Palpation can be described as either light or deep.

With *light palpation*, the skin is pressed with the fingertips of the dominant hand approximately 0.5 to 1 inch (Fig. 18-2). A gentle, circular motion of the hand

over the area is added. Pressure is exerted and released. Continuous pressure would dull the tactile discrimination senses (Fuller & Schaller-Ayers, 1990). Light palpation is used to check skin temperature and moistness, detect abnormal masses, and locate tender or painful areas. The presence of pain or tenderness is best monitored by observing the patient's facial expression while palpating.

Deep palpation involves compression of an area to a depth of 1.5 to 2 inches and requires significantly more pressure than light palpation (Fig. 18-3). The fingers are also placed at a greater angle to the body than in light palpation. One or both hands may be used, depending on the structure being examined. When both hands are used, the fingertips of one hand are placed over the fingertips of the other hand. The top hand presses and guides the bottom hand (Fuller & Schaller-Ayers, 1990). The purpose of deep palpation is to locate organs and determine their size and to detect abnormal masses. Usually only advanced practitioners use deep palpation to assess patients.

Different parts of the hand are more suitable during palpation for different tactile sensations. The fingertips are concentrated with nerve endings and can sense fine differences in texture and consistency. The fingertips are used to discriminate a raised versus a flat skin lesion or to evaluate an arterial pulse. The skin over the dorsum of the hand is sensitive to temperature because this skin is thin and nerve density is great. Skin temperature over a specific area is best evaluated by comparing its tempera-

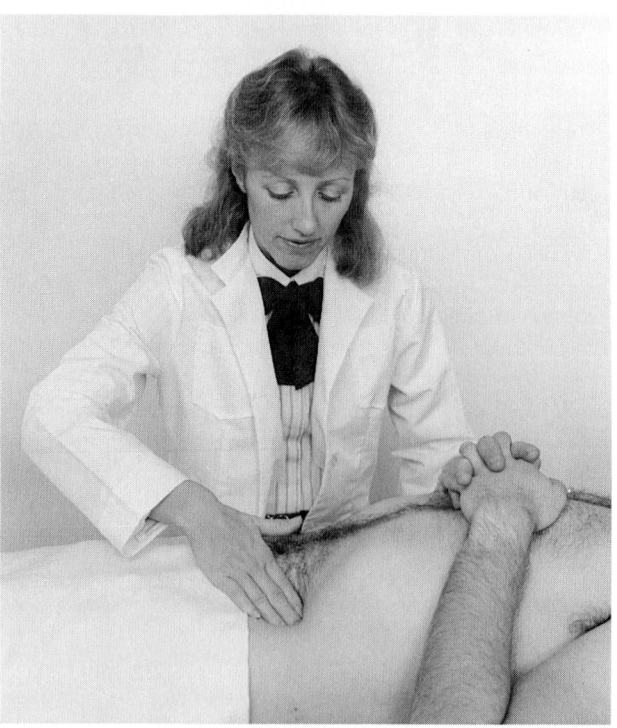

Figure 18–2. Light palpation. The fingertips are moved in a circular motion, depressing the body surface 0.5 to 1 inch.

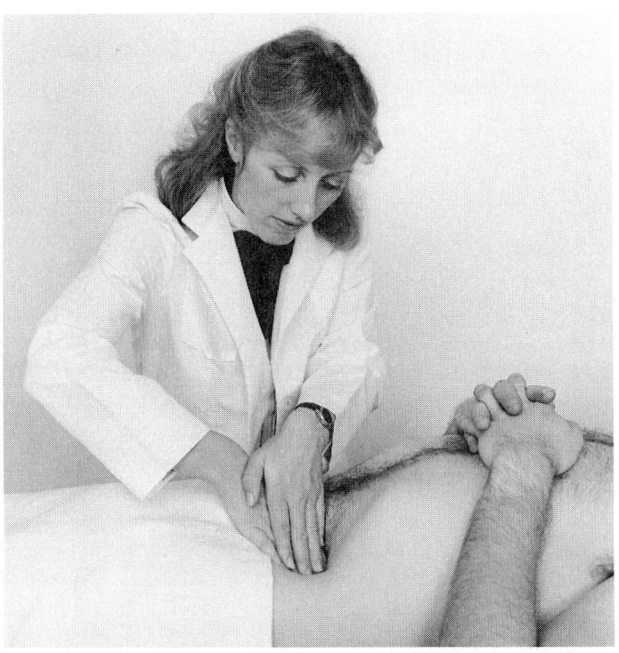

Figure 18–3.   Deep palpation. the fingers are held at a greater angle to the body surface than in light palpation, and the skin is depressed 1.5 to 2 inches.

ture to adjacent areas. The palm of the hand is sensitive to vibration and is useful in locating a vibration associated with a heart murmur.

Effective palpation requires patient relaxation because tensed muscles block access to underlying tissue. The patient's ability to relax can be enhanced if the hands of the nurse are warmed and actions are explained to the patient before he or she is touched.

Percussion

Percussion, which uses the sense of hearing, is the act of striking a body surface with the hand in order to interpret the sound produced. The propagation of sound waves is determined by the density of the medium in which they are traveling. The number of substances of different density that sound must travel through also affects the transmission of the sound. Sound required to traverse skin, muscle, fat, bone, fluid, and air moves less well than through any single medium. This is the reason

for percussing *between* the ribs and tensing the skin under the finger.

Percussion provides information about the nature of an underlying structure. It is used to outline the size of an organ, most commonly the heart and liver. Percussion is also used to determine if a structure is air-filled, fluid-filled, or solid. This has application in percussion of the lungs, bladder, and abdomen.

Five characteristic sounds are produced by percussion: resonant, hyperresonant, tympanic, dull, and flat. The degree to which sound propagates is called **resonance.** Air is resonant; solid tissue is not. As a standard, percussion of normal lung tissue is called *resonant,* emphysematous lung tissue is *hyperresonant,* the gastric air bubble is *tympanic,* the liver is *dull,* the thigh is *flat.* Flat means not at all resonant. The specific qualities of each of these sounds are given in Table 18-1.

Percussion may be performed directly or indirectly (Fig. 18-4). *Direct percussion* is accomplished by tapping an area directly with the fingertip of the middle finger or thumb. *Indirect percussion* interposes a finger, the **pleximeter,** between the area to be percussed and the finger creating the vibrations, the **plexor.** The steps for indirect percussion are:

1. Rest the tip of the nondominant middle finger (the pleximeter) flatly against the skin over the area to be percussed.
2. Poise the rest of the hand above the surface and not touching the surface.
3. Flex the dominant hand and position it over the pleximeter in a horizontal position.
4. Using the tip of the dominant middle finger (the plexor), strike the pleximeter, aiming for the space between the fingernail and the distal interphalangeal joint. (The plexor fingernail should be short to facilitate percussing with the tip, not the pad, of the finger.)
5. Deliver several sharp successive blows, quickly withdrawing the plexor.
6. Identify the percussion sound (see Table 18-1).
7. Proceed to the next area, moving from more resonant to less resonant areas.

Labeling the percussion note is often difficult. The most helpful observations consist of change in the sound

TABLE 18–1

Characteristics of Percussion Tones

Tone	Quality	Pitch	Intensity	Location
Flatness	Extreme dullness	High	Soft	Sternum, thigh
Dullness	Thudlike	Medium	Medium	Liver, diaphragm
Resonance	Hollow	Low	Loud	Normal lung
Hyperresonance	Booming	Very low	Very loud	Emphysematous lung
Tympany	Musical, drumlike	High	Loud	Air-filled stomach

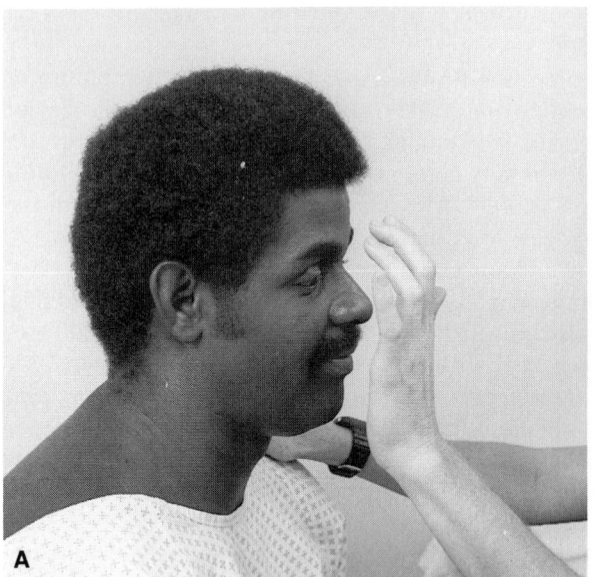
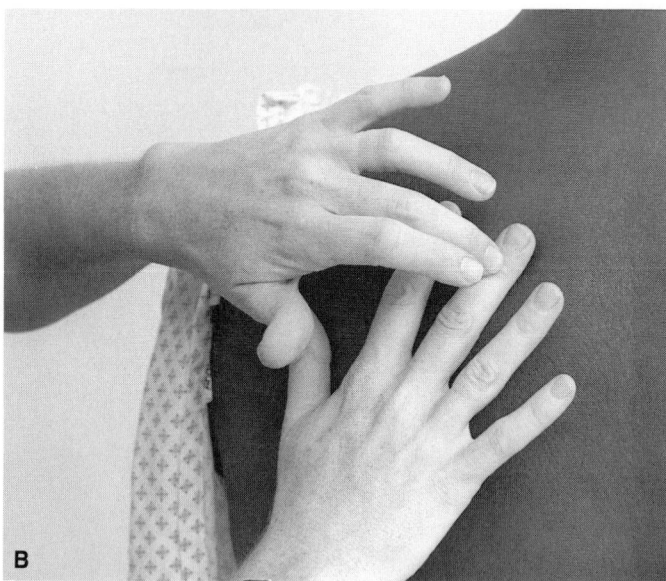

Figure 18–4.   Two percussion methods.   **A.**   Direct percussion is performed by using the fingers of one hand to strike the surface.   **B.**   Indirect percussion is performed with two hands, using the finger of one hand as a plexor and the finger of the other hand as a pleximeter.

from one area to another. A change from resonant to dull is easier to appreciate than the reverse. Whenever possible, percuss first a resonant area and move toward dullness to define borders.

Auscultation

Auscultation is the art of listening for sounds of movement within the body. The heart and blood vessels are auscultated for the sound of moving blood; the lungs are auscultated for moving air.

Four properties are used to describe sound: frequency, intensity, duration, and quality. **Frequency** is the measure of vibration, expressed in cycles per second. Many cycles per second or a high frequency produces a high-pitched sound; few cycles per second produce low-pitched sounds. **Intensity** describes the loudness of sound and is measured in decibels. Breath sounds over the trachea are loud, whereas most heart sounds are soft. How long the sound lasts is the *duration*. An abnormal heart sound may be described according to its duration within the cardiac cycle. *Quality,* sometimes called timbre, is harder to define. It reflects the musical characteristic of a sound. Blowing, squeaking, and humming are adjectives frequently used in describing the quality of a sound.

An instrument called the stethoscope is used to aid auscultation. The **stethoscope** collects and amplifies sound, selects frequencies, and screens out extraneous sound. The head of the stethoscope applied to the skin collects the sound from beneath it. Most stethoscopes have two types of heads, a diaphragm and a bell (Fig. 18-5). The diaphragm is a flat piece that is applied firmly

against the skin and responds best to high-frequency sounds and excludes low-frequency ones. The bell is funnel- or cup-shaped and allows high-frequency sounds to escape and collects low-pitched sounds. The bell should simply be allowed to rest on top of the skin. If too much pressure is applied, the skin is stretched and a diaphragm effect is produced. Table 18-2 contrasts using the bell and diaphragm. The conduit of the stethoscope is a combination of rubber or plastic, and metal. Leaks in the conduit allow sound to escape. The most common leak is a poor fitting earpiece, either too large or too small. Comfort is a good guide to properly sized ear-

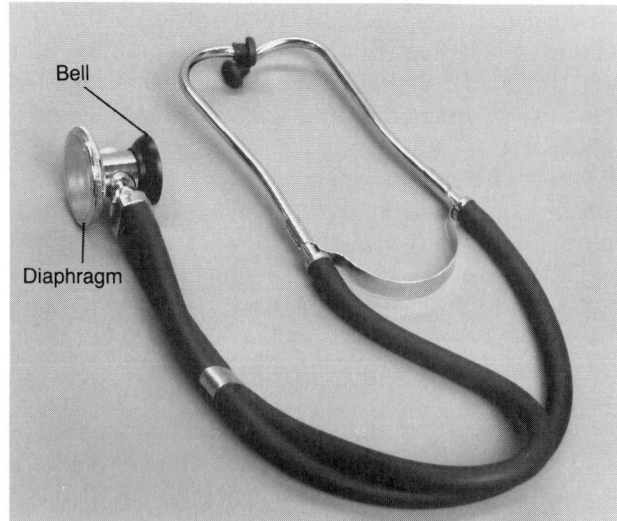

Figure 18–5.   The bell of the stethoscope is used to auscultate low-frequency sounds, and the diaphragm is used to auscultate high-frequency sounds.

TABLE 18–2

Stethoscope Diaphragm and Bell Usage

	Technique	Purpose	Example
Diaphragm	Press firmly against the skin	Detects high-pitched sounds	Breath sounds, normal heart sounds, bowel sounds
Bell	Lay lightly on the skin	Detects low-pitched sounds	Abormal heart sounds, bruits

pieces. The earpieces of the stethoscope should fit snugly, occluding the ear canal and screening out environmental noise. It is essential that the room be as quiet as possible during auscultation. Extraneous sounds that can confuse the examination may be heard through a stethoscope. Avoid creating extraneous noise from bed linen or clothing rubbing against the stethoscope, bumping the stethoscope tubing, or moving the chestpiece while auscultation. If a patient has body hair over the area of auscultation, wetting it with water reduces the crackling sound that hair creates.

Odors

Smell is a sense occasionally useful in physical examination. Halitosis (bad breath) may indicate poor oral and dental hygiene. The ketones of diabetic acidosis create a fruity odor to the breath. Body odor may indicate poor hygiene related to an inability to care for oneself. Certain infected wounds also have an odor.

ASSESSMENT OF INDIVIDUAL ASPECTS OF FUNCTIONAL HEALTH

The remainder of this chapter discusses the information and skills needed to conduct a basic patient assessment, organized according to functional health. Each functional pattern describes an aspect of human performance or ability that contributes to the overall health of the person.

The nurse's goal in assessing each pattern is to identify:

- Patient's normal functional pattern
- Risk factors for dysfunction
- Presence of any dysfunction
- Patient's satisfaction with functional abilities
- Patient's adaptations to dysfunctional patterns
- Effect of dysfunction on performance of daily activities.

For clarity, discussion of functional health assessment follows a consistent format. First, an overview of the pattern is presented, followed by an outline of the major assessment parameters that should be considered. Next, subjective data related to the pattern are discussed, including a list of suggested interview questions. Finally, objective data are presented, providing a list of appropriate data along with a detailed explanation of how the physical examination is performed.

Assessment skills described in this chapter are intended for a nurse generalist. In some situations, nurse specialists are trained to perform more advanced assessment techniques. Chapters in Section II of this text address the concept of each functional health pattern in depth. Each chapter contains a section on nursing assessment related to the functional area.

ASSESSMENT OF HEALTH PERCEPTION AND HEALTH MANAGEMENT

The major health problem in the United States and Canada is chronic disease, such as heart disease, cancer, and stroke. For those under 25 years of age, accidents cause the majority of deaths, followed by suicide (National Data Book, 1986). Control of these health problems depends directly on modification of a person's behavior and habits of living. Death and disability in middle age are premature and preventable.

Prevention necessitates eliminating habits that many people enjoy: overeating, overindulgence in alcohol, smoking cigarettes, and driving fast. Prevention also implies doing things that require special effort: exercising regularly, eating a healthy diet, submitting to regular physical examinations, wearing automobile seatbelts, and striving for a harmonious life. The solution to many problems of ill health in modern Western society involves people taking responsibility for their own health. Assessment of a person's health perception and health maintenance reveals knowledge, behavior, and attitudes toward preventing disease and living a healthy lifestyle. Unit VI contains chapters concerned with health maintenance and health management.

Subjective Data

Interviewing the patient assists the nurse in obtaining subjective information concerning the patient's perception of his or her health and methods used to maintain health and wellness. The major concerns of this assessment should include the patient's perception of health status, preventive health practices, compliance with medical treatment, and patient safety. Numerous lifestyle choices reflect a health-valuing and health-promoting attitude. Similarly, many behaviors strongly suggest a disregard or lack of knowledge pertaining to practices or habits known to contribute to illness, accidents, and disease.

During a health assessment, the nurse should discuss the patient's health promotion activities, such as exercise programs, weight control, routine medical and dental examinations, wearing seatbelts and motorcycle helmets, and stress management. The nurse should inquire about alcohol and drug use, including the use of recreational drugs. The patient's overall compliance in following health-related advice should be assessed.

A detailed allergy history should be obtained for every patient, including food, pollen, insect, and any environmental allergens. The nurse should inquire specifically about allergies to medications and the specific type of reaction that was experienced. Patients often confuse a medication side-effect, such as nausea, with an allergic reaction.

Selected sample interview questions for eliciting the patient's perception and management of health include:

- How would you describe your overall state of health?
- What health problems have you had in the past?
- Have you ever been advised to change any aspect of your lifestyle?
- What things do you do to stay healthy?
- What health professionals do you visit on a routine basis: physician; dentist; ophthalmologist; gynecologist?
- How much alcohol do you drink per day?
- What prescription medications do you take? Indicate dose, frequency, and the last time you took this medication.
- What nonprescription medications do you take?
- Do you or have you ever used recreational drugs?
- Do you have allergies? Describe what you are allergic to and describe the type of reaction you have.

Objective Data

Although direct observation of a patient's health practices is usually not possible, some objective data reflecting effort (or lack of effort) toward health promotion may be found through specific measurable consequences of health behavior. Examples of such behavior include: the blood sugar level of a diabetic patient; the number of pounds lost by an overweight patient; blood pressure measurement of a hypertensive patient; the number of clinic appointments a patient has kept or canceled; the number of hospital admissions for the same health problem. Some home health nurses count a patient's pills to estimate if medications are being taken correctly.

ASSESSMENT OF ACTIVITY AND EXERCISE

Activity and exercise describe the wide range of physical activities that people initiate and perform to maintain life, health, and well-being. Mobility, the ability to move about freely, is an important component of activity and exercise because it affects independence and daily living. Mobility and physical activity are necessary for many functions in daily living, including the ability to care for oneself, to work, to maintain a home, to obtain resources, and to engage in social and recreational activities. In addition, physical exercise is important for promoting health and preventing complications associated with inactivity.

Collection of subjective and objective data concerning musculoskeletal function, respiratory function, and cardiovascular function is important in the assessment of activity and exercise. Body movement depends on the normal functioning of the bones and muscles of the body, and how well movement is coordinated by the nervous system. The respiratory and cardiovascular systems work together to supply the muscles of the body with oxygen and energy and to ensure that waste products produced during activity can be transported to other parts of the body for removal. Dysfunction of the musculoskeletal, respiratory, or cardiovascular system affects functional capacity to perform normal activities requiring exercise.

Assessment of activity and exercise focuses on the patient's mobility status, energy level, activity tolerance, oxygenation, circulation, and ability to perform self-care activities. For clarity in discussing assessment of activity and exercise, the assessment has been divided into mobility and self-care assessment, respiratory assessment, and cardiovascular assessment.

Mobility and Self-Care Assessment

Assessment of activity and exercise should reveal if any restrictions to mobility or self-care exist. For many patients, only a brief discussion is necessary. Many other patients, however, experience mild to severe deficits as a result of conditions such as neuromuscular disease, orthopedic trauma or deformity, spinal cord injury, cerebral vascular accident (stroke), brain tumor, or chronic respiratory or cardiac disease. For such patients, a detailed evaluation is necessary.

When a patient's mobility or self-care functions are compromised, a daily living assessment should be performed. A daily living assessment includes evaluation of the ability to perform self-care skills (bathing, toileting, dressing, grooming, and eating) and simple motor activities (sitting, standing, walking, climbing stairs, and opening doors). Depending on the patient's living situation, an assessment of some home maintenance skills may also be appropriate. These skills include cooking, shopping, housekeeping (making a bed, cleaning, vacuuming, washing dishes), laundry, paying bills, and using the telephone. The architecture of a home, particularly the presence of stairs, can complicate independent activity and should be considered. The daily living assessment provides key information about a person's ability to live independently or the amount of assistance that is required to do so. More information on daily living assessment is provided in Chapter 28.

Mobility assessment is preventive as well as descriptive. Patients with impaired mobility are at risk for accidents and injury. Elderly people, particularly those who have fallen in the past, are most susceptible. A thorough assessment of risk factors is necessary for instituting appropriate safety precautions.

Subjective Data

Interviewing the patient to assess normal activity patterns and any restrictions of activity or exercise is important. A program of regular physical activity is important at every age and should be discussed with every patient. Participation in sports and recreational activities contributes not only to physical but psychological well-being. The nurse should determine if the patient has any pain or discomfort associated with exercise, and if there are desirable activities that the patient is unable to participate in. Energy level also affects the desire and ability to be physically active. Fatigue is frequently associated with cardiac and respiratory disease, anemia, and cancer.

Suggested patient interview questions related to mobility and self-care include:

- Do you need any assistance with bathing, dressing, eating, or toileting?
- Do you need any assistance with cooking, cleaning, shopping, or other jobs around your home?
- Describe your activities on a routine day. How much physical exercise do you get? What recreational activities do you enjoy?
- Do you have any trouble walking?
- Do you experience any pain or discomfort during physical exercise?
- Does the condition of your feet or legs limit your activity in any way?
- Have you noticed any change in your activity level over the last 6 months? Is there anything you are no longer able to do?
- Have you fallen or injured yourself within the last year?

Objective Data

Objective data useful in evaluating a patient's mobility status include: gait and balance, muscle strength, coordination, and joint mobility. For additional information on assessing mobility status, refer to Chapter 29.

Gait and Balance. Gait is a manner of walking. Balance refers to stability and equality between both sides of the body. An evaluation of gait and balance contributes to the assessment of a patient's mobility as well as risk for injury due to falling. Gait and balance abnormalities may also indicate dysfunction or disease in other body systems, particularly the brain, spinal cord, muscles, and skeleton. A patient may acquire a slowed, cautious, or unnatural gait as an unconscious means of protection from pain, weakness, or loss of balance.

Gait and balance may be observed during many activities that naturally occur during a health assessment. The nurse should assess the patient's balance as he or she walks into the room, moves around in bed, rises from the sitting position, or rolls onto his or her side. To assess gait, the nurse asks the patient to walk a distance of about 10 feet down a hallway. A normal gait is quick, springy, and rhythmic, with the arms naturally swinging back and forth. Characteristics of abnormal gait include the following: slow, measured steps; limping; leaning to one side; shuffling of the feet; shorter steps taken on one side compared to the other; wide outward swinging of one leg; a wide gait or stance; leaning the trunk forward; lifting the knee higher than normal with each step; and short, hurrying steps. If the patient uses any assistive devices for ambulation, such as a cane, crutches, walker, prosthesis, or brace, he or she should be assessed while using the aid. The nursing assessment should focus on coordination, stability, comfort, and safety.

Foot pain is a common cause of decreased mobility. The patient's feet should be inspected for the presence of bunions, corns, calluses, ingrown toenails, spurs, and ulcers.

Muscle Strength. A nurse should perform a simple screening of motor function in the arms, because arm movement and strength are essential for many self-care activities. Deficits should be reported to the physician or a nurse specialist for a more comprehensive and detailed assessment of muscle function.

Simple techniques for assessing overall motor strength of the arms include the following:

- Ask the patient to close both eyes and hold his or her arms straight in front with palms up for 20 to 30 seconds. If the hand drifts down or the forearm pronates, motor weakness is present in that arm.
- Ask the patient to hold each arm out and maintain it in this position against efforts made to depress it. Note the strength in each arm.
- Ask the patient to raise both arms over the head with palms forward. Note whether this position can be maintained for 20 to 30 seconds. Assess whether the patient is able to maintain arms in this position against force exerted on each arm to bring it down to the side.

It is expected that muscle strength is slightly greater in the dominant arm. Notable differences in strength or overall difficulty in performing these tests reveal problems with movement or weakness in the arms.

Joint Mobility. Joint movement is also important to activity and exercise function. All joints should have appropriate range of motion. Often the nurse can observe this by watching the extent and ease with which a person moves extremities. If the patient complains of stiffness or does not move an area of the body, the nurse should evaluate joint mobility by moving each joint through full range of motion and noting any limitations in movement. Refer to Chapter 29 for additional information on assessment of joint mobility.

Respiratory Assessment

Subjective Data

Functional respiratory assessment should focus on four major areas: risk factors for lung disease (such as smoking or occupational exposure to pollutants); signs and symptoms of respiratory dysfunction (such as cough, sputum production, and dyspnea); impact of respiratory status on activities of daily living; and adaptive measures that the patient uses for any respiratory dysfunction that is present. Suggested interview questions that can help to elicit this information include:

- Do you have any breathing difficulties? Have you noticed any change in your breathing?
- Do you now or have you ever smoked? How much and how long?
- Do you have a history of any respiratory disease such as asthma, bronchitis, pneumonia, or tuberculosis?

- Have problems with your breathing required you to change your lifestyle? Are there things you can no longer do?
- What things make your breathing better? What makes it worse?
- Do you take any medications or treatments for your breathing? How effective do you believe they are?
- Do you cough? When? Do you bring up sputum? How much? What does it look like?
- Do you have any allergies that cause problems with your breathing?

Objective Data

Objective data concerning respiratory function are collected through inspection, percussion, palpation, and auscultation of the chest. Data concerning breathing patterns, evaluation of the thorax, and assessment of breath sounds are important in evaluating respiratory function. Anatomic landmarks assist the nurse in proper location and in interpretation of findings.

Anatomic Landmarks of the Chest and Lungs. Anatomic landmarks and imaginary reference lines are used during the assessment of structures that lie within the thorax (chest) (Fig. 18-6). The lines and landmarks of the chest are used during lung auscultation and percussion to define the specific area of the lung being examined. These landmarks and reference lines also provide a standard vocabulary for use in describing and documenting assessment findings. Anatomic lines and landmarks are described for the anterior, posterior, and lateral chest wall.

The major anatomic landmarks on the *anterior chest wall* are the suprasternal notch, the sternal angle (or angle of Louis), the clavicles, the ribs, and the intercos-

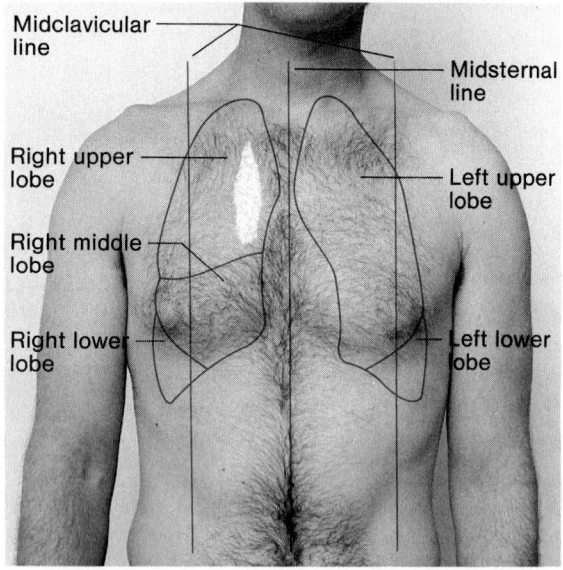
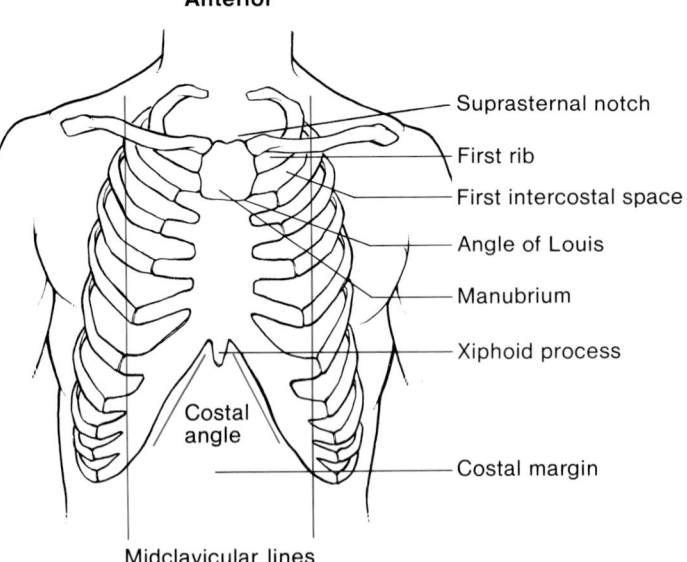

Figure 18-6. Landmarks of the anterior, posterior, and lateral chest wall.

tal spaces (see Fig. 18-6). The suprasternal notch is located at the base of the throat and defines the superior border of the manubrium. The sternal angle is the slight rise over the sternum where the manubrium and body of the sternum connect.

Three imaginary reference lines are used on the *lateral chest wall:* the anterior, posterior, and midaxillary lines (see Fig. 18-6). The anterior axillary line begins at the anterior axillary fold and runs downward along the anterior lateral wall of the chest. The posterior axillary line begins at the posterior axillary fold and runs downward.

The midaxillary line is drawn midway between the anterior and posterior lines, beginning at the midaxilla.

The landmarks on the back, or *posterior chest wall,* are the spinous processes of the vertebrae and the two scapula. The three vertical reference lines are the vertebral (or midspinal) line and the two scapular lines (see Fig. 18-6). The vertebral lines run vertically down the spinous processes of the vertebrae. The scapular lines run parallel to the vertebral line, through the inferior angle (lower edge) of the scapula. The spinous processes of the vertebrae can be identified by first locating the

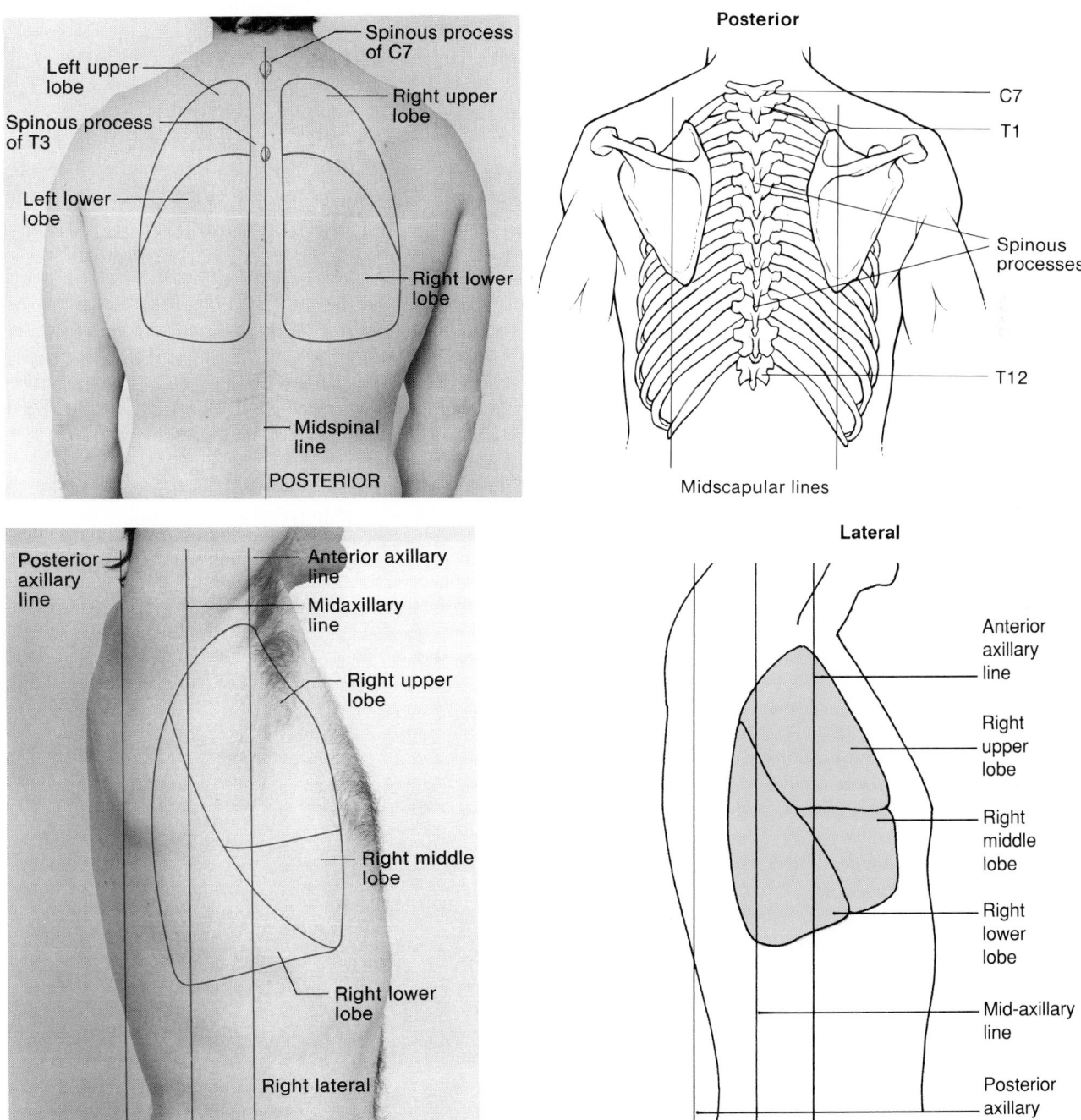

Figure 18–6   *(Continued)*

seventh cervical vertebrae (C7). To do this, the nurse asks the patient to flex his or her head forward. The most prominent spinous process that can be palpated at the back of the neck is the seventh cervical vertebrae. If two vertebrae appear equally prominent, they are the seventh cervical vertebrae with the 1st thoracic vertebrae directly below it. The processes of T4 through T12 angle downward so that they overlie the vertebrae below. For example, the spinous process of T6 overlies the seventh thoracic vertebrae and is adjacent to the seventh rib.

Inspection. Inspection related to the respiratory examination focuses on four general areas: configuration of the thorax; breathing patterns; signs of labored breathing; and observation of the skin and nails.

The shape of the thorax is best examined by having the patient sit upright with the chest area unclothed. The *anterior-posterior (AP) diameter* is a term used to describe the distance between the sternum and the vertebral column, drawn as a straight line through the thorax. In the normal adult, the AP diameter is approximately one half of the lateral diameter (or width) of the chest. One of the most common abnormalities of thorax configuration is seen in patients with chronic obstructive pulmonary disease (COPD). These patients exhibit a "barrel-shaped" chest in which the AP diameter enlarges and approximately equals the lateral diameter. Other thoracic abnormalities include: kyphosis, an exaggerated convex curve of the spine; scoliosis, lateral deviation of the spinal curve; and kyphoscoliosis, a combination of abnormal lateral and convex curvature of the spine. The presence of any of these conditions may deform the rib cage, impede lung expansion, and interfere with breathing.

Normal breathing is silent, effortless, and occurs at a rate of 12 to 20 times per minute in adults. Careful observation of the patient's breathing should normally reveal a pattern that is smooth, regular, symmetric, and rhythmic. Abnormal breathing patterns are discussed in Chapter 19.

While observing the patient's breathing pattern, the nurse should look for indications of respiratory distress or increased effort in breathing. Symptoms such as nasal flaring, facial straining, and pursed-lip breathing indicate abnormal respiratory effort. Abnormal effort during inspiration is evidenced by active, visible use of the scalene and sternomastoid muscles of the neck and shoulders. These muscles are called accessory muscles. Contraction of the abdominal muscles, which assists upward movement of the diaphragm, may also be observed. During inspection of the patient's breathing, observe the intercostal space. Airway obstruction or decreased lung compliance may result in retraction of the intercostal spaces during inspiration, whereas some respiratory diseases (such as emphysema) can cause bulging of the intercostal spaces during expiration.

The color and appearance of the skin and nails may reflect insufficient delivery of oxygenated blood to the tissues due to respiratory dysfunction. With normal supply of oxygen, the nailbeds, the tongue, and the lips appear pinkish-red in color. Hypoxia (decreased supply of oxygen to the tissues) changes this color to a grayish, bluish, or purplish tone. When this change in color is confined to the nailbeds and lips, it is called peripheral cyanosis; when it progresses to the tongue and mucous membranes of the mouth, it is called central cyanosis. Central cyanosis indicates a significant problem with oxygenation of body tissues and can be caused by respiratory, cardiac, or metabolic problems.

Clubbing of the nails is a sign of chronic hypoxia. To determine if nail clubbing is present, the nurse examines the contour of the nail and adherence of the nail to the nailbed. When viewed in profile, normal fingernails present an angle of 160 degrees between the nailbed and the finger (Fig. 18-7). With clubbing, swelling flattens the angle to 180 degrees or less. With advanced clubbing, the nail becomes less adherent to the base of the nail and feels spongy. The nails and fingertips appear large and swollen and are sometimes described as "drumsticklike."

Palpation. Palpation is used in respiratory assessment to evaluate painful or abnormal areas on the chest wall, to test for symmetry of chest expansion, and to detect tracheal deviation. Light palpation with the fingertips is used to examine any areas on the chest where the patient has complained of discomfort, or where visible abnormalities are present.

Normal chest expansion during inspiration is symmetric, indicating equal expansion of both lungs. To evaluate chest symmetry, the nurse stands behind the

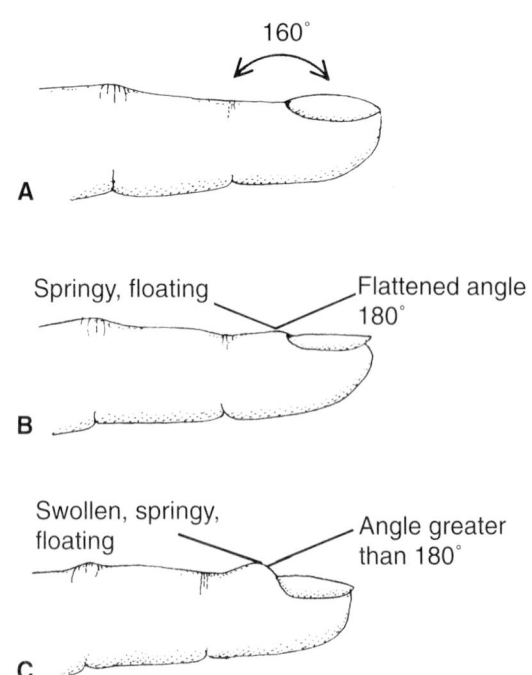

Figure 18–7. Clubbing of the nails. **A.** Normal nails. **B.** Early clubbing. **C.** Late clubbing.

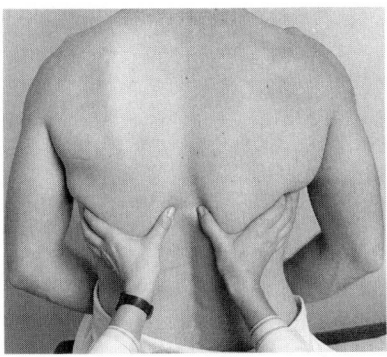

Figure 18–8. Palpation of thoracic excursion. In the posterior approach, the nurse's hands are placed at the level of the 10th rib and observed for equal outward movement as the patient inhales.

patient; places his or her thumbs at the level of the 10th rib and wraps the hands around the lateral rib cage (Fig. 18-8). The patient is asked to inhale deeply, and the nurse observes his or her thumbs for equal, outward movement.

The trachea is normally in a straight, vertical position. Many lung disorders, such as masses and pneumothorax, can cause a shift in the trachea from its normal midline position. The trachea may be checked for deviation in several ways. The nurse may stand behind the patient and reach across the patient's shoulders, placing the index finger on each side of the trachea in the suprasternal notch. The trachea may also be palpated anteriorly by placing the index finger along one side of the trachea and noting the space between it and the sternomastoid (Fig. 18-9). The other side is also compared (Bates, 1991). The trachea and surrounding area are palpated; the space on either side of the trachea and the ends of the suprasternal notch should be equal.

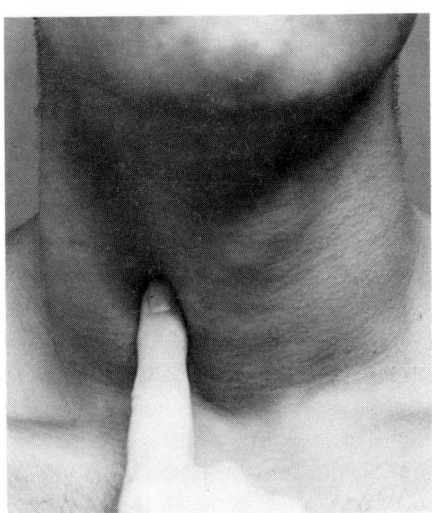

Figure 18–9. The nurse may examine for tracheal deviation anteriorly by placing the index finger along side the trachea and noting the space between the trachea and sternomastoid.

Percussion. Percussion of the chest is a technique used to determine whether the underlying tissue is air-filled, fluid-filled, or solid. Percussion reveals a hollow, loud, low-pitched sound when the lung is air-filled. Diagnostically, chest percussion has largely been replaced by examination of the chest by x-ray. Percussion is usually performed only by advanced practitioners in special circumstances and is not routinely done during respiratory assessment.

Auscultation. Lung auscultation involves listening with a stethoscope over the anterior and posterior chest wall for variations in breath sounds that may indicate improper aeration of lung segments or the presence of an obstruction. Breath sounds are created by the movement of air in the tracheobronchial tree with each inspiration and expiration.

Normal Breath Sounds. Breath sounds are classified as bronchial, bronchovesicular, and vesicular. They are described according to location, ratio of inspiration to expiration, intensity, and pitch. The normal anterior location for each of the three types of breath sounds is described in Table 18-3.

Bronchial Breath Sounds. Bronchial breath sounds are loud and high-pitched, with a hollow quality often compared to the sound of air blowing through a pipe. Expiration is longer and louder than inspiration with bronchial breath sounds. They are normal when heard over the trachea but indicate a lung abnormality when heard elsewhere. Abnormal bronchial sounds may be associated with pneumonia, pleural effusion, tumor, or atelectasis.

Vesicular Breath Sounds. Vesicular breath sounds are normally heard over all areas of the lung tissue except over or near the major airways. Vesicular sounds are described as soft and breezy, with inspiration markedly longer than expiration.

Bronchovesicular Breath Sounds. Bronchovesicular breath sounds are intermediate in character between bronchial and vesicular sounds. They are described as breezy, but softer and lower pitched than bronchial sounds. Inspiratory and expiratory times are approximately equal. Bronchovesicular sounds are normally heard in two areas only: on the anterior chest over the bifurcation of the main bronchi in the first or second intercostal spaces and posteriorly between the scapula. Like bronchial sounds, bronchovesicular sounds should not be detected elsewhere over the chest.

Adventitious Breath Sounds. Adventitious breath sounds are abnormal sounds that occur from air passing through narrowed airways or fluid, or from an inflammation of lung pleura. The major adventitious breath sounds are crackles (rales), rhonchi, and wheezes. These sounds are often superimposed over normal breath sounds and take much practiced listening to discern. Adventitious breath sounds are described in detail in Chapter 30.

TABLE 18–3

Normal Breath Sounds from Anterior Location

Location	Description	Ratio of Inspiration to Expiration	Intensity	Pitch
Bronchial	Blowing, hollow sounds over the trachea	Inspiration / Expiration	Expiration is longer and louder	Expiration is higher
Bronchovesicular	Intermediate sounds over first and second anterior intercostal spaces and posteriorly between scapula	Inspiration / Expiration	Medium and similar	Medium and similar
Vesicular	Soft and breezy sounds over all lung area except airways	Inspiration / Expiration	Inspiration markedly longer and louder	Inspiration is higher

Bronchial breath sounds

Scapula

Intercostal space

Bronchovesicular breath sounds

Vesicular breath sounds

How to Listen to the Lungs. Auscultation of the lungs is facilitated by having the patient sit upright. The patient must inhale more deeply than usual through the mouth. The nurse listens to a full inspiration and expiration at each stethoscope location and notes during which phases of the respiratory cycle any abnormalities occur. The nurse should not try to listen through clothing because the sounds will be distorted or muffled. The nurse should establish a pattern for auscultation that moves from one side of the chest to the other so that he or she can make comparisons and identify abnormalities more easily. Only the diaphragm of the stethoscope should be used, pressing it firmly against the skin, for listening to breath sounds.

The upper lobes project forward so they are best heard on the anterior wall but may also be auscultated on the upper back. The lower lobes tilt backward and, therefore, are auscultated on the posterior and lateral chest wall. The right middle lobe is auscultated only from the anterior chest wall. When auscultating breath sounds, it is important to observe the patient carefully and ensure that hyperventilation does not occur. To avoid this, many nurses auscultate each lung segment once, repeating auscultation in multiple locations (as shown in Procedure 18-1) only if abnormalities are found. If this is necessary, the patient should be provided with rest periods as needed. Refer to Procedure 18-1.

PROCEDURE 18–1. Auscultating Breath Sounds

■ Purpose
1. To listen for variations in breath sounds that may indicate the presence of airway obstruction or disease process.

■ Assessment
- Determine if the patient is distracted by an immediate need (e.g., pain, need to void, and so forth). Attend to that need first.
- Explain to the patient what you plan to do and approximately how long it will take.
- Provide for privacy so patient is not concerned about being viewed or overheard. Visitors and family members may be asked to leave the room.
- Ensure that the room is warm and quiet.

■ Equipment
Stethoscope

■ Procedure
1. Wash hands.
   Note: Moderately warm water increases circulation to warm your hands; this decreases discomfort to patient during examination.
2. Assist the patient to an upright sitting position. Lift patient gown to expose chest.
   Rationale: Upright position improves chest excursion. Breath sounds are distorted or muffled if assessed through clothing.
3. Warm diaphragm of stethoscope by holding between hands for a short time.
   Rationale: To decrease discomfort to patient from cold stethoscope on chest.
4. Ask patient to breathe deeply through the mouth. Patient should breathe slowly.
   Rationale: Mouth breathing enhances volume of breath sounds; nasal breathing decreases volume and can simulate adventitious sounds. Slow breathing rate is necessary to avoid hyperventilation.

Auscultate Anterior Chest
5. Place diaphragm of stethoscope about 1 inch below the middle of the right clavicle, making sure it lies between the ribs. Listen to one full inspiration and exhalation. Repeat the process at the corresponding site on the left side.
   Rationale: Placement of stethoscope over intercostal space improves sound quality. Representative sounds of the right and left upper lobes are audible here.
6. Note normal and adventitious breath sounds at each point on the chest as you proceed.
   Rationale: Movement of air through airways pro-

duces characteristic sounds. Abnormal sounds are indicative of airway disturbances.
7. Move stethoscope downward about 1.5 to 2 inches along midclavicular line. Note sounds; move scope laterally to opposite side.
   Rationale: Air movement through other (larger) airways of upper lobes can be heard here. Listening to sounds at corresponding points on opposite sides of sternum allows you to compare similar lung fields.
8. Move scope downward another inch or two along midclavicular line to fifth intercostal space. (This space lies just below the nipple line on males, approximately across from the head of the xiphoid process of the sternum.) Note sounds, then move to same spot on opposite side.
   Rationale: Right middle lobe and corresponding segments on left can he heard here.

Auscultate Posterior Chest
9. Instruct patient to lean forward and cross arms in front.
   Rationale: This position separates scapulae and facilitates listening to posterior breath sounds.
10. Begin by auscultating the area about 2 inches below the shoulders and 2 inches to the right of the spine. Note sounds, and move to corresponding point on left.
   Rationale: These positions allow the nurse to compare breath sounds of posterior segments of upper lobes.

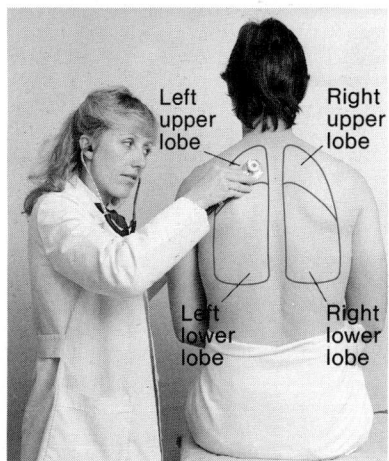

Step 10

(continued)

PROCEDURE 18–1. Auscultating Breath Sounds (continued)

11. Move scope directly downward 2 or 2.5 inches; note sounds, then move scope laterally and listen on right.
    Rationale: Superior segments of lower lobes are audible here.
12. Repeat process, moving downward 2 to 2.5 inches; listen to corresponding opposite side.
    Rationale: Each placement of stethoscope allows you to hear sounds of different segments of lung.
13. Move scope downward to area just below scapula. Listen on right and left. Listen also to areas laterally along lower rib cage.
    Rationale: Lower lobes end at level of 10th thoracic vertebra (about 1.5 inches below scapulae) and follow the contour of the lower ribs. Their large size and the fact that many clinical problems can affect the lower lobes make lateral assessment essential.

14. Replace patient's clothes and assist to comfortable position.
15. Discuss your findings with patient.
    Rationale: Provides an opportunity for patient feedback on effectiveness of therapies. Provides directions for patient teaching if new therapies are to be initiated (e.g., cough, deep breathing, incentive spirometry).
16. Record assessment findings. Be specific as to description and location of adventitious sounds.

■ **Lifespan Considerations**

Newborn and Infant
- Newborns have difficulty maintaining body temperature. Uncover only body area that you are directly assessing.
- At 8 to 12 months of age, infants become fearful of strangers. Spend several minutes becoming acquainted with the child before examining.

Toddler and Preschooler
- Children 2 to 5 years of age are often afraid of examining equipment. Letting them handle the stethoscope and using a "This is a game" approach often allay the fear.
- Auscultate breath sounds before performing any invasive examination, which may cause the child to cry.

School Age and Adolescent
- Older children are modest. They may or may not want a parent to be with them during the examination; give the child the choice. Protect modesty through use of gowns or drapes.

Older Adult
- A lengthy physical examination may be exhausting for the older adult and may need to be completed in phases.
- The older adult may become easily chilled. Provide warmth through adequate draping or gowning.

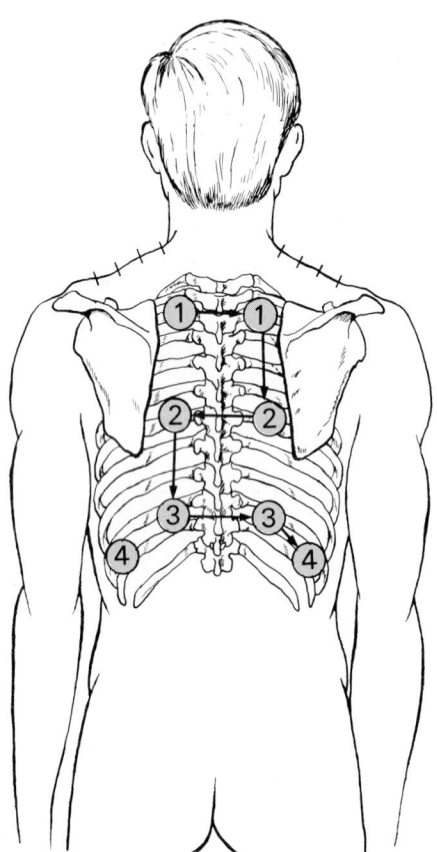

Steps 11, 12, and 13

Cardiovascular Assessment

Activity and exercise are impeded when the heart cannot work effectively to pump blood, or when the vasculature is unable to supply the perfusion of blood that is needed by the tissues of the body. Assessment of cardio-vascular status is an essential component of health assessment for every patient.

Subjective Data

The major thrusts for assessment of cardiovascular function include risk factors for cardiovascular disease (such as hypertension, elevated cholesterol, or smoking); signs and symptoms of cardiovascular dysfunction (such as pain, dizziness, or palpitations); the impact of cardiovascular dysfunction on activities of daily living; and specific adaptations to cardiac or circulatory impairment.

Interview questions to help elicit this information might include:

- Do you have any family history of heart or blood vessel disease, such as heart attack, stroke, high blood pressure, or diabetes?
- Have you been told that you have high blood pressure or elevated blood cholesterol? Do you smoke? Are you diabetic?
- Have you ever experienced chest pain or discomfort? If so, describe in detail.
- Have you experienced any of the following, either at rest or during physical exertion: dizziness, heart palpitation (fluttering), shortness of breath, leg pain, or cramping?
- Do you take any medications for a heart or circulatory problem? If so, give specific information regarding the medication.
- Have heart or circulatory problems interfered with your normal activities? If so, what modifications have you had to make?

Objective Data

Objective data about cardiovascular status are obtained by assessing vital signs, assessing the heart, and assessing arteries and veins. In most cases, assessment of the patient's vital signs is the first objective information gathered in a health assessment. Significant deviation from normal heart rate and blood pressure may be the first indicator of a serious problem in circulatory func-

tion. The techniques for accurate vital sign measurement are discussed in Chapter 19.

Landmarks for Cardiac Assessment. The **precordium** is the area on the anterior chest overlying the heart and its great vessels. Knowledge of the location of structures within the precordium is necessary to perform effective cardiac assessment.

There are four major areas on the precordium for examining the heart (Fig. 18-10). Each area corresponds to one of the heart's four valves and is located as follows:

- Aortic area—second intercostal space to the right of the sternum
- Pulmonic area—second intercostal space to the left of the sternum
- Tricuspid area—fifth intercostal space, left of the lower sternal border
- Mitral (or apical) area—fifth intercostal space, just medial to the midclavicular line.

Inspection, palpation, and auscultation are the three basic techniques used to assess the precordium and vasculature. Percussion may be used to estimate the size of the heart, but this method has generally been replaced by x-ray examination.

Inspection. The entire precordium should be inspected for movement. Inspection can be enhanced by using tangential light across the chest and by observing the heart at eye level. Normally, the only movement seen is in the mitral valve area. A visible pulsation occurs with ventricular contraction as the left heart strikes the anterior chest wall. This pulsation is called the *point of maximal impulse* (PMI). It is not abnormal if the PMI is not seen, as often occurs in patients with thick chest walls or large breasts. Abnormal movements over the precor-

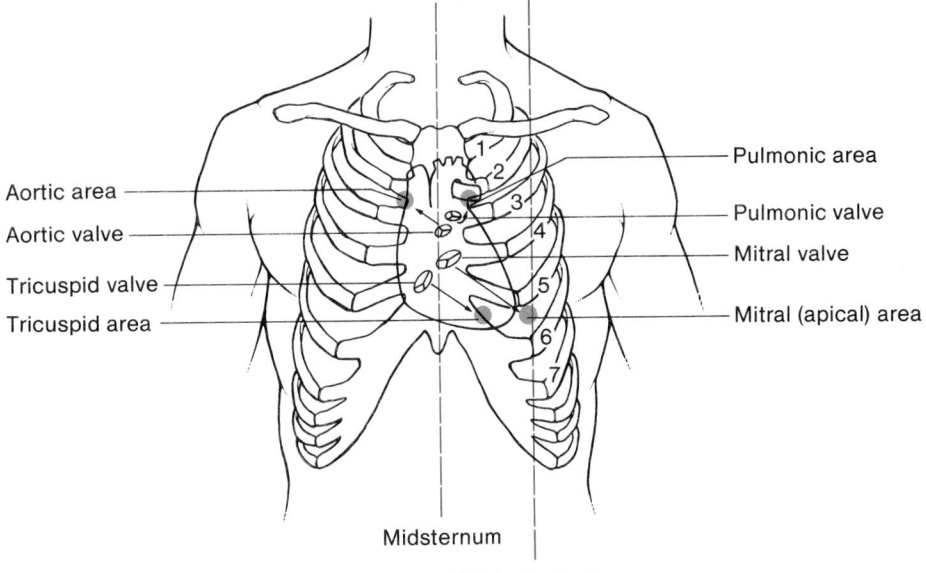

Figure 18–10. Heart sounds are referred from valvular points of origin to the auscultatory or precordial landmarks. Sound travels in the direction of blood flow and may be heard some distance from the valve.

Aortic area
Aortic valve
Tricuspid valve
Tricuspid area

Pulmonic area
Pulmonic valve
Mitral valve
Mitral (apical) area

Midsternum
Midclavicular line

dium include: forceful movement around the area of the PMI, called a heave; anterior movement of the sternum, called a lift; or small areas of pulsation in the intercostal spaces or around the sternum.

Inspection can also be used to assess peripheral circulation. Skin should be examined for color and temperature. Observed varicosities (swollen twisted veins) can indicate venous problems.

Palpation. Palpation follows and complements inspection. The nurse should palpate in each of the four precordial areas, noting any vibrations (termed *thrills*) or pulsations. The fingertips are the most sensitive to pulsation; the heel and ulnar surfaces of the hand are most sensitive to vibration. The nurse should feel for the PMI in the mitral area and note its exact location and size. The normal PMI is a light tap, located at the medial to midclavicular line, confined to the area of one intercostal space. Pulsations or vibrations over the aortic, pulmonic, or tricuspid areas are usually abnormal.

Palpation is also important in peripheral vascular assessment. Skin temperature is best evaluated using the back of the hand. The evenness of skin temperature is important. Symmetric coolness or warmth may be normal; unilateral coolness may indicate decreased blood flow; unilateral warmth may indicate local infection. Generalized cool skin accompanied by pallor and moistness may indicate peripheral vasoconstriction due to circulatory shock. In a cardiovascular assessment, arterial pulses should also be palpated, noting rate, rhythm, amplitude, and symmetry. Assessment of significant arterial pulses is explained in Chapter 19.

Palpation is also used to assess capillary refill. Capillary refill time is a simple test of circulatory status using the nailbeds. The nurse presses down on the nailbed until it turns white and notes how quickly the color returns when pressure is released. Normal refill time is 1 to 2 seconds; prolonged capillary refill indicates poor circulation.

Auscultation. Valuable information can be acquired by listening to heart sounds. Learning the basic techniques of cardiac auscultation is enhanced by using a consistent pattern for auscultating the precordium and by concentrating on one heart sound or phase in the cardiac cycle at a time. Refer to Procedure 18-2.

Normal Heart Sounds. Normal heart sounds include S_1 and S_2. Systole (ventricular contraction) is the period of time from the beginning of the first heart sound (S_1) to the beginning of the second heart sound (S_2). Diastole (ventricular relaxation) is the period of time from the beginning of the second heart sound to the beginning of the next ventricular contraction.

The first heart sound coincides with the beginning of systole when the mitral and tricuspid valves close. The mitral valve usually closes slightly before the tricuspid valve, however, a single sound is usually heard. When an

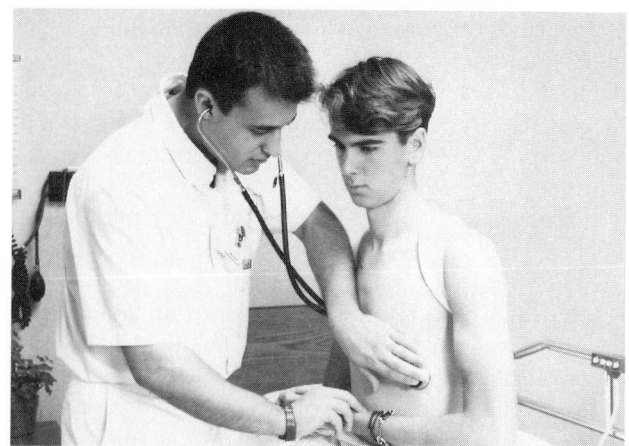

Figure 18–11. The nurse determines the S_1 sound by comparing it to the radial pulse.

audible difference in closure of the two valves is detected, the first sound is said to be split. Because the force generated in the left ventricle is much greater than the right ventricle, the first heart sound is dominated by the mitral valve and is best heard in the apical area (Fig. 18-11).

The second heart sound coincides with the beginning of diastole when the aortic and pulmonic valves close. Aortic valve closure slightly precedes and dominates the second heart sound, therefore, the second heart sound is best heard in the aortic area. During inspiration, when filling of the right ventricle is enhanced, right ventricular systole is prolonged; this often creates splitting of the second heart sound. Because pulmonic closure is a soft sound, a split S_2 usually can only be detected in the pulmonic area.

The first and second heart sounds are high-pitched sounds heard best using the diaphragm of the stethoscope. When the heart rate is slow, it is easy to differentiate the two sounds. Systole is shorter than diastole, so two "paired" sounds (S_1 then S_2) are heard, followed by a pause. When the heart rate is faster, the pause is less distinctive or even absent. To clarify S_1 from S_2 in this situation, the nurse feels the patient's carotid pulse when listening to the heart. The carotid pulse and S_1 occur almost simultaneously.

Extra and Abnormal Heart Sounds. The third heart sound, also referred to as S_3, is an extra sound occurring early in diastole as the ventricle rapidly fills. It can be normal in healthy children or young adults, but in older people it often signifies congestive heart failure. The third sound is best heard in the mitral area using the bell of the stethoscope. An S_3 is a soft, low-pitched sound, making it difficult to hear. Placing the patient in a left side-lying position may increase its audibility. The presence of a third heart sound is an important clinical finding that should be sought if a patient is at risk for congestive heart failure.

The fourth heart sound, also referred to as S_4, is an

PROCEDURE 18–2. Auscultating Heart Sounds

■ Purpose
1. To assess normal and abnormal functioning of the heart valves.
2. To detect cardiac problems.

■ Assessment
- Determine if the patient is distracted by an immediate need (e.g., pain, urge to urinate). Attend to that problem first.
- Explain to the patient what you plan to do and approximately how long it will take.
- Provide for privacy so patient is not concerned about being viewed or overheard. Visitors and family members may be asked to leave the room.
- Ensure that the room is warm and quiet.

■ Equipment
Stethoscope with a bell-shaped and flat-disc diaphragm.

■ Procedure
1. Wash hands.
   Note: Moderately warm water increases circulation to warm your hands; this decreases discomfort to patient during examination.
2. Assist the patient to supine position. You may want to reexamine the patient in the upright sitting position. Lift the patient gown to expose chest.
   Rationale: Some heart sounds may be accentuated in certain positions.
3. Warm diaphragm of stethoscope by holding between hands for a few moments.
   Rationale: To decrease discomfort to patient from cold stethoscope on chest.
4. Listen in the mitral area using the diaphragm (see Fig. 18–10). Identify the first and second heart sounds. Count the heart rate, noting whether the rhythm is regular or irregular. If the rhythm is irregular, count the heart rate for a full minute. Also note whether the irregularity has a pattern, or whether it is totally unpredictable.
5. Listen in the aortic area using the diaphragm. Concentrate first on S_1, then S_2, noting if splitting occurs. Shift your concentration to systole and then diastole; listen for extra sounds, such as murmurs.
   Rationale: The diaphragm of the stethoscope transmits the high-pitched sounds of S_1 and S_2. Murmurs are best heard over the valvular areas in the direction the blood is flowing through the heart.
6. Listen in the pulmonic area, still using only the diaphragm. Repeat the sequence described in step 5, concentrating on S_1, S_2, systole, and diastole. Compare the loudness of S_2 in the aortic and pulmonic areas.

Rationale: Loudness of S_2 in the aortic area relates to the systemic arterial blood pressure and can be louder than normal in adults with hypertension. Loudness of S_2 in the pulmonic area relates to the pulmonary artery pressure and may be louder than normal in patients with chronic obstructive pulmonary disease. It is abnormal for the pulmonic S_2 to be louder than the aortic S_2 in adults over 40 years of age.

7. Move the diaphragm to the tricuspid and mitral areas.
8. Return to the aortic area, this time using the bell of the stethoscope. As before, concentrate individually on S_1, S_2, systole, and diastole.
9. Repeat the same process, using the bell, in the pulmonic, tricuspid, and mitral areas. Especially in the mitral area, concentrate during diastole to detect the presence of a third or fourth heart sound.
   Rationale: The lower pitched sounds of the mitral and tricuspid valves, as well as an S_3, S_4, are best transmitted through the bell of the stethoscope.
   Note: To increase your ability to hear an S_3 or mitral murmur, have the patient lie on the left side while you auscultate with the bell. An S_3 often disappears when the patient sits up.
10. Replace the patient's clothes. Assist to a comfortable position.
    Rationale: To provide comfort and warmth.
11. Record your assessment findings describing the intensity, quality, and location of the sounds.

■ Lifespan Considerations

Newborn and Infant
- Newborns have difficulty maintaining body temperature. Uncover only body area that you are directly assessing.
- At 8 to 12 months of age, infants become fearful of strangers. Spend several minutes becoming acquainted with the child before examining.

Toddler and Preschooler
- Children 2 to 5 years of age are often afraid of examining equipment. Letting them handle the stethoscope and using a "This is a game" approach often allay the fear.
- Auscultate heart sounds before performing any invasive examination, which may cause the child to cry.

School Age and Adolescent
- Older children are modest. They may or may not want a parent to be with them during the examination; give the child the choice. Protect modesty through use of gowns or drapes.

(continued)

PROCEDURE 18–2. Auscultating Heart Sounds *(continued)*

- An S_3 is normal in children and young adults.

Older Adult
- An S_3 may indicate heart failure in older adults. An S_4 may be present with coronary artery disease or hypertension.

- A lengthy physical examination may be exhausting for the older adult and may need to be completed in phases.
- The older adult may become easily chilled. Provide warmth through adequate draping or gowning.

---

extra sound occurring late in diastole, just before the first heart sound. It coincides with atrial contraction when blood is actively propelled into the ventricle. The fourth heart sound is thought to result from a stiffened left ventricle and is frequently associated with hypertension and coronary artery disease. The fourth sound is low-pitched, best heard using the bell of the stethoscope over the mitral area. The development of an S_4 is not as serious as an S_3 and does not necessarily indicate heart failure. Figure 18-12 illustrates where the third and fourth heart sound occur in the cardiac cycle.

Murmurs are vibrating sounds produced from turbulent blood flow through the heart, especially across the valves. The more common causes for a murmur include partially obstructed flow through a valve opening (stenosis), increased blood flow across a normal valve, backward (regurgitant) blood flow due to a leaky (incompetent) valve, blood flow into a dilated chamber, and blood flow through an abnormal opening between heart chambers. Murmurs resemble a blowing or swishing noise and may occur during systole or diastole. They may be low-pitched or high-pitched, so both the bell and diaphragm of the stethoscope are appropriate for detecting murmurs. When a murmur is heard, it should be noted whether it occurs during systole (between S_1 and S_2) or during diastole (after S_2), and where it is heard on the precordium. Diastolic murmurs are almost always caused by heart disease; systolic murmurs may be related to heart disease but are frequently benign.

Bruits are abnormal arterial sounds, similar to murmurs, caused by increased turbulence of blood flow. Bruits can be detected by placing the stethoscope over major blood vessels, such as the femoral artery, carotid artery, or the abdominal aorta. Bruits occur when an artery is partially obstructed or distended, which prevents blood flow from moving straight through the vessel.

ASSESSMENT OF NUTRITION AND METABOLISM

Assessment of nutrition and metabolism collects data concerning dietary habits and metabolic needs. Information reflects how well the body is able to ingest, digest, absorb, and metabolize food, and use it to maintain tissue integrity and fluid and electrolyte balance, and to fight infection.

Subjective Data

Assessment of nutrition and metabolism requires specific information about the patient's normal diet and careful observations of the physical features that reflect nutritional state. The nutrition-metabolism assessment should focus on normal food and fluid intake, alterations in normal eating patterns, how dietary changes have impacted daily living, and the development of medical problems secondary to altered nutritional status.

Interview questions to focus a nutrition-metabolism assessment might include some of the following:

- Describe what you eat on a typical day.
- How much fluid do you drink each day?
- Are you on a special diet? If so, is this difficult for you to follow?
- Is the added expense of your diet a problem for you?

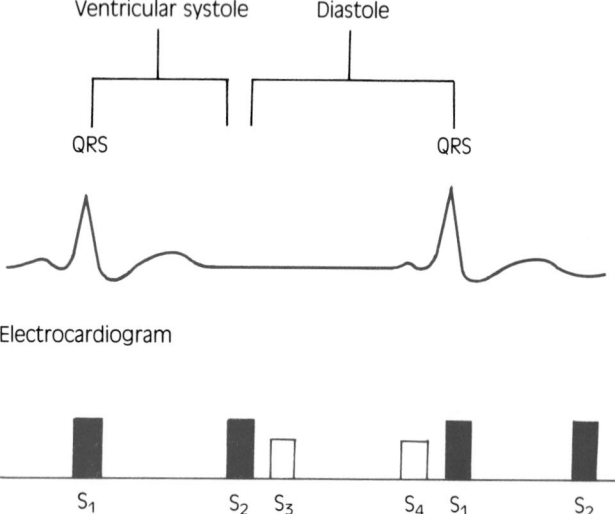

Figure 18–12.   Occurrence of S_3 and S_4 heart sounds in the cardiac cycle.

- Do you (or think you need to) reduce your intake of fat, calories, sugar, caffeine, or salt?
- Have you noticed any change in your weight over the last 6 months? Year? 5 years?
- Are you content with your weight? Have you ever tried to gain (lose) weight?
- Do you prepare your own meals?
- Do you have any problems chewing, swallowing, or digesting food?
- Do you frequently develop infections?
- Do you think you heal well?
- Do you have any skin problems?
- Do you have any dental problems?

Objective Data

Objective data are used to validate subjective information obtained during the patient interview. Objective data collected for nutrition and metabolism pattern include height and weight measurement, assessment of the mouth and teeth, assessment of the abdomen, and assessment of the skin.

Height and Weight. Weight measurement, especially when compared to height, can provide important information regarding nutritional status. Standardized tables have been developed (e.g., Metropolitan Height and Weight Tables for Men and Women, Ages 25 to 59) that recommend ideal body weight for men and women (Table 18-4). Such standardized tables are also available to evaluate growth in children (see Appendix A). Such tables provide a baseline for evaluating the patient's weight. Deviations from normal body size, ranging from obesity to severely underweight, can influence not only nutritional state, but other health patterns, such as exercise–activity and self-concept.

TABLE 18–4
Height and Weight Tables

Height (in)	(cm)	Weight					
		Small Frame		Medium Frame		Large Frame	
		(lb)	(kg)	(lb)	(kg)	(lb)	(kg)
Men							
61	154	128–134	58–61	131–141	59–64	138–150	63–68
62	157	130–136	59–62	133–143	60–65	140–153	64–69
63	159	132–138	60–63	135–145	61–66	142–156	64–71
64	162	134–140	61–64	137–148	62–67	144–160	65–73
65	164	136–142	62–64	139–151	63–69	146–164	66–74
66	167	138–145	63–66	142–154	64–70	149–168	68–76
67	170	140–148	64–67	145–157	66–71	152–172	69–78
68	172	142–151	64–69	148–160	67–73	155–176	70–80
69	175	144–154	65–70	151–163	69–74	158–180	72–82
70	177	146–157	66–71	154–166	70–75	161–184	73–84
71	180	149–160	68–73	157–170	71–77	164–188	74–85
72	182	152–164	69–74	160–174	73–79	168–192	76–87
73	185	155–168	70–76	164–178	74–81	172–197	78–89
74	187	158–172	72–78	167–182	76–83	176–202	80–92
75	190	162–176	74–80	171–187	78–85	181–207	82–94
Women							
57	145	102–111	46–50	109–121	49–55	118–131	54–59
58	147	103–113	47–51	111–123	50–56	120–134	54–61
59	150	104–115	47–52	113–126	51–57	122–137	55–62
60	152	106–118	48–54	115–129	52–59	125–140	57–64
61	154	108–121	49–55	118–132	54–60	128–143	58–65
62	157	111–124	50–56	121–135	55–61	131–147	59–67
63	159	114–127	52–58	124–138	56–63	134–151	61–69
64	162	117–130	53–59	127–141	58–64	137–155	62–70
65	164	120–133	54–60	130–144	59–65	140–159	64–72
66	167	123–136	56–62	133–147	60–67	143–163	65–74
67	170	126–139	57–63	136–150	62–68	146–167	66–76
68	172	129–142	59–64	139–153	63–69	149–170	68–77
69	175	132–145	60–66	142–156	64–71	152–173	69–79
70	177	135–148	61–67	145–159	66–72	155–176	70–80
71	180	138–151	63–69	148–162	67–74	158–179	72–81

Based on lowest mortality, ages 29 to 59 years. From Metropolitan Life Insurance Co., 1983. Adjusted for height in bare feet. Figures allow 5 lb of clothing for men, 3 lb of clothing for women.

Weight measurement can also be used to evaluate fluid status or the response of the patient to medical treatment (e.g., diuretic therapy to treat congestive heart failure). Rapid weight gain or loss is due to the gain or loss of body fluid rather than body fat.

Weight measurement can be done on a variety of scales; the choice depends mainly on the status of the patient. An upright scale is appropriate for the patient with normal mobility who can step onto a platform and maintain balance while weight is determined. A chair scale is used when a patient can transfer to a chair but is unable to support the body in a standing position for accurate weight measurement. A bed scale is used for the patient who is too weak or immobile to use other scales safely. Special infant scales are used to determine the height and weight of babies. Scales can be calibrated in terms of pounds or kilograms, with some scales providing both measures of weight. To convert from pounds to kilograms, divide by 2.2; to convert from kilograms to pounds, multiple by 2.2.

For most patients, height and weight measurements are obtained on admission to a health-care agency. When daily or frequent weights are required to evaluate patient progress, weight is measured at the same time each day (usually before breakfast), using the same scale. Refer to Procedure 18-3.

Height is measured with a measuring stick attached to a standing scale. The patient stands erect without shoes on the scale, and the height is determined by lowering the sliding arm until it rests on the patient's head. Height can be measured in inches or centimeters. To convert inches to centimeters multiply by 2.54; to convert centimeters to inches divide by 2.54.

Mouth Assessment. Examination of the mouth includes the buccal mucosa, teeth, lips, gums, and tongue (Fig. 18-13). A bright light and a tongue blade are used to inspect the mucous membranes, teeth, and gums. The nurse should not insert his or her fingers into the patient's mouth. If necessary, a piece of gauze can be used to displace the tongue. Mucous membranes should appear pink and moist. The nurse should observe for le-

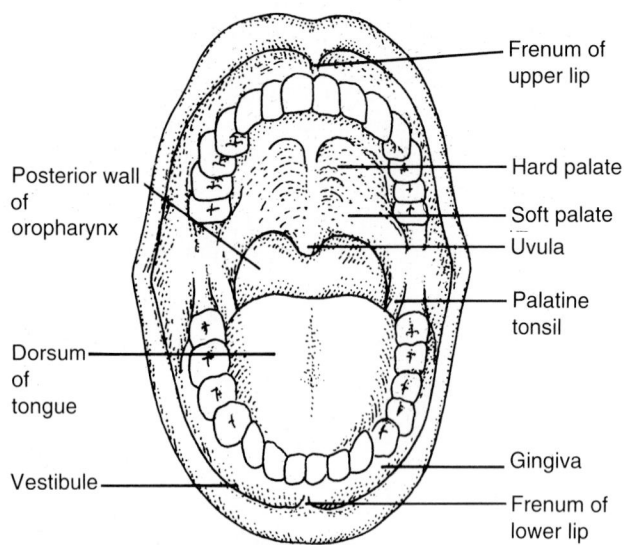

Figure 18–13. Structures of the mouth.

sions in the mouth or on the gums, especially if the patient complains of pain or has ill-fitting dentures. The teeth should be inspected for stability and overall hygiene. A major concern when examining the mouth is to detect any abnormalities that might impede the patient's ability to chew, swallow, or enjoy food.

Abdominal Assessment. Basic abdominal assessment consists of inspection, auscultation, and light palpation. Techniques performed by advanced practitioners include abdominal percussion (to estimate the size of the liver and spleen and to identify the presence of air in the stomach and bowel) and deep palpation (to estimate the size of the liver and spleen and to detect abnormal masses).

Landmarks for Abdominal Assessment. The abdomen is divided, for descriptive purposes, into four quadrants (see Procedure 18-4). The upper and lower quadrants are separated by an imaginary horizontal line through the umbilicus. The right and left quadrants are separated

(Text continues on page 326)

TABLE 18–5

Organs in the Four Abdominal Quadrants*

Upper Right Quadrant	Upper Left Quadrant	Lower Right Quadrant	Lower Left Quadrant
Liver	Left lobe of liver	Lower lobe of right kidney	Lower lobe of left kidney
Gallbladder	Stomach	Cecum	Sigmoid colon
Duodenum	Spleen	Appendix	Section of descending colon
Head of pancreas	Upper lobe of left kidney	Section of ascending colon	Left ovary
Right adrenal gland	Pancreas	Right ovary	Left fallopian tube
Upper lobe of right kidney	Left adrenal gland	Right fallopian tube	Left ureter
Hepatic flexure of colon	Splenic flexure of colon	Right ureter	Left spermatic cord
Section of ascending colon	Section of transverse colon	Right spermatic cord	Part of uterus (if enlarged)
Section of transverse colon	Section of descending colon	Part of uterus (if enlarged)	

*The uterus and urinary bladder fall in the lower midline.

PROCEDURE 18–3. Measuring Weight

■ Purpose

1. To provide baseline data from which to assess total fluid balance or nutritional status.
2. To provide baseline data to determine drug dosages or information for diagnostic testing with dye or radioactive injections.

■ Assessment

- Assess necessity for baseline, daily, or weekly weight measurements.
- Review previous weight measurements, if available.
- Identify time of day previous weights were measured. Weights can vary considerably during a 24-hour period so it is important that serial weights be done at the same time each day. Most hospitals weigh patients in the early morning. Check hospital policy.
- Assess patient's mental and physical status to determine if a standing, sitting, or bed scale is appropriate.

■ Equipment

An appropriate scale
Note: Use the same scale each time you weigh the patient.
Protector towel or plastic sheet

■ Procedure

1. Have patient void before weighing.
   Note: A full bladder, wet gowns, saturated dressings affect the measurement.
2. Patient should wear same clothing for each weigh. Slippers or shoes are removed before measurement.
3. Place protection on scale.
   Rationale: To prevent transfer or microorganisms.
4. Check that scale registers zero. Adjust as necessary.

■ Procedure

Weight with Chair Scale

1. Place scale beside patient and lock wheels.
   Rationale: To prevent accidental falls.
2. Transfer patient onto chair.
   Note: If arm of chair is removable, unlock and remove before transfer. Lock back into place after transfer to provide security and prevent accidental falls.
3. Read digital display or adjust counterweights to determine patient's weight.
4. Transfer patient back to bed or wheelchair.
5. Clean the scale according to agency policy.

■ Procedure

Weight with Standing Scale

1. Assist patient onto scale. Patient must stand in *center* of platform and not lean or hold onto supports.
   Rationale: Depending on type of equipment, movement may cause inaccurate weight.
2. Read digital display or adjust counterweights to determine patient's weight.
3. Assist patient from scale. Dispose of protector sheet.

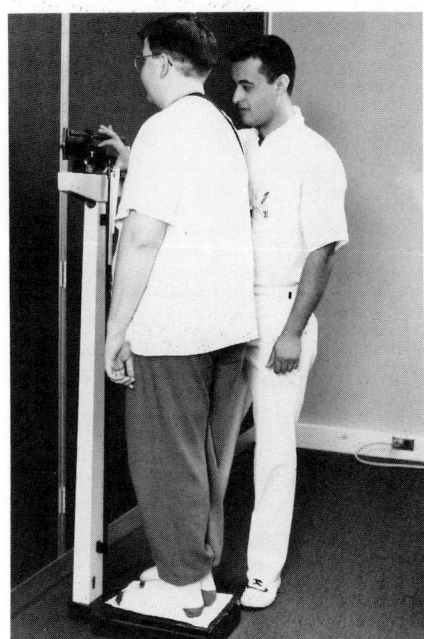

Step 2

■ Procedure

Weight with Bed Scale

1. Elevate patient's bed to level of stretcher scale.
2. With one or two assistants, turn patient with back toward the scale.
3. Roll scale toward the bed, lock wheels in place, and lower stretcher onto bed.
4. Roll patient onto stretcher.
5. Attach stretcher arms to stretcher and gradually elevate stretcher about 2 inches above mattress surface.

(continued)

PROCEDURE 18–3. Measuring Weight *(continued)*

Note: Inform patient before elevating. Reassure that he will not fall but his head may feel lower than his body.

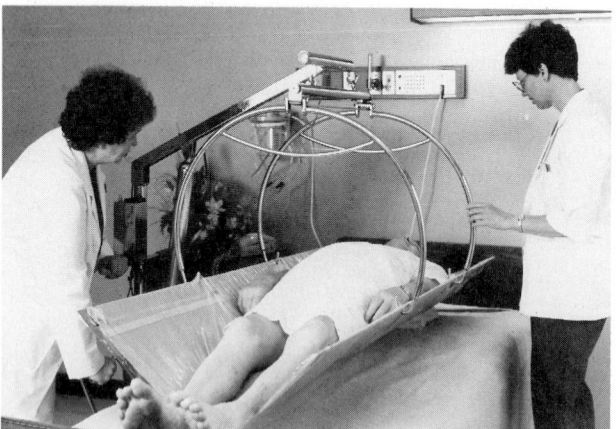

Step 5

6. Determine that stretcher is not touching any equipment. Lift all drains and tubing away from stretcher. *Rationale: Equipment alters measurement and affects accuracy.*
7. Read digital display for patient's weight. *Note:* This is a good time to change patient's linen as they are elevated off the bed.

8. Gradually lower stretcher to the bed. Remove stretcher arms and transfer patient off stretcher. Remove stretcher.
9. Unlock bed scale wheels and move away from bed.
10. Assist patient to comfortable position.
11. Clean stretcher and scale according to agency policy.
12. Record weight and note any extra linen or equipment weighed with the patient.

■ **Lifespan Considerations**

Infants
• Infants are usually weighed nude. Be careful that room temperature is warm because infant's body temperature can fluctuate severely because of their immature thermoregulatory system.
• Infants often roll and kick. The nurse's hand should always be within 1 to 2 inches of the child's body to prevent accidental falls.

■ **Home Care Modifications**
• Patients requiring serial weights are encouraged to keep a written log of their weights.
• If visual problems restrict the patient's ability to read the scale, family members may be able to assist.
• Patients are instructed to weigh at the same time each day, usually in the morning before breakfast, and to wear similar weight clothing for each measurement.

PROCEDURE 18–4. Auscultating Bowel Sounds

■ **Purpose**
1. To determine the presence or absence of intestinal peristalsis.

■ **Assessment**
• Plan to auscultate the abdomen before palpating or percussing if performing a complete abdominal examination. Stimulation of the abdominal wall may alter bowel mobility.
• Determine if the patient is distracted by an immediate need (e.g., pain, urge to urinate). Attend to that problem first.
• Provide for privacy so patient is not concerned about being viewed or overheard.
• Ensure that the room is warm and quiet.
• If the patient has a nasogastric tube with suction, turn off the suction during auscultation because the sound will confuse your assessment.

■ **Equipment**
Stethoscope

■ **Procedure**
1. Wash hands and warm stethoscope diaphragm. *Rationale: Cold hands or stethoscope may cause contraction of the abdominal muscles, which may be heard during auscultation.*
2. Ask the patient when he or she last ate. *Rationale: Bowel sounds may be increased shortly after eating or if a meal is long overdue.*
3. Assist patient to a supine position with abdomen exposed.

(continued)

PROCEDURE 18–4. Auscultating Bowel Sounds (continued)

4. Visually divide the abdomen into four quadrants using the umbilicus as the center-cross landmark (See Table 18-5).

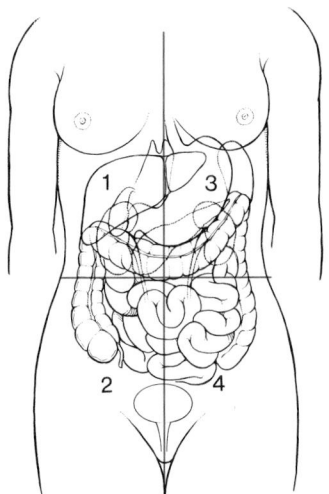

Step 4

5. Place the stethoscope diaphragm in each of the four quadrants. Listen for pitch, frequency, and duration of bowel sounds at each site.
   Rationale: Active bowel sounds are irregular, gurgling noises, occurring every 5 to 20 seconds.

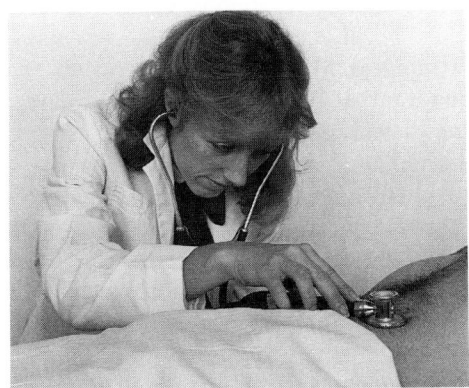

Step 5

6. If bowel sounds are not heard, listen for 3 to 5 minutes in all quadrants before concluding that they are absent.
   Rationale: Bowel sounds are very irregular and require assessment to continue longer to confirm that they are absent and not hypoactive. Absent or hypoactive bowel sounds indicate inhibited intestinal motility.

7. Place stethoscope bell over the epigastrum. Listen for sounds associated with pulse rate.
   Rationale: A bruit is created by blood flow through the abdominal aorta. It may be normal or associated with irregularities of the arterial system.

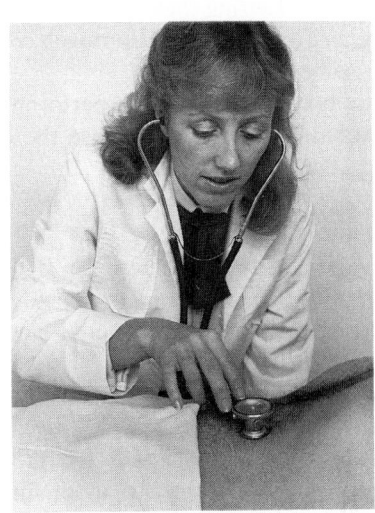

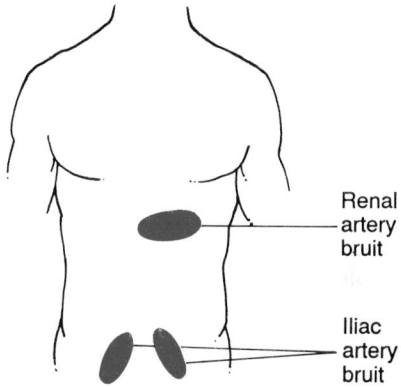

Renal artery bruit

Iliac artery bruit

Step 7

8. Proceed with the rest of physical examination or cover the patient's abdomen and assist to a comfortable position.

9. Document your findings.

■ **Lifespan Considerations**

Newborn and Infant

• Newborns have difficulty maintaining body temperature. Uncover only body area that you are directly assessing.

(continued)

PROCEDURE 18-4. Auscultating Bowel Sounds (continued)

- At 8 to 12 months of age, infants become fearful of strangers. Spend several minutes becoming acquainted with the child before examining.

Toddler and Preschooler
- Children 2 to 5 years of age are often afraid of examining equipment. Letting them handle the stethoscope and using a "This is a game" approach often allay the fear.
- Auscultate bowel sounds before performing any invasive examination, which may cause the child to cry.

School Age and Adolescent
- Older children are modest. They may or may not want a parent to be with them during the exam; give the child the choice. Protect modesty through use of gowns or drapes.

Older Adult
- A lengthy physical exam may be exhausting for the older adult and may need to be completed in phases.
- The older adult may become easily chilled. Provide warmth through adequate draping or gowning.

---

by an imaginary vertical line between the xiphoid and symphysis pubis. Structures underlying each of the four quadrants are listed in Table 18-5 and pictured in Procedure 18-4.

Inspection. During inspection, the contour, skin, and movement of the abdomen are noted. The patient is observed at eye level from the side, from the foot of the bed, and from directly over the abdomen. Tangential lighting is used across the abdomen to accentuate subtle changes.

The contour of the abdomen can be evaluated by placing the patient supine and viewing at eye level from the side. It is described as flat, rounded, or scaphoid (concave). A flat contour is seen in well-nourished and muscularly competent people. A rounded abdomen is normal in a young child, but in adults it is generally caused by poor muscle tone or excessive fat. A scaphoid contour is prevalent in thin patients and may indicate malnutrition. The nurse should note symmetry of the abdomen (asymmetry is abnormal) and the position of the umbilicus. It is usually in the center of the abdomen, flush with the abdominal wall, or only slightly inverted or everted.

The abdominal skin should be similar in color and texture to skin on other areas of the body. Note the presence and location of scars, rashes, lesions, petechiae (small red, hemorrhagic spots), or striae. **Striae** are streaks from rapid or prolonged stretching of the skin. Recent striae are pink or blue; they turn silvery white with age. Pregnancy, ascites, and weight loss are common causes of striae. Fine veins may normally be visible on the abdomen, especially in the inguinal area; distended, prominent veins are abnormal and are frequently associated with liver disease.

Visible movement over the abdomen is not uncommon. Wavelike movements of intestinal peristalsis may be seen in thin patients. A normal aortic pulsation is frequently visible in the epigastrium. Rise and fall of the abdomen synchronized with respiration are frequently seen, especially in men.

Auscultation. The nurse should always auscultate the abdomen before palpating (or percussing, if performed), because movement or stimulation may alter motility of the bowel and increase the sounds. Bowel sounds are created as air and fluid mix in the intestine. Normal peristaltic sounds occur every 5 to 20 seconds (refer to Procedure 18-4).

The nurse should auscultate all four quadrants. Bowel sounds are usually best heard in the right lower quadrant near the area of the ileocecal valve. The diaphragm of the stethoscope is used because bowel sounds are relatively high-pitched. If the patient has a nasogastric tube attached to suction, turn off the suction during auscultation because the sound of the suction interferes with accurate assessment. Only after listening to a quadrant for 5 minutes and hearing no sounds can the nurse conclude absence of bowel sounds. Clinically, this becomes impractical because some bowel assessments could take up to 20 minutes. Most nurses listen for 1 to 2 minutes at each quadrant. If bowel sounds are not detected after this time, bowel tones are known to be hypoactive and thus charted.

Increased frequency and loudness of bowel sounds are called borborygmi. Borborygmi reflect increased intestinal peristalsis, which may be related to diarrhea, laxatives, emotional upset, or intestinal obstruction. Borborygmi heard before a meal are better known as "stomach growling."

Light Palpation. Light palpation is performed to obtain information about pain or discomfort and to detect abdominal masses. The nurse should palpate all four quadrants, reserving the area of suspected pain or abnormality until last. Relaxation of the abdominal wall is necessary for an accurate assessment. The nurse can promote relaxation by positioning the patient with knees slightly flexed and arms to the sides or across the chest. The nurse uses four fingers and palms as a unit to press lightly and smoothly in a circular motion, depressing the skin approximately 1 inch. The nurse should monitor for pain or tenderness by watching the patient's face while the nurse palpates. The location and approximate size of any abnormal masses should be noted.

Skin Assessment. The skin is examined through inspection and palpation. It is assessed for color, turgor, edema, perspiration, injuries, and skin lesions. The skin should also be observed for past injuries: calluses, stains, scars, needle marks, and insect bites. The grooming of the patient's hair and nails should be noted.

Skin Turgor. The amount of fluid in the tissues is assessed by checking skin turgor and inspecting for edema. The nurse can check for skin turgor by pinching a small area of skin and noting how quickly it returns to position when released. If skin turgor is poor, the skin remains elevated or slowly resumes position. Poor skin turgor may indicate dehydration, but may also occur with normal aging or with weight loss.

Edema. Edema is fluid accumulation in the tissues. The degree of edema is estimated by noting how long the tissue remains indented when pressed. Edema is assessed in dependent areas such as the hands, feet, ankles, and lower legs. The nurse should press firmly with the thumb, for at least 5 seconds, behind the medial malleolus, over the dorsum of the foot, and over the shin. When a patient is bedridden, the dependent areas are the back and sacrum. A grading system, ranging from +1 to +4 is often used to record edema. Edema of +1 is described when indentation of the skin disappears immediately after releasing pressure. With +4 edema, the indentation remains a minute or longer after releasing pressure.

Skin Lesions. A skin lesion is an abnormality in the structure of the skin as a result of injury or disease. Every lesion should be described in terms of size, color, type, and location. Lesions may be measured with a metric ruler to ensure accurate size determination. Refer to Chapter 34 for a complete description and graphic representation of different types of lesions.

ASSESSMENT OF ELIMINATION

Elimination is the excretion of waste products from the body through the gastrointestinal and urinary systems. Elimination assessment focuses on determining the adequacy of bowel and bladder function, observing characteristics of feces or urine, identifying risk factors that may contribute to problems in elimination, assessing the impact bowel or bladder dysfunction has on daily living, and understanding the patient's methods of management and coping for any bowel or bladder dysfunction.

Urinary Elimination

Subjective and objective data are collected to assess urinary function, identify risk factors, and identify management strategies for coping with bladder dysfunction.

Subjective Data

The collection of subjective information should focus on the patient's normal urinary pattern and any recent changes in the normal urinary pattern. Questions the nurse may use to elicit this information from the patient include:

- Describe your urinary habits. How frequently do you urinate? What is the amount and color of your urine?
- Have you noticed any changes in your urinary pattern (i.e., frequency of voiding; quantity of urine)?
- Do you experience any problems with urination such as pain, dribbling, difficulty beginning urination, or difficulty controlling urination?
- Have you ever had bladder surgery or a urinary catheter? If so, describe.
- Have you ever noticed blood in your urine?
- Has a problem with urinary elimination affected your daily activities?
- Describe how you manage any current problems with urinary elimination.

Objective Data

Objective data concerning urinary elimination are obtained through inspection of the urine and the lower abdomen and light palpation and percussion of the urinary bladder.

Inspection. Assessment of the bladder for distention due to urinary retention is warranted when a patient complains of lower abdominal (or bladder) discomfort or reports a history of difficulty urinating, or when a prolonged time has elapsed since the last voiding occurred. The bladder is inspected for signs of distention, which appears as a swelling of the lower abdomen, just above the symphysis pubis. Observation of urinary distention may be difficult in the obese person. When the bladder contains less than 500 mL of urine, no bulge is present on inspection.

Inspecting voided urine of the patient provides additional data concerning urinary elimination status. Urine is normally pale yellow to colorless, aromatic, and without sediment. For additional information about assessment of urine, refer to Chapter 37.

Percussion. Percussion of the lower abdomen follows inspection to determine the presence of a distended bladder. Percussion begins at the umbilicus and proceeds toward the symphysis pubis. When the bladder is empty or contains only a small amount of urine, a hollow note is heard when the bladder is percussed; percussion over a full bladder produces a duller sound.

Light Palpation. Light palpation can provide additional data when bladder distention is suspected. Again, the nurse palpates from the umbilicus to the symphysis pubis, using the fingertips of both hands. With light palpation, the abdomen feels tense when the bladder is full. Often the patient exhibits signs of sensitivity or discomfort when the full bladder is being palpated. Palpation can stimulate voiding.

Bowel Elimination

Assessment of bowel elimination completes data collection for the elimination pattern. Collection of subjective and objective data should focus on normal bowel habits, risk factors for bowel dysfunction, and the impact of bowel dysfunction on daily activities.

Subjective Data

Bowel function is considered a private matter, but it is important for the nurse to develop comfort in asking patients questions regarding their bowel status. Interviewing the patient can elicit information concerning normal bowel habits and any current or past problems in bowel status, as well as the impact of the elimination pattern on daily living. Sample questions to elicit this information include:

- How often are your bowel movements? When was your last bowel movement?
- Have you noticed any recent change in your bowel pattern?
- What is the color and consistency of your stools? Have you ever noticed blood in your stool?
- Do you consider your bowel pattern normal?
- Do you have any difficulty maintaining bowel regularity?
- What do you do to keep regular? Certain foods? Laxatives? Enemas?
- Have you ever had bowel surgery? If so, describe.

Objective Data

Inspection of the feces, abdominal examination, and rectal examination provide objective data concerning bowel elimination. Abdominal assessment has already been outlined in detail in the section entitled "Assessment of Nutrition and Metabolism."

Inspection. The abdomen is observed for distention, which can signify that decreased peristalsis is present in the intestines. When distention is present, the abdomen appears larger than usual, and in severe distention, the skin appears stretched and taut. The patient may be able to verify that the abdomen does appear larger than usual. Inspection of the perirectal area should reveal intact skin without excoriation or redness.

Inspection of normal stool reveals soft formed, light or dark brown feces. Stool characteristics and tests for the presence of blood are presented in detail in Chapter 38.

Palpation. In addition to being part of the abdominal assessment, palpation is used to evaluate the rectum for abnormalities or the presence of stool. To palpate the rectum, a lubricated, gloved index finger is inserted in the rectum and directed toward the umbilicus. The presence of internal or external hemorrhoids, polyps, or abnormal masses should be documented. Frequently, a rectal examination is performed to detect the presence and consistency of stool in the rectum. Hard, dry stool may indicate the presence of a fecal impaction, which may require manual removal.

ASSESSMENT OF SLEEP AND REST

Assessment of sleep and rest focuses on normal sleep patterns of the patient, alterations from the normal sleep pattern, and satisfaction with quality of rest and sleep.

Subjective Data

Information is collected from the patient concerning sleep habits, problems with obtaining adequate rest or sleep, and any aids that are used to induce sleep. Suggested questions to elicit this information include:

- How many hours per day do you normally sleep? What time do you usually go to bed and get up?
- Do you nap during the day? When? How long?
- Do you generally feel rested and energetic during the day?
- Are you satisfied with your sleep pattern?
- Do you have difficulty going to sleep? Staying asleep?
- Do you do anything to help induce sleep? Do you ever take medications for sleep?
- Do you anticipate problems sleeping while you are in the hospital?

Objective Data

Most of the data indicating a dysfunctional sleep pattern are subjective, although a few objective signs may support subjective data. Frequent yawning, decreased attention span, and dark circles or puffiness around the eyes may be related to sleep deprivation. Continual dozing during the day may also occur when the amount or quality of sleep is inadequate.

ASSESSMENT OF COGNITION AND PERCEPTION

Perception involves acquiring information about the environment through our senses, (sight, hearing, touch, taste, and smell). Cognition involves intellectual abilities such as memory, reasoning, thinking, and motivation. The goal in assessment of cognition and perception is to identify impairments in sensory function and to evaluate cognitive function, comfort, pain, language, and communication. Deficits in any of these areas may increase the person's susceptibility to injury and interfere with the ability to live independently.

For assessment purposes, cognition and perception are divided into three areas: cognitive function, sensory function, and pain. Each of these areas impacts on the others so the interrelationships among data must be considered, as well as specific subjective and objective information.

Cognitive Function

Cognitive function refers to a person's ability to think, which is primarily evaluated through written and verbal communication. Factors that contribute to cognition include awareness, thought processes, memory, language, judgment, and attention span. Whereas significant impairment in cognitive abilities is readily noticeable upon first interaction, it often requires repeated assessments over a period of time to detect subtle changes or minor deficits in cognitive ability.

Subjective Data

Subjective data for appraising mental abilities are gathered throughout the health assessment, from the context of a patient's conversation and the degree of cooperation given during the physical examination. The nurse assesses whether the patient has difficulty understanding or answering questions or following directions. The patient's responses to questions are evaluated in terms of clarity and appropriateness. The patient should be able to express any health concerns in a coherent, clear manner.

Possible questions to further elicit information concerning a person's cognitive and communication ability include:

- Explain what your doctor has told you about your health.
- How much formal education have you received?
- Would you say learning is "easy" or "hard" for you?
- Describe the last experience you had in learning something new. How do you believe you learn best?

- Are you able to remember recent events? Events in the distant past?
- Can you tell me your full name? What is today's date? Where are you right now?
- Describe how you feel when faced with a decision to make. Is making decisions easy or difficult for you?

Objective Data

Objective data concerning the cognitive abilities of the patient are obtained through the neurologic examination.* This examination also obtains information on sensory function. The neurologic examination is a systematic method of assessing the integration of brain function and motor response. Abnormalities often reflect impairment to the brain or spinal cord. If a patient is fully alert and oriented, the nurse may only perform a full neurologic assessment to obtain a baseline. In many agencies, comprehensive detailed neurologic testing is performed by advanced practitioners. See Procedure 18-5 for a detailed description of how to perform a neurologic assessment.

Level of Consciousness. Consciousness is awareness and responsiveness to the surrounding environment. Impairment in consciousness is evaluated on a continuum. At the highest level of consciousness, a person responds to environmental stimuli with appropriate verbal and motor activity. The person is attentive, cooperative, and completely oriented to self, time, and place. Impaired consciousness may initially be demonstrated by loss of orientation and inability to follow simple commands. At the lowest level of consciousness, the comatose state, painful stimuli are necessary to induce a verbal or motor response.

The Glasgow Coma Scale provides the nurse with a standardized assessment tool, with which subtle changes in consciousness states can be detected quickly (Table 18-6). This tool is used when serial assessments are done

(Text continues on page 333)

* The neurologic system is responsible for numerous functions such as memory/consciousness, reception of sensory impulses, coordination, and initiating muscle movement. A complete neurologic assessment comprises an integration of assessments of cognitive–sensory and activity–mobility patterns. Deficits in any of these functional areas may increase the patient's susceptibility to injury and interfere with the ability to live independently.

TABLE 18-6

Glasgow Coma Scale

Best Eye-Opening Response		Best Verbal Response		Best Motor Response	
Purposeful and spontaneous	4	Oriented	5	Obeys commands	6
To voice	3	Disoriented	4	Localizes pain	5
To pain	2	Inappropriate words	3	Withdraws to pain	4
No response	1	Incomprehensible sounds	2	Flexion to pain	3
Untestable	U	No response	1	Extension to pain	2
		Untestable	U	No response	1
				Untestable	U

PROCEDURE 18–5. Assessing the Neurologic System

■ Purpose

1. To obtain baseline information about the patient's neurologic status.
2. To assess the patient's orientation to their environment.
3. To evaluate the patient's cognitive function and ability to make judgments.
4. To assess the integrity of motor and sensory pathways and the patient's ability to ambulate safely.

■ Assessment

1. Determine if the patient is distracted by an immediate need (e.g., pain, urge to urinate). Attend to that need first.
2. Explain to the patient what you plan to do and approximately how long it will take. A complete neurologic assessment can be very lengthy. The nurse must decide how extensive the assessment should be based on the patient's diagnosis, level of consciousness, and physical disabilities. An efficient nurse learns how to integrate components of the neurologic assessment with other parts of the patient's functional assessment (i.e., cranial nerves assessed during head and neck examination, mental status evaluated during nursing history, and reflexes tested during musculoskeletal assessment.
3. Ask significant others if they have noted memory loss or changes in behavior of patient.
4. Question patient about presence of headache, seizures, dizziness, visual changes, or numbness/tingling of any body parts.
5. Review medication history for any drugs that may alter level of consciousness or cause behavioral changes (i.e., analgesics, sedatives, antidepressants, antipsychotics, or central nervous system stimulants).

■ Equipment

May need all or part of equipment depending on comprehensiveness of assessment.

Sterile safety pin or hypodermic needle
Sterile cotton applicator
Vials of hot and cold water
Tongue blade
Penlight
Vials of coffee, vanilla, or clove extracts
Vials of salt, sugar, lemon solutions
Snellen chart
Tuning fork
Reflex hammer

■ Procedure

Cognitive/Sensory Assessment

1. Assess the level of consciousness by asking direct questions that require a verbal response. Note appropriateness of response and emotional state.
   Rationale: Alterations in mental status may be demonstrated by irritability, decreased attention span, inability or unwillingness to cooperate, and an abnormal perception of the environment.
2. Evaluate patient's speech patterns.
   Rationale: Normally, speech should be clear, well-paced, and coherent. Language should seem appropriate for educational and socioeconomic level.
3. Observe general appearance: hygiene, appropriateness of clothing to setting and weather.
4. If patient responses are inappropriate, ask direct questions related to person, place, and time (e.g., "What is your name?" "Where are you right now?" "What city do you live in?" "What day is this?").
   Rationale: Measures patient's orientation to immediate environment. As consciousness deteriorates, patients become disoriented to person, place, and time.
   Note: Be sure patient's inappropriate response is not caused by a communication or language problem.
5. If patient doesn't or inappropriately responds to orientation questions, give simple commands (e.g., "squeeze my fingers" or "wiggle your toes"). If there is no response to verbal commands, test response to painful stimuli by applying firm pressure on patient's sternum or finger nailbed with your thumb.
   Rationale: Level of consciousness can vary from fully alert and oriented, to unable to follow commands, to unresponsiveness to external stimuli.
   Note: Avoid pinching patients skin to elicit a pain response.
6. Document level of consciousness objectively by stating specific patient responses to verbal or tactile stimulation.
   Note: Use of Glasgow Coma Scale (see Table 18-6) helps charting of frequent level of consciousness testing. Assessments are more objective and consistent.
7. Assess function of cranial nerves as noted in Table 18-7.
   Note: An increase in intracranial pressure (ICP) puts direct pressure on the optic nerve (C-II). The osculomotor (C-III), trochlear (C-IV), the abducents (C-VI) exit the brain stem at the level of the tentorial notch. When ICP increases and the brain

(continued)

PROCEDURE 18–5. Assessing the Neurologic System *(continued)*

shifts downward, changes in the functions of these nerves are noted.

8. Assess sensory pathways:
   a. Patient's eyes are closed during all sensory tests.
      Rationale: Tests are valid only if patient doesn't see where stimulus strikes skin.
   b. Apply stimuli to skin in a random unpredictable order while comparing one side or body to the other.
      Rationale: Sensations should be felt equally on both sides of the body. Random stimuli prevent patient from anticipating and correctly guessing where stimulus is.
   c. Patient should verbally state when he or she feels a particular stimulus. If an area of altered sensation is detected, note which spinal cord segment is affected by referring to a dermatome chart.

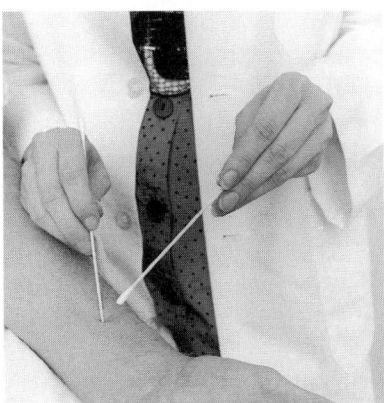

Step 8

9. Test pain sensation first by lightly touching pointed then blunt end of sterile pin to proximal and distal aspects of the arm and legs.
   Rationale: Assesses intactness of spinothalamic tract. If pain sensation is intact, nurse may omit tests for temperature.

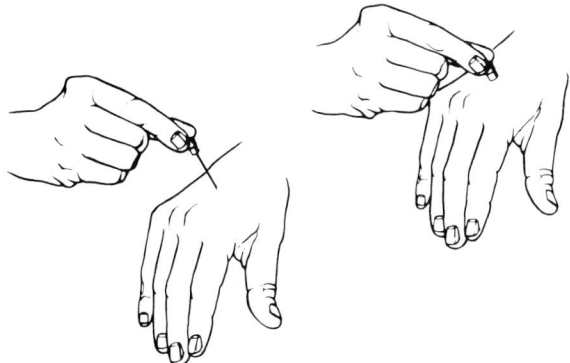

Step 9

10. Test temperature sensation by touching skin with vials of hot, then cold, water.
    Note: Patient should identify hot versus cold sensation.

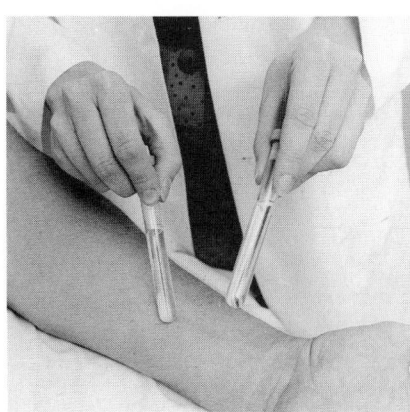

Step 10

11. Lightly stroke proximal and distal aspects of patient's arms and legs with a cotton ball. Ask patient to tell you when and where each stroke is felt.
    Rationale: Testing the patient's perception of light touch and the following tests of vibration and position assess intactness of the posterior column. Loss of any of these sensations may indicate a lesion of the posterior column on the same side as the loss.

2. Apply a vibrating tuning fork to the distal interphalangeal joint of fingers and great toe. Ask pa-

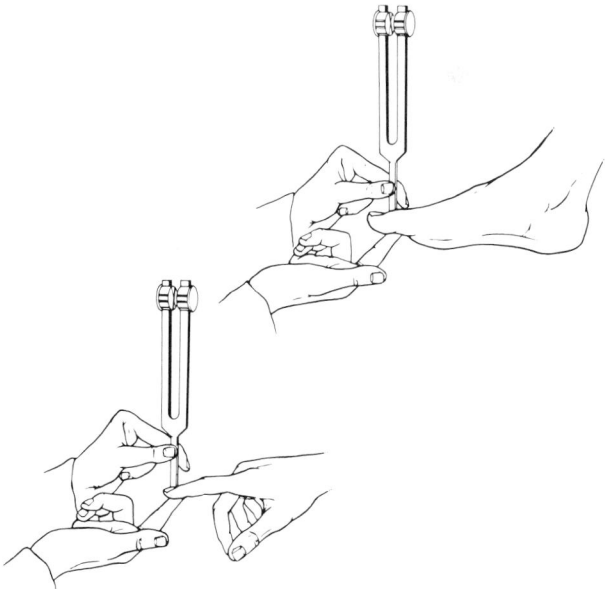

Step 12

(continued)

PROCEDURE 18–5. Assessing the Neurologic System *(continued)*

tient to describe what he or she feels and when it stops.

Note: If patient doesn't feel vibration, move the tuning fork proximally to the next joint until sensation is felt.

13. Grasp patient's finger. Move finger up and down asking patient to identify position. Repeat procedure with toes.

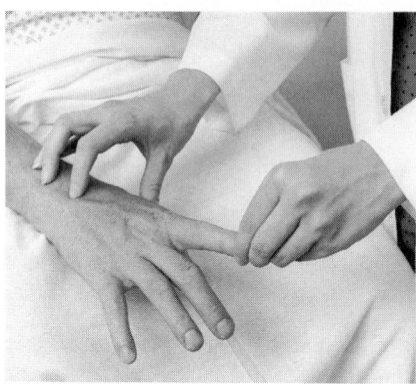

Step 13

Activity-Mobility Assessment

14. Inspect arm and leg muscles for atrophy, tremors, fasiculations, or other abnormal movements.

15. Assess strength of specific muscle groups by having patient extend or flex individual joints against resistance provided by examiner's hands. Test biceps, triceps, wrist leg muscles, and ankle. Evaluate for symmetry of same muscle groups.

16. Ask patient to close eyes and hold arms in front of body with palms up. Hold position for 30 seconds and observe for pronation of hands or drifting of arms.

Note: Notice if weaknesses are on one or both sides.
Rationale: Detects presence of deformities, reduced mobility of joints, or decreased muscle strength. Upper and lower extremities of dominant side are usually stronger than nondominant side.

17. Evaluate coordination and balance by:
a. Performing a series of rapid alternating movements (RAMS).
1) Have patient pat upper thigh by rapidly alternating his or her palm and the back of the hand.
2) With dominant hand, have patient touch his or her thumb to each finger on that hand as quickly as possible.
3) Have patient use his or her dominant fore-

finger to first touch your forefinger, then his or her nose. Instruct patient to repeat this many times as fast as he or she can.

Note: Difficulty performing any of these tests may suggest further evaluation for cerebellar disease is indicated.

b. Romberg test: Ask patient to stand with feet together, arms at sides. Have patient maintain this position for 30 seconds with eyes open, then 30 seconds with eyes closed. Assess for swaying.

Note: Stay close to patient to assist in case he or she begins to fall.
Rationale: Patients with cerebellar disease may not maintain balance with eyes open or shut; problems with proprioception cause difficulty only with eyes shut.

c. Ask patient to walk across the room. Observe gait for symmetry, rhythm, limping, shuffling, or other abnormalities.
Rationale: Changes in gait may be characteristic of specific neurologic diseases.

18. Assess deep tendon reflexes (see Table 18-8).
a. Compare symmetry of reflex on each side of body.
b. Extremity to be tested should be completely relaxed and slightly extended.
c. Reflex hammer should be held loosely and allowed to swing freely into an arc.
d. Tap tendon briskly.
e. Document reflexes by grading 0–4+ on stickman.
0 —no response
1+—diminished reflex (may be normal)
2+—normal
3+—brisker than normal (may be normal)
4+—hyperactive—upper neuron disorder suspected

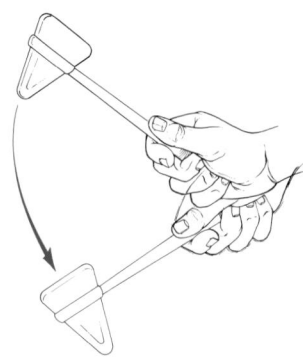

Step 18

(continued)

PROCEDURE 18–5. Assessing the Neurologic System (continued)

■ Lifespan Considerations

Newborn and Infant
The infant at birth has litte or no voluntary control over muscular movements. Much of the infant's motor activity is seen as mass responses to stimuli and built-in reflexes as described below:

Rooting Reflex
- Infant turns head toward a warm object placed against his or her cheek.
- Function is to help the infant locate the mother's breast when nursing.

Sucking
- Swallowing and gagging reflexes—well developed in normal infants at birth.

Moro Reflex
- In response to loud noise or sudden movement, infant extends arms in tense, quivering embrace and often cries.

Tonic Neck Reflex
- When relaxed or asleep on back, infant has head turned to one side with arm and leg of that side extended, while extremities of opposite side are flexed.

Toddler and Preschooler
- Children are often fearful of strangers and examining equipment. Spend several minutes becoming acquainted with the child. Allowing them to handle the equipment before examining and using a "This is a game" approach often helps allay the fear. There are several screening tools available such as the Denver Development Test, which is designed to evaluate cognitive and psychomotor skills of infants and children of varying ages.

Older Adult
- A lengthy examination may be exhausting for the older adult and may need to be completed in phases.
- Arthritic changes in joints may limit range of motion and physical mobility and should be considered in evaluating assessment data.

---

for high-risk patients (e.g., brain tumor, after brain surgery, after a cerebral vascular accident). The patient is scored according to the best response given, and the results are documented appropriately in the patient's record. The nurse is able to detect subtle changes in consciousness state by reviewing the scale and noticing deviations from baseline.

Reading Ability and Memory. Reading ability and memory are specific aspects of cognitive functioning that are vital to effective patient teaching. In most cases, the patient's level of formal education, occupation, and verbal skills provide sufficient data to make a valid judgment. If limited reading ability is suspected, the nurse should ask the patient to read aloud a short passage from the newspaper or a patient education pamphlet and paraphrase what was read. Short-term memory can be evaluated by asking the patient to recall events in the day, such as activities, visitors, or meals eaten. Long-term memory is reflected in the ability to provide historic information about family, health problems, or hospitalizations.

Sensory Function

The purpose of assessing sensory status of the patient is to determine functioning of the five senses: vision, hearing, touch, taste, and smell. Assessment should also include the impact sensory deficits have on daily activities and any devices the patient uses to cope with sensory impairment.

Sensory losses may be congenital but are often associated with the normal aging process. Elderly patients should be assessed carefully for sensory deficits because many adaptive techniques are available to improve the safety, pleasure, and independence of their lives. Physical examination of the senses is usually not performed in a basic health assessment, unless evidence of impaired function is uncovered during the patient interview. Physical examination of the senses routinely is part of health screening examinations.

Subjective Data

Patients are usually aware of sensory loss and can verbalize specific deficits to the nurse when questioned. During the interview, the nurse should observe the patient for signs of sensory impairment, such as asking questions to be repeated, watching lips closely during speech, squinting to improve vision, or holding reading material at arm's length.

Questions concerning sensory status include:

- Do you wear glasses or contact lenses to improve your

vision? For distance or near vision? Do you use other visual aids such as a magnifying glass or large print books?

- Have you noticed any recent changes in your ability to see close or distant objects?
- Do you have difficulty seeing at night?
- Do vision problems interfere with any of your normal activities (such as shopping, paying bills, or driving)?
- Have you sustained any injuries or falls related to an inability to see clearly?
- Do you have any devices to augment your hearing, such as a hearing aid or telephone amplifier? Are you satisfied with their use?
- Do you avoid or feel uncomfortable around people because of difficulty hearing?
- Do you have a history of prolonged exposure to loud noises such as combat, factory noises, construction work, or rock music?
- Have you noticed any difficulty in your ability to smell or taste?
- Are you particularly sensitive to any smells?
- Do you experience any numbness or lack of sensation in your hands or feet?
- Do you have difficulty regulating the temperature of your bath?
- Have you ever been injured without being aware at the time?

Objective Data

Objective data that provide valuable information about sensory function include: use of sensory aids, tests for visual acuity, tests for auditory acuity, cranial nerve assessment, and sensory assessment. Many of these data are specialized and not routinely collected in basic nursing assessment, unless deficits in normal function have been detected or the patient is at risk for dysfunction.

Sensory Aids. The use of glasses, contact lenses, hearing aids, and other assistive devices should be documented in the patient's health assessment. The proper care of such devices should also be solicited and written in the patient's record. This ensures proper use and care of expensive devices during the patient's stay in a health-care agency.

Visual Assessment. The Snellen "E" or alphabet test is used for assessing distant visual acuity. The patient is positioned 20 feet from the Snellen chart (Fig. 18-14), which has been placed at eye level. Each eye is tested separately and both eyes together. The nurse covers one of the patient's eyes without applying pressure and instructs the patient to keep both eyes open. The nurse directs the patient to identify the smallest line that can be seen, reading the letters or imitating the direction of the "E." Each line on the Snellen chart is marked with the number of feet from which a person can normally read

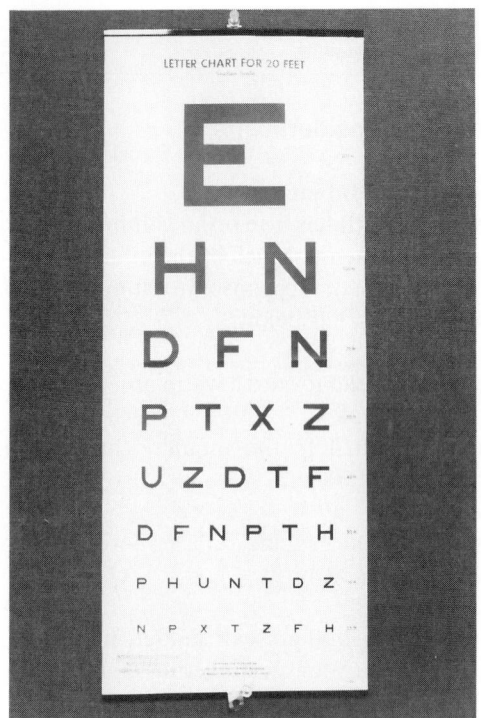

Figure 18–14. Snellen eye chart.

that line. The patient's distance from the chart (20 feet) is compared to the number by the line the patient can read. For example, if the patient can read the 100 foot line, visual acuity would be reported as 20/100. Any person with less than 20/20 acuity should be referred to an ophthalmologist or optometrist for evaluation.

To test near vision, the nurse can hold newsprint 14 inches from the patient's face. If the patient is unable to focus well enough to read, experiment with the distance to determine if improvement occurs by moving the print closer or farther away. Visual problems with close objects occur more frequently after the age of 40.

Advanced practitioners may be trained to examine the eye with an ophthalmoscope (Fig. 18-15).

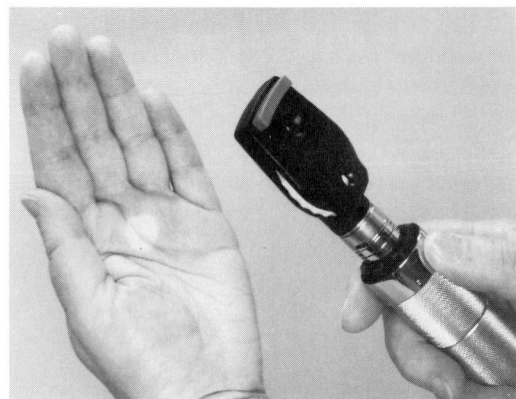

Figure 18–15. Ophthalmoscope.

Auditory Assessment. Assessment of auditory function can occur simply during normal conversation. During the interview, the nurse should lower his or her voice to assess the patient's ability to hear. Hearing loss is suggested in a patient who turns a particular ear or leans toward the speaker, hears only when able to see the speaker's face (evidence of lip-reading), or speaks in a loud or distorted voice. People with hearing loss may avoid social settings because conversation is especially difficult in groups with background noise. Other physical symptoms associated with hearing loss are tinnitus (ringing in the ears) and vertigo (dizziness).

If hearing loss is suspected, the external ear canal should be examined before specialized tests are performed. Using an otoscope (Fig. 18-16), the canal is visualized after the pinna has been pulled up, out, and back to straighten the ear canal. The canal is inspected for inflammation or cerumen (ear wax). A build-up of cerumen can temporarily impede normal hearing.

Weber's test and the Rinne test, in which a tuning fork is used, can be performed to further evaluate hearing loss. Weber's test is used to evaluate lateralization of sound (Fig. 18-17A). The tuning fork is activated and placed at the top of the patient's head. Normally vibrations can be heard equally in both ears, but in conduction deafness, the vibrations may be best heard in the affected ear, whereas in sensorineural loss, the sound lateralizes to the unaffected ear.

The Rinne test discriminates between bone conduction and air conduction of sound (see Fig. 18-17B). The tuning fork is struck, and its stem is placed in front of the ear and then firmly against the mastoid process. Normally, the person should hear the sound of the tuning fork when it is placed in front of the ear, indicating air conduction of sound is greater than bone conduction. When the sound is not detected until the tuning fork is placed on the mastoid process, bone conduction of sound is greater than air conduction due to a conductive hearing loss.

Cranial Nerve Assessment. Intact cranial nerve function is important for normal sensory functioning. Vision

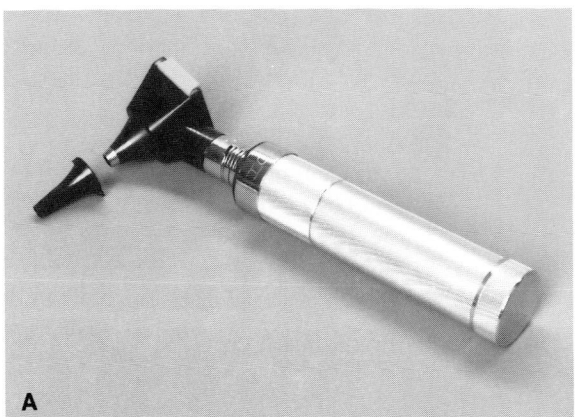
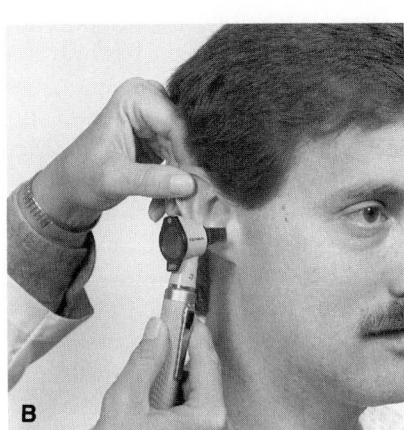
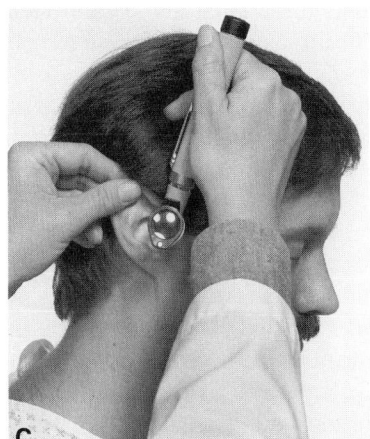

Figure 18–16. Ear examination. **A.** Otoscope. **B.** Method used for otoscopic examination of a cooperative patient. **C.** Method used for otoscopic examination of an uncooperative patient and children.

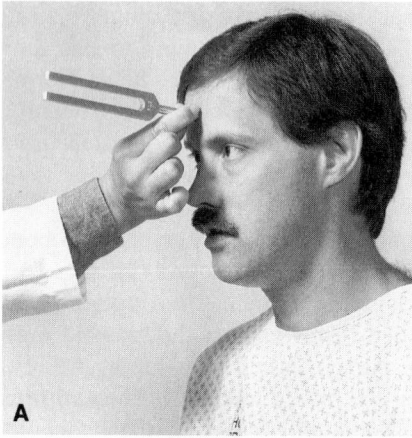

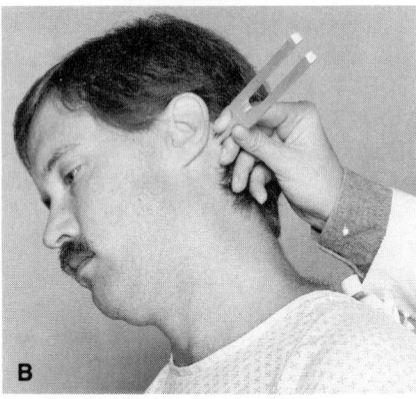

Figure 18–17. Hearing tests using a tuning fork. **A.** Weber's test. **B.** Rinne test.

depends on normal functioning of cranial nerves II, III, IV, and VI. Cranial nerve VIII is important for hearing, and cranial nerve I is important for the sense of smell. Other cranial nerves are important in the coordination of facial movement or reflex activity. During an initial neurologic assessment, or at specific intervals for high-risk patients, normal functioning of the cranial nerves is checked. Table 18-7 lists the cranial nerves and techniques the nurse can use to assess their functioning.

Sensory Assessment. Loss of tactile sensation may occur with a variety of conditions such as diabetes, peripheral vascular disease, spinal cord injury and brain trauma, tumor, or vascular lesion. Patients with decreased tactile sensations are at risk for injury from hot or cold, prolonged pressure, or shearing force. Sensory perception is evaluated by observing the patient's response to light touch, vibration, and pain. With the patient's eyes closed, various areas of the body can be touched with a wisp of cotton to assess light touch, a tuning fork to test vibration, and a pin to test pain. Water of different temperatures can be used to assess temperature discrimination. Documentation should include the inability to sense stimuli and the affected location of the body.

Deep Tendon Reflexes. Testing deep tendon reflexes may be indicated in certain high-risk patients. The nurse uses a reflex hammer to tap various tendons in the body to see if this action elicits the appropriate reflex arc through the spinal cord. Normally, a brisk contraction of the muscle occurs. Common reflexes that may be tested include the biceps, the triceps, the patellar, and the Achilles. Refer to Table 18-8 for explanations of the procedure used to test these reflexes.

Three significant variations from the normal reflex pattern can occur (McHugh & McHugh, 1990). First, reflexes on the same side of the body may be different. Second, cortical damage may affect reflexes on one side of the body and not the other. Finally, there can be a difference in the reflex pattern above and below the waist if spinal cord compression has occurred. Abnormal reflex patterns should be brought to the attention of the physician.

Pain Assessment

Pain is a sensory and emotional experience in which a person experiences or reports to experience severe discomfort or uncomfortable sensations. Pain has two components: a sensory component, which is neurophysiologic, and a perceptual component, which is cognitive and emotional. Theories of pain are discussed in depth in Chapter 40.

Acute illness, chronic disability, surgical intervention, and treatment modalities can all cause the patient pain. Pain can limit normal function and affect wellness in all health patterns.

Accurate assessment of pain is necessary to identify and treat the underlying cause of pain. Assessment permits the nurse to better understand the patient's pain experience.

Subjective Data

The pain experience is personal and subjective, thus the patient interview is the best way to collect information to assess pain. Pain assessment should include asking the patient to describe the location, intensity, quality, onset, and chronology of their pain experience. Factors that influence the pain experience and methods of effective pain management should also be determined. Lastly, the impact the pain experience has on daily life and other health patterns should be explored. Some patients are reluctant to discuss and describe their pain experience because of personal beliefs or values.

Questions helpful in soliciting subjective information concerning the patient's pain experience include:

• Are you experiencing any pain or discomfort? If so, describe the location, intensity, when it first occurred, and what seemed to cause it.

TABLE 18–7

Cranial Nerve Function and Assessment

Number	Name	Function	Method of Assessment
I	Olfactory	Sense of smell	Ask patient to identify different mild aromas, such as vanilla, coffee, chocolate, cloves.
II	Optic	Vision	Ask patient to read Snellen chart.
III	Oculomotor	Pupillary reflex	Assess pupil reaction to penlight.
		Extraocular eye movement	Assess directions of gaze by holding your finger 18 inches from patient's face. Ask patient to follow your finger up and down and side to side.
IV	Trochlear	Lateral and downward movement of eyeball	Assess directions of gaze. Test with cranial nerve II.
V	Trigeminal	Sensation to cornea, skin of face, nasal mucosa	Lightly touch cotton swab to lateral sclera of eye to elicit blink. Measure sensation of touch and pain on face using cotton wisp and pin.
VI	Abducens	Lateral movement of eyeball	Assess directions of gaze. Test with cranial nerve III.
VII	Facial	Facial expression	Ask patient to smile, frown, raise eyebrows.
		Taste—anterior two thirds of tongue	Ask patient to identify different tastes on tip and sides of tongue: sugar (sweet), salt, lemon juice (sour).
VIII	Auditory	Hearing	Assess ability to hear spoken word.
IX	Glossopharyneal	Taste—posterior tongue	Ask patient to identify different tastes on back of tongue as above.
		Swallowing	Place a tongue blade on posterior tongue while patient says "ah" to elicit a gag response.
		Movement of tongue	Ask patient to move tongue up and down, and side to side.
X	Vagus	Swallowing	Assess with cranial nerve IX by observing palate and pharynx move as patient says "ah."
		Movement of vocal cords	
		Sensation of pharynx	
XI	Spinal accessory	Head and shoulder movement	Ask patient to turn head side to side and shrug shoulders against resistance from examiner's hands.
XII	Hypoglossal	Tongue position	Ask patient to stick out tongue to midline, then move it side to side.

• What factors seem to aggravate (relieve) the pain?
• Describe your methods of managing the pain? Do you use medication, heat or cold therapy, TENS unit, and so forth, to help decrease pain?
• Do you take any medications to help decrease pain? If so, give name, dose, frequency, and length of time you have taken this medication.
• Have you ever used relaxation techniques to manage discomfort? If so, how effective are they?
• Has your pain limited your ability to perform normal daily activities such as exercise, working, or attending social events?
• Has your pain negatively affected your ability to relate to those people who are close to you?

Objective Data

Objective data are not always available to document the experience of pain. Acute pain stimulates the sympathetic nervous system and produces the following objective symptoms: increased blood pressure, increased pulse, increased respiratory rate, dilated pupils, and diaphoresis. Observing the patient's body position and facial features also gives clues to the presence of pain.

Grimacing, guarded positioning, tense body posture, refusal to move a body part, muscle spasms, or rubbing a body part can all indicate the presence of pain despite verbal denial. A "facial mask of pain," in which the patient's facial expression is flat or fixed, the eyes appear dull, and fatigue is evident, commonly occurs in chronic pain. Emotional expression such as crying, moaning, or yelling also can occur during pain.

ASSESSMENT OF SELF-PERCEPTION AND SELF-CONCEPT

Self-perception and self-concept pattern focuses on the content and feelings associated with a person's self-evaluation. The components of self-concept include one's sense of power, acceptance and value by others, and competence in physical, intellectual, and social dimensions (Panicucci, 1983). Self-concept is influenced by the way others evaluate and interact with a person throughout the lifespan. Body image, the mental picture and feelings about one's body, is an important component of self-concept.

During a basic health assessment, the goal in assessing

TABLE 18–8

Assessment of Deep Tendon Reflexes

Reflex	Procedure		Normal Response
Biceps	Flex patient's arm at the elbow with his or her forearm resting on the thigh, palm up. Place your thumb on the base of the biceps tendon in the antecubital fossa. Strike your thumb with the reflex hammer.	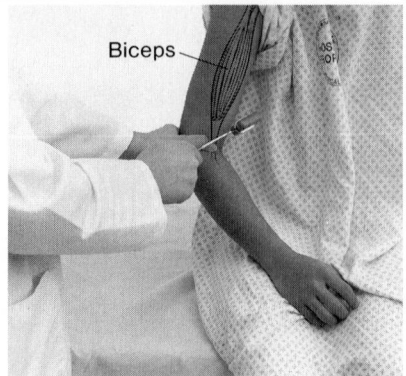	Flexion of forearm at the elbow
Triceps	Hold patient's arm across his or her chest, flexing the elbow at a 90-degree angle. Support wrist as patient allows forearm to become limp. Strike the tendon just above the olecranon process.	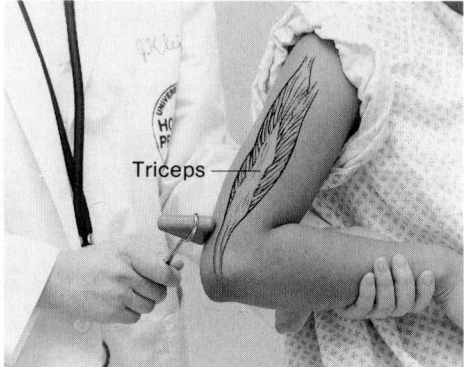	Extension at the elbow
Patellar	Patient sits upright with legs hanging loosely over side of bed. If patient remains supine, support back of knee while leg is flexed at a 45-degree angle. Strike patellar tendon just below patella.	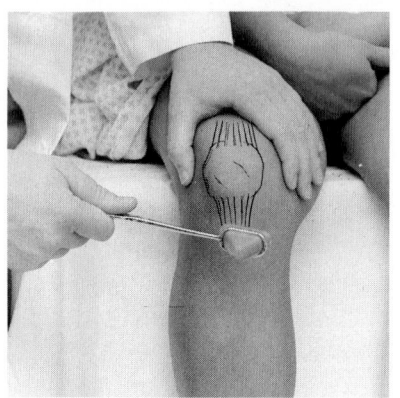	Extension of lower leg at the knee
Achilles	Patient's knee should be slightly flexed while foot is dorsiflexed. Strike Achilles tendon 1 inch above heel.	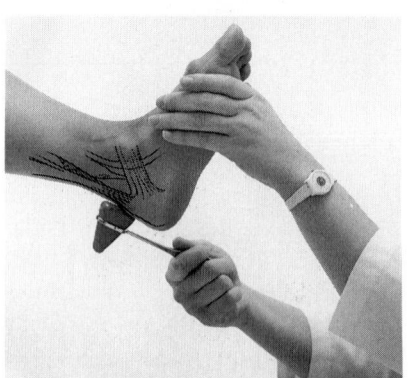	Plantar flexion

the self-perception is to describe the patient's general view of self and his or her satisfaction with that image. Patients whose primary health problem directly relates to a disturbance in self-concept, such as psychiatric, chemically dependent, abused, or anorexic patients, require an extensive evaluation by a mental health specialist. However, many illnesses alter one's self-concept due to changes related to physical strength, appearance, and loss of control. For this reason, consideration of self-concept should be integrated into the health assessment of every patient.

Subjective and supporting objective data should be collected concerning normal self-concept, recent changes in self-concept, and the presence of conditions (e.g., burns, skin disorders, colostomy, mastectomy, or obesity) that could threaten or alter body image.

Subjective Data

Possible questions that help the patient describe self-perception include:

- How would you describe yourself?
- What do you consider to be your strengths and weaknesses?
- Most of the time, do you feel good or not so good about yourself?
- How do you feel about your appearance?
- How has your illness changed the way you feel about yourself?

Objective Data

Nonverbal cues to a person's self-concept are reflected in eye contact, personal grooming and appearance, posture, body movements, mood, emotions, voice and speech pattern. Low self-concept may be reflected in poor eye contact, inattention to personal grooming, and body language that conveys embarrassment or shame.

Formal Assessment Tools. Some paper and pencil tests have been developed to assist with self-concept assessment. Rosenberg's Self-Esteem Scale (Rosenberg, 1979), Piers-Harris Self-Concept Scale (Piers & Harris, 1969), and the Locus of Control Scales (Wallston, et al., 1978) are examples.

ASSESSMENT OF ROLES AND RELATIONSHIPS

Assessment of roles and relationships describes the quality of a person's family and social roles. Significant relationships may exist among the immediate family and extended family, with individual friends in the workplace, or in the community. Most people fill a variety of roles: husband or wife, parent, worker, student, col-

league, friend, coach, advisor. These roles may be rewarding and stimulating, or they may be overwhelming and stressful.

The goal in a basic health assessment is to identify the patient's major roles in the family, at work, and in social life, and to identify the patient's relative satisfaction or dissatisfaction with each role. The assessment should also indicate how health problems or hospitalization may interfere with a person's ability to fulfill role expectations and maintain relationships. Whereas this information normally is obtained from the patient, it is often helpful (and sometimes necessary) to consult other members of the family unit to obtain meaningful data.

Information obtained in the assessment should focus on the patient's family configuration and occupation, recent or anticipated changes in the roles or relationships of the patient, and the patient's level of satisfaction with current roles and relationships.

Subjective Data

Within the family unit, important information includes who shares the household, what responsibilities or dependencies each member has, and the presence of specific problems, such as issues related to parenting, caring for elderly parents, or marital discord. The illness of a family member may necessitate shifting responsibilities within the family, such as financial support, child care, cooking, and home maintenance. Chronic illnesses often involve the patient in long and sometimes permanent dependence on others. It is important to evaluate the specific circumstances of that dependence, the patient's attitude, and the patient's coping ability.

Roles and relationships related to work are an important area to assess. Factors such as job-related stress, insufficient time for leisure activities, unsafe work environment, job insecurity, inadequate pay, or lack of recognition may negatively affect physical and psychological well-being.

A change in one's relationships may contribute to the cause or exacerbation of an illness. The nurse should explore areas in which recent change has occurred, such as divorce, death, or illness of a family member, loss of a job, change in job status or pay, increase in job responsibility, or transition from student to worker.

Suggested questions to help obtain this information from the patient include:

- Describe your family and home situation.
- Do family members depend on you? What affect does your illness have on your family? How are they managing in your absence?
- Are there any family problems you have difficulty handling?
- What kind of work do you do? Are you satisfied with your job? Do things generally go well for you at work?
- Does your state of health affect your ability to work?

- Have you experienced any recent changes in your relationship with family, coworkers, or others?
- Do you believe your neighborhood and community are supportive?

Objective Data

Objective data are obtained by watching the interactions of the patient with family members and others. Verbal interactions and nonverbal communication can support what the patient has discussed in the interview. Observing visitors, cards, and flowers can help to validate that the patient has positive relationships with others. Likewise, the absence of visitors and communication from others might suggest the lack of positive relationships.

Repeated unexplained injuries, such as bruises, burns, and fractures, should be noted with suspicion of possible abusive relationships. Frequently, people involved in abusive relationships verbally deny that abuse has occurred.

ASSESSMENT OF COPING AND STRESS TOLERANCE

Stress is an event that disrupts or challenges a person's equilibrium. Although stress is most readily conceptualized as negative, positive life changes also challenge a person and therefore create stress. Examples of positive stressors include marriage, pregnancy, job promotion, and a long-awaited vacation. Whether something is a stressor depends largely on a person's perception of the event. Each person's response to stress is unique. The way in which a person reacts, and hopefully adapts, to stress is called a coping behavior. Coping behaviors may be adaptive, producing relief from stress and even growth, or they may be maladaptive and lead to further disintegration and disorganization.

Serious illness, hospitalization, and surgery are universally perceived as stressful events. A variety of behavioral response patterns may be manifested in response to the stress of illness, such as anxiety, denial, questioning, ambivalence, suspicion, hostility, regression, loneliness, rejection, depression, and withdrawal (Lambert & Lambert, 1985).

In assessing coping and stress tolerance, the goal is to identify and acknowledge current stressors the patient is experiencing, determine how the patient has handled stressful events in the past, and identify current methods the patient is using to cope.

Subjective Data

Subjective data concerning coping and stress tolerance can be obtained through the interview, which can consist of open-ended or specific questions. Another technique is to ask the patient to describe a stressful event that has occurred in the past and his or her response to it. Such a description can help the nurse to identify past stressors as well as how the patient managed the situation. The manner in which past life crises were handled is often a good predictor of how present or future situations will be managed. Suggested questions for interviewing the patient regarding coping and stress tolerance include:

- What are you most concerned about right now? How does the situation make you feel?
- How has your health status affected the stress you feel?
- What do you usually do to relieve stress and tension? Medications, drugs, alcohol, exercise?
- With whom do you talk things over when you are upset or worried? Are they available to help you now?
- Can you recall another time in your life that was similarly stressful for you? How did you work through that difficult time?

Objective Data

The nurse can collect objective data from the patient by observing for symptoms indicating sympathetic stimulation or by having the patient fill out a stress assessment tool, which objectifies the current stress level.

Sympathetic Stimulation. Stress activates the sympathetic nervous system, which produces certain physiologic effects. Sympathetic stimulation may increase the force and rate of the heart beat, increase respiratory rate and depth, decrease blood flow to the skin resulting in pallor and diaphoresis, and increase blood flow to the muscles. These symptoms may be pronounced in the event of a sudden stressful event. When a person is exposed to chronic stress, the symptoms may be less sudden and less dramatic. The sympathetic response to stress is detailed further in Chapter 47.

Stress Assessment Tools. Holmes and Rahe (1967) developed an assessment tool to evaluate the amount of stress a person is experiencing due to current life stressors. These researchers attempted to rank order and weigh the stress value of certain life events, such as the death of a spouse, personal injury or illness, pregnancy, changing jobs, or a family vacation. Each life event was appointed a stress unit value. People are asked to indicate which life events have occurred during the last year, and the scores are tabulated. High scores, indicating high stress, correlated with high rates of illness. See Table 18-9 for Holmes and Rahe's Social Readjustment Scale.

TABLE 18–9

Holmes and Rahe's Social Readjustment Scale

The patient selects from the scale life events that have occurred during the past year. Add the stress unit values associated with each event to determine the final score.

Life Event	Stress Unit Value	Life Event	Stress Unit Value
Death of spouse	100	Children leaving home	29
Divorce	73	Trouble with in-laws	29
Marital separation	65	Outstanding personal achievement	28
Jail term	63	Spouse begins or stops work	26
Death of close family member	63	Begin or end school	26
Personal injury or illness	53	Change in living conditions	25
Marriage	50	Revision of personal habits	24
Fired at work	47	Trouble with boss	23
Marital reconciliation	45	Change in work hours or conditions	20
Retirement	45	Move or change in residence	20
Change in health of family member	44	Change in schools	20
Pregnancy	40	Change in recreation	19
Sexual difficulties	39	Change in church activities	19
Gain of new family member	39	Change in social activities	18
Business readjustment	39	Mortgage or loan less than $10,000	17
Change in financial status	38	Change in sleeping habits	16
Death of close friend	37	Change in number of family gatherings	15
Change to different line of work	36	Change in eating habits	15
Arguments with spouse	35	Vacation	13
Mortgage, or loan more than $10,000	31	Christmas	12
Foreclosure of mortage or loan	30	Minor law violations	11
Change in responsibilities at work	29		

Score interpretation:

150–199	Mild stress
200–299	Medium stress
300+	High stress: Associated with high rates of illness

(Adapted from Holmes, T. H. & Rahe, R. H. (1967, August). The social readjustment rating scale. *Journal of Psychosomatic Research, 11*(2), 213–218.)

ASSESSMENT OF SEXUALITY AND REPRODUCTION

Sexuality is the behavioral expression of sexual identity. It may involve, but is not limited to, sexual relationships with a partner. Sexual expression is a complex integration of physiologic, psychological, and social aspects of human nature. Physical illness and its treatment may influence sexual function. For example, impotence is frequently associated with diabetes mellitus, alcoholism, chronic renal disease, and several drug therapies. Patients may question their own desirability after such surgeries as mastectomy, radical neck dissection, ostomy, and hysterectomy.

Although it is increasingly more acceptable in society to discuss sexual matters, most patients and nurses are hesitant in addressing this subject during a health interview. Sexuality is, however, such an integral aspect of human nature that to ignore it would be neglecting a vital component of health. The subject of sexuality should be introduced early in the patient–nurse relationship, ideally in the context of a comprehensive health assess-

ment. Including sexuality in the initial patient contact conveys to the patient that sexual health is an appropriate, legitimate concern. The sexual assessment is not meant to illuminate nonexistent problems. Rather the patient is, in effect, given permission and encouragement to present sexually related questions.

The areas for assessment of sexuality and reproduction include reproductive functioning, sexual role and satisfaction with that role, and potential for alteration in sexual role or function. The impact of the patient's current health status on sexual role and functioning should also be discussed.

Subjective Data

The best approach to obtaining a sexual history is to introduce subjects of least sensitivity first. The nurse should begin by focusing on chronologic events such as puberty, menstruation, menopause, and reproductive history. The nurse can invite the patient to elaborate on any problems or expectations in these areas. The nurse can also determine the patient's knowledge and compliance with preventive health practices such as breast self-examination, regular Pap smear, and testicular and prostate examination.

A sexual assessment is appropriate at every age and should be adapted to correlate with the patient's developmental level. Many adolescents are concerned with changes in their bodies and early sexual experience. The nurse can use this opportunity to educate, support, and guide the adolescent in matters involving sexuality. Married people may have concerns about their own sexuality, as well as concerns related to parenting and sex education for their children. Many elderly patients enjoy sexual relations throughout their lives and may desire acknowledgement and discussion of their concerns.

Selected questions to elicit information concerning the sexual–reproductive pattern include:

- (Adolescents) Many (boys, girls) at your age have questions about dating, becoming intimate, contracting a disease, or getting pregnant. What questions do you have?
- (Women) At what age did you begin menstruating? How long is your typical menstrual cycle? What was the date of your last menstrual cycle? Do you have any problems related to menstruation?
- (Women) How many times have you been pregnant? How many children do you have?
- (Women) Do you examine your breasts? How often?
- What method of contraception do you use? Is this method acceptable to you and your partner?
- Have you ever been diagnosed as having a sexually transmitted disease (syphilis, gonorrhea, genital herpes, chlamydia, or AIDS)?
- Many (men, women) in your situation have questions about how their illness or surgery will affect the sexual aspects of their lives. What questions do you have?
- Has your (illness, surgery, disability) interfered with your being a (mother, wife, husband, father)?
- Has anything changed your ability to function sexually?

Objective Data

Objective data concerning sexual–reproductive function can be obtained through examination of the breasts and the reproductive organs. Breast examination is important in early detection of breast cancer. Breast examination should be conducted as a joint activity of the patient and the nurse, with the nurse's primary role as educator. Although breast cancer is rare in men, a brief examination of the male breast is also appropriate. Examinations of female internal reproductive organs is not commonly part of the basic health assessment unless the nurse is working in a specialized area such as labor and delivery.

Inspection. The patient should be taught to inspect the breasts during any breast examination. The nurse

should instruct the patient to stand before a mirror and observe the breasts in three different positions: with the arms to the side; with the arms clasped behind the head and the hands pressing forward; and leaning forward with hands pressing firmly on the hips. Normal breasts appear rounded, and essentially symmetric, although one breast is often slightly larger than the other. The skin should be smooth and intact with the areola darker in color, round, and symmetric. The nipple should be everted and without discharge or lesions. Abnormal findings with inspection include flattening, bulges or changes in breast size, marked asymmetry, redness, dimpling, and edema.

Inspection of the female external reproductive organs includes the labia minora, the labia majora, clitoris, and vaginal opening. The color of these organs should be pink, with some blue or brown pigments occasionally seen. Bright red color or obvious areas of excoriation are abnormal and often occur in the presence of infection. Normal vaginal secretions, which are white, colorless, and odorless, may be noted. Foul smelling, purulent drainage is abnormal.

Inspection of the external male reproductive organs include the glans, foreskin and shaft of the penis, and the scrotum. The man may be circumcised or uncircumcised. If uncircumcised, the foreskin must be gently retracted during the examination to inspect the glans and the urethral opening. The size of the penis can vary among men, but inspection should reveal no lesions or abnormal discharge. Smegma is a normal white discharge that may collect around the glans, especially in the uncircumcised man. The scrotal sac is wrinkled in appearance, with the left scrotal sac usually hanging lower than the right.

Palpation. Palpation is used in examining the reproductive structures to determine possible underlying abnormalities in the breast or scrotum. The breast should be palpated with the patient in the supine position with hands behind the head. Palpate each breast for tenderness, nodules, or masses. The nurse should use three or four fingers, pressing the flat part of the fingers in small circles, moving the circles slowly around the breast. A sequential pattern of palpation should be followed so that all areas in the breast are included. Begin at the outer edge of the breast gradually working toward the nipple (Fig. 18-18). Also the area between the breast and the axilla should be examined. The final step in breast examination is gentle squeezing of the nipple to check for discharge.

Self breast palpation should be performed with the woman standing and lying down, with the arm of the breast being examined over the head. Teaching of breast self-examination is illustrated in Chapter 48. The woman can be taught the skills during the health assessment by the nurse.

Palpation of the male genitalia is performed to detect

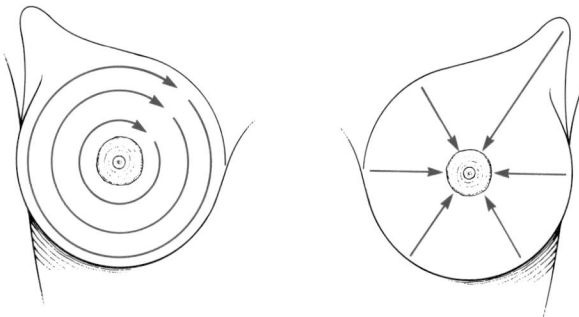

Figure 18–18. Breast examination. Begin at the outer edge and gradually work toward the nipple. **A.** Clockwise approach. **B.** Spoke approach.

the presence of the testicle in each scrotal sac and the absence of pain, swelling, or growths. The testicles should feel round, smooth, and freely movable within the scrotum. Testicular self-examination is discussed and illustrated in Chapter 48.

ASSESSMENT OF VALUES AND BELIEFS

Assessment of values and beliefs is also referred to as a spiritual assessment because it focuses on the spiritual dimension of life. Spirituality may be defined as the quality that transcends the physical world, permeates and unifies a person's entire being, and gives life purpose, meaning, and importance. Spirituality usually, but not always, involves a belief and relationship with a higher being or God. Values and beliefs emerge from a person's sense of spirituality and guide the opinions about what is right, good, proper, and meaningful. Values help determine choices about the conduct of one's life, including health-related decisions concerning personal practices, treatments, and even life or death. The spiritual realm is one aspect of being human that often comes into focus during illness or crisis.

Illness, injury, loss, aging, and disability are spiritual as well as physical and emotional experiences. Serious or life-threatening illness often triggers a person's first encounter with mortality. Crisis often provides the motivation to question one's life, goals, and what is important.

Because body, mind, and spirit are intertwined, distress in any one area affects the health of the whole person. Spiritual distress can adversely affect a person's response to illness and treatment, and the ability to cope effectively with the crisis. Conversely, spiritual contentment can have an equally positive influence. Prayer and other religious practices are stabilizing forces in many peoples' lives. Prayer can affirm God's presence, inspire courage, and lessen feelings of abandonment. A nurse who understands a patient's spiritual beliefs is better prepared to support coping strategies and provide the resources that are spiritually helpful to the patient.

Assessment of values and beliefs focuses on the significance of religious affiliation and religious practices; the spiritual needs of the patient and the resources available to meet those needs; and the relationship between spiritual beliefs and the present state of health.

Subjective Data

Spiritual values, like sexual values and practices, are emotionally laden for both the nurse and the patient. It is advisable to discuss this pattern toward the end of the assessment along with other psychological issues. By this time, the nurse has become established as a sensitive, helpful professional and has a sense of the patient's willingness to share personal information. Mention of spiritual beliefs may arise during the discussion of coping–stress tolerance pattern. If this occurs, the nurse can smoothly direct the conversation toward the value–belief pattern.

The following interview questions may be used to discuss the value–belief pattern:

- Is religion or God significant to you? If yes, can you describe how?
- Are there any religious practices that are important to you? What religious books or symbols are helpful? Is prayer helpful to you?
- Has being sick made any difference in your relationship with God or your practice of your faith?
- Would you like to speak with a chaplain (priest, minister, rabbi)?

Objective Data

Assessment of the value–belief pattern depends primarily on subjective data. However, visible expression of spiritual values is sometimes present. The nurse may notice religious articles such as a Bible, prayer book, or rosary in the room of a hospitalized patient. The nurse may also observe the patient in prayer, either alone or with family, friends, or clergy.

CONCLUDING THE ASSESSMENT

The nurse should bring formal closure to his or her interaction with the patient when the assessment is completed. The nurse summarizes the findings and evaluates the patient's primary problems and concerns. The patient may want to add to or correct the nurse's conclusions. Sharing this information validates the nurse's impressions and clarifies any misunderstandings between the nurse and the patient. The nurse should explain, particularly to the hospitalized patient, that assessment of his or her condition and needs is ongoing. The nurse should encourage the patient to volunteer additional or new information as changes occur. Assessment findings

Nursing Research

Selected Nursing Research Studies

Barnfather, J. (1989, Winter). Evaluation of two assessment techniques for adaptation to stress. *Nursing Science Quarterly, 2*(7), 172–182.

Beyea, S., et al. (1989, September/October). Assessing elders using the functional health pattern assessment model. *Nurse Education 14*(5), 32–37.

Derdiarian, A. K. (1990, January–February). Effects of using systematic assessment instruments on patient and nurse satisfaction with nursing care. *Oncologic Nursing Forum, 17*(1), 95–101.

Levin, R. F., et al. (1989). A comparison of assessment and diagnostic competencies of B.S. and A.D. nurses. *Classif Nurs Diagn Seventh Conference*, pp. 447–452.

Takahashi, J. J., et al. (1989, November). Preoperative nursing assessment: a research study. *AORN Journal, 50*(5), 1022, 1024–1029, 1031–1032.

Wilbur, J. E. (1989, September–October). Evaluation of health assessment skills. *Journal of Continuing Education Nurs, 20*(5), 212–216.

Possible Topics for Nursing Inquiry

- How often do staff nurses use percussion to determine bladder distention on postoperative patients?
- How does patient's perception of nurse interviewer differ when nurse sits rather than stands during the collection of subjective data?
- What role does intuition play in directing advanced practitioner versus beginning practitioner in interviewing technique during admission assessment?
- What is the significance of privacy in obtaining subjective data during a patient interview?
- How does the functional health approach compare with the body systems approach to nursing assessment in obtaining accurate information to support nursing diagoses?
- How effective is clinical simulation in refining physical assessment techniques?

should be documented in the patient's chart by the nurse in a legible, concise fashion according to agency protocol. Chapter 10 discusses documentation.

LIFESPAN CONSIDERATIONS

In planning and focusing a functional health assessment, it is important to consider developmental and age-related factors. The nurse should be knowledgeable about common problems of each age group, so that appropriate screening measures that permit early detection can be included. It is also important to be aware of the cognitive development of the person so that questions can be phrased appropriately. Understanding the emotional development of the patient helps the nurse plan the examination to be less traumatic and anxiety provoking.

Newborn and Infant

Nursing assessment is made shortly after birth and at 24 hours of age. If parents are present during the assessment, the nurse should explain what the examination includes and why it is being performed. Whenever possible, parents should be reassured that findings are normal. Permitting parents to see their newborn and participate can help parent bonding and allay fears.

During the first year of life, the infant is frequently examined by a nurse for well-baby examinations. This is a wonderful opportunity to educate the parents on a variety of infant care topics. It is important to assure parents of the wide range of normal growth and development and to allow time to discuss any concerns they may have about their child.

Keeping the newborn infant properly covered during the physical examination is important to prevent a drop in body temperature. During the first year of life, head and chest circumference are measured, the baby is weighed, and reflexes are tested. When examining any infant, it is important to finish inspection and auscultation before doing any invasive procedure. Such techniques can frighten the child or cause pain, which may induce the infant to cry. The nurse should encourage the parent to hold the infant during the examination to decrease fear and help the child feel more secure. The infant should never be left on an examining table without being properly guarded. Infants can move quickly and fall. The infant must be properly restrained when the nurse is looking into his or her ears, eyes, nose or throat, so that quick movements do not result in injury.

Safety Alert

- Always hold an infant on an examining table and restrain during invasive assessment procedures to avoid injury upon sudden movement of the child.
- Never palpate the abdomen of a patient complaining of sudden, severe abdomial pain because this could rupture an inflamed appendix causing peritonitis.
- When listening to breath sounds, give the patient rest periods to avoid hyperventilation because this could cause dizziness and syncope.
- Never palpate both carotid arteries at the same time because blood flow to the brain can be occluded.
- Don't leave confused or unstable patients alone on an examining table because they may try to get down and fall.

Toddler and Preschooler

The young child is often afraid to be examined and may associate physical examination with the discomfort of invasive procedures or getting injections. Encouraging the parent to assist by holding and comforting the child during the examination can be helpful. The nurse should explain in simple terms what he or she plans to do; demonstrating how equipment works can help alleviate some anxiety in this age group (Fig. 18-19A). Allowing the child to touch the stethoscope or see the shinning light of the otoscope can help prepare the child for examination procedures. For some children, it may be helpful to use a puppet (see Fig. 18-19B) or allow them to role play examining a doll or stuffed animal. It is important not to lie to children. If the child is going to experience pain, it is best to say, "This will hurt for a while, but you can squeeze your mom's hand and yell as loud as you want." Whenever possible, the nurse should perform uncomfortable procedures immediately so that anxiety does not escalate.

School Age and Adolescent

As the child ages, more of the assessment questions can be directed specifically to the child. The nurse should use vocabulary that the child can understand when asking questions or explaining procedures. The nurse should encourage the child to ask questions. Whenever possible, the child should be given simple choices. The child can be distracted during the examination through conversation or playing simple games. Some children are

ticklish, especially when the abdomen is examined. Children at this age can be modest, so proper draping and measures to ensure privacy are important.

Adolescence is a period of rapid physical and emotional development. During this time period, the youth is often examined alone, unaccompanied by a parent. Sensitive questioning and honestly answering any questions the teen asks develop good rapport. Because sexual maturation occurs during this period of time, the examination includes examination of sexual organs and appropriate health teaching. The nurse should discuss any concerns the adolescent has about the maturation process.

Adult and Older Adult

By the time the person has reached adulthood, multiple exposures to physical examination and assessment have

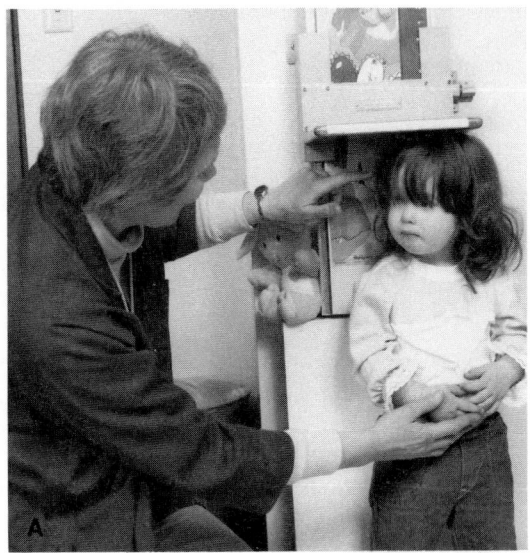

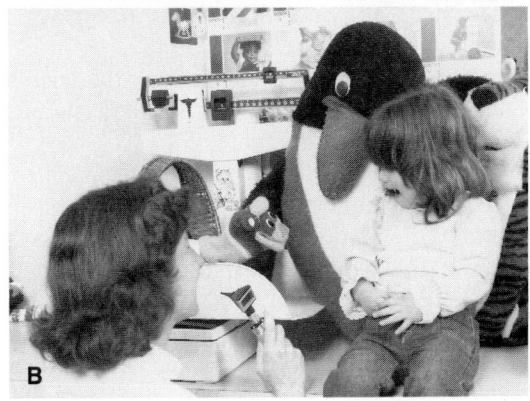

Figure 18–19.   Assessment of a toddler.   **A.** Even the simple activity of weighing or measuring a child should be explained first. The nurse holds a protective hand in front of the child in case the child makes a sudden movement.   **B.** The nurse uses a hand puppet to distract the child while performing other routine procedures.

occurred. Some adults still are apprehensive and feel invasion of privacy during assessment procedures. It is important to prepare the patient for all procedures and provide for privacy. Health teaching regarding desirable screening measures, such as breast self-examination, testicular self-examination, and routine gynecologic examinations, should be included in the health examination for the adult.

During later years of adulthood, a person may have chronic health problems that necessitate adaptation of the physical assessment. Arthritic joints or decreased mobility may make getting onto an examination table more difficult. Holding various positions required for examination, especially for long periods of time, may be tiring. Lengthy examinations may be fatiguing and should be planned when the patient is well rested, if possible. Hearing loss may necessitate speaking more loudly and clearly to facilitate communication. The elderly person can easily become chilled, so proper draping in a warm examination room is important for patient comfort.

Key Concepts

- A functional health assessment is the collection of subjective and objective data concerning functional ability.
- The purpose of the functional health assessment is to identify normal functional abilities, risk factors that can contribute to dysfunction, and actual dysfunctional states or problems.
- Adequate psychological and physical preparation of the patient is important for effective assessment.
- The nurse uses interviewing techniques to obtain subjective (patient perception) data concerning each functional health pattern.
- Objective data are collected through the techniques of inspection, palpation, percussion, and auscultation during the physical examination.
- The focus of a functional health assessment by the nurse is to determine normal and abnormal aspects of function, the patient's degree of satisfaction with function, the patient's adaptation to dysfunctional patterns, and the effect of function on performing activities of daily living.
- Assessment of health-perception and health-management should focus on the patient's perception of health status, preventive health practices, compliance with medical treatment, and safety.
- Assessment of activity and exercise should focus on mobility, self-care, energy level, activity tolerance, oxygenation, and circulation.
- Objective data are collected concerning musculoskeletal function in the areas of gait and balance,

muscle strength, joint mobility, independence in self-care activities, and any assistive devices that are used.
- Respiratory and cardiac function are evaluated through inspection, palpation, percussion, and auscultation using normal landmarks of the thorax.
- Assessment of nutrition and metabolism should focus on food and fluid intake in relationship to metabolic demands, skin integrity, and wound healing.
- Assessment of elimination should focus on normal excretory function (bowel and bladder) and specific management to assist normal function.
- Assessment of cognition and perception should focus on cognitive functions such as memory, language, reasoning, problem solving, pain level, and sensory-perceptual capabilities such as vision and hearing.
- Assessment of sleep and rest involves eliciting the patient's perception of sleep, rest, and relaxation.
- Assessment of self-perception and self-concept focuses on the patient's perception of self, such as body image and sense of worth.
- Assessment of roles and relationships describes the quality of a person's family, work, and social roles.
- Assessment of coping and stress tolerance describes current stressors the patient is experiencing, past coping methods, and the effectiveness of current coping methods.
- Assessment of sexuality and reproduction describes reproductive function, sexual role, and the impact of current health status on sexual role function.
- Assessment of values and beliefs includes the significance of religious affiliation and religious practices, resources available to meet the spiritual health needs of the patient, and the relationship between spiritual beliefs and the current state of health.
- Lifespan considerations are important in individualizing assessment techniques to obtain important information from the patient.

References

Bates, B. A. (1987). *Guide to physical examination and history taking* (4th ed.). Philadelphia: J. B. Lippincott.
Fuller, J. & Schaller-Ayers, J. (1990). *Health assessment: A nursing approach.* Philadelphia: J. B. Lippincott.
Holmes, T. H. & Rahe, R. H. (1967). The social readjustment rating scale. *Journal of Psychosomatic Research, 11*(2), 213–218.
Lambert, V. A. & Lambert, C. E. (1985). *Psychosocial care of the physically ill: What every nurse should know* (2nd ed.). Englewood Cliffs: Prentice Hall.
McHugh, J. & McHugh, W. (1990, August). How to assess deep tendon reflexes. *Nursing '90, 20*(8), 62–64.
National Data Book and Guide to Sources. (1986). *Statistical abstract of the United States* (106th ed.). Washington, D.C.: U.S. Department of Commerce, Bureau of the Census.
Panicucci, C. L. (1983). Functional assessment of the older adult in the acute care setting. Symposium on Gerontologic Nursing in Acute Care. *Nursing Clinics of North America, 18*(2), 355–363.
Piers, E. V. & Harris, D. B. (1969). *Piers-Harris children's self-concept scale.* Nashville: Counselor Recording and Tests.
Rosenberg, M. (1979). *Concerning the self.* New York: Basic Books.
Wallston, B. S., Wallston, K. A., & DeVellis, R. (1978, Spring). Development and validation of the health locus of control (HCL) scales. *Health Education Monograph, 6*, 160–170.

Bibliography

Barnfather, J. S., et al. (1989, Winter). Evaluation of two assessment techniques for adaptation to stress. *Nursing Science Quarterly, 2*(7), 172–182.

Beyea, S., & Matzo, M.: (1989, September–October). Assessing elders using the functional health pattern assessment model. *Nurse Educator, 14*(5), 32–37.

Brigdon, P., & Todd, M.: (1990, January). In search of the perfect assessment. *Professional Nurse, 5*(4), 181–184.

Collinsworth, R., & Boyle, K.: (1989, December). Nutritional assessment of the elderly. *Journal of Gerontologic Nursing, 15*(12), 17–21, 38, 39.

Carlson, K. (1989, November). Assessing a child's chest. *RN, 52*(11), 26–32.

Calloway, C. K. (1990, April). Zeroing in on chest pain. *Nursing '90, 20*(4), 44, 45.

Derdiarian, A. K. (1990, January–February). Effects of using systematic assessment instruments on patient and nurse satisfaction with nursing care. *Oncology Nursing Forum, 17*(1), 95–101.

Fuller, J. & Schaller-Ayers, J. (1990). *Health assessment: A nursing approach.* Philadelphia: J. B. Lippincott.

Gabriel, R. M., & Kirschling, J. M.: (1989). Assessing grief among the bereaved elderly: A review of existing measures. *Hospice Journal, 5*(1), 29–54.

Gordin, P. C. (1990, January–February). Assessing and managing agitation in a critically ill infant. *MCN, 15*(1), 26–32.

Halloran, E. J. (1988, November–December). Computerized nurse assessments. *Nursing and Health Care, 9*(9), 496–499.

Kaufman, J. (1990, June). Nurse's guide to assessing the twelve cranial nerves. *Nursing '90, 20*(6), 56–58.

Levin, R. F., et al. (1987). A comparison of assessment and diagnostic competencies of B.S. and A.D. nurses. *Classification of Nursing Diagnoses.* Proceedings of the Seventh Conference of the North American Nursing Diagnosis Association. St. Louis: North American Nursing Diagnosis Association, pp. 447–452.

McConnell, E. A. (1990, March). Assessing abdominal pain in a postoperative patient. *Nursing '90, 20*(3), 86–88.

Morrison-Beedy, D., & Robbins, L.: (1989, December). Sexual assessment of the aging female. *Nurse Practitioner, 14*(12)35, 38, 39, 42+ .

Mulhearn, S. (1989, October). The nursing process: Improving psychiatric admission assessment. *Journal of Advanced Nursing, 14*(10), 808–814.

Rosenberg, A., et al. (1989, November–December). Neurological assessment of the multiple trauma patient. *Orthopedic Nursing, 8*(6), 49–55.

Rossi, L. (1987). Organizing data for nursing diagnosis using functional health patterns. *Classification of Nursing Diagnoses.* Proceedings of the Seventh Conference of the North American Nursing Diagnosis Association. St. Louis: North American Nursing Diagnosis Association, pp. 97–101.

Takahashi, J. J., et al. (1989, November). Preoperative nursing assessment: A research study. *AORN Journal, 50*(5), 1022, 1024–1029, 1031, 1032.

Thompson C. (1989, December). The nursing assessment of the patient with cardiac pain on the coronary care unit. *Intensive Care Nursing, 5*(4), 147–154.

Tripp, S. (1984). Development of a nursing diagnosis health assessment tool. Proceedings of the Fifth Conference of the North American Nursing Diagnosis Association. St. Louis: North American Nursing Diagnosis Association, pp. 425-332.

Wilbur, J. E. (1989, September–October). Evaluation of health assessment skills. *Journal of Continuing Education in Nursing, 20*(5), 212–216.

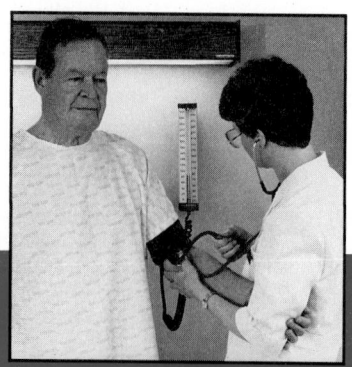

Vital Sign Assessment

19

Body Temperature
    Factors Affecting Body Temperature
    Factors Affecting Body Temperature Measurement
    Assessing Temperature
        Sites
        Equipment
        Scales
        Methods
Pulse
    Characteristics
    Factors Affecting Pulse Rate
    Assessing the Pulse
        Sites
        Methods
        Equipment
        Assessing Pulse Characteristics
Respirations

Factors Affecting Respirations
Assessing Respirations
    Characteristics
    Methods for Measuring Respiratory Rate
Blood Pressure
    Physiologic Factors Determining Blood Pressure
        Blood Flow
        Resistance
    Factors Affecting Blood Pressure
    Assessing Blood Pressure
        Sites
        Equipment
        Methods
        Abnormalities
Lifespan Considerations
Documenting Vital Signs
Key Concepts

Vital signs—body temperature (T), pulse (P), respirations (R), and blood pressure (BP)—are the foundation for clinical decision-making. The vital signs indicate the function of the body's homeostatic mechanisms. Assessment of a patient begins by measuring and interpreting the vital signs.

Typical or normal values for vital signs have been established for patients of various ages (Table 19-1). During initial measurement of a patient's vital signs, the values are compared to the normal ranges to determine any variation that might indicate illness. When several sets of vital signs have been obtained, this information forms a baseline against which subsequent measurements can be compared. Isolated vital sign values are not as helpful; the nurse should evaluate a series of values and establish trends for the patient. Vital sign trends that deviate from normal are much more significant than isolated abnormal values.

The tasks involved in measuring vital signs are simple and easily learned, but interpreting the measurements and incorporating them into ongoing care and assessment requires knowledge, problem-solving skill, and experience. Although vital signs are often part of routine care, they provide valuable information and should not be taken lightly.

The frequency with which vital signs are assessed should be individualized for each patient. For example, very ill patients have their vital signs monitored more frequently than patients who are less ill. Young patients and elderly patients also have their vital signs checked more frequently. Patients seen in outpatient settings, wellness clinics, or psychiatric institutions may require infrequent vital sign checks. Most inpatient settings have a policy regarding the minimum frequency of vital sign assessment. In addition, physicians order vital signs to be checked at specific intervals, based on the patient's condition. Ultimately, however, the nurse caring for the patient is the best judge of how often vital signs should be obtained.

BODY TEMPERATURE

Humans are warm-blooded creatures, which means they can maintain internal body temperature without regard to the outside environment. The body's tissues and cells

TABLE 19–1

Normal Vital Signs Ranges

	Pulse	Respirations	Temperature (° F)	Blood Pressure (mm Hg)	
				Systolic	*Diastolic*
Newborn (> 96 hours)	70–190	30–60	96–99.5	60–90	20–60
Infant (> 1 month)	80–160	30–60	99.4–99.7	74–100	50–70
Toddler	80–130	24–40	99–99.7	80–112	50–80
Preschooler	80–120	22–34	98.6–99	82–110	50–78
School-age	75–110	18–30	98–98.6	84–120	54–80
Adolescent	60–90	12–20	97–99	94–140	62–88
Adult	60–100	12–20	97–99	90–140	60–90
Older adult (> 70 yrs)	60–100	12–20	96–99	90–140	60–90

are best able to function within a relatively narrow temperature range. The body's surface or skin temperature can vary widely with environmental conditions and physical activity. Despite these fluctuations, the temperature of the inside of the body, the **core temperature,** remains relatively constant, unless the patient develops a febrile illness. The body's organs require this constant internal temperature for optimal functioning.

Although the normal adult temperature ranges from 36.1°C to 37.2°C (97°F to 99°F) taken orally, body temperature can fluctuate with exercise, changes in hormone levels, and extremes of external temperature. Rectal temperatures are usually higher than oral temperatures by 0.6°C (1°F) (Guyton, 1986). Oral temperatures, taken correctly, are thought to best reflect the core temperature (Erickson, 1980).

Regulation of the body temperature requires the coordination of many body systems. For the core temperature to remain normal, heat production must equal heat loss. The hypothalamus, part of the central nervous system, is the body's built-in thermostat. It can sense small changes in body temperature and stimulates the necessary changes in the nervous system, circulatory system, skin, sweat glands, or shivering mechanism to maintain homeostasis. Chapter 36 describes the regulation of body temperature in detail.

Factors Affecting Body Temperature

Several factors can affect body temperature and knowing these factors helps the nurse accurately assess the significance of body temperature variations.

Age. Infants have unstable body temperatures because their thermoregulatory mechanisms are immature. Temperature instability continues into adolescence and then stabilizes. Normal temperature drops as a person ages (Kurtz, 1982): it is not uncommon for an elderly person to have a body temperature as low as 35°C (95°F), especially in cold weather. When evaluating low-grade temperatures in the elderly and identifying those at risk

for hypothermia, it is important to remember that lower temperatures are associated with older age.

Environment. Ordinarily, changes in environmental temperatures do not affect core temperature because of our internal regulatory mechanisms (Kolanski, 1981), but exposure to extremely hot or cold temperatures can alter body temperature. The degree of change is related to the temperature, humidity, and length of exposure. It is also influenced by the body's thermoregulatory mechanisms; for example, infants and the elderly often have diminished control mechanisms (Kolanski, 1981). When the body is exposed to temperatures below 33°C (91.4°F), the body's ability to adjust is impaired (Vick, 1984), and the body cannot maintain a normal temperature. As the core temperature drops to 25°C (77°F), death may occur.

Time of Day. Body temperature normally fluctuates throughout the day. Temperature is usually lowest from 1 to 4 AM and highest from 4 to 6 PM. A person's body temperature can vary as much as 2°C (1.8°F) from early morning to late afternoon (Samples, 1985). In the past it was believed that this variation was related to variation in muscle activity and digestive processes, which are usually minimal in the early morning while people sleep. However, it has been found that there is no direct relationship between circadian rhythm and body temperature (Vick, 1985). In some humans, the situation is reversed and body temperature is increased at night and decreased during the day. There is even greater variation in body temperature at various times of the day in infants and children.

Exercise. Body temperature increases with exercise because exercise increases heat production. Strenuous exercise can temporarily raise the temperature as high as 40°C (104°F) (Guyton, 1986).

Stress. Emotional or physical stress can elevate body temperature. When stress stimulates the sympathetic nervous system, circulating levels of epinephrine and

---

Safety Alert

- Do not take oral temperatures in infants, young children, or unconscious or irrational patients, since they cannot follow directions and may bite down or choke on the thermometer.
- Do not take rectal temperatures in infants, since rectal perforation or mucosal damage may occur.
- If a glass thermometer accidently breaks, avoid contact with the mercury and call environmental services (or the designated group) for safe disposal.
- When taking a rectal temperature, to prevent trauma lubricate the thermometer generously and insert gently, especially if hemorrhoids are present.
- When palpating the carotid artery, palpate in the lower half of the neck to avoid stimulating the

carotid sinus, which can result in bradycardia and syncope.
- Do not palpate bilateral carotid pulses simultaneously, since this can seriously impair blood flow to the brain.
- When checking for orthostatic hypotension, assist the patient from a lying to a sitting to a standing position and monitor carefully for dizziness or difficulty maintaining balance. If the patient appears unsteady, return the patient to the supine position immediately.
- When using an automatic blood pressure device for serial blood pressure readings, check the cuffed limb frequently to ensure adequate arterial perfusion and venous drainage between measurements.

---

norepinephrine are increased. As a result, the metabolic rate is increased, which in turn increases heat production. Stressed or anxious patients may have an elevated temperature without underlying pathology.

Hormones. Women usually have greater variations in their temperature than do men. Progesterone, a female hormone secreted at ovulation, increases body temperature by 0.3°C to 0.6°C (0.5°F to 1°F) above baseline temperature. By measuring their temperature daily, women can determine when they ovulate; this is the basis for the rhythm method of birth control. Thyroxine, epinephrine, and norepinephrine also elevate body temperature, by increasing heat production (Shaver, 1991).

Factors Affecting Body Temperature Measurement

Smoking. If body temperature is measured orally immediately after a patient has been smoking, the measurement may be altered by -0.2 ± 0.2°F (Woodman, Perry, & Simms, 1967).

Oxygen Administration. For years it was thought that the increased air current directed at the nasal passage decreased the temperature of the mouth. But numerous studies have found minimal differences (-0.4 ± 0.69°F) in patients receiving oxygen by mask or cannula (Dressler, 1983; Lim-Levy, 1982; Yonkman, 1982).

Drinking Hot or Cold Liquids. Drinking hot or cold liquids may cause slight variations in oral temperature readings; the most marked variation is found after drink-

ing ice water (-0.2°F to -1.6°F) (Woodman, Perry, & Simms, 1967).

Assessing Temperature

Temperature measurement is a routine part of vital sign evaluation. It is done to establish a baseline so that comparisons can be made as a disease progresses or therapies are instituted. The reliability of a temperature value depends on choosing the correct equipment, selecting the most appropriate site, and using the correct procedure. The nurse must ensure that the thermometer is placed correctly and is left in place the appropriate length of time.

Sites

Nurses should use their judgment in selecting the route by which temperature is measured. The three sites most commonly used are the mouth, rectum, and axilla. In most clinical situations, any of the three sites is satisfactory if proper technique is used and normal variations are considered for the different sites. Additional sites are the esophagus and pulmonary artery, both of which are considered core temperatures. Normal temperature varies within a person, from person to person, and from site to site (Table 19-2).

Oral. The most common site for temperature measurement is the oral route. Advantages of this route include easy access and patient comfort. Because the temperature measurement could be affected if the person has had hot or cold liquids or has been smoking, the

TABLE 19–2

Normal Temperatures for Adults Obtained from Different Sites

Oral	Axillary	Rectal	Esophogeal/ Pulmonary Artery
37°C	36.5°C	37.5°C	37.3°C
98.6°F	97.6°F	99.5°F	99.2°F

nurse should wait 30 minutes before placing the thermometer in these situations. This allows the mouth temperature to return to baseline.

The oral route is contraindicated in some situations. It should not be used in people who cannot follow instructions to keep their mouths closed, who are mouth breathing, or who might bite down and break the thermometer. Oral temperature assessment, especially with a glass thermometer, may not be prudent or safe in infants, young children, unconscious patients, irrational patients, or patients with seizure disorders.

Rectal. The rectal route is believed to be the most reliable, as few factors can artificially influence the reading. Rectal temperatures are recommended for patients who cannot have their temperatures taken orally, or when an oral temperature changes quickly or unexpectedly. Care should be taken to avoid placing the thermometer into fecal material, as this may falsely elevate the temperature reading. This route is contraindicated in patients with diarrhea, those who have undergone rectal surgery, or those with diseases of the rectum. It is also contraindicated in infants, as it may cause trauma to the rectal mucosa. Some adult patients may be uncomfortable having their temperature taken rectally, so careful explanation of the rationale for this route is important.

Axillary. The axillary route is considered the least accurate and least reliable of all the sites because the temperature obtained using this route can be influenced by a number of factors. For example, if the patient has recently bathed, the temperature may reflect the temperature of water used. If friction was used to dry the skin, the friction may influence the temperature. The axillary route is the recommended route for infants and children and is the route of choice in patients who cannot have their temperatures measured by the oral or rectal route.

Equipment

Several types of thermometers are available. Traditionally, all temperature monitoring was done using a glass mercury thermometer, but advances in technology have provided quicker, more sanitary methods.

Glass Mercury Thermometer. The glass thermometer used to be the most commonly used type of thermometer, and it is still used in many homes. It is a slender glass tube that is sealed at one end and has a bulb of mercury at the other end. It should be handled only at the sealed end because touching the mercury bulb could influence the temperature reading. The tube is calibrated in degrees, using the Celsius or Fahrenheit scale. Exposing the bulb to heat causes the mercury to expand and rise to a point on the scale. The mercury stabilizes at this point and does not fall unless the thermometer is shaken vigorously. The temperature is read by holding the thermometer at eye level and noting the location of the mercury on the scale. Figure 19-1 shows the correct way to hold a thermometer to obtain an accurate reading.

Two types of glass thermometers are shown in Figure 19-2. The tip of the oral thermometer is slender and allows for maximal exposure to the oral mucosa. The rectal thermometer tip is blunt to decrease the risk of trauma to the rectal mucosa. Often the tips are color-coded (blue for oral and red for rectal) to avoid mixups. The oral thermometer may also be used for axillary temperature measurement.

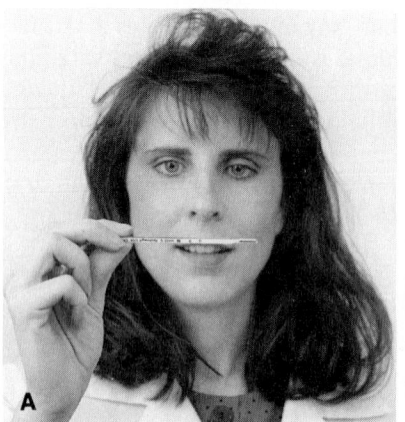
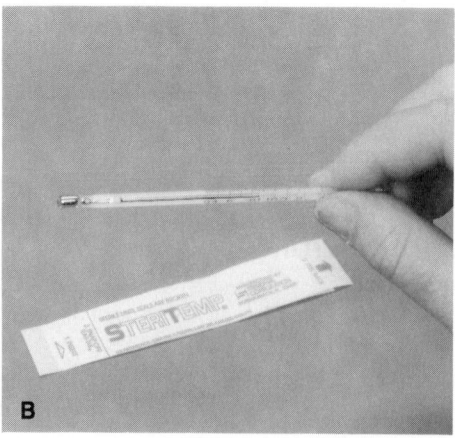

Figure 19–1. To read a glass thermometer correctly, the nurse holds it at eye level **A** and turns it to note the location of the mercury on the scale **B.**

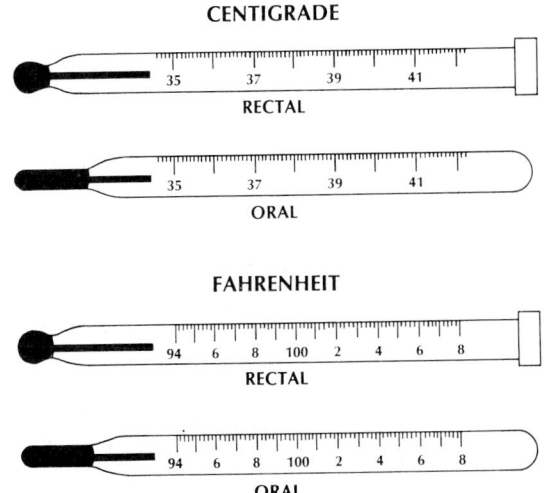

CENTIGRADE

RECTAL

ORAL

FAHRENHEIT

RECTAL

ORAL

Figure 19–2. The two glass thermometers on the top use the centigrade scale to measure temperature; the two on the bottom use the Fahrenheit scale. Note the blunt bulbs on the rectal thermometers and the long thin bulbs on the oral thermometers.

Electronic Thermometers. The electronic thermometer is the most widely used thermometer in hospitals today. There are many types on the market but all have similar characteristics (Fig. 19-3). The thermometer consists of a battery-powered display unit and a temperature-sensitive probe connected to the display unit by a thin cord. When used, the probe is covered by a disposable plastic sheath to prevent the transmission of infection. These thermometers provide a reading in less than 60 seconds and are thought to be most accurate if placed in the sublingual pocket (Erikson, 1980). Results may be displayed in Celsius or Fahrenheit; some thermometers can display both. The electronic thermometer is ideally suited for use with children because the sheath is un-

breakable and the time necessary for accurate measurement is short.

Disposable Paper Thermometers. Single-use paper thermometers (Fig. 19-4) are thin strips of chemically treated paper. They have raised dots that change color to reflect the temperature, usually in less than a minute. These thermometers are available in Celsius or Fahrenheit scales.

Temperature-Sensitive Strips. Temperature-sensitive strips, the newest piece of equipment for measuring temperature, can be used to obtain a general indication of body surface temperature. They are usually placed on the forehead or abdomen; the skin under the strip must be dry. After a specified length of time, the strip changes color. On one brand, a green "N" indicates a normal temperature, a brown "N" indicates a transition phase, and a blue-green "F" indicates an elevated temperature. The transition phase reflects the onset of a high temperature in the area where the strip was placed. The strip is removed and discarded after the color change has been noted. This method is particularly useful at home. Because children under 2 years of age still have immature thermoregulatory systems, any variation from normal should be confirmed using a standard thermometer.

Scales

Temperature can be measured on the Celsius or Fahrenheit scale (Fig. 19-5). The scale used varies from institution to institution. Nurses do not routinely have to convert from one scale to the other, because individual institutions generally use only one scale. But if conversion is necessary, simple formulas can be used. To change Celsius into Fahrenheit, multiply the Celsius reading by 9/5 and add 32 to the result.

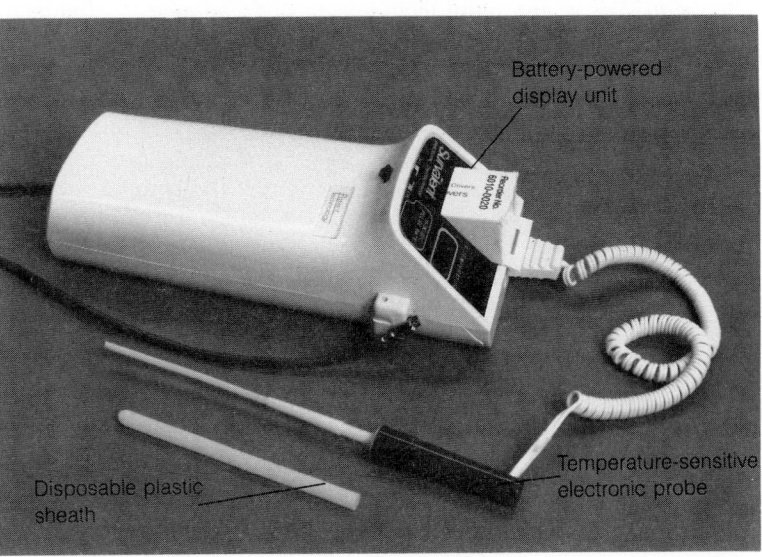

Battery-powered display unit

Disposable plastic sheath

Temperature-sensitive electronic probe

Figure 19–3. Electronic thermometer.

$$F = (9/5 \times C°) + 32°$$

For example:

$$F = (9/5 \times 37°) + 32° = (66.6°) + 32° = 98.6° \, F$$

To change Fahrenheit into Celsius, subtract 32 from the Fahrenheit reading and multiply the result by 5/9.

$$C = (F° - 32°) \times 5/9$$

For example:

$$C = (102° - 32°) \times 5/9 = (70) \times 5/9 = 38.8° \, C$$

Methods

The nurse is responsible for taking temperatures, documenting the results, and reporting abnormal values to the physician. After selecting the most appropriate method of measurement, the nurse should gather the necessary equipment and explain the procedure to the patient. See Procedure 19-1 for specific details on how to obtain a temperature measurement using each of the different routes and equipment.

PULSE

Contraction of the ventricles of the heart ejects blood into the arteries. The force of the blood entering the aorta from the left ventricle causes stretching or distention of the elastic aortic wall. As the aorta first expands then contracts, a pulse wave is created that travels along the blood vessels. The pulse wave or pulsation can be felt as a throb or tap where the arteries lie close to the skin surface.

Characteristics

Characteristics of the pulse include rate or frequency, rhythm, and quality. Rate or frequency refers to the

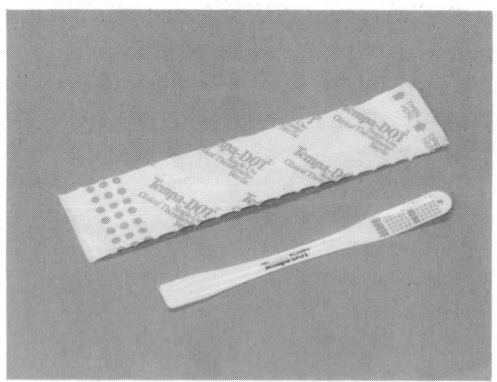

Figure 19-4. Disposable paper thermometer. The dots change color to indicate temperature.

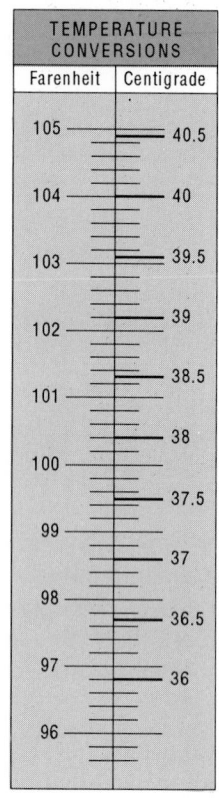

Figure 19-5. Temperature conversion chart.

number of pulsations per minute. Pulse rhythm refers to the regularity with which pulsation occurs. Pulse quality refers to the strength of the palpated pulsation.

The rate and rhythm of the pulse are established by specialized cells that make up the conduction system of the heart. The stimulus for contraction of the heart normally starts as an electrical impulse in the sinoatrial node (SA node) of the right atrium. In adults, the SA node initiates the impulse 60 to 100 times per minute. The electrical impulse then spreads quickly through the conduction system to the remainder of the heart so that the heart muscle fibers contract in a synchronous fashion. Irregularities of heart rhythm usually indicate a failure in the conduction system or origination of an impulse in a site other than the SA node.

The quality of the arterial pulse is determined by factors such as the force with which blood is ejected from the ventricles, the amount of blood ejected with each heartbeat (the **stroke volume**), and the patency and compliance or elasticity of the arteries.

Factors Affecting Pulse Rate

Age. The average pulse rate of an infant ranges from 100 to 160 beats per minute. The heart rhythm in infants and children often varies markedly with respiration, increasing during inspiration and decreasing with expiration. The normal range of the pulse in an adult is 60 to

PROCEDURE 19-1. Assessing Body Temperature

■ Purpose
1. Obtain baseline data against which future measurements can be compared.
2. Screen for alterations in temperature.
3. Evaluate temperature response to therapies.

■ Assessment
- Identify patient's baseline temperature.
- Assess for clinical signs and symptoms of temperature alteration.
- Assess for factors that influence body temperature:
  - Ingestion of hot or cold food or liquids in last 15 minutes
  - Smoking within last 15 minutes
  - Recent exercise
  - Age, hormones, drugs that cause variations in body temperature.
- Determine site most appropriate for temperature measurement.

■ Equipment
Appropriate thermometer
Plastic thermometer sheaths or tissues to wipe thermometer
Water-soluble lubricant and disposable gloves (for rectal temperature)
Pen and vital sign documentation record
Gloves

■ Procedure
1. Wash hands. Explain the procedure to the patient.
2. If using a mercury thermometer, put on disposable gloves.
   Rationale: Gloves protect nurse's hands from body secretion contamination. Unnecessary with electronic thermometer because nurse never touches oral probe.
3. Remove thermometer from storage container and rinse in cold water. Wipe dry with tissue.
   Rationale: Storage solution is irritating to mucosa. Cold water is used to rinse thermometer because hot water would cause mercury to expand and break thermometer.
4. Hold thermometer at eye level.
5. Check temperature reading on thermometer. If reading is not below 35°C, shake down by holding thermometer at end away from bulb between thumb and forefinger, and snap wrist sharply. Place plastic sheath on electronic thermometer.
   Rationale: Thermometer must be at eye level to accurately read mercury. Mercury must be below patient's

body temperature before use in order to register accurately.

■ Procedure

Assessing Oral Temperature
1. See steps 1 to 5.
2. Place thermometer probe in patient's mouth in the posterior sublingual pocket (at the right or left of the frenulum at the base of the tongue).
   Rationale: Sublingual pocket has large superficial blood vessels that reflect heat of core body temperature.

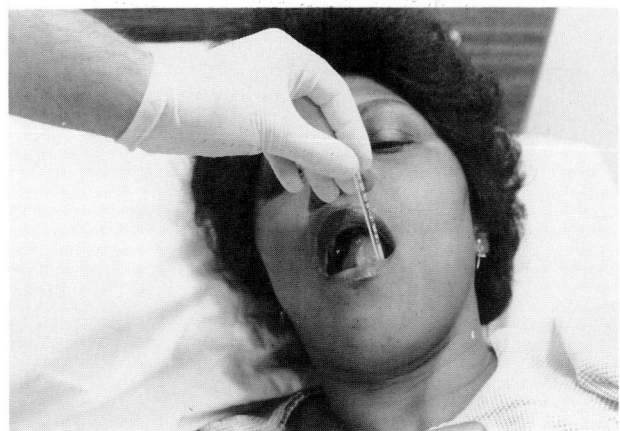

Step 2

3. Ask patient to maintain thermometer position with lips closed.
   Rationale: Maintains correct placement of thermometer in sublingual pocket.
4. Leave in place 3 to 5 minutes with mercury thermometer, or 10 to 20 seconds with electronic thermometer. Check agency policy regarding recommended time interval.
   Rationale: Research results vary as to amount of time needed to register accurate temperature.

■ Procedure

Assessing Axillary Temperature
1. Close bedroom door or unit curtains, assist patient to comfortable position, and expose axilla.
2. Insert thermometer into middle of axilla; fold patient's arm down and place across chest.
   Rationale: Maintains correct position of thermometer against blood vessels in axilla.

(continued)

PROCEDURE 19–1. Assessing Body Temperature *(continued)*

3. Hold thermometer in place 9 minutes in adults, 5 minutes in children.
Rationale: Research now indicates there is no significant difference in accuracy between axillary and rectal temperature, if the thermometer is left in place for the recommended period of time.

■ **Procedure**

Assessing Rectal Temperature
1. Close bedroom door or bed curtains. Assist patient to Sim's position with upper leg flexed. Expose only anal area.
Rationale: Privacy is essential to reduce embarrassment from exposing buttocks. Lateral position exposes anal area for thermometer placement.
2. Apply water-soluble lubricant liberally to thermometer probe tip.
Rationale: Facilitates insertion of thermometer without irritating or traumatizing the rectum.
3. Separate patient's buttocks with one hand to expose anus.
4. Ask patient to take a deep, slow breath. Insert thermometer into anus in direction of umbilicus, for an infant 1/2″, for an adult, 1 1/2″. Do not force.
Rationale: Deep, slow breath allows patient to relax external sphincter. Insertion depth allows adequate exposure of mercury bulb against blood vessels in rectal wall.
5. Hold in place 3 to 5 minutes according to agency policy.
Rationale: Holding thermometer prevents rectal damage or perforation from patient moving with thermometer in place.
6. If using an electronic thermometer, discard the sheath and read the digital display.
7. If using a mercury thermometer, wipe off secretions with a tissue. Hold the thermometer at eye level and rotate it slowly until mercury column is visible. Note upper end of column as the temperature reading.
Rationale: Reading at eye level ensures accuracy.

8. Wash mercury thermometer in soapy, tepid water. Rinse and replace in storage container.
Rationale: Mechanically removes organic material that may inhibit the action of the disinfectant in the storage container.
9. Remove gloves and wash hands.
Rationale: Reduces transmission of microorganisms.
10. If using electronic thermometer, replace in battery charging unit.

■ **Lifespan Considerations**

Infants and Children
• When taking rectal temperature in an infant or child, do not allow the child to roll over or kick due to risk of thermometer advancing and perforating rectum. Have assistance if necessary, or select an alternate site for temperature evlauation.
• Axillary temperature is the perferred site in infants and children because it is easily accessible, there is little danger of mercury poisoning from thermometer breakage in mouth, and there is no chance of rectal perforation and possible resultant periotonitis.
• If attempting to take rectal temperature in a newborn but the thermometer will not advance, the rectum may not be patent.

Older Adults
• Older adults may have difficulty flexing their legs and assuming the left lateral position. Thermometer may be inserted with both legs straight.

■ **Home-Care Modifications**
If family members need to assess temperature of patient, they may need to know:
• how frequently to monitor temperature.
• when to notify home-care nurse or physician.
• not to measure temperature orally in children under 6 years of age, or in confused or unconscious patients.
• to wash the thermometer in tepid, soapy water, and to store it dry.

100 beats per minute. The normal pulse ranges for various age groups are shown in Table 19-1.

Autonomic Nervous System. Stimulation of the parasympathetic nervous system results in a decrease in the pulse rate. Normally there is a certain amount of parasympathetic control of the heart to maintain the pulse

rate below 100 beats per minute. Conversely, stimulation of the sympathetic nervous system results in an increased pulse rate. Sympathetic nervous system activation occurs in response to a variety of stimuli including pain, anxiety, exercise, fever, and ingestion of caffeinated beverages, and in response to changes in intravascular volume.

Medications. Certain cardiac medications, such as digoxin, decrease heart rate. Medications that decrease intravascular volume, such as diuretics, may cause a reflex increase in pulse rate. Other medications mimic or block the effects of the autonomic nervous system. For example, atropine inhibits impulses to the heart from the parasympathetic nervous system, causing increased pulse rate. Other medications, such as propranolol, block sympathetic nervous system action, resulting in decreased heart rate.

Assessing the Pulse

The pulse is an important part of vital signs measurement. The baseline pulse rate and rhythm are established during the initial nursing assessment and are used for comparison with future measurements.

Sites

The pulse can be assessed in any location where an artery lies close to the skin surface and can be compressed against a firm underlying structure such as muscle or bone. The most commonly assessed pulses are the temporal, carotid, apical, brachial, radial, femoral, popliteal, pedal, and posterior tibial (Fig. 19-6).

Temporal. The temporal artery courses across the temporal bone of the skull. The pulsation of the temporal artery is most easily palpated just in front of the upper part of the ear.

Carotid. The sternomastoid muscles, which stand out when the jaw is forcefully clenched, run from below the ear to the clavicle and sternum. Beneath them lie the carotid arteries. The artery is most easily palpated along the medial border of the sternomastoid muscle in the lower half of the neck. Palpating the carotid arteries in the upper part of the neck may result in stimulation of the carotid sinus, which causes a reflex drop in pulse rate. The carotid pulse best represents the quality of pulsation in the aorta because of its proximity to the central circulation.

Apical. The contraction or beating of the heart ventricles can also be palpated with the hand or auscultated with a stethoscope placed over the area of the left ventricle. Normally this area is at the level of the fifth intercostal space at about the midclavicular line.

Brachial. The brachial artery lies between the groove of the biceps and triceps muscles in the inner aspect of the upper arm. The brachial pulse is most easily palpated with the patient's arm flexed at the elbow and supported by the examiner to prevent muscle contraction, which may obscure the pulse.

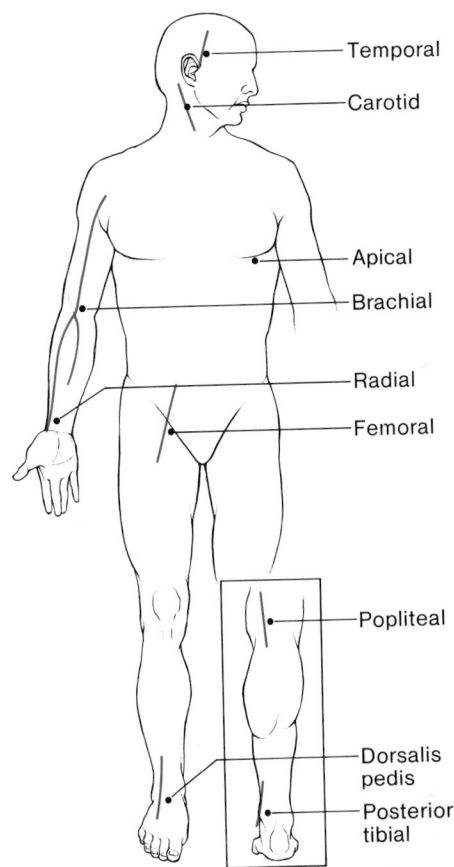

Figure 19–6. Pulse sites. The inset shows the left leg. The posterior tibial pulse is on the medial aspect of the ankle.

Radial. The radial artery pulse is the site most commonly assessed in the clinical setting. The radial pulse is palpated on the thumb side of the inner aspect of the wrist.

Femoral. The femoral pulse is palpated in the anterior, medial aspect of the thigh, just below the inguinal ligament, about halfway between the anterior superior iliac spine and the symphysis pubis. Deep palpation may be required to detect the femoral pulse beneath the subcutaneous tissue.

Popliteal. The popliteal pulse is palpable behind the knee in the lateral aspect of the popliteal fossa (the hollow area at the back of the knee joint). The pulse is best assessed with the knee flexed and the leg relaxed. The patient may be supine or prone.

Pedal. The pedal pulse or dorsalis pedis pulse can be felt on the dorsal aspect of the foot (the area of the foot that is on top in a standing position). The pulse is palpated lateral to the tendon that runs from the great toe toward the ankle. The dorsalis pedis pulse may be congenitally absent in some patients.

Posterior Tibial. The posterior tibial pulse is located behind the malleolus (the rounded protuberance of bone) of the inner ankle. The pulse is palpated by hooking the fingertips behind the bone.

Methods

Palpation. The pulse is palpated with the first and second, or second and third fingers of one hand. Light pressure is initially used to locate the area of strongest pulsation. More forceful palpation may then be used to count the rate, determine the rhythm, and assess the quality of pulsation. The number of pulses is counted for 15, 30, or 60 seconds and multiplied as necessary to yield pulses per minute. The time interval used to assess the pulse depends on the patient's condition and the norms of the institution. Patients with irregular pulse rates or abnormally slow or fast pulse rates are best assessed for a full minute. Patients with a regular rhythm and normal rate may be assessed for a shorter time. Fifteen-second intervals may be used when the pulse is assessed frequently, as during recovery from anesthesia.

Regardless of the time interval selected, the initial pulsation is counted as zero. Pulses at or after completion of the time interval are not counted. Counting the first pulse as one or counting pulses after the period of assessment results in overestimation of the pulse. The error is multiplied when intervals of less than 60 seconds are used to assess the rate. Counting even one extra pulsation in a 15-second pulse assessment results in overestimation of the pulse rate by four. Procedure 19-2 gives detailed instructions on taking a pulse.

Auscultation. The apical pulse provides the most accurate assessment of the pulse rate and is the preferred site of assessment whenever the peripheral pulses are difficult to assess or the rhythm of the pulse is irregular.

Apical pulse assessment is done by placing the diaphragm of the stethoscope over the apex of the heart. The sounds heard are due to vibrations caused by the opening and closing of the cardiac valves. Each heartbeat consists of two sounds. The first, S_1, is caused by closure of the mitral and tricuspid valves separating the atria from the ventricles. The second sound, S_2, is caused by the closure of the pulmonic and aortic valves. The sounds are often described as a muffled "lub-dub." Together they constitute one heartbeat. To determine the apical pulse, the heartbeats are counted for a full minute.

Equipment

Stethoscope. Auscultation of the apical pulse requires a stethoscope. The stethoscope should have snugly fitting ear pieces and thick-walled tubing about 12 inches long for optimal sound transmission (Bates, 1991). The stethoscope should be equipped with a bell and a diaphragm.

Doppler. Peripheral pulses that cannot be detected by palpation may be assessed with an ultrasonic Doppler device (Fig. 19-7). The transmitter of the device is placed over the artery to be assessed. A conductive gel is first applied to the skin to reduce resistance to sound transmission. High-frequency waves directed at the artery from the transmitter are disturbed by the pulsating flow of blood and are reflected back to the ultrasound device. The sound disturbances (Doppler shifts) are amplified and heard through ear pieces or a speaker attached to the device.

Doppler assessment of the pulse is generally used to determine the adequacy of flow to an area when occlusive vascular disease threatens the blood supply. Doppler may also be useful in situations of cardiopulmonary collapse where peripheral vasoconstriction makes pulses difficult to palpate.

Assessing Pulse Characteristics

The pulse is assessed for rate, rhythm, and quality. Pulse rate and rhythm are routinely assessed; pulse quality is assessed less often or in exceptional circumstances when abnormalities may be anticipated.

Rate. In adults, the normal rate is 60 to 100 pulsations per minute. Adult pulse rates above 100 beats per minute are called **tachycardia.** Sympathetic nervous system activation results in an increased pulse rate. Tachycardic rates may also occur when the impulse for cardiac contraction comes from an abnormal site in the heart that stimulates the heart to beat faster.

An abnormally slow pulse rate is called **bradycardia.** In adults, a pulse rate below 60 is considered bradycardic. Bradycardia may be the normal resting heart rate in a trained athlete. Disease of the SA node may result in bradycardia due to poor impulse formation. Bradycardia may be caused by enhanced parasympathetic nervous system activity, as occurs with stimulation of the carotid sinus.

Rhythm. Normally, cardiac contractions occur at evenly spaced intervals, resulting in a regular rhythm. Infants and children often have increased pulse rates during inspiration and decreased rates during expiration; this is called *sinus arrhythmia.* This tendency decreases with aging.

Heart disease, medications, or electrolyte imbalances may alter the normal rhythmic beating of the heart, causing an irregular pulse. An irregular pulse rhythm that still has a consistent pattern of pulsation is called *regularly irregular.* An example is pulsus bigeminus, in which a normal heartbeat initiated in the SA node is followed by a heartbeat initiated in a different part of the heart. The second beat is early and often weaker than the first, resulting in a regularly irregular pulse.

If there is no pattern to the pulse, it is called *irregularly irregular.* Irregularly irregular pulses may be detected in

PROCEDURE 19–2. Obtaining a Pulse

■ Purpose
1. Obtain a baseline measure of heart rate and rhythm.
2. Evaluate the heart's response to various therapies and medications.
3. Peripheral pulse may be palpated to assess local blood flow to an extremity.

■ Assessment
- Review medical history to determine risk factors for alterations in pulse rate (heart disease, postoperative, fluid or electrolyte imbalances, pain, hemorrhage).
- Assess for physical signs and symptoms of alteration in cardiac or vascular status (dyspnea, chest pain, palpitations, syncope, edema, cyanosis).
- Identify factors that influence pulse (age, medications, fever, exercise).
- Identify site most appropriate for pulse assessment.
- Review previous and baseline pulse assessments, if available.

■ Equipment
Wristwatch with second hand
Vital sign flow sheet and pen
Doppler and jelly (optional, for hard-to-palpate pulses)
Stethoscope

■ Procedure

Radial Pulse
1. Wash hands and explain the procedure to patient.
2. Position patient comfortably with forearm across chest or at their side with wrist extended.
   Rationale: Relaxed position of lower arm with wrist extended allows easier artery palpation.
3. Place fingertips of your first three fingers along the groove at base of thumb, on patient's wrist.
   Rationale: Fingertips are the most sensitive part of the hand for palpating pulses. Do not use the thumb to palpate: it has a strong pulse that may be felt and confused with the patient's.
4. Press against radial artery to obliterate pulse, then gradually release pressure until pulsations are felt.
   Rationale: Moderate pressure is needed to accurately assess rate and regularity of pulse.
5. Assess pulse for regularity and strength.
6. If pulse is not easily palpable, use Doppler:
   a. Apply conducting gel to end of probe or to radial site.
      Rationale: Doppler works by ultrasound, which transmits sound better with the airtight seal provided by gel.
   b. Press "on" button and place probe against skin on

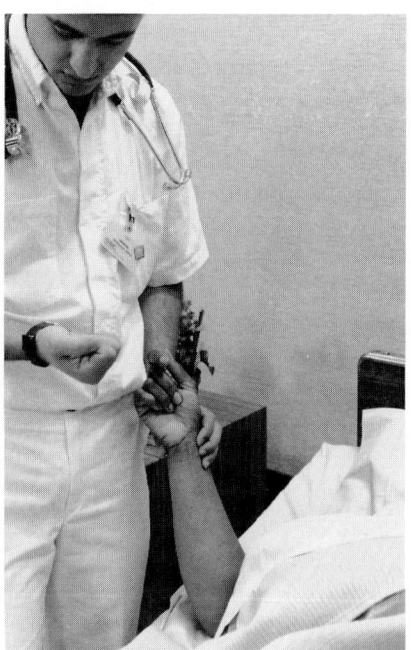

Step 3

pulse site. Reposition slightly using firm pressure until pulsating sound is heard.
7. If pulse is regular, count pulse for 15 seconds and multiply by four. If pulse is irregular, count for a full minute.
   Rationale: If pulse is irregular, a longer counting period ensures a more accurate pulse rate determination.

■ Procedure

Apical Pulse
1. Position patient in supine or sitting position with sternum and left chest exposed.
   Rationale: Allows easy access for selection of auscultory site. Rustling from clothing or bed linens will not distract from hearing pulse.
2. Warm diaphragm of stethoscope by holding in the palm of your hand for 5 to 10 seconds.
   Rationale: Cold metal or plastic diaphragm can startle the patient when placed directly on the chest.
3. Insert the ear pieces of stethoscope into your ears and place diaphragm over apex of patient's heart. The heartbeat is usually heard loudest at the fifth intercostal space, near the midclavicular line.
4. Assess the heartbeat for regularity and arrhythmias.
   Rationale: Frequent irregularities within 1 minute may indicate inadequate caridac perfusion.
5. If rhythm is regular, count the heartbeat for 30 sec-

(continued)

PROCEDURE 19–2. Obtaining a Pulse *(continued)*

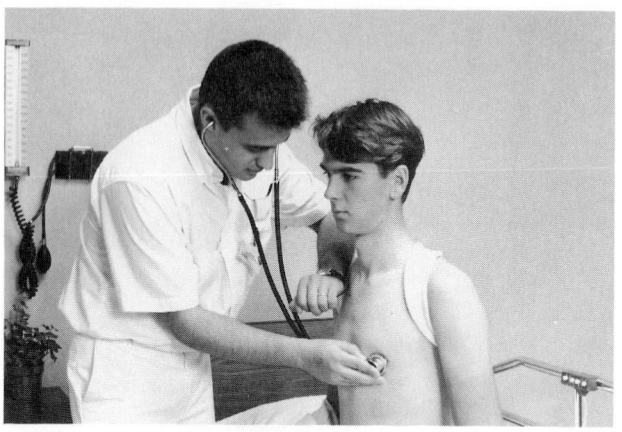

Step 3

onds and multiply by two. Count for a full minute if the rhythm is irregular.
Rationale: Heart rate is more accurate counted over a longer period if the rate is irregular.

6. Replace patient's gown and assist in returning to a comfortable position.

7. Share results of assessent with patient, if appropriate.
Rationale: Promotes patient's understanding of health and response to therapies.

8. Document pulse on vital signs record.

■ **Lifespan Considerations**

Infants and Children
• Newborns and children under 2 years of age have weak radial pulses. Apical pulses are assessed for heart rate.
• The apex of the heart on an infant is at the third to fourth intercostal space, to the left of the midclavicular line.
• Crying greatly increases the pulse rate. Crying can be decreased by taking the pulse while the child sits in a parent's lap, or by distracting the child with toys.

Older Adults
• If patient is taking cardiac medications such as digitalis preparations or beta blockers, or if patient has a history of cardiac arrhythmias, a more accurate assessment of heart rate and rhythm is obtained using the apical pulse site.

■ **Home-Care Modifications**
• Pulse may need to be assessed at home if patient is taking various cardiac medications. The caregiver or patient must be taught how to locate and count the pulse, as well as to keep a diary of daily pulse rate to take to health-care appointments.
• Digital pulse rate devices are available for home use.

---

a condition known as atrial fibrillation. In atrial fibrillation, the atria of the heart do not contract in a synchronous fashion, and the impulse for the heartbeat does not come from the SA node. Consequently, the time interval between successive ventricular contractions varies and an irregularly irregular pulse is detected.

When an abnormal pulse rhythm is noted, the examiner should consider using the auscultatory method to obtain an apical pulse rate. The examiner must also determine whether irregularity of the pulse is a new finding for the patient. Many people have chronically irregular pulse rhythms, but a new finding of pulse irregularity requires immediate investigation to determine the causes and to assess the need for treatment.

Quality. Pulse quality generally refers to the strength of pulsation and may be rated on a numerical scale (Table 19-3). The normal quality of the pulse is described as full or strong, and easily palpated. Weak pulses are easily obliterated by the examiner's fingers and may be described as thready. A bounding pulse is stronger than normal and difficult to obliterate. Pulse quality reflects the stroke volume, the compliance or elasticity of the arteries, and the adequacy of blood delivery. When stroke volume is decreased, as in severe

hemorrhage, the pulse is often thready and may be difficult to palpate in the peripheral arteries. In cardiopulmonary failure, the pulse is usually palpated more easily in the central areas such as the carotid or femoral arteries. With aging, the arteries lose elasticity and the pulse becomes more bounding. The combination of rapid pulse rate and increased stroke volume with exercise results in a pulse that can be felt by the person and is sometimes called a pounding heart.

Peripheral pulses should be palpated bilaterally to compare quality. Equality of pulsation provides information about local blood flow. For example, partial occlusion of a right femoral artery would result in weaker femoral, popliteal, dorsalis pedis, and posterior tibial pulses on the right than on the left. Bilateral pulse comparison is used to monitor for complications after procedures invasive to the arteries, such as arteriography. After an arteriogram, during which a large artery is punctured and injected with radiographic dye, the normal clotting to seal the artery may cause total arterial occlusion. Weakened or absent pulses distal to the puncture site would signal an occlusion.

Pulse Deficits. In some situations, stroke volume may vary from beat to beat during cardiac contraction, result-

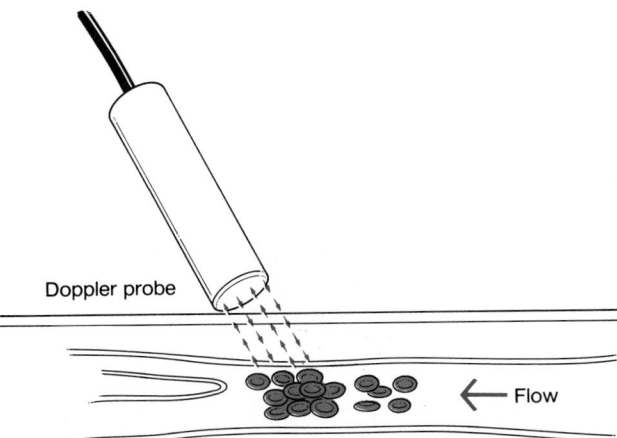

Figure 19–7. Doppler sound generation. The transmitting crystal emits an ultrasound beam through the skin to a vessel and moving red blood cells. The red cells reflect the ultrasound beam to the receiving crystal. Adapted from Durbin, N. (1983). The application of Doppler techniques in critical care. *Focus on Critical Care*, *1010*(3), 44–46.

ing in a pulse wave so weak that it cannot be perceived by palpation at a peripheral site. It is important to recognize this situation because it provides information about the heart's ability to adequately perfuse the body. When some of the ventricular contractions do not perfuse, there is a difference between the apical and peripheral pulses—a **pulse deficit.** The presence and magnitude of the pulse deficit can be determined by having two nurses simultaneously measure the apical and radial pulses. Both nurses should use the same watch or clock to count the pulse for a full minute. The difference between the pulses is then documented. When a pulse deficit is present, the radial pulse rate is always lower than the apical pulse rate. See Procedure 19-3 for details on determining pulse deficit.

RESPIRATIONS

Respiration is a term used to summarize two different but related processes: external respiration and internal respiration. External respiration is the process of taking oxygen into the body and eliminating carbon dioxide from the body. Internal respiration refers to the use of oxygen, the production of carbon dioxide, and the exchange of these gases between the cells and the blood.

The respiratory system is made up of four parts:

- The lungs, which are responsible for gas exchange
- The thoracic cavity, which includes the chest wall and the respiratory muscles
- The control center in the brain
- The nerves and nerve tracts that connect the brain and the muscles.

All these parts must be functioning for the respiratory system to be able to maintain homeostasis.

At rest, the normal respiratory rate of an adult is 12 to 20 breaths per minute. Normal **tidal volume** (the amount of air moving in and out with each breath) is 500 mL, or 6 to 8 L/min (Ganong, 1989).

The process of inspiration is active. Inspiratory muscles contract, resulting in increased intrathoracic volume as the lungs are pulled into a more expanded space. The pressure in the airway becomes negative and air flows in. At the end of inspiration, natural lung recoil occurs, the airway pressure becomes slightly positive, and the air flows out as the muscles relax. Expiration is basically a passive process.

Normal breathing is automatic and involuntary. In people with healthy respiratory systems, the normal stimulus to breathe is hypercarbia, an increased carbon dioxide level. Chemoreceptors throughout the body sense changes in carbon dioxide levels and stimulate the respiratory center, which increases or decreases respiratory rate and depth accordingly. A decreased oxygen level also has the effect of increasing respiratory rate and depth.

There are two separate centers in the nervous system for control of breathing. Voluntary control of breathing is possible, and the center for voluntary control is in the cerebral cortex. Spontaneous, involuntary respirations are controlled by a rhythmic discharge of impulses from the brain to the nerves that innervate the respiratory muscles. The rate of these discharges is regulated by alterations in the arterial levels of carbon dioxide and oxygen. Breathing stops if the spinal cord is cut above the level of the phrenic nerve (Ganong, 1989). Chapter 30 provides an in-depth explanation of respiratory control.

Factors Affecting Respirations

Several factors can affect respiratory rate, rhythm, and depth, and familiarity with these factors allows the nurse to accurately assess the significance of alterations.

Age. Normal growth from infancy to adulthood results in a larger lung capacity. As lung capacity increases, lower respiratory rates are sufficient to exchange air. As

TABLE 19–3

Scale to Rate Pulse Quality

0	No pulse detected
1+	Thready, weak pulse, easily obliterated with pressure; pulse may come and go
2+	Pulse difficult to palpate, may be obliterated with pressure
3+	Normal pulse
3+	Bounding, hyperactive pulse; easily palpated and cannot be obliterated

PROCEDURE 19–3. Assessing Pulse Deficits

■ Purpose
1. Evaluate the effectiveness of cardiac contractions by determining if there is a difference between apical and radial heart rates.

■ Assessment
- Identify patients at risk for unequal apical and radial heart rates (history of heart disease, elderly patients).
- Assess for physical signs and symptoms of altered cardiac status (dyspnea, palpitations, syncope, cyanosis).
- Review baseline pulse assessments, if available.

■ Equipment
Wristwatch with second hand
Stethoscope
Vital sign documentation sheet and pen
Second examiner

■ Procedure
1. Explain procedure to patient. Introduce second examiner. Position patient comfortably.
   Rationale: Ensures patient comfort and cooperation.
2. Remove clothing as necessary to select stethoscope placement site. Warm diaphragm of stethoscope by holding in hand. Place stethoscope over apex of heart.

Rationale: The heartbeat is usually heard best at the fifth intercostal space, near the midclavicular line.
3. Second examiner places fingertips over radial artery pulse site.
4. Place a watch where both examiners can clearly observe the second hand. Both examiners agree to start counting when the second hand reaches a predetermined number.
   Rationale: A pulse deficit will be accurate only if apical and radial heartbeats are counted simultaneously.
5. Count the apical and and radial rate for a full minute.
   Rationale: Accuracy is increased by counting heart rate for 60 seconds.
6. Reposition patient and adjust clothing.
7. Document the apical and radial heart rates.

■ Lifespan Considerations

Infants and Children
- Pulse deficit tends to be a problem of the older adult and is rarely evaluated in childen.

Older Adults
- If radial pulse is weak and difficult to count, repeat procedure for a second minute to check accuracy of radial pulse.

---

a person continues into older age, lung elasticity decreases. With this decrease in lung capability, the respiratory rate once again increases to allow for the same exchange of air.

Medications. Narcotics can impair the ability to voluntarily inspire, and the respiratory rate may decrease. Other drugs, depending on their action, may alter rate, rhythm, and depth in other ways.

Stress. Stress or strong emotion can change a person's respiratory pattern. Stress can increase both the rate and depth of respirations.

Exercise. When people exercise, their tissues need more oxygen. Also, extra carbon dioxide and heat are being produced and must be eliminated. The body responds to these needs by increasing the rate and depth of respirations.

Altitude. The oxygen content of the air decreases as the altitude increases. To compensate for the decreased oxygen content, the rate and depth of respirations at higher elevations increase to improve the supply of oxygen available to the body tissues.

Sex. Because men normally have a larger lung capacity than women, men may have a lower respiratory rate than women.

Body Position. When the body is slumped or stooped, gas exchange can become impaired. As a result, the rate and depth of respiration may be increased.

Fever. When a person has a fever, the respiratory system provides an avenue for the release of extra heat. Since heat can be lost from the lungs, the result is an increased respiratory rate. Also, as the metabolic rate increases with the temperature, respiratory rate is affected. Respiratory rate can increase as much as four breaths per minute with every 0.6°C (1°F) increase in temperature above normal (Guyton, 1986).

Assessing Respirations

Respirations should be assessed in every vital sign evaluation. A normal baseline for each patient should be established so that comparisons can be made. The assessment should include respiratory rate, rhythm, depth, and quality.

Respirations are the easiest of all the vital signs to assess. Perhaps because of this, the assessment of respiratory rate, rhythm, and depth is often done sloppily. The respiratory assessment can provide valuable information, and a thorough assessment of a patient's respirations is vital in gathering clues to his or her condition. When assessing a patient's respiratory status, the nurse should keep in mind the patient's normal pattern, the influence of any disease conditions, and the influence of any therapies that could affect the patient's respiratory status.

Characteristics

Rate. Respiratory rate changes with age. At rest, the normal respiratory rate for an infant is 30 to 60 breaths per minute, decreasing to 12 to 20 breaths per minute for an adult. **Tachypnea** is an abnormally fast respiratory rate (usually above 20 breaths per minute). **Bradypnea** is an abnormally slow respiratory rate (usually less than 12 breaths per minute). **Apnea,** the absence of respirations, is often described by the length of time in which there are no respirations (for instance, a 10-second period of apnea). Continuous apnea is synonymous with respiratory arrest and is not compatible with life.

Rhythm and Depth. Respirations should be regular in rhythm and depth. Regularity refers to the pattern of inspiration and expiration. Expiration is normally twice as long as inspiration. Depth is assessed by observing the movement of the chest wall. Several abnormal patterns may be found on the physical examination (Table 19-4).

Biot's respirations are a cyclic pattern of breathing in which periods of shallow breathing alternate with periods of apnea. This respiratory pattern is seen in patients with meningitis, encephalitis, head trauma, brain abscess, and heatstroke.

Cheyne–Stokes respirations are a cyclic pattern of breathing in which periods of respirations of increased rate and depth alternate with periods of apnea. Common conditions causing Cheyne–Stokes respirations include congestive heart failure, drug overdoses, increased intracranial pressure, and meningitis. Cheyne–Stokes respirations are the most common abnormal pattern assessed (Guyton, 1986).

Kussmaul respirations are a pattern of breathing characterized by respirations of increased rate (more than 20 breaths per minute) and increased depth. This abnormal pattern is most commonly associated with metabolic acidosis and renal failure.

Apneustic respirations are a pattern of breathing characterized by a long inspiratory period that is gasping in nature followed by a short expiratory period. This pattern is commonly seen in patients with central nervous system disorders.

Quality. Respirations are usually automatic, quiet, and effortless. When assessing respirations, the nurse

TABLE 19–4
Abnormal Breathing Patterns

Abnormal Breathing Pattern	Description	Conditions
Bradypnea	Respiratory rate below 12 BPM	Neurologic disturbances, electrolyte disturbances, narcotic or barbiturate overdose, post-anesthesia
Tachypnea	Persistent respiratory rate above 20 BPM	Trauma, injury, stress, pain; respiratory, cardiac, liver disease
Biot's Apnea	Cyclic breathing pattern characterized by shallow breathing alternating with periods of apnea	Neurologic problems (meningitis, encephalitis), head trauma, brain, abscess, heatstroke
Cheyne–Stokes Apnea	Cyclic breathing pattern characterized by periods of respirations of increased rate and depth alternating with periods of apnea	Congestive heart failure, drug overdose, increased intracranial pressure
Kussmaul Duration 1 Minute	Increased rate (above 20 BPM) and depth of respirations	Metabolic acidosis, diabetic ketoacidosis, renal failure

should be attentive to changes from the normal quality. Abnormalities in quality are usually characterized as problems with effort or noise.

Dyspnea describes respirations that require excessive effort by the patient. Respirations can be painful and labored. Patients may report being unable to catch their breath. Dyspnea can occur at rest or with activity; dyspnea that occurs with activity is called exertional dyspnea. Healthy people who are not in good physical condition may experience exertional dyspnea.

Breathing can also be noisy. A number of terms are used to describe the different types of noisy respirations that the nurse can hear without a stethoscope.

Stridor is a harsh inspiratory sound that can sound like crowing. It may indicate an upper airway obstruction. It is commonly heard in children with croup or after aspiration of a foreign object.

Wheezing is a high-pitched musical sound. It is usually heard on expiration but may be heard on inspiration. It is associated with partial obstruction of the bronchi or bronchioles, as in asthma.

Sighs are breaths of deep inspiration and prolonged expiration. Everyone sighs, and sighing aids in the expansion of alveoli. However, more frequent sighing may indicate stress or tension.

Methods for Measuring Respiratory Rate

Patients must be unaware that the nurse is doing a respiratory assessment, because if they are conscious of the procedure they may alter their breathing pattern or rate. Often, nurses assess the respiratory rate after taking the radial pulse, while still holding the patient's wrist. With an infant or young child, respirations should be assessed before the temperature is taken so that the child is not crying, which would alter the respiratory status. See Procedure 19-4 for details on assessing respirations.

BLOOD PRESSURE

Blood pressure is the force that blood exerts against the walls of the vessels. The pressure in the systemic arteries is most commonly measured in the clinical setting. Blood pressure is stated in millimeters of mercury (mm Hg).

Physiologic Factors Determining Blood Pressure

The contractions of the heart result in a pulsating flow of blood into the arteries. The pressure is highest when the ventricles of the heart contract and eject blood into the aorta and pulmonary arteries. The blood pressure measured during ventricular contraction (cardiac systole) is the **systolic blood pressure.** During ventricular relaxation (cardiac diastole), blood pressure is due to elastic recoil of the vessels and the measured pressure is the **diastolic blood pressure.** The mathematical difference between the measured systolic and diastolic blood pressures is the **pulse pressure.** For instance, a systolic pressure of 120 mm Hg and a diastolic pressure of 80 mm Hg results in a pulse pressure of 40 mm Hg.

Blood pressure is a function of the flow of blood produced by contraction of the heart and the resistance to blood flow through the vessels (Kaplan, 1988). The pressure, flow, and resistance relationship is described mathematically as pressure equals flow multiplied by resistance ($P = F \times R$).

Blood Flow

Blood flow is essentially equal to cardiac output. Cardiac output is the product of stroke volume (the amount of blood pumped from each ventricle with each heartbeat) and heart rate. A stroke volume of 70 mL and a heart rate of 72 beats per minute results in a cardiac output of 5040 mL/min, or about 5 L/min. Average cardiac output in a resting man is 5.5 L/min (Ganong, 1989).

Decreased stroke volume due to poor cardiac pumping (as occurs with a failing heart) or reduced blood volume (as in severe hemorrhage) may result in decreased cardiac output. Bradycardia may also cause decreased cardiac output. Conversely, a rapid heart rate and larger stroke volumes would be expected to increase cardiac output. The magnitude of change in cardiac output created by increases or decreases in one of the factors (heart rate or stroke volume) is influenced by the concurrent response of the other factor. For example, if stroke volume falls to 40 mL, the cardiac output stays in the normal range if the heart rate simultaneously increases to 100 beats per minute ($40 \times 100 = 4000$ mL, or 4 L). A person with a heart rate of 50 beats per minute can maintain a normal cardiac output only if the stroke volume is 80 mL or more ($50 \times 80 = 4000$ mL or 4 L). An increase in heart rate in response to a decrease in stroke volume to maintain a normal cardiac output is an example of a compensatory response.

Resistance

Resistance to blood flow is caused by the friction among the cells and other blood components, and between the blood and the vessel walls. The friction within the blood components reflects the viscosity of the blood and is largely due to the number and shape of the blood cells. Normally, the number and type of blood constituents do not vary greatly, and viscosity is a constant factor in determining resistance.

Friction between the blood and the vessel walls varies with the dimensions of the vessel lumen. The most important lumenal dimension is the diameter (Guyton, 1987). The diameter of the blood vessel is controlled by contraction and relaxation of the smooth muscle in the vessel walls.

PROCEDURE 19–4. Assessing Respirations

■ Purpose

1. Assess respiratory status by evaluating rate and quality.
2. Evaluate the influence of medications and therapies on respiration.

■ Assessment

- Identify risk factors for altered respiratory status (chest trauma, respiratory disease, smoking history, respiratory depressant medications).
- Assess for physical signs and symptoms of altered respiratory status (cyanosis, clubbed fingers, reduced level of consciousness, pain during inspiration, dyspnea, coughing).
- Review pertinent laboratory studies (arterial blood gases, complete blood count).
- Determine baseline respiratory rate.

■ Equipment

Watch with second hand
Vital signs documentation sheet and pen

■ Procedure

1. After assessment of pulse, keep your fingers resting on patient's wrist and observe or feel the rising and falling of chest with respiration. *Do not* explain procedure to patient.

Rationale: Explaining procedure may make patient self-conscious about respirations and could cause him or her to alter respiratory pattern.

2. When one complete cycle or inspiration and expiration has been observed, look at second hand of watch and count the number of complete cycles. If rate is regular in an adult, count 30 seconds and multiply by two. In children under 2 years of age or in adults with an irregular rate, count for a full minute.
Rationale: Children normally have irregular respiratory patterns.
3. Note depth and rhythm of respiratory cycle.
Rationale: Respiratory characteristics give additional data about alterations in respiratory status.
4. Discuss findings with patient, if applicable.
5. Document results.

■ Lifespan Considerations

Infants and Children

- A crying child's respiratory rate cannot be accurately assessed. Count respirations when the child is sleeping, if possible. If the child is crying, attempt to quiet him or her before assessing respirations. If the child cannot be quieted, write "crying" on the recording sheet.

Factors Affecting Blood Pressure

Age. Blood pressure measurements in normal newborns indicate a positive correlation between birth weight and blood pressure. In one study of newborns in the first 12 hours of life, direct blood pressure measurements averaged about 51/41 mm Hg for newborns weighing less than 2000 g and 62/51 mm Hg for newborns weighing more than 3000 g (Kitterman, 1969).

Blood pressure gradually increases throughout childhood and correlates with height and weight as well as age. This makes it difficult to identify abnormal blood pressure levels for children at various developmental stages, but it has been proposed that a diastolic pressure consistently above the 95th percentile for age indicates a need for diagnostic evaluation (Pruitt, 1987).

In adults, there is a trend toward gradually increasing systolic and diastolic blood pressure with aging. In part, this trend is due to increased systemic vascular resistance, reflecting arterial narrowing and decreased vessel elasticity due to atherosclerotic vessel disease. The increase in systolic blood pressure is proportionally greater than the increase in diastolic blood pressure;

therefore, pulse pressure widens. Normal blood pressures for various age groups are shown in Table 19-1.

Autonomic Nervous System. The autonomic nervous system influences heart rate, cardiac contractility, systemic vascular resistance, and blood volume. Increased sympathetic nervous system activity results in increased heart rate, stronger contraction of heart muscle, changes in vascular smooth muscle tone, and increased blood volume due to retention of water and sodium. The cumulative effect is increased blood pressure. Therefore, factors that enhance sympathetic nervous system activity (such as pain, anxiety, fear, smoking, and exercise) result in increased blood pressure readings.

Exceptions occur when sympathetic nervous activity cannot keep up with a stressor. An example is a patient with severely diminished blood volume resulting from hemorrhage. Activation of the sympathetic nervous system occurs to maintain adequate blood pressure, but this may not be enough to compensate for the volume loss. Measured blood pressure may be quite low, although sympathetic nervous system activity is markedly increased.

Medications. Any medication that alters one or more of the previously described determining factors may cause a change in blood pressure. Examples are diuretics, which decrease blood volume; cardiac medications, which affect the rate or contractile force of the heart; narcotic analgesics, which reduce pain and sympathetic nervous system activity; and specific antihypertensive agents.

Normal Fluctuations. Blood pressure fluctuates from minute to minute in response to a variety of stimuli. Increased ambient temperature causes blood vessels near the skin surface to dilate, decreasing both resistance and blood pressure. Blood pressure also fluctuates with the respiratory cycle, increasing during expiration and decreasing during inspiration.

In addition to minute-to-minute fluctuations, there is a discernible circadian pattern to blood pressure. Investigators performing direct, continuous monitoring of blood pressure have documented a consistent variation in blood pressure throughout the day. One study revealed a peak pressure at about 10 AM, a plateau through the late afternoon, and a gradual fall in pressure during the night, with lowest pressures recorded at about 3 AM. Blood pressure then gradually rose during the early morning, with a sharp increase between 7 and 10 AM (Pruitt, 1987).

Assessing Blood Pressure

Blood pressure may be measured directly with a catheter placed into an artery. Direct measurement provides a continuous reading of blood pressure and is used in critical-care settings. However, blood pressure is usually measured by indirect methods, using an inflatable cuff to temporarily occlude arterial blood flow through one of the limbs. As the cuff is deflated and flow returns, the blood pressure can be determined by palpation, auscultation, or oscillations. Procedure 19-5 gives detailed instructions for measuring blood pressure.

Sites

Upper Extremity. The blood pressure is usually measured in the arm with a cuff wrapped around the upper part of the limb and the flow auscultated or palpated at the brachial artery. Blood pressure may also be determined by auscultation or palpation of the radial artery in the wrist with an appropriate-sized cuff applied to the forearm.

Lower Extremity. The cuff may be wrapped around the thigh or above the ankle. Thigh pressure measurement requires a larger cuff. The patient is placed in a flat, prone, or supine position with the cuff centered mid-thigh, over the popliteal artery. Blood flow is auscultated or palpated at the popliteal fossa. A systolic blood pressure measured in the thigh is generally 10 to 40 mm Hg higher than that measured in the arm. To measure blood pressure in the ankle, the patient is placed in a flat, supine position and a standard arm cuff is placed just above the malleolus. The posterior tibialis or dorsalis pedis pulse may be auscultated or palpated as the cuff is deflated.

Equipment

Sphygmomanometer. A sphygmomanometer consists of an inflatable bladder enclosed in a nondistensible cuff. The bladder is connected to an inflating mechanism such as a bulb or pump, a valve for deflation, and a manometer (Fig. 19-8). The manometer may be a gravity mercury or aneroid type.

Mercury manometers consist of a vertical glass tube marked in 2-mm increments. Cuff pressures are transmitted through the tubing into the manometer and force the mercury to rise in the glass tube. The surface tension of the mercury in the tube causes the top of the mercury column to be curved. The pressure reading is made from the top point of the curved surface, or meniscus, of the mercury. The manometer must be at eye level to ensure an accurate reading. Particulate matter or air bubbles in the glass tube distorts readings. Enough mercury must be present in the reservoir to maintain the meniscus at zero with the cuff deflated. The air vent at the top of the glass tube must be clean and allow free passage of air, or the mercury will be unable to rise and fall smoothly in the tube.

Aneroid manometers have a circular gauge marked in 2-mm increments. The pressure transmitted from the cuff causes movement of a metal bellows within the manometer, and this movement is indicated by a needle on the gauge. Aneroid manometers require yearly calibration with a properly functioning mercury manometer or other pressure standard. Checks of manometer function should be made throughout the range of pressure measurement to ensure the device's accuracy. Aneroid manometers with a stop peg at the zero point or an external reset are not recommended, as it is impossible to verify the accuracy of the manometer.

The tubing and hand bulb must be free of cracks or holes and connections must be airtight to prevent leaks that cause poor transmission of pressure. The deflation valve must function smoothly to allow the operator to control the rate of deflation.

Stethoscope. A stethoscope is necessary for the auscultatory method of blood pressure measurement. The stethoscope should have snugly fitting ear pieces and thick-walled tubing about 12 inches long for optimal sound transmission. The stethoscope should be equipped with a bell and a diaphragm.

PROCEDURE 19–5. Obtaining Blood Pressure

■ Purpose

1. Evaluate the patient's hemodynamic status by obtaining information about cardiac output, blood volume, peripheral vascular resistance, and arterial wall elasticity.
2. Obtain baseline measurement of blood pressure.
3. Monitor the hemodynamic response to various therapies or disease conditions.

■ Assessment

- Assess blood pressure on initial patient examination and whenever status changes.
- Identify factors that may alter blood pressure (medications, exercise, age, emotional conditions, smoking, postural changes).
- Assess best site for obtaining blood pressure.
- Determine correct size of blood pressure cuff.
- Review previous blood pressure readings, if available.

■ Equipment

Stethoscope
Sphygmomanometer with bladder and cuff
Documentation record and pen

■ Procedure

1. Wash hands, explain procedure to patient, assist patient to a comfortable position with forearm supported at heart level and palm up.
   Rationale: Variations in blood pressure can occur with patient in different positions. Blood pressure increases when the arm is below heart level and decreases when above heart level. Diastolic blood pressure may increase 10% if arm is unsupported, secondary to isometric exercises used to support arm.
2. Expose the upper arm completely.
3. Wrap deflated cuff snugly around upper arm with

center of bladder over brachial artery. Lower border of cuff should be about 2 cm above antecubital space (nearer the antecubital space on an infant).
Rationale: Placing bladder directly over brachial artery ensures proper compression of artery during cuff inflation.

4. If using a mercury manometer, the manometer should be vertical and at eye level.
   Rationale: Prevents distortion and promotes accurate reading of mercury level.
5. Palpate brachial or radial artery with fingertips. Close valve on pressure bulb and inflate cuff until pulse disappears. Inflate cuff 30 mm Hg higher. Slowly release valve and note reading when pulse reappears.
   Rationale: Identifies approximate systolic blood pressure reading, to prevent underestimating systolic blood pressure should patient have an auscultatory gap.

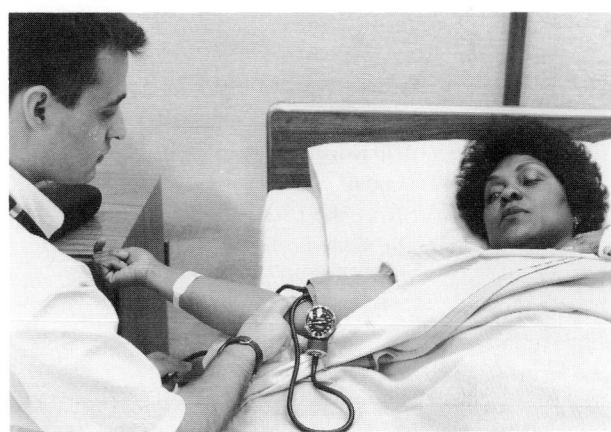

Step 5

6. Fully deflate cuff and wait 1 to 2 minutes.
   Rationale: Waiting period prevents falsely high readings by allowing blood trapped in the vein to be recirculated.
7. Place stethoscope ear piece in ears. Repalpate the brachial artery and place stethoscope diaphragm or bell over the site.
8. Close bulb valve. Inflate cuff to 30 mm Hg above reading where brachial pulse disappeared.
   Rationale: Ensures accurate assessment of systolic blood pressure.

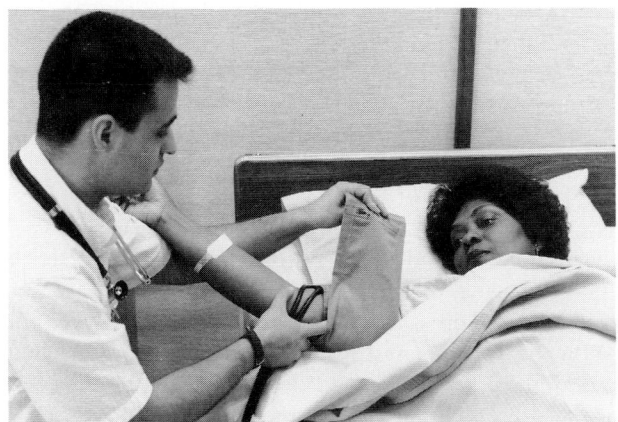

Step 3

(continued)

PROCEDURE 19–5. Obtaining Blood Pressure *(continued)*

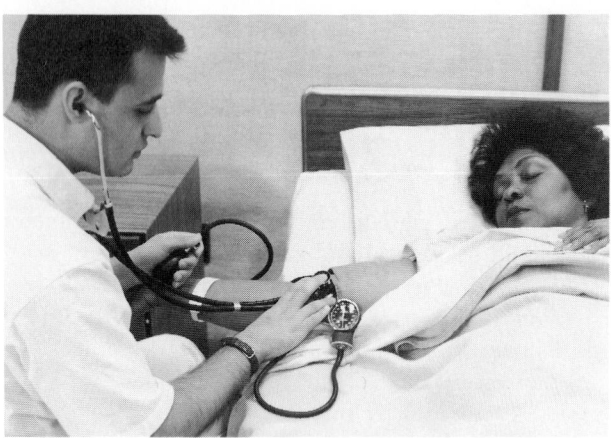

Step 7

9. Slowly release valve so pressure drops about 2 to 3 mm Hg per second.
   Rationale: Inaccurate measurements may occur if deflation rate is faster.
10. Identify manometer reading when first clear Korotkoff sound is heard.
    Rationale: Indicates systolic pressure reading.
11. Continue to deflate and note reading when sound muffles or dampens (fourth Korotkoff) and when it disappears (fifth Korotkoff).
    Rationale: American Heart Association recommends using the fifth Korotkoff sound as diastolic pressure in adults, fourth Korotkoff in children. In adults, if fourth and fifth Korotkoff are 10 mm Hg or greater apart, note all three readings.
12. Deflate cuff completely and remove from patient's arm.
13. Record blood pressure. Record systolic (e.g., 130) and diastolic (e.g., 80) in the form 130/80. If three pressures are to be recorded, use the form 130/80/40 (40 is the fifth Korotkoff). Abbreviate RA or LA to indicate right or left arm measurement.
14. Assist patient to comfortable position and discuss findings with patient, if appropriate.
    Rationale: Encourages patient understanding of

health status and promotes compliance with therapies.

■ **Lifespan Considerations**

Infants and Children
- Selection of proper-sized cuff and bladder is important for obtaining accurate blood pressure measurements in children and adults alike. The bladder width should be 40% of the circumference of the limb.
- In infants, Korotkoff sounds may be too faint for accurate measurement. Accurate assessment of systolic pressure can be obtained by using a Doppler (ultrasonic device).
- When blood pressure is monitored in children, take respirations and pulse rate first, since they are the least invasive and least likely to cause the child anxiety. Temperature should be the last vital sign measured because it the most invasive.
- Blood pressure varies according to age; see Table 19-1.

Older Adults
- Adults with hypertension are prone to auscultatory gaps in blood pressure. Estimation of systolic pressure using the brachial artery palpation technique will prevent inaccurate readings secondary to auscultatory gap.

■ **Home-Care Modifications**
- Patients with hypertension may be taught to monitor their blood pressure at home.
- A variety of monitors for home use is available. They include digital printouts with time and date for accurate record-keeping.
- Teach the patient:
  - to avoid caffeinated beverages, smoking, and exercise for 30 minutes before measurement
  - to use the same arm and body position for each measurement.
  - at what measurements the patient should alert the nurse or physician.

Doppler. The Doppler method is useful during low flow states or when the blood pressure is difficult to auscultate by stethoscope. The method involves the use of an ultrasonic device that transmits and receives high-frequency sound waves (see Fig. 19-7). A standard cuff is used to occlude an artery while the ultrasound transducer is placed over the artery distal to the site of occlusion. Arterial wall motion creates Doppler shifts in the ultrasonic frequency, which are received and amplified

by the ultrasound unit. Systolic blood pressure is the point at which continuous pulsatile flow is heard. Diastolic blood pressure may be difficult to identify reliably with the Doppler but is considered the point at which continuous flow is heard.

Electronic Methods. Automated devices are frequently used to monitor blood pressure indirectly during anesthesia, in the critical-care area, and postoperatively.

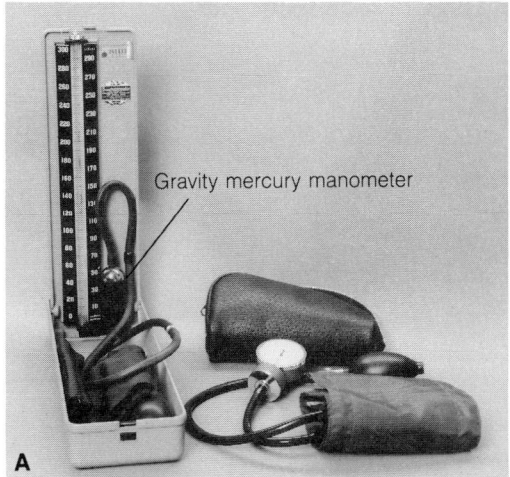 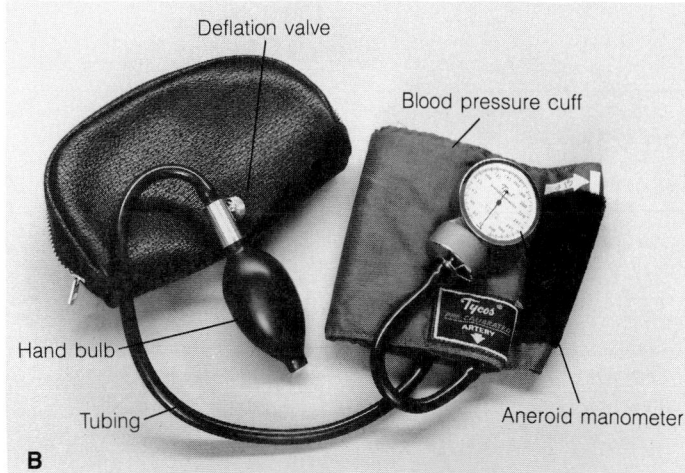

Figure 19–8. Sphygmomanometers. **A.** Gravity mercury. **B.** Aneroid.

The electronic units determine blood pressure by analyzing the sounds of blood flow or measuring oscillations. In either case, a cuff attached to the machine is automatically inflated to occlude the artery. The sounds of blood flow are detected by a microphone in the cuff. Oscillatory devices measure blood pressure by microcomputer analysis of oscillations (the amplitude of the pulsations) transmitted from the artery to the cuff (Hahn, 1985). Systolic, diastolic, and mean arterial blood pressure and heart rate are displayed on the monitor.

Methods

Baseline blood pressure ideally is measured with the patient in a resting state. Therefore, the patient should be in a warm, quiet environment and at least one-half hour should be allowed to elapse after smoking, exercising, or eating. Sometimes blood pressure must be measured when the patient is anxious or in pain, but the readings may differ from those made if the patient were in a basal state.

Proper Cuff Size. The American Heart Association has made specific recommendations about cuff size and application (Table 19-5). Using an inappropriate size or placement may lead to an erroneous reading. This is a common error: one study documented that "miscuffing" occurred in 32% of blood pressure measurements (Manning, 1983).

Cuff size is based on the circumference of the limb being used. The width of the cuff bladder should be 40% of the circumference of the midpoint of the limb. An average adult arm requires a bladder 12 to 14 cm wide. The bladder length should be 80% of the limb circumference, or about twice the bladder width (Fig. 19-9).

The cuff should be applied snugly around the limb, with the bladder centered over the artery. Using a too-small cuff or one that is loosely applied results in spuriously high readings. Using a too-large cuff results in spuriously low readings.

Proper Position. Blood pressure should be measured with the arm at heart level. Elevating the arm above

TABLE 19–5

Recommended Bladder Dimensions for Blood Pressure Cuff

Arm Circumference at Midpoint* (cm)	Cuff Name	Bladder Width (cm)	Bladder Length (cm)
5–7.5	Newborn	3	5
7.5–13	Infant	5	8
13–20	Child	8	13
24–32	Adult	13	24
32–42	Wide adult	17	32
42–50†	Thigh	20	42

* Midpoint of arm is defined as half the distance from the acromion to the olecranon.
† In patients with very large limbs, the indirect blood pressure should be measured in the leg or forearm.
From Frolich, E., Grim, C., Labarthe, D. et al. (1987). *Recommendations for human blood pressure determinations by sphygmomanometers.* American Heart Association.

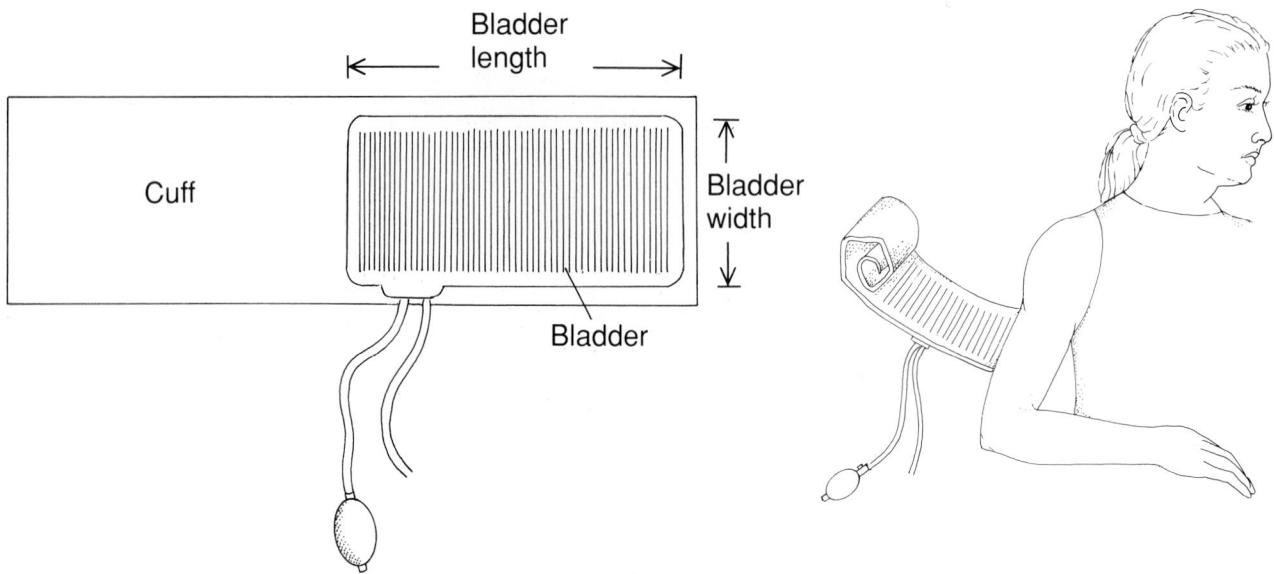

Figure 19–9. Proper cuff size is important in obtaining accurate blood pressure measurements. The bladder length should be 80% of the limb circumference or about twice the bladder width.

heart level results in a falsely low measurement; positioning the arm below heart level results in a falsely high reading. When the patient is flat, the arm is approximately at heart level. If the patient is sitting or standing, the forearm should be supported at the horizontal level of the heart (generally considered the level of the fourth intercostal space, where the ribs join the sternum). Failure to support the arm causes the patient to contract the arm muscles, elevating the blood pressure.

Correlation with the Respiratory Cycle. The intrathoracic pressure changes that occur during a normal respiratory cycle affect the heart and great vessels. Consequently, blood pressure is lower during inspiration than expiration. Exaggerated decreases in systolic blood pressure with inspiration (called pulsus paradoxus or **paradoxical blood pressure**) occur in diseases such as cardiac tamponade, constrictive pericarditis, emphysema, hypovolemic shock, and pulmonary embolus (Braunwald, 1988). Consistently measuring blood pressure at end expiration eliminates variability of readings due to respiratory changes.

Venous Congestion. An inflated cuff reduces venous blood return to the heart in the extremity. Increased venous pressures are transmitted back to the arterial side of the circuit and arterial pressures are transiently elevated. Slow, prolonged, or frequent cuff inflation promotes venous congestion. The cuff should be inflated rapidly when taking a reading and deflated completely after measurement. At least 2 minutes should elapse before sequential cuff inflation on any one limb. Elevat-

ing the arm above the head between cuff measurements speeds venous return to the heart.

Auscultation. When the blood pressure is determined by the auscultatory method, an inflatable cuff is used to temporarily occlude flow through a limb. As the cuff is deflated and blood flow returns, the **Korotkoff sounds** can be heard with a stethoscope placed over the artery. Five distinct phases are identifiable (Fig. 19-10, Table 19-6). The onset of the Korotkoff sounds of phase I is the recorded systolic pressure. Diastolic pressure is indicated by the onset of phase V sounds in adults and phase IV sounds in children.

Because the Korotkoff sounds are low in frequency, the bell of the stethoscope is best used for auscultation, although most practitioners use the diaphragm. If the sounds are inaudible with the diaphragm, the nurse can try the stethoscope bell. Care must also be taken not to press the head of the stethoscope too firmly against the skin, as this may partially occlude blood flow and alter the reading.

An **auscultatory gap** is the absence of Korotkoff sounds between phases I and II (Nelson, 1984). Failure to identify an auscultatory gap may result in underestimation of the systolic blood pressure or overestimation of the diastolic pressure. An auscultatory gap can be detected by palpating the brachial or radial pulse while inflating the cuff. The cuff should be inflated about 30 mm Hg above the number where palpable pulsation disappears. In addition to detecting an auscultatory gap, palpation gives an initial estimate of systolic blood pressure and eliminates the need to inflate the cuff to ex-

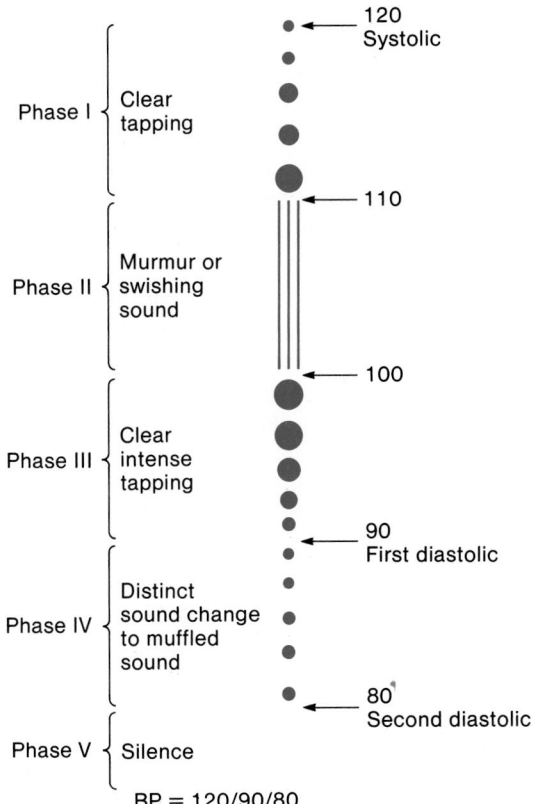

Phase I — Clear tapping

120 Systolic

110

Phase II — Murmur or swishing sound

100

Phase III — Clear intense tapping

90 First diastolic

Phase IV — Distinct sound change to muffled sound

80 Second diastolic

Phase V — Silence

BP = 120/90/80

Figure 19–10.   Five phases of Korotkoff sounds.

tremely high pressures in people with normal or low blood pressure. When an auscultatory gap is detected, the systolic and diastolic pressures are recorded as usual and the magnitude and range of the auscultatory gap is also noted (for instance, 196/90; auscultatory gap from 184 to 150).

Palpation. When Korotkoff sounds are inaudible, blood pressure may be estimated by palpation. The cuff

is applied and inflated as previously described and the brachial or radial artery palpated during cuff deflation. Systolic blood pressure is the point at which pulsation returns. Diastolic blood pressure is difficult to determine reliably with palpation, but is indicated by a snap or whipping palpable vibrations. Palpated blood pressure is usually recorded as a systolic reading over "P" for palpated (for instance, 110/P).

Abnormalities

Hypertension.   **Hypertension** is the condition in which blood pressure is chronically higher than normal. Although the natural trend in industrialized societies is for increased blood pressure with aging, hypertension is a dangerous disease associated with increased risk of death. One study demonstrated decreased morbidity and mortality with specific pressure-reducing medical therapy for people with diastolic blood pressure above 90 mm Hg (Hypertension Detection and Follow-Up Program Cooperative Group, 1979). Therefore, adults of any age with blood pressure above 140/90 mm Hg should be evaluated for hypertensive disease. Hypertension is covered in greater detail in Chapter 31.

Orthostatic Hypotension.   In an adult, moving from a flat, horizontal position to a vertical position results in pooling of blood in the lower extremities. People with a healthy, intact autonomic nervous system reflexively compensate for the volume shift by increasing the rate and force of myocardial contraction and vasoconstriction, thus maintaining adequate blood pressure. Even with normal compensation, however, systolic blood pressure usually falls and heart rate increases with position change.

Inadequate reflex compensation to position change results in **orthostatic hypotension.** Symptoms of orthostatic hypotension are those of decreased cerebral perfusion such as dizziness, weakness, blurred vision, and syncope as well as marked changes in blood pressure and heart rate. Orthostatic blood pressure changes may indicate failure of autonomic nervous system protective reflexes or hypovolemia. Hypovolemia or impaired vasoconstriction is signaled by decreased blood pressure and increased heart rate. Autonomic nervous system dysfunction is indicated by decreased blood pressure without marked increases in heart rate (Underhill, 1989).

There is disagreement in the literature about the magnitude of change in blood pressure and heart rate necessary to diagnose orthostatic hypotension. Schatz (1984) defined normal orthostatic changes as a drop in systolic blood pressure of 10 to 15 mm Hg and a heart rate increase of 5 to 25 beats per minute. Changes indicative of orthostatic hypotension are a drop in systolic blood pressure of 20 to 30 mm Hg and a drop in the diastolic measurement of 10 to 20 mm Hg. Robertson and Robertson (1985) described normal response to posture

TABLE 19–6

Korotkoff Sounds

Phase	Description	Recording
I	Initiated by the onset of faint, clear tapping sounds of gradually increasing intensity.	Recorded as systolic pressure.
II	Sound has a swishing quality.	
III	Marked by crisper, more intense sounds.	
IV	Characterized by muffled, blowing sounds.	Recorded as diastolic pressure in children.
V	Absence of sound.	Recorded as diastolic pressure in adults.

change as a systolic blood pressure decline of about 10 mm Hg, a diastolic increase of 5 mm Hg, and a heart rate increase of 5 to 20 beats per minute. Abnormal changes are any fall in diastolic blood pressure accompanied by signs or symptoms of diminished blood flow to the head. Neither of these sources discussed the implications of heart rate changes when assessing response to orthostasis.

Moore and Newton (1986) documented an average heart rate increase of 12.6 beats per minute between supine and standing positions in healthy young adults. Vargas and Lye (1982) noted that older subjects have a blunted heart rate response to posture change.

There are also procedural discrepancies among various studies. It is unknown how much time should elapse after a position change before blood pressure and heart rate are measured. Moore and Newton (1986) recommended letting 2 minutes elapse before checking blood pressure and at least 45 seconds before checking the heart rate. Stephen (1987), studying older adults, recommended letting 1 minute elapse after position change before measuring blood pressure and heart rate.

The person experiencing postural hypotension is at risk for falling. Therefore, checking postural vital signs is one way of screening to ensure patient safety. Patients with chronic orthostatic hypotension should be instructed to change positions slowly, moving from a lying to a sitting to a standing posture and allowing several minutes to elapse before proceeding to the next position.

Orthostatic blood pressure should be measured in patients exhibiting symptoms of dizziness, blurred vision, or weakness when changing position, patients taking diuretic medications, and those with a history of volume loss. Systematic, consistent technique in assessing blood pressure and heart rate response to position change provides the best data for determining and monitoring therapy.

The initial measurement of blood pressure and heart rate is made with the patient in a flat, supine position. The patient should remain in this position for at least 2 minutes before the nurse measures the blood pressure and heart rate. The cuff is then left in place, and the patient is assisted to a sitting position with his or her legs dangling over the side of the bed or examining table.

Nursing Research

Selected Nursing Research Studies

Abrams, L., et al. (1989). Effects of peripheral IV infusion on neonatal axillary temperature measurement. *Pediatr Nurs, 15*(6), 630–632.

Campbell-Heider, N., et al. (1988). Nurses' attitudes toward conventional and automated vital signs measurement methods. *Med Instrum, 22*(5), 257–262.

Hahn, W. K., et al. (1989). Blood pressure norms for healthy young adults: Relation to sex, age, and reported parental hypertension. *Res Nus Health, 12*(1), 53.

Hellmann, R., et al. (1989). The influence of talking on diastolic blood pressure readings. NLN Publication #15-2232, 78–82.

Neff, J., et al. (1989). Effect of respiratory rate, respiratory depth, and open versus closed mouth breathing on sublingual temperature. *Res Nurs Health, 12*(3), 195–202.

Robichaud-Ekstrand, S., et al. (1989). Comparison of electronic and glass thermometers: Length of time of insertion and type of breathing. *Can J Nurs Res, 21*(1), 61–73.

Schron, E. B., et al. (1989). The systolic hypertension in the elderly program: Implications for nursing practice and research. *Prog Cardiovasc Nurs, 4*(4), 135–145.

Possible Topics for Nursing Inquiry

- In patients who have no rectums, are temperatures obtained from the stoma accurate?
- What criteria do nurses use to determine the frequency of monitoring patients' temperatures?
- When assessing for orthostatic hypotension, how long should the patient maintain each position before blood pressure and pulse are measured?
- What constitutes significant changes in systolic and diastolic blood pressure and heart rate when a patient moves from a supine to a sitting position?
- Can diastolic blood pressure be accurately and reliably determined via Doppler or palpation?
- How often do nurses use the palpation method for determining auscultatory gap when monitoring blood pressure in acute-care settings?
- What is the validity and accuracy of respiratory rate measurement in a typical acute-care setting?
- What is the effect of eating versus fasting on pulse rate?
- Is taking an apical pulse for a full minute more reliable in accurately measuring pulse rate when an irregularity of rhythm is noted?

Another 2 minutes are allowed to elapse before the second measurement of blood pressure and heart rate. The patient should be asked whether any symptoms of dizziness, lightheadedness, dimming of vision, or weakness are present. The patient is assisted to a standing position, and after 2 minutes blood pressure and heart rate are measured. Again, the patient is asked to report symptoms of decreased cerebral perfusion.

Patients experiencing severe orthostatic hypotension may be unable to tolerate a standing position long enough for the nurse to obtain the blood pressure and heart rate. If the patient becomes severely symptomatic while standing, he or she should be returned to bed without completing the measurements.

The blood pressure and heart rate values are recorded, as well as the position of the patient when the values were obtained. Any symptoms of diminished ce-rebral perfusion are also documented. See Procedure 19-6 for a step-by-step description.

LIFESPAN CONSIDERATIONS

Knowledge of developmental considerations is important for the nurse who is measuring and interpreting vital signs. Normal ranges for the vital signs across the lifespan are summarized in Table 19-1.

Newborn and Infant

Temperature, pulse, and respirations fluctuate widely in newborns. Thermoregulatory mechanisms are immature in newborns, and ambient temperature may markedly affect their body temperature. Pulse and respiration

---

PROCEDURE 19–6. Assessing for Orthostatic Hypotension

■ Purpose
1. Assess the compensatory status of the cardiovascular system to changes in body position.

■ Assessment
• Identify patients at risk for postural drops in blood pressure:
  • history of saline depletion
  • inadequate vasoconstrictor mechanisms secondary to prolonged bedrest
  • autonomic insufficiency secondary to spinal cord injury or drugs (digoxin, beta-adrenergic blockers, calcium channel blockers).
• Assess patient for complaint of dizziness or lightheadedness during position changes.
• Review serum electrolytes, if available, for saline imbalances.
• Review baseline blood pressure measurements, if available.

■ Equipment
Stethoscope
Sphygmomanometer
Watch or clock with second hand
Vital sign documentation record and pen

■ Procedure
1. Wash hands. Explain procedure to patient.
2. Position patient supine with head of bed flat for 2 minutes.
   Rationale: To allow blood pooled in lower extremities to reenter circulation.
3. Check and record supine blood pressure and pulse.

Rationale: Provides baseline information with which to compare measurements after position changes. Pulse rate is assessed to help differentiate the cause of postural hypotension. During position changes, if pulse rate rises as blood pressure falls, secondary to sympathetic stimulation, the cause may be decreased venous return to the heart or saline imbalances. If the pulse does not increase when the blood pressure falls, the cause may be related to the lack of sympathetic response.

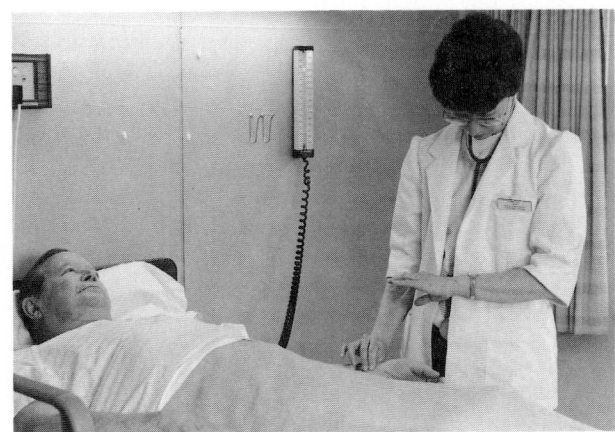

Step 3

4. Assist patient to a sitting position with legs dangling over the edge of the bed. Wait 2 minutes and check blood pressure and pulse rate.
   Note: The waiting period is a convenient time to auscultate the patient's lung fields.

(continued)

PROCEDURE 19–6. Assessing for Orthostatic Hypotension (continued)

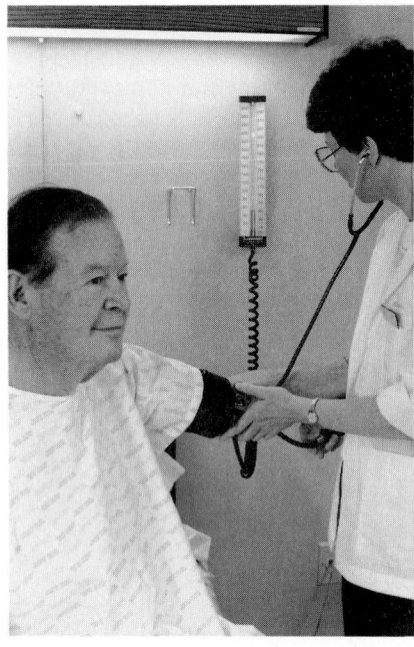

Step 4

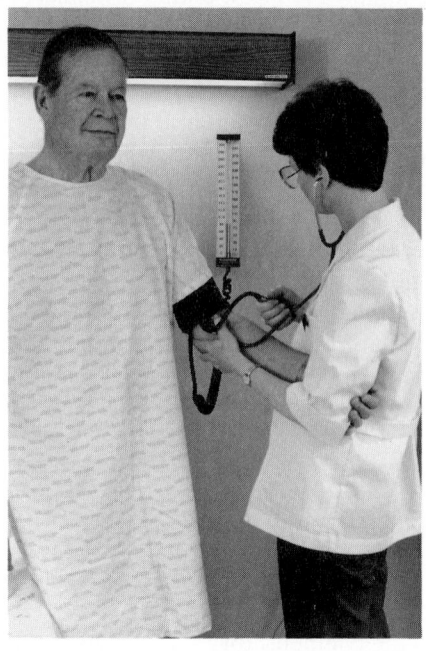

Step 5

5. Assist patient to standing position. Wait 2 minutes and check blood pressure and pulse rate. Be alert to signs and symptoms of dizziness.
   Rationale: If blood pressure drops significantly, the patient may become lightheaded and may need to be returned to bed before test completion.
6. Assist the patient back to a comfortable position.
7. Record measurements and any symptoms that accompanied the postural change.

Rationale: A drop of 15 mm Hg in systolic pressure or a drop of 10 mm Hg in diastolic pressure should be reported.
8. Discuss findings with patient, if appropriate.
   Rationale: If there is a significant postural blood pressure drop, advise the patient to sit on the edge of the bed for several minutes before walking to avoid dizziness and possible falls.

Patient Teaching

Instruct the patient as follows:

- If you are monitoring your own vital signs, make sure you know and understand normal ranges and when it is important to contact a health-care provider.
- Keep a chart of specific vital sign measurements so you can show it to the physician for identifying trends.
- Never leave a small child alone when taking his or her temperature. You may need to restrain the child to prevent injury and to obtain an accurate measurement.

- Keep the thermometer in the sublingual pocket of the mouth when obtaining an oral temperature.
- Inform the nurse whether you drank a hot or cold beverage recently, or whether you smoked within 30 minutes of an oral temperature measurement.
- When monitoring your pulse, palpate the radial artery for a full minute to determine rate and rhythm.
- If you plan to monitor your blood pressure at home, compare various types of monitoring equipment to determine the most cost-effective system for your needs.

increase rapidly above resting values when a newborn is active, crying, or startled. The apical pulse is the most reliable method of assessing heart rate, since peripheral pulses are faint and difficult to palpate and accurately count. Healthy newborns may exhibit periodic apnea (Nelson, 1987). Blood pressure is not routinely assessed in the newborn or infant because the information obtained is unreliable.

Safety considerations are important when monitoring the vital signs of the newborn or infant. Axillary temperatures are preferred, since rectal temperature monitoring can cause mucosal tearing or perforation and an oral thermometer cannot safely be held in the infant's mouth. Infants move quickly, so it is important to protect them from falling or injury during vital sign monitoring.

Toddler and Preschooler

As a child enters the second year of life, vital signs fluctuate less. The pulse rate decreases to a normal range of 80 to 120 beats per minute, and respirations fall to 22 to 40 breaths per minute. Normal blood pressure ranges from a systolic pressure of 80 to 112 mm Hg over a

diastolic pressure of 50 to 80 mm Hg. Blood pressure is routinely monitored after the age of 3 years.

The toddler and preschooler may become fearful of procedures involving vital sign measurement, and at this age verbal explanations do little to allay fears. Permitting the child to play with a stethoscope or to push the button on the electronic thermometer may help to calm the patient's fears. Having the parent hold and talk to the child can be comforting when the child is frightened.

Safety concerns continue to be important in this age group. Temperature monitoring should be done using the axillary route until the child is 4 or 5 years old and can follow directions about holding the thermometer in the sublingual pocket. It is not safe to use an oral glass mercury thermometer in children in this age group, because inadvertently biting down on the thermometer could cause breakage, lacerations, and possible mercury poisoning.

Child and Adolescent

The broad range of normal values reflect the wide variability in children's vital signs. In general, temperature, pulse, and respirations gradually decrease through child-

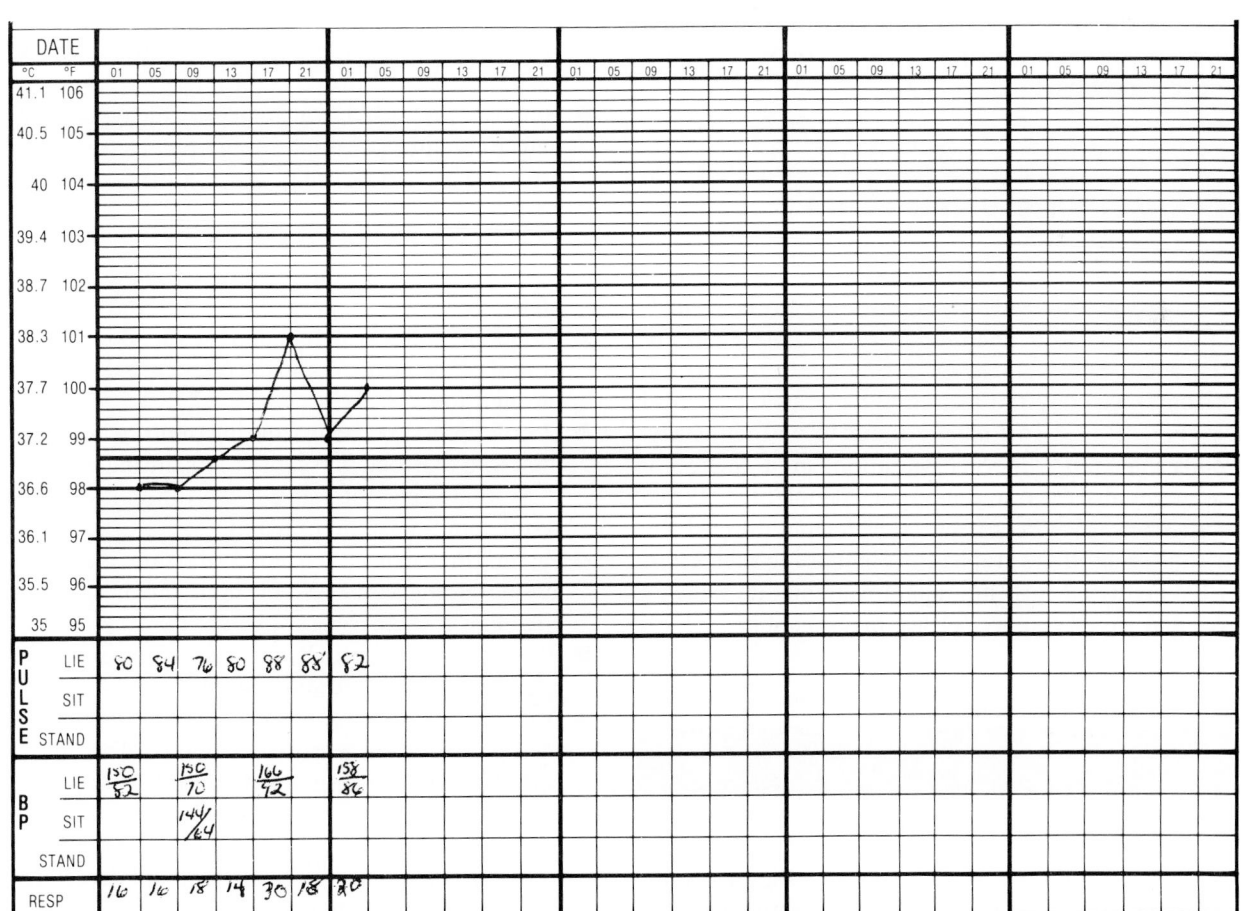

Figure 19–11.   Vital signs graphic flowsheet.

hood, but blood pressure increases and is correlated with height and weight (Nelson, 1987).

Children in this age group are familiar with vital sign assessment and seldom exhibit fear during monitoring. Health teaching about normal values and the reason for taking vital signs helps to educate the child. A child may try to experiment by putting the thermometer under hot water or near a light source, so any unlikely temperature readings should be validated.

Adult and Older Adult

Vital signs usually stabilize during young adulthood. As adults age, the effects of lifestyle and chronic diseases become evident in the vital signs. Respiratory rate and pattern are influenced by chronic respiratory disease and exposure to pollutants such as cigarette smoke. Cardiovascular diseases may cause changes in the heart rate and rhythm. The incidence of hypertension increases with age: half of all adults over age 64 have hypertension (Roben, 1986). Conversely, orthostatic hypotension is common in the elderly, although the actual incidence is unclear. It is also uncertain whether orthostatic hypotension occurs as a result of the normal aging process or is seen only in elderly people with existing disease states (Mader, 1989). Older adults also have lower normal ranges for body temperature (Kolanski, 1981).

Often adults ask the nurse about the values obtained during monitoring. This is an excellent opportunity for patient education.

DOCUMENTING VITAL SIGNS

The nurse is responsible for documenting the vital signs that have been assessed and for reporting any abnormalities to the physician in a timely fashion. Vital signs are often documented in a graph format, with time as the horizontal axis and the measured value as the vertical axis (Fig. 19-11). This allows trends to be seen easily. Trends may reflect normal variations or a change in response to disease or therapy. For example, the normal trend is toward a decreased body temperature in the early morning. If the graph shows increasing values during the night and early morning, this trend may indicate fever and would require further investigation.

Key Concepts

- Temperature, pulse, respirations, and blood pressure are considered the vital signs, because significant deviations from normal ranges are not compatible with life.

- Vital sign assessment is an important nursing function that permits the nurse to detect alterations from normal and evaluate patient progress.
- Body temperature can be monitored in three sites: oral cavity, rectum, and axilla.
- Factors that can affect body temperature include age, environmental conditions, time of day, exercise, stress, and hormone level.
- Smoking, drinking hot or cold liquids, or administering oxygen can alter body temperature measurement.
- Equipment to monitor body temperature includes glass mercury thermometers, electronic thermometers, chemically treated paper thermometers, and temperature-sensitive strips.
- As the heart contracts and ejects blood into the circulation, pulsations can be palpated at various arterial sites in the body.
- Evaluation of the pulse should include rate, rhythm, and quality.
- Factors such as age, autonomic nervous system stimulation, and medications can affect the pulse.
- An irregular pulse should be counted for a full minute, preferably at the apical site.
- A pulse deficit occurs when a cardiac contraction creates a pulse wave that is weak and not palpable at peripheral sites.
- Respiratory rate, rhythm, and depth can be altered by age, medications, stress, exercise, altitude, sex, body position, and the presence of a fever.
- Abnormal breathing rates include tachypnea (more than 20 breaths per minute), bradypnea (less than 12 breaths per minute), and apnea (interval of absent respirations).
- Abnormal breathing patterns include Biot's respirations, Kussmaul respirations, and apneustic respirations.
- Blood pressure is a function of the flow of blood produced by the heart and the resistance to blood flow through the vessels.
- Systolic pressure occurs during ventricular contraction, and diastolic pressure occurs during ventricular relaxation. Pulse pressure is the difference between systolic and diastolic pressure.
- Factors that can affect blood pressure include age, autonomic nervous system input, medications, and circadian rhythms.
- Blood pressure is usually measured indirectly using a sphygmomanometer and a stethoscope.
- Auscultation of blood pressure reveals five different phases known as Korotkoff sounds. The first Korotkoff sound corresponds to systolic pressure, the fifth (fourth in children) to diastolic pressure.
- Selecting proper cuff size, keeping the arm at heart level, avoiding venous congestion, and detecting the presence of an auscultatory gap are important steps in obtaining accurate blood pressure readings.

■ Orthostatic hypotension occurs when a person experiences a decrease in blood pressure when changing from a supine to an upright position.

■ Normal variations in vital signs occur throughout the lifespan.

References

Bates, B. (1991). *A guide to physical examination and history taking* (5th ed.). Philadelphia: J. B. Lippincott.

Braunwald, E. (1988). *Heart disease: A textbook of cardiovascular medicine* (3rd ed.). Philadelphia: W. B. Saunders.

Dressler, D., Smejkal, C., & Ruffolo, M. (1983). A comparison of oral and rectal temperature measurements in patients receiving oxygen by mask. *Nursing Research, 32,* 373.

Durbin, N. (1983). The application of Doppler techniques in critical care. *Focus on Critical Care, 1010*(3), 44–46.

Erickson, R. (1980). Oral temperature difference in relation to thermometer and technique. *Nursing Research, 29,* 157.

Ganong, W. F. (1989). *Review of medical physiology* (13th ed.). Los Altos, CA: Lange Medical Publications.

Guyton, A. (1986). *Textbook of medical physiology* (7th ed.). Philadelphia: W. B. Saunders.

Guyton, A. (1987). *Human physiology and mechanisms of disease* (4th ed.). Philadelphia: W. B. Saunders.

Hahn, G. D. (1985). Clinical monitoring in anesthesia: Applied technology in monitoring blood pressure. *AANA Journal, 53,* 149.

Hazinski, M. F. (1984). The cardiovascular system. In J. Howe, E. J. Dickason, D. A. Jones, et al. (Eds.), *The handbook of nursing.* New York: John Wiley & Sons.

Hypertension Detection and Follow-Up Program Cooperative Group. (1979). Five-year findings of the hypertension detection and follow-up program. *Journal of the American Medical Association, 242,* 2562.

Kaplan, N. M. (1988). Systemic hypertension: Mechanisms and diagnosis. In E. Braunwald (Ed.), *Heart Disease* (3rd ed.). Philadelphia: W. B. Saunders.

Kirkendall, W. M., Feinleib, M., Freis, E. D., et al. (1980). *Recommendation for human blood pressure determination by sphygmomanometers.* American Heart Association.

Kitterman, J., Phibbs, R. H., & Tooley, W. H. (1969). Aortic blood pressure in normal newborn infants during the first 12 hours of life. *Pediatrics, 44,* 959.

Kolanski, A., & Gunter, L. (1981). Hypothermia in the elderly. *Geriatric Nursing, 2,* 362.

Kurtz, K. J. (1982). Hypothermia in the elderly: The cold facts. *Geriatrics, 37,* 85.

Lim-Levy, F. (1982). The effect of oxygen inhalation on oral temperature. *Nursing Research, 31,* 150.

Mader, S. L. (1989). Aging and postural hypotension. *Journal of the American Geriatric Society,, 37,* 129.

Manning, D. M., Kucherirka, C., & Kaminiski, J. (1983). Miscuffing: Inappropriate blood pressure cuff application. *Circulation, 68,* 763.

Moore, K. I., & Newton, K. (1986). Orthostatic heart rates and blood pressures in healthy young women and men. *Heart & Lung, 15,* 611.

Nelson, W. E., Behrman, R. E., & Vaughan, V. C. (1987). *Nelson's textbook of pediatrics* (13th ed.). Philadelphia: W. B. Saunders.

Nelson, W. P., & Egbert, A. M. (1984). How to measure blood pressure—accurately. *Primary Cardiology, 10,* 14.

Pruitt, A. W. (1987). Systemic hypertension. In W. E. Nelson, R. E. Behrman, & V. C. Vaughan (Eds.), *Nelson's textbook of pediatrics* (13th ed). Philadelphia: W. B. Saunders.

Rattery, E. B., & Miller-Craig, M. W. (1978). Information derived from direct 24-hour recordings. In D. L. Clement (Ed.), *Blood pressure variability.* Baltimore: University Park Press.

Roben, N. (1986). Hypertension. In D. L. Carnevali & M. Patrick (Eds.), *Nursing management for the elderly* (2nd ed.). Philadelphia: J. B. Lippincott.

Robertson, D., & Robertson, R. M. (1985). Orthostatic hypotension—diagnosis and therapy. *Modern Concepts of Cardiovascular Disease, 54,* 7.

Samples, J., Van Cott, M., Long, C., et al. (1985). Circadian rhythms: Basis for screening fever. *Nursing Research, 34,* 377.

Schatz, I. J. (1984). Orthostatic hypotension: Diagnosis and treatment. *Hospital Practice, 19*(4), 59.

Shaver, J. (1991). Assessment of reproductive function. In M. Patrick, S. Woods, R. Craven, et al. (Eds.), Medical-surgical nursing (2nd ed.). St. Louis: J. B. Lippincott.

Stephen, S. A. (1987). *Effect of postural changes on arterial blood pressure and heart rate in healthy older adults.* Unpublished master's thesis, University of Washington.

Underhill, S. L. (1989). History-taking and physical examination of the patient with cardiovascular disease. In S. L. Underhill, S. L. Woods, E. S. Sivarajan, et al. (Eds.), *Cardiac nursing* (2nd ed.). Philadelphia: J. B. Lippincott.

Vargas, E., & Lye, M. (1982). Physiological responses to postural change in young and old healthy individuals. *Experimental Gerontology, 17,* 445.

Vick, R. (1984). *Contemporary medical physiology.* Menlo Park, CA: Addison-Wesley.

Woodman, E., Perry, S., & Simms, L. (1967). Sources of unreliability in oral temperatures. *Nursing Research, 16,* 276.

Yonkman, C. (1982). Cool and heated aerosol and measurement of oral temperature. *Nursing Research, 31,* 354.

Bibliography

Abrams, L., Buckholz, C., McKenzie, N. S., et al. (1989). Effects of peripheral IV infusion on neonatal axillary temperature measurement. *Pediatric Nursing,* 15:630–632.

Campbell-Heider, N., Campbell-Heider, N., & Knapp, T. R. (1988). Nurses' attitudes toward conventional and automated vital signs measurement methods. *Medical Instrumentation, 22,* 257–262.

Cooper, J. W. (1989). High blood pressure monitoring guidelines: Diuretics. *Nursing Homes, 38*(3), 7–9.

Frolich, E., Grim, C., Labarthe, D., et al. (1987). *Recommendations for human blood pressure determination by sphygmomanometers.* American Heart Association.

Hahn, W. K., Brooks, J. A., & Hite, R. (1989). Blood pressure norms for healthy young adults: Relation to sex, age, and reported parental hypertension. *Research in Nursing and Health, 12*(1), 53.

Hellmann, R., et al. (1989). The influence of talking on diastolic blood pressure readings. National League for Nursing Publ #15-2232, 78–82.

Leigh, B., Guisinger, D., & Fech, J. (1989). Blood pressure screening in the workplace. *American Association of Occupational Health Nurses Journal, 7*(1), 14–17.

Neff, J., Ayoub, J., Longman, A., et al. (1989). Effect of respiratory rate, respiratory depth, and open- versus closed-mouth breathing on sublingual temperature. *Research in Nursing and Health, 12,* 195–202.

Preparing to take a patient's blood pressure. *Nursing '89, 19*(6), 65.

Robichaud-Ekstrand, S., & Davies, B. (1989). Comparison of electronic and glass thermometers: Length of time of insertion and type of breathing. *Canadian Journal of Nursing Research, 21*(1), 61–73.

Schron, E. B., Davey, J. A., Jensen, J. M., et al. (1989). The systolic hypertension in the elderly program: Implications for nursing practice and research. *Progress in Cardiovascular Nursing, 4*(4), 138–145.

Sheehan, M. M. (1990). Blood pressure monitoring. *Nursing '90, 20*(4), 79–81.

Tifft, C. P. (1989). Management of orthostatic hypotension. *Hospital Medicine, 25*(3), 25–28.

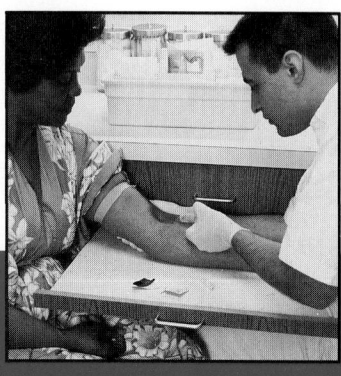

Diagnostic Tests and Procedures

LEARNING OBJECTIVES

Upon completion of this chapter, the student will be able to do the following:

- Discuss the nursing responsibilities before, during, and after laboratory and diagnostic procedures.
- Describe the collection of blood samples or other specimens for laboratory analysis.
- Discuss the significance of various laboratory tests.
- Identify common noninvasive viewing tests used to visualize body organs or functions
- Discuss how information about functional health status gained from laboratory or diagnostic procedures can be used to individualize patient care.

KEY TERMS

Angiography	Hemoglobin	Radioisotope
Ascites	Leukocytosis	Radiopaque
Barium	Leukopenia	Roentgenogram
Biopsy	Lumbar puncture	Thoracentesis
Blood gases	Mammography	Thrombocytopenia
Coagulation studies	Myelogram	Thrombocytosis
Culture	Nuclear scan	Ultrasonography
Endoscopy	Paracentesis	Venipuncture
Fluoroscopy		

20

The Nurse as a Facilitator for Diagnostic Testing
  Patient Preparation
  Responsibilities During Testing
  Responsibilities After Testing
  Using Data to Individualize Care
Laboratory Tests
  Blood Specimen Collection
    Venipuncture
    Arterial Puncture
    Capillary Puncture
    Blood from a Central Venous Catheter
  Hematologic Tests
    Complete Blood Count
    Erythrocyte Sedimentation Rate
    Blood Coagulation Studies
    Blood Chemistry Studies
    Blood Lipid Studies
    Serum Enzymes
    Serum Drug Levels
    Arterial Blood Gases
  Urine Testing
    Urine Specimen Collection
    Routine Urinalysis
    24-Hour Urine Collection

  Culture and Sensitivity Testing
    Blood Culture
    Urine Culture
    Sputum Culture
    Swab Culture
Diagnostic Tests
  Noninvasive Viewing Techniques
    X-rays (Radiography)
    Ultrasonography
    Magnetic Resonance Imaging
  Invasive Viewing Techniques
    Endoscopy
    Angiography
  Aspiration Diagnostic Procedures
    Biopsy
    Lumbar Puncture
    Thoracentesis
    Paracentesis
  Diagnostic Procedures That Evaluate Electrical
    Conduction
    Electrocardiography
    Electroencephalography
Lifespan Considerations
Key Concepts

Diagnostic and laboratory tests involve procedures that provide information about part or all of the body. Diagnostic tests make use of specialized equipment designed to visualize or evaluate normal body function. Ultrasound, x-rays, or visualization of internal body organs through scopes are examples of diagnostic procedures. Laboratory tests include procedures that require the collection of specimens from the patient (for example, blood, urine, or sputum). Once these specimens are obtained, they are studied for abnormalities in the laboratory.

Information obtained from diagnostic or laboratory tests is used to diagnose specific illnesses or conditions, or to follow the progress of treatment. The nursing role in diagnostic and laboratory testing has a broader focus. For example, in addition to benefiting from the information obtained to assess a patient's health status, the nurse facilitates diagnostic and laboratory procedures by ob-

taining samples, preparing and supporting the patient, performing postprocedure assessments, and sharing the results of the procedures with the physician. Finally, the nurse uses the data obtained in diagnostic or laboratory procedures to assess function, dysfunction, or patients at risk for dysfunction to individualize nursing care.

Individualized patient care results when information obtained through the diagnostic or laboratory tests is used by the nurse to help the patient manage simple tasks of daily living (Carnevali, 1983). For example, chest x-rays are often obtained to diagnose and follow the course of treatment for pneumonia. The nurse is not expected to read or interpret the chest x-ray, or suggest changes in treatment based on the x-ray findings. Rather, the nurse uses the information obtained from the x-ray report to plan optimal positioning of the patient. The x-ray report describes the portion of the lung affected by pneumonia and by poor air exchange. Knowing that both air flow and blood flow are gravity-dependent, the nurse positions the patient with the non-affected side down to maximize air flow and blood flow to the healthy lung tissue. Thus, the nurse is using the x-ray information to promote oxygenation in a patient.

Laboratory data also can be used to individualize care and to help the patient meet daily living needs. For example, a nurse who becomes aware of a patient's low hemoglobin value (the oxygen-carrying component of the red blood cell), plans activity sessions with frequent rest periods for the patient. This planning ensures that the oxygen supply is sufficient to meet the demands of the body.

An overview of common diagnostic and laboratory tests is provided in this chapter. General rather than specific nursing responsibilities associated with the procedures are outlined. In addition, common nursing implications of the diagnostic and laboratory tests are described. (In-depth information on important tests can be found in chapters in Section II.)

THE NURSE AS A FACILITATOR FOR DIAGNOSTIC TESTING

Patient Preparation

The nurse frequently plays a key role in preparing the patient for laboratory and diagnostic tests. The nurse may have responsibility for scheduling the procedure, for patient teaching, for witnessing signatures for informed consent, for physically preparing the patient, or for obtaining the supplies and equipment. See Procedure 20-1, "Preparing the Patient for Diagnostic Tests."

Patient Scheduling. The nurse may schedule laboratory and diagnostic procedures. Once the physician's order is verified, the nurse is responsible for ensuring that a requisition has been prepared for the ordered test and that the requisition is directed to the appropriate department or facility.

Whenever possible, tests involving the same specimens or similar procedures are grouped together. For example, tests involving a venipuncture for sampling of blood are ordered to be done at the same time to avoid unnecessary resampling. Tests requiring fasting are usually grouped together to avoid requiring the patient to fast on numerous occasions. X-ray procedures also may be scheduled at the same time to avoid many trips to the x-ray facility.

Each patient should be considered individually, however, when tests are scheduled. The nurse must consider that scheduling too many consecutive procedures may overtire the elderly, the severely ill, or patients with chronic health problems. Fasting may be difficult for patients with diabetes mellitus; tests should be scheduled early in the morning for these patients to avoid potential complications.

Tests may need to be ordered in the proper sequence for optimal results. For example, tests using barium (a contrast medium used to visualize the digestive tract) can interfere with other internal body-viewing techniques, and should be scheduled to take place after these other tests are completed.

Laboratory and diagnostic procedures often are performed on an outpatient basis. In this situation, the patient or the patient's caretaker may do the scheduling. To avoid confusion, the nurse provides the patient with details of the test, information about scheduling, and the telephone number. It is helpful to provide this information in written form; when patients encounter difficulties or become confused, they may neglect to have important tests done.

Patient Teaching. Explanations about the testing procedure can help relieve the patient's anxiety, ensure cooperation, and assist the patient in coping with an uncomfortable or painful procedure. Often, diagnostic procedures are performed to determine what is causing the patient's current symptoms. It is not unusual for the patient to imagine the worst, fearing that the test may

---

Patient Teaching

Instruct the patient as follows:

- NPO means nothing by mouth; determine from the nurse which meals to omit, whether or not water can be taken, how to take necessary medications, and when normal intake of foods or fluids can be resumed.
- If a sputum specimen is to be collected, avoid touching the inside of the sputum-collection container with your fingers, tongue, or lips when coughing the specimen into the container.
- Be sure you understand what is expected of you before all procedures, particularly if you must remain motionless during any part of the examination.
- Be clear on signs of inflammation and the necessity of reporting these signs if you have undergone invasive procedures.
- Do not use deodorants, powders, perfumes, or creams on the day you are having a mammogram.
- Save *all* urine during 24-hour urine collections.
- Tests involving radioisotopes will not cause you to become radioactive.
- Keep the limb immobilized before and following angiographic examinations. It is also necessary to report numbness and tingling following the examination.

■ **Purpose**

1. Decrease anxiety and increase patient cooperation with a procedure.
2. Ensure that diagnostic test will provide good test results without untoward effects.

■ **Assessment**

- Review patient's history of drug or food allergies (especially important for dye injection studies or when procedures require premedication).
- Assess patient's knowledge of the procedure.
- Assess patient's ability to follow directions and cooperate before and during the test.
- Evaluate patient's physical ability to tolerate the procedure.
- Assess need for nursing staff to accompany patient to procedure.
- Obtain and document patient's baseline vital signs.
- Identify correct name band on patient's wrist.

■ **Equipment**

Signed permission for diagnostic procedure.
Pajama bottoms and hospital gown.
Patent intravenous access (if necessary for procedure).
Supplies and equipment specific to procedure.

■ **Procedure**

1. Identify the specific procedure or procedures to be performed.
2. Obtain a written consent for invasive procedures after the physician has explained the study to the patient.
   Rationale: Patients should be informed of the reason for the procedure, what to expect during the procedure, and what are the associated risks. The patient's signing of the consent must be observed and signed by a witness.
3. If more than one procedure is ordered, they should be scheduled in an order least traumatic to the patient and which will produce the most accurate results.
   Rationale: Tests that need to be repeated due to inaccurate results are traumatic and costly to the patient, and can delay needed treatment. Rescheduled procedures often mean an extended hospital stay.
4. Identify specific preparations needed to be performed before the procedure (i.e., enemas, NPO status, ingestion of contrast material).
5. Provide instruction to the patient and significant others regarding the procedure and rationale for any special preparations or dietary/fluid restrictions required by the study.
6. Monitor dietary or fluid restrictions.
   Note: Patients who have NPO diagnostic procedures scheduled for several consecutive days may become

dehydrated. Encourage them to eat and drink well when not NPO. Consider scheduling a rest day between procedures if possible.
7. Continue to provide psychological support to the patient as needed.
8. When a patient who routinely takes special medications (i.e., cardiac medications, anticonvulsants, anticoagulants, diabetic medications) is NPO obtain physician orders regarding the administration of his or her medications before the procedure.
   Rationale: Holding essential medications may alter therapeutic blood levels of the drug. Giving medications with a sip of water may not interfere with the outcome of the procedure.
9. Immediately before the procedure:
   a. Have patient urinate unless contraindicated by the study.
   b. Reidentify any patient allergies and identiband.
   c. Remove hairpins, contact lenses, jewelry and fingernail polish if required by procedure.
   d. Administer and document premedication if ordered.
   e. If transported with intravenous line, assess that IV is patent and remaining volume is sufficient.
   f. Supervise transfer from bed to wheelchair or gurney. If transported to gurney, side rails or safety belt should be fastened.
   g. Provide blanket.
   Rationale: All of these interventions are directed toward patient safety or comfort.
10. Accompany patient during transport if required by patient's physical or emotional status.

■ **Lifespan Considerations**

Infants and Children

- It is often difficult to explain a procedure so a child can understand. Role-playing, puppets, or showing the equipment are useful techniques for patient teaching.
- Children under 12 should never be left alone in a strange department.
- Allow parents to accompany child to procedure, or have child bring a "security object" (i.e., blanket, stuffed animal) to decrease his or her anxiety.
- Painful procedures should never be done at the bedside of children under 12 years of age. The bedside should be kept a "safe place" for them at *all* times.

Patients with Mental or Sensory Impairments

- Patients who have mental or sensory impairments often have established a trusting relationship with their nurse. They may have difficulty communicating with or relating to people they don't know well. Accompany these patients to other departments whenever possible.

reveal a serious or life-threatening disease. Careful patient teaching may help alleviate these fears. Conversely, the patient also should be informed that not all questions can be answered by performing a specific test; some tests may raise as many questions as they answer.

Most patient teaching occurs before the procedure (Fig. 20-1); but some information can be offered during the testing. Explanations are made in terms the patient can understand. Children present a unique situation; methods such as role-playing or showing the equipment may be helpful. For all age groups, time is allowed for questions after explanations. When the patient is anxious, information may need to be repeated several times before the patient is able to process the important content. Explanations need to be age-appropriate, factual, and individualized for patients with special needs (e.g., patients who are hearing- or vision-impaired). An interpreter should be used for patients who do not understand or read English.

The nurse should be prepared to answer such questions as: what will they do? Where will the test be done? Will it be painful? How long will it take? Will I be able to go to work (school, home) after the test is completed? When will I know the results of the test? Clear, direct answers to these questions will help to prepare the patient emotionally and physically for the procedure.

In many agencies, printed information on common diagnostic procedures is available. After the patient has had time to read the information, the nurse can clarify points and answer questions. When the nurse is not knowledgeable regarding a particular procedure, the department performing the test can be contacted for information.

Informed Consent. Before any diagnostic procedure, the patient should possess adequate and accurate information to make the decision whether or not to have the procedure performed. Most patients agreeably submit to diagnostic studies because they hope to learn the reason for pain or discomfort. The patient also expects that the test will provide information about how the problem can be treated and resolved.

When the patient has been informed about what the procedure entails, the risks and benefits of the procedure, and the alternatives to the procedure, the patient has received the information necessary for him or her to give informed consent for the procedure. It is important to consult agency protocol to identify those procedures that require a *written* statement of informed consent. Informed consent is discussed in Chapter 3 and a sample consent form is printed in Chapter 23.

If the adult patient should indicate a lack of understanding about a procedure or is unsure regarding the decision to undergo the procedure, the nurse should not attempt to assist the patient in making a decision; instead, the physician should be contacted. When the patient is a child or is incapable of understanding the pro-

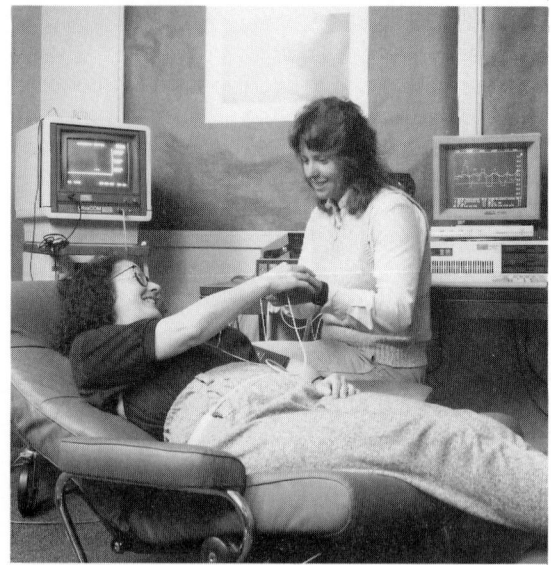

Figure 20–1. Patient teaching before testing.

cedure, his or her representative should be the one to indicate understanding.

Physical Preparation. Many procedures require specific physical preparation of the patient (preprocedure protocols) to ensure accurate test results. Frequently, the nurse explains preprocedure protocols to the patient and conveys the importance that they be followed. The protocols are usually found in written form and will be available for many inpatient and outpatient studies.

Fasting is commonly required before many examinations. The patient receives a "nothing by mouth" (NPO) order for a specified period before the procedure (usually overnight or a period of hours). When an NPO patient is receiving routine medication (e.g., medication to control blood pressure or anticonvulsant medication), however, it is important to verify if the medications can be given with a small sip of water or by means of an alternate route.

Other preprocedure preparations of the patient may require nursing assistance. Cleansing of the bowel is a common preparation when the gastrointestinal tract is the focus of the study. For some studies, the patient may need to be "scrubbed" (involving a specific protocol for skin cleansing) or shaved before the procedure. Although it is desirable most of the time for the patient to have an empty urinary bladder, some tests may require that the bladder be full. Medication, often a sedative, may be ordered to be administered at a specific time before the test.

Collection of Supplies. Some procedures do not require that the patient be transported to another department; instead, the tests are performed at the bedside. In this situation, it is usually the nurse's responsibility to obtain the supplies and equipment. Often, supplies for a specific procedure are prepackaged, and only sterile gloves or local anesthetic agents may be needed in addition to the prepackaged kit.

Responsibilities During Testing

The nurse may be called on to assist the physician or the technician performing the diagnostic test. Setting up equipment, providing equipment and specimen-collection containers as they are needed, ensuring the maintenance of sterility, administering medication, and providing for patient safety are some of the typical tasks that a nurse may perform. Once the procedure is complete, the nurse documents all the functions.

In some situations, the nurse will perform the procedure. Again, the nurse will gather and arrange equipment, maintain a sterile field, administer prescribed medication, and ensure patient safety.

Patient Assessment. Patient assessment is necessary to detect any changes in status during the procedure. Vital signs and observations such as the patient's affect, skin color, and mental status are recorded before the procedure, and serve as baseline data. Allergies and laboratory data pertinent to the study are noted.

During the procedure the patient is observed for adverse effects. If possible, records are made of vital signs and other observations at specific intervals. Changes in vital signs or in other baseline parameters are acted on immediately. For example, a decreasing blood pressure, an increasing pulse, pallor, diaphoresis, and complaints of light-headedness or dizziness could indicate shock. In this situation, intervention would be directed at correcting the change; monitoring of vital signs and other indicators would continue during the intervention phase. The whole sequence should be recorded on specific forms prepared for monitoring purposes.

Patient Support. Supporting the patient during the procedure is an important function that may be performed by a family member or by the nurse. When children undergo procedures, the parent is encouraged to remain with the child whenever possible. Being allowed to keep a special blanket or a stuffed animal may also help reduce a child's anxiety. Activities such as holding the patient's hand or quietly standing next to the patient may be all that is needed.

The nurse can also offer emotional support with statements about what to expect (e.g., "You may feel some stinging as the doctor injects the anesthetic," or "We are nearly finished"). Attending to the elderly patient's physical comfort by supporting a tired limb or by making sure that the patient is warm enough, can also be comforting.

Patient Positioning. It is often the nurse's responsibility to position the patient during diagnostic procedures. Positioning can be a matter of simply assisting the patient into a position of comfort, or, in many situations, assisting the patient into the specific position indicated for the test or procedure. In the course of this chapter, preferred positions for certain tests are discussed.

Common positioning postures include: prone (face down), supine (lying on back), high Fowler's (head of

---

Safety Alert

- Use Universal Precautions for all tests involving collection of body fluids.
- Determine whether or not the patient is allergic to iodine before cleansing the skin with a povidone–iodine antiseptic before venipuncture.
- In order to avoid hematoma formation when an evacuation tube is used for venipuncture, pull the tube off the evacuation tube needle before withdrawing the needle from the vein.
- Apply pressure over the puncture site after all venipunctures. If bleeding continues, have the patient elevate the area and continue to hold pressure.
- Apply pressure over the puncture site for at least 5 minutes when arterial blood gases are drawn.
- Do not draw blood from an extremity into which intravenous fluids are infusing. Tests may not be accurate.
- Restrain an infant on an examination table during invasive procedures to avoid injury should the child move suddenly.
- Determine if the patient is allergic to iodine whenever a test involving contrast dyes is anticipated.
- Closely monitor vital signs and watch for bleeding after all invasive tests involving the vascular system.
- Assure that all clothing with metal fastenings, all jewelry, and any metal hairpins have been removed before magnetic resonance imaging examinations (MRI).
- After angiographic examinations, including cardiac catheterization, monitor peripheral pulses distal to the catheter puncture site to assure arterial circulation has not been impaired. The temperature and color of the skin on the extremity should be compared to the opposite extremity.
- Encourage fluids after studies involving contrast dye unless fluids are contraindicated. Fluids will help the kidneys to excrete the dye.
- Do not leave confused patients alone on an examination table because of the possibility of fall should they try to get down unassisted.

bed elevated 90°), semi-Fowler's (head of bed elevated 45°), dorsal recumbent (supine with legs flexed and rotated outward), lithotomy (supine with legs flexed in an elevated position), knee–chest position, Trendelenburg's (supine with head lower than feet), lateral or side-lying position, and Sims' (semiprone between a prone and side-lying position). These positions are illustrated in Figure 20-2. Postions commonly used to routinely position the patient in bed are discussed in more detail in Chapter 29.

Once positioned, the patient may require assistance in maintaining that body position. Certain positions can cause fatigue, especially when limbs are not adequately supported. The nurse should support the patient and use pillows to increase comfort and decrease fatigue. The elderly or other people with limited joint mobility may experience pain or discomfort when an extremity must be manipulated or held stationary. Some positions may cause breathing difficulties for those with respiratory problems. Infants and young children, who are unable to understand the necessity of remaining still, need to be restrained to ensure safety during the testing procedure.

Responsibilities After Testing

Patient Assessment. Vital signs and other observations described above function as baseline assessment

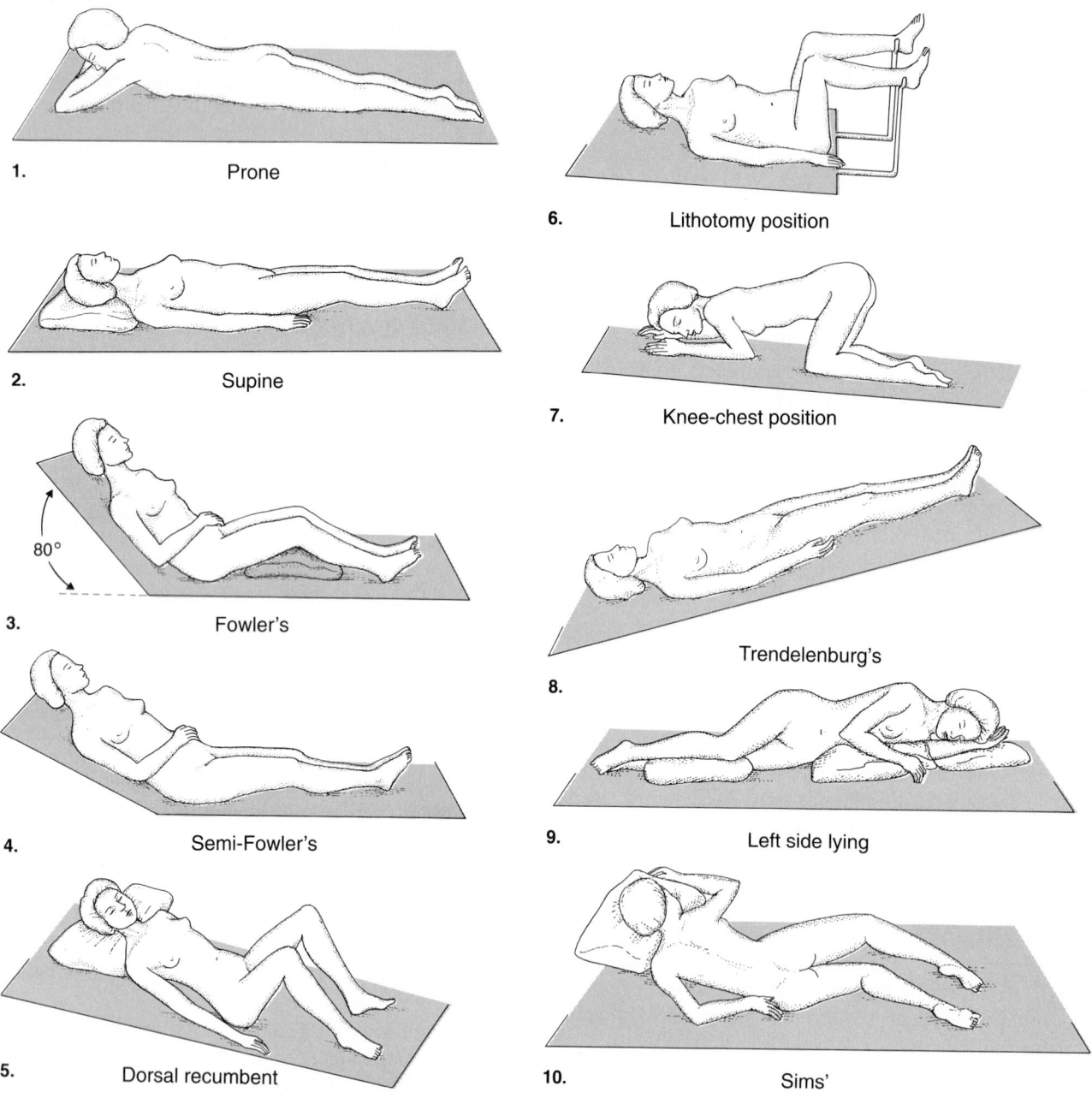

1. Prone

2. Supine

3. Fowler's

80°

4. Semi-Fowler's

5. Dorsal recumbent

6. Lithotomy position

7. Knee-chest position

8. Trendelenburg's

9. Left side lying

10. Sims'

Figure 20–2. Body positions used during diagnostic tests, surgery, or during patient care delivery.

data. Postprocedure data are compared to baseline. After the procedure is complete or the patient returns from the procedure, the nurse continues to assess the patient's status. It is important to be well informed about specific, possible complications for each procedure. Observations will be directed at detecting such problems promptly. The frequency of assessment may be determined by agency protocol. All significant changes from baseline data should be reported immediately to the physician.

Specimen Collection and Equipment. During many diagnostic procedures, specimens are collected and transported immediately to the laboratory for analysis. The nurse may be responsible for ensuring that the specimen is collected in the appropriate container, labeled properly, and transported to the laboratory. Universal precautions, which include the wearing of gloves, are followed to avoid contact with body fluids (e.g., by means of needle puncture or spilling of specimen). It is wise to send the specimen to the laboratory before the area is cleaned to avoid inadvertent disposal of the specimen.

Cleaning the work area after a diagnostic procedure may be the responsibility of the nurse. Care should be taken to dispose of needles and other sharp objects in a designated receptacle to avoid accidental injury and exposure of other health-care workers.

Documentation. It is important to document the diagnostic or laboratory test. The type of procedure, the name of the person performing the procedure, the date and time of the procedure, a summary of patient assessments before, during, and after the procedure, and collection and disposition of specimens should be recorded. The patient's response should also be documented, particularly any complications during or after the procedure (e.g., pain, nausea, fatigue).

Using Data to Individualize Care

The nurse uses the information obtained through laboratory and diagnostic testing to assess the functional health of the patient and to plan individualized care. The use of test results to help plan nursing care may be the most important aspect of diagnostic and laboratory testing.

Individualizing care based on functional health is a natural consequence of laboratory and diagnostic testing, and one that defines the nurse as a patient advocate. For example, blood tests may reveal that a patient has dysfunctional urinary elimination because of kidney failure. In this situation, the nurse reviews the patient's medications that are eliminated by the kidney and watches for signs of toxicity. Another example of the nurse individualizing care based on test data is the identification of a patient at risk for skin breakdown or poor wound healing, by noting a low serum albumin level; this

patient may require increased attention to nutrition or a pressure support mattress to ensure skin integrity and good healing of wounds. Finally, a test such as cardiac catheterization may reveal extensive coronary heart disease (CHD). The nurse, aware of the potential problems with oxygenation, may appraise the patient's heart rate during activity to assess the patient's response to exercise. Table 20-1 lists selected laboratory and diagnostic tests for each functional health pattern.

LABORATORY TESTS

Although specimens for laboratory tests may be obtained either at the bedside or in the laboratory, the assay of blood, urine, and other body samples takes place in the laboratory. Protocols for sample collection ensure that specific amounts of samples are collected and analyzed under standard conditions. After laboratory assay, the nurse may be responsible for communicating any abnormal results to the physician. In addition, the nurse uses the information gathered through laboratory testing to plan the patient's care.

Using Laboratory Reference Ranges. The nurse examines the patient's records thoroughly each day for the results of diagnostic laboratory testing. Often, changes in the patient's condition (deterioration or improvement) can be reflected in changes in laboratory values. For this reason, normal reference values for common laboratory tests are provided in this text (see the Appendix). Caution should be exercised in comparing the patient's values to the reference values, however; normal values for some laboratory tests will vary between laboratories because of regional differences in patient characteristics and differences in measurement technique.

Blood Specimen Collection

The sampling of blood for laboratory assay is performed either by laboratory phlebotomists or by nursing personnel. Venous blood is most commonly used for blood tests. Venous blood can be obtained by means of a venipuncture or through an intravenous catheter placed into a central vein. Arterial blood is less commonly assayed; it can be obtained with arterial puncture or through an indwelling arterial catheter. Capillary blood is obtained using a lancet. Gloves are worn during all blood collection procedures in accordance with Universal Precautions for avoiding contact with body fluids (CDC, 1987).

Venipuncture

The procedure for blood sampling known as **venipuncture** involves puncturing the vein with a needle for the

TABLE 20–1

Relationship of Selected Laboratory and Diagnostic Procedures to Functional Health

Functional Pattern	Test	Functional Pattern	Test

Health Perception–
Health Management
	Diagnostic tests
	  Mammogram
	  Pap smear
	  Biopsy
		Nutritional–Metabolic	Laboratory tests
			  Hematocrit
			  White blood count
			  WBC differential
			  Sedimentation rate
			  Electrolytes
			  Protein (albumin)
			  Blood glucose
			  Blood lipid studies
			  24-hour urine collection
			  Culture and sensitivity tests
			Diagnostic tests
			  Barium enema
			  Upper GI series
			  Abdominal ultrasound
			  Endoscopy
			  Liver biopsy
			  Bone marrow biopsy
			  Paracentesis
			  Cholangiogram, Cholecysto-
			    gram, ERCP

Elimination	Laboratory tests
	  Urinalysis
	  Urine culture and sensitivity
	  Stool culture and sensitivity
	  Blood urea nitrogen (BUN)
	  Creatinine
	Diagnostic tests
	  Sigmoidoscopy
	  Barium enema
	  Pelvic ultrasound
	  Renal biopsy
	  IVP (kidney x-ray with
	    contrast)
	  Cystoscopy
		Activity–Exercise	Laboratory tests
			  Hemoglobin
			  Hematocrit
			  Blood coagulation studies
			  Blood lipid studies
			  Serum enzymes
			  Arterial blood gases
			Diagnostic tests
			  X-rays (chest; extremities)
			  Lung perfusion scan
			  Angiography
			  Cardiac catheterization
			  Thoracentesis
			  Electrocardiogram
			  Exercise treadmill testing
			  Bronchoscopy

Sleep–Rest	Diagnostic tests
	  Electroencephalogram
		Cognitive–Perceptual	Laboratory tests
			  Electrolytes
			  Blood glucose
			  Blood chemistries
			  Arterial blood gases
			Diagnostic tests
			  Computed tomography
			  Magnetic resonance imaging
			  Cerebral angiography
			  Electroencephalogram
			  Lumbar puncture
			  Myelogram

Self–Perception	None—Assessment of pattern
	  based mainly on
	  subjective data
		Role Relationship	None—Assessment of pattern
			  based mainly on
			  subjective data

Sexuality–Reproductive	Laboratory tests
	  Hormone levels
	  Pregnancy tests
	Diagnostic tests
	  Pelvic ultrasound
	  Mammography
		Coping–Stress Tolerance	None—Assessment of pattern
			  based mainly on
			  subjective data

Values–Beliefs	None—Assessment of pattern
	  based mainly on
	  subjective data		

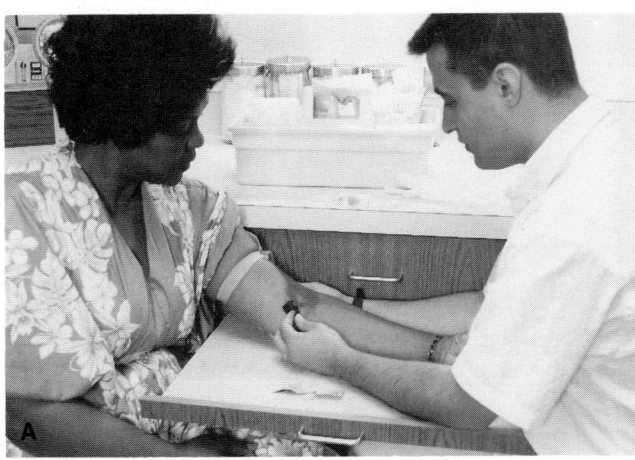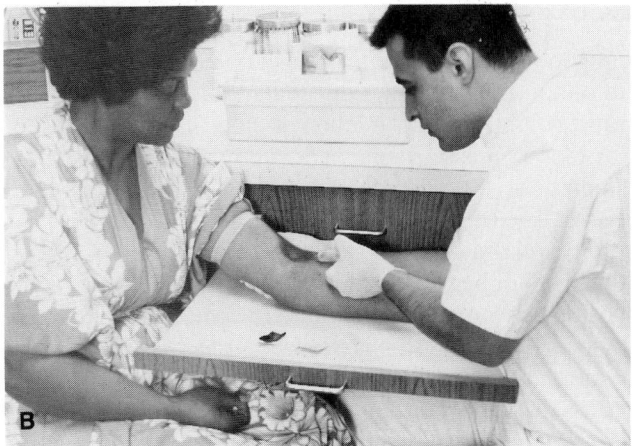

Figure 20–3. Venipuncture. **A.** Cleansing the site. Betadine, which is used for cleansing, darkens the arm, but can be removed after the procedure. **B.** Aspirating blood with the vacuum tube.

purpose of blood withdrawal. Aseptic technique is used during the procedure to prevent the transfer of microorganisms into the blood stream. The most common sites for venipuncture are the antecubital area (basilic, median cubital, or cephalic veins), or the dorsal surface of the hand (the dorsal metacarpal, basilic, or cephalic veins).

Venipuncture sampling begins with the application of an occluding tourniquet. The tourniquet should not be so tight as to eliminate distal arterial blood flow; a pulse should be palpable "downstream" from the tourniquet. Areas of inflammation and bruising and scarred areas are avoided. Specimens should not be withdrawn from a limb into which fluids or medications are infusing intravenously (Goe, 1989a).

Once a suitable vein is located, the tourniquet may be released (for patient comfort) while the site is prepared. The method for skin preparation may vary from institution to institution. One method involves cleansing the skin with a povidone–iodine solution, which is allowed to remain on the skin for 1 to 2 minutes before it is removed by an alcohol swab (Fig. 20-3A). The alcohol is allowed to dry to prevent contamination of the specimen. The tourniquet is reapplied and gloves are donned to prevent contact with blood.

Blood is drawn using a needle and a syringe or with an evacuated collection tube (a vacuum tube which, when attached to the venipuncture needle, "pulls" the blood from the punctured vein) (Fig. 20-3B). The needle, with the bevel (the flat, slanted edge of the needle) directed upward, is passed through the skin into the vein (Fig. 20-4). Two approaches to a venipuncture can be used: a direct (the skin and vein are penetrated in one motion) or an indirect approach (the needle punctures the skin parallel to the vein and is then directed laterally into the vein). Practitioner preference usually determines which venipuncture approach is chosen. Once the penetration of the vein produces a show of blood in the syringe, the

desired amount of blood is then aspirated (Goe, 1989a). After the needle is removed from the site, pressure is applied for 1 to 2 minutes to stop the flow of blood. An adhesive bandage may be applied.

Arterial Puncture

Arterial sampling is performed to evaluate blood gases, which indicate the metabolic, oxygen, and ventilatory status of the patient. In most agencies, personnel must receive special training and become certified for arterial puncture. The nurse who performs arterial blood sampling should be aware of several important points: the radial artery at the wrist is the preferred arterial site because it is superficial and easily palpable, but occasionally the brachial or femoral arteries are used; a heparinized syringe is employed (in some settings, the syringe may be glass); on collection of the sample, pressure should be applied over the puncture site for at least 5 minutes; and finally, the arterial specimen should be transported immediately to the laboratory, on ice (Goe, 1989a).

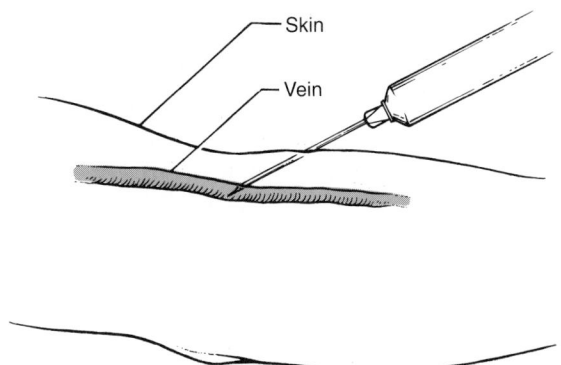

Figure 20–4. During the venipuncture procedure, the needle with an upward bevel is passed through the skin.

Capillary Puncture

Finger or heel pricks with a lancet or autolet can be used to obtain small samples of capillary blood for analysis. Most commonly, this method of blood sampling is used for blood glucose, hematocrit, peripheral blood smear studies, or for phenylketonuria (PKU) tests in newborns.

Obtaining a capillary sample can be aided by warming the finger or heel or placing the extremity in a dependent position to improve blood flow. To acquire the capillary blood sample, the skin is cleansed, usually with alcohol. Gloves are donned and the point of the lancet or autolet is briskly pierced through the skin (Fig. 20-5). If a finger is used, the side of the finger pad, rather than the center, is pricked; this is less painful for the patient. Likewise, the side of the heel should be selected for infants. When a drop of blood appears on the surface of the skin, it can be collected in a capillary blood tube or on a reagent strip. The autolet or lancet is disposed of according to the hospital policy for disposition of needles to avoid injury to health-care workers.

When capillary puncture is used to obtain blood to evaluate blood glucose levels, the blood sample is placed on a reagent strip. Blood glucose can be determined by visually interpreting the color changes on the reagent strip, or by placing the strip in a battery-operated device which can compute blood glucose from the sample (see Procedure 20-2, "Measuring Blood Glucose by Skin Puncture").

Blood from a Central Venous Catheter

The use of a central venous catheter allows access to the patient's blood supply for long-term intravenous infusions and for frequent blood sampling. This method of blood sampling avoids venipuncture and allows for frequent, speedy blood collection. Commonly, central venous catheters are used for cancer patients (who will receive chemotherapy and follow-up evaluation for an extended period of time), for patients on long-term antibiotic therapy, and for patients who are receiving total parenteral nutrition (TPN).

Central venous catheters include "triple-lumen", Groshong, Hickman, and other types of venous access devices, which are placed through the subclavian vein into the superior vena cava. Frequently, these catheters have more than one lumen; consequently, blood can be withdrawn through one lumen while fluids infuse through another. The larger lumen should be reserved for obtaining blood samples in a multiple-lumen catheter. Agency protocol should be consulted before sampling through a central venous catheter. It is recommended that a 2- to 3-mL sample be discarded from the catheter before obtaining blood for analysis. Samples for most studies can be obtained in this manner; however, sampling for coagulation studies has not been shown to produce reliable results (Goe, 1989a).

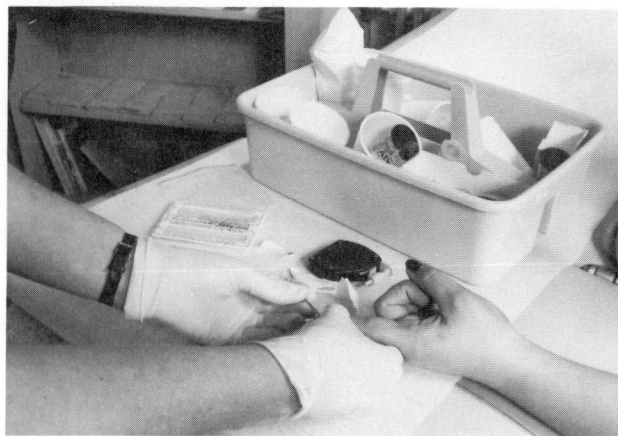

Figure 20–5. In capillary puncture, the finger is cleansed and pricked.

Hematologic Tests

Diagnostic laboratory tests for hematologic values are common. Anemias, bleeding or coagulation problems, hemolytic disorders, or nutritional disorders can be identified through assessment of blood values. A few of the most common hematologic studies—complete blood count (CBC), the erythrocyte sedimentation rate (sed rate; ESR), blood coagulation studies, blood chemistry and lipid studies, serum drug and enzyme levels, and arterial blood gases—are examined briefly in the following discussion. For more complete information, refer to Chapters 31 and 35.

Complete Blood Count

The complete blood count, or CBC, is one of the most commonly performed laboratory tests. The components of the CBC are the blood cells, which are formed in the bone marrow and are suspended in plasma. Blood cells and plasma make up the blood volume of the individual, about 8% of the body weight (Ganong, 1986). The blood cells accounted for in a CBC are the red blood cells (erythrocytes or RBCs), the white blood cells (leukocytes or WBCs), and platelets. Also examined are the WBC differential (Diff), hematocrit (Hct), hemoglobin (Hb), the morphology (shape or structure) of the cells, and activity (appropriate function) of the blood cells. The Appendix contains CBC reference ranges.

Red Blood Cell Count. The RBC count is expressed in the number of RBCs per microliter (μL) of whole blood. Red blood cells are produced in the bone marrow in response to a chemical produced in the kidney (erythropoietin). Increased RBCs in the blood suppress the production of new RBCs.

Hemoglobin. The protein compound in RBCs that is responsible for carrying oxygen to and carbon dioxide

PROCEDURE 20–2. Measuring Blood Glucose by Skin Puncture

■ Purpose
1. Monitor blood glucose levels at the bedside for patients who are at risk for hypo- or hyperglycemia.
2. Monitor the effectiveness of insulin administration.

■ Assessment
• Review the physician's order to determine the time and frequency of glucose monitoring.
   Note: The procedure should be performed before meals since carbohydrate ingestion will alter blood glucose levels.
• Assess the patient's medical history to determine if the patient is at risk for complications from skin punctures (i.e., bleeding disorders, anticoagulant therapy, or low platelet count).
• Assess the skin area to be used for puncture (fingers, toes, heels). Avoid areas with open lesions or ecchymosis.
• Assess the patient's understanding of the purpose of the procedure and the patient's physical and emotional ability to learn the procedure and perform it independently.

■ Equipment
Alcohol or povidone–iodine swab
Sterile lancet or autolet
Cotton balls
Blood glucose reagent strip
Glucose testing meter
Disposable gloves

■ Procedure
1. Have the patient wash hands with soap and warm water.
   Rationale: The fingertips are the most common skin puncture sites in adults. Washing not only decreases the chances of infection but, due to the warm water, promotes vasodilation of the puncture site.
2. Position patient at rest in a comfortable posture.
3. Remove the reagent slip from the container and handle according to the manufacturer's instructions.
   Rationale: The glucose meter may need recalibration or "rezero-ing."
4. Place the reagent slip with test pad up on a dry surface.
   Rationale: Moisture on the test pad could alter the final test results.
5. Choose the finger to be punctured, massage gently, and hold in a dependent position.
   Rationale: The dependent position and stimulation will help increase circulation to the puncture site.

6. Wipe the puncture site with alcohol (or a povidone–iodine swab). Allow the site to dry completely.
   Rationale: If tracked into the puncture site, alcohol may cause stinging and could hemolyze or dilute the blood sample.
7. Don gloves.
8. Remove the cover of the lancet or autolet. Place the autolet against the side of the finger and push the release button. If a lancet is used, it should be held perpendicular to the side and should pierce the site quickly.

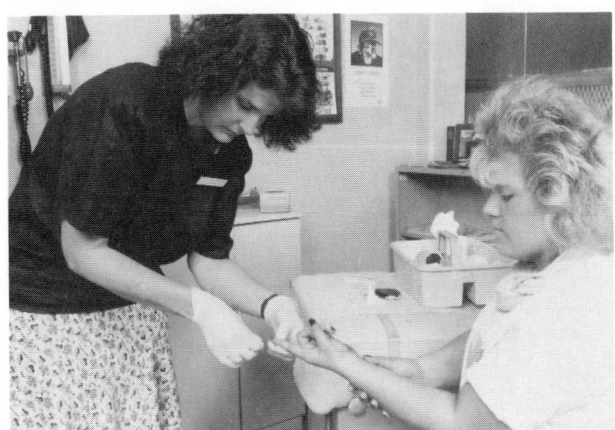

Step 8

9. Wipe the initial drop of blood with a cotton ball.
   Rationale: The first drop of blood may contain more serous fluid than blood cells and lead to a false glucose reading.
10. Squeeze the puncture gently or massage the skin toward the site to obtain a large drop of blood. Hold the reagent strip next to the drop of blood and allow the blood to cover the test pad completely. Do not smear the blood.
    Rationale: Smearing or incomplete coverage of the test pad will lead to false glucose readings.
11. Start the timing (usually 60 seconds) using the glucose meter, or a watch if the meter is not available.
    Rationale: For most glucose meters and for optional testing techniques using reagent strips, blood must be in contact with the test pad at least 60 seconds to ensure accurate results.
12. Following the manufacturer's instruction, wipe the blood from the test pad with a cotton ball after the specified period of time.

(continued)

PROCEDURE 20–2. Measuring Blood Glucose by Skin Puncture *(continued)*

13. Place the reagent strip into the glucose meter. After the recommended period of time, read the results. If a glucose meter is not available, compare the color of the test pad with the color strip on the side of the reagent strip container.
Rationale: Accurate timing of the test ensures a correct reading of the glucose level.

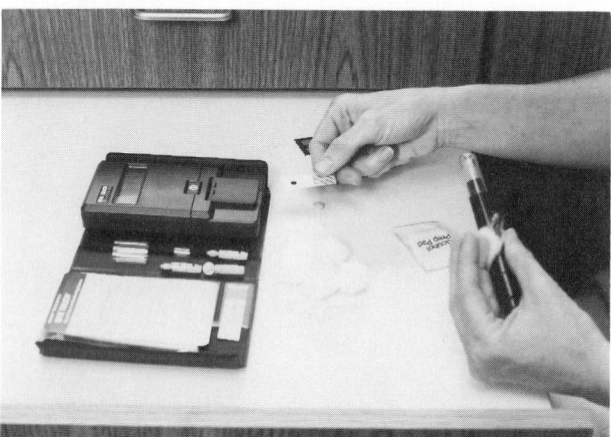

Step 13

14. Turn off the glucose meter. Dispose of used equipment in the appropriate manner.
Rationale: The lancet or autolet should be disposed of in a used-needle receptacle to avoid inadvertent punctures by others.

■ **Lifespan Considerations**

Infants
• The heel is the most common site for skin puncture. The nurse may want to use a heel-warming device or may wrap a warm, moist towel around the foot before the skin puncture to promote vasodilation.

Children
• Children are especially apprehensive about any type of skin puncture. The use of distraction techniques and allowing parents to be present may increase the child's cooperation with the procedure.

■ **Home Care Modifications**
• Handwashing alone before skin puncture is sufficient to cleanse the skin when the test is performed at home.

---

from the tissues is the **hemoglobin** (Hb) molecule. When Hb is low, anemia is present.

Hematocrit. The percent of RBCs in 100 mL of total blood volume is the hematocrit (Hct) level (consequently, a Hct of 39% means that there are 39 mL of RBCs in 100 mL of whole blood). Since Hct reflects the relationship between plasma and RBCs, the Hct can increase and decrease with alterations in fluid volume or in RBC number. See Chapter 32 for more information.

White Blood Cell Count. The WBCs defend against foreign substances in the body, such as bacteria, parasites, or other particles. The WBC count reflects the number of WBCs per 1 μL of whole blood. An elevated WBC count (**leukocytosis**) usually indicates infection in the body, but can follow severe tissue injury. A low WBC count (**leukopenia**) can accompany diseases of the bone marrow, or immunosuppression (unresponsiveness of the body's natural immune system) due to chemotherapy or AIDS. Leukocytosis or leukopenia can be best interpreted through examination of the WBC differential.

WBC Differential. The differential count is a list of the relative number of each type of WBC in the blood. There are five different types of leukocytes that can be seen under the microscope when a peripheral blood smear is examined (see Appendix). The most common type of leukocyte

is the neutrophil, which responds to infection and inflammation in the body. Other types of leukocytes include eosinophils (seen in allergic reactions), basophils (which play a role during anaphylaxis), lymphocytes (seen in viral conditions), and monocytes (which migrate to areas of injury to ingest damaged cells and foreign particles). Refer to Chapter 35 for more information on interpreting WBC differential results.

Platelet Count. Platelets, like the red and white blood cells, also are formed in the bone marrow. The disklike shape of these cells helps them to aggregate and form a plug at bleeding sites. A very low number of platelets (a condition known as **thrombocytopenia**) increases bleeding time; an excessive number of platelets (**thrombocytosis**) is found after some surgeries or hemorrhage, and is often associated with anemia or infection.

Erythrocyte Sedimentation Rate

The ESR measures the speed at which anticoagulated erythrocytes settle in a long, narrow tube. Inflammation and infection will affect the protein content of the erythrocytes, making them heavier. Consequently, the speed of settling depends on the size of the clumps in which the affected cells aggregate (gather). The faster the settling, the higher the ESR. The ESR is a nonspecific indicator of inflammatory disease. Although many factors affect the ESR, it is considered a test with neither disease nor organ specificity (Goe, 1989a).

Blood Coagulation Studies

Coagulation studies evaluate the ability of the blood to clot. Bleeding disorders, as well as medication-induced anticoagulation (clot prevention), can be assessed with coagulation studies. The type of test chosen is considered a diagnostic study if bleeding is a problem. If anticoagulation is the goal of medication therapy, tests specific to the particular anticlotting mechanism affected by the drug are chosen. Common blood coagulation studies include platelet count (see above), bleeding time, platelet aggregation, partial thromboplastin time (PTT or aPTT), and prothrombin time (Protime; PT) (see Appendix B).

Blood Chemistry Studies

Homeostatic mechanisms in the body are responsible for maintaining the body's stable state through regulation of cellular activity. Among the homeostatic mechanisms are the regulation of blood chemistries: the electrolytes and other chemical substances in the blood that affect cellular activity. Measurement of electrolytes and other chemical constituents in the blood may be one of the most frequent tests performed to evaluate the status of the patient (see the Appendix for reference ranges for common chemistry studies).

Electrolytes. When electrolytes are ordered, a sample of blood is analyzed for sodium, potassium, carbon dioxide, and chloride levels. The levels of these constituents are stable in the healthy person, but may become unbalanced in several disease states (including diseases of the lungs, kidneys, and heart), and in relation to the body's fluid-volume status. Since the electrolyte balance in the body can change rapidly, certain values may be measured several times daily.

Blood Glucose. The next most common test performed is probably measurement of blood glucose. Glucose is formed from the digestion of carbohydrates, and is used by cells as a source of energy. Entry of glucose into the cells is facilitated by insulin, a hormone secreted by the pancreas. Blood glucose testing is used to detect disorders in the process of carbohydrate breakdown and glucose metabolism. Measurement of blood glucose can be done with a venipuncture sample or with capillary blood (see Procedure 20-2, "Measuring Blood Glucose by Skin Puncture"). Blood glucose analysis may be performed on the fasting person (fasting blood sugar; FBS) or at specified times during the day.

Chemistry Profiles. Frequently, blood chemistry tests are ordered in groups (profiles or panels) and use a single venous sample. A typical profile may include the measurement of electrolytes, glucose, and blood urea nitrogen

(BUN). Occasionally, larger panels are obtained and contain (in addition to the electrolytes, glucose, and BUN) results of calcium, magnesium, inorganic phosphate, creatinine, and protein values, including total protein, albumin, globulin, and the albumin/globulin ratio (A/G ratio). Reference ranges for these tests are given in the Appendix. See Chapter 32 for more information on how to relate these tests to functional and dysfunctional patterns.

Blood Lipid Studies

Blood lipid studies measure the level of fat in the blood. Since a strong relationship has been demonstrated between high blood lipid levels and atherosclerosis (Lipid Research Clinics Trial Results, 1984), blood lipid studies are performed to identify people with hyperlipoproteinemia (high blood lipids). Evaluation of the amount of total cholesterol, low-density lipoproteins (LDL), and high-density lipoproteins (HDL) is important for accurate identification of people at risk for coronary heart disease (CHD).

Current guidelines identify an optimal cholesterol level as less than 200 mg/dL (Report of the NCEP, 1988). Total cholesterol can be sampled in a nonfasting individual (Goe, 1989b). If the total cholesterol level is found to be elevated, a second test may be done to evaluate LDL and HDL. Since LDLs carry blood cholesterol to the cells of the body, high LDL levels are directly related to an increased risk of CHD. On the other hand, increased levels of HDL may have a protective effect, as HDL removes cholesterol from cells and transports it to the liver, where it is secreted in bile (Goe, 1989b). See Chapter 31 for more information on blood lipid levels.

Serum Enzymes

Enzymes are protein substances that enter into energy-producing reactions within cells. When cells are damaged, either through disease or injury, enzymes are liberated into the blood, where they are detected through enzyme assay. The testing of blood for the presence of enzymes is useful for detecting abnormalities in the bones, liver, kidney, brain, muscles, and most commonly in the heart.

Isoenzymes (subfractions of enzymes) may be specific to certain organs and therefore a more specific indicator of where cell destruction has occurred. For example, a rise in creatine kinase-MB (CK-MB; an isoenzyme of creatine kinase) is 96% to 99% specific for myocardial injury and indicates that a myocardial infarction has occurred (Lott & Stang, 1980). The rise in enzyme levels after myocardial injury follows a predictable time-table, and consequently permits the diagnosis of specific injury through the assessment of enzymes within that time-frame (Goe, 1987).

Commonly measured serum enzymes and some of the organs in which the enzymes are found include creatine kinase (CK, CPK; heart, muscle, or brain); lactic dehydrogenase (LD, LDH; liver, lung, kidney, or heart);

aspartate amino transferase (AST, SGOT; liver, heart, skeletal muscle, kidney, or brain); serum aminotransferase (ALT, SGOT; primarily liver); alkaline phosphatase (ALP, alk phos; liver and bone); and amylase (pancreas or salivary glands).

Serum Drug Levels

Serum drug levels are obtained to determine the effectiveness of drug therapy or to identify toxic levels. Information about the serum concentration of drugs is most commonly used to monitor the blood levels of cardiac medications (e.g., digoxin, quinidine, or procainamide), antibiotics (e.g., gentamycin and tobramycin), or theophylline. It is important to remember that serum drug levels should be interpreted in the context of the patient's signs and symptoms. When serum drug levels exceed therapeutic ranges, the physician should be notified.

Arterial Blood Gases

Arterial **blood gases,** obtained from an arterial sample of blood, are used to evaluate the metabolic and respiratory status of the patient. The pH of blood as well as the partial pressure of oxygen and carbon dioxide are measured. The bicarbonate level is usually calculated from the results. These parameters can be altered by changes in respiratory pattern, changes in activity, changes in oxygenation, changes in renal status, or changes in other factors such as shock or an elevated blood glucose level. Blood gases are drawn when there has been no change in oxygen delivery or activity level for at least 15 minutes (see the Appendix for reference values for arterial blood gases; also see Chapters 30 and 32).

Urine Testing

The analysis of urine is an important indicator of a person's health status. Alterations in metabolism, infection, renal disease, and fluid volume problems can be confirmed by examination of the urine.

Urine Specimen Collection

Urine samples are collected for routine analyses, for identification of bacteria, and for special 24-hour examination. Specimens are voided into a clean container for routine urinalysis. Once labeled, the specimen must be rapidly transported to the laboratory, since any bacteria will multiply rapidly if the specimen is left at room temperature. When culture for identification of bacteria is desired, a clean-voided procedure or catheterization is performed. Specimens for urinalysis also can be taken from an indwelling urinary catheter by aspirating urine from a special port with a needle and syringe. Refer to Chapter 37 for details regarding different procedures for urine specimen collection.

Routine Urinalysis

Routine urinalysis (UA) is a common procedure performed on admission to the hospital and during physical examination. The UA is usually performed in the laboratory. Reported information includes the urine color and turbidity; pH and specific gravity; presence of protein, glucose, or ketones; and the presence of bacteria, blood cells, and sediment. Any bacteria or red or white cells greater than five cells (viewed in a high-power field) should be considered abnormal (Fischbach, 1988).

24-Hour Urine Collection

Occasionally, urine is collected for 24-hour analysis for urine metabolites to evaluate the patient for abnormalities in metabolism, kidney function, or hormone activity. Catecholamines (epinephrine and norepinephrine), electrolytes, proteins, creatinine, cortisol, porphyrins, amylase, or vanillymandelic acid (VMA) are most commonly assayed.

The container used for storage of the urine during the 24-hour period is supplied by the laboratory and may contain chemical preservatives. Care should be taken to avoid skin exposure to these caustic chemicals when urine is poured into the container.

During the collection period, each of the patient's urine voidings are collected (by means of a collection "hat" placed in the toilet, a bedside commode, or a bedpan) and poured into the collection container, which has been labeled with the patient's name and the date. The *exact time* of the first collection is noted and each voiding during the next 24 hours is collected and poured into the collection container in the same manner. The container usually is kept in a refrigerator or on ice during the entire collection period. Once the *exact* 24-hour period has passed, the container of urine is taken to the laboratory, where it is again refrigerated until analysis.

Culture and Sensitivity Testing

Culture refers to the growth of microorganisms in a specialized growth media under precise conditions (heat, moisture, nutritive ingredients, oxygen). Sensitivity (susceptability to specific antimicrobial drugs, e.g., antibiotics) can be determined during the culturing process. The culture and sensitivity testing of collected specimens are performed when a microorganism is suspected during routine examination of a specimen, or after a **Gram stain** analysis in which bacteria are stained to allow tentative identification of suspected organisms.

Testing for culture and sensitivity can be performed on a number of specimens, such as blood, urine, or sputum.

These specimens are collected using techniques designed to prevent contamination of the specimen with other substances. Once collected, each specimen is labeled and transported to the laboratory immediately to prevent multiplication of bacteria within the specimen.

Blood Culture

When the origin of a fever or other signs of infection are not readily identified, the culturing of blood is indicated. Blood cultures identify pathogenic organisms within the blood (bacteremia). The blood is drawn with the usual venipuncture technique and is placed immediately into specialized tubes containing culture media. Usually more than one specimen is drawn from more than one site. If the site and timing of sampling is not specified by the physician, samples may be drawn 10 minutes apart from two different sites. The sampling should be performed while the patient is febrile and before treatment with an antibiotic or an antipyretic. Although preliminary results may be available within 24 hours, a period of a week or more may be necessary before an organism can be identified (Goe, 1989a).

Urine Culture

The urinary tract (bladder, ureter, urethra, and kidney) is a common site of bacterial infection, particularly in the elderly. A urine culture is indicated when the UA white cell count is greater than five cells per high-powered microscopic field. The urine is collected with a sterile (catheterization) or clean-voided procedure. Early morning specimens should be obtained because bacterial count is highest in the morning (Fischbach, 1988). Whenever possible, specimens should be collected before the administration of antibiotics.

Sputum Culture

Sputum is cultured to identify organisms and diagnose conditions such as bronchitis, viral or bacterial pneumonia, or tuberculosis. Whenever possible, the specimen should be collected in the early morning (before eating or oral hygiene). The specimen must be coughed up from pulmonary bronchi (and not the mouth or postnasal region). The sputum specimen is collected in a sterile container and is transported immediately to the laboratory. Occasionally, a specimen must be obtained through nasotracheal suctioning when a patient cannot cough effectively.

Swab Culture

Specimens can be obtained by swabbing areas where infection is suspected (e.g., the throat or wounds). Culture kits with a swab and culture media inside a flexible plastic tube usually are provided for swab cultures. The swab is placed quickly and gently into the region to be cultured and then placed immediately into the inner, media-containing tube of the culture kit. The inner tube is then crushed by applying pressure to the flexible outer container surrounding the inner tube. The specimen is labeled with the patient's name and immediately transported to the laboratory. Culture results are usually available within 48 hours.

DIAGNOSTIC TESTS

Diagnostic examinations may be performed for a variety of reasons, ranging from the ruling out or diagnosis of suspected disease to evaluation of current treatment modalities. A single diagnostic test or a series of tests may be required for complete evaluation of a particular patient's symptoms.

This section includes a description of general categories of diagnostic tests. The discussion covers noninvasive viewing techniques, invasive viewing techniques, tests that entail the examination of body tissues or fluid, and tests that evaluate neural or muscle electrical conduction. Information included in this section about the procedures can be used by the nurse to teach and inform the patient, for preparing the patient, for supporting the patient, and for assessing of the patient. Individualization of patient care will be based on information gained from the examination. Table 20-2 discusses ways in which diagnostic procedures can affect normal function.

Noninvasive Viewing Techniques

A number of noninvasive procedures have the capability of visualizing organs within the body and detecting structural abnormalities. The oldest and most common noninvasive procedure is the **roentgenogram,** or x-ray. Many new, more sophisticated diagnostic techniques such as computed tomography, ultrasound, and magnetic resonance imaging have been developed in the last decade to better permit visualization of internal structures. Occasionally, noninvasive viewing procedures are coupled with invasive techniques, such as the injection of dye to enhance visualization of internal structures (Hughes, 1986).

X-rays (Radiography)

X-rays (radiographs) visualize internal structures on film by directing roentgen rays (short gamma rays) from an x-ray machine toward body tissues. Underlying structures of differing densities permit varying amounts of the x-ray to penetrate the tissues and form an image on the x-ray film. Soft tissues, such as organs and muscle, visualize poorly and appear as gray forms. Dense tissues such as bone appear white and are the most clearly defined. Empty space, such as an empty bladder, appears black on film. Differential absorption of x-rays

TABLE 20–2

Potential Alteration in Normal Function Secondary to Diagnostic Procedures

Health Pattern	Potential Disruption
Nutritional–Metabolic	NPO status may increase potential for inadequate nutrition or fluid volume deficit
	Bowel preparation may contribute to fluid volume deficit
	Invasive procedures increase risk for infection
Activity–Exercise	Bedrest or restricted activity may be required post-procedure
	Fatigue is common
	Increased potential for shock with many invasive procedures
Elimination	Increased potential for constipation after using barium
	Bowel preparation before a procedure can cause diarrhea
	NPO and resulting fluid volume deficit can decrease urine output
Sleep–Rest	Necessary preparation and anxiety can interrupt sleep
Cognitive–Perceptual	Pain or discomfort commonly occur with invasive procedure
	Confusion can occur when procedure prep causes fluid volume deficit electrolyte imbalances
Self-Perception	Embarrassment common with some procedure (e.g., sigmoidoscopy)
	Scars or invasive techniques may affect self-image
Role–Relationship	Testing may necessitate absence from work, school, or social activities
	Tests may interfere with ability to carry out normal activities as wife–husband or mother–father
	Expense of tests may be a burden on the family provider
Sexuality–Reproductive	Some tests (e.g., fluoroscopy) are unsafe during pregnancy
	Fatigue and anxiety may interfere with normal sexual response
Coping–Stress	Anxiety concerning discomfort during the procedure and the test results are common for most diagnostic procedures
	Hospitalization may be necessary for some procedures
Values–Beliefs	Some people may question the necessity or ethical validity of certain prescribed tests

allows diagnoses by noting abnormalities in the projected image on the film. X-rays are commonly used to identify fractures, abnormal growths, structural abnormalities, or the abnormal presence of fluid.

Radiology facilities are available in hospitals, clinics, physicians' offices, and some community diagnostic and laboratory centers. X-rays are obtained frequently on an outpatient basis on a physician's direction. In the hospital setting, patients usually are transported to the radiology department for x-rays; however, if the patient cannot be moved safely, some portable x-rays can be obtained in the patient's room.

Simple, routine x-rays (e.g., chest x-rays or abdominal x-rays) take place in the radiology department and require no preparation other than removal of clothing, jewelry, or metal in the area to be examined. Female patients should be queried as to whether they are pregnant and the date of their last menstrual period so that the reproductive area can be protected from x-rays when pregnancy is a possibility. All patients should be reassured that x-rays cause no pain or sensation as they pass through the body. In addition, most patients want to be reassured that the amount of radiation exposure will be minimal. The nurse may or may not accompany the patient to the radiology department. During the procedure, all personnel leave the room during filming to limit their exposure to radiation.

The patient will be positioned (by the nurse or technician) depending on the view that is needed. It may be helpful if the nurse communicates any limitations in mobility or positioning to the radiology personnel. For example, some patients, particularly the elderly, may find it uncomfortable to assume necessary positions for extended periods of time. Finally, long waits in the x-ray department may be very fatiguing for some individuals.

X-rays Using Contrast Media. Frequently, a contrast medium, usually a **radiopaque** (opaque to x-rays) dye, is used to allow better visualization of soft tissues or to permit observation of organ motion. The procedure for administration of the contrast medium can vary according to the test being performed. When the gastrointestinal (GI) tract is being studied, the contrast medium **barium** can be swallowed for an upper GI series or administered rectally for a barium enema examination.

Radiopaque dye also can be injected directly into the venous circulation. In this situation, the noninvasive x-ray procedure is coupled with an invasive technique. When circulating dye reaches the organ to be studied, the organ is clearly outlined, in contrast to the shades of gray normally produced on x-ray. To ensure that a concentrated amount of dye reaches the target organ, a catheter may be inserted into the venous circulation and advanced to the proximity of the organ before dye is injected.

Some contrast media are iodine-based; consequently, sensitivity to iodine should be determined before the procedure. This information can be obtained by the nurse, who obtains information about all known allergies, including allergies to fish or to iodine, and determines if there have been past reactions to diagnostic procedures using contrast dyes. Reactions to iodine for sensitive people can be minor or severe, including itching, hives, pallor, wheezing, hypotension, and loss of consciousness (Stafford, 1987).

It is important to inform the patient that some people may experience a burning sensation or a hot flush as the dye is injected. This reaction is normal. The patient should also be informed to report all sensations to the personnel in the radiology department. Table 20-3 provides a complete list of diagnostic procedures using contrast media.

Fluoroscopy. **Fluoroscopy** is a type of x-ray procedure used to visualize movement within the body. Fluo-roscopy can be performed at the bedside using portable equipment, but usually takes place in the radiology department. Fluoroscopy may be used to permit continuous observation of the gastrointestinal tract and is often used during placement of catheters (e.g., pacemaker catheters; feeding tubes) to visualize organ structures and facilitate manipulation of the catheter.

The patient is placed on a specialized table through which x-rays can pass. The x-rays are projected "live" onto a fluoroscopy screen, much like the projection of a television image; recordings are made of the moving picture. Occasionally, the patient is given contrast medium, which projects black on the screen.

The patient should be informed that tests involving fluoroscopy are performed in a darkened room to permit better visualization. Fluoroscopy exposes the attending personnel as well as the patient to more irradiation than a standard x-ray. Consequently, most tests or procedures will be performed rapidly to prevent unnecessary exposure; this may require that the patient be asked to restrain movement for an extended period.

Mammography. **Mammography** involves x-ray examination of the breast to screen for cancer and to evaluate palpable breast masses or cysts (Dodd, Goodson, & Marchant, 1987). Performed in the radiology department or on an outpatient basis, mammography involves a specialized x-ray technique using xerographic plates instead of film. This method requires lower levels of radiation to obtain reliable images. Occasionally, tests requiring the injection of dye into the mammary ducts or scans that detect subtle variances in tissue temperature will be performed after mammography.

The patient who is to have a mammogram should be instructed not to use creams, perfumes, powders, or deodorants the day of the examination; these products interfere with images. The nurse should also provide the patient with information regarding the frequency of repeat mammography: currently it is recommended that

---

TABLE 20–3

Diagnostic Procedures Using Contrast Media

Procedure	Area Visualized
Arteriogram	Circulation through arteries
Arthrogram	Joint cartilage and surfaces of the joint
Barium enema	Large intestines
Barium swallow	Pharynx and esophagus during swallowing
Bronchogram	Bronchi and pulmonary tree
Cerebral angiogram	Circulation to the brain
Cholangiogram	Bile ducts
Cholecystogram	Gallbladder
Endoscopic retrograde cholangiopancreatogram (ERCP)	Pancreatic ducts, liver, and biliary tree
Intravenous pyelogram (IVP)	Kidneys and ureters
Myelogram	Spinal cord, spinal canal, and spinal roots
Upper gastrointestinal series (UGI)	Esophagus, stomach, and duodenum

women who are 35 to 40 years old have a baseline mammogram; women 40 to 49 years of age should repeat mammography every 1 to 2 years; and women over the age of 50 should have annual mammograms. High-risk women may have more frequent mammography.

Radioisotope Scanning. Some diagnostic radiology examinations scan the body after the introduction of radioactive isotopes. This type of examination, known as a radioactive or **nuclear scan,** may take place in the nuclear medicine or radiology departments, and can be helpful in evaluating organ function and identifying disease. Organ function, organ size, or the presence of abnormal structures in the thyroid, heart, brain, lungs, spleen, bone marrow, bones, and kidneys can be detected through nuclear scans.

The patient can be informed that a **radioisotope** is a radioactive chemical which can be used safely in diagnostic testing. Some of these substances pass uniformly through normal tissue, but collect in higher concentration in rapidly growing tissues such as cancerous tumors. Other radioisotopes have an affinity for certain body organs; for example, radioactive iodine is picked up by the thyroid (Seigal, 1986). Still other radioisotopes gather in vascular areas of organs such as the heart while remaining conspicuously absent in areas that are ischemic and deprived of blood.

Very small quantities of radioisotopes are administered either orally or intravenously. Occasionally, agents also are administered to block the absorption of the substance by nontarget organs or tissues. After a short waiting period (minutes to 1 or 2 hours) while the isotope is assimilated, the body is scanned. The scanner visualizes the transit and uptake of the isotope in the body, and the image is recorded on a photographic plate.

During the procedure, some patients may experience anxiety and claustrophobia because the equipment is large, noisy, and placed close to the body. There is no danger to the patient. When explaining the procedure to the patient, it is important for the nurse to stress that radiation exposure is minimal (usually no more than with a standard x-ray), and that there is no possibility that the patient will become radioactive. The scanning itself is not painful, but some discomfort may be experienced because of the necessity to remain still for long periods of time. Because of their potential for causing damage to developing fetuses, radioactive scans should be avoided by pregnant women (Jankowski, 1986).

Computed Tomography. Computed tomography (CT) is performed in the radiology department. CT scans (also referred to as CAT scans) take multiple, thin, cross-sectional images of organs by directing a narrow beam of x-rays at the organ. A computer then generates a multidimensional image, which can reveal abnormalities. After initial scanning, a contrast medium may be used to improve imaging, and additional scans may be obtained.

CT scans are able to discern minor differences in the density of soft tissues. This information is used to diagnose such problems as tumors, benign growths, infarction, bleeding into tissues, and abscess formation (Hsu, 1986).

Very low doses of radiation are used in CT scans; radiation exposure is less than that of a normal x-ray, even when many images are obtained. The testing takes more time than an ordinary x-ray examination—up to an hour—and the patient must remain still during the procedure. Children and restless adults may require sedation. Of concern to some patients is the feeling of claustrophobia experienced as the bulky CT scanner appears to "surround" the body during examination.

Ultrasonography

Ultrasonography (ultrasound) is a noninvasive technique that uses high-frequency sound waves. Ultrasound procedures are performed both at the bedside and in specialized areas in the ultrasound or radiology department. During an ultrasound, a small instrument called a transducer converts electrical energy to sound waves, which are directed toward structures of the body and are then deflected back to the transducer and recorded. For this reason, ultrasounds are often called echograms (or "echoes"). Body tissues of differing densities deflect sound waves uniquely, enabling differentiation of tissues. The pattern of sound waves can be viewed on an oscilloscope, and a photograph can be made.

Ultrasound is used to provide information about the size, consistency, and shape of internal structures; abnormalities such as masses, edema, inflammation, stones, and free fluid are also identified (Haughey, 1981). A number of body organs such as the heart, liver, gallbladder, and thyroid can be scanned using ultrasound. Ultrasound also is used frequently to evaluate the size of the fetus and placenta during pregnancy (Katerndahl, 1982) (Fig. 20-6). Because sound is poorly conducted by air, ultrasound is not very helpful in diagnosing lung abnormalities. A Doppler stethoscope can be used with ultrasound to detect blood clots or peripheral vascular disease (Massey, 1986).

The ultrasound procedure requires no contrast medium. A coupling agent (mineral oil or gel) is used on the patient's skin to facilitate good contact between the transducer and the skin. The patient must lie still during the procedure; sedation may need to be ordered for the very young or restless. Consent forms are usually not required, since ultrasound is noninvasive, involves no radiation exposure, and is associated with no complications or side effects.

Ultrasonography should be performed before any procedures that require contrast medium, or any procedures that involve the introduction of air or gas into an organ (e.g., sigmoidoscopy); such tests could alter the clarity of the ultrasound. The patient may be kept NPO

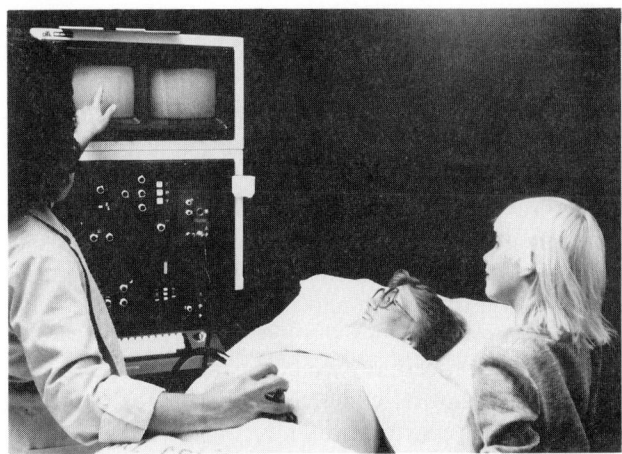

Figure 20–6. Ultrasound is frequently used in pregnancy. Parents and their children are delighted to see the fetus on the screen and to observe its heartbeat and movements.

for 8 to 10 hours before an abdominal ultrasound to reduce any gas present in the intestines. For some examinations, particularly those involving the pregnant uterus, the patient may be asked to have a full bladder, since a full bladder helps to elevate pelvic organs and provide better visualization. In this situation, the patient should be asked not to void for 3 to 4 hours before the test.

Magnetic Resonance Imaging

Magnetic resonance imaging (MRI) is the most recent technologic advance in noninvasive viewing techniques. The technique uses a bulky piece of equipment which is usually located in or adjacent to the radiology department. The MRI procedure uses a strong magnetic field and radio waves to produce images of bones, joints, muscles, organs, and to evaluate blood flow. Magnetic resonance imaging can detect deviations in the pumping action of the heart, lesions or masses in fluid-filled soft tissue, or abnormalities in blood vessels. Tissues absorb and deflect electromagnetic energy differently depending on their physiochemical composition. Computers then detect and analyze abnormal findings.

There are two advantages of MRI: radiation is not used and contrast media are not necessary to clarify images. The expense of MRI and the necessity for cooperation from the patient, who must remain motionless during the fairly lengthy scan time, are considered disadvantages. Magnetic resonance imaging also cannot be used on any patients with metal implants or cardiac pacemakers (Engler & Engler, 1986), since the strong magnet used in the procedure can actually dislodge metal within the body.

Most MRI scans require minimal patient preparation. Abdominal or pelvic scans require the patient to be NPO for 4 to 6 hours before the procedure. All patients should have empty bladders. All clothing with metallic closures must be removed; all metallic objects should be removed from pockets and hair before the procedure. A consent form may be required before the procedure. Like the CT scanner, the MRI machinery is large and encloses the patient (Fig. 20-7); consequently, some patients may experience claustrophobia. It is also helpful to inform patients that a rhythmic knocking may be heard during the procedure.

Invasive Viewing Techniques

Directly accessing a body organ or cavity may be necessary to obtain information that cannot be obtained through noninvasive means. Common invasive diagnostic procedures include endoscopy, angiography, and cardiac catheterization.

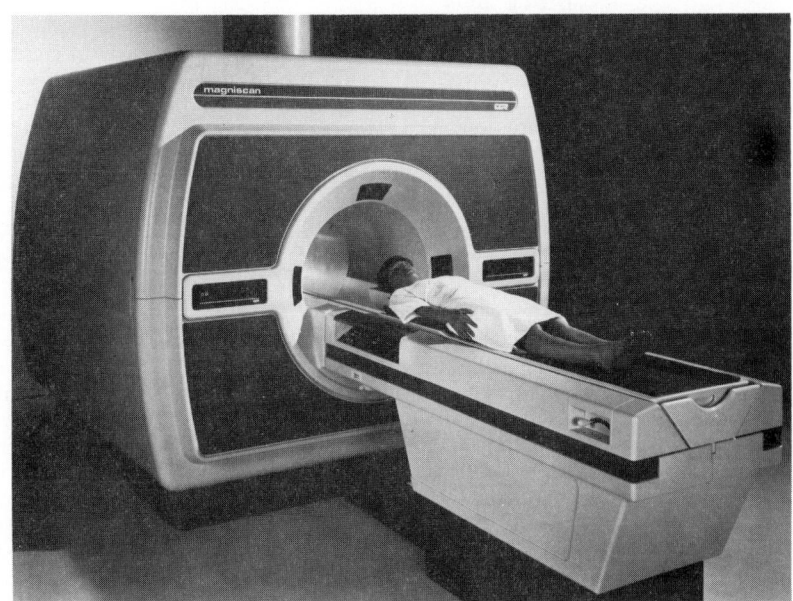

Figure 20–7. Patient is shown on the gantry of a Thomson-CGR Magniscan 5000 superconductive magnet. (Courtesy of Thomson-CGR Corporation.)

Endoscopy

Visualization of a body organ or cavity by means of a scope is referred to as **endoscopy.** Endoscopy may be performed on an inpatient or an outpatient basis, in a special treatment room located in the radiology department or in surgery or, rarely, at the bedside. Endoscopy may aid in providing information regarding structure or function of a particular body part. The physician examines areas directly through the scope, or views images on a television screen directly connected to a camera within the scope. Specific endoscopic examinations are named for the organ or part of the body visualized (e.g., bronchoscopy visualizes the bronchus and sigmoidoscopy examines the sigmoid colon). See Table 20-4 for a listing of common endoscopic procedures. More specific information regarding endoscopic procedures is given in Chapters 33 and 38.

During the procedure, special instruments called endoscopes are used to visualize interior parts of the body. In the past, these instruments were rigid metal or synthetic tubes. Fiberoptic scopes represent a tremendous advance over these earlier devices. The distant tip of the scope may have an opening through which anesthesia can be given or lavaging fluids infused and suctioned. Fiberoptic scopes can be inserted through normal body openings (e.g., mouth or anus) or inserted through small surgical incisions. Tissue can be removed during endoscopy for biopsy. Examinations can be performed under both local and general anesthesia; the choice depends on which area of the body is being examined. Most procedures take less than 1 hour.

Nursing care before and after endoscopic procedures can vary depending on the specific procedure performed. It is important that the nurse explain the procedure to the patient before the examination. If the examination is to be performed on an outpatient basis, the preparation for the examination must be discussed thoroughly, with provision of written material as available. Informed consent may be necessary for some examinations, and the agency policy manual should be consulted.

Before the actual examination, baseline vital signs and assessments are obtained. Frequently, the patient is kept NPO; laxatives or an enema may be given for lower GI visualizations. Sedation may be administered before the procedure to help relax the patient.

After the procedure, vital signs are monitored; any significant changes, complaints of pain, or abnormal bleeding are reported promptly, since endoscopy can cause perforation or other trauma to the visualized organ. After some endoscopic procedures, the ability to swallow must be assessed before the patient eats or drinks; local anesthesia used in procedures involving the upper GI (Fisher & Kaplan, 1983) or respiratory tracts can temporarily paralyze the trachea or esophagus.

Angiography

Angiography, performed in the radiology department, permits visualizations of the vascular system. Angiography is helpful in evaluating patency, blockage, or aneurysm (dilation weakness of a blood vessel). Angiography can allow studying of blood flow to the heart, brain, kidney, lungs, and lower extremities (Massey, 1986). Under fluoroscopy, an intravenous catheter is placed in either the femoral or brachial artery and is threaded to the area to be studied. After administration of a contrast dye, x-rays and cineography are taken of the vessels being studied.

Before the procedure, the patient is usually kept NPO. Once the procedure is explained by the physician,

TABLE 20-4
Endoscopic Procedures

Procedure	Area Visualized
Arthroscopy	Internal structure of a joint
Bronchoscopy	Bronchus and bronchial tree
Colonoscopy	Large intestine (sigmoid through cecum)
Colposcopy	Cervix and vagina
Cystoscopy	Urinary bladder, urethra, and prostatic urethra
Endoscopic retrograde cholangiopancreatography (ERCP)	Common bile ducts and pancreatic ducts
Upper GI endoscopy or Esophagogastroduodenoscopy (EGD)	Esophagus, stomach, and upper duodenum
Fetoscopy	Fetus in utero
Laparoscopy	Abdominal (peritoneal) cavity to visualize pelvis and adjacent organs
Mediastinoscopy	Mediastinal structures, organs, and lymph nodes
Sigmoidoscopy	Sigmoid colon, rectum, and anal canal

informed consent is obtained. Allergies to contrast media or to iodine are assessed before the procedure.

Postprocedure care includes maintenance of a pressure dressing over the arterial access site for a period of 6 to 8 hours. Vital signs are monitored frequently, and frequent assessments are made of the access site and peripheral arterial pulses distal to the access site. Any bleeding, excessive swelling, or signs of decreased circulation or sensation to the extremity distal to the access site should be reported promptly to the physician. The patient is kept on bedrest and the extremity is kept immobile for 6 to 12 hours after the procedure. Since the dye is excreted by the kidneys, the patient should be encouraged to drink large amounts of fluids to help eliminate the dye.

Coronary Angiography (Cardiac Catheterization). Cardiac catheterization is an angiographic procedure performed in the radiology department to assess the blood flow through the coronary arteries, to evaluate congenital structural defects, or to evaluate heart valve dysfunction (Cabaniss, 1986). After the angiographic approach under fluoroscopy, dye is injected into the coronary arteries, pressures in various areas of the heart are measured, and movement of the flow of blood through the chambers of the heart can be observed.

Before the procedure, all current laboratory work, particularly coagulation studies and hematocrit, should be recorded on the patient's chart. Allergies should be assessed. Informed consent should be obtained after discussion with the physician. The patient may be NPO or restricted to clear liquids before the procedure. After the procedure, nursing care is the same as that for other angiographic procedures. In addition to observing and reporting bleeding and changes in circulatory status, any chest pain should be reported to the physician immediately.

Aspiration Diagnostic Procedures

Aspiration diagnostic tests may be performed at the bedside or in the operating room. Aspiration is performed to obtain specimens for examination or to withdraw fluid that has abnormally collected in a body cavity. Usually, a special aspiration needle with a stylet and an outer, hollow-bore needle is used. The stylet is used to pierce the skin and then is withdrawn, leaving the outer needle in place through which tissue and fluid can be withdrawn. Biopsy (Dodd, 1987), lumbar puncture, paracentesis, and thoracentesis are examples of aspiration diagnostic examinations.

The patient undergoing aspiration diagnostic examination may experience discomfort associated with piercing the skin and obtaining specimens. Aseptic technique must be observed to prevent introduction of bacteria through the entry wound. Gloves should be worn during handling of body fluids.

Biopsy

Biopsy involves an excision of a small amount of tissue for microscopic examination. A biopsy may be performed to rule out or confirm cancer or to identify the nature of organ dysfunction. Frequently, biopsies are performed in surgery, but tissue for examination can be obtained by needle aspiration at the bedside. Liver biopsy, renal biopsy, and bone marrow aspiration are three biopsy procedures that may be done at the bedside.

Liver Biopsy. When liver dysfunction is suspected, a liver biopsy may be performed to identify cellular changes within the liver (Liu & Hughes, 1986). Since blood clotting depends on proper liver function, any liver dysfunction can alter normal clotting and result in excessive bleeding. Consequently, blood coagulation studies are performed and evaluated before liver biopsy. If the laboratory results show an increase in bleeding time or prothrombin time, the physician may order vitamin K (aquamephyton) to be administered before the biopsy is performed.

Before the procedure, an informed consent is signed. The patient may be NPO. Sedation and a local anesthetic are used during the procedure; the patient should be informed that some discomfort will be experienced as the local anesthetic is injected. The patient assumes a supine position with the right hand under the head, which is turned to the left. A biopsy needle is inserted aseptically, usually between the sixth and seventh ribs. A small amount of liver tissue is withdrawn (the patient may experience some pressure as the specimen is removed). While the biopsy specimen is obtained, the patient may be instructed to take a deep breath and hold it. The deep breath elevates the diaphragm and prevents chest wall movement, thus minimizing the risk of inadvertent trauma to the diaphragm or lung.

After a liver biopsy, it is important to check vital signs and assess frequently for signs of bleeding. A pressure dressing is applied to the biopsy site and movement is limited to prevent bleeding. The patient may be instructed to lie on the right side, often on a small towel, to provide extra pressure to the site. Potential complications of liver biopsy include hemorrhage, pneumothorax, and peritonitis.

Renal Biopsy. A renal biopsy is performed to verify abnormalities in the nephron of the kidney (the functional unit of the kidney responsible for making urine) (Kirkpatrick & Sirmon, 1986). The procedure is similar to that performed for liver biopsy but the biopsy needle is inserted through the flank (posteriorly, between the ilium and the lower rib area) and into the kidney. Because the kidney is highly vascular, postprocedural bleeding is a possible complication. Monitoring of vital signs, applying a pressure dressing, and careful assessment of the patient are indicated. After renal biopsy, the urine is assessed for blood; the comparison of serial specimens will ascertain that any blood in the urine is decreasing in amount.

Bone Marrow Biopsy. Red and white blood cells and platelets are produced in the bone marrow. Should the patient's hematologic studies reveal abnormal cell numbers or certain abnormalities in the structure of these cells, a bone marrow biopsy may be performed to rule out or diagnose anemias or cancer (e.g., leukemia, multiple myeloma, Hodgkin's disease), or to evaluate the effectiveness of chemotherapy. The iliac crest or the sternum are commonly chosen for biopsy in adults. The tibia is the preferred site for biopsy in small children; little marrow is found in the iliac crest or sternum of children.

After explanation of the procedure and the signing of informed consent, the patient is positioned in the supine position for a sternal puncture, or in the prone position for puncture of the iliac crest. Usual sterile procedures are performed, including draping of the area and preparation of the area with an antiseptic such as a povidone–iodine solution. The patient should be informed that the aspiration of marrow can be painful, but that it is important to remain still during the procedure. The bone is punctured with appropriate equipment and approximately 0.2 to 0.5 mL of marrow is aspirated. Concurrently, a venous blood sample is obtained.

After the biopsy procedure, the patient is assessed for signs of bleeding or infection. Vital signs are monitored closely. Bedrest is usually maintained for an hour, after which normal activities may be resumed.

Lumbar Puncture

A **lumbar puncture,** or spinal tap, is performed to obtain samples of cerebrospinal fluid (CSF), to assess for infection, bleeding, or tumors, or to obtain CSF pressure measurements in situations where blockage of CSF circulation is suspected (Hsu, 1986). The procedure can be performed at the bedside, in the radiology department, or in special procedure areas. A lumbar puncture also may be performed to administer anesthesia, antibiotics, chemotherapy, or to perform specialized examinations such as a **myelogram** (an x-ray examination of the spinal cord using contrast dye).

After the procedure is explained to the patient, informed consent is obtained. Fasting is usually not required, but the patient is encouraged to empty the bowel and bladder before the procedure. To separate the vertebrae as much as possible, the patient is positioned in a side-lying position with legs flexed and head bent toward the chest (Fig. 20-8). Aseptic technique is maintained throughout the procedure to prevent infection.

To gain access to the CSF, a needle within a stylet is placed between the vertebrae of the spinal column into the subarachnoid space. The space between the third and fourth lumbar vertebrae (*Diagnostics,* 1986) is usu-

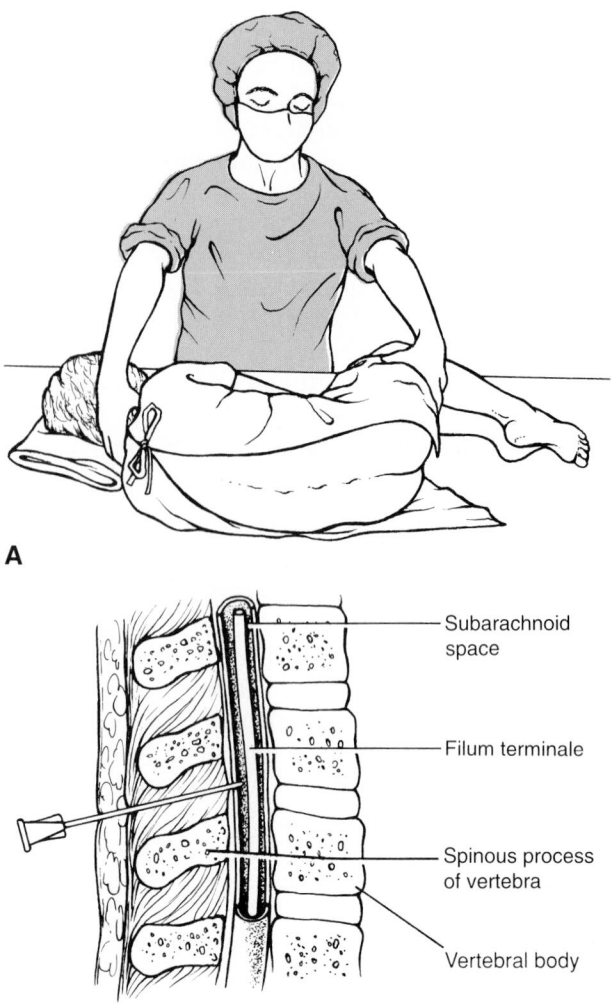

A

Subarachnoid space

Filum terminale

Spinous process of vertebra

Vertebral body

B

Figure 20–8. Lumbar puncture. **A.** Positioning of child for lumbar puncture. **B.** Location of puncture in the spinal column.

ally chosen because it contains spinal fluid but is below the level of the spinal cord. Once spinal fluid is obtained, it is evaluated for appearance and the presence of cells, protein, or glucose; CSF may also be cultured for the presence of bacteria.

Once the procedure is completed, pressure is applied to the puncture site for a brief period; an adhesive bandage may be applied over the site. The site should be assessed for the leakage of CSF or any signs of inflammation. Assessment of vital signs and neurologic status should be performed according to agency protocol. Severe headaches can occur after the procedure if air was introduced at the time of the procedure or if a significant amount of CSF was lost. Occasionally, the patient is instructed by the physician to lie flat for a specified period of time; other physicians may ask that the patient's head remain elevated at a specified angle. The patient may be encouraged to drink lots of fluids after the procedure to replace lost CSF and minimize discomfort from headache.

Thoracentesis

Thoracentesis, performed at the bedside, is a procedure performed to aspirate fluid from the pleural cavity surrounding the lungs. Normally this space contains a minimal amount of fluid that lubricates the pleural lining around the lung; occasionally, more fluid can collect. A small amount of fluid can be removed from the pleural space for laboratory analysis (Mengert & Albert, 1989). Larger amounts of fluid that have collected in the pleural space due to infiltration or infection may be removed, restoring space for lung expansion and improving respiratory function.

The procedure is explained to the patient and an informed consent is obtained. The patient is positioned upright and asked to bend forward; leaning over a bedside table may be suggested (Fig. 20-9). This position widens the spaces between the ribs to permit easier access to the pleural space. The area is cleansed and draped, and a local anesthetic is administered. The aspiration needle is inserted and fluid is withdrawn through a syringe. Occasionally, a catheter is inserted, the needle is withdrawn, and the fluid is allowed to flow through the catheter into a sterile, closed container. During the procedure, the patient is observed carefully for alterations in pulse or respiratory rate, changes in skin color, or difficulty breathing.

After the fluid is aspirated, the catheter or needle is removed and a sterile dressing coated with petroleum jelly is applied firmly to the site. Vital signs continue to be monitored and the patient is observed closely for changes in respiratory status. Breathing after the pro-

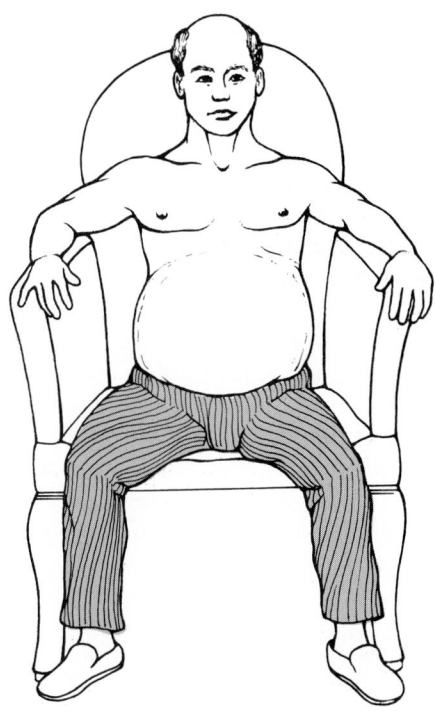

Figure 20–10. Positioning for paracentesis.

cedure is usually easier; however, pneumothorax can occur should the needle accidentally puncture the lung. Changes in respiratory pattern, bloody sputum, or severe coughing should be reported to the physician.

Paracentesis

Paracentesis is a bedside procedure intended to remove fluid from the peritoneal space in the abdomen. Like the pleural space, the peritoneal space normally contains only a small amount of lubricating fluid. Large amounts of fluid (e.g., 1000 to 2000 mL) can accumulate in the peritoneal space in certain disease states, however, including liver failure, renal failure, and cancer. The large accumulation of fluid, also known as **ascites,** can press on the diaphragm and make breathing difficult for the patient. Pressure from ascites can also interfere with gastrointestinal function.

An informed consent is obtained from the patient after explanation of the procedure. The patient's weight is recorded before the procedure, and abdominal girth may be measured. The patient is encouraged to void before the procedure, since an empty bladder will decrease the likelihood that accidental perforation of the bladder will occur.

The patient having a paracentesis is placed in a sitting position with support for the back (Fig. 20-10). If the patient cannot tolerate a sitting position, the bed should be placed in a high Fowler's position. The upright position allows most of the fluid to gravitate to the lower abdomen for easy removal. Strict aseptic conditions are used to puncture the abdomen at a site generally halfway between the symphysis pubis and the umbilicus. A large-

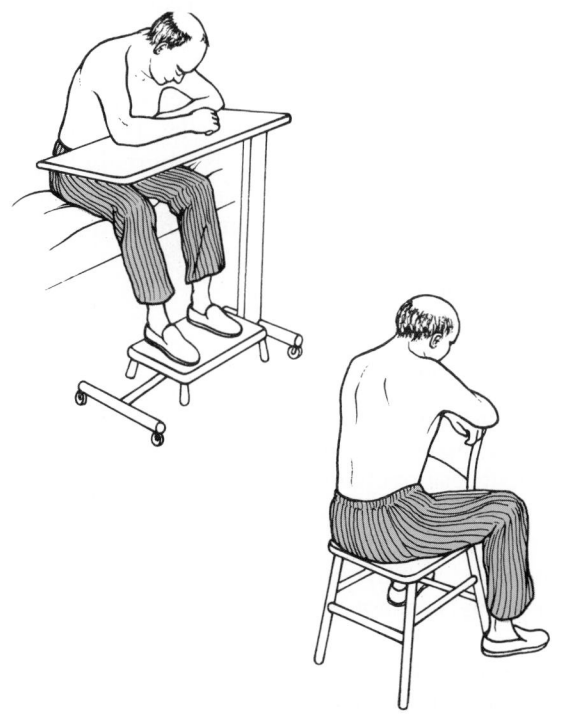

Figure 20–9. Positioning for thoracentesis.

bored abdominal paracentesis needle (sometimes referred to as a trocar) is used. Once the inner stylet is removed from the needle, a catheter is attached, which permits fluid to flow freely from the abdomen.

Once the procedure is completed, a bulky dressing may be applied to the puncture site, since there is usually some leakage of fluid after the procedure. Vital signs are monitored after the procedure. In addition, electrolytes may be monitored frequently. If a very large amount of fluid is withdrawn, pressure changes can occur that will affect blood flow. Additionally, since the fluid contains protein and electrolytes, the fluid and electrolyte status of the patient may be affected. For these reasons, some physicians limit the amount of fluid withdrawn at any one time during paracentesis. Another possible complication is the possible puncture of organs during the procedure, so the patient is observed for early signs of shock.

Diagnostic Procedures That Evaluate Electrical Conduction

Studies that evaluate electrical impulses supply information regarding the functioning of body organs, commonly skeletal muscle, the heart, or the brain. Electrodes (electrical sensors) are applied to specific areas of the body to measure the strength, tone, velocity, or direction of electrical impulses. These impulses are displayed on an oscilloscope or printed on a paper graph. The most common diagnostic procedures used to evaluate electrical conduction are the electrocardiogram (EKG or ECG) and the electroencephalogram (EEG).

Electrocardiography

The **electrocardiogram** is a recording of the electrical impulses generated by the heart. The ECG can be obtained on an inpatient or scheduled on an outpatient basis. For hospitalized patients, the ECG is usually obtained in the patient's room, using portable equipment. A technician usually obtains the ECG, although nurses also obtain tracings in some agencies (Fig. 20-11).

The ECG is capable of identifying abnormalities such as arrhythmias (irregular disturbances in heart rhythm), injury from a myocardial infarction, enlargement of heart chambers, and, occasionally, electrolyte imbalance. Should a patient complain of chest pain, an ECG is usually ordered to rule out the heart as a source of the pain. See Chapter 31 for information on how to relate the ECG to functional and dysfunctional patterns.

Obtaining an ECG involves the application of electrodes to the arms, legs, and chest. Clothing is removed from areas where the electrodes are to be placed. A conducting medium, usually a gel, is applied to the skin surface underneath the electrode. The patient will feel no unusual sensation as the recording is obtained. Occa-

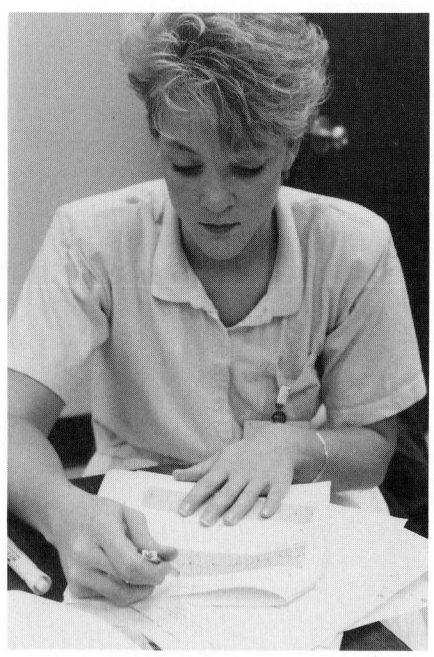

Figure 20–11.   Nurse interpreting ECG tracing.

sionally a patient may be asked to refrain from consuming food or beverages containing caffeine for 24 hours before a scheduled ECG, since caffeine is a stimulant and can affect heart rate and rhythm. The patient should be asked for a list of all current medications, since the ECG requisition may require specific information regarding the patient's medications. After the procedure, the patient should be assisted in removing any gel used on the skin before dressing.

Exercise Tolerance Testing.   The maximal exercise capacity and functional impairment can be assessed through exercise tolerance testing (ETT, stress EKG). This test employs the use of a wide, motorized belt (treadmill) on which the patient walks. The speed and slope of the treadmill apparatus is adjusted every few minutes according to an established protocol. The patient is monitored with a continuous ECG tracing and blood pressure determinations. The test usually lasts about 30 minutes.

Electroencephalography

An **electroencephalogram** is a recording of the electrical activity in the brain. The EEG can be scheduled on an outpatient basis or obtained in the hospital. In the hospital, it is most desirable to obtain the EEG in a quiet area reserved for this procedure; however, with portable equipment, the EEG can be performed at the bedside when patients cannot be moved.

During an EEG, a regular pattern of waves is recorded with scalp electrodes and a multichannel, high-amplification recorder (electroencephalograph). The recording is particularly useful in identifying brain activity responsible for epilepsy. The absence of electrical activity in the brain is used to support the diagnosis of brain death (Hsu, 1986).

Ideally, the patient's hair should be free of oils, creams, or sprays when an EEG is to be obtained; however, this is not always possible. When the study is to be made during sleep, sleep may be limited the night before the test. Food and fluids should be ingested normally, since hypoglycemic states can affect brain patterns. The patient may be asked to avoid stimulants such as coffee or tea on the morning of the test.

Electrodes are placed on the scalp with paste (tiny needles are sometimes employed). Sedation may be ordered before the test to stimulate sleep. The test itself is painless and the patient will experience no electric shocks or any unusual discomfort. Occasionally, the patient will be asked to hyperventilate, to view moving patterns or cards, or to watch revolving lights to determine if brain patterns change with these activities. The study takes approximately an hour, unless a sleep EEG is required. After the test, the sedated patient will be allowed to rest until the sedation has worn off. The patient's hair may need to be washed to remove the electrode paste.

LIFESPAN CONSIDERATIONS

At each stage of life there are distinct ways of reacting to health-related issues. The age-related developmental stage of a patient will affect the diagnostic and laboratory testing process. The needs of the patient before, during, and after diagnostic and laboratory procedures must be considered. In addition, the age of the patient may have an influence on the interpretation and individualization of the information obtained from the test.

Newborn and Infant

The newborn is entering the world with basic trust. The parents of the newborn are in the process of bonding, and generally experience a strong protectiveness. Parents should not be excluded from the testing environment unless their presence is deleterious to the process. When they are present, the nurse should explain why the test is being performed and what the test includes.

Some general principles apply to the newborn infant: if testing includes exposure of the infant to the environment, the procedure should be performed as quickly as possible to prevent excessive body cooling and a drop in body temperature. A heel-stick is the preferred method of obtaining blood; occasionally, femoral artery samples are needed. If the test requires that the infant not be fed for a period of time, the infant should be observed for signs of dehydration.

During the first year of life, the infant has learned to experience fear of strangers and strange environments.

Parents should be encouraged to hold the infant whenever possible for the procedure. If this is not possible, the infant should be restrained on the examination table to prevent sudden, quick movements during the procedure. After the procedure, the parent should be allowed to hold the child warmly and closely. Since the skin

---

Nursing Research

Selected Nursing Research Studies

Anderson, D. O. et al. (1989) Psychological preparation for cardiac catheterization. *Heart and Lung, 18*(2), 154–163.

Fegley, B. J. (1988). Preparing children for radiographic procedures: Contingent versus non-contingent instruction. *Research in Nursing and Health, 11*(1), 3–9.

Flam, B., et al. (1989). Effects of preparatory information of a myelogram on patients' expectations and anxiety levels. *Patient Education and Counseling, 14*(2), 115–126.

Heidrich, S. M., et al. (1989). Effects of fetal movement, ultrasound scans, and amniocentesis on maternal–fetal attachment. *Nursing Research, 38*(2) 81–84.

Hjelm-Karlsson, K. (1989). Comparison of oral, written, and audio-visually based information as preparation for intravenous pyelography. *International Journal of Nursing Studies, 26*(1), 53–68.

Lawrence, P. A., et al (1989). Accuracy of nurses in performing capillary blood glucose monitoring. *Diabetes Care, 12*(4), 298–301.

Possible Topics for Nursing Inquiry

- What difference in the patient's perception of anxiety occurs when preprocedure instructions are given verbally rather than written?
- What is the variability in blood values in samples obtained with an evacuation collection tube rather than with a needle and syringe?
- What is the significance of privacy in a patient's perception of dignity during procedures that expose body parts?
- Is bedtime blood glucose testing done most commonly before or after the evening snack?
- What is the effect of music during invasive procedures in reducing perceived pain or anxiety?
- What is the average length of time between collection of a urine sample and receipt of the sample in the laboratory?

is fragile, tape should not be used to secure dressings. Any observations to be made of the child after the procedure should be carefully explained to the parents.

Toddler and Preschooler

The toddler is becoming autonomous. Events are "processed" and assimilated into the child's world. The parent is closely involved with the child's happiness. The toddler tends to resist external control and may loudly proclaim unhappiness with being restrained. Consequently, it may be difficult for the parent to see the child restrained and struggling. Explanations about the test should be given completely and carefully to the parent, the test should be performed quickly, and the parent should be allowed to hold and comfort the child if possible.

The preschooler has more developed language skills. This child has become familiar with play and with fantasy. These skills can be useful in helping the child work through fears associated with testing procedures. Playing with doctor or nurse dolls or using dramatic play with role reversal (the child is the doctor; the parent the child) can help the child process feared or traumatic events. Allowing the child to keep a security blanket or favorite toy during the procedure may also be helpful.

Before the test, the child should be allowed to touch instruments if possible. If questions are asked, it is important to reply with simple, honest explanations. If the child asks if the procedure will hurt, the nurse should say something like, "Yes, it will hurt for a very short time, but it is alright if you yell as loud as you want." At this point, it is important to perform the procedure immediately and quickly so that the fear does not become overwhelming for the child. After the test the child should be comforted. Instruments and equipment should be removed from the environment immediately as these children want to explore their world and need to be protected from possible accidents.

Child and Adolescent

The school-aged child is rapidly becoming less dependent on parents, but continues to "cuddle" in times of stress. During this developmental stage the child learns right from wrong and has a strong sense of morality. It is also a period of rapid growth. Modesty may be evident.

Since language skills are developed, instructions and information about testing procedures should be directed at the child in easily understood language. Sometimes cooperation can be enhanced if the child is offered simple choices (e.g., "which arm" or "when"). The parent should be encouraged to support the child. The natural modesty and privacy of the child should be protected.

The adolescent has entered a period marked by confusion. At the same time, the adolescent is searching for identity. Since this age group is very active, injury may lead to a number of diagnostic and laboratory tests. The youth may prefer to have tests done unaccompanied by a parent. Nevertheless, the parent must be responsible for giving informed consent for invasive procedures until the child is of "legal" age. Consequently, both must be involved in discussions.

Adult and Older Adult

By the time the person is an adult, a number of diagnostic and laboratory tests may have occurred. However, fear, pain, and anxiety continue to be associated with tests for diagnostic purposes. Careful teaching and support from the nurse can help the patient deal with these feelings.

The older adult presents numerous problems related to laboratory and diagnostic testing. Explanations of tests are processed slowly and may take more time. The significance of the test may be associated with fear of debilitating or chronic illness. Blood sampling may be difficult: an appropriate site for venipuncture may be difficult to find; veins are fragile and hematomas may form easily; and skin is fragile and easily torn with application and removal of tape. It may be difficult for the older adult to maintain a position for a very long period. Since some preparations require a period of abstinence from food or drink, dehydration is a potential problem. Some test results may vary with age, and careful interpretation should be made of results. Finally, preparations for tests may be fatiguing, and an opportunity for rest should be provided frequently.

Key Concepts

- Diagnostic and laboratory testing includes procedures that examine all or part of the body.
- The nurse facilitates diagnostic and laboratory testing by preparing the patient, including scheduling, teaching, ensuring informed consent, physically preparing the patient, or obtaining necessary supplies and equipment.
- The nurse may have responsibilities during the procedure that include offering support to the patient, assessing the patient, and collecting or assisting with collection of the specimen.
- After the procedure, the nurse may be required to offer additional support and to assess the patient for complications. Also at this time, the nurse documents the procedure, including the patient's response to the procedure.
- Whereas information obtained from diagnostic and laboratory tests is used by the physician to diagnose specific illnesses or conditions, or to follow the progress of treatment for medical problems, the nurse will

relate the information to functional and dysfunctional health states and will use it to individualize the care of the patient.

■ Adequate psychological and physical preparation of the patient and support of the patient during diagnostic and laboratory testing ensures the patient's cooperation as well as adequate test results. The nurse should consider the patient's lifespan stage, including developmental tasks.

■ The physician is responsible for obtaining informed consent. The nurse may witness the signature of the patient.

■ Blood specimen collection includes venipuncture, arterial puncture, capillary puncture, and, occasionally, obtaining blood from central venous catheters

■ Hematologic tests measure substances in the blood.

■ Urine testing evaluates metabolic processes within the body.

■ Diagnostic studies include procedures that allow organ systems or functions to be visualized and recorded. Some examinations are invasive and require entering a natural body opening or call for a puncture or an incision; other procedures are considered non-invasive.

■ Noninvasive viewing techniques include radiographs (x-rays), fluoroscopy, mammography, radioisotope scanning, computed tomography, ultrasonography, and magnetic resonance imaging.

■ Invasive studies include endoscopy, angiography, biopsy, and puncture of body cavities.

■ Some examinations measure the electrical activity within the organ. Examples of these examinations include electrocardiography and electroencephalography.

■ After diagnostic and laboratory testing, the nurse may be required to monitor the patient closely for any signs of complications secondary to the procedure.

■ The nurse often is responsible for communicating results of laboratory and diagnostic tests to the physician.

References

CDC 91987). Recommendations for prevention of HIV transmission in health care workers. *Morbidity and Mortality Weekly Report, 36,* 25–185.

Cabaniss, C. (1986). Cardiovascular disorders. In P. Liu (Ed.), *Blue Book of Diagnostic Tests.* Philadelphia: Saunders.

Carnevali, D. L. (1983). *Nursing care planning: Diagnosis and management* (3rd ed.). Philadelphia: J. B. Lippincott.

Diagnostics (2nd ed.). (1986). Springhouse, PA: Springhouse Corporation.

Dodd, G., Goodson, W., & Marchant, D. (1987). Optimizing Dx of breast lumps. *Patient Care, 15,* 43–58.

Engler, M., & Engler, M. (1986). The hazards of magnetic resonance imaging. *American Journal of Nursing, 6,* 650.

Fischbach, F. (1988). *A manual of laboratory diagnostic tests* (3rd ed.). Philadelphia: J. B. Lippincott.

Fisher, R., & Kaplan, W. (1983). The role of gastrointestinal endoscopy. *Medical Times, 111*(2), 31.

Ganong, W. F. (1986). Circulating body fluids. In W. F. Ganong (Ed.), *Review of medical physiology* (12th ed.) (pp. 421–423). Los Altos, CA: Lange Medical.

Goe, M. R. (1989a). Laboratory tests using blood and urine. In S. L. Underhill, S. L. Woods, E. S. Sivarajan Froelicher, & C. J. Halpenny (Eds.), *Cardiac nursing* (2nd ed.) (Ch. 25). Philadelphia: J. B. Lippincott.

Goe, M. R. (1989b). Hyperlipoproteinemia. In S. L. Underhill, S. L. Woods, E. S. Sivarajan Froelicher, & C. J. Halpenny (Eds.), *Cardiac nursing* (2nd ed.) (Ch. 57). Philadelphia: J. B. Lippincott.

Goe, M. R. (1987). Creatine kinase enzyme determination: Implications for cardiovascular nursing. *Progress in Cardiovascular Nursing, 2,* 44–52.

Haughey, C. W. (1981). What to say and do when your patient asks about CT scans. *Nursing 81, 11*(12):72–77.

Hsu, C. (1986). Neurologic disorders. In P. Liu (Ed.), *Blue book of diagnostic tests.* Philadelphia: Saunders.

Hughes, J. (1986). Radiologic applications. In P. Liu (Ed.), *Blue book of diagnostic tests.* Philadelphia: Saunders.

Jankowski, C. (1986). Radiation and pregnancy: Putting the risks in proportion. *American Journal of Nursing, 86,* 260–265.

Katerndahl, D. (1982). Obstetric and gynecologic application of ultrasound. *Postgraduate Medicine, 71*(4), 177.

Kirkpatrick, W., & Sirmon, M. (1986). Renal disorders. In P. Liu (Ed.), *Blue book of diagnostic tests.* Philadelphia: Saunders.

Lipid research clinics coronary primary prevention trial results: II. The relationship of reduction in incidence of coronary heart disease to cholesterol lowering. (1984). *Journal of the American Medical Association, 251*(3), 365–374.

Liu, P., & Hughes, J. (1986). Alimentary and hepatobiliary disorders. In P. Liu (Ed.), *Blue book of diagnostic tests.* Philadelphia: Saunders.

Lott, J. A., & Stang, J. M. (1980). Serum enzymes and isoenzymes in the diagnosis and differential diagnosis of myocardial ischemia and necrosis. *Clinical Chemistry, 26,* 1241–1250.

Massey, J. (1986). Diagnostic testing for peripheral vascular disease. *Nursing Clinics of North America, 21,* 207–217.

Mengert, T., & Albert, T. (1989). Pulmonary therapeutics. In Larson and Ramsey (Eds.), *Medical therapeutics: A pocket companion.*

Report of the national cholesterol education program expert panel on detection, evaluation, and treatment of high blood cholesterol in adults. (1988). *Archives of Internal Medicine, 148,* 36–39.

Stafford, C. (1987). Reactions to drugs and diagnostic agents. *Postgraduate Medicine, 82*(6), 179–183.

Bibliography

Newman, F., Ogburn-Russell, L., & Rutledge, N. (1987). Magnetic resonance imaging: The latest in diagnostic technology. *Nursing 87,* (1), 45–47.

Tilkian, S. M., Conover, M. B., & Tilkian, A. G. (Eds.). (1987). *Clinical implications of laboratory tests* (4th ed.). St Louis: C. V. Mosby.

UNIT V
Selected Clinical Nursing Therapeutics

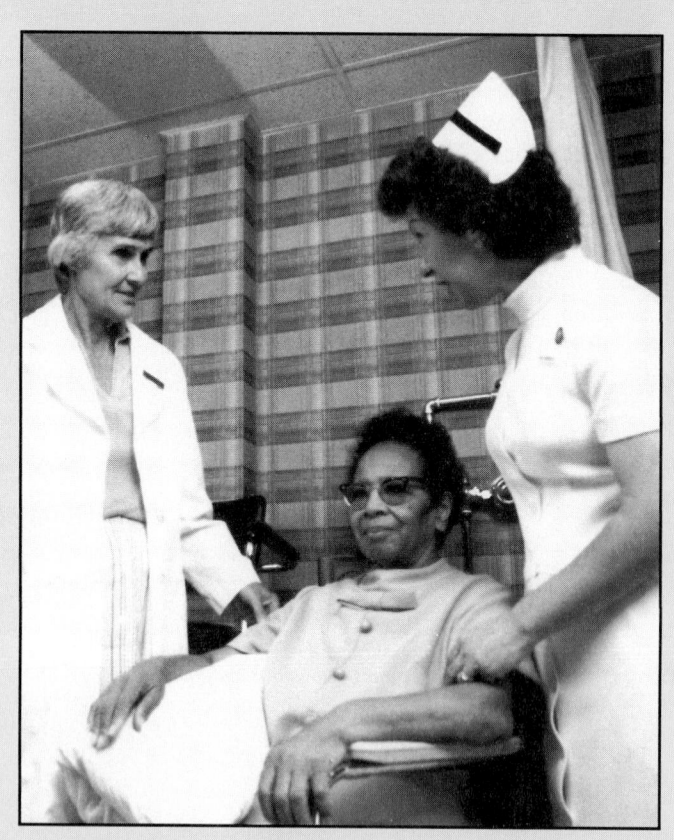

CHAPTERS

21 Patient Teaching

22 Asepsis

23 Perioperative Nursing

24 Medication Administration

U nit V focuses on nursing responsibilities associated with common clinical situations that provide the basis for many aspects of nursing care: patient teaching, asepsis, caring for the patient before and after surgery, and medication administration.

Patient teaching, the subject of the first chapter, is a fundamental nursing responsibility. Nurses teach patients and families both formally and informally and during almost every patient encounter.

The next two chapters discuss medication administration and nursing care of the patient who is having surgery. Both depend on basic skills and knowledge of patient teaching and asepsis. Care of the surgical patient involves much patient teaching both before and after surgery and also requires application of the principles of medical and surgical asepsis. Similarly, medication administration uses aseptic principles and often requires teaching the patient about self-administration, drug actions, and side effects. Additionally, both involve nursing interventions resulting from physician orders as well as independent nursing actions.

Unit V provides the knowledge base and skills needed for providing holistic nursing care in situations that are the basis for many patient encounters and for patients at any point on the health–illness continuum.

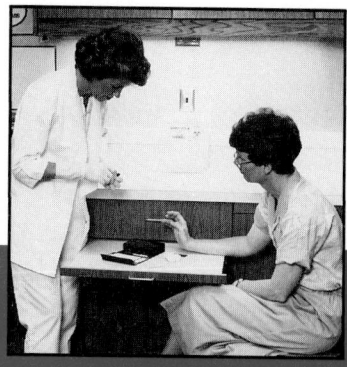

Patient Teaching

LEARNING OBJECTIVES

Upon completion of this chapter, the student will be able to do the following:

- List, in order, the steps in the theory of how people learn.
- Name and define factors that inhibit and facilitate learning.
- Define the three types of illness-prevention teaching activities.
- State why education programs must be individualized.
- Describe patient education in terms of the nursing process.
- Explain the abilities, needs, and motivations of different age groups as they pertain to learning.

KEY TERMS

Affective	Learning	Psychomotor
Cognitive	Motivation	Stimulus
Compliance	Noncompliance	

21

Teaching–Learning Process
  Sequence of Events in Learning
  Domains of Knowledge
    Psychomotor
    Cognitive
    Affective
  Learning Styles
Patient Teaching to Promote Health and Function
  Preventive Health Education
  Patient Teaching for Acute Problems
    Preoperative Teaching
    Postoperative Teaching
  Patient Teaching for Chronic Problems
Assessment for Learning
  Assessing Learning Needs
    Priorities
    Realistic Approach
    Cultural and Language Needs
    Baseline Knowledge
  Assessing Learning Readiness
    Motivation
    Compliance

  Sensory and Physical State
  Literacy Level
Nursing Diagnoses and Patient Goals
  Planning for Learning
  Appropriate Family and Friend Involvement
Implementation of Patient Teaching
  Sensitivity
  Environment Control
  Structured Teaching Sessions
  Audiovisual Aids
  Communication
  Repetition
  Teaching Methods
    Psychomotor
    Cognitive
    Affective
  Teaching Strategies
Evaluation of Learning
Documentation of Patient Teaching
Lifespan Considerations
Key Concepts

Because of changes in health-care payment, the trend today is to discharge patients "sicker and quicker." Effective patient education ensures that the responsibility for care is transferred safely to the patient. Nurses have become the primary patient teachers, and they also coordinate and reinforce information from other health-care professionals.

A hospital stay seems to be an excellent opportunity for well-meaning health-care professionals to impart as much wisdom as possible to the patient. But in reality the stress of illness and hospitalization hinders learning. Even the most positive hospital experience (i.e., the easy birth of a healthy baby) can be extremely stressful. Because of this stress, the patient may not hear or understand the teaching. Therefore, effective patient education almost always involves outpatient follow-up.

Throughout this chapter, the term *patient* is used to

mean the learner. The learner usually is the patient, but if the patient cannot participate in self-care, the learner becomes the relative, friend, or employee willing to take on the care.

Nurses doing patient education can influence but not control their patients, because learning and changing are voluntary actions. Nurses "encourage and assist individuals to take positive and responsible actions to improve their health" (DuBrey, 1982). No matter how important the nurse believes certain actions and attitudes are, the choice is the patient's. The nurse never takes for granted that the patient's beliefs are the same as his or hers; even beliefs that the nurse finds hard to understand must be respected.

Patient education is seldom the formal process experienced in school. Much patient teaching takes place informally during nursing care. During any patient-care activity, the patient or family may ask questions, and this curiosity indicates a degree of motivation that must be honored. At these times, patient education can be extremely effective.

Patient education consists of more than handouts, pamphlets, and videotapes. It requires a therapeutic relationship, as discussed in Chapter 17. This fact was recognized by Florence Nightingale. Every time a nurse empowers a patient toward autonomy and self-care, some autonomy and power is reflected back to the nurse and the profession of nursing.

TEACHING—LEARNING PROCESS

Learning is the acquisition of a skill or knowledge by practice, study, or instruction. Learning theory has changed over the centuries. According to an early, teacher-centered theory, learning required a disciplined mind, and the goal was to memorize a great deal of facts. Later, student-centered theorists believed that learning could be done in a completely intuitive way: by encouraging self-direction, an active unfolding of knowledge would occur. Still others claimed that learning must build on prior knowledge and experience: the teacher actively imparts new ideas, while the learner passively associates them with related ideas to grasp principles (Rankin, 1990).

Nursing students have experienced all of these theories at work. It is impossible to learn anatomy without memorizing a great number of facts. Dealing with people, especially patients, always has an intuitive component. Pharmacology builds on the student's knowledge of pathophysiology, chemistry, anatomy, physiology, and mathematics.

Sequence of Events in Learning

It is believed that people learn by accomplishing certain sequential events (Fig. 21-1). According to Gagne (1974), first the learner receives a **stimulus** to learn. The stimulus, which may be internal or external, is an incen-

tive that rouses the mind or spirit. The actual learning is characterized by motivation, comprehension, and acquisition. Memorizing is done with retention and recall. Response manifests as generalization, performance, and feedback.

Domains of Knowledge

Knowledge can be acquired in three different domains: psychomotor, cognitive, and affective learning.

Psychomotor

Psychomotor refers to the muscular movements that result from some sort of knowledge. This is the easiest knowledge to measure because it can be physically demonstrated. Teaching a new mother to breastfeed is an example of psychomotor learning. When she can successfully and independently breastfeed her infant to the physical satisfaction of both, she has demonstrated her psychomotor learning.

The nurse is often responsible for teaching a patient to perform a certain skill independently (for instance, effective handwashing or good body mechanics). Principles are taught, the nurse demonstrates the skill, the patient practices the skill, any questions are answered, and followup resources are identified. Because time is important, the process should be started early, as soon as the need is identified. A *return demonstration* is when the nurse observes the patient performing the new skill; this is a valuable tool for evaluating psychomotor learning. The effective use of return demonstrations requires a sharp eye and praise from the nurse. The nurse should focus on the patient's progress rather than commenting on deficits.

Cognitive

Cognitive refers to rational thought (knowing as opposed to feeling). Cognitive learning is a logical thinking experience and results in a changed way of thinking.

Moving from the simple to the complex is likely to

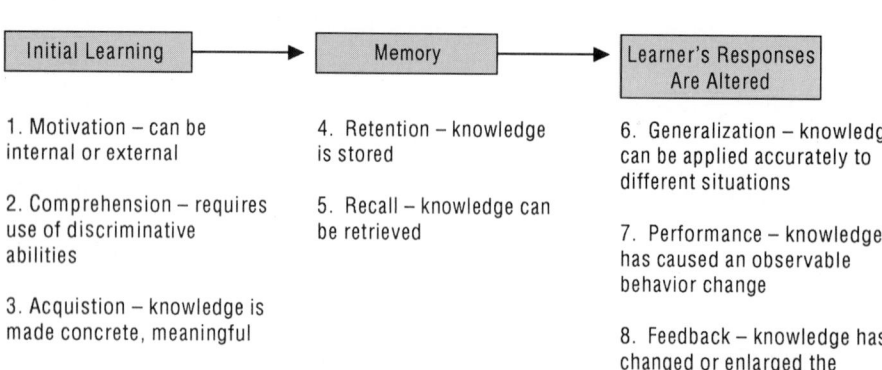

Initial Learning	Memory	Learner's Responses Are Altered
1. Motivation – can be internal or external	4. Retention – knowledge is stored	6. Generalization – knowledge can be applied accurately to different situations
2. Comprehension – requires use of discriminative abilities	5. Recall – knowledge can be retrieved	7. Performance – knowledge has caused an observable behavior change
3. Acquistion – knowledge is made concrete, meaningful		8. Feedback – knowledge has changed or enlarged the learner's point of view

Figure 21–1. The sequential events in the learning process.

yield the best results. Ideally, the nurse starts with basic facts and concepts and moves to a discussion of how they are related. Finally, the patient learns to apply the material correctly in different situations.

In the schoolroom, written examinations are an efficient and effective method of testing this sort of learning. But outside of the schoolroom, written tests are often not the best evaluation tool because patients may feel intimidated by them. Verbal feedback can be effective. Ask the patient questions that break down and reassemble the information. Give the patient different theoretical situations in which to apply the information.

Teaching the new mother the anatomy and physiology of the breast as a mammary organ is an example of cognitive learning. When she can discuss the physiology of her milk supply, the let-down reflex, and the way these two work together, she has demonstrated her cognitive knowledge.

Affective

Affective is an emotional reaction (feeling as opposed to knowing). Affective learning results in changed beliefs, attitudes, or feelings. Sensitivity is important when doing affective teaching because the line between counseling and teaching may be blurred. Whether a loss or a gain, change is stressful and the patient needs emotional support. Cognitive and affective learning are more difficult to measure than psychomotor learning because the learning is focused on thoughts and feelings.

Teaching the new mother that breast milk is a healthy food for her newborn is an example of affective teaching. The nurse would know that learning had occurred if the patient said she planned to breastfeed because it was a healthy choice for her baby.

Learning Styles

The McBer Learning Styles Grid (McBer & Co., 1985) is one way to express how people prefer to learn and deal with ideas (Fig. 21-2). The horizontal axis represents the continuum of "doing" as opposed to "watching," the vertical axis the continuum of "feeling" (intuitive learning) as opposed to "thinking" (logical thought). A brief test is given and a number is assigned for each of these two preferences that expresses the degree to which the person prefers one or the other. Seldom does a person prefer solely one or the other, and under different circumstances preferences may vary. However, the test indicates the person's general preferences and the personal style that he or she brings to the learning experience.

Once these preferences are elicited, the learner is assigned to the corresponding quadrant:

Quadrant A learners enjoy "tinkering" (hands-on learning, generally without instruction).

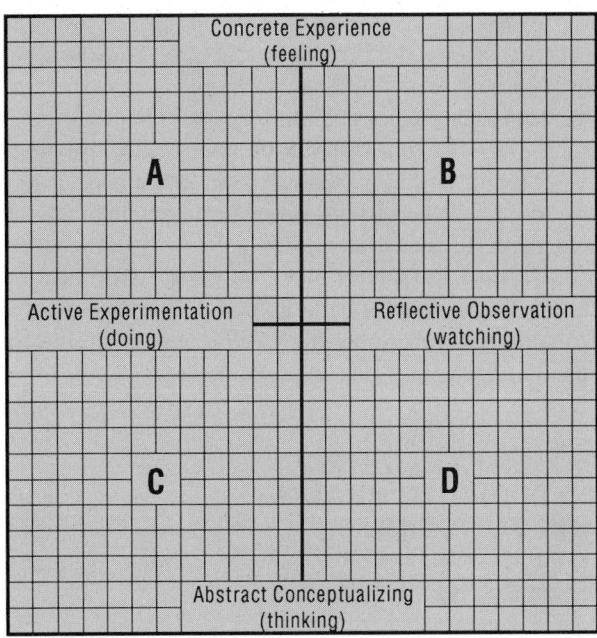

Figure 21-2.   The McBer Learning Styles Grid plots how people prefer to learn. Learners are scored on two learning characteristics, a general preference to do or watch and a general preference to feel or think. People who score into Quadrant A are those who prefer to learn intuitively, with "hands on" experience. Quadrant B represents people who also prefer intuitive learning but would apt to observe rather than do. Quadrant C represents a "hands on" learner who prefers that data be given in an orderly way, for example, written instruction. Quadrant D represents the learner who prefers to learn by watching but likes data in an orderly, rational way.

Quadrant B learners prefer to see concrete situations, perhaps several times and from several points of view.
Quadrant C learners prefer hands-on experience and enjoy receiving information in a logical sequence (i.e., written instruction).
Quadrant D learners enjoy watching step-by-step demonstrations. They can combine divergent ideas into a logical whole.

During patient care, it is unlikely that the nurse will be able to explore the patient's learning style in great detail. But the nurse should remember that the same material must be presented in different ways to different patients. For instance, if the nurse is demonstrating a psychomotor skill and the patient reaches over and takes the tools from the nurse's hands, the nurse should realize that this patient has a "doing" learning preference. Another patient may ask the nurse to demonstrate a skill repeatedly, reflecting a "watching" style. Whether the nurse chooses to talk the patient through a procedure or to demonstrate many times depends on the patient's preference.

Another clue to learning style is the patient's response to written instructions. If the patient responds positively by studying and asking questions, learning is probably occurring. But if the directions sit on the bedside stand unread, the patient may prefer a more intuitive, face-to-face approach. A possible opener could be, "I want to check out what you know about wet-to-dry dressings. Let's talk about it." Teaching the intuitive learner may take more time because he or she prefers human contact over written instructions.

Sometimes, no matter how creative the approach, the patient shows no interest in learning. This is probably a problem of motivation, which will be discussed later in this chapter.

PATIENT TEACHING TO PROMOTE HEALTH AND FUNCTION

Preventive Health Education

Preventive education, the most effective way to promote function, falls into three categories:

Primary education means teaching the skills necessary to stay healthy or to avoid disease. Teaching healthy eating habits is an example (Fig. 21-3).

Secondary or preventive teaching means teaching the knowledge and skills for early detection or prevention of disease or dysfunction. Breast self-examination for early detection of breast cancer is an example.

Tertiary education deals with an already recognized disease process. Teaching the patient with essential hypertension about the importance of taking daily antihypertensive medications and getting routine blood pressure checks is an example of tertiary education.

Preventive education is further discussed in Chapter 26. The nurse should be knowledgeable about preventive education programs that are available in the hospital or community.

Patient Teaching for Acute Problems

Acute problems cause anxiety. Although a limited amount of anxiety can aid learning and help the patient pay attention (Redman, 1988), anxiety levels often surpass this point, especially in the hospital. If extreme anxiety and fears are not addressed first, a well-planned patient education presentation is a waste of time. If the patient's counseling needs are beyond the nurse's abilities, professional resources may be needed (i.e., psychiatric clinical nurse specialist, psychologist, or psychiatrist).

Table 21-1 lists important teaching opportunities during hospitalization. Patient education in an acute situation includes preoperative and postoperative teaching.

Preoperative Teaching

The purpose of preoperative teaching is to give the necessary facts while remaining sensitive to the patient's emotional needs. Key information includes an orientation to the hospital, explanations of preoperative procedures and initial postoperative procedures, and anything else the patient needs to know to decrease anxiety. Structured instruction in turning, coughing, and deep breathing can be combined with information about what the patient can expect and how to help in the recupera-

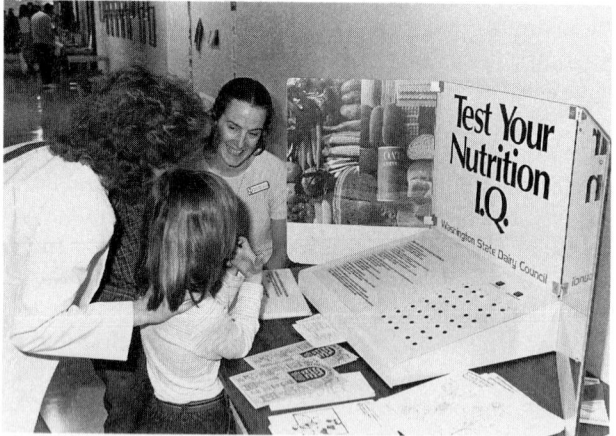

Figure 21–3. Nurses teach people how to stay healthy by testing their knowledge of normal nutrition. (Courtesy of Overlake Hospital Medical Center, Bellevue, WA.)

TABLE 21–1

Important Teaching Opportunities During Hospitalization

Opportunity	Possible Learning Need
Admission	Unit policies, how to work call light and bed, specific treatments that have been ordered and why
New medication	Action of drug, possible side effects, frequency, and any special considerations
Diagnostic procedure	Preparation that is necessary before procedure, what will be experienced during procedure, any restrictions or special considerations after procedure
Surgery	Preoperative preparation, postoperative protocols (e.g., deep breathing, leg exercises), pain control, how to get out of bed and turn easily
Discharge	Limitations on activity or diet, procedures such as wound care, when to call the physician

tion. Explaining what to expect can help decrease the patient's anxiety, especially about pain and pain relief.

Different patients require different amounts of knowledge. For example, a nurse is preparing two 40-year-old women scheduled for hysterectomies. One is a biology researcher with a doctoral degree, the other a dancer and choreographer. The researcher is interested in the techniques and expected timetables for the surgery and finds comfort in exploring these subjects. The dancer worries about scarring, body image, and pain. The first patient takes an intellectual approach, the second a physical, body-centered approach. Applying the learning styles chart in Figure 21-2, the nurse could approach the researcher from the Quadrant C point of view and the dancer from Quadrant B. These patients are undergoing the same operation, but because they are two different types of learners, they have different learning needs.

Postoperative Teaching

The focus of postoperative education is on hospital recovery, home recovery, and followup resources. The nurse will probably deal less with anxiety and more with acute pain and practical going-home issues. Effective pain management greatly enhances postoperative teaching. Encourage the patient to ask for pain medication as needed or to use patient-controlled analgesia as needed. Encouraging the patient to do small things independently as early as possible can aid learning, especially for the "hands-on" learner. Increasing independent functioning also enhances the recovering patient's self-concept and helps him or her feel more "normal."

Patient Teaching for Chronic Problems

The patient with an acute problem may be anxious, but the patient with a chronic problem is more likely to be depressed or fatigued. A degree of self-neglect may indicate depression: chronic illness is so relentless that it is hard for the patient to stay motivated. Some of the most common education areas for chronically ill patients are cancer, pulmonary disease, cardiovascular disease, diabetes, and mental health (Redman, 1988).

Imparting knowledge to these patients can involve teaching skills (psychomotor) or facts (cognitive), and often the nurse is also in a position to teach the value of improved self-care (affective). Therefore, the nurse is often a counselor as well as a teacher. Chronically ill patients must be approached from where they are, not from where the nurse thinks they should be. Preaching only prompts the patient to think, "What do you know? Have you ever been sick like me?" The nurse who listens actively to the patient and proceeds accordingly stands a much better chance of changing the patient's attitude, possibly resulting in improved self-care.

ASSESSMENT FOR LEARNING

Nursing assessment in patient education focuses on external and internal factors. External factors shape the nurse's perception of the patient's learning needs, and internal factors show the patient's readiness to learn. These assessments are usually done simultaneously.

Assessing Learning Needs

The educational assessment begins with defining what the patient needs to know or do to function more independently. The classic example is the need to gain knowledge or perform a certain skill before safe hospital or home-care discharge. For example, parents must be able to care independently for their infant's colostomy before the infant can be discharged to their rural home, or a couple must show the visiting nurse that they can function independently with the wife's new paraplegia before routine nursing visits are stopped. Table 21-2 gives examples of appropriate teaching for each functional health area.

Priorities

Patients often have more needs than resources, so priorities must be set in an effort to have the most impact for the limited resources available. Teaching a patient basic skills in the hospital but arranging home nursing visits for followup teaching would be the result of priority-setting. Because time is usually the scarcest resource, assessment and priority-setting *must* begin at admission.

When possible, the nurse should ask the patient to identify his or her learning needs. This process sets priorities and helps the nurse judge the patient's motivation level. When the patient is motivated, the learning is much more likely to result in attitude or behavioral change.

Realistic Approach

The nurse who takes a realistic approach sets priorities and tries not to teach too much. Consider the following:

- The patient's energy level. Physical weakness can make people unable to learn (Anderson, 1990).
- The patient's age. Educational goals for children, adolescents, and adults are different, and these patients require different teaching styles.
- The patient's lifestyle. If you foresee the need for followup care, will the patient be able to gain access to it?
- The patient's emotional state. The patient may be too anxious or depressed to learn. It is not uncommon for those who have received an emotional shock (for instance, a diagnosis of cancer) to go through a period of

TABLE 21–2

Examples of Patient Teaching for Functional Health Patterns

Health Pattern	Example of Possible Teaching
Health perception/ health management	Breast self-examination, importance of regular physical examinations and immunizations
Activity/exercise	Importance of regular exercise, how to use ambulation devices (e.g., crutches, walker), deep breathing and coughing, leg exercises
Nutrition/metabolic	Healthy diet, dietary restrictions, wound care, how to monitor temperature, total parenteral nutrition at home
Elimination	How to maintain regular bowel function, Kegel exercises to decrease stress incontinence, self-catheterization
Cognitive/perceptual	Pain management (e.g., how to use patient-controlled analgesia), how to use memory aids, importance of regular eye and ear examinations
Sleep/rest	Importance of getting adequate rest, aids to promote sleep
Self-concept	Normal body changes, methods of promoting self-esteem
Role/relationship	Assertiveness training, parenting classes
Coping/stress	Biofeedback, relaxation techniques
Sexuality	Prenatal classes, contraception
Values and beliefs	Patient's rights, "do not resuscitate" options

denial, followed by painful periods of realization and depression.

Cultural and Language Needs

Religion, health beliefs, language, and sex-role stereotyping are important factors for the nurse to consider when planning patient education. Not all groups share certain mainstream health-care norms and values; for instance, Jehovah's Witnesses do not believe in accepting blood transfusions, most Islamic sects do not donate or receive organs, and many Native Americans and Chinese people have folk-medicine beliefs that they practice and trust. People who do not speak English require an interpreter. Working effectively with these people requires the nurse to have an open, accepting attitude.

When a patient from a different culture needs to be educated about nutrition, a registered dietitian (RD) may be able to help. RDs often are familiar with cultural food beliefs and can tailor a plan for that patient's needs.

In many cultures, women are the only ones to prepare food or care for the sick. Therefore, the nurse must identify and include these women in any dietary or health teaching.

Baseline Knowledge

The nurse must compare the patient's current knowledge, attitudes, and skills with those necessary for independent functioning. "Tell me what you know about (relevant topic)" can be a useful opener, but avoid making the patient feel tested: feeling tested can be intim-

idating and can harm the nurse–patient relationship. "When did your symptoms first appear?" may be a gentler lead, as most people are willing to talk about their symptoms, and this can lead to further inquiry. For example, what the patient did when the symptoms appeared can tell a great deal about baseline knowledge. Asking about family history may not only supply data about baseline knowledge but also about cultural beliefs and attitudes. Finding out about previous patient-education experiences may give some indication about where teaching can begin.

Assessing Learning Readiness

Motivation

Motivation provides drive or incentive. It is a powerful determinant of success in patient education (DuBrey, 1982) and therefore is closely related to compliance. Motivation can be affected by many things: financial problems, inconvenience, denial, lack of social support, nonacceptance of the disease, anxiety, fear, shame, or negative self-concept. Motivation can change from day to day. Patients who use their illness to get attention may not be motivated to get and stay well.

When assessing motivation, it is important to learn what the patient values. The patient who associates a health-care goal with something already valued will probably be more motivated. For instance, a pregnant diabetic woman is generally motivated to achieve good blood-sugar control because her efforts increase the chances for a healthy baby.

Motivation is difficult to assess. There may be verbal cues (a patient who says, "My wife takes care of all that") or nonverbal cues (lack of attention, missing appointments). Noticing motivational signs during assessment is vital, because a misjudgment could waste time. Imagine carrying out lengthy patient teaching, only to find on evaluation that the patient learned little because he was anxious about the hospital bill!

Compliance

Assessing the patient's history of **compliance** or **noncompliance** (adherence or nonadherence to the recommended plan) is important. "What have you done in the past for your nausea?" may yield different answers from the patient and family members. Unless a written record is available, past compliance may be hard to assess. "People often find it hard to take blood pressure pills twice a day, every day. Has this ever been a problem for you?" can also be a useful lead when assessing compliance. Giving the patient an agenda can also be useful: "As I listen to you, it sounds like we need to talk about wound care and diet. What do you think?"

Sensory and Physical State

The patient's sensory abilities and physical state affect his or her learning readiness, and the teaching plan must be modified accordingly. For example, a patient with poor vision or compromised fine-motor skill may be unable to give a subcutaneous injection safely. A patient with intermittent claudication (muscular pain brought on by exercise) may be unable to perform physical exercise. A woman who has just given birth may be too tired to learn anything.

Literacy Level

One out of five Americans read at or below a fifth-grade level (Doak, 1985). They may not understand most written directions, videotapes, or even some audiotapes. Most patient-education materials are aimed at people who read at a high-school level or above, so a huge segment of the population is confused by this material but is too ashamed to admit it.

Illiteracy is found in every walk of life, among all races, and at all socioeconomic levels. A person's appearance and use of spoken language do not indicate his or her literacy. Many people with low literacy levels have average intelligence and can speak articulately. A roughly dressed laborer may be able to read well, but a professionally dressed person may be unable to read at a functional level. Educational level gives only a rough estimate of literacy.

How can the nurse determine the patient's literacy level? Direct testing would be the most accurate way

(Doak, 1985), but this is impractical. Here are some less accurate, but expedient, methods:

- Check the level of the patient's pleasure reading, if any.
- Give the patient something to read and later ask for a description of the contents, in his or her own words.
- If possible, offer the patient several options for learning methods (reading, watching, or listening). When in doubt, use the lower-literacy material. When teaching stressed people, it is better to start with simpler material and add complexity later.

NURSING DIAGNOSES AND PATIENT GOALS

It is wise to include at least one patient-education nursing diagnosis on the care plan; the most useful are Knowledge Deficit, Noncompliance, and Self-Care Deficit. The first two diagnoses are still in a working stage by NANDA and may be changed. The nursing diagnosis states the general area of knowledge deficit, which is more clearly delineated in the goals and outcome criteria sections of the care plan.

Planning for Learning

The display shows the patient-education part of a sample care plan. Without a written plan, teaching is likely to be haphazard and ineffective. Having a written plan also serves as a useful reference for evaluation and fosters communication with other professionals, so they may take part in the teaching.

Patient-centered, patient-involved goals are the most effective. It is human nature to commit only to something in which we have some involvement or influence. Including the patient in the planning process often shows the nurse clearly what the patient is willing or unwilling to do, clarifying goals for the patient and nurse.

Be brief and realistic in writing goals and outcome criteria. Do not promise overly optimistic outcomes. For example, make it clear to a pregnant diabetic that tight blood-sugar control does not *guarantee* a healthy baby, but definitely increases the odds. Create measurable goals with a timeframe. Anderson (1990) suggests this form for writing a goal statement:

Who + Does + What + How + When = Goal.

Example: Patient + will demonstrate + dressing change + unassisted + before discharge.

Find out if prepackaged written materials or audiovisual aids are available. Are there any resources for the nonreader?

Remember the resources available to you and the patient when setting priorities. For example, it would be ideal for the newly diagnosed diabetic to know all the

Sample Teaching Plan

Data	Initials	Nursing Diagnosis	Goals/Nursing Orders	Date	Initials	Outcome/ Evaluation
8/29	KM	Knowledge Deficit, wound care, related to lack of instruction	Mr. B will demonstrate wound care independently by discharge, including:			
			1. Demonstrating wet-to-dry technique	9/1	KM	1. Demonstrated adequate technique.
			2. Naming the signs and symptoms of wound infection	8/30	CJ	2. Named increased temperature, pain, redness, and swelling.
			3. Stating how to reach emergency resources	9/2	KM	3. Stated 555-1234 for consulting nurse, 911 for ambulance.
			4. Stating the time and date of his first followup clinic appointment	9/2	CJ	4. Showed card data 9/5, 10 A.M., Dr. Smith

details of the American Diabetes Association diet before hospital discharge, but this is completely unrealistic. It is more important for the patient to know basic dietary guidelines and how to inject insulin safely, how to recognize and treat low blood sugar reactions, and how to check blood sugar. In this case, as in almost all cases, making sure the patient knows about followup outpatient resources is vital.

Outpatient education is often more effective than inpatient education for several reasons. Outpatients are generally less stressed and therefore are better able to learn. They have lived at home with the change for a period of time and bring practical, everyday questions to the session. Just attending an outpatient education session indicates a willingness to learn, and as stated previously motivation is a strong indicator of educational success.

Appropriate Family and Friend Involvement

Whenever possible, include family and friends in patient education. Their support is a strong indicator of patient success (DuBrey, 1982). A statement such as, "I'm here

because my wife made me come" indicates denial on the patient's part and also tells the nurse about the wife's attitudes and influence. Never assume that because someone is a blood relative, he or she automatically wants to participate in patient education or care. Friends are often as supportive as family members. For example, male homosexual AIDS victims are often cared for by partners and friends in family-like groups.

IMPLEMENTATION OF PATIENT TEACHING

When implementing patient teaching, the nurse should consider the following variables that can affect learning.

Sensitivity

Because low-level needs must be met before higher-level functions, such as learning, can start (Rankin, 1990), begin by seeing to patient comfort, easing acute symptoms such as pain, hunger, thirst, nausea, or dyspnea. Give the patient a chance to use the toilet. Offer pain medication and determine that the patient is comfortable. Less is learned during the acute phase of an illness; learning becomes more fruitful as recovery occurs.

Anger, fear, anxiety, worry, grief, and guilt block learning. Be sensitive to patient distress and be ready to modify the plan accordingly. Use supportive body language and statements. No matter how thorough planning has been, last-minute changes may be needed.

After assessing the patient's sensory and physical state, the nurse may conclude that it is an inappropriate time to begin teaching.

A young woman visits a diabetes education clinic, ostensibly to help get her Type I diabetes under better control. During the interview, it becomes clear that the patient has adequate knowledge to control her blood sugar. It becomes equally clear that she is under tremendous emotional stress: she was the victim of a date rape 6 months before. She apparently had been in a state of denial about the assault that she could no longer sustain. The emotional stress, not a lack of knowledge, rendered her unable to control her blood sugar.

The nurse abandons the teaching plan. The most appropriate nursing intervention is to find appropriate, immediate mental health services for the patient.

Environment Control

Anyone who has ever tried to study in a room that was too hot, cold, dim, bright, noisy, or distracting knows that environmental comfort affects learning. During patient-education sessions, the nurse tries to make the environment conducive to learning. If necessary, unin-

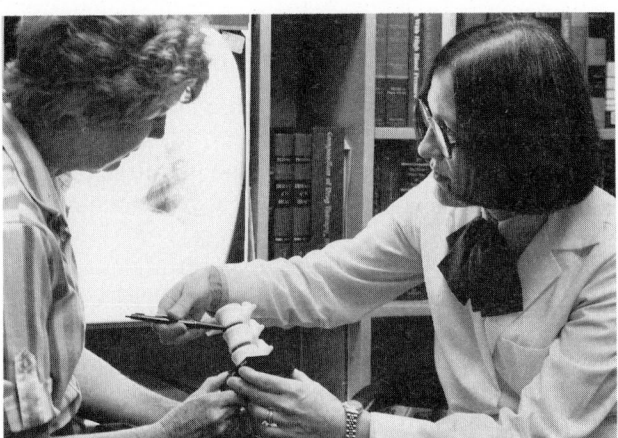

Figure 21–4. The nurse uses a replica of the vertebrae to explain to the patient where her disc problem is and how surgery will repair it. (Courtesy of Overlake Hospital Medical Center, Bellevue, WA.)

volved visitors are sent away temporarily. Privacy is often important: closing the curtains in a semiprivate room, sitting close to the patient, speaking quietly, and facing the patient all contribute to a greater sense of privacy. The patient's comfort is the most important factor. The patient may feel more comfortable with certain belongings in sight or the heat at a higher temperature than the nurse would choose.

For the hospitalized patient, the best times for teaching are often in the morning after the physician's rounds, after lunch, or in the evening, depending on visitors. Sessions should be limited to 20 to 30 minutes to avoid tiring the patient. The nurse should warn the patient about any time restraints. Saying, "I have 20 minutes to talk" communicates clearly the nurse's time limit, minimizing the chance that the patient will feel slighted.

Structured Teaching Sessions

Trying to teach too much at once can block learning (Anderson, 1990). It is important to be selective with information. Lecturing is appropriate only when addressing a group; discussion is much more effective when teaching a small group or one person. Listening to the patient's response gives excellent feedback about his or her progress.

As discussed earlier, people have different learning styles. Some prefer to do and others prefer to watch. When teaching a psychomotor skill, the nurse should be sensitive to those who like to do. A demonstration may have been planned, but if the patient reaches out to touch the materials, the nurse may consider talking the patient through the skill instead. Children learn through play and are generally an energetic and eager group of "doers." But if the child prefers to watch, a demonstration instead of instructive play may be best.

Audiovisual Aids

Audiovisual aids are not a substitute for human contact. They are best used to reinforce or supplement face-to-face teaching (Fig. 21-4). Videotapes, slide-tape programs, pamphlets, or handouts can be useful for subjects that are taught often, such as insulin injections or breastfeeding. Let the patient decide which aid would be best, if more than one form is available. A followup discussion that includes an evaluation of the learning is imperative; without this, there is no way to tell how effective learning has been.

Communication

Good communication is necessary for effective patient teaching. Chapter 17 discusses communication in the nurse–patient relationship in more detail. Active listening requires the nonverbal communication techniques of silence, attending, and observing (DuBrey, 1982). If a patient is comfortable and believes that he or she has the nurse's undivided attention, learning is greatly enhanced.

Participation is the best measure of involvement (Anderson, 1990). Getting a person to participate can be done by *leading*, making a pointed, specific statement such as, "Your son has been readmitted to the hospital. I wonder if this isn't hard on the whole family." Pointed, specific questions can accomplish the same thing: "What bronchodilators does your son take and how do they work for him?"

The patient who rambles needs to be *focused*: "You mentioned earlier that you fear going into labor. Would you like to talk about it?"

To *clarify* understanding, the nurse repeats what she or he hears the patient saying and asks if it is accurate. To clarify with an AIDS patient, for example, the nurse might ask, "Am I right? You've been hooking up all of your own total parenteral nutrition for the last year?"

Reflecting or *restating* (repeating back the patient's words) can also serve as a valuable communication tool. While expressing a great deal of personal feeling about death, that same AIDS patient could stop talking and begin to brood. The nurse could gently probe by quoting the patient's earlier statement: "You'd rather die than go on like this?"

Repetition

The realities of today's health care—short hospital stays, limited home-care opportunities, and very ill patients—provide less time for patient teaching. It becomes imperative to set priorities and repeat information. When cognitive or affective learning is the goal, try repeating the information in different ways. For example, if the patient has been learning a therapeutic diet, ask what would be appropriate food choices in different restaurants, on a picnic, or at a party. Have the patient repeat back the information several times. Ask the patient how his or her daily routines will be affected by this new learning, and check to see if the taught routines are being integrated into activities of daily living. Ask patients to practice and demonstrate psychomotor skills several times before discharge. Repetition may point out deficits in learning that would not be evident in a single evaluation session.

Because discharge instructions can seem overwhelming to the patient, the nurse should clarify important concepts, review factual information, and have the patient repeat the knowledge and practice the skills.

Teaching Methods

Methods of teaching differ in the three domains of knowledge.

Nursing Research

Selected Nursing Research Articles

Bove, P. A., et al. (1989). Investigation of the methods used to teach blood-pressure measurement techniques. *Health Values, 13*(3), 36–44.

Fegley, B. J. (1988). Preparing children for radiologic procedures: Contingent versus noncontingent instruction. *Research in Nursing and Health, 11*(1), 3–9.

Hjelm-Karlsson, K. (1989). Comparison of oral, written, and audiovisually based information as preparation for intravenous pyelography. *International Journal of Nursing Studies, 26*(1), 53–68.

Johnson, M. L., et al. (1990). Dietary practices, nutrition knowledge, and attitudes of coronary heart disease patients. *Health Values, 14*(1), 3–8.

Parfitt, J. M. (1990). Humorous patient teaching: Effects on recall of postoperative exercise routines. *AORN Journal, 52*(1), 114–120.

Stanford, L. (1987). Testicular self-examination:

Teaching, learning, and practice by nurses. *Journal of Advanced Nursing, 12*(1), 13.

Yount, S. T., et al. (1990). Preoperative teaching: A study of nurses' perceptions. *AORN Journal, 51*(2), 572.

Possible Topics for Nursing Inquiry

- What is the impact of shortened stays on teaching techniques used by nurses?
- How much do nurses know about written information available for patients from community agencies?
- How effective are return demonstrations as an evaluation tool for patient learning?
- Is the McBer learning grid useful for individualizing teaching to patients in a clinical setting?
- How significant is family involvement in patient compliance after discharge?
- How effective is videotaped preoperative instruction on patient's learning of postoperative exercises?

Psychomotor

Psychomotor methods involve the muscular motions needed to learn a skill. The nurse assembles the appropriate equipment (i.e., dressings, syringes); having the necessary supplies at hand can save time and prevent interruptions. Written material can be referred to during the session and can be kept by the patient, serving as a reminder the first few times the patient practices the skill independently. Approach the skill step by step, allowing for the patient's questions and comments. Many adults are intimidated by learning a new skill, so encouragement and praise almost always improve performance. Comments such as, "Lots of people have that same concern" or "I've had many patients with that same problem" help the patient feel less isolated.

Cognitive

Since this domain of learning involves expanding knowledge, it is important to organize material from the simple to the complex. Introduce the patient to the basic concepts and give definitions. Then help the patient to integrate these concepts into something meaningful and beneficial to health. The most common error is to try to teach too much. It is far better to teach some basic ideas well than to overload the patient with many hard-to-remember facts.

Affective

Trying to change a person's values and feelings is a challenging job for the educator. When trying to modify an attitude or emotional response, the nurse must keep a nonjudgmental, nonthreatening attitude. Acknowledging the patient's power to accept or reject the material can empower the patient and sometimes can lead to more healthy decision-making. The nurse who states emphatically the rightness of his or her position and the wrongness of the patient's loses all credibility and influence. Listen carefully to what the patient *does* value, and work from there.

For example, a nurse is trying to encourage a depressed, noncompliant paraplegic to join a support group. The patient is too depressed to be involved in self-care, but does seem to have a strong sense of contributing as a family member. Gently approach the patient with the idea that better physical and mental health would enable him to better contribute to his family's well-being. The patient may begin to assign a higher value to health when it is tied to better family functioning.

Teaching Strategies

Choosing the right strategy for patient education can make the experience more enjoyable for nurse and pa-tient. If possible, use a variety of strategies to enhance learning and retention. Combining modalities such as seeing, hearing, and touching promotes better learning than using only one modality.

Lectures are most commonly used with a group of learners. They are most effective when teaching facts (cognitive learning) but are less effective for psychomotor or affective learning. A simple lecture (a one-way communication from teacher to learner) is much more effective when combined with discussion. Learners who are eager to contribute may be stifled by a lecture. Be sensitive to see if the patient appears bored, anxious, or easily distracted.

Values clarification can be a useful tool for affective learning. The nurse must first know what the patient's value system is to begin with. A nonjudgmental discussion about people's perceptions of themselves and their world can help the patient see more accurately the consequences of certain actions and perhaps stimulate change in that value system. Sometimes it does not stimulate any change; the nurse must respect this.

A question-and-answer session is an opportunity for the patient to focus learning by asking questions. It can be useful with individual patients or groups. Discussion involves learners more deeply in the learning process because it requires participation. Cognitive and affective learning can be enhanced by this strategy.

Demonstrations are particularly useful for psychomotor learning (Fig. 21-5). Explaining the skill while slowly demonstrating it leads into talking the patient through the procedure for the first few times. Videotapes or audiotapes can be used, but human contact is almost always preferable. Repeated practice can be used to help the patient move toward independent functioning. Return demonstrations help the nurse evaluate learning. Praise the patient's learning while noting any areas for improvement.

Role-playing, or acting out feelings or knowledge, is especially useful for teaching affective behavior to adults or children. It can be used to work through past, present, or anticipated emotional trauma. The patient reacts based on his or her experience while the nurse stands by to offer guidance and feedback. The learner may need to repeat the role-playing several times before internalizing it.

Testing, oral or written, is best used for cognitive and psychomotor learning. Return demonstrations can also be considered a test. Informal oral testing is better than formal written testing because of literacy concerns and because many people are intimidated by written tests. Affective learning cannot be tested because no answer is right or wrong. Tests are useful as assessment tools (pretests) or as evaluation tools to check the patient's progress.

Simulation is a technique to evaluate if the patient can apply learning in different situations. Offer a scenario to the patient and ask what the best choice(s) would be. For example, the nurse could evaluate dietary learning by

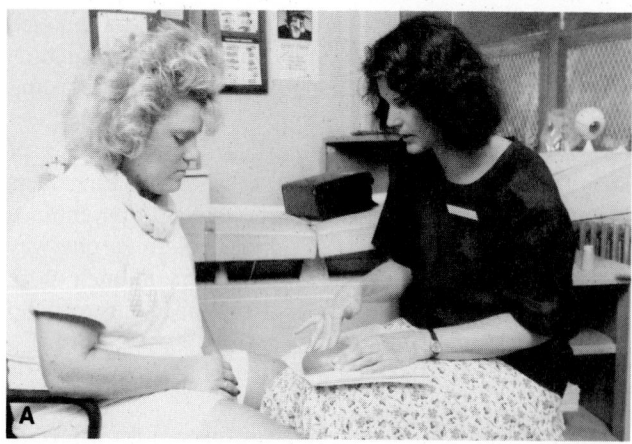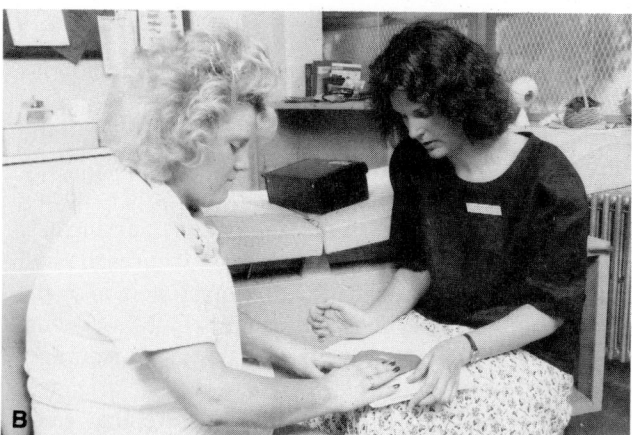

Figure 21–5. **A.** The nurse uses a visual aid to help her teach breast self-examination. **B.** The patient is then asked for a return demonstration to evaluate skill attainment. (Courtesy of University of Washington School of Nursing, Seattle, WA.)

asking the patient what would be the best choices in various restaurants, or could evaluate diabetic sick-day care by posing different sick-day scenarios.

EVALUATION OF LEARNING

Evaluation of learning is most effective when it is systematic, practical, and ongoing. Measurable, clearly stated goals streamline evaluation. If the patient participated in goal formation, he or she is likely to be able to do much of the evaluation.

This final phase depends heavily on what has preceded it. If evaluation becomes unclear, review the goals. Were they realistic for the patient's abilities, timeframe, and resources? Were they clearly stated and measurable?

Feedback from the nurse to the patient is most effective when it enhances the patient's self-concept and motivates him or her to higher learning (Rankin, 1990). Asking the patient to repeat or demonstrate what has been learned to family members is one way to accomplish this, especially with children. Remind the patient of the progress made rather than what is still left to be done.

Evaluation can be done in several ways: by written tests, questionnaires, oral tests, or return demonstrations.

Written tests are time-consuming, intimidating, and not always specific to the patient (DuBrey, 1982). They are useful only if:

- The patient is literate (do not take this for granted).
- Clear educational objectives have been mutually agreed on.
- It is necessary to measure a broad sample of factual information.
- A skilled test-writer has prepared the test.

As in the classroom, written tests are most useful in evaluating cognitive learning.

Questionnaires can be useful for long-term followup of education, but they have drawbacks. They must be prepared by a skilled author who understands what is to be measured.

Oral tests are usually more expedient and less intimidating than written ones. Questions can be informally phrased, and the patient usually gives immediate, specific, and useful feedback. It is best to stay as casual as possible, since the higher the patient's anxiety about being tested, the less likely it is that the evaluation will be accurate. Evaluation of the patient's verbal response can be useful in testing cognitive learning, but affective learning in the form of an attitude change is difficult to measure.

The *return demonstration* is a way of testing skill performance. How accurately and independently the patient can perform a skill is almost always a clear indication of learning. Psychomotor skills can be evaluated with this method. The nurse should give feedback about parts done well along with areas for improvement.

DOCUMENTATION OF PATIENT TEACHING

Documenting patient education is as important as documenting any other aspect of patient care. Documentation of patient education serves several purposes (Anderson, 1990):

- It communicates the plan and progress to other health-care professionals.
- It fulfills the nursing job description as delineated by local, state, and national licensing agencies.
- It provides a legal record.

Documentation must contain the subject matter, the patient's response, and any necessary break in the process (for example, if after evaluation the nurse found it necessary to return to the planning stage). Well-documented patient education can serve as a record of methods that did or did not work, and can give some indication of patient compliance over time.

LIFESPAN CONSIDERATIONS

Changes across the lifespan affect the patient's learning needs and abilities. When planning patient teaching, consider the patient's developmental level to individualize the teaching and promote optimal learning.

Newborn and Infant

Newborns and infants learn by interacting with their environment. During this period of rapid development, the baby is learning a great deal (for example, how to recognize his or her mother, how to follow objects as they move, how to hold toys). The nurse should encourage an environment rich in appropriate stimuli to foster normal cognitive development.

During this stage, the infant is not ready for formalized teaching; instead, any necessary teaching is given to parents and caregivers. Teaching the parents about various aspects of child care helps promote positive parent–child bonding.

Toddler and Preschooler

Because toddlers and preschoolers are accustomed to learning from and communicating with their parents, the parents are usually the most effective teachers. Play is the way children learn, so using dolls or toys as models can be effective and can be continued at home (Fig. 21-6). In fact, learning is more successful if it can be continued at home and added to existing home routines (Anderson, 1990).

Children age 2 to 5 like to be spoken to with their parents listening. They are likely to have many questions and may ask some of the same ones many times. Their questions should be answered immediately, directly, and in language they can understand. Preschoolers are generally energetic and restless, so try to limit the session to 10 minutes (Anderson, 1990). Let the child handle machines or supplies as soon as possible. Children of this age can understand some anatomy, so when possible use models and correct anatomic names.

Trust is vital. If the preschooler asks, "Will it hurt?" and you say, "No" and it does, you have lost credibility with the child and learning is hindered.

Preschoolers, compared to toddlers, have learned to

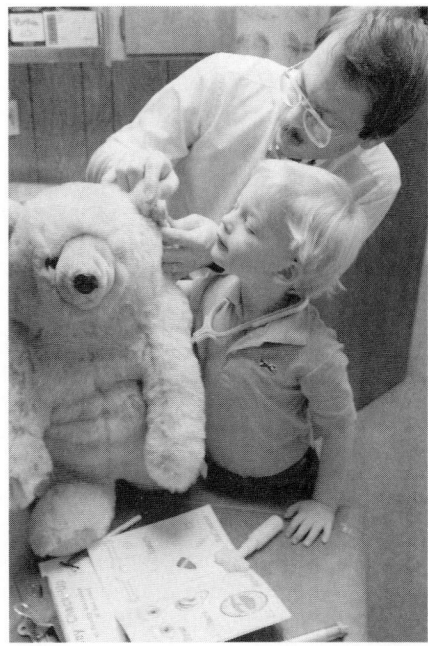

Figure 21–6.   Teaching should be individualized for the age of the patient. Demonstrating on a friendly stuffed animal and using age-appropriate coloring books makes learning fun for this preschooler. Teaching used in the health-care facility can be carried through at home. (Courtesy of Overlake Hospital Medical Center, Bellevue, WA.)

do many more things (using the toilet, eating, and dressing, for example), and they are usually proud of these things. Young children are extremely egocentric: they think the world revolves around them and that all events relate to them. Teaching should be related to the child's specific life experiences when possible.

Learning should be evaluated frequently to ensure that the child understands. A preschooler usually enjoys displaying new knowledge, giving the nurse the chance to praise the child repeatedly and offer rewards such as stickers, picture books, or rubber stamps.

Child and Adolescent

School-age children are usually eager to learn. They can understand cause and effect ("If I don't stay off my leg, it won't heal as quickly and it'll be longer before I can play outside at recess"). Include children in educational planning, allowing them to help set goals. Being accustomed to a classroom atmosphere, they understand the scheduling of work and play.

All questions should be answered immediately and truthfully, or the nurse loses credibility. Trust is vital to learning and also to establishing a relationship where the child feels comfortable enough to express fears and concerns.

Educational content can be more sophisticated for this

group than for the preschooler. Coloring books for teaching anatomy work well. Written material is fine at the proper reading level, keeping in mind that the hospitalized child may regress. Procedures must be explained directly to the child with the parents in the background. Sessions should be no longer than 30 minutes.

"Winning" is important for school-age children, so success framed as such is generally highly valued. Use of charts with stickers to mark progress is effective with this group.

Adolescents generally enjoy complete, open, and honest explanations to their questions. Their peers are usually more influential than parents, teachers, or nurses. It is fine to include peers in a teaching session; in fact, general health-care information may be thrown in for the benefit of these visitors (Fig. 21-7). A sensitive, caring attitude is essential to educate adolescents effectively. To maintain the adolescent's trust, confidences must be kept; if a confidence must be broken, tell the patient who you must tell and why.

Adolescents must be included in any educational planning because their struggle for independence makes them averse to having anything imposed on them. They are more likely to comply when alternatives and consequences are explained (Anderson, 1990). Ask the patient what he or she needs to know. Find out the value system associated with the illness, and work from the youngster's point of view. Adolescents are generally sophisticated learners, able to understand broad concepts and assimilate much information (Anderson, 1990). They are oriented to the present, however, and are more in tune with immediate advantages than with long-term results.

This age group is accustomed to teaching sessions of 45 to 50 minutes in school, and this is probably the maximum effective length. It may be better not to include parents in the session to encourage patient autonomy and heighten self-concept; parents can be informed

later. Literature to review between sessions can be useful with this group.

Adult and Older Adult

Adults tend to be motivated by activities that enhance or maintain their self-esteem (Anderson, 1990). Self-direction and achievement generally boost self-esteem; dependence and error generally decrease it. Adults tend to take errors personally, thinking poorly of themselves if they think they are taking too long to grasp a concept.

Adult learners respond well to a straightforward teaching approach and can apply the knowledge immediately. Try to provide a comfortable, informal, friendly learning environment where the patient can feel appreciated.

Young adults usually have plenty of energy and take good health for granted. Learning must be practical, as these people generally lead busy lives. When setting educational goals with patients from this group, take a practical approach, if possible explaining how the change will improve day-to-day life. Adults of this age are often motivated by the thought of maintaining their functioning to care for their children.

In general, middle-aged adults are more aware of health problems and do not take good health for granted

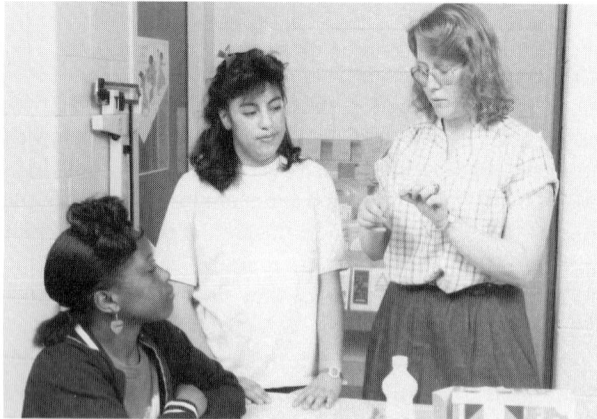

Figure 21–7. Adolescents respect each other's attitudes. Teaching adolescents in small peer groups is helpful in getting a message across.

Principal Teaching Methods

Psychomotor (skill)

1. Skill demonstration
2. Talking the learner through the skill
3. Repeated practice

Cognitive (knowledge)

1. Lecture
2. Discussion (factual questions and answers)
3. Simulation (application of knowledge in different contexts)
4. Independent study
5. Tests

Affective (values)

1. Discussion and values clarification
2. Role-playing
3. Simulation
4. Discussion (factual questions and answers)

the way younger adults do. Still capable of learning and changing, people in this age group sometimes lack the self-confidence to try something new. Middle-aged adults should be involved in all aspects of the teaching plan, as they are usually familiar with the concepts of goal-setting and achievement (Anderson, 1990). These people have a broad base of life experience, and teaching goals will more likely be met if they are given time to assimilate new knowledge into old. Approach learning directly, explaining all rationales fully. Try to keep sessions under 1 hour, and allow time for the patient to practice skills in private.

Middle-aged people enjoy praise as much as anyone else. Evaluate the patient in a supportive atmosphere, stressing how much progress has been made. Gently correct misconceptions, and be sensitive to the patient's fears and anxieties.

The elderly are the fastest-growing segment of our population. General adult learning principles apply to this group, but the elderly do require some special considerations.

Tips for Teaching the Elderly Learner

- Use a brightly lit, glare-free room.
- Use visual aids with large, well-spaced letters and primary colors.
- Eliminate extraneous noise.
- Face the learner.
- Speak in slow, low tones.
- Limit sessions to 20 to 30 minutes.
- Watch for cues indicating inadequate hearing such as leaning forward, cupping an ear, frowning when trying to hear, or starting a separate conversation.
- Relate new material to the past or past experiences in a meaningful way.
- Supply one idea at a time. Use frequent summaries and positive feedback.
- Provide a written or recorded summary of the session.

Medication Teaching

- Be sure the patient knows what each medication does, how many to take, and when.
- Discuss what to do if the patient misses a dose. (Containers that hold a week's worth of medications can be a boon to accuracy and consistency.)
- Be sure the patient has written medication instructions in appropriate size, form, and language.

Motivation to learn may be low if the patient feels that life is near the end. Two motivational strategies to try are:

- Show the patient how the new knowledge will improve the quality of his or her life, regardless of its length.
- Show how the new knowledge could improve the patient's independence.

A high quality of life and independence are usually highly valued by the elderly.

Physiologic changes that normally occur with aging may hinder learning. Vision may decrease because of cataracts; smaller, less-reactive pupils; or a decrease in color perception. The ability to hear high-pitched sounds usually decreases, although low-pitch hearing may be intact. Rapid speech may become unintelligible because the elderly often take longer to process what they hear. Hearing loss can be a source of shame and frustration for the elderly learner, causing withdrawal and worsening feelings of isolation.

The elderly often suffer from *short-term memory loss.* Do not assume there is memory loss, but be sensitive to it. When it does exist, it is usually associated with meaningless learning, complex learning, or new information that has required a reassessment of old learning (Anderson, 1990). If new information conflicts with old, time is needed to reexamine the old learning; this may cause some anxiety and may act as a barrier to new learning. The elderly learner has large stores of information, so scanning for recall may take longer.

Generally, older learners need more time to learn psychomotor skills. Often they compensate by putting a great deal of effort into accuracy.

Key Concepts

- Patient education is a dynamic process used to empower the patient toward autonomy and self-care.
- For financial, legal, ethical, and humanitarian reasons, the responsibility for patient education usually falls to nurses.
- The nurse assesses the patient's learning needs and readiness to learn, then forms a teaching plan. The plan is then implemented, the learning evaluated, and the process documented.
- Determining whether the learning will be primarily psychomotor, cognitive, or affective affects the entire process.
- People have varying learning styles, and different age groups require different approaches.
- In patient education, the nurse can influence but not control. Education must be patient-centered.

References

Anderson, C. (1990). *Patient teaching and communication in an information age.* Albany: Delmar Publishers, Inc.

Doak, C. C., et al. (1985). *Teaching patients with low literacy skills.* Philadelphia: J. B. Lippincott.

DuBrey, R. J. (1982). *Promoting wellness in nursing practice.* St. Louis: C. V. Mosby.

Gagne, R. M. (1974). *Essentials of learning for instruction.* Hinsdale: Dryden Press.

McBer & Co. (1985). *Learning-style inventory.* Boston: Author.

Rankin, S. H., & Stallings, K. D. (1990). *Patient education.* Philadelphia: J. B. Lippincott.

Redman, B. (1988). *The process of patient education* (6th ed.). St. Louis: C. V. Mosby.

Bibliography

Brannon, L., & Feist, J. (1988). *Health psychology, an introduction to behavior and health.* Belmont, CA: Wadsworth Publishing Co.

Falvo, D.R. (1985). *Effective patient education, a guide to increased compliance.* Rockville, MD: Aspen.

Gerber, K. E., & Nehemkis, A. M. (1986). *Compliance, the dilemma of the chronically ill.* New York: Springer.

Haggard, A. H. (1989). *Handbook of patient education.* Rockville, MD: Aspen.

Springhouse Corp. (1987). *Patient teaching.* Springhouse, PA: Nursing '87 Books.

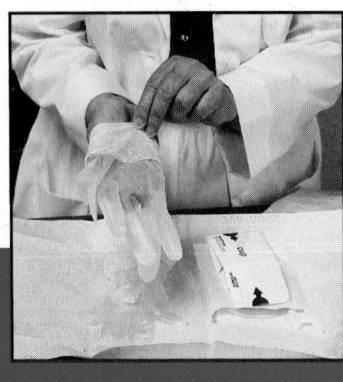

Asepsis

LEARNING OBJECTIVES

Upon completion of this chapter, the student will be able to do the following:

- Identify the chain of infection and give examples of ways infection can occur.
- Describe factors that increase infection in various settings.
- Discuss the role of various agencies and health personnel in infection control.
- Identify ways a caregiver can increase protection from infectious exposure.
- Identify ways a caregiver can decrease infection exposure for patients.
- Differentiate between medical and surgical asepsis.
- Incorporate good hand-washing as an integral part of practice.
- Differentiate appropriate use of cleaning, disinfection, and sterilization.
- Discuss different systems of isolation.
- Identify age-related considerations in preventing the transmission of infectious disease.

KEY TERMS

Antiseptic
Asepsis
Bactericidal
Bacteriostatic
Communicable disease
Contamination
Disinfection
Infectious disease
Nosocomial infection
Pathogen
Sepsis
Sterilization
Universal precautions
Virulence

22

Role of Microorganisms in Infection
  Agents Causing Infection
  Chain of Infection
    Infectious Agent
    Source
    Portal of Exit
    Mode of Transmission
    Portal of Entry
    Susceptible Host
  Progress of an Infection
  Nosocomial Infections
    Risk Factors in Nosocomial Infection
     Development
  Infection Hazards in Nonacute Care Settings
Infection Control
  Recognition of Factors
  Regulatory Agencies
    Infection Control Committee
    Reporting Infectious Disease
  Employee Health
    Monitoring and Counseling of Personnel
    Transmissible Diseases
    Significant Exposure
    Work Restriction
  Waste Disposal
Aseptic Practices
  Categories of Asepsis
    Medical Asepsis
    Surgical Asepsis

  Handwashing
  Cleaning, Disinfection, and Sterilization
    Cleaning
    Disinfection
    Sterilization
    Levels of Disinfection and Sterilization
    Factors Affecting Disinfection and Sterilization
     Effectiveness
  Use of Barriers
    Masks
    Gowns, Caps, and Shoe Coverings
    Gloves
    Private Rooms
    Equipment and Refuse Handling
  Isolation Systems
    Universal Precautions
    Category-Specific Isolation
    Disease-Specific Isolation
    Body-Substance Isolation
    Protective (Reverse) Isolation
    Nursing Considerations
  Surgical Asepsis
    Principles of Surgical Asepsis
    Skin Preparation
    Surgical Handwashing
    Sterile Gloves
  Lifespan Considerations
Key Concepts

Regardless of where they practice, preventing the transfer of microorganisms is a concern of every nurse. In homes, schools, clinics, industry, hospitals, and extended care facilities, nurses strive to teach about, prevent, and treat infections. Promoting healthy lifestyles and preventive health practices is an important focus as the nurse tries to prevent infection for all patients.

A sea of microorganisms live and multiply on every surface we touch and in the air we breathe. They grow on our skin and flourish in our digestive tracts. Often microorganisms help produce food and maintain the ecology of the planet. Most of the time humans and microorga-

nisms live in harmony. When this balance is upset, microorganisms are capable of causing infection. **Asepsis** means to make free from disease-producing organisms.

Infectious disease is the most common reason people contact a health-care provider, accounting for more physician office visits than any other cause. Worldwide, many preventable infectious diseases are common, resulting in great suffering and the loss of many lives. The economic costs of preventing and treating infection is very great.

This chapter discusses some nursing practices aimed at providing a safe and therapeutic environment designed to protect patients, family members, and health-care providers from acquiring infections. Future chapters on skin integrity and wound healing (see Chap. 34) and infection (see Chap. 35) provide additional information on specific infectious diseases as well as diagnostic and treatment procedures.

ROLE OF MICROORGANISMS IN INFECTION

Microorganisms that are capable of harming people are called **pathogens** or pathogenic; they produce disease. When these organisms enter and multiply within body tissues, they destroy normal physiologic body processes. The organisms or their toxins disrupt normal cell function or kill the cells entirely. **Sepsis,** a term that means poisoning of tissues, is often used to describe the presence of infection. When the infection or the products of infection are carried throughout the body by the blood it is known as *septicemia. Aseptic* is the opposite of septic, or to be without disease-producing organisms.

Infection (in the strictest sense of the word) means the process of causing to become diseased. Unfortunately, in common usage "infected" and "septic" are used interchangeably. In most instances when a patient is said to be infected, it means he or she has a disease caused by microorganisms. When the patient is referred to as septic, it means he or she is displaying the manifestations of microbial destruction of tissues, such as high fever or hypotension.

Infectious disease refers to the pathology or pathologic events that result from the invasion and multiplication of microorganisms in a host. Toxins and enzymes produced by the microorganisms cause tissue injury. This injury produces manifestations of infection, namely, fever; rashes; malaise; nausea and vomiting; diarrhea; purulent discharge from wounds; hot, reddened, tender area around wounds or puncture sites; aches and pains; or total body collapse.

A major portion of the health-care practitioner's time, energy, and talent is devoted to developing and maintaining good practices to control the spread of microorganisms. These practices, known as aseptic techniques, are used in the broader context of infection control.

Aseptic techniques start and end with handwashing. They include the processes of cleaning, disinfection, and sterilization. The use of barriers against the spread of microorganisms, such as gloves, masks, hair coverings, and gowns, as well as patient isolation, are part of aseptic practice.

Agents Causing Infection

There are four groups of microorganisms that are potentially pathogenic to humans. They include bacteria, viruses, fungi, and parasites. Brief descriptions are given here. (For more information, see Chap. 35.)

Bacteria. Bacteria are single-celled, independent living microorganisms, some of which are capable of causing disease in humans. Bacteria may be airborne, food- or waterborne, soil- or vectorborne, or sexually transmitted. They differ in size and shape, growth and replication requirements, and the method by which they inflict harm to the host. Some are capable of producing metabolic toxins, which they secrete into the host organism's system (exotoxin producers). Others can produce poisons that are contained in their cell walls and released after the death of the microorganism (e.g., gram-negative endotoxin producers). In addition, all bacteria are capable of causing diminished organ function by invading tissues and initiating inflammation.

Viruses. Viruses are particles of nucleic acid and protein that are often membrane-bound. They reproduce inside living cells and cause a variety of diseases. Some infections are acute and controlled by the host's defense mechanisms; others spread throughout the body and cause severe tissue damage or result in chronic illness.

Fungi. Fungi are single-celled organisms that include molds and yeasts. *Candida albicans,* present in normal human flora, can develop into a yeast infection of the mouth, skin, vagina, and intestinal tract in the immunocompromised adult. Fungal infections of the hair, skin, and nails also frequently occur in humans. Fungi also infest and destroy plant life and cause fermentation in food and milk.

Parasites. Parasites are multicellular organisms that live on another organism without contributing anything to the host. Examples of parasites include protozoa, helminth, and arthropod species. Protozoa are free-living microorganisms that commonly thrive in water and often are contracted by humans through unsanitary conditions surrounding food preparation or handling. Sexual contact, insects, and domestic animals can also carry parasites to humans. Malaria and sleeping sickness are examples of diseases caused by protozoa. Helminths are worms that infect the gastrointestinal tract or other body tissues of humans. Examples of helminths include tapeworms, hookworms, or trichinae (or pork worm). Arthropods include mites, fleas, and ticks, which often are responsible for skin diseases and systemic disease.

Chain of Infection

The life cycle of pathogenic organisms is frequently described as an uninterrupted chain of events. For organisms to spread disease they must grow, reproduce, and move from one source to another. Nursing interventions are directed at stopping the transmission from the source to the patient, and at controlling other links in the chain.

The illness produced by microorganisms is called an infection. Infections may be localized to one site, such as a wound, or they may be systemic. Before they occur, a series of conditions must be met. This "chain of infection" includes the infectious agent, the source, the portal of exit, the mode of transmission, the portal of entrance, and a susceptible host (Fig. 22-1).

Infectious Agent

The first link in the chain of infection is the microbial agent, which may be a bacterium, a virus, a fungus, or a parasite. Characteristics that affect the ability of the infectious agent to cause disease include pathogenicity, virulence, invasiveness, and specificity. *Pathogenicity* is the ability of the organism to harm and cause disease. **Virulence** involves the vigor with which the organism can grow and multiply. *Invasiveness* describes the ability of the organism to enter tissues, whereas *specificity* refers to the attraction of the organism to a specific host, which may include humans. The more pathogenic, virulent, and invasive the organism is, the more likely that normal body defenses can be overcome, causing an infection to occur.

These capacities are determined by the structure or chemical composition of the microorganisms, which include the organism's ability to attach to skin and mucous membranes, the production of enzymes that counteract the immune system's response to invasion, and the production of toxins.

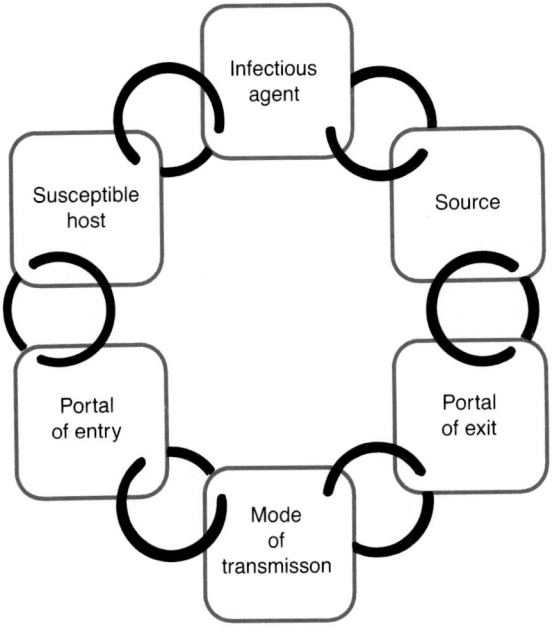

Figure 22–1. The chain of infection.

Source

The source of organisms, also called reservoirs, are various elements in the environment. Inanimate objects, human beings, and animals are all sources. Inanimate objects may include medications, air, food, water, blood, or any other material in which organisms can find nourishment or lie dormant and survive. Human sources include other patients, hospital personnel, visitors, or the patients themselves. Patients may become infected from people who have active disease, people in the incubation portion of their own disease, or people who harbor the pathogens but have no symptoms of disease (known as carriers). Animals are often sources of disease for human beings. Insects and rats have been responsible for historic epidemics in the past and continue to spread disease today. A person's own bacterial flora may cause contamination. Endogenous microorganisms from the patient's gastrointestinal tract cause disease if they become established in the lungs or a wound.

Portal of Exit

Portal of exit provide a means for the microorganism to leave the source. Sputum, emesis, stool, urine, blood, wound drainage, or secretions from genitals all permit microorganisms to exit from the source. Animal discharge or bloodborne organisms carried by mosquitoes can also provide a means of escape.

Mode of Transmission

The four main routes of transmission are contact, vehicle, airborne, and vectorborne. Contact transmission is the most frequent means of transmitting infections in hospitals. Table 22-1 lists common infections and describes their mode of transmission.

Contact Transmission. Contact transmission is by direct, indirect, or droplet contact. *Direct contact* involves physical transfer of organisms between a susceptible host and an infected or colonized person. Hospital personnel can transfer organisms to patients during patient care such as bathing, dressing changes, and inserting invasive devices. *Indirect contact* occurs when a susceptible host is exposed to a contaminated object such as a dressing, a needle, or a surgical instrument. *Droplet contact* occurs when mucous membranes of the nose or mouth or conjunctiva are exposed to secretions of an infected person who is coughing, sneezing, or talking. It is considered contact instead of airborne because droplets seldom travel more than 3 ft.

Vehicle Transmission. Vehicles are contaminated items that transmit pathogens. Food can carry *Salmonella,* water can carry *Legionella,* drugs can carry bacteria from contaminated infusion supplies, and blood can carry hepatitis.

TABLE 22–1

Common Infections and Their Means of Transmission by Infective Material

Disease	Infective Material	Mode of Transmission
Chickenpox	Respiratory and lesion secretions	Contact: Direct, indirect, droplet
Common cold—Rhinovirus	Respiratory secretions	Contact: Droplet
Diarrhea	Feces	Contact: Direct, indirect
Gonorrhea	Discharge	Contact: Direct (sexual)
Hepatitis A	Feces	Contact: Direct, indirect
Herpes	Lesion secretions	Contact: Direct, indirect
Influenza	Respiratory secretions	Contact: Droplet
Measles	Respiratory secretions	Contact: Droplet
Mumps	Respiratory secretions	Contact: Droplet
Rubella	Respiratory secretions	Contact: Droplet
Urinary tract infection	Urine	Contact: Direct, indirect
Wound infection	Pus	Contact: Direct, indirect
Pneumonia	Respiratory secretions	Contact: Direct, indirect (sometimes droplet)

Airborne Transmission. Airborne transmission occurs when fine particles are suspended in the air for a long time, or when dust particles contain pathogens. Air currents widely disperse organisms, which can be inhaled by or deposited on the skin of a susceptible host.

Vectorborne Transmission. Vectors are living animals, such as rats or insects, that carry pathogens. This type of transmission is of great concern in tropical areas where mosquitoes transmit diseases such as malaria.

Portal of Entry

The portal of entry permits the organism to gain entrance into the host. Pathogens can enter a susceptible host through orifices of the body such as the mouth, nose, ears, eyes, vagina, rectum, or urethra. Breaks in the skin or mucous membranes from wounds or abrasions increase opportunity for the organism to enter the host. Modern medicine's practice of placing tubes for long-term intravenous or gastric feedings and drainage of body cavities further increases the number of potential routes of entry into the body, thus increasing susceptibility to infection.

Susceptible Host

A host is a person whose own body defense mechanisms are unable at the time of exposure to withstand the invasion of pathogens. The body has numerous defense mechanisms that naturally resist entry and multiplication of pathogens. These factors are discussed in detail in Chapter 35. When infectious disease occurs in humans, the agent of infection has overcome the ability of the body to resist infection. A primary focus of nursing practice is identifying patients with compromised defenses and working to enhance their defenses.

Progress of an Infection

When the signs and symptoms of a disease are apparent, the disease is said to be clinical. Many infections are subclinical, in that the patient and other observers note no symptoms of disease even though the organism is present in the body and causes antibodies to be formed and immunity gained (Alcamo, 1986).

The course of an infection that results in a disease state is a dynamic series of events that express competition between the host and the invading organism. Disease is usually a result of the organism's growth and multiplication inside the host. The exception for this is when the disease is caused by the release of toxins, such as in food poisoning and botulism. The pattern for most diseases follows a predictable course, which includes the incubation period, the prodromal period, acute illness with symptoms, and the convalescent period. The timeframe during which a disease can be passed from one person to another is known as the communicable period. Figure 22-2 illustrates the progress of the infection in the case of measles.

Incubation Period. The incubation period is the time between entrance of the pathogen and the appearance of symptoms. The length of this period varies depending on the number of organisms absorbed, the time they require to grow and multiply, their virulence, and the resistance of the host. The point of entry may also be a factor.

Prodromal Period. The prodromal period is characterized by nonspecific symptoms such as nausea, fever, general weakness, or aches and pains. Although prodromal symptoms are nonspecific, the cluster of symptoms and their order of appearance often help in the diagnosis of the disease.

Acute Phase of Illness. The acute phase of an illness occurs when specific symptoms appear. Depending on

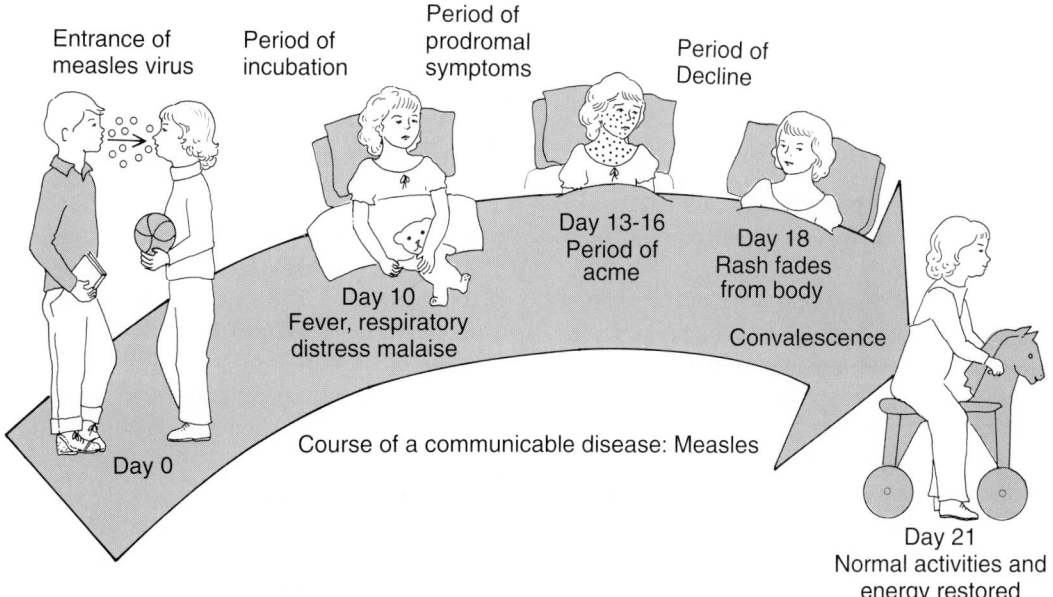

Figure 22–2.   The course of a communicable disease—measles. Day 0: Entrance of the virus by absorption of respiratory droplets from another child's sneeze and incubation begins. Day 10: Fever, respiratory distress, malaise. Day 13: The period of acme begins with the appearance of the body rash. Day 16: The rash covers the body at its peak, then begins to fade, first the face and then the trunk as the period of decline takes place. Day 18: The body begins to return to normal. Day 21: Normal activities and energy restored. The period of communicability is from 4 days before the rash to 4 days after. (Modified from Alcamo, I. E. (1987). *Fundamentals of microbiology*, 2nd edition (p. 546). Menlo Park, CA: Benjamin/Cummings Publishing Company.)

the pathogen, there is a cluster of symptoms and often laboratory analysis that can identify the disease. The period during which the symptoms subside is included in this phase. The acute phase of an illness may be preceded by a crisis period followed by rapid recovery or a slow recuperation.

Convalescent Period. Convalescence is a period that completes the progress of an infection. The body systems return to normal, and appetite and energy return. Antibodies begin to be present in the person's blood.

Communicable Period. If the causative agent of the disease is transmissible between one person and another, the disease is said to be a **communicable disease.** If the agent passes with ease from one host to the next, it may be called a *contagious disease*. Not all diseases are contagious. For example, tetanus can be contracted in an isolated event when a person sustains a puncture wound. Childhood diseases (measles, mumps, chickenpox) are classic examples of communicable diseases. Infections in patients in hospitals are not necessarily contagious, but because of the large number of patients with lowered

host defenses, such infections are more easily transmitted than they would be in the community.

An infected person may be contagious during the incubation period, the acute phase, or the convalescent period, depending on whether or not organisms are being shed into the environment. When the agent is not present in body secretions, but hidden within the host's cells, the infection is called *latent*. When the agent is being shed from the host's body in respiratory secretions, feces, blood, urine, or is cultured from body tissues, the infection is communicable. The period of communicability begins after the agent has multiplied sufficiently for shedding to begin and lasts as long as the level of shedding is sufficient for transmission. Diseases spread more rapidly if they have a short latent period (Garner & Simmons, 1983). Unfortunately, the latent period is almost always shorter than the incubation period; thus the person is usually shedding microorganisms before any signs and symptoms are apparent. Periods of communicability vary with the disease and the control of microorganisms within the infected person's tissues. Because of the uncertainty of the period of communicability and the lack of identifiable infection in some people, all body secretions should be considered as potentially containing infectious agents (Alcamo, 1986).

Nosocomial Infections

Nosocomial infections are infections associated with health-care delivery. The term is most commonly applied to those infections acquired in acute care hospitals, although extended care facilities, psychiatric institutions, and outpatient care facilities are included in the scope of this definition. At times, the patient is exposed to the infection while in the hospital but the disease itself does not become apparent until after discharge.

About 6% of all hospital patients get nosocomial infections. The incidence has not changed in the last 15 to 20 years (Castle & Ajemian, 1987). There have been declines in some types of infections, but they have been replaced with increases in infections seen in compromised patients. As people live longer and more extensive surgeries are performed and more technology is used, rates could be expected to rise in the future (Castle & Ajemian, 1987).

The urinary tract is the most common site for nosocomial infection, accounting for 40% of hospital-acquired infection. Other common infections are surgical wound infections (25%), respiratory tract infections (15%), infections of the skin and subcutaneous tissues (15%), and septic thrombophlebitis and bacteremias

from intravascular infusion or monitoring devices (5%) (Schaffner, 1987).

Risk Factors in Nosocomial Infection Development

The longer the patient is in the hospital, the greater the risk of infection. Exposure to the hospital environment changes the patient's own body flora. The risk factors that contribute to the development of nosocomial infections can be grouped into three categories: environment, therapeutic regimen, and the resistance of the patient. They interact in varying patterns of importance, but all must be considered when attempts are made to decrease the patient's risk. Figure 22-3 illustrates sources of microbial contamination.

Environment. Although the modern hospital has come a long way since Lister and Nightingale, it is still a reservoir of organisms that pose a threat to an increasing number of patients who have decreased resistance to infection. The sources of these organisms include the air, other patients, families and visitors, contaminated equipment, food, and hospital personnel.

Therapeutic Regimen. Multiple factors that are part of the therapy used to cure the patient can also contribute to the patient's risk of infection. Steroids, immunosuppression, cancer therapy, and prolonged antibiotic

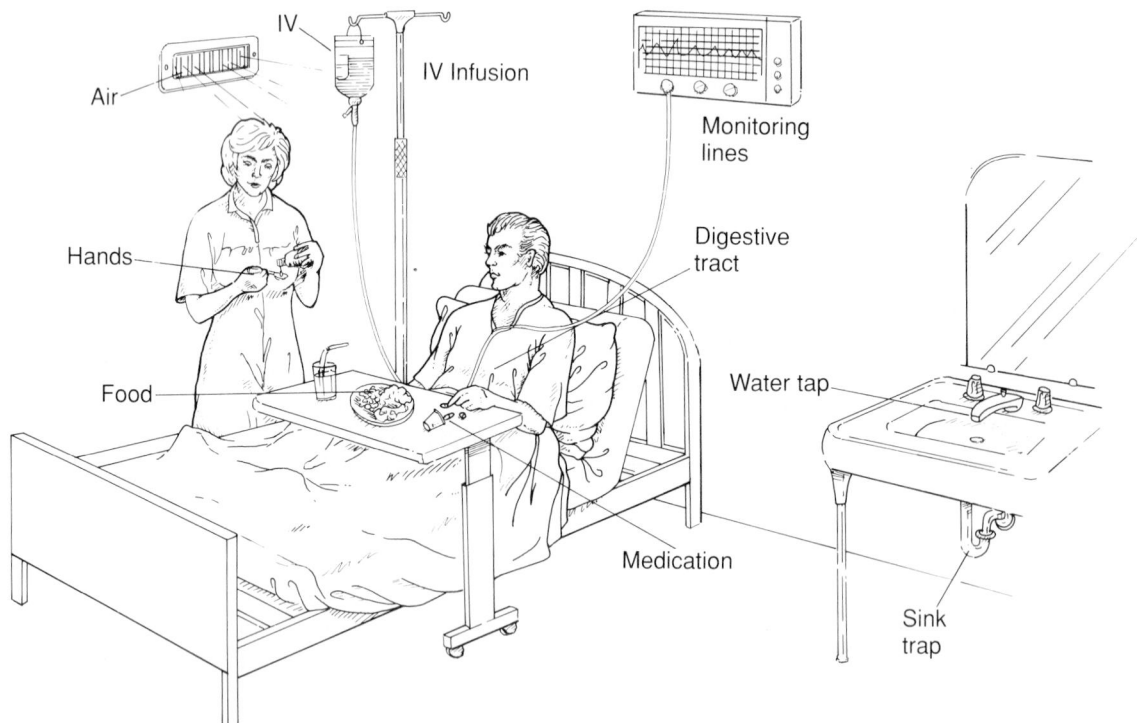

Figure 22–3. Sources of microbial contamination in the hospital environment. Transfer of contamination by hands of hospital personnel is prevalent.

use predispose the patient to infection. Equipment such as arterial or venous catheters and indwelling urinary catheters invades body orifices and provides routes for bacterial invasion into the body. Prolonged intravenous and gastrointestinal tube feedings are also invasive and may be contaminated with improper use. Inadequate dressing techniques for wounds can provide media for bacterial growth. Identifying treatments that pose risk and discontinuing their use as soon as possible decrease the chance of nosocomial infection.

Resistance of the Patient. Many changes in the physical or psychological status of the patient can impact resistance to infection. Any break in the integrity of the skin or mucous membranes increases the chance of infection. Stress, fatigue, poor nutrition, and chronic illness can also decrease the patient's ability to ward off infection. Adequate hygiene (e.g., bathing, handwashing after toileting) is important to decrease microorganisms on the skin that could contribute to infection risk.

Infection Hazards in Nonacute Care Setting

Although the most severe infections are seen in association with hospitalization, there are infection risks in other health-care delivery sites.

Ambulatory Care Settings. Patients come to ambulatory care settings for diagnosis or treatment of health problems. Frequently, such procedures involve invasive techniques increasing the risk of infection. Waiting rooms may contain many people with active infections. This is especially true of pediatric populations. Infection risk is increased because children frequently play with toys provided or interact as they wait to be seen by the physician. All equipment such as thermometers and devices used to examine body orifices must be cleaned and disinfected after each use to avoid cross-contamination.

Home Care. Many patients are being discharged to home care more quickly, and more sophisticated invasive treatments are being performed in the home setting. Indwelling urinary catheters, intravenous infusions for medications or nutrition, and extensive open wounds and drainage collection systems are seen more frequently in the home setting. The nurse is frequently responsible for teaching people in the home how to perform prescribed procedures in an aseptic manner. The nurse often teaches individuals how to care for family members with communicable illness and to prevent its spread.

Schools. Classrooms, athletic departments, and health clinics in schools pose the risk of infection to children and their teachers. Schools often employ nurses to teach health classes and to develop and monitor infec-

---

Safety Alert

- Never recap a needle or other sharp instruments after use on a patient. This could cause an accidental fingerstick and expose a health-care worker to infection.
- Place sterile objects on dry surfaces and avoid splashing liquids when pouring. Moisture may cause contamination.
- Never assume that an object is sterile. Always check the integrity of the packaging and the label for an expiration date.
- Discard sterile supplies if not used immediately. Opened, unused sterile objects do not remain sterile.
- Develop a habit of frequent handwashing whenever appropriate. Unwashed hands are the most frequent mode of transmission of microorganisms in health-care settings.
- Wear gloves for contact with all body substances from any patient. To avoid possible infection exposure, touch nothing wet that comes from a body surface with bare hands.
- Provide patients with washcloths and soap to wash their hands after toileting and before eating to prevent self-contamination with endogenous flora.

---

tion control practices. The incidence of communicable illness is high among children who are grouped together for study and play. Children are often unaware of their illness and have not yet learned good hygiene practices to prevent infection transmission. The school nurse is often the first one to identify a potential outbreak of a communicable disease and is responsible for evaluating children who may be infectious to stop the spread of infection and obtain proper treatment for the infected child.

Workplace. Employees in the workplace are exposed to, and can expose their coworkers to, infections. Working conditions and materials that workers use may have infectious risks. Farmers and other people who work with animals have a high risk of contacting diseases carried by animals. Sinks, bathrooms, lunchrooms, and food utensils may be sources of infection in the workplace. Many industries employ nurses who screen employees for communicable diseases and who collaborate with building maintenance personnel to maintain hygienic conditions and supervise waste disposal.

Extended Care Facilities. Nursing homes, psychiatric care facilities, drug and alcohol treatment centers, and group homes for the mentally or physically impaired have a high risk for infection. Often such institutions are understaffed with personnel who do not have extensive training in infection control. Their residents are often incapable of maintaining their own personal hygiene and are frequently debilitated from chronic medical conditions. Communicable diseases are common in these facilities, and the patients' underlying medical problems often place them at risk for delays in early recognition of infections. Elderly patients often do not mount a febrile response to infection, and their increasing agitation or confusion in response to an infection may be dismissed as a sign of old age. Immunization status of the elderly and other facility residents may not be up-to-date.

INFECTION CONTROL

Acute-care hospitals have organized infection control programs. The Joint Committee on Accreditation of Healthcare Organizations (JCAHO) mandates an active infection control program and an appointed infection control practitioner who surveys the institution for active cases of infection and documents the occurrence of nosocomial infections. The infection control practitioner is usually a nurse with advanced training in infection control practices and methods for tracking the source and spread of infections (epidemiologic studies). In addition, each department in the hospital must have written policies and procedures for the control of infection. The caregivers in individual departments as well as support personnel (e.g.,. housekeepers, transport personnel) must have periodic educational updates, usually on an annual basis, on infection control.

Several studies have demonstrated cost saving with good infection control (Beyt, Troxler, & Cavaness, 1985; Dixon, 1987). Approximately one third of nosocomial infections can be prevented with effective infection control programs. None of these studies begins to quantify the benefits of increased quality of life that result when infection is avoided.

Recognition of Factors

The essential first step in combating infections is to recognize situations, areas, procedures, and patients who present a high chance of producing infectious complications and, if possible, to make provisions to alter them.

Rates of nosocomial infections vary according to:

Type of hospital: tertiary care (referral hospitals) and large municipal teaching hospitals have higher rates of infection than smaller community hospitals.

Infection control programs: hospitals with organized, efficient surveillance programs have lower rates of infection.

Area of the hospital: intensive care units, premature nurseries, special care areas such as dialysis and transplant units are high-risk areas. The laboratory and central service are also high-risk areas.

Type of patient: patients who are very young or very old, the neutropenic patient, those with burns or trauma are among high-risk patients.

Documentation: how well a hospital documents the incidence of infection with adequate cultures and laboratory techniques impacts infection control.

Regulatory Agencies

Several agencies are involved in the control of institutional safety designed to protect the patient, staff, and community from infectious disease. Local, state, regional, provincial, and national groups require reporting of specific infections. Physician's offices, school nurses, health clinics, extended-care facilities, and various acute care facilities must report episodes of infection to these agencies. The agencies compile statistics on the incidence of the disease in the area and provide the practitioner with information on control and treatment.

Both the Centers of Disease Control (CDC) and JCAHO publish guidelines for storage, cleaning and disinfection, and use of equipment and supplies. JCAHO sets requirements to which hospitals must adhere to obtain accreditation. The CDC does basic research on infectious disease and conducts large multicenter studies on data gathered by local centers. *Morbidity and Mortality Weekly Report* from the CDC outlines statistics on infectious disease. The World Health Organization (WHO) receives information about communicable disease from all countries and compiles this information into periodic reports.

Infection Control Committee

The infection control program of the hospital, compelled by JCAHO regulations, requires the existence of an infection control committee. The committee is composed of members from various hospital departments: physicians, nurses, and personnel representing the laboratory, housekeeping, central supply, diagnostic imaging, and quality assurance officers. The committee annually reviews all policies and procedures of all hospital departments for current information on infection control. A person from the committee, usually a nurse, is appointed to be in charge of surveillance, analyzing, and reporting infectious diseases. This person is called the infection control practitioner or the hospital epidemiologist. This person gathers all data on the occurrence of infections in the hospital, reports required information to the local health department, and brings the information to the committee for review. The committee makes recommendations for changes in hospital policies, revises procedures as necessary, and reviews individual practitioner infection rates. In addition, the infection control nurse is often involved in employee education programs.

Reporting Infectious Disease

The infection control practitioner or hospital epidemiologist is responsible for reporting diseases to appropriate agencies as required by law. The guidelines as to what is a reportable disease vary from location to location and from time to time. These variations are based on differences in the occurrence of disease in various climates, the consequences of the disease in terms of morbidity and mortality, and interest about the results of current control efforts. Health departments can mandate how urgently the reports are needed. Each local board designates whether the report must be made by a "same day as discovery" phone call or by written report. Good communication and rapport between clinical agencies and regulatory agencies are necessary to optimize infection control and prevent severe outbreaks of infectious disease.

Employee Health

Millions of people work in hospitals and health-care agencies. Some hospitals have started personnel health service programs as part of their infection control program or employee benefit package. The objectives of the program include stressing maintenance of sound habits of personal hygiene, good health practices in diet, exercise, and rest, and individual responsibility in infection control; monitoring and investigating potentially harmful infectious exposures and outbreaks of infections among personnel; providing care to personnel for work-related illnesses or exposures; identifying the infection risks related to employment and instituting appropriate preventive measures; and containing costs by preventing infectious disease that results in absenteeism and disability (Williams, 1983).

Monitoring and Counseling of Personnel

When they become employed, people often have to provide an immunization and health history and undergo a screening physical examination. Laboratory testing may also be required. Almost all institutions require a personal health and safety education lecture as part of the orientation process and on an annual or semiannual basis. Some institutions require laboratory screening for high-risk diseases and offer their employees routine immunization programs. A mechanism for prompt diagnosis and management of job-related illnesses and provision for prophylaxis of preventable diseases is important to ensure health of all employees.

Access to health counseling about infections is especially important for women of childbearing age. Personnel who are or who might become pregnant need to know about potential risks to the fetus due to work assignments and about preventive measures that reduce

TABLE 22–2

Risk of Transmission to Fetus and Recommendations for Pregnant Employees' Interactions with Patients Having Communicable Infectious Diseases

Patient Disease	Period of Risk of Congenital Transmission	Employee Susceptibility*	Recommendations†
HIV	Unknown—most probably entire pregnancy	S	B
Chickenpox/zoster	High risk if rash appears within 7 days of delivery	S	A
Cytomegalovirus	Low risk of symptomatic disease transmission	S	B
Enterovirus	High risk of ECHO viruses at time of delivery, lower for coxsackie viruses	S	‡
Hepatitis B	High risk with third trimester infection of mother	I, S	B, C, D
Herpes simplex	Low risk; infection during delivery is more likely	S	C or A
Influenza	Low risk	S	A
Measles	Low risk	I, S	A, C
Mumps	Undefined	I, S	A, C
Rubella	Very high risk during first 3 months	I or S	A
Syphilis	High risk at any time during pregnancy	S	C
Toxoplasmosis	Highest in third trimester	S	C
Tuberculosis	Rare, insufficient data to quantify risk	S or I	A

* S, susceptible; I, immune.
† A. Do not enter patient's room.
B. No direct patient care.
C. Direct patient care using appropriate isolation precautions.
D. Seronegative pregnant women may wish to transfer out of a high-risk area for the duration of pregnancy.
‡ During third trimester follow recommendation B.
Adapted from Sherertz, R. J., & Hampton, A. L. (1987). In R. J. P. Wenzel (Ed.), *Hospital employee health. Prevention and control of nosocomial infection* (p. 193). Baltimore: Williams & Wilkins.

those risks. Pregnant nurses may not be allowed to care for patients who have diseases that pose risks to the unborn baby. Among the diseases that pose particular risk to the fetus if contracted by the mother are rubella, hepatitis B, cytomegalovirus, and AIDS. Table 22-2 summarizes infections that pose risk to pregnant employees and their implications for fetal transmission.

Transmissible Diseases

The CDC Committee on Infection Control in Hospital Personnel has divided infections that commonly occur in hospitals and are transmissible between patients and staff into two groups. Category I infections are transmitted both to and from personnel and patients. Category II infections are transmitted primarily from infected patients to personnel. CDC guidelines include preventive measures, diagnostic and epidemiologic methods, and recommendations for prophylaxis after exposure, as well as guidelines for work restriction because of illness (Williams, 1983). Table 22-3 lists some infectious processes and their relative risk of transmission between patients and personnel.

Because hospital personnel are at risk of contracting and transmitting vaccine-preventable diseases, maintaining current immunization status is a good health practice. Employees who work in high-risk areas, such as pediatric wards, dialysis units, or transplant units, can be required to prove their immunization currency as a condition of employment. Chapter 26 contains a list of available vaccines and their effectiveness. The cost of vaccination may be borne by the institution or by the employee, depending on individual personnel policies and benefits (Castle & Ajemian, 1987).

Significant Exposure

Institutional policies and employee restrictions are designed to prevent exposure to and contracting of an infectious disease. A "significant" exposure is investigated to protect the employee, the patient, and the institution. Many institutions carry their own employee insurance and, both for humanitarian and economic reasons, they must protect their employees. The significance of an exposure is determined by the type and duration of exposure, with consideration of the mode of

TABLE 22–3

Risk of Infection Transmission between Patients and Hospital Personnel*

Disease	Transmission Route	
	Patient to employee	*Employee to patient*
HIV	?	?
Chickenpox/disseminated zoster (shingles)	High	High
Conjunctivitis/viral	High	High
Cytomegalovirus	Low	?
Hepatitis A	Low	Rare
Hepatitis B†	Low	Rare
Hepatitis non-A, non-B	Low	?
Herpes simplex‡	Low	Rare
Influenza	Intermediate	Intermediate
Measles	High	High
Meningococcal infection	Rare	?
Mumps	Intermediate	Intermediate
Pertussis	Intermediate	Intermediate
Respiratory syncytial virus	Intermediate	Intermediate
Rotavirus (viral gastroenteritis)	Intermediate	Intermediate
Rubella	Intermediate	Intermediate
Salmonella/Shigella	Low	Low
Scabies	Low	Low
Staphylococcus aureus	?	Rare
Streptococcus, group A	?	Rare
Syphilis	Low	?
Tuberculosis§	Low to high	Low to high

* Even though the risk of transmission may not be considered high for all patient populations, the consequences to the patient or to the staff member may be high.
† Proof of immunity may be required as a condition of employment in some special care areas, such as dialysis units, to protect the employee.
‡ Some institutions require relief from work in special care units, such as the operating room, nursery and delivery rooms, burn units, and transplant units.
§ Proof of freedom from an active disease is a legal requirement in most states as a condition of employment.
? Insufficient data available to comment.
Adapted from Shererty, R. J., & Hampton, A. L. (1987). In R. J. Wenzel (Ed.), *Hospital employee health. Prevention and control of nosocomial infections* (p. 179). Baltimore: Williams & Wilkins.

transmission, whether the host was susceptible, and whether precautions were taken. Exposures to hepatitis, rubella, meningococcal meningitis, tuberculosis, varicella (chickenpox), and AIDS are commonly investigated by the infection control nurse. Most exposure requires a timely reporting, by way of an incident report, by staff members to expedite prophylaxis (if any is available) and to qualify for labor and industry insurance coverage if an illness results (Castle & Ajemian, 1987; Williams & Garner, 1986). If an employee contracts an infectious disease, it must be reported to the local health department.

Needlesticks. One of the most frequently occurring, potentially serious exposures to disease for health-care personnel is from needlestick injuries that may carry organisms that cause bloodborne diseases, such as hepatitis or AIDS. Accidental needlesticks account for nearly one third of all health-care accidents. In 1987 there were 800,000 reported needlestick injuries resulting in an expense of millions of dollars for accident work-ups alone. Liability and treatment for infected personnel drove the costs into the billions of dollars for employers and insurers (Baxter, 1988). Every year, 100 to 200 health-care workers die from hepatitis B.

Approximately 40% of all needlestick injuries result from recapping needles after their contact with blood from a patient (e.g., after an injection, drawing blood, or starting an IV). In the past, used needles were recapped or bent or broken after use to prevent accidental contamination by housekeeping personnel. The CDC strongly advises all institutions to educate their employees as to the dangers of these practices (Fig. 22-4). Puncture-proof, plastic units (Fig. 22-5) into which needles can be safely deposited (uncapped) immediately after their use are provided in all patient care areas (News-AJN, 1988).

Gloves. The use of clean gloves for starting and discontinuing all intravenous catheters, drawing blood specimens, suctioning, emptying urinary drainage bags, or dealing with any high-risk body fluid must become a standard of practice for all personnel. Gloves cannot protect all personnel in every situation, but increased use of gloves for contact with all mucous membranes, nonintact skin, and moist body substances, in combination with good handwashing practices makes a difference in cross-contamination between patients and staff.

Work Restriction

An ill health-care employee should not be in contact with patients if that illness poses a threat to the patient or other personnel. Caregivers with diseases characterized by profuse coughing, sneezing, or frequent diarrhea should probably stay home from work and care for themselves. Hospitals should have well-defined policies directed at restricting or limiting work for personnel with a potentially transmissible disease. See Table 22-4 for a list of conditions requiring relief from direct patient contact or partial work restriction.

Health-Care Worker with AIDS. Personnel considered to have any of the clinical features associated with the AIDS spectrum should be counseled about the risks they pose to patients and to themselves in the work environment. There is no evidence that any health-care worker infected with the AIDS virus has transmitted the infection to a patient; however, there is potential risk. Health-care workers who perform invasive procedures in which a needlestick or scalpel injury would provide

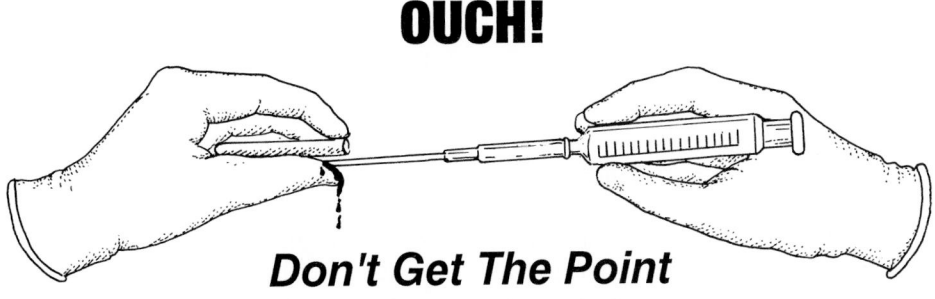

Figure 22-4. Sample needlestick hazard poster.

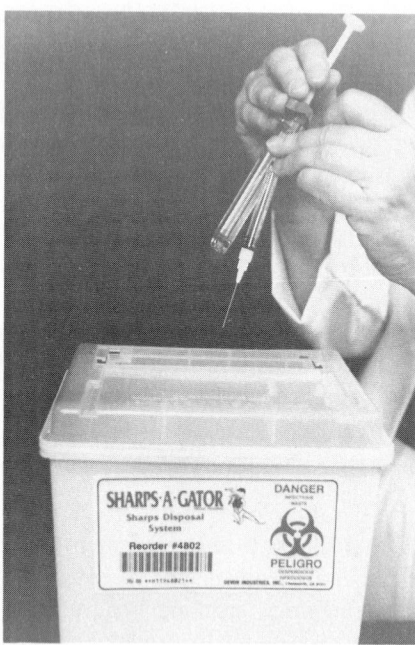

Figure 22–5. Disposal container for contaminated sharps.

exposure of their blood to that of the patient's pose the greatest risk. All personnel with AIDS should wear gloves for direct contact with mucous membranes or nonintact skin of all patients. Any health-care worker with AIDS and exudative lesions or weeping dermatitis should refrain from all direct care and handling patient care equipment until the lesions clear (CDC, 1988a).

The AIDS virus impairs the immune system, making people with the AIDS virus more likely to acquire infectious diseases or experience more serious complications. These staff members should be counseled about potential risks to themselves and may be prohibited from working in acute care settings by individual institutions.

Waste Disposal

Health-care facilities produce tons of waste daily. Several regulatory agencies are involved in identifying and directing acceptable practices for collecting, transporting, and disposing of wastes. Rules and regulations are set by the JCAHO, the Department of Social and Health Services (DSHS), the Environmental Protection Agency (EPA), the Occupational Safety and Health Administration (OSHA), and local health departments. All these agencies have partial jurisdiction over waste disposal.

Local health agencies and the JCAHO require hospitals to develop programs to dispose of wastes categorized as infectious, injurious, or hazardous to employees, patients, visitors, the general public, and the environment. Table 22-5 lists common materials within each category of institutional waste for which proper waste disposal

protocol must be followed. Hazardous waste from health-care facilities comes from radiology, the laboratory, and pharmacy, in addition to nursing units. Most of the waste produced by hospitals is not infectious, injurious, or hazardous. Safe waste includes paper, plastic, metal, or glass products used for a multitude of purposes within the health-care agency.

There is a great deal of controversy about hospital waste products, much of it caused by the public's fear of the AIDS virus. The CDC has maintained that hospital waste in general is no more infective than residential waste. There is no current evidence that hospital waste has contributed to disease in the community (CDC, 1987); however, public concerns about the disposal of hypodermic syringes, blood, and fecal material have provoked board of health reviews of institutional policies. It is to be anticipated that there will be more consistent and rigid regulations in the future. Current CDC recommendations are for incineration or autoclaving of infective waste before disposing in a sanitary landfill. Liquid body fluids (blood, urine, aspirated body fluids) can be flushed down a drain connected to a sewer system. This practice has been questioned recently by the media and some political bodies.

Another public health concern is the use of disposable diapers for infants and geriatric patients. Although most commercial packages advise rinsing the diaper in the toilet before disposal into garbage containers, it is known that there is little institutional or residential compliance with this advice. The result is millions of tons of carefully wrapped feces lying in sanitary landfills in non-biodegradable plastic.

Studies continue to assess the potential health risks of medical wastes, and new regulations will emerge. The staff member who handles this waste conscientiously at the bedside by bagging and labeling all waste and who transports it to the proper receptacle in the dirty utility room saves others from potential harm and contributes to controlling the considerable cost involved in waste disposal.

ASEPTIC PRACTICES

Aseptic practices are those techniques used to keep objects or people free from microorganisms. The dramatic reduction in the incidence of disease that occurred during the late 1800s and early 1900s was largely due to understanding that microorganisms caused disease and that these organisms could be controlled. The established control methods include: physical agents, such as disinfectants, which are used on agents outside the body; chemical agents, such as antiseptics, which are used on inanimate objects as well as on the body surface; and chemotherapeutic agents, such as antibiotics, which are used to combat microorganisms on body surfaces and inside the body.

TABLE 22–4

Infectious Conditions Requiring Work Restriction

Condition	Infection	Duration of Restriction
Skin lesions that are infected or draining	Impetigo Infected sebaceous cysts Boils Hangnails	Until lesions resolve
Purulent discharges	Sinusitis Conjunctivitis Pharyngitis	Until discharge ceases

Gastroenteritis	Causing:
	    Diarrhea
	    Vomiting
		Until stool is formed

Upper respiratory tract infections	Accompanied by:
	    Fever
	    Purulent sputum
		Until acute symptoms resolve

Diagnosed communicable disease	Chickenpox	Until all lesions dry and crust
	Hepatitis	Until antigenemia resolves
	Measles	Until 7 days after the rash appears
	Mumps	Until 9 days after onset of parotitis
	Pertussis	From the beginning of the catarrhal stage until 7 days after start of therapy
	Rubella	Until 5 days after the rash appears
	Shingles	Until lesions dry and crust
	Tuberculosis	Until sputum shows no growth on smears. Approximately 2 weeks after start of therapy

Herpes simplex	With open lesions excluded from:
	    Nursery
	    Delivery room
	    Operating room
	    Burn units
	    Transplant unit
	    Oncology unit
		Until lesions heal

Data from Williams, W. W., & Garner, J. S. (1987). In J. V. Bennett & P. S. Brockman (Eds.), *Personnel health services hospital infections* (2nd ed). Boston: Little, Brown and Williams, W. W. (1983). Guideline for infection control in hospital personnel: CDC guidelines. *Infection Control, 4*(4), 326–349.

Categories of Asepsis

The two major categories of aseptic practice are medical asepsis and surgical asepsis. Nurses practice these techniques to ensure patient safety and comfort and to prevent the spread of infection.

Medical Asepsis

Medical asepsis refers to measures taken to control and reduce the number of pathogenic organisms present. It is also known as "clean technique." Aseptic measures used to prevent the spread of organisms from place to place include handwashing, gloving, gowning, and disinfecting to help contain microbial growth.

Surgical Asepsis

Surgical asepsis refers to "sterile technique." To be sterile, an object must be free of all microorganisms. Sterile technique is used to prevent the introduction or spread of pathogens from the environment into the patient. Sterile technique is employed when a body cavity is entered with an object that may damage the mucous membranes, when surgical procedures are performed, and when the patient's immune system is already compromised. Procedures that require sterile technique include insertion of intravenous catheters, giving injections, urinary catheterization, dressing changes, irrigation of drainage tubes that enter sterile parts of the body, and all operative procedures.

Patients whose immune systems are compromised may require the use of sterile technique and supplies more than patients with adequate host defenses. Premature infants, burn patients, transplant recipients, and patients receiving chemotherapy or radiation are examples of groups for whom sterile technique may be employed more frequently. Asepsis, regardless of type, begins and ends with effective handwashing.

TABLE 22–5
Categories of Institutional Waste

Infectious Waste	Injurious Waste	Hazardous Waste
Blood and blood products	Needles	Radioactive materials
Pathology laboratory specimens	Scalpel blades	Chemotherapy solutions and their containers
Laboratory cultures	Lancets	Caustic chemicals
Body parts from surgery	Broken glass	
Contaminated equipment (e.g., dialysis materials and suction receptacles)	Pipettes	
	Aerosol cans	
Food		
Infant and adult diapers—unrinsed		

Handwashing

Even with the new emphasis on gloving for contact with patient secretions, nothing is more effective in preventing the spread of infections than handwashing. It is also the least expensive method of decreasing the risk of infecting one's self or others.

Contact transmission is the most common form of contamination in patient care. Contact is often from the hands of personnel or the patients themselves. Hospitals have high concentrations of virulent pathogens. Any patient contact poses the risk of contamination of the caregiver's hands with microorganisms that become transient flora until the hands are washed. Caregiver's hands are common vehicles for transfer of pathogens from patient to patient, from contaminated articles to patients, and from their own body flora. Experts say that proper handwashing can reduce nosocomial infection rates by 50%, yet studies have demonstrated that handwashing is the least practiced infection control measure in hospitals (Castle & Ajemian, 1987).

Equipment necessary for handwashing (soap, running water, and paper towels) is inexpensive and should be readily available to all health-care providers. High-risk areas, such as the nursery, critical care, transplant or burn units, and operative suites, may also require the use of antiseptic cleansing agents, nail files or sticks, and antiseptic-impregnated scrub brushes.

Hands should be washed before and after every patient care contact. The use of gloves during patient care does not eliminate the need for handwashing. Hands should be washed in the following situations:

- At the beginning and end of shift of work
- Before contact with a patient
- Between contact with different patients
- Before and after contact with wounds, dressings, specimens, or bedclothes
- Before performing any invasive procedures
- Before administering medications
- After contact with any patient secretion or excretion
- Before and after using the bathroom or blowing nose

Medical and surgical asepsis vary in the technique for proper handwashing. Handwashing for surgical asepsis is longer and more methodic, and often special antimicrobial agents may be used. These variations are usually defined by institutional protocols. During a surgical scrub of the hands, the hands are held higher than the elbows to avoid contamination from water running back from the forearms to the hands. This is not required when the handwashing is done to ensure medical asepsis (Procedure 22-1). Antiseptics should be used during surgical scrubs, before invasive procedures, and routinely in some high-risk areas. Studies have demonstrated that effectiveness of handwashing is determined by adequate friction, thoroughness of surfaces cleansed, and minimum duration of use, rather than the particular cleansing agent employed (Larson, 1987).

Most long-term flora on the hands reside in the nailbed and under the fingernails. Special attention is required for these areas, and soft sticks or fingernails from the opposite hand may be used to clean them. Fingernails should be kept short, and nail polish should be avoided because cracked or chipped nail polish can harbor bacteria that cannot be reached by ordinary handwashing. Artificial fingernails present a similar reservoir for infectious agents. Ideally, rings should be removed before handwashing and placed in pockets or pinned to the uniform during patient care so that potential places harboring bacteria can be minimized. Nurses who wear a thin wedding band may slide it up on the finger so the area under the ring can be properly cleansed.

If hands become dry or cracked or develop dermatitis, the caregiver is less apt to wash the hands as often as necessary. This is a frequent complication for people with sensitive skin. Switching to another soap or antiseptic solution, thorough drying after every washing, and using skin lotion may help. Gloves should be worn during patient care when the nurse's skin is abraded.

Handwashing technique should be learned by all caregivers, the patient, and their family members. Patients should be provided with materials to wash their hands

PROCEDURE 22–1. Handwashing

■ Purpose
1. Reduce the numbers of resident and transient bacteria from the hands.
2. Prevent transfer of microorganisms from the hospital environment to the patient and from the patient to hospital personnel.

■ Assessment
- Inspect hands for breaks or cuts in skin or cuticles.
- Identify appropriate times for handwashing before and after patient contact.
- Identify need to repeat handwashing if hands become contaminated during a procedure.

■ Equipment
Warm, running water
Soap. Most hospitals supply liquid soaps, containing a germicidal agent, in dispensers at each sink.
Paper towels.

■ Procedure
1. Remove all rings except a plain wedding band. Push watch 4 to 5 inches above wrist.
   Rationale: Microorganisms lodge in the irregular surfaces of jewelry.
2. File nails short. Refrain from wearing nail polish or fake fingernails.
   Rationale: Microorganisms harbor under long nails, which are hard to clean. Microorganisms may hide in cracked nail polish crevices or along adhesive edges of paste on nails.
3. Turn on the water and adjust temperature to warm. Do not splash water or lean against the wet sink.
   Note: Faucets may be controlled by your hands or may be operated by knee levers or foot pedals.
   Rationale: Warm water removes less protective oils from the skin than hot water and reduces chapping of hands from frequent handwashing. Microorganisms need moisture to thrive. Avoid water splashing and sink contact on clothing to prevent contamination of uniform.
4. Hold hands lower than elbows and thoroughly wet hands and lower arms under running water.
   Rationale: Hands are more contaminated than lower arms; water should flow from least to most contaminated areas.
5. Apply soap. If bar soap is used, rinse bar before lathering and rinse bar again before returning it to the dish.
   Rationale: To reduce the number of surface bacteria present on the soap bar.

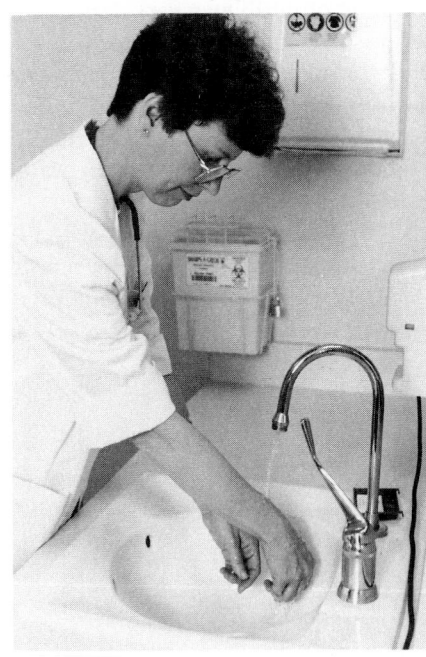

Step 4

6. Rub palms, wrists, and back of hands firmly with circular movements. Interlace fingers and thumbs, moving hands back and forth. Continue using plenty of lather and friction for 15 to 30 seconds on each hand.

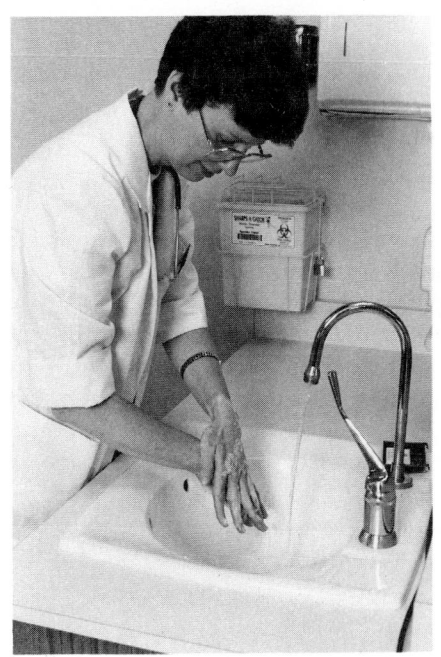

Step 6

(continued)

PROCEDURE 22–1. Handwashing *(continued)*

Note: Timing of scrub may vary depending on purpose of wash.
Rationale: Mechanically loosens and removes dirt and microorganisms on all hand surfaces.

7. Clean under fingernails using fingernails of other hand and additional soap. Use orangewood stick if available.

8. Rinse hands and wrists thoroughly with hands held lower than forearms.
Rationale: Washes away microorganisms and dirt and prevents recontamination of clean skin surfaces.

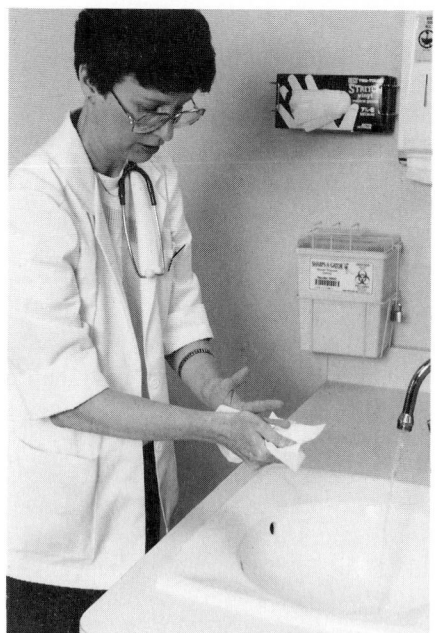

Step 9

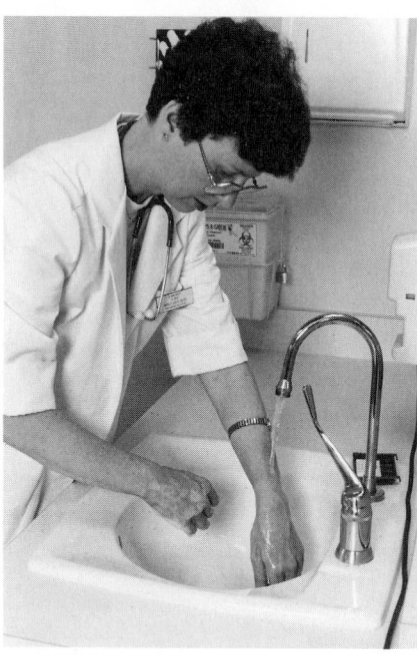

Step 8

9. Dry hands and arms thoroughly with paper towel, wiping from fingertips toward forearm. Discard in proper receptacle.
Rationale: Drying hands prevents chapping and cracking of skin. Dry from cleanest area (fingertips) toward least clean to reduce chances of contamination.

10. Turn off water using clean, dry paper towel on faucets.
Rationale: Prevents transfer of microorganisms from faucet to hands.

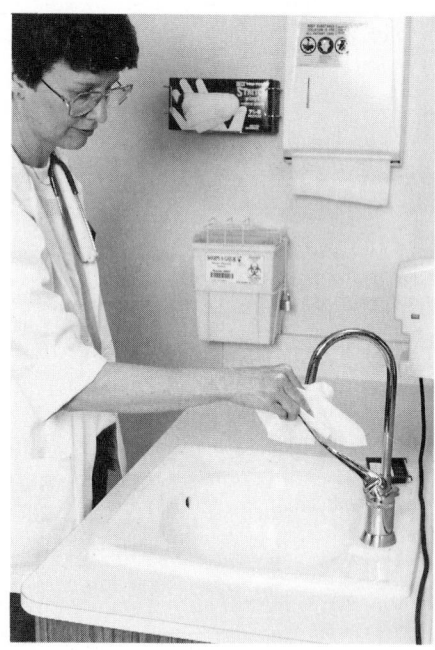

Step 10

■ **Home-Care Modifications**

• Visiting nurse should bring to patient's home bactericidal soap in a plastic container and paper towels.

• If running water is unavailable, disposable washcloths or alcohol may be used as an alternative to handwashing. Both these agents are drying to the hands if used often.

after toileting, and all visitors should be instructed to wash their hands before contact with the patient and before leaving the patient's room. The paramount importance of adequate handwashing cannot be stressed too often, no matter how unsophisticated it may seem, if caregivers desire to control infection.

Cleaning, Disinfection, and Sterilization

The methods used to control microorganisms include physical methods, chemical methods, and chemotherapeutic agents. Physical methods for controlling microorganisms include cleaning by scrubbing surfaces, the use of heat and cold to exceed the growth temperature of the organism, and the use of ultraviolet light, ionizing radiation, or ultrasound vibration. Chemical methods use solutions in various strengths to kill the organisms or prevent their growth and multiplication. Chemotherapeutic agents, such as antibiotics, also kill or retard the growth of pathogens after their administration.

A chemical used on lifeless objects is called a *disinfectant*. If the object is living, the chemical is called an antiseptic. Solutions that are disinfectants at higher concentrations may be diluted to be used as antiseptics on living objects. A chemical is **bactericidal** if it kills microorganisms; an agent that prevents bacterial multiplication but does not kill all forms of the organism is called **bacteriostatic.**

The method used for a particular procedure depends on characteristics of the object and the organism. To be useful, the method chosen must kill or retard growth of the pathogens without damaging the material or person being treated. Additional factors in method selection include the amount of time required to kill the organism and the stability of the agent being used.

Cleaning

Cleaning refers to the physical removal of visible dirt and debris by washing, dusting, or mopping surfaces that are contaminated. Soap is used for mechanical cleaning. It is manufactured from fats and chemicals that cause it to form a lather that emulsifies fats and lifts off dirt and other materials that can be rinsed away.

Contamination refers to an unclean condition where microorganisms are actually or potentially present. *Decontamination* refers to the removal of potentially pathogenic microorganisms using a process that makes the item safe to handle before other procedures are performed. Cleaning precedes disinfection and sterilization.

After patient discharge, all patient rooms should be cleaned as though the patient were infected. Furniture and floors should be cleaned with a disinfectant detergent. Walls, blinds, and curtains should be washed if they are visibly soiled. Disinfectant fogging is no longer

recommended. Terminal cleaning of patient rooms should also be directed toward all items that were in direct contact with the patient. All nondisposable items (urinals, bedpans, thermometer holders, and so forth) should be bagged, labeled, and sent for decontamination. All disposable items should be discarded even if unopened (Lynch & Cummings, 1987).

Disinfection

Disinfection refers to the processes used to reduce the numbers of microorganisms that are potential pathogens from the surface of an object, usually by chemical or physical means. These processes do not necessarily remove all potential of infection because spores may remain that are capable of growing at a later time. Agents used in chemical disinfection are registered and regulated by the EPA. Until 1982 they also tested new products, but for budgetary reasons have discontinued that practice. Chemical disinfectants used in the healthcare setting include alcohol, chlorine and chlorine compounds, formaldehyde, glutaraldehyde, and hydrogen peroxide. **Antiseptics** are used to retard bacterial growth on living organisms. Most commonly antiseptics are used for handwashing, as skin preparation before invasive procedures, and to pack or irrigate wounds. Antiseptics used commonly for skin and wound care include povidone-iodine, sodium hypochlorite (Dakins), chlorhexidine gluconate (Hibiclens), acetic acid, hydrogen peroxide, and alcohol. Table 22-6 lists common disinfectants and antiseptics along with their common uses. The CDC has published information on the use of these chemicals in relation to objects and humans and the desired level of disinfection for their use (Simmons, 1983).

Sterilization

Sterilization is the complete destruction of all microorganisms, leaving no viable forms of organisms including spores. Sterilization processes are caustic because they require extremes of heat, potent chemicals, or gas that cannot be used on body tissues. Any process used to sterilize equipment must be effective in killing organisms, but not destructive to the equipment.

The two most popular methods are steam sterilization and gas sterilization with ethylene oxide.

Steam Sterilization. Supersaturated steam under pressure is the most widely used and dependable method of sterilization. It is nontoxic, inexpensive, and sporicidal, and it rapidly penetrates fabrics. Moist heat destroys microorganisms by the irreversible coagulation and denaturation of enzymes and structural proteins. Chemical indicators, which change color when the object being steriled has been exposed to steam penetration for a specific period of time, are placed on the outside and inside of their package. This enables the health-care worker to know when sterilization of an object has been effective.

Gas Sterilization. Ethylene oxide is used to sterilize medical products that cannot be steam sterilized. It is a colorless gas that can penetrate plastic, rubber, cotton, and other substances. Articles must be left to release the gas through aeration before they are used. Liquids may not be sterilized using this process because ethylene oxide is absorbed and not released. The main disadvantages of this type of sterilization are expense and the required length of time (2 to 5 hours).

Other sterilization methods include dry heat, which is used on products such a sharp instruments or petroleum products, which can be damaged by moist heat. Ionizing radiation by electron accelerators and gamma rays is used on several medical products including tissue for transplantation, drugs, and pharmaceuticals. Microwave ovens are under study for use in hospital sterilization processes (Castle & Ajemian, 1987; Rutala, 1987).

Levels of Disinfection and Sterilization

There are different levels of disinfection of body sites and of equipment used for patient treatment. Hospital policies identify whether cleaning, disinfection, or steril-ization is indicated based on an item's intended use and on other factors such as cost and the area in the hospital where the item is to be used. Many equipment items used in patient care have the potential of harboring microorganisms that cause disease. It is impractical and unnecessary to sterilize all such items. Items can be grouped in categories to help identify proper methods of disinfection or sterilization. Modifications may be necessary in any of the categories when these items are to be used for high-risk patients.

Any item entering sterile tissues or the vascular system must be sterile. This category would include surgical instruments, cardiac and urinary catheters, implants, intravenous fluids, and needles. Most of these items are purchased as sterile or are sterilized by autoclaving. If the items could be destroyed by heat used during auto-claving, ethylene oxide gas or chemical solutions may be used.

Any item that may come in contact with mucous membranes or skin that is not intact must be free of all microorganisms with the exception of spores. Intact mucous membranes are generally resistant to bacterial spores but are susceptible to viruses and tubercle bacilli. Respiratory therapy and anesthesia equipment, thermometers, and gastrointestinal endoscopes are included in this category. These items can be disinfected with high-level disinfectants. It is usually necessary to rinse

---

TABLE 22–6
Common Disinfectants and Antiseptics

Agent	Kills	Uses
Disinfectants		
Alcohol	Bacteria, not spores, virus, fungi	Thermometers, endoscopes, medication vials
Chlorine	Most microbes	Countertops and floors
Formaldehyde (formalin)	Bacteria, spores, fungi, virus	Hemodialysis units
Glutaraldehyde	Bacteria	Endoscopes, anesthesia and respiratory equipment
Antiseptics		
Povidone-iodine	Bacteria	Skin decontamination, wound packing, and irrigation
Sodium hypochlorite (Dakin's)	Bacteria, yeasts	Wound irrigation and packing
Chlorhexidine gluconate (Hibiclens)	Gram-positive organisms	Skin scrubs and irrigation
Acetic acid	*Pseudomonas*	Cleaning, packing, irrigating wounds
Hydrogen peroxide (3%)	Decomposes necrotic tissue	Irrigates wounds, cleans pus and necrotic tissue
Alcohol	Bacteria	Skin prep before injections
Hexachlorophene	Bacteria	Handwashing, skin prep; wash off to avoid neurotoxicity

items thoroughly to decontaminate them before they are disinfected; after disinfection, they are dried and wrapped to prevent dust exposure.

Because intact skin is an effective barrier to most microorganisms, items that come in contact with intact skin need not be sterile. Items such as bedpans, blood pressure cuffs, linens, bedside tables, and room furniture can be cleaned and reused.

Factors Affecting Disinfection and Sterilization Effectiveness

Many factors can affect the effectiveness of disinfection and sterilization. Thorough cleansing of objects used on patients is the most important requirement for sterilization and disinfection to be successful. Organic matter contained in blood, pus, or fecal material coagulated on the surface of an object may interfere with antimicrobial activity by acting as a physical barrier.

The number and location of microorganisms affect the length of time it takes to destroy them; the larger the number of microorganisms, the longer it takes. The item must have all surfaces exposed to the disinfecting agent. This may require disassembly of equipment so that all cracks and crevices are exposed and so total immersion in a solution is possible.

Varying resistance of microorganisms occurs because of properties of the organisms themselves. The strategy chosen must aim to kill the most resistant form of the organism. For example, to kill bacterial spores, a higher concentration of solution and a longer period of exposure may be necessary.

Various methods are used to produce sterile conditions on instruments and equipment used in patient care. Boiling, soaking, baking, and steaming were traditional methods and are still useful for home care. With the development of plastic and rubber products and the use of high technology instruments, more objects need to be protected from destruction by moisture or heat. Chemical, gas, or ultraviolet methods are more common in the disinfection and sterilization of many modern products. Both the concentration of the agent and exposure time are critical factors in ensuring adequate treatment, so manufacturers' guidelines must be followed.

Use of Barriers

The techniques used to prevent the transfer of pathogens from one person to another are forms of isolating the host from microorganisms. These methods are referred to as barrier nursing. Its aim is to contain pathogens by establishing aseptic barriers around the patient and personnel. The most commonly used barriers are masks, gowns, gloves, private rooms, waterproof disposal bags for linen and trash, labeling and bagging of contaminated equipment and specimens, and control of airflow into sterile areas and out of contaminated areas. With the advent of AIDS, goggles have been added to the list, as well as check valves on masks used in mouth-to-mouth resuscitation. The most important aspect of barrier methods is the awareness of the staff about the need to prevent cross-contamination of people, equipment, and supplies.

Some research facilities are testing the effectiveness of laminar flow units, which totally isolate immune-suppressed patients from the environment. Plastic curtains are assembled in a box around a patient's bed and connected to a system that filters the air entering the enclosed space. Ports with sleeves for covering the caregivers' arms are built into the sides of the unit.

Masks

Masks prevent transmission of infectious agents through the air. Masks protect the wearer from inhaling large-particle droplets that are transmitted by close contact and generally travel only a short distance (up to 3 ft) and small-particle droplets that remain suspended in air and may travel further. Masks lose their effectiveness when they are wet or worn for long periods of time. They also are ineffective when they are not changed after caring for each patient.

Gowns, Caps, and Shoe Coverings

Gowns should be worn when the caregiver's clothing is likely to be soiled by infected material. Gowns should be changed when they become moist and should be worn only once and discarded. Caps are used to cover the hair, and special covers are available for shoes. New products are being developed to be used in high-risk areas (e.g., labor and delivery, emergency room) to shield body parts from accidental exposure to contaminated body secretions (Procedure 22-2).

Gloves

Gloves protect personnel from acquiring infected organisms on their hands. They also reduce the likelihood that personnel will transmit their own or other patients' microbial flora from their hands to another patient. Gloves are a major barrier to contact transmission when they are changed between patients, and when hands are washed and dried before and after gloving. Clean, nonsterile gloves should be worn when direct contact with moist body substances from any patient is anticipated. Gloves should be changed between patients or when they become torn or grossly soiled. Gloves should not be washed and reused.

Private Rooms

Separation of patients into private rooms decreases the chance of transmission of infection by all routes. Airborne infections always require private rooms. Patients

(Text continues on page 448)

PROCEDURE 22–2. Donning and Removing a Mask and Gown

■ **Purpose**
1. Prevent spread of microorganisms from the nurse to the patient.
2. Prevent contamination of the nurse's clothing from the patient.

■ **Assessment**
• Identify when gowning or masking is appropriate.
• Examine uniform for obvious soiling.

■ **Equipment**
Clean, dry gown and mask. Gowns are to be used once and discarded for laundry or disposal.

■ **Procedure**

Donning Mask
1. Wash hands.
   Rationale: Prevents spread of microorganisms.
2. If required, position mask over mouth and nose. Bend nose bar over bridge of nose. Secure strings or elastic.
   Note: Mask should never be allowed to hang around neck. Mask should be changed if used longer than 30 minutes because effectiveness is dramatically reduced after that time.

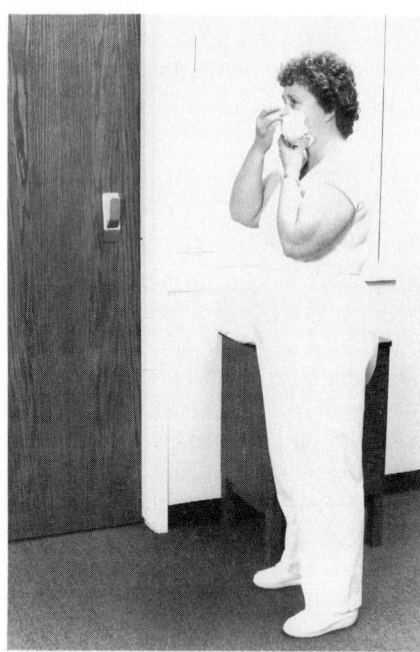

Step 2A

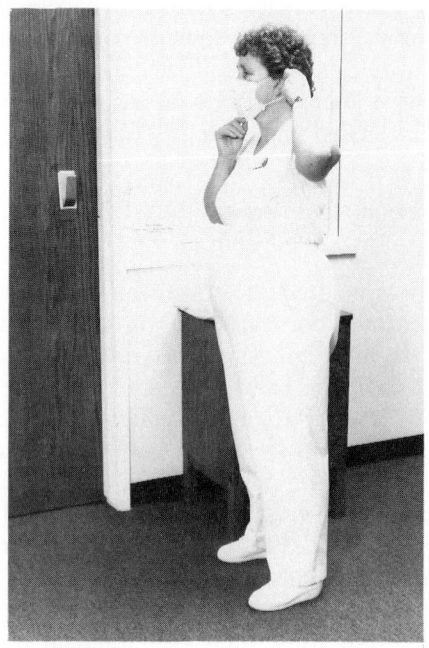

Step 2B

■ **Procedure**

Donning Clean Gown
1. Grasp gown by collar allowing it to unfold.
2. Place arms through sleeve and pull gown over shoulders.
3. Fasten neck ties. Overlap the gown at the back and fasten waist ties.
   Rationale: Overlapping back ensures uniform is completely covered at the back.

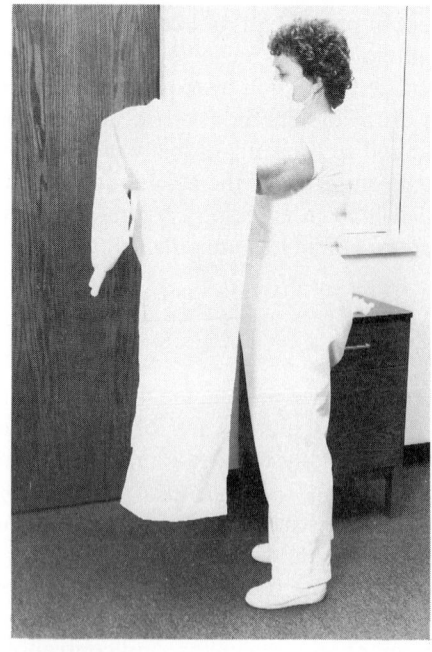

Step 2A

(continued)

PROCEDURE 22–2. Donning and Removing a Mask and Gown *(continued)*

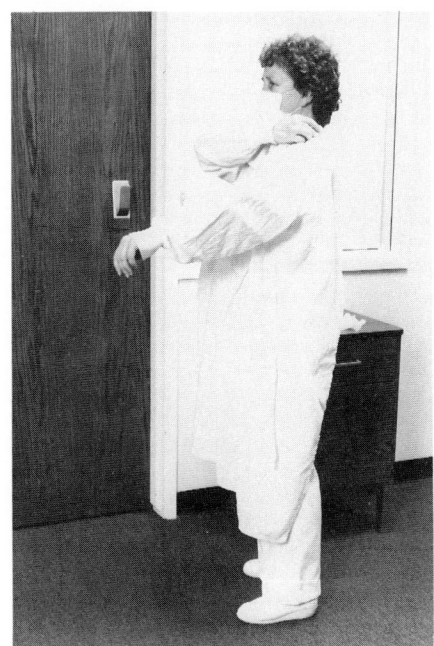

Step 2B

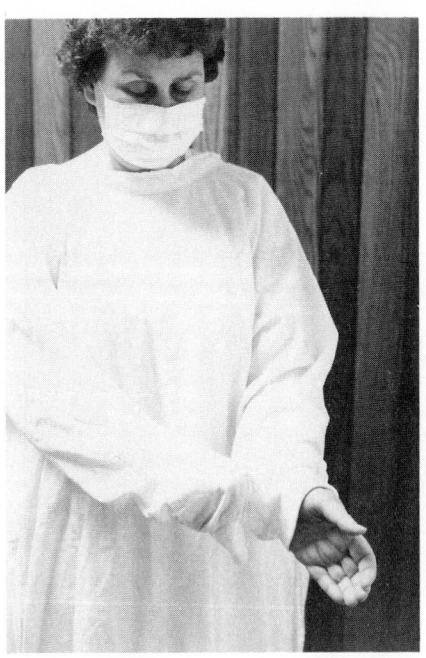

Step 4A

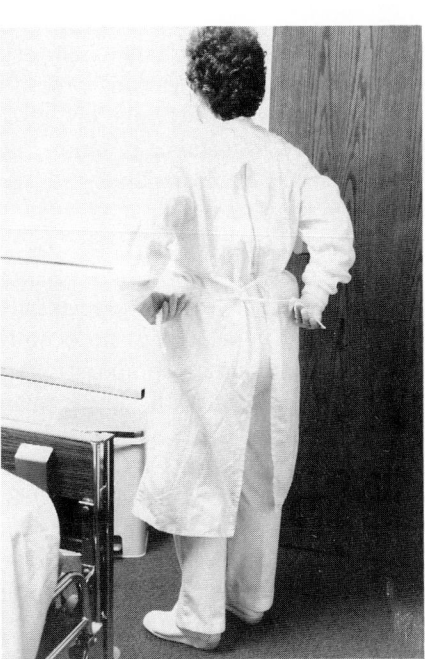

Step 3

■ **Procedure**

Removing Contaminated Gown
1. Untie waist ties and let hang freely.
2. Wash hands.
3. Untie neck ties and let gown fall forward off shoulder.

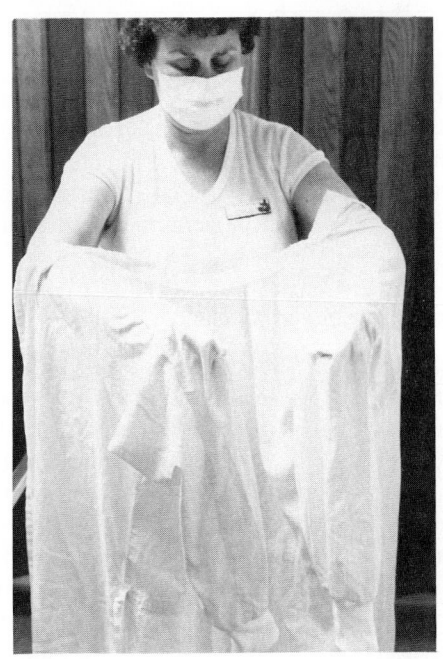

Step 4B

4. Slide arms out of gown working from the inside.
5. Holding gown away from your body, fold contaminated side of gown toward the inside.
   Rationale: Turning gown inside out reduces spread of microorganisms and protects uniform from contamination.

(continued)

PROCEDURE 22–2. Donning and Removing a Mask and Gown (continued)

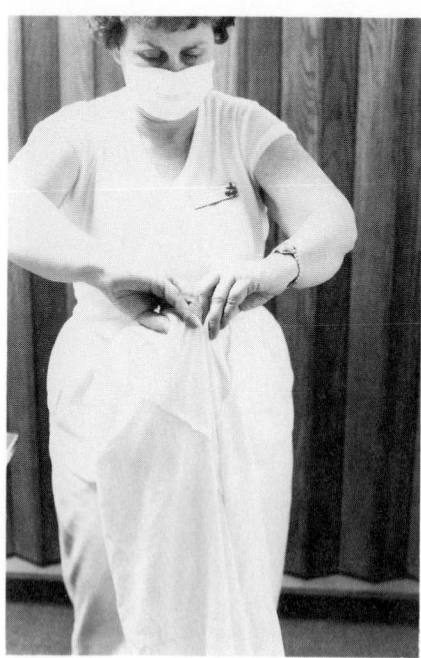

Step 5

6. Discard in appropriate receptacle.
7. Remove and discard mask.
8. Wash hands.

with poor hygienic habits or those who are incontinent should be placed in private rooms. High-risk groups include children under the age of 5, patients with altered mental status, and patients with large draining wounds or blood loss that cannot be contained in dressings.

Equipment and Refuse Handling

Special handling of articles and linen soiled by all bodily fluids is indicated. These articles should be placed in impervious bags before they are removed from the patient's bedside. Bagging in watertight containers is indicated to prevent exposure of personnel and to prevent contamination of the environment. The outside of the bag should not be contaminated when placing the articles inside it. Each hospital has procedures for labeling and decontaminating exposed articles. Items visibly soiled with body substances should be rinsed and placed in plastic bags or clearly marked containers in dirty utility rooms before returning them to the central processing areas.

Isolation Systems

Isolation means to place a patient apart from others to prevent the spread or contraction of infection. Isolation procedures have been used in some form for centuries.

Protective isolation is used to protect a high-risk person from exposure to pathogens. Various precaution systems, namely, category-specific isolation, disease-specific isolation, and body-substance isolation, have been developed to prevent the transmission of pathogens from an infected person to others.

The first two manuals published by the CDC, entitled *Isolation Techniques for Use in Hospitals*, recommended only the category-specific isolation precaution system. In the 1980s, increased episodes of nosocomial infections (especially among immunocompromised patients) and the AIDS epidemic fostered the development of two new systems, disease-specific isolation and body-substance isolation. In addition, the CDC called for universal blood and body-fluid precautions in 1988 (CDC, 1988a).

Body-substance isolation and universal precautions recommended by the CDC direct health-care providers to protect themselves and others from potential exposure to infectious agents by considering all patients as potentially infected. **Universal precautions** involve the application of precautions to blood and all body fluids containing traces of blood from all patients regardless of patient diagnosis. Universal precautions are intended to protect providers from bloodborne pathogens, whereas body-substance precautions apply to all infectious agents whatever their mode of transmission (e.g., contact, airborne, or vehicleborne). The CDC recommends universal precautions for blood and body fluids of all

Universal Precautions

Prevention of Transmission of HIV, HBV, and Other Bloodborne Pathogens in Health-Care Settings

Under universal precautions, blood and certain body fluids of all patients are considered potentially infectious for human immunodeficiency virus (HIV), hepatitis B virus (HBV), and other blood-borne pathogens. Blood is the single most important source of HIV, HBV, and other bloodborne pathogens in health-care settings. Infection-control efforts for HIV, HBV, and other bloodborne pathogens must focus on preventing exposure to blood as well as delivery of HBV immunization.

Epidemiologic evidence has implicated only blood, semen, vaginal secretions, and possibly breast milk in transmissions. Although the risk is unknown, universal precautions also apply to tissues and to cerebrospinal fluid, synovial fluid, pleural fluid, peritoneal fluid, and amniotic fluid. Universal precautions do not apply to feces, nasal secretions, sputum, sweat, tears, urine, and vomitus unless they contain visible blood.

Health-care workers must consider *all* patients as potentially infected with bloodborne pathogens and must adhere rigorously to infection-control precautions for *all* patients.

General Precautions
- Consider *all* patients as potentially infected.
- Wear gloves when touching blood, body fluids containing blood, and body fluids to which universal precautions apply; for handling items or surfaces soiled with blood or applicable fluids, and for performing venipuncture and other vascular access procedures. Change gloves after each contact with a patient.
- Use protective barriers (i.e., wear masks, protective eyewear or face shields and gowns or aprons) when performing procedures that may produce blood or body fluid droplets or splashes.
- Wash hands and skin surfaces immediately and thoroughly if contaminated with blood or other body fluids to which universal precautions apply.
- Take precautions to prevent injuries from needles, scalpels, and other sharp instruments during procedures, when cleaning instruments, during disposal, or when handling. To prevent needlestick injuries, needles should not be recapped, purposely bent or broken by hand, removed from disposable

syringes, or otherwise manipulated by hand. After they are used, disposable syringes and needles, scalpel blades, and other sharp items should be placed in puncture-resistant containers for disposal.

Special Considerations
- Health-care workers who have exudative lesions or weeping dermatitis should refrain from all direct patient care and from handling patient-care equipment until the condition resolves.
- Pregnant health-care workers are not known to be at greater risk of contacting HIV infection than health-care workers who are not pregnant; however, if a health-care worker develops HIV infection during pregnancy, the infant is at risk of infection resulting from perinatal transmission. Because of this risk, pregnant health-care workers should be especially familiar with and strictly adhere to precautions to minimize the risk of HIV transmission.

Precautions for Invasive Procedures
(Here an invasive procedure is defined as any surgical entry into tissues, cavities, or organs or repair of major traumatic injuries.) General blood and body fluid precautions listed above, combined with the precautions listed below, should be the *minimum precautions for all such invasive procedures.*
- All health-care workers who participate in invasive procedures must routinely use appropriate barrier procedures to prevent skin and mucous membrane contact with all patients' blood and other body fluids.
- Gloves and surgical masks must be worn for all invasive procedures.
- Protective eyewear or face shields should be worn for all procedures that commonly result in generation of droplets or splashing of blood, body fluids containing blood, and other applicable body fluids.
- Gowns or aprons made of materials providing an effective barrier should be worn during invasive procedures likely to result in the splashing of blood or other pertinent body fluids.
- All health-care workers who perform or assist in vaginal or cesarean delivery should wear gloves and gowns when handling the placenta or the infant until blood and amniotic fluid have been removed from the infant's skin. Gloves should be worn until post-delivery care of the umbilical cord.

(continued)

Universal Precautions *(continued)*

- If a glove is torn or a needlestick or other injury occurs, the glove should be removed and a new glove used as promptly as patient safety permits; the needle or instrument involved in the incident should also be removed from the sterile field.

From Centers for Disease Control. (1987). Recommendations for prevention of HIV transmission in health care settings. *Morbidity and Mortality Weekly Report, 36* (Suppl), 25; and Centers for Disease Control. (1988). Update: Universal precautions for prevention or transmission of human immunodeficiency virus, hepatitis B virus, and other bloodborne pathogens in health-care settings. *Morbidity and Mortality Weekly Report, 37,* 24.

---

patients in addition to either disease-specific or category-specific isolation.

Body-substance isolation developed at Harborview Medical Center of Seattle and at the University of California in San Diego uses protective barriers, gloves, masks, gowns, and goggles to shield providers from contact with all moist body secretions. This system eliminates patient isolation except for patients with airborne infections or for those people who cannot control their own body secretions.

Universal Precautions

Health-care providers are directed by the CDC to consider all patients as potentially infected with bloodborne pathogens such as HIV (AIDS) and HBV (hepatitis). The CDC recommends that their precautions be universally applied to blood or body fluids containing traces of blood from all patients regardless of their diagnosis (CDC, 1988a). Universal precautions also apply to semen and vaginal secretions as well as tissue extracted by biopsy or during operative procedures. Cerebrospinal fluid (CFS), synovial fluid, peritoneal fluid, and amniotic fluid require precautions because they may have been contaminated by the patient's blood during needle insertion while obtaining the specimen. The CDC excludes feces, nasal secretions, sputum, sweat, tears, urine, and vomitus from the high-risk category of carrying bloodborne pathogens unless they contain visible blood. Saliva and human breast milk require precautions when there is intensive exposure such as dentistry and breast milk banks.

Universal precautions recommend gloves when exposure to blood or body fluids containing blood is anticipated. Masks and goggles should be worn when any splattering of blood or body fluids is anticipated during procedures. Gowns should be worn to avoid soiling of uniforms and the exposure of the caregiver's skin when gross contamination is possible (CDC, 1988a).

Category-Specific Isolation

Category-specific isolation protocol groups diseases according to their routes of transmission. Seven groups

include most diseases that have similar epidemiology. The advantage of this system is simplicity. This system can be applied early in the hospital stay before an exact diagnosis is known. Because it is more general, this system is easier to implement. Its main disadvantage is that the system may lead to overisolation because more precautions are employed than are necessary for every disease in the category. This can add to hospital costs and may decrease caregiver compliance with the prescribed precautions.

The seven isolation categories are described below (Garner & Simmons, 1983). A category ending in the term "isolation" is used when a private room is necessary, whereas the term "precaution" is used when a private room is optional. Cards for each category are commercially printed in specific colors with instructions

---

Respiratory Isolation
Visitors—Report to Nurses' Station Before Entering Room

1. **Private Room** – *necessary*; door must be kept closed.
2. **Gowns** – not necessary.
3. **Masks** – must be worn by all persons entering room if susceptible to disease.
4. **Hands** – must be washed on entering and leaving room.
5. **Gloves** – not necessary.
6. **Articles** – those contaminated with secretions must be disinfected.
7. **Caution** – all persons susceptible to the specific disease should be excluded from patient area; if contact is necessary, susceptibles must wear masks.

Figure 22–6. Category-specific sign for respiratory isolation.

for those who care for the patient or entering their room. (Fig. 22-6 shows an example of the card providing directions for respiratory isolation.)

Strict Isolation. Strict isolation is designed to prevent transmission of very contagious or virulent infections that are spread by both air and contact. All barriers are used every time the room is entered (Procedure 22-3).

Contact Isolation. Contact isolation is designed to prevent transmission by close or direct contact with a patient who has a highly transmissible disease.

Respiratory Isolation. Respiratory isolation is designed to prevent transmission by droplet transmission through the air.

Tuberculosis Isolation. Tuberculosis isolation is designed to prevent small particle transmission of microorganisms suspended in the air from patients with active cases of tuberculosis.

Enteric Precautions. Enteric precautions are designed to prevent the transmission of infections by direct or indirect contact with feces.

Drainage–Secretions Precautions. Drainage–secretions precautions are designed to prevent transmission of infections by direct or indirect contact with purulent secretions or body cavity drainage.

Blood–Body Fluid Precautions. Blood–body fluid precautions are designed to prevent transmission by infected blood or body fluids. Body fluids include saliva, semen, peritoneal fluid, tears, and other body cavity aspirates.

Disease-Specific Isolation

More than 160 specific diseases are listed in the CDC guidelines for disease-specific isolation. These diseases are considered likely to occur in U.S. hospitals. Disease-specific isolation depends on accurate identification of the infective organism. These precautions are aimed at interrupting the mode of transmission by identifying which secretions, excretions, body fluids, or tissues are or might be infective. Each specific disease is identified as to whether a gown, gloves, mask, or private room is required. Cards are available for posting outside patient rooms with spaces available to write in directions for caregivers and visitors. The health-care provider is required to make decisions based on the patient's age, mental status, and overall status concerning minimum precautions necessary to prevent transmission of the organism. It is presumed that young children require more precaution than adults because often they are not toilet trained and may not comply with instructions.

Similar adjustments may be necessary for people who become confused.

Disadvantages of disease-specific isolation precautions include the increased responsibility of decision-making by the health-care provider; isolation also may be delayed until the organism is identified by laboratory means. This delay may actually exceed the period of greatest infectivity of the patient. It may also presume that body fluids are sterile when they may also harbor pathogens (Garner, 1986). Advertising the diagnosis of the patient outside the patient's room, especially in the event of AIDS or sexually transmitted diseases, may breach patient confidentiality.

Body-Substance Isolation

Infection-control practitioners were aware of the shortcomings of both of these major isolation systems and were concerned about noncompliance of caregivers with infection control measures, unacceptable rates of nosocomial infections, and the appearance of an epidemic of AIDS infection. Originally, body-substance isolation was developed to control cross-infection of patients in intensive care units, but this method also proved promising to limit the spread of the AIDS virus.

Two basic premises underlie this method of infection control. First, infection may be present before a diagnosis is made. Infection control measures often are initiated too late to prevent transmission. Second, the risk of transmitting or contracting infection from most organisms is from direct contact of the organism by the caregivers hands, or by equipment that has been soiled by potentially infectious bodily secretions. These premises lead to the conclusion that all body substances may harbor pathogens, and contact with them must be avoided. The cardinal rule of body-substance isolation is never to touch with bare hands anything wet that comes from a body surface or body cavity (Fig. 22-7). Gloves are worn for all contact with mucous membranes, nonintact skin, and moist body substances at all times. Body substances include blood, urine, feces, sputum, saliva, wound drainage, or aspirated body fluids. Gloves are not necessary for contact with unsoiled articles or intact skin.

Gowns are worn when personal clothing may be soiled with the patient's body fluids. Masks are worn for anticipated contact with respiratory droplet secretions, or while suctioning. Protective eyewear is added when secretions are likely to splash. Cards are available to remind staff of universal precautions and can be located in all patient rooms. In addition, "STOP" cards are used to identify rooms of patients with airborne communicable diseases.

Body-substance isolation has the advantage of being simple, and there is no delay in instituting this form of isolation until the causative agent is found. The infection control committee usually examines all three systems of isolation and decides which system is to be used through-

PROCEDURE 22–3. Practicing Strict Isolation Technique

■ Purpose
1. Prevent transfer of pathogens spread by airborne and contact methods.

■ Assessment
- Determine epidemiology of disease to determine if strict isolation is mandatory.
- Note that patient is in a private room with door closed.
- Identify and assemble supplies necessary to complete care in patient unit.

■ Equipment
Isolation cart outside room containing mask, clean gown, disposable clean gloves, plastic bags for linen, plastic bags for transport of specimens

■ Procedure

Entering a Strict Isolation Room
1. Wash hands.
2. If clock is not available in room to use when taking patient's pulse, remove watch and seal in plastic bag.
3. Don mask, gown, gloves in hallway or anteroom. Pull cuff of gloves up over gown sleeves.
   Rationale: Provides uninterrupted covering for protection of wrist and arm.
4. Carry supplies into patient unit. Close door.
   Rationale: Prevents airborne pathogens from leaving patient unit.
5. Provide nursing care as necessary.

Exiting a Strict Isolation Room
6. Place contaminated linen into a cloth or plastic bag, and close bag. Carry to doorway where second, nongloved health-care worker holds a large bag with cuff folded down over his or her hands. Place first bag into second bag, being careful not to touch outside of second bag. Ungowned worker immediately closes bag and labels as isolation linen.
   Rationale: Double-bagging technique is used to contain pathogens and protect hospital personnel from contamination.
7. Remove contaminated, disposable, or recyclable supplies from room using double-bagging technique.
8. Untie waist ties of gown. Remove gloves and discard in patient's room. Wash hands. Untie neck ties.
   Rationale: Waist ties on gown are considered very contaminated. Neck ties should be untied only with clean hands to prevent contamination of hair.
9. Remove gown by folding toward inside without touching the outside surfaces. Discard in room. Remove mask, and discard in room.
   Rationale: Prevents transmission of pathogens by leaving all contaminated articles inside room.
10. Use clean, dry paper towel to open inside door handle. Leave room and close door from outside with bare hands.
    Rationale: Paper towel protects hand from becoming contaminated from inside door handle.
11. Wash hands.
    Note: Visitors may enter and leave room with instructions and supervision from nursing staff.

■ Lifespan Considerations

Infants and Children
- Parents should be encouraged to participate in their child's care with unrestricted visitation hours and given instruction in the isolation procedure.
- Toys should be made of materials that can be easily disinfected. They must be cleaned if they fall to the floor, which is considered one of the most contaminated areas of the room.

---

out the agency. The three systems of isolation are compared in Table 22-7.

Protective (Reverse) Isolation

Protective (reverse) isolation is used to prevent infection for people whose body defenses are known to be compromised. Patients who are neutropenic (neutrophils $<500/cm^3$) as a result of chemotherapy, radiation therapy, or immunosuppressive medications are prime candidates. Patients with extensive burns or dermatitis are at high risk. Such a patient is placed in a private room, ideally one with a laminar flow unit, which directs airflow outward and away from the patient. All people coming in contact with the individual must wear gowns, gloves, and masks. Meticulous handwashing is also employed by everyone entering the room. Food and equipment coming into the patient's room are treated at the highest level of disinfection. All of these measures help to ensure that the environment of the patient stays as free from pathogens as possible, thus decreasing the chance that infection occurs in these high-risk people.

PATIENT CARE

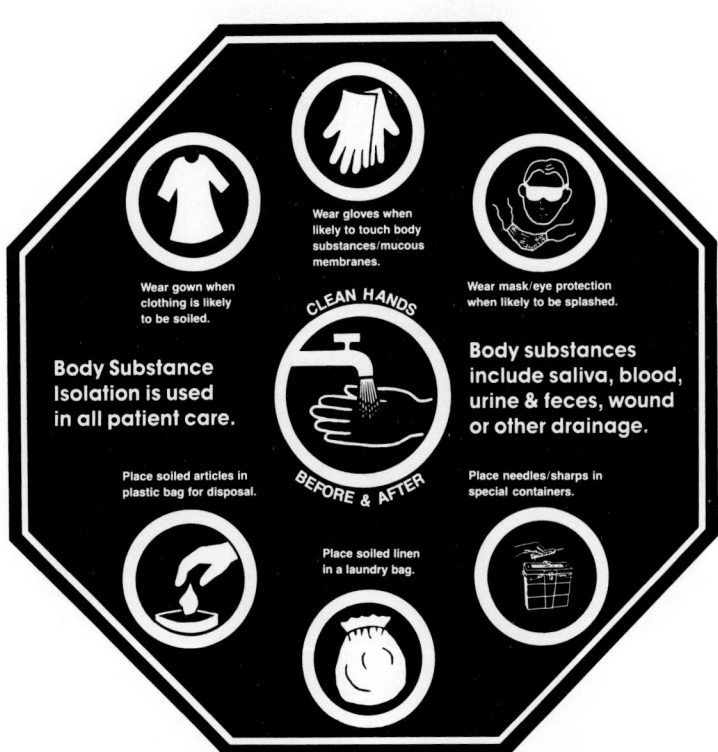

Figure 22–7.   Body substance isolation sign.

Body Substance Isolation

Nursing Considerations

To isolate means to set apart from others. Psychological effects of being separated from staff and loved ones occur when isolation is employed. Patients spend more time alone. The bodies, hands, and faces of caregivers are covered. Patients may mistakenly feel they are dirty or untouchable, especially if they have diseases that are considered socially unacceptable. Lack of social interaction can be psychologically injurious, especially to children and their parents. Nursing goals should be directed at preventing the spread of microorganisms while maintaining the patient's social support.

Transporting of patients with infections should be avoided whenever possible. If transport to other departments is necessary, the patient's gown and dressings should be changed before leaving the room. If the infection is transmitted by the airborne route, the patient should wear a mask and the transporters should be immune to the disease whenever possible.

Isolation systems are also costly in terms of equipment, supplies, and the time required by caregivers. Even more expensive are breaks in isolation technique that result in infection. All personnel, physicians, nurses, technicians, students, and housekeepers are responsible for complying with isolation precautions. All personnel are responsible for tactfully calling observed

infractions to the attention of those who do not comply. Compliance is best obtained by using a consistent, simple system; educating the staff; and instilling a sense of personal responsibility in all caregivers.

Surgical Asepsis

Surgical asepsis, or sterile technique, is defined as those practices that produce or maintain equipment and areas that are free from all microorganisms. The purpose of sterile technique is to prevent the introduction of microorganisms from the environment into the patient. Surgical asepsis is used during:

- Surgical operations
- All procedures that invade the bloodstream
- Procedures that cause a break in skin or mucous membranes (e.g., intramuscular injections)
- Dressing changes and wound care
- Procedures involving inserting catheters or devices into sterile body cavities (e.g., bladder)
- Care for high-risk groups (e.g., transplant recipients, burn patients, or immunosuppressed patients)

When all organisms and their spores are destroyed, the item is deemed sterile. In surgical asepsis, any item

TABLE 22–7

Comparison of Category-Specific, Disease-Specific, and Body-Substance Isolation Precautions

	Category-Specific	Disease-Specific	Body-Substance
Isolation precautions	Seven categories, each with a different set of precautions	Individualized for each disease	Universal precautions for all body fluids
Instruction card for door or cubicle	Separate, preprinted, color-coded card for each category	All-purpose black and white card to be individualized for each patient	All-purpose red, black, and white sign for all patients. In addition, STOP sign cards are used to identify rooms of patients with airborne diseases.
Advantages	Simpler system; less diagnostic information needed to assign precautions Less decision-making needed to assign precautions	Minimizes unnecessary precautions; may reduce cost of placing patient on isolation precautions May encourage compliance, especially by physicians	Recognizes the potential colonization of all body substances No decision-making is necessary for the use of barriers other than recognition of the potential for exposure to body substances. Cross-contamination between patients is minimized because gloves are changed between patients and no surface touches two people.
Disadvantages	Unnecessary precautions taken for some diseases May increase cost of isolation	Requires more skill and responsibility to assign precautions Requires more diagnostic information about disease to assign precautions	None currently recognized. Cost is not acknowledged as a factor. No barriers are used other than those indicated to avoid soiling by obvious body secretions.

Adapted from Garner, J. S. (1986). Isolation precautions. In J. V. Bennett & P. S. Brachman (Eds.), *Hospital infections* (2nd ed.; p. 147). Boston: Little, Brown.

not sterile is called "contaminated." To be sterile, an item must have been processed at the highest level of disinfection. These items are clearly labeled as sterile on their packaging. The packaging must not be torn, punctured, wet, or outdated. During any sterile procedure, care must be taken to keep all sterile equipment sterile.

Principles of Surgical Asepsis

Surgical asepsis starts with thorough planning and preparation of the environment, supplies, and personnel. Surgical asepsis can be carried out in many settings. The operating room is an area where surgical asepsis is carried out extensively. Staff members in the operating room require special training in maintaining technique for various operative procedures. Operative suites are specially constructed rooms that provide for no-touch handwashing at sinks controlled by foot pedals, have special airflow patterns, and control traffic into and out of areas.

Good personal hygiene is basic behavior for all per-

sonnel. Staff members who are ill with respiratory infections or who have conditions which cause diarrhea, vomiting, or skin lesions should not participate in sterile procedures. Street attire is not worn in the operating room or other hospital areas where sterility is important. Shoes can be covered with shoe covers, and beards and hair can be covered by caps and masks. Jewelry should not be worn on the hands.

General principles of surgical asepsis are discussed in Table 22-8.

Skin Preparation

Skin preparation reduces microorganisms present on the skin. The skin cannot be sterilized. Chemicals used to sterilize objects would kill dermal cells. Chemical disinfection of the skin is called degermation.

The bacteria on the skin are both transient and resident flora. The transient microorganisms are held in place by sweat, oil, and debris. They can be removed easily with soap and water, and by the friction of scrub-

TABLE 22–8
Principles of Surgical Asepsis

Technique/Principle	Rationale
Moisture may cause contamination. • Handle liquids carefully near sterile fields to prevent splashing. • Place wet objects on sterile, water-impermeable surfaces, such as sterile basins.	Microorganisms travel more easily through moist environments. When a sterile surface becomes moist, microorganisms may be transmitted from an unsterile surface by capillary action.
Never assume that an object is sterile. • Check to see that it is labeled as sterile. • Always check the integrity of the packaging. • Always check the expiration date on the package. • If there is any doubt about the sterility of an object, it should be considered unsterile.	Commercially prepared products are labeled as sterile on their packaging. Special indicators are used to show that objects have completed their sterilization process, such as tapes on the outside of packages or chemically impregnated paper inside containers. Packages that are torn, punctured, or moist cannot be considered sterile. All packaging materials should have clearly visible dates that indicate when sterility cannot be guaranteed. Items that have passed that date cannot be used.
Always face the sterile field.	The area defined as sterile for the purposes of the procedure is the "field." Objects that are out of the line of vision may be inadvertently contaminated and their sterility is never guaranteed.
Sterile articles may touch only sterile articles or surfaces if they are to maintain their sterility.	Anything considered unsterile may transfer microorganisms to the sterile object it touches. An object used on an unsterile surface, such as swabs used in cleaning the skin, must be used once and then discarded because skin cannot be sterilized. Keep unsterile objects away from the field.
Sterile equipment or areas must be kept above the waist and on top of the sterile field. • Drapes hanging over the edge of the table are not considered sterile.	Waist level is the limit of good visual field. By defining only the top of the field as sterile, maximum visibility of all sterile objects used in the procedures is ensured.
Prevent unnecessary traffic and air currents around the sterile area. • Close doors. • Unfold drapes or wrappers slowly. • Do not sneeze, cough, or talk excessively over the sterile field. • Do not reach across sterile fields.	Microorganisms cannot be completely excluded from the air even with the best filtration and air flow designs. Movement creates air currents that circulate organisms in the air. Masks do not contain all organisms expelled from the oral or nasal cavities and become moistened more quickly from talking. Move around a sterile field or turn the field slowly by reaching under the drapes if an object is not convenient to a sterile person.
Open, unused sterile articles are no longer sterile after the procedure.	Once the protective wrappings have been removed, the article is being contaminated by the air. Even if it is untouched and resting on a sterile surface, it must be discarded or resterilized before it is used. Liquids opened during the procedure that remain in their original container are also considered to be contaminated.
A person who is considered sterile who becomes contaminated must reestablish sterility.	If a "scrubbed" person punctures the gloves or is contaminated accidentally by touching an unsterile object, he or she must change the contaminated article. If a scrubbed person leaves the area of the sterile field, he or she must go through the procedure of rescrubbing, gowning, and gloving.
Surgical technique is a team effort. • A collective and individual "sterile conscience" is the best method of enhancing sterile technique.	Staff members must rely on one another to maintain sterile technique. Persons who are considered sterile must have access to sterile supplies delivered to them by circulators in the operating room or prepared by themselves at the bedside. Team members must be open to critiques by other members about their technique and respond to their suggestions that objects of their clothing have been contaminated or that they have contaminated an object. Periodic review of procedures and infection control surveillance reports enhance everyone's sterile technique.

bing. Resident flora adhere to epithelial cells and extend into hair follicles and glands in the skin. Resident flora vary on different locations of the body.

Antiseptic agents are used in skin preparation and surgical scrubs to reduce the number of transient microorganisms. They do not penetrate into the dermis, nor are they able to remove all resident flora. The mechanical action of scrubbing and rinsing with water helps remove organisms from deeper layers of the skin, but a portion of these bacteria remain. When surgical gloves are worn, especially for extended periods, resident flora grow and replicate from deeper skin layers. Any puncture or tear of gloves during sterile procedures allows these organisms to contact an open wound. Torn gloves must be immediately changed to reduce the chance of contamination.

The objective of surgical scrubs and skin preparation of the patient is to remove dirt, oil, and microorganisms from the skin; to reduce bacterial counts to a minimum; to avoid abrading the skin; and to leave a layer of antimicrobial material on the skin that inhibits the growth of microbes for an extended period of time.

Preparation of the patient's skin consists of several steps. The first is washing with soap and water, or a bath or shower before the planned procedures. Removal of hair with depilatory creams, clipping with sterile scissors, or shaving may be necessary. If shaving is ordered, it should not be performed more than 2 hours before the surgical procedure because tiny nicks in the skin may predispose the patient to infection. After the skin is cleansed and hair has been removed, the skin is scrubbed with an antimicrobial agent. For surgical procedures, this may take place in the operating room.

Surgical Handwashing

Surgical hand scrubs differ from general handwashing that the nurse performs during most patient encounters in both technique and length. A disposable scrub brush or sponge is usually used, but some agencies use equipment that can be resterilized. Sterile nail cleaners made of plastic or metal should also be available. Antiseptic soap containers that dispense the solution by knee or foot pressure must be located above or next to a splashproof sink. Some of the disposable brushes are impregnated with antimicrobial scrub solutions. The solution of choice in most institutions is an iodophor solution.

There are two methods of gauging adequacy of hand scrubs, the time method and the stroke method. In the time method, the fingers, the hand, and the arms are scrubbed for a standard period of time, usually 5 or 10 minutes, depending on agency protocol. In the stroke method, a standard number of strokes are used for each surface of the fingers, the hands, and the arms. For example, nails may receive 30 strokes, while other areas of the hands and arms may receive 20 strokes. The fingers are considered to have four sides, and each side

Nursing Research

Selected Nursing Research Studies

Goldwater, P. N., et al. (1989, January). Impact of recapping device on venipuncture-related needle stick injury. *Infect Control Hosp Epidemiol, 10*(1), 21–25.

LeClair, S. M., et al. (1988, August). Survey of nursing personnel attitudes toward infections and their control in the elderly. *American Journal of Infection Control, 16*(4), 159–166.

Pottinger, J., et al. (1989, December). Bacterial carriage by artificial versus natural nails. *American Journal of Infection Control, 17*(6), 340–344.

Mayet, F. M., et al. (1989, January). Choice or habit? A surgical glove study. *National News, 26*(1), 19–20.

Pritchard, V., et al. (1988, September 7). Patient handwashing practice. *Nursing Times, 84*(36).

Weinstein, S. A., et al. (1989, October). Bacterial surface contamination of patients' linen: Isolation precautions verses standard care. *American Journal of Infection Control, 17*(5), 264–267.

Possible Topics for Nursing Inquiry

- Does handwashing practice increase in frequency when signs are displayed in prominent locations reminding caregivers to wash their hands?
- Do caregivers customarily provide patients with materials to wash their hands after toileting or before meals?
- Does the institution of isolation procedures increase the patient's perception of social distance from significant others?
- Does the use of barrier precautions diminish the caregiver's attention to improving host defense mechanisms in the patient?
- How do various recapping devices compare in preventing needlestick injuries?

as well as the webs between the fingers is scrubbed with circular motion and firm pressure. The arm is divided into thirds. Each one third is scrubbed up to 2 inches above the elbow, using circular strokes. The stroke method ensures that all skin surfaces are exposed to the same amount of scrubbing and solution. The time method does not ensure equal attention to all areas.

Before starting the scrub, all nail polish should be removed. Fingernails should be short and without sharp edges that can puncture surgical gloves. The hands should be free of lesions, cuts, or abrasions because traumatized skin can harbor bacteria. Hands should always be held higher than the level of the elbows and away from the body to allow water to run off at the elbows. Water running down the arms to the hands can cause contamination. Hands must be thoroughly dried. This procedure for surgical hand scrubbing should be written, well illustrated, and prominently posted in the scrub area.

Sterile Gloves

Sterile gloves are required for all procedures that require surgical technique. Gloves are worn to prevent contamination of wounds, equipment, supplies, and the site of invasive procedures. Sterile gloves are donned after the hands have been thoroughly cleaned.

In the operative suite or during invasive procedures, the practitioner may use either a closed method or open method for donning gloves. The closed method is preferred when sterile gowns are used for the procedure. The sterile gown is donned, the hands are slid into the sleeves until the cuff seam is reached, and the dominant hand is used to pick up a cuffed glove for the other hand. The glove is drawn over the nondominant hand, and the sleeve is pulled onto the wrist. The dominant hand is gloved in the same manner using the sterile glove on the other hand. For procedures performed at the bedside, it is more common to use the open method of gloving (Procedure 22-4).

Lifespan Considerations

Age-related factors are important to consider in preventing the transmission of infection. Age affects the immune system, making some age groups more susceptible to infection. Activities also vary among different age groups, changing exposure patterns to infection. The groups people associate with at various ages harbor different organisms that pose risk to those who do not yet have immunity.

Newborn and Infant

Prevention of infection of the newborn begins by protecting the fetus from infection exposure during pregnancy. Infection in the mother can be transmitted to the fetus during pregnancy. The result may be minor or major congenital anomalies or fetal death, depending on the time of exposure and the organism involved. In general, the earlier in pregnancy the mother is infected, the more severely the fetus is affected. A very mild or asymptomatic infection in the mother may have serious consequences for the unborn infant. Very early in pregnancy when exposure is most dangerous, the mother may be unaware that she is pregnant. All women of childbearing age should have up-to-date immunizations, and those trying to get pregnant should avoid exposure to infectious disease whenever possible. Adequate prenatal care is important in decreasing maternal infection.

Newborn infants have an immature immune system. They lack maternal antibodies for most diseases and are not yet capable of producing their own. At about 2 months of age, infants appear to begin developing some body defense mechanisms. At 6 months of age, infants start to produce their own gamma globulin (that fraction of blood protein that contains antibodies), and they become more resistant to some organisms. The most frequent mode of transmission of organisms is from direct contact from the skin and hands of caregivers and, to a lesser extent, through contaminated infant formula. Teaching all caregivers the importance of scrupulous handwashing and general good hygiene has been shown to decrease infection in this age group (Donowitz, 1987). Immunizations are begun during the infant period and continue on through childhood. It is important to provide parents with an immunization schedule and to teach parents the importance of this method of preventing many contagious diseases.

Toddler and Preschooler

Body defenses continue to develop as the infant reaches toddlerhood. Despite better defenses against infection, young children frequently become infected because normal behavior at this age fosters transmission of microorganisms. Children of this age often are not yet toilet trained and have poor personal hygiene. Playing on the floor, continually putting objects in their mouth, and even playing with their bodily secretions all contribute to exposure to potential pathogens. Increased exposure to groups of children in a day-care or preschool setting is another factor affecting the spread of infection. Upper respiratory tract and subsequent ear infections are common among this population.

In the very young child, it is important to begin teaching hygiene practices that help to limit infectious exposure during their entire lifetime. Proper handwashing after using the bathroom and before meals is an important habit for the young child to develop. When children of this age are exhibiting signs of infection, they should be isolated from other children so that infection transmission can be minimized.

School Age and Adolescent

During the middle school years, the incidence of many infections decreases. Direct contact and airborne infections are more common in the winter months because

(Text continues on page 460)

PROCEDURE 22–4. Applying and Removing Sterile Gloves

■ Purpose
1. Prevent transfer of microorganisms from hands to sterile objects or open wounds.

■ Assessment
- Identify appropriate time to wear sterile gloves.
- Inspect glove package to determine whether it is dry and intact.
- Assess that nails are filed short and all jewelry is removed from hands.
- Examine ungloved hand for presence of open cuts or lesions, which may harbor microorganisms and prevent the nurse from participating in a procedure.

■ Equipment
Packaged sterile gloves in correct size
Flat working surface

■ Procedure

Applying Gloves
1. Wash hands.
   Rationale: Reduces the number of microorganisms that could be transferred if gloves accidently puncture or tear.
2. Remove outside wrapper by peeling apart sides.
   Rationale: Protects inner package from inadvertently opening and contaminating the gloves.
3. Lay inner package on clean, flat surface above waist level. Open wrapper from the outside keeping gloves on inside surface.
   Rationale: Objects below waist level are considered contaminated. Inner surface of wrapper is considered sterile.
4. Grasp inside edge of right cuff with thumb and first

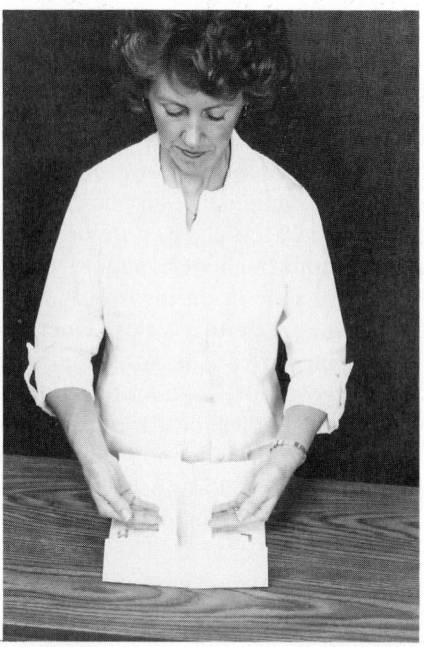

Step 3A

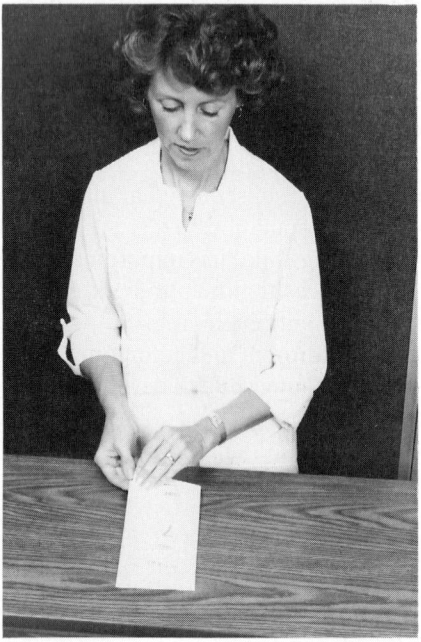

Step 2

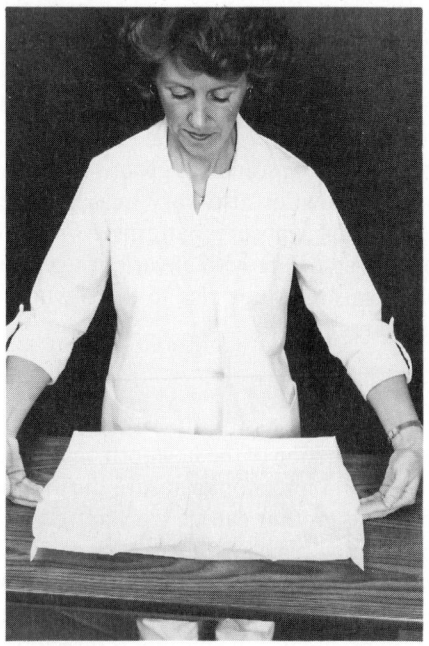

Step 3B

(continued)

two fingers of left hand. Holding hands above waist, insert right hand into glove. Adjust fingers inside glove after both gloves are on.
Rationale: Inner edge of cuff unfolds against skin of hand and is not sterile once applied. Contamination occurs if ungloved hand contacts gloved hand.

5. Slip gloved hand underneath second gloved cuff still in pakage, and pull over left hand.
   Rationale: Sterile cuff protects fingers of gloved hand from becoming contaminated.
6. Keeping hands above waist, adjust glove fit, touching only sterile areas.

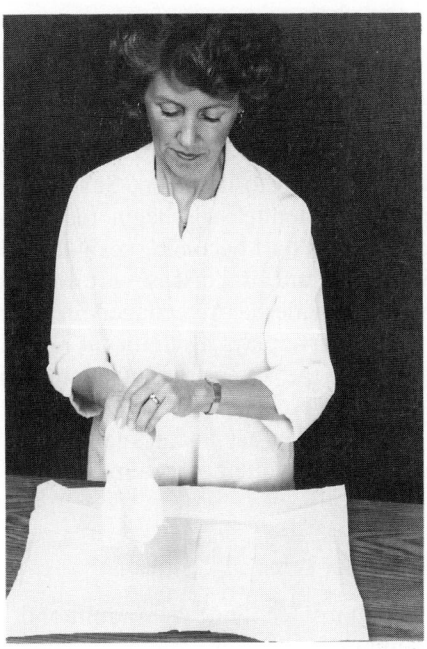

Step 4

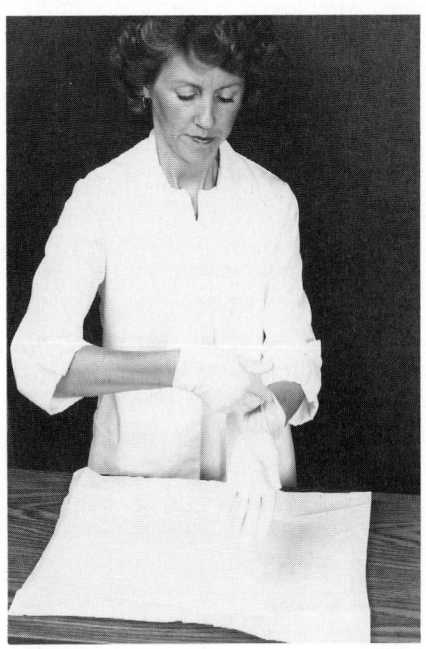

Step 5B

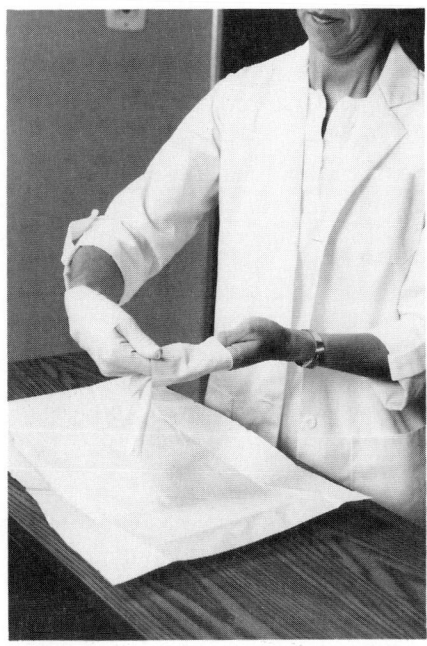

Step 5A

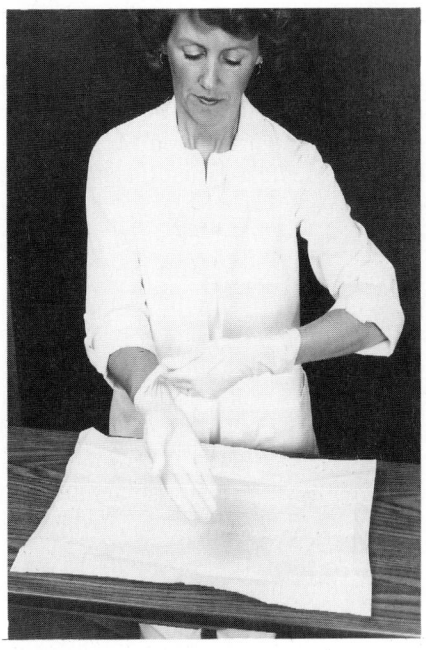

Step 6

(continued)

PROCEDURE 22–4. Applying and Removing Sterile Gloves *(continued)*

Rationale: Prevents potential contamination while ensuring a smooth fit over fingers.

Removing Gloves
7. With right hand, grasp outer surface of left glove just below thumb. Peel off without touching exposed wrist.
Rationale: After use, outer surface of gloves is contaminated and could transfer microorganisms to the nurse's wrist.

8. Place ungloved hand under thumbside of second cuff and peel off toward the fingers, holding first glove inside second glove. Discard into appropriate receptacle.
Rationale: Folding contaminated glove surfaces toward the inside minimizes the chances of contacting microorganisms.
9. Wash hands.

---

children crowd into school rooms and engage in indoor recreational activities. Skin eruptions such as impetigo and infestations of lice occur in this age group because personal hygiene aids, clothing, and sports equipment are shared.

Adolescence brings new elements of exposure. Athletic injuries are common and pose infectious risk. Accidents become more frequent in this age group and often predispose a person to infection. Sexually transmitted diseases and mononucleosis begin to rise in this age group when teens start becoming sexually active. Respiratory infections and viral diseases are common because many group activities keep teenagers in close quarters.

The school nurse plays a significant role in detecting and preventing the spread of infections among older children and adolescents. Health teaching is also important in preventing injury and sexually transmitted diseases among this population group.

Patient Teaching

Instruct the patient as follows:

- Cover your mouth when coughing or sneezing and properly dispose of paper tissues to avoid the transmission of infection through respiratory secretions.
- Wash your hands carefully and thoroughly, especially after using the bathroom or before eating.
- Boil items for 10 minutes or use a dilute solution of bleach to decrease bacteria counts when necessary.
- Learn the signs of infection so you can contact the health-care provider promptly, thus avoiding unnecessary spread of infection.
- Symptoms of infection may be less pronounced as you age so that an infection may be present without a significant increase in temperature.
- Traveling to a foreign country or to a different location (primitive woodlands and mountains) may increase your risk for some infections, and precautions such as boiling drinking water may be necessary.
- Preserve your intact skin because this provides the best barrier to invasion of pathogens into the body.

Adult and Older Adult

By the time most people reach adulthood, they have acquired immunity to many communicable diseases. Infection as a complication of injury continues to be a threat, as do sexually transmitted diseases. As adults increase their independence and travel, especially to foreign countries, they may be exposed to new infectious organisms.

As the adult ages, the incidence of infection as a complication of chronic disease increases. The effects of longstanding cardiovascular disease, diabetes, drug and alcohol abuse, and cancer can predispose the adult to infection. Elective surgical procedures can also pose an infection risk.

In working with adult populations, the nurse can stress preventive health practices to reduce the risk of chronic disease states and thus decrease potential infection risk. Monitoring to ensure current immunizations for the adult is also important because adults frequently forget to update immunization as necessary.

The risk of infection is greatly increased in elderly people due to an increase in debilitating chronic diseases, malignancy, and waning immunologic responses in this age group. The elderly are predisposed to serious infections because of decreased nutritional status, decreased activity level, poor circulation, frequent breaks in skin integrity, and impaired mechanical clearance mechanisms. Sometimes old diseases such as tuberculosis and herpes zoster can be reactivated, and there is an increased incidence of staphylococcal and streptococcal infections among the elderly.

Severely disabled elderly people are at particular risk because they are often unable to perform their own personal hygiene. Immobility and incontinence also greatly increase infection risk. Approximately 5% of those beyond the age of 65 are in extended-care facilities. Patients are often housed in crowded rooms, and they frequently have invasive devices such as Foley catheters. Limited staffing as well as high staff turnover makes it difficult to institute infection control programs. Accidents, especially falls, are more common as a person's functional abilities decrease. Medications, such as sedatives, can also indirectly contribute to increased infection risk.

Hospitalized elderly patients develop nosocomial infections at two to five times the rate of younger patients. They have higher rates of pneumonia, urinary tract infections, bacteremia, and surgical wound infections during the hospitalization where they are often treated with vigorous courses of antibiotics. They are often returned to their nursing facilities on continuing antibiotic regimens. This can lead to the development of antibiotic-resistant organisms in nursing homes. When these patients, who are potential reservoirs for transmission to other patients in their nursing home, are readmitted to acute-care hospitals, they become reservoirs for the new facility. Thus, they may require several acute-care admissions and pass on more virulent organisms with each roundtrip (Garibaldi & Nurse, 1986; Gross & Levine, 1987).

Key Concepts

- Agents that cause infection are everywhere in the environment, on body surfaces, in food, and in products used in normal activities of daily living.
- Intact skin and mucous membranes are major barriers against organisms and infection transmission.
- A communicable disease is caused by an organism that is transmissible from one person to another.
- Infections in patients in hospitals are not necessarily easily passed from one person to another (contagious); but because of the large number of patients with lowered host defenses, diseases are transmitted more easily than in the community.
- Because of the uncertainty of the period of communicability and the lack of identifiable infection in some patients, all body secretions should be considered contaminated.
- The chain of passage of infectious organisms from person to person, from object to person, and from reservoirs in the environment can be broken with infection control practices.

- The incidence of infections associated with health-care delivery (nosocomial infections) can be decreased with good infection control practices.
- Regulatory agencies at local, state, regional, and national levels are involved in the control of infection and institutional waste to protect patients, staff, and the community.
- The infection control committee, with the aid of the infection control nurse, is responsible for developing and administering the infection control program of health-care facilities.
- Employee health programs to monitor and counsel personnel are important components of institutional and community infection control programs.
- Effective infection control measures have a favorable cost–benefit ratio.
- Contact transmission of infectious organisms on the hands of caregivers is the most frequent mode of transmission of infection in health-care facilities.
- Handwashing is the single most important infection control practice.
- Handwashing techniques should be learned by all caregivers, the patient, and family members.
- Institutional waste disposal methods are important factors in infection control programs.
- Aseptic practices are those techniques used to keep people or objects free from microorganisms.
- Isolation procedures and barrier nursing practices are important in preventing the spread of infection.
- Gloves should be worn whenever there could be contact with the patient's body secretions.
- Cleaning, disinfection, and sterilization can be accomplished by various methods and agents.
- Sterile technique is used to prevent the introduction of microorganisms from the environment into the patient.
- An item is sterile when all organisms and their spores are destroyed on the object.
- Manufacturers' instruction manuals must be consulted to ensure adequate exposure to the appropriate concentration of an agent to produce sterility of objects and to prevent damage to costly equipment.
- Infectious exposure and risk of contracting infectious disease change during a person's lifespan.

References

Alcamo, I. E. (1986). *Fundamentals of microbiology* (2nd ed.). Reading, MA: Addison-Wesley.

Baxter Healthcare Corporation (1988). *A point of concern*. Product information. Mission Viejo, CA: ICU Medical Inc.

Beyt, B. E., Troxler, S., & Cavaness, J. (1985). Prospective payment and infection control. *Infection Control, 6*(4), 161.

Castle, M. & Ajemian, E. (1987). *Hospital infection control: Principles and practice* (2nd ed.). New York: John Wiley and Sons.

Centers for Disease Control (1986). Update: Universal precautions for prevention and transmission of human immunodeficiency virus, hepatitis B virus and other blood-borne pathogens in health-care settings. *Morbidity and Mortality Weekly Report,* November.

Centers for Disease Control (1987). Recommendations for prevention of HIV transmission in health-care settings. *Morbidity and Mortality Weekly Report, 36*(2S), 3–17s.

Centers for Disease Control (1987). Reports on AIDS. *Morbidity and Mortality Weekly Report.*

Centers for Disease Control (1987). Acquired immunodeficiency syndrome (AIDS): Recommendations and guidelines. *Morbidity and Mortality Weekly Report.*

Centers for Disease Control (1988a). Recommendations for prevention of HIV transmission in health-care settings. *Morbidity and Mortality Weekly Report, August.*

Dixon, R. E. (1987). Costs of nosocomial infections and benefits of infection control programs. In Wenzel, R. P. (Ed.), *Prevention and control of nosocomial infections* (pp. 19–25). Baltimore: Williams & Wilkins.

Donowitz, L. G. (1987). Infection in the newborn. In Wenzel, R. P. (Ed.), *Prevention and control of nosocomial infections* (pp. 481–493). Baltimore: Williams & Wilkins.

Garibaldi, R. A. & Nurse, B. (1986). Infections in the elderly. *American Journal of Medicine, 81*(Suppl 1A), 53–58.

Garner, J. S. & Simmons, B. P. (1983). Guidelines for isolation precautions in hospitals: CDC guidelines. *Infection Control, 4*(4), 249–325.

Garner, J. S., and Simmons, B. P. (1986). Isolation precautions. In Bennett, J. V., and Bachman, P. S. (Eds.). *Hospital infections* (2nd ed., pp. 143–150). Boston: Little Brown.

Gross, P. A. & Levine, J. F. (1987). Infections in the elderly. In Wenzel, R. P. (Ed.). *Prevention and control of nosocomial infections* (pp. 541–559). Baltimore: Williams & Wilkins.

Larson, E. (1987). Skin cleansing. In Wenzel, R. P. (Ed.), *Prevention and control of nosocomial infections* (pp. 250–256). Baltimore: Williams & Wilkins.

Lynch, P. & Cummings, M. J. (1987). Body substance isolation. Information packet obtained by personal communication from Harborview Medical Center, Seattle, WA.

News-AJN (1988). AIDS precautions changing practice. *American Journal of Nursing, 88*(3), 372–390.

Rutala, W. A. (1987). Disinfection, sterilization, and waste disposal. In Wenzel, R. P. (Ed.), *Prevention and control of nosocomial infections* (pp. 257–282). Baltimore: Williams & Wilkins.

Schaffner, W. (1987). The global impact of hospital-acquired infections. In Wenzel, R. P. (Ed.), *Prevention and control of nosocomial infections* (pp. 13–18). Baltimore: Williams & Wilkins.

Simmons, B. P. (1983). CDC guideline for hospital environment control. *American Journal of Infection Control, 11*, 96–115.

Williams, W. W. (1983). Guidelines for infection control in hospital personnel: CDC guidelines. *Infection Control, 4*(4), 326–349.

Williams, W. W. & Garner, J. S. (1986). Personnel health services. In Bennett, J. V. & Bachman, P. S. (Eds.), *Hospital infections* (2nd ed.; pp. 17–38). Boston: Little, Brown.

Bibliography

Belkin, N. L. (1988, February). Surgical gowns and drapes as aseptic barriers. *American Journal of Infection Control, 16*(1), 14–18.

Centers for Disease Control (1981). Antiseptics, handwashing, and handwashing facilities: Guidelines activity. Atlanta: Hospital Infections Branch, Center for Infectious Disease—Department of Health and Human Services.

Centers for Disease Control (1984). National nosocomial infection surveillance. *CDC Surveillance Summaries, 33*(255), 95.

Centers for Disease Control (1988). What to do to stop disease in child day care centers: A kit for child day care directors. HE 20.7008:C 43/kit.

Cools, H. J. M. et al (1988, August). Infection control in a skilled nurse facility: A six-year survey. *Journal of Hospital Infection, 12*(2), 117–124.

Davis, A. T. (1985). Responses to infections in childhood. In Youmans, G. P., Patterson, P. Y., & Sommers, H. M. (Eds.), *The biologic and clinical basis of infectious diseases* (3rd ed.; pp. 113–122). Philadelphia: W. B. Saunders.

EHP writes infection control manual for pregnant employees. (1989, November). *Hospital Employee Health, 8*(11), 142–143.

Fedson, D. S. (1987). Immunization for health care workers. In Wenzel, R. P. (Ed.), *Prevention and control of nosocomial infections* (pp. 116–174). Baltimore: Williams & Wilkins.

Feigin, R. D. (1987). Opportunistic infections in the compromised host. In Feigin, R. D. & Cherry, J. D. (Eds.), *Textbook of pediatric infectious diseases* (2nd ed.; pp. 769–786). Philadelphia: W. B. Saunders.

Ferwerda, H. E. (1989, September). Getting on top of infection control problems. *American Journal of Nursing, 89*(9), 1191.

Ford, C. D. (1990, January–February). Disposal of sharps: implications and control. *Journal of Intravenous Nursing 13*(1), 42–47.

Ford-Jones, E. L. (1987). The special problems of nosocomial infection in the pediatric patient. In Wenzel, R. P. (Ed.), *Prevention and control of nosocomial infections* (pp. 494–540). Baltimore: Williams & Wilkins.

Fox, J. P. (1987). Epidemiology of infectious diseases. In Feigin, R. D. & Cherry, J. D. (Eds.), *Textbook of pediatric infectious diseases* (2nd ed.; pp. 4–69). Philadelphia: W. B. Saunders.

Gallucci, B. B. & Schaidt-Rokosky, J. (1991). Immune responses. In Patrick, M., Woods, S. L., Craven, R. F., et al. (Eds.), *Medical surgical nursing: Pathophysiological concepts* (pp. 186–201). Philadelphia: J. B. Lippincott.

Gold, R. (1985). Immunization. In Mandell, L. A. & Ralph, E. D. (Eds.), *Essentials of infectious diseases* (pp. 101–112). Boston: Blackwell Scientific Publications.

Goldwater, P. N. et al (1989, January). Impact of a recapping device on venipuncture-related needlestick injury. *Infection Control Hospital Epidemiology 10*(1), 21–25.

Grazier, S. (1988, October). The loneliness barrier . . . patients in isolation. *Nursing Times 84*(41), 44–45.

Hapgood F. (1987). Viruses emerge as a new key for unlocking life's mysteries. *Smithsonian 18*(8), 116–127.

Hoeprich, P. (1989). Infectious diseases: A modern treatise of infectious processes (4th ed.). Philadelphia: J. B. Lippincott.

Jackson, M. M. et al (1989, November). Infection prevention and control in the era of the AIDS/HIV epidemic. *Seminars in Oncology Nursing 5*(4), 236–243.

Jackson, M. M. & Lynch, P. (1986). Ambulatory care setting. In Bennett, J. V. & Bachman, P. S. (Eds.), *Hospital infections* (2nd ed.; pp. 325–333). Boston: Little, Brown.

LaForce, F. M. (1987). The control of infection in hospitals: 1750–1950. In Wenzel, R. P. (Ed.), *Prevention and control of nosocomial infections* (pp. 1–12). Baltimore: Williams & Wilkins.

Larson, E. (1984). Current handwashing issues. *Infection Control 5*, 15–17.

Larson, E. (1989, July). Handwashing: It's essential—even when you use gloves. *American Journal of Nursing 89*(7), 934–941.

LeClair, S. M. et al. (1988, August). Survey of nursing personnel attitudes toward infections and their control in the elderly. *American Journal of Infection Control 16*(4), 159–166.

Ledger, W. (1988, October). Surgical asepsis in labor and delivery. *Infection Control Hospital Epidemiology 9*(10), 469–470.

Lemmink, J. A. (1987). Infection control—When a surgical wound becomes infected. *RN 50*(9), 24–29.

Makulowich, G. (1988, June). Gowns and goggles—New uses in the age of AIDS. *AIDS Patient Care 2*(3), 22–24.

Mayet, F. M. et al. Choice or habit? A surgical glove study. *NAT News 26*(1), 19–20.

McFarlane, A. (1990, February). Why do we forget to remember handwashing? *Professional Nurse 5*(5), 250, 252.

McFarlane, A. (1989, April). Infection control: Reducing the risk to medical patients. *Professional Nurse 4*(7), 344, 346–348.

Mooney, B. R. & Armington, L. C. (1987). Infection control: How to prevent nosocomial infection. *RN 50*(9), 21–23.

Mullen, R. J. et al. (1989, June). *MMWR* (Suppl) 38(S-6), 3–37.

Patterson, P. Y. (1985). Introduction to infectious diseases. In Youmans, G. P., Patterson, P. Y., & Sommers, H. M. (Eds.), *The biologic and clinical basis of infectious diseases* (3rd ed.; pp. 1–5). Philadelphia: W. B. Saunders.

Petersdorf, R. G. & Dale, O. C. (1987). Infections in the compromised host. In *Harrison's principles of internal medicine* (11th ed.; pp. 764–770). New York: McGraw-Hill.

Pottinger, J. et al. (1989, December). Bacterial carriage by artificial versus natural nails. *American Journal of Infection Control 17*(6), 340–344.

Preston, G. A., Larson, E. L., & Stamm, W. E. (1981). The effect of private isolation rooms on patient practices, colonization and infection in an intensive care unit. *American Journal of Medicine 30,* 614.

Pritchard, V. et al. (1988). Patient handwashing practice. (Sept. 7–13). *Nursing Times, 84*(36), 68, 70, 72.

Pugliese, G. et al. (1989, February). Prevention of human immunodeficiency virus infection: Our responsibilities as health care professionals. *American Journal of Infection Control 17*(1), 1–22.

Reid, E. (1988, July). Breast milk banks and HIV. *Midwife Health Visitor and Community Nurse 24*(7), 287, 289–290.

Shererty, R. J. & Hampton, A. L. (1987). Infection control aspects of hospital employee health. In Wenzel, R. P. (Ed.), *Prevention and control of nosocomial infections* (pp. 175–204). Baltimore: Williams & Wilkins.

Weinstein, S. A. et al. (1989, October). Bacterial surface contamination of patients' linen: Isolation precautions versus standard care. *American Journal of Infection Control 17*(5), 264–267.

Williams, W. L. (1984). Nosocomial infections. In Rytel, M. W. & Mogabgab, W. J. (Eds.), *Clinical manual of infectious diseases* (pp. 215–239). Chicago: Year Book Medical.

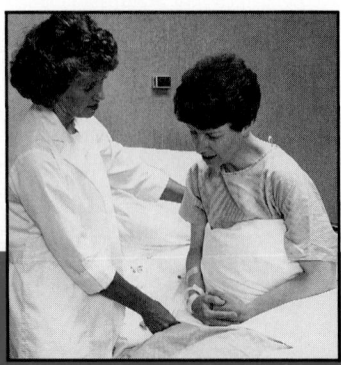

Perioperative Nursing

LEARNING OBJECTIVES

Upon completion of this chapter, the student will be able to do the following:

- Discuss three phases of perioperative management.
- Discuss the impact of surgery on functional health.
- Identify lifespan considerations for the patient having surgery.
- Identify appropriate common NANDA nursing diagnoses for the preoperative, intraoperative, and postoperative phases.
- Describe appropriate preoperative patient teaching.

- Discuss emotional support, safety, and asepsis during the intraoperative phase.
- Identify appropriate nursing assessments in the recovery facility and during the postoperative period.
- Identify common postoperative complications and appropriate nursing care to promote normal function.
- Develop an appropriate discharge plan for the surgical patient.

KEY TERMS

Anesthesiologist	Intraoperative	Postoperative phase
Elective surgery	phase	Preoperative phase
Emergent surgery	Malignant	Regional anesthetic
General anesthetic	hyperthermia	Urgent surgery

23

Surgical Intervention
Classification of Surgery
Surgical Facilities
  Clinic or Physician's Office
  One-Day Surgical Centers
  Hospitals
Phases of Perioperative Nursing
  Preoperative Phase
  Intraoperative Phase
  Postoperative Phase
Impact of Surgery on Functional Health
  Health Perception and Health Maintenance
  Exercise and Activity
  Nutrition and Metabolism
  Elimination
  Sleep and Rest
  Cognition and Perception
  Self-Concept
  Roles and Relationships
  Coping
  Sexuality
  Values and Beliefs
Lifespan Considerations
Preoperative Nursing
Nursing Assessment
Nursing Diagnoses and Patient Goals
Nursing Interventions
  Preoperative Teaching

  Informed Consent
  Patient Preparation
  Preoperative Checklist
Evaluation
Intraoperative Nursing
Nursing Assessment
Nursing Diagnoses and Patient Goals
Nursing Interventions
  Emotional Support
  Patient Safety
  Anesthesia Monitoring
  Asepsis
  Wound Closure
  Transport to the Recovery Facility
Evaluation
Postoperative Nursing
Nursing Assessment
  Assessment in the Recovery Facility
  Assessments During the Postoperative Period
Nursing Diagnosis and Patient Goals
Nursing Interventions
  Nursing Interventions in the Recovery Facility
  Nursing Interventions on the Surgical Recovery Unit
  Discharge Planning and Home Care
Evaluation
Key Concepts

Surgery is a means of treating injury and disease. The goal of surgery is to return the patient to the highest level of functioning and health possible, as soon as possible, within the limits imposed by the injury or disease state. Generally, surgery is performed because it is the treatment that has been chosen by the surgeon and the patient as the best means to achieve the desired goal.

In modern culture surgery has become a common method of treating disease and promoting health. In the last few decades the complexities of surgery have increased greatly, and entire organ systems can be transplanted to replace nonfunctioning body parts. All surgical procedures can potentially affect functional abilities of the person in every health pattern. The impact can be great and permanent or brief and temporary. Perioperative nurses provide specialized care to the surgical patient, promoting the return to optimal functional capacities.

Perioperative nursing involves the period before, during, and after any surgical procedure. During this time, the nurse plays an integral role, using the nursing process to individualize care and meet the surgical patient's specific needs.

Perioperative nursing is a continually challenging nursing specialty that requires knowledge, technical skill, creativity, leadership, and excellent communication skills. To meet the constantly changing needs of the surgical patient in this age of ever-increasing technology, the professional nurse must continually upgrade knowledge and skill through self-education and participation in educational inservice. As with all specialties in the nursing profession, the importance of teamwork and cooperation among colleagues cannot be overemphasized. This spirit of teamwork is especially important and relevant for the perioperative nurse.

SURGICAL INTERVENTION

Classification of Surgery

There are many specific reasons why surgery may be performed. Surgery may be performed to find out why a problem or set of symptoms is or has been occurring. Surgery may also be performed to alleviate pain, prolong life, improve mobility, provide for vascular access for medications or nutrition, improve function, or improve appearance. General classifications of surgery according to purpose are provided in Table 23-1.

The urgency with which surgery must be performed differs for each individual situation. **Emergent surgery** involves a situation in which surgery must be performed immediately to preserve function of a body part or the life of the patient. An example of emergent surgery is the repair of severe bleeding from a major vessel (rupture of aorta) or the repair of a perforated appendix. **Urgent surgery** occurs when a decision for surgery is indicated for a health problem but the surgery does not need to be performed immediately to preserve life or function. Examples of urgent surgery include gall bladder removal, repair of fractures, or removal of cancerous growths. **Elective surgery** includes those surgical procedures that are performed based on the desire of the patient but not needed to preserve life or function. An example of an elective surgical procedure is cosmetic surgery.

Surgical Facilities

The facility chosen for surgery depends on the type and complexity of the procedure and the availability of necessary supplies and equipment. For example, if the planned surgical procedure requires laser or radiation technology, or if the patient requires intensive care nursing, the chosen facility needs to have the required technical equipment and personnel available. Facilities where surgery is commonly performed include a clinic or physician's office, a one-day surgical center, or a hospital.

Clinic or Physician's Office

Surgery performed in a clinic or physician's office is usually limited to minor surgical procedures such as diagnostic procedures, oral procedures, gynecologic procedures, or removal of lesions from the skin. Procedures done in these facilities usually require either no anesthesia, local anesthesia, or regional blocks. Surgery performed in these facilities is the least expensive, since complex equipment is not used and inpatient recovery is not needed.

One-Day Surgical Centers

One-day surgical centers, also known as outpatient surgical centers, ambulatory surgical units, or surgi-centers have recently developed and proliferated in an attempt to keep rising surgical costs down. These facilities admit patients for the day of surgery and are usually affiliated with, and located in or near hospitals.

Because one-day surgical centers can save time and money, many hospitals are moving toward performing an ever-increasing number of surgeries in these centers. Some hospitals with well developed one-day surgery programs may do over 50% of their caseloads in these centers (Gruendemann & Meeker, 1987). One-day surgery centers are limited to procedures and patients suitable to this short-stay program. Patients must be assessed in terms of their anesthetic and surgical risk and in terms of their ability to safely and adequately care for themselves after discharge from the short-stay facility. These centers also provide a special challenge to perioperative nurses and recovery room nurses, who must provide optimal care and patient teaching to patients within a limited amount of time.

Hospitals

Hospitals are comprehensive facilities for all types of surgery and postsurgical recovery. These facilities have necessary equipment and personnel available to perform surgeries requiring intensive monitoring, complex technology, and prolonged recovery. Hospitals provide a wide range of services and have extensive emergency backup systems, should these be necessary, but are generally more expensive than either the one-day surgery centers or clinics. Cost containment may prevent admission to a hospital for minor surgical procedures, since insurance companies may not be willing to reimburse the cost of inpatient hospital care.

Phases of Perioperative Nursing

Perioperative nursing includes three distinct phases: the preoperative phase (this phase begins when the decision for surgical intervention is made and ends when the patient is transferred to the operating room), the intraoperative phase (this phase begins when the patient is transferred to the operating room and ends when the patient is admitted to the recovery facility), and the postoperative phase (this phase begins when the patient

TABLE 23–1

Types of Surgery Based on Purpose and Urgency

Classification	Purpose	Examples
Purpose		
Diagnostic	Confirmation of suspected diagnosis	Biopsy, culture, endoscopy, fluid tap
Explorative	Confirms the type and extent of a disease process	Laparotomy, joint exploration
Reconstructive	Repairs physical deformities or improves physical appearance	Rhinoplasty, mammoplasty, skin grafting
Curative	Diseased or damaged body organ or structure is removed or repaired and the patient is cured	Appendectomy, hysterectomy, fixation of fractures
Transplant	Diseased or damaged body organs and structures replaced with donated or artificial organs	Heart, kidney, cornea, bone, liver, lung, pancreas, or skin transplants
Palliative	Alleviates pain or other disease symptoms, slows progression of diseases but does not cure	Tumor debulking, nerve blocks, placement of feeding tubes
Urgency		
Emergent	Preserves function of body parts or life of patient	Repair of severe bleeding from major vessel
Urgent	Indicated for health problem but immediacy not necessary to preserve function of life	Gallbladder removal, repair of fractures, removal of cancerous growth
Elective	Based on patient's desire but not needed to preserve life or function	Cosmetic surgery

is admitted to the recovery facility and ends when the patient has recovered from the surgical experience). In each of these phases, the nurse plays an integral role, using the nursing process to individualize care and meet the surgical patient's specific needs.

Preoperative Phase

The **preoperative phase** includes all the activities necessary to prepare the patient properly for surgery. It begins when the decision for surgery is made and ends when the patient is transferred to the operating room. Proper preoperative evaluation by the nurse, the anesthesiologist, and the surgeon is essential to plan adequately for the designated procedure. This evaluation includes all functional health patterns. A thorough medical history is also taken to ensure patient safety. The history and evaluations include the following areas: cardiac and respiratory system assessments, medication history, previous anesthetic experiences, fluid and electrolyte status, allergies, mobility limitations, nutritional status, oral status, dental status, integumentary status, and emotional state. Additionally, the patient's learning requirements need to be assessed and preoperative teach-

ing needs to be accomplished. The operative consent form is completed in this phase. The patient's psychological needs are also addressed at this point. Preoperative management is discussed in detail later in this chapter.

Intraoperative Phase

The **intraoperative phase** includes those activities that occur from the time the patient is transferred to the operating room until the time the patient is transferred to the recovery facility. It includes both the time spent in the preoperative area (holding room) and the time spent in the operating room itself. In the holding area, the final preparations for the patient's surgery are completed. The final assessment is accomplished and the intravenous lines are inserted, if this has not already been done. These activities may be completed by the holding room nurse or the anesthetist, depending on the particular hospital's protocol. A regional block (spinal, subarachnoid block, epidural block, or other block) may be administered if this is the anesthetic of choice. While these activities are being done, the scrub nurse and circulating nurse are preparing the sterile instruments, supplies, and the remainder of the necessary equipment, medications, and nonsterile supplies that are required for the successful and efficient completion of the surgical procedure. All these activities require precise timing and cooperation among the people involved.

During the procedure, the anesthetist or the nurse (for procedures requiring local anesthesia) closely and frequently monitors the patients' vital signs, intravenous fluids, urine output, medications, blood loss, and anesthetic agent being used for the particular procedure. Depending on the procedure, the blood gas values and electrolyte values may also be frequently monitored. The scrub nurse closely follows the procedure and assists the surgeons with the sterile instruments, sterile supplies and equipment, and the sterile sutures. The circulating nurse closely monitors all activities, maintains accurate written records, and ensures the continued sterility of the procedure and the safety of the patient. At the end of the procedure, the circulating nurse, the surgeons, and the anesthetist provide for the safe and timely transport of the patient into the recovery area (recovery room, intensive care unit, or patient unit).

Postoperative Phase

The **postoperative phase** involves those activities that occur from the time the patient is transferred from the operating room until he or she has progressed beyond the acute phase of his or her recovery. This phase requires the nurse to monitor a number of parameters closely and frequently, including maintenance of an adequate airway, vital signs, blood gases and electrolyte values (as appropriate), level of consciousness, blood loss, assessment for hemorrhage, intravenous fluid administration, level of regional block (if used), emotional state, level of pain control, and tolerance of the procedure. Further along in the recovery phase, the nurse continues to assess respiratory status, bowel status, incision status, and the patient's tolerance to fluids and foods. The patient's learning needs are also addressed in the recovery phase, and the patient is encouraged to participate in care, as appropriate, in preparation for self-care after discharge. As the patient progresses in recovery, increased independence will, it is hoped, occur. When the patient is ready for discharge, complete discharge directions and instructions for follow-up care are given. These discharge instructions are usually given to both the patient and a family member or significant other.

Impact of Surgery on Functional Health

Surgery can have a significant impact on a person's life. These changes can influence many areas of a person's functional health. This section discusses how these changes can affect functional health and how nurses can make positive contributions toward maximizing a patient's health and function.

Nursing Research

Selected Nursing Research Studies

Biley, F. C. (1989). Nurses' perception of stress in preoperative surgical patients. *Journal of Advocate Nursing, 14*(7), 575–581.

Davis, M. J., et al. (1990). Vital signs of class 1 surgical patients. *Western Journal of Nursing Research, 12*(1), 28–37.

Heidenreich, T., et al. (1990). Postoperative temperature measurement. *Nursing Research, 39*(3), 153–155.

Mansorn, A. M. (1989). Needlestick injuries in the OR: Facts and preventions. *Today's OR Nurse, 11*(11), 15–17, 26–28.

Parfitt, J. M. (1990). Humorous preoperative teaching: Effects on recall of postoperative exercise routines. *AORN Journal, 52*(1), 114–120.

Yount, S. T., et al. (1990). Preoperative teaching: A study of nurses' perceptions. *AORN Journal, 51*(2), 572, 574–575, 577–579.

Possible Topics for Nursing Inquiry

- How does preoperative teaching retention compare when preoperative instruction occurred 1 week before surgery versus 1 day before surgery?
- How do antimicrobial showers versus antimicrobial skin scrubs compare in preventing wound infections postoperatively?
- How effective is using music during preoperative period in the sugical holding area to decrease patient anxiety?
- What is the incidence of compliance with leg exercises among postoperative patients?
- What are the effects of parents' presence in the surgical holding area with children under 12 on the family coping postoperatively?
- What are the indicators for proper time to remove skin staples postoperatively to ensure optimal wound healing?
- How useful is hypnotic suggestion in the reduction of postoperative nausea for patients having abdominal surgery?

Health Perception and Health Maintenance

The impact of surgery on health perception and health maintenance can involve many aspects of safety. Safety considerations include both psychological safety and physical safety. Psychological safety is a feeling of comfort, security, and well-being. It can be enhanced by feelings of trust and confidence in the patient's caregivers; nurses can do much to promote these feelings. Providing emotional support and promoting an understanding of procedures greatly facilitates this process. When possible, the person's significant others should be included in the explanation of surgical procedures. Physical safety considerations include safety with anesthesia, safety with medications, chemical and electrical safety, procedural safety, safety with special equipment (such as lasers and radiation units), safety in surgical positioning, and safety in moving and transporting patients.

Exercise and Activity

Depending on the nature of the surgery, the impact of surgery on exercise and activity levels can be significant. Such alterations in activity levels may be either temporary or permanent. The woman who is to have a breast biopsy in an ambulatory surgery center will probably need to curtail her regular activities for only a few hours, whereas the person who is to have an operation on a fractured leg will need to alter activity levels for several weeks to several months, depending on the extent of rehabilitation needed to return the person to his or her previous level of functioning. Both of these patients will experience relatively temporary changes in their activity levels. However, permanent changes in a person's activity level may also occur as a result of surgery. A person who has a leg amputated secondary to trauma or peripheral vascular disease will need to make permanent changes in his or her activity pattern. All three of these patients will benefit greatly from well planned and well executed nursing interventions directed at returning them to their highest possible level of functional activity. Accurate assessments, in-depth patient preparation and teaching (as time allows), excellent technical skills, and intensive follow-up care are all important aspects of providing optimal care for the patient to minimize the adverse effects of surgery on activity level.

Nutrition and Metabolism

Nutrition and metabolic activity are additional areas of functional health that can be significantly altered by surgery. As Chapter 33 discusses, it is beneficial for the patient to be in an optimal nutritional state to undergo surgery safely and successfully. This optimal nutritional state benefits the patient in several ways, including promoting wound healing, increasing resistance to infection, promoting physical and psychological well-being, maintaining an adequate energy level, and maintaining an optimal fluid and electrolyte balance. After surgery, a diet with sufficient amounts of protein and vitamins A and C is especially useful in rebuilding tissues and in promoting wound healing. Adequate amounts of carbohydrates and fat are also important to avoid depleting protein stores.

Additionally, it is necessary to assess the patient having surgery for metabolic disorders, including diabetes, Cushing's syndrome, adrenal disorders, thyroid disorders, renal insufficiency, and steroid or other medication therapies. Preoperatively, it is necessary to perform a thorough assessment of the patient for the presence and extent of these conditions and to provide treatment. This helps to minimize complications both intraoperatively and postoperatively.

Thermoregulation. It is not uncommon for the surgical patient to experience an undesirable alteration in body temperature regulation (Hathaway, 1988). Hypothermia can occur secondary to a number of factors, including decreased ambient temperature in the operating room, vasodilation secondary to the use of certain anesthetic agents, blood loss, prematurity, advanced age, intravenous fluid administration, exposure of body surface area, cool skin preparation solutions, and decreased consciousness leading to a decreased ability to maintain body temperature. There are many interventions that help alleviate body heat loss, including providing warm blankets, using warming blankets (electric), warming skin preparation solutions and intravenous solutions, and minimizing body surface exposure.

Another problem of body temperature alteration is **malignant hyperthermia,** a hypermetabolic state resulting from the use of certain anesthetic agents, including certain inhalation agents and muscle relaxants (Kneedler & Dodge, 1987). It is often fatal, and it is therefore important to identify susceptible patients. It has been identified as an inherited disease and, therefore, those people who have had cases of malignant hyperthermia identified in their families are particularly susceptible. This disease is manifested by a sudden, rapid increase in body temperature (possibly by as much as 1°F per minute). Consequently, in addition to identifying susceptible individuals, it is important to monitor body temperature closely during surgery for all patients, and to have emergency medications and equipment immediately available.

Another example of hyperthermia is fever associated with an infectious process or trauma. It is beneficial to treat an infection before surgery (if possible) to place the patient in the optimal state of health. This promotes healing and lessens the chances that the infection will spread or become systemic. Infection can also occur postoperatively. The patient should be monitored carefully for this potential postoperative complication so that immediate treatment can be instituted.

Elimination

Elimination is another area of functional health that is significantly affected by surgery. Both bladder and bowel elimination can be affected. Before surgery, the patient is usually placed on NPO (nothing by mouth) status. This results in both decreased urinary function and decreased bowel function.

An adequate urinary output indicates adequate renal function and cardiac output. Even when the patient is NPO, the urine output should be *at least* 30 mL per hour (Wells, 1987). The patient may have an indwelling urinary catheter placed in the bladder preoperatively. If a urinary catheter is not in place, the patient should void immediately before going to the operating room to help prevent bladder distention during or after the procedure. Emptying the bladder also helps to make the abdominal organs more visible during abdominal surgery procedures. Intraoperatively, the urinary output is monitored closely for all patients with indwelling catheters. Patients who are undergoing shorter procedures (less than 2 to 4 hours) may not have a urinary catheter. For both patients with urinary catheters and those without, blood pressure and fluid and electrolyte balance are carefully monitored intraoperatively, since these measurements yield helpful information in the evaluation of adequate renal function and adequate fluid circulation. Postoperatively, urinary output should continue to be closely monitored. In this stage, an inadequate output could indicate hypovolemia, hemorrhage, electrolyte imbalance, inadequate circulation, hypoxia, or impending shock. Patients without a urinary catheter should void within 8 hours of the surgical procedure.

Bowel function may also be altered by the surgical experience. When the patient has been placed on NPO status preoperatively, bowel function is less active. In addition, the patient may be required by the physician to have "enemas until clear" or to take laxatives. These help to cleanse the bowel of fecal material. This is especially important for patients undergoing gastrointestinal surgery, to help prevent the possible spillage of bowel contents intraoperatively, which could lead to peritonitis. In the postoperative phase, bowel activity may take several days or longer to resume its normal functioning. This delayed bowel activity is caused by a combination of factors, including decreased food and fluid intake, decreased dietary bulk, pain medications, decreased physical activity, stress, lack of a normal routine, decreased privacy, and decreased intestinal peristalsis.

A complication that can sometimes occur after gastrointestinal surgery is paralytic ileus. Paralytic ileus is a condition in which there is significantly decreased bowel functioning. Intestinal peristalsis may temporarily cease altogether. The bowel becomes distended, is partially paralyzed, and bowel sounds are usually absent. This condition may occur postoperatively secondary to a lack of peristaltic activity partially due to bowel manipulation during surgery. It can be painful to the patient. Paralytic ileus usually responds to treatment with a nasogastric tube, bowel rest, and intravenous therapy (Drain & Cristoph, 1987).

Nursing interventions to assist the patient through these changes in bowel and bladder functioning are important in helping the patient to undergo the surgical procedure successfully and to return to an optimal level of functioning. Some of these interventions may include appropriate patient preparation (both physical and emotional), patient teaching to help the patient and family understand the procedure and the recovery process, administering necessary medications and treatments, helping the patient to rest, promoting comfort, encouraging increased activity as appropriate, and promoting an appropriate diet and fluid intake as tolerated. Additionally, monitoring the patient's vital signs, electrolyte and fluid balance, and appropriate laboratory values is also beneficial to the success of the procedure and the recovery process.

Sleep and Rest

The functional area of sleep and rest can be significantly affected when a person undergoes a surgical procedure. The surgical patient may experience a disruption in normal sleep–rest pattern due to preoperative preparation activities, changes in schedule, stress or anxiety related to the impending procedure, medication therapy, physical or emotional pain, anxiety due to separation from family and significant others, money worries and job uncertainties, and changes in normal diet and activity level. Nursing interventions can be helpful in promoting rest. Some of these interventions include providing a restful environment, relieving patient anxiety through patient teaching and emotional support, making referrals to other health professionals as appropriate (social workers, mental health professionals, financial counselors, chaplains, clinical nurse specialists), and administering medications and treatments as appropriate. It is often helpful to administer a medication to help the patient sleep (sedative) the night before surgery. The patient may also be given a medication to promote rest and relaxation (such as diazepam) as part of the preoperative medication regime.

Postoperatively, adequate sleep and rest are important both for wound healing and emotional well-being. Growth hormone, which promotes protein synthesis and collagen formation, is released in greater amounts during periods of rest (Drain and Cristoph, 1987). Therefore, sufficient rest promotes wound healing. The patient who is able to rest sufficiently and maintain adequate amounts of REM (rapid eye movement) sleep is better able to handle the stress associated with surgery and recovery. Adequate periods of rest and sleep need to be planned, and a quiet, restful environment should be maintained.

Cognition and Perception

Pain perception, confusion, and sensory deficit are three of the areas in which alterations in cognition and perception may be manifested by the surgical patient.

Pain. Pain may be experienced either preoperatively or postoperatively, or both. Pain, which has both a physical component and a psychological component, may occur preoperatively secondary to a disease process or to a traumatic injury. It could also occur postoperatively secondary to a surgical incision or procedure. Psychological pain may manifest itself in the form of stress, anxiety, or actual physical pain associated with a surgical procedure or disease process. Nursing interventions are vital in helping patients to cope with pain. Some of these interventions may include medication therapy, positioning, physical therapy, relaxation techniques, psychological support, distraction techniques, and referrals to other health professionals as appropriate. It is also helpful to maintain a restful and comfortable environment.

Confusion. Confusion may be experienced by patients either preoperatively or postoperatively. Patients may be confused secondary to medication therapy, unfamiliar surroundings and people, sensory overload, electrolyte imbalances, pain, anxiety, or sleep deprivation. Nursing interventions to assist confused patients include orienting and reorienting patients to unfamiliar surroundings and people, maintaining a safe and comfortable environment, promoting increased visual and auditory input (radio, television, calendars, pictures of significant others) during waking hours, promoting a quiet and restful environment during the hours set aside for sleep and rest, and monitoring medication therapy.

Sensory Deficits. Sensory deficits may also contribute to a significant change in normal functioning for the hospitalized patient. As discussed above, confusion may be associated with decreased sensory input. The patient may become confused as to time of day, day of the week, or what year it is. Patients may become forgetful or uncooperative due to lack of stimulation. It is therefore important to promote sensory stimulation. Interventions may include radio, television, diversional activities, reading materials, physical therapy, occupational therapy, exercise classes, informational classes, and various other stimulating activities appropriate to the patient's condition.

Self-Concept

Self-concept is another area of functional health that can be dramatically affected by surgery. Self-concept reflects a person's sense of self-worth, and involves attitudes, feelings, and beliefs. For many people, self-concept may be closely related to physical appearance. Physical appearance may be altered by a surgical procedure. This alteration may be minor, such as a small scar, or it may be major, such as a limb amputation or a radical neck dissection. However, the degree of alteration depends on the patient's perception of it. Surgical alterations may also involve removal of certain organs (such as the uterus, breast, lung, portions of the colon, esophagus, or other organs), which may result in significant emotional and psychological changes. These alterations may affect a person's self-image and self-concept, and may require intensive, long-term rehabilitation, both physical and emotional.

In addition to providing the patient with the necessary technical care, teaching, extensive rehabilitation, and emotional support, nursing interventions may also include referral to agencies and support groups that can be beneficial to the patient after surgery and discharge from the acute-care facility. Some of these groups include the American Cancer Society and its numerous affiliates, the American Heart Association, and the American Red Cross. These organizations can assist with individual and family coping with the change in self-image through support groups. They can also assist with educational needs, financial and housing services, transportation services, and physical care needs. These organizations provide an invaluable service to the patient and the community.

Roles and Relationships

Another important area of functional health that can be affected by a surgical procedure is that of roles and relationships. Personal, family, and business relationships may all be affected by surgery and the separation that surgery may entail. Changes in these relationships may be either temporary or permanent. Procedures from which one quickly recovers generally allow a person to resume previous relationships without any long-range changes or conflicts. Chronic illnesses and major procedures may lead to changes in role relationships which could take considerable time to be adapted to. Secondary to illness, a person may need to make major changes in lifestyle, which could have a major impact on role relationships. Some of the lifestyle changes that may become necessary due to surgery include dietary alterations, medication, changes in activity level and energy level, changes in mobility, changes in sleeping patterns, changes in usual sexual practices, and changes in recreational activities. A prolonged recovery period that necessitates a long separation can be problematic for a person's role as a husband or wife and as a parent. Additionally, a prolonged recovery may create problems in a person's work relationships. In addition to the stress this separation may cause, a person may also be troubled by financial worries.

The appropriate nursing interventions may depend on the specific role relationship that is creating the conflict.

TABLE 23–2

Surgical Procedures Affecting Appearance, Mobility, and Functioning

Physical Appearance	Mobility	Functioning
Radical neck surgery	Bone fractures	Vaginectomy
Mastectomy	Dislocations	Hysterectomy
Amputations	Back surgeries	Prostatectomy
Facial surgeries	Amputations	Ostomies
Oral surgery	Casts, immobilizers	Oral surgeries

Providing the patient and family members with emotional support and appropriate patient teaching can positively affect role relationships. Additionally, it may be beneficial to make a referral to another health team professional, such as financial counselor, mental health professional, nurse specialist, chaplain, rehabilitation specialist, or dietitian.

Coping

Surgery, even minor surgical procedures, entails significant stress. Coping behaviors and stress tolerance are closely related to how a person defines stress and how that person has managed stress in the past. It is important to identify stress management strategies that have been effective in the past, because these strategies may be effective again in the future. It is also important to keep in mind that stress tolerance and coping behaviors are an individual matter, and that what is effective for one person may not be effective for another. Nursing interventions to assist a person in coping and managing stress include identifying and promoting effective stress management strategies and coping behaviors, providing emotional support and patient teaching for the patient and family, and making referrals to other health professionals as necessary.

Sexuality

Sexuality is an area of functional health that may be either temporarily or permanently affected by surgery. Separation, prolonged convalescence, and actual surgical alterations may all significantly affect a person's sexuality and sexual identity. This impact may be physical, psychological, or both. Physical changes that may affect a person's sexuality include surgeries that alter physical appearance, surgeries that limit mobility, surgeries that alter reproductive capacity, and surgeries that limit physiologic functioning.

Table 23-2 lists surgeries that may affect a person's physical appearance, mobility, and functioning. Some of these changes are permanent, whereas others are temporary. Although any of the surgeries listed may affect a person's psychological as well as physical functioning, some have been noted to be particularly significant in regard to sexual functioning. These surgeries include ostomies, urinary diversion procedures, mastectomies, hysterectomies, and prostatectomies. In addition, some procedures may lead to impotence in men. These procedures include certain types of prostatectomies, orchiectomies, and certain urinary diversion procedures. While these procedures may leave a man impotent, surgically corrective procedures may be available to restore sexual functioning.

In terms of nursing interventions, it is important for the patient to be fully informed of options regarding surgery or alternative forms of treatment. Additional nursing interventions include performing a thorough assessment of the potential sexual or psychological impact, and providing patient teaching, technical skills, emotional support, and referrals as appropriate. It is also important for the patient to understand clearly the depth and scope of any limitations imposed by the surgical procedure. It can sometimes be uncomfortable for the patient to discuss sexual matters with the nurse or physician. Therefore, it is important for the nurse or physician to create as open and comfortable an environment as possible, and initiate discussion when appropriate.

Values and Beliefs

The value–belief system is significant in that it guides our personal choices and life decisions. Important aspects of the value–belief system are a person's cultural background, philosophy, and religious orientation. These aspects of a person's belief system affect the choices made with regard to surgery and treatment options. There are many examples of how the value–belief system may affect surgical decisions. One example is that of abortion. The decision as to whether or not to have an abortion is significantly affected by a person's cultural and religious beliefs. Another example is that of blood transfusions. Some religions prohibit their members from receiving blood products. This is a significant factor for a person who has experienced major trauma, major blood loss, or major surgery. Choices a person is required to make should be made only when the person is fully informed of the alternatives and the expected consequences of any decisions. After arrival at a decision, the person needs expert care, knowledgeable teaching, and emotional support. Additionally, the services of the chaplain may also be useful at this time. Even if the health professional disagrees with the person's decision, it is important to remain nonjudgmental and supportive.

Lifespan Considerations

People undergoing surgical procedures have different needs related to their age and developmental level. For each of these needs, it is important for the nurse to make appropriate assessments and to plan and perform the appropriate interventions.

Newborn and Infant

For the newborn or infant, the separation from his or her parents during a surgical experience may be a traumatic situation. The infant's ability to understand what is going on is limited, and he or she may perceive it as a strange, frightening, and lonely experience. It is therefore important for the nurse to hold the infant caringly, to provide a stuffed animal or other toy as appropriate, and to promote a calm, comfortable environment. It is also important to provide careful explanations to the parents and to include them in the care of the infant as much as possible.

There are also significant physiologic factors to consider when performing surgery on an infant. The infant's ability to tolerate blood loss and alterations in temperature is significantly less than an adult's (Hathaway, 1988). It is therefore mandatory to monitor these two factors closely and to make every attempt to minimize both blood loss and heat loss from the body. Additionally, an infant's skin is sensitive, and it is important to select skin preparation solutions, tape, and dressings that are gentle to the skin. Instruments, equipment, and medications are another important consideration. All of these items need to be appropriate to the infant's size and physiologic status.

Toddler and Preschooler

Many of the same factors that apply to the infant also apply to the toddler or preschooler age group. At this age, separation anxiety may be more significant because the child is more aware of his or her surroundings. Although the child has an expanded capacity to understand what is going on, the situation may still be perceived as frightening and lonely. It is important to provide careful explanations to the parents and to elicit their cooperation as needed. It is useful to have all instruments and equipment ready in the operating room before the child is brought in. This helps shorten the waiting time before anesthetic induction and helps to maintain a calm, quiet environment. It may also be useful to have the parents hold the child while medications are being administered. Another method of medication administration sometimes used to help a child undergo anesthesia is to insert medication as a suppository to promote relaxation and anesthesia before the child is brought into the operating room. This causes sufficient relaxation so that other procedures are not perceived as quite so frightening. If possible, it is also helpful to remove the child's clothing, apply the grounding pad, and apply the monitors after the child is asleep. As with the infant, it is important to use instruments and equipment that are of appropriate size and medications that are of appropriate dosage. Again, as with the infant, minimizing blood loss and temperature loss are significant factors in promoting a safe and efficient surgical experience.

Another important consideration for both the infant and the toddler is the planning of a safe recovery phase. A crib with siderails can be useful in helping to provide a safe environment. Sometimes, soft restraints may also be useful. It is important to monitor the child's airway and vital signs carefully, and to keep the child warm. It is also useful in many situations to have the child's parents in the recovery room as the child regains awareness of surroundings. This helps to keep the child calm and help ensure cooperation with the necessary procedures.

Child and Adolescent

Older children, including school-aged children and adolescents, may have an increased understanding of surgery and many of the activities that a surgical procedure will entail. They benefit (along with their parents) from a more detailed preoperative teaching program. Many hospitals now include a tour of the operating room for school-aged children and adolescents. The child who has seen the operating room, the operating table, the anesthesia machine, and the mask used to administer an anesthetic is generally not as frightened as the child who has not had this experience. The child can be involved in the administration of anesthesia by holding the mask or counting as the anesthesia is administered. Simple choices, such as which arm the child would prefer the intravenous (IV) tube in, may help to give the child a better sense of control. The older child is more likely to cope better with separation from parents than the infant or preschooler.

The adolescent having surgery also has special needs. Teenagers often are concerned with body image and possible disfigurement. Adolescents may vary markedly in their ability to cope with the stress of the surgical experience. In striving toward attaining identity and independence, the adolescent may attempt to hide feelings. In addition to providing extensive teaching both to the adolescent and their family, it is important for the nurse to demonstrate support and acceptance of the adolescent's feelings and behavior.

For children of all ages, it is important to prepare instruments, supplies, and equipment with the size of the child or adolescent in mind. The dosages of medications to be given also depend on the young person's size and weight, and should be calculated accordingly.

Adult and Older Adult

Considerations previously discussed in the section on the impact of surgery on functional health patterns apply to many adults and older adults. Additionally, certain adults may require special considerations when having surgery, due to visual alterations, auditory alterations, altered mobility, or alterations imposed by chronic disease.

When the adult is visually impaired, it is helpful for the patient to keep glasses on until just before anesthesia is administered. Visual orientation helps to decrease fear and gain confidence. Contact lenses should be removed before transport to the operating room. Visual impairment should be noted on the chart, so that operating room personnel are aware of this significant deficit.

Elderly patients may also have hearing impairments. It is important to allow the hearing-impaired adult to keep hearing aids on, or to speak in a loud voice until anesthesia is delivered. Being able to hear members of the health-care team helps to alleviate fear, help ensure successful teaching, and help keep the patient oriented to the environment.

Patients with altered mobility may require individualized planning for positioning during the surgical experience. Special considerations may be necessary when the patient has limited joint mobility, obesity, extreme thinness or fragility, or back problems. Specific positions necessary for surgical procedures (such as the lithotomy, prone, and side-lying positions) may require modification or the use of special padding, positioning devices, or restraints to assist in the maintenance of required positions.

Alterations imposed by chronic illness, which frequently are present in older adults, require specific planning and special monitoring during the surgical experience. Respiratory insufficiency and cardiovascular problems may affect a person's ability to tolerate certain anatomic positions (e.g., head-down positions may impede breathing for a person with respiratory problems). Kidney or liver dysfunction can affect excretion and metabolism of anesthetic agents. The elderly person with severe chronic organ dysfunction is a greater surgical risk, permitting only essential surgical procedures.

PREOPERATIVE NURSING

The preoperative phase begins when the decision for surgery is made and ends when the patient arrives in the operating room. The nurse uses the nursing process to individualize and provide safe care during this period.

Nursing Assessment

Nursing assessment during the preoperative phase is critical because it provides information that directly affects the patient's safety and well-being throughout the entire surgical experience. The nurse assesses the patient in each of the functional health patterns. This data collection process includes obtaining information from a number of sources, including the interview and physical assessment of the patient, information from the history and physical examination, information from diagnostic studies and laboratory reports, and information obtained directly from physicians, nurses, and other health professionals.

Some of the most significant information to be assessed from the patient's medical chart includes the hematology report, allergy history, chronic disease history, current cardiovascular and respiratory status, history of past surgeries and anesthesia, height and weight, and the results of diagnostic studies. The rationale for obtaining this data preoperatively is given in Table 23-3.

The collection of physical data is an integral part of the preoperative assessment for many health-care providers. The physician completes an in-depth medical history and physical examination of the patient. The anesthesiologist, or in many cases the nurse anesthetist, completes a preanesthetic assessment form, such as the example given in Figure 23-1. Data collected on this form are particularly important and useful to the anesthesia department in preparing to administer the selected anesthetic agents in a safe and prudent manner. The nurse also completes an in-depth interview and physical assessment of the patient during the preoperative period. Information obtained assists the nurse in identifying potential and actual nursing diagnoses and individualizing the perioperative nursing care.

Another important focus of the preoperative assessment is the learning needs of the patient and the family. Patient teaching is begun during the preoperative period, but teaching is significant to a positive surgical experience during all phases of the surgical experience. Table 23-4 lists factors to be assessed when formulating a teaching plan for the perioperative patient.

Nursing Diagnoses and Patient Goals

Preoperative nursing assessment allows the nurse to identify potential and actual problems for the surgical patient. Common problems for the patient before surgery include knowledge deficit, ineffective individual coping, pain, and sleep pattern disturbance. These problems, stated as nursing diagnoses, are listed in Table 23-5, along with appropriate patient-centered goals.

Nursing Interventions

Nursing interventions in the preoperative period include patient teaching, ensuring informed consent, and adequate physical and psychological preparation of the patient.

TABLE 23–3
Preoperative Assessment Data

Assessment Data	Rationale
Interview and Physical Assessment	
Proposed surgery	To individualize patient teaching and preoperative preparation
History of previous surgery	To recognize and avoid problems encountered in previous surgery
History of allergies	To avoid administering medications that would elicit an allergic response
Patient preferences	To provide individualized care, decrease stress, and avoid potential problems
Chronic disease history	To provide competent care and necessary medications for patients with chronic conditions, including diabetes, thyroid disorders, cardiac arrhythmias, cancer, respiratory insufficiency, renal insufficiency, and bleeding disorders
Smoking history	To identify increased risk for postoperative respiratory complications
Current respiratory and cardiac status	To assess for safe anesthetic and medication administration, to minimize postoperative complications
Current height and weight	To determine body surface area for calculating proper drug dosage
Vital signs	To detect abnormalities and provide baseline data
Mobility restriction	To plan for patient's surgical positioning needs and safe transport
Laboratory and Diagnostic Test Data	
Blood studies (hematocrit, hemoglobin, WBC, sodium, potassium, coagulation studies)	To evaluate patient for actual or potential problems with anemia, infection, fluid and electrolyte imbalance, cardiac arrhythmias, or bleeding disorders
Urinalysis	To evaluate for adequate renal function and the absence of urinary tract infection
Electrocardiogram	To evaluate for normal cardiac function and the absence of cardiac arrhythmias
Chest x-ray	To evaluate respiratory status
Type and cross-match	To identify blood type and match with potential donor blood should a transfusion of blood be necessary

Preoperative Teaching

Preoperative teaching helps patients understand what will occur during each phase of the surgical process and how they can participate in their own recovery. Additionally, preoperative teaching helps decrease the patient's anxiety. Preoperative teaching should include a general orientation and explanation of the surgical experience. Discussion of preoperative activities to ready the patient for surgery and postoperative care to help promote optimal postoperative function and recovery should be included. Whenever possible, family members should be included in the preoperative teaching sessions.

Preoperative teaching often takes place after the patient has been admitted to the surgical unit. The trend in recent years has been to admit a greater number of patients on the morning of surgery. When this happens,

there is often little time available for patient teaching, and the patient may be anxious and unable to process the information given. Some surgical centers have patients preadmitted a few days or a week before their scheduled surgery. In an outpatient setting, the nurse can begin preoperative teaching, in addition to obtaining a nursing history and necessary laboratory specimens. Audiovisual material may be available for the patient to view. Frequently, the patient is sent home with written material explaining what will happen before, during, and after surgery, and how the patient can best help in his or her own surgical recovery. When the patient is admitted for surgery, any questions can be answered.

General Information. General orientation to the surgical experience should include:

DATE	TIME	WARD	HR	BP	R	T	WT(Kg)	HT

DIAGNOSIS

PROPOSED OPERATION

ALLERGIES

MEDICATIONS

HISTORY

FAMILY HISTORY

PREVIOUS ANESTHETICS

PERTINENT PHYSICAL EXAM.

RELEVANT LAB/EKG/X-RAY RESULTS

ANESTHESIA PLAN

ASA   1   2   3   4   5   E

PLAN AND RISKS DISCUSSED WITH PATIENT   Y   N

PATIENT CONSENTS TO PLAN   Y   N

AMOUNT BLOOD ORDERED

PREMEDICATION

SIGNATURE

SIGNATURE

UNIVERSITY OF WASHINGTON HOSPITALS
HARBORVIEW MEDICAL CENTER
UNIVERSITY OF WASHINGTON MEDICAL CENTER
SEATTLE, WASHINGTON

PRE-ANESTHETIC ASSESSMENT

WHITE—MED. RECORD
CANARY—DEPT. COPY
PINK—RESIDENT COPY

UH 0004   REV MAR 89

Figure 23–1. Example of a preanesthetic form.

TABLE 23–4

Preoperative Patient Learning Assessment

Assessment	Rationale
Review history and physical, nursing history, and lab values; consult with health-care professionals; interview patient	This information will provide the data base that is imperative in developing a plan and providing competent care
Assess patient and family's readiness to learn	A receptive patient and family will retain more information
Assess patient's cognitive level	This will help to determine appropriate teaching techniques and depth of content
Assess patient's environment	An appropriate learning environment which is stress-free, relaxed, and comfortable will enhance learning
Assess patient's current knowledge level regarding surgical procedure and preoperative and postoperative care	This assessment information will help determine appropriate level of teaching

- The expected time the procedure will begin
- How long it will take
- When the patient will probably return to his or her room
- Where the family and friends of the patient can wait during the surgery
- How the patient will be transported to the operating room
- What type of medications and anesthesia will be administered
- Other factors specific to the surgical procedure.

If the patient will be transferred to an intensive care unit after surgery, a tour of the unit is often provided for the patient and family.

Preoperative Protocols. The nurse should fully explain all preoperative activities and the reason they are important for a successful surgical outcome. Explanations should be provided for any procedure that must be performed preoperatively, such as bowel preparation, skin preparation, and the insertion of urinary or intra-venous catheters or nasogastric tubes. The patient should be informed of any dietary or fluid restrictions, including NPO status.

Postoperative Protocols. Preoperative teaching also provides the patient with information concerning what conditions will be like after surgery. Frequently, patients have many specific questions such as "How much pain will I have?" or "What will my scar look like?" It is often better to ask patients what questions or concerns they have about their upcoming surgery and to deal with these issues before proceeding with the information that should be presented to each surgical patient.

Preoperatively, it is helpful to explain to the patient what tubes (IVs, catheters, nasogastric tubes) will be in place during the postoperative period, the size and location of the incision, what medications will be ordered to control pain and nausea, and activities that the patient will participate in to promote recovery and prevent complications.

The patient should be taught and given time to demonstrate turning, deep breathing, using the incentive

TABLE 23–5

Selected Preoperative Nursing Diagnoses and Patient Goals

Nursing Diagnosis	Patient Goal
Knowledge deficit; regarding perioperative procedures and diagnostic studies related to lack of instruction	Patient will verbalize understanding of perioperative care
Ineffective individual coping related to anxiety and stress associated with the impending surgical procedure	Patient will demonstrate effective coping before, during, and after surgery
Pain related to disease process or injury	Patient will experience adequate control of pain
Sleep pattern disturbance related to preoperative activities and anxiety	Patient will maintain sufficient rest prior to surgery

spirometer, coughing, getting out of bed using good body mechanics, performing leg exercises, and (when appropriate) using a patient-controlled analgesia (PCA) machine. Since these procedures are frequently used for a wide variety of patients in addition to the surgical

---

Patient Teaching

Instruct the patient as follows:

- Familiarize yourself with the following information: what time surgery is scheduled, how long it will take, how long you will be in the recovery facility, and where family members should wait during the surgery.
- Do not drink or eat anything after midnight of the evening before surgery (or as designated by the physician's order).
- Make sure you understand everything involved in preoperative preparation (e.g., antimicrobial scrubs, enemas).
- Tell the nurse when you are uncomfortable or nauseous, because the physician will order something for pain and nausea as needed (PRN) following surgery.
- Have the nurse explain the reason for any tubes, drains or catheters (IVs, NG tubes, hemovacs) that may be in place during the postoperative period.
- Practice preoperatively turning, deep breathing, coughing, leg exercises, and how to get out of bed.
- Practice (under the nurse's guidance) using any special equipment that will be used during the postoperative period (e.g., incentive spirometer, PCA [patient-controlled analgesia machine]).

---

patient, specific guidelines are included in appropriate clinical chapters; these are listed in Table 23-6

Informed Consent

The informed consent obtained before any surgical procedure is an important medical legal document. In most hospitals it is the responsibility of the surgeon to explain fully the proposed surgical procedure to the patient and obtain informed consent. Informed consent is part of the physician's legal responsibility, which involves providing the patient with all the information needed to make the decision to undergo surgery. This information needs to be discussed in language the patient can understand. If the patient does not speak or understand the physician's language, an interpreter should be used. The information that the surgeon usually discusses includes describing the proposed surgery, the possible risks and benefits of the procedure, the reason why the surgery is indicated, the probability of success, the consequences of nonsurgical treatment or no treatment, and any other information that will help the patient reach an informed decision. The patient also has the right to ask any questions, and to withdraw consent at any point before the surgery begins. An example of a consent form appears in Figure 23-2.

The nurse may also be involved in obtaining consent, usually by witnessing the signature of patient on the consent document. The nurse should be knowledgeable concerning the agency's policy regarding informed consent, and ensure that this policy is strictly followed. If the patient seems unsure or indicates lack of understanding, the nurse should notify the physician so that more information can be provided. It is the responsibility of the nurse to make sure the informed consent contains all correct, necessary information, is properly signed and witnessed, and is part of the patient's medical record before the surgical procedure.

In addition to the proposed procedure, the consent form also lists the name of the surgeon and assisting surgeons, possible complications (e.g., hemorrhage,

---

TABLE 23–6

Preoperative Patient Teaching of Postoperative Protocols

Procedure	Rationale	Related Chapter
Turning, getting out of bed	Improve postoperative mobility to mimimize impact of immobility	Chapter 29: Body Mechanics and Mobility
Deep breathing, coughing, use of incentive spirometer	Improve postoperative gas exchange and prevent respiratory complications	Chapter 30: Oxygenation: Respiratory Function
Leg exercises	Improve venous return and prevent deep venous thrombosis postoperatively	Chapter 31: Oxygenation: Cardiac Function and Tissue Perfusion
Using patient-controlled analgesia	Optimal pain control postoperatively	Chapter 40: Pain Perception and Comfort

I HEREBY AUTHORIZE DR. _J.I Montgomery_ , AND SUCH ASSISTANTS AS MAY BE DESIGNATED, TO PERFORM:

Appendectomy
(NAME OF TREATMENT PROCEDURE)

AND ANY OTHER RELATED PROCEDURES OR FORMS OF TREATMENT, INCLUDING APPROPRIATE ANESTHESIA, TRANSFUSIONS THAT THEY DEEM NECESSARY FOR THE WELFARE OF_____

Melissa Conroy
(NAME OF PATIENT)

I CONSENT TO THE ADMINISTRATION OF ANESTHESIA AND/OR SUCH DRUGS AS MAY BE NECESSARY. I UNDERSTAND THAT ALL ANESTHETICS INVOLVE RISKS OF COMPLICATION, SERIOUS INJURY, OR, RARELY, DEATH FROM BOTH KNOWN AND UNKNOWN CAUSES.

I CONSENT TO THE EXAMINATION AND RETENTION FOR SCIENTIFIC PURPOSES AND STUDY BY THE UNIVERSITY OF WASHINGTON MEDICAL STAFF OF ALL TISSUES AND ORGANS REMOVED DURING THE COURSE OF THE ABOVE TREATMENT WITH PRIVILEGE OF ULTIMATE DISPOSAL RESTING WITH SAID MEDICAL STAFF.

I UNDERSTAND THAT THE EXPECTED RESULTS OF SAID TREATMENT CANNOT BE GUARANTEED. THE PHYSICIANS, SURGEONS, OR DENTISTS OF THE UNIVERSITY OF WASHINGTON HAVE DISCUSSED TO MY SATISFACTION THE FOLLOWING:

A. THE NATURE AND CHARACTER OF THE PROPOSED TREATMENT/PROCEDURE.

B. THE ANTICIPATED RESULTS OF THE PROPOSED TREATMENT/PROCEDURE.

C. THE RECOGNIZED ALTERNATIVE FORMS OF TREATMENT/PROCEDURE.

D. THE RECOGNIZED SERIOUS POSSIBLE RISKS, AND COMPLICATIONS OF THE TREATMENT/PROCEDURE AND OF THE RECOGNIZED ALTERNATIVE FORMS OF TREATMENT/PROCEDURE, INCLUDING NON-TREATMENT.

E. THE ANTICIPATED DATE AND TIME OF THE PROPOSED TREATMENT/PROCEDURE.

MY PHYSICIAN HAS OFFERED TO ANSWER ALL INQUIRIES CONCERNING THE PROPOSED TREATMENT/PROCEDURE. I UNDERSTAND THAT I AM FREE TO WITHHOLD OR WITHDRAW CONSENT TO THE PROPOSED TREATMENT/PROCEDURE AT ANY TIME.

WITNESS	SIGNATURE OF PERSON GIVING CONSENT
J.I Montgomery, M.D.	_Melissa Conroy_
DATE SIGNED _1/20/92_ TIME _12:45_ ☐ A.M. ☒ P.M.	RELATIONSHIP TO PATIENT (If Applicable)

☐ PLEASE CHECK IF THIS IS A TELEPHONE MONITORED CONSENT.

NO TREATMENT WILL BE PERFORMED UNTIL THIS CONSENT HAS BEEN EXECUTED. THIS CONSENT WILL BE PERMANENTLY FILED IN THE PATIENT'S MEDICAL RECORD.

UNIVERSITY OF WASHINGTON HOSPITALS

HARBORVIEW MEDICAL CENTER
UNIVERSITY HOSPITAL

SPECIAL CONSENT TO TREATMENT
(DIAGNOSTIC & SURGICAL PROCEDURES, ANESTHESIA,)
(MEDICAL TREATMENT & OTHER PROCEDURES)

UH 0173   REV JAN 83   • 1-83-617

Figure 23–2.   Example of a consent form.

nerve palsies, loss of function, coma, death), alternative treatments, and consequences of nontreatment. The consent should specifically list the surgical site (e.g., the left or right eye, knee, kidney, or ear). The consent needs to be signed and dated by the surgeon, the patient, and a witness. If the patient is underage, or not mentally or physically competent to give consent, the consent needs to be obtained from the patient's parents, spouse, legal guardian, or next-of-kin. It is important that the patient not take any medications that might alter judgment or perception before the consent is signed. Many drugs that are commonly administered as preoperative medications, such as narcotics or barbiturates, can alter cognitive abilities and invalidate informed consent.

Patient Preparation

The nurse is responsible for preparing the patient physically and emotionally to ensure optimal condition for the surgical experience. Patient preparation includes the following, as ordered by the physician or indicated by agency policy: placing the patient on NPO status, starting an intravenous line, placing a nasogastric tube, preparing the intestinal tract, preparing the skin, and administering preoperative medications.

NPO Status. Food and fluids are restricted for any patient receiving a general anesthetic. The patient is usually put on NPO status after midnight of the evening before surgery, or, if the surgery is scheduled for late in the day, the patient is NPO for 8 hours before the scheduled surgery. It is important for the patient to have an empty stomach to help ensure safe anesthetic administration and prevent aspiration. If the surgical patient is receiving important medications (antihypertensive agents, anticonvulsant agents, antiarrhythmic agents) that should not be suddenly discontinued, the nurse should clarify with the physician how and if these medications should be administered. Some physicians permit medications to be taken with a sip of water in certain situations, whereas other situations necessitate giving important medications parenterally. Insulin orders for diabetic patients should also be clarified.

Intravenous Access. Intravenous access in any surgical patient is important to provide fluid and electrolyte replacement and provide access to administer intravenous medications. Vascular access may be through a peripheral line or a central line, or in certain cases both may be indicated. The IV may be started in the preoperative period to ensure adequate hydration status. For those patients who are well hydrated, IV insertion may be delayed until the patient is in the operating room. For any surgical patient, a large-gauge (e.g., 18) intravenous device should be used in case a blood transfusion is necessary during the surgery or postoperative period.

Nasogastric Decompression. For selected surgical patients, a nasogastric tube may be inserted to decompress stomach contents. Nasogastric decompression may be necessary for patients who have not been NPO before surgery, due to the sudden onset of their problem. Nasogastric decompression is also indicated when surgery is performed on the stomach or the intestines.

Bowel Preparation. Enemas, suppositories, laxatives, and antibiotics (e.g., neomycin) may be given preoperatively to help cleanse and sterilize the colon. This is done to decrease the possibility of bowel content spillage intraoperatively, which could lead to peritonitis and other complications. Bowel preparation is most important when surgery is performed on the intestines, but is often necessary for general abdominal surgery.

Skin Preparation. The purpose of skin preparation preoperatively is to decrease the number of microorganisms present on the skin, thus decreasing the chance of infection. Depending on the type of surgery, the hospital policy, and the surgeon's preference, the patient may need shaving, clipping of body hair, scrubbing of the surgical area, or showering with antimicrobial soap. Usually, the skin preparation focuses on the area that will be involved in the surgery itself, and wide margins around that area. Common sites of skin preparation are illustrated in Figure 23-3. A surgical "prep," or shaving the hair in the affected area, was a common preoperative procedure until recently. Shaving hair on or near the surgical site is no longer recommended, since tiny breaks in skin integrity can increase the risk of infection postoperatively. It has recently been recommended by the Centers for Disease Control that hair be clipped or a depilatory cream used for removal (Garner, 1986). When shaving is necessary, it is usually done in the operating room immediately before the surgical procedure, since surgical shaves performed hours before the procedure are associated with increased incidence of infection.

Preoperative Medications. A sedative is often ordered the evening before surgery to help decrease anxiety and induce sleep. Preoperative medications given just before surgery may be given for a number of purposes, including to promote relaxation, to decrease nasal and salivary secretions, to assist anesthetic delivery, to relieve pain, and to promote sedation. The trend in recent years has been to give fewer medications preoperatively, except for antibiotics. When giving any preoperative medication, it is important to administer the medication on time so that maximum effect can be coordinated with the time of surgery. The preoperative medications are usually ordered to be given "on call" (when the operating room calls and says to administer the medication) from the operating room. The aim is that the medication be given approximately 1 hour before the surgical procedure ac-

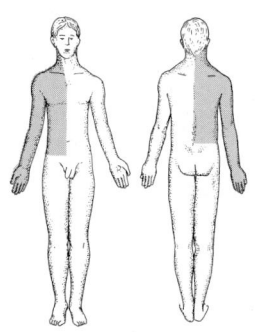

Shoulder prep. Shave fingertips to hairline, midline chest to midline spine on operative side, and to iliac crest, including axilla.

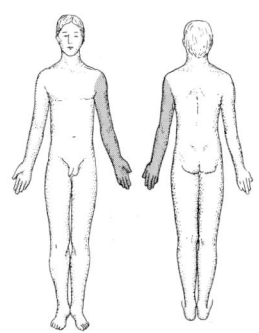

Hand prep. Shave fingertips to shoulder. Trim and clean fingernails. Use brush on hand and nails.

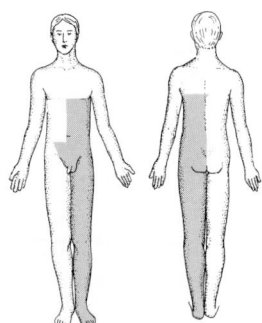

Hip prep. Shave toes to nipple line and at least 3 inches beyond midline back and front. Complete pubic shave. Clean and trim toenails. Use brush on foot and nails. Hip fractures—all preps done in the operating room.

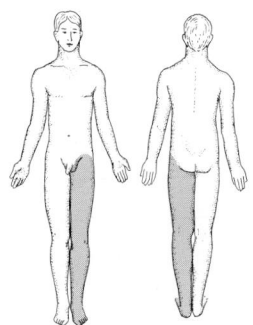

Knee and lower leg prep. Shave entire leg, toes to groin. Clean and trim toenails. Use brush on foot and nails.

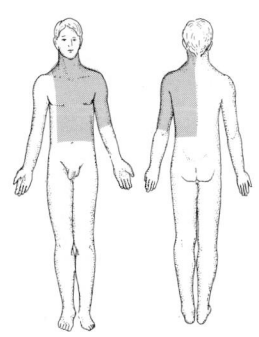

Mastectomy prep. Shave from upper neck to iliac crest, from nipple line on unaffected side to midline of back (affected side). Prep axilla and entire arm to elbow on affected side.

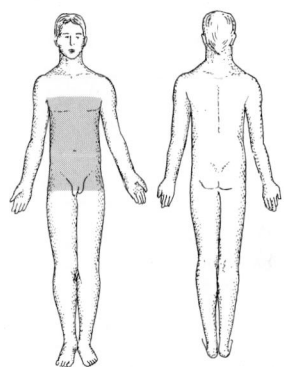

Abdominal prep. Shave from 3 inches above the nipple line to upper thighs, including pubis.

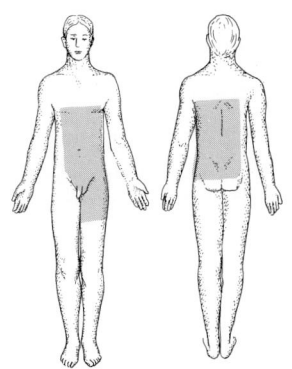

Flank prep (as for renal procedures, adrenalectomy, sympathectomy). Shave from nipple line to pubis and 3 inches beyond the midline in back. Shave pubic area. Shave upper thigh on the affected side.

Figure 23–3. Common sites of preoperative skin preparation.

tually begins, so that optimal drug blood levels will occur during the surgery (Gruendemann & Meeker, 1987). Whenever medications that can impede cognition are administered, the patient is kept in bed with the side-rails up.

Preoperative Checklist

Many hospitals use a preoperative checklist on the day of surgery to summarize the patient's preoperative preparation and ensure that all information is in the patient's

PREOPERATIVE CHECK LIST

Insert this list in the front of the chart when operation is scheduled.
EACH ITEM must be checked by unit R.N. and O.R. R.N. If not applicable, write NA.
When completed by O.R. R.N., place check list under Report of Operations.

DATE:	UNIT	SURGERY (Initial Only)	COMMENTS/INSTRUCTIONS
1. Pre-op teaching _____			
2. ID band correct and on unaffected side _____			
3. Allergies/sensitivities YES___ NO___ Band on YES___ NO___			Allergy sticker on front of chart.
4. Consent signed & witnessed _____			No abbreviations
Sterilization consent signed and witnessed _____			
5. H & P: chart___ dictated_____			
6. Old chart sent to surgery_____			
7. Lab: Hct:____ K+____ if ordered Other _____			If abnormal K+, write in red.
8. NPO Status: Date and time of last food_____ last fluid_____			
9. Blood: In lab _____ Autologous _____ UWB _____ URBC _____ Type & Hold _____			
10. EKG (60 or over) Yes ___ No___			
11. Chest x-ray YES____ NO____			
12. Voided: Time_____ Foley _____			
13. Vital signs charted _____ Wts charted, if ordered _____			
14. Preop Meds Given Yes___ NO___ CABG Pt. on O$_2$, Yes___ NO___ Versed given Yes___ NO___ Resp. rate charted Yes___ NO___			
15. Removed\Noted Dentures ____ Contacts____ Hearing Aids____ Make-Up ____ Jewelry ____ Glasses ____ Clothing ____			CABG patients MUST have rings removed.
16. Additional Information: Blind ____ Deaf____ Need interpreter _____ Prep on unit ____ Pacemaker ____			Note mobility problems
17. Family notified of time change_____ Family directed to waiting area _____			Note which waiting area
18. Addressograph on chart_____			

Final chart check and chart placed in unit designated location.

Time Checked _____ Staff Nurse Signature _____

Transportation: Time Left Unit _____
                Time Arrived in OR _____

Transporter Signature _____

Final chart check by OR R.N. Signature _____

6000-70CP (1/89)   **REVISED (1/90)**

Figure 23–4. Example of a preoperative checklist.

record before transport to the operating room. Figure 23-4 is an example of a preoperative checklist. The checklist usually includes the information listed in Table 23-7. The preoperative checklist provides a quick check to make sure that all patient preparation activities have been completed. The nurse usually checks off each item as it is completed, and then signs the form in the appropriate place. It is important for the nurse to make sure that all activities that require the patient to be out of bed (such as showering and voiding before surgery) are accomplished before any preoperative medications that can alter the level of consciousness are administered. After such medications are given, the patient should be instructed to stay in bed with the siderails up. This helps ensure patient safety, since dizziness or disorientation could occur after such medications have been administered. When all the preparation for surgery has been completed, the preoperative checklist filled, and documentation completed according to agency protocol, the patient is ready for transport to the operating room.

Evaluation

During the preoperative evaluation, the nurse determines whether the patient's preoperative goals were met. As the nurse performs interventions in the preoperative phase, continual evaluation of the patient's response occurs and is documented in the patient's chart. This information is essential in formulating an individualized plan of care for succeeding phases in the surgical experience.

Selected outcome criteria are provided for each of the general preoperative patient goals.

Goal
Patient will verbalize understanding of perioperative care.

Possible Outcome Criteria
- Patient asks questions about impending surgical procedure during preoperative preparation.
- During preoperative preparation, patient describes what will happen during surgery.
- After teaching, patient demonstrates effective turning, coughing, deep breathing, and leg exercises, and states why they are important in postoperative recovery.

Goal
Patient will demonstrate effective coping regarding stress of surgery.

Possible Outcome Criteria
- During preoperative teaching, patient discusses fears and concerns regarding the surgical procedure.
- Patient verbalizes decreased fear and anxiety after patient teaching.
- Patient verbalizes coping strategies or support system to be used to control stress and anxiety of surgical experience.

Goal
Patient will demonstrate adequate control of pain.

Possible Outcome Criteria
- Patient verbalizes an acceptable pain level during the preoperative period.
- Patient completes presurgical activities without limitation due to pain.

TABLE 23–7
Information on a Preoperative Checklist

Types of Information	Rationale
Allergies	To prevent allergic reactions
Current vital signs	To provide preoperative vital sign baseline
Units of blood available	To enable blood transfusion to take place in the event of blood loss
Preoperative medications given	To ensure preoperative relaxation and other desired medication effects will occur
Jewelry and dentures removed	Jewelry and dentures are removed to prevent their loss or damage and promote patient safety during surgery
Skin preparation completed	To document the completion of antimicrobial scrubs and shaving to help prevent infection
Availability of x-rays	To document availability since x-rays are used by the surgical team
Availability of past records (old chart)	To document availability since these records are often needed as reference by the surgical team
Voided	To help prevent intraoperative or postoperative bladder distention
Valuables secured	To prevent damage or loss of patient's valuables
Nurses' signature	To document the completion of all required preoperative activities

Goal
Patient will maintain sufficient rest before surgery.

Possible Outcome Criteria
- Patient verbalizes feeling adequately rested morning of surgery.
- Patient maintains a restful sleep the night before surgery, as observed by the nurse during the night.
- Patient participates in normal presurgical activities without feeling excessive fatigue, as observed by the nurse.

INTRAOPERATIVE NURSING

The intraoperative phase begins when the patient is transferred into the holding area of the operating room (Fig. 23-5), and ends when the patient is transferred to the designated recovery facility (ambulatory recovery facility, recovery room, or intensive care unit). In the intraoperative phase, the nurse continues to individualize care through use of the nursing process.

The nurse should provide a warm, caring environment and offer appropriate emotional support. In some hospitals, a limited number of family members may stay in the holding area with the patient until the patient is transferred into the operating room.

Nursing Assessment

Assessment is continual in the intraoperative period because of the dynamic status of the patient and the potential for serious complications. Assessment begins when the patient is brought to the holding area and continues throughout the surgical procedure. In addition to planning for the intraoperative needs of the patient, assessment allows the nurse to begin to plan for the recovery phase of the surgical experience. It is the responsibility of the operating room nurse to communicate specific assessment data to the recovery facility, so that the patient's individualized needs can be anticipated.

In the holding area, final assessments of the patient before surgery are completed. The holding area nurse and the operating room nurse will check the following: the patient's name band, that jewelry and dentures have been removed, patient's allergies, appropriate dress of the patient, surgical consent obtained, NPO status, appropriate records and paperwork, laboratory and diagnostic study results on the chart, blood availability, preoperative medication administration, and any additional physician's orders.

When the patient arrives in the operating room, the operating room nurse reviews the patient's record, noting diagnostic studies, medical and nursing history, vital signs, and laboratory values (hematocrit, hemoglobin, white blood count, electrolyte values). A brief assess-

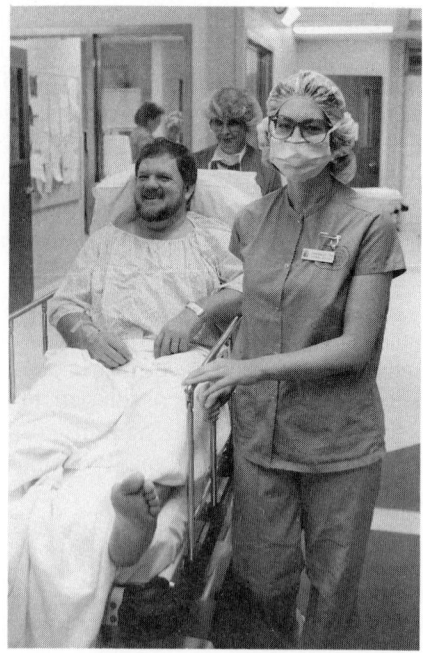

Figure 23–5. The patient is transferred from his unit to the holding room before admission to the actual operating room. In the holding area further assessments are made by the nurse.

ment is conducted to determine the patient's physical and emotional status. Tubes such as intravenous lines and urinary catheter are checked for patency. The comfort and pain level of the patient is determined, as well as his or her communication ability, emotional needs, and ability to cope with the planned surgery. Any questions the patient may have are identified and answered.

During surgery, continual assessment takes place. All patients will have the following parameters monitored, as appropriate to the procedure and the individual patient's condition: blood pressure, heart rate, respiratory rate, temperature, oxygen saturation, electrocardiogram (EKG), arterial pressure, central line pressures, laboratory values (hematocrit, blood glucose level, sodium, potassium, arterial oxygen and carbon dioxide, blood pH, and clotting factors), urinary output, and blood loss. The blood pressure, heart rate, respiratory rate, temperature, oxygen saturation, and EKG are monitored continuously and recorded on the patient's chart. Continuous monitoring is necessary to detect and treat any abnormalities immediately.

Nursing Diagnoses and Patient Goals

From assessment data, the nursing diagnoses and the patient goals can be identified. Although diagnoses and goals vary depending on the individual patient, some of the common problem areas during the intraoperative period include Ineffective Coping, High Risk for Injury, High Risk for Infection, and Altered Tissue Perfusion.

TABLE 23–8

Selected Intraoperative Nursing Diagnoses and Patient Goals

Nursing Diagnosis	Patient Goal
Ineffective individual coping related to anxiety associated with the surgical procedure	Patient will demonstrate effective coping behaviors
High risk for injury related to equipment, electrical, or physical hazards during surgery	Patient will maintain injury-free status during the surgical procedure
High risk for infection related to breaks in asepsis or individual risk factors	Patient will maintain an infection-free wound site postoperatively
Altered tissue perfusion due to blood loss during the surgical procedure	Patient will maintain adequate blood flow to all body tissues during the surgical procedure

Possible nursing diagnoses and patient goals for the intraoperative period are listed in Table 23-8.

Nursing Interventions

Nursing intervention during the intraoperative period focuses on providing emotional support, providing a safe environment and preventing injury, providing anesthesia or monitoring the patient during anesthetic administration, maintaining asepsis, and promoting wound healing. These interventions are carried out by either the scrub nurse or the circulating nurse.

The scrub nurse wears a sterile gown, mask, headgear, and gloves and protects her shoes with a disposable cover. The scrub nurse hands the surgeon required instruments, sponges, drains, and other equipment, anticipating what will be needed (Fig. 23-6). Anticipation helps keep to a minimum the time the patient is under anesthesia and the time the wound is open. Other responsibilities include preparing the sterile tables before

surgery. Before the surgeon closes the wound, the nurse accounts for all equipment to ensure that nothing remains inside the surgical site. The scrub nurse must have a thorough understanding of the principles of asepsis, anatomy, and tissue care; an awareness of surgical objectives; knowledge and skills to anticipate needs of other members of the surgical team; and the ability to reach decisions and perform interventions in an emergency situation (Smeltzer & Bare, 1992).

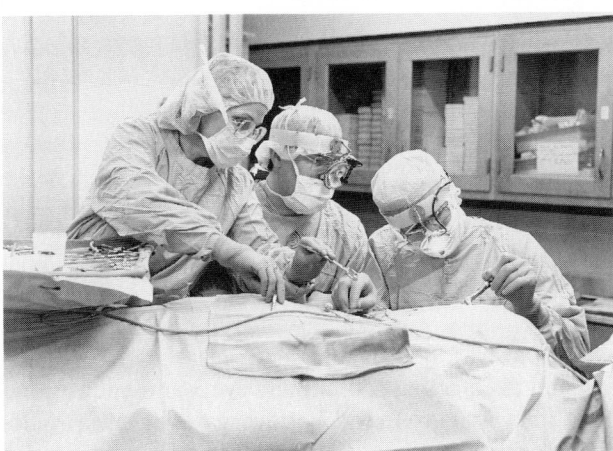

Figure 23–6. The scrub nurse anticipates the needs of the surgeon and hands him the instruments. (Photo by Cynthia Taylor. Courtesy of the University of Washington, Seattle, WA.)

Safety Alert

- Instruct the patient to stay in bed with siderails up to avoid injuries from falls after preoperative medications which affect cognition have been administered.
- Make sure all patients going to the operating room have the correct identification band, to avoid mistaken identity when the patient is not alert.
- Make sure any allergies are clearly identified to avoid possible allergic reactions.
- Position patients carefully and pad bony areas well during surgery.
- Postoperatively check circulatory status frequently to detect impairment promptly, thus avoiding nerve and muscle damage.
- Check all equipment and monitors used in the operating room before each use, to ensure proper functioning and prevent potential patient injury.
- Maintain strict surgical asepsis at all times in the operating room to prevent infection.
- Monitor temperature throughout the surgical procedure, noting any sudden rise in temperature (which could indicate malignant hyperthermia) so that treatment can be initiated promptly.

The circulating nurse manages the operating room and protects the safety and health needs of the patient (Smeltzer & Bare, 1992). Protection involves controlling the environment for cleanliness, temperature, humidity, and lighting. The circulating nurse ensures that the patient's rights are protected. It is the circulating nurse who greets the patient in the operating room and positions and drapes the patient in preparation for surgery. Coordinating activities of related personnel (laboratory, x-ray, etc.) and monitoring aseptic practices are also the circulating nurse's responsibilities (Smeltzer and Bare, 1992). The circulating nurse assists the scrub nurse in counting sponges and instruments after surgery.

Emotional Support

Providing emotional support for the patient in the operating room can be vital to the success of the procedure. While some patients may be awake only a short period of time (half an hour or less) before anesthetic induction, other patients are awake during the entire procedure. It is helpful to elicit the patient's cooperation, and it is important to make the patient as comfortable as possible. This allows the patient to tolerate the procedure in a calmer, more relaxed manner, resulting in better outcomes. Providing appropriate information and explanations for each phase of the procedure helps prevent unexpected, stressful surprises for the patient and promotes a more relaxed, cooperative environment. Often, a relaxed patient requires less medication during the intraoperative phase (Smeltzer & Bare, 1992).

It is also important for the nurse to provide emotional support for the patient's family. This is accomplished by answering any questions they may have, providing them with information on the progress of the procedure, and giving more detailed information if indicated and time permits. It is also important to let the family know when the procedure is completed, how long the patient will be in the recovery facility, and where the patient will go after discharge from the recovery facility. For outpatients who are to be discharged home after their surgical procedure, the intraoperative nurse may also be involved in planning for discharge and in discharge teaching.

Patient Safety

While safety is important in all phases of the surgical experience, the following areas are particularly important in the intraoperative phase: equipment safety, electrical safety, chemical safety, radiation safety, and safe transporting and positioning of patients.

Equipment Safety. The operating room nurse routinely checks and maintains equipment used during surgical procedures. Safety policies for patient care equipment should include the following principles:

- Establishment of written procedures for the use of equipment
- Special classes and education for those persons certified to operate and care for equipment
- Establishment of routine, periodic maintenance programs for equipment that meet or exceed manufacturers' recommendations
- Inspection of equipment (such as connectors, grounding pads, and settings) before each patient use
- Availability of current, written instructional materials to all persons certified to use the equipment
- Available professional assistance if equipment problems should arise
- Written documentation of the use, settings, and care of special equipment.

Electrical Safety. One of the most significant potential hazards to the patient in the operating room is electricity. Electrical equipment is used in many surgical procedures. Some of the more common electrical devices include lasers, x-ray machines, electrosurgical units (electrocautery), video equipment, physiologic monitors, electronic microscopes, heart bypass machines, cell savers, blood warmers, heating–cooling blankets, ultrasonic devices, cryosurgery units, and surgical spotlights. Appropriate operating room personnel should know how to use the equipment safely, how to check the equipment for proper functioning, and how to report problems, especially emergent problems such as fire or explosion. The most common potential threats to patient safety related to electrical devices are electric shock and burns. It is important that operating room personnel know how to prevent these problems and how to activate the emergency system should they occur. The safety principles of patient-care equipment previously discussed should also apply to all electrical equipment. Additionally, personnel using electrical equipment should be familiar with the safe use of backup systems should a power failure occur.

Chemical Safety. Chemical safety is another important area of patient safety in the operating room. It is important that staff be aware of chemical hazards, read and follow warning labels, and follow all safety precautions. Some of the more common chemical hazards in the operating room include ethylene oxide used for sterilizing purposes (an eye irritant, also potentially explosive and flammable), alcohol used as a disinfectant (flammable), methyl methacrylate used as a bone cement (an eye and respiratory tract irritant, also potentially flammable and explosive), housekeeping chemicals used for cleaning and disinfecting (potentially eye, skin, and respiratory tract irritants), and various gases (such as halothane, nitrous oxide, forane, nitrogen, and carbon dioxide) used both for anesthetic purposes and/or for gas-powered equipment (potentially combustible and asphyxiating) (Kneedler and Dodge, 1987). It is important that personnel working with these chemicals have knowledge of their potential hazards, how to use them safely, and what to do should an accident occur.

Radiation Safety. Radiation hazards in the operating room include the portable x-ray machine, fluoroscopy, diagnostic radiology, radiation implants, and other forms of radiation therapy. Radiation is potentially hazardous in that it changes or modifies body cells and can lead to genetic defects, thyroid disorders, leukemia, and other forms of cancer. It is important that all personnel who work with radiation sources strictly adhere to the policies and procedures set forth by the hospital's radiation safety officer. Such practices include the use of monitoring badges, lead aprons, and other shielding devices. It is also important to keep in mind the principle of distance. The amount of radiation exposure decreases inversely with the square of the distance from the source, and it is recommended to maintain a maximal distance from the source.

Positioning. The proper positioning of the patient is another important safety consideration in the operating room. The responsibility for positioning is a shared one. The anesthesiologist, the surgeon, and the circulating nurse all participate in placing the patient in the proper position for the surgical experience. The ideal position can be defined as the position that provides the best possible exposure for the surgeon, the best possible exposure for airway management and monitoring for the anesthetist, and the best possible position for the physiologic safety of the patient. Proper positioning is vital to prevent nerve and muscle damage, which can be temporary or lead to permanent dysfunction (Gruendemann, 1987). It is important to use adequate padding for all body prominences and joints to avoid pressure areas and to provide optimal functioning of the respiratory, nervous, and circulatory systems. Some of the more commonly used surgical positions include supine, Trendelenburg, reverse Trendelenburg, lithotomy, sitting, prone, and lateral or side-lying. Illustrations of selected surgical positions are provided in Chapter 20. Patients in each of these positions require special padding or support devices to ensure physiologic safety.

Draping. Proper draping of the surgical area helps to maintain asepsis by creating a sterile field, thus limiting exposure to microorganisms. Drapes are used to cover other areas of the body, exposing only the incisional area. Often, drapes are cloth or paper and fastened into place. Newer plastic adhesive drapes form a complete transparent seal over the skin into which the incision is made.

Anesthesia Monitoring

Monitoring patient status during and after anesthesia is an important responsibility for the nurse in the operating room or in the recovery facility. Knowledge concerning

specific anesthetic agents is important to focus assessment parameters.

The administration of anesthesia may be performed by an anesthesiologist or a certified professional nurse. Both of these professionals have specialized education and skills in the administration of anesthetic agents and in monitoring patients during surgical and other procedures. An **anesthesiologist** is a physician who has specialized education in the administration of anesthesia. A certified registered nurse anesthetist (CRNA) is a registered nurse who has received specialized education and certification in the administration of anesthesia. Both professionals are also skilled in the management of pain and in the placement of vascular access lines.

Anesthesia may be classified as general anesthesia or regional anesthesia. **General anesthesia** effectively produces analgesia, relaxes muscles, and results in a sleeplike state. **Regional anesthesia** decreases sensation and pain to selected parts of the body.

General Anesthesia. General anesthesia may be administered either by the inhalation method or the intravenous method. Inhalation agents (gases) are delivered from the anesthesia machine and tubing via a face mask, endotracheal tube, or endonasal tube. Some of the inhalation agents most commonly used include nitrous oxide, oxygen, halothane, enflurane, and forane. Intravenous agents can also be delivered through an established vascular access. Some of these agents include barbiturates (thiopental), narcotics (morphine, meperidine, fentanyl), tranquilizers (diazepam), and phencyclidines (ketamine).

Muscle relaxants, such as succinylcholine chloride, are also commonly administered during surgical procedures (Wells, 1987). Muscle relaxants are especially beneficial during wound closure. When an abdominal incision is to be closed by the surgeon using sutures, relaxed and non-tense abdominal muscles result in a wound that is easier to suture by allowing the wound edges to be approximated (brought together) in their relaxed state.

Close monitoring of the patient is necessary during induction and use of general anesthesia. There are four stages of anesthesia, as shown in Table 23-9, beginning with onset of anesthesia or analgesia and ending with the toxic stage. Patients who are receiving general anesthesia normally go through the first three stages. The type of anesthesia may vary the transition. These stages are observed by the anesthetist; however, the nurse may assist in assessment by taking vital signs. As the patient emerges from anesthesia, the sequence of stages is reversed.

Regional Anesthesia. Regional anesthesia can be a useful alternative to general anesthesia. Instead of placing the entire body in a sleep-like condition, regional

TABLE 23–9

Stages of Anesthesia

	Reflexes	Heart Rate	Respiration	Blood Pressure	Eyes
I. Analgesia amnesia	Present	Normal	Slow rate Increased depth	Normal	Some dilation Reacts to light
II. Dreams and excitement (frequently bypassed with intravenous induction agents)	Active	Increased	Irregular breathing Breath holding	Increased	Pupils widely dilated and divergent
III. Surgical Involves four planes; plane 2 and plane 3 best for surgery	In progression of loss Lid reflex Pharyngeal (swallowing) Laryngeal (can tolerate oral airway, suctioning and then intubation) Gag and corneal reflexes lost	Decreased	Progressively depressed until apneic	Normal to decreased	Early plane: constricted pupils, then slightly dilated and centrally fixed
IV. Toxic Extreme depression	No reflexes	Weak and thready	Completely flaccid	Decreased	Widely dilated pupils

From Patrick, M. L., et al. (1991) Medical–surgical nursing: Pathophysiological concepts (p. 376). Philadelphia: J. B. Lippincott.

anesthesia affects only selected parts of the body. This type of anesthesia can be used for surgeries of the lower extremities (feet, ankle, knees, hips) and other localized operative sites, such as the fingers, hands, nose, eyes, or ears. Regional anesthetics have the advantage of minimizing the pulmonary and gastrointestinal complications (pulmonary congestion, atelectasis, nausea, and vomiting) that sometimes occur with general anesthetics. Patients receiving regional anesthetics also often experience shorter recovery periods from the anesthetic experience as compared to patients receiving general anesthetics. If the patient and the procedure are appropriate for regional anesthesia, it is generally considered the method of choice (Gruendemann & Meeker, 1987). Specific methods used to provide regional anesthesia, including topical, nerve blocks, local injection, spinal, epidural, caudal, and other other regional blocks, are described in Table 23-10.

TABLE 23–10

Regional Anesthesia

Type of Regional Anesthesia	Definition and Uses	Examples of Use
Topical	The direct application of an anesthetic agent to skin or mucosal surfaces (mouth, throat, nose, cornea)	Often used before injections (nerve blocks, epidurals) or endotracheal tube placement
Nerve or nerve bundle block (local)	The injection of a local anesthetic agent into a nerve bundle or the nerve supply of the operative site	Breast biopsy, node biopsy, ear procedure, cataract extraction, or cornea transplant
Epidural or peridural	The injection of a local anesthetic agent into the potential space outside the dura	Lower extremity surgery (foot, ankle, knee), lower abdominal procedures, or for postoperative pain relief
Spinal	The injection of a local anesthetic agent into the subarachnoid space	Useful for surgeries below the xyphoid process, or abdominal surgery

Asepsis

Maintaining asepsis to avoid microorganism contamination of the surgical site is the responsibility of the nurse as well as all members of the surgical team. The Association of Operating Room Nurses (AORN), the professional organization for perioperative nurses, has established guidelines for maintaining asepsis and for sterilization of equipment, instruments, and supplies (AORN, 1987). These guidelines are highlighted in the accompanying display.

Additional policies and procedures have been established in the operating room to ensure asepsis (Fig 23-7). Every operating room nurse should be familiar with agency policies concerning the surgical hand scrub, surgical cleaning and preparation of the patient's skin before surgery, special considerations for cleaning the operating room environment and disposing of waste products, processing methods for the sterilization of instruments and supplies, and methods for draping the surgical patient and establishing the sterile field.

Guidelines for Maintaining Asepsis

- All items within a sterile field should be sterile. Items of questionable sterility should be re-sterilized. All sterile packages should be inspected for damage to package integrity. They also need to be protected from moisture, tearing, sharp objects, or other threats to the integrity of the wrapping material. In addition, they must be unwrapped and dispensed according to acceptable sterile procedure.
- The gowns and gloves used by the scrubbed personnel should be sterile. They must be donned in the correct manner and scrubbed personnel need to be cautious always to maintain the sterility of their gowns at the level of the sterile field and their gloves. Therefore, the arms and hands of the scrubbed personnel must be maintained between the level of the sterile field (table) and the scrubbed person's shoulder level.
- Tables and ring stands draped with sterile drapes should be considered sterile only at the table level. Drapes need to be impervious to moisture soaking through them in order to remain sterile. Items dropping over the sides of the table need to be considered unsterile.
- Scrubbed personnel must remain close to the sterile field and unscrubbed personnel must stay at least 1 foot away from the sterile field. Scrubbed personnel should move around a sterile field in such a way as to maintain the sterility of the sterile field. Unscrubbed personnel should not move between two sterile fields.

Wound Closure

The nurse often assists the surgeon in wound closure, and may be directed to remove wound closure devices during the postoperative period. The type of material used for wound closure has an affect on wound healing. Sutures, staples, or clips may be used to close a wound. At times, a combination of closure methods may be employed; for example, a patient may have absorbable sutures closing the viscera and staples approximating wound edges.

Sutures. Suture is defined as the material used to sew an incision together. Sutures can be either absorbable (e.g., catgut or chromic) or nonabsorbable (e.g., synthetic nylon or polypropylene, silk). Nonabsorbable sutures must be removed after the incision has healed. Absorbable sutures absorb into the skin, so that removal is not necessary. The type of suture used depends on the size and location of the wound being closed, how strong the suture material needs to be for the type of wound being repaired, the desired cosmetic result, and the surgeon's preference. Generally the least amount of suture and smallest size of suture, as appropriate to the wound, results in the most optimal wound closure. Sutures represent a foreign body that can potentially lead to infections, such as stitch abscesses.

Staples. The use of skin staples is also an effective method of wound closure. Skin staples are made of stainless steel and look like paper staples flat against the skin. Skin staples are minimally reactive to the body as a foreign substance, and therefore minimize the risk of infection. A staple gun is used to place staples to close the incision. The use of skin staples also reduces tissue handling because staples provide for faster wound closure than sutures. Skin staples are usually removed using a staple remover within the first week after surgery, after incisional healing has occurred.

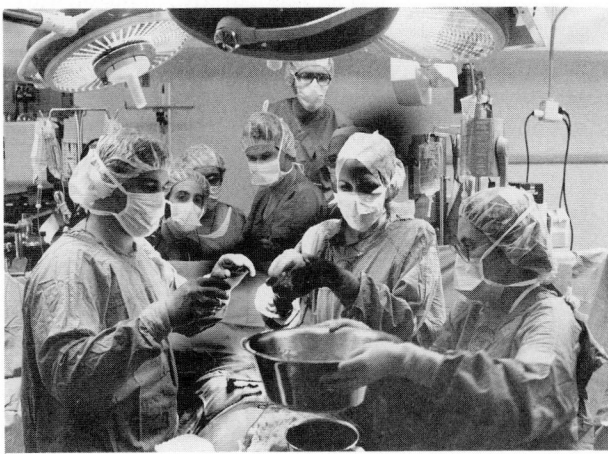

Figure 23–7. Asepsis is maintained as a heart transplant is performed. (Photo by Joe Freeman. Courtesy of the University of Washington, Seattle, WA.)

Clips. Skin clips can also be used for incisional closure. Clips, which are larger than staples and protrude up from the incision in a clamp-like fashion, are also made of stainless steel. Clips approximate skin edges and are removed by pinching the top of the clip together, releasing the section of the clip that approximates the skin edges.

Transport to the Recovery Facility

When the intraoperative phase of the surgical procedure has been completed, the circulating (nonscrubbed) nurse, the anesthetist, and the surgeon safely transport the patient to the recovery facility. They each complete their written documentation and provide the recovery facility with this written report of the surgical experience. The nurses in the recovery facility have been notified of the patient's impending arrival and have prepared for the patient accordingly.

Evaluation

As the nurse performs interventions during the intraoperative period, the results are being evaluated and revised as needed. Intraoperative evaluation is focused on the individual patient goals. Selected outcome criteria are provided, but the nurse should individualize outcome criteria for each surgical patient.

Goal
Patient will demonstrate effective coping behaviors.

Possible Outcome Criteria
• Patient asks appropriate questions of the anesthetist, nurse, and surgeon when in the operating room.
• Patient communicates effectively with the anesthetist, the nurse, and the surgeon before receiving the anesthesia.
• Patient remains alert and cooperative in the operating room before receiving the anesthesia.

Goal
Patient will maintain injury-free status during the surgical procedure.

Possible Outcome Criteria
• Patient experiences no skin injury due to electrical devices or surgical equipment.
• Patient experiences no nerve or muscle damage from inadequate padding or positioning during surgery.

Goal
Patient will experience an infection-free wound site postoperatively.

Possible Outcome Criteria
• Patient's wound site does not appear inflamed or have purulent drainage within 4 hours of surgery, as observed by nurse.
• Patient's wound site appears well approximated and shows evidence of normal wound healing 24 hours postsurgery.

Goal
Patient will maintain adequate blood flow to all body tissues during the surgical procedure.

Possible Outcome Criteria
• Patient's vital signs remain normal during the surgical procedure.
• Patient's hematocrit and hemoglobin remain within preoperative baseline range during surgical procedure.

POSTOPERATIVE NURSING

The postoperative phase begins when the patient is transferred into the recovery facility and ends when the patient has recovered from the surgical intervention. This phase could be short (less than a day) or long (several months or longer), depending on the nature and extent of the procedure and the patient's ability to recover from it. The nurses in the recovery facility, the nurses in the postsurgical unit, and the nurses in extended-care or home-care settings all use the nursing process during the postoperative period to individualize patient care.

Nursing Assessment

Systematic assessment is needed during the postoperative period to detect quickly any surgical complications and individualize nursing care to promote optimum recovery from the surgery.

Assessment in the Recovery Facility

Assessments are made frequently during the immediate postoperative period. The recovery room nurse usually obtains a verbal report from the operating room staff, and reads written documentation of the surgery and the physician's postoperative orders. Information that is important for planning care includes the type and extent of the surgical procedure performed, the type of anesthesia used, the dosage and time medications were given, the amount of blood lost, whether or not the patient is still intubated, and any surgical or anesthetic complications that may have occurred. It is also important to know whether the patient is an inpatient or an outpatient. Important assessments during the immediate postoperative period are listed in Table 23-11.

Assessment of cardiovascular function is necessary to

TABLE 23–11

Assessments and Interventions in the Immediate
Postoperative Period (Recovery Room)

Focus Area	Assessments and Interventions
Respiratory	Check airway patency and monitor respiratory rate and depth, breath sounds, skin color, and chest expansion
Cardiac	Monitor blood pressure and other vital signs at least every 15 minutes
Neurologic	Monitor pupillary response; monitor muscle strength to determine muscle relaxant reversal, if used
Dressings	Monitor for integrity of dressings and for hemorrhage or hematoma formation
Pain management	Monitor for both subjective and objective manifestations of pain, administer analgesics as appropriate
Renal function	Monitor amount of urinary output for patients with indwelling catheter (at least 30 mL per hour); for patients with a urinary catheter, monitor for bladder distention

detect bleeding promptly. Vital signs are usually monitored every 15 minutes, or more frequently if the patient's condition warrants it. The pulse rate is assessed for rhythm and rate. Both the blood pressure and pulse are evaluated for trends rather than absolute values. A decreasing blood pressure along with an increased pulse rate is significant in the postoperative patient, since it can indicate hemorrhage or shock. Certain anesthetic agents and muscle relaxants can also cause hypotension. The patient's skin should be evaluated for color (e.g., pale or cyanotic), temperature, and diaphoresis. Pale, cyanotic, cool, or clammy skin can indicate impaired tissue perfusion, possibly due to shock. The dressing is also observed for bleeding, which, when present, may be circled on the dressing with the time indicated. When evaluating incisional bleeding, it is also important to check for drainage under the patient, where bleeding can go unnoticed. Catheters, drains, and chest tubes are also evaluated for the type of drainage and the amount of blood present. Laboratory values, such as hematocrit, may also be requested during this period to help evaluate circulatory status.

Respiratory function should be assessed during the immediate postoperative period to detect promptly any signs of hypoxia or airway obstruction. Respiratory rate and depth should be evaluated and compared to baseline data. Hypoxia may be first detected as apprehension, anxiety, or restlessness. Loud, irregular respirations may indicate obstruction of the airway due to the presence of vomit or accumulated secretions, or positioning so that the tongue falls to the back of the throat.

Neurologic assessment is performed to assess recovery from the anesthetic agent. Return of reflexes, indicated by swallowing and gagging, occurs when anesthesia effects are ending. Level of consciousness changes as the anesthetic agent wears off. Initially, the patient is unconscious and does not respond to verbal or tactile stimuli. As the anesthetic agent begins to wear off, the patient will respond to loud noises or to his or her name being called. Finally, the patient becomes oriented to person and place. During this period of time the patient may still appear sleepy, and will fall into a sleep when not stimulated.

The nurse also assesses the patient's fluid balance, urinary output, and pain level during the immediate postoperative period. The patency of all tubes and drains and the proper working of all equipment should be ascertained.

Assessment During the Postoperative Period

During the rest of the postoperative recovery period, the nurse performs systematic functional assessment. Table 23-12 lists possible postoperative complications and appropriate nursing assessments for each functional health pattern.

The nurse individualizes assessment based on the individual patient and the surgery that was performed. Assessment is also individualized based on the length of time since the surgery has occurred. During the first few days after surgery, assessments may focus on pain, tissue perfusion, and respiratory function, whereas later in the postoperative course, ability to perform self-care and manage at home after discharge may be more important. An overview of functional health assessment is provided in Chapter 18. More detailed information concerning assessment of each functional health pattern is provided in clinical Chapters 25 through 49.

Nursing Diagnoses and Patient Goals

Nursing assessment during the postoperative period permits identification of actual and high-risk postoperative problems. The general goal for any postoperative patient is to prevent or minimize complications and return the patient to optimal functioning. While the specific nursing diagnoses and goals vary from patient to patient, some of the more common nursing diagnoses and goals are listed in Table 23-13.

Nursing Interventions

Nursing interventions in the postoperative period include nursing management in the recovery facility, in the postsurgical recovery unit, and discharge planning for home care.

TABLE 23–12

Postoperative Functional Health Assessment

Function	Potential Complication	Assessments
Health perception/ health maintenance	Injury secondary to equipment or body positioning or inadequate recovery from anesthesia	Skin, CMS (color, movement, sensation) patent airway, safe environment (siderails up)
Activity/exercise	Hemorrhage/shock	Vital signs, color, bleeding from wound, hematocrit, urine output
	Atelectasis	Respiratory rate and depth, breath sounds, color, arterial blood gases, temperature
	Deep vein thrombosis	Circulation, calf pain or swelling
	Pulmonary emboli	Respiratory rate and depths and other vital signs, breath sounds
Nutrition/metabolism	Wound infection	Temperature and other vital signs, observe wound for redness, warmth, swelling and purulent drainage
	Poor wound healing dehiscence evisceration	Observe wound
	Fluid volume deficit	Postural blood pressure and pulse, intake and output, weight, skin turgor
	Nausea/vomiting	Bowel sounds, abdominal distention
	Malignant hyperthermia	Monitor temperature and other vital signs
	Hypothermia	Monitor temperature
Elimination	Urinary retention	Urine output, (especially first 8 hours after surgery), bladder distention or discomfort
	Paralytic ileus	Absent bowel sounds abdominal distention
	Constipation	Lack of stool, abdominal distention, hypoactive bowel tones
Sleep/rest	Sleep deficit	Sleep duration and quality
Cognition/perception	Pain	Pain level and pain relief after medication
	Confusion	Orientation to person, place, time; level of consciousness
Self-concept	Altered self-concept	Assess reaction to wound, drains tubes, etc.
Role relationships	Altered role relationship	Assess perception of alteration in roles or relationships
Coping	Ineffective coping	Assess anxiety, stress, and lack of coping
Sexuality	Altered sexual function	Assess impact on sexuality and sexual function
Values–beliefs	Spiritual distress	Assess surgery or recovery period affects on spiritual belief or values

Nursing Interventions in the Recovery Facility

Assessment and continual monitoring of the patient's condition until the effects of the anesthetic have subsided and the physiologic status of the patient has stabilized are the primary responsibilities of the nurse in the recovery facility. The nurse provides a safe environment for the patient so that injury does not occur.

The nurse maintains a patent airway for the patient through positioning, suctioning, and care of the endotracheal tube, if it is still in place. Fluid replacement and blood administration may be necessary to maintain adequate circulating volume. Pain medications are frequently administered to control postoperative discomfort. As the patient regains consciousness, the nurse begins to encourage deep breathing and moving to improve ventilation and circulation.

For the patient to be discharged from the recovery facility, certain conditions must be met. These conditions usually include stable vital signs, airway control, control of bleeding and wound drainage, normal thermal state, absence or control of any anesthetic or surgical

complications, full or nearly full recovery from the anesthetic, adequate respiratory function, orientation to the environment, adequate fluid balance and urinary output, and ability to request assistance if needed (Drain & Cristoph, 1987). If the patient is to be discharged home, in addition to the previously listed criteria, the patient needs to be fully awake, able to use the bathroom, able to eat, and able to walk. Discharge teaching for the patient also needs to be completed, and a responsible family member or friend needs to be available to accompany the patient home.

After the inpatient has met the recovery facility's discharge criteria, transfer to the postsurgical nursing unit may occur. The recovery nurse gives report to the nurse responsible for the surgical patient. This report includes the type of surgery performed and the patient's tolerance of the procedure, the type of anesthesia used, vital signs, intravenous lines, blood loss, blood and/or fluid replacement, dressings, tubes and drains, urinary and drainage output, medications administered, level of pain and method of pain management used, and any complications that occurred. If there are family mem-

TABLE 23–13

Postoperative Nursing Diagnoses and Patient Goals

Nursing Diagnosis	Patient Goal
High risk for aspiration related to anesthesia, decreased level of consciousness	Patient will not aspirate
Impaired gas exchange related to anesthesia, decreased mobility, pain, pain medications	Patient will demonstrate adequate oxygenation of body tissues
Altered tissue perfusion related to loss of blood, postoperative edema, anesthetic agents, immobility	Patient will maintain adequate circulation of blood to all body tissues
High risk for fluid volume deficit related to loss of fluids during surgery, decreased oral intake, and abnormal drainage postoperatively	Patient will maintain adequate fluid volume
High risk for infection related to surgical wound, invasive lines, decreased nutritional status	Patient will not develop infection postoperatively
Hyperthermia related to anesthetic agents	Patient will maintain temperature within normal limits
Urinary retention related to anesthesia, immobility, and edema	Patient will void within 8 hours of surgery and without difficulty thereafter
Constipation related to anesthesia, pain medication, decreased mobility	Patient will resume normal bowel function when normal diet orders are resumed
Pain related to surgical trauma, inflammation, edema, and invasive procedures	Patient will verbalize that postoperative pain is well controlled
High risk for activity intolerance related to pain, fatigue, and tubes catheters, and drains	Patient will maintain optimal state of mobility, progressively increasing activity daily
Anxiety related to pain, separation from family, job, and normal activities	Patient will demonstrate adequate coping during the postoperative period
Knowledge deficit related to lack of instruction in postoperative activities to prevent complications and promote return to normal function	Patient will participate in postoperative activities to prevent complications
Impaired home maintenance management related to decreased mobility and decreased energy	Patient will manage normal daily activities in the home setting with necessary assistance from family and friends

bers or friends waiting in the surgery waiting area, they should be informed that the patient is being transferred to another unit.

Nursing Interventions on the Surgical Recovery Unit

Nursing interventions in this phase of postoperative recovery are aimed at preventing postoperative complications and promoting optimal return to normal function. Nursing interventions build on the patient teaching done in the preoperative period, and should be individualized for each surgical patient. A brief overview of nursing intervention is provided here, but in-depth information is provided in selected clinical chapters throughout this text.

Mobility and Self-Care. During the early postoperative period the patient may require assistance with mobility and self-care. Encouraging the patient to progressively increase mobility and independence in self-care helps prepare the surgical patient for discharge. Early ambulation is indicated for most surgical patients to minimize potential complications. Activity orders are individualized for the patient by the physician. The patient usually dangles (sits on the side of the bed with legs dangling over the side) on the evening of surgery, or may get out of bed and sit in a chair for a brief period of time. Administering pain medication before activity and teaching the patient how best to get out of bed will increase patient comfort. The nurse should encourage the patient to ambulate progressively longer distances each postoperative day. Standby assistance should be provided if the patient is weak or unsteady when ambulating. If the patient complains of dizziness or becomes diaphoretic when ambulating, the patient should be returned to bed.

Adequate hygiene after surgery is important to ensure patient comfort. If the patient has many tubes and has had major surgery, a bed bath is often given on the first postoperative day. Any solutions used to prepare the skin before surgery (e.g., Betadine) should be cleaned off. Antiembolic hose (TEDS) should be removed at the time of the bath and the skin inspected. The patient should always be encouraged to provide as much self-care as possible. The surgical patient often may shower if surgical dressings and IV sites are covered with a protective, waterproof barrier. Care should be taken when the patient is showering, since the warm water can promote vasodilation and hypotension.

Respiratory Maintenance. Aggressive treatment, especially in the immediate postoperative period, is needed to minimize atelectasis and prevent possible respiratory complications. Deep breathing and coughing, turning and positioning, early and aggressive ambulation, and the use of incentive spirometry are all helpful in preventing postoperative respiratory complications. Refer to Chapter 30 for detailed descriptions of these interventions.

Circulatory Maintenance. Venous stasis due to immobility increases the incidence of clot formation in the lower extremities. If clots lodge in the pulmonary circulation (a pulmonary embolus), gas exchange can be severely curtailed and death may occur. Leg exercises, frequent turning and positioning, the use of antiembolic stockings, adequate hydration, and early ambulation all decrease the risk of deep vein thrombosis.

Hydration and Nutrition. Intravenous fluids are used during the postoperative period to provide adequate hydration until the patient can take fluids orally. Fluid volume deficit can occur due to excessive loss of fluids and inadequate fluid replacement. Postural blood pressure should be monitored on all postoperative patients to detect fluid volume deficits. The amount of time IV fluids are required to be administered depends on the surgery and the individual patient. Before IV fluids are discontinued, normal bowel tones should be present, indicating normal intestinal peristalsis has returned after the surgery. The return of peristalsis may be slower if surgery has been performed on the gastrointestinal tract.

Progressive dietary intake is ordered postoperatively depending on the patient's recovery. Frequently, the physician may order diet as tolerated (DAT), and the nurse orders the appropriate diet based on assessment of the patient. After the return of peristalsis, a clear liquid diet is ordered, progressively followed by a full liquids, soft diet, and a regular diet. As the diet is advanced, the nurse continually assesses the patient for nausea, vomiting, abnormal bowel tones, or abdominal distention. The presence of abnormal findings may necessitate a change in diet orders.

Elimination. Nursing interventions are important to promote normal urinary and bowel elimination. During the postoperative period, the patient is expected to void within 8 hours of surgery. The postoperative patient may be unable to void because of edema, trauma, medications, or the inability to ambulate to the bathroom. An order for intermittent catheterization may be necessary to treat urinary retention in the immediate postoperative period. An indwelling catheter may be indicated for patients having urologic or gynecologic surgery. Urine output should be at least 30 mL per hour during the postoperative period; urine volumes less than this should be reported to the surgeon. When low urine output occurs, challenging the patient with increased IV fluid or administering diuretics may be necessary to ensure adequate urine output.

Bowel elimination can also be affected by the surgery. Normal bowel movements are not expected until normal intestinal motility has returned and the patient has resumed eating. Rectal tubes and return flow enemas may be ordered to help relieve intestinal gas and promote the passing of flatus. Constipation can occur postoperatively due to decreased activity, side effects of medication (especially pain medication), fluid volume deficit, and fear of painful evacuation. When the patient has started eating, stool softeners are frequently ordered. The nurse should encourage activity, adequate fluid intake, and a diet that promotes normal bowel evacuation. When a bowel movement has not occurred 3 days after resuming normal dietary intake, laxatives, suppositories, and enemas may be necessary.

Wound Care. Wound assessment, aseptic care of the wound, and monitoring wound drainage systems are all important nursing interventions. The nurse inspects dressings regularly and notes the amount and type of wound drainage (wound healing is discussed in detail in Chapter 34). Some surgeons prefer to change the first postoperative dressing. When changing a dressing for the first time, the nurse carefully removes dressing material to avoid inadvertent removal of drains. Symptoms of wound infection (redness, warmth, or purulent drainage) should be reported to the physician. Removal of sutures, staples, and clips is often the responsibility of nursing personnel.

Comfort and Rest. Pain management is an important nursing intervention during the postoperative period. The nurse uses nonpharmacologic interventions such as positioning, back massage, distraction, and emotional support to help the postoperative patient feel more comfortable. The nurse also administers pain medications as needed to control postoperative discomfort. Teaching the patient to recognize and report the occurrence of pain is important for pain management. If the dose, frequency, or medication ordered by the physician for pain control is ineffective, the physician should be notified.

Rest is important to promote healing. Hypnotics and barbiturates may be ordered during the postoperative period to help ensure rest. The nurse can provide a quiet, comfortable environment that encourages sleep and rest. Whenever possible, nursing activities, especially during the night, should be grouped together to allow for uninterrupted periods of rest.

Discharge Planning and Home Care

Discharge needs may vary depending on the surgical procedure and the individual patient. While many patients recover sufficiently to be discharged home, other patients may need to be transferred to an extended-care facility. Some patients who have sufficiently recovered from their surgical procedure to be discharged home, may need the assistance of visiting nurse service.

Many hospitals have developed special discharge procedures and forms that the nurse uses when preparing the patient for discharge. Discharge concerns for the surgical patient include pain management, wound care and dressing changes, monitoring for infection, dietary needs, bowel and bladder function, activity restriction, recommended sexual activity, and ability to perform self-care activities. The patient must be taught to manage any special equipment that is required at home and perform necessary procedures (such as dressing changes) independently. The patient needs to know where to buy needed supplies and how to arrange for specialized equipment. A limited number of supplies may be given to the patient to assist until the family can purchase necessary items.

The patient's family or caregiver should be included in the patient teaching session, and written guidelines should be given. For example, these guidelines may include calling your health-care provider: if your temperature is over 100°F, if you notice increased drainage, if your incision site becomes red or swollen, or if you experience increased pain in the operative area. Guidelines for activity level and activity restrictions (e.g., carrying anything that weighs more than 10 pounds, driving a car, abstaining from sexual intercourse for 6 weeks) should also be included. Verbal and written instructions for any prescribed medications should be given, and time provided to answer any questions. Instructions concerning a follow-up appointment with the surgeon, along with a phone number, should be given to the patient.

The nurse should explore with the patient what assistance he or she will have after discharge and how he or she plans to manage once home. Asking questions such as, "How do you envision your first few days home from the hospital?" may help to identify how the patient will cope after discharge. When the identified plan does not seem realistic, the nurse can help the patient explore alternative approaches or encourage the recruitment of family or friends for help.

EVALUATION

During postoperative evaluation, the nurse determines whether goals have been met. Goals and outcome criteria relate to preventing postoperative complications and returning the patient to optimal functioning. The more common postoperative nursing diagnoses and goals are listed in Table 23-13. Outcome criteria for four of these goals are presented here, but individualized care is important postoperatively.

Goal
Patient will resume normal bowel function when normal diet orders are resumed.

Possible Outcome Criteria
- Patient verbalizes decrease in abdominal pains caused by decreased intestinal peristalsis.
- Patient reports normal bowel movement 24 hours after regular diet resumed.

Goal
Patient will verbalize that postoperative pain is well controlled.

Possible Outcome Criteria
- During postoperative period, patient requests pain medication before pain becomes severe.
- Patient practices good positioning and other pain relief measures, as observed by nurse during postoperative period.

Goal
Patient will obtain optimal state of mobility, progressively increasing activity daily.

Possible Outcome Criteria
- Patient stands at bedside, with nurse's help if appropriate, the evening of surgery.
- Patient walks to bathroom, with nurse's help, by 24 hours after surgery.
- Patient walks 24 feet in hallway second day after surgery.

Goal
Patient will demonstrate adequate coping during the postoperative period.

Possible Outcome Criteria
- Patient discusses surgical experience with the nurse during postoperative period.
- Patient talks to family during their first visits, as reported by family.
- Patient states positive atittudes about reality of returning to home and work before discharge.

Key Concepts

- Perioperative nursing provides individualized care for the surgical patient during the preoperative, intraoperative, and postoperative phases of the surgical experience.
- Surgery may be performed in a variety of clinical facilities, including the physician's office or clinic, one-day surgical centers, or hospitals.
- Surgical procedures can affect all functional health areas.
- Lifespan considerations are important when individualizing care for the surgical patient.
- Preoperative teaching is important to minimize postoperative complications and decrease patient anxiety.
- Informed consent must be obtained before any surgical procedure.
- Preoperative preparation of the patient includes NPO status, starting IV access, bowel preparation, skin preparation, administering preoperative medications, and, at times, inserting a nasogastric tube.
- Nursing personnel in the operating room provide emotional support, provide a safe patient environment, and maintain asepsis.
- Anesthesia may be administered by a nurse with special preparation (CRNA).
- General anesthesia produces a sleep-like state, whereas regional anesthesia decreases pain and sensation in certain areas.
- Sutures, staples, or clips may be used to approximate wound edges and promote healing.
- Continual nursing assessment is important in the recovery facility to promptly detect complications and monitor recovery from anesthesia.
- Nursing care during the postoperative period is focused on preventing surgical complications and promoting optimum return of normal function.
- Complications that can occur during the postoperative period include hemorrhage, shock, atelectasis, deep vein thrombosis, pulmonary emboli, wound infection, fluid volume deficit, nausea, vomiting, malignant hyperthermia, hypothermia, urinary retension, paralytic ileus, sleep deficit, pain, confusion, altered self concept, altered role relationships. altered coping, and altered sexual function.
- To prepare for discharge, the patient should be taught activity restrictions, how to care for the incision, and what symptoms warrant contacting a physician

References

The Association of Operating Room Nurses, Inc. (1987). *AORN standards and recommended practices for perioperative nursing*. Denver, CO: Author.

Drain, C., & Cristoph, S. (1987). *The recovery room: A critical care approach to post anesthesia nursing* (2nd ed.). Philadelphia: W. B. Saunders.

Garner, J. S. (1986). CDC guidelines for prevention and control of nosocomial infections: Guidelines for prevention of surgical wound infections, 1985. *American Journal of Nursing, 14*(4), 71–80.

Gruendemann, B., & Meeker, M. (1987). *Alexander's care of the patient in surgery* (8th ed.). St. Louis: C. V. Mosby.

Gruendemann, B. (1987). *Positioning plus: A clinical handbook on patient positioning for perioperative nurses*. Chatsworth, CA: Devon.

Hathaway, R. G. (1988). *Nursing care of the critically ill surgical patient*. Rockville, MD: Aspen.

Kneedler, J., & Dodge, G. (1987). *Perioperative nursing care: The nursing perspective* (2nd ed.). Boston: Blackwell.

Smelzter, S., & Bare, B.G. (1992). *Textbook of medical–surgical nursing* (7th ed.). Philadelphia: J. B. Lippincott.

Wells, M. P. (1987). *Decision making in perioperative nursing*. Philadelphia: B. C. Decker.

Bibliography

Carpenito, L. J. (1989). *Nursing diagnosis: Application to clinical practice* (3rd ed.). Philadelphia: J. B. Lippincott.

McConnell, E. A. (1987). *Clinical considerations in perioperative preventive aspects of care*. Nursing: Philadelphia: J. B. Lippincott.

Patrick, M. L., Woods, S., Craven, R., et al. (1991). *Medical–surgical nursing: Pathophysiological concepts*. Philadelphia: J. B. Lippincott.

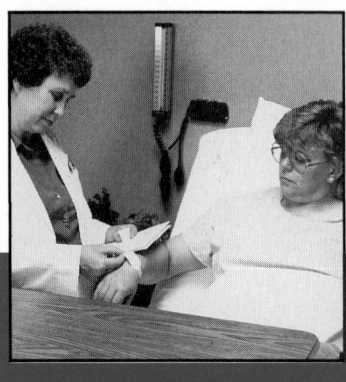

Medication Administration

LEARNING OBJECTIVES

Upon completion of this chapter, the student will be able to do the following:

- Describe essential components in a drug order.
- Discuss pharmacokinetic principles of drug action.
- Describe variables that affect drug action.
- List the five rights to ensure proper drug administration.
- Calculate proper drug dosage from different systems of drug measurement.
- Discuss important information concerning medication

to assess from the patient on admission and before medication administration.
- Individualize a teaching plan to improve patient compliance.
- List two nursing diagnoses for the patient managing self-medications.
- Describe recommended guidelines and procedures for oral, subcutaneous, and intramuscular medication administration.

KEY TERMS

Absorption	Intradermal	Pharmacodynamics
Buccal	Intramuscular	Pharmacokinetics
Distribution	Intravenous	Subcutaneous
Drug	Medication	Sublingual
Excretion	Metabolism	Transdermal

24

Drugs and Medications
  Names of Drugs
  Types and Forms of Drugs
  Sources of Information About Medications
  Medication Standards
  Systems of Medication Distribution
  Nonprescription and Prescription Medications
  Components of a Drug Order
  Types of Orders
  Systems of Drug Measurement
    Metric System
    Apothecaries' System
    Household System
Legal Aspects of Medication Administration
  Laws Affecting Drugs and Medications
  Drug Enforcement Agencies
  The Nurse's Role
    Nurse Practice Acts
    Institutional Medication Policies
  The Patient's Rights
  Substance Abuse
Principles of Drug Action
  Pharmacokinetics
    Absorption
    Distribution
    Metabolism
    Excretion
  Pharmacodynamics
    Therapeutic Effects
    Side (Adverse) Effects
  Factors Affecting Drug Action
Medication Assessment
  Information Collected on Admission
    Medication History
    Allergies
    Medical History
    Pregnancy and Lactation Status
  Assessment Before Medication Administration
    Medication Record
    Diet and Fluid Orders
    Laboratory Values
    Physical Assessment
  Assessment of Knowledge and Compliance
    Compliance
    Knowledge

Nursing Diagnoses
  Diagnostic Statement: Noncompliance
    Definition
    Defining Characteristics
    Related Factors
  Diagnostic Statement: Knowledge Deficit
    Definition
    Defining Characteristics
    Related Factors
  Related Nursing Diagnoses
Medication Administration
  Process to Ensure Safety
    Interpretation of the Order
    Calculating Medication Dosages
    Administering Medications According to the "Five Rights"
    Medication Errors
    Documentation of Medication Administration
  Oral Medications
    Advantages
    Contraindications
    Forms of Oral Medications
    Routes of Oral Medication
  Topical Medications
    Medications Applied to the Skin
    Ophthalmic Medications
    Otic Medications
    Nasal Medications
    Rectal Medications
    Vaginal Medications
  Inhaled Medications
  Parenteral Medications
    Advantages and Disadvantages
    Equipment
    Medication Preparation Techniques
    Intradermal Injections
    Subcutaneous Injections
    Insulin Administration
    Heparin Administration
    Intramuscular Injections
    Intravenous Administration
  Discharge Planning and Home Care
Evaluation
Lifespan Considerations
Key Concepts

The nurse's role in administering medications has become increasingly complex and diversified. The responsibility for administering the correct medication and dosage by the specified route, using proper technique, and taking appropriate precautions was once all that was expected of the nurse. Today these important functions constitute only part of safe medication administration; the level of knowledge and skill now demanded of the nurse is much broader. In addition to delivering pills and giving injections, the nurse must observe and interpret the patient's response to therapy, and recognize medication incompatibilities and interactions. The nurse must also be knowledgeable about the actions and side effects of medications, as well as be aware of the moral, ethical, and legal aspects of drug therapy. The nurse must be familiar with sources of medication information and know when to use them. Finally, the nurse must be able to recognize unsafe or unclear medication orders, and know what to do when such an order is encountered.

This chapter will discuss general principles of medication administration. Its purpose is not to provide information about specific drugs, but rather to identify the essential prerequisite knowledge the nurse must have to administer drugs safely to patients. Legal aspects of medication administration will be considered, and a brief description of pharmacokinetics, or drug action, is also presented. Finally, various aspects of assessment, preparation and administration of medications, and patient teaching will be discussed.

DRUGS AND MEDICATIONS

The term drug is often used interchangeably with medication, but there is a specific difference between them. A **drug** is any substance that alters physiologic function, with the potential for affecting health. A **medication** is a drug administered for its therapeutic effects. Thus, all medications are drugs, but not all drugs are medications. To administer medications effectively and safely, the nurse must possess a broad range of general and specific knowledge.

Names of Drugs

Medications or drugs can be known by any of four names. The **chemical name** of a medication describes the constituents that make up its molecular structure. It describes in chemist's terms the placement of atoms or atomic groupings. An example of a chemical name is that of the anti-inflammatory agent ibuprofen, i.e., 2-(4 iso-butylphenyl) propinoic acid.

The **generic name** is the name assigned by the manufacturer before a new medication becomes official. This name is simpler than the chemical name, from which it is

often derived. Examples of medications known by their generic names include morphine sulfate, cephradine, and ethacrynic acid.

The **official name** is the name under which it is listed in one of the official FDA publications, such as the National Formulary or United States Pharmacopeia.

The brand name or **trade name** is a registered name assigned by the manufacturer. Brand names are proper nouns; their first letter is capitalized and they are marked with a circled R. Some medications are manufactured by several companies and so may be known by several different brand names. An example is ampicillin sodium (official name): this drug is marketed under the names Omnipen-N, Polycillin-N, SK Ampicillin-N, and Totacillin-N.

Types and Forms of Drugs

Medications are classified in many ways, for example according to their clinical composition, clinical actions, or their therapeutic effect on body systems. For example, some agents used to fight cancer cells are known by the general classification "antineoplastic (i.e., anticancer) agents." Drugs that act to open bronchial tubes narrowed by asthma are called "bronchodilators." Each broad medication category has a set of characteristics common to all drugs within the classification. By understanding general drug classifications, the nurse will find it easier to learn about the actions, side effects, and precautions needed for unfamiliar drugs. Table 24-1 lists classes of medications used to support or improve functional abilities.

Medications are prepared in a variety of forms. Pills and powders, liquid forms for drinking or injection, suppositories, creams, ointments, and inhalants are some of the forms in which medications are manufactured. Table 24-2 lists different drug preparations. The most desirable form of medication for any given patient is determined by several factors; the disease process being treated, the age of the patient, the ability of the patient to swallow, the availability of personnel trained in special techniques of administration, and the amount of medication that must be delivered are only some of the considerations that must be made in deciding on appropriate medication forms. In addition, the same medication may be prepared in different dosage concentrations. Because of the wide variety of available forms and dosages of medications, it is important that the nurse pay close attention to the medication order, and administer the specified form.

Sources of Information About Medications

A fundamental rule of safe drug administration is "never administer an unfamiliar medication." Before giving any

TABLE 24–1

Classes of Medications to Promote Normal Function

Health Pattern	Drug Class	Action
Activity and exercise	Antihypertensives	Decreases blood pressure
	Antiarrhythmics	Increases regularity of heart rhythm
	Cardiotonics	Increases strength of cardiac contraction
	Antianginals	Increases coronary blood flow
	Anticoagulants	Decreases clot formation
	Bronchodilators	Opens airways
Nutrition and metabolism	Antibiotics	Decreases or prevents infection
	Antiemetics	Decreases nausea
	Antacids	Decreases gastric acidity
	Insulin	Decreases blood sugar
	Corticosteroids	Decreases inflammation
	Thyroid	Regulates metabolic rate
	Vitamins and minerals	Supplements inadequate dietary intake
Elimination	Laxatives	Promotes stool evacuation
	Antidiarrheals	Decreases diarrhrea
	Diuretics	Increases urine production
Sleep and rest	Sedatives, hypnotics	Induces sleep
Cognition and perception	Analgesics	Decreases pain
	Antipsychotics	Decreases psychotic symptoms (e.g., hallucinations)
Coping and stress tolerance	Antianxiety agents	Decreases anxiety
	Antidepressants	Decreases depression
Sexuality and reproduction	Ovarian hormones	Provides hormone replacement Provides birth control

drug, the nurse must first understand the condition of the patient for whom a medication is ordered. This knowledge, and knowledge of the ordered medication, form the basis for knowing why (and whether) the drug is appropriate for that patient. The nurse should be familiar with dosage ranges of the drug being given, its expected therapeutic effects, and its possible adverse actions.

Although the nurse is expected to remember a great deal of information about drugs, the tremendous number and variety of available medications make reliance on memory impractical and potentially dangerous. For this reason, the nurse must know how and when to consult standard resources to find out information about medications.

The subject of pharmacology involves detailed information. With so many new medications being introduced on the market, the subject seems to grow ever greater in scope and complexity. It is important that nurses develop a "habit" of looking up medications in reference sources and foster an awareness of latest developments.

There are many different sources of information on dosages, therapeutic effects and side effects of medications, and nursing care during and after medication administration. Package inserts or brochures provide detailed information on the medication product contained in a packaged unit. These inserts contain material on all clinically significant aspects of a medication's desirable and adverse effects, along with dosage and method of administration. The information printed contains information that must be approved by the Food and Drug Administration (FDA).

Several reference books can be used to gain a better understanding of a medication or class of medications. *The Physicians' Desk Reference* (PDR; Medical Economics Data, Oradell, NJ) is published annually as a compendium that supplies information on approximately 2500 medications; the information is provided by the drug manufacturers. Included in the PDR are pictures of the different medications.

The American Medical Association Drug Evaluations is a less comprehensive book published previously by the former Council on Drugs. The Department of Drugs works in collaboration with the American Society for Clinical Pharmacology and Therapeutics to provide authoritative and unbiased information on medications to professionals in medicine, nursing, and pharmacy. The compendium contains detailed evaluative monographs on over 1300 separate medications and compounds, as well as discussions of groups of related medications.

The American Hospital Formulary Service is available by subscription from the American Society of Hospital Pharmacists, Washington, DC. Both individual monographs on single generic medications and full and descriptive statements on groups of medications with simi-

TABLE 24–2
Drug Preparations

Type of Preparation	Description
Oral Preparations	
Capsule	Gelantinous container to hold powder or liquid medicine
Elixer	Liquid preparation of medication with alcohol base
Emulsion	Suspension within an oil base
Enteric coated	Coating which causes absorption in intestines rather than stomach
Lozenge (troche)	Tablet held in the mouth to be dissolved
Powder	Finely ground drug; frequently mixed with liquid before administration
Spansule	Time-released capsule which dissolves more slowly to provide an effect over a long period of time
Suspension	Medication in liquid which must be shaken before administration because it separates
Syrup	Medicine dissolved in sugar and water
Tablet	Compressed hard disk of powdered medication; may be scored for easy breaking
Tincture	Potent solution with alcohol base made from plants, dosage usually small
Topical Preparations	
Cream	Nongreasy, semisolid preparation for topical application
Gel or jelly	Translucent or clear semisolid substance which liquefies when applied to the skin
Liniment	Oily liquid used on the skin
Lotion	Emollient liquid, which may be a clear solution or a suspension, which is applied to the skin
Ointment	Drug combined with oil base for external application
Paste	Thick ointment used for local application to the skin
Suppository	Medicine contained within a gelatinous base (shaped for easy insertion into the body) which dissolves at body temperature, slowly releasing the drug
Transdermal patch	Medicine which is contained in a patch, which, when applied to the skin, permits gradual but controlled absorption

lar actions and uses are included in the service. The medication descriptions are presented in sections organized on the basis of pharmacologic properties. The medications are indexed by common brand names, generic name, and therapeutic class. Medication forms most commonly used by hospitals are also listed.

The latest developments in medication therapy are published in current journals such as the *American Journal of Nursing* (AJN) and *RN Magazine*. AJN began a monthly newsletter, *Nurses' Drug Alert* (Powers, New York, NY) as part of its journal format, and it is available by itself in monthly issues. This newsletter updates the nurse clinician on new medications, medication reactions, and clinical situations. Another newsletter, *Medical Letter,* is published biweekly and provides evaluations of the effectiveness and potential toxicity of medications.

Many hospital pharmacies also provide newsletters with up-to-date information about medication side effects and interactions, as well as new medications added to the formulary. Information about specific medications

that emphasizes nursing implications can also be obtained in nursing reference guides and textbooks.

Medication Standards

Because medications may vary, the standards guiding medication quality are usually created and controlled by the government. The official list of medication products in the United States is listed in two texts, the *United States Pharmacopeia* (USP) and the *National Formulary* (NF). The corresponding book of standards in Canada is the *British Pharmacopeia*. The USP and NF describe medication products according to their source, physical and chemical properties, tests for purity and identity, method of storage, category, and normal dosages. Both references provide invaluable information for practicing nurses.

Medications may vary according to their properties: purity, potency, bioavailability, efficacy, and safety and toxicity. Medication standards must provide an appropriate range of quality for these properties. Such standards for those properties are discussed in Table 24-3.

Systems of Medication Distribution

There are three types of systems used to ensure the safe storage and administration of medications: the stock supply, the unit dose supply, and the self-administered supply. Each of these systems of medication distribution vary from one institution to another, depending on their procedures and policies.

Patient-care areas in hospitals have a designated area where medications for patients are prepared. Some institutions have a central room with locked cupboards containing supplies, whereas others may use mobile medication carts with locked drawers or locked wall cabinets near the patients' rooms. In some institutions, there are satellite pharmacy units on a particular floor servicing several patient-care areas. In accordance with narcotic control laws, narcotic medications are kept in locked drawers in all patient-care areas.

Stock Supply. A stock supply system in a patient-care area provides large quantities of frequently prescribed medications for that particular unit; these are stored in locked cupboards in a storage room. Individual doses are dispensed and administered by the nursing staff, who measure individual doses from the large stock bottles or packaged containers. Examples of stock supply medications are narcotics and saline solution.

Unit Dose. A unit dose system involves the pharmacy in prepackaging and prelabeling an individual patient dose. This individual unit dose is a prescribed amount of medication dispensed at a specified time.

This type of system is gaining popularity because it provides a double-check mechanism, ensuring patient safety. Pharmacists and nurses both participate in administering medications and evaluating their effects. The pharmacist can provide information to the nurse about potential medication interactions or contraindications. This system also has been found to save valuable nursing time.

Self-Administered Medications. The self-administered medication (SAM) system supplies each patient with his or her prescribed doses and quantities for a given period of time. Each medication is supplied in a separate container and is to be used for one patient only. Medications can be stored at the patient's bedside, allowing the patient to administer his or her own medications. The Sam system can be used along with the stock or unit dose systems. For example, a patient may have sublingual nitroglycerin supplied by the SAM system and other medications supplied by the unit dose system. This combination allows the nitroglycerin to be used immediately if chest pain occurs.

This method of administration allows greater opportunity for the patient to become involved in his or her own care. It also lessens the time the nurse spends administering medications, allowing more time for care and management of patients.

TABLE 24–3

Properties of Medications Controlled by Standards of Quality

Property	Summary of Pertinent Information
Purity	1. A truly pure drug contains only one specific chemical agent. Pure drugs are rarely attainable. 2. Additives may be needed to facilitate formulation or change absorption. 3. Dusts or other contaminants from the environment may enter the drug. 4. The kind and concentration of extraneous substances allowed are specified by standards of purity.
Potency	1. Potency is generally dependent on the concentration of active drug. 2. When active ingredients are unknown, potency is measured by testing in animals (bioassay). 3. When active ingredients are known, potency is measured by chemical assay.
Bioavailability	1. The degree that a drug can be absorbed and transported by the body to its active site determines bioavailability. 2. Factors influencing bioavailability include particle size, crystalline structure, solubility, and polarity. 3. Blood or tissue concentrations at a specified time following administration are commonly used to measure bioavailability.
Efficacy	1. The effectiveness of the drug in promoting desirable clinical changes is called efficacy. 2. Objective measures are rarely available for determining efficacy; data are usually interpreted subjectively. 3. Double-blind studies are needed to establish efficacy as distinguished from placebo effect.
Safety/toxcity	1. The incidence and severity of adverse reactions attributable to the use of a drug determines the safety of that drug. 2. No active drug is free of toxicity. 3. The difference between therapeutic and toxic dosages determines the margin of safety of a substance. 4. When considering use of a drug, its adverse reactions must be weighed against its benefits.

Adapted from Spencer, R. T., et al. (1989). Clinical pharmacology and nursing management (3rd ed.) (p. 19). Philadelphia: J. B. Lippincott.

Nonprescription and Prescription Medications

Nonprescription Medications. Many drugs are available to the public without need for a written order from a physician. They are sold over-the-counter (OTC) because they are generally regarded as safe enough for use without medical or nursing supervision. Common examples of OTC drugs include cold remedies and mild analgesics such as aspirin. Control over the safety, effectiveness, and advertising of nonprescription medications is maintained by the FDA.

Nonprescription medications are considered safe when used as directed. The dangers of these readily available medications lie in their misuse, which can lead to dangerous side effects. Overuse can cause cumulative drug effects. Some people persist in self-medicating with nonprescription drugs, and delay seeking professional help, which can result in a minor problem developing into a major one because of early mistreatment. There is also danger of serious drug interactions. It is essential for the nurse to determine which (if any) nonprescription medications the patient has been taking, and ensure that no medications are taken without the physician's knowledge.

Prescription Medications. Some medications may have a narrow margin of safety between therapeutic and toxic doses, may produce serious side effects, or require close monitoring to determine their effectiveness in individual patients. These medications require medical supervision and must be ordered with a formal written order. A prescription is a legal order for the preparation and administration of a medication. Physicians and dentists are legally responsible for prescribing therapeutic agents. In some states, nurse practitioners and physician assistants may also prescribe some medications.

Components of a Drug Order

The physician conveys an order by specifying the name of the patient, the name of the medication, amount and frequency of the dose, and the route of administration. Included with this directive is the date and time the prescription was written and the signature of the prescribing physician. In most hospitals or health agencies, orders are written on a form specifically intended for the physician orders. These orders are a permanent part of the patient's chart. The patient's first and last name must be written with the medication order to avoid confusion between two patients with the same last name. The patient's identification or admission number can be written with the order as further identification.

The year, month, day, and time of day are also part of the written order (e.g., 1/19/92; 9 am). The time of day should include the abbreviation AM or PM to eliminate confusion between morning and afternoon times. Some

hospitals use military time or the 24-hour clock (e.g., midnight = 0000 hours, 6 PM = 1800 hours). Including the time of day on the written order also clarifies when certain orders (e.g., narcotics) automatically terminate.

Abbreviations are commonly used in the medication order. Certain standard abbreviations are used to indicate the amount and frequency of a medication dosage; these abbreviations are considered legal and can be used in the patient's chart. The more commonly used abbreviations are listed in Table 24-4.

Medication Name. The name of the medication can be written in most settings using the generic or trade name. The name should be written clearly, since many medications are very similar in spelling but very different in drug action. When the medication name is not clear, the physician should be contacted for clarification.

Medication Dosage. Medication dosage can be written in the metric, apothecaries', or household measurement system. The frequency and the strength of the dose is also indicated. If a medication is dispensed in only one dosage, the physician may indicate the number of tablets or pills to be taken. Two examples of these directives are: Digoxin 0.25 mg once a day, or Isocal (1/2 strength) 240 mL three times a day.

Route of Administration. The method of administration is commonly abbreviated as a part of the written order. Many medications can be given by several routes (e.g., orally [PO], intravenously [IV], intramuscularly [IM]). If an order specifies a certain route for medication administration, and the patient's condition changes, making the ordered route inappropriate or possibly unsafe, the nurse must notify the physician so that the route of administration can be changed.

Signature. Since the written order is considered a legal request, the signature of the physician must be written following the written order. An unsigned order is considered invalid and should not be carried out until the physician's signature has been secured.

Types of Orders

Standing Order. The standing order is a directive that should be carried out for a specified number of days or until another order is written to cancel it. In many hospitals or health agencies, the standing orders must be reviewed and rewritten within a specified time frame, or they will be cancelled automatically.

P.R.N. Orders. A p.r.n. order does not indicate a specific time for administration of a medication, but rather gives parameters so that the medication can be administered *as it is needed*. Pain medications, nausea medications, and laxatives are often ordered on a p.r.n.

TABLE 24–4

Common Abbreviations Used in Medication Orders

Abbreviation	Meaning	Abbreviation	Meaning
a or a.	before	no.	number
a.c.	before meals	noct.	night
ad lib	as desired	OD	right eye
alt.h.	alternate hours	os	mouth
AM	in the morning; before noon	OS	left eye
A.D.	right ear	OU	both eyes
A.S.	left ear	oz	ounce
A.U.	each ear	p or p.	after; per
aq.	water	p.c.	after meals
b.i.d.	twice a day	per os, PO	by mouth
c	with	PM	afternoon; evening
cap., caps.	capsule	p.r.n.	as needed, according to necessity
cc	cubic centimeter	q.	each, every
d	day	q.h.	every hour
D/C, dc	discontinue	q.i.d.	four times a day
dil.	dilute	q. 1 h.	every one hour
dist.	distilled	q. 2 h.	every two hours
DS	double strength	q. 3 h.	every three hours
EC	enteric coated	q. 4 h.	every four hours
elix.	elixir	q. 6 h.	every six hours
et	and	q. 8 h.	every eight hours
ext.	external, extract	q. 12 h.	every twelve hours
fl, fld	fluid	q.o.d.	every other day
g, gm, Gm	gram	q.s.	as much as needed, quantity sufficient
gr	grain	qtts	drops
gtt	drop	qt	quart
H	hypodermical	R. or PR	rectally, per rectum
h., hr	hour	Rx	take, prescription
h.s.	at bedtime	s	without
IM	intramuscular	sc	subcutaneously
inj.	injection	sol. or soln.	solution
IV	intravenous	SQ	subcutaneous
IVPB	IV piggy back	stat.	immediately, at once
kg	kilogram	tab.	tablet
L	liter	tbsp, T	tablespoon
lb	pound	t.i.d.	three times a day
liq.	liquid	tinct., tr	tincture
mcg	microgram	tsp, t	teaspoon
mEq	milliequivalent	ung.	ointment
mg	milligram		

basis. This directive requires the nurse to use good judgment as to when a medication is needed and when it is safe to administer.

One-Time Order. The one-time or single order is written for when a medication is to be given only once. A preoperative medication, to help calm the patient and dry secretions before surgery, is an example of a one-time order.

Stat Order. A stat order (from the Latin *statim*, "immediately") is a single order for a medication that must be given immediately. An example of this order is Lasix 20 mg IV stat.

Telephone and Verbal Orders. At times the nurse and physician may discuss a patient's condition over the phone and decide to change the patient's medication regimen. Since the physician is not available to write and sign the order, the nurse may write the order on the physician's order sheet. This type of order is usually designated on the sheet as a "TO (Telephone Order) by Dr. –," and signed by the nurse. It is important for the nurse to repeat the order to the physician before it is written down to ensure accuracy. The order must be co-signed by the physician within a specified time, usually within 48 hours. Similar rules are followed for verbal orders.

Systems of Drug Measurement

Calculation of medication dosages requires a knowledge of the three systems of measurement: the metric system, the apothecaries' system, and the household measures system. All three of these systems are used currently in

TABLE 24–5

Approximate Volume and Weight Equivalents: Metric and Apothecaries' Systems

Metric		Apothecaries'
Volume		
1 milliliter (mL)	=	15 minims
4 milliliters (mL)	=	1 fluidram
15 milliliters (mL)	=	1/2 fluid ounce
30 milliliters (mL)	=	1 fluid ounce
500 milliliters (mL)	=	1 pint
1000 milliliters (mL) or 1 liter (L)	=	1 quart
Weight		
milligram (mg) or 1/1000 grams (g)	=	1/60 grain (gr)
60 milligrams (mg) or 0.06 grams (g)	=	1 grain (gr)
1 gram (g) or 1000 milligrams (mg)	=	15 grains (gr)
4 grams (g)	=	1 dram (ʒ)
30 grams (g)	=	1 ounce (oz)
0.45 kilograms (kg)	=	1 pound (lb)
500 grams (g)	=	1.1 pound (lb)
1000 grams (g) or 1 kilogram (kg)	=	2.2 pounds (lb)

North America, although the metric system is used with increasing frequency.

Metric System

The metric system was introduced in Europe in the late 18th century and is widely used throughout the world. Most European countries and Canada have adopted the metric system. The United States uses all three systems but is committed to converting to the metric system by the Metric Conversion Act of 1975. This act does not specify a date by which this conversion will take place, however. The USP uses only the metric system for weights and measures.

The metric system is based on the decimal system, which is organized in units of tens. The basic units can be multiplied or divided to form secondary units or subdivisions. Calculations of multiples are done by moving the decimal to the right, and divisions are done by moving the decimal to the left.

The basic units used in the metric system include the liter (L)—volume of fluids, the gram (g or Gm)—weight of solids, and the meter (m or M)—measure of length. The subdivisions of the metric basic unit, derived from Latin, are designated with prefixes as follows: deci ($^1/_{10}$ or 0.1 of the unit), centi ($^1/_{100}$ or 0.01 of the unit), and milli ($^1/_{1000}$ or 0.001 of the unit). Multiples of the metric basic unit, derived from Greek, are designated with prefixes as follows: deka (10 times the unit), hecto (100 times the unit), and kilo (1000 times the unit).

Metric equivalents, in volume and weight, are used in medication administration and are listed in Table 24-5. The unit of length, the meter, is not used to compute dosage of medication; rather, it is used for measurements related to the area of a patient's body (abdominal girth, calf circumference), size of wounds, size of areas saturated with drainage, size of skin reactions to medications (tuberculin test), or the size of the area to which medication is applied topically (nitroglycerin ointment).

In clinical practice, the subdivisions milligram (mg) and microgram (μg), and the multiple of the gram, the kilogram (kg), are solely used as measurements of weight. Secondary units of the liter are expressed in milliliters (400 mL), or as decimals (1.5 L) rather than fractions.

Apothecaries' System

The apothecaries' system is the oldest of the three systems of measurement, dating from 1617. Although the apothecaries' system is slowly being replaced by the metric system, its units of measure are used in everyday life. Fluids such as juice and milk are bought in pints and quarts, gasoline is bought in gallons, distances are measures in inches, feet, or miles, and body weight is measured in pounds.

In the apothecaries' system the basic unit of weight is the grain (gr), followed in ascending order with the scruple, the dram, the ounce, and the pound, although the scruple and the dram are seldom used for measurement. The basic unit of volume is the minim (m), followed by the fluidram, the fluid ounce (oz), the pint, the quart, and the gallon. Equivalent measures are listed in Table 24-5.

The symbol for the unit of measure usually is followed by the quantity, expressed by lower-case Roman numerals (i.e., ʒii). An exception to this rule is in using fractions of a unit, where the fraction comes after the abbreviation or word but is expressed in Arabic numerals (i.e., gr $^1/_4$) When the unit of measure is written as a word or an abbreviation, the quantity is expressed in Arabic numerals and precedes the unit of measure (i.e., 2 oz).

Household System

The household system is used primarily for measurements in the home, such as teaspoons, tablespoons, cups, glasses, and drops. Pints and quarts are also household measures but are defined as apothecaries' measures. The household system of measurement is the least accurate of the three systems. Equivalent units of the metric, apothecaries', and household system are listed in Table 24-6.

LEGAL ASPECTS OF MEDICATION ADMINISTRATION

People have long recognized the power of various substances to promote healing. We have also known that these same substances must be used carefully because they have the potential to cause harm and even death. For this reason the job of administering drugs has been relegated to only a relative few in society.

In the interest of public safety, laws have been passed to ensure that medications used in this country are safe, and that they are administered only by qualified people. Agencies have been established to enforce these laws.

Laws Affecting Drugs and Medications

Legislation through the federal government of the United States is directed to regulate and control the manner in which medications are manufactured and marketed. A summary of medication legislation is given in Table 24-7.

The earliest federal legislation was the Pure Food and Drug Act of 1906. This law allowed the government some control in preventing the marketing of many worthless and dangerous drugs. It was later amended to require pharmaceutical companies to accurately label the indications and uses of medications to eliminate false and misleading claims.

Although this law was enacted to ensure the safety of medications, it was limited in its ability to control pre-marketing substance testing. In 1937, reports of illness and death in patients receiving the Elixir of Sulfanilamide aroused public interest (Hahn, et al., 1986). A drug manufacturer replaced the anti-infective chemical sulfanilamide with diethylene glycol, which had not been tested for toxicity in laboratory animals. Many patients died as a result of this switch in chemicals. Because of this tragic incident, the public placed pressure on Congress to pass new legislation to ensure greater safety of prescription medications.

The FDA, an agency of the Department of Health and Human Services, was organized to regulate the manufacture and sale of medications to protect the public's health. This regulatory agency implemented the Federal Food, Drug, and Cosmetic Act of 1938, which gave the FDA the power of enforcement to regulate the effectiveness of all medications. This act mandated that drug manufacturers perform toxicity tests in laboratory animals before seeking FDA approval to market any medication. The law also established procedures by which the FDA could keep a medication from being marketed, or order its recall if the medication was inadequately tested or deemed dangerous for use in patients.

Further amendments were made to tighten control over the quality of all marketing medications. The Durkham–Humphrey Amendment of 1952 was written to clarify which medications could be sold with or without a prescription. After the thalidomide incident of 1962, in which series birth defects were caused by the mother taking thalidomide while pregnant, the Kefauver–Harris Amendment was written, requiring that all medications be proven for safety and efficacy before being approved for marketing.

Once a medication has proven reasonably safe after preclinical toxicity tests in animals, the FDA requires the effects of the medication on humans to be investigated clinically in three phases before it can be marketed.

TABLE 24–6

Equivalent Measures of Volume: Metric, Apothecaries', and Household

Metric		Apothecaries'		Household
0.06 milliliters (mL)	=	1 minim (m)	=	1 drop (gtt)
1.0 milliliter (mL)	=	15 minims (m)	=	15 drops (gtt)
5 milliliters (mL)	=	1 fluidram (f₃)	=	1 teaspoon (tsp)
15 milliliters (mL)	=	4 fluidrams (f₃)	=	1 tablespoon (Tbl)
30 milliliters (mL)	=	1 fluid ounce (f₃)	=	2 tablespoons (Tbl)
180 milliliters (mL)	=	6 fluid ounces (f₃)	=	1 teacupful
240 milliliters (mL)	=	8 fluid ounces (f₃)	=	1 glassful
500 milliliters (mL)	=	1 pint (pt)	=	1 pint (pt)
1000 milliliters (mL)	=	1 quart (qt)	=	1 quart (qt)
4000 milliliters (mL)	=	1 gallon (gal)	=	1 gallon (gal)

TABLE 24-7

United States Legislation Affecting the Clinical Use of Medications

Year Enacted	Law	Impact
1906	Pure Food and Drug Act	Prevented the marketing of adulterated drugs; required labeling to eliminate false or misleading claims.
1938	Federal Food, Drug and Cosmetic Act of 1938	Mandated tests for drug toxicity and provided means for recall of drugs; established procedures for introducing new drugs; gave FDA the power of enforcement.
1952	Durham–Humphrey Amendment	Tightened control of certain drugs; specified drugs to be labeled "may not be distributed without a prescription."
1962	Kefauver–Harris Act	Tightened control over the quality of drugs; gave FDA regulatory power over the procedure of drug investigations; stated that efficacy as well as safety of drugs had to be established.
1970	Controlled Substances Act	Defined drug abuse and classified drugs as to their potential for abuse; provided strict controls over the distribution, storage, and use of these drugs.
1983	Orphan Drug Act	Provided incentives for the development of drugs for treatment of rare diseases.

The FDA also has jurisdiction on all antibiotics, which must meet the standards of purity and potency. The Division of Biological Standards of the National Institutes of Health, a division of the Public Health Service, regulates biologic products such as vaccines, antitoxins, immune serums, immunologic diagnostic aids, and blood derivatives.

The Federal Trade Commission (FTC) regulates the advertising of nonprescription medications. The Wheeler–Lea Act of 1938 mandated that the FTC protect the public from false advertising and from deceptive practices. Control over advertising to the medical profession is under the jurisdiction of the FDA as a result of the Kefauver–Harris Amendments.

Recent changes in Medicare and Medicaid laws have also had an effect on medication administration. Reimbursement of hospitals by the government (through Medicare and Medicaid) has decreased in recent years, forcing hospitals to enact cost-saving measures. To save money, hospital pharmacies no longer stock multiple medications with similar actions. Premixed forms of medications are used more often than before, as are generic forms of drugs. Some medications such as antibiotics are now discontinued automatically after a specified period of time, unless the physician reorders them.

Drug Enforcement Agencies

As a result of the continuing spread of drug abuse and increasing public concern in the late 1960s, Congress enacted the Comprehensive Drug Abuse Prevention and Control Act of 1970, which replaced the Harrison Narcotic Act of 1914 and the Drug Abuse Amendments of 1965. Title II of this 1970 law is called the Controlled Substances Act (CSA), which categorizes controlled substances into five schedules (I, II, III, IV, and V) according to their extent of abuse potential and medical usefulness. Table 24-8 describes the five schedules. Some of these controlled substances include narcotics, amphetamines, barbiturates, and tranquilizers. Under this law it is illegal to possess a controlled substance without a valid prescription, and the law also limits the number of times the prescription can be filled. The primary reasons for the CSA was to prevent drug abuse and dependence, to provide treatment and rehabilitation for people dependent on drugs, and to strengthen drug abuse laws.

In the hospital setting, narcotics are kept in a locked drawer or box as an additional safety measure. Narcotics may be ordered only by physicians registered with the Department of Justice, Bureau of Narcotics and Dangerous Drugs. A record must be kept for each narcotic administered. There are various types of narcotic control sheets provided by individual hospital pharmacies; there is, however, information that is generally required: the name of the patient receiving the narcotic, the date and hour the narcotic was given, the amount of the narcotic used, the name of the physician prescribing the narcotic, and the name of the nurse administering the narcotic. A narcotic count is done at specified times

TABLE 24–8

Five Schedules of Controlled Substances Categorized by the Controlled Substances Act

Schedule	Characteristics	Dispensing Restrictions	Examples*
I	• High abuse potential • No accepted medical use—for research, analysis or instruction only • May lead to severe dependence	• Approved protocol necessary	Heroin, marijuana, tetrahydro-canabinols, LSD, mescaline, peyote, levomoramide, race-moramide, benzylmorphine, and others
II	• High abuse potential • Accepted medical uses • May lead to severe physical and/or psychological dependence	• Written Rx necessary—only emergency dispensing permitted without written Rx • Only required amount may be prescribed • No Rx refills allowed • Container must have warning label	Opium, morphine, hydromor-phone, meperidine, codeine, oxycodone, methadone, secobarbital, pentobarbital, amphetamine, methylpheni-date, methaqualone, and others
III	• Less abuse potential than drugs in Schedules I and II • Accepted medical uses • May lead to moderate/low physical dependence or high psychological dependence	• 34-day supply limit • Written or oral Rx required • Rx expires in 6 months • No more than 5 Rx refills allowed • Container must have warning label†	Preparations containing limited quantities of opium, codeine, hydrocodone, morphine, dihy-drocodeine or ethylmorphine, and nonnarcotic drugs such as: derivatives of barbituric acid except those that are listed in another schedule, glutethi-mide, methylprylon, chlor-phenterminel, mazindol, paregoric, and others
IV	• Low abuse potential compared to Schedule III • Accepted medical uses • May lead to limited physical or psychological dependence	• Written or oral Rx required • 34-day supply limit • Rx expires in 6 months • No more than 5 Rx refills allowed • Container must have warning label†	Barbital, phenobarbital, chloral hydrate, meprobamate, fen-fluramine, chlordiazepoxide, diazepam, oxazepam, chloraze-pate, flurazepam, lorazepam, dextropropoxyphene, penta-zocine, and others
V	• Low abuse potential compared to Schedule IV • Accepted medical uses • May lead to limited physical or psychological dependence	• May require written Rx or be sold with Rx (Check state law)	Medications, generally for relief of coughs or diarrhea, contain-ing limited quantities of certain narcotics

Courtesy Winthrop Laboratories, New York, NY. Modified from Ruggieri, N. L. Drug Therapy 10(12):58–64, 1980 and the DEA pharmacist's manual—an informational outline of the Controlled Substances Act of 1970. U.S. Dept. of Justice, Washington, D.C., June 1980. (Data apply to federal CSA and Uniform Controlled Substances Act; state laws may differ.)

*The examples cited constitute a partial listing. Individual hospital counsel should be consulted for a complete list for a particular state.

† Caution: Federal law prohibits the transfer of this drug to any person other than the patient for whom it was prescribed.

such as at each change of shift. The type and amount of narcotics issued by the pharmacy for that particular unit are counted and any narcotic administered during that previous shift must be on the narcotic control sheet. Before administering a narcotic, the nurse should verify the count in the narcotics drawer and sign the narcotic control sheet to indicate that the medication has been removed. If all or part of a dose is discarded, a nurse should find a second nurse to witness the discarding of the dose and to countersign the control sheet. At the end of the shift, one nurse should record the amount of each narcotic on the narcotic control sheet while the other nurse counts the narcotics out loud. Any discrepancies must be identified and corrected before the nurse leaves the unit; if the discrepancy cannot be resolved, it must be reported to the nursing supervisor or pharmacy.

The Nurse's Role

Legal responsibilities for nurses administering medica-tions include practicing within the scope of the state's nurse practice act, and following the institution's medica-tion administration policies.

Nurse Practice Acts

The administration of medications by nurses is con-trolled by nursing legislation. Nurse practice acts, estab-lished to describe legitimate nursing functions, vary from state to state. It is important that nurses are in-formed about how their state's nurse practice act defines the boundaries of their functions. Each nurse must also recognize their individual limits of knowledge and skill.

Under current nurse practice laws, nurses are responsible for their own actions regardless of the physician's written order. If an order is ambiguous or inappropriate, it is the nurse's responsibility to clarify the medication order with the prescribing physician. If the nurse is not satisfied with the physician's response and believes the order is incorrect or unsafe, it is his or her responsibility to notify the charge nurse or head nurse. Nurses have the right and responsibility to decline to administer a medication if they feel it jeopardizes patient safety.

The nurse is also expected to practice in a safe and prudent manner. The nurse is responsible for being knowledgeable about the medication's actions, indica-tions and contraindications, relation to the patient's disease process, and any adverse effects of the drug. He or she must also know appropriate dosages and dosage schedules, routes and methods of administration, and actions to take in the event of an adverse patient response.

Dispensing medications (i.e., preparing a medication that someone else will deliver) is not a legal practice for registered nurses in most states. Whereas physicians prescribe and pharmacists dispense therapeutic agents, it is the nurse's legal domain to administer medications in a safe and timely manner.

Institutional Medication Policies

Nurses work in a variety of settings, including schools, hospitals, nursing homes, and private industries. Each institution develops and oversees its own policies concerning administration of drugs by nurses and these rules can vary widely.

At some institutions, only registered nurses may administer medications. At others, graduate nurses, licensed practical (or vocational) nurses, or nursing students may be allowed to administer medications. Restrictions may be placed on the types of medications they can give, or on the degree of supervision or experience required. Each institution is governed by its own policies and procedures, and it is the responsibility of the nurse and nursing student to be aware of practice within their institution.

The Patient's Rights

Often the patient has little or no knowledge of pharmacology and medications. Thus, patients must rely on the

Patient Rights According to the Patient's Bill of Rights

1. To be informed of the drug's name, purpose, action and any possible adverse side effects.
2. To refuse any medication.
3. To have a qualified person, i.e., nurse or physician assess your medication history including allergies.
4. To have complete information about the experimental use of any drug and to refuse or consent to its use.
5. To receive labelled medications safely.
6. To receive appropriate therapy adjunctive to the drug therapy.
7. Not to be given unnecessary medications.

From the American Hospital Association, 1973, p. 82.

expertise of the nurse for proper administration of their medications. Patients look to the nurse as a teacher: many of them need to take medications at home, so an essential nursing function is teaching the patient how and when to take home medications. The nurse is thus vested with tremendous responsibility.

The patient has the right to expect safe and appropriate drug administration by the nurse. To accomplish this, the nurse must observe the "five rights": the right drug, in the right dose, at the right time, by the right route, to the right patient. As simplistic as these general rules sound, full compliance with them requires great depth of knowledge by the nurse. These rights are discussed more fully in the "Implementation" section of this chapter.

In addition to these five rights, the patient has the right to refuse to take medications. Under these circumstances it is the duty of the nurse to explain to the patient as fully and clearly as possible the importance of taking the medication. When a patient refuses to comply with prescribed medication therapy, the patient's physician must be notified.

Substance Abuse

The illegal use of drugs by any health professional jeopardizes both patient welfare and professional credibility. The chemically impaired nurse cannot be relied on always to exercise optimal clinical judgment. It is important for the addicted nurse to be identified, so that he or she can obtain treatment, and to ensure patient safety.

Stringent rules and procedures help to prevent diversion of patient medications to hospital personnel. It is the duty and legal obligation of each nurse to maintain accurate medication records, and to report any discrepancies. Nurses are further required by law (and by concern for patient welfare) to report any known diversion of controlled substances by fellow employees.

PRINCIPLES OF DRUG ACTION

Practicing nurses must have an understanding of the ways by which drugs and medications exert their effects. **Pharmacokinetics** is the phase of drug action that describes the process by which a drug moves through the body and is eventually eliminated. **Pharmacodynamics** is the physiologic and biochemical effects of a drug on the body. In addition to pharmacokinetics, a number of variables affect drug action in individuals.

Pharmacokinetics

Pharmacokinetics involves the absorption, distribution, metabolism, and excretion of a medication. Each medication has its own characteristic rate and manner by which it is absorbed by body tissues, delivered to reac-

tive cells, transformed to harmless substances, and removed from the body. The effects and the effectiveness of all medications depend on these four primary factors.

Absorption

Absorption is the process by which a medication enters the bloodstream. The rate at which any drug is absorbed depends on several factors. First, the route of administration affects how quickly and how completely a medication is absorbed. For example, drugs injected directly into the bloodstream are absorbed almost immediately, whereas drugs taken orally can take longer periods to be absorbed. Drug solubility is also a factor affecting absorption; medications in solution are more rapidly absorbed than drugs in timed-release capsules.

The site of administration can either inhibit or promote drug absorption. Tissues rich in capillary blood flow accelerate absorption. Conversely, poor circulation impedes absorption.

Finally, the acid–base environment of body fluids can affect drug absorption. Acidic medications break down (or dissociate) more slowly in an acidic environment, such as the stomach, whereas alkaline medications dissociate more slowly in the small intestine. Slower dissociation causes slower absorption.

Distribution

Once the medication has entered the body and has been absorbed, it must be delivered to the target cells and tissues by the circulatory system, a process called **distribution.** The effectiveness of a medication depends on its concentration at the reactive site. Some medication will be bound to plasma proteins, thus decreasing the total amount of medication available to the tissues. As with absorption, distribution depends on effective circulation.

Certain medications have greater affinity for a specific type of tissue than others. Iodine, for example, accumulates readily in the thyroid gland, but minimally in other tissues. By contrast, alcohol seems able to enter many types of tissue.

Metabolism

After the medication has been distributed to the cells and interacts with them, it undergoes chemical changes. These changes are necessary to convert it to a less active, more readily excretable form. The process by which the drug is thus deactivated is called biotransformation, or simply **metabolism.**

Metabolism of medications takes place mainly in the liver, but can also occur in the blood plasma, kidneys, the intestinal mucosa, and the lungs. Alterations in liver function, including diminished liver function that occurs with aging, can affect the rate at which drugs are metabolized.

Nursing Research

Selected Nursing Research Studies

Allan, E. L., & Barker, K. N. (1990). Fundamentals of medication error research. *American Journal of Hospital Pharmacy, 47,* 555–571.

Edmund, M., Khakoo, R., McTaggert, B., & Solomon, R. (1988). Effect of bedside needle disposal units on needle recapping frequency and needlestick injury. *Infection Control and Hospital Epidemiology, 9*(3), 114–116.

Epperson, E. L. (1984). Efficacy of 0.9% sodium chloride with and without heparin for maintaining indwelling intermittent injection sites. *Clinical Pharmacy, 3,* 626–629.

Fuqua, R. A., & Stevens, K. R. (1988). What we know about medication errors: A literature review. *Journal of Nursing Quality Assurance, 3*(1), 1–17.

Gardner, C. (1987). Risk management of medication errors: Part I. *NITA,* 187–196; Part II: 266–278.

Hamilton, R. A., Plis, J. M., Clay, C., et al. (1988). Heparin sodium versus 0.9% sodium chloride injection for maintaining patency of indwelling intermittent infusion devices. *Clinical Pharmacy, 7,* 439–443.

Maki, D., & Will, L. (1984, April). *Colonization and infection associated with transparent dressings for central venous catheters: A comparitive trial.* Paper presented at the meeting of the Surgical Infection Society, Montreal, Quebec.

Possible Topics For Nursing Inquiry

- Do environmental factors such as temperature or air quality affect the absorption or effectiveness of medications?
- How is compliance with medication regimes affected by different types of patient teaching?
- What is the rate of compliance with medications following patient discharge teaching from the hospital?
- How often is intravenous site care necessary to reduce risk of infection?
- What is the minimum amount of blood volume required to discard from a central venous catheter to obtain blood samples for laboratory tests?
- Can intravenous catheters be flushed with normal saline to maintain patency?
- Does cleansing the skin with alcohol have an affect on infection rates after subcutaneous injections?

Excretion

Drug metabolic by-products are removed from the body by **excretion.** After a medication has been broken down, or metabolized, the resultant products are excreted from the liver in bile, which is dumped into the intestine. Some of the drug's metabolites are excreted in feces, but many are reabsorbed through the intestinal wall and reenter the circulation. Some drugs (such as alcohol and anesthetic gases) are excreted by the lungs. The great majority of drugs are excreted by the kidneys, with the remnants of the original drug becoming components of urine.

Pharmacodynamics

Drug activity is the result of chemical interactions between a medication and the cells of the body to produce a biologic response. Drugs act by manipulating a body process. They can inhibit or stimulate a process, or can replace a missing element. Most drugs interact with a cellular component to initiate a series of biochemical and physiologic changes that result in the drug's effect. The cellular component that interacts with the drug molecules is termed a receptor cite (Malseed & Harrigan, 1989). Drugs can affect a cell membrane, a cellular enzyme, or certain intracellular components.

The biochemical and physiologic effects can be local or systemic. Local effects can be seen in the application of moisturizing lotion to chapped skin. An example of systemic effects are those of some analgesics (pain medications), which can affect the nervous system, the heart, and the gastrointestinal tract.

Medication effects are monitored by changes in the patient's clinical condition. Physical or psychological symptoms generally improve, or laboratory tests show improvement, when medications are effective. In addition to clinical observations, medications are often monitored by laboratory measurements of their level in the blood.

Therapeutic Effects

The desired and intentional effects of a medication are called its therapeutic effects. These effects vary with the nature of the medication, the length of time the patient has been receiving the medication, and the patient's physical condition. Interactions with other medications can also affect a drug's therapeutic action. The onset of action of medications varies widely and, thus, time needed for therapeutic effects to become evident also varies (Fig. 24-1).

Side (Adverse) Effects

Every medication is prescribed to accomplish a therapeutic goal, so each drug is carefully chosen for its thera-

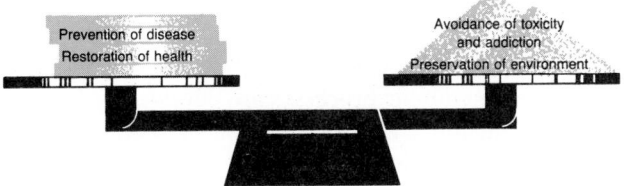

Figure 24–1. The proper use of medications attempts to strike a balance between risks and benefits.

peutic effects. Practically all medications produce additional effects other than their primary therapeutic effect. These additional medication effects are called side effects. Many of these effects are minor and essentially harmless.

Some side effects can be ignored, but others are undesirable. Some are important because they are potentially harmful. These adverse effects may result from the secondary effects of a medication, from toxicity or cumulative medication effects, from individual patient sensitivity, or from idiosyncratic reactions (Rodman, 1985).

Secondary Reactions. Secondary reactions to a medication occur due to the multiple actions of a drug within the body. These effects vary from minor to major importance to the patient. Minor secondary effects may be disturbing to the patient who does not expect them. The patient who has been given phenazopyridine (Pyridium) to treat painful urination should be warned that the urine will turn red while the medication is being taken. Common medication side effects that may necessitate discontinuation of the medication include nausea and vomiting, changes in gastrointestinal function (e.g., gastric bleeding, diarrhea), and changes in level of consciousness, such as excitation or somnolence (Spencer et al., 1989).

Sometimes unpleasant secondary effects may be present after initial doses of a medication, but they may subside with subsequent doses. Bothersome secondary effects of a medication may be tolerated by a patient if they are far outweighed by the therapeutic effects. In some cases, there may be little choice other than to accept secondary effects of a drug, especially when no alternative medication is available, and when lack of treatment will result in death. Chemotherapy agents used to treat cancer are a prime example of this dilemma.

For some patients, the secondary effects of a medication may lead to life-threatening problems, such as liver or kidney damage, or bone marrow suppression. If the physician and nurse are aware of medication side effects, and if the patient is closely monitored, important secondary effects of medications can often be identified early and appropriate intervention can be instituted.

Medication Toxicity. Medication toxicity is described as a deleterious effect a medication has on various tissues of the body. It results from overdosage, ingestion of a medication intended for external use, and a buildup of the medication in the blood due to impaired metabolism and excretion. Careful attention must be given specifically to the dosage as well as to monitoring for toxicity. Some medications can produce toxic effects almost immediately, whereas some toxic effects are not apparent for days or weeks.

Cumulative Effects. Cumulative effects of a medication occur when the patient is unable to metabolize or break down a medication before the next dose is given. Unless the medication dosage is adjusted, the amount of the medication builds up in the patient's body. In some cases, this cumulative effect is desirable, such as with medications used to prevent depression.

Tolerance. Tolerance to a medication can occur in patients who develop a decreased response to a medication, requiring an increase in the dosage to achieve therapeutic effect. Some medications that produce tolerance include tobacco, ethyl alcohol, opiates, and barbiturates.

Hypersensitivity Reactions. Hypersensitivity reactions occur when a patient is unusually sensitive to the therapeutic effects or to the secondary effects of a medication. An estimated therapeutic dosage of medication may be too large for the individual patient and may result in a degree of action that is greater than desired. For example, a middle-aged man of normal body weight usually requires 75 to 100 mg of meperidine to relieve pain; rarely, a man of similar age and body size may respond with pain control of long duration and excessive somnolence. Usually, if the medication dose or the medication dosing interval are decreased, the medication may be administered safely.

Idiosyncratic Effects. Idiosyncratic effects are the unpredictable and inexplicable symptoms caused by a genetic defect in the patient that alters the way he or she responds to a medication. These symptoms are completely different from what is expected and may occur the first time a medication is administered. Patients may not react as expected or may overreact to a particular medication.

One genetic defect that results in idiosyncratic medication reactions occurs in black men who are given antimalarial medications. Five to ten percent of black men lack an enzyme that protects the integrity of the red blood cell membrane; when a susceptible man is given the antimalarial medication primaquine, his red blood cells are hemolyzed. When a patient belongs to a known risk group, blood tests can be used to screen for the genetic defect that causes an idiosyncratic medication reaction (Rodman, 1985).

Allergic Reactions. Allergic reactions result from an immunologic reaction to a medication to which the patient has already been sensitized. A foreign substance or antigen has been introduced into the body, and the body responds by producing antibodies. Patients respond to certain medications as they would to this foreign substance, and develop symptoms of an allergic reaction. These symptoms can be mild or severe. A mild allergic reaction can produce symptoms such as skin reactions (urticaria), pruritus, angioedema, rhinitis, nausea, vomiting, and diarrhea. Mild reactions can occur within minutes of medication administration to 2 weeks after the administration of a medication. Skin reactions, including hives, rashes, and lesions, usually improve soon after the medication is discontinued (Rodman, 1985). Severe allergic reactions produce symptoms such as wheezing, dyspnea, hypotension, and tachycardia, and occur immediately after the medication is given. A severe allergic reaction is called an anaphylactic reaction and requires immediate medical intervention, since it can be fatal. Treatment includes discontinuation of the medication responsible and administration of intravenous fluids, steroids, and antihistamines.

Medication Interaction. Medication interaction occurs when the effects of a medication are altered by the concurrent presence of other medications or food (Fig. 24-2). This interaction of medications may result in potentiation or synergism, which increases a drug's effects. Interaction can also result in antagonism, where drug effects are decreased. In some cases a drug will precipitate from solutions if mixed with other incompatible medications. Sometimes a drug is influenced by foods; an example of food–drug interaction is the deactivation of the antibiotic tetracycline by dairy products.

The nurse must be aware of drug interactions with other medications and foods to protect the patient from their harmful effects. Incompatibility charts and the hospital pharmacist are valuable resources for providing this information.

Factors Affecting Drug Action

A number of variables can alter the effects of medications. Among these are the age of the patient, weight, height, gender, genetic factors, environment, time of administration, organ system function, and psychological condition.

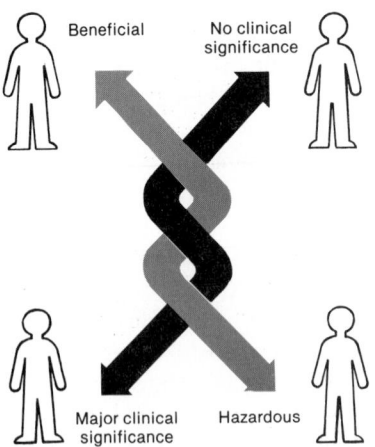

Figure 24–2. Drug interactions may vary.

Age. Developmental factors greatly affect the action of medications. During the first years of life, tissues, organs and metabolic processes are developing. Factors in the infant that affect drug action include increased total body water volume, decreased body fat, decreased plasma proteins, relative lack of gastric acid, changing metabolic rate, and immature renal and liver function. Care must be taken to arrive at an appropriate medication dose for each infant, considering these variables. During this early period, medication may also affect developing tissues—for example, when the antibiotic tetracycline is given to very young children, permanent staining of teeth may occur.

Many physiologic changes occur in older adults that affect their response to medications. Changes such as decreased lean body mass and total body water, increased body fat, more alkaline gastric secretions, and decreased gastric and intestinal motility, all affect drug action in the body. In addition, many older people have chronic health problems involving the liver, the kidneys, or the cardiovascular system; the cumulative effect of these changes usually is that decreased doses of medications need to be administered at less frequent intervals. Side effects and adverse medication reactions are more common in older adults because of physiologic changes that have occurred, chronic disease states that are often present, and multiple medications that are often ordered for the older adult.

Weight. The patient's body weight must be considered when administering any medication. The greater the body weight, the greater the mass of body tissues and thus the larger the dose of medication required. A person's weight may be used to estimate the appropriate beginning dosage for a medication.

Height. Height and weight can be used to estimate body surface area. Dosages of drugs, including anesthetics, may be based on estimates of body surface area.

Gender. There are two main reasons that men and women respond to medications differently: differences in fat and water distribution, and differences in hormones. Although women weigh less than men, they have proportionally more adipose tissue; men have more body fluid than women. Some medications are more soluble in fat, whereas others are more soluble in water. Generally, men absorb some medications more readily than women.

Genetic Factors. Because of genetic factors, a patient may metabolize a medication differently or respond to a specific medication with abnormal sensitivity. These reactions, called idiosyncratic reactions, were discussed earlier in this chapter.

Time of Administration. The time of administration of oral medications can affect their speed and duration of action. An empty stomach facilitates absorption of an oral medication, thus enhancing its efficacy. Some medications, such as ferrous sulfate, irritate the gastric mucosa of the stomach and must be taken with or after meals.

Organ System Function. Predictable medication effects depend on properly functioning organs. The presence of liver, kidney, or cardiovascular dysfunction, as well as a number of other organic or glandular conditions, can seriously alter the effects of a medication on the body. Because of their respective importance in medication metabolism and excretion, decreased liver or kidney function can result in cumulative drug effects (Coutts, 1986). Decreased cardiac output, heart failure, or circulatory problems can alter delivery of medications to body tissues.

Glandular dysfunctions such as thyroid disorders or diabetes can have profound effects on medication action, and the nurse must be knowledgeable about the effects these types of disorders have on a wide variety of medications. The complexity of these effects makes the consultation of drug resources (such as the PDR) a practical necessity.

Psychological State. The patient's psychological status can affect the action of psychoactive medications. For example, analgesics relieve pain and sedatives decrease anxiety by acting on the nervous system; patients who are experiencing extreme anxiety often require larger doses of either of these types of drugs to relieve symptoms than do patients with much lower anxiety levels.

MEDICATION ASSESSMENT

To administer medications safely to any patient, it is important to collect information during the initial assessment. In addition to this baseline data, a medication-specific assessment should be part of the ongoing nursing assessment to determine drug effectiveness and promptly identify side effects. Assessment is also necessary to individualize appropriate patient teaching to help ensure patient compliance with pharmacologic therapy.

Information Collected on Admission

Important information to elicit from the patient during the initial interview includes a medication history, allergies, medical history, and pregnancy and lactation status.

Medication History

During the admission interview, the patient should be asked the names, dosages, dosage schedules, and the action of the medications routinely taken before admission. Whenever possible, the nurse should discuss the medication history with the family present. A family member may provide information that is not volunteered by the patient, such as "mother doesn't take her water pill in the evening because she doesn't like to go to the bathroom at night." Some patients bring their medications with them from home. Nurses need to ascertain whether the physician would like the patient to continue taking these medications. In many hospitals all medications brought in by the patient are sent home with family members or are stored in a secure location until the patient is discharged. Some agencies permit patients to keep their own medications at the bedside once they have been checked and labeled by the pharmacy department and an order has been obtained from the physician. The physician should be alerted about all medications the patient has been taking, so that necessary medications can be ordered for the patient. This is especially important if the patient is taking antidiabetic agents, anticonvulsant medications, or cardiovascular medications.

The nurse should also discuss the use of any over-the-counter medications by the patient. A question such as "do you take any medications that you buy without a prescription" may be helpful in eliciting this information. A patient may consider a medication such as aspirin, acetaminophen, or a laxative so common that they do not remember to include them when asked to list medications. In particular, eye drops, nasal sprays, skin lotions, and food additives may not be considered medications by the patient.

When patients are taking multiple medications, when they cannot remember the names of all the medications they are taking, or when their medication profile does not match their clinical status, the patient or family should be asked to bring all bottles of medications in for the nurse to evaluate. Access to the patient's medication bottles allows the nurse to make a complete list of ordered prescription medications, and may allow the nurse to notice actual or potential medication problems. The nurse should note whether prescriptions have expired, whether all medications are stored separately in correctly marked containers, and if the number of pills in the bottle seems correct considering the date and specifics of the prescription.

Allergies

During the admission interview, a patient should be asked about allergies to any medication. If the patient indicates any medication allergies, the nurse should ask follow-up questions about the allergic symptoms noted with each drug. This information allows the nurse to differentiate between a medication that caused a true allergic response and a medication that caused unpleasant side effects. In some situations medications that caused unpleasant side effects, such as nausea, may be used.

All stated patient allergies should be written on the patient's record, on the cover of the patient's chart, and in any other locations mandated by hospital policy. The record should also include the patient's reaction to each medication. Hospitalized patients should have all allergies listed on a wrist band and on all medication administration records.

Medical History

Before administering any medication to a patient, the nurse should be aware of the patient's medical diagnosis and general medical history. The presence of renal, hepatic, cardiac, respiratory, endocrine, or neurologic dysfunction is important to ascertain before administering any medication. The nurse can use this information to identify those patients at greater risk for drug toxicity or those patients who may require extra care in drug administration.

Drug or alcohol abuse is also important to determine before medication administration. The patient who has frequently used narcotics or alcohol may require higher doses of sedatives or narcotics to obtain the desired effect. Patients who have a history of drug abuse or addiction are more likely to become drug dependent when given narcotics, sedatives, or tranquilizers. Use of aspirin in the alcoholic patient may predispose the patient to gastric irritation and bleeding. The use of normal doses of acetaminophen in alcoholic patients may occasionally cause severe hepatic or renal dysfunction (Kaysen, et al., 1985; Seeff, et al., 1986).

Pregnancy and Lactation Status

A patient's pregnancy or lactation status is important to determine before medication administration. Drugs known to cause birth defects in the developing fetus are called teratogenic. The use of any drug known to be teratogenic or which has not been thoroughly evaluated should be avoided during pregnancy. In certain rare instances (e.g., a pregnant patient with difficult-to-control epilepsy), the use of a potentially harmful drug during pregnancy may be indicated. The physician should discuss the risks and benefits of such treatment with the patient before administration of the drug, and this discussion should be documented in the patient's record. Late in pregnancy, hepatotoxic medications should be avoided, since there is an increased risk of incurring liver damage (Coults, 1986).

A medication may be excreted through breast milk and ingested by a nursing infant. Most medications are excreted in low dosages that do not affect a nursing infant, but certain medications such as some narcotics, antibiotics, anticoagulants, anticonvulsants, histamine

antagonists, and tranquilizers can be excreted in amounts great enough to affect the infant (Spencer, et al., 1989). If a woman must receive a medication that is excreted in large concentrations in breast milk, she should bottle-feed her infant.

Assessment Before Medication Administration

Before the administration of any medication, the nurse should assess the patient medication record, current diet and fluid orders, scheduled diagnostic tests or surgical procedures, and the physical status of the patient.

Medication Record

Before giving a patient any medication, the nurse should check the patient's current medication administration record. The patient may have several medications ordered to treat the same problem. Checking the patient's medication record allows the nurse to see which medication has been used most recently and whether it is time for the medication to be administered. Knowing a patient's current medications also allows the nurse to avoid giving a medication that may interfere with or add to the effect of another medication the patient has received.

Diet and Fluid Orders

A patient may have fluids and food withheld in preparation for surgery or for a diagnostic test. When a patient is ordered to have nothing by mouth (NPO), most oral medications are usually not given. When the patient is receiving important medications that should not be discontinued abruptly (e.g., blood pressure medication, digoxin, anticonvulsants), the physician should be contacted concerning alternative orders for medication administration. In some situations, physicians order that oral medications be administered with a small sip of water even though a patient is NPO.

When a diabetic patient is NPO the nurse should contact the physician concerning specific orders for diabetic medications. Patients taking oral hypoglycemics still produce some endogenous insulin, so the physician may hold these agents if they are NPO for short periods of time. The patients' blood glucose level is monitored regularly, and insulin may be needed if blood glucose levels rise above normal. When insulin-dependent diabetic patients are NPO, they should have their insulin doses adjusted and their blood glucose levels monitored frequently. If the insulin-dependent patient is NPO for longer than 4 hours, infusion of IV dextrose solutions and continuous IV insulin facilitate efficient, safe care. It is important that patients receiving insulin have scheduled tests or surgery on time to avoid glucose imbalance.

Laboratory Values

Laboratory tests may be used to monitor serum drug levels, medication effects, and medication side effects. Dosages of medications such as digoxin, gentamicin, phenytoin, and theophylline are monitored through serum levels to determine proper dosage for the patient. The nurse is responsible for assessing these serum drug levels and notifying the physician when values outside the therapeutic range are obtained. This permits the physician to change the medication dosage to ensure therapeutic effects without causing undesirable toxicity.

Laboratory tests may also be used to monitor the direct effects of a medication. Medications such as iron, potassium, and thyroid preparations that are given to maintain a body substance, may be monitored by drawing serum concentrations. Anticoagulants are also monitored for therapeutic effect by drawing venous blood to determine the coagulation status of the patient.

Common or serious side effects of medications may be monitored using laboratory tests. Many diuretics are potassium-wasting, hence potassium levels are drawn to detect hypokalemia. Many types of chemotherapy cause leukopenia (decreased numbers of white blood cells) or thrombocytopenia (decreased numbers of platelets); thus, blood counts are monitored before and after chemotherapy. When medications are known to cause kidney dysfunction, laboratory tests of kidney function (serum creatinine and blood urea nitrogen) are done at regular intervals. When medications can potentially cause liver damage, laboratory tests of liver function (SGOT, SGPT) are frequently evaluated (Henrietta, 1987).

Physical Assessment

Before giving a medication, the nurse should quickly assess the patient's physical status to judge the patient's ability to take the medication. Variables that influence the ability to take a medication include the ability to swallow, normal gastrointestinal motility for oral medications, and presence of adequate muscle mass and venous access for parenteral medications. If the medication is likely to have an effect on vital signs or on the function of a body system, vital signs or appropriate body systems are assessed before medication administration.

Ability to Swallow. Before administering an oral medication, a nurse must be sure that the patient has an adequate swallowing reflex. If the nurse has a suspicion that a patient is not able to swallow, he or she should give the patient several sips of water. If the patient coughs or chokes when given the water, the medication should not be given and the patient's physician should be informed.

Gastrointestinal Motility. The patient who has recently undergone major surgery or who has gastrointestinal dysfunction may not be able to absorb oral medications. If a nurse suspects that a patient's gastrointestinal function is abnormal, he or she should perform a quick abdominal assessment before giving an oral medication. If the patient's abdomen is distended and firm, and if bowel sounds are hyperactive or absent, gastrointestinal dysfunction is present. The patient's physician should be contacted to check if oral medications should be given.

Adequate Muscle Mass. Premature infants or debilitated patients may have very limited amounts of lean muscle mass. If an irritating medication is given into subcutaneous (SC) tissue or into a very small muscle, pain, inadequate absorption of medication, or tissue damage could occur. The patient's physician should be contacted to determine if another route of medication administration could be used.

Adequate Venous Access. Before giving an IV medication, the nurse should be sure that the IV catheter is located in an adequate vein. The catheter insertion site should be checked for temperature, redness, swelling, and pain. If the catheter is being used to infuse IV fluids, the infusion rate should be fast enough to deliver the IV medication in a time limit appropriate to the specific medication.

Vital Signs. Blood pressure, heart rate, and respiratory rate may be affected by medications. Before giving a medication that may affect one of the vital signs, the nurse should measure and record that value. Blood pressure should be measured before administering antihypertensive medications or before administering coronary vasodilators (nitroglycerin, isosorbide dinitrate). If the patient's systolic blood pressure is low (usually less than 90 or 100 mg Hg systolic), the medication may be withheld. Counting apical heart rate is necessary before giving digitalis, a medication that slows the heart rate. If the heart rate, when counted for 1 minute, is slow (usually less than 60 beats/minute), the medication may be withheld. Respiratory rate should be counted before giving a medication, such as a narcotic, that may affect the rate.

Body System Assessment. Medications are often used to treat a dysfunctional body system. In order to assess the effect of a medication, the nurse needs to assess the appropriate body system before giving the medication. For example, bronchodilators can be inhaled by a patient with chronic obstructive lung disease to treat bronchospasm. Before beginning the treatment, the nurse should assess the patient's respiratory system. This quick assessment includes counting the respiratory rate, asking the patient to rate his or her ease of breathing, noting the use of accessory respiratory muscles, and auscultating the patient's breath sounds. After the treatment, the assessment is repeated. The nurse can judge the effect of the treatment by noting any changes in assessment findings and by noting the length of time the change lasts.

Assessment of Knowledge and Compliance

Many factors influence whether a patient will comply with prescribed medication. Nursing assessment can provide a knowledge base to assist the nurse in better understanding whether the patient is likely to comply with the physician's drug order. Assessment can also provide the basis for individualized patient teaching to help ensure patient compliance.

Compliance

Compliance with a medication routine means that the patient takes the medication as prescribed. Lack of compliance occurs in many ways, such as when the patient fails to take any of the prescribed drug, fails to take the proper number of doses of the drug, takes extra doses of the drug, fails to follow the dosage schedule as prescribed, discontinues the medication prematurely, excessively uses a PRN order, or takes medications that were ordered previously for another condition. Compliance with a medication routine is more likely to occur when the patient understands and agrees with the rationale for using the medication, the routine for taking the medications, and the desired effect of the medications. Simple medication routines that are tailored to the patient's lifestyle are more likely to be followed.

A patient's attitude about medical care and about a specific medication can influence the patient's compliance with drug therapy. The nurse can begin by asking general questions such as "Do you feel that these medications will help you get better?" The nurse should also be alert to comments made by the patient that indicate lack of confidence in the prescribed drug treatment.

Lifestyle and financial considerations also affect compliance with drug therapy. The patient who has a regular income, health insurance, and a stable home situation is more likely to be able to afford to pay for medications and be able to organize routines to remember to take them. When a patient does not have a home, an income, or health insurance, buying, storing, and remembering to take medication regularly can be difficult.

Knowledge

Patient knowledge about a prescribed medication may vary with each individual patient and depends on many factors. Some patients desire and receive detailed information about the medications they are taking, whereas other patients want and receive minimal information. The nurse should determine what the patient needs to know to safely take the medication, and then ask questions to elicit this information. Inadequate knowledge or gaps in important knowledge areas should be clearly documented so that an individualized teaching plan can be formulated.

Assessment of cognitive ability is important for individualizing the teaching plan and determining whether the patient can independently manage self-medication. Cognitive impairment, confusion, and psychiatric disorders may increase the potential for noncompliance. Learning disabilities may necessitate creative teaching to help ensure understanding and compliance with therapy. It is often helpful to include family members or the caregiver in the teaching sessions. For confused or cognitively impaired patients, the nurse may need to check the patient's mouth to see that the pill has been swallowed.

NURSING DIAGNOSES

Noncompliance and Knowledge Deficit are NANDA nursing diagnoses that often are applicable to the patient who is managing self-medication. In addition, medication side effects can contribute to many other significant problems for the patient.

Diagnostic Statement: Noncompliance

Definition

Noncompliance is a patient's informed decision not to adhere to a therapeutic recommendation (NANDA, 1990).

Defining Characteristics

Behavior indicative of failure to adhere (by direct observation or by statements of patient or significant others); objective tests (physiologic measures, detection of makers); evidence of development of complications; evidence of exacerbation of symptoms; failure to keep appointments; failure to progress (NANDA, 1990).

Related Factors

Patient value system: health beliefs, cultural influences, spiritual values; patient–provider relationships (NANDA, 1990).

Diagnostic Statement: Knowledge Deficit

Definition

Knowledge deficit is the state in which an individual experiences a deficiency in cognitive knowledge or psychomotor skill regarding the condition or treatment plan (NANDA, 1990).

Defining Characteristics

Verbalization of the problem; inaccurate follow-through of instruction; inaccurate performance of test; inappropriate or exaggerated behaviors, e.g., hysterical, hostile, agitated, apathetic (NANDA, 1990).

Related Factors

Lack of exposure; lack of recall; information misinterpretation; cognitive limitation; lack of interest in learning; unfamiliarity with information resources (NANDA, 1990).

Related Nursing Diagnoses

Medication administration can increase the potential for the occurrence of many nursing diagnoses. High Risk for Infection is an appropriate diagnosis when administering parenteral medications to some patients or when administering medications that decrease bone marrow function, and High Risk for Injury is an appropriate diagnosis when administering medications that can cause syncope or alter cognition. Many medications can alter normal bowel function, causing Diarrhea or Constipation, and some can cause Altered Sexuality Patterns, Sexual Dysfunction, and Sleep Pattern Disturbance. Impaired Home Maintenance Management may occur when medication regimes are very complex and difficult to manage independently.

MEDICATION ADMINISTRATION

A series of events have taken place before the nurse administers medications. This series and those that follow are illustrated in Figure 24-3.

Process to Ensure Safety

Knowledge and skill are important in ensuring patient safety during medication administration. To administer medications safely, the nurse must:

- Accurately interpret the physician's order.
- Accurately calculate the amount of drug to give for the prescribed dose.
- Develop a systematic and safe procedure, using the "five rights" for drug administration.
- Document medication administration according to agency policy.

Interpretation of the Order

The nurse is responsible for safe interpretation of the medication order. When a new order is written by the physician, the nurse must be able to read the specifics of the written order. When the order is illegible, misinterpretation of the intended medication request can easily occur. If the written order is not completely clear or contains unusual abbreviations, the nurse should consult the physician for clarification. Clarification of the written order may also be necessary if important information, such as the route or frequency, is omitted from the medication order.

The nurse should also evaluate whether the amount and route ordered is likely to be safe for the patient. The nurse needs to know, or look up, the dosage range, the route of administration, contraindications, and side effects before giving any medication. If the nurse questions the safe use of any prescribed medication, he or she has the legal responsibility to consult with the physician rather than administer a medication that could potentially cause harm.

Calculating Medication Dosages

Medication orders are usually written in metric units of measurement, and medications are usually supplied in

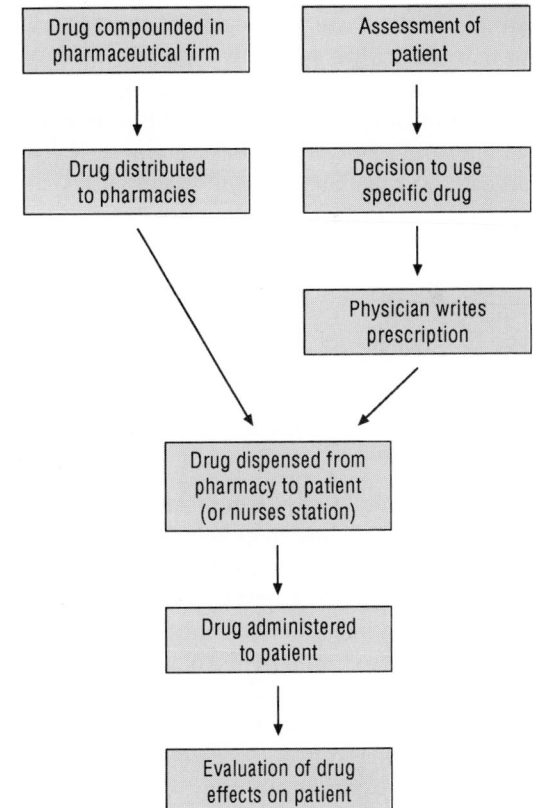

Figure 24–3. Series of events in drug therapy. Adapted from Spencer, R. T., Nichols, L. W., Lipkin G. B., et al. (1989). *Clinical Pharmacology and Nursing Management* (3rd ed.). Philadelphia: J. B. Lippincott.

metric units of measurements. Occasionally, liquid medications or commonly used oral medications may be ordered in apothecary or household units of measurement. If a medication is ordered in one unit of measurement and supplied by the pharmacy in another unit of measurement, the nurse must calculate the amount of medication needed in the measurement system ordered.

If the calculated dosage of a medication seems unusual (e.g., if it consists of more than three tablets, a fraction of less than one-half tablet, or more than one unit dose of a liquid medication), or if the nurse has any doubts about the accuracy of his or her calculation, he or she should ask another nurse or a pharmacist to check the dosage calculation (Spencer, et al., 1989). Calculations of dosages of medications with important or toxic side effects (including heparin and insulin) should also be double-checked by another nurse or pharmacist.

Conversions Within a System. If the medication is ordered and supplied in the same measurement system, the nurse can use the following formula to calculate the amount of medication needed:

Dosage ordered $\times$

$$\frac{\text{Volume on hand}}{\text{Dose on hand}} = \text{Volume to be given}$$

Conversions within the metric system can be done using this formula or can be calculated simply by remembering that the metric system is based on units of ten. Equivalents are computed by multiplying or dividing, moving the decimal point to the right or left, respectively. There are only three basic units in the metric system used to calculate medication dosages: the gram (g), the milligram (mg), and the microgram (μg). The equivalents among these three units are: 1 gram (g) = 1000 milligrams (mg) = 1,000,000 micrograms (μg).

To change grams to milligrams, the grams are multiplied by 1000 (since there are 1000 milligrams in 1 gram), or the decimal point is moved three places to the left. An example of this conversion in an equation is: 800 mg = 0.8 g.

Conversions from One System to Another. Use of the metric system of measurement is becoming more common, although the need to convert from one system to another continues to exist. For example, a patient's order may specify grains but the medication is dispensed from the pharmacy in milligrams. Nurses must have the knowledge of commonly used equivalents to help them convert from one system to another. It is important to note that conversion from one system of measurement to another system results in an approximate equivalent, not an equal answer. Refer to Tables 24-5 and 24-6 for common conversion equivalents. Knowledge of volume conversion may be necessary when using liquid medications.

Knowledge of approximate weight equivalents for the metric and apothecaries' systems is necessary in situations that involve converting a patient's body weight from kilograms to pounds, or when converting grams and milligrams to grains, and vice versa.

When converting units of weight from the metric system to the apothecaries' system, the nurse must remember that a milligram is smaller than a grain. When smaller units are converted to larger units, the result is a smaller number. If the physician orders the dose of medication in grains and the medication available is dispensed in grams, then the grams must be converted to grains. An example of this conversion is to change 15 milligrams to grains. It is known that 60 milligrams is approximately equal to 1 grain; therefore, the equation can be computed as follows:

$$
\begin{aligned}
\text{miligrams} &: \text{grains} = \text{milligrams} : \text{grains} \\
60 &: 1 = 15 : X \\
60\,X &= 15 \\
X &= 15 : 60 \text{ or } 15/60 \\
X &= 0.25 \text{ grain or } 1/4 \text{ grain}
\end{aligned}
$$

Conversely, when converting from a larger unit (grains) to a smaller unit (milligrams), the result is a larger number. An example of this conversion is to change 10 grains to milligrams. The equation is computed as follows:

$$
\begin{aligned}
\text{grains} &: \text{milligrams} = \text{grains} : \text{milligrams} \\
1 &: 60 = 10 : X \\
1/60\,X &= 10 \\
X &= 10 \times 60 \\
X &= 600 \text{ milligrams (mg) or} \\
&\quad 0.6 \text{ gram (G)}
\end{aligned}
$$

These same rules apply when converting pounds to kilograms and vice versa. The pound is a smaller unit than the kilogram, therefore the computation is made by dividing (so the result will be a smaller number). If a patient weighs 180 pounds (lbs), how many kilograms does this convert to? It is known that 2.2 pounds is approximately equal to 1 kilogram. The equation is computed as follows:

$$
\begin{aligned}
\text{pounds} &: \text{kilograms} = \text{pounds} : \text{kilograms} \\
2.2 &: 1 = 180 : X \\
2.2\,X &= 180 \\
X &= 180 : 2.2 \text{ or } 180/2.2 \\
X &= 81.8 \text{ kilograms (kg)}
\end{aligned}
$$

To convert kilograms to pounds, the conversion is made by multiplying by 2.2 (so the result is a larger number). An example of this equation is as follows:

$$kilograms \ : \ pounds \ = \ kilograms \ : \ pounds$$
$$1 \quad : \quad 2.2 \quad = \quad 60 \quad : \quad X$$
$$2.2 \ X \quad = \quad 60$$
$$X \quad = \quad 60 \times 2.2$$
$$X \quad = \quad 132 \ pounds \ (lbs)$$

Calculating Children's Dosages. Calculation of children's dosages are most often calculated using the child's weight or body surface area. When necessary, they can be determined by several different formulas. Calculation of the adult dosage is reduced in proportion to the age or weight of the child. There is no one completely satisfactory method of computing a child's dose from an adult's; these formulas should be used as guides. Keep in mind that most drugs are ordered specifically for a child and are not computed from an adult dose. The nurse must take into account the wide varieties in the size of a child and the individual metabolic rate, which influences the therapeutic dose. Observing the child's response to the medication may determine if the dosage of the medication needs to be adjusted for the benefit of the individual child.

The most common formula for determining dosages for children is Clark's Rule. This formula is based on the assumption that the average adult weighs 150 pounds:

$$\frac{Weight \ of \ child \ in \ pounds}{150} \times Usual \ adult \ dose$$
$$= Child's \ dose$$

Another method of determining medication dosages for children, called Young's Rule, is based on the age of the child in years. This formula is stated as follows:

$$\frac{Age \ of \ child \ in \ years}{Age \ of \ child \ + \ 12} \times Usual \ adult \ dose$$
$$= Child's \ dose$$

Intravenous Medication Calculations. Intravenous medication calculations are calculated to ensure the proper infusion rate for IV medications. To infuse a medication over a set time period, the nurse needs to calculate the appropriate rate of flow for the medication. Intravenous flow rates are calculated in drips/minute. To calculate IV drip rate, the nurse can use the following formula:

$$\frac{mL \ of \ solution}{Hours \ to \ administer} \times \frac{Drops \ per \ mL \ (drip \ rate \ factor)}{60 \ (min/hr)}$$
$$= Drops \ per \ minute$$

The amount, type, and infusion rate of IV medication are ordered by the physician. The drip rate factor varies with the type and brand of IV tubing. Two general types of IV tubing, macrodrip and minidrip tubing, are available. Macrodrip (large-drop) tubing is often used to administer piggyback medications. Macrodrip tubing is made so that each drop of solution equals a fraction of a milliliter. The drip rate factor of macrodrip tubing varies with the brand of the tubing; most Cutter brand macrodrip tubing is made with a drip rate factor of 20 drops/mL; most Abbot brand macrodrip tubing is made with a drip rate factor of 15 drops/mL; and most Travenol brand macrodrip tubing is made with a drip rate factor of 10 drops/mL. The drip rate factor of a specific type of macrodrip tubing is found on the outside of the tubing package. All brands of minidrip tubing have the same drip factor, 60 drops/mL. Because the drop rate per milliliter (60) is equal to the number of minutes per hour, the formula for calculating drip rate when using minidrip tubing may be simplified to mL/hour = drops/minute.

Administering Medications According to the "Five Rights"

After the nurse has validated the order and calculated the proper drug dose, accurate administration of a medication can be assured by following the "five rights" of medication administration. Each time a medication is administered it is important to be sure that the right patient is given the right medication, in the right dose, by the right route, at the right time.

The Right Patient. The first "right" of administering medications, the right patient, means that the medication is given to the patient for whom it is intended (Fig. 24-4).

Incorrect identification of patients can occur when a nurse is busy, when patients of similar names are located in the same areas of an institution, and when patient identification procedures are not followed. Errors can be avoided if the nurse identifies the patient by name and checks the name band against the patient's medication record before giving him or her medications. The institution's "name alert" policy should be followed whenever patients with similar names are located in the same unit. Name alert procedures involve a special way of identifying patients with similar names and a way of alerting other departments of the patients' name similarity.

"Five Rights" of Medication Administration

- Identify the *right patient*
- Select the *right medication*
- Give the *right dose*
- Give the medication at the *right time*
- Give the medication by the *right route*

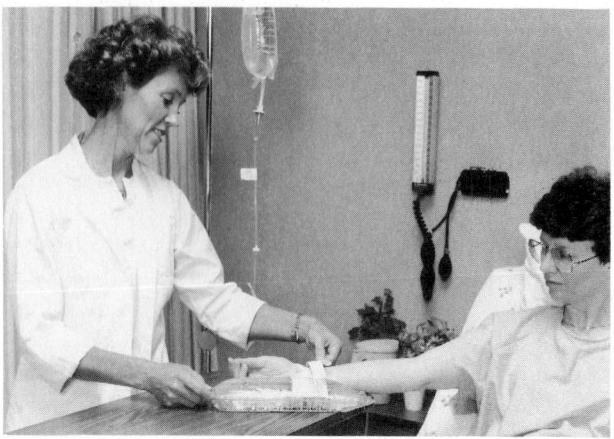

Figure 24–4. No matter what the administration route, the nurse must always check that he or she has the right patient. The nurse checks the medication record, the unit dosage, and the patient's identification bracelet. If the patient is conscious, the nurse also asks the patient to state his or her name.

The Right Medication. The second "right" of administering medications, the right medication, means that the medication given is the medication that was ordered, and that the medication ordered is appropriate for the individual patient. Medication errors may occur when a pharmacist incorrectly dispenses a medication that is similar in shape and color to the ordered medication (Heiftz, et al., 1987); when a pharmacist or nurse incorrectly dispenses or administers a medication whose name is similar to the medication ordered (Lakshmanan, et al., 1986); when the physician orders a medication that isn't appropriate for the individual patient; when the nurse or physician administers a medication that they have not prepared; or when a nurse incorrectly identifies a medication. The risk of giving the wrong medication can be decreased by using a "unit dose medication" system; by only administering medications that have been prepared and labeled by the nurse, or medications that have been prepared and labeled by the hospital pharmacist; by checking the medication label with the medication order; by knowing the generic and trade names of a medication and the reason it is being given to the patient; and by listening for patient clues. Patient clues, such as statements like "this doesn't look like the same pill I've taken before," should alert the nurse to recheck the medication order.

The Right Dosage. The third "right" of administering medications, the right dosage, means that the medication is given in the dose ordered and that the dose ordered is appropriate for the individual patient. Incorrect dosages of medications may be given if a physician orders a dose that is not appropriate for an individual patient; if a pharmacist dispenses or if a nurse administers an incorrect amount of medication; or if a pharma-

cist, nurse, or secretary transcribes an order incorrectly onto the patient's medication record. These errors may be avoided if the nurse and pharmacist are aware of the usual dosages ranges of medications; if the nurse double-checks with the physician whenever questions concerning the accuracy of a dosage arise; if the nurse and pharmacist correctly calculate the amount of medication required; and if the nurse double-checks medications transcribed onto a patient's medication record with the physician's orders before beginning administration of a new medication and whenever a new medication record is started. The nurse should be alert for clues that suggest that the medication dosage may not be correct, and should double-check medication dosages whenever a patient suggests that the dosage that he or she is used to taking is different from the dose the nurse is administering; when multiple tablets are needed to supply a single medication dose (Spencer 1989); when large or abrupt changes in medication dosages are ordered; and when the amount of medication supplied by the pharmacist does not match the amount needed for the ordered doses.

The Right Route. The fourth "right" of administering medications, the right route, means that the medication is given by the ordered route and that the ordered route is safe and appropriate for the individual patient. The physician's medication orders should always specify the route of administration. If a route is not specified or if the route ordered seems inappropriate, the nurse should check with the physician to clarify which route should be used. Other actions that help to ensure that a medication is given by the proper route include knowing the usual route/routes of administration of a medication, knowing the safety of administering a medication via the ordered route, and double-checking route of administration before administering a medication.

The Right Time. The fifth "right" of administering medications, the right time, means that the medication is given at the time ordered. Medication policies defining the meaning of "on time" vary with institutions; usually a medication is said to be given "on time" if it is given within 30 minutes or 1 hour before or after the dose is scheduled to be given. Many factors influence the schedules used to administer medications. These factors include: a medication may be more effective if given on an "around-the-clock" schedule when given in IV form, but may be appropriate to give during waking hours in the oral form; a medication that interacts with food may need to be given before meals; a medication that causes gastric irritation may need to be given with meals; and routine medication administration schedules vary between institutions. The nurse needs to be aware of the scheduling requirements of the medication he or she is giving and the routine scheduling times used at his or her institution. The nurse also should be aware of the situations in which medication scheduling problems frequently occur. Medication scheduling problems are more likely to occur when different units within an institution use different routine administration schedules; after patient transfer from one unit or facility to another; or when a limited number of doses of medication are ordered. Before giving a medication, the nurse should always check the medication record to note when the medication was last administered, and, when necessary, the total number of doses administered.

Medication Errors

A medication error has occurred when a medication is not administered as ordered; when the medication is administered according to the order, but the medication order is not safe or appropriate for the individual patient; or when the documentation in a patient's chart does not reflect that a medication was administered as ordered. The most common medication errors are related to documentation errors: the medication was given, but not charted. Another documentation error is failure to note the site where a parenteral injection was given. Other common medication errors include: an IV medication was administered at the wrong rate; the dose of medication administered was not the dose ordered; a medication was given at the wrong time; the wrong medication was administered; and a medication was charted, but was not given. Errors of medication substitution are more common with the increased use of generic name medications, and the nurse must be sure that the name of the medication supplied is the same as, not just similar to, the name of the medication ordered. Other less common errors are: the medication was given by the wrong route; a medication was given to a patient with a known allergy to that medication; and a medication was given to the wrong patient (Nakato, 1987).

Documentation of Medication Administration

The medication policies of an institution define the time and type of medication charting that is done. Medication charting is usually done immediately after a medication is given. Medication documentation includes the time, route, dosage, site of administration (for intradermal, subcutaneous, or intramuscular injections), and the nurse's initials and signature (Fig. 24-5).

Specific documentation is also required if a medication has not been given. In many agencies the normal time of administration is circled when a medication has been held. It is important to indicate why the medication was not given; at times, this can simply be a matter of indicating NPO next to the designated time for administration. At other times, the reason is more complex and an explanation needs to be written in other appropriate places in the chart.

Some medications (e.g., insulin or heparin) may have separate flow sheets on the chart on which medication administration must also be charted. Frequently this flow sheet contains laboratory data or other pertinent information. Such a flow sheet permits a health-care provider to visualize patterns in management over time. When numerous injections are administered, a chart documenting the location of each injection is provided, to ensure adequate site rotation. Whenever injections are administered, the site used should be included in documentation.

The nurse is also responsible for documenting the therapeutic and side effects of any medication administered. For example, if a narcotic is administered for pain, the amount of pain relief obtained by the patient should be documented. If a patient develops a rash after the administration of an antibiotic, the onset and type of rash should be described in detail.

A medication error is documented by charting the medication, as it was given, in the patient's medication record; by making note of the error in the progress notes; and by filling out a quality assurance or unusual incident form.

Oral Medications

Medications that are given by mouth are designed to be swallowed (oral route), to be held under the tongue until they dissolve (sublingual route), to be administered through tubes, or to be held in the side of the mouth until they dissolve (buccal route). Refer to Procedure 24-1, "Administering Oral Medications."

(Text continues on page 526)

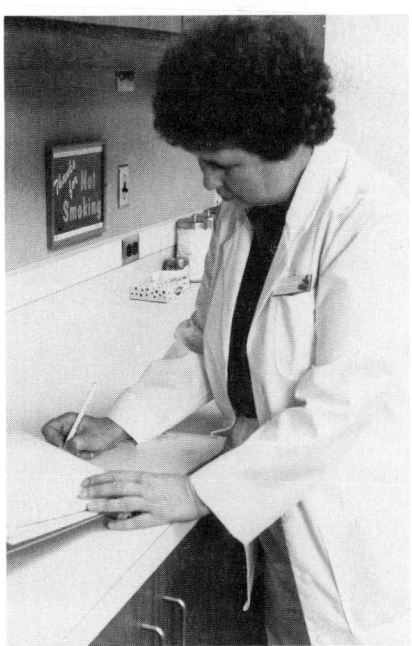

Figure 24–5.   Documentation of medication administration is an important part of the nurse's role.

PROCEDURE 24–1. Administering Oral Medications

■ **Purpose**

1. Provide a safe, effective, economical route for administering medications.
2. Provide a sustained drug action with minimal discomfort.

■ **Assessment**

- Review medication orders for accuracy and completeness. An order should include patient's name, drug name, dosage, route, and time.
- Review drug inserts, pharmacology textbooks, or *Physician's Desk Reference* for any unfamiliar drugs that are ordered.
- Assess patient's allergy history.
- Assess patient's ability to take oral medications.
  - level of consciousness, cooperativeness.
  - presence of swallow reflex.
  - symptoms of nausea and vomiting.
  - recent gastrointestinal surgery, or bowel obstruction.
  - presence of nasogastric tube to suction.
  - current diet order.
- Identify any pre-administration assessments of pulse, blood pressure, that must be done.
- Identify that correct medication and dosage is available at the time scheduled.

■ **Equipment**

Medication kardex or record.
Medication cart.
Disposable medication cups.
Water, juice, or milk.
Mortar and pestle (optional for crushing pills).

■ **Procedure**

1. Wash hands.
   Rationale: Reduces transfer of microorganisms from hands to medication.
2. Arrange medication kardex or cards next to medication cart or cabinet, medication trays and cups.
   Rationale: Organizing work space saves time and reduces chance of errors.
3. Prepare medications for only one patient at a time.
   Rationale: Prevents errors during preparation.
4. Remove ordered medication from cart or shelf. Compare label on medication with medication kardex or card. If there is a discrepancy, recheck the patient's chart and physician's orders.
   Rationale: Cross-checking label against transcribed order decreases errors.
5. Calculate correct drug dosage if necessary.

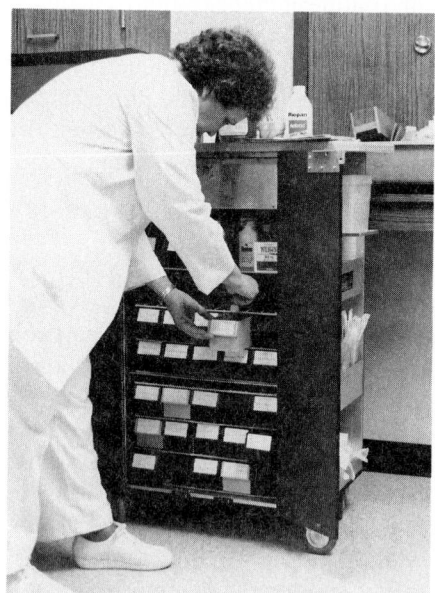

Step 4

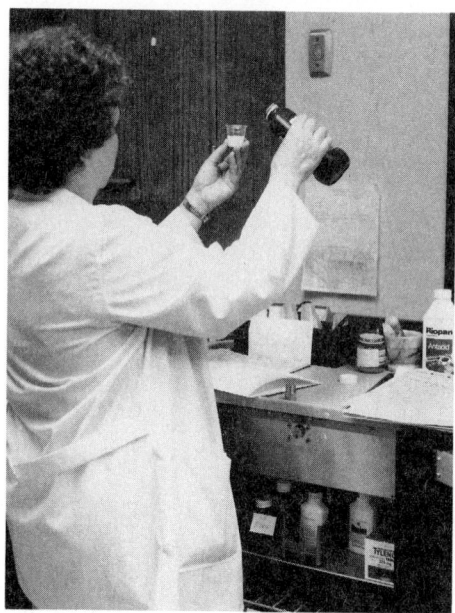

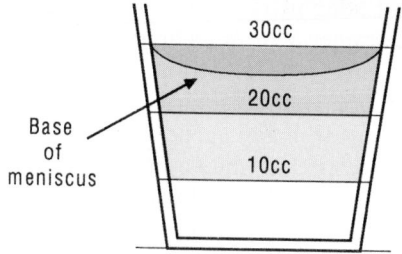

Base
of
meniscus

30cc

20cc

10cc

Step 6D

(continued)

PROCEDURE 24–1. Administering Oral Medications *(continued)*

6. Preparing medications:
   a. Unit dosage: Place packaged medication directly into medicine cup or lay on tray without unwrapping.
   b. Medications from a multidose bottle: Pour tablets or capsules into the container lid and transfer into medicine cup. Extra tablets can be returned to the bottle. Do not touch medications.
      Rationale: Maintains cleanliness of drugs.
      Note: If patient has trouble swallowing tablets, grind with mortar and pestle until smooth. Mix powder in small amount of custard or applesauce. *Do not* crush enteric coated tablets, as the contents are irritating to gastric mucosa. Consult pharmacist or physician.
   c. Liquid medications: Remove cap and place on counter top upside-down to prevent contamination. Hold bottle so label is against palm of hand.
      Rationale: This prevents soiling of label when pouring medication.
   d. Hold mediation cup at eye level and fill until bottom of meniscus is at desired dosage. Discard excess poured liquid from cup into sink. Do not pour back into bottle.
      Rationale: Permits accurate measurement and prevents contamination of medication in bottle.
   e. Oral narcotic: Compare previous drug count on narcotic record with current supply. Place drug in medication cup and record information on narcotic record.
      Rationale: Strict monitoring is required of all controlled substances.
7. Compare prepared medication with medication kardex (or card) and container label.
   Rationale: Reckecking label reduces medication errors.

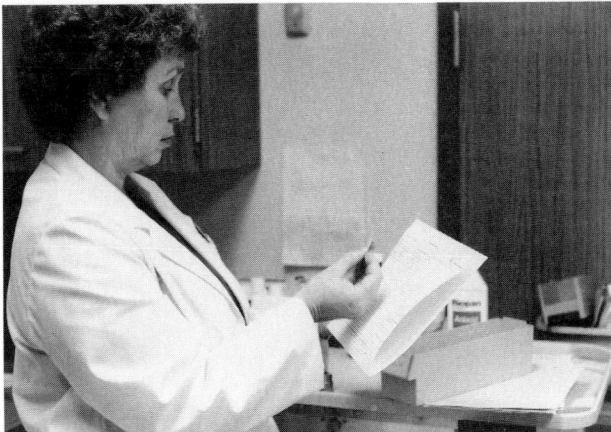

Step 7

8. Reread label and place medication container or unused drug back on cart or shelf.
   Safety Alert: Medications are checked three times before administering to the patient:
   a. when removing container from the storage area.
   b. after placing medication into cup.
   c. before returning container back to storage area (unless using unit dosage system).
9. Take medication directly to patient's room. Do not leave unattended.
10. Ask patient to state his or her name and compare name on medication card or record with name on patient's identification band.
    Rationale: Ensures administration of drugs to proper patient.

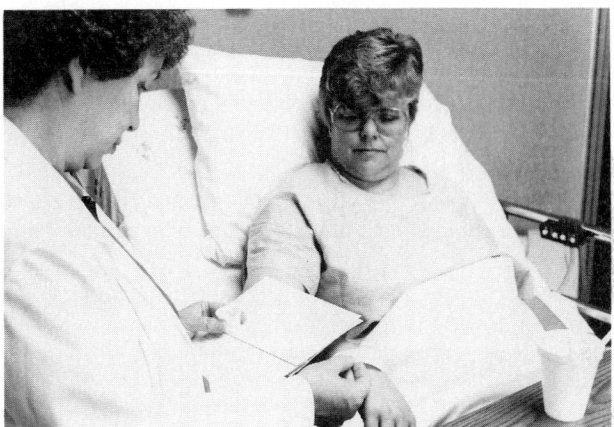

Step 10

11. Complete any preadministration assessment (i.e., blood pressure, pulse) required by specific medication.
    Rationale: Medications having a direct action such as decreasing pulse rate or blood pressure require assessment to determine if medication can be given safely at that time.
12. Explain purpose of medication to patient.
    Rationale: Accordance with patient's rights and will improves compliance.
13. Assist patient to sitting position.
    Rationale: Position assists swallowing and prevents aspiration.
14. If using unit dose medications: Read label, unwrap medication, and place in cup. Give medication cup and glass of water or juice to patient.
15. If patient is unable to hold the medication cup; place pill cup to lips and introduce medication into his mouth.
    Rationale: Prevents contamination of medication.

(continued)

16. Stay with patient until all medications are swallowed. You may need to look inside patient's mouth to be certain.
    Rationale: The nurse is responsible that patient receives ordered medications.
    Note: If tablet or capsule falls on the floor, discard and repeat preparation.
17. Dispose of soiled supplies and wash hands.
18. Record time medication was administered and any preadministration assessment data which were collected.

■ **Lifespan Considerations**

Infants and Children

- Tablets and capsules are not a recommended form of oral medication in children under 5 years of age because they may not be swallowed safely. Liquid preparations are available for most oral medications. Some liquid drugs come with a calibrated dropper for measuring small amounts of medication for infants. Do not interchange droppers between different medications. *Rationale: Different companies use different sized droppers and medications may be inaccurately measured.*
- Play techniques may encourage a child's cooperation in swallowing medications.
- Always let the child know that you have medicine, not candy.

Older Adults

- Normal physiologic changes with aging that may influence a patient's ability to take oral medications include decreased salivation and elasticity of oral mucosa, resulting in a dry mouth, and delayed esophageal clearance, which may impair swallowing. A liquid form of medication may be necessary.
- Additional changes with aging are decreases in stomach peristalsis and gastric acidity, and decreased colon motility.

■ **Home-Care Modifications**

- Assess patient or family member's knowledge of drug therapy.
- Assess patient's sensory function (sight, hearing, touch) to determine if special teaching or administration strategies are required. Have patient wear eyeglasses or hearing aid during teaching sessions.
- Assess patient's ability to read. Patient may be unable to read prepared booklets or medication label.
- Patient and/or family members should be instructed in purpose of medications, dosage schedule, common side effects, who to call with problems, and what to do about missed doses.
- Give guidelines for drug safety, as appropriate: discarding outdated drugs, keeping drugs out of reach of children, refrigerating medications.
- Devise learning aids if needed. Examples include calendars for each week that contain separate ziplock bags with medications to take at specific times; egg cartons with color-coded sections for medications to take at specific times. Commercial drug-scheduling divided containers are available to provide 1 week of medication at a time.

Advantages

Advantages of giving medications by mouth include: it is usually the simplest and easiest way to take medications; minimal discomfort is experienced; it usually has the fewest side effects of any route; and oral medications tend to be less expensive and more widely available than medications given by other routes.

Contraindications

Medications should not be given by mouth when a patient is unable to swallow or when a patient is nauseated or vomiting. If the patient is unable to swallow water or fluids, oral medications should be discontinued or should be given by another route. Relative contraindications to giving oral medications include NPO status and gastric suction. If a patient is NPO before a test or surgery, the physician may continue selected oral medications. These ordered medications would be given with sips of water. If the patient is NPO after major surgery, oral medications are usually held or administered by another route until intestinal function has returned. Usually, patients being treated with gastric suction have oral medications held or given by another route. Occasionally, a physician may order a specific medication to be administered through a nasogastric tube and may order the gastric suction discontinued for a specified period of time (usually 30 minutes) after medication administration.

Forms of Oral Medication

Oral medications, commonly termed PO (from the Latin *per os,* "by mouth") are supplied in liquids, capsules, and tablets. Liquid medications are commonly used for small children or for adults who are not able to swallow pills easily. Liquid medications vary in the ingredients used to formulate them; syrups usually contain sugar, elixirs usually contain alcohol. Capsules contain medication particles, powder, or liquid inside a gelatin case. Tablets are made of medication combined with ingredients that bind them together; they may be coated with sugar or films to make them less likely to break apart. Medications whose ingredients are irritating to the stomach may be covered with an enteric coating, which remains intact until it comes in contact with alkaline intestinal secretions. Medication in sustained-release capsules and tablets is specially treated to be slowly absorbed.

Routes of Oral Administration

Oral Administration. Methods of preparing and administering oral medications are designed to ensure that the medication moves to the back of the patient's throat, moves down the esophagus, and is properly absorbed. Whenever taking any oral medications, the patient should be standing, sitting, or should have the head of his or her bed elevated. If the patient is able to swallow liquids, but is not able to move liquids to the back of his or her mouth, liquid medications may be administered using a syringe with a piece of rubber tubing attached. The medication is drawn up through the tubing into the syringe; the tubing is inserted into the side of the patient's mouth and the medication is slowly injected into the back of the mouth. Antifungal liquid medications (Mycostantin) that work through contact with the mucous membranes in the mouth are given by the "swish and swallow" technique: the patient puts the liquid in his or her mouth, moves the liquid back and forth in the mouth several times, and swallows it.

Several techniques may be used to administer medications to the patient who is able to swallow soft foods, but is not able to swallow whole capsules or tablets. A capsule can be opened and the contents can be added to a small amount of the patient's food, such as ice cream or applesauce. Most tablets, except enteric-coated and sustained-release tablets, can be crushed and added to soft foods. Enteric-coated tablets should not be crushed, as this may allow the irritating medication to come in contact with the stomach and result in gastric irritation. If a sustained-release medication is crushed, all its medication will be absorbed at the same time, resulting in higher than expected initial levels of medication and in shorter than expected duration of medication action.

Even patients with normal swallowing reflexes may have problems swallowing and moving tablets or capsules down their esophagus. Drug-induced esophagitis, an inflammation of the esophagus, may occur if a tablet or capsule lodges in the esophagus and begins to dissolve there. Several techniques help to aid movement of a

tablet or capsule through the esophagus and to prevent drug-induced esophagitis. The patient should be in a semi-Fowler's, sitting, or standing position when taking medications, and should not return to a flat, recumbent position for at least a minute and a half after taking a capsule or pill (Neuman, 1985). Whenever possible, the patient should drink about 100 mL of fluid after swallowing a capsule or tablet (Pagliaro, 1986). If a patient senses that a medication is "stuck in his or her throat," a small portion of a soft food, such as a banana, should be offered to help to move the medication through the esophagus (Neuman, 1985). If the feeling persists, the physician should be notified.

Hospitals provide calibrated medicine glasses and droppers to aid in obtaining accurate measurement of prescribed doses of liquid medications, as shown in Figure 24-6. When measuring liquids, it is important for the nurse to hold the measuring container at eye level. The other hand is used to pour the medication to the indicated level. An elliptical curve, called the meniscus, is produced because the solution tends to cling to the side of the measuring container. It is the lower part of the meniscus that should rest on the calibration line of the dose being measured (see Step 6d in Procedure 24-1).

Calibrated medicine droppers may be supplied with the medication. It is important to use the dropper supplied because the dose of the medication depends on the size of the opening in the dropper, the angle at which the dropper is held, and the viscosity of the solution.

Administration Through Tubes. Oral medications may be administered through nasogastric or gastric tubes or through nasointestinal or jejunal tubes. When giving oral medications through gastric or intestinal tubes, care should be taken to decrease the risks of patient aspiration and of clogging the feeding tube. The

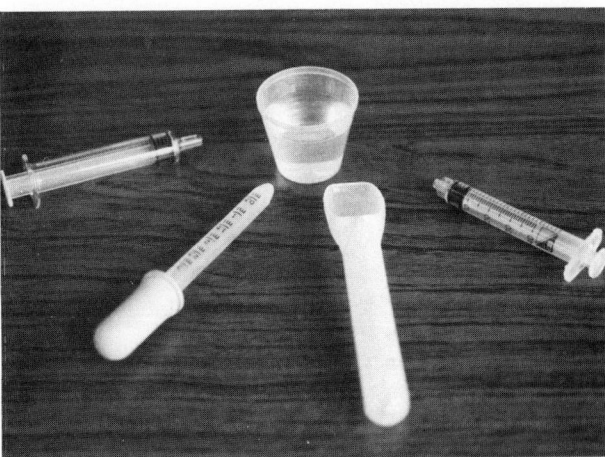

Figure 24–6. Devices used to measure liquid medications accurately: (left to right) oral syringe, dropper, medicine cup, spoonlike device, injection syringe without needle.

risk of aspiration, movement of food into the lungs rather than into the stomach, is decreased if the patient is properly positioned. The patient should be in a semi-Fowler's or Fowler's position whenever receiving food or medications, and the head of the patient's bed should remain elevated for at least 30 minutes after medications are administered (Pagliaro & Pagliaro, 1986). A feeding tube may become clogged if medications solidify in it. Hydrophyllic gels, such as Metamucil, should not be given through feeding tubes, as gels tend to attract water and solidify within the feeding tube (Spencer, et al., 1989).

Most liquid medications can be given through feeding tubes. Tablets may be given a feeding tube if they can be crushed into fine particles and dissolved in water. Before and after administering a medication, the feeding tube should be irrigated with 15 to 30 mL of saline or water. If it becomes difficult to instill fluid into the tube, the tube can be irrigated with 30 to 50 mL of warm water or carbonated beverage. These fluids may help to dissolve food or medication particles within the tube and may restore tube patency.

Sublingual Administration. The **sublingual** tablet is placed under the tongue and allowed to dissolve (Fig. 24-7). If the patient's mucous membranes are dry, 1 mL of saline or water should be used to wet the membranes underneath the tongue so that absorption can occur (Rasler, 1986). Sublingual tablets should not be swallowed.

Buccal Administration. The **buccal** route has not been used frequently for medication administration. Recently, pharmaceutical companies have released a variety of medications for buccal administration, including sustained-release nitroglycerin, narcotics, antiemetics,

tranquilizers, and sedatives (Wong, 1987). Buccal medications should be placed underneath the upper lip or in the side of the mouth (Fig. 24-8); buccal medications should not be chewed, swallowed, or placed under the tongue (Forget-me-nots, 1985).

Topical Medications

Topical medications include medications that are placed on the skin surface or in body cavities.

Medications Applied to the Skin

Medications are usually applied to the skin to treat local (skin) conditions or to treat systemic conditions. Medications used to treat local skin conditions or infections are prepared in irrigation solutions or in creams or lotions. When transdermal medications are placed on the skin, the medications is absorbed through the skin, and they have systemic (total body) effects.

Irrigation Solutions. Irrigation solutions, such as normal saline, Dahkin's Solution (dilute bleach), or provoiodine, may be used to clean a wound. These solutions should be applied using a large (50 mL) syringe and gentle pressure. Use of a smaller syringe may generate pressure that is high enough to harm granulation tissue (Cooper, et al., 1983).

Creams and Lotions. Creams and lotions may be used to treat a skin or wound infection, to treat a skin disease, or to decrease symptoms of skin disorders. Antibiotic creams, such as silvadene or neosporin, may be applied to clean skin surfaces. These medications may be

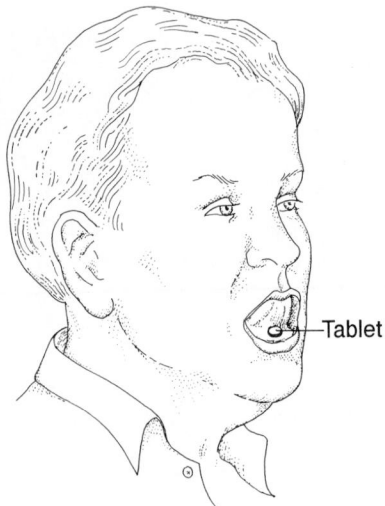

Figure 24-7. In sublingual administration, the patient is told to place the tablet under the tongue and allow it to dissolve. The tablet should not be swallowed.

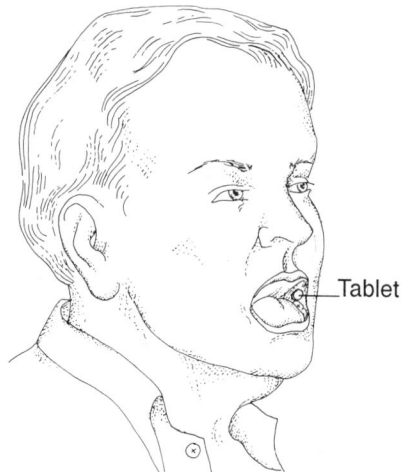

Figure 24-8. In buccal administration, the patient places the tablet at the side of the mouth (as shown) or under the upper lip. The patient should not place the tablet under the tongue or swallow it.

applied using a sterile swab, a sterile tongue depressor, or fingers covered with sterile gloves. Antibiotic creams should be applied in a thin layer; thick coatings of creams increase patient cost and make the medication more likely to have a systemic effect.

Transdermal Medications. **Transdermal** medications, those designed to be absorbed through the skin for systemic effects, are prepared in a medication patch form or in gel form. The medication patches are made using special membranes that allow medication to be slowly absorbed. These patches allow controlled amounts of medication to be supplied over a 24- to 72-hour period. Patients should be cautioned to remove one patch and clean the skin underneath the patch, before applying another patch. Nitroglycerin and scopolamine transdermal patches are in common use (Fig. 24-9). Patients using scopolamine should be cautioned not to use more than one patch at a time; use of multiple scopolamine patches has resulted in death. Nitroglycerin gel is applied to nitroglycerin paper that is marked with half-inch increments, and the gel is applied to the measuring paper using a continuous motion. Large variations in dosage can result if thick bands of nitroglycerin are applied or if more than one layer of nitroglycerin is applied. The nitroglycerin paper and nitroglycerin are applied to a skin surface and are taped to the skin using paper tape. If a dose of nitroglycerin ointment is applied before surgery, it should be applied on an easily visible area of skin, such as the forehead or chest.

Ophthalmic Medications

Solutions or ointments may be placed in the eye to treat eye irritation, infections, and glaucoma. The lower eyelid is gently retracted and the solutions or ointments are placed in the conjunctival sac (Fig. 24-10). Care should be taken to avoid touching the eye or eyelid with the tip of the ointment tube or dropper. The patient should be instructed not to rub his or her eye after medication is applied.

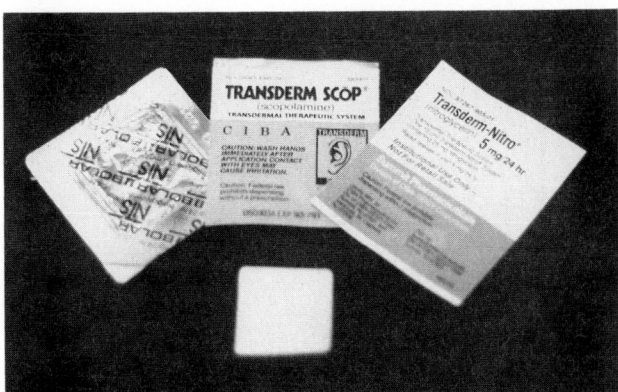

Figure 24–9. Scopolamine and nitroglycerin transdermal patches.

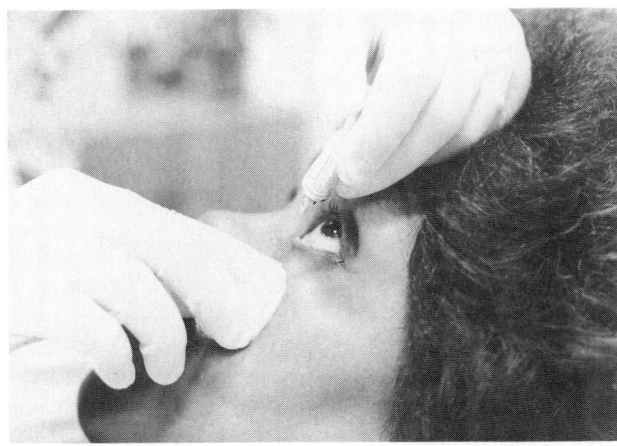

Figure 24–10. Instillation of ophthalmic medication. The lower eyelid is gently retracted and medication deposited in the conjunctival sac.

Otic Medications

Solutions may be dropped into the ear to treat external ear infections or to soften and remove ear wax. Solutions used in the ear should be at room temperature; use of hot or cold solutions in the ear may cause vertigo, nausea, and pain (Spencer, et al., 1989). The patient should lie on his or her unaffected side. The nurse gently pulls the pinna of the ear to straighten the ear canal, and drops the ordered amount of medication into the center of the ear canal (Fig. 24-11) The nurse then gently presses the area near the front of the ear several times to encourage movement of the solution down into the ear canal, and has the patient remain on his or her side for 5 to 10 minutes after the ear drops are administered.

Nasal Medications

Solutions are usually sprayed into the nose to treat nasal congestion. The patient should sit up and lean his or her head back. The nurse holds the bottle of medication in one hand, with the top of the bottle placed just inside the nares, and with the spray applicator top aimed toward the midline of the nose. The nurse squeezes the bottle while the patient inhales. Over-the-counter nasal sprays may contain decongestant and adrenergic medications (medications that stimulate the sympathetic nervous system); frequent use can cause systemic effects such as increased heart rate and increased blood pressure. Rebound nasal congestion, causing symptoms of nasal congestion that are as bad as or worse than original symptoms, commonly occur if decongestant nasal sprays are used for longer than several days.

Rectal Medications

Medication in suppository form (medication incorporated into a small, cylindrically shaped, waxy base) may be placed in the rectum to treat systemic complaints or to

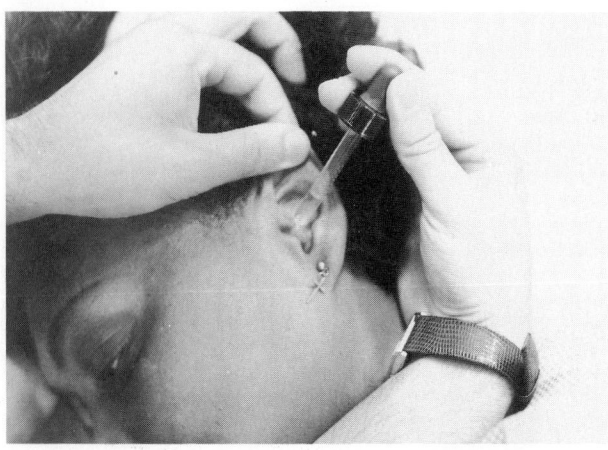

Figure 24–11. Instillation of otic medication. The pinna of the ear is gently pulled to straighten the ear canal and lukewarm drops deposited.

encourage bowel movements. Antiemetic suppositories may be used to treat nausea when other routes are not appropriate. The technique used to place suppositories is shown in Figure 24-12.

Liquid medications may be instilled into the rectum using an enema to encourage bowel movements or to treat patients with elevated potassium levels. Enema fluids are usually given in volumes of about 100 mL and are usually meant to be retained by the patient for 10 to 30 minutes. An enema of resin-containing fluid may be used to remove potassium from the bowel of a patient with an elevated potassium level. The procedure for administering small-volume enemas is discussed in Chapter 38.

Vaginal Medications

Medications given vaginally come in a variety of forms: foams, jellies, liquids (douches), creams, tablets, or suppositories. These medications may be used for contraception, to help kill any bacteria in the vaginal area before gynecologic surgery, to treat vaginal itching or

infection, or to induce labor. Prostaglandin vaginal suppositories are given to cause uterine contractions and induce labor in women after fetal demise (when death of the fetus occurs early in a pregnancy). The technique for instilling vaginal suppositories and tablets is shown in Figure 24-13.

Inhaled Medications

Inhaled medications may be used to induce anesthesia during surgery and to treat respiratory disorders. Anesthetic medications are administered by anesthesiologists or nurse anesthetists through an anesthesia machine. Inhaled medications given by nurses may be delivered through a mechanical ventilator, through a hand-held nebulizer, or through a metered-dose inhaler. Liquid medications are added to a receptacle in the ventilator or the nebulizer and changed into a gas form when air or oxygen flows over them. A metered-dose inhaler is a small device that a patient holds in his or her hand and presses when he or she inhales (see Fig. 30-5). Each time it is pressed, the metered-dose inhaler releases a set dose (metered dose) of medication. Inhaled medications have a rapid effect on the lungs and are rapidly absorbed by the systemic circulation. Bronchodilator medications, used to open lung airways and to promote easier breathing, are frequently part of the therapy for patients with chronic obstructive lung disease. The patient's respiratory status (reported ease of breathing, breath sounds, respiratory rate, and use of accessory respiratory muscles) should be assessed before and after he or she receives any inhaled medication.

Parenteral Medications

Medications that are given by injection or infusion are given by the parenteral route. Parenteral medications may be injected into intradermal (ID) tissue, subcutaneous (SC) tissue, intramuscular (IM) tissue, or

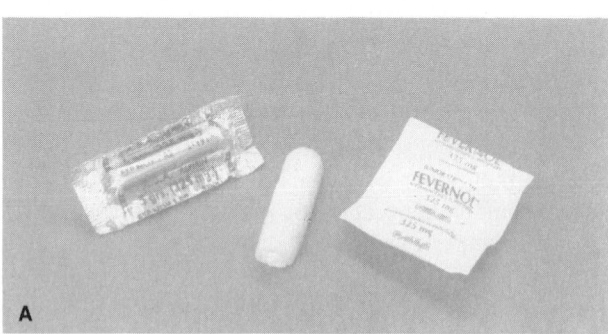

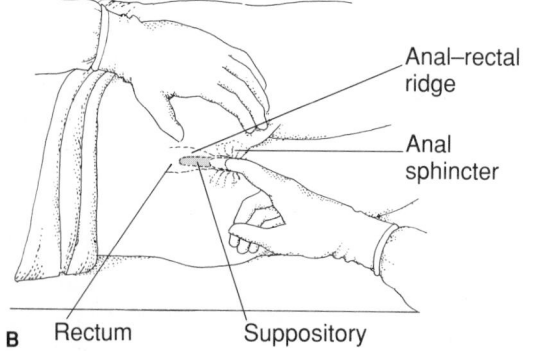

Figure 24–12. Insertion of rectal suppositories. **A.** Prepackaged suppositories. **B.** The suppository is inserted past the internal anal sphincter against the rectal wall.

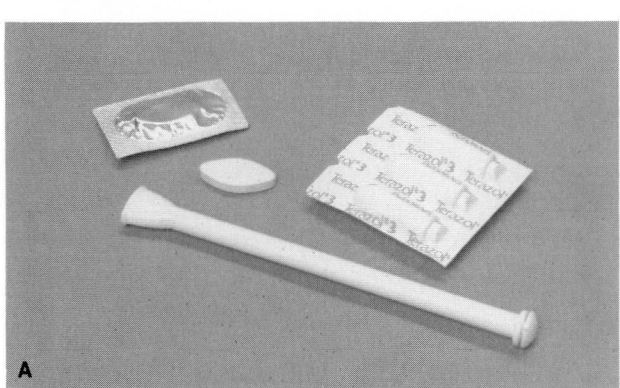 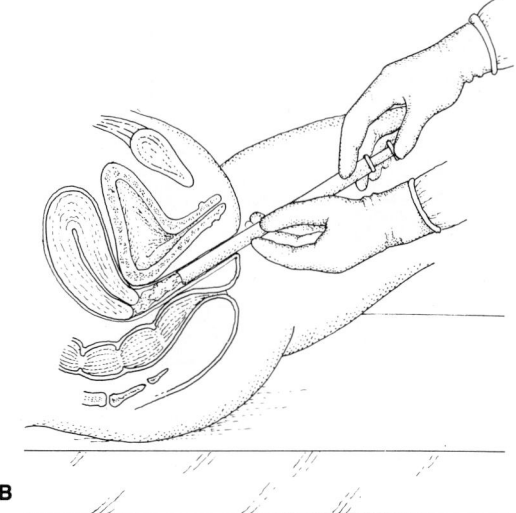

Figure 24–13. Insertion of vaginal medication. **A.** Vaginal suppository and applicator. **B.** Insertion of vaginal cream using applicator.

intralesional tissue; into venous (IV) or arterial circulation; or into intraspinal or intra-articular spaces. The ID, SC, IM, and IV routes will be discussed in this chapter.

Advantages and Disadvantages

Medications given by a parenteral route usually are absorbed more completely and have a faster onset of action than medications given by other routes. Parenteral medications are injected through the skin; bypassing the skin barrier makes infection more likely to occur if aseptic technique is not used when preparing and administering parenteral medications. Complications may occur if parenteral medications are not given into the tissue site or space intended. Tissue damage may occur if the pH, osmotic pressure, or solubility of the medication is not appropriate to the tissue where the medication is given. Specialized equipment required for parenteral administration usually makes medications given by these routes more expensive than medications given by other routes.

Equipment

Equipment needed to administer parenteral medications includes a container for the medication and a system to deliver the medication. Medications used for ID, SC, or IM injections are usually supplied in vials, ampules, or prefilled syringes.

Vials. Vials are plastic or glass containers that may hold one or more doses of medication (Fig. 24-14A). The vial is opened by removing a plastic cap that covers a rubber diaphragm at the top of the container. A needle is

used to pierce the center of the diaphragm, and the correct amount of medication is withdrawn into a syringe.

Medications that are not stable for long periods of time may be supplied in a vial in powdered form. An appropriate diluent (sterile liquid specified by the medication manufacturer) is mixed with the powder to reconstitute it.

Ampules. Ampules are thin-walled glass containers that hold a single dose of a liquid medication (Fig. 24-14B). Ampules are shaped like a bowling pin; an ampule has a wide base, a narrow neck, and pointed top. Before the ampule is opened, all medication should be moved into the ampule base. Medication can be moved from the top to the base of the ampule by gently tapping the top of the ampule with the finger. To open the ampule, the nurse holds an alcohol pad over the neck of the ampule with his or her thumb, then holds the top and bottom of the ampule still with his or her hands, while pushing on the ampule with a thumb. See Procedure 24-3 for illustrations. Care should be taken not to cut the hands when opening the ampule or when withdrawing medication from it.

Syringes. Syringes, usually made of plastic, consist of a barrel, a plunger, and a syringe tip (Fig. 24-15). The plunger fits snugly within the syringe barrel. Moving the plunger out of the barrel allows fluid or air to be moved into the syringe; pushing the plunger into the barrel allows fluid or air to be moved out of the syringe. A needle is attached to the syringe tip (the narrow end of the syringe); syringes may be packaged with or without an attached needle. Needle gauge (size) varies from 14 to

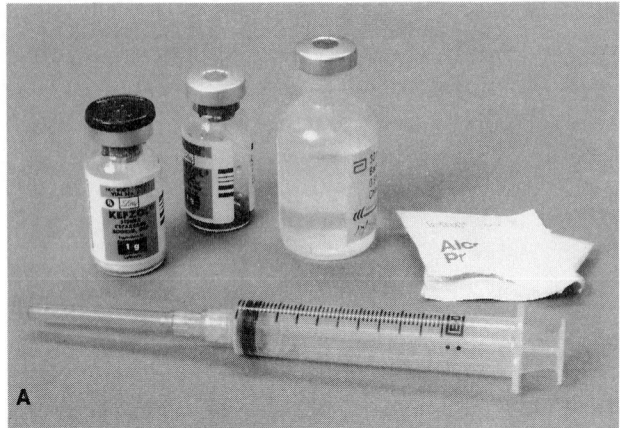 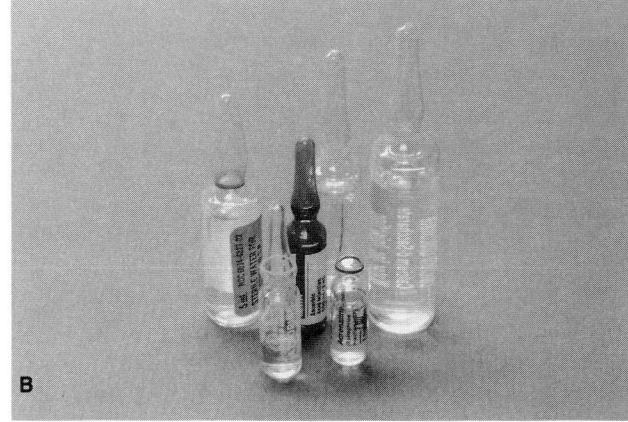

Figure 24–14. Containers for medication. **A.** Vials. **B.** Ampules.

29; the needles with the smallest gauge (that is, the smallest diameter) are labeled with the largest number. Needle length varies from 0.5 to 3 inches (Fig. 24-16).

The three common types of syringes are tuberculin syringes, insulin syringes, and standard syringes. Tuberculin syringes are 1-mL syringes, calibrated with 0.1-mL markings, and supplied with a small-gauge (25- to 28-gauge), short-length (0.5 to 0.625 inch) needle. Tuberculin syringes are used to administer tuberculin, rubella, or sensitivity (allergy) tests. Insulin syringes, calibrated in units of insulin (100 units of insulin per 1 mL), are used to administer insulin. Insulin syringes are made in ⅓-mL, ½-mL, or 1-mL sizes, with very small-gauge needles (26- to 29-gauge) attached to them. Standard syringes are supplied in 3-mL, 5-mL, or 10-mL sizes. Standard syringes may be supplied without needles or may be supplied with 18-, 21-, 23-, or 25-gauge needles

that are 0.5 to 3 inches long. Intramuscular injections are usually administered to adults using a 3- or 5-mL syringe with a long (1.5 to 2 inch), medium-sized (21- or 23-gauge) needle. Larger-gauge needles are used to administer viscous medications or to mix intravenous medications.

Prefilled syringes, prepared by a medication manufacturer or by an institution's pharmacy, may be used to supply medications. One system of prefilled syringes that has been in widespread use is the tubex system. Medications, such as narcotic analgesics and heparin, are supplied in a cartridge with an attached needle. The needle and cartridge fit into a metal or plastic injector device (Fig. 24-17). Air and any extra medication are expelled from the syringe and the medication is injected. Because the needle is fused to medication cartridge, needle gauge or length cannot be changed; the nurse

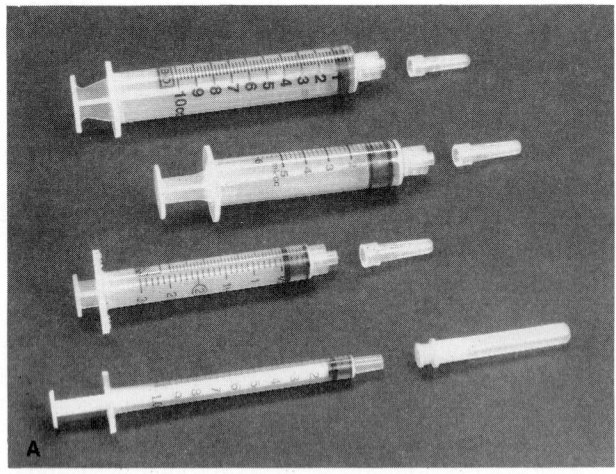 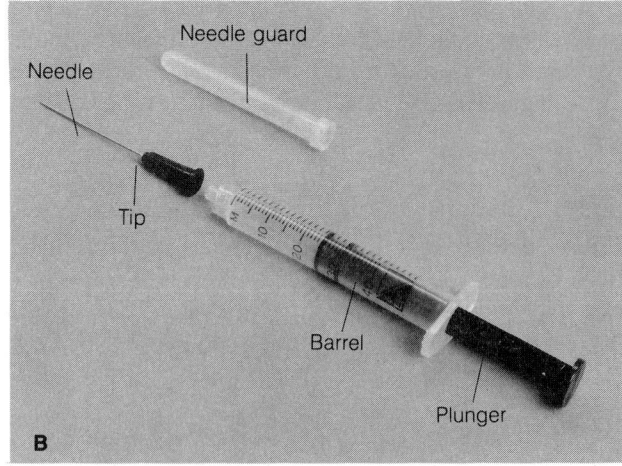

Figure 24–15. **A.** Syringes (from top to bottom): 10 mL, 5 mL, 3 mL, and tuberculin. **B.** Syringe parts and needle.

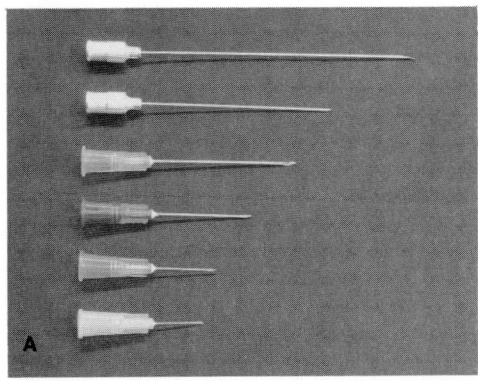 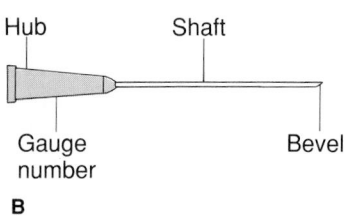

Figure 24–16. Needles. **A.** Different gauges and lengths. **B.** Parts of a needle.

must use the needle supplied even if it is not the most appropriate size for an individual patient. A second disadvantage of the prefilled syringe system is that medications supplied in this form are usually more expensive than medications supplied in vials.

Medication Preparation Techniques

Before administering a parenteral medication, it may need to be drawn up into a syringe, be reconstituted, or mixed with another medication.

Drawing up Medications. Drawing up medications is the process of moving medications from an ampule or vial into a syringe. If drawing up medication from an ampule, the nurse first opens the ampule, then removes the needle cap from a syringe. The needle is placed directly into the open ampule, and the syringe plunger is pulled back until all the medication from the ampule is added to the syringe. Air is usually drawn into the syringe along with the liquid medication. To rid the syringe of air, the syringe is held with the needle pointed upwards. If any medication has adhered to the top of the syringe in the air bubble, the barrel of the syringe is tapped until the liquid moves down the syringe barrel to

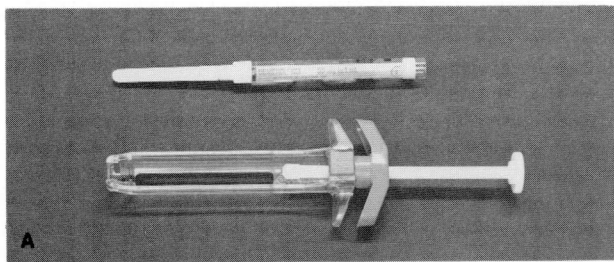

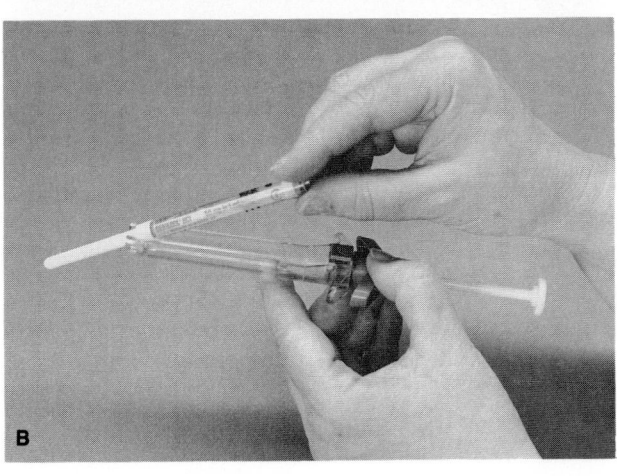

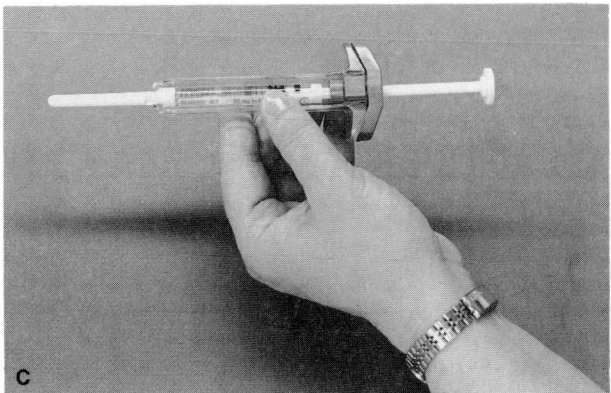

Figure 24–17. Prefilled syringes. **A.** Prefilled medication cartridge and injector device. **B.** Screwing the cartridge into the injector device. **C.** Ready for injection.

join the rest of the medication. The air and any volume of unneeded medication should be slowly expelled.

Reconstituting Medications. Reconstituting medications is accomplished by adding the proper diluent to a powdered medication. Vials of powdered medications may be packaged along with vials of the proper type and volume of diluent. The manufacturer's directions written on the medication box or vial should be read to learn the amount and type of diluent to add. To reconstitute the medication, the nurse first removes the caps from both the medication and diluent vials, and cleans the tops of both vials with an alcohol wipe. The diluent is drawn up into the syringe and injected into the medication vial. The nurse holds the medication vial in his or her hand and mixes the medication and diluent until the medication has dissolved. He or she then draws the reconstituted medication into a syringe, removes any air and unneeded medication from the syringe, and administers as directed.

Mixing Medications. Mixing medications together in the same syringe may allow a patient to receive fewer injections at a lower cost. Medications may be mixed together if they are compatible with each other. The compatibility of medications (the ability to mix medications without their constituents or their actions being affected) is studied by pharmaceutical companies. Information about medication compatibility is usually discussed in the medication insert and in medication references. Medications are mixed in a syringe by first drawing up one medication into the syringe. Any air and unneeded medication are expressed out the syringe. The ordered volume of the second medication is slowly added to the syringe containing the first medication. If the medication is added rapidly, too much of the second medication may be drawn up. If too much of the second medication is added, the syringe and medications must be discarded. Refer to Procedure 24-2, "Drawing up Two Medications in a Syringe."

Equipment Disposal. Disposal of equipment in a careful manner helps to decrease the risk of inadvertent exposure to a patient's blood. After administering an injection, the syringe and needle should be placed in a needle disposal box. Recapping a needle (placing the protective cap back onto the needle) or breaking the needle off increase the risk that the nurse will inadvertently poke him- or herself with the used needle. These practices should be avoided.

Intradermal Injections

Intradermal injections are given into the dermis, the layer of tissue located underneath the skin surface (Fig. 24-18A). Allergy or tuberculin skin tests are administered by intradermal injection. Most frequently, intra-

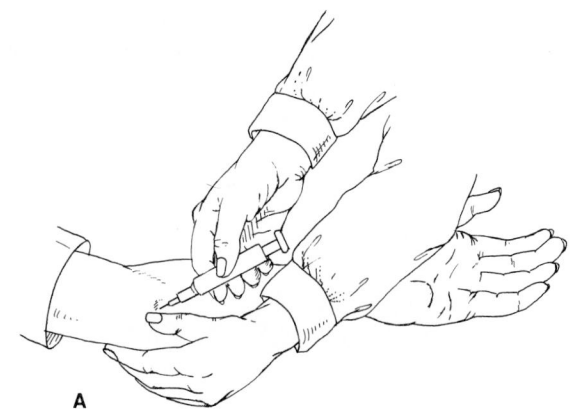

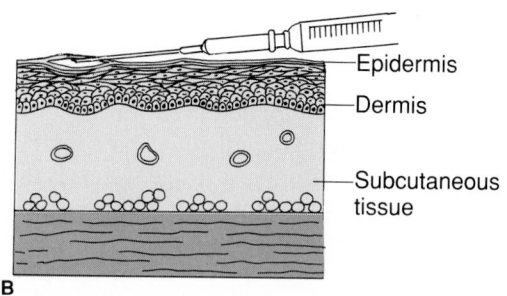

Figure 24–18.   A. For intradermal injection, the syringe is held almost parallel to the skin with the bevel up. **B.** A small volume of medication is deposited right under the skin, forming a small bleb.

dermal injections are given into the inner forearm area, but sites in the upper chest, upper arm, and across the scapula may also be used. Intradermal injections are usually administered using a 1-mL syringe and a small-gauge needle (25- to 28-gauge). The skin is cleaned using an alcohol wipe. The syringe is held, with the bevel of the needle up, almost parallel to the skin. The needle is inserted until all of the bevel lies under the skin. Small volumes of medication (usually 0.25 mL or less) are injected slowly (Fig. 24-18B). The site of testing is documented, and the site is examined 48 hours after the injection is given.

Subcutaneous Injections

Subcutaneous injections are given into the subcutaneous tissue, the layer of fat located below the dermis and above the muscle tissue (Fig. 24-19). When a medication is injected into subcutaneous tissue, absorption is usually slow, sustained, and complete. Small amounts (0.5 to 1 mL) of medication may be injected subcutaneously using a syringe with a short (0.5- to 0.625-inch), small-gauge (25 to 28) needle. Subcutaneous injections may be administered into the upper arm, the upper back, the abdomen, the upper buttocks, and the thigh (Fig. 24-20).

Speed of absorption varies with the site selected: medications injected into the abdomen are absorbed most

PROCEDURE 24–2. Drawing up Two Medications in a Syringe

■ Purpose
1. Minimize the number of injections a patient receives.
2. Prevent contaminating one vial of medication with medication from the other vial.

■ Assessment
• Review drug literature to ensure compatibility of the two medications.

■ Equipment
Medication order or card.
Two vials of ordered medication.
Sterile 1 to 3 mL syringe with appropriate gauge and length needle.
Antiseptic swabs.
Additional needle (optional).

■ Procedure
1. Wash hands.
2. Cleanse tops of both vials with antiseptic.

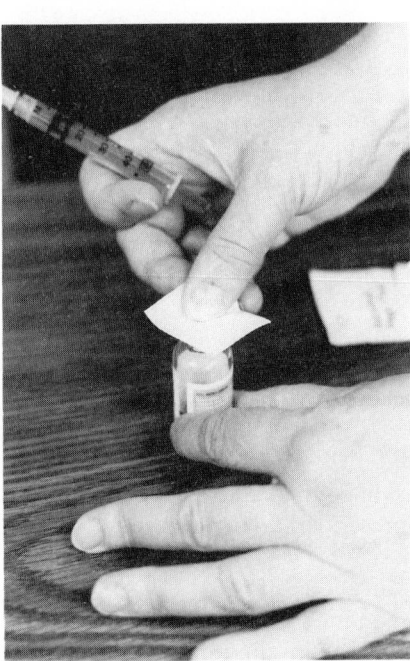

Step 2

3. With syringe, aspirate volume of air equal to medication dose from first medication (Vial A).
4. Inject air into Vial A, being careful that needle does not touch solution.
   Rationale: Air in vial creates positive pressure to facilitate solution withdrawal. The same needle will

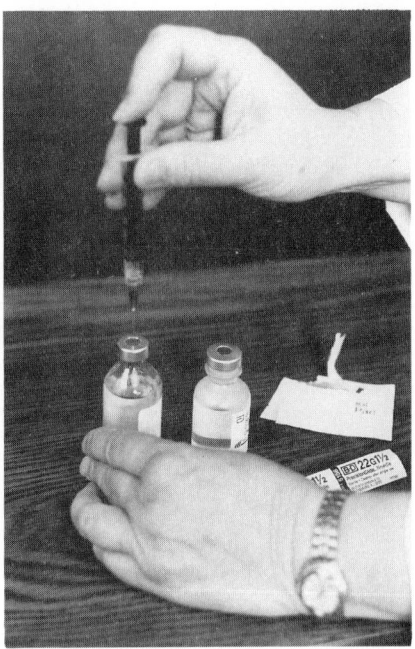

Step 4

be used to withdraw medication from second vial, so it must not have medication from Vial A on it.
5. Remove syringe from Vial A.
6. Aspirate volume of air equal to the medication dose from second medication (Vial B). Inject air into Vial B.

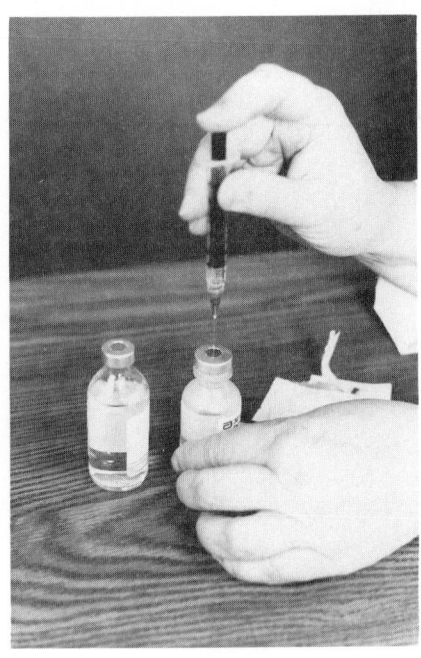

Step 6

(continued)

PROCEDURE 24–2. Drawing up Two Medications in a Syringe (continued)

7. Invert Vial B and withdraw required volume of medication into syringe.

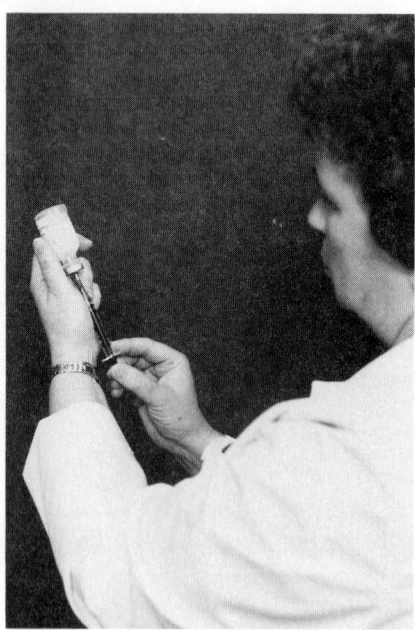

Step 7

8. Expel all air bubbles and withdraw needle from vial B.
9. Attach new sterile needle to syringe.
   Rationale: Prevents medication adhering to needle from Vial B from contaminating medication in Vial A.

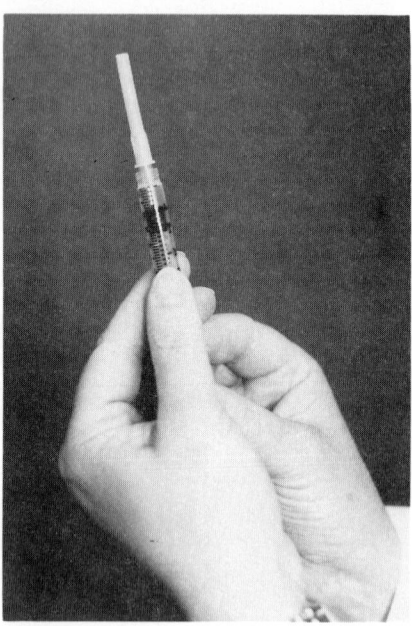

Step 9

10. Determine what total combined volume of medication would measure on syringe scale.
    Rationale: Prevents accidental withdrawal or excess medication from Vial A.
11. Insert needle into Vial A, invert vial, and carefully withdraw required volume of medication.

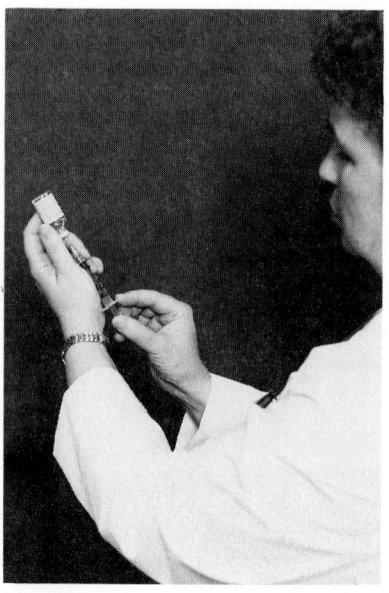

Step 11

12. Withdraw needle from Vial A.
13. Check medication and dosage before returning or discarding vials.
14. Wash hands.

Modification for Insulin:

■ **Equipment**
U-100 insulin syringe.
Vials of prescribed U-100 insulin.

■ **Procedure**
1. Wash hands.
2. In preparing insulins in suspension, gently rotate vials between palms of hands to mix solution.
   Rationale: Medication separates from solution during storage. Mixing ensures accurate concentrations of medications throughout solution. Shaking vigorously causes frothing and may make accurate insulin measurement more difficult.
3. Follow steps 2 to 7 above.
4. Regular insulin is the first insulin drawn into the syringe.

(continued)

PROCEDURE 24–2. Drawing up Two Medications in a Syringe *(continued)*

Rationale: Ensures insulin will always be drawn up in the same order to prevent errors and prevents contamination of vial containing regular insulin, which may be used in emergency treatment.

5. Follow steps 8 to 15 above. Extreme care must be taken to prevent contamination of regular insulin vials with insulins containing modifying proteins (intermediate or long-acting).

6. Have another nurse cross-check insulin dosage against physician's order while drawing up medication.
   Rationale: Prevents errors in insulin drug administration, which could potentially be very serious.

---

rapidly, medications injected into the arms are absorbed at an intermediate rate, and medications injected into the thigh are absorbed at the slowest rate (Berelowitz, 1987). Sites of abnormal subcutaneous tissue, such as areas lying underneath burns, birthmarks, inflamed tissue, or scars produce unpredictable medication absorption and should be avoided. Absorption may be slow or incomplete if subcutaneous medication is administered to a patient with generalized edema, severe peripheral vascular disease, or to a patient in cardiogenic shock (Spencer, et al., 1989). Medication absorption may be faster than expected when subcutaneous injections are administered to patients with little subcutaneous tissue, such as premature infants or cachectic adults. If a patient has little subcutaneous tissue, abnormal subcutaneous tissue, or abnormal blood flow to subcutaneous tissue, the nurse should check with the physician to see if an alternate route of administration can be used.

Nonirritating, water-soluble medications, such as narcotics, may be administered by subcutaneous injection.

Heparin and insulin are the most common medications given subcutaneously. See Procedure 24-3 for guidelines for administering subcutaneous injection.

Insulin Administration

Insulin is administered subcutaneously to regulate blood glucose levels. When administering insulin, an insulin syringe (1-mL syringe with 26- to 27-gauge, 0.5-inch needle) is used. The needle on an insulin syringe is not detachable. The syringe is calibrated in units; most syringes today contain 100 units per mL and are referred to as U-100 syringes. When administering insulin, the number of units prescribed is measured in the syringe. It is important to use U-100 strength insulin with a syringe that has been calibrated 100 units per mL. Low-dose

(Text continues on page 541)

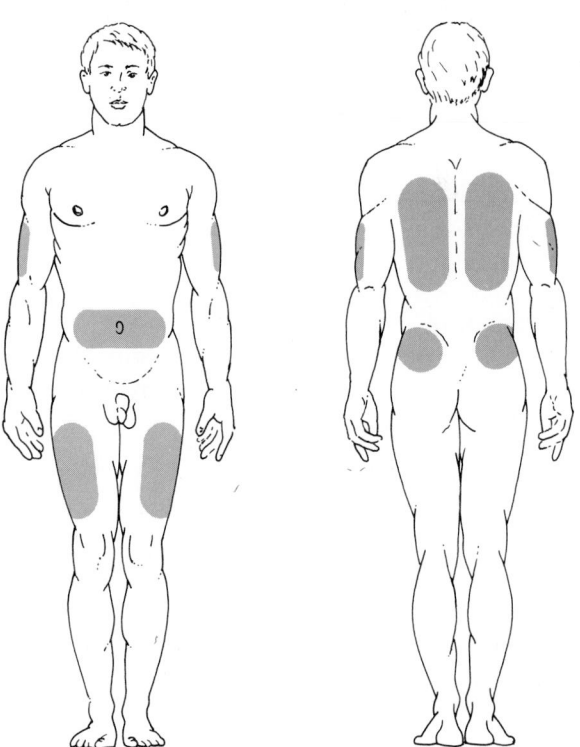

Figure 24–19. Subcutaneous injection deposits medication in subcutaneous tissue at a 45° or 90° angle.

Figure 24–20. Sites used for subcutaneous injections.

PROCEDURE 24–3. Administering Subcutaneous Injections

■ Purpose
1. Ensure more rapid absorption and action of a drug than can be achieved orally.
2. Administer drugs to patients unable to take oral medications (i.e., unconscious, nausea/vomiting, NPO status).
3. Administer medications that are not active by the oral route, or are inactivated by the digestive enzymes (i.e., heparin, insulin).

■ Assessment
- Review patient's medical history, medication history, and allergy status.
- Assess for contraindication to receiving subcutaneous injections. Circulatory shock or localized body areas of reduced tissue perfusion would interfere with drug absorption.
- Assess for anxiety related to fear of injections.
- Review chart for documentation of previous injection sites. Note rotation schedule when administering insulin or heparin.
- Inspect administration site for lesions, rash, ecchymosis, lipid dystrophy, etc.
- Refer to drug literature to determine appropriateness of medication and dosage, common side effects, and nursing implications.

■ Equipment
Medication card or order.
Antiseptic swabs.
Vial or ampule of ordered medication.
Sterile gauze or cover for opening an ampule.
Sterile syringe and needle. 1 to 2-mL syringe with 25 to 27-gauge ½-inch needle. A 1-inch needle may be used on very obese adults. The correct needle length is half of the skin fold width.

■ Procedure
1. Check medication order. See Procedure 24-1 "Administering Oral Medications," steps 1 to 5.
2. Wash hands.
3. Assemble needle and syringe.
4. Remove needle guard.
5. Vials:
   a. Rotate vial between palms to disperse medication.
   b. Cleanse top of medication vial with alcohol swab.
   c. Pull back barrel on syringe to an amount of air equal to the medication dosage to be withdrawn.
   d. Insert needle into vial and inject air.
   e. Invert vial and withdraw the desired volume of medication.

Rationale: Injected air prevents creation of negative pressure within the vial so medication can be easily withdrawn.
6. Ampules:
   a. Flick upper stem of the ampule with fingernail several times.
   Rationale: Releases medication trapped in upper chamber of ampule.
   b. Wrap a sterile gauze or alcohol wipe around ampule neck and break off top at neck by snapping it away from you.
   Rationale: Protects fingers from broken glass.

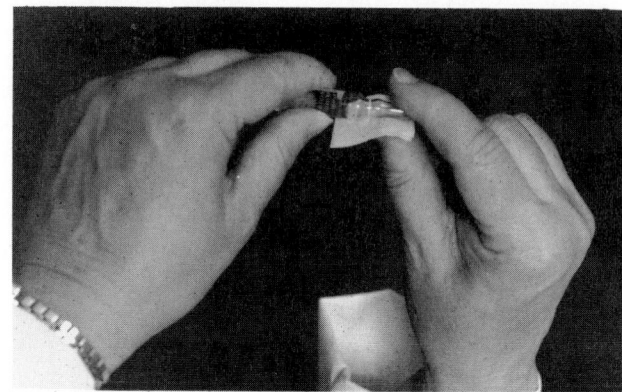

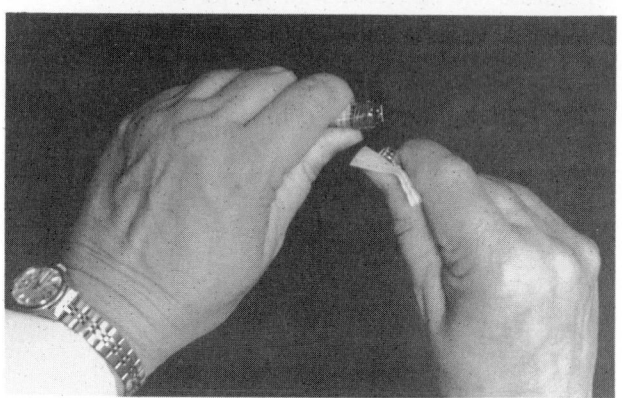

Step 6B

   c. Insert needle into ampule and withdraw required dosage of medication. Ampule may need to be held on its side to withdraw all the medication.
   d. Dispose of used ampule in appropriate container.
   Rationale: Prevents broken glass from cutting other health care workers.

(continued)

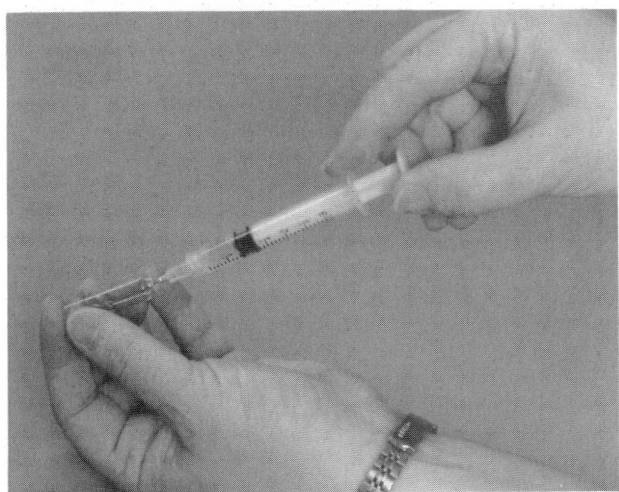

Step 6C

7. Cover needle with guard.
Note: In some agencies, a filter needle is used to draw medications from vials and ampules. The filter needle must be replaced by a regular subcutaneous needle before injecting medication into the patient.
Rationale: Filter needle traps rubber or glass fragments from being drawn up with the medication. Needle change prevents trapped particulate from being injected into patient.
8. Recheck drug and dosage against medication order or card for accuracy.
Note: If administering insulin, complete cross-check with another nurse.
Rationale: Prevents drug errors.
9. Explain procedure to patient and identify patient by name and identification bracelet.
10. Select injection site that is free from tenderness, swelling, scarring, inflammation.
Rationale: Injection into skin areas with abnormal characteristics could impair drug absorption or increase change of absscess or infection.
11. Some authorities recommend gloving nondominant hand.
Rationale: Maintains universal precautions should blood leak from injection site.
12. Cleanse site with antiseptic swab in circular motion from center toward outside. Allow area to dry thoroughly.
Rationale: Cleanses site from cleanest toward more contaminated areas.
13. Remove needle cap and expel air bubbles from syringe. Hold syringe in dominant hand.

14. Place nondominant hand on either side of injection site. Spread or pinch skin to stabilize site.
Rationale: Pinching the skin is thought to lessen the pain of needle insertion by desensitizing the area. Spreading the skin creates a firmer surface for needle insertion. Recommendations to support either technique vary.

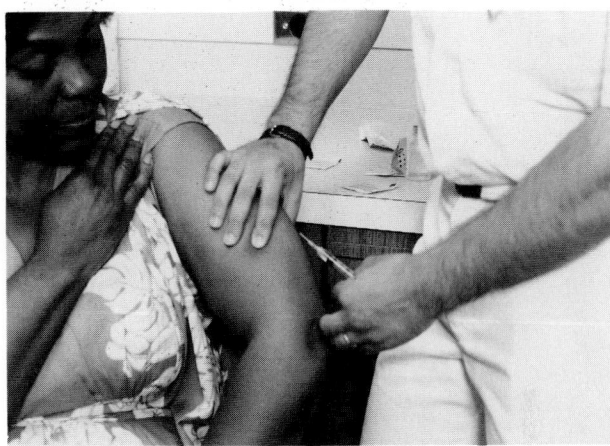

Steps 14 and 15

15. Hold syringe between thumb and forefinger of dominant hand. Inject needle quickly at a 45- to 90-degree angle depending on the amount of adipose tissue. Release pinched skin.
Rationale: Quick insertion minimizes discomfort.
16. Aspirate by slowly pulling back on plunger. If blood appears in syringe, withdraw needle, discard syringe and prepare a new injection.

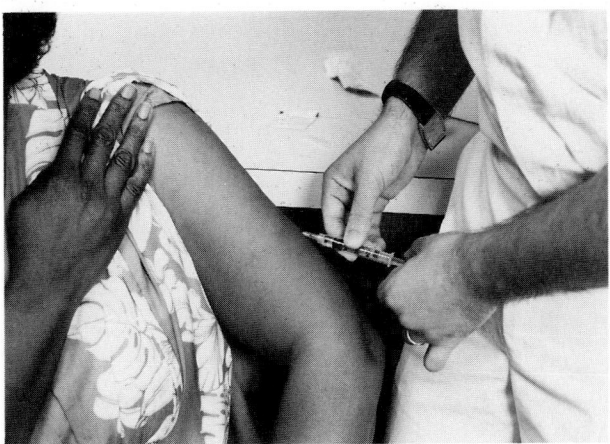

Step 16

(continued)

PROCEDURE 24–3. Administering Subcutaneous Injections *(continued)*

17. If no blood appears, inject medication with slow, even pressure.
    Note: See "Variations for Administering Heparin."
    Rationale: Aspiration of blood indicates needle is placed intravenous.
    Rationale: Subcutaneous medications are intended to be absorbed slowly from the subcutaneous tissues and may be dangerous if injected directly into the vein.

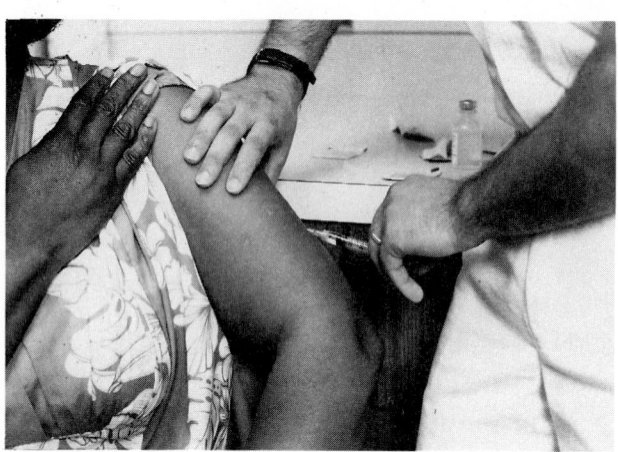
Step 17

18. Remove needle quickly while pressing antiseptic swab over site.
    Rationale: Patient discomfort is minimized by supporting tissues while needle is withdrawn.

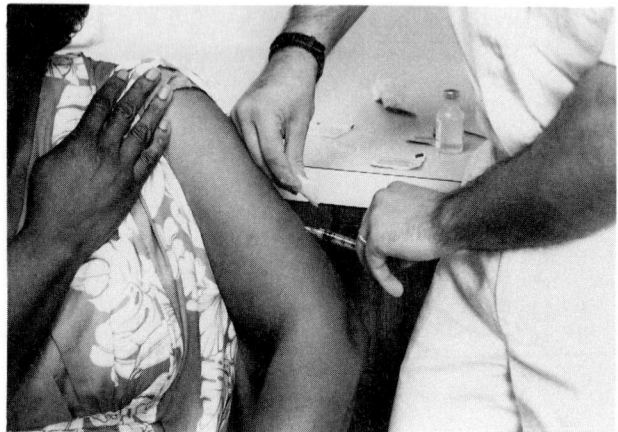
Step 18

19. Gently massage site with antiseptic swab.
    Rationale: Massage stimulates circulation to the injection site and may facilitate drug absorption.
    Note: See "Variations for Administring Heparin."

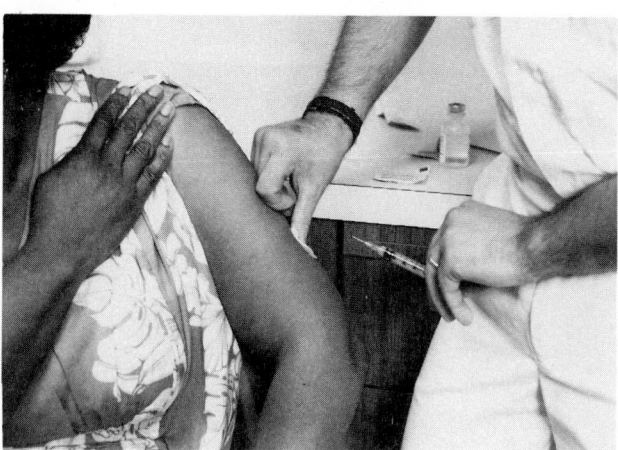
Step 19

20. Assist patient to position of comfort.
21. Do not recap needle. Dispose of syringe and needle in appropriate container.
    Rationale: Protects nurse and other health-care workers from accidental needle injury.
21. Wash hands.
22. Record according to agency protocol.

■ **Procedure**

Variations for Administering Heparin

1. Select a site on the abdomen on either side of the umbilicus.
   Rationale: There are no major muscle groups or muscle activity in this area so the chance of hematoma is reduced.
2. Due to the anticoagulant properties of heparin, pinching the site, aspirating for blood, and massaging the tissues are contraindicated.

■ **Lifespan Modifications**

Infants and Children

• Infants and children up to about 5 years of age shold be restrained for injections. Quick movement by the child once the needle is injected could break the needle shaft. An assistant is usually required to help restrain the child. Tell the child, "I will help you to hold still," to convey you are asking for cooperation.
• Painful procedures should not be done in the child's bed, which is a "safe zone." Parents also are regarded as "safe protectors" and should not help restrain the
(continued)

PROCEDURE 24–3. Administering Subcutaneous Injections *(continued)*

child during a painful procedure. Let the parent comfort the child after the injection.
• Praise, bandaids, and "good kid" stickers are effective rewards for children for a job well done.

■ Obese Adult
• Obese patients have a layer of fatty tissue above the subcutaneous layer. Select appropriate needle length to deliver medication to the subcutaneous skin layer. Pinching the skin at the site and injecting the needle below the tissue fold may also facilitate delivering medication to the subutaneous layer.

■ Home-Care Modifications
• If a visually impaired patient must self-administer injections, family members or the home health nurse can preload several syringes and place them in the refrigerator. This increases the patient's independence.
• A patient requiring multiple or daily injections should develop a pattern of site rotation to minimize trauma and scarring of body tissues.
• In some settings the patient may be taught not to cleanse the skin with alcohol or aspirate when giving self-injections.

---

insulin syringes (0.5 mL; 50 units) permit better visualization when small dosages (less than 10 units) of insulin are given.

If subcutaneous injections of insulin are given repeatedly into the same site, unpredictable insulin absorption and lipodystrophy (dimpling in the skin due to atrophy of subcutaneous tissue) may occur. Each injection should be given about 1 inch (the width of a thumb) from the last injection site. Areas that feel numb or are located within 1 inch of scars, burns, or irritated tissue should be avoided. Site rotation should be planned and well documented to prevent repeated use of the same site. Injection of cold insulin has also been related to lipodystrophy formation; insulin need not be refrigerated for short-term use. It is helpful to observe patients injecting insulin because technique problems can influence dose administration and absorption.

Heparin Administration

When heparin is administered subcutaneously, the purpose is the prevention of deep-vein thrombosis, which could cause pulmonary emboli. Because subcutaneous injections of heparin frequently cause hematoma formation, precautions are necessary. Subcutaneous injections of heparin are given in the abdomen, to avoid highly vascularized areas (e.g., arms and legs), which have an increased incidence of hematoma formation. A variety of techniques have been suggested to decrease the incidence of hematoma formation, including using an alcohol wipe to clean any heparin off the needle before injection; insertion of the needle at a 90-degree angle to the skin; injection of heparin without aspirating to check for blood return; and use of an air lock (0.2 mL of air) to prevent tracking of heparin through the subcutaneous tissue. None of these techniques has been shown to

significantly decrease the risk of post-injection hematoma formation (Hanson, 1987). Care should be taken not to cause trauma during or after the injection; thus, pinching the skin, moving the needle, or rubbing the site after the injection, should be avoided.

Intramuscular Injections

Intramuscular injections are given into the muscle layer, beneath the dermis and SC tissue (Fig. 24-21). Medications administered by IM injection usually are absorbed at an intermediate rate, slower than IV administration

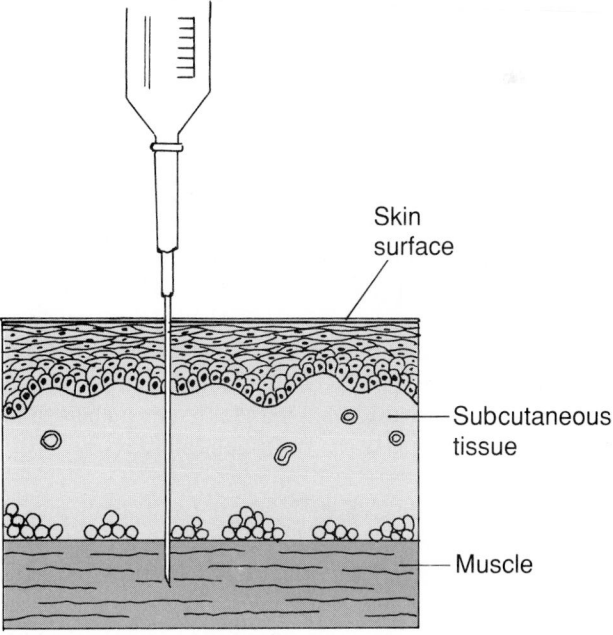

Figure 24–21.   The intramuscular injection deposits medication into the muscle at a 90° angle.

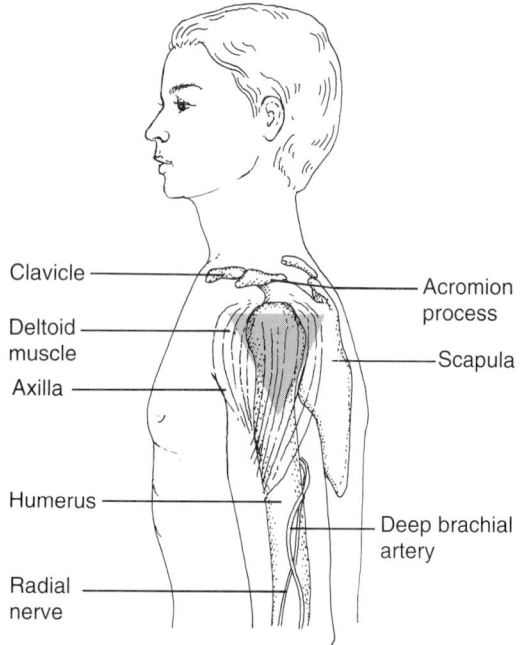

Figure 24–22. Deltoid muscle injection site. The site is located by imagining a line extending 2.5 to 5 fingerbreadths from the acromion process. A triangle is formed that indicates the injection site.

and more rapid than SC administration. A larger volume of medication per injection and a wider variety of medications may be administered into IM sites than into SC sites. Medications in solution or suspension may be injected into IM sites; those given by this route include antibiotics, antiemetics, narcotics, and vaccines. Intramuscular injections are administered using a 3- to 5-mL syringe with a 19- to 25-gauge, 1- to 3-inch needle. The larger-gauge needles are used when the medication solution is very thick; longer needles are used for larger adults. A 23-gauge, 1.25-inch needle is a commonly used size for IM injections for average-sized adult patients. Procedure 24-4 discusses administering IM injections.

Intramuscular injections may be administered into sites in the upper arm (deltoid muscle), the hip (ventral gluteal), the thigh (vastus lateralis or rectus femoris), and the buttocks (dorsogluteal). Site choices are influenced by the age of the patient, the medication to be injected, the amount of medication to be injected, and the general condition of the patient. Injections should not be given into abnormal muscle tissue, such as tissue underneath burns, scars, or inflamed areas.

The Deltoid Site. The deltoid site has a small amount of muscle mass with little overlying subcutaneous fat; medication injected into this site is absorbed rapidly. The deltoid site is used infrequently because the muscle is small and because it lies close to the radial nerve and the brachial artery. If the site must be used, the risk of injury to the radial nerve and brachial artery can be decreased if the site is located carefully, using anatomic landmarks. The deltoid site is located by drawing an imaginary line two to three fingerbreadths (2.5 to 5 cm) below the lower edge of the acromion process of the scapula. The injection is given into the thickest area of muscle that lies over the mid-axillary line (Fig. 24-22). To give the injection, the needle is angled slightly toward the acromion process or inserted at a 90-degree angle. Children under the age of 18 months have poorly developed deltoid muscles and should not receive IM injections into this site. The deltoid muscle in children from 18 months to 15 years of age is large enough to accommodate 0.5 mL of medication. Patients older than 15 years may receive injections of 0.5 to 2 mL into the deltoid (Pagliaro, 1986).

The Rectus Femoris and Vastus Lateralis Sites. Injection sites in the thigh, the vastus lateralis and rectus femoris sites, offer rapid rates of medication absorption. Because these muscles contain no large blood vessels or nerves, they are safe injection sites to use for IM injections for most patients. The rectus femoris site is the site of choice for infants and children, but may also be used for adults. The rectus femoris site is located one-third of the distance from the knee to the greater trochanter of the femur, in the center of the anterior thigh (Fig. 24-23). An injection is administered into this site by lifting the

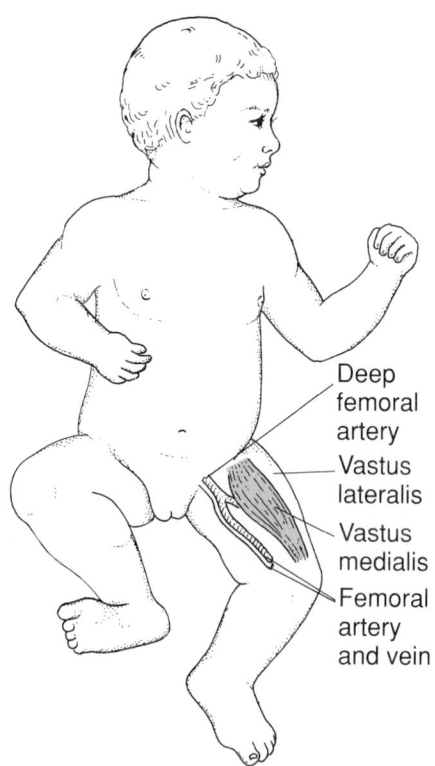

Figure 24–23. Rectus femoris site used in children. It is located one-third of the distance from the knee to the greater trochanter of the femur in the center of the anterior thigh.

PROCEDURE 24–4. Administering Intramuscular Injections

■ **Purpose**
1. Administer medication deeply into muscle tissue, without injury to the patient.
2. Administer a medication with absorption and onset of action quicker than the oral route and that may be irritating to the subcutaneous tissues.

■ **Assessment**
- Review patient's medical history, medication history, and allergy status.
- Assess for contraindications to receiving intramuscular injections; circulatory shock, reduced blood flow or muscle atrophy.
- Assess for anxiety related to fear of injection.
- Review chart for documentation of previous injection sites, if patient is receiving multiple injections.
- Refer to drug literature to determine appropriateness of medication and dosage, common side effects, and nursing implications.
- Assess adipose tissue and muscle mass of patient to determine needle size.

■ **Equipment**
Medication card or order.
Antiseptic swabs.
Vial, ampule, or tubex of medication.
Syringe or tubex: 2 to 3 mL for adult; 1–2 mL for child.
Sterile needle 1.5- to 3-inch, 21- to 23-gauge for adult; 0.5- to 1-inch, 25- to 27-gauge for children.

■ **Procedure**
1. Prepare needle, syringe, and medication by following steps 1–7 of Procedure 24-3, "Administering Subcutaneous Medications."
2. If medication is known to be irritating to subcutaneous tissues, replace needle after withdrawing medication.
   Rationale: Prevents medication adhering to outside of needle from irritating and burning subcutaneous tissues as needle passes into muscle.
3. Select appropriate injection site by inspecting muscle size and integrity. Consider volume of medication to be injected.
   Rationale: Larger muscles can absorb larger volumes of medication.
4. Assist patient to a comfortable position and expose only the area to be injected. Don gloves, especially on nondominant hand.
   Rationale: Promotes comfort and privacy. Maintains universal precautions if blood leaks from injection site.

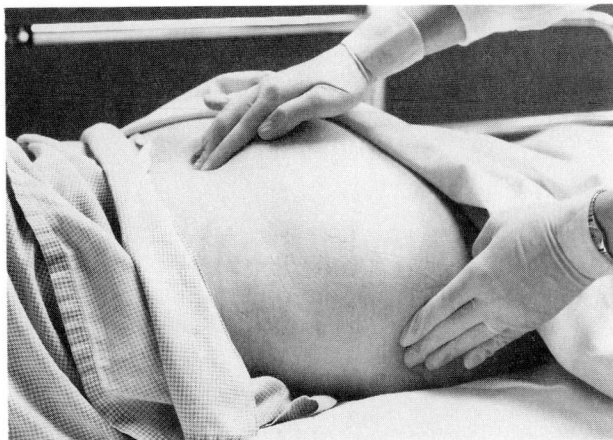
Step 5A: Using anatomic landmarks.

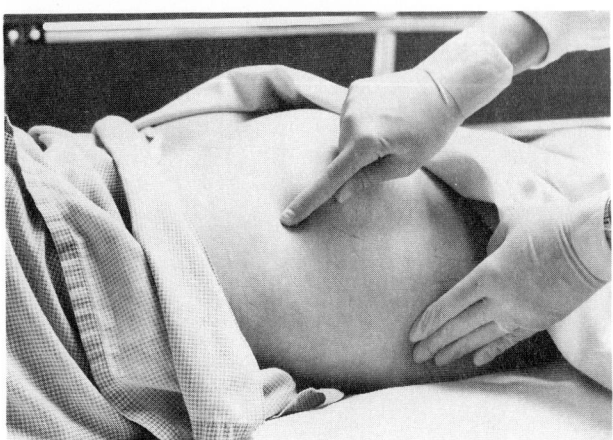
Step 5B: Locating the exact injection site.

5. Use anatomic landmarks (5*A*) to locate the exact injection site (5*B*) (see Figs. 24-22 to 24-26).
   Rationale: Injection into proper site prevents trauma to bones, nerves, or blood vessels.
6. Cleanse the site with antiseptic swab, wiping from center of site and rotating upward.
7. Remove needle cover.
8. Expel air bubbles from syringe.
9. Hold syringe between thumb and forefinger of dominant hand (like a dart).
10. Spread skin at the side with nondominant hand.
    Rationale: Facilitates needle insertion by firming skin surface and flattens tissue so needle penetrates into muscle.
    Note: If patient has very small muscle mass, may pinch muscle before insertion.
11. Insert needle quickly at a 90-degree angle.
    Rationale: 90-degree angle enables needle to reach deep muscle layers (see Fig. 24-21). Rapid needle insertion minimizes patient discomfort.

(continued)

PROCEDURE 24–4. Administering Intramuscular Injections (continued)

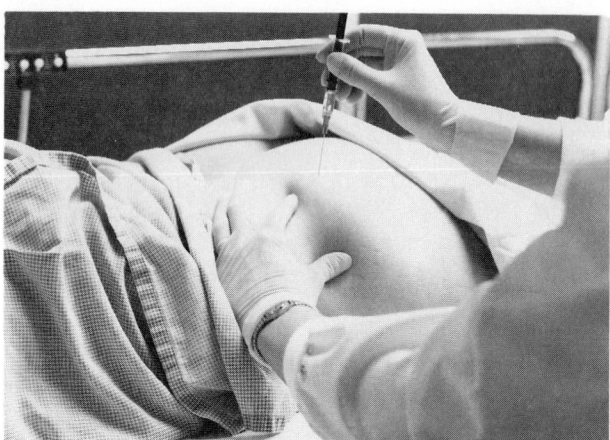

Step 10

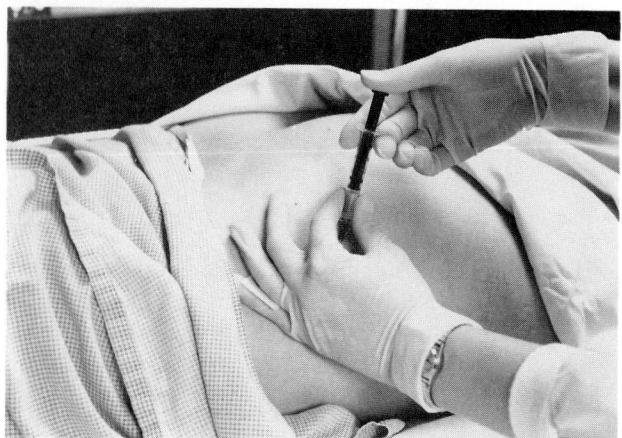

Step 12B

Note: If blood appears in syringe, remove needle, dispose of syringe, and prepare new medication.
Rationale: Aspiration of blood indicates needle placement intravascularly.

13. Withdraw needle while pressing antiseptic swab above site.
Rationale: Minimize discomfort by supporting tissues during needle withdrawal.

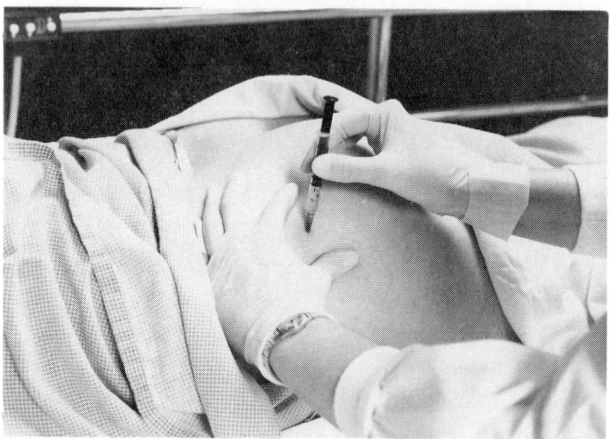

Step 11

12. Stabilize syringe barrel by grasping with nondominant hand. Aspirate slowly by pulling back on plunger with dominant hand. If no blood appears, inject medication slowly.

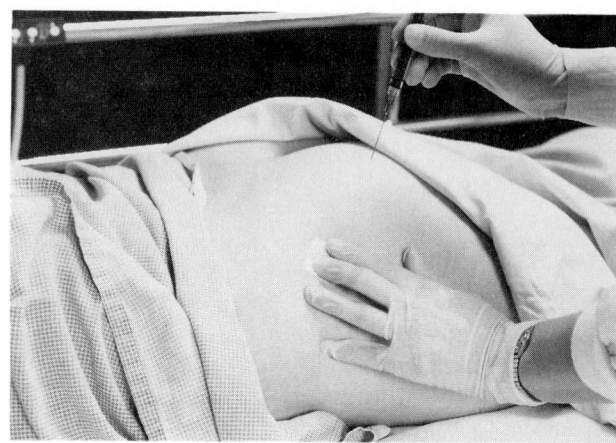

Step 13

14. Gently massage site.
Rationale: Stimulates local circulation and speeds drug absorption.

15. Do not recap needle. Dispose of equipment in proper receptacle.
Rationale: Protects nurse and health-care workers from accidental needle injury.

16. Wash hands.

17. Record medication and patient response according to agency protocol.

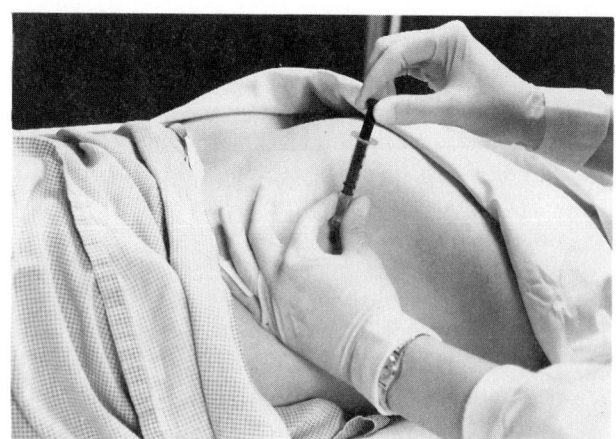

Step 12A

(continued)

PROCEDURE 24–4. Administering Intramuscular Injections *(continued)*

■ **Procedure**

Variations for Air Lock Injection Technique
1. When preparing medication for injection:
   a. Withdraw desired volume of medication into syringe and expel all excess air.
   b. Holding syringe so needle points up, pull back plunger to visually inspect total volume of medication in syringe. Note that there is approximately 0.2 mL more solution than necessary for accurate dosage
      Rationale: "Dead space" of needle and needle hub contain this additional medication when giving an injection without the air lock. The patient does not receive the 0.2 mL of solution.
   c. Expel the volume of solution not required in the prescribed dosage. Pull back plunger and visually inspect syringe for correct dosage.
      Rationale: When using air lock technique, the additional medication would not be trapped in the needle and hub space, but be injected into the patient. The patient would receive more medication than was ordered.
   d. Expel all excess air from syringe, leaving only 0.2 mL air.
      Rationale: It is believed that the air lock technique clears excess medication from the needle following

injection. *This technique is thought to prevent medication from leaking into the subcutaneous tissues and skin surface as the needle is withdrawn, preventing irritation and staining.*
2. When preparing for injection, the needle must enter patient at a 90-degree angle to the floor.
   Rationale: Ensures that the air bubble follows the solution and maintains the "air lock."

■ **Procedure**

Variations for Z-track Injections
1. When preparing the injection site: pull the skin and subcutaneous tissues about 1 to 1.5 inches to one side of the selected site (see Fig. 24-27).
   Rationale: Creates a zig-zag track through the tissues, which prevents back-leak of medication when needle is withdrawn.
2. Insert the syringe at a 90-degree angle.
3. Aspirate and administer medication while continuing traction on skin.
4. Leave needle inserted an additional 10 seconds.
   Rationale: Allows medication to disperse and muscle to begin absorption.
5. Remove needle, release traction on skin.
   Rationale: Zig-zag pathway seals medication into the muscle tissue.

---

muscle away from the bone and inserting the needle at a right angle to the muscle. Short needles (1 inch long or shorter) should be used to administer injections into the rectus femoris site in children. Infants and toddlers can tolerate injections of 0.5 to 1 mL into the rectus femoris muscle; preschool-aged children can tolerate injections of 1.5 mL into the rectus femoris site (Pagliaro, 1986).

The vastus lateralis site is used for IM injections for older children and adults. In children, the vastus lateralis site is located in the middle third of the area between the greater trochanter and the knee on the medial outer aspect of the thigh. In adults, the vastus lateralis site is the area located between one handbreadth above the knee and one handbreadth below the greater trochanter on the medial outer portion of the thigh (Fig. 24-24). Children less than 15 years of age can tolerate injections of up to 2 mL into the vastus lateralis site; adults can tolerate injections of up to 5 mL into the vastus lateralis site (Pagliaro, 1986).

The Ventrogluteal Site. The ventrogluteal site on the lateral hip is a site free of major blood vessels, nerves, and fat. To locate the ventrogluteal site, the heel of the

opposite hand (for right hip nurse must use left hand; for left hip nurse must use right hand) is placed over the greater trochanter, with the index and middle fingers angled towards the anterior superior iliac spine and toward the iliac crest, respectively. The injection is given in the center of the triangular area thus formed, with the needle directed at a 90-degree angle to the skin or with the needle angled slightly towards the iliac crest (Fig. 24-25). Toddlers should not receive injections into the ventrogluteal site; muscles in this site are not well developed until a child begins to walk. After the age of 3 years, volumes of up to 1 mL may be injected into the ventrogluteal site; preschool-aged children can be given 1.5 mL; school-aged children can be given 2.0 mL; and older children and adults can be given up to 2.5 mL into the ventrogluteal site (Pagliaro, 1986).

Elderly and debilitated patients who have lost muscle mass elsewhere often have enough muscle in the ventrogluteal site to allow safe administration of IM injections. If adequate muscle mass is not visualized, the nurse palpates the ventrogluteal site. If adequate muscle mass is not felt, the nurse checks with the physician to see if medications can be administered by another route.

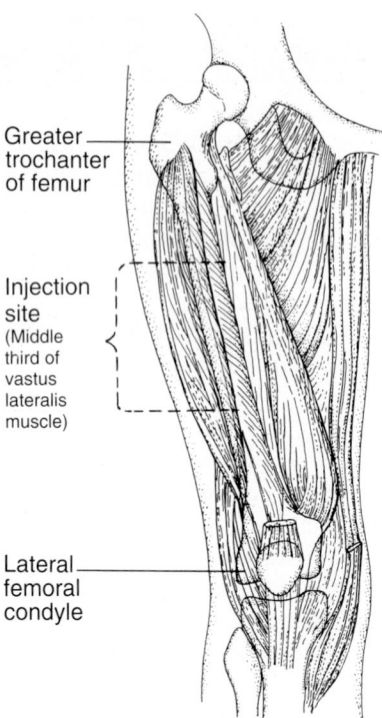

Figure 24–24. Vastus lateralis site for injection. The thigh is divided into thirds; the middle third is the injection site.

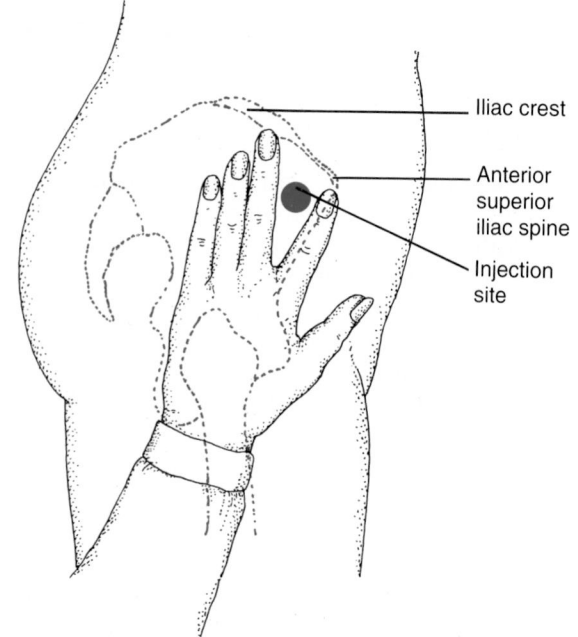

Figure 24–25. Ventrogluteal site injection. The heel of the hand is placed over the greater trochanter and the middle fingers reach toward the iliac crest where the index finger is angled toward the anterior superior iliac spine. The injection is given in the center of the resulting triangle.

The Dorsogluteal Site. The dorsogluteal site of the buttocks has been used commonly for IM injections. To locate the dorsogluteal site, the index fingers are used to locate the greater trochanter and the posterior superior iliac spine. An imaginary line is drawn between these landmarks, and the injection is given lateral and superior to the midpoint of this line drawn between the greater trochanter and the posterior superior iliac spine (Fig. 24-26). The needle is inserted at a 90-degree angle to the skin. Problems with the dorsogluteal site include: medication given into this site is slowly absorbed; the sciatic nerve and gluteal artery lie close to the site; infants of less than 18 months and debilitated adults may not have enough muscle mass to allow a safe injection into this site; and the thick layer of fat present over this site in many people may make it difficult to reach muscle tissue consistently. Some adult patients of normal size and weight who are given IM injections into the dorsogluteal site might receive the injection in SC fat. Researchers found that more than 95% of the women and 85% of the men they studied would have received IM injections into the SC fat if injections were given into the dorsogluteal site with 1.5-inch needles (Cockshott, et al., 1982). Use of the gluteal site should be limited to medications that can be safely given into SC fat; irritating medications and medications that must be more rapidly and consistently absorbed, such as hepatitis B vaccine, should be given into the vastus lateralis or ventrogluteal sites. Children of less than 3 years of age can be given injections of up to

1 mL into the dorsogluteal site; children of 3 to 6 years of age can be given 1.5 mL; children of 6 to 15 years of age can be given 2 mL; and children of more than 15 years of age and adults can receive injections of 2 to 4 mL into the dorsogluteal site (Pagliaro, 1986). The pain and bleeding that may occur when injections are administered into the dorsogluteal site are less likely to occur if the patient is positioned lying prone, with his or her toes pointing inward.

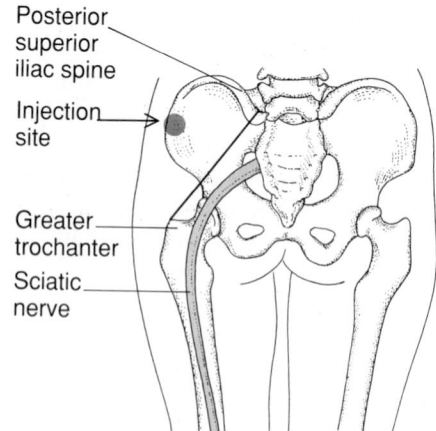

Figure 24–26. Dorsogluteal site for IM injection. The injection is given lateral and superior to the midpoint of an imaginary line drawn between the greater trochanter and posterior superior iliac spine.

Most medications that are appropriate for IM injection can be given using the technique described in Procedure 24-4. Medications that cause irritation of subcutaneous tissue (such as hydroxyzine) or that discolor subcutaneous tissue (such as iron) should be given by the Z-track method (Fig. 24-27). The variation using the Z-track method is given in Procedure 24-4. If these techniques are not followed or if site selection is not accurate, complications can occur; complications related to IM injections are listed in Table 24-9

Intravenous Administration

Intravenous medications are given in catheters inserted into veins. Advantages of using the IV route to administer medications include: the onset of medication action is usually rapid; predictable, therapeutic blood levels of medications can be obtained; the route can be used when gastrointestinal dysfunction or compromised peripheral circulation make medication absorption unpredictable by oral or IM routes; medications that cannot be given by other routes may be delivered intravenously; and larger doses of medications can be administered by this route than by IM injection. The disadvantages of this route include the high cost of treatment, the difficulty of ad-

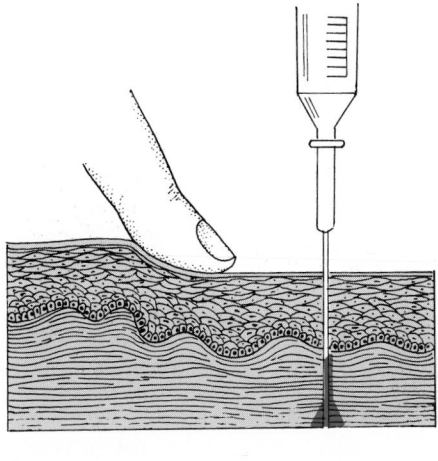

A

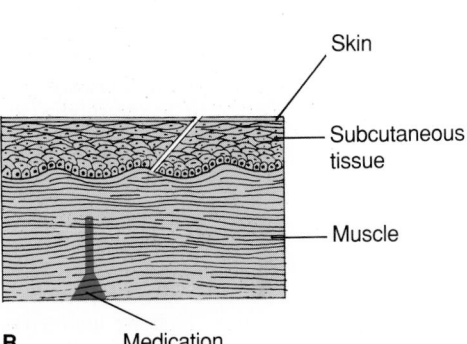

Skin

Subcutaneous tissue

Muscle

B   Medication

Figure 24–27. Z-track method. **A.** Pull skin and subcutaneous tissue 1 to 1.5 inches to side of injection site while injecting medication. **B.** Release traction to allow skin to fall back, sealing medication in site.

ministering IV medications outside of hospital settings, the difficulty of maintaining patent peripheral IV catheters in patients with limited numbers of adequate venous sites, and the increased risk of complications with this route. The complications related to IV administration of medications are given in Table 24-10.

Intravenous medications should be prepared and packaged in a sterile manner and should not be prepared in an oil or aqueous suspension. Intravenous administration of a medication that is not sterile, such as an oral medication, may cause an infection within the vein (phlebitis), or may cause a generalized infection (sepsis). Medications prepared in oil or water suspension contain large particles suspended in a solution. If a medication suspension is given intravenously, the large medication particles may act as emboli and lodge in small veins. A wide variety of medications can be given intravenously. Categories of medications that are given commonly by the IV route are antibiotic, narcotic, antiarrhythmic, and antiulcer medications. Intravenous catheters are placed in the peripheral or the central circulation.

Intravenous medications can be administered directly into the vein or through various access devices that have been placed in a vein after venipuncture. Peripheral IV catheters or heparin locks are used for short-term therapy, whereas central venous access devices (Hickman or Groshong catheters) are employed for more long-term therapy. Venous access devices are discussed more completely in Chapter 32. Intravenous medications may be given by IV push (bolus), by intermittent infusion (IV piggyback), or by continuous infusion. Intravenous pain medication may be self-delivered by the patient using a patient-controlled analgesia (PCA) device.

The IV Push Technique. The IV push technique is used to administer medications that must be given rapidly to have the desired therapeutic effect or medications that are incompatible with intravenous fluids (e.g., phenytoin). If a medication ordered to be given IV push is not prepackaged in a syringe, the nurse needs to draw up the medication into a syringe. A 3- or 5-mL syringe with a short (1 inch), 20-gauge needle can be used for giving most IV push medications. Medications whose total volume is less than 1 mL should be drawn up in a 1-mL syringe to allow more accurate measurement of medication volume. Some IV push medications may be ordered in volumes of greater than 5 mL. Intravenous push medications may be given into a continuously infusing IV or into a capped IV port (a "heparin lock"). The rate of medication infusion may be ordered by the physician; more commonly, the exact rate of infusion is not specified. The nurse should check in a medication reference manual for the infusion time recommended by the pharmaceutical company. Once the nurse knows the recommended total infusion time, he or she can calculate the infusion rate by dividing the total volume of medication

(Text continues on page 550)

TABLE 24–9

Complications Associated with Administration of Intramuscular Medications

Complication	Signs/Symptoms Associated with Complication	Causes	Nursing Measures Used to Decrease Risk of or to Avoid Complications
Pain with injection	Pain with injection	Muscle tense during injection Medication irritating to IM tissue Inadvertent tracking of medication or alcohol through SC tissue	Encourage patient to relax muscles during injection. Use Z-track technique when administering medications that are irritating to SC tissue. Change needle after drawing up medication. Use an air lock when giving irritating medications. Let alcohol skin prep dry before giving injection.
Damage to SC or IM tissue, including sterile abscesses (collection of undissolved medication), SC tissue discoloration, hematomas, and muscle contractions	Tissue nodules (lumps) or indurations (indentations), bruising, brown discoloration, or pain in IM injection site. Muscle contracture (in infants) characterized by difficulty crawling 4 weeks to 1 year after receiving IM injections (Pagliaro, 1986).	Multiple injections given into same area Injection given into abnormal tissue Injection of drug that is not water-soluble (e.g., dilantin or valium) IM administration of heparin IM route used for patient with a low platelet count SC deposition of iron supplements (e.g., Imferon)	Give an injection at least 1 inch away from location of recently administered injections or from scars, burns, or areas of abnormal SC or IM tissue. Rotate injection sites (give injections at least 1 inch away from recent injection.) Record sites used for all injections. As soon as possible, change from IM route to another route of medication administration. Be sure that medication is recommended for IM administration. Check with physician before administering IM injection to a patient whose platelet count is less than 30,000/mL. Don't administer IM injections into atrophied muscle. The risk of knee contractures for infants is decreased if passive range-of-motion exercises are done, and if warm soaks and massage are applied to the thighs (Pagliaro, 1986). Iron supplements (e.g., Imferon) should be given using the Z-track technique.
Nerve injury	Shooting pain down limb (Pagliaro, 1986), temporary or permanent paralysis	Nerve struck during injection Medication injected close to nerve	Careful visual location of site followed by palpation of site landmarks and boundaries. Avoid use of deltoid and dorsogluteal sites whenever possible.

(continued)

TABLE 24–9
(continued)

Complication	Signs/Symptoms Associated with Complication	Causes	Nursing Measures Used to Decrease Risk of or to Avoid Complications
Bone injury	Pain or bone damage	Bone struck during IM injection	Avoid use of deltoid site whenever possible. Use a short needle (1.25-inch) when giving injections into the deltoid or ventrogluteal sites. Use visual inspection and palpation to locate injection sites.
Speed shock (rapid absorption of medication)	Unexpectedly rapid onset of action of medication. May lead to increased heart rate and respiratory rate, decreased level of consciousness, and cardiovascular collapse	Medication administered directly into a vein or artery	After inserting needle into muscle, aspirate (pull back on plunger of syringe) to check for blood. If blood appears in syringe barrel, remove syringe and needle and discard. Draw up another dose of medication and administer in a new site.
Infection of muscle or bone	Muscle or bone pain in injection site, skin redness or warmth, localized swelling	Introduction of organism into tissue or bone during injection	Follow strict aseptic technique when administering IM injections.

TABLE 24–10
Complications Associated with Intravenous Administration of Medications

Complication	Signs/Symptoms Associated with Complication	Causes	Nursing Measures Used to Decrease Risk of or to Avoid Complications
Speed shock	Headache, tightness in chest, shock, cardiac arrest (Pagliaro, 1986)	Medication administered more rapidly than intended	Know time period recommended for medication administration. If administering by IV bolus technique, time infusion with a watch with a second hand. If administering by continuous drip or intermittent drip methods, regulate drip rate accurately. Check rate of infusion of medication at least several times per hour. Any medications with serious or toxic side effects when given too rapidly should be infused using an infusion control device. All medications that are titrated or must be infused at a consistent rate should be administered using an infusion control device.

(continued)

TABLE 24–10
(continued)

Complication	Signs/Symptoms Associated with Complication	Causes	Nursing Measures Used to Decrease Risk of or to Avoid Complications
Catheter insertion site infection or systemic infection	Redness, warmth, or pain at catheter insertion site; fever, increased leukocyte count, organisms present on blood culture samples, chills, shaking, increase in body temperature	Break in aseptic technique when preparing or administering IV medications. Contamination of IV catheter site when IV dressing is changed. IV equipment changed infrequently. Contaminated IV solution.	Catheter securely taped to skin. Check catheter insertion site at least once per shift and before and after infusion of medications. Change IV tubing every 48 to 72 hours.
Extravasation (medication administered outside of the vein lumen)	Pain, swelling at distal end of catheter, slowed rate of infusion, increase in size of one extremity (with IV) over the other extremity, severe tissue sloughing	Catheter migrated out of vein during patient movement.	Avoid placing IV catheter close to patient's wrist or elbow, whenever possible. Catheter securely taped to skin.
Thrombophlebitis	Redness and warmth along cannulated vein, burning pain. Slow flow rate. When palpated, vein feels hard, cord-like	Trauma to vein during catheter insertion or from catheter movement. Irritation of vein resulting from medication administered	Catheter securely taped to skin. IV site inspected at least once per shift. Whenever possible, irritating medications should not be infused into the small veins of the hands and forearms. Whenever possible, avoid placing catheters near the wrist or elbow. If placement in these areas is necessary, decrease catheter movement by securing arm to an arm board. Check catheter insertion site at least once per shift and before and after infusion of IV medications.

that is ordered by the recommended total time of infusion. Generally, IV push medications are given over a period of at least 1 minute.

The Intermittent Infusion Technique. The intermittent infusion technique (also called IV "piggyback") is the most common technique for infusing IV medications. It is used to administer medications that need to be infused over an intermediate length of time (usually, 30 minutes to 1 hour) and medications that are not stable for long periods of time. Medications administered by intermittent infusion are supplied in bags that contain 50 to 250 mL of IV fluid. These bags of fluid contain the medication dissolved in normal saline or in 5% dextrose in water (D_5W). The pharmacist who prepares the medication labels the bag with the patient's name, the name

of the medication, the type of IV fluid, and the suggested rate of infusion (see Procedure 24-5).

The nurse administering the medication is responsible for making sure that the medication supplied is the medication ordered; the medication, as ordered, is safe for the individual patient; the IV catheter is patent (the catheter is still in the vein; the catheter site is not reddened or swollen); and the medication is infused at the proper rate. Decisions about the safety of administering a medication to an individual patient are made with a knowledge of the usual dose and dosage range of the ordered medication, the patient's size and weight, the reason that the medication is ordered for the patient, and any other conditions that might influence the way the medication affects the individual patient.

Intermittent infusions of medications may be given

PROCEDURE 24–5. Administering IV Medications Using Intermittent Infusion Technique

■ **Purpose**

1. Maintain therapeutic levels of medication in the patient's blood.
2. Dilute irritating intravenous solutions.
3. Prevent complications associated with bolus administration by delivering medication over a longer period of time.
4. Prevent combining medications that are incompatible.

■ **Assessment**

- Review physician's order for type of medication, dosage, schedule, and if particular intravenous solution is needed.
- Assess patency of existing intravenous line.
- Inspect insertion site for infiltration or phlebitis.
- Determine patient's drug allergy status.

■ **Equipment**

Medication Kardex or card.
Medication prepared and labeled in a 50–250-mL sterile infusion container.
IV infusion set.
21- or 23-gauge sterile needle.
Alcohol or betadine swab.
20-mL syringe of sterile NaCl. (Optional: If medication is incompatible with primary infusing intravenous solution.)
(Heparin lock). Two sterile syringes and needle with 3 mL normal saline each, and a sterile syringe with 1 mL heparin flush solution (10 μ heparin per mL).

■ **Procedure**

1. Wash hands.
   Rationale: Reduces transmission of microorganisms.
2. Connect infusing tubing to medication container (see Procedure "Changing Intravenous Solution and Tubing").
   Rationale: Primed intravenous tubing prevents air bubble from entering patient's vein.
3. Connect capped, sterile needle to end of infusing set.
   Rationale: Cap maintains sterility of needle before connecting it to the primary intravenous line.
4. Confirm patient's identity by asking his or her name, and by looking at identiband.
   Rationale: Prevents administering medication to wrong patient.
5. Hang medication bag at or above level of primary IV solution.
   Rationale: This is not always necessary, but may be needed to regulate medication flow to the patient.

6. Wipe injection port, nearest IV insertion site, on primary IV tubing with antiseptic.
   Rationale: Prevents contamination with microorganisms during needle insertion.
7. Remove needle cover from medication tubing and insert into injection port of primary intravenous line. Secure with tape.
   Note: If medication is not compatible with primary IV solution, clamp primary IV tubing above injection port, insert needle with 20-mL syringe of NaCl and flush IV line. Remove needle. Insert needle attached to medication tubing and secure with tape.
   Rationale: Prevents reactions and precipitation of uncompatible solutions.
8. Regulate flow of medication solution. Most medications infuse over 20 to 60 minutes. Check pharmacy directives. Monitor periodically.
   Note: Primary IV line may need to be clamped for medication solution to infuse. Some infusion sets include backcheck valves that stop primary IV solution flow while medication infuses, then automatically open when medication infusion stops.

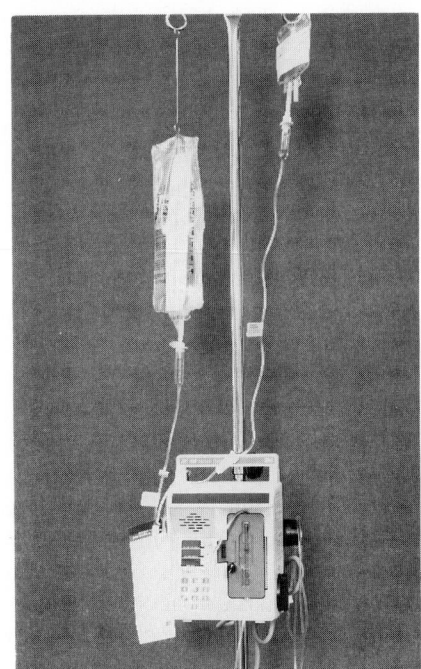

Step 8

9. When medication has infused, turn off flow clamp. Regulate primary infusion as necessary.
   Rationale: Medication infusion may alter flow rate of primary solution.
10. Discard medication solution container, tubing, and

(continued)

needle or leave hanging with needle covered for future use, as dictated by agency policy.
Rationale: Medication line establishes a potential route for microorganisms to enter the primary IV. Protective needle covers and changing tubing every 48 to 72 hours, according to agency policy, decreases the chance of contamination.

11. Wash hands.
12. Document medication administration and add IV volume to IV intake.

■ **Procedure**

Using a Heparin Lock

1. Perform steps 1 to 6 of above procedure.
2. Insert needle of the 3-mL NaCl syringe into port. Aspirate for blood return.
   Rationale: Blood return ensures that intravenous catheter is in the vein. Sometimes there is no blood return even though the catheter is patent.
3. Inject 2–3 mL of NaCl. Do not force solution.
   Rationale: Establishes patency of IV catheter, and flushes heparin from the catheter.
4. Remove needle and discard in appropriate receptacle.

5. Insert needle of medication tubing into injection port. Secure and regulate flow as described above.
6. When medication has infused, turn off clamp and remove needle.
7. Cleanse port.
8. Insert needle of second NaCl syringe and inject 2 to 3 mL NaCl. Discard.
   Rationale: Flushes remaining medication from the catheter and prevents incompatibilities with heparin.
9. Insert needle of heparin flush solution. Inject slowly. Remove and discard.
   Rationale: Anticoagulant action of heparin prevents blood in IV catheter from clotting.
10. Wash hands.
11. Document medication administration and add IV volume to IV intake.

■ **Lifespan Considerations**

Infants and Children

• Infants receive much smaller volumes of fluid than adults. Intravenous medications should be infused through a volume control IV unit to avoid potentially serious fluid overload.

---

when a patient does not require administration of continuous IV fluids. The patient's IV catheter may be converted to a heparin lock. The heparin lock, a small, dead-end connector, is attached to the proximal end of an IV catheter. One to 3 mL of solution is instilled ("flushed") through the heparin lock every 8 hours or after any medication is infused through the heparin lock, to maintain catheter patency. The fluid used to flush heparin lock catheters is usually a solution of 10 U/mL heparin; normal saline or more concentrated solutions of heparin (100 U/mL) may also be used.

The Continuous Infusion Technique. The continuous infusion technique is used to infuse medications that need to be given continuously in order to have their desired effect (e.g., heparin or theophylline), or medications that are toxic if given over short periods of time (e.g., multivitamins or cisplatin). Medications ordered by continuous infusion are supplied in IV bags containing 250 to 1000 mL of IV fluid.

Macrodrip or minidrip IV tubing, with or without leur-lock connections and in-line filters, are used to connect the IV medications and fluids to the IV catheter. Leur-lock tubing, made with connections that screw together, is usually used for administering medications or fluids into central catheters. Tubing made with an in-line filter is used to give medications and fluids into central

catheters. Before giving a medication through IV tubing with an in-line filter, the nurse should check if medication is affected by the filter. Some medications are filtered out of solution by an in-line filter; if one of these medications is infused through a catheter tubing with an in-line filter, the patient would not receive any medication.

If the patient is receiving more than one continuously infusing IV, and if the ordered medication is compatible with other IV medications and fluids the patient is receiving, the second IV may be connected to a medication infusion port of the first IV so that the medications infuse into the same catheter. The ordered IV drip rate is calculated and the rate of infusion is regulated. An IV timing tape, a tape marked with the time that the IV is started, intermediate infusion times, and the time that the IV is ordered to be completed, can act as a quick reference to check if the IV is infusing at the ordered rate. Refer to Chapter 32 for specific information concerning calculation and regulation of IV drip rates. The rate of flow of continuously infusing IV fluids should be checked at least once per hour to ensure that the rate has not changed with a change in patient position or catheter patency.

If an IV has infused at a rate that is faster or slower than the ordered rate, a prompt correction of IV rate may allow the actual infusion time to be close to the ordered infusion time. Intravenous fluids or medications that infuse 1 to 2 hours earlier or later than ordered are generally considered to be medication errors. If a medication must be delivered at an exact rate or over a set period of time, an infusion controller pump may be used; these machines monitor and control the rate at which a medication is infused by counting the drops infused or by monitoring the IV volume infused.

Patient-Controlled Analgesia (PCA). Patient controlled analgesia devices permit the patient to administer narcotics intravenously as needed for pain control. A PCA machine is programmed to deliver a set amount of narcotic through a syringe into tubing that is connected to a continuously infusing IV. Specific dosages and time intervals can be programmed into the machine to prevent overdosage; medication is delivered when the patient pushes a control button. Refer to Chapter 40 for more information on patient-controlled analgesia.

Discharge Planning and Home Care

Medication routines that are specific to the patient and integrated into daily routine are more likely to be followed. To tailor medication routines and patient teaching to the individual patient, the nurse should assess the patient's physical and psychosocial status, financial situation, usual daily routine before the current illness, and the patient's learning style and manner of coping with previous medical regimes. This information can generally be gathered informally, by talking with the patient and family. By informing the patient and family of an intent to make the medication routines "practical so that they can work," the nurse is likely to elicit useful information.

The physical condition of the patient may influence the ability to take medications as prescribed. The physical senses of sight and hearing often deteriorate with disease or with advancing age. Does the patient see and hear well enough to follow daily medication routines? A diabetic patient with retinopathy and blurred vision may not be able to draw up insulin accurately in a syringe. The ability to perform fine motor movements may also change with illness or advancing age. The coordinated motor movements needed to administer injections can be learned by most people, but the nurse should expect to spend more time teaching this technique to elderly patients. Patient assessments also include making a judgment about the patient's ability to comprehend, follow, and remember instructions. A neurologic deficit that may limit a patient's ability to follow a medical routine may or may not be easy to recognize. Overt signs of aphasia (inability to speak or comprehend) or anomia (inability to remember the names of objects) can be easy to recognize; more subtle forms of neurologic dysfunction may be perceived as "vagueness" or "lack of atten-

tiveness" by the nurse. When the nurse is concerned about a patient's ability to comprehend and retain information, asking the patient to restate instructions several hours after hearing them may help clarify whether the patient has the cognitive ability to self-administer medications safely.

The psychosocial condition of the patient influences his or her ability to take medications correctly. People living in situations without supportive friends or family members may be less likely to follow medical regimes. If the nurse is aware of the situation, he or she can help the

---

Patient Teaching

Instruct the patient as follows:

- Learn the name, purpose, dose, and common side effects of any prescribed medications you are taking.
- Take every prescribed dose, even if you start to feel better before the medication is finished.
- Take only the prescribed dose of medication—increasing the dosage will not always increase the desired effect, and in many cases may be dangerous.
- Study possible food or drug interactions to your prescribed medications. Find out whether the drug should be taken with meals or on an empty stomach.
- Learn symptoms that necessitate contacting a health-care professional.
- Keep all medications in their original prescription containers and store according to specifications.
- Check expiration dates and discard when expired; old medications may lose potency and be ineffective.
- Never take medications prescribed for another individual. Never give your prescribed medications for another's use.
- Do not take medications in the dark or when you are groggy, since drug errors may occur.
- If remembering to take prescribed medications is a problem, keep a check-off chart or use a special dispensing unit to improve compliance.
- Keep all medications out of reach and in child-proof containers to avoid accidental ingestion.
- Keep a list of all current medications so accurate information can be given to any health-care provider.
- Whenever possible, provide the patient with written information on essential content for future reference.

patient problem-solve, help the patient get family support or counseling, and simplify the medication routine to fit the patient's situation.

The patient's financial situation may limit his or her ability to obtain the medication or to take the medication as prescribed. Patients with limited resources should be placed on the least expensive, simplest medication routine possible. The nurse should make sure that the patient understands the possible consequences of discontinuing medications.

The complexity of a medical routine may make compliance difficult for the individual patient. Medication regimes that involve multiple dosing intervals of multiple medications, or through-the-night dosing, may be difficult to remember. The nurse should consider, given the patient's abilities and limitations, whether safe self-administration of medications can occur. If the nurse has concerns about the patient's ability to take medications safely, the patient's physician should be consulted to see if the medication routine can be simplified or if help can be obtained for the patient at home. After discussing the planned home medication routines with the patient, it is helpful to ask the patient his or her plan for taking the medications. If the patient does not have a plan for taking the medications, techniques such as prefilled medication boxes, calendars with the medications written on them, or storage of medications in places that prompt the patient to remember them may be useful (Forget-me-nots, 1985).

Priorities for teaching can be guided by thinking, "what does this patient need to know to take his or her medications safely?" Information should be presented in nontechnical language, in both written and discussion formats. Brief, practical information about the following topics is usually appropriate: the name of the medication; the reason for taking the medication; how and when to take the medication; how long to take the medication; the foods, drinks, prescription or over-the-counter medications that may affect the action of the medication; any activities that may be affected when taking this medication; and the usual side effects of the medication and their treatment. If a medication is being given to improve a bothersome symptom, for example a metered-dose inhaler used to treat shortness of breath, specific warnings about using more than the ordered dosage should be included. Without this warning, a patient may feel "if a little is good, more is better," and may take excessive amounts of medication.

Whenever possible, begin teaching the patient about discharge medications early during his or her hospital stay. Teaching about administration techniques that require learning psychomotor skills, such as giving insulin injections, should be begun at least 24 hours before patient discharge. The patient is unlikely to learn a complex psychomotor skill unless frequent demonstrations of the skill occur during hospitalization.

Likelihood of compliance with medication routines

can be difficult to predict. Patients who are very unlikely to comply with medication routines can be easy to spot; included in this group are people with ongoing substance abuse problems, or complex or unstable living arrangements. Compliance with medication regimes is lower than one might expect among other groups of people. Twenty percent of people may not fill initial prescriptions; 40% to 60% of people may stop taking their medications early. Average long-term compliance with medication regimes used to prevent complications (such as antihypertensives) is about 50%. Matching medication routines and teaching materials to the individual patient; frequent, ongoing outpatient compliance checks; encouraging involvement of family or friends in assisting the person with medication compliance; and discussing compliance issues with the patients, may help increase rates of compliance.

EVALUATION

Assessing the patient's response to medications is an important function of the professional nurse. Evaluation should include therapeutic effects obtained from the medication, unexpected adverse effects from the medication, the patient's compliance with the medication regime, and the patient's knowledge level concerning prescribed medications.

The nurse can ask the patient if the prescribed medication seems to be working. Subjective feelings of improvement are important indicators of therapeutic effect for many medications. The nurse can also use physical assessments (e.g., vital signs, lung auscultation) to see if physical improvement in status has occurred. Laboratory test values provide additional objective data useful in evaluating many medications.

The nurse should be knowledgeable about side effects for any drug administered. Signs of toxicity or unpleasant side effects should be documented and reported to the physician.

Assessment of the patient's understanding and compliance with drug therapy is also an important part of evaluation. Having the patient verbally describe the dose, frequency, action, and side effects of each medication is one way to evaluate knowledge level. Patients administering injections for the first time should demonstrate their skill in injection technique before discharge. Patients should be able to explain how they plan to purchase, store, and take their medication after discharge.

LIFESPAN CONSIDERATIONS

Medication administration techniques are affected by developmental stage and age-related factors.

Newborn and Infant

Special considerations are important when giving oral, SC, IM, and IV medications to newborns and infants. Liquid forms of oral medications should be used for newborns and infants; if these are not available, the medication should be crushed and dissolved in water. A syringe can be used to draw up and give oral medications. Medications should be given on an empty stomach unless otherwise noted; infant formulas may alter medication absorption and the infant is less likely to "spit up" medications if before feedings.

Parenteral medications should be given to newborns and infants with special care. The SC route is rarely used for administering medications to infants and newborns; SC injections can be difficult to administer to the newborn or premature infant who has little or no subcutaneous tissue. If the route must be used, the nurse should discuss technique concerns with the infant's physician. The physician may choose to have injections given into intradermal tissue. Once medication action, dosage, and length of action are determined, they will probably remain constant if technique remains consistent.

Intramuscular injections of 0.5 to 1 mL of medication can be administered into the rectus femoris site of infants of less than 2 years of age. Newborns and infants are given IV medications with the following guidelines:

- The smallest possible amounts of medication are used.
- Infusions are monitored using electronic flow devices.
- IV sites in the hand, scalp, forearm, foot, or central circulation are used (Teitell, 1984).
- Careful assessment of catheter site condition is performed frequently.
- The site is protected and the child is restrained, as needed.

Teaching concerning medication administration is geared toward caregivers. Teaching should encompass the reason the child is receiving the medication, the proper medication dosage, the method of measuring the dosage, the dosage schedule in relationship to feedings, how long to continue the medication, the desired effect of the medication, what to do if the child spits up the medication, and signs and symptoms of common important medication side effects. If an infant spits up a volume of medication that looks like the total dose, within 5 to 10 minutes after receiving it, the medication should usually be repeated.

Toddler and Preschooler

Children in this age group are beginning to explore their world, learning about themselves and their environment. Because this time is one of exploration, accidental medication poisoning is a particular risk. Parents should be encouraged to store all medications in a protected area, out of the child's reach; make sure that medications are packaged in containers with childproof caps; and make sure that children are aware that medications are not candy.

The toddler or preschool-aged child who is given medication may have multiple concerns: a fear of the unknown or unfamiliar, a fear of pain, fear of being separated from family, or a fear of loss of control. Procedures should be explained in simple terms, appropriate to the child's past experiences and level of understanding. Attempts should be made to assure the child that the medication is not given as a punishment. Whenever possible, allow the child to make choices about therapy. Effective teaching materials for toddlers and preschoolers include texts fashioned like coloring books and dolls or puppets (Streckfuss, 1985). Dolls and puppets can be used to demonstrate a procedure and, if necessary, the child can return the demonstration on the doll.

Physical changes during this period also have implications for medication administration. Oral medications are still given in liquid form or, if necessary, tablets are crushed and mixed with food. Children younger than 3 years old have straighter, stiffer external auditory canals than do older children and adults. To administer ear drops to this age group, the pinna of the ear is pulled down and back before dropping medication into the ear canal. The preferred site for administering IM injections to toddlers is the rectus femoris site; injections of up to 1.5 mL of medications may be given. Preschoolers can receive injections of up to 0.5 mL into the deltoid site, up to 1.5 mL into the rectus femoris site, ventral gluteal, or dorsogluteal sites, and up to 2 mL into the vastus lateralis site (Pigliaro, 1986). Many young children are very fearful of injections, and the injection should be given as promptly as possible to avoid escalation of anxiety and fear. The child must be carefully restrained, often by another person, to ensure safety during the procedure.

Child and Adolescent

As the child matures and develops, more teaching and responsibility for medication administration can be directed at the child. Most school-aged children can swallow tablets and capsules. To increase compliance, the dosage schedule should avoid school hours whenever possible. When medication administration is necessary during school hours, most schools require that medications be deposited with the school nurse in the original prescription container.

Many school-aged children are still fearful of injections, and worry about crying or loosing control when injections are administered in groups. Even though children of this age can understand the importance of remaining still during an injection, sudden movement often occurs as the needle pierces the skin. Support of the extremity or judicious positioning helps ensure safety during the injection procedure. By the time a child has reached school age, all injections sites may be used, since all muscles have adequately developed.

Teaching during the adolescent years should emphasize the importance of not taking any prescription medication that has not specifically been ordered for the person. The adolescent should be questioned concerning the use of illegal drugs or alcohol, both of which often interact with prescribed medications.

Adult and Older Adult

As adults age, the need for more medications to treat chronic health problems may become a reality. Compliance with complex medication schedules can be difficult, especially for the older person who has cognitive deficits. Most adults can swallow tablets, but neurologic problems can interfere with swallowing ability.

Physical conditions, such as cachexia or obesity, may influence which IM sites are chosen for adults. The cachectic adult may retain muscle mass in the ventrogluteal site longer than in other IM sites. The least desirable IM site for an obese adult is the dorsogluteal site, where the presence of a thick fat layer often causes the medication to be deposited in the subcutaneous tissue. Visual deficits may make reading drug information and prescription labels more difficult. Decreased fine motor skill and tactile sensation may increase the difficulty of administering eye drops or insulin injections.

The elderly person is at increased risk for drug toxicity because of altered renal excretion and hepatic metabolism of drugs. Decreased circulation can affect absorption of ingested drugs. The elderly should be watched more carefully for drug toxicity, especially when renal or liver disease is present.

Drug misuse can occur when medications are saved to be used at a future time; elderly people may also share their own prescription drugs with a friend who complains of similar symptoms. Older patients on a fixed income may find that the expense of many medications stresses an already limited budget. Although these problems can occur among all age groups, the frequency is increased among elderly populations due to their increasing dependence on medications to improve health and functioning.

Key Concepts

- Medication administration is a significant nursing responsibility that requires a good understanding of pharmacologic principles, assessment skills, and ability to individualize patient teaching.
- A drug is a substance that alters physiologic function, and a medication is a drug that is administered for its therapeutic effects.
- Medications can be identified by four different names: chemical name, generic name, official name, and brand name.
- Drug references are available to provide the healthcare professional with specific information on each medication. It is the responsibility of the nurse to use reference drug sources to be knowledgeable about each drug administered.
- Medication distribution systems include the stock supply, the unit dose, and self-administered medication system (SAM).
- A drug order must include the patient's name, the date and time of the order, the name of the medication, the dose, the frequency, the route of administration, and the physician's signature.
- Types of drug orders include standing orders, PRN orders, one-time orders, stat orders, and telephone and verbal orders. It is the nurse's responsibility to interpret accurately and carry out safely the physician's orders.
- Three systems of measure are used in calculation of drug dosage, namely, the metric system, the apothecaries' system, and household measure. It is the responsibility of the nurse to calculate drug dosage accurately within a given system and from one system to another.
- Federal legislation controls the way medications are manufactured, marketed, and controlled. The nurse must practice within the state's Nurse Practice Act and the agency's policies and procedures concerning medication administration.
- To ensure patient safety, the nurse must follow the "five rights" (right drug, in the right dose, at the right time, by the right route, to the right patient) whenever a medication is administered.
- Drug activity is the result of chemical interactions between a medication and the cells of the body, which produce a biologic or physiologic response. This response can be altered by drug absorption, distribution of the drug, metabolism of the drug, or excretion of the drug.
- Many factors, such as age, weight, gender, time of administration, and organ system function can affect drug action.
- Therapeutic effects are the desired effects obtained from medication administration. In addition, side effects such as secondary effects, toxicity, cumulative effects, tolerance, hypersensitivity reaction, idiosyncratic reaction, allergic reaction, or drug or food interactions can occur.
- Assessment when the patient first enters the health-

care facility to obtain baseline information concerning medications, assessment before any administration of medications, and assessment to individualize patient teaching concerning medications, are important to ensure patient safety.

■ Nursing diagnoses related to medication administration may include Noncompliance or Knowledge Deficit.

■ Many forms of medications, such as tablets, capsules, syrups, and elixers are appropriate for oral administration. Oral medications may be swallowed, administered through gastric or intestinal tubes, or given via the sublingual or buccal route.

■ Topical medications include medications that are applied to the skin or inserted in a body cavity. Solutions, creams, lotions, and transdermal patches are applied to the skin. Topical medications can be inserted into the eye, ear, nose, rectum, and vagina.

■ Parenteral medications are given by injection or infusion into intradermal tissue, subcutaneous tissue, intramuscular tissue, or into venous or arterial circulation.

■ Sites commonly used for intramuscular injections include the deltoid, ventral gluteal, vastus lateralis, rectus femoris, and the dorsogluteal muscles. Anatomic landmarks must be used to identify each site properly.

■ Intravenous medications enter the venous circulation by IV push, intermittent infusion, or continuous drip. The patient may control the delivery of intravenous medications through the use of a patient-controlled analgesia device.

■ Developmental concerns are important for the nurse to consider when administering medication.

References

Berelowitz, M. (1987). *Insulin bioavailability: Its relevance to clinical practice.* Princeton, NJ: Squibb-Novo.

Cockshott, W. P., Thompson, G. T., Howlett, L. J., et al. (1982). Intramuscular or intralipomatous injections? *New England Journal of Medicine, 307,* 356.

Cooper, D. M., Watt, R. C., & Alterescu, V. (1983). *Guide to wound care.* Libertyville, IL: Hollister.

Coutts, R. T. (1986). Drug metabolism and elimination. In A. M. Pagliaro & L. A. Pagliaro (Eds.), *Pharmacologic aspects of nursing.* St. Louis: C. V. Mosby.

Forget-me-nots. (1985). *American Journal of Nursing, 85,* 167.

Hahn, A. B., Oestreich, S. J. K., Barkin, R. L., et al. (1986). *Mosby's pharmacology in nursing.* St. Louis: C. V. Mosby.

Hanson, M. J. S. (1987). Hematoma associated with subcutaneous heparin administration. *Focus on Critical Care, 14*(6), 62.

Heifetr, S., Day, D., & Ipp, E. (1987). Inadvertent chlorpropamide hypoglycemia—No longer once in a blue moon? (letter) *New England Journal of Medicine, 316,* 223.

Henrietta, G. (1987). Lab tests you can't overlook: Part I. *Nursing '87, 11,* 56.

Kaysen, G. A., Pond, S. M., Roper, M. H., et al. (1985). Combined hepatic and renal injury in alcoholics during therapeutic use of acetaminophen. *Archives of Internal Medicine, 145,* 2019.

Lakshmanan, M. C., Hershey, C. O., & Breslau, D. (1986). Hospital admissions caused by iatrogenic disease. *Archives of Internal Medicine, 146,* 1931.

Lesser, P. B., Vietti, M. M., & Clark, W. D. (1986). Lethal enhancement of therapeutic doses of acetaminophen by alcohol. *Digestive Diseases and Sciences, 31,* 103.

Malseed, R. T. & Harrigan, G. S. (1989). *Textbook of Pharmacology and Nursing Care.* Philadelphia: J. B. Lippincott.

Nakato, D. (1987). *Ten most common medication errors: Their cause and prevention.* Unpublished manuscript.

NANDA (1990). *Taxonomy I Revised 1990, with official nursing diagnoses.* St Louis, MO: North American Nursing Diagnosis Association.

Neumann, H. H. (1985). Drugs and esophagitis: One banana makes a swallow (letter). *Journal of the American Medical Association, 254,* 3424.

Pagliaro, A. M. (1986). Preparation, administration, and monitoring of medications. In A. M. Pagliaro & L. A. Pagliaro (Eds.), *Pharmacologic aspects of nursing.* St. Louis: C. V. Mosby.

Pagliaro, L. A., & Pagliaro, A. M. (1986). Age-dependent drug selection and response. In A. M. Pagliaro & L. A. Pagliaro (Eds.), *Pharmacologic aspects of nursing.* St. Louis: C. V. Mosby.

Rasler, F. E. (1986). Ineffectiveness of sublingual nitroglycerin in patients with dry mucous membranes (letter). *New England Journal of Medicine, 314,* 181.

Rodman, M. J., Karch, A. M., Boyd, E. H., et al. (1985). *Pharmacology and drug therapy in nursing* (3rd ed.). Philadelphia: J. B. Lippincott.

Scherer, P. (1987). New drugs. *American Journal of Nursing, 84,* 448.

Seeff, L. B., Cuccherini, B. A., Zimmerman, H. J., et al. (1986). Acetaminophen hepatotoxicity in alcoholics: A therapeutic misadventure. *Annals of Internal Medicine, 104,* 399.

Spencer, R. T., Nichols, L. W., Lipkin, G. B., et al. (1989). *Clinical pharmacology and nursing management* (3rd ed). Philadelphia: J. B. Lippincott.

Strechfuss, B. L. (1985). Pediatric I.V. care. *National Intravenous Therapy Association, 8,* 75.

Teitell, B. C. (1984). Considerations for neonatal I.V. therapy. *NITA, 7,* 521.

Wong, D. L. (1987). Lozenges can be "lifesavers." *American Journal of Nursing, 87,* 1129.

Bibliography

Bell, D. S. H., & Clements, R. S. (1986). *Intensive insulin therapy: Rationale and methods.* Princeton, NJ: Squibb-Novo.

Benet, L. Z., & Pagliaro, L. A. (1986). Pharmacokinetic considerations in drug response. In A. M. Pagliaro & L. A. Pagliaro (Eds.), *Pharmacologic aspects of nursing.* St. Louis: C. V. Mosby.

Campbell, R. K. (1986). *Diabetes and the pharmacist* (2nd ed.). Elkhart, IN: Ames.

Fielo, S., & Rizzolo, M. A. (1985). The effects of age on pharmacokinetics. *Geriatric Nursing, 6,* 328–331.

Fraunfelder, F. (1986). Ocular beta-blockers and systemic effects. *Archives of Internal Medicine, 146,* 1073–1074.

Frid, A., Gunnarsson, R., Guntner, P., et al. (1988). Effects of accidental intramuscular injection on insulin absorption in IDDM. *Diabetes Care, 11*(1), 41.

Garden, J., & Freinkel, R. (1986). Systemic absorption of topical steroids. *Archives of Dermatology, 122,* 1007.

Hodler, C., & Alexander, J. (1990). A new and improved guide to IV therapy. *American Journal of Nursing, 90,* 43–47.

Hull, R. L. (1987). Prospective changes in drug administration. *Nursing '87, 17*(1), 54.

Kenner, C. V., Guzzetta, C. E., & Dossey, B. M. (1985). *Critical care nursing: Body-mind-spirit* (2nd ed). Boston: Little, Brown.

Kimmerle, R., & Rolla, A. (1985). Iatrogenic Cushing's syndrome due to dexamethasone nasal drops. *American Journal of Medicine, 79,* 535.

King, A. J., & Krumlovsky, F. A. (1986). Cafergot substitution for carafate (letter). *New England Journal of Medicine, 314,* 1642.

Lenox, A. C. (1990). IV therapy: Reducing the risk of infection. *Nursing '90, 20*(3), 60–61.

Lewis, L. W. (1988). *Fundamental skills and concepts in patient care* (4th ed.). Philadelphia: J. B. Lippincott.

Northrop, C. E. (1986). Don't keep packaging problems under wraps. *Nursing '86, 16*(11), 43.

Northrup, C. E. (1986). Don't overlook discharge teaching about drugs. *Nursing '86, 16*(11), 43.

Nova, G. (1987). Dialyzable drugs. *American Journal of Nursing, 87,* 933.

Ramsey, R. (1988). Adjusting drug dosages for critically ill elderly patients. *Nursing '88, 18*(7), 47–49.

Shaw, N., & Lyall, E. (1985). Hazards of glass ampoules. *British Medical Journal, 291,* 1391.

Thatcher, G. (1985). Insulin injections: The case against random rotation. *American Journal of Nursing, 85,* 690.

Viall, C. D. (1990). Your complete guide to central venous catheters. *Nursing '90, 20*(2), 34–41.

Wiggins, M. S., & Sesin, P. (1990). Guidelines for administering IV drugs. *Nursing '90, 20*(4), 145–152.

section two

Human Function and Clinical Nursing Therapeutics

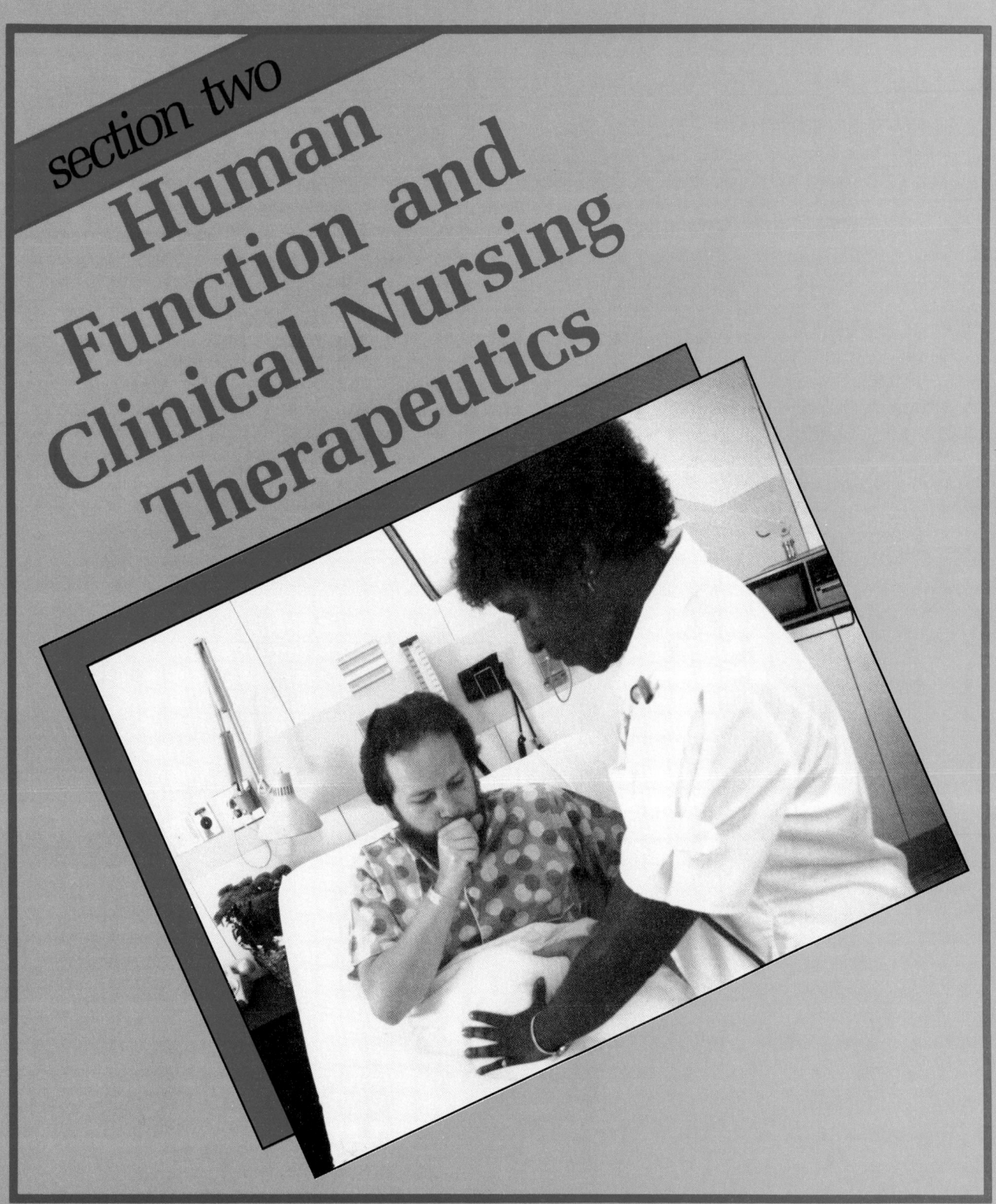

UNIT VI
Health Perception and Health Management

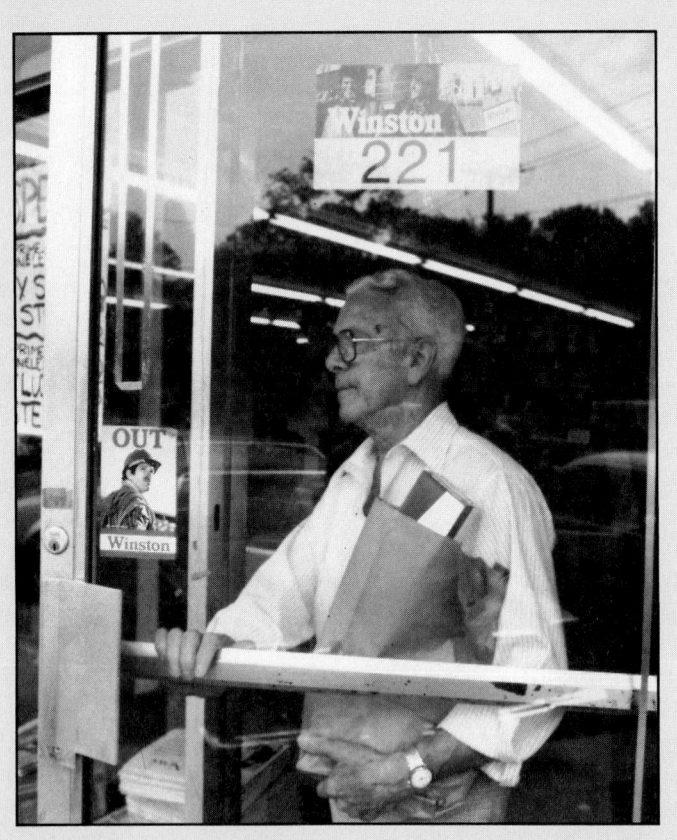

CHAPTERS

25 Safety

26 Health Maintenance

27 Home Maintenance Management

The chapters in Unit VI focus on patients' perceptions of their own health and their health promoting practices. To take full advantage of patient strengths, the nurse needs to know what a patient has done or will do to maintain, support, or restore health and function. The first chapter discusses the concepts and principles of safety and details nursing care for patients with safety needs. In addition to creating a safe environment within the health care facility, the nurse explores the safety of the patient's own environment and identifies risks and hazards that represent a threat to the patient's safety.

The next chapter explores the patient's health and wellness status. Health promoting practices and resources are discussed so the nurse has a knowledge base from which to assess and intervene for patients with altered health maintenance. Patient teaching is also emphasized for patients exhibiting health-seeking behaviors.

The final chapter in this unit focuses specifically on the patient's home environment. The concept of home maintenance management is explored and assessing the patient's and family's ability to maintain the home is discussed. Finally, holistic nursing interventions for promoting or supporting home maintenance management are emphasized; these are critical for effective discharge planning.

The chapters in this unit explore essential concepts and skills today's nurses need to evaluate patients' ability to care for themselves at home.

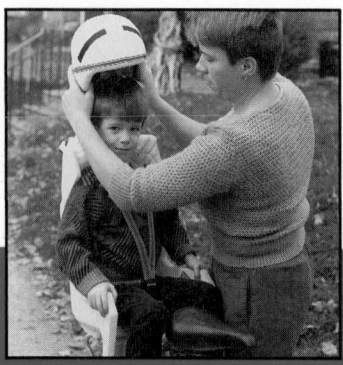

Safety

LEARNING OBJECTIVES

Upon completion of this chapter, the student will be able to do the following:

- Recognize the importance of safety.
- Identify intrinsic and extrinsic factors that affect safety.
- Relate special safety considerations to developmental stages.
- Discuss factors that create a potential for altered safety.
- Describe common problems resulting from altered safety.
- Identify individual safety patterns through assessment.
- Identify high-risk individuals for safety dysfunction through assessment.
- Define and characterize the appropriate nursing diagnoses for altered safety.
- Discuss nursing interventions to promote a safe health-care environment.
- List patient teaching topics to promote safety.
- Identify nursing interventions for altered safety.
- Describe discharge planning and home care concerns.

KEY TERMS

Asphyxiation	Poisoning	Restraints
Electrical shock	Pollution	Suffocation
Ground		

25

Normal Safety Function
  Characteristics of Safety
  Normal Functional Pattern
  Factors Affecting Safety
    Intrinsic Factors
    Extrinsic Factors
  Lifespan Considerations
Altered Safety Function
  Potential for Altered Safety
  Manifestations of Altered Safety
    Falls
    Fires
    Burns
    Poisoning
    Suffocation
    Electrical Shock
    Radiation Injury
    Infection
    Stress-related Illnesses
    Motor Vehicle Accidents
  Impact of Safety Dysfunction on Activities of Daily
      Living
    Fear
    Isolation
    Nutritional Deficits
    Loss of Sleep and Rest
    Poor Self-Concept
Assessment
  Subjective Data
    Functional Pattern Identification
    Risk Identification
    Dysfunctional Identification

  Objective Data
    Assessment of the Neurologic System
    Assessment of the Integumentary System
    Assessment of Mobility
Nursing Diagnoses and Patient Goals
  Diagnostic Statement: High Risk for Injury
    Definition
    Defining Characteristics
    Related Factors
  Related Nursing Diagnoses
  Patient Goals
Implementation
  Nursing Interventions to Promote Health and
      Safety Function
    Orientation to the Patient Unit
    Fire Safety
    Electrical Safety
    Radiation Safety
    Infection Control
    Fall Prevention
    Childhood Safety
    Burn Prevention
    Poison Prevention
    Motor Vehicle Safety
  Nursing Interventions for Altered Safety Function
    Fire Evacuation
    Emergency Care in Accidental Poisoning
    Cardiopulmonary Resuscitation
    Filing an Incident Report
  Discharge Planning and Home Care
Evaluation
Key Concepts

Accidents are the fourth leading cause of death in the United States. In people aged 1 to 37 years, accidents were the leading cause of death in 1986 (National Safety Council, 1989, p. 8,22). The leading categories of accidents resulting in death were motor vehicle accidents, falls, drowning, and fires and burns. Accidents may also result in injury, permanent disability, pain, and emotional distress.

Safety is important on every level of human interaction. It is an individual, community, national, and worldwide concern.

Rarely will any person experience a truly danger-free environment. Consequently, the promotion of safety involves awareness and implementation. Traditionally, nursing's realm of safety care involved only the hospital environment. However, nursing care today involves a scale both broad and specific. Maintaining a safe health-care environment remains one of the nurse's important roles, but teaching the patient and family about safety precautions at home and in the workplace and community has become an important nursing action.

Nurses work in many different environments, some hazardous. The nurse must act to minimize his or her own potential for injury. Safety habits for the patient and nurse will ensure an optimal therapeutic environment and promote health.

NORMAL SAFETY FUNCTION

Safety and security are essential needs of basic human functioning. Safety and security are second in priority only to physiologic needs in Maslow's hierarchy of needs (Maslow, 1970). Safety not only prevents harm and injury, it allows one to feel secure in one's actions. Stress may be reduced and general health is promoted. Safety allows other basic human needs, such as love, belonging, and self-esteem to be met, and personal goals to be accomplished. A positive outlook on life will result in better mental health as well.

Characteristics of Safety

Characteristics of safety are illustrated in Figure 25-1.

Pervasiveness. Safety is pervasive in our lives; it affects everything we do. Subconsciously we are concerned with safety in all our activities: eating, breathing, sleeping, working, and playing. Consciously we take responsibility or neglect responsibility for our own safety.

Perception. A person's perception of safety and danger influences the incorporation of safety into life's activities. Safety measures are effective only as far as hazards are accurately perceived. Safety factors are not innately understood, but are learned. With maturity, one comes to recognize possible dangers and realizes the importance of practicing safety. Parents, teachers, health-care workers, and laws help in the perception process.

Management. Once a person recognizes dangers in the environment, he or she takes measures to prevent those dangers, and thus practices safety. Prevention is a major characteristic of safety. Self-care is involved in safety practices, but one should learn to manage safety in such a way that safety is provided for other persons as well.

Normal Functional Pattern

The complex physiologic and psychologic systems of the human body work together to allow a person to avoid or minimize injury. Reflexes withdraw the hand from the

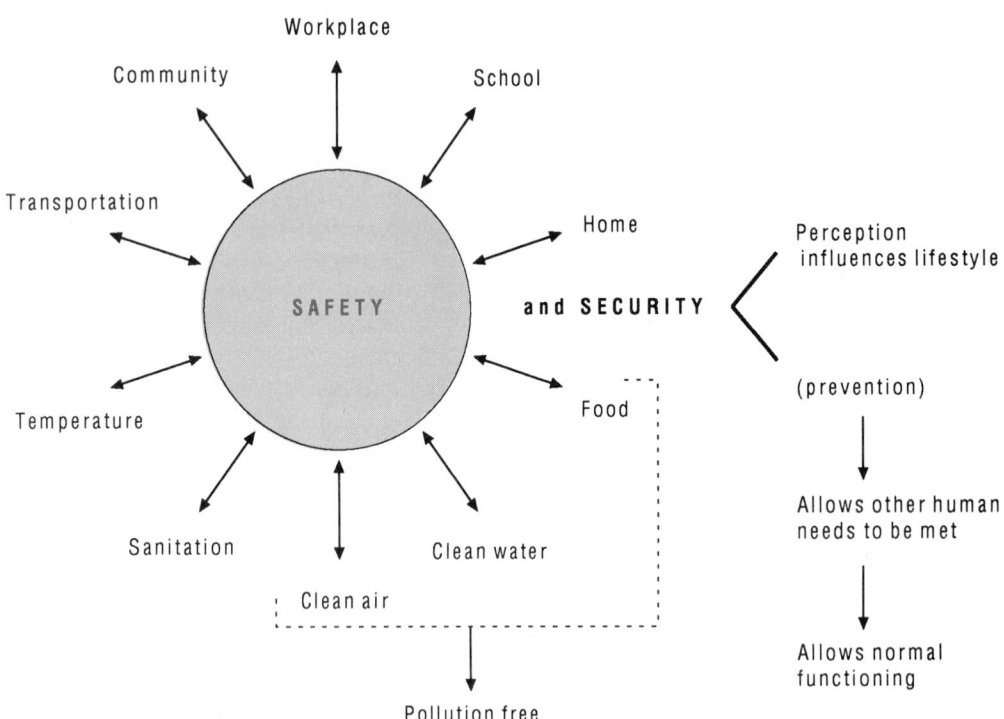

Figure 25–1. Characteristics of safety (pervasiveness, perception, and management) help the individual function normally.

flame before conscious thought can move the hand. A loud noise causes a startle reaction and an immediate increase in level of alertness. The sensation of pain provides important feedback that an activity or situation is dangerous. Normal functional patterns of safety involve the person's awareness of threats and conscious and unconscious responses to avoid harm.

Factors Affecting Safety

A person's full participation in safety promotion and avoidance of harm depends on intrinsic and extrinsic factors.

Intrinsic Factors

Cognition and Perception. Complex cognitive and perceptual functions, such as judgment, orientation, and socially appropriate behaviors, depend on the accumulation and accurate interpretation of information. The abilities to think clearly, recall past problems and solutions, imagine feasible solutions to current problems, and act to solve problems are cognitive functions needed to promote safety. Perception of danger based on past experience and accumulated knowledge is also essential to promoting safety. Alterations in cognition and problem-solving may result from a variety of contributing factors, including head injury, cerebrovascular accident, inadequate perfusion, drug use, medications, and central nervous system disease.

Activity and Exercise. Activity and exercise condition one's body to react quickly in an emergency. Deficient activity and exercise may place people at increased risk for many health conditions such as obesity or osteoporosis, as well as impair their ability to protect themselves from outside hazards. Inadequate activity and exercise may result from lack of motivation, neurologic impairment, pain, or sedentary lifestyle.

Nutrition and Metabolism. Adequate nutritional intake promotes general health. People who suffer from inadequate or inappropriate nutritional intake or metabolic disorders such as diabetes mellitus may experience fatigue, weakness, or chronic illnesses that place them at high risk for injury. Inadequate nutrition may result from lack of knowledge about nutrition, poor dentition, chronic nausea, or inability to shop for or pay for food.

Physiologic Factors. Chronic or pre-existing health conditions may alter one's ability to function safely. Promotion of safety depends on intact neurologic, cardiovascular, and musculoskeletal systems, and on the proper functioning of many other physiologic processes.

In terms of safety, a functioning neurologic system consists of peripheral nerves that sense hazards in the environment, the spinal cord for relaying impulses that allow the reflex arc to function, and the brain to coordinate activities, process information, and initiate responses. A functioning cardiovascular system provides oxygen and nutrients to the rest of the body as needed for quick response. Musculoskeletal integrity is essential for normal posture and movement. Disruption inhibits mobility and the ability to respond to hazards, as well as raising the risk of accidents.

Neurologic impairment that may alter safety can be caused by head injury, medications, alcohol and drugs, stroke, spinal cord injury, degenerative diseases such as Parkinson's disease and Alzheimer's disease, and brain tumors. Cardiovascular dysfunction that may impair safety can be caused by hypertension, congestive heart failure, congenital cardiac anomalies, or peripheral vascular disease. Musculoskeletal alteration that impairs safety can be caused by fractures, osteoporosis, muscular dystrophy, or arthritis.

Sensory Abilities. Any disturbance in communication ability or any sense impairment is a safety concern. Impaired sight, hearing, smell, or sensation prevent a person from seeing an obstacle in his or her path, hearing a fire alarm, smelling a toxic gas, or feeling the hot bath water. Sensory dysfunction is common in the elderly and those with complications of diabetes mellitus or other chronic diseases.

Age. Age can compromise safety because of inadequate knowledge and experience or physiologic limitations. Just as the very young do not possess the knowledge of potential hazards or the coordination to protect themselves from injury, the aged experience slowed cognitive functioning as well as slowed reflexes that put them at risk for falls and other accidents.

Lifestyles and Habits. Some people are more prone to safety problems because of inherent lifestyle patterns and unhealthful habits. A person's lifestyle might involve risk-taking or impulsive behavior such as walking alone at night or high-speed driving. They may enjoy potentially dangerous sports such as skydiving or mountain climbing, and may not follow usual safety precautions.

Habits such as cigarette smoking, use of alcohol and illicit drugs, sexual promiscuity, and poor dietary practices also impair safety. These practices may result from ignorance of risks, addiction, or lack of concern for health and safety.

Previous Experience. Previous experience with danger and safety promotion will affect perception and behavior in future situations. A person who was injured in a fire in the past is likely to practice fire prevention in the home. Conversely, a person with little previous experience with danger or safety promotion may not share the concern for safety. For example, immigrants from warm climates may not dress appropriately for cold winter weather and are at risk for hypothermia and frostbite.

Fatigue. Fatigue may be responsible for poor perception of danger, poor judgment, and poor problem-solving. Careless driving, irresponsible taking of medication, and inadvertent overexposure to sunlight may result. Fatigue arises from poor sleep habits, lifestyle patterns, stress, or a variety of medical conditions.

Coping and Stress Tolerance. Psychologic factors such as anxiety and depression alter one's ability to perceive safety hazards, express concerns, and follow safety precautions. The hospitalized patient may be anxious about surgery and not process information about postoperative procedures; this could result in injury or complications following surgery.

Coping mechanisms used in times of stress, such as denial or rationalization, may also alter safety. Personality factors such as impulsiveness, distrust, or shyness also affect safety promotion. Psychologic factors may be inborn, learned, or the result of mental illness.

Extrinsic Factors

Home Environment. One's home environment may be safe or may contain many hazards. A safe home environment features adequate ventilation, a reliable heating system, a nonskid bathtub surface, well maintained electrical appliances and electric cords, sturdy stepstools and ladders, and careful labeling and storage of all potentially toxic substances. Foods and medications should be discarded on their expiration date. Fire escape routes should be practiced and smoke alarms must be functioning and appropriately located (Fig. 25-2).

Workplace. The workplace may include hazards that are obvious or invisible. From the secretary who works in an office with asbestos ceiling tiles, to the salesman driving long hours on the road, to the fisherman on an ice-coated ship deck, safety must be a concern of every worker. The Occupational Safety and Health Administration (OSHA) is required to investigate worker complaints (Stanevich, et al., 1989), and many states have enacted worker right-to-know legislation that requires employers to notify workers of occupational hazards.

Safety concerns inherent to some occupations include noise, dust and air pollution, working at heights, dangerous machines, and exposure to toxic substances. These factors are dangerous when usual safety precautions such as wearing protective gear are not followed by the worker, or the worker is unaware of the hazard.

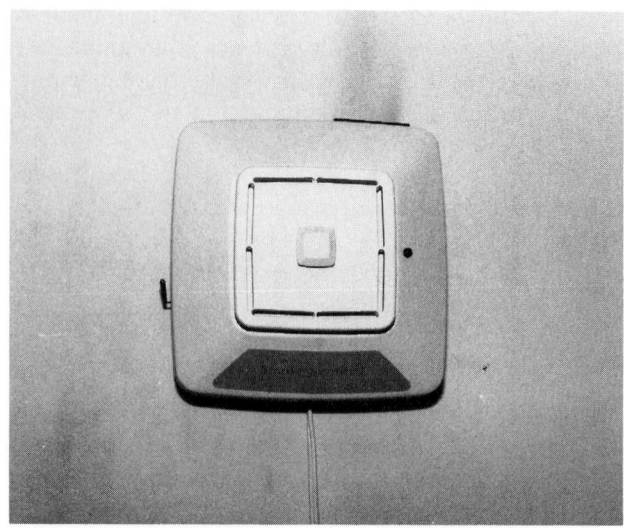

Figure 25–2.   Smoke alarms may be electric or battery-operated. They should be checked regularly to be sure they are functional; this is especially true of battery-operated alarms. There should be one on every floor near a potential source of fire or at the top of steps.

Community. The community in which one lives, works, shops, and plays may present safety concerns. Noise (e.g., from trains and planes), crime, poor lighting, presence of landfills, busy intersections, dilapidated houses, cliffs, and unprotected creeks are hazards. The community should be free from most of these hazards to lend a feeling of safety and security. Nevertheless, these hazards are found in many rural and urban areas today.

Sanitation. Sanitation affects safety. Lack of sanitation in the form of a clean water supply, sewage system, absence of insects and rodents, and refrigeration of food supply may result in the danger of increased spread of disease and infection. Sanitation is often lacking in impoverished areas.

Clean Air and Water. Pollution, the presence of harmful or unnatural substances in air, water, and land, affect the safety of people for years to come. Radon, a gas resulting from natural radioactive decay processes, has been linked to lung cancer and may be present in excess in many of our homes (Loken, et al., 1989). Increasing government and public awareness of environmental issues has led to many clean-up programs for known pollutants and safety guidelines to prevent further pollution. Safety risks from pollutants may be hidden for many years following their emission into the environment. Pollution results from ignorance about its risks or lack of concern for environmental safety.

Thermoregulation. The temperature of the outdoor as well as indoor environment affects safety. Extremes in temperature or other climate conditions such as wind, humidity, snow, rain, or ice present a hazard to people. Inappropriate dress or protection increases the safety risk. Indoor thermoregulation problems may result from inadequate finances or lack of help in maintaining a heating or cooling system in the home.

Lifespan Considerations

Safety concerns are individualized to fit developmental stages. The diverse physiologic and psychologic capabilities across the lifespan put different age groups at risk for different injuries. Interventions are geared toward specific age-related concerns.

Newborn and Infant

Because they lack life experience and the necessary musculoskeletal and neurologic maturity, the newborn and infant may be susceptible to burns, falls, and accidents. Their ability to thermoregulate is immature (Freiberg, 1987, p. 134), and their ability to satisfy basic needs depends on inarticulate cries and nonverbal communication. Without a clear means of communication and with limited ability to respond to environmental challenges, the newborn and infant depend on caregivers to create a safe environment where normal growth and development can occur without injury. Safety in the environment is a major parenting task.

Infants are curious; they explore the environment by pulling things and placing almost anything in their mouths. Dangling cords, tablecloths, plastic bags, and bottles and cans are tempting objects for exploration. A safe environment for the newborn and infant should include a comfortable temperature range; nonrestrictive, nonflammable, but adequate clothing; warm bath water; clean air; safe toys; guard rails at staircases and steps; protection with locked, padded rungs or rails for cribs or changing tables; covered electrical outlets; and appropriate car seats for automobile travel (Fig. 25-3).

Toddler and Preschooler

Falls, bumps, and bruises are common occurrences at this age of exploration and exuberance. The increasing mobility of the toddler and preschooler, along with the lack of life experience and still immature neurologic and musculoskeletal systems, are potentially hazardous. The

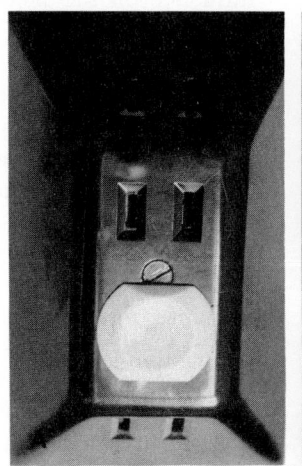
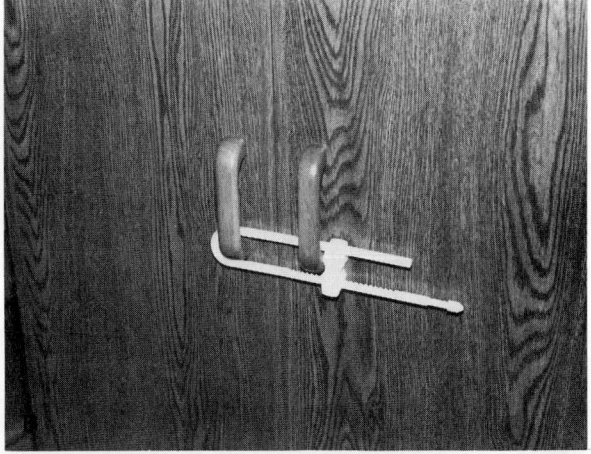
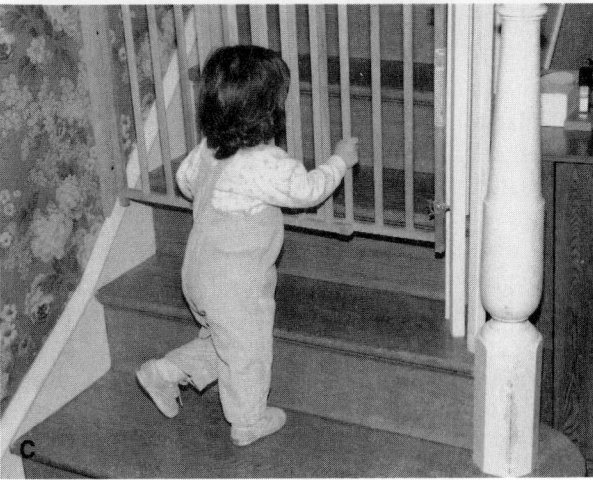

Figure 25–3. Examples of some safety features to "child-proof" a home: electric outlet cover (**A**), locks on cupboard doors (**B**), and rails across stairs (**C**).

parents of the toddler and preschooler must anticipate the wide-ranging interests of their explorer. Once upright, the toddler can reach up to a new source of interesting items. Curiosity still reigns; pets and other animals become new, moveable objects of exploration. Life experiences begin to accumulate, however, and learning of safe and dangerous behaviors begins. Setting a safe example is an important first step for the parents of the toddler and preschooler.

Improving eye–hand coordination, increasing strength, and increasing speed characterize the toddler and preschooler. This age group delights in opening and closing doors, turning knobs, climbing furniture, and all sorts of active play. Although these young children usually are able to communicate basic needs in words or actions, parents must still ensure a comfortable environmental temperature, adequate, nonflammable, nonrestrictive clothing, and warm bath water. The bathtub should have a nonskid mat or decals to prevent slipping when standing up.

Toddler toys must be sturdy, free of sharp or rough edges, and free of small, removable, or breakable parts that could be swallowed or damage an eye. Tricycles, push cycles, rocking horses, and other active toys that use large muscle groups are enjoyed by toddlers and preschoolers but should be used under supervision until the child understands the safety limits of the toy.

Toddlers need guard rails at staircases and steps, but as the transition to preschooler occurs, children begin to learn safety rules and gain motor control. Preschoolers usually can avoid bumps and learn to climb safely up and down stairs. Preschoolers also benefit from learning about safety zones; a safety zone is a safe place to stand or sit when a potentially dangerous activity is underway. For instance, a kitchen should have a safety zone where the child may watch activity but is out of the reach of stove, oven, or knives.

Outside the home, toddlers and preschoolers initially need supervision but, with caregiver guidance, will learn about playing out of the way of automobile traffic and avoiding strange animals.

The preschool years are also ones of increasing social interaction. The rules of safe social interaction are often learned by trial and error, and striking out may occur. Usually the natural exuberance of this age is to blame rather than any malicious intent; however, parents may help their preschooler by teaching cooperation and sharing. This is also the age at which caution toward strangers should be encouraged. Identification bracelets, fingerprinting, and frequent photographs are recommended by some law enforcement agencies.

Fire safety is a family concern when children reach this age. Learning about matches, electric cords, stoves, and ovens is important for the curious preschooler who might by tempted to experiment. The whole family should regularly practice crawling on the floor and using escape routes in case of fire. Local fire departments often have useful information about planning alternative escape routes.

Child and Adolescent

Physiologic maturity is almost complete for the school-age child. Motor control of large muscles and rapidly developing fine motor control enable the school-age child to accomplish complex tasks. Learning occurs at an astounding rate. Life experiences accumulate and are used to make judgments about the appropriateness of behaviors. The expanding world of the school-age child demands flexible responses and presents opportunities for independent action.

Children in this age group can make their needs known verbally, and often have reflexes that are quick enough to protect them from burns, falls, and other accidents. New activities will require new skills, and this age group may learn to ski, ride horseback, swim, bicycle, sail, or participate in team sports. Safety precautions are important. Helmets should be worn when cycling, riding, or playing contact sports, lifejackets when sailing or boating. All children should be taught to swim or at least float and tread water. The buddy system is an important outdoor and water safety strategy to learn.

Safe examples set by parents continue to be a major influence on the school-age child. A home that uses alcohol in moderation, keeps guns locked away, and uses discussion rather than force to resolve conflict will demonstrate the safety habits needed for later years.

Growth and development spurt during adolescence. Physical maturity of the musculoskeletal system is nearing completion, and the nervous and cardiovascular systems are fully mature (Freiberg, 1987, p. 344). While life experience is accumulating rapidly, so are new responsibilities. The autonomy of the adolescent develops in response to social and societal pressures. Driving a car, coping with drugs, beginning to explore sexuality, babysitting, working after school, and developing expertise are all adolescent activities that require judgment and independent action. As opportunities are explored, the adolescent may know a behavior is unsafe but social pressure may persuade him or her to act against better judgment. Supportive parents who allow discussion and expression of conflict provide a home environment that is safe for the adolescent.

Adult and Older Adult

With physical maturity complete, the adult moves at will in a world full of potential dangers. Accidents at home, in the workplace, and during sports are too common. Safety habits may become rusty, and overconfidence or ignorance can still place the adult in the path of danger.

Motor vehicle accidents continue to be a major cause of adult deaths, and were the leading cause of accidental death for people aged 1 through 78 years in 1986

(National Safety Council, 1989, p. 25). Use of safety belts with shoulder harnesses is mandatory in some states, as is the use of helmets on motorcycles. For the outdoor enthusiast the buddy system is still the best safety measure. Boaters, hikers, skiers, hunters, and mountain climbers are lost every year when they travel alone. Every sport has experts who can share safety information with beginners, often through clubs or associations of enthusiasts.

Advancing age entails some loss in physical function and, often, losses of acuity of sensory–perceptual function. The older adult may have impaired eyesight, impaired hearing, decreased proprioception, and decreased sensitivity to touch. The ability to thermoregulate may be impaired; the elderly are at a higher risk than younger adults for hypothermia and heat stroke (Kane, Ouslander, & Abrass, 1989, p. 321). Reflex responses slow and the musculoskeletal system may lose flexibility and strength. Various conditions such as arthritis, osteoporosis, or congestive heart failure may limit the older adult's ability to endure sustained physical activity. Medications taken to control conditions such as high blood pressure or Parkinson's disease may result in orthostatic hypotension and the potential for falling. Some of the elderly experience cognitive impairment, with a severity ranging from mild memory losses to a dementia that prevents safe independent living. The principles of a safe environment for the older adult follow the same general guidelines as for all ages: comfortable temperature range; adequate clothing; bath water of the right temperature (the setting on the hot water heater may need to be turned down); adequate ventilation; lighting that allows for safe navigation throughout the house at all times of day; nonskid surfaces on stairs, in the kitchen, and bathroom (throw rugs should be removed); and stable supports for climbing (firm stair rails, grab bars if needed).

ALTERED SAFETY FUNCTION

Potential for Altered Safety

The patient-care and outside environments possess the potential for altered safety in many forms. Nurses at work, patients in the hospital, families at home, or laborers on a job site are at risk for hazards, invasive trauma, disease, and pollution. These potentially compromise individual or community safety.

Hazards. When hazards exist, the potential for altered safety function also exists. Hazards in the home include poorly lighted stairways, throw rugs, slippery floors, cluttered areas, and unstable ladders, all of which may lead to falls. The risk of falls is compounded when an aged person or person with impaired mobility encounters these hazards. Other hazards in the home in-

Hazards in the Home

- Poor lighting inside or outside
- Uneven walking areas
- Steps with broken concrete
- Steps without handrails
- Loose mats on steps
- Cluttered steps or clutter near head of stairs
- Slippery tub or shower
- Extension cords across open spaces where people may trip
- Throw rigs on slippery floors
- Chairs with wide legs at the base
- Folding chairs or outdoor chairs that topple easily when poorly balanced
- Insecure stools or stepladders
- Standing on chairs rather than stools or stepladders
- Items placed precariously on closet shelves
- Bookcases or heavy pieces of furniture that might topple
- Defective smoke detectors
- Oily or dirty rags bunched together, especially near heat
- Stacks of old newspapers or boxes in basement or garage
- Flammable liquids in illegal containers
- Items used often in the kitchen placed over the gas stove
- Loose-fitting clothes worn while cooking
- Water temperatures that are too hot and may burn
- Defective wiring
- Overload of outlets or frayed cords
- Smoking in bed or alone at night in living room
- Electrical appliances in the bathroom where they may fall in the bathtub or sink
- Obstructed doorways or pathways in case of fire
- Many medications, or unlabeled medications, in medicine cabinet
- Unlocked cupboards or cabinets with potential poisons
- Poisonous plants where children can reach them
- Unsafe sexual practices
- Pets that may harm children, the elderly, or visitors
- Cigarette smoking in a closed area in the presence of nonsmokers
- Plastic bags where children will find them
- Cribs near windows or near venetian blind cords
- Unsupervised children in the bathtub
- Poor hygiene, especially in the bathroom and kitchen
- Improper food preparation
- Rodents or insect infestation

clude medications and household cleansers left within reach of children, careless smoking, and lack of supervision of infants and children at play. People are often unaware of hazards in the home until accidents occur.

The patient-care environment contains many hazards as well. Accidents such as falls, fires, and poisoning occur due to problems with equipment, procedural errors, and impairment of the patient. Examples of equipment problems are a wheelchair with nonlocking wheels that causes a fall when a patient attempts to sit down, or a malfunctioning heating pad unit that causes a fire. The frequent use of oxygen in patient rooms increases the risk of fire, hence smoking is prohibited wherever oxygen is in use. Many hospitals have adopted totally smoke-free environments to promote safety and health. Procedural errors such as not checking patient identification bands before administering medication or not monitoring intravenous infusion rates may cause harm to patients as well. Falls or burns may be suffered by the patient impaired by medication that causes central nervous system depression, sensory dysfunction such as blindness or hearing loss, decreased mobility due to neurologic or musculoskeletal illness, language or other communication barrier, or confusion due to mental or physical illness.

Procedures and policies for patient care and equipment operation have been developed in hospitals to minimize hazards. They should be reviewed periodically to promote safety of the patients and staff. Nursing assessment of factors that put patients at risk for accidents should help identify safety concerns and the precautions necessary to minimize risks.

Invasive Trauma. Invasive trauma in the home may occur when electrical safety is ignored. Overloading of outlets, use of appliances with frayed cords, or allowing an infant or child to play with plugs or near electrical outlets may result in electrical shock or burns. New parents are often unaware of these household risks for their children and are amenable to safety education by nurses.

The hospital environment contains electrical hazards for both the nurse and patient. With heavy use or misuse, equipment may develop flaws that result in excessive leakage of electricity. A potentially dangerous electrical circuit may be created by the nurse who simultaneously touches a damaged or ungrounded electrical appliance and the patient with wet skin or a central intravenous line. The patient with a skin surface broken by wounds, invasive lines, abrasions, or punctures, or with wet skin, is more vulnerable to electric current flow. Such patients should be considered electrically sensitive and the nurse must remember to avoid creating a potentially hazardous circuit. The use of faulty or ungrounded electrical equipment also increases the risk of electrical shock.

Patients and staff are also at risk for invasive trauma in the form of radiation when safety function is altered.

Radiation is used in diagnosis and treatment in many patient-care facilities. X-ray machines and pharmaceuticals for injection or implantation emit small doses of radiation into the environment. While the patient receives the intended dose of radiation, nurses and x-ray technicians are exposed to small doses repeatedly. Safety precautions for staff include distancing and shielding themselves from the radiation source and measuring accumulated dose. Regular inspection and servicing of equipment and licensing of x-ray and pharmacy technicians helps minimize risks to the patients and staff.

Disease. Disease is pervasive in the health-care environment. Not only are patients being diagnosed, monitored, and treated for diseases that brought them there, they are exposed to additional disease in the environment. Disease in the form of microorganisms such as viruses, bacteria, fungi, and parasites create the potential for altered safety. Infection may result, especially if the patient is compromised by fatigue, stress, poor nutrition, or other conditions that impair immunity. Patients are at risk for infection (termed nosocomial infection when acquired in the health-care environment) when safety precautions are not carried out. Medical and surgical asepsis are the primary safety precautions for preventing disease in the health-care environment. Handwashing is the basis for medical asepsis (see Chap. 22). Nurses are at risk for contacting infection, as well.

Viruses such as herpes, cytomegalovirus (CMV), and human T-lymphotropic virus (HTLV), along with multiresistant bacteria and yeast, all cause dangerous infections in susceptible people. To prevent the spread of these organisms in health-care settings the Centers for Disease Control have developed an approach entitled *Universal Precautions* (Centers for Disease Control, 1988). This approach considers contaminated any body substance—urine, stool, saliva, blood, sputum. All hospital staff must act to protect themselves and other patients from body substances by wearing disposable gloves when handling any of these substances. If aerosolization is suspected, goggles, mask, and gown must be worn. Nurses should be especially careful when bathing patients, as any open or fluid-filled lesion is a potential source of pathogenic organisms. Each hospital will have an infection control manual to help guide the nurse in caring for patients in a safe, protective manner. Many hospitals are also adopting special signs as a means of educating staff and the public (see sample signs in Chap. 22).

The ability of an organism to overwhelm the body's defenses is facilitated by injury or unsafe behaviors outside the health-care environment as well. Unsafe sex is associated with gonorrhea, genital warts, syphilis, and AIDS. Sharing of needles by intravenous drug abusers is associated with hepatitis B and AIDS. Use of contaminated water and food is associated with typhoid fever, hepatitis A, and parasite infections. Poor hygiene is

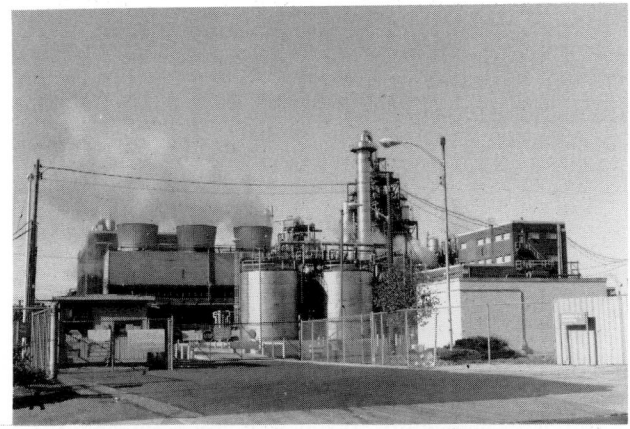
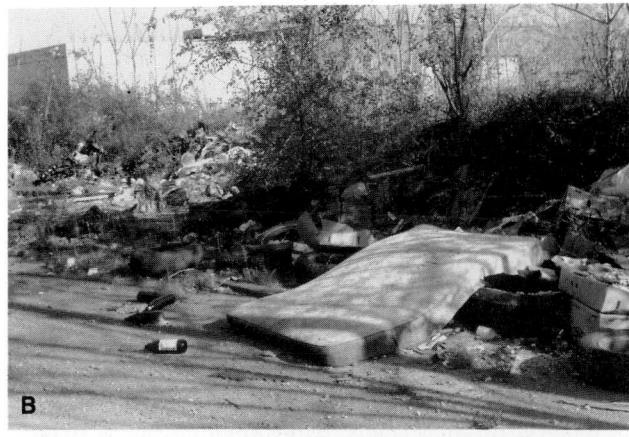

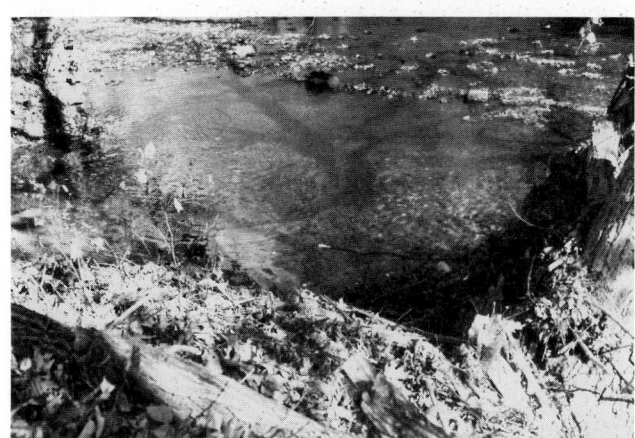
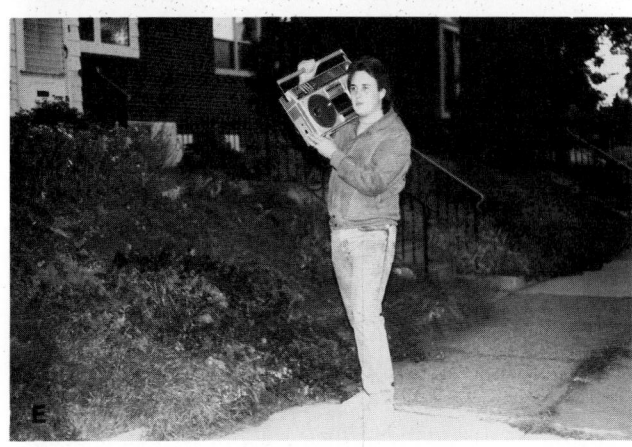

Figure 25–4.   There are various kinds of pollution that alter personal and community safety: air (**A**), land (**B**, **C**), water (**D**), and noise (**E**).

associated with urinary tract infections, colds, and tuberculosis. Being bitten by an infected tick can result in Lyme disease. Safety precautions that help reduce the risk of these infections include safer sexual practices, proper sanitation of public water supply, proper cooking and preparing of food, and control of rodent and insect infections.

Pollution.   Pollution may occur in the form of air, water, land, or noise pollution, all of which potentially alter

safety (Fig. 25-4). Toxic substances in the air, water, or ground, frequently the by-products of manufacturing, have been found to increase the risk of cancer. Air pollution increases the risk for and severity of respiratory problems such as asthma and chronic bronchitis. Allergy symptoms are often worsened by poor air quality due to pollution. Polluted water affects our food supply and may lead to the spread of disease and infection. Noise pollution from airplanes, trains, heavy automobile traffic, loud music, or public stadiums may harm people by increasing stress and impairing hearing.

Safety precautions on local and national levels are needed to protect people from pollution.

Disregard for Safety. Disregard for safety by individuals or groups may impair the safety of many. A person may engage in unsafe driving practices and potentially injure others in automobile accidents. Bicycle, skateboard, and other recreation and sports accidents also occur due to disregard for safety. Disregard may be intentional or due to ignorance of risks and safety precautions. Employers may disregard safety and cause harm to workers or the general population; this occurs when safety gear is not supplied for operating dangerous machinery, when toxic waste is not disposed of properly, or when a product is sold with potential safety flaws. Nurses can increase public awareness about automobile safety by stimulating discussion with patients who have been involved in motor vehicle or bicycle accidents. Safety precautions such as following safe driving speed for road conditions, use of infant car seats, use of seat belts, avoidance of alcohol when driving, and use of bicycle helmets can minimize risk.

Manifestations of Altered Safety

Altered safety is manifested in a variety of accidents and illnesses. Any accident or illness that causes harm and could have been prevented is a manifestation of altered safety. Accidents include falls, fires, burns, poisoning, suffocation, electrical shock, radiation exposure, and motor vehicle accidents. Illnesses attributed to altered safety include infection, respiratory problems, allergies, and the effects of pollution.

Falls

Falls are common both inside and outside the health-care environment. Falls are also common in the very young and the ill or disoriented. Falls often result in pain, permanent disability, and even death; in the elderly, they may result in hip fracture. Falls were the second leading cause of accidental death overall in the United States in 1986, and the leading cause of accidental death in people aged 79 and over (National Safety Council, 1989). Variables that increase a patient's risk for falls include weakness, decreased mobility of the lower extremities, sleeplessness, incontinence, confusion, depression, and substance abuse (Easterling, 1990).

A common scenario for falls in the health-care environment involves the elderly or impaired hospitalized patient who falls on the way to the bathroom at night. The patient may be disoriented at night and not see the way clear of obstacles cluttering the path from the bed to the bathroom.

Falls at home commonly involve stairways. Poor lighting, obstacles on the stairs, or slippery or poorly repaired steps contribute to falls in the home.

Fires

Fires are potentially lethal in the health-care environment and in the home. They may be caused by careless smoking practices, faulty electrical equipment, or by not attending to food cooking on the stove. Patients in the health-care environment are especially at risk for injury since they may be incapacitated and unable to flee the area without assistance.

Four classes of fires exist, based on the type of material burning:

1. Class A: paper, wood, cloth.
2. Class B: flammable liquids, such as fuel oil, cooking oil or grease, paint, solvents; or gases, such anesthesia gases.
3. Class C: electrical fires.
4. Class D: combustible metals.

Firefighting measures vary according to fire classification.

Flammable gases such as oxygen and anesthetic agents contribute to the risk of fires in the health-care environment. Commonly used electrical equipment such as monitors, heating or cooling units, or respiratory therapy equipment may malfunction or be used improperly, causing sparks that ignite linens easily in the presence of oxygen. Burns may also be sustained from cardioversion during resuscitation efforts. Regular servicing of and education about electrical equipment as well as strict smoking policies in the health-care environment may help reduce the risk of fires.

Grease fires originating from careless cooking practices are common in the home. Stoves in use may be left unattended and splattering grease may easily be ignited by a high flame. These fires may spread to curtains, kitchen cabinets, and clothing. Children left unsupervised near stoves contribute to the risk of kitchen fires.

Burns

Burns are a major cause of injury and death in the home for infants and children (National Safety Council, 1989). They also occur in the health-care environment due to scalds and fires. The person with sensory impairment is at risk for scalds from hot water or steam. A diabetic with peripheral neuropathy may step into very hot bath water and not feel the excessive temperature.

Children may sustain burns in the home by playing with matches or candles, pulling a teakettle off the stove, being fed formula that is too hot, or playing outdoors without sunscreen.

Poisoning

Poisoning occurs through the ingestion, inhalation, or absorption of potentially hazardous substances (Fig. 25-5). Poisoning compromises the cardiovascular, respi-

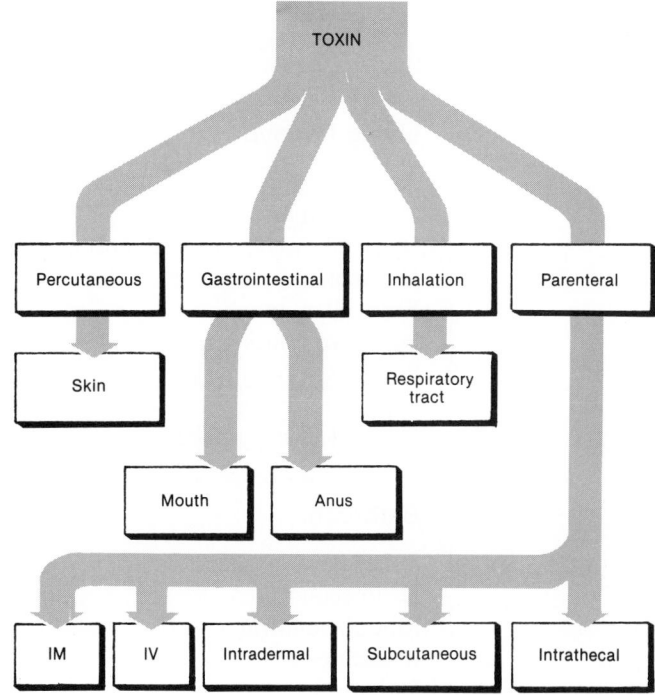

Figure 25–5. Routes by which toxins may enter the body.

ratory, central nervous, hepatic, gastrointestinal, or renal systems through chemical reactions. Toddlers and young children are at risk for poisoning, as are adults with sensory impairment and communication barriers.

In the home children may ingest household cleansers or medicines such as acetaminophen or aspirin. Adolescents and young adults frequently experiment with alcohol and drugs and may overdose inadvertently or attempt suicide. The older adult may ingest an overdose of medication due to difficulty reading the label from poor eyesight, illiteracy, or language barrier, or due to mental impairment. Plants, pesticides, and paint products are also potential household poisons. Improper storage and labeling of medications and household products contribute to poisoning accidents (see the display on Common Home Topics).

Poisoning may occur in the health-care environment when pharmaceutical products are administered improperly. They may be given to the wrong patient, in excessive dosage, or by the wrong route. Cardiac medications, narcotics, cancer chemotherapy, and intravenous medications are all potentially lethal. Short cuts taken in preparing and administering medications contribute to errors.

Suffocation

Suffocation or **asphyxiation** occurs due to drowning, smothering, strangling, airway obstruction, or from entrapment in a confined space. Drowning was the third most common cause of accidental death in United States in 1986 (National Safety Council, 1989), and usually occurs in children.

Suffocations in the home include the infant suffocating in a pillow or blanket, toddlers strangling by a shoulder harness or clothesline, older adults choking on poorly chewed meat, the child trapped in an abandoned refrigerator, and the infant drowning in a bathtub. Drownings occur in bodies of water, pools, bathtubs, and even large pails of water. Lack of supervision, hazardous swimming conditions, careless boating and water sports, and impairment by drugs and alcohol contribute to the risk of drowning.

Suffocation in the health-care environment frequently occurs because of airway obstruction, either by choking on foreign objects or aspiration of fluid into the small airways of the lungs. Impairment of chewing and the gag reflex, usually occurring in the older adult or neurologically impaired patient, cause airway obstruction. Improperly fitting dentures and overzealous feeding of the neurologically impaired patient lead to choking and aspiration.

Electrical Shock

Electrical hazards from electrical equipment and outlets are common in the home and health-care environments. Lighting and electric power lines in the community create a threat as well. **Electrical shock** occurs when a current travels to the ground through the body rather than through electrical wiring, or from static electricity that builds up on the surface of the body. A macroshock may cause superficial and deep burns, muscle contractions, and cardiac and respiratory arrest.

In the health-care environment electrical shock is a danger because of the abundant electrical equipment in

---

Common Home Toxins

Living Room/Den	**Kitchen/Laundry**
Air freshener	Scouring powder, ammonia
Glass cleaner	Oven cleaner, drain cleaner
Rug and upholstery shampoo	Dishwashing detergent
Houseplant insecticides	Moth balls
Flea collar, bomb	Bleach
Furniture polish	Metal polish
Permanent ink markers	Insect spray, rodent killer
Typewriter correction fluid	Laundry detergent
Carbonless copy paper	Spot remover

Bathroom	**Garage/Basement**
Toilet bowl cleaner	Latex, oil-base paints
Disinfectant	Paint stripper
Mildew remover	Wood preservative
Medicines	Adhesives, glues, epoxys
Hairspray	Herbicides, insecticides
Hair color	Insect repellents, poisons
Home permanent	Fertilizers
Nail polish/remover	Gasoline, fuels
Lice/flea shampoo	Other chemicals

---

proximity to the patient. Water from a spilled water pitcher, diaphoretic skin, or a leaking intravenous line increase the conduction of electricity. The lack of use of three-pronged plugs to ground electrical equipment contributes to electrical shocks. A **ground** is an electrical connection with a large conducting body (e.g., the earth) that allows dissipation of the electrical charge.

In the home, the use of frayed cords or overloaded outlets, use of electrical appliances near the sink or bathtub, or lack of supervision of children near uncovered electrical outlets or electrical appliances, present hazards.

Radiation Injury

Radiation injury may occur from excessive exposure to radiation used to diagnose or treat illness in the heathcare environment, or from leakage of radiation into the community from power plants and industrial sources. Radiation can injure the skin, reproductive organs, bone marrow, gastrointestinal tract, and other parts of the body. The risk of injury is increased by closer proximity and longer exposure to radiation.

In the health-care environment the potential for radiation injury exists when a nurse must care for patients with radioactive implants, or when technicians or nurses must restrain a patient during radiography. Failure to use lead shielding for staff and patients and not following radiation safety procedures for care of patients with implants contributes to the risk of injury.

In the community, nuclear accidents and exposures have occurred. Large groups of people are at risk for injury. Psychologic stress may be incurred even if physical injury is avoided. Federal agencies such as the Nuclear Regulatory Commission are primarily responsible for establishing and enforcing guidelines for radiation safety.

Infection

Infection may occur in the hospital or at home when safety against the transmission of microorganisms is altered. Infectious illnesses include gastroenteritis, hepatitis, tuberculosis, sexually transmitted diseases, and Lyme disease. Practices in the home that place a person at risk for infection are unsafe sex, lack of immunization, improper food preparation, and poor hygiene. Community problems such as water supply contaminated by sewage or tick infestations near residential areas may also cause infection. Nosocomial infections include urinary tract infections, pneumonia, hepatitis, and gastroenteritis. Debilitated patients, patients on mechanical ventilators, and those with chronic illnesses are at risk for nosocomial infection. Poor handwashing practices, lack of asepsis for invasive procedures, and lack of isolation precautions contribute to nosocomial infections.

Respiratory problems may result from unsafe air pollution levels in the community or occupational exposure to dust, asbestos, or other airborne substances. Passive smoke inhalation from living or working with those who smoke cigarettes is a recently recognized potential cause of respiratory disease. Cigarette smoking and asbestos exposure have been linked to lung cancer, and smog and dust worsen respiratory allergy symptoms and cause chronic bronchitis. Coal dust from mining causes fibrosis of the lungs, known as "black lung." The Occupational Safety and Health Administration establishes guidelines to prevent injury to workers from pollutants.

Stress-related Illnesses

Stress-related illnesses include peptic ulcer disease, anxiety, depression, and psoriasis.

Fear of the environment, caused by feeling unsafe and insecure at home and in the health-care environment, can lead to stress-related illnesses. Unfamiliar surroundings, invasive procedures, and absence of close family members and friends contribute to patient stress in the health-care environment. Competent, caring nurses can alleviate much of the patient's stress. Stress-related illnesses can develop over time outside the health-care environment due to noise, crime in the community, and fear of environmental hazards. Community action groups help people work together to overcome these safety concerns, and thus avoid undue stress.

Motor Vehicle Accidents

Motor vehicle accidents often occur because of hazardous driving practices. They may involve one or more drivers or passengers, as well as bicycle riders, skateboarders, and pedestrians.

Motor vehicle accidents are the leading cause of accidental death in the United States, causing 49,000 deaths in 1988 (National Safety Council, 1989). Motor vehicle accidents also cause permanent disability, pain, and suffering. Factors that contribute to the risk of motor vehicle accident deaths include lack of defensive driving techniques, failure to use helmets by bicycle riders and skateboarders, and use of alcohol and other substances that cause impairment while driving. At least 24,000 people die and 534,000 are injured in alcohol-related motor vehicle accidents each year. More than half of fatalities from motor vehicle accidents are alcohol-related (National Safety Council, 1989).

Impact of Safety Dysfunction on Activities of Daily Living

There are many people who, intentionally or as a result of physiologic dysfunction, behave in unsafe ways. Depending on the source of safety concerns, the activities of daily living of the person will be affected correspondingly. The inability of a person to safely complete activities of daily living is an indicator of the need for nursing intervention. Interferences with ability to perform personal hygiene, prepare meals, participate in activities, and engage in usual vocational or career activities may be the outcomes of the manifestations of altered safety. Loss of income or increased expenses may result from lost workdays and from the need to purchase equipment or to hire people to assist with care or other activities of daily living.

Fear

The person who does not feel safe and secure may fear many activities essential for daily living. Fear of falls, fires, accidents on the job, or crime in the community may impair normal functioning. Fear may be generated from real or imagined safety hazards, and may actually contribute to altered safety by increasing stress and anxiety. Emotional tension may impair perception and judgment, making a person accident-prone.

Isolation

Altered safety may lead to social isolation. Rather than risk harm from potential safety hazards, the person may avoid activities and contact with others. Staying at home where the person feels safest isolates him or her from support systems as well.

Nutritional Deficits

Nutritional deficits may arise from contaminated food and water that are not safe to consume, fear of disease from polluted or contaminated food or water, or inability to shop for food due to fear of crime or falls outside the home. Many older adults have difficulty shopping for food and preparing balanced meals, resulting in weight loss and vitamin and iron deficiencies.

Loss of Sleep and Rest

Altered safety may result in loss of sleep and rest due to anxiety and fear of potential danger. The person remains vigilant to safety hazards in the environment, preventing normal relaxation activities and proper sleep at night. Lack of sleep leads to poor job performance and loss of interest in recreation and sex.

Poor Self-Concept

Altered safety may impair one's self-concept. The person may believe that he or she is accident-prone and therefore not performing well at his or her job or sports activities and not worthy of enjoying his or her usual activities. Problems in self-concept and self-esteem can lead to substance abuse and personality disorders (Freiberg, 1987, p. 387).

ASSESSMENT

Assessment of a person's ability to function safely involves careful investigation of intrinsic and extrinsic aspects of their lives. Questions about safety require people to reveal the ways they act in the privacy of their home as well as in public. The nurse who builds trust by being nonjudgmental and supportive will elicit the most accurate information.

Subjective Data

Assessment of the person with a potential for altered safety begins with a careful investigation of the person's concerns or perception of hazards, including the person's accident and injury history. The accident-prone person will often report a history of falls, bruises, broken bones, burns, cuts, scratches, and restricted activity. The pattern of past injuries is important; accidents are often related to periods of emotional stress, fatigue, or diminishing health. People may share their fears about unsafe behaviors and concerns about the potential for injury. Many people are aware of their unsafe behaviors and will share this information if nonjudgmental assistance is offered.

Functional Pattern Identification

Current safety practices or plans for management of hazards are part of the assessment. The nurse may ask the following questions:

Does the person use appropriate restraints when in a
  car?
Can the person read traffic signs and danger warnings?
  Does the child have a childproofed home?
Does the person have up-to-date immunizations?

Keeping in mind the special concerns for each age group allows the nurse to direct questions appropriately. Recent changes in the environment (home, school, workplace), the support system (divorce, a change in caregivers, death of family member), or developmental stage (transition from infant to toddler) should alert the nurse to explore these areas. Data may need to be gathered not only from the patient, but also from his or her family, caregivers, referring health professionals, and others to obtain a clear picture of his or her safety. Soliciting data from sources other than the patient must be done with the patient's permission, unless the patient is underage or declared incompetent. This ensures patient confidentiality and promotes trust.

Risk Identification

Current safety concerns must take into account the patient's reason for seeking health care. A recent change in health status related to cognition, perception, sensation, or activity–exercise pattern may recently have placed the patient at high risk for injury. The nurse should explore these areas fully and also question the patient about occupation, home environment, lifestyle and habits, and lack of knowledge of safety practices that may put them at risk. What medications does the patient take? Are there side effects such as drowsiness or dizziness that may contribute to injury?

It is also the responsibility of the nurse to assess for injuries related to abuse or neglect. This is a skill that requires sensitivity and the ability to question the probability of explanations offered for injuries. Often it is essential to confer with other health professionals, and a diagnostic work-up may be ordered (see section on Physiologic Assessment). If injuries seem disproportionate to the reported cause or occur with unexpected frequency,

---

Nursing Research

Selected Nursing Research Studies

Brink, S. G., et al. (1989). A hospital-based infant safety-seat program for low-income families: Assessment of population needs and provider practices. *Health Education Quarterly, 16*(1), 45–56.

Lofgren, R. P., et al. (1989). Mechanical devices on the medical wards: Are protective devices safe? *American Journal of Public Health, 79*(6), 735–738.

Ryden, L. A., et al. (1989). Occupational low-back injury in a hospital employee population: An epidemiologic analysis of multiple risk factors of a high-risk occupational group. *Spine, 14*, 315–320.

Wright, B. A., et al. (1990). Frequent fallers: Leading groups to identify psychological factors. *Journal of Gerontologic Nursing, 16*(4), 15–19, 41–42.

Possible Topics for Nursing Inquiry

What factors contribute to the increased risk for falling in hospitalized elderly patients?
What risk factors contribute to the potential for back injuries in caregivers?
Do cultural factors have a relationship with usage of infant safety seats in motor vehicles?

further investigation is warranted. No age group is immune to abuse or neglect, and people with higher dependency needs are at higher risk. The nurse should keep in mind that the highest risk groups include children, the elderly, the developmentally disabled, and the debilitated.

Dysfunctional Identification

Nurses may determine dysfunctional patterns of safety when the person reports serious, preventable injury, or a recent change in ability to participate safely in the activities of daily living. A dysfunctional pattern may also be evident in the presence of unsafe behaviors, observed by the nurse or described by the patient. By virtue of specialized knowledge, the health-care team may determine that the person is at risk for injury, illness, or infection because of unsafe behaviors or physiologic dysfunction. It must be noted that unless the patient shares a concern for preventing injury, illness, or infection, there may be no agreement on the existence of a dysfunctional pattern. The nurse must help the patient realize the importance of safety before safety dysfunction can be changed.

As part of the nursing health history, the nurse asks about previous injuries, accidents, and hospitalizations. The nurse should find out about the cause of these accidents and if any unsafe behavior or hazards have been rectified. For example, a patient may report a history of burns from a fire. What was the cause of the fire? If smoking in bed contributed to the injury, have careless smoking practices been altered? If not, does the patient realize the potential for further problems?

Objective Data

Objective data contribute to safety function assessment. Through physical assessment techniques, the nurse assesses for injuries and risk factors for injury. Physical assessment should focus on the neurologic system, skin integrity, and mobility.

Assessment of the Neurologic System

Assessment of the neurologic system for safety function includes determination of mental status, sensory function, reflexes, and coordination.

Assessment of mental status begins with observation of the patient's appearance and general behavior. For the purposes of safety promotion, the nurse must focus attention on the patient's ability to detect danger and rapidly avoid hazards. It is important to note any impulsive behavior or examples of behavior that suggest impaired or unsafe judgment. Determine the patient's level of alertness, orientation to time, person, and location, attention span, and basic cognitive function by asking simple questions. Decision-making can be determined

by asking "what if" questions appropriate to the patient's age and life experiences.

After assessment of mental status, examination of sensory function allows the nurse to verify the accuracy and quality of sensory input. Testing should at least include sensitivity to pinprick and light touch of the extremities. If sensation is impaired, the patient is deprived of important information that may warn of danger or ongoing injury.

Assessment should include testing of the special senses—vision, hearing, taste, and smell. Impaired taste or smell may prevent the patient from detecting spoiled food or a natural gas leak. Alterations in visual acuity may prevent the patient from differentiating pills, detecting uneven terrain or stairs, and reading traffic signs or telephone numbers. Impaired hearing acuity has profound implications. The gag reflex should also be tested before feeding a patient with decreased alertness or muscle strength. A review of important withdrawal reflex arcs will provide clues to the patient's ability to respond reflexively to potentially harmful stimuli by pulling away from danger. Reflex arcs to test include biceps, triceps, knees, and ankles. Coordination is important to prevent falls. Coordination can be tested by observing the patient's gait and repetitive motions.

Many times in the hospital the nurse observes changes in the patient's awareness and sensitivity to the environment. The patient with delirium may have limited awareness of the environment and poor integration of information. He or she may move inappropriately to discontinue intravenous medication lines, feeding tubes, or ventilation tubing. Ongoing neurologic assessment of some patients is essential.

Assessment of the Integumentary System

A brief physical examination of the integument (see Chap. 18) will provide important clues to the patient's history of accidents or injury. The skin should be inspected for bruises, cuts, scratches, and scars. The location and distribution of the lesions should be carefully noted and correlated with the patient's explanation of their origin. A bath is an excellent opportunity for the nurse to assess the integument while providing a refreshing comfort measure.

Assessment of Mobility

Mobility is assessed by inspection and palpation of the patient's muscles, joints, and bones. Range-of-motion testing of joints, muscle strength testing of the extremities, and observation of ambulation is important in determining risk for altered safety. Any joint showing limitation in range of motion and any muscle group showing weakness places the person at a disadvantage when trying to avoid hazards. For example, the person with arthritis in the knees may be safely active on level surfaces but unable to use stairs in an emergency. Observation of posture and gait can also provide valuable information.

Cardiovascular integrity as it relates to safety is assessed through determination of the person's mobility and activity tolerance, and the presence of any conditions that impair function. If a person can only walk 50 feet before chest pain (exertional angina) becomes severe, the ability to accomplish many daily tasks is limited. If this person lives more than 50 feet from the emergency exit of his or her apartment building, escape during a fire may be impossible. Activity tolerance is usually stated as distance or duration of activity (walking, standing) before fatigue or other symptoms interrupt the activity; it is an important assessment in discharge planning for the person's safety outside the hospital environment.

Information about activities of daily living may be gathered from caregivers and family but should be supplemented by direct observation whenever possible. The nurse should observe the person moving from bed to chair or commode (and back) when appropriate; for the more mobile person, the nurse should observe him or her walking from bedroom to bathroom, front door, kitchen, and telephone locations.

Toileting includes the ability to safely get on and off a toilet or commode. Weakness or pain in the hips may create a need for a raised toilet seat to make access safer. The nurse should assess for safe footing and transfers (position changes) in showers or at the sink, and the need for grab bars or special benches if standing is difficult. Some people can get into the bathtub but are unable to get out without assistance.

Because assessment of the ability to dress safely is difficult in the hospitalized person who is only allowed a hospital gown, it is recommended that the nurse observe the person dressing in street clothes some time before discharge. Putting clothes on in the correct sequence, maintaining balance, and avoiding pinching with zippers or shoelaces are assessed.

NURSING DIAGNOSES AND PATIENT GOALS

The accepted nursing diagnosis involving alterations in safety is high risk for injury. The nurse uses data from the subjective and objective assessments to determine if the patient is at high risk for injury.

Diagnostic Statement: High Risk for Injury

Definition

High risk for injury is a state in which the individual is at risk for injury as a result of environmental conditions interacting with the individual's adaptive and defensive resources (NANDA, 1990).

Defining Characteristics

Presence of risk factors such as

Internal. Biochemical, regulatory function (sensory dysfunction, integrative dysfunction, effector dysfunction, tissue hypoxia); malnutrition; immune–autoimmune; abnormal blood profile (leukocytosis/leukopenia; altered clotting factors; thrombocytopenia; sickle cell, thalassemia; decreased hemoglobin); physical (broken skin, altered mobility); developmental age (physiologic, psychosocial); psychologic (affective, orientation) (NANDA, 1990).

External. Biologic (immunization level of community, microorganisms); chemical (pollutants, poisons, drugs, pharmaceutical agents, alcohol, caffeine, nicotine, preservatives, cosmetics, dyes); nutrients (vitamins, food types); physical (design, structure, and arrangement of community, building, and/or equipment); mode of transport/transportation; people/provider (nosocomial agents, staffing patterns, cognitive, affective, and psychomotor factors) (NANDA, 1990).

Related Factors

See those listed under Defining Charcteristics above.

Related Nursing Diagnoses

Other nursing diagnoses may be evident in people at risk for safety or in those who have manifested safety dysfunction. Such nursing diagnoses include High Risk for Aspiration, Ineffective Breathing Pattern, Fatigue, High Risk for Infection, High Risk for Poisoning, Post-Trauma Response, Social Isolation, High Risk for Suffocation, and High Risk for Trauma. Safety dysfunction also affects the person's ability to perform activities of daily living. Nursing diagnoses in these situations may include Impaired Home Maintenance Management, Altered Nutrition: Less Than Body Requirements, Altered Role Performance, Situational Low Self-Esteem, Sleep Pattern Disturbance, and Impaired Social Interaction. Psychologic reactions may include nursing diagnoses such as Anxiety, Defensive Coping, Fear, and Hopelessness.

Patient Goals

Long-term goals for the person at risk for injury include:

The patient will identify actual and high-risk environmental hazards.
The patient will demonstrate safety habits appropriate to selected environments (home, health-care setting, workplace, community).

The patient will experience a decrease in the frequency and severity of accidents.

These goals must be individualized to reflect the unique needs of the person at risk. Once individualized, long-term goals are supported by specific nursing interventions.

IMPLEMENTATION

Nursing interventions to promote safety are based on the data gathered in the assessment and the resulting nursing diagnosis and patient goals. They may be thought of as falling into two broad categories: providing a safe environment in the health-care facility, and providing safety education.

Nurses promote these safety interventions wherever they practice. For example, school nurses function as safety educators for school-age children. Children should be taught how to say no to drugs and how to tell anybody when they don't want to be touched. In many states school nurses are required to report suspected child abuse. School nurses may also identify children who seem accident-prone. These children may have a neuromuscular or sensory–perceptual basis for their accidents, and should be evaluated. Screening for problems with vision and hearing is especially important.

The occupational health nurse may be involved in safety education and accident prevention at the worksite. Adults often need to be taught the proper body dynamics for lifting heavy loads. For the sedentary worker, principles of body alignment and stretching may help to prevent muscle strain from poor posture. Proper lighting may improve productivity as well as prevent eye strain.

Occupational health nurses act to identify hazardous materials in the workplace and appropriate worker protection (adequate ventilation, protective clothing and eyewear), as well as developing instructional safety promotion programs to prevent back injury, on-the-job accidents, and illness.

Community health nurses may help the older adult safety-proof his or her home against falls by removing loose rugs and obstacles in hallways and stairwells. Community health nurses often educate members of the community about safety promotion through health fairs and lectures.

All nurses may act as community activists and advocates for environmental safety in such areas as clean air and water, safe, well-lighted pedestrian walkways, and laws supporting seat belt and helmet use.

> **Selected Nursing Interventions for Common Problems**
>
> **Falls**
>
> - Nonskid floors
> - Patient teaching regarding ambulation and activity
> - Orientation to patient unit
> - Nightlight, bedrails
>
> **Fires**
>
> - Limited smoking facilities
> - Patient teaching
> - Fire drills and development of fire-fighting skills
> - Knowledge of location of emergency equipment, phone numbers, and evacuation routes
>
> **Electrical Shock**
>
> - Equipment used with dry hands only
> - Spilled fluid mopped up
> - Grounded electric plugs
> - Equipment damage reported
>
> **Poisoning**
>
> - Patient teaching
> - Safe medication preparation and administration
> - 5 Rs
>
> **Motor Vehicle Trauma**
>
> - Patient teaching
> - Seatbelts
> - Approved carseats
> - Safe driving

Nursing Interventions to Promote Health and Safety Function

Nurses and patients interact in environments that contain some unique hazards. It is important for the nurse to provide for patient safety in the hospital or clinical environment as well as help the patient develop personal safety habits. The Centers for Disease Control and the OSHA provide guidelines for promotion of safety. Each accredited health-care setting must have an ongoing safety program.

The same safety practices used in the health-care environment can be used in the home. These include electrical safety, fire safety, and prevention of falls, burns, accidents, and infectious disease.

Orientation to the Patient Unit

The patient is placed at a higher risk for injury in the health-care environment because of its unfamiliarity and the procedures the patient undergoes. The nurse is responsible for protecting the patient from environmental hazards. It is also the nurse's responsibility to anticipate and minimize, as much as possible, the adverse consequences of procedures and treatments. Many nursing policies and procedures are intended to protect the patient, and a familiarity with these policies assist the nurse in the health-care environment.

Initial nursing actions to promote safety and security for the patient are introduction of staff to the patient and orientation of the patient to the immediate environment. Orientation includes use of call-light system and bed controls, location of personal care supplies in the bedside stand, location of bathroom, operation of lights, and schedule of unit activities. The nurse should ensure that the room is uncluttered and free of obstacles between the bed and the bathroom. Use of a night light and bedside rails is standard. Each patient should be instructed as to activity limitations and assisted with ambulation as needed. The nurse who talks to the patient and answers questions in a calm, confident, caring manner increases the security of the patient.

Fire Safety

Hospital safety programs emphasize reducing fire hazards by strictly limiting smoking, using nonflammable materials whenever possible, and practicing fire drills and firefighting skills.

In the patient-care area each nurse should become familiar with emergency phone numbers, the locations of fire alarms, fire extinguishers and fire hoses, shut-off valves for oxygen and other flammable gases, evacuation equipment, and exits. Posted wall maps should show evacuation routes.

Fire extinguishers are designed to fight specific types of fires and are labeled appropriately; see Table 25-1 for descriptions of various fire extinguishers. Nurses can review these topics with children and adults as appropriate.

Electrical Safety

Nurses must also protect themselves and patients from dangerous shocks by keeping hands dry when manipulating machinery, mopping up spilled fluid, ensuring all plugs are grounded (three-pronged), and reporting any equipment damage. Regular servicing of electrical equipment should be maintained in the patient-care environment.

Radiation Safety

When radiation is in use in the health-care environment, the location is marked by an international symbol (Fig. 25-6). Radioactive implants or ingestion of radioactive materials may make the patient a source of radioactive contamination. Nurses routinely wear radiation detection badges to assist the institution's radiation safety officer in monitoring exposure levels. These badges are collected regularly and the exposure levels are calculated to assure that staff are staying within safety limits of exposure.

The three cardinal rules of radiation protection are:

1. Minimize time of exposure to the source.

TABLE 25–1

Correct Fire Extinguishers to Use with Specific Classes of Fires

Class and Type of Fire	Type of Fire Extinguishers
Class A	Water (stored pressure, gas cartridge, soda acid, pump)
(Paper, wood, cloth)	Multipurpose dry chemical (stored pressure, gas cartridge)
	Loaded stream
Class B	Carbon dioxide
	Regular dry chemical (stored pressure, gas cartridge)
(Flammable liquids, such as fuel oil, cooking oil or grease, paint, solvents; or gases, such anesthesia gases)	Multipurpose dry chemical (stored pressure, gas cartridge)
Class C	Multipurpose dry chemical (stored pressure, gas cartridge)
(Electrical fires)	Carbon dioxide
	Liquified gas
Class D	Special dry powder
(Combustible metals)	

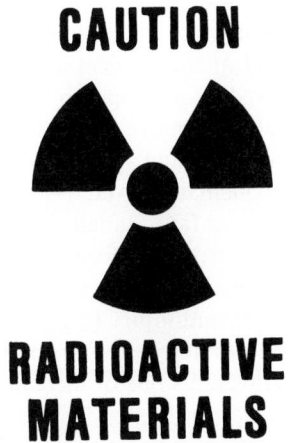

CAUTION

RADIOACTIVE
MATERIALS

Figure 25–6. International Radiation Symbol.

2. Maximize distance from the source.
3. Use appropriate shielding.

Nursing care of radiation therapy patients must be well organized so that necessary assistance and support can be given in an efficient manner without needless exposure of the nurse. Usually, lead shields or lead aprons are available if close contact with the patient is required. Generally, gloves should be worn to prevent skin contact with any body substances (urine, stool, saliva, blood). Patients may be encouraged to do as much of their own care as possible. A private room with private bath is essential to prevent accidental exposure of other patients. Linens should be kept in the room until the radioactive source is removed. Soiled linens, excreta, and other waste may require special labeling and disposal.

After cessation of therapy the radiation safety officer will sweep the room with a radiation detector to assess for spills or contamination. After clearance the room may be cleaned and linens sent to the laundry. If the patient is to go home while receiving radiation therapy through an ingested substance (e.g., iodine-131), the hospital radiation safety manual will list directions for protection of the family, caregivers, and home environment.

Although the risk of radiation injury in the community is low, nurses should teach people about the sources and effects of radiation. Greater public awareness and understanding of radioactive waste and nuclear power can lead to stricter regulation of radiation used in industry, and, therefore, a safer community and less psychologic stress.

Infection Control

Infection control is a high priority in the health-care environment. Most hospitals have full-time staff, usually nurses, devoted to teaching and implementing infection control practices throughout the hospital. The principle of asepsis helps prevent the spread of microorganisms from place to place and person to person. Handwashing, disinfection, sterilization, isolation precautions, and immunization are practices carried out in the health-care environment to control infection (see Chap. 22).

Immunization against infections (communicable diseases) is important for children, adults, and health-care workers. Influenza and hepatitis B vaccines are frequently offered to health-care employees working in close contact with patients or with patients' blood, respectively. Because there is no immunization for tuberculosis, health-care workers are usually tested yearly for exposure. If a person has been infected with tuberculosis, treatment is implemented to prevent active illness and spread to others.

The nurse plays an important role in advocating timely vaccination of at-risk people. Childhood vaccination programs are mandatory in many states and should provide the child with protection from diphtheria, polio, measles, mumps, rubella, pertussis (whooping cough), and tetanus. Some of these vaccinations require booster doses throughout life. Currently the recommendation for a tetanus booster is once every 10 years (Plotkin & Mortimer, 1988, p. 590). Adults should be reminded of this and tetanus status should be evaluated periodically, especially when a wound has been incurred. Vaccinations for influenza are often suggested for the elderly and for people with underlying chronic disease. The influenza vaccine is changed annually to anticipate the most likely virulent strains, and may need to be an annual event for those at risk. The pneumococcal vaccine is recommended for persons over 65 or those between 2 and 65 with asplenia, chronic illness, or immunosuppression due to illness or therapy (Plotkin & Mortimer, 1988, p. 288).

Nurses should also teach sexually active adolescents and adults safe sex practices to prevent sexually transmitted diseases. These practices include abstinence, limiting the number of partners, using condoms and other barrier contraceptives, and using spermicide containing honoxynal-9 (Burns, 1988). Women should receive regular gynecologic check-ups and men and women should seek medical attention for possible exposure to or at the first sign of sexually transmitted disease.

Fall Prevention

In the health-care environment the nurse must ensure the patient's safety from falls (see display). The room needs to be kept free of clutter, well lit during transfers and ambulation, and side rails and grab bars must be firmly anchored (Fig. 25-7A). The floor must be non-skid, either carpeted or free of liquid. Wheelchairs, beds, commode chairs, or shower chairs must have working brakes (Fig. 25-7B), be free of any sharp edges, and have a support surface that is comfortable. Patients with orthostatic hypotension should be taught to change position slowly to allow for blood pressure stabilization.

Considerations in Preventing Falls in the Health-Care Environment

Environmental

Is the bed in the lowest position?
Are the bed wheels locked?
Are the wheelchair brakes on?
Is there a night light available in the room?
Are there any obvious physical hazards in the room (wet floors, cords)?
Are the items needed by the patient within easy reach (water glass, tissues)?

Patient

Can the patient demonstrate correct use of the call light?
Is the call light within reach of the patient?
What kind of footwear does the patient use?
Is the patient aware of prescribed activity?
Does the patient demonstrate physical or mental limitations (previously identified or new)?
Is the patient receiving medications that may have side effects contributing to falls (e.g., hypnotics, sedatives, psychotropics, analgesics, diuretics)?
Is the patient receiving other medications or treatments that could potentially contribute to falls?

The use of physical restraints is not necessarily advocated. Physical **restraints** are defined as any manual method or physical or mechanical device, material, or equipment, attached or adjacent to the person's body that the person cannot remove easily, that restricts freedom of movement or normal access to one's body (Omnibus Budget Reconciliation Act, 1989). Restraints do not specifically prevent falls (Janelli, 1989; Powell, Mitchell-Pedersen, Fingerote, & Edmund, 1989), yet restraints may be deemed necessary to limit physical activity of a patient to prevent injury (e.g., from a fall) or to prevent movement that would disrupt therapy (e.g., pulling out an intravenous line or mechanical ventilator tubing).

Restraints, if used, must be used cautiously to prevent agitation, preserve dignity, prevent physical injury from the restraining device, and avoid abuse of a patient's right to move about freely. Health-care institution guidelines should be followed regarding the use of restraints, and the reason for their application must be described in the patient's care record. Nurses may apply restraints in an emergency without a physician's order; however, an order should be obtained as soon as possible. The nurse should also use direct supervision and communication as much as possible to reassure and reorient the patient.

Types of restraints include a jacket or vest restraint, which is worn on the patient's chest and tied to the bed frame or legs of a chair, a belt restraint on stretchers or wheelchairs used in transporting, mitt or hand restraints that prevent confused patients from using their hands, wrist or ankle restraints that immobilize one or more limbs, and mummy restraints that are wrapped around a

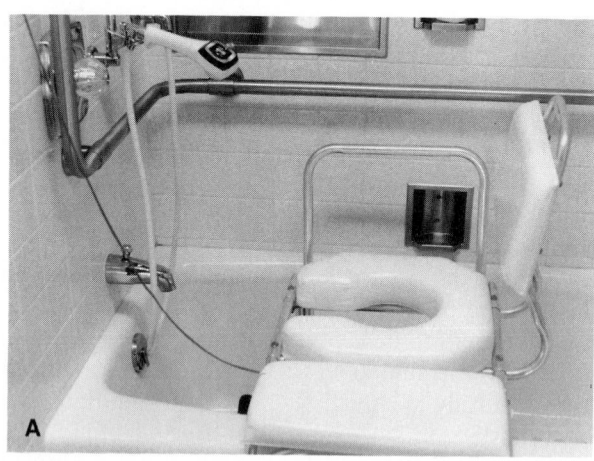
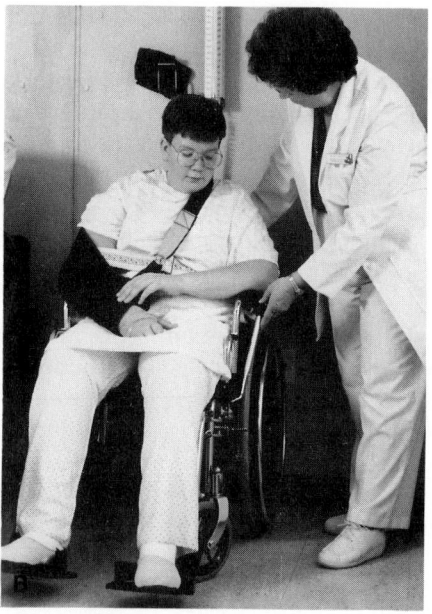

Figure 25–7. The health care facility must provide safety for the patient. **A:** This shower protects the patient with grab bars, safety rails, shower seat, and transfer seat. **B:** The nurse checks wheelchair brakes for safe use.

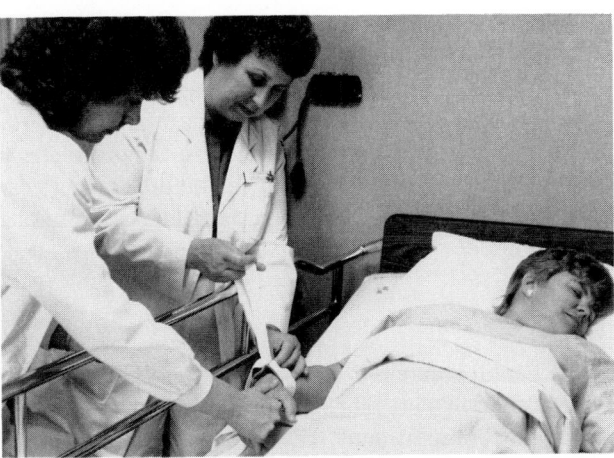

Figure 25–8. Wrist restraints are used at times for patient protection. They are an aid if the patient is inclined to pull out tubes.

child's body to prevent movement during a procedure. Figure 25-8 illustrates a wrist restraint.

Nurses should educate parents about the potential for infants to fall. Prevention includes not leaving an infant unattended in a bath, bed, or table where he or she may roll or fall off, keeping the crib side rails up, using guard rails or gates at the top and bottom of the stairs when the infant crawls, and supervising the child in a walker, jumper, swing, or high chair. Nurses should teach adults, especially older adults, to remove throw rugs, make sure stairways are well lighted and repaired, remove clutter from stairways and walkways, install handrails wherever needed, avoid use of unstable ladders and step stools, never attempt to do anything beyond reach or physical ability, and clean up damp areas promptly (Fig. 25-9).

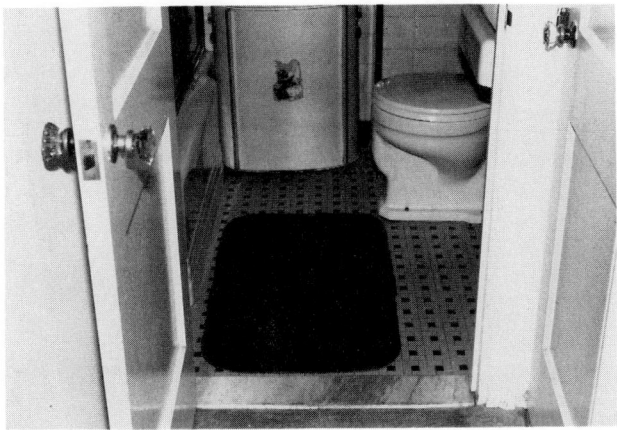

Figure 25–9. Throw rugs are a major source of falls. Rugs should have a backing that will not slip; otherwise the rug should be removed. If a person falls in the bathroom there are many places that could cause damage to the head.

Childhood Safety

The care of children in the health-care environment requires special safety precautions to prevent injury in unfamiliar surroundings. High staff-to-patient ratios, use of cribs and beds with side rails, carpeting on floor, play areas with age-appropriate toys and furnishings, locked medications and supply rooms, and protected exits contribute to safety.

Parents should be made aware of the need to child-proof the home, as well as closely supervise the child in any potentially hazardous area outside the home (see Patient Teaching display). Parents should be taught to use only cribs and other infant equipment approved by the U.S. Consumer Products Safety Commission or other regulatory agency. The use of older equipment that is worn or poorly designed may present a hazard.

Toys should be age-appropriate. Toys with small pieces should be kept out of the reach of infants to prevent suffocation by choking. Sharp edges and missile-type toys also present a hazard to younger children. Parents should be taught that plastic bags can be used in play and may

---

Patient Teaching: Childproofing the Home

Instruct the patient as follows:

- Cover unused electrical outlets with safety plugs to prevent fingers from being poked into them.
- Place electrical cords and handles of pots and appliances out of reach to avoid having appliances or substances pulled over.
- Secure screens on all windows within reach of a toddler on a chair.
- Place all plastic bags out of reach to avoid accidental suffocation.
- Cover controls of appliances with tamper-proof locks or covers to prevent burns and other injuries.
- Keep matches and cigarette lighters out of reach to prohibit fires caused by accident or curiosity.
- Lock up potentially toxic substances to deter accidental swallowing.
- Keep hot water temperature at <115°F to prevent scalds and burns.
- Place nonskid mats in showers or tubs and bath mats on floor.
- Remove doors from unused refrigerators and freezers to prevent entrapment and asphyxiation.
- Fence yards for outdoor play within safe perimeters.

cause suffocation. Pillows and restrictive blankets should not be used with infants to prevent suffocation. Food should be prepared appropriately for infants and toddlers to prevent choking, and bottles should not be propped to prevent aspiration by infants. Pacifiers should not be hung around an infant's neck and care should be taken when using harness restraints to prevent choking.

Nurses should make parents aware that drowning not only occurs in pools, but also in bathtubs and other sources of water around the home. Pools should be fenced in, and children of all ages should be supervised at pools and beaches. Children should wear life jackets for boating and fishing, and should be warned not to ice skate or play on ice unless ice thickness is proven safe. Infants and toddlers should never be left unattended in the bathtub or kiddie pools. Pails or basins of water should not be left in an infant's or toddler's reach.

Children should be taught bicycle safety. Helmets should be worn to protect against head injury in the event of a fall (Fig. 25-10). Proper signalling and illumination of self and bicycle at night are important for accident prevention. Parents should be taught to check for small children riding low vehicles before driving a car out of a driveway or parking space. Children should be warned about riding in streets or near driveways.

Burn Prevention

In the health-care environment, burns can be prevented by testing bath water for temperature when the patient has sensory impairment, checking heating pads, heat lamps, and other electrical equipment for proper function, assisting patients in handling hot beverages as needed, and not allowing patients to smoke in bed.

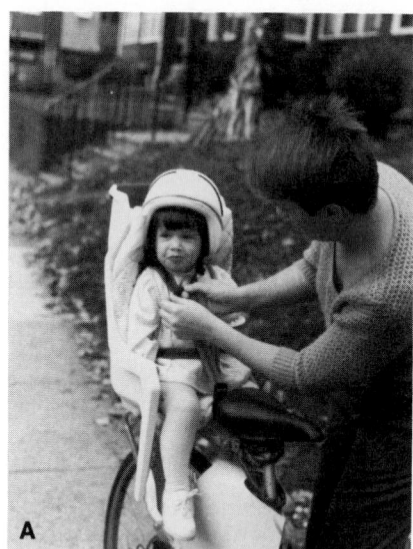
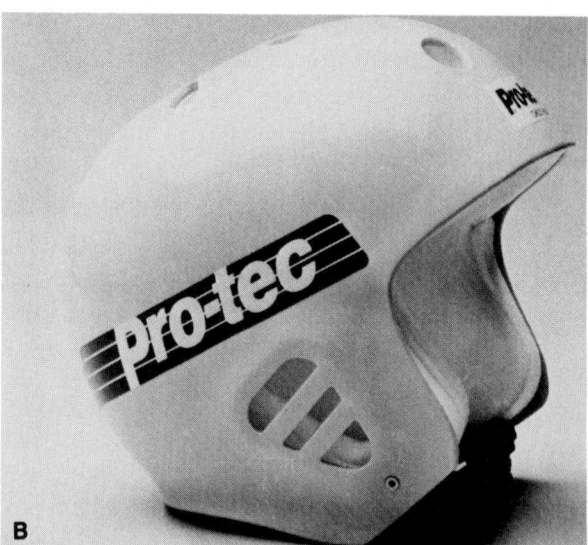
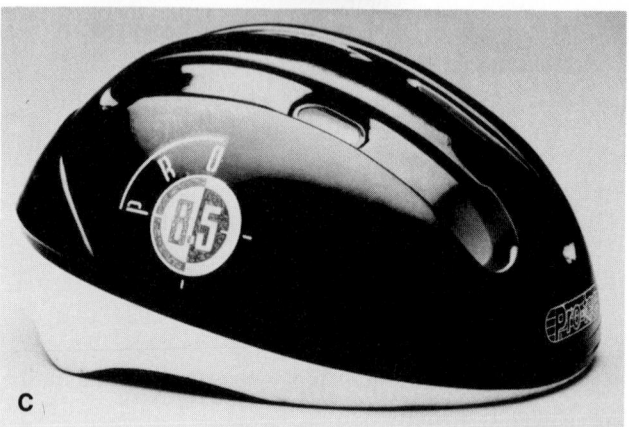
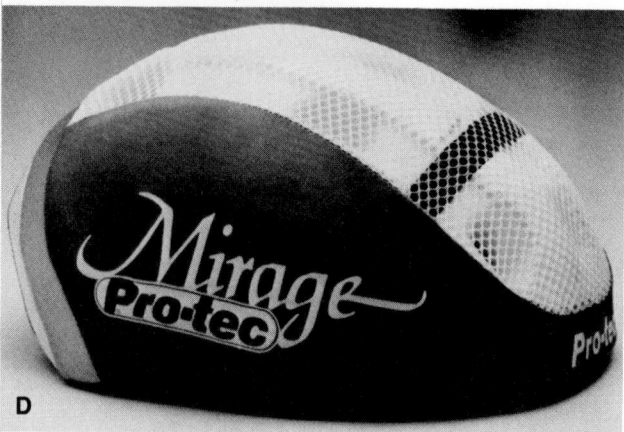

Figure 25-10. Wearing helmets should be part of bicycle safety teaching. If children learn to wear helmets when they are young, it will be easier for them to continue to use them through adolescence and adulthood. Different types of helmets are provided. **A:** A child's helmet, worn by the child on the back of the bicycle. **B, C,** and **D:** Are adult helmets. (Helmet photos courtesy of PRO-TEC, Inc.)

Nurses should teach patients with sensory impairment to monitor water temperature at home as well. The thermostat on the hot water heater may need to be adjusted. Parents should keep pot handles turned away from the front of the stove top where young children might reach. Young children should never be left to play unsupervised in the kitchen, near burning fireplaces, barbecue grills, or containers of gasoline. Parents should be taught to apply sunscreen to children playing outdoors to prevent sunburn.

Adults should be taught to never smoke while using lighter fluid to start a charcoal fire or when filling lawn-mowers with gasoline. Smoking in bed or late at night in a chair may be hazardous. Smoking materials should be properly extinguished.

Poison Prevention

Poison prevention in the health-care environment can be accomplished primarily through safe medication preparation and administration practices. Nurses are responsible for checking that physician's orders for medications are signed and updated appropriately and that they have been transcribed accurately. Identification of the patient by checking the identification band worn by the patient is essential before administering any medication. Any significant side effects should be documented and reported to the physician.

Nursing intervention for poison prevention in the home involves education of parents (see Patient Teaching display). All medications, including over-the-counter products, should be stored in childproof containers out of the reach of children. Parents should not treat medications as candy. Household cleansers and other potentially toxic products should be stored in child-proofed or locked cupboards or on shelves out of children's reach. All household chemical products should be kept in their original containers with warning labels and emergency information intact.

All poisonous house plants should be kept out of young children's reach and children should be supervised outdoors. Some poisonous plants include azaleas, buttercups, daffodils, mistletoe berries, philodendrons, poinsettias, potato sprouts, tomato greens, and tulip bulbs. Older children should be taught never to eat berries, mushrooms, seeds, or plants grown in the wild.

Nurses should teach people to keep poison control center phone numbers posted near telephones. An integrated system of local centers across the United States and Canada can provide emergency information whenever a substance is ingested, inhaled, or splashed in the eyes or on the skin.

Motor Vehicle Safety

Nursing intervention for motor vehicle safety involves patient education about potential hazards and safety

---

Patient Teaching: Preventing Childhood Poisoning

Instruct the patient as follows:

- Keep all medications and toxic products in original containers.
- Keep childproof caps on toxic products if children live in the home or are frequent visitors.
- Keep all medications, including vitamins, out of the reach of children, in a locked chest.
- Keep household chemical products out of the reach of children.
- Do not treat medicines as candy.
- Do not take or give medicine in the dark.
- Read labels carefully before using drugs or toxic products.
- Keep emergency poison control telephone numbers handy.
- Have emergency drugs in the home—syrup of ipecac and Epsom salts.
- Use toxic chemical products in a well-ventilated area.
- Do not mix common household cleaning products.
- Destroy all old medications.
- Destroy unused medications by flushing down toilet or washing down sink, rather than by throwing in trash.
- Use childproof containers when available.
- Identify any poisonous houseplants, and keep seeds, bulbs, leaves, and fruits of such plants away from children.

From Spencer, R. T., et al. (1989). *Clinical pharmacology and nursing management* (3rd ed.) (p. 48). Philadelphia: J. B. Lippincott.

---

measures. Use of seat belts has greatly decreased morbidity and mortality on the highways (National Safety Council, 1989). Most states now have mandatory seat belt laws in effect.

Infants and children should be properly restrained in automobiles as well, using approved car seats (Fig. 25-11). Infants weighing up to 18 or 20 pounds need to be in a rear-facing car seat, semi-reclined with their heads well supported. Toddlers and preschoolers (20–60 lbs.) should be secured in a forward-facing car seat. Children over 60 pounds need to wear a properly applied lap/shoulder harness (Slota, 1990).

Motor vehicle safety also includes maintaining a safe driving speed for road and weather conditions. Nurses have many opportunities to educate the public about the effects of alcohol on a driver. Any substances that can impair alertness and reaction time, such as antihistamines, should be avoided while driving motor vehicles.

Adolescents should be taught about the danger of riding with friends who are impaired by alcohol or drugs.

Nursing Interventions for Altered Safety Function

When safety is not maintained, harm to a person or group occurs. In the health-care environment, specific nursing interventions are carried out when preventive measures fail. Nursing interventions for altered safety function include fire evacuation, emergency first aid for poisoning, administration of obstructed airway and cardiopulmonary resuscitation techniques, and filing an incident report.

Fire Evacuation

In the event of a fire in the patient-care area, nurses are responsible for determining which patients are in immediate danger. Ambulatory patients should be directed toward exits to wait in a safe area or enlisted to help evacuate bedridden patients. Stretchers and wheelchairs should be used, and, if necessary, patients can be carried or dragged on sheets. Elevators should not be used in the event of a fire. The fire alarm should be activated and the hospital switchboard notified of the fire's location. The local fire department will be notified automatically. If the fire is small, a fire extinguisher can be used, but other interventions should not be neglected because small fires can quickly flare up out of control. Windows and doors should be closed and oxygen turned off in the area to reduce the fire's oxygen supply. Patients should be evacuate in surrounding areas, if necessary, and given wet washcloths to breathe through to reduce smoke inhalation.

Health-care facilities are required to have fire evacuation plans with exits clearly marked. Additional staff from the facility and firefighters will respond quickly to help nurses evacuate patients. Nurses should never attempt to extinguish fires if the patients' or their own safety is in jeopardy. Evacuation of patients requiring mechanical ventilation can be accomplished by manual respiration with an ambubag. Tubes connected to suction must be clamped before disconnection and intravenous fluids should be transported with the patient.

Emergency Care in Accidental Poisoning

In the health-care environment, ingestion of dangerous substances, overdosage, or incorrect medication can be treated as in the home. The patient's physician should be notified, but if the substance is potentially toxic, the poison control center should be notified without delay. The center will require information about the specific poison (the ingredients section on the label may provide this information), quantity ingested, person's age and weight, and apparent symptoms. The nurse may be instructed to induce vomiting with syrup of ipecac if the patient is not unconscious or convulsing, or if the substance was not a strong corrosive or petroleum product. The patient should be positioned on his or her side or with his or her head placed between his or her legs to prevent aspiration. The nurse may gather urine, vomitus, or blood samples as instructed.

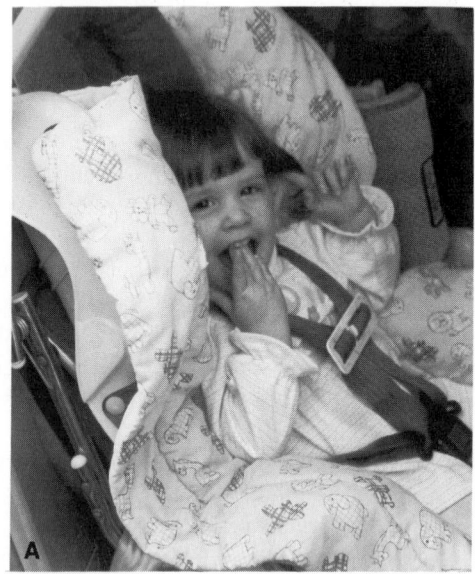 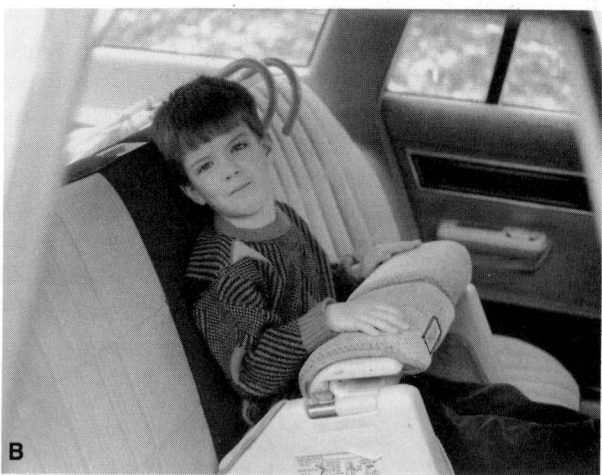

Figure 25–11.   Carseats are designed for infants (**A**), and toddlers and pre-schoolers (**B**).

**Doses for Inducing Emesis
with Syrup of Ipecac**

Pediatric

6–12 months—administer 10 mL orally.
Over 1 year—administer 15 mL orally, followed by
one to two glassfuls of whatever fluid the child will
tolerate (ipecac is not effective on an empty stomach). Maintain activity level. Results should occur
within 30 minutes.

Adult

Administer 30 mL. The same procedure as above
is applied to the adult victim.

From Spencer, R. T., et al. (1989). Clinical pharmacology and nursing
management (3rd ed.) (p. 48). Philadelphia: J. B. Lippincott.

If poisonous substances have been instilled into the
eye or on the skin, immediate irrigation with lukewarm
water for 10 to 15 minutes may reduce harmful effects.
Clothing should be removed from the skin. The person
should be instructed to blink as much as possible during
eye irrigation.

Cardiopulmonary Resuscitation

If a patient chokes, aspirates, or is found cyanotic and
apneic, the nurse is responsible for initiating resuscitation efforts; see Chapter 31 for the procedure for obstructed airway and cardiopulmonary resuscitation.
Electrical shock may also lead to cardiac arrest requiring
cardiopulmonary resuscitation (CPR).

Filing an Incident Report

An incident report is filed when an accident occurs in the
health-care environment. It is a confidential document
filed with the institution's legal, insurance, or quality
assurance department for internal use only. In it, the
nurse describes how an accident occurred, what the
effects to the patient were, and what was done for the
patient. Incident reports are commonly used for falls and
medication errors.

In addition to filing an incident report, the nurse must
enter on the patient's medical record a description of the
accident and effects on the patient. The patient's physician should be notified of the accident and will document
the patient's condition, as well. The nurse does not make
note of the incident report on the medical record since it
is used internally. The incident report can be reviewed
by the institution's attorneys in the event of a lawsuit and
it may be collected by the risk manager to see if trends of
accidents in the workplace are developing.

Discharge Planning and Home Care

In the health-care setting the nurse is responsible for
identifying areas in which the person is unsafe when
performing essential activities of daily living. The nurse
must devise a discharge plan that prepares the patient,
home caregivers, and the home itself for optimal safety
in performing the activities of daily living. Although
other health professionals, such as social workers, occupational therapists, and physical therapists may be involved in the discharge planning process, the nurse is
often considered the most accurate source of information about the patient's function in the arena of activities
of daily living. The therapists may observe the patient
during therapy sessions, but the nurse can assess the
person's functioning at the end of the day when fatigue
has its greatest effect on performance.

The nurse has the opportunity to observe the patient
engaging in transfers and mobility, toileting, hygiene,
eating and feeding, and dressing. The observations
made during assessment and throughout the patient's
hospital stay allow the nurse to anticipate the measures
that need to be taken to promote safety in these activities
at home (Fig. 25-12). Nursing interventions to promote
safe performance in the home involve patient education
and are carried out throughout hospitalization.

The nurse who is working with a newly disabled patient helps the health-care team anticipate the environmental changes that may be needed after discharge.
Often the patient or family/caregivers are asked to draw
a floor plan of the house, noting especially the width of
doorways, configuration of the bathroom and kitchen,
stairs approaching the home and within the home, and
access to transportation from the home. Special equipment in use by the patient during the hospitalization may
need to be used in the home, and hospital beds, wheelchairs, tub benches, and mechanical lifts may not fit in
the home. Early identification of the patient's post-discharge equipment needs will help the family/caregivers
to modify the home before the patient is discharged.

Essential to the overall safety picture is the support
system. Actively involved caregivers or supportive
friends can provide assistance in assessing the availability of the caregivers, their level of desired participation,
and their own capacity for safe judgment. The nurse
should identify who will be providing care, and whether
they will be available occasionally, part-time, or 24 hours
a day. The nurse must ask what care the caregivers can
provide: assistance with mobility and transfers, with
other activities of daily living (toileting, hygiene, dress-

Home Safety Guidelines

Throughout the Home

Electrical cords in good repair

Only one electrical fixture per plug

Upholstered furniture away from heat sources: baseboards, space heaters, etc.

Fireplaces screened

Smoke detectors with operational power sources

Adequate lighting

Minimal clutter

Loose carpeting tacked down

Stair edges marked with tape or contrasting paint (especially in areas of poor lighting—basement, outdoors)

Sturdy handrails by all stairs

Safety glazing or glass in all glass doors and panels: visible decals will decrease chance of accidental collision

Bathroom

Nonskid backing on bathmat

Nonskid mat or decals for tub or shower

Grab bars for toilet and tub if needed

Expired medications discarded

Hot water heated to <115°F

Kitchen

Fire extinguisher in working order

Adequate ventilation

Liquid fuels stored away from heat sources (e.g., charcoal lighter fluid)

Expired foods discarded

Refrigerator adequately cooling to prevent spoilage

Pilot lights lit (gas stove or oven)

Miscellaneous

Ladders in good repair with nonskid surface on feet and steps

Bicycles in good repair with reflectors working and working brakes

Doors removed from unused refrigerators and freezers

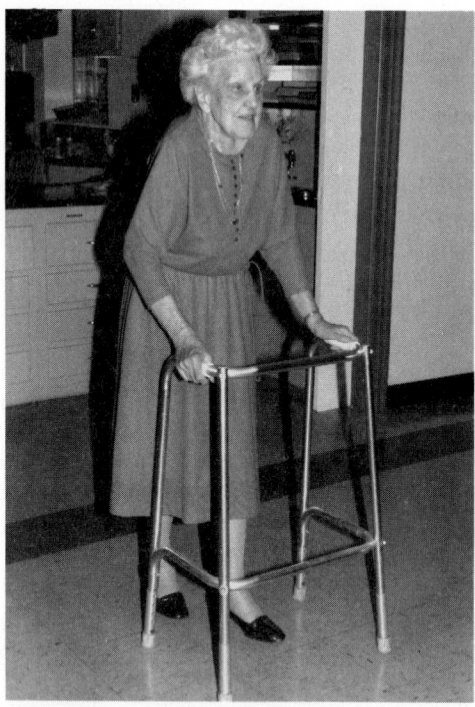

Figure 25–12. Use of a walker promotes safety when walking. The nurse may observe the patient and her ability to use the walker before she is discharged.

ing, eating), with laundry, shopping, and bill paying, or with supervision during inactive times. Prior to discharge, the nurse should determine what training the caregivers need in order to safely provide care. Discharge teaching plans should include this caregiver training.

Whenever the nursing assessment has identified that the person is unsafe in an activity of daily living, and interventions to educate the patient in the needed safety habits have not succeeded, the nurse must incorporate any available caregivers into the plan for safe discharge. When possible, it is recommended that the caregivers come to the health-care setting and observe and practice under the guidance of health professionals. This may include attending therapy sessions, or even sleeping overnight to better understand the needs of the patient around the clock. When caregivers are unable to come to the hospital, a home health referral will allow a home health nurse to visit patient and caregivers in the home and provide training there.

Some communities offer a service that will call the single older adult daily and will respond to a call-for-help signal activated on a medallion worn around the neck. This system or a buddy system of telephone calls can provide a quick response to accidents for the older adult.

Nursing Management Plan
The Patient at Risk for Injury

Nursing Diagnosis: High risk for injury related to sensory and integrative dysfunction manifested by altered mobility and faulty judgment.

Patient Goal: Patient will demonstrate safety habits in performance of activities of daily living and injury prevention.

Patient Outcome Criteria

- Patient uses nurse call light system for assistance to bathroom at each need to use facilities immediately after instruction by the nurse.
- Patient demonstrates safety practices in dressing and hygiene.
- Patient uses over-the-bed lights, nonskid slippers each time when transferring to chair or out of bed.
- Patient identifies modification for home safety (removal of throw rugs, installation of handrails in hallway, better lighting of hallway and stairway) 12 hours after nurse's instruction about home safety.

Nursing Interventions	Scientific Rationale
1. Position bed in lowest position.	1. To minimize distance to floor if patient falls.
2. Place patient call light within reach of hand and give instructions.	2. To allow patient to call for help.
3. Explain all safety modifications of the patient's room: removal of clutter, providing a clear path to bathroom, use of a night light, brakes on bed and chairs, placement of call light.	3. To increase patient and family awareness of safety promotion strategies.
4. Perform frequent visual checks of patient.	4. Patient may attempt to get out of bed or chair without calling for assistance.
5. Use safety belt in all transfers if the patient is unsteady or has difficulty with balance.	5. To allow for control/monitoring of patient movement without trauma to any body part.
6. Evaluate the patient's ability to use toilet; obtain raised toiled seat and/or grab bars if indicated.	6. Patients with hip muscle weakness may be unable to rise from low toilet seat. Grab bars may assist the weak person to move slowly and safely.
7. Assist patient to perform hygiene at sink with large mirror; encourage patient to scan the whole visual field.	7. Mirror provides patient with visual reinforcement of activity.
8. Discuss floor plan of home with patient and support person. Make suggestions for modifications that will lead to a safer environment.	8. To start patient and support person in planning for the patient's safety when discharged.

EVALUATION

The effectiveness of nursing interventions to promote safety is determined through nursing observation and feedback from patient caregivers and health-care professionals in the community. During the period of hospitalization, the nurse is constantly evaluating the effectiveness of interventions by the ease with which the patient accomplishes necessary activities of daily living and the absence of accidents.

Nursing interventions have the long-term goals of identification of actual and potential environmental hazards, demonstration of safety habits, reduction in frequency and severity of accidents, and development of safe compensatory strategies for physical deficits. To measure the progress toward these goals, the nurse may question the patient and caregivers (using "what if" and "what would you do if" questions), ask for and evaluate performance of selected safety habits (for example, transfers in and out of the bathtub), gather data on the frequency and type of accidents, and evaluate the effectiveness of compensatory strategies (are they using the suggested strategies, is the patient satisfied, does the strategy make the activity easier, safer, faster to accomplish?). Any accident, fall, scrape, or bruise requires analysis by the nurse to identify the cause and the best means to prevent recurrence. The nurse has a fundamental responsibility to promote patient safety around the clock, and every opportunity for interaction with the patient is an opportunity to promote and evaluate safety habits.

Examples of outcome criteria that measure the achievement of patient goals are given below.

Goal

The patient will identify actual and high-risk environmental hazards.

Possible Outcome Criteria

- Patient verbalizes difficulty in walking to bathroom in the health-care facility within 24 hours of being admitted as a patient/resident.
- Patient expresses fear of falling over obstacles at home prior to discharge.

Goal

The patient will demonstrate safety habits in performance of ADLs and injury prevention.

Possible Outcome Criteria

- Patient uses nurse call light system for assistance to bathroom at each need to use facilities immediately after instructions by the nurse.
- Patient uses over-the-bed lights, nonskid slippers, and glasses when transferring to chair at first and subsequent times out of bed.
- Patient identifies modification for home safety (removal of throw rugs, installation of handrails in hallway, better lighting of hallway and stairway) 24 hours after nurse's instruction about home safety.
- Patient demonstrates safety practices in dressing and hygiene.

Goal

The patient will experience decreased frequency and severity of accidents.

Possible Outcome Criteria

- Patient practices safety precautions, as evidenced by absence of falls or accidents in 48 hours before discharge.

Key Concepts

- Safety is a basic human need that is essential in the health-care environment, home, and community.
- Intrinsic factors that affect safety include cognition and perception, activity and exercise, nutrition and metabolism, physiologic factors, sensory abilities,

age, lifestyle and habits, previous experience, fatigue, and psychologic factors.

- Extrinsic factors that affect safety include home environment, community environment, the workplace environment, sanitation, pollution, and thermoregulation.
- Manifestations of altered safety include falls, fires, burns, poisoning, suffocation, electrical shock, radiation injury, infection, allergies, respiratory problems, stress-related illness, and motor vehicle accidents.
- Infants, older adults, and those impaired by illness or medications are at risk for falls.
- Falls in the health-care environment are frequently associated with walking to the bathroom.
- Nursing interventions to promote health and safety function involve providing a safe health-care environment and patients' education.
- It is important for nurses to educate parents about the developmental capabilities of infants and children and the special safety precautions needed for their care.
- Nurses must be familiar with interventions for altered safety function such as fire evacuation and filing an incident report.

References

Burns, E. A., Robinson, J. C., & Scherger, J. E. (1988). Which barrier contraceptive for whom? *Patient Care, 22*(15), 109–139.
Centers for Disease Control. (1988). Update: Universal precautions for prevention of transmission of human immunodeficiency virus, hepatitis B virus, and other blood-borne pathogens in health care settings. *Morbidity and Mortality Weekly Report, 37,* 377–388.
Easterling, M. L. (1990). Which of your patients is headed for a fall? *RN, 53*(1), 56–59.
Freiberg, K. L. (1987). *Human development: A life-span approach* (3rd ed.). Boston: Jones and Bartlett.
Janelli, L. M. (1989). Physical restraints: How little we know. *Nursing Homes, 38*(1/2), 10–12.
Kane, R., Ouslander, J., & Abrass, I. (1989). *Essentials of geriatrics.* New York: McGraw-Hill.
Loken, S., & Loken, T. (1989). Radon: Detection and treatment. *Nurse Practitioner, 14*(11), 45–46, 48, 51.
Maslow, A. H. (1970). *Motivation and personality* (2nd ed.). New York: Harper and Row.
NANDA (1990). *Taxonomy I revised 1990, with official nursing diagnoses.* St. Louis, MO: North American Nursing Diagnosis Association.
National Safety Council. (1989). *Accident facts.* Chicago: Author.
Omnibus Budget Reconciliation Act (OBRA). (1990). Regulations and Interpretive Guidelines (draft). Health Care Financing Administration.
Plotkin, S. A., & Mortimer, E. A. (1988). *Vaccines.* Philadelphia: W. B. Saunders.
Powell, C., Mitchell-Pederson, L., Fingerote, G., & Edmund, L. (1989). Freedom from restraint: Consequences of reducing physical restraints in the management of the elderly. *Canadian Medical Association Journal, 141*(6), 561–564.
Slota, M. C. (1990). Child passenger safety in the car: Are we involved enough? *Critical Care Nurse, 10*(4), 72–74, 77–79.
Spencer, R. T., et al. (1989). *Clinical pharmacology and nursing management* (3rd ed.). Philadelphia: J. B. Lippincott.
Stanevich, R. S., & Stanevich, R. L. (1989). Guidelines for occupational safety and health program. *American Association of Occupational Health Journal,* 205–214, 242–244.

Bibliography

Dallaire, L. B., & Burke, E. V. (1989). A new program for reducing patient falls. *Nursing 89, 19*(1), 65.

Driscoll, A. (1989). To recap or not—preventing needlesticks. *Professional Safety, 34*(1), 27–29.

Escher, J. E., O'Dell, C., & Gambert, S. R. (1989). Typical geriatric accidents and how to prevent them. *Geriatrics, 44*(5), 54–56, 66, 68–69.

Halpern, J. S. (1990). Bicycle helmets for children. *Journal of Emergency Nursing, 16*(1), 36–40.

Injury-proofing the school-age child. (1989). *Patient Care, 23*(15), 178.

Jacobs, B. B. (1989). Accidental death, injury in America, and injury control: Three reports from the National Academy of Sciences and the sequence of solutions. *Emergency Care Quarterly, 5*(2), 63–73.

Kids and small objects: A dangerous combination. (1990). *Patient Care, 24*(3), 128, 131.

Ryden, L. A., Molgaard, C. A., Babbitt, S., et al. (1989). Occupational low-back injury in a hospital employee population: An epidemiologic analysis of multiple risk factors of a high-risk occupational group. *Spine, 14,* 315–320.

Sloan, K. A. (1990). The safety seal injury prevention program: A response to the epidemic of injury and death in children. *Journal of Emergency Nursing, 16*(2), 83–89.

Stepnick, A., & Harrison, B. S. (1990). Safety needs and AIDS: A model care plan. *Home Health Care Nurse, 8*(2), 25–31.

Tideiksaar, R. (1989). Home safe home: Practical tips for fall-proofing. *Geriatric Nursing, 10*(6), 280–284.

Vandewater, D. A. (1990). Safety-proofing an elder's home: A checklist. *Perspectives, 14*(1), 5.

Varas, R., Carbone, R., & Hammond, J. S. (1988). A one-hour burn prevention program for grade school children: Its approach and success. *Journal of Burn Care and Rehabilitation, 9*(1), 69–71.

Veach, S. L. (1990). Advocating bicycle helmet use: A nursing issue. *Imprint, 37*(2), 141–142.

Wilson, D., & Molloy-Martinez, T. (1989). Promoting driving safety for teens and adults. *Nurse Practitioner, 14*(10), 28, 30–31, 34–36.

Wilson, M. H. (1989). Preventive care for childhood injury. *Patient Care, 23*(15), 79–81, 84, 86.

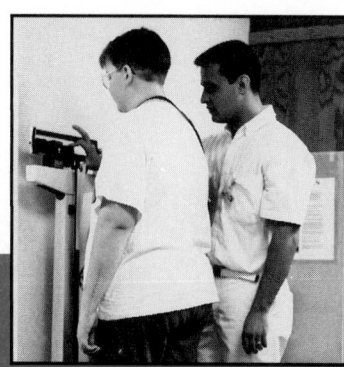

Health Maintenance

LEARNING OBJECTIVES

Upon completion of this chapter, the student will be able to do the following:

- Describe the characteristics essential for normal health.
- Give examples of health-promotion and illness-prevention behaviors.
- Describe important lifespan development considerations for health maintenance.
- Recognize major factors that affect motivation and health maintenance.
- Explain how the environment, poverty, and unhealthy lifestyles or habits may alter health maintenance.
- Characterize manifestations of altered health maintenance.
- Obtain subjective data through a nursing history to assess health-maintenance.
- Provide appropriate information about common illnesses that may result from altered health maintenance.
- List resources for patient-teaching information on health-maintenance.
- Value health-promotion concepts and act as a role model for patients.

KEY TERMS

Health-maintenance activities	Health-promotion activities	Illness-prevention activities

26

Normal Health Maintenance
  Characteristics of Normal Health Maintenance
    Perception
    Motivation
    Management
  Normal Functional Health Maintenance
    Health Promotion
    Illness Prevention
    Combination of Promotion and Prevention
  Factors Affecting Health Maintenance
  Lifespan Considerations
Altered Health Maintenance Function
  Potential for Altered Function
    Environment
    Poverty
    Unhealthy Lifestyle and Habits
  Manifestations of Altered Function
    Chronic Illnesses
    Accidents and Injuries
    Childhood and Developmental Problems
    Psychosocial Problems
  Impact of Dysfunction on Activities of Daily Living
Assessment
  Subjective Data
    Functional Pattern Identification

    Risk Identification
    Dysfunctional Identification
  Objective Data
    Physical Assessment
    Diagnostic Tests
Nursing Diagnoses and Patient Goals
  Diagnostic Statement: Altered Health Maintenance
    Definition
    Defining Characteristics
    Related Factors
  Diagnostic Statement: Health-Seeking Behaviors
    Definition
    Defining Characteristics
  Related Nursing Diagnoses
  Patient Goals
Implementation
  Nursing Interventions to Promote Health and
    Function
    Education About Common Illnesses
    Self-Examination Techniques
    Routine Health Care
  Nursing Interventions for Altered Function
  Discharge Planning and Home Care
Evaluation
Key Concepts

Florence Nightingale believed the following:

- Health is the ability to use well every power one has.
- Preventable disease should be a crime.
- It is cheaper to promote health than to care for illness.
- Goals of nursing should include health maintenance, health teaching, and disease prevention.

Modern nurses still address these issues. They have the potential and the responsibility to help people, families, and communities in maintaining and improving health. The nursing activities of health education and patient teaching focus on enhancing a person's ability to engage in effective health behavior. Although nurses may promote healthy behaviors, it is the patient's option to accept or reject those behaviors.

Health maintenance has become an increasingly pop-

ular concept and has contributed to the growth of health maintenance organizations (HMOs). HMOs are based on the belief that it is easier and more economical to maintain health than to treat illness. Consumers of care in HMOs prepay for health care; regular examinations, immunizations, health teaching, and other health-related activities are a prime focus of the organization. There are several well-established HMOs that are freestanding organizations, and several health insurance groups have organized similar programs.

NORMAL HEALTH MAINTENANCE

Health-maintenance activities are the behaviors that a person in stable health uses to maintain or improve that state of health over time. To understand health maintenance, one must recall the concepts of health and wellness (see Chap. 11). Health and wellness involve assuming responsibility for oneself, making informed choices, having self-worth, and managing stress. Health maintenance, then, is the continuity of those beliefs and behaviors.

Health-care workers may define health and wellness in one way, but a patient may define it differently. Ultimately, a person's understanding of health depends on how that person defines health. If a person believes that health means being free of disease, the parameters of health are narrow. If a person believes that health is the optimal functioning of biologic, psychosocial, and spiritual factors with the environment, however, the meaning of health becomes broad.

Characteristics of Normal Health Maintenance

To maintain our level of health and to strive for higher levels of well-being, one often must alter the health habits and our environment. This may involve seeking new support people. Normal health maintenance requires three characteristics (Fig. 26-1):

- Perception of health
- Motivation to change direction if necessary
- Adherence to management goals.

Perception

A person's ability to maintain a desired level of health depends on that person's perception of the existing health status and knowledge to manage positive health behaviors. For example, many elderly people mistakenly believe that joint pain is a normal part of aging and therefore do not seek medical attention. When asked about their health status, these people may say they are in good health, forgetting about or ignoring the joint pain.

The person who believes that health is a gift from God may believe that there is little that can be done to improve health. The person's perception, then, influences how he or she rates personal health and influences the options available for management.

Motivation

The person's perception and understanding of health determines the accountability and responsibility that he or she assumes for health. This self-awareness reveals

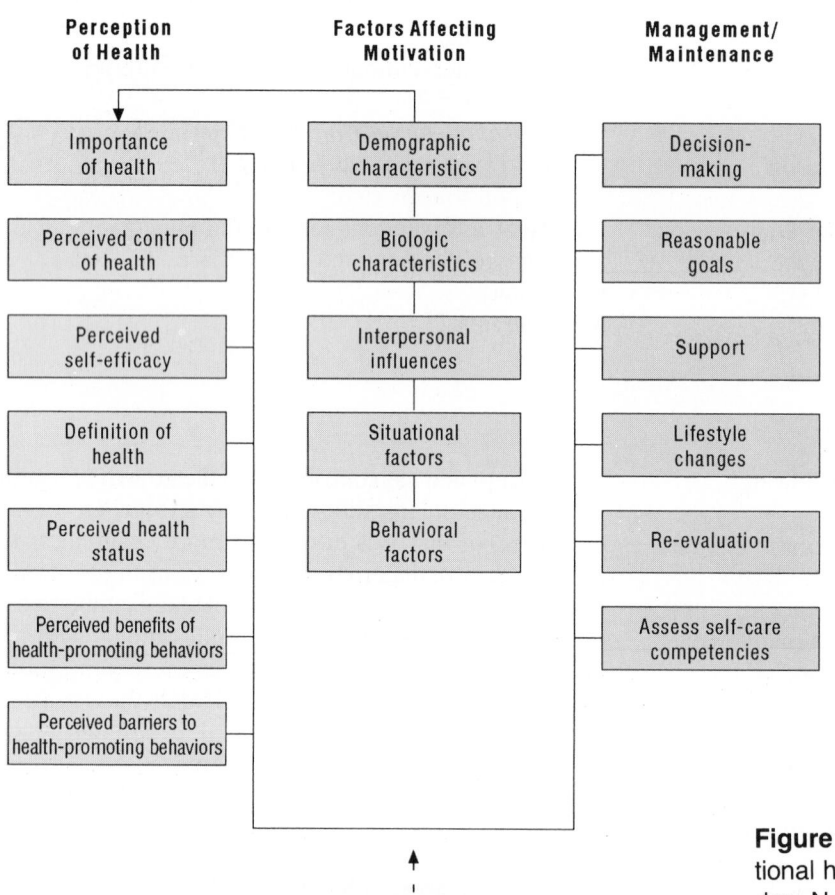

Figure 26–1. Characteristics of normal functional health maintenance. Adapted from Pender, N. (1987). *Health promotion in nursing practice* (2nd ed.). Norwalk, CN: Appleton & Lange.

the person's level of motivation for changing his or her health behaviors. When a person is strongly motivated toward realizing an optimal level of wellness, the person will actively seek the health information, teaching, and activities that help achieve that goal. A person less strongly motivated may not succeed in achieving those goals and behaviors, no matter what the nurse counsels.

Because each person defines health in relation to personal expectations and values, the degree of motivation for change depends on those expectations and values. Motivation is internally generated: although the nurse can support and enhance motivation, the patient is the ultimate determinant.

Biologic capabilities influence both the initiation of motivation in the person and the person's potential for success. For example, even a person who is highly motivated toward a healthy lifestyle with optimal nutrition, regular exercise, and stress management may not succeed in achieving wellness because of the limitations of his or her genetic inheritance.

Management

Reducing health risks is not always easy. Reducing risks usually entails making a decision to change our lifestyle and to break old habits (for instance, quitting smoking, losing weight, controlling alcohol intake, and exercising regularly). Often it is far easier to continue the risky behavior, hoping the worst does not happen. Taking the initiative to change our lives is sometimes motivated by situational factors (such as marriage, pregnancy, or a friend's newly diagnosed lifestyle disease) and new awareness that a behavior is risky.

Once we make the decision and take the initiative to change, setting goals that are realistic and achievable is the next step. Momentary overenthusiasm may cause us to set goals that are unrealistic and difficult to achieve, and this may lead to failure. For example, a man who has a problem controlling his alcohol intake may set the goal of never having another alcoholic drink, but does not seek support and keeps putting himself in situations where he is tempted to drink. For this person, the goal is unrealistic and needs to be modified.

Adapting and adhering to new health behaviors can be trying and frustrating. During the transition, people may need social support to comply with their goals. Social support can be obtained from nurses and other health-team members, friends, family, and support groups such as Alcoholics Anonymous, Weight Watchers, Parents Without Partners, and Parents Anonymous. In some situations changes may be needed in the person's social life. For instance, someone who takes illicit drugs probably has friends who do, too. The person who wants to stop using drugs may need to seek new friends as well as a new lifestyle.

Managing health-maintenance goals is similar to the nursing process: an assessment of the need for change is completed, goals are set, plans for intervention are made, and outcomes are evaluated and reconsidered. The selected health behaviors may be continued, or different health behaviors may be selected if the first selections are not useful or possible.

Normal Functional Health Maintenance

The basic components of health maintenance are health promotion and illness prevention. **Health-promotion activities** are approach behaviors that seek to expand the potential for health; **illness-prevention activities** are avoidance behaviors (Pender, 1987; Duncan & Gold, 1986). Approach behaviors require a decision to make positive changes in an effort to increase our level of wellness. We use avoidance behaviors to avoid illness, rather than to promote health per se. The two behaviors often overlap.

Health Promotion

Put simply, people use health-promotion activities to feel better. Health-promotion behaviors enhance our overall well-being; examples are increasing dietary fiber, avoiding artificial food additives and refined carbohydrates, developing regular patterns of exercise and sleep, controlling stress, seeking wellness information, establishing and maintaining friendships, and being environmentally concerned. People who use health-promotion behaviors want to move beyond the absence of disease in their lives toward high-level wellness by evaluating their lifestyle, learning about options, and striving to become all they can be. Health promotion is not about any particular disease or condition: people using health-promotion behaviors do so to pursue their highest level of wellness, not to prevent a specific disease.

Illness Prevention

People use preventive behaviors to protect themselves from certain diseases or conditions. Illness prevention is targeted at three levels (Table 26-1), but because the third level is directed at restoring health after illness, it is not considered a health-maintenance activity.

Primary illness prevention includes activities and lifestyle factors directed toward high-level wellness, such as adequate nutrition, regular exercise, and stress management. Maintaining health is the primary mode for preventing illness.

Secondary prevention includes screening clinics such as well-child assessments and checks for blood pressure and uterine and breast cancer. The goal of these clinics is to identify abnormalities within a population. The clinics tend to have one focus and refer those with abnormal results elsewhere for follow-up.

TABLE 26–1

Three Levels of Illness Prevention

Level	Description	Examples
Primary prevention	Seeks to prevent a disease or condition at a prepathological state; to stop something from ever happening	Immunizations, fluoride supplements, car seat restraints, oral contraceptives, and education in elementary schools about drug addiction
Secondary prevention	Seeks to identify specific illnesses or conditions at an early stage with prompt intervention to prevent or limit disability; to prevent catastrophic effects that could occur if proper attention and treatment were not provided	Physical assessments, developmental screening, vision screening, breast and testicular self-examinations, pregnancy testing
Tertiary prevention	Occurs after a disease or disability has occurred and the recovery process has begun. Intent is to halt the disease or injury process and assist the individual in obtaining an optimal health status.	Habilitation for handicapped children, support groups such as Reach for Recovery and Alcoholics Anonymous, cardiac rehabilitation, health education for a newly diagnosed diabetic

Combination of Promotion and Prevention

Health-promotion and illness-prevention activities may be difficult to differentiate (Table 26-2). Daily jogging may be a health-promotion behavior for one person and an illness-prevention behavior for another. A person who begins to jog because of a risk of cardiovascular disease and then continues because he feels better may switch from illness-prevention to health-promotion behavior. A person may be involved with health promotion and all three levels of illness prevention. For example, a woman with diabetes mellitus may give herself insulin (tertiary prevention), perform a monthly breast self-examination (secondary prevention), brush her teeth daily (primary prevention), and exercise regularly to feel good (health promotion).

Factors Affecting Health Maintenance

Many factors influence health maintenance, either positively or negatively. These factors affect what people believe about health as well as what healthy and unhealthy practices they perform.

Cognition and Perception. Cognitive and perceptual factors include what health means to a person, how important it is, and how the person perceives control over health, self-efficacy, health status, benefits, and barriers. The more we value health, the more likely we are to participate in health-promoting and health-maintaining behaviors.

Values are influenced by peers, family, and society (Orem, 1980; Pender, 1987; Steiger & Lipson, 1985). A person may believe that health is controlled primarily by himself or herself (internal) or by factors beyond his or her control (external). People with an internal perception of control are more likely to engage in health-seek-

ing behaviors on their own, but people with an external perception of control are more likely to do so with social pressure (Steiger & Lipson, 1985; Pender, 1987; Wernet & Weiss, 1987).

The person's belief about self-efficacy or the ability to accomplish a certain behavior affects his or her willingness to try the behavior. As the person's mastery of behaviors increases, he or she may be more likely to engage in additional activities. Success with one activity can motivate the person to try other activities (Gillett, 1988; Sennott-Miller & Miller, 1987).

People may define health negatively (not being ill) or positively (an optimal state of well-being). That definition influences how the person perceives health and the mechanics of maintaining health (Murray & Zentner, 1985). People who see themselves as having a positive health status may be more likely to continue behaviors that promote and maintain that level of health. However, two people with the same health status may have different perceptions of that health status. Those who see the benefits of health behaviors are more likely to begin or continue those behaviors; those who see the effects as negative or neutral are less likely to do so (Murdaugh & Hinshaw, 1986).

People with a low perceived barrier to health behaviors are more likely to pursue healthy behaviors than those with a high perceived barrier. Barriers can be time, finances, access, convenience, attitude, culture, and social support (Murdaugh & Hinshaw, 1986).

Age and Development. Age may have a significant impact on the person's ability to manage his or her health status. A 25-year-old woman with arthritis or diabetes mellitus may perceive her health status as low and may not engage in proper health-maintenance practices, but an 80-year-old woman might see such conditions as acceptable and might carry out practices to promote optimum health.

TABLE 26–2

Normal Functional Health Maintenance

Health perception and health maintenance	• Has a personal perception of health and all it entails • Has a strong motivation for an optimal level of wellness • Sets health goals and seeks help in managing them • Has sufficient financial resources to maintain health • Maintains a safe environment at home and work • Performs activities of daily living
Nutrition and metabolism	• Has sufficient knowledge of nutrition • Plans daily menu carefully • Obtains and digests appropriate amounts of nutrients to promote optimal nutrition • Protects body against infection • Maintains homeostatic thermoregulation
Elimination	• Maintains a regular schedule for elimination • Understands body processes in digestion and elimination • Practices hygiene after elimination
Activity and exercise	• Maintains good hygiene through self-care • Uses good body mechanics in ADLs • Maintains optimum motor function • Uses leisure hours in a healthy manner • Uses oxygen efficiently
Cognition and perception	• Demonstrates optimum cerebral function • Builds knowledge and skills
Sleep and rest	• Develops quality sensory perception • Maintains a regular sleep pattern • Maintains balance of work and rest • Provides time for relaxation
Self-perception and self-concept	• Displays activities appropriate for developmental level • Demonstrates positive self-concept • Has a stable body image • Recognizes and cherishes personal identity as unqiue • Recognizes uniqueness of other people
Roles and relationships	• Demonstrates functional verbal and nonverbal communication • Participates in social interactions • Builds and maintains meaningful relationships • Has intrinsic mechanisms or support persons to help with coping during grieving
Sexuality and reproduction	• Has valid knowledge about sexual functioning and human sexuality • Accepts sexual functions and sexuality as normal • Recognizes and accepts personal sexual feelings • Maintains healthy lifestyle during pregnancy
Coping and stress tolerance	• Makes decisions reflecting understanding of personal limitations • Protects self against overwhelming situations and changes • Manages to keep in touch with personal needs while balancing life's roles with minimal conflict
Values and beliefs	• Expresses respect for all life and the quality of life • Maintains realistic goals for self based on value decisions • Demonstrates a zeal for life • Provides for spiritual sustenance

Developmental level also affects a person's ability to manage health. Although infants and young children must rely on their parents and guardians for health maintenance, school children can learn proper behaviors and may be able to carry them out independently or with little supervision. Common problems in older adults may also affect health maintenance. For example, loss of teeth may preclude proper nutrition, arthritis may affect the ability to exercise, or slowed cognitive processes may affect safety practices. In these cases, increasing age hinders health maintenance.

Past Experience. A person's past experience with health and the health-care system, both positive and negative, affect health maintenance. If a person had a negative experience with an agency or program, he or she may refuse to participate again even if no alternatives are available. If a particular health practice (for instance, a low-calorie diet) worked well for the patient or a family member in the past, the patient is likely to participate again. Also, a person's health maintenance may be affected by a relative's or friend's experience (for instance, a family history of cancer or a close friend who had a heart attack).

Lifestyle and Habits. A person's lifestyle and habits strongly affect health maintenance. For example, a student living in a dormitory may have a busy school schedule and may work part-time. She may find little time for regular exercise, a balanced diet, and adequate sleep; instead, she grabs vending machine snacks, stays up late studying, and spends her leisure time socializing with friends. A person whose lifestyle conveniently incorporates adequate sleep, exercise, and nutrition may more easily achieve good health maintenance.

Economics. Unfortunately, economics plays a large role in health maintenance. Poor people may be unable to afford nutritious food and adequate housing. They may not receive routine medical care and screenings and may seek health care only when a serious illness develops. Homeless children do not receive immunizations, dental care, or the usual safety and security required for health promotion. Wealthier people have greater financial access to medical care, nutritious food, and preventive programs such as aerobics classes and health lectures.

Culture, Values, and Beliefs. The culture in which a person was raised influences his or her health beliefs and practices, including diet, child-bearing and child-rearing customs, self-medication, and alternate therapies. A language barrier may prevent people from entering the health-care system. Religious beliefs and personal or family values also affect health maintenance. Some people place great value on physical health to achieve spiritual health. Others may have religious beliefs that pro-

hibit certain medical practices and treatments. A belief that health is solely God's will and cannot be altered may hinder health maintenance.

Roles and Relationships. People who are comfortable in their roles and relationships with others often form strong support systems and use available resources to promote health. Having role models and relationships with others who have good health-maintenance practices may benefit one's own health maintenance.

Coping and Stress Tolerance. The coping mechanisms that people use to handle everyday events may help or harm their health. Stress-reducing techniques such as relaxation breathing or imagery promote health; other coping mechanisms, such as denial and use of alcohol, may lead to health problems.

Lifespan Considerations

Health-maintenance opportunities begin before conception and continue until we die. Characteristics of development at various stages call for specific health-maintenance behaviors.

Newborn and Infant

Health maintenance begins during the prenatal period. Low birth weight and congenital defects—which put infants at risk for additional health problems—have been linked to lack of prenatal care, poor nutrition, and use of alcohol and drugs during pregnancy.

Because their immune systems are immature, infants are at risk for infectious diseases, so immunizations are of primary importance. The nervous system develops rapidly and bones, muscles, and other organ systems grow during infancy, so proper nutrition and regular medical check-ups are important.

Toddler and Preschooler

Toddlers and preschoolers develop and learn through exploration and imitation. Curiosity and lack of experience predisposes them to accidents and injuries. Exposure to other children in day-care centers, school, or play groups puts them at risk for infection. Safety practices, proper sleep and nutrition, and regular immunization schedules are important for health maintenance. Toddlers and preschoolers begin to learn healthy and unhealthy practices by imitating their parents.

Child and Adolescent

School children begin to form beliefs about health. They are still primarily influenced by their parents, but teachers and friends become increasingly important. Peer influence is so strong for adolescents that they may

Nursing Research

Selected Nursing Research Studies

Dynes, M. (1988). Orem's model used for health promotion: Directions for research. *Advances in Nursing Science, 11*(1), 13–22.

Gillett, P. (1988). Self-reported factors influencing exercise adherence in overweight women. *Nursing Research, 36*(1), 25–29.

Johnson, C., Nicklas, T., Arbeit, M., et al. (1988). A comprehensive model for maintenance of family health behaviors. The "Heart Smart" family health promotion program. *Family and Community Health, 11*, 1–7.

Speake, D., Cowart, M., & Pellet, K. (1989). Health perceptions and lifestyles of the elderly. *Research in Nursing and Health, 12*, 93–100.

Walker, S., Sechrist, K., & Pender, N. (1987) The health-promoting lifestyle profile: Development and psychometric characteristics. *Nursing Research, 36*(2), 76–81.

Woods, N., Laffrey, S., Duffy, E., et al. (1988). Being healthy: Women images. *Advances in Nursing Science, 11*(1), 36–46.

Possible Topics for Nursing Inquiry

- What are cultural indicators of health-seeking behaviors among families of shool-age children?
- What is the relationship between self-reported health practices and assessments of health states?
- What motivational factors have a correlation with positive health-maintenance behaviors?

adopt unhealthy practices, such as smoking or drinking alcohol, to fit in.

School children may begin to develop problems such as obesity, high cholesterol levels, and poor stress management that can become symptomatic in adulthood. Physical and intellectual development are rapid. Health-maintenance concerns include proper nutrition, sleep, and exercise; safety; and learning to deal with stress and frustration.

Adolescents must deal with sexual development and confirmation of their identity. Peer influence, a struggle for independence, and the physical changes accompanying sexual development make adolescence a time for experimenting with healthy and unhealthy practices. Safe driving, preventing sexually transmitted diseases and pregnancy, avoiding drugs and alcohol, and maintaining mental health are primary health-maintenance concerns during adolescence.

Adult and Older Adult

With rapid physical and intellectual growth completed and health beliefs ingrained, the adult should now enjoy productive and satisfying years. The adult may now be at risk for heart disease, cancer, and stroke, however, depending on his or her health beliefs and practices and genetic factors. The responsibilities of raising a family, holding a job, and being a productive member of society may lead to addictions or stress-related illnesses. Health-maintenance concerns include exercise, nutrition, self-examinations, health screening, stress management, and reduction or cessation of alcohol and smoking.

Health maintenance focuses more on secondary prevention as the adult ages. Exercise, nutrition, social stimulation, and regular medical check-ups are important because of the normal physiologic changes of aging and the increased risk of illness in older adults. Using medications safely and identifying community resources and support groups are also important health-maintenance considerations.

ALTERED HEALTH MAINTENANCE FUNCTION

Potential for Altered Function

Numerous factors, together or separately, may disrupt health maintenance.

Environment

Pollution, nearby highways, lack of safe play areas, inadequate housing, and unsanitary conditions lead to poor health maintenance and set the stage for illness. The work environment may lead to health-maintenance problems if conditions include long working hours, poor ventilation, poor lighting, lack of nutritious food, and sedentary or repetitious tasks.

Poverty

Poverty is often associated with poor health maintenance. Poverty may cause homelessness or may force people to live in overcrowded conditions with poor sanitation and heating. Children may sleep poorly if they share beds with other family members. Nutrition may be inadequate, leading to poor school performance. Unemployment and dropping out of school cause boredom, and boredom and frustration about such conditions often lead to substance abuse and crime. A knowledge deficit about health maintenance, lack of motivation to improve practices, and difficulty obtaining adequate resources are some of the reasons for increased morbidity and mortality rates in the lower socioeconomic group.

Unhealthy Lifestyle and Habits

People with an unhealthy lifestyle and habits are considered to have poor health maintenance. Unhealthy habits include lack of exercise, poor diet (in terms of fiber, cholesterol, fat, and protein content), use of cigarettes, use of alcohol (except in moderation), use of illegal drugs or abuse of prescription drugs, multiple sexual partners, lack of sleep, lack of contraception, poor dental hygiene, and disregard for safety. Although most people can have some unhealthy habits without suffering health problems, all unhealthy habits carry some increased risk for illness. Repeated, multiple unhealthy habits usually lead to at least one preventable health problem.

An example of someone with an unhealthy lifestyle is John Davis, a salesman who works 70 hours a week. He spends most of his time traveling, drinks five to seven cups of coffee daily, and does not exercise. He dines out every night and has a heavy meal, usually of red meat, and three or four cocktails each evening. He is under increasing stress to obtain new clients and smokes two packs of cigarettes a day.

Manifestations of Altered Function

Altered health maintenance may result in mental or physical problems. Common manifestations include chronic illnesses, childhood injuries and developmental problems, and psychosocial disruptions. Some manifestations are the result of prolonged exposure to poor health maintenance (for instance, smoking that leads to lung cancer). However, other conditions may be the result of a one-time exposure, such as the adolescent who becomes pregnant after failing to use contraception just one time.

Chronic Illnesses

Many chronic illnesses have been linked to altered health maintenance. Hypertension and cardiovascular disease are associated with diet, stress, cigarettes, and obesity. The Framingham study identified risk factors for cardiovascular disease that are the basis for most cardiac prevention and rehabilitation programs (Dawber, 1980). Such risk factors as cigarette smoking, sedentary lifestyle, high-cholesterol diet, obesity, and stress can be modified, but family history cannot. People with multiple risk factors are at a much greater risk for coronary artery disease and myocardial infarction.

Cancer has been linked to a number of practices we now consider poor health maintenance, although the exact cause is unknown. A low-fiber diet is associated with colon cancer, cigarette smoking is directly related to lung cancer, and excessive exposure to ultraviolet light causes skin cancer. A direct cause-and-effect relationship has not been established in many cancers, but continuing research will ultimately reinforce health-maintenance beliefs. Practices once considered healthy and desirable (such as eating large amounts of red meat and sunbathing) have now fallen out of favor because of research findings.

Gastrointestinal illnesses are also related to altered health maintenance. Stress contributes to the development of peptic ulcer disease and colitis. Gastritis may be caused by ingesting alcohol and other irritants. Obesity is considered an illness in itself because the person's general health is poor and the risk of other chronic conditions is increased. Obesity may have a genetic component, but is directly related to diet and exercise patterns.

Musculoskeletal and dermatologic illnesses also result from altered health maintenance. Osteoporosis, which often occurs in postmenopausal women, has been linked to inadequate calcium intake during adulthood and lack of exercise as the woman ages. Psoriasis, eczema, and other rashes are aggravated by stress and dietary factors.

Accidents and Injuries

Many accidents and injuries are preventable and are often caused by single episodes of altered health maintenance. They may result when safety practices are disregarded. Accidents, a leading cause of death and disability, include motor-vehicle accidents, falls, drowning, and job-related injuries. Injuries include sprains, strains, fractures, lacerations, burns, and other trauma.

Unwanted pregnancy and transmission of sexually transmitted diseases can be considered accidents as well because they may result when safe sex and contraception practices are disregarded. Adolescents who become pregnant are at higher risk for having babies with low birth weight and additional health problems. Unwanted pregnancies and sexually transmitted diseases can cause psychological distress and may isolate the victim from society.

Childhood and Developmental Problems

Problems that children experience because of altered health maintenance include tooth decay, infectious diseases, growth retardation, and learning difficulties. Tooth decay results from poor dental hygiene and ingesting sugary food and beverages. Infectious diseases such as mumps, measles, rubella, polio, diphtheria, and meningitis result from lack of immunization. Growth retardation and improper neurologic and musculoskeletal development may result from inadequate nutrition. Obesity may begin in infancy from an improper diet. Learning and intellectual development may be slowed by poor nutrition and lack of discipline and sleep.

Psychosocial Problems

Psychosocial problems may result from specific illnesses caused by altered health maintenance, or from a more general loss of well-being. Addiction is both a psychological problem and a physical illness. Behavioral changes often occur in the addict, including abusive and violent behavior, withdrawal, and mood swings. Other psychosocial manifestations of altered health maintenance include anxiety, depression, and social rejection. Anxiety often accompanies unhealthy lifestyles that include stress, excessive caffeine intake, lack of sleep, alcohol consumption, and cigarette smoking. These people worry about their health, but do not improve their health maintenance. Depression may accompany obesity.

Family and friends may reject people who show disregard for their own health. Today, society values people who lead healthy lifestyles. Many smokers feel like outcasts in today's nonsmoking environments.

Impact of Dysfunction on Activities of Daily Living

Altered health maintenance may marginally or greatly affect activities of daily living (ADLs). Poor sleep habits can affect a person's ability to work or a child's school performance. Poor nutrition reduces the energy a person has to carry out ADLs. Ingesting alcohol impairs the drinker's cognitive and physical performance. Cigarette smoking can impair oxygenation and lead to frequent respiratory infections, making ADLs more difficult to perform.

Any illness, injury, or other problem not prevented by health-maintenance activities disrupts a person's usual level of functioning. An athlete, for example, tries to maintain optimum health by getting enough sleep, not smoking, eating a nutritious diet, and doing physical conditioning. Any disruption in these health-maintenance activities would place him or her at a disadvantage in competition. Similarly, anyone with altered health maintenance does not perform ADLs optimally.

ASSESSMENT

The nurse's assessment of a patient's health maintenance tends to be more abstract than other physical assessments such as thermoregulation and respiratory function. The objective of this assessment is to evaluate how well the patient can manage his or her own health behaviors and those of the family, and to identify deficiencies, risks, potential for improvement, and motiva-

tion to change. Information about other functions, such as nutrition, mobility, and values, is used in the health-maintenance assessment. Much of this assessment is done through the health history interview, observations, and validation of self-assessment techniques.

Subjective Data

Subjective data are obtained in an organized interview. During the interview, the nurse should note the patient's verbal and nonverbal communication and should use observation skills to guide the data collection. Subjective data are used to identify the patient's normal functional patterns of health maintenance, risk factors for altered health maintenance, and active health-maintenance dysfunction. Data are collected from sources such as the patient, family members or significant others, parents (if a child), and medical records.

Functional Pattern Identification

All patients can be assessed for health maintenance, even if no problems are suspected. Information on normal patterns of health maintenance helps reinforce the patient's state of health, and information can also be gained on areas that need further work. For example, the nurse may learn while discussing exercise that the patient walks three times a week for 20 minutes and places high value on cardiovascular health. This information could be used to encourage the patient to walk four times a week.

Questions the nurse must answer include (Gordon, 1987):

What is the patient's perception of his or her health status?
How does the patient define health?
What value does the patient place on health?
How could the patient's health be improved?
What is the patient doing to maintain his or her health?
What prevents the patient from engaging in a desired health behavior?
How much control does the patient have over his or her own health?
What is the patient's perceived ability to perform health behaviors?

The patient's perception of his or her health and ability to manage health is important. The nurse should validate all information obtained in this area, because miscommunication can hurt the patient–nurse relationship and can create barriers for health behavior.

Risk Identification

Cues from the nursing history can alert the nurse to risk factors, which are traits that increase the patient's vulnerability to a certain condition or disease. Risk factors can be classified as genetic background, age, biologic characteristics, personal habits, and environment. They vary in intensity, and multiple risk factors may interact to develop additional risk factors (Pender, 1987). The intensity of the risk factor can be modified by behaviors such as dieting, exercising, avoiding tobacco, genetic testing, or leaving a particular environment or situation.

Risk identification can be done with the help of several assessment tools. A computer program called *Healthier People,* developed by the Centers for Disease Control and Emory University, helps the patient and nurse identify risk factors; another computer program, *Health-Predict: Personal Health Analysis,* is available from Compuhealth Associates, St. Louis, Missouri. *The Health Hazard Appraisal* (Health Care Service, Inc., 1981) and *Lifestyle Assessment Questionnaire* (University of Wisconsin at Stevens Point, 1981) are risk appraisals that are sent to the respective company for scoring. A self-test for risk appraisal is *Health Style: A Self-Test,* by the U.S. Department of Health and Human Services, Office of Disease Prevention and Health Promotion (DDHS Publication #D 81-50155).

These risk appraisals are designed to help the patient and nurse identify common threats to health and to motivate behavioral change. Some items are difficult for the patient to answer, however; errors may result if the patient cannot answer or selects an inappropriate answer. These appraisals are not a substitute for a nursing assessment (Berlin, et al., 1990).

Dysfunctional Identification

A dysfunction is any behavior that alters health maintenance. In many cases, the patient perceives the dysfunction and may or may not want to change, or the patient may learn that a behavior is dysfunctional through health education. Many people are unaware of their dysfunctional behavior; for instance, someone immunized in 1965 for measles may not know that adequate immunity was not obtained. As researchers learn more about risks to health, nurses must transmit that information to patients.

Identifying dysfunction goes beyond identifying risk factors. The nurse assesses not only the risk factor, but how that factor has altered the patient's health maintenance. For example, when assessing the patient's diet, the nurse might ask:

How do you feel when you skip breakfast?
Have you had your blood pressure checked since you stopped restricting your salt intake?
I see that you eat two or three eggs each morning for breakfast. Have you ever had your cholesterol level checked? Have you ever had signs of cardiovascular disease, such as chest pain?

By asking such questions and having the patient describe the possible effects of risky practices, the nurse identifies actual health-maintenance dysfunctions.

Objective Data

Objective data include results of the physical assessment and diagnostic tests that focus on general health management and prevention. Objective data are used to identify the patient's health maintenance through screening techniques.

Physical Assessment

There is no specific physical assessment skill for health maintenance; instead, data obtained from the assessments of other functional health patterns are used (Fig. 26-2).. The screening assessments in Table 26-3 can be pooled to comprehensively assess health maintenance.

During the physical assessment, the patient's self-examination skills (for example, breast or testicular self-examination) must be validated to ensure that he or she is effectively performing each skill. Patients who engage in risky behavior should be assessed for their ability to spot potential abnormalities; for example, smokers should be able to perform oral screening, and intravenous drug users should be able to assess for phlebitis.

Many patients have health-assessment equipment at home, such as scales, thermometers, or machines to measure blood pressure or monitor blood glucose levels

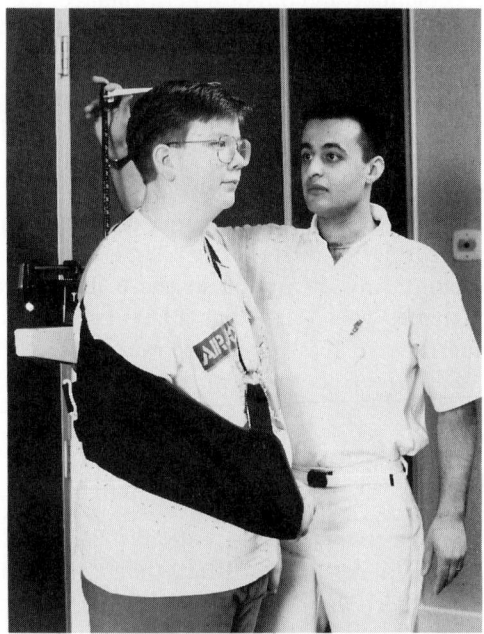

Figure 26–2. The adolescent undergoes a growth spurt, which the nurse monitors as a part of health assessment.

TABLE 26-3

Selected Health Assessment Across the Lifespan

Infant and Preschool Child

Health history and family history: initially and then update as needed.

Vision: *Infancy*—follows objects, corneal light reflex, turn to light

Toddler—cornreal light reflex, cover test

Preschool—Snellen E, screenings as for toddler

Hearing: *Infants*—startle reflex (birth), tracking sounds (3–6 months), recognizes sounds (6–8 months), location of sound (8–12 months)

Preschool—pure tone audiometry beginning at age 4 years. Inability to cooperate and understand instructions hinders this screening in younger children.

Speech: Assess in infancy and early preschool with Denver Developmental Screening Test (DDST) and Denver Articulation Screening Examination (DASE) for children 2.5 to 6 years.

General development: DDST ages newborn to 6 years can be done along with physical assessments.

Congenital hip dislocation: newborn though age 23 months

Blood pressure: before age 1 year, then yearly. Flush technique may be used.

Dental: *Infancy*—presence of teeth and oral care, screening by dentist at age 2 years and then every 6–12 months

General physical assessment: at ages 1, 2, 4, 6, 9, 12, 18, 24 months, then yearly, including height and weight

Urine: phenylketonuria (PKU) before age 4 weeks; glucose and protein at same time as physical assessment

Nutrition: same as for physical assessment

Blood: sickle cell if indicated at 6 months; hemoglobin or hematocrit at 9 months and then every 6 months through 24 months, yearly thereafter

Tuberculin: baseline at 23 months if at risk, secondary to endemic status; repeat before beginning school year

School-Age Child

Health-history: update

Vision: visual acuity every 1–2 years

Hearing: pure tone audiometry ages 6, 8, and 11 years

Dental: assessed by dentist every 6–12 months

General physical assessment: including blood pressure, general development, height, weight, and nutrition every year

Urine: glucose, protein yearly

Blood: hematocrit or hemoglobin every 1–3 years as indicated by nutritional status and history

Tuberculin: if in an at-risk environment, every 1–3 years

Adolescent

Health history: update

Vision: visual acuity every 1–2 years; usually odd year age (i.e., 13, 15)

Hearing: pure tone audiometry ages 14 and 18 years

General physical assessment: including blood pressure, general and sexual development, height, weight, nutrition every 1–2 years

Scoliosis: age 11 and then yearly through age 14 or completion of growth spurts

Self-examination technique: *Girls*—breast at age 14–15 years. *Boys*—testicular at age 14–15 years.

Urine: analysis every 3 years

Blood: hemoglobin or hematocrit every 1–3 years, others as indicated

Dental: by dentist every 6–12 months

Young Adult (19–39 years)

Health history: update as needed

Vision: visual acuity every 1–5 years, glaucoma every 3 years beginning at age 35

Hearing: gross screening yearly

Physical assessment: including risk appraisal, height, weight, and nutrition every 3–5 years

Blood pressure: every 2–3 years

Dental: every 6–12 months

Self-examinations: *Women*—breast every month with professional evaluation every 1–2 years. *Men*—testicular monthly.

Mammogram: women, once between 35 and 39 years

Pap smears: women, every 3 years after two successive normal results

Urine: complete analysis every 5–10 years

Blood: cholesterol every 5–10 years, blood glucose every 10 years, hematocrit—women every 3–5 years, men every 5–10 years

Tuberculosis: establish baseline, repeat as needed if in high-risk environment

Middle Adult (40–60)

Health history: update as needed

Vision: visual acuity every 5 years, glaucoma every 3 years

Hearing: every 3–5 years, more frequently if in noisy environment

General physical assessment: every 2–3 years including height, weight, and nutrition

Blood pressure: every 2–3 years

Dental: every 6–12 months

Women only: self breast examination monthly, with professional evaluation every 1–2 years, mammogram every 1–2 years, Pap smear every 1–3 years

Urine: complete analysis every 5–10 years

Blood: cholesterol, blood glucose, hematocrit every 5 years

Other: stool guaiac yearly, sigmoidoscopy for bowel cancer every 5 years beginning at age 50, baseline EKG, and medication evaluation

Older Adults (60 and over)

Health history: update as needed

Vision: acuity and glaucoma every 2–3 years

Hearing: every 3–5 years

Blood pressure: yearly

General physical assessment: every 2–3 years including height, weight, and nutrition

Cancer screenings: stool guaiac yearly, sigmoidoscopy every 5 years. Women only—cervical/uterine every 1–3 years depending on risk, monthly self breast examination, mammogram yearly. Men only—prostate every 1–2 years.

Urine: complete analysis every 2 years

Blood: chemistry, lipid, and CBC every 2–3 years

Dental: every 6–12 months

Other: EKG as indicated or at risk, medication evaluation

(Fig. 26-3). Inspecting the equipment for accuracy and assessing the patient's ability to use the equipment safely increases the accuracy and reduces the risk of injury or incorrect data. The patient should know what to do with the data obtained: does he or she know normal and abnormal readings? If abnormal data are obtained, when should a professional be consulted?

Diagnostic Tests

Many diagnostic tests can be used to assess health maintenance, including urine tests for protein and glucose, a complete blood count for hematocrit and hemoglobin, an electrocardiogram, a chest x-ray, a stool test for occult blood, and a mammogram (see Table 26-3). Some screening tests may be initiated independently by nurses; others require a physician's order. Some tests are performed on the nursing unit, others in a laboratory. Some, such as cholesterol screening and mammograms, can be obtained from a community agency. Agency policies vary on physician's orders, written consent, and protocols. Nurses should review all diagnostic test results and incorporate them into the health-maintenance assessment.

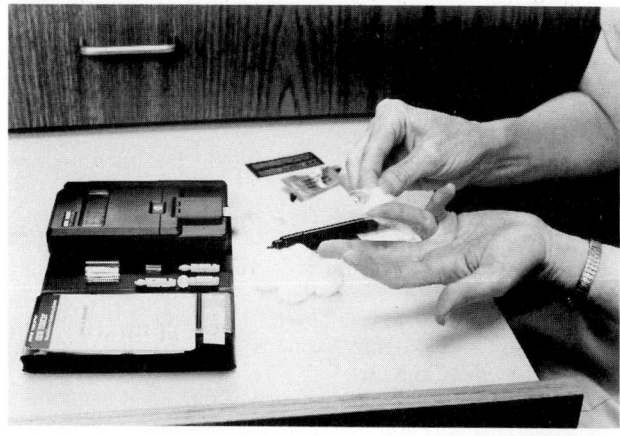

Figure 26–3. Equipment for monitoring blood glucose increases the health-maintenance abilities of the person with diabetes.

NURSING DIAGNOSES AND PATIENT GOALS

NANDA lists two diagnoses of altered health maintenance: Altered Health Maintenance and Health-Seeking Behaviors.

Diagnostic Statement: Altered Health Maintenance

Definition

Altered Health Maintenance is the inability to identify, manage, and/or seek out help to maintain health (NANDA, 1990).

Defining Characteristics

Demonstrated lack of knowledge regarding basic health practices; demonstrated lack of adaptive behaviors to internal/external environmental changes; reported or observed inability to take responsibility for meeting basic health practices in any or all functional pattern areas; history of lack of health-seeking behavior; expressed interest in improving health behaviors; reported or observed lack of equipment, finances, and/or other resources; reported or observed impairment of personal support systems (NANDA, 1990).

Related Factors

Lack of or significant alteration in communication skills (written, verbal, and/or gestural); lack of ability to make deliberate and thoughtful judgments; perceptual/cognitive impairment; ineffective individual coping; dysfunctional grieving; unachieved developmental tasks; ineffective family coping; disabling spiritual distress; lack of material resources (NANDA, 1990).

Diagnostic Statement: Health-Seeking Behaviors

Definition

Health-Seeking Behaviors is a state in which an individual in stable health is actively seeking ways to alter personal health habits and/or the environment to move toward a higher level of health. Stable health status is defined as age-appropriate illness prevention measures achieved; patient reports good or excellent health; and signs and symptoms of disease, if present, are controlled (NANDA, 1990).

Defining Characteristics

Major. Expressed or observed desire to seek a higher level of wellness.

Minor. Expressed or observed desire for increased control of health practice; expression of concern about effect of current environmental conditions on health status; stated or observed unfamiliarity with wellness community resources; demonstrated or observed lack of knowledge in health-promotion behaviors (NANDA, 1990).

Related Nursing Diagnoses

Nursing diagnoses closely related to health maintenance include, High Risk for Infection, High Risk for Injury (trauma, poisoning, suffocation), Knowledge Deficit, and Noncompliance.

Although Knowledge Deficit is an accepted nursing diagnosis, more often it is considered to be a related or contributing factor (Jenny, 1987).

Noncompliance is a situation in which the patient has expressed a desire to comply but does not do so because of barriers or an informed decision not to adhere to recommendations (Carpenito, 1989; McLane, 1987). This nursing diagnosis must be used carefully to ensure that the patient is not labeled "noncompliant" before complete data collection is done.

Patient Goals

Although goals must be individualized for each patient, common goals include the following:

The patient will identify areas for improvement in health maintenance.
The patient will adopt appropriate health-seeking behaviors.
The patient will maintain or improve current health status.

IMPLEMENTATION

The purpose of nursing interventions is to help the patient reach and maintain a desired health status. Most interventions are educational and explore alternatives in health practices. Such education can take place in acute-care settings, the home, school, workplace, or outpatient clinics.

The nurse uses the teaching-learning process to educate the patient about self-care (Fig. 26-4). The nurse shares knowledge with the patient and leads the patient through the learning process. Both nurse and patient should assess the patient's knowledge deficit and set priorities and objectives. The nurse lets the patient set the pace and creates a supportive learning environment. Nurse and patient both evaluate the process by observing progress toward goals.

Nursing Interventions to Promote Health and Function

Nursing interventions to promote proper health maintenance include:

• Educating patients about common illnesses

• Teaching self-examination techniques
• Encouraging routine physicals, health screenings, and immunizations.

Education about Common Illnesses

Teaching patients about common illnesses can help improve health maintenance and prevent illness. Nurses should know how to teach patients about hypertension, heart disease, cancer, osteoporosis, sexually transmitted diseases, lung disease, and childhood infectious diseases. Patient education involves teaching patients about risk factors for and warning signs of common illnesses. Information should be appropriate for the patient's age and likelihood of developing an illness. For example, adults and older adults should be taught about hypertension and heart disease; adolescents and sexually active adults who are not monogamous must be warned about sexually transmitted diseases; young parents should be advised about childhood infectious diseases. Patients can also be referred to agencies such as the American Cancer Society for information.

Hypertension and Heart Disease. Hypertension and heart disease share some risk factors. Patients should be told that the hereditary predisposition cannot be altered, but other risk factors can be altered and can prevent such illness. Eliminating risky behaviors such as smoking, eating a high-fat and high-cholesterol diet, high sodium intake, being overweight, and lack of exercise may pre-

---

Selected Nursing Interventions for Common Problems

Health Promotion

• Explore beliefs regarding health and the patient's expectations.
• Encourage modification of lifestyle through smoking cessation and diet modification.
• Promote a regular program of exercise.
• Identify mechanisms for stress management.
• Teach patient about common illnesses and risk factors appropriate to the age of the patient.
• Encourage routine assessment of health maintenance practices, such as health screening and immunizations.
• Teach patient self-examination techniques for early detection of dysfunction.
• Encourage contact with resources and support services to assist the patient with health maintenance.

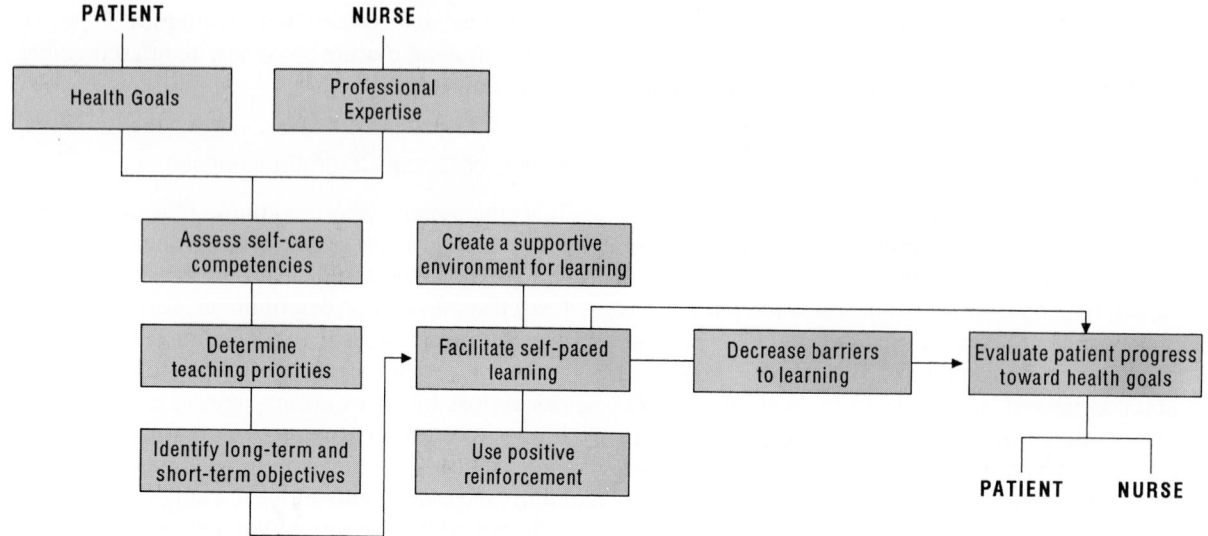

Figure 26–4. The self-care education process. Adapted from Pender, N. (1987). *Health promotion in nursing practice* (2nd ed.) Norwalk, CN: Appleton & Lange, p. 195.

Patient Teaching

Instruct the patient as follows:

- Reduce cholesterol intake by using low-fat dairy products and skim milk, fish, poultry with skin and fat removed, egg whites only, and unsaturated vegetable oils.
- Avoid red meat, egg yolks, fried foods, shellfish, cream sauces and soups, butter, lard, ice cream, and desserts made with whole milk and eggs.
- Avoid constipation by drinking at least eight 8-oz. glasses of fluid a day; increasing fruits, vegetables, and whole grains in diet; establishing regular exercise; and responding to the urge to defecate.
- If a balanced diet is eaten, don't take vitamin and mineral supplements; however, pregnant women and other patients with special needs should consult their physician.
- Perform relaxation breathing by inhaling deeply to the count of 4, holding your breath for 4 seconds, then exhaling to the count of 6. This exercise can be performed anywhere to relieve tension and can be repeated as needed.
- Exercise vigorously (raising the pulse rate) at least three times a week for 20 to 30 minutes to promote cardiovascular fitness. However, stop and consult a doctor for chest pain, dizziness, shortness of breath on mild exertion, or joint or muscle pains that persist.

Symptoms of Myocardial Infarction

Cardinal symptom is persistent chest pain. May be described as heaviness, squeezing, or crushing; may radiate to left side of jaw or neck or left shoulder or arm.

Other Symptoms

- Anxiety
- Dizziness
- Sweating
- Nausea
- Shortness of breath

vent subsequent illness. Healthy diet and exercise information should be given. Patients with one or two risk factors should learn the symptoms of myocardial infarction and should be advised to seek medical attention immediately if they occur, because identification of early signs and prompt medical intervention reduce mortality.

Cancer. Because cancer comes in many forms and can invade virtually any body tissue, there are many risk factors and warning signs. Cancer education and screening programs have traditionally been age- and sex-related, but an increasing number of younger women are suffering breast and lung cancer. Therefore, the nurse must inform a wide variety of patients about the risks and warning signs of cancer; education should begin in

Seven Warning Signs of Cancer
Changes in bowel or bladder habits
A sore that does not heal
Unusual bleeding or discharge
Thickening or lump in breast, testicle, or elsewhere
Indigestion or difficulty swallowing
Obvious change in wart or mole
Nagging cough or hoarseness

childhood and carry on into old age. Risks include diet, sun exposure, cigarette smoking, exposure to asbestos, and pollution. Patients should be taught practices that are believed to prevent cancer, such as eating a high-fiber diet, using sunscreen, and avoiding chemical products associated with cancer.

Osteoporosis. Patients, especially women, should be taught that practices to prevent osteoporosis begin in childhood with adequate calcium intake. Calcium intake must be maintained throughout adulthood. Older women should learn the importance of weight-bearing exercise and estrogen replacement (for postmenopausal women) to decrease bone decalcification.

Self-Examination Techniques

Self-examination of the breasts, testicles, and skin are important health-maintenance practices. They should be started by age 18, but patients can be taught the techniques earlier if they want to learn. Education includes a demonstration by the nurse and a return demonstration by the patient to ensure competency. Patients should know what they are looking for, and should learn that breast and testicular masses may be benign or malignant. Any mass, no matter how small, should be brought to the physician's attention to aid in early diagnosis and treatment. Skin lesions that do not heal, are multicolored, or change color, shape, or texture are suspicious. Skin cancers occur often in sun-exposed areas and in people with fair complexions, but everyone should carefully inspect all skin surfaces. See Chapter 48 for more information on breast and testicular self-examination.

Routine Health Care

Part of health maintenance is the routine assessment by health-care providers. Well-baby visits, yearly physicals, prenatal care, health screenings, and immunization programs are examples of routine health care. These visits can identify areas of strength and weakness in health maintenance, and education can be provided to improve

health-maintenance practices, if necessary. The content of the physical examination may vary according to the patient's age, family history, and previous health status. The nurse should encourage patients to comply with routine health-care visits and to seek care sooner if problems arise.

Health screenings include blood pressure measurement, cholesterol screening, blood sugar testing, vision and hearing assessment, obesity screening, and stool testing for blood. Screenings are often aimed at high-risk populations, but all patients should be encouraged to participate. Screenings take place in hospitals, physicians' offices, clinics, schools, workplaces, community agencies, and even shopping malls. The nurse can provide information about screenings and the implications of their results.

Immunization programs are health-maintenance concerns for children and adults (Fig. 26-5). All new parents should be familiar with the immunization schedule for their children; adults often do not realize that children need periodic immunizations for protection from specific infectious diseases throughout their lifespan. The nurse should review immunization histories, particularly for tetanus, rubella, and measles, and advise patients appropriately.

Nursing Interventions for Altered Function

Nursing interventions for altered function also tend to be educational in nature and may include information about smoking cessation, diet modification, exercise programs, stress management, and alcohol and drug rehabilitation. The nurse may lead a program on smoking cessation or diet modification, for example, or may simply provide background information and referrals to such programs.

The primary nursing goal is to help the patient assume responsibility for self-care in these areas. To help a

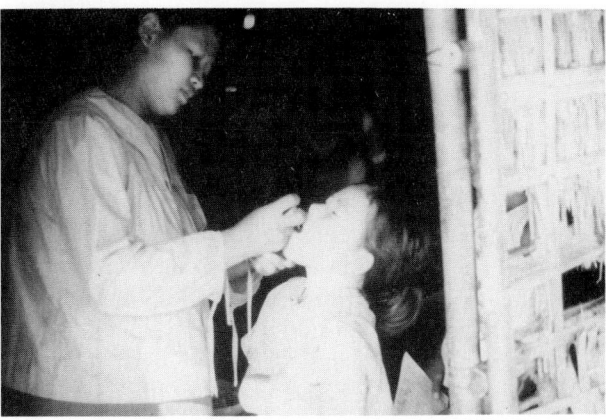

Figure 26–5. A refugee worker administers polio vaccine in a refugee camp school, Khao I Dang, Thailand. (Photo courtesy Sherry Riddick.)

patient assume responsibility, the nurse not only imparts knowledge but also may need to change the patient's attitudes and instill motivation. Motivation to change may be increased by teaching the patient the potential outcomes of altered health-maintenance practices. The nurse also provides emotional support to patients making changes in their health maintenance.

Interventions also address related and contributing factors as a way to correct the disruption. Barriers to health protection and promotion (such as misinformation or lack of transportation or health insurance) guide the type of interventions used. A patient with financial problems can be referred to a public clinic and the Department of Social Services. Giving the patient information about public or volunteer transportation may solve transportation problems. Patients who cannot afford an exercise or diet program may borrow books and videotapes from a public library or attend free community lectures.

Discharge Planning and Home Care

By discharge, the patient or caregiver should be able to competently manage the patient's health needs. Discharge planning begins during the admission process. The nursing management plan should reflect the patient's educational needs for discharge. Goals are set and prioritized so that essential information is taught first and reinforced during the hospitalization. Nurses can enlist the help of other members of the health-care team, such as a dietitian to help with meal planning or a clinical nurse specialist to provide information on smoking cessation. Family members and significant others must be included in the teaching so that they can offer support after discharge. Reference materials such as printed menus for a low-cholesterol diet should be provided.

If the patient needs extensive care or continuing help, additional interventions are indicated; for instance, the patient may be referred to a home-health agency for in-home nursing assistance. Home-health nurses can help patients to monitor their health status and to manage diet and exercise. Often, however, patients can take responsibility for health maintenance with additional support and contact with the health-care provider or referral agency on an outpatient basis. A home-health nurse or public-health nurse may assist the patient who is learning new skills or who needs reinforcement or continuation of learning.

EVALUATION

Nursing interventions related to health maintenance are successful if the nurse and patient agree that progress has been made toward the identified goals. Progress is easily measured by establishing outcome criteria. The following are general goals and outcome criteria for patients with altered health maintenance, although goals and outcome criteria are always individualized.

Goal
Patient will identify areas for improvement in health maintenance.

Possible Outcome Criteria

Patient identifies at least three problems in health maintenance (e.g., overweight, sedentary lifestyle, cholesterol level above normal) by this afternoon.

Goal
The patient will adopt appropriate health-seeking behaviors.

Possible Outcome Criteria
- Patient asks for information about weight-loss programs at the next meeting.
- At the next meeting, patient reports scheduling walks for 30 minutes four times a week.
- At the next meeting, patient uses the stairs instead of the elevator and parks his or her car in the lot rather than using valet parking.
- Patient and spouse read a complete book on low-cholesterol diets within the next week.
- Patient says he or she will eliminate high cholesterol foods from diet beginning immediately.

Goal
The patient will maintain or improve current health status.

Safety Alert

- Advise patients beginning exercise programs to start slowly and proceed cautiously, never overexerting themselves. Pregnant patients and those with a history of cardiac problems, diabetes, arthritis, or hypertension should consult their physician before initiating an exercise program.
- Advise patients that dieting for weight loss must sill meet the patient's nutritional needs. Make sure meals contain foods from all five groups (meat, breads, fruits, vegetables, and dairy products) and that no meals are skipped.
- Warn patients against trying fad diets, exercise regimens, or other advertised "health" products or services that offer quick results. They are often a waste or money and may be dangerous.

Possible Outcome Criteria
- Patient loses 5 pounds in 3 weeks.
- Patient says he or she feels better and has more energy in 3 weeks.
- Patient reduces his or her cholesterol level by 10% in 1 month.

If no progress towards the goal occurs, the nurse and patient need to reassess the goal. Conclusions may be:

- The goal was too difficult to attain, and appropriate adjustments should be made.
- The patient did not want the goal, but agreed to it out of courtesy or because of intimidation or fear.
- Barriers exist, and interventions are needed to reduce them.
- The goal was established without the patient's knowledge.
- The goal was established on insufficient information; additional information is needed to establish a desired goal.

After conclusions are reached, the patient and nurse can then mutually decide whether to readjust previous goals, establish new goals, or terminate goals related to health maintenance.

Key Concepts

- Health-maintenance activities are those behaviors that the person in a stable state of health uses to maintain or improve that state of health over time.
- A person's ability to maintain health depends on his or her perception of health, motivation to change, and adherence to management goals.
- How a person perceives health depends on personal, cultural, and religious beliefs.
- Health promotion and illness prevention are components of health maintenance. Health promotion is characterized by approach behaviors, illness prevention by avoidance behaviors.
- Environmental factors, poverty, and unhealthy lifestyle and habits create a potential for altered health maintenance.
- The manifestations of altered health maintenance are chronic illnesses, accidents and injuries, childhood

---

Nursing Management Plan
The Patient with Health-Seeking Behavior

Nursing Diagnosis: Health-seeking behaviors as evidenced by lack of knowledge of testicular self-examination and a desire to learn.

Patient Goal: Patient will learn testicular self-examination techniques.

Patient Outcome Criteria

- Patient lists risks of and needs for regular self-examinations immediately after nurse's explanations.
- Patient demonstrates effective self-assessment skills on return demonstration immediately after instruction.
- Patient distinguishes normal from abnormal findings in discussion with nurse immediately after teaching session.
- Patient performs monthly assessments as reported back to nurse at regular examinations.

Nursing Intervention	Scientific Rationale

1. Develop a teaching plan
   a. Testicular cancer rates, risks, and survivor rates when treated early
   b. Skill
   c. Normal and abnormal findings
	1. Individualized teaching plans meet unique learning needs as related to the diagnosis.

2. Provide written material for information	2. To allow patient to refer back to material and not rely on memory alone
3. Demonstrate skill initially and on return	3. Demonstration aids in learning of new skills whereas return demonstration aids in validating proficiency of skill acquisition
4. Assess performance with routine assessments	4. Reinforces need for health-promoting behavior

and developmental problems, and psychosocial problems.

- Two categories of alteration in health maintenance are approved by NANDA as nursing diagnoses: Altered Health Maintenance and Health-Seeking Behaviors.
- The nurse can diagnose and treat health maintenance alterations; most nursing interventions involve patient teaching of appropriate health behaviors and knowledge to manage self-care.
- Nursing interventions to promote health and function include education about risk factors for and warning signs of common illnesses.
- Routine health care including prenatal care, well-baby visits, immunizations, yearly physicals, and health screenings can be nursing interventions to promote health and function.

References

Berlin, J., Thorington, B., McKinlay, J., et al. (1990). The accuracy of substitution rules for health risk appraisals. *American Journal of Health Promotion, 4*(3), 214–219.

Carpenito, L. (1992). *Nursing diagnosis: Application to clinical practice* (4th ed.). Philadelphia: J. B. Lippincott.

Dawber, T. R. (1980). The Framingham study: The epidemiology of atherosclerotic disease. Cambridge: Harvard University Press.

Duncan, D., & Gold, R. (1986). Health promotion: What is it? *Health Values, Achieving High-Level Wellness, 10*(3), 47–48.

Edelman, C., & Mandle, C. (1986). *Health promotion throughout the lifespan.* St. Louis: C. V. Mosby.

Gallagher, L., & Kreidler, M. (1987). *Nursing and health: Maximizing human potential throughout the life cycle.* Norwalk, CN: Appleton & Lange.

Gillett, P. (1988). Self-reported factors influencing exercise adherence in overweight women. *Nursing Research, 37*(1), 25–29.

Gordon, M. (1991). *Manual of nursing diagnosis: 1991–1992.* New York: McGraw-Hill.

Hill, L., & Smith, N. (1985). *Self-care nursing.* Englewood Cliffs, NJ: Prentice-Hall.

Jenny, J. (1987). Knowledge deficit: Not a nursing diagnosis. *Image, 19*(4), 184–185.

McLane, A. (Ed.). (1987). *Classification of nursing diagnoses: Proceedings of the seventh conference.* St. Louis: C. V. Mosby.

Murdaugh, C., & Hinshaw, A. (1986). Theoretical model testing to identify personality variables affecting preventive behaviors. *Nursing Research, 35*(1), 19–23.

Murray, R., & Zentner, J. (1985). *Nursing assessment and health promotion through the lifespan* (3rd ed.). Englewood Cliffs, NJ: Prentice-Hall.

Murray, R., & Zentner, J. (1985). *Nursing concepts for health promotion* (3rd ed.). Englewood Cliffs, NJ: Prentice-Hall.

NANDA (1990). *Taxonomy I revised 1990, with official nursing diagnoses.* St. Louis, MO: North American Nursing Diagnosis Association.

Pender, N. (1987). *Health promotion in nursing practice* (2nd ed.). Norwalk, CN: Appleton & Lange.

Pender, N. (1987b). Health and health promotion: The conceptual dilemmas. In M. Duffy & N. Pender (Eds.), *Conceptual issues in health promotion: A report of proceedings of a Wingspan Conference.* Indianapolis: Sigma Theta Tau International.

Pender, N., & Pender, A. (1986). Attitudes, subjective norms, and intentions to engage in health behaviors. *Nursing Research, 35*(1), 15–18.

Richmond, J. (1979). *Healthy people.* Washington, DC: U. S. Government Printing Office, DHEW (PHS) Publication No. 79-55071.

Sennott-Miller, L., & Miller, J. (1987). Difficulty: A neglected factor in health promotion. *Nursing Research, 36*(5), 268–272.

Smith, J. (1983). *The ideal of health: Implications for the nursing profession.* New York: Teachers College Press.

Steiger, N., & Lipson, J. (1985). *Self-care nursing: Theory and practice.* Bowie, MD: Brady Communications.

World Health Organization. (1947). The constitution of the World Health Organization. *World Health Organization Chronicles,* 1:29.

Young, W. (1987). *Introduction to nursing concepts.* Norwalk, CN: Appleton & Lange.

Zindler-Wernet, P., & Weiss, S. (1987). Health locus of control and preventive health behavior. *Western Journal of Nursing Research, 9*(2), 160–175.

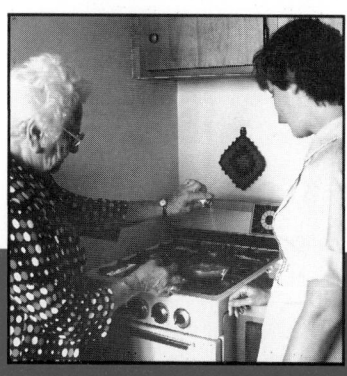

Home Maintenance Management

27

Normal Home Maintenance Management
  Environment
  Characteristics of Normal Home Maintenance
      Management
    Balance
    Growth Promotion
    Resources and Support Systems
  Normal Home Maintenance Functional Pattern
  Factors Affecting Home Maintenance Management
    Health Promotion and Safety
    Cognition and Perception
    Mobility
    Nutrition
    Elimination
    Roles and Relationships
    Coping and Stress Tolerance
    Lifestyle and Habits
    Economic Resources
    Family and Social Supports
    Community Resources
  Lifespan Considerations
Altered Home Maintenance Management
  Potential for Altered Home Maintenance
      Management
    Health Promotion and Safety Deficits
    Cognitive and Sensory Deficits
    Decreased Mobility
    Altered Nutrition
    Insufficient Family or Social Supports
    Insufficient Community Resources
  Manifestations of Altered Home Maintenance
      Management
    Verbal Expression
    Inability to Function Safely
    Lack of External Supports and Resources
    Family Stress

Poor Environmental Conditions
    Homelessness
Assessment
  Subjective Data
    Functional Pattern Identification
    Risk Identification
    Dysfunctional Identification
  Objective Data
    Functional Deficits
    Home Assessment
    Community Resource Assessment
Nursing Diagnoses and Patient Goals
  Diagnostic Statement: Impaired Home
      Maintenance Management
    Definition
    Defining Characteristics
    Related Factors
  Related Nursing Diagnoses
  Patient Goals
Implementation
  Nursing Interventions to Promote Health and
      Function
    Enhancement Internal Resources
    Patient Teaching
    Discharge Planning
  Nursing Interventions for Altered Home
      Maintenance Management
    Health-Care Options and Placement
    Contracting
    Resources
    *Discharge Planning in Impaired Home
        Maintenance Management*
      Home Care
      Community Support
Evaluation
Key Concepts

All of us have a perception of ourselves in relation to the world and of our ability to maintain ourselves in that world. Independence is often linked to the ability to manage and care for ourselves at home. *Home maintenance management* (HMM) is the ability to independently maintain a safe, growth-promoting immediate environment. This involves the ability to care for our basic needs and to manage the complex activities necessary for independent functioning in our highly complex society.

The example of a young single mother with two children living in a two-bedroom apartment in the suburb of a large Midwestern city will illustrate this concept. Many factors are important in enabling independent management for this mother. A safe, affordable shelter is required. Adequate financial resources are necessary to purchase food, clothing, and medical care and to pay for utilities. Household tasks such as cleaning and washing clothes are important in maintaining a healthy environment. The mother must be able to perform normal daily activities such as hygiene, cooking, dressing, and grooming, not only for herself but also for her children. Mobility, or the ability to move freely both within and outside the home environment, is important to perform many necessary tasks. The cognitive ability to understand how to organize work, manage financial responsibilities, and ensure safety within the home is essential. Transportation is necessary to purchase food, keep appointments within the community, and participate in social activities.

Alterations in health often affect a person's ability to manage independently at home. Sometimes independence can be maintained with adequate support from the family or the community. For example, a 68-year-old woman may be able to return to her home after surgery if her daughter stays with her for the first week. In more complex situations, many community resources may be needed to support independent living at home. When home management is no longer feasible, the patient may need to be placed in a facility to provide adequate support.

As a person moves or is moved from one environment to another, it is important to consider his or her ability to carry out functions of daily living in the new environment. Understanding the person in relation to the home or other living environment is important in developing plans for care that maximize the person's ability to maintain himself or herself in a safe home environment.

NORMAL HOME MAINTENANCE MANAGEMENT

Environment

A person's *environment* is his or her physical, psychological, or social surroundings. It may be the hospital room, the home, the neighborhood, the family, or a support system of friends. To maintain a safe, growth-promoting environment, the person must have adequate shelter, adequate nutrition, a safe environment, and nurturing to allow for growth. This ability is complex and dynamic.

Characteristics of Normal Home Maintenance Management

Balance

HMM is influenced by a balance between what the person *needs* to do and what the person can do for himself or herself. The person must be able to perform both **activities of daily living** (ADLs), such as bathing, grooming, dressing, feeding, and toileting, and **demands of daily living** (DDLs), such as responsibilities (self-imposed or imposed by others) for housing, pets, job, or home environment. Internal resources (e.g., strength, knowledge, endurance, and motivation) and external resources (e.g., friends, family, money, or professional services) are available to each person. Carnevali's balance model (Fig. 27-1) shows how ADLs and DDLs need to be balanced with internal and external resources (Carnevali, 1984). Also important to this balance is the relationship between the person's competence and the demands of an activity (Lawton, 1985). For instance,

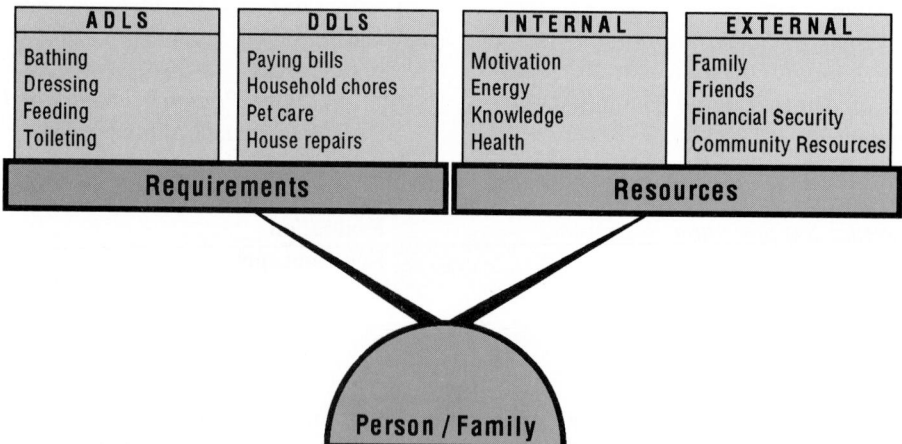

Figure 27–1. Balance model, showing the need to balance requirements (ADLs, DDLs) and resources (internal and external) to achieve home maintenance management.

does the person have the knowledge to perform ADLs? The strength?

Another model, the person and environment fit model, also helps us understand HMM (Fig. 27-2). This model emphasizes the importance of how well a person and his or her environment are matched. For example, a child in a friendly preschool environment is matched well with the activities and general surroundings. The child appears to fit well into this environment.

Growth Promotion

A safe home environment provides basic needs such as shelter, nutrition, safety, and nurturing to allow growth. This growth includes all family members. Depending on the family, the environmental needs may vary: growth promotion for a toddler differs from growth promotion for a wheelchair-bound person. In some families, there may be a variety of needs over several generations.

Resources and Support Systems

Resources include both internal and external ones, as discussed above. A homemaker, for instance, must have strength to lift and move objects; a knowledge of safety, cleanliness, and nutrition; physical and emotional endurance; patience; and motivation to perform ADLs and DDLs. External resources include family members who cooperate; friends for emotional support; money to buy food, clothing, cleaning materials, and transportation; and professional services as needed.

Support systems can include community agencies and organizations that provide needed services. Police and fire services are necessary for a safe community. Transportation to shops, medical services, and entertainment can be provided for the person who cannot provide his or her own transportation. Meals on Wheels brings food to the homebound and the elderly. Churches and synagogues provide a variety of support services.

Rubenstein (1985) noted that the "presence of social supports is necessary for most individuals so that they may live their lives as they wish." Similarly, Horowitz (1985) commented that "older people give as well as receive services from their families and a balanced exchange characterizes the majority of intergenerational relations at any point in time."

Normal Home Maintenance Functional Pattern

Normal HMM occurs when a person can independently maintain a growth-promoting environment. The home is comfortable and safe, and the person performs self-care and hygiene tasks, interacts with others, meets financial obligations, and engages in activities from which he or

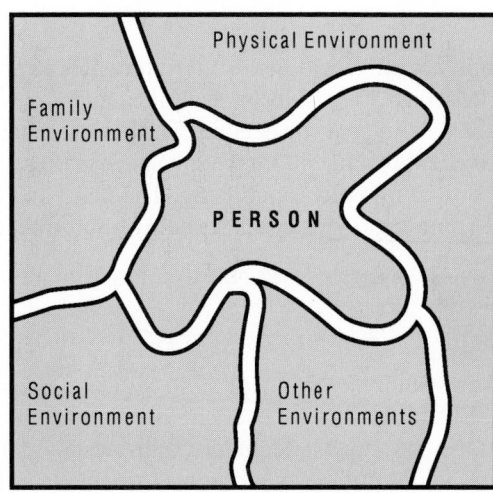

Figure 27–2. Person and environment fit model illustrates the importance of environment–person match for home maintenance management.

she derives personal enjoyment and a sense of worth. Although some people may have personal deficits, they can adjust to their situation through their own resourcefulness or the assistance of others.

Factors Affecting Home Maintenance Management

Internal resources (a person's functional abilities) and external resources (family and social supports and community resources) affect a person's ability to manage successfully in the home. For more detailed information, see the appropriate clinical chapters throughout this textbook.

Health Promotion and Safety

Living at home requires continual attention to promoting one's own health in whatever way is appropriate. For a healthy adult, that may mean exercising three times a week; for a person with advanced respiratory disease, it may mean taking medication and breathing as instructed. Maintaining a safe environment by reducing the potential for injury is essential for living at home.

Cognition and Perception

The ability to interpret sensory cues and problem-solve appropriately are critical for living at home. Cognitive ability is needed to process the information presented in patient teaching. Hearing, sight, touch, and smell are important in maintaining orientation and in interacting effectively with others and the environment.

Mobility

The ability to move within the environment is important in HMM (Fig. 27-3). Mechanical aids, such as wheelchairs or walkers, may be needed. The patient must have enough strength and endurance to engage in those activities essential for daily functioning. The heart and lungs must be able to provide enough energy for normal activities.

Nutrition

A person's ability to buy, cook, and eat nutritious meals is another factor in independent home management. The ability to chew adequately and swallow so that aspiration does not occur promotes safe intake of food. The person's desire and motivation to eat and to follow a recommended diet are also important.

Elimination

The ability to independently manage toileting (getting to the bathroom facilities, managing clothing, lowering oneself safely onto the toilet, cleaning the perineal area, and washing one's hands) is important in HMM. Lack of bowel or bladder control requires additional resources if the patient is to remain at home.

Roles and Relationships

People need to be able to communicate needs and desires to others to meet many demands of living and to mobilize external resources. Communication is important within the family to foster positive relationships and promote self-esteem. Social isolation can occur when communication is limited.

Coping and Stress Tolerance

Coping ability is important, especially in our complex world. Think for a moment how a simple task such as shopping for groceries has grown in complexity, now that many stores offer dozens of choices in each food category. The ability to cope with day-to-day stresses in a way that promotes safety and growth fosters the ability to manage independently at home.

Lifestyle and Habits

There is great variability in expectations regarding HMM. For example, one family may value a spotless home; another may feel more comfortable with clutter. One family may eat home-cooked meals together; another may eat out often or snack during the day. Some families have a traditional approach to HMM, in which the mother cooks and does housework and the father does home repairs, mows the lawn, and takes out gar-

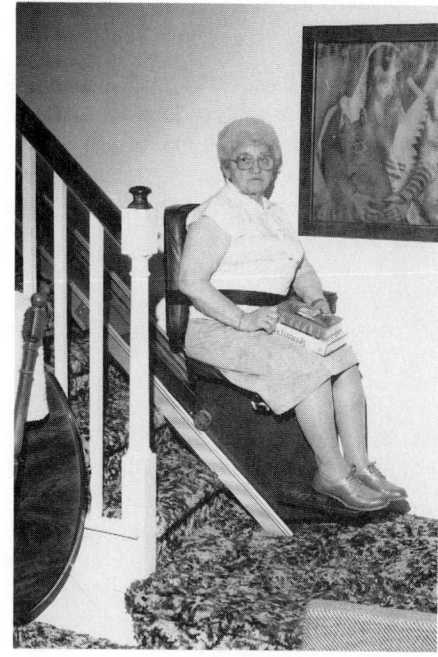

Figure 27–3. This woman with arthritis and a heart condition can manage living in a two-floor house because she uses a "Stair Ride."

bage. Often these expectations are learned early in life from the family and community.

Economic Resources

Money is needed for such necessities as food, clothing, and shelter. Appropriate money management, such as paying bills on time and budgeting, is an important skill. A steady source of income offers security that allows planning and fosters HMM.

Family and Social Supports

Family and friends become important external resources for people with deficits in functional abilities. Family members or friends can volunteer to provide services: for example, children may shop for an elderly relative, cut the grass, and do home repairs. When functional deficits are great, the support must increase. A family member may come every day to prepare meals and supervise daily activities.

Community Resources

The availability, accessibility, and acceptability of technical and professional resources in the community can affect HMM. Services such as hospice care, home health care, a crisis telephone line, a business that rents hospital equipment, and Meals on Wheels affect the person–environment fit and thus are important in HMM.

If functional deficits can be counterbalanced with appropriate community services, the effect on HMM is decreased. A resource-rich community with, for instance, support services for family caregivers and programs to transport wheelchair-bound people provides extra support to keep patients at home.

Lifespan Considerations

Age and developmental level affect HMM. As people mature, they acquire skills and abilities to permit greater independence in HMM.

Newborn and Infant

Newborns and infants depend on their caregivers for all their basic needs and for a safe environment in which they can grow and develop. The birth of a child can add stress to the family, making HMM more difficult for the parents. A mother coming home from the hospital with her newborn may be depleted of internal resources, limiting the energy she has to perform household chores and to care for herself and her infant. This is a time when using external resources (such as the father, grandparents, or neighbors) can keep the house running smoothly and allow the mother to care for and nurture the infant properly.

Toddler and Preschooler

Tremendous physical growth occurs in the first few years of life, which allows the young child to move around more purposefully in the environment and communicate needs more clearly. Independence in a home environment is still not feasible for this age group. Children learn by actively exploring their surroundings, and their environment needs to be made safe so that injuries do not occur. Physical maturation permits the toddler, and especially the preschooler, to perform some ADLs independently, such as eating, toileting, and dressing (Fig. 27-4). Assistance may still be needed with bathing, fastening buttons, doing up zippers, and tying shoes.

Some children in this age group are given increased responsibility around the house. Usually this starts with simple tasks such as putting away toys. Some parents also encourage young children to participate in household chores such as feeding pets or emptying wastebaskets. Such chores help set the stage for further responsibility for home maintenance management at later ages.

Child and Adolescent

The school-age child has independent self-care skills and usually assumes greater responsibility for household chores. In many families, everyone participates in tasks. Chores appropriate for a school-age child include keep-

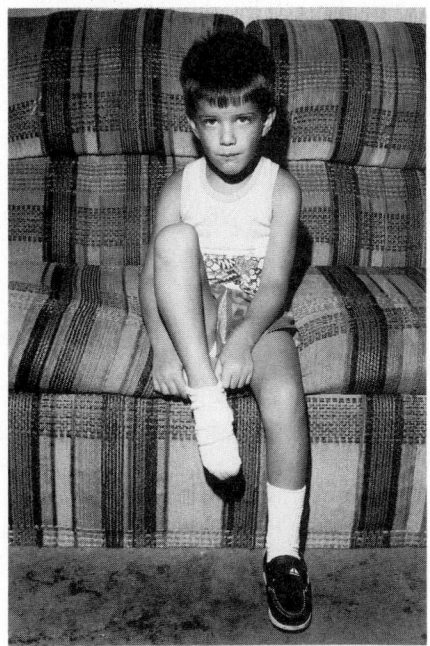

Figure 27–4. Preschoolers learn to dress themselves.

ing his or her room tidy, helping with the dishes or setting the table, vacuuming, sweeping, dusting, doing yard work, and caring for pets. Some children show an interest in food preparation and may work with an adult to help prepare meals. Children can often independently prepare simple meals that do not need cooking, such as sandwiches. In some families children receive allowances, which helps them learn how to manage money responsibly.

As the child approaches adolescence, greater independence is achieved. The preadolescent or adolescent may stay home alone while parents are away or working. The number of children left to manage independently has increased dramatically in recent years, as more mothers have joined the work force. Guidelines about what the child may do and how to handle emergencies should be made clear.

Adolescents may begin to work outside the home, often as papercarriers or babysitters. When babysitting, the adolescent is responsible for maintaining a safe environment for others. Getting a driver's license is another rite of passage that may increase the adolescent's responsibility, because he or she can run errands, go to a job, and get to appointments.

Some adolescents are legally emancipated and do not live with their parents. In such situations several concerns arise. The adolescent's cognitive and developmental abilities may not be balanced with HMM tasks. Family situations may support or hinder the adolescent's ability to manage independently. Often adolescents flee a negative home situation in which there was abuse and little opportunity to learn management skills, or a young woman who is pregnant may feel forced out of her parents' home. Adolescents may find it impossible to stay in school and support themselves financially. With limited education, any jobs the adolescent may get are low-paying and offer few benefits such as medical insurance.

Adult and Older Adult

A developmental task of early adulthood is to emancipate from parents, which usually means moving away. Often this occurs for the first time when the young person leaves for college or the armed services or gets a full-time job. The young adult must master many tasks, such as shopping for food, cooking, balancing a checkbook, and buying and maintaining a car. In recent years, there has been a trend toward delayed emancipation; some adults live with their parents into their 30s. Adult children often move back into their parents' home after a divorce or financial setback.

During early adulthood, marriage and the birth of children add to the complexity of HMM. Buying a house also brings many new responsibilities. Health for many young adults is usually good, so HMM is relatively easy and uncomplicated.

As children grow and leave home, parents may need to move to a smaller house or apartment to lighten their HMM responsibilities. Retirement may cause financial burdens that affect HMM. As the adult ages, chronic health conditions that hinder the ability to manage independently in the home become more common. Cognitive changes may impair safety, especially when the older person lives alone.

According to a 1989 survey, more than 20% of adults over age 65 have difficulty with at least one ADL or with walking. With increased age, especially over 80 years, difficulties with ADLs increase dramatically. Bathing is the most common ADL problem, followed by transferring between bed and chair, dressing, toileting, and feeding (DHHS, 1990a).

ALTERED HOME MAINTENANCE MANAGEMENT

Altered HMM may occur as a result of decreased functional abilities, insufficient family or social supports, or insufficient community resources. For each condition across the life span, prevalence (the number of people with the condition) may be high although incidence (the number of new cases of the condition) is low because of the longevity of the health problem.

Figure 27-5 shows that the total number of Americans needing home care increases with age. The high prevalence of physical conditions in the elderly has implications for the development of long-term nurse–patient relationships and for continuity of care in the health-care delivery system.

Potential for Altered Home Maintenance Management

Physical deficits or chronic debilitating diseases that decrease the patient's ability to perform ADLs can lead to difficulty in managing a home (Carpenito, 1989). Factors affecting the ability to manage at home include the medical diagnosis of a chronic debilitating or limiting condition, the medical prognosis for the condition, and the need for treatments and complex medication regimens.

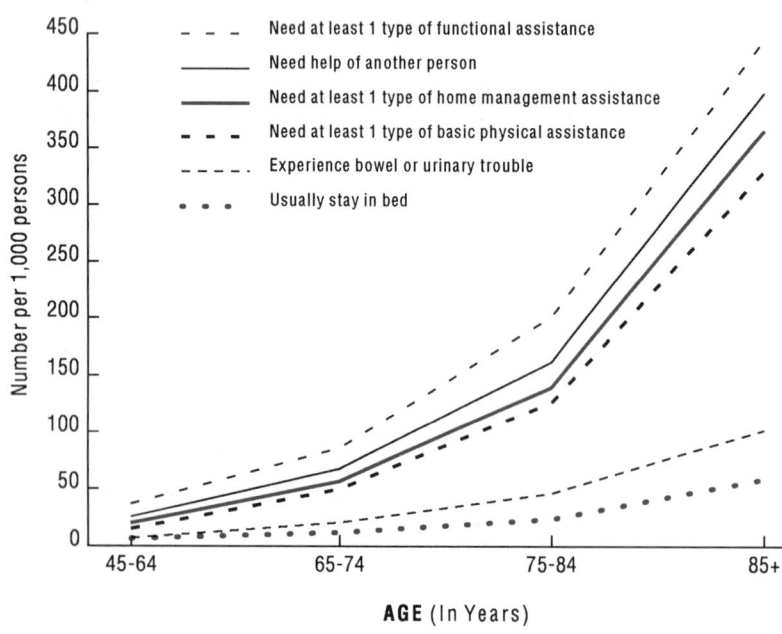

Figure 27–5. The number of people who need home care per 1000 adults 45 years of age or over. From U.S. Department of Health and Human Services. (1986). *Americans needing home care, United States. Vital and Health Statistics, Series 10, No. 153. DHHS Publication No. 86-1581. Hyattsville, MD; National Center for Health Statistics.*

Health Promotion and Safety Deficits

Injury potential, alterations in health maintenance, and knowledge deficit regarding self-care procedures are important in HMM. Injury potential becomes a risk factor if the safety of any person is threatened; an example of this is a stairway without railings, on which children could fall and hurt themselves. Alterations in health maintenance due to health beliefs, a change in financial situation, or lack of supervision can also impair a person's ability to live at home. If a person cannot learn to manage necessary diets or treatments, his or her ability to promote health at home is impaired.

Cognitive and Sensory Deficits

Sensory loss, especially blindness, can hinder the ability to manage independently at home. The loss of sight can decrease independent functioning and can increase the risk for injury. Severe pain can also hinder HMM because it can decrease the person's ability to carry out daily activities and functions.

An alteration in thought processes, if not responsive to treatment, can profoundly affect the ability to manage at home. Dementia (e.g., Alzheimer's disease) is a progressive condition in which memory loss and confusion greatly affect the patient's functional abilities. The severely confused person cannot live independently and may not be able to live safely with the family owing to the need for continual care. Mental illness such as schizophrenia and substance abuse also may impair the patient's ability to manage at home without significant support from family or community resources.

Decreased Mobility

Many medical problems (e.g., arthritis, neurologic impairments, fractures, respiratory disease, cardiovascular disease, cancer) can impair the patient's mobility and alter self-care abilities. Minor mobility problems may make housework or home repairs difficult; limited mobility may also hinder the patient's ability to get out of the house safely in case of a fire or emergency. The inability to do grooming, toileting, and personal hygiene tasks may impair the person's ability to live independently. The inability to maintain home hygiene and cleanliness may pose health and safety risks.

Altered Nutrition

The inability to provide adequate nutrition impairs the patient's ability to manage independently. Buying and cooking food and cleaning up require energy. Depression can decrease the desire to eat properly, especially when the patient lives alone. Lack of financial resources may also hinder proper nutrition. Physical changes affect mastication and swallowing also contribute to the potential for impaired HMM.

Insufficient Family or Social Supports

Family and social supports can compensate for functional deficits, and the extent to which family members and friends are interested or able to help is a crucial factor affecting HMM. Their coping abilities and reserves, commitment and ability to be caregivers, and functional health are factors in the balance and fit equation. Busy adults may need their energy for their own home and family; they may not have time to meet the needs of an older person or a person with special needs.

Insufficient Community Resources

HMM may be hindered by community and service deficits—lack of community agencies that provide supportive health and social services to assist the person in managing in the home. Some chronically mentally ill and developmentally disabled people cannot manage their finances or maintain hygienic living conditions without community assistance. Their environmental conditions may be stable, but without daily supervision from professionals or family they would be evicted and could become homeless.

Manifestations of Altered Home Maintenance Management

Verbal Expression

Patients probably know whether they can maintain an adequate, safe home environment. They may express this difficulty, or they may request advice or assistance. They may present financial difficulties and seek financial assistance. Patients with cognitive deficits may be unable to verbalize their concerns or remember their functional limitations, however.

Inability to Function Safely

Functional impairments, lack of family or social supports, or lack of community resources can hinder a person's ability to function safely at home. People living alone who have decreased functional abilities manifest impaired HMM as:

- Decreased ability for self-care or care of family members
- Decreased maintenance of safe and clean living space
- Decreased maintenance of economic obligations
- Decreased cognitive functioning and ability to respond appropriately to environmental stimuli.

Lack of External Supports and Resources

People with decreased family, social, or community resources and decreased internal resources may manifest altered or impaired HMM in any of the following ways:

- Decreased ability or availability of caregivers to perform self-care activities
- Decreased assistance in meeting financial obligations
- Inability to reach available resources
- Unavailability of community resources or services specific to the patient's needs.

Family Stress

Family members of the patient with functional health deficits may show signs of not being able to maintain the patient or themselves at home. Caregivers responsible for round-the-clock supervision of the patient may show signs of stress, reduced ability to cope, alterations in functional abilities, and financial loss. Physical or verbal abuse may signal severe family stress.

Poor Environmental Conditions

Unhealthy or unsanitary living conditions indicate impaired HMM. Filth, rodents, infestation, or environmental hazards are visual cues to an unhealthy environment. Lack of running water, heat, or proper storage facilities for food also are seen in poor living conditions.

Homelessness

The homeless are people or families who have no regular shelter to live in and often move (Bachrach, 1987). Conditions contributing to homelessness include alcoholism, drug addiction, chronic mental illness, unemployment, personal crises leading to displacement from home, financial cuts in public assistance programs, and a decrease in available low-cost housing (Imperato, 1987). Generally, the homeless are chronic mentally ill people who have been discharged from mental-health facilities and do not have access to adequate community services (Imperato, 1987).

Homeless people subsist on public assistance, free shelters, food lines, or money obtained by begging. Because of the lack of shelters, homeless people are particularly vulnerable to assault and robbery, infectious and communicable diseases, and social isolation. Exposure to the elements, especially to extreme cold, can lead to severe health problems and death. In addition, homelessness has serious adverse affect on maternal and child health; homeless children are less likely to be fully immunized, and homeless women have a high incidence of low-birth-weight infants (Vermond, 1987).

ASSESSMENT

Functional assessment of HMM should encompass the functional abilities of the patient, family, home, and community. Subjective information is collected to assess how the patient normally manages at home, what the home is like, and what family support is available.

Subjective Data

Interviewing the patient, family, or other caregivers provides valuable information about the patient's ability to manage at home, risk factors contributing to decreased ability to manage at home, and identification of actual HMM problems.

Functional Pattern Identification

The patient's competencies, capabilities, concerns, deficits, and limitations must be explored to understand how the patient manages at home. The display provides key questions that can be used to elicit this information.

Assessment starts by asking the patient to describe his or her ability to manage self-care tasks such as bathing, dressing, grooming, and eating. Document the patient's ability to carry out household chores independently or with assistance. The patient can describe how functional limitations are handled at home and whether management has been satisfactory. Determine whether the patient needs aids such as walkers, oxygen equipment, or a hospital bed. Assess medications and treatments and the patient's compliance with the specified regimen.

Family and social supports are also important to document. The patient should verbalize adequate assistance from family members, neighbors, or community resources. The patient should have a realistic plan in place should an emergency such as fire occur. Telephone numbers of emergency help should be posted near the telephone, and the patient should know about appropriate community agencies.

Risk Identification

Rarely is a single factor the cause of impaired HMM. The relationship between functional impairments and available internal and external supports determines the risk for impaired ability to manage at home. The greater the functional impairment, the greater the risk; the fewer available supports, the greater the risk. Common risk factors associated with impaired HMM include:

Home Management

- How will you manage at home on a day-to-day basis?
- What treatments will you be doing at home?
- What medications will you be taking at home?
- What do you want it to be like at home?
- What kinds of problems do you think you will have at home?

- Multiple or catastrophic illnesses
- Limited social or physical functioning
- Repeated hospital admissions within 6 months
- Age over 80, especially women
- Age over 70 with a disability
- Lack of social or family support and living alone.

The presence of these risk factors does not automatically indicate impaired HMM; the importance of the risk factors for each patient must be determined. During the entire assessment it is important to be continually aware of cues that would indicate cognitive impairments, such as repeating the same question or giving vague answers that are not consistent. People with cognitive impairments are often unable to manage in the home but rarely are able to realistically identify their own limitations.

Community deficits also can contribute to decreased ability to manage at home. Incidence is greater in the following situations:

- Unsafe neighborhoods
- Inadequate housing for the disabled
- Refusal of agencies to accept difficult clients
- Inadequate home health services
- Lack of volunteer programs
- Long waiting lists for services (especially nursing homes)
- Lack of affordable housing

Dysfunctional Identification

Assessment data about the patient's functional abilities and the support available from family or others are important to diagnose impaired HMM. A dysfunctional pattern can be identified when the patient or family verbalizes the inability to perform daily tasks and manage at home. People with impaired HMM cannot perform self-care and hygiene tasks, do not engage in activities and interactions with others, and do not do things from which they would otherwise derive enjoyment and a sense of worth. Bills go unpaid; the house may be in disrepair.

It is important to assess family support to determine how well a person can function at home. Family assessment can be done with questionnaires covering a broad range of topics, including therapeutic competencies, emotional competencies, family living patterns, use of community resources, physical independence, knowledge of health condition, and use of hygiene and health care (Choi, Josten, & Christensen, 1983). The most significant factors to assess are barriers to home care and the ability of the family members to provide care. The display lists questions that can be used to obtain this information.

Assessing family support focuses on family characteristics that show decreased family involvement with or

---

> **Key Questions for Assessment of Family and Social Support of the Person with Impaired Home Maintenance Management**
>
> - How much can you rely on friends and relatives?
> - What help will you have at home?
> - How much do you think your friends and relatives understand your health and medical problems?
> - Whom would you like me to talk to about your health and medical problems?
> - How do you think your spouse and friends will handle or cope with your being home?

---

support for the patient. To assess family involvement with the patient, ask directly how much support family members are willing and able to provide. Observe for evidence of family visits. Look for evidence of family concern, such as cards and presents. Observe family communication patterns and dynamics. Families differ in their reaction to illness of a family member. The prognosis and severity of the illness can affect family interactions and subsequent involvement with the patient. Chronic illness can lead to rejection of the patient and can impair family dynamics (Levine, Leventhal, & Nguyen, 1985).

Assess the ability and willingness of the caregiver to perform, or to help the patient perform, any therapeutic treatments. Caregiving often consists of bathing, dressing, toileting, transferring, feeding, housekeeping, shopping, preparing meals, managing finances, and providing transportation (Stephens & Achritianson, 1986; Kane & Kane, 1981). Therefore caregivers must be assessed for their ability, willingness, and capability to carry out these activities. Wound dressing changes, ostomy care, home parenteral therapy, and physical therapy may require additional time and energy.

Other subjective data about the caregiver include the caregiver's comments about the emotional and physical strains of providing care or an overload of responsibility. Objective signs of physical exhaustion, stress, and limited coping help to support such subjective data.

Objective Data

Objective data can be collected from the patient to support verbalized functional abilities. In addition, assessing the home and available community resources allows the nurse to individualize interventions. Medical records may be reviewed to determine past behavior (for example, compliance with prescribed therapies or keeping medical appointments).

Functional Deficits

General observation of the patient can provide important information. Poor grooming, dirty clothing (especially with cigarette burns), or clothing inappropriate for the weather can indicate a self-care deficit. Clothing that hangs loosely, coupled with a gaunt appearance, may indicate difficulty providing appropriate nutrition. Note any inarticulate or difficult-to-follow stories, unusual emotional affect, inability to follow instructions, expression of self-harm, or display of anger or frustration.

Observing the patient doing activities such as bathing, feeding, toileting, and walking provides objective data as to his or her ability to perform these tasks safely without undue fatigue. When complex procedures are necessary (e.g., wound care, stoma management, glucose monitoring, insulin injections), observe the patient or caregiver performing the task to determine his or her knowledge level and ability to manage necessary skills.

Home Assessment

The patient's house is important enough to be considered a separate assessment element. This assessment is often performed by a community health nurse. A comprehensive home assessment includes safety, sanitation, mobility, temperature, and personal space (Sargis, Jennrich, & Murray, 1987). The display summarizes home assessment.

- Learn whether the house is rented or owned, since this determines whether modifications are feasible.
- Look for smoke or fire alarms, adequate lighting, flat door sills, and adequate security.
- Determine whether the house is infested with vermin or rodents.
- Ask about sewer and garbage services.
- Determine the source of water and the condition of the plumbing.
- Assess for adequate and safe cooking and food storage equipment. Although rural and urban areas differ in the types of sanitation measures, sanitation should not be a source of disease.
- Assess for easy access throughout the house. Handrails on tubs and staircases, wide doorways for wheelchair access, and flat, even floors contribute to easy mobility. There should not be scatter rugs, and halls should be uncluttered.
- Determine the adequacy of heating and cooling systems. Inadequate temperature control can lead to hypothermia or hyperthermia.

Do not overlook the personal aspects of a home. The presence of mementos, pictures, or religious items in a well-kept house reflects self-esteem. A nice garden, sewing equipment, or a workshop provides additional information on the person's home activities (Thomas, 1985). A person with impaired HMM may not be able to continue such self-actualizing activities. Being aware of the patient's past gives the nurse a more complete understanding of the person and how the current health condition has changed the person's way of living. For example, an active 80-year-old man who gardens daily may interpret a broken hip as devastating, but a sedentary man who enjoy watching television and doing crossword puzzles may find the same situation a minor nuisance.

Community Resource Assessment

The purpose of community assessment is to identify resources that can be used for people with impaired HMM. A comprehensive community assessment is not needed to diagnose impairments, but being familiar with community resources allows the nurse to develop a more

---

Summary of Home Assessment for Impaired Home Maintenance Management

Subjective Data (asked of patient)

Ownership: rent hotel room, apartment, or house; own; live with others
Access: ground floor, stairs
Condition:
  Utilities: heat, water, telephone, electricity
  Hygiene: housekeeping habits
  Sanitation: rodents, sewer, infestations
  Safety: handrails

Objective Data

From patient chart
Phone: own phone number or message phone

From home visit
Neighborhood: crime potential, located near environmental hazards
Access: ground floor, condition of stairs and sidewalk, proximity to public transportation
Utilities: type of utilities available and in service, cooking arrangements
Hygiene: odors, facilities for cleaning, appropriateness of food storage
Sanitation: presence or evidence of vermin or rodents
Safety: short electrical cords, handrails, fire alarms, stable rugs

---

Summary of Community Assessment for Impaired Home Maintenance Management

Subjective Data

Knowledge of services
Previous use of services
Satisfaction with previous service or agency

Objective Data

Access to services (home delivery, distance to reach service)
Outpatient services (clinics, equipment vendors)
Agencies offering health education program (American Cancer Society, American Heart Association, American Lung Association, American Red Cross)
Agencies offering direct care services (area agency on aging, local public health department, mental health department, visiting nurse association; Meals on Wheels; day-care centers for children, elderly, mentally ill, or mentally handicapped)
Volunteer services (Gray Panthers, church groups, specialized community-based services and agencies)

---

realistic and individualized nursing care plan for the patient. The nurse needs information about the economic stability of the community, the patient's neighborhood, the social and health resources available in the community, and the community's cultural norms. An overview of community assessment is presented in the display. The presence of services as recorded in service directories is one way to objectively validate what the patient describes. Nurses should be familiar with available emergency care, equipment rental stores, and visiting nurse services, and should know where welfare and Medicare offices are located.

NURSING DIAGNOSES AND PATIENT GOALS

The nurse uses data from the assessment to determine the presence of conditions that disrupt normal HMM. Impaired HMM is a broad diagnosis that includes both management and maintenance aspects of living at home. Interdisciplinary professional communication is required for resolving this nursing diagnosis and assisting the patient toward outcome goals.

Diagnostic Statement: Impaired Home Maintenance Management

Definition

Impaired HMM is the inability to independently maintain a safe, growth-promoting immediate environment (NANDA, 1990).

Defining Characteristics

Subjective. Household members express difficulty in maintaining the home in a comfortable fashion; household requests assistance with home maintenance; household members describe outstanding debts or financial crises (NANDA, 1990).

Proposed Nursing Diagnoses Related to Impaired Home Maintenance Management

Nursing diagnoses approved by NANDA are still being developed. Practitioners and researchers have proposed additional nursing diagnoses, some relevant to impaired HMM. Gould and Wargo (1987) developed and proposed the following nursing diagnoses especially relevant to patients with impaired HMM:

1. Actual or potential alteration in meeting basic human needs
2. Impaired adjustment related to reluctance to separate from the health-care agency
3. Impairment of lifestyle and role expectations related to chronic disease process
4. Impairment of home management of disease process due to cognitive, psychological, or physical limitations, requiring a nursing specialist consultation.

In a study of nursing diagnoses, 104 nurses were asked to generate health-promotion nursing diagnoses (Frenn, et al.). Of the 76 health-promotion nursing diagnoses, several apply to patients with impaired HMM:

1. Effective or ineffective community resource use
2. Effective or ineffective risk factor management
3. Potential for injury from environmental hazards
4. Effective or ineffective leisure management
5. Accepted or unresolved independence or dependence
6. Resource deficit.

Objective. Disorderly surroundings; unwashed or unavailable cooking equipment, clothes, or linen; accumulation of dirt, food wastes, or hygienic wastes; offensive odors; inappropriate household temperature; exhausted or anxious family members; lack of necessary equipment or aids; presence of vermin or rodents; repeated hygienic disorders, infestations, or infections (NANDA, 1990).

Related Factors

Individual/family member disease or injury; insufficient family organization or planning; insufficient finances; unfamiliarity with neighborhood resources; impaired cognitive or emotional functioning; lack of knowledge; lack of role modeling; inadequate support systems.

Related Nursing Diagnoses

Any nursing diagnosis indicating impaired functional capabilities, such as Activity Intolerance, Self-Care Def-

icit, Impaired Physical Mobility, Incontinence, High Risk for Injury, or Altered Nutrition, can often be seen in the patient who has impaired HMM (Table 27-1). Also, the patient's inability to care for himself or herself at home can increase Anxiety, Fear, Ineffective Individual or Family Coping, and Self-Esteem Disturbance. Noncompliance and Knowledge Deficit are also associated with impaired HMM.

Patient Goals

The basic goal for the patient with impaired HMM is to live in a supportive environment that has been agreed on by the patient, family, and health-care providers. Patient goals can be written in terms of rehabilitation or restoration of independence. **Rehabilitation** goals should be written for patients who are expected to regain some level of physical or cognitive functioning through training rather than through health improvement. In devel-

TABLE 27–1
Effects of Selected Nursing Diagnoses on Daily Life

Functional Cluster	ADL	DDL	IR	ER	Fit
Health Perception and Health Management					
Knowledge deficit: treatments		X	X		
Knowledge deficit: medications		X	X		
High risk for injury	X		X		X
Altered health maintenance	X	X			X
Nutrition and Metabolism					
Altered nutrition	X				
Altered elimination	X	X			X
Fluid volume deficit		X			
Activity and Exercise					
Impaired mobility	X	X		X	X
Self-care deficit	X	X		X	X
Activity intolerance	X	X			X
Pain		X	X		
Circulation and Respiration					
Impaired gas exchange		X		X	
Ineffective breathing patterns		X			X
Altered tissue perfusion		X			
Sensory/Perceptual					
Visual alterations	X				X
Auditory alterations	X				X
Tactile alterations	X				X
Roles and Relationships					
Impaired social interactions			X	X	X
Hopelessness		X	X		X
Powerlessness		X	X		X
Altered thought processes	X	X	X		X
Impaired verbal communication		X	X	X	

ADL, activities of daily living; DDL, demands of daily living; IR, internal resources, ER, external resources.

oping goals for the patient, it is important to decide whether rehabilitation or independence is the best way to ensure a safe, nurturing environment.

When forming goals for the patient, consider the following:

- The level of functioning to be achieved or maintained
- The extent of independence expected
- The level of family involvement
- The level of support services available to the patient living in the community.

Possible goals include:

The patient/caregiver will overcome the functional deficit(s) that contribute or lead to impaired HMM.
The patient will return to a safe home environment.
The patient will continue to live at home.
The caregiver will care for the patient at home.

IMPLEMENTATION

Nursing Interventions to Promote Health and Function

Enhancing internal resources, patient teaching, and discharge planning help promote the ability to function safely at home.

Enhancement of Internal Resources

The patient's internal resources are enhanced by improving his or her physical or psychocognitive abilities; examples are physical exercise, cognitive therapy, or group activities. Treatments or medications that promote the patient's comfort and mobility indirectly enhance his or her internal reserves of strength and endurance. Psychological support and encouragement help increase the patient's motivation and confidence.

Patient Teaching

Patient teaching is a powerful tool to promote the patient's ability to live safely at home. Teaching can focus on knowledge needed to improve functional abilities or limit dysfunction (Fig. 27-6). Some teaching topics are:

- Medications
- Dietary modifications
- Medical equipment and procedures to be used at home
- Ambulation techniques to improve safety
- Community resources and how they can be reached
- Home safety measures (i.e., removing clutter, installing handrails by tubs and stairs, improving lighting)
- Solving anticipated problems

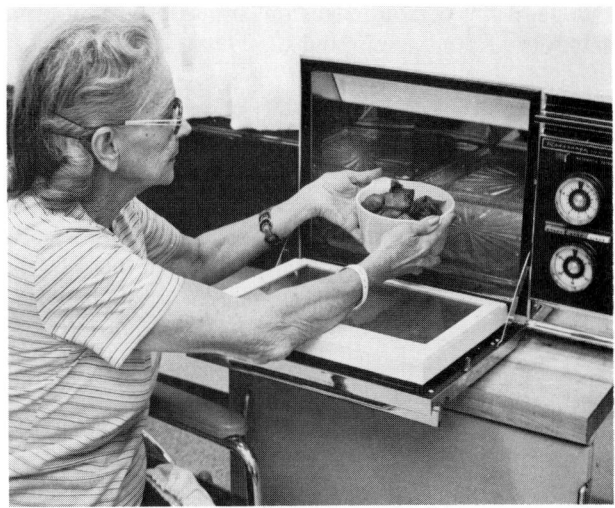

Figure 27-6. Fast no-mess cooking in a microwave oven can encourage those who live alone or are on modified diets to prepare meals that meet their nutritional needs.

Discharge Planning

Discharge planning is the activity that facilitates the patient's transition between different settings (McKeehan, 1981). The **discharge planner** is the health or social services professional who is responsible for coordinating the transition and who acts as a link between the hospital and the community (Runner-Heidt, 1984). The discharge planner is often a nurse.

Discharge planning does not solve all the problems of impaired HMM, but it can reduce readmissions, reduce residual effects of the health condition through continuity of care, and improve patient and family satisfaction with health care. Discharge planning is discussed in more depth later in this chapter.

The key elements of discharge planning for the patient are transition and continuity of care, and the key elements of discharge planning for the nurse are coordination, facilitation, and negotiation.

Transition. When people undergo transitions, their assumptions about themselves change, and they develop new assumptions that allow them to adapt (Schlossberg, 1981). As a nursing concern related to adaptation, transition is particularly obvious when a patient moves between settings, such as from the hospital to home, or from home to a long-term care facility (Chick & Meleis, 1986). But the physical move is only one type of transition the patient actually makes: the related change of assumptions may involve self-concept, role performance, mobility, self-care, or communication with family members. For example, a mother with terminal cancer may be experiencing the transition from her role as a caregiver to the role of a care recipient. Balance and fit change as the person makes the transition from old to new settings and assumptions.

Continuity of Care. **Continuity of care** is both an ideal and a necessity. Continuity of care is the provision of health services without disruption, regardless of the patient's movement between settings. From the patient's perspective, it involves having a home health nurse visit the day the patient is discharged from the hospital or having the physician's office contact the local pharmacy about the patient's medication needs. When health services are disrupted, the patient may experience a relapse, requiring additional health care or hospitalization. Thus, continuity of care helps to maintain the patient's health status and reduces health-care costs.

Organizational, policy, and financial realities can work against achieving continuity. Communication between health professionals about a patient's needs may not occur. For any patient requiring some health or social service at home, a nursing goal ought to be continuity of health or social service care. Discharge plans started at admission can help ensure continuity of care through early, expedient referrals to community services and agencies.

Coordination. *Coordination* is the act of assembling and directing activities so that services are provided harmoniously. The result of coordination is a team working together with a unified purpose; health professionals work with other health professionals and with the patient. Payment based on diagnosis-related groups has led to shorter hospital stays, and as a result nurses must coordinate health and social services for post-discharge needs (Phillips & Cloonan, 1987).

One way to coordinate services is to initiate and conduct team conferences and family conferences, preferably before the patient is discharged or the patient's problems have become too complex. At a team conference, discussion focuses on planning care for the patient. At a family conference, professionals and the family gather to discuss family issues related to the patient. Both types of conferences provide an opportunity for patients, family, and health-care professionals to plan care and set goals.

Facilitation. *Facilitation* is making something easier and smoother, eliminating problems and barriers. To facilitate the patient's transition, the discharge planner must anticipate patient needs and plan ahead. Anticipating discharge needs begins at admission with assessment for impaired HMM. The nurse must take into account the different settings and patient needs and resources (Clemen, Eigsti, & McGuire, 1981; Wells, 1985).

Negotiation. This is the process by which goals are determined between the nurse, patient, and family. The most elaborate care plan is doomed to failure if attempts

to achieve the goals are hampered by the patient, family, or a health-care professional. Negotiation need not be a formal process. It may result in a *contract,* an agreement between the nurse and patient that delineates the roles and responsibilities of each. Contracts are discussed further below.

For example, the home-care priorities of a young mother with a respirator-dependent infant may differ from those of the nurse. Negotiating with the mother over which goals and objectives have priority has two effects. The mother will be more willing to work with the nurse to attain goals, and she will feel more in control of her situation. For this case, the goal of "negotiate care priorities" would be appropriate for the nurse.

Nursing Interventions for Altered Home Maintenance Management

Impaired HMM has consequences for the patient and those involved professionally and personally. At least three major consequences of impaired HMM have direct intervention implications. Nurses planning patient care need to be aware of these consequences, since each has nursing implications:

The patient who cannot manage at home may need supportive care, such as a visiting nurse or a home-health aid.

The patient's health problems may require greater family involvement with and support of the person. This requires considering the family as a unit for decision making and for caregiving.

The patient, especially one with chronic mental illness, may become homeless.

In addition to these consequences of impaired HMM, the nurse may face ethical problems and interpersonal conflicts. The brief section on ethical considerations is intended to foster introspection by nurses rather than provide solutions.

Health-Care Options and Placement

With each functional health problem that alters balance and fit, a different level of deficit is manifested. The level of deficit determines the level of assistance needed with daily activities, which determines the level of health care required to stay at home. The *level of care* refers to the intensity and permanence of care required to maintain, restore, or promote health.

Levels of care range from minimal to extensive (Fig. 27-7). Each level of care is related to a type of health care service. At the low end of the continuum is intermittent, temporary, or minimal care. Low-level care can be provided by temporary homemaker services to a healthy

---

Selected Nursing Interventions for Common Impaired HMM Problems

Impaired Self-Care, Difficulties with New Medications, Altered Mobility

- Patient teaching

Severe Functional Deficit

- Decisional control; placement in a care facility or in-home services

Powerlessness, Helplessness, Frustration with Limitations

- Contracting

Need for Continuity of Care in Home

- Discharge planning

Limited Financial Resources, Limited Cognitive Ability to Obtain Community Resources

- Advocacy

---

nent, or intensive. An example of high-level care is 24-hour nursing care for a quadriplegic with a tracheostomy. High-level care services include hospices, high-technology home care, rehabilitation, long-term care, or skilled nursing facilities. If the patient is homebound, moderate or high-level care may be appropriate depending on the patient's abilities, external resources, and the home environment.

The base of Figure 27-7 indicates the severity and permanence of impaired HMM. A person living at home and using a walker for ambulation steadiness has low impaired HMM and needs a low level of care. At the other extreme, a person with no family support and a severe chronic debilitating condition, such as advanced Parkinson's disease, has severely impaired HMM and needs a high level of care. Figure 27-7 also shows that the placement decision relates to the complexity and range of impairments that may affect HMM.

Some patients may be so disabled and have such severely impaired HMM that they cannot leave home. These patients are called **homebound.** They usually require direct health care, indirect care, and case management.

The specific type of service chosen is based on both the deficits manifested and the preferred place for receiving care. The interdisciplinary team of physician, nurse, family, and social worker decides whether the patient should receive care at home or in a health-care facility. Placement decisions are affected by the presence or absence of family supports. (The term "placement" reflects the attitude that a provider makes the decision and controls care, but ideally placement occurs with the full understanding of the patient and the family.) Widowhood, living alone, and childlessness are related to nursing-home placement (Horowitz, 1985). The most

patient recovering from hip surgery, for example; other low-level care services are adult or child day-care centers. Moderate levels of care include home health care, residential care, and respite care. At the other end of the continuum is high-level care, which is continual, perma-

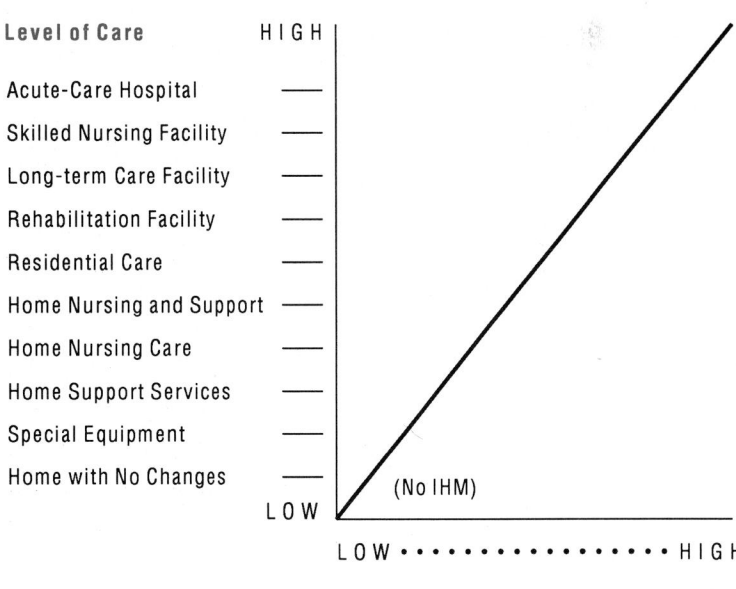

Figure 27–7. Relationship between level of care and impaired home maintenance (IHM) severity. Graph shows the more severe the IHM, the greater the level of care that is required.

common recipients of home and community services are very old women, people who have difficulty with several ADLs, people living alone, and Medicaid recipients.

Although the physician, nurses, and social workers may prefer one type of service or level of care, the reality is that placement is often influenced by insurance coverage. Medicare, available to those over age 65, is a federally funded health insurance plan administered by the Social Security Administration. Medicaid, funded by the Federal and state governments, provides financial assistance to the disabled or financially needy. Other constraints affecting placement are the limited number of nursing-home beds and home health agencies. All these constraints force nursing care plans to be both economically realistic and scientifically sound. For example, to qualify for Medicare-covered home health care, patients must be confined to their homes and must require skilled nursing care for an acute or postacute condition.

Family as Resource. According to Horowitz (1985), "the support available from families is one of the most critical factors in preventing or delaying nursing home utilization" and distinguishes those who enter nursing homes from those who remain at home. Family supports and family decisions must be considered in the diagnosis of impaired HMM. When a family member cannot provide self-care, other family members face a choice: they can help the person remain at home, or they can place the person in a health-care facility.

The family member who cares for the patient is called the **caregiver.** Often the caregiver is an adult child or spouse caring for a parent or spouse who has some degree of physical, mental, emotional or economic impairment that limits independence and makes ongoing assistance necessary. The prevalence of caring for parents has increased and is discussed in the health care literature as parentcaring. Caregiving includes providing emotional support, direct health services, and financial support; mediating with health and social service organizations; and sharing a household (Horowitz, 1985). It includes tasks such as bathing, toileting, feeding, preparing food, maintaining a home, and housekeeping.

When one family member has a severe disability and severely impaired HMM, the strain on caregivers can be great. The family may feel unable to provide the necessary care. Poor families with many existing problems may already be experiencing extreme stress (Aleman, 1983) and may be unable to take on the added responsibility of caregiving. A patient in such a family would experience poor balance and poor fit with the family situation.

Each family must decide how to care for the affected family member. The family, especially the caregiver, needs information on respite care, levels of care that are

alternatives to home care, and realistic prognostic information. This information is important in making family choices. Those managing the affairs of an older person need to be aware of potential challenges (Anthony, 1987).

Family dynamics vary widely, and the nurse must be sensitive to family patterns and facilitate the decision-making process without being judgmental. At times, families may make decisions that appear to the nurse as unloving, irresponsible, overly protective, or self-sacrificing. But the nurse must refrain from judging the decision while still taking action to meet the patient goals. Involving the family in the placement decision (to the extent that the family wants to be involved) is as important as accepting their decision.

Contracting

The limitations inherent in impaired HMM may contribute to feelings of helplessness, hopelessness, stress, or disempowerment. One way to minimize such feelings is to negotiate a contract with the patient or caregiver about the identified responsibilities. A contract is a written agreement that results from negotiating the assignment of those responsibilities (Spradley, 1985). The sense of control and empowerment achieved through the contract enhances the patient's internal resources (specifically, motivation and commitment). The nurse and the patient or caregiver discuss who will be responsible for what, and reach a consensus. The consensus on responsibilities is then written down so that each party can be held accountable.

Resources

Nursing interventions designed to promote HMM generally focus on enhancing the patient's internal or external resources or on enhancing the patient's fit with the environment.

Enhancing external resources is done either through direct involvement with the patient and agencies or indirectly through community activism. Direct involvement includes arranging services for the patient or family, such as respite care for caregivers, or advocating for the patient if needed services are unavailable. Indirect involvement includes fundraising or volunteering for community agencies, or working for candidates who support community resources.

The physical aspects of promoting HMM include providing mechanical devices (walkers, portable oxygen tanks) that allow the patient or caregiver to better manage with a functional deficit at home. It may be necessary to alter the physical environment (installing wheelchair ramps, electric beds, handrails in the bathroom) to ease access, increase mobility, or increase safety.

Discharge Planning in Altered Home Maintenance Management

Levels of Discharge Planning. Every patient deserves some formal assessment of post-discharge needs and a nursing action to meet those needs to the fullest extent possible. Even a patient with such severely impaired HMM that a nursing-home placement is planned deserves a discharge plan related to family involvement or anticipatory guidance.

Discharge plans vary depending on patient needs and the nursing interventions required to minimize impaired HMM. All patient goals and nursing orders must be developed from the perspective that human responses to health and illness occur regardless of health-care delivery settings. In general, the more complex the transition for the patient, the more complex the discharge plan needs to be. The three levels of discharge planning are summarized in Table 27-2.

Basic Discharge Plan. The least complicated and most common discharge plan is teaching the patient about self-care or HMM. Patient teaching for impaired HMM does not involve simply following a standardized teaching protocol. The teaching must anticipate problems the patient will experience at home. For instance, when discharging a newborn with an apnea monitor to a home in which there are already three little children, the nurse must teach the parents to check that the monitor parameters have not been changed by the other children.

Simple Referral. The second type of discharge plan involves referring the patient to community resources (for instance, a smoker to a smoking cessation clinic, a high-risk mother to the local health department, a caregiver to a respite service). A **referral** is a request for a service that is outside the scope of the referring professional. The nurse acts as the discharge planner and must know both the community resources and the patient's ability to reach those resources. Knowledge of the community resources is based on the community assessment and on personal knowledge. Knowledge of the patient's ability to reach resources is based on the functional health pattern assessment.

Complex Referral. The third and most complex type of discharge plan involves referring the patient to the dis-charge planner. The nurse may choose to involve the discharge planner because referring the patient to an appropriate community resource can be time-consuming and complex (Gikow, 1981). This type of discharge planning is particularly appropriate for patients with multiple risk factors for impaired HMM (Rasmusen, 1984).

This third level of discharge plan involves interdisciplinary collaboration and coordination. The discharge planner takes responsibility for coordinating the activities necessary to transfer the patient from one setting to another. However, referring the patient to the discharge planner does not absolve the nurse of responsibility. The nurse must follow up and evaluate if the discharge planner has acted and if the patient is satisfied with the discharge plan. The nurse may need to reinforce plans made by the discharge planner.

A referral to the discharge planner is appropriate for coordinating placement of the patient in a skilled nursing facility or a long-term care facility. The discharge planner can also coordinate and initiate services the patient will need if discharged to home (e.g., a visiting nurse).

Discharge Preparation. The nurse is responsible for ensuring that the inpatient with impaired HMM is prepared for discharge, or that the family has received necessary information and assistance.

Physical Considerations. Physical interventions for the inpatient with impaired HMM include direct physical care related to the patient's health problems. For example, occupational therapy is one type of physical intervention that prepares the patient for returning home with a disability that limits his or her ADLs. The nurse's role is to reinforce what the patient has learned in occupational therapy.

The nurse may recommend changes in the home based on a home assessment done either by interviewing the patient or by visiting the home. Common physical changes include installing ramps and handrails, moving furniture to make room for a rented hospital bed, or installing equipment such as oxygen tanks and suction machines. If a severely disabled patient is expected to return home, a home visit should be made before discharge.

TABLE 27–2

Levels of Discharge Planning

Discharge Plan Level	Nursing Interventions	People Involved
Basic, universal	Self-care and illness teaching	Nurse, patient, caregiver
Simple referral	Refer to community resources Coordinate for continuity	Nurse, patient, caregiver
Complex referral	Refer to discharge planner Facilitate coordination Negotiate outcomes	Nurse, discharge planner, family

---

Patient Teaching

Instruct the patient as follows:

- Familiarize yourself with community resources to help meet your needs after discharge.
- Learn about community support groups that may offer emotional support and assistance after discharge.
- Learn about new medications you will be taking after discharge. Ask for written information to which you can refer.
- Follow instructions and demonstrate procedure you will perform at home after discharge.
- Learn symptoms that are significant and warrant contacting the physician.
- Learn about any activity restriction or diet restrictions that must be followed after discharge.
- Familiarize yourself with new equipment you will be using at home after discharge.
- Learn how to contact help should an emergency arise. Have the number of your physician and the emergency room handy, and know how to contact emergency personnel (e.g., 911) if necessary.

Psychocognitive Considerations. Psychological interventions are designed to meet educational, psychological, and coping goals. Education should focus on matters that contribute to impaired HMM. Topics to be included in predischarge teaching are who to call for help and when, self-care (such as wound care), and health maintenance topics appropriate for the patient's specific health problems.

Anticipatory guidance is information given about a situation before the situation occurs so that the patient can develop problem-solving and coping strategies. Anticipatory guidance is an important psychological intervention because it prepares the patient for decisions to be made at home and for the extent of self-care required after discharge.

Family Considerations. Social and family interventions are developed to meet social support and resource goals. Referrals may be made to social workers and the discharge planner. A *social worker* is trained to assess and help people regarding public assistance, social or family crisis, and access to social service programs. The social worker may be asked to see the patient for financial or insurance matters or for counseling. A patient may develop a fear of going home, especially if he or she lives alone or feels isolated; involving social supports in care is an important nursing intervention. Family conferences, another nursing intervention, can be held before the patient is discharged.

Home Care

Home care, when feasible, is ideal, but the nurse must consider family and community support, the home environment, and the patient's condition. Home health care is defined as "all the services and products that maintain, restore, or promote physical, mental, and emotional health that are provided to patients in their homes" (Spradley, 1985). Home care, even when extensive, is less costly than inpatient services. Home health care aims to support families and patients to prevent admission to a facility, provide respite care, maintain or restore impaired health, or provide follow-up services (Spradley, 1985). Home care has been found to play a role in recovery from illness and in permitting the very old person to continue living at home (Shapiro, 1986).

Ethical Considerations. In planning home care for a patient with impaired HMM, four ethical considerations are relevant:

- Respect
- Beneficence
- Justice
- Fidelity (Haddad, 1987)

Everyone deserves *respect* based on his or her worth and dignity. Respect is demonstrated by providing autonomy and informed consent. When there is a discrepancy between the preferences of the health-care provider, the family, and the patient, ethical problems of paternalism (the attitude of knowing what is best for the patient) and lack of respect exist.

Beneficence is the principle of doing good. In an effort to provide the best possible health care, the nurse may actually be providing care against the patient's wishes. Beneficence dilemmas often manifest as paternalism, used in the name of doing good for the patient. For the patient with impaired HMM, nurses and physicians may think that they know what would be the best placement or service. But if the nurse is left with the sense that the patient's wishes are not being met, there may be an ethical dilemma with respect or beneficence.

In times of economic constraints, *justice* is likely to be a major ethical dilemma. Fair, equitable distribution of benefits is inherent in justice. Nurses are continually faced with justice dilemmas. An older, belligerent, and unmotivated alcoholic who is dying of cirrhosis and requires home care might not receive the same intensity of care as a developmentally delayed, respirator-dependent infant born to a middle-class couple who had been trying to have a family for many years.

Fidelity refers to keeping promises. When a nurse provides care in a less-structured setting such as the home, she or he may make promises in an effort to be nice, but those promises may not be realistic. Nurses who negotiate contracts with patients must be prepared to fulfill those contracts.

Nursing Research

Selected Nursing Research Studies

Berne, A. S., Data, C., Mason, D. J., et al. (1990). A nursing model for addressing the health needs of homeless families. *Image, 22*(1), 8–13.

Given, G., Strommel, M., Collins, C., et al. (1990). Responses of elderly spouse caregivers. *Research in Nursing Health, 13,* 77–85.

Luker, K. A., & Chalmers, K. K. (1989). The referral process in health visiting. *International Journal of Nursing Studies, 26,* 173–185.

Magilvy, J. K., Brown, N. J., & Dydyn, J. (1988). The experience of home health care: Perceptions of older adults. *Public Health Nursing, 5*(3), 140–145.

Pallett, P. J. (1990). A conceptual framework for studying family caregiver burden in Alzheimer's-type dementia. *Image, 22*(1), 52–57.

Pesznecker, B. L., Zerwekh, J. V., & Horn, B. (1989). The mutual participation relationship: Key to facilitating self-care practices in clients and families. *Public Health Nursing, 6*(4), 197–203.

Stiller, S. B. (1988). Success and difficulty in high-tech home care. *Public Health Nursing, 5*(2), 68–75.

Van Ort, S., & Woodtli, A. (1990). Home health care: Providing a missing link. *Journal of Gerontology Nursing, 15*(9), 4–9.

Possible Topics for Nursing Inquiry

- How can preventive health-care services be provided to homeless families with school-age children?
- As caregivers become burned out and the patient's health status deteriorates, what factors become important in their decisions about placement of the patient?
- Is there a difference in the health and functional patterns between patients with whom a contract was negotiated and patients with whom no contract was negotiated after 1 year of home care?
- To what extent is information about patients exchanged between agencies providing different services to homebound patients?
- From the perspective of the patient and caregiver, what community services are lacking in rural, suburban, and urban areas?

Discussing ethical problems with an ethicist, member of the clergy, or supervisor can help. Remember that the role of a nurse is that of a patient advocate. The patient's preferences must take the highest priority.

Case Management. People who are not patients in a health care facility but are receiving health care are outpatients. Nursing interventions with outpatients are likely to consist of direct physical care, indirect health care, monitoring the patient status, or case management. **Case management** is an approach to providing care in which the patient's services are coordinated by one designated health provider. Nurses are in ideal positions to be case managers of patients with impaired HMM since they make home visits to provide care, make ongoing assessments of patients, and can act to coordinate services.

Meeting Physical Needs. With relatively short lengths of stay in hospitals, patients are going home with increasingly complex health needs. As a result, there has been an increase in the use of high-technology equipment at home (Taylor, 1985). Direct physical care is provided at home by visiting nurses and home health aides trained in the basics of personal care. Wound care, intravenous administration of antibiotics and hyperalimentation, and supervision of medications are common nursing activities in the home. Common high-technology therapies in the home are respiratory care, parenteral or enteral nutrition, intravenous therapy, dialysis, and biotelemetry (Haddad, 1987).

Many patients who live at home cannot prepare meals due to physical limitations. Meals can be delivered by Meals on Wheels. Table 27-3 shows that for many common physical limitations, there are community resources to assist the patient to remain at home safely.

Other physical interventions may be making small but important changes in the house. Color-coding medication bottles enhances the ability to self-medicate. Removing color can be equally important, however; for instance, eliminating confusing color patterns in the home simplifies visual cues necessary to locate objects in a room (Schafer, 1985).

Ongoing education about self-care, treatment, and medications is a major psychocognitive intervention for homebound patients. Nurses should allow patients to express their frustrations due to lifestyle alterations. Communication is critical in making psychological inter-

TABLE 27–3

Matching Community Resources and Impaired Home Maintenance Manifestations

Impaired Home Maintenance Manifestation	Possible Community Resources
Difficulty arranging transportation to employment, volunteer site, senior center, medical appointment, etc.	Carpools with neighbors, families of other older people, fellow volunteers or workers City provisions for older people: reduced bus fares, taxi scrip, "Trans-Aide" Volunteer services: Red Cross, Salvation Army, church organizations for emergency or occasional transportation
Living alone and fearing accidental injury or illness without access to assistance	Telephone check-up services through local hospitals, or friends, neighbors, or relatives Postal alert: register with local senior center; sticker on mailbox alerts letter carrier to check for accumulation of mail Newspaper delivery: parents of the delivery person can be given an emergency phone number if newspapers accumulate Neighbors can check pattern of lights on/off
Needs assistance with personal care such as bathing and dressing	Private pay for hourly services: home aides from private agencies listed in phone book Visiting nurse association: services include aide services when nurses are used Medicaid/Medicare: provisions for home aides are limited to strict eligibility requirements, but such care is provided in certain situations Student help: posting notices on bulletin boards at nursing schools can yield inexpensive helpers Home sharing: sharing the home with another person who is willing to provide this kind of assistance in exchange for room and board
Needs occasional nursing care and/or physical therapy	Visiting nurse: services provided through Medicare or Medicaid or sliding-scale fees; must be ordered by a physician Home health services: private providers listed in phone book; also nonprofit providers, Medicare and Medicaid reimbursement for authorized services
Difficulty cooking meals, shopping for food, and arranging nutritious diet	Home-delivered meals: Meals on Wheels delivers frozen meals once a week, sliding fees Nutrition sites: meals served at senior centers, churches, schools, and other sites Cooperatives: arrangements with neighbors to exchange a service for meals, food shopping, etc.
Not enough contact with other people: insufficient activity or stimulation; loneliness and boredom	Senior centers: provide social opportunities, classes, volunteer opportunities, outings Church-sponsored clubs: social activities, volunteer opportunities, outings Support groups: for widows, stroke victims, and general support Adult day care: provides social interaction, classes, discussion groups, outings, exercise
Difficulty doing housework	Homemaker services for those meeting income eligibility criteria Service exchanges with neighbors and friends (i.e., babysitting exchanged for housework help) Home helpers: hired through agencies or through employment listings at senior centers, schools, etc. Home sharing: renting out a room or portion of the home, reduced rent for help with housework
Forgetful about financial affairs; eyesight too poor for balancing checkbook and reading necessary information	Power of attorney given to friend or relative for handling financial matters Joint checking account with friend or relative for ease in paying bills Volunteer assistance available from the American Red Cross, Salvation Army, church groups, senior centers, other organizations
Needs assistance with will, landlord–tenant concerns, property tax exemptions, guardianship, etc.	Senior citizens' legal services Lawyer referral service offered by the county bar association City/county aging programs: hot lines for information and assistance in phone book

(From Hooyman, N. (1983). Social support networks in services for the elderly. In Whittaker, J. K. & Garbino, J. (eds.), *Social support networks: Informal helping in the human services.* New York: Aldine Publishing Company, 145–146.)

ventions. Nurses with specialized education in psychological nursing manage cases of people with mental illnesses who live in the community (Grau, 1986).

Meeting Caregiver and Family Needs. Most commonly, social and family interventions are directed at the caregiver. Interventions include educational and support programs, burden-reducing programs, psychotherapeutic interventions, and self-help groups (Gallagher, 1985). It is important for the nurse to determine the caregiver's routine: "Caregivers must experiment for long periods before a satisfactory procedure for managing the problem is worked out. Once it is established, therefore, it is rigidly adhered to" (Archbold, 1982). Maintaining the routine becomes a parameter for other nursing interventions (Schafer 1985; Norris, 1986).

A major and increasingly important family intervention is **respite care,** which provides a temporary break for the caregiver from the responsibility of caring for the patient. Families must balance their caring, giving roles with meeting their own needs.

For decreased social contacts and isolation, the nurse may refer the patient to adult day-care centers, group meals, church activities, senior centers, or support groups (Hooyman, 1983). By focusing too much on a caring role, nurses can actually contribute to the isolation of patient and family (Coombs, 1984).

Community Support

If in the community assessment the nurse has noted a lack of a particular resource or support service, it is within his or her role as a nurse to become active in the community to develop the needed services. Working with the housing authority, supporting political candidates whose platforms reflect social consciousness, or volunteering for community-based health projects are examples of a few ways that nurses can intervene at the community level to indirectly affect the lives of those with impaired HMM.

EVALUATION

Patients with impaired HMM often have a chronic illness or a progressive disease that leads to additional impairment. To evaluate the effectiveness of nursing interventions, goals must have been appropriately set for the patient's condition and prognosis. Improvement may not be a realistic goal with chronic illness or progressive disease. For example, the physical health of a person with terminal cancer will not improve; thus, impaired HMM will not resolve until death.

Meeting patient goals can be taxing and frustrating for the nurse. Goals may not have been met because of factors outside the realm of nursing responsibility, such as medical complications that decrease the resources and abilities to perform ADLs. Other goals that initially seemed realistic and attainable may not be met due to nurse-related problems. Unclear communication between the patient and health and social service professionals is one such problem. Communication problems can result in decreased patient compliance with medical and nursing treatments. Communication problems between nurses and other health professionals can result in decreased collaboration and coordination. Other problems include choosing inappropriate criteria for measuring nursing accomplishments, overinvolvement with the patient, and general burnout (Eliopoulos, 1982). Table 27-4 lists some reasons for unmet goals.

The following is a list of sample goals and outcome criteria for patients with impaired HMM.

Goal
The patient/caregiver will overcome the functional deficit(s) that contribute or lead to impaired HMM.

Possible Outcome Criteria
- Within 24 hours, patient/caregiver expresses desire to maintain self or other at home.
- Within 24 hours, patient/caregiver identifies the major factors that restrict self-care.
- By third day, patient expresses readiness and willingness to learn alternate ways to perform skills necessary for home living.
- By third week, patient demonstrates to nurse or occupational therapist the ability to perform tasks related to home living.
- By discharge, caregiver eliminates major safety hazards from the home, as relayed to the nurse.

Goal
The patient will return to a safe home environment.

Possible Outcome Criteria
- Within 2 days, patient demonstrates ability to understand simple verbal directions.
- Within 1 week, patient/caregiver agrees to perform responsibilities as outlined in contract.
- By discharge, patient/caregiver demonstrates ability to correctly and confidently perform treatments or procedures to be continued at home.
- By discharge, patient expresses satisfaction with preparatory arrangements.
- By discharge, patient/caregiver identifies at least two people or community service agencies who can answer questions and provide additional referrals.
- By discharge, patient/caregiver expresses willingness to make financial arrangements for home care.
- After discharge, patient/caregiver uses the home care support service needed and available, as described at next appointment.

TABLE 27–4
Some Reasons for Unmet Home Maintenance Goals

Patient/Caregiver/Community Factors	Nurse-Related Factors
Worsening medical condition	Poor communication with patient
Constraints of the health-care system	Poor communication with other health or social service professionals
Lack of insurance for needed services	Inappropriate goals or criteria selected
Lack of needed service in the community	Overinvolvement with patient or family
Lack of patient commitment to the care plan	Time constraints on developing plan and intervening
Caregiver stress and burnout	

Nursing Management Plan
The Patient With Impaired Home Maintenance Management

Nursing Diagnosis: Impaired home maintenance management related to activity intolerance and living alone, as manifested by inability to perform instrumental activities of daily living and decreased ability to perform self-care.

Patient Goal: The patient will continue living in the home environment.

Patient Outcome Criteria

- At initial interview, patient expresses commitment to continued living at home.
- The patient demonstrates how to contact emergency services before discharge.
- The patient demonstrates an ability to meet financial obligations before discharge.
- During first month at home, patient uses Meals-on-Wheels, home health aide, and church home visitation program on a regular basis, as reported to healthcare worker.
- The patient demonstrates an ability to perform ADLs during regular home visits.

Nursing Intervention	Scientific Rationale
1. Discuss the options regarding living at home and the patient's preferences. Develop a contract based on those preferences.	1. Patient's participation in decision-making enhances the patient's commitment to carrying out the contract. A contract facilitates communication and enhances efficiency for those involved.
2. Review financial obligations with the patient and assess the patient's ability to pay bills and keep records.	2. With the potential for impaired cognitive functioning and with the complexity of billing systems, the patient's ability to keep financial records and to make financial decisions affects the patient's ability to remain at home.
3. Refer to the community services necessary to support the patient's living at home.	3. Referrals to community services are most successful if made by professionals with a patient data base and with a responsibility to coordinate the services provided to the patient.
4. Assess the patient for social isolation, depression, or anxiety related to living alone. Refer to support groups as appropriate.	4. When people are unable to leave the home and have social contacts, affective disorders may develop.
5. Assess for specific patient teaching needs related to living at home and then provide (or arrange to provide) that education. Periodically evaluate the knowledge retention.	5. Patient teaching is most effective if tailored to the immediate knowledge needs. Knowledge retention may deteriorate with changes in physical status.

Goal

The patient will continue to live at home.

Possible Outcome Criteria

- By 1 month after discharge, patient/caregiver expresses desire for continued home living.
- By 2 months after discharge, patient/caregiver continues to use available community resources that support continued living at home.
- By 3 months after discharge, patient/caregiver demonstrates continued ability to carry out responsibilities as contracted.
- By 3 months after discharge, patient/caregiver participates in learning and demonstrating new skills necessary for continued home living.
- By 3 months after discharge, patient/caregiver seeks additional or alternative sources for financing home care.

Goal

The caregiver will participate in caring for the patient at home.

Possible Outcome Criteria

- Within 1 week, caregiver lists at least three signs of stress he or she may experience as a caregiver and can name two ways to relieve stress.
- Within 2 weeks, caregiver participates in decision-making about care and placement of patient.
- Within 2 weeks, caregiver demonstrates adequate physical strength to perform home care tasks.
- Two weeks before discharge, caregiver identifies physical barriers at home that must be changed before patient arrives home.
- By discharge, caregiver lists signs or symptoms of changes in patient status requiring immediate medical attention, and describes steps to take in such an event.
- By discharge, caregiver describes alternate plans for patient care if he or she cannot provide the necessary care or supervision.

Key Concepts

- Home maintenance management is the ability to independently maintain a safe, growth-promoting environment. Environment may be the hospital room, the home, the neighborhood, or the friend and family support system.
- Changing environments is stressful. It is important to consider whether the patient can continue activities of daily living in the new environment.
- Impaired home maintenance management is an imbalance between what the patient *needs* for home maintenance and what the patient can *provide* for himself or herself.

- The person and environment fit refers to the degree of match between the person's functional abilities and the resources within the patient's environment.
- The ability to maintain a safe, nurturing home environment depends on the person's physical and emotional development.
- Impaired Home Maintenance Management is a nursing diagnosis appropriate for a wide range of functional deficits.
- The family's needs must be considered at all times in planning and implementing nursing interventions, because family members are often the primary caregivers for the patient after discharge from the hospital.
- The nature of health problems and functional deficits that lead to impaired HMM is such that most patients will not improve in health. Thus, realistic patient goals must be established that make use of existing patient and family strengths.
- Possible consequences of impaired HMM include out-of-home placement, family strains, and homelessness.

References

Aleman, A. R. (1983). Nursing care with the multiproblem poor family. *Home Healthcare Nurse, 1*(2), 34.

Anthony, T. M. (1987). Caretaker, take care. *Geriatric Nursing, 8,* 78.

Archbold, P. G. (1982). An analysis of parent-caring by women. *Home Health Care Services Quarterly, 3*(2), 5.

Bachrach, L. L. (1987). Geographic mobility and the homeless mentally ill. *Hospital & Community Psychiatry, 38*(1), 27.

Carnevali, D. L. (1984). The nursing domain for diagnostic reasoning. In D. L. Carnevali, P. H. Mitchell, N. F. Woods, et al., *Diagnostic reasoning in nursing.* Philadelphia: J. B. Lippincott.

Carpenito, L. J. (1989). *Nursing diagnosis: Application to clinical practice* (3rd ed.). Philadelphia: J. B. Lippincott.

Chick, N., & Meleis, A. I. (1986). Transitions: A nursing concern. In P. L. Chinn (ed.), *Nursing research methodology: Issues and implementation.* Rockville, MD: Aspen.

Choi, T., Josten, L., & Christensen, M. L. (1983). Health-specific family coping index for noninstitutional care. *American Journal of Public Health, 73,* 1275.

Clemen, S. A., Eigsti, D. G., & McGuire, S. L. (1981). *Comprehensive family and community health nursing.* New York: McGraw-Hill.

Coombs, E. M. (1984). A conceptual framework for home nursing. *Journal of Advanced Nursing, 9,* 157.

Eliopoulos, C. (1982). Chronic care and the elderly: Impact on the client, the family and the nurse. In T. Wells (ed.), *Aging and health promotion.* Rockville, MD: Aspen.

Gallagher, D. E. (1985). Intervention strategies to assist caregivers of frail elders: Current research status and future research directions. *Annual Review of Gerontology and Geriatrics, 5,* 249.

Gikow, F. F. (1981). How to determine appropriate community services for the elderly. *Nursing and Health Care, 6,* 322.

Gould, E. J., & Wargo, J. (1987). *Home health nursing care plans.* Rockville, MD: Aspen.

Grau, L. (1986). Britain's community psychiatric nursing team. *Geriatric Nursing, 7,* 143.

Haddad, A. M. (1987). *High-tech home care: A practical guide.* Rockville, MD: Aspen.

Hooyman, N. (1983). Social support networks in services to the elderly. In J. K. Wittaker & J. Garbarino (eds.), *Social support networks: Informal helping in the human services.* New York: Aldine.

Horowitz, A. (1985). Family caregiving to the frail elderly. *Annual Review of Gerontology and Geriatrics, 5,* 194.

Imperato, P. J. (1987). New York's homeless. *New York State Journal of Medicine, 87*(1), 1.

Kane, R. A., & Kane, R. L. (1981). *Assessing the elderly: A practical guide to measurement.* Toronto: Lexington Books.

Lawton, M. P. (1985). Activities and leisure. *Annual Review of Gerontology and Geriatrics, 5,* 127.

Levine, H., Leventhal, E. A., & Nguyen, T. V. (1985). Reactions of families to illness: Theoretical models and perspectives. In D. C. Turk & R. D. Kerns (eds.), *Health, illness and families: A lifespan perspective.* New York: John Wiley & Sons.

McKeehan, K. (1981). *Continuing care.* St. Louis: C. V. Mosby.

NANDA (1990). *Taxonomy I revised 1990, with official nursing diagnoses.* St. Louis, MO: North American Nursing Diagnosis Association.

Norris, C. M. (1986). Restlessness: A disturbance in rhythmicity. *Geriatric Nursing, 7,* 302.

Phillips, E. K., & Cloonan, P. A. (1987). DRG ripple effect on community health nursing. *Public Health Nursing, 4*(2), 84–88.

Rasmusen, L. A. (1984). A screening tool promotes early discharge planning. *Nursing Management, 15*(5), 39–45.

Runner-Heidt, C. M. (1984). Where does the discharge planner go from here? *Home Healthcare Nurse, 2*(4), 30–35.

Sargis, N. M., Jennrich, J. A., & Murray, K. M. (1987). Housing conditions and health: A crucial link. *Nursing and Health Care, 8,* 335.

Schafer, S. C. (1985). Modifying the environment. *Geriatric Nursing, 6,* 157.

Schlossberg, N. K. (1981). A model for analyzing human adaptation to transition. *Consulting Psychology, 9*(2), 2.

Shapiro, E. (1986). Patterns and predictions of home care use by the elderly when need is the sole basis for admission. *Home Health Care Services Quarterly, 7*(1), 29–43.

Spradley, B. W. (1985). *Community health nursing: Concepts and practice* (2nd ed.). Boston: Little, Brown & Co.

Spradley, B. W., & Dorsey, B. (1985). Home health care. In B. W. Spradley: *Community health nursing: Concepts and practice* (2nd ed.). Boston: Little, Brown & Co.

Stephens, S. A., & Achritianson, J. B. (1986). *Informal care of the elderly.* Lexington, MA: Lexington Books.

Taylor, M. B. (1985). The effects of DRGs on home health care. *Nursing Outlook, 33,* 288.

Thomas, S. D. (1985). Assessing and adapting the home environment. In M. O. Hogstel (Ed.), *Home nursing care for the elderly.* Bowie, MD: Prentice-Hall.

U.S. Department of Health and Human Services. (1986). *Americans needing home care.* Vital and Health Statistics, Series 10, No. 153. DHHS Publication No. (PHS) 86-1581. Hyattsville, MD: National Center for Health Statistics.

Vermund, S. H., Belmar, R., & Drucker, E. (1987). Homelessness in New York City: The youngest victims. *New York State Journal of Medicine, 87*(1), 3.

Wells, M. I. (1983). Discharge planning: Closing the gaps in continuity of care. *Nursing '83, 13*(11), 45.

Bibliography

Hayes, J. C. (1986). Patient symptoms and family coping: Predictors of hospice utilization patterns. *Cancer Nursing, 9,* 317.

Hillman, S. (1986). Assessing the patient in the home environment. In S. Stewart-Siddall (Ed.), *Home health care nursing: Administrative and clinical perspectives.* Rockville, MD: Aspen.

Holing, E. V. (1986). The primary caregiver's perception of the dying trajectory: An exploratory study. *Cancer Nursing, 9,* 29.

Keating, S. B., & Kelman, G. B. (1988). *Home health care nursing.* Philadelphia: J. B. Lippincott.

Perlman, R., & Giele, J. Z. (1983). An unstable triad: Dependents' demands, family resources, community supports. *Home Health Care Services Quarterly, 3*(3/4), 12.

Rubenstein, R. L. (1985). The elderly who live alone and the social supports. *Annual Review of Gerontology and Geriatrics, 5,* 165.

U.S. Department of Health and Human Services. (1986). *Current estimates from the National Health Interview survey, United States, 1985.* Vital and Health Statistics, Series 10, No. 160. DHHS Publication No. (PHS) 86-1588. Hyattsville, MD: National Center for Health Statistics.

U.S. Department of Health and Human Services. (1990a). *Functional status of the non-institutionalized elderly: Estimates of ADL and IADL difficulties.* National Medical Expenditure Survey Research Findings, DHHS Publication No. (PHS) 90-3462.

U.S. Department of Health and Human Services. (1990b). *Use of home and community services by persons ages 65 and older with functional difficulties.* National Medical Expenditure Survey Research Findings, DHHS Publication No. (PHS) 90-3466.

UNIT VII
Activity and Exercise

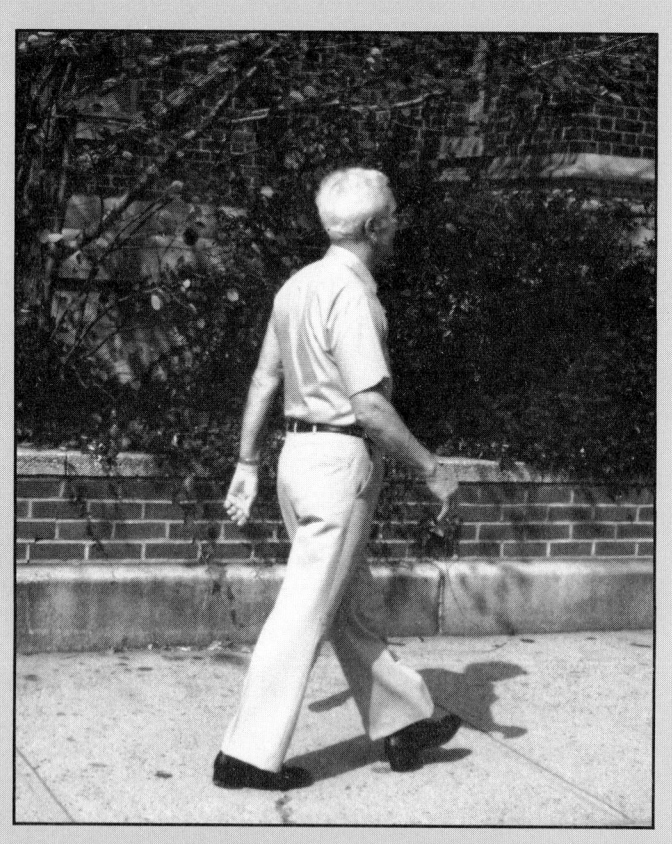

CHAPTERS

28 Self-Care and Hygiene

29 Body Mechanics and Mobility

30 Oxygenation: Respiratory Function

31 Oxygenation: Cardiac Function and Tissue Perfusion

Activity and exercise is a vital area of human function that includes both the ability and the desire to expend energy. Unit VII discusses this area of human function and explores body mechanics and mobility, respiratory and cardiac function, and the area of self-care, which involves activities that require energy expenditure.

The first chapter explores self-care and hygiene. Assessment focuses on how well the patient can meet his or her own self-care needs. Holistic nursing interventions are aimed at assisting the patient with self-care activities to the degree necessary to support independent function. The next chapter considers body mechanics and mobility, two major components of energy expenditure, as factors in patient care from the perspectives of both the nurse and the patient. The assessment emphasis is on evaluating a patient's ability to move around in his or her environment to meet daily needs. Nursing interventions to promote health and function focus on helping the patient engage in activity in safe, effective ways. The chapter also explores nursing interventions for patients with altered mobility.

The last two chapters in this unit discuss respiratory and cardiac function. The ability to engage in energy consuming activities is influenced by both areas of function. These chapters explore concepts and nursing care related to the basic human need for adequate oxygenation.

This unit considers patient activity and energy use. These functions are essential for the patient to maintain activities of daily living.

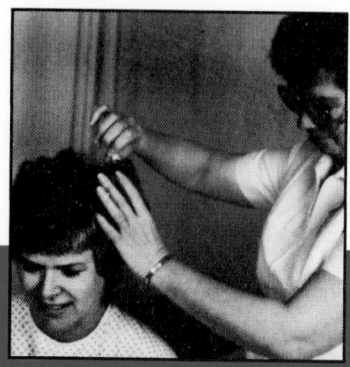

Self-Care and Hygiene

LEARNING OBJECTIVES

Upon completion of this chapter, the student will be able to do the following:

- Discuss the importance of self-care and hygiene in health and illness.
- Identify several physiologic factors that may alter self-care.
- Identify environmental factors that complicate independence in self-care.
- Identify behavioral factors that affect independence in self-care.
- Discuss important subjective and objective areas of assessment in identifying self-care deficits.
- Identify defining characteristics for the four areas of self-care deficit (bathing/hygiene, dressing, feeding, toileting).
- Describe nursing goals for each of the four areas of self-care deficit.
- List outcome criteria for each of the four areas of self-care deficit.
- Describe interventions for each of the four areas of self-care deficit.
- List beneficial patient teaching for each of the four areas of self-care.

KEY TERMS

Caries	Condom catheter	Plaque
Cerumen	Gingiva	Tartar
Commode	Pediculosis	Urinal

28

Normal Self-Care Function
  Characteristics of Normal Self-Care
    Bathing and Hygiene
    Hair Care
    Feet and Nail Care
    Eyes, Ears, and Nose Care
    Oral Care
    Feeding
    Toileting
    Dressing and Grooming
  Normal Self-Care Functional Patterns
  Factors Affecting Normal Self-Care
    Neuromuscular Function
    Energy
    Cognition and Perception
    Intact Senses
    Motivation
    Culture, Values, and Beliefs
    Environment
  Lifespan Considerations
Altered Self-Care Function
  Potential for Altered Self-Care
    Decreased Energy
    Acute Illness and Surgery
    Pain
    Neuromuscular Impairment
    Sensorimotor Deficits
    Cognitive Dysfunction
    Dysfunctional Environment
    Emotional Disturbance and Depression
  Manifestations of Altered Self-Care
    Poor Hygiene and Grooming
    Inability to Demonstrate Self-Care Activities
    Verbalization of Reluctance to Perform Self-Care
Assessment
  Subjective Data
    Functional Pattern Identification
    Risk Identification
    Dysfunction Identification
  Objective Data
Nursing Diagnoses and Patient Goals

Self-Care Deficit, Bathing/Hygiene
  Definition
  Defining Characteristics
  Related Factors
Self-Care Deficit, Dressing/Grooming
  Definition
  Defining Characteristics
  Related Factors
Self-Care Deficit, Toileting
  Definition
  Defining Characteristics
  Related Factors
Self-Care Deficit, Feeding
  Definition
  Defining Characteristics
  Related Factors
Related Nursing Diagnoses
Patient Goals
Implementation
  Nursing Interventions to Promote Health and Self-Care
  Nursing Interventions for Altered Self-Care
    Scheduled Care
    Nurse–Patient Relationship
    Bathing and Skin Care
    Perineal Care
    Backrubs
    Care of Feet and Nails
    Hair Care
    Shaving
    Oral Care
    Eye Care
    Ear Care
    Feeding
    Toileting
    Dressing
    Care of Unit Environment
  Discharge Planning and Home Care
Evaluation
Key Concepts

S elf-care and hygiene refers to a person's ability to care for himself or herself by performing the primary care functions of bathing and general body hygiene, dressing, feeding, and toileting. Because these activities are basic to healthy functioning, they are often taken for granted. The ability to independently perform appropriate self-care and hygiene practices greatly enhances the patient's health status and emotional well-being. When patients cannot perform these activities because of illness or injury, however, their health and well-being are jeopardized. Proper nutrition and care of skin, teeth, hair, and nails promote good health by helping to protect the body from infection and disease and by allowing the person to feel good and have a positive self-image. The ability to perform self-care allows the person to remain independent, has a positive influence on self-concept and self-image, and gives him or her a sense of control.

The nurse can play a crucial role in helping patients learn or relearn self-care techniques. Because nurses focus on patients' response to health and illness rather than on the disease itself, helping patients gain or regain independence in self-care is one of the more important goals of nursing. When illness or injury interferes with the ability to perform self-care, the nurse assists or performs tasks the patient cannot manage, or offers support to family members or other caregivers. But the main focus is to help patients achieve as much independence in self-care as possible.

NORMAL SELF-CARE FUNCTION

This section describes the activities that are included in self-care and hygiene practices.

Characteristics of Normal Self-Care

Bathing and Hygiene

Skin (discussed in Chap. 34) is the first line of defense against microorganisms and infection entering the body. This is why keeping skin intact and healthy is so important. Increased perspiration interacts with bacteria on the skin to cause body odor, which can be offensive, and excess sebum can promote bacterial growth. Regular bathing removes excess oil, perspiration, and bacteria from the skin surface. This is particularly important when the skin is compromised by an injury or illness, leaving the body more susceptible to infection (for example, an open wound or skin breakdown due to pressure sores).

Bathing also increases circulation (from the friction of a washcloth) and helps maintain muscle tone and joint mobility (from the movement of limbs during the bath). In addition, bathing provides relaxation and comfort and gives most people a sense of well-being. A warm or hot

---

> **Benefits of Bathing**
>
> - Cleanses body secretions, microorganisms, debris, and perspiration from skin
> - Stimulates circulation
> - Mobilizes joints
> - Provides relaxation, physical and emotional comfort
> - Provides opportunity to evaluate skin status and observe for signs of physical problems or deterioration
> - Provides opportunity for positive patient–nurse interaction

---

bath increases circulation by dilating blood vessels near the skin surface, allowing more blood to flow to the skin.

Bathing allows the nurse to assess the patient's physical condition, noting injured areas, bruises, rashes, or any other unusual signs. Bathing can also promote conversation between the patient and the nurse, facilitating a trusting, satisfying relationship.

Hair Care

Shampooing removes dirt and oil from the hair and scalp. It also increases scalp circulation. For most people, having their hair shampooed is relaxing. Clean hair makes patients feel good about their appearance and enhances feelings of self-worth. Daily brushing and combing of hair is important in maintaining the health of the hair by distributing oil across the hair shafts and massaging the scalp, which stimulates circulation. Neatly groomed hair also promotes a good self-image.

Feet and Nail Care

Healthy feet are important because they are crucial in helping people to stand and walk. Feet are usually washed along with the rest of the body when showering or bathing. Nails are trimmed as needed. There are many tiny bones, ligaments, and muscles in the foot, and comfortable, properly fitting shoes are essential to healthy feet. Shoes should accommodate the size and shape of the foot and should be large enough so that toenails do not rub on the shoes, causing skin breakdown or ingrown nails.

Many people ignore their feet until problems occur. The feet are vulnerable to injury because of their increased exposure and susceptibility to skin breakdown. Mobility can be jeopardized by seemingly minor problems such as ingrown nails, ill-fitting shoes, swollen feet, corns, or abrasions.

Eyes, Ears, and Nose Care

Under normal conditions, the eyes require little care because the lacrimal fluid bathes the eyes continually and the lids and lashes prevent foreign material from entering the eye. Special care may be needed for patients who wear glasses, contact lenses, or prostheses, those who have other visual problems, or those who use eye medications.

Ears need little attention, although the external ear should be cleansed while bathing. Patients wearing hearing aids may need special care. Some people may have excess accumulation of ear wax (**cerumen**), which often requires careful removal. A sharp object, such as a hairpin or toothpick, should never be used to extract wax, as this can damage the tympanic membrane. Not even cotton-tipped applicators should be used on the inner ear, as they can force wax further into the ear canal.

Nostrils can be cleaned by gentle blowing with both nostrils open. Closing one nostril while blowing can force foreign material into the eustachian tube or cause other damage to the inner canal.

Oral Care

The mouth and teeth play vital roles in the mastication (chewing) and digestion of food. The muscles in the cheeks aid in chewing. The tongue has taste buds that allow us to discern different flavors of foods and helps mix saliva with food for food breakdown and digestion. The tongue also aids in swallowing, moving the food toward the pharynx.

Teeth (Fig. 28-1) are composed of the crown, the dentin, the pulp cavity, the neck, and the root. The crown, the hard surface exposed outside the gum, is covered with enamel. The dentin under the enamel covers the pulp cavity, which houses the blood vessels and nerves. The neck and root are below gum level.

Proper care of teeth and gums helps prevent gum deterioration and tooth loss. Cavities in the enamel (**caries**) are caused by deposits of **plaque,** a substance that forms and hardens on the teeth and is composed primarily of bacteria and saliva. Bacterial enzymes from the plaque combine with carbohydrates from food and organic acids to ferment and break down enamel. Caries form more often when food and plaque remain on the teeth for long periods of time. Plaque and food particles can be removed by daily brushing, flossing, and rinsing. When plaque remains on the teeth over a period of time, it hardens into **tartar,** which cannot be removed by simple brushing; it must be scraped off by a professional with dental instruments.

Fluoride in small amounts strengthens teeth during their formation and helps prevent caries. Fluoride is added to most water-treatment systems at the appropriate concentration (1.0 parts per million) (Valentine, 1988). Where fluoride is not added, parents may want to

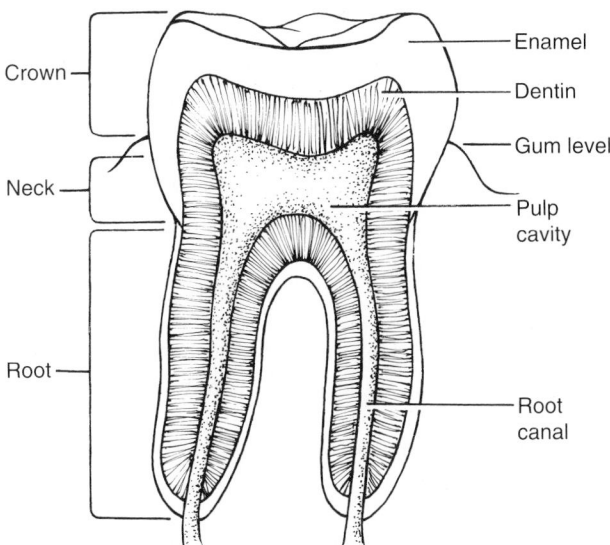

Figure 28–1.   Parts of a tooth.

ask the dentist how to give children appropriate supplements of fluoride until the age of 14.

Healthy gums are important because they provide support for the teeth. The gums are made up of the oral mucosa (**gingiva**), which covers the bone supporting the tooth; the alveolar bone, which forms sockets around the teeth; and the periodontal ligament, which joins the teeth to the bone. Inflammation in these tissues, called gingivitis or periodontitis, can be caused by local irritation from bacteria, plaque, tartar, food impaction, or mechanical, chemical, or thermal extremes.

Proper oral hygiene includes daily brushing, flossing, and rinsing of teeth, and care of dentures or other appliances. Regular dental check-ups are important to ensure the health of the teeth and gums.

Feeding

The ability to feed oneself may be the most important self-care skill in terms of independence. Independence or even partial independence in making food choices and being able to feed oneself can be immensely gratifying and can enhance self-concept for patients of all ages. Feeding requires the desire to make food choices and eat, the energy and muscular coordination to move food from the plate to the mouth, and the ability to chew and swallow.

Toileting

Normal toileting includes feeling the urge to void and, independently or with assistance, moving to the toilet or bedpan, rearranging clothing, voiding, and effectively cleaning areas of excretion. Chapters 37 and 38 give detailed descriptions of normal urinary and bowel function.

Dressing and Grooming

Dressing oneself includes being able to get clothes from the closet or drawers, put them on, manage fasteners (such as zippers and buttons), and put on socks and shoes. Normal dressing and grooming patterns include the daily brushing and combing of hair. Depending on cultural or personal preferences, some women wear makeup every day, and for many women shaving underarm and leg hair is an important part of grooming. For men, shaving can be extremely important to their physical appearance and self-image. Some men feel as though they are not properly groomed without shaving every day, while others do not need to shave every day. Some men experience skin irritation if they do not shave daily. The amount of beard growth may dictate how often shaving is needed. Men with beards or mustaches may need to trim them periodically and must be careful to remove spilled food particles from them.

Normal Self-Care Functional Patterns

Self-care and hygiene techniques vary depending on cultural or personal preferences, but in general patterns include a proper diet, normal toileting, daily bathing or cleansing of the skin and perineal areas, daily brushing, flossing, and rinsing of the teeth, special care for dentures or other oral appliances, brushing or combing of hair, and other grooming preferences. Men may shave or trim facial hair; women may put on makeup. Some people prefer to bathe in the morning, whereas others bathe before going to bed.

Other areas that require attention and care are the hair, feet, and nails. The hair should be shampooed as frequently as needed to keep it clean, depending on its texture and oiliness. People with dry hair may need to moisturize their hair with conditioners or other commercial products.

Shoes should be comfortable and fit properly. Toenails should be trimmed so that they do not rub against the shoes. Fingernails should be cleaned and trimmed periodically.

Most people dress and groom themselves in the morning, soon after arising. Clothes may need to be changed during the day depending on activities and weather.

Factors Affecting Normal Self-Care

Many of us take self-care activities for granted because they seem simple and are accomplished on a routine basis throughout life. But many factors influence whether or not a person can perform these tasks that are important to daily living. Self-care requires adequate neuromuscular functioning, muscle strength, mobility, fine motor control, adequate energy levels, and intact sensory capabilities. Cognitive functioning, psychological factors (motivation, mental status), and sociocultural factors (values, cultural grooming practices) also influence the performance of self-care activities.

Neuromuscular Function

Self-care activities such as swallowing, getting to the toilet, and dressing require a well-functioning neuromuscular system. To accomplish these tasks, the central nervous system sends messages to the peripheral nervous system and the muscle fibers to coordinate the necessary fine and gross motor activity. Normal muscle strength and normal contraction and relaxation of muscles is also needed.

Fine motor control allows the person to have command of small, precise movements (usually of the hands). Fine motor control requires coordination of muscle groups to facilitate activities such as cutting food, opening a milk carton, buttoning a shirt, applying makeup, and wiping after toileting. *Gross motor activity* involves the coordinated movement of large muscle groups (e.g., climbing in and out of the bathtub, walking or driving to the grocery store, carrying groceries home, getting on and off the toilet). Normal alignment, awareness of the body's spatial position (proprioception), and balance are needed to coordinate these large motor movements. Newborns and infants, in whom these motor skills are not developed, and people with compromised motor abilities from illness or injury cannot do these tasks without assistance.

Energy

Energy must be available at the cellular level for muscle movement to occur. Adequate energy stores prevent fatigue during self-care. This energy level requires adequate nutrition and the ability to break down food so it can be absorbed and used by the cells. This process also requires adequate oxygen, so respiration plays a significant role. The circulatory system delivers nutrients, oxygen, and other substances to the cells to produce adenosine triphosphate (ATP), a nucleotide used to store energy, and removes waste products produced by cellular metabolism.

Cognition and Perception

The ability to perceive and understand methods of self-care is important in achieving independence. People with normal cognitive and perceptive abilities are usually motivated to perform self-care. However, those with limited cognitive abilities may be unaware of the need for self-care, may not know appropriate methods of achieving it, or may be unable to assess what they can safely perform independently. They can be trained to perform some basic self-care skills, but the training requires a great deal of time, with much repetition of the skills and appropriate feedback. They can be taught to wash, dress, and toilet independently in a familiar setting, but they may require assistance with more complex tasks, such as shopping for groceries.

Intact Senses

Senses that function normally help a person to maintain independence in self-care activities. Sight is particularly important because it permits a person to locate and use objects. People with impaired sight can make adjustments to their environment to help them find objects and move about, but they may have difficulty in unfamiliar environments. Touch and taste can signal unsafe conditions, such as temperatures that are too hot or too cold. Hearing may not be essential to performing self-care activities, but impaired hearing can interfere with understanding verbal instructions and cues.

Motivation

Motivation can be a powerful factor in achieving independence in self-care. Even though a person is physically capable of self-care, he or she must be motivated to perform self-care and must feel that self-care is important. People with a positive self-image and those who perceive themselves as worthy of attention and care have a greater motivation to attend to self-care.

Culture, Values, and Beliefs

Self-care routines and practices are largely a reflection of what one learns from one's family or from the community in which one grows up. Habits formed around how frequently one bathes, brushes teeth, changes clothes, or what one eats are usually learned early in life from family members, friends, and peers within the community. Such preferences may vary widely from person to person and culture to culture. For instance, many Americans do not feel clean unless they bathe daily and use a deodorant, but people in other cultures consider bathing once a week to be normal, and do not feel the need to mask natural body odors. Some people are extremely sensitive regarding their privacy during bathing; others are used to communal baths. Some people worry if they do not have a bowel movement each day; others are content with one every other day or even less frequently. Nurses should be aware of the vast differences in family customs and personal preferences in relation to self-care practices.

Environment

The environment in which people learn and practice self-care activities greatly influences those practices. For example, in a household without running water, family members may bathe only once every 2 or 3 days, and the children may bathe together. Financial resources can influence diet and eating habits as well as grooming practices or whether one can afford grooming products. Food buying practices can be greatly influenced by what food stores are available in the community and whether there is available transportation (either public or private). Television and print advertising have a large impact on the products people use and consume and on their food-buying and grooming practices.

Lifespan Considerations

Normal developmental stages impact self-care throughout the lifespan. Considering the patient's age helps the nurse understand self-care needs and plan appropriate interventions.

Newborn and Infant

Newborns participate in self-care only by crying and letting others know when they need to be fed or diapered. They need to be fed, bathed, dressed, and groomed by a caregiver. Newborns are born with sucking, rooting, and swallowing reflexes that allow them to ingest milk and liquids. They communicate hunger by crying and indicate satiety by falling asleep. By 3 to 4 months, infants begin to develop eye–hand coordination, and by 5 to 6 months many children can grasp and eat pieces of food. As gross motor function develops around 7 to 9 months, children can hold a spoon, drink from a cup with help, and drink with a straw. At 9 to 12 months, children can usually pick up finger food and feed themselves, can hold and drink from a bottle, drink from a cup with some spilling, and spoon-feed themselves with quite a bit of spilling. By 18 months, most children can spoon-feed themselves without spilling (Bellack & Bamford, 1984).

Infants are totally dependent on caregivers for toileting. They usually develop the ability to control elimination of urine and feces after the first year of life when neuromuscular function has matured in the infant. Urination may occur as frequently as 20 times a day, and the daily amount varies between 250 and 500 mL. Stools are also frequent and can be soft or liquid. Keeping the skin as dry and clean as possible helps preserve its integrity.

Changing an infant's diaper is relatively easy in early infancy and becomes more difficult as the child becomes more active. During a diaper change, an infant should never be left unattended in a place where he or she could roll or fall.

Toddler and Preschooler

Self-care abilities increase considerably during this stage, particularly in feeding and toileting. As gross motor development increases in toddlers and preschoolers, they gain more mastery of their environment.

Toddlers' eating patterns are erratic, but most toddlers can drink well from a cup and use a spoon without spilling (Bellack & Bamford, 1984). Small portions of easy-to-handle food are appropriate.

Many children achieve daytime bowel and bladder control between ages 2 and 3. Staying dry through the night is usually achieved by age 4, but some children still wet the bed at night until age 5.

Preschoolers (ages 4 to 5) can manage most aspects of bathing and grooming with some support, but children under age 4 need support in wiping, handwashing, and dressing and undressing.

During illness or stress, most children regress in their toileting and feeding habits. Children who are toilet-trained commonly revert to wetting their pants or the bed at night when ill or hospitalized. Older children who can feed themselves may want to be fed or drink from a bottle again. *Regression* is a common coping mechanism, especially for toddlers and preschoolers. During a stressful period, a child may revert from the most recently learned behavior to an earlier behavior that is more comfortable and satisfying. This "time-out" behavior permits the child to withdraw, conserve energy, and regain control. Regression is a normal reaction, and caregivers should understand and permit it.

Child and Adolescent

Although independent in self-care, some school-age children and adolescents may require reminders to bathe, brush their teeth, and change clothes appropriately. They still need direction and encouragement to eat healthy foods and use appropriate table skills. As the child approaches adolescence, self-care activities become more important as the body begins to mature and physiologic changes start to occur.

Hormonal changes in adolescents result in the growth of body hair. Both sexes develop pubic and axillary (underarm) hair. Boys develop facial hair and may begin shaving. Sebaceous glands become more active and often produce excess oil on the skin. Many adolescents suffer minor skin problems and some experience acne, which can be psychologically devastating to the adolescent's self-image. Sweat glands become fully developed and functional, and adolescents may need to begin using a deodorant or antiperspirant. Daily bathing and shampooing becomes important to counteract body odor.

Along with these physiological changes, adolescents undergo extreme psychological and emotional changes. Adolescence is a time of burgeoning independence, self-discovery, and beginning to develop one's own identity and define oneself as a person. Girls and boys become interested in looking attractive to the opposite sex. Dressing and grooming practices are heavily influenced by the behaviors of peers, because adolescents want to be accepted by others. Teenagers are also influenced by advertisements and television and often copy hairstyles or clothes worn by movie personalities or popular music celebrities.

Adult and Older Adult

Self-care is usually independently performed by young and middle-aged adults. By this age, people have established self-care techniques that enhance their appearance and health. Busy lifestyles that include working and raising families may leave little time for self-care and health maintenance, but regular exercise and a proper diet are important to this age group to maintain healthy, strong bodies. The literature in the last 10 years is full of research showing the influence of exercise, diet, and stress on health in this age group.

The elderly pose special problems in self-care. Skin becomes drier and less elastic and resilient because glands reduce their production of oil. The skin usually becomes discolored, and brown spots, called liver spots, may appear on the hands and feet. Hair becomes thinner and grows more slowly, and hair loss is common. Men and women experience changes in hair color. Teeth may gradually deteriorate from periodontal disease or caries, and many elderly people wear dentures. The oral mucosa tends to become drier as saliva production lessens; some elderly people experience receding gums.

The feet of the older adult require special attention, since they generally are at risk for foot problems related to reduced peripheral blood flow from arteriosclerosis or poor circulation. Poor circulation makes the feet more vulnerable to infection and skin breakdown, particularly after trauma. Some older adults are not mobile enough to care for their feet and may be unable to inspect them easily.

Older adults may need to care for appliances such as hearing aids, glasses, dentures, contact lenses, or artificial eyes. Reduced circulation and decreased muscular flexibility may impair the older person's agility and increase the time needed to perform tasks. Healing is often slower. Bones are often brittle and more vulnerable to fractures when falls occur. The elderly are generally at greater risk for injury due to decreased perception and altered sensation. This age group has the greatest number of people with physically disabling chronic diseases that require alterations in activities of daily living.

ALTERED SELF-CARE FUNCTION

Nurses often encounter deficits in self-care; in fact, one study found that self-care deficit was the third most common nursing diagnosis (Gordon, 1987). In hospital and community nursing, "self-care deficits are usually produced by activity intolerance, impaired mobility, uncompensated short-term memory deficits (as in Alzheimer's disease) and uncompensated cognitive or sensorimotor deficits" (Gordon, 1987). Problems with self-care range from short-term and simple to long-term and complex.

Potential for Altered Self-Care

Decreased Energy

Acute or chronic illness or injury can jeopardize independence in self-care by decreasing energy levels. Compromised respiratory or cardiac function reduces the body's ability to provide sufficient energy to the cells. Impairment of the cardiac system results in diminished delivery of nutrients and oxygen to the cells and removal of waste products of metabolism. Diseased lungs cannot provide adequate levels of oxygen to maintain cell metabolism. In both situations the person's energy level declines, resulting in fatigue and decreased ability to carry out self-care. Decreased energy and weakness can also result from disruption in diet, infection, disturbed gastrointestinal function, or fluid and electrolyte imbalance, or can be a response to a medication.

Acute Illness and Surgery

People who have undergone surgery or who have been acutely ill often need assistance with self-care. The amount of help needed varies depending on the illness or surgery, the patient's general health, and any sociocultural expectations. Drowsiness and confusion are common from analgesics, fluid and electrolyte imbalance, and hypoxemia. Nausea and vomiting add to the general malaise and produce a lack of motivation to perform self-care. Postoperative patients may experience weakness as a result of anesthesia, hypovolemia, lowered hematocrit level, and atelectasis, all of which may temporarily decrease cellular oxygen. Weakness combined with pain also impedes self-care. Casts, splints, IV lines, incisions, urinary catheters, nasogastric tubes, surgical drains, and anxiety constitute encumbrances to mobility and interfere with the ability to perform activities of daily living.

Pain

Patients may experience so much pain that they are unable to care for themselves. The ability or willingness to move may be significantly curtailed. Care-givers should be aware that most of the medications taken for pain (analgesics) also cause drowsiness and lightheadedness, hence patients taking such medications should be closely monitored during self-care activities to avoid falls. If patients are not taking analgesics, engaging in grooming and self-care activities may serve as a distraction from the pain (Foster, 1986). Some patients find bathing or being bathed a relaxing experience that can help distract from the pain.

Neuromuscular Impairment

Conditions such as stroke, spinal cord injury, and some nervous system disorders (parkinsonism, cerebral palsy, myasthenia gravis, and muscular dystrophy) may cause permanent neuromuscular impairment and are serious threats to independent self-care. Many of these conditions produce muscle weakness, muscle atrophy, lack of coordination, spasticity, partial or total paralysis, and joint contractures that make walking, talking, eating, and using the extremities extremely difficult or impossible. However, many people with these conditions can progress to a high level of independence in self-care with the aid of appliances or other creative alterations.

Injury to upper or lower extremities can render a person unable to perform self-care functions owing to immobility from casts, splints, or pain and weakness. These people need assistance from nurses or family members or special aids.

Sensorimotor Deficits

People who suffer sensorimotor deficits because of surgery, injury, or infection may need assistance in self-care. Those who have lost some sight may need help with eating or getting to the bathroom. If the visual impairment is prolonged or permanent, the patient may learn to compensate by making adjustments to the environment. For example, placing food and utensils on a tray in a consistent manner makes it easier for a visually impaired person to eat independently. Furniture can be arranged so that the person does not bump into objects or fall on the way to the bathroom. Hearing-impaired people may have difficulty carrying out self-care activities because they cannot hear instructions or verbal cues. Devising alternate methods of cuing and communicating proper instructions can help them to perform self-care independently.

Cognitive Dysfunction

Patients with a decreased level of consciousness or confusion due to injury or illness must be carefully assessed to determine how much assistance will be needed for self-care. Although these patients may be physically capable of feeding, dressing, bathing, and toileting, they may not be alert enough to know when these activities need to be performed or how to perform them safely. The nurse plays an important role in helping such patients to achieve and resume the highest level of self-care possible. The range of cognitive deficits is vast. Patients with minor deficits need to be reminded to provide self-care, but those with severe disabilities (such as severe head trauma or injuries) are often totally dependent on others and mechanical aids for self-care. Patients with cognitive deficits need to be carefully and individually assessed to determine what self-care skills they can accomplish or learn to accomplish with assistance.

Dysfunctional Environment

Some people, because of poverty or poor living conditions, may not have access to the facilities needed for appropriate self-care. Homeless people, migrant workers, and the rural poor often do not have access to proper resources, putting them at risk for self-care deficits. They may not have access to adequate bathroom facilities or running water to bathe properly and wash their clothes. They may not have enough food to ensure a proper diet or adequate cooking facilities to prepare a nutritious meal.

People in wheelchairs may have problems finding wheelchair-accessible facilities, putting them at risk for self-care deficits. For example, bathrooms must be designed so that wheelchairs can move in and out of stalls. Sinks must be at the right height for a wheelchair-bound person. Home alterations may be necessary to allow the person to perform self-care; see Chapter 27 for more details on home maintenance management.

The attitudes of other people can affect self-care independence. A caregiver may want to do something "for" the disabled person that he or she can really do independently. The caregiver may do this to save time and effort, but performing a task independently to the fullest extent possible enables the patient to gain independence and self-confidence and bolsters self-concept.

Emotional Disturbance and Depression

Emotional factors can result in self-care deficits. The inability to perceive reality appropriately due to side effects of medication, an unfamiliar environment, psychosis, or schizophrenia may cause inattentiveness to the need for personal care. Such people are highly distractible and have short attention spans, making them unable to concentrate on such basic needs as eating, grooming, and toileting. Severe dysfunction may be reflected by wearing inappropriate, or no, clothes in public or refusing to eat due to a fear of being poisoned.

Autism is characterized by an inability to respond to external stimuli and preoccupation with inner thoughts, daydreams, delusions, and hallucinations. A person with such a severe disorientation to the environment requires a great deal of assistance or prompting to carry out activities of daily living.

Depressed people may lack the energy or interest to care for themselves and may be poorly groomed, poorly nourished, or constipated. In addition, poor grooming may exacerbate feelings of depression. Self-care problems in older people may be greatly complicated by depression, resulting in disruption in self-care.

Manifestations of Altered Self-Care

Different degrees of deficit concerning ability to perform self-care can be seen in different people. Some deficits are temporary, whereas other are permanent.

Indications that deficits are present are poor grooming and hygiene, inability to demonstrate self-care skills, or verbalization of reluctance to perform self-care.

Poor Hygiene and Grooming

Visual cues indicating poor hygiene and grooming are readily apparent. There may be an offensive body odor. The skin may be soiled, dry, or flaky, or may have rashes and excoriated areas. Hair may be oily, unwashed, and uncombed. Nails may be dirty and broken. Clothes may be soiled, torn, or inappropriate. Inspection of the mouth may reveal sores, caries, inflamed gums, plaque buildup, and stained teeth. Mouth odor, or halitosis, is common. Soiling of pants with urine or feces may indicate difficulty in toileting.

Inability to Demonstrate Self-Care Activities

Inability to demonstrate gross and fine motor coordination needed for self-care activities indicates impaired ability to perform these functions independently. Gross motor abilities are needed to get to the bathroom, bathe, dress, and eat. Fine motor skills are required to fasten garments, apply makeup, open food containers, and cut food. The patient should be able to perform self-care activities without cuing and without excessive fatigue.

Verbalization of Reluctance to Perform Self-Care

If the patient expresses reluctance or fear to perform self-care activities, a deficit is present. Some patients may be reluctant due to depression, altered cognition, or dependent personality, others due to fatigue or fear of pain. Some people may fear that they will be unable to perform the activity successfully. Other patients may lack interest in self-care because their value system does not attach significance to conventional grooming activities.

ASSESSMENT

To determine which self-care activities the patient can perform, the nurse does a systematic assessment.

Subjective Data

By asking questions, the nurse can learn what the patient considers normal self-care activity and areas where the patient perceives difficulties. These questions are designed to elicit the patient's feelings about the problem, what he or she sees as the solution, and his or her level of motivation to alter self-care ability. If family members are present, they may give their perceptions of the patient's self-care abilities.

Functional Pattern Identification

Interviewing the patient permits the nurse to collect information about normal self-care patterns. Questions to elicit this information are listed in the display. Such information helps to determine how the patient normally manages self-care and what his or her feelings and values are about self-care. Determining normal self-care patterns permits the nurse to promote independence and optimal functioning.

This information can be used to individualize patient care. Bathing can be scheduled in the morning or evening, according to patient preference. Oral care can be provided before or after breakfast, with cold or warm water. Patients who sleep late may want to delay self-care activities, but others prefer to wash and apply makeup before seeing anyone.

Normal self-care patterns can be categorized according to the assistance required by the patient (Table 28-1). Level 0 reflects complete independence; at the other extreme, Level 4 reflects complete dependence on others.

Risk Identification

As the nurse gathers self-care information from the patient, she or he identifies factors that could put the patient at risk for self-care deficits. The nurse should observe and interview the patient for the following risk factors:

- Pain
- Immobility or limited use of an extremity
- Mental confusion or decreased mental alertness
- Decreased visual acuity or other sensory deficits
- Inability to control bowel or bladder function
- Decreased energy levels or fatigue
- Socioeconomic factors that might impair self-care

The patient's responses should be corroborated by a physical examination. For example, if the patient says he does not have problems with bathing and shampooing, but the nurse observes skin breakdown, body odors, and dirty fingernails, this would indicate that the person is at risk for self-care deficits.

Subjective Questions to Assess Self-Care

- How do you manage bathing/hygiene, dressing, eating, toileting?
- Describe the way in which you bathe, perform hygiene, dress, eat, toilet on your best days.
- Describe the way in which you bathe, perform hygiene, dress, eat, and toilet on your worst days.
- Are you satisfied with your ability to bathe, dress, eat, and toilet?
- Describe any factors that interfere with bathing, dressing, eating, and toileting.
- What goals and expectations do you have for these activities?
- Do you foresee alterations in your ability to care for yourself?
- What are the important daily activities for you?
- Can you pursue these important daily activities as much as you desire?
- Describe any factors interfering with the activities mentioned?
- How strong is your desire to participate in self-care?
- Is your desire for independence strong enough to withstand pain, inconvenience, and possible failure in performing self-care functions?

Where indicated, these questions should be asked separately for each of the areas of bathing and hygiene, dressing, eating, and toileting.

TABLE 28–1

Levels of Self-Care

Level	Description	Example
Level 0	Is independent in self-care activities	Healthy college student who lives in an apartment
Level 1	Uses equipment or devices to perform self-care activities independently	Elderly man who uses a cane for extra support during walking
Level 2	Requires assistance or supervision from another to complete self-care activities	Postoperative patient who needs help in bathing first day after surgery
Level 3	Requires assistance or supervision from another, as well as devices or equipment	Patient who ambulates using a walker and needs contact supervision
Level 4	Is completely dependent on another to perform self-care activities	Comatose patient who requires complete care by nursing staff

Dysfunctional Identification

The nurse should be familiar with the signs of dysfunctional patterns. The nurse can use an Index of Activities of Daily Living, developed by Katz (1963, 1983), to aid in this assessment and determine the level of functional independence in self-care practices of feeding, continence, transferring, going to the toilet, dressing, and bathing (Table 28-2). This standardized assessment guide allows the nurse to compare self-care deficits with normal patterns. Katz believed that loss of self-care is a natural part of aging and proceeds in an orderly fashion, with more complex activities being lost first. He also argued that people regain functional self-care abilities in patterns similar to the development of these skills in children. For example, they achieve feeding and continence skills first, then transfer and toileting abilities, and finally dressing and bathing abilities.

Objective Data

The nurse can validate information obtained during the patient interview by objectively observing the patient as he or she engages in self-care functions. The nurse should look for several specific factors:

- Evidence of inability to manage self-care (i.e., poor grooming, body odor, lice, skin lesions, poor nutrition)
- Ability to process sensory input by hearing, sight, smell, and touch
- Evidence of disabilities, such as impaired vision, weakness, cognitive deficits, immobility or spasticity,

---

Physical Assessment for Self-Care Deficits

- Body temperature, pulse rate, respiration rate (before, during, and after activity), breath sounds, blood pressure
- Height and weight
- Gait and posture
- Range of motion
- Muscle firmness
- Strength of hand grip
- Status of mouth and teeth
- Skin and nails (i.e., bony prominences, lesions, color, temperature, texture)
- Food or fluid intake

---

or mental lethargy (sometimes laboratory data can give explanations for weakness or lethargy)
- Manual dexterity
- Use of sensory or mechanical aids (i.e., glasses or contact lenses, dentures, hearing aid, cane or walker, condom catheter, raised toilet seat, or special eating utensils)

Assess the patient's cardiopulmonary response before, during, and after each self-care activity by assessing pulse rate, respiratory rate, and quality of breathing, and observing for changes in skin color. At the same time, note any alterations in the patient's normal physical status (see display).

TABLE 28–2

Index of Independence in Activities of Daily Living*

ADL	Independent	Dependent
Bathing (sponge, shower, or tub)	Needs assistance only in bathing a single part (such as back or disabled extremity) or bathes self completely	Needs assistance in bathing more than one part of body; needs assistance in getting in or out of tub or does not bathe self
Dressing	Gets clothes from closets and drawers; puts on clothes, outer garments, braces, manages fasteners (act of tying shoes is excluded)	Does not dress self or remains partly undressed
Toileting	Gets to toilet, gets on and off toilet, arranges clothes, cleans organs of excretion (may manage own bedpan at night or may not be using mechanical supports)	Uses bedpan or commode or needs assistance getting to and using toilet
Transfer	Moves in and out of bed and chair independently (may be using mechanical supports)	Needs assistance in moving in or out of bed and/or chair; does not perform one or more transfers
Continence	Has self-control of urination and defecation	Has partial or total incontinence in urination or defecation; partial or total control by enemas, catheters, or regulated use of urinals and/or bedpans
Feeding	Gets food from plate into mouth; precutting of meat and preparation of food (as buttering bread) are excluded from evaluation)	Needs assistance in feeding; does not eat at all or uses parenteral feeding

Independence means without supervision, direction, or active personal assistance, except as noted below. This is based on actual status and not on ability. A patient who refuses to perform is considered as not performing, even though he or she is deemed able.

To formulate realistic goals and interventions, the nurse must assess the resources available to the patient. This can mean internal resources (psychological, intellectual, and emotional factors) and external resources (living arrangements, finances). Table 28-3 lists external and internal resources and their influence on self-care.

NURSING DIAGNOSES AND PATIENT GOALS

Self-care deficit is manifested as actual or potential problems with self-care. The nurse determines the existence and extent of self-care deficit through patient assessment.

NANDA-accepted nursing diagnoses are Bathing/Hygiene, Dressing/Grooming, Feeding, and Toileting Self-Care Deficits. The diagnosis Self-Care Deficit is broad and can be used for problems involving a variety of body systems.

Self-Care Deficit, Bathing/Hygiene

Definition

A state in which the individual experiences impaired ability to perform or complete bathing/hygiene activities for oneself (NANDA, 1990).

TABLE 28–3
Assessment of External and Internal Resources

Factor	Influence
External Resources	
Housing (location, design, access by elevators/stairs, special equipment, kitchen and bathroom facilities, access to telephone, how many people share facilities)	• Mobility around home • Ability to shop for and prepare food • Access to bathroom for self-care
Air and water	• Availability of water for bathing and drinking • Air quality for breathing • Hot water for bathing
Neighborhood (proximity of shops, hospitals/clinics; available transportation)	• Ability to obtain groceries • Access to health care and assistance
Financial resources	• Ability to purchase food and self-care products • Ability to afford health care
Support network and community resources (family and friends, support groups and volunteers such as Meals on Wheels, home health care)	• Help with shopping, getting to doctor's appointments, self-care, and meal preparation
Government and social services	• Financial or material assistance for supplies and special equipment
Internal Resources	
Inner strength	• Ability to handle physical, mental, and emotional work
Endurance	• Stamina or "staying power" to cope with physical, mental, or emotional difficulties
Sensory input	• Ability to attend to and process environmental stimuli to provide a safe environment when attending to self-care needs
Cognitive abilities	• Amount and use of knowledge regarding self-care
Desire	• Will or motivation to participate in self-care
Courage	• Willingness to take risks and bear hardship to achieve self-care independence
Skills	• Abilities regarding psychomotor functions, dexterity, or communication and interpersonal relationships
Communication	• Ability to make others understand and make needs known

Defining Characteristics

Inability to wash body or body part; inability to obtain water; inability to regulate temperature or flow of water (NANDA, 1990).

Related Factors

Intolerance to activity, decreased strength and endurance, pain, discomfort, perceptual/cognitive impairment, neuromuscular impairment, depression, and severe anxiety (NANDA, 1990).

Self-Care Deficit, Dressing/Grooming

Definition

A state in which the individual experiences impaired ability to perform or complete dressing/grooming activities for oneself (NANDA, 1990).

Defining Characteristics

Impaired ability to fasten clothing; inability to maintain appearance at a satisfactory level (NANDA, 1990).

Related Factors

Activity intolerance, decreased strength and endurance, pain, discomfort, perceptual/cognitive impairment, neuromuscular impairment, depression, and severe anxiety (NANDA, 1990).

Self-Care Deficit, Toileting

Definition

A state in which the individual experiences impaired ability to perform or complete toileting activities for oneself (NANDA, 1990).

Defining Characteristics

Inability to get to toilet or commode, to sit on toilet or commode, to manipulate clothing for toileting, to carry out proper toilet hygiene, to flush toilet or to empty commode (NANDA, 1990).

Related Factors

Impaired transfer ability, impaired mobility, intolerance to activity, decreased strength and endurance, pain, dis-

---

Nursing Research

Selected Nursing Research Studies

Berlowitz, D. R., & Wilking, S. V. W. (1989). Risk factors for pressure sores. *Journal of the American Geriatrics Society, 37,* 1043–1050.

Harrell, J. S., & Damon, J. F. (1989). Prediction of patients' need for mouth care. *Western Journal of Nursing Research, 11,* 748–756.

Lindell, M. E., & Olsson, H. M. (1989). Lack of caregivers' knowledge causes unnecessary suffering in elderly patients. *Journal of Advanced Nursing, 14,* 976–979.

Loomes, S. (1988). Is it safe to lie down in the hospital? *Nursing Times, 84*(49), 63–65.

Ohwaki, S., & Zingarelli, G. (1988). Feeding clients with severe multiple handicaps in a skilled nursing care facility. *Mental Retardation, 26,* 21–24.

Schnelle, J. F., Traughber, B., Sowell, V. A., et al. (1989). Prompted voiding treatment of urinary incontinence in nursing home patients. *Journal of the American Geriatrics Society, 37,* 1051–1057.

Swindale, J. E. (1989). The nurse's role in giving preoperative information to reduce anxiety in patients admitted to hospital for elective minor surgery. *Journal of Advanced Nursing, 14,* 899–905.

Watson, R. (1989). A nursing trial of urinary sheath systems on male hospitalized patients. *Journal of Advanced Nursing, 14,* 467–470.

Webster, R., Thompson, D., Bowman, G., et al. (1988). Patients' and nurses' opinions about bathing. *Nursing Times, 84*(37), 54–57.

Possible Topics for Nursing Inquiry

- Do differences in self-care deficit exist between patients who are admitted to the hospital for acute problems and those who have chronic problems with acute exacerbations?
- Does consistent help with bathing and toileting from the time of admission affect the level of self-care deficit at discharge?
- Would hospitalized patients experience less self-care deficit if a card describing the amount of help required for self-care were posted on the wall above the bed and updated each shift?
- What is the relationship between self-care ability and level of depression for hospital patients and for chronically ill patients in the community?

comfort, perceptual/cognitive impairment, neuromuscular impairment, depression, and severe anxiety (NANDA, 1990).

Self-Care Deficit, Feeding

Definition

A state in which the individual experiences impaired ability to perform or complete feeding activities for oneself (NANDA, 1990).

Defining Characteristics

Inability to cut food; inability to bring food from receptacle to mouth (NANDA, 1990).

Related Factors

Intolerance to activity, decreased strength and endurance, pain, discomfort, perceptual/cognitive impairment, neuromuscular impairment, depression, and severe anxiety (NANDA, 1990).

Related Nursing Diagnoses

Other nursing diagnoses frequently exist along with self-care deficit, including Impaired Skin Integrity (related to inability to clean oneself after toileting and provide hygiene); Altered Nutrition: Less than Body Requirements and Fluid Volume Deficit (related to inability to feed oneself); Altered Oral Mucous Membrane (related to inability to manage mouth care and feed oneself); Ineffective Individual Coping (related to depression over limitation of self-care abilities); Anxiety (related to inability to reliably reach the toilet); Powerlessness (related to difficulty in maintaining usual schedule); and Altered Family Processes (related to stress).

Patient Goals

The following general areas may be included in formulating goals for patients with the four self-care deficits:

Patient will participate as completely as possible in hygiene measures.
Patient will increase level of independence in eating safely.
Patient will participate in dressing himself or herself.
Patient will manage toileting as independently as possible.

In practice, goals are highly personalized and specific. Because of their personal nature, goals reflect the wishes of the patient and the stage of illness. For example, a chronically ill person who looks at death as a release may have a different response to the prospect of working to become more independent than a person who has a favorable prognosis for complete recovery.

IMPLEMENTATION

Nursing Interventions to Promote Health and Self-Care

The nurse should emphasize to all patients the importance of increasing their independence in self-care. Patient education is a cooperative venture that requires the nurse's knowledge, patience, and effort and the patient's motivation to learn. Some people have an innate desire to be independent and therefore a willingness to learn. Others are inclined to be dependent and are reluctant to learn or relearn how to care for themselves.

Some patients may be unaware of proper methods of bathing and hygiene, eating habits, dressing and grooming practices, and toileting practices that promote optimum health. The nurse can demonstrate and explain healthy practices and provide reminders or teaching aids. Necessary equipment (i.e., toothbrush, toothpaste, rinse basin, and water) should be made available, or the nurse may need to instruct the patient how to floss the teeth or how to wash the perineum thoroughly.

Nursing Interventions for Altered Self-Care

People with self-care deficits often must learn new skills or methods of overcoming or coping with difficulties. The nurse can be instrumental in teaching new skills and nurturing the desire for self-care independence. Careful assessment of patient values and interests often reveals motivating factors that might encourage a patient to achieve independence.

It is important to communicate carefully when providing assistance or teaching patients in self-care. Explain techniques as simply as possible, avoiding technical or medical terms the patient may not understand. Learning or relearning self-care skills often takes time and effort. Be patient, supportive, and reassuring. When the patient is unsuccessful, do not criticize; when the patient is successful, regardless of how small or insignificant the task may seem, provide reinforcement and encouragement. Be careful not to provide care for patients that they can perform for themselves, as this fosters dependence and a helpless role.

Nurses should be aware that some degree of regression in self-care is normal during illness, particularly in children and the elderly. They may have temporary problems with incontinence or may not attend to self-care due to weakness, fatigue, or anxiety.

Selected Nursing Interventions for Common Self-Care Problems

Self-Care Deficit: Bathing

- Plan hygiene when the patient is well rested
- Gather supplies as necessary—basin, water, soap, toilet articles
- Offer pain medication if necessary before hygiene
- Encourage sitting by sink or in shower when endurance is limited
- Work with occupational therapy to teach relearning of skills when new cognitive or physical impairments occur
- Use verbal cuing if necessary; praise accomplishments
- Assist with hygiene that cannot be performed independently

Self-Care Deficit: Feeding

- Have patient sit in chair or high Fowler's position in bed
- Medicate as necessary for pain or nausea before meals
- Provide opportunity for oral care and make sure dentures are in place
- Plan rest periods before and after meals
- Provide an environment free from unpleasant odors or sights that may have a negative impact
- Provide assistance with organizing food tray as needed (e.g., open containers, cut meat, or verbally cue patients who are able to do so)
- Provide appropriate foods (e.g., finger foods, thickened liquids) as needed
- Provide utensils that aid feeding (e.g., plates with rims, straws, special spoons and forks)

- Use verbal cueing and positive encouragement
- Work with speech therapy or occupational therapy to individualize teaching plan for patients with new physical or cognitive impairments

Self-Care Deficit: Dressing/Grooming

- Provide rest period before dressing or grooming activities
- May need to space different grooming activities throughout the day to avoid fatique
- Assemble all necessary clothing or grooming aids
- Clothing should be loose fitting and easy to fasten (e.g., sweat suits, Velcro fasteners)
- When possible perform activities in sitting position
- When patient is unable to perform activities independently, ask perferences so they can feel involved
- Work with occupational therapy to individualize teaching for patients with new physical or cognitive impairments

Self-Care Deficits: Toileting

- Encourage routine toileting to avoid urgent need to reach toilet facillities
- Provide patient with needed supplies (e.g., bedpan, urinal, toilet tissue, washcloth for cleansing hands)
- Ensure clear access to toilet or bedside commode by removing clutter
- Encourage clothing that is easy to remove
- Provide equipment to ensure safety (call light, railings, raised toilet seat, adequate lighting)
- Provide ambulation aids or bedside commode if ambulation is difficult

---

Scheduled Care

Patients with self-care deficits need the nurse's assistance in performing hygiene. For the patient's comfort and the nurse's planning for the shift schedule, specific types of hygienic care are given at regular intervals; see the display. Hygienic procedures should be individualized according to personal and cultural preferences.

Nurse–Patient Relationship

Providing assistance with self-care activities gives the nurse an opportunity to develop a trusting, satisfying relationship with the patient. Many of these activities, such as bathing, shampooing, or combing the hair, are relaxing and soothing to the patient. Pleasant conversation during these activities can enhance feelings of comfort and self-worth. These activities give hospitalized or long-term care patients a chance to interact with people.

Some patients are anxious or embarrassed about needing assistance with bathing, grooming, dressing, and toileting. The nurse must be sensitive to the patient's preferences and respect the patient's sense of privacy and modesty. Curtains should be pulled around beds and doors closed when bathing or dressing patients to ensure privacy. Some patients are sensitive to having these activities performed by someone of the opposite sex.

The environment in the hospital or long-term care facility should promote self-care independence. Supplies or equipment should be available, such as a bedpan or a walker if the patient needs support in getting to the bathroom.

Safety Alert

- Hold infants and small children firmly and attend to them when on a high changing table.
- When assisting a patient to a bedside commode from bed, lock the bed and the commode firmly before moving to prevent falls.
- To avoid burns, check the water temperature carefully for patients with diminished ability to perceive extremes in temperature (older patients, anyone with decreased circulation to the legs).
- Encourage patients with balance problems to use handrails in the bathroom.
- Avoid cutting toenails of diabetics or other patients with poor circulation to the legs. Filing is usually safe.
- To prevent falls, find sturdy shoes and check the floor for water spills when helping a patient ambulate.
- To prevent aspiration of food, sit patients upright in bed or in a chair before meals.
- Raise the siderails on both sides of the bed if you must leave even for a brief time.

Bathing and Skin Care

There are two types of baths: cleansing baths and therapeutic baths. *Cleansing baths* are needed to keep the skin free of secretions, microorganisms, perspiration, and debris. All body parts should be cleansed, but areas requiring particular attention to prevent skin breakdown, odors, or discomfort are the face, hands, axillae, back, and perineum. *Therapeutic baths* soothe skin irritation or promote healing (Table 28-4).

Methods of Bathing. There are several methods of bathing, depending on the patient's condition and abilities:

- Tub bath
- Stand-up shower
- Sit-down shower with shower chair
- Bed bath (partial or complete)
- Partial bath at a nearby sink or washbasin

Selecting the appropriate method should take into account the patient's energy level and need to conserve energy for other activities; surgical dressings or body parts that may need to be kept dry; the patient's preference; and the need to encourage independent self-care.

Some methods are easier for the patient to perform independently or with limited assistance. If the nurse provides the needed equipment, some patients can

Scheduling Hygiene Care

Early-Morning Care

Comfort measures and preparation for the day
- Bedpan, urinal, or assistance to bathroom
- Preparation for diagnostic tests or early surgery
- Washing hands and face
- Oral care
- Preparation for breakfast

Morning Care (AM Care)

Comfort measures and after-breakfast care
- Bedpan, urinal, or assistance to bathroom
- Bath, shower, or bathing
- Back massage
- Hair care and shaving
- Oral care
- Care for feet and nails
- Dressing
- Bed linen change
- Straightening bedside unit
- Positioning (bed or chair)

Afternoon Care

After tests, after lunch, and before visitors
- Bedpan, urinal, or assistance to bathroom
- Washing hands and face
- Oral care
- Bed linens and repositioning if needed

Hour-of-Sleep (HS) Care

Comfort measures and bedtime
- Bedpan, urinal, or assistance to bathroom
- Washing hands and face
- Oral care
- Back massage
- Bed linens (change soiled linens, fluff pillow, pull out wrinkles)
- Bedclothes
- Straightening unit (place needed night objects within reach)

Types of care depend on the patient's abilities and the health-care facility's policies. Care should be individualized and self-care should be promoted as much as possible.

Safety Alert: Bathing

- Check and adjust water temperature to avoid burning.
- Use caution when moving in and out of the bathtub or shower. Use handrails and other means of support.
- Prevent chilling the patient by closing the door to cut drafts, using warm water, and increasing the room temperature if possible. Dry exposed parts quickly and cover areas not being bathed (if a bed bath or partial bath).
- Monitor adults frequently when they are bathing or showering. If any doubt exists about a patient's ability to tolerate the procedure while standing, use a shower chair or help the patient bathe at the bedside.
- Avoid vigorous rubbing to dry skin, as this can facilitate skin breakdown in those with compromised circulation or those with less elastic skin tone (i.e., the elderly). Patting dry is best.
- Use nonslip surfaces and handrails in bathroom and shower stalls.
- Move slowly when changing body positions to permit circulation changes and avoid falls. Using leg exercises to stimulate circulation before rising from a sitting position will also help prevent dizziness and falls.
- Never leave infants or young children unattended in or near the bathtub or shower.

---

bathe themselves, although assistance may be needed to reach the back and feet. In assessing which type of bath should be used, the nurse should take into account not only the patient's abilities but also the method that allows him or her the most independence in self-care. Tub baths or showers are more effective for cleansing and ensuring that the skin is thoroughly rinsed, but require more mobility and agility. It has been reported that oxygen requirements for showering are significantly greater than those for a tub bath or bed bath (Johnson, Watt, & Fletcher, 1982). Patients who suffer dizziness, weakness, or mental confusion should not be allowed to take stand-up showers. Obese patients may find it difficult to maneuver into a bathtub and might risk falling. For these patients, a shower may be more appropriate.

The usual time of day for bathing varies greatly. Some people prefer to bathe in the morning; others find an evening bath to be relaxing and an inducement to a good night's sleep. It is not always possible to satisfy personal preferences, but patients appreciate the opportunity to wash their face and hands in the morning before breakfast and before going to sleep at night. The frequency of bathing should be determined by the patient's needs. The comatose patient or the patient who has excessive body excretions or wound drainage requires bathing every day (sometimes more frequently) to avoid skin irritation, breakdown, and infection.

Proper washing techniques to ensure asepsis include washing from clean areas to dirty areas, when possible. Washing extremities from distal to proximal stimulates circulation and venous blood return. Preventing excess skin dryness is important in promoting the health and integrity of skin. See Procedures 28-1 and 28-2.

(Text continues on page 660)

TABLE 28–4

Types of Therapeutic Baths

Type	Purpose	Nursing Considerations
Sitz bath	To cleanse, soothe, and reduce inflammation of perineal or vaginal area after childbirth, vaginal or rectal surgery, or from local irritation of hemorrhoids and fissures	Water temperature depends on the patient's condition and personal preference but is usually 105°–113°F.
Hot-water bath	To relieve muscle spasms and soreness by total immersion	Water temperature should be 113°–114.8°F but may be individualized to patient condition and preference. Be alert for vasodilation with resultant orthostatic blood pressure drop, and for scalding of skin.
Warm-water bath	To cleanse, promote relaxation, and relieve tension	Water temperature is adjusted to patient preference.
Cool-water bath	To relieve muscle tension or to decrease body temperature in febrile patients	Water should be tepid (98.6°F), not cold. Alcohol added to the water enhances cooling through evaporation from skin surfaces. Avoid chilling; shivering may increase body temperature.
Soaks	To soften and loosen secretions during dressing changes, or to reduce pain and swelling or itching of inflamed or irritated skin	Medications or topical agents may be added to the water. Hot, warm, or cold water is applied to an isolated body part.

PROCEDURE 28–1. Bathing a Patient in Bed

■ **Purpose**
1. Cleanse the skin, control body odors, and promote self-esteem.
2. Stimulate circulation.
3. Provide an opportunity for assessment of skin and physical mobility.
4. Provide range-of-motion exercises for joints.
5. Promote relaxation and comfort.

■ **Assessment**
- Assess patient's ability to perform self-care and amount of assistance needed. Evaluate activity tolerance, cognitive function, musculoskeletal function, and level of discomfort to determine type of bath.
  Note: Patient should be encouraged to be as independent as possible but should not become fatigued. Pain should not be intensified.
- Assess patient preferences for bathing (i.e., frequency, time of day, type of skin-care products).
- Review chart to determine what other procedures or therapies the patient is receiving to coordinate scheduling and prevent fatigue.
- Identify patients with special considerations for bathing:
  - Elderly: susceptible to dry skin.
  - Immobilized patients: pressure areas on dependent and bony parts; need for range-of-motion exercises to joints.
  - Patients with altered sensation: risk for burns from hot water.
  - Obese or diaphoretic patients: excessive perspiration or moisture on skin surfaces that rub against each other provides medium for excoriation and bacterial growth.
- Review history for precautions regarding movement or positioning.
- Assess patient's knowledge and practice of hygiene to determine learning needs.

■ **Equipment**
1. Two bath towels.
2. Two washcloths.
3. Bath blanket.
4. Washbasin with warm water (110°–115°F). Test by measuring with bath thermometer or by placing several drops on your inner forearm.
5. Soap, soap dish, or liquid nonsoap cleanser.
6. Personal skin-care products (deodorant, powder, lotions, cologne).
7. Clean gown or pajamas.
8. Bedpan or urinal.
9. Laundry bag.
10. Disposable clean gloves for perineal care.

■ **Procedure**
1. Close curtains around bed or shut room door.
   Rationale: Provides privacy.
2. Help patient to use bedpan, urinal, or commode, if needed.
   Rationale: Patient will be more comfortable and relaxed after elimination.
3. Close window and doors to decrease drafts.
   Rationale: Promotes patient comfort and minimizes chilling.
4. Wash your hands.
   Rationale: Reduces transmission of microorganisms.
5. Raise bed to high position. Lock siderail up on opposite side of bed from your work.
   Rationale: Avoids strain on nurse's back and prevents patient from falling out of bed.
6. Remove top sheet and bed spread and place bath blanket on patient. Help patient move closer to you, and remove gown.
   Rationale: Bath blanket provides for patient comfort and warmth. Bringing patient closer to you prevents undue muscle strain.
   Note: If top linen is to be reused, place it on back of chair; otherwise, place it in laundry bag.
   Note: If patient has an IV line, remove gown from arm, lower IV container, and slide it through gown with tubing. Rehang IV container and check flow rate.

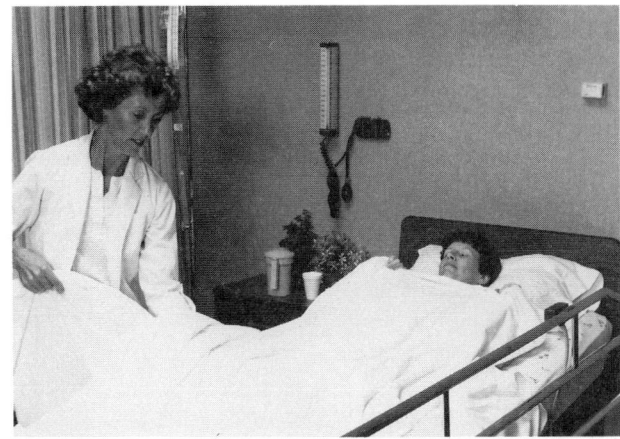

Step 6A

(continued)

PROCEDURE 28–1. Bathing a Patient in Bed *(continued)*

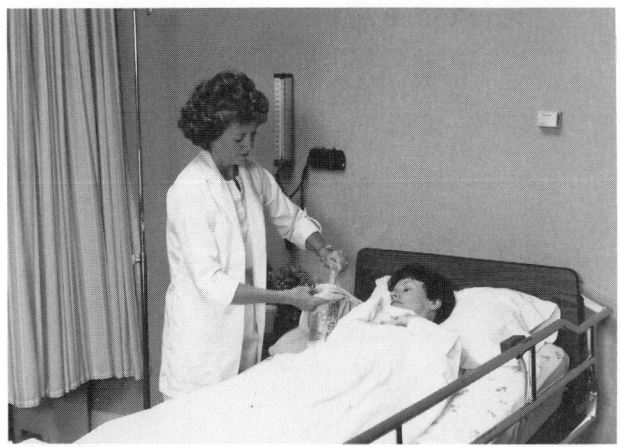

Step 6B

7. Lay towel across patient's chest.
8. Wet washcloth and fold around your finger to make a mitt.
   a. Fold washcloth in thirds.
   b. Straighten washcloth to take out wrinkles.

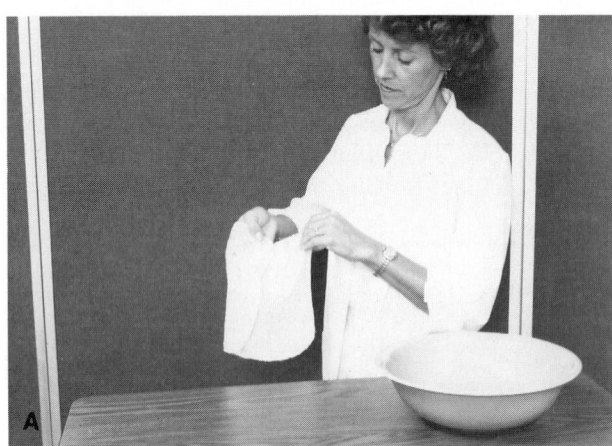

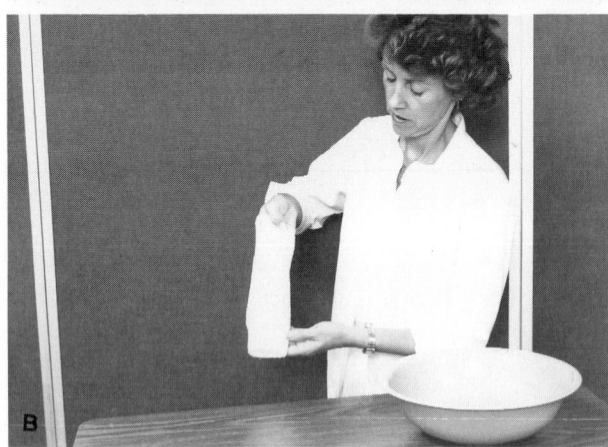

Step 8A and B

c. Fold washcloth over to fit hand.
d. Tuck loose ends under edge of washcloth on palm.
Rationale: Mitt retains heat and water better than a loosely held washcloth. Prevents water from dripping on patient.

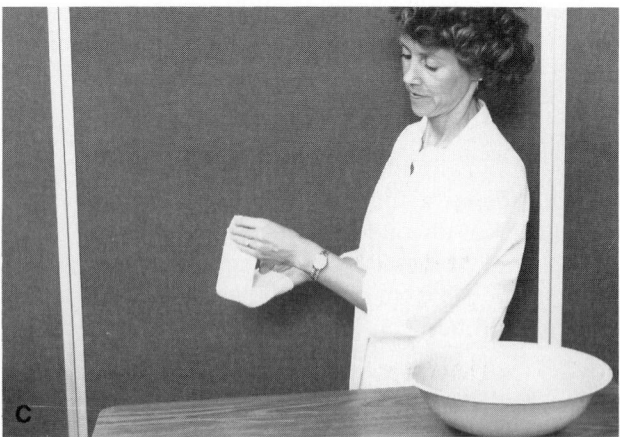

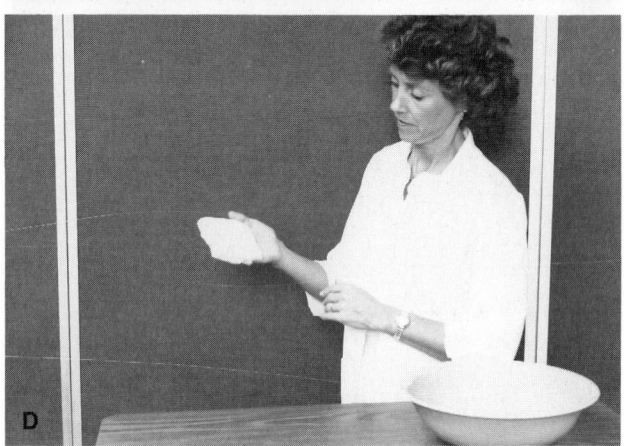

Step 8C and D

9. Cleanse eyes with water only, wiping from inner to outer canthus. Use separate corner of mitt for each eye.
   Rationale: Washing eye from inner to outer canthus prevents secretions from entering and irritating nasolacrimal ducts. Using separate corners for each eye prevents transfer of microorganisms from one eye to the other.
10. Determine if patient would like soap used on face. Wash face, neck, and ears.
    Rationale: Soap can be very drying, especially to the face.
    Note: Avoid letting soap bar sit in washbasin, or water will become too soapy for rinse. Liquid non-

(continued)

PROCEDURE 28-1. Bathing a Patient in Bed (continued)

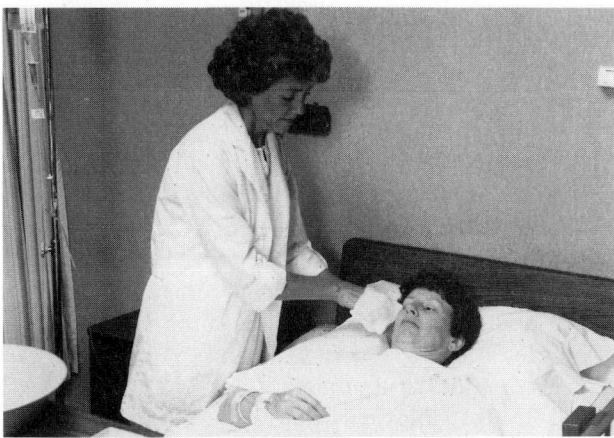

Step 9

detergent cleansing agents are available in many institutions to mix directly into bath water. These products are nondrying and need not be rinsed from the skin.

11. Fold bath blanket off arm away from you. Place towel lengthwise under arm. Wash, rinse, and dry the arm using long firm strokes from the fingers toward the axilla. Wash axilla.
Rationale: Stroking from distal to proximal stimulates circulation and facilitates venous blood return.

12. (Optional) Place bath towel on bed and put washbasin on it. Immerse patient's hand and allow to soak for several minutes. Wash, rinse, and dry hand well. Repeat on other side. Apply lotion.
Rationale: Soaking softens cuticles and loosens dirt under nails.

13. Repeat for hand and arm nearest you.

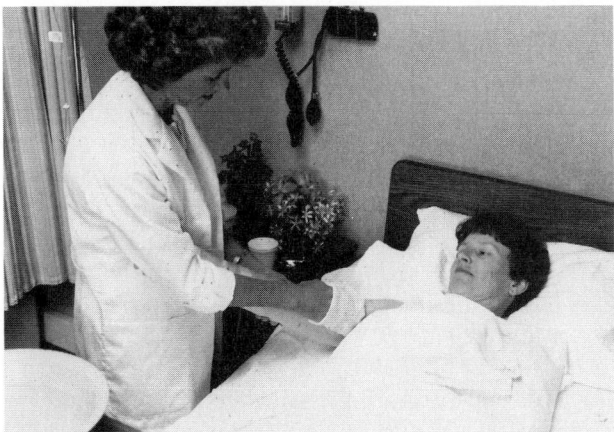

Step 13

14. Apply deodorant or power according to patient preferences. Avoid excessive use of powder or inhalation of powder.

Rationale: Hygiene products control excess body moisture and odor. Excessive powder can cause caking, which leads to skin irritation; inhalation can cause respiratory difficulty.

15. Assess temperature of bath water and change water if necessary. If you leave bedside, lock siderails up to prevent accidental falls.

16. Place bath towel over chest. Fold bath blanket down to below umbilicus.
Rationale: Maintains warmth and prevents unnecessary exposure of body parts.

17. Lift bath towel off chest and bathe chest and abdomen with mitted hand using long, firm strokes. Give special attention to skin under the breasts and any other skin folds, if patient is overweight. Rinse and dry well.
Note: A light dusting of bath powder under the breasts or between skin folds absorbs excess moisture and prevents skin maceration and irritation.

18. Help patient don a clean gown.

19. Expose leg away from you by folding over bath blanket. Be careful to keep perineum covered.
Rationale: Prevents unnecessary exposure of body parts.

20. Lift leg and place bath towel lengthwise under leg. Wash, rinse, and dry leg using long, firm strokes from ankle to thigh.
Rationale: Washing from distal to proximal stimulates circulation and facilitates venous blood return.

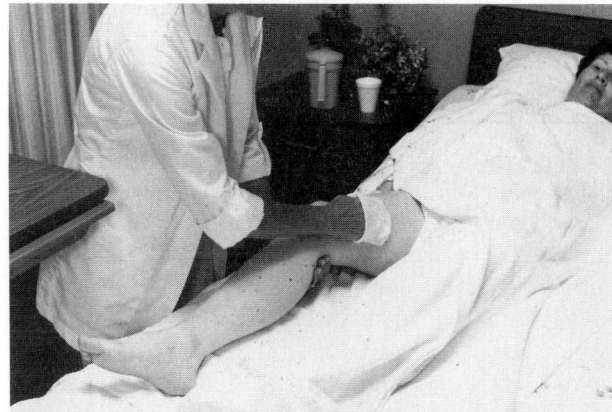

Step 20

21. Wash feet or place in basin of water as for hands. Rinse and dry well. Pay special attention to space between toes.
Note: Trim or file toenails after soaking if necessary.

22. Repeat for other leg and foot.

23. Assess bath water for warmth. Change water if necessary.

(continued)

PROCEDURE 28–1. Bathing a Patient in Bed (continued)

24. Assist patient to side-lying position. Place bath towel along side of back and buttocks to protect linen. Wash, rinse, and dry back and buttocks. Give a backrub with powder or lotion.

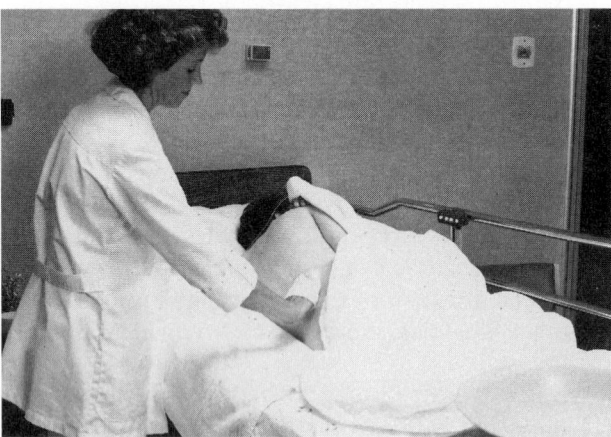

Step 24

Rationale: Stimulates circulation and promotes comfort.
Note: Wear disposable, clean gloves when cleansing anal area.

25. Assist to supine position. Assess if patient can wash genitals and perineal area independently. If unable to, drape with bath blanket so that only genitals are exposed. Don disposable, clean gloves, wash, rinse, and dry genitalia and perineum (see text for instructions).
26. Apply powder, lotion, cologne according to patient preference.
27. Assist with hair and mouth care.
28. Make bed with clean linen.
29. Clean equipment and return to appropriate storage area.
30. Wash your hands.
31. Chart significant observations.

Age-Related Considerations. Newborns are bathed only with warm water to preserve the bacteriostatic acid mantle on the skin. Careful covering of the newborn and careful drying are important to maintain body temperature. Because the infant's thermoregulatory mechanisms are immature, it is important not to leave a child with wet skin exposed for more than a short time. Sponge baths are given to infants to avoid excessive wetting of the umbilical cord until it falls off. When the area is well healed, infants are often bathed daily in a small tub or sink, using mild soap. Babies are slippery when wet. Provide firm head support and ensure that all supplies are at hand. Never leave infants and young children alone in the bath or on a changing table. Because newborns and infants urinate and defecate frequently, the perineal area should be washed frequently during diaper changes.

Using powder on infants is discouraged because it carries the risk of aspiration; lotions and non–water-soluble lubricants are preferred. If parents want to use powder, they should apply only a small amount to their hands and avoid application near the baby's head.

Toddlers and older children can bathe in a tub or shower but must be monitored carefully for safety and the thoroughness of washing. School-aged children can manage most aspects of bathing and grooming with minimal support. Toys provide a source of enjoyment for most younger children during a bath.

Many adolescents bathe and groom meticulously without reminders because appearance is important to their self-esteem. Some adolescents accept help willingly, appreciating the opportunity to be well-groomed, but others may be uncomfortable needing assistance in intimate activities such as bathing, dressing, and toileting. Recognizing this feeling and providing privacy helps to minimize discomfort.

Many older adults need special treatment to prevent and treat dry skin (see the display). Dry skin is increased by inadequate fluid intake, too-frequent bathing with

---

Techniques to Avoid Excessive Skin Dryness

- Avoid bathing too frequently. Twice a week is sufficient.
- Avoid using harsh soaps and detergents on clothes.
- Use liquid, nondetergent cleansing agents rather than soap.
- Avoid astringents or alcohol-based solutions for cleaning the skin.
- Use lubricants containing lanolin immediately after washing or bathing to prevent moisture loss.
- Add oil to the rinse water for bed linens and underwear.
- Drink six to eight glasses of water per day.
- Keep water in open containers in the room or use a humidifier to help keep moisture in the room.

PROCEDURE 28–2. Assisting with the Bath or Shower

■ Purpose
Same as Procedure 28-1.

■ Assessment
Same as Procedure 28-1.

■ Equipment
1. One bath towel.
2. One washcloth.
3. Soap, soap dish, or liquid (nonsoap cleanser).
4. Personal skin-care products (deodorant, powder, lotions, cologne).
5. Clean gown or pajamas.
6. Laundry bag.

■ Procedure
1. Place towel or disposable bath mat on floor by tub or shower.
   Rationale: Prevents slipping and falls, as well as transfer of microorganisms from floor to feet.
2. Help patient to bathroom.
3. Place "occupied" sign on bathroom door.
   Rationale: Maintains privacy. Doors are not usually locked, so nurse can come in to assist patient.
4. Fill bathtub halfway with warm water (105°F). Test water or have patient test water. If taking shower, turn shower on and adjust temperature.
   Rationale: Testing temperature before entering water prevents burns.
5. Help patient into shower or tub, providing necessary assistance.
   Note: Many patients can bathe or shower independently, others may need varying degrees of help. Instruct patient in use of safety bars and call bell signal. Shower chairs are available so patient can sit during shower to prevent fatigue (see Fig. 25-7).
6. Check on patient within 15 minutes. Wash any areas he or she could not reach.
   Rationale: Prolonged exposure to warm water may cause vasodilation and pooling of blood. This can result in lightheadedness or dizziness.
7. Help patient out of tub or shower. Assist with drying.

Note: If patient is unsteady, drain water before getting patient out of tub to prevent falls.
8. Assist patient with dressing and grooming.
9. Help patient to room.
10. Return to bathroom to clean tub or shower according to agency policy. Discard soiled linen. Place "unoccupied" sign on door.

■ Lifespan Considerations

Newborn and Infant
- An infant should not be submerged in water until the umbilical cord has fallen off (around 7 to 10 days of age) to prevent infection.

Child
- Children under age 8 should not be left unattended in a bath to prevent drowning.
- Children often enjoy washing themselves but require supervision to be sure it is done thoroughly.

Adolescent
- Sebaceous glands become active during puberty. Special cleansing agents may be necessary to treat facial acne. Antiperspirants and more frequent baths will control body odors.

Older Adult
- The older adult is susceptible to dry skin due to reduced sebaceous gland activity, epidermal thinning, and decreased fluid intake. Lotions, bath oil, and decreased use of soap can reduce the drying effects of aging.
- The older adult may have decreased sensation and is at risk for burns from hot water.

■ Home-Care Modifications
- Patients at risk for falling should be instructed to apply lotions and oils after the bath and not put them in bath water. Oils can make the bathtub or shower surfaces more slippery.
- Safety devices such as tub bars, nonskid tub surfaces, and bathroom carpeting can be installed to reduce the chance of falls and promote independence.

---

soaps or detergents, and the use of defatting solutions such as alcohol on the skin. Use practices that reduce skin dryness, and teach the patient to do the same (see the display).

Because it is thinner and more fragile, the skin of many elderly people requires special care to prevent skin breakdown. To maintain skin integrity avoid vigorous rubbing while drying, applying constant pressure to a body part for long periods of time, and falls or other accidents. Older people have less effective temperature-regulating ability, so avoid chilling them. Cover the areas not being bathed, dry the exposed part quickly, use warm water, close the room door, and increase the temperature in the room. To prevent falls, have the patient move slowly to permit the circulatory system to adjust to position changes. Leg exercises stimulate circulation and can be used before rising from a sitting position, helping to prevent dizziness and falls. Due to the skin's reduced ability to perceive sensations, elderly patients may need help to determine a safe water temperature.

Perineal Care

If the patient cannot perform adequate perineal and genital care, the nurse must do so. Cleansing of the perineum and genitals is usually a part of the bath but may need to be done more frequently if the person is incontinent of urine and/or feces or has drainage in the perineal area. The nurse can teach perineal and genital care while bathing the patient.

For women, perineal care involves cleansing the upper inner thighs, the labia majora, and the folds between the labia majora and minora. Wipe from front to back to avoid contaminating the vagina or urethra with microorganisms from the anus (Fig. 28-2A). For men, perineal care involves washing the upper inner thighs, the penis, and the scrotum, and in uncircumcised men retracting the foreskin and washing the glans penis (Fig. 28-2B). For both sexes, the buttocks are cleansed after the genitals, from a side-lying position.

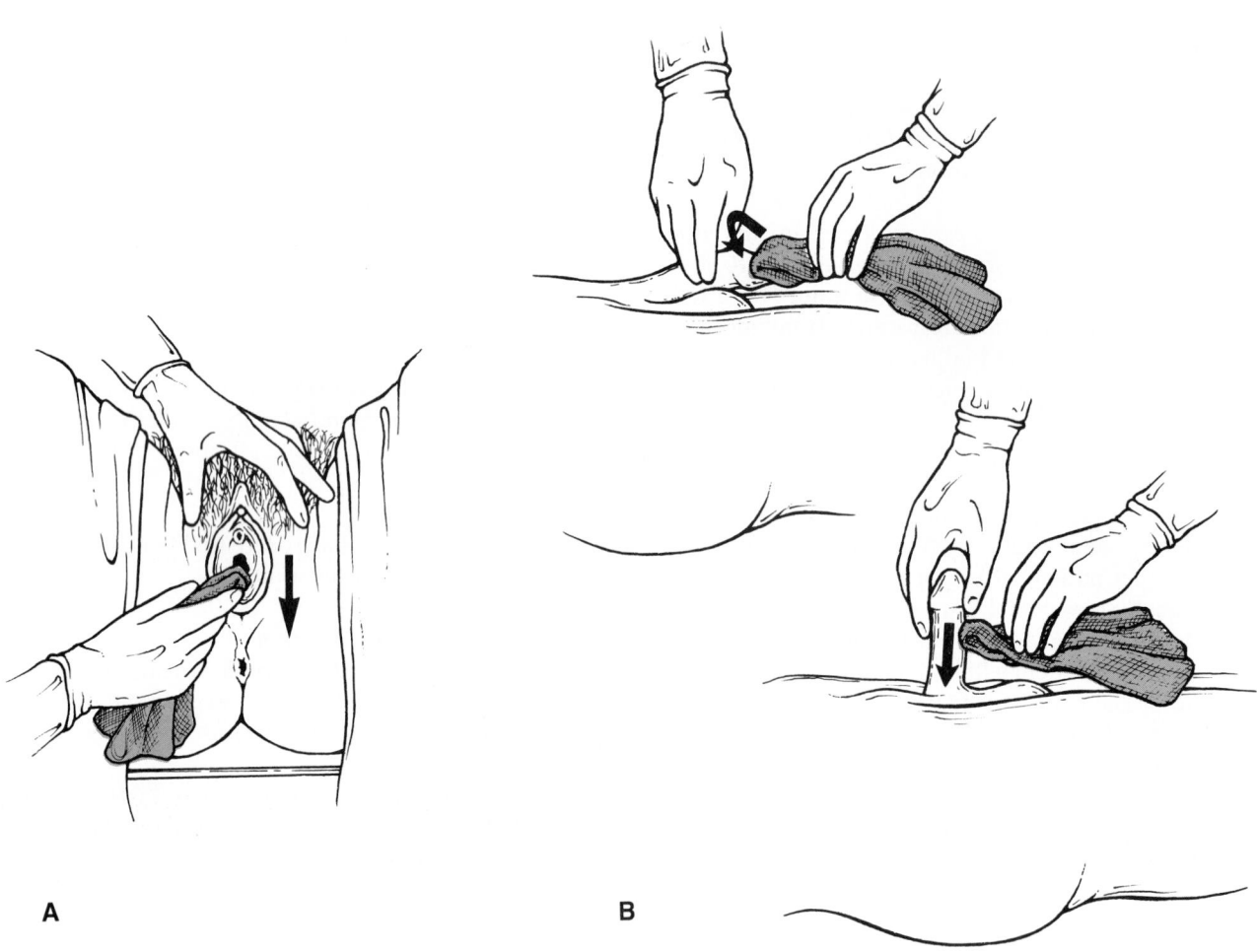

A

B

Figure 28–2. Perineal care. **A:** Female. The labia are spread to expose the urethral meatus and the vaginal orifice. The area is cleansed from the pubic area toward the anus in one stroke. This is repeated several times, always using a clean area of the washcloth. **B:** Male. The tip of the penis is cleansed from the urethral meatus downward in a circular motion. The penile shaft is cleansed from the tip downward toward the scrotum.

Avoid temperature extremes, as perineal tissue is more sensitive than other skin. Pouring water over the perineum while the patient sits on the toilet or a bedpan is a comfortable way of rinsing for the patient who cannot use a tub or shower, or between baths. Certain people are at greater risk for infection and irritation of these areas, including patients with indwelling catheters; those with perineal, rectal, or lower urinary tract surgery; incontinent patients; and women after childbirth. Perineal care is routinely performed frequently by or for these people.

Many patients can do their own perineal care with minimal assistance. A nurse giving perineal care to a patient of the opposite sex should be direct and professional to help allay embarrassment. Gloves must be worn during perineal cleansing of all patients and while handling items that may contain exudate from the perineal area, because organisms may enter the nurse's circulation through lesions (open sores, cuts, or burns).

Backrubs

Backrubs are given to patients with limited mobility to provide comfort and to enhance the blood supply to the skin and muscles. The degree of pressure used varies and should be determined by observing the patient's response or verbal cues. For the most relaxing effect, both hands should maintain contact throughout the procedure. Avoid direct pressure over bony prominences to avoid damaging the underlying tissue. A lubricant (cream or lotion) permits the hands to glide over the skin. Some young people with oily skin find alcohol a cooling and refreshing lubricant, but it is drying to the skin and can cause cracking and skin breakdown in dehydrated patients and older adults.

If possible, the patient should assume a prone position for a backrub. If this is contraindicated or inconvenient, use the side-lying position. Remember good body mechanics; the nurse should also be in a comfortable position. With immobile patients, it may be effective to perform a partial backrub after turning the patient from one side to the other to enhance circulation to the lateral aspect of the hips. See Procedure 28-3.

Care of Feet and Nails

Feet and nails often need special attention. Assess the appearance of the feet and attend to any problems. Table 28-5 lists common foot problems, causes, and treatment. The color and temperature of the skin gives clues to the quality of perfusion (blood flow). Cold feet with a dusky skin color may signal poor circulation. People with diabetes mellitus, elderly people, and patients with poor circulation are at special risk for foot difficulties, so good foot care and education about self-care is essential. Combining teaching with carrying out or assisting with care is a good way to motivate a person

with foot problems. The feet of people with peripheral vascular disease must be protected from trauma during foot care, so avoid cutting nails too short and cutting into calluses. Some hospital policies forbid nurses from cutting the toenails of diabetic patients or people with peripheral vascular disease, because healing is slow and there is a high risk of infection. These patients often have toenails that are thick, distorted, and difficult to cut safely, but the nails can be safely filed. See Procedure 28-4.

Hair Care

Shampooing. Shampooing cleans the hair and scalp and helps get rid of excess secretions. It promotes circulation to the scalp and provides a relaxing, soothing experience for the patient. The nurse can use this opportunity to inspect the hair for dandruff or lice. Shampooing can be done while the patient sits in the shower chair, leans back over the sink, leans forward over a pan of water on the bedside table, lies on a stretcher over a sink (if unable to sit), or in bed with a tray to drain the water. Protect the patient from fatigue and chilling. See Procedure 28-5.

Brushing and Combing. Combs are usually provided for patients in the hospital, but brushes often must be brought from home. Patients who can brush and comb their hair should be given the equipment and encouraged do so independently, but patients who cannot comb their own hair need assistance (Fig. 28-3). Brushing hair massages the scalp, stimulating circulation, and facilitates oil distribution along the hair shaft more effectively than combing. Patients with long hair who must spend an extended period of time in bed need a hairstyle that minimizes matting; combing the hair daily, braiding it, or tying it back helps. If tangles occur, hair is divided into small sections, brushed, and then combed. Tightly curled hair usually requires a wide-toothed comb or a

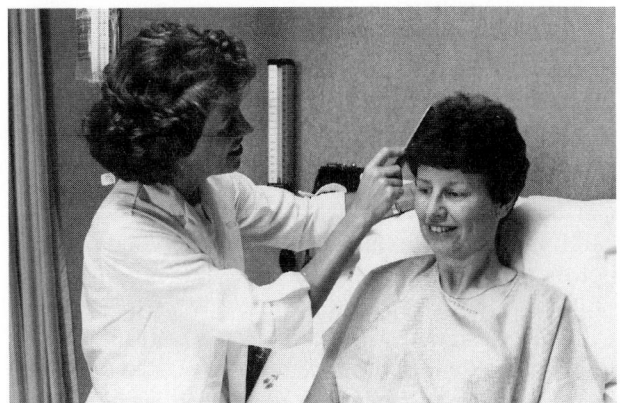

Figure 28–3. The nurse assists with grooming by combing the patient's hair.

PROCEDURE 28–3. Massaging the Back

■ **Purpose**

1. Stimulate circulation to the skin.
2. Relieve muscle tension.
3. Promote comfort and relaxation.

■ **Assessment**

- Assess patient for muscle fatigue or stiffness, complaints of back discomfort or tension.
- Identify patients with impaired physical mobility who may benefit from back massage.
- Assess skin for localized areas of redness on the back, shoulders, or hips.
- Assess patient's desire for back massage.
- Identify conditions that may contraindicate backrub (rib and vertebral fractures, burns, or open wounds).
- Determine any limitations to positioning.

■ **Equipment**

1. Bath blanket.
2. Bath towel (to absorb excess moisture).
3. Lotion, powder, or alcohol. Lotion is used to lubricate the skin and prevents friction during massage. Powder reduces friction and prevents "sticky" feeling on diaphoretic patients. Powder and lotion are not used together. Alcohol cools the skin, but can be drying.

■ **Procedure**

1. Help patient to side-lying or prone position.
2. Expose back, shoulders, upper arms, and sacral area. Cover remainder of body with bath blanket.
   Rationale: Prevents unnecessary exposure and chilling.
3. Wash hands in warm water. Warm lotion by holding container under running warm water.
   Rationale: Prevents startle response and muscle tension from cold lotion and hands.
   Note: Alcohol is applied cold, but warn the patient before application.
4. Pour small amount of lotion into palms.

5. Begin massage in sacral area with circular motion. Move hands upward to shoulders, massaging over scapulae in smooth, firm stroke. Without removing hands from skin, continue in smooth strokes to upper arms and down sides of back to iliac crest. Continue for 3 to 5 minutes.
   Rationale: Continuous, firm pressure promotes relaxation and stimulates circulation.

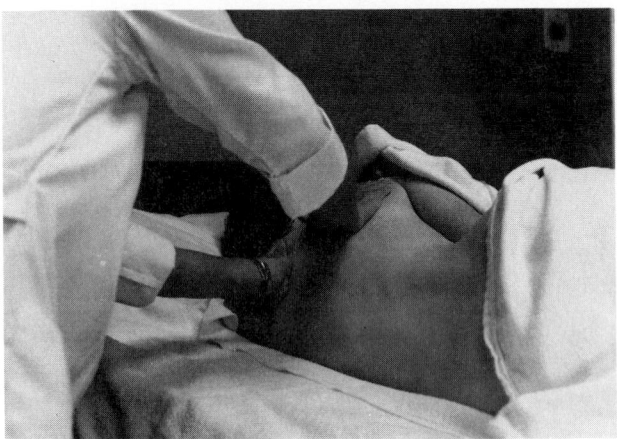

Step 5

6. While massaging, assess for whitish or reddened areas that do not disappear, and broken skin areas.
   Note: Provide additional massage to reddened areas to stimulate circulation.
7. If additional stimulation is desired, *petrissage* (kneading) over the shoulders and gluteal area and *tapotement* (tapping) up and down the spine can be done.
8. End massage with long, continuous, stroking movements.
   Rationale: Stroking is the most relaxing of the massage movements.
9. Pat excess lubricant dry with towel. Retie patient's gown and assist to comfortable position.
10. Wash your hands.

---

pick and a firm-bristled brush. Combing with the fingers can loosen tangles. With Afro hairstyles, hair is combed carefully to avoid breaking. A lubricating conditioner or petroleum jelly may be used.

Lice. Infestation with lice is called **pediculosis.** Lice found on the hair of the head, eyebrows, eyelashes, and beard is known as pediculosis capitis; on the body, pediculosis corporis; and in the perineal area, pediculosis pubis.

Head lice and pubic lice attach their eggs, called nits,

to hairs with a tenacious substance that makes them hard to remove. Nits, which may be visible with a light and magnifying glass, resemble shiny ovals. To the naked eye they appear similar to dandruff. Lice live on the skin and their bites cause itching. Inflamed bites can be seen along the hairline. Body lice suck blood from the skin and tend to live in the clothing, making them hard to detect. Clues to the presence of body lice are scratching and hemorrhagic lesions on the skin.

The usual treatment for pediculosis is gamma benzene hexachloride (Kwell), which comes in lotion, cream, and

TABLE 28–5

Common Foot Problems

Type	Description	Possible Causes	Treatment
Calluses	Flattened thickening of epidermis, often on bottom or side of foot over a bony prominence	Tight shoes or inadequate padding in shoes	Soften by soaking in warm water and abrade with pumice stone.
Corns	Cone-shaped lesion (thickening of epidermis), usually on 4th or 5th toe over a toe joint	Pressure from tight shoes	Softer, better-fitting shoes or foam protective pads. Keratolytic agents with salicylic acid applied to keratinous skin.
Plantar warts	Round or irregular, flattened by pressure, surrounded by cornified epithelium. Often painful.	Virus, but may be worsened by inadequate circulation or pressure from tight shoes	Remove by curettage, freezing with solid carbon dioxide, or application of salicylic acid.
Bunions (hallax valgus)	Inflammation and thickening of bursa of the great toe joint. Enlargement of the joint and displacement of toe.	Heredity, degenerative bone and joint disease, and tight shoes or high heels	Surgical intervention or symptomatic relief by wearing shoes wide at the front.
Ringworm, tinea pedis (athlete's foot)	Redness, scaling, and cracking of skin, especially between toes	Fungus, worsened by moist, unventilated environment	Apply antifungal powder or ointment. Daily changing of socks; wear 100% cotton socks to absorb moisture.
Ingrown nails	Inflammation, swelling, and pain of tissues at edge of nail	Improper trimming of nails, poorly fitting shoes	Prevent by trimming nails straight across and wearing well-fitted shoes. Pain and inflammation treated with anti-inflammatory agents. Surgical removal of nail may be required.
Foot odor	Excessive foul odor of feet	Possibly from fungal foot infections; exacerbated by hot, moist environment	Decrease excess moisture: use deodorant foot powders, 100% cotton socks, well-ventilated shoes.

shampoo form. Lice can be treated by showering with Kwell. Because of the heavy hair growth of the area, pubic lice are often difficult to remove; the shampoo may be applied and left on for 12 to 24 hours. Linens and clothing used by the patient must be washed in hot water. Blankets, furniture, and carpets can be sprayed with insecticide. People with whom the patient has had sexual or intimate contact should also be treated.

Dandruff. Dandruff is a chronic, diffuse scaling of the epidermis of the scalp. It is characterized by itching and flaking of whitish scales, which are annoying and embarrassing to the person. Frequent brushing and daily shampooing with a keratolytic shampoo may control the problem, but persistent, severe cases may require medical attention.

Shaving

Shaving may be important to men to make them feel good about their physical appearance. Most men with-

out beards shave every day, and receiving help with shaving can boost the patient's morale. To avoid cuts, soften the beard with warm towels before shaving. Use soap lather or shaving cream, pull the skin taut, and shave in the direction in which the hair grows to decrease irritation (Fig. 28-4). Men with decreased energy and fine motor skills find it easier to use electric shavers, and some hospitals provide electric shavers for patients. Patients at risk for excessive bleeding (i.e., those with

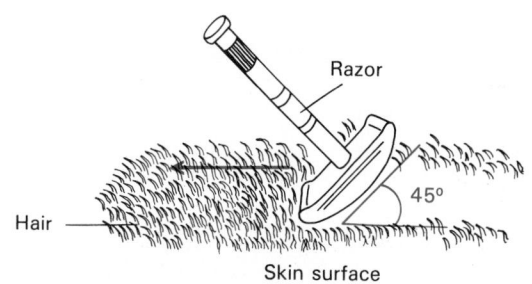

Figure 28–4. Shave in the direction of hair growth.

PROCEDURE 28–4. Performing Foot and Nail Care

■ Purpose
1. Maintain skin integrity around nails.
2. Provide for patient's comfort and sense of well-being.
3. Maintain foot function.
4. Encourage self-care.

■ Assessment
- Note patient's gait for limping or unusual position. Unnatural gait can be caused by painful feet, or bone and muscle disorders.
- Assess footwear worn by patient. Socks should be worn to absorb excess perspiration and avoid fungal infections.
- Identify patients at risk for foot or nail problems:
  - Diabetes is associated with changes in micro-circulation to peripheral tissues. The diabetic patient is at high risk for infection from breaks in skin integrity and may also have decreased sensation to pain as a result of neuropathies.
  - Elderly patients' ability to perform foot and nail care may be impeded by poor vision, obesity, or musculoskeletal conditions that limit their ability to bend and maintain balance.
  - Cerebrovascular accident may alter the patient's gait due to foot drop, muscle weakness, or paralysis.
  - Conditions associated with foot and ankle edema (renal failure, congestive heart failure) interfere with blood flow to surrounding tissues and impede proper shoe fit.
- Determine patient's ability to perform self-care.
- Inspect nails and skin of fingers, toes, and feet. Assess areas between toes for dryness and cracking.
- Assess patient's knowledge of foot and nail care practices.
- Review agency policy for trimming nails. Many agencies require a physician's order to perform nail trimming on high-risk patients.
- Identify patients going to surgery. Nail polish must be removed so nailbeds can be assessed for changes in oxygenation.

■ Equipment
1. Waterproof pad.
2. Washcloth, towels.
3. Washbasin, warm water, soap.
4. Lotion.
5. Disposable gloves.
6. Nail clippers, file.
7. Orange stick.
8. Polish remover (if necessary).

■ Procedure
1. Wash your hands.
2. Help patient to chair if possible. Elevate head of bed for bedridden patient.
3. Remove colored nail polish if patient is scheduled for surgery. Review agency policy to determine if patient may wear clear nail polish.
   Rationale: Colored nail polish prevents observation of the nail beds for changes in color associated with poor oxygenation.
4. Fill washbasin with warm water (100°–104°F). Place waterproof pad under basin. Soak patient's hands or feet in basin.
   Rationale: Warm water softens nails, increases local circulation, and reduces inflammation.
   Note: Diabetic patients may have decreased sensation in their extremities. Test water temperature carefully to prevent burns.
5. Place call bell within reach. Allow hands or feet to soak for 10 to 20 minutes.
   Rationale: Softening allows easier removal of dead epithelial cells and reduces possibility of nails cracking during trimming.

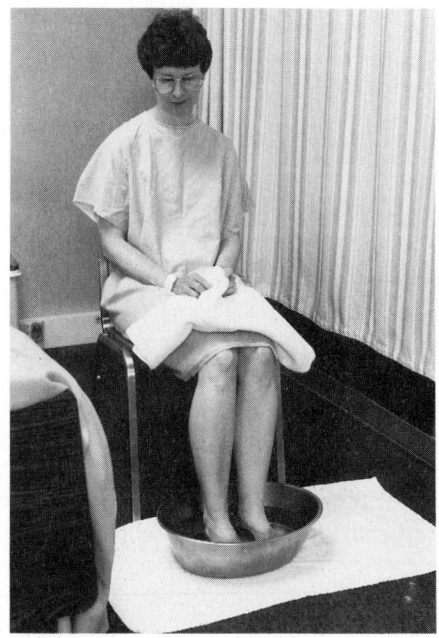

Step 5

6. Dry the hand or foot that has been soaking. Rewarm water and allow other extremity to soak while you work on the softened nails.
   Rationale: Increases efficiency.

(continued)

PROCEDURE 28–4. Performing Foot and Nail Care (continued)

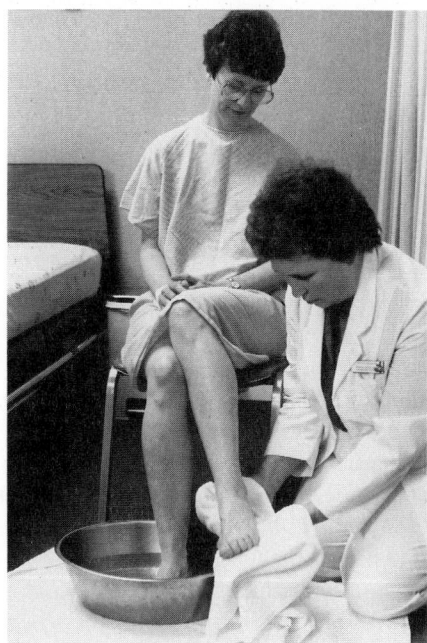

Step 6

7. Gently clean under nails with orange stick.
   Note: If nails are thickened and yellow, patient may have fungal infection. Wear disposable gloves to prevent transmission of infection.

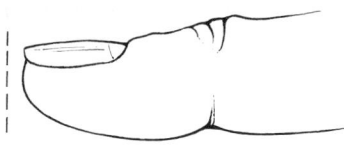

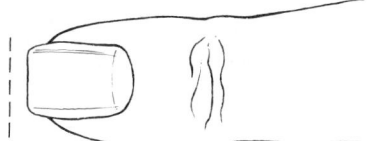

Step 8

8. Beginning with large toe or thumb, clip nail straight across. Shape nail with file. File rather than cut nails of patients with diabetes or circulatory problems. *Rationale: Trimming straight across prevents splitting of nail and injury to tissues around the nail.*
   Note: Patients with severely hypertrophied nails should be referred to a podiatrist or foot clinic for care.
9. Push cuticle back gently with orange stick. *Rationale: Reduces inflamed cuticle and hang nail formation.*
10. Repeat procedure with other nails.
11. Rinse foot or hand in warm water.
12. Dry thoroughly with towel. *Rationale: Removing excess moisture inhibits bacterial growth.*
13. Apply lotion to hands or feet.
14. Help patient to comfortable position.
15. Remove and dispose of equipment.
16. Wash your hands.

■ Lifespan Considerations

Infant
- Parents must learn to care for nails to prevent the infant from scratching himself or herself. The nails should be cut straight across using blunt scissors. It is easiest to trim the nails when the baby is asleep.

Child
- Nail-biting is often a concern in school-age children. It may be a learned behavior or a symptom of nervous tension. Bad-tasting over-the-counter preparations are available to paint on the nails as a reminder not to bite. Other measures may include positive reinforcement and rewards for "good" days with no nail-biting.

Older Adult
- Elderly patients may have dehydrated epidermal cells and decreased sebaceous gland secretion from normal physiologic effects of aging. This predisposes them to fungal infections and breaks in skin integrity.

bleeding disorders or those taking anticoagulants or large doses of aspirin) should use an electric razor rather than a safety razor to avoid cuts. Some men like to use an aftershave lotion. Men with beards or mustaches may need help in trimming them and in keeping them clean and free from food particles. Facial hair can be washed during a bath or shower. Mustaches or beards are shaved off only at the patient's request.

Shaving underarm and leg hair is an important part of grooming for many women. This is done using basically the same shaving technique as for men.

Oral Care

Brushing the teeth and cleansing and rinsing the mouth are comfort measures. Patients find that having their teeth brushed and mouth cleaned induces feelings of

PROCEDURE 28–5. Shampooing Hair of a Bedridden Patient

■ **Purpose**
1. Promote comfort and self-esteem.
2. Apply medication to scalp and hair.

■ **Assessment**
• Assess condition of hair and scalp.
• Determine agency policy about shampooing hair of bedridden patients. Some agencies require a physician's order.
• Assess activity level of patient and identify positioning restrictions.
• Assess patient's preference for hair-care products. Determine whether medicated shampoo has been ordered and is available.

■ **Equipment**
1. Comb and brush.
2. Hair dryer (optional).
3. Two bath towels, one washcloth.
4. Shampoo (cream rinse is optional).
5. Water pitcher.
6. Plastic shampoo basin.
7. Washbasin or bucket.
8. Bath blanket.
9. Waterproof pads.
10. Cotton balls (optional).
11. Hydrogen peroxide (optional, to cleanse matted blood from hair).

■ **Procedure**
1. Place waterproof pads under patient's head and shoulders and remove pillow.
   Rationale: Prevents soiling and wetting of bed linen.
2. Raise bed to highest position.
   Rationale: Reduces strain on nurse's back.
3. Remove any pins from hair. Comb and brush hair thoroughly.
   Rationale: Removes tangles, distributes scalp oils through hair, and results in thorough cleansing.
4. Lay bed to flat position.
5. Place shampooing basin under head. Place bath towel around shoulders and folded washcloth where neck rests on basin.
   Rationale: Shoulder padding protects patient from becoming wet. Washcloth protects neck from strain and discomfort.
6. Fold bed linens down to waist. Cover upper body with bath blanket.
   Rationale: Provides for patient warmth and protects linen from water.
7. Place washbasin under spout of shampoo basin on a chair or table at the bedside.

Rationale: Allows water to run away from face and head into a receptacle.
Note: Plastic trash bags are often used to collect water runoff.
8. Place dampened washcloth over patient's eyes.
   Rationale: Protects eyes from soapy water.
   Note: Cotton balls may be placed in patient's ears to keep water from collecting in the ear canal.
9. Using water pitcher, wet hair thoroughly with warm water (approximately 110°F). Check temperature by placing small amount of water on your wrist. A bath thermometer may be used.
   Rationale: Prevents burns to face and scalp.
10. Apply small amount of shampoo.
    Note: Before shampooing, hydrogen peroxide may be used to dissolve matted blood in hair. Peroxide normally feels bubbly and warm. Reassure patient that it will not bleach hair.
11. Massage scalp with fingertips while making shampoo lather. Start at hairline and work toward neck.
    Rationale: Massage stimulates circulation to the scalp; systematic lathering ensures thorough cleansing.

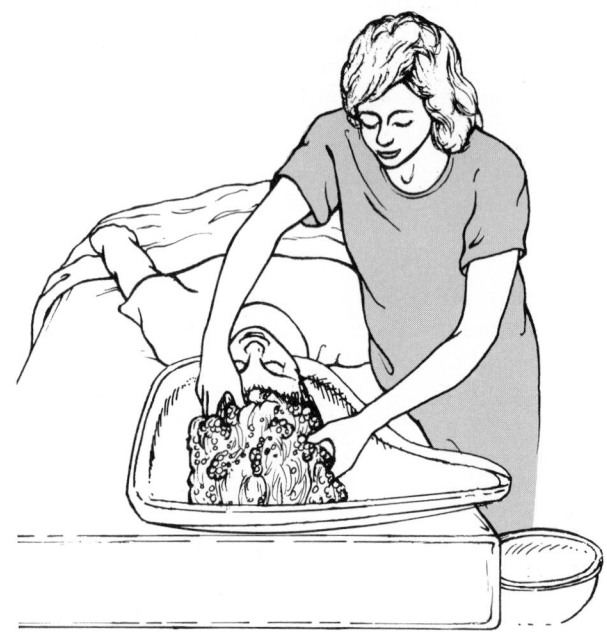

Step 11

12. Rinse hair with warm water. Reapply shampoo and repeat massage.
13. Rinse hair thoroughly with warm water.
    Note: Clean hair "squeaks" when rubbed between fingers.

(continued)

PROCEDURE 28–5. Shampooing Hair of a Bedridden Patient (continued)

Rationale: Soap residue in hair may dry and irritate hair and scalp.

14. Apply small amount of conditioner per patient request. Rinse well.
    Rationale: Conditioner prevents drying and makes combing easier.

15. Squeeze excess moisture from hair. Wrap bath towel around hair. Rub to dry hair and scalp. Use second towel if necessary.

16. Remove equipment and wet towels from bed. Place dry towel around patient's shoulders.
    Rationale: Prevents chilling of patient.

17. Dry hair with hair dryer. Comb and style.

18. Help patient to comfortable position.

19. Dispose of soiled equipment and linen.

■ Lifespan Considerations

Infant

- Shampooing is usually done during daily bath to prevent seborrhea, a gray, scaly scalp condition (cradle cap).

- Prewarm the room and use warmed towels to prevent chilling infant during bath.

Child

- Pediculosis infestations are common in school-age children. Assess hair carefully for nits (lice eggs).

Adolescent

- Many adolescents shampoo their hair daily. Offering to shampoo their hair may improve their self-esteem and help them feel better than many other nursing interventions.

Older Adult

- Many older adults have decreased subcutaneous tissue and chill quickly. Prewarm towels and thoroughly dry hair after a shampoo to prevent chilling.

- Older adults may have decreased sensation to heat. Use a hair dryer cautiously on a low heat setting to prevent burning the scalp.

---

well-being. Rinsing is soothing to the patient with a dry mouth. An unclean mouth can harbor bacteria that can multiply and cause other problems. See Procedure 28-6.

Nurses can assist patients who can perform brushing and flossing by providing the necessary equipment. They may need to assist or perform these functions for patients unable to do so. Assisting patients with mouth care gives the nurse an opportunity to teach proper techniques and to stress their importance. By encouraging regular brushing and flossing, the nurse can contribute to the prevention of caries and periodontal disease and help prevent the loss of teeth. Doing oral care also permits the nurse to assess the oral cavity.

Brushing and Flossing. Patients who can brush and floss without help should be encouraged to do so. If the patient cannot get out of bed to use the sink, provide the necessary equipment and hold the basin for spitting (Fig. 28-5).

For patients with natural teeth, use a soft-bristled toothbrush with a rounded, even brushing surface and a nonabrasive toothpaste. Brush holding the toothbrush at a 45° angle to the teeth for the outside of all teeth and the inside of the back teeth. Brushing should begin with

the tips angled slightly into the groove around the teeth. In this position, the teeth should be brushed with small rotating motions over two or three teeth at a time. The

(Text continues on page 672)

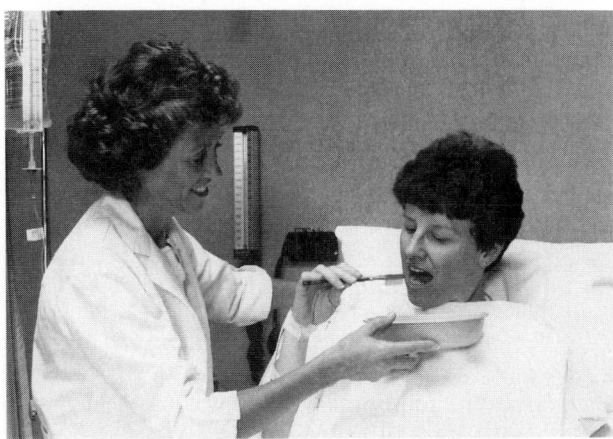

Figure 28–5. Some patients may be able to provide their own oral care but are not able to ambulate to use the sink. In such cases, the nurse assists with equipment as needed.

PROCEDURE 28–6. Providing Oral Care

■ **Purpose**
1. Cleanse tooth surfaces to prevent odor and caries.
2. Maintain hydrated, intact oral mucosa.
3. Promote self-esteem and comfort.

■ **Assessment**
• Inspect lips, buccal membrane, gums, palate, and tongue for lesions or inflammation.
• Assess for presence of caries or halitosis (bad breath).
• Identify patients at risk for oral hygiene complications:
   • Dehydration, NPO status, nasogastric tubes dry the oral mucosa.
   • Oral airways accumulate secretions and irritate the mucosa.
   • Chemotherapy often results in stomatitis and ulcerations.
   • Anticoagulant therapy or clotting disorders predispose the patient to gum bleeding.
   • Oral surgery or trauma may contraindicate tooth brushing; special rinses may be ordered.
• Determine patient's ability to assist with procedure.
• Assess patient's risk for aspiration.

■ **Equipment**
1. Toothbrush (sponge-ended swabs may be used for patients at risk for bleeding).
2. Toothpaste.
3. Cup with water, straw.
4. Emesis basin.
5. Washcloth, towel.
6. Mouthwash (optional).
7. Dental floss.
8. Disposable gloves (if the nurse provides oral care).

■ **Procedure**
1. Wash your hands.
2. Close bedside curtains or room door and explain procedure to patient.
3. Help patient to a sitting position. If patient cannot sit, help to a side-lying position.
   Rationale: High or semi-Fowler's or side-lying position helps prevent choking and aspiration.
4. Place towel under patient's chin.
   Rationale: Reduces chances of soiling bed linens and gown.
5. Moisten toothbrush with water. Apply small amount of toothpaste.
6. Hand toothbrush to patient or don disposable gloves and brush patient's teeth as follows:
   a. Hold toothbrush at a 45° angle to the gum line.
   b. Using short, vibrating motions, brush from the

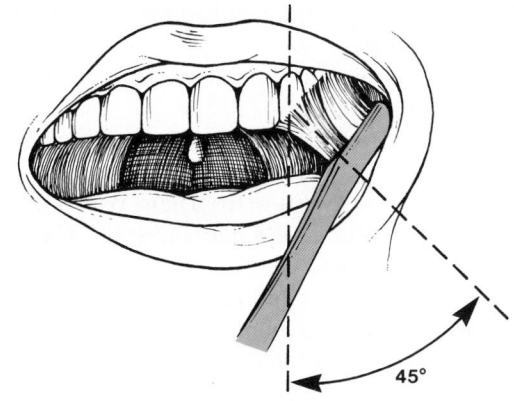

Step 6A

gum line to the crown of each tooth. Repeat until outside and inside of teeth and gums are cleaned. *Rationale: Angle of toothbrush allows brush to reach all tooth surfaces and to penetrate and cleanse under the gum line, where plaque and tartar accumulate.*
   c. Cleanse biting surfaces by brushing with a back-and-forth stroke.
   d. Brush the tongue lightly. Avoid stimulating the gag reflex.
   Rationale: Bacteria accumulate and grow on the tongue surface and must be removed.
   Note: If patient is anticoagulated or has a clotting disorder, use a very *soft toothbrush or a sponge-ended swab to prevent gum bleeding.*
7. Have patient rinse mouth thoroughly with water and spit into emesis basin (Fig. 28-5).
   Note: If tongue is heavily coated, prepare a mixture of half-strength hydrogen peroxide and have patient hold in mouth for a few seconds and then spit out. The coating will gradually dissolve. Repeat every 1 to 2 hours.
8. Remove emesis basin, set aside, and dry patient's mouth with washcloth.
9. Floss patient's teeth.
   Rationale: Flossing removes particulate matter trapped between the teeth and below the gum line.
   a. Cut 10-inch piece of dental floss. Wind ends of floss around middle finger of each hand.
   b. Using index fingers to stretch the floss, move the floss up and down around and between lower teeth. Start at the back lower teeth and work around to the other side.
   c. Using thumb and index fingers to stretch the floss, repeat procedure on upper teeth.
   d. Have patient rinse mouth thoroughly and spit into emesis basin.

(continued)

PROCEDURE 28–6. Providing Oral Care *(continued)*

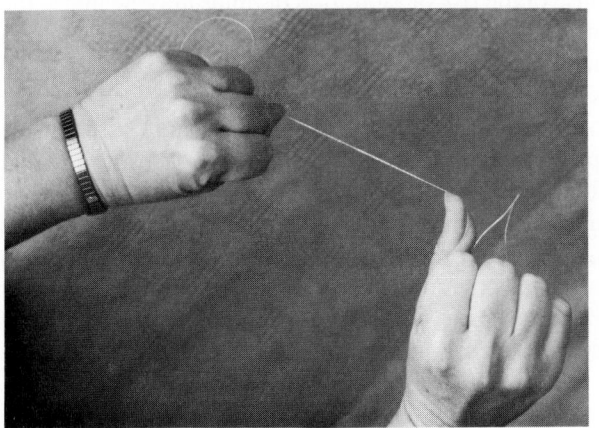

Step 9A

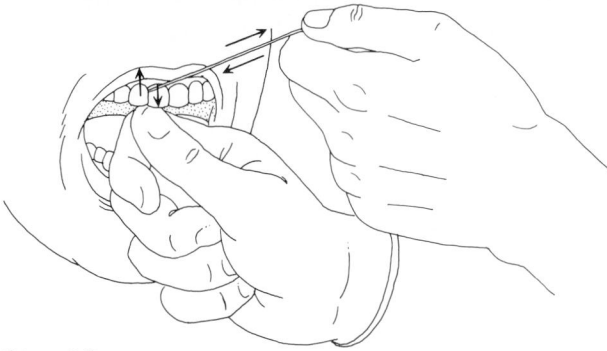

Step 9C

10. Remove basin, dry patient's mouth.
11. Remove and dispose of supplies. Help patient to comfortable position.
12. Wash your hands.

■ Procedure

Variation for the Unconscious Patient
1. Always explain the procedure to the patient.
2. Place patient in a side-lying position with head of bed lowered so saliva runs out of mouth by gravity. *Rationale: Prevents aspiration.*
3. Place towel or waterproof pad under patient's chin.

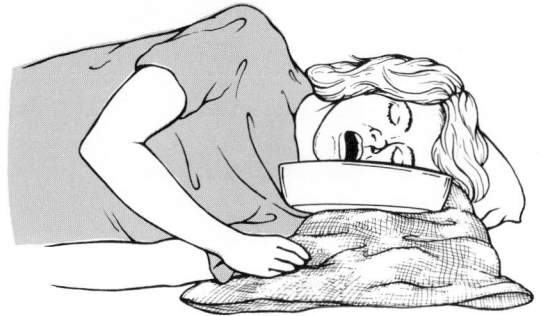

Step 4

4. Place emesis basin against patient's mouth or have suction catheter positioned to remove secretions from mouth.
5. Use padded tongue blade to open teeth gently. Leave in place between the back molars. *Never* put your fingers in an unconscious patient's mouth. *Rationale: Unconscious patients often respond to oral stimulation by biting down.*
6. Brush teeth and gums as directed above, using toothbrush or padded tongue blade.

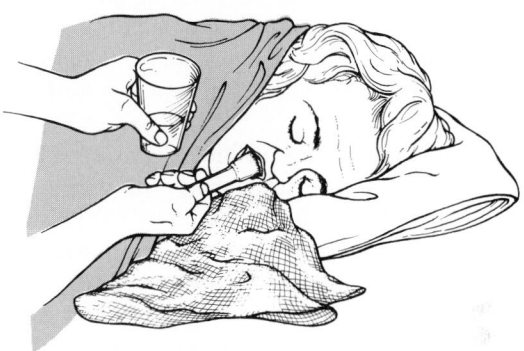

Step 6

7. Swab or suction to remove pooled secretions. A small bulb syringe or syringe without needle may be used to rinse oral cavity.
8. Apply thin layer of petroleum jelly to lips to prevent drying or cracking. *Note: Lemon glyerin swabs can be drying to the oral mucosa if used for extended periods.*

■ Lifespan Considerations

Infant
- A dry gauze or washcloth can be used to remove accumulated secretions from an infant's gums.
- A small, soft-bristled brush is used after first teeth have erupted.

Child
- Children under 3 or 4 years of age may not understand what "rinse" or "spit" means. Do not offer them water to rinse with if they are NPO because they will swallow the rinse.
- Children or teens wearing braces need special attention to remove food particles from the wires.

Older Adult
- Many older adults wear full or partial dentures. Be sure dentures are removed regularly and cleansed. Special denture cleansers are available. The gums or any remaining teeth should be brushed well.

bristles on the front of the brush are used to clean the inside of the front teeth in a rotating movement. The chewing surfaces can be cleaned with a brisk back-and-forth motion, taking care not to traumatize the gingival tissue. Brushing of the tongue is important to remove microorganisms and debris. The tongue is brushed toward the throat (with the grain), lightly toward the teeth, and on the sides.

For the patient who has difficulty grasping the small handle of an ordinary toothbrush, an electric toothbrush can be used because it has a larger handle that is easier to grasp and requires less manipulation. The handle of a regular toothbrush can be built up with tape, a bicycle handlebar grip, or a split rubber ball.

Flossing finishes the task of removing plaque and debris from between teeth. Unwaxed dental floss is used. The floss should be long enough so that a new section of the floss can be used when it becomes frayed. Avoid traumatizing the gums.

Other nursing measures include cleansing and moisturizing the oral mucosa by rinsing with water, saline, half-strength hydrogen peroxide, dilute mouthwash, or an anesthetic mouthwash. Patients with drainage and/or lesions in the oral cavity and those who cannot take fluids by mouth may need rinsing and cleansing as often as every 2 hours. Such patients may have dry lips; a water-based lubricant or petroleum jelly can be applied.

Oral Care in the Comatose or Unconscious Patient. Feeding tubes, nasogastric tubes, and constant breathing through the mouth can dry mucous membranes. Because of the risk of aspiration of fluids into the lungs, the unconscious patient should be turned on the side during mouth care so that fluids can drain easily. Brush the external surfaces of the teeth in the usual way. To protect your fingers, place a padded tongue blade between the upper and lower teeth toward the back on one side. Then, using a toothbrush, cotton-tipped applicator, or gauze on a tongue blade, clean the interior of the teeth and the chewing surfaces. To prevent aspiration, use only small amounts of cleaning solution, such as saline or dilute hydrogen peroxide. A suction device can also be used to remove the fluid safely. See Procedure 28-6.

Denture Care. Determine immediately whether the patient wears dentures. Encourage the patient to wear the dentures, which improve eating, talking, and appearance and may boost the patient's self-image.

Dentures collect the same debris, plaque, and tartar as do natural teeth. If the patient cannot care for the dentures, the nurse needs to do so, using a brushing technique similar to that for natural teeth. A soft toothbrush is recommended because hard-bristled brushes can produce grooves in dentures. Soap and water is effective, although a mild commercial cleaning agent can

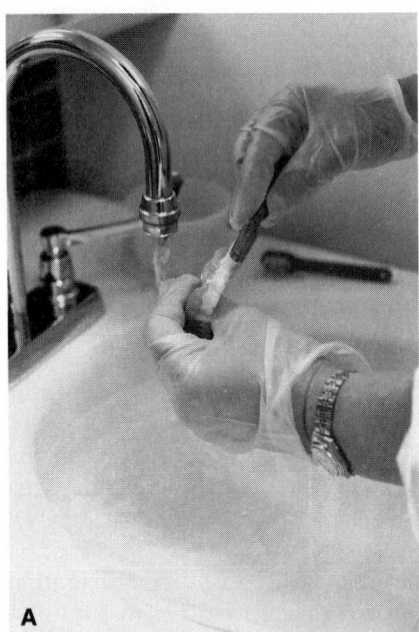 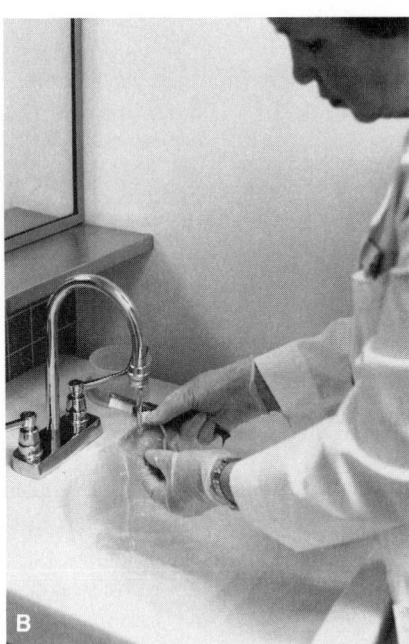 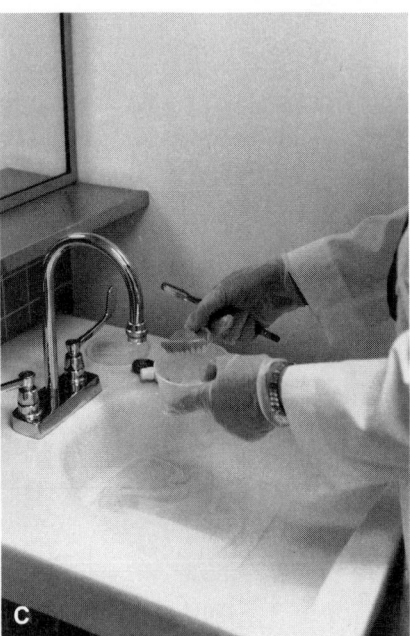

Figure 28–6. Denture care. **A:** Dentures are brushed as though the nurse were brushing natural teeth. **B:** Dentures are rinsed. **C:** To prevent damage, dentures should be stored in a plastic container when not in use or when carried to and from the sink.

be used. Dentures must be protected from breakage. Keep them in a denture cup while carrying them to the sink, wash them in a plastic pan, and store them in a covered container if not worn continuously (Fig. 28-6).

The patient should rinse the mouth before reinserting the dentures. Gums and tongue should be cleansed with a soft brush when the dentures are out. Massaging the gums with a brush or thumb and forefinger helps to stimulate circulation and toughen the oral mucosa. Dentures should be removed at night so that tissues are exposed to air (Renn, 1989).

Older patients should be taught the five signs and symptoms of oral cancer, emphasizing self-examination. Teach the finger massage technique for stimulation of alveolar mucosa and gingiva to promote healthy tissues. Review and teach denture care.

Eye Care

Some patients need help with eye care, particularly those who have had eye surgery, injury, or infection, or unconscious patients who have lost the blink reflex. The nurse must make an assessment of eye problems (see the display). Observations include noting whether the eyelids are edematous, crusted with secretions, or inflamed with sties and whether the lacrimal ducts are inflamed, tearing excessively, or are crusted with secretions. The sclera are examined for discoloration and the conjunctiva for inflammation and degree of redness. Pupil constriction or dilation and response to light and coordination of eye movements also are assessed.

Patients with eye inflammation, draining, or crusting need help cleaning these secretions from the eyes. Eyes should be cleansed with a washcloth or cotton ball soaked with saline or sterile water. Clean from the inside of the eye toward the outside. If infection is not suspected, use a different part of the washcloth for each eye; if infection is present, use a different cloth for each eye. This reduces the potential for spreading infectious debris from one eye to the other.

Eyeglasses and Contact Lenses. Determine if a visual aid is used, and locate the aid and encourage its use. Safeguarding these aids contributes to the patient's independence and safety.

Glasses should be cleaned daily, but patients do not often ask for this kind of help. Glass lenses can be washed under warm water, but plastic ones should be washed with a special cleaning solution. Both can be dried with facial tissue or a lens cloth. Store glasses in a secure place where the patient can reach them. When patients are too ill to manage these activities, are going to surgery or other treatment, or have other physical limitations to self-care, the nurse must take responsibility for glasses. Note their location in the nurses' notes; this allows the nurse on the next shift or the next unit to which the patient is transferred to find them.

Contact lenses are a common alternative to glasses. These concave plastic discs cover the pupil and float on the tear layer. Contact lenses are widely worn; therefore, it is imperative to check for their presence in patients who are unconscious or confused.

Contact lenses may be hard, soft, or gas-permeable hard or soft. Hard lenses are made of rigid plastic that does not absorb air or liquid. Because they restrict oxygen supply to the cornea, their use is limited to 14 hours per day. Some kinds of soft lenses are worn during the day and removed at night, but others can be worn for as long as 14 to 30 days. Disposable contact lenses are a recent innovation that lessen care.

Red conjunctiva, excess tearing, and burning pain are symptoms of lens overwear. Secretions and foreign matter (dust, pollen) accumulate under the lenses as they are worn. These substances are irritating to the eye and result in distorted vision and increased risk of infection. Since all contact lenses decrease the flow of oxygen to the cornea to some extent, corneal damage can occur if they are left in place for too long.

Contact lenses must be cleaned and disinfected after removal, using the appropriate method for the type of lens. If the patient cannot do so, the nurse must remove and care for the lenses (Fig. 28-7). To care for soft lenses, a cleaning solution is used to loosen and remove film and debris. Rinsing is required after cleaning, using a rinsing and disinfecting solution to remove loosened deposits. The lenses are then covered with rinsing solution for storage. Before insertion, each lens is rinsed again with the rinsing solution to ensure removal of particulate matter. Recommended care includes a weekly heat or

(Text continues on page 676)

Assessment for Eye Problems

- Does the patient use eyeglasses or contact lenses or have an artificial eye?
- How does the patient rate visual acuity?
- Is the patient experiencing eye problems now?
- Are eyelids edematous, crusted with secretions, inflamed with sties?
- What is the appearance of the lacrimal ducts? Are they inflamed, tearing excessively, not tearing at all, or crusted with secretions?
- Are sclera discolored?
- Are conjunctiva inflamed, pale?
- Are pupils dilated, constricted, responsive to light?
- Are eye movements coordinated?

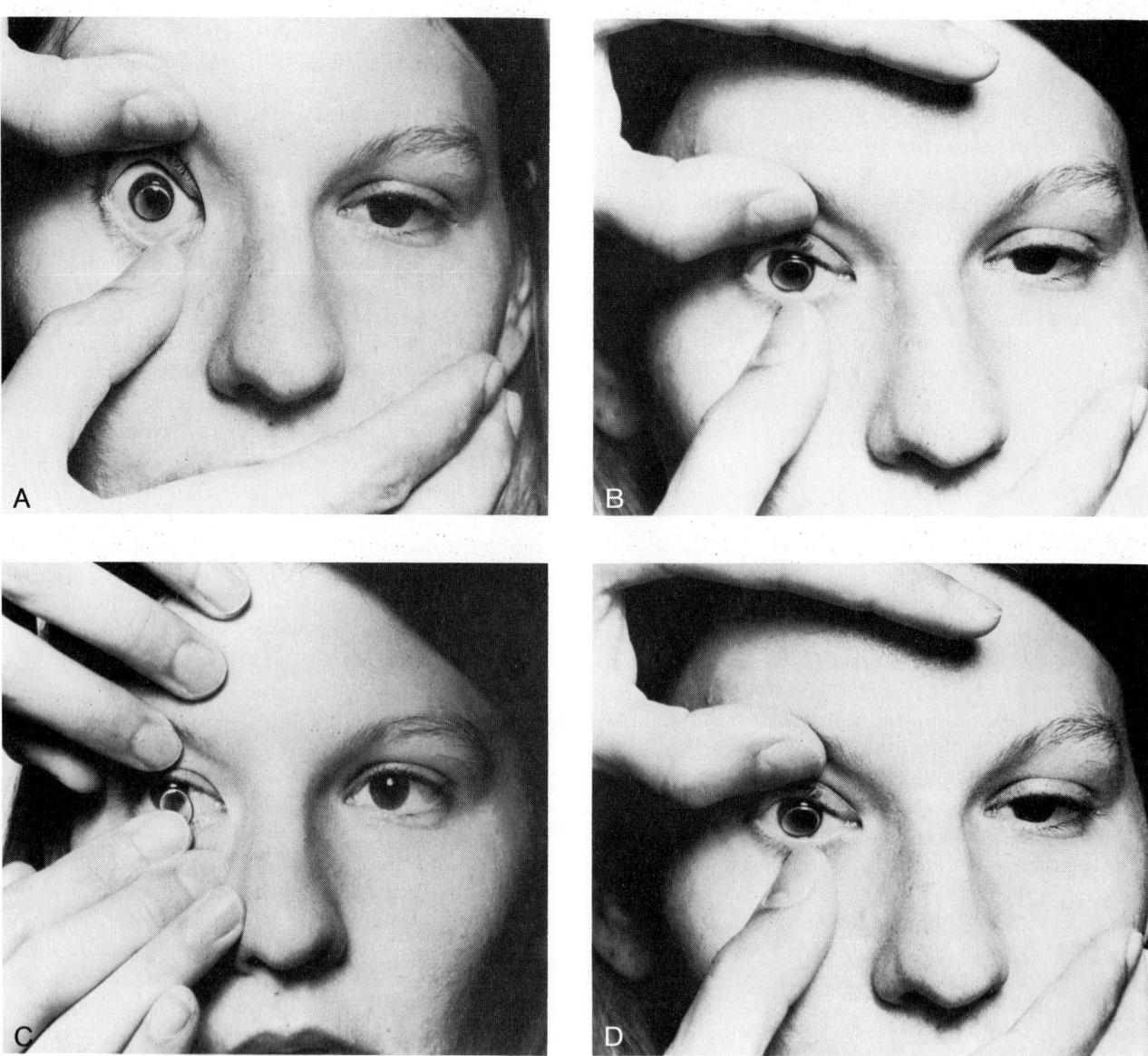

Figure 28–7. Removal of contact lenses. Primary Stages in Hard Lens Removal: **A:** After the eyelids have been separated and the hard contact lens has been correctly positioned over the cornea, widen the eyelid margins beyond the top and bottom edges of lens. **B:** After the lower eyelid margin has been moved near the bottom lens edge and then the upper eyelid margin has been moved near the top lens edge, you are ready to move under the bottom edge of the lens by pressing slightly harder on the lower eyelid while moving it upward. **C:** After the lens has tipped slightly, move the eyelids toward one another; this causes the lens to slide out between the eyelids. Possible Lens Positions: **D:** Directly over the cornea. This normal wearing position of a contact lens is also the correct position for removing it. If the lens cannot be removed, however, slide it onto the sclera. Here the lens can remain with relative safety until experienced help is available; other white areas of the eye to the side or above the cornea might also be used. If the lens is to be removed, however, slide it to a position directly over the cornea. A lens in this position—or a similar one anywhere around the periphery of the cornea—should be moved as soon as possible. If the lens is to be removed, slide it to a position directly over the cornea; if the lens cannot be removed immediately, slide it onto the sclera. Soft Contact Lens Removal: **G:** With clean hands, pull down the lower lid with the middle finger and place the index fingertip on the lower edge of the lens. Slide the lens down to the white part of the eye. **H:** Compress the lens lightly between the thumb and index finger. Bring thumb and index finger together in a "pinching" motion, causing the lens to double-up between and allowing air underneath. Remove the lens from the eye. Suction Cup: **I:** Contact lenses may also be removed by pressing gently on the lens with a small suction cup to break the suction. (Panels A to H courtesy of American Optometric Association).

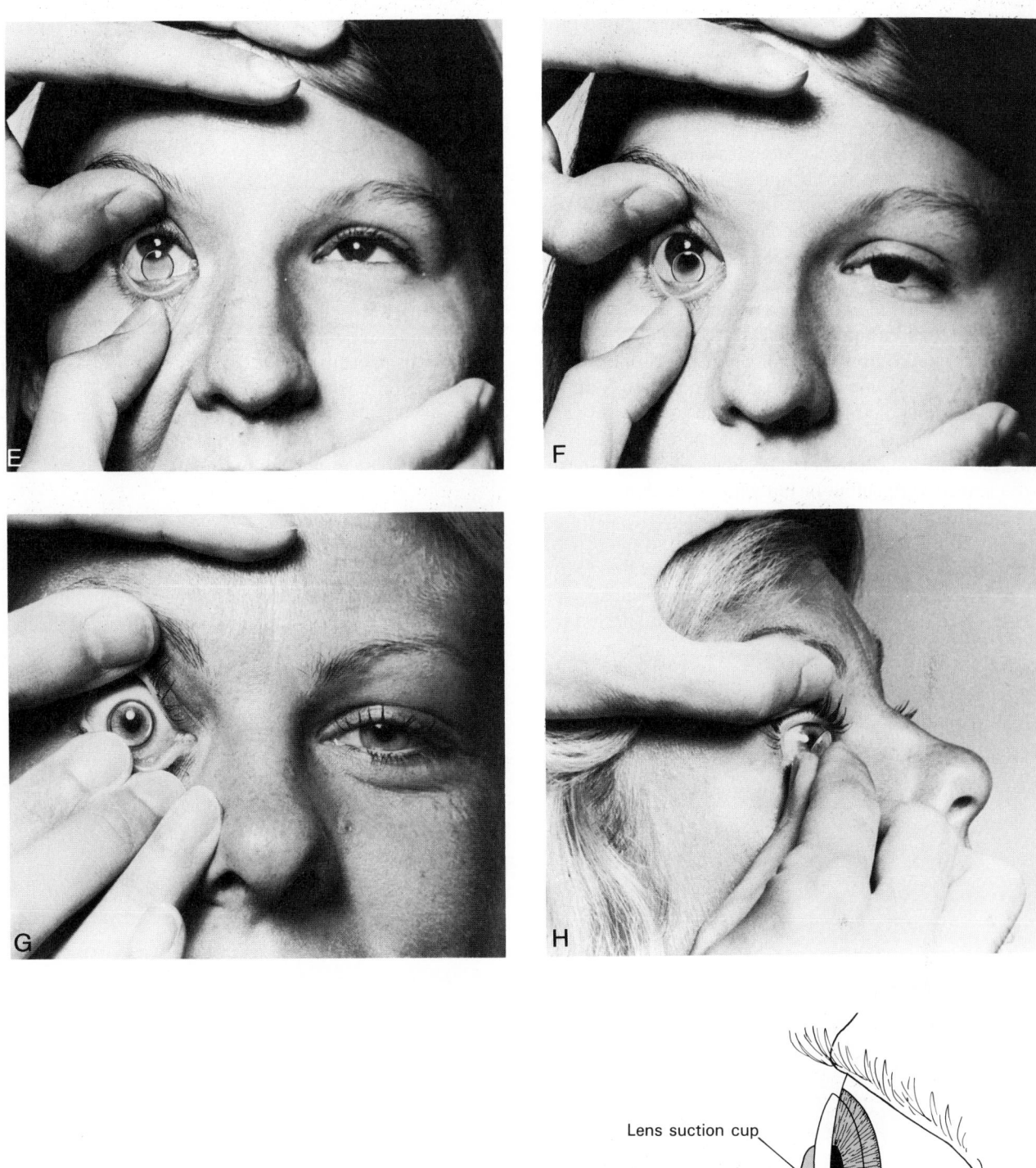

Lens suction cup

Contact lens

Figure 28–7. (continued)

chemical cleaning of lenses to remove accumulated protein, lipids, and mucin.

Artificial Eyes. Artificial eyes are made of glass or plastic. Some are permanent, but others require daily removal for cleaning. Most patients prefer to provide eye care for themselves, but the nurse may need to assist by removing the artificial eye if there is evidence of inflammation, if the patient is scheduled for surgery, or if the patient is dependent due to injury or immobility.

To remove an artificial eye, pull down on the lower eyelid and exert slight pressure below the eyelid to overcome the suction holding the eye in place. To ease removal, a small bulb syringe or medicine dropper bulb may be used to create a suction great enough to counteract the suction holding the eye in the socket. The eye can be cleaned with saline and stored in saline or water in a covered, labeled container. The edges of the eye socket are cleaned with saline or tap water and should be inspected for redness, swelling, or drainage. Because of the proximity of the eye to the sinuses and underlying brain tissue, infection in this area is of great concern.

To reinsert the eye, pull down on the lower lid and slip the eye into the socket, lifting the upper lid to permit the eye to slide in.

Eye Care in the Comatose Patient. Comatose patients are at risk for corneal ulceration, which can cause blindness. When the blink reflex is lost, eyes may remain open and become dry. To prevent these complications, eyes are kept moist and protected from the air. Liquid tear solution (methylcellulose) or saline can be instilled to prevent drying, or the eyes can be closed and covered with a protective shield.

Ear Care

Healthy ears require little care. Check the external ear for inflamed tissue, drainage, and discomfort. Clean the auricles with a washcloth-covered finger. Excessive cerumen can be removed with the twisted end of a clean washcloth while pulling the auricle down, or by irrigation if this method fails. Emphasize the danger of using bobby pins, cotton-tipped applicators, toothpicks, or other sharp objects to remove cerumen. Bobby pins or toothpicks can rupture the tympanic membrane or traumatize the ear canal; cotton-tipped applicators can push the wax further in and block the ear canal.

Care of Hearing Aids. A hearing aid is a sound-amplifying device powered by batteries. The aid contains a microphone that picks up sound waves, changes them into electric signals, and transmits them; an amplifier for magnifying sound; a receiver that transforms the electric signals back to sound energy; and an ear mold that channels the sound to the tympanic membrane. There are several kinds of hearing aids (see Fig. 28-8 and the display).

Hearing aids are expensive and significant to their owners. These devices must be handled and stored safely. Note the type of device, how the patient cares for it, how well it functions, and what problems the patient

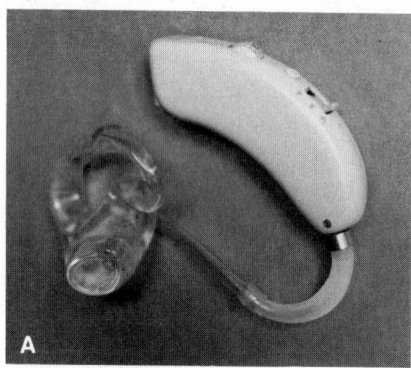

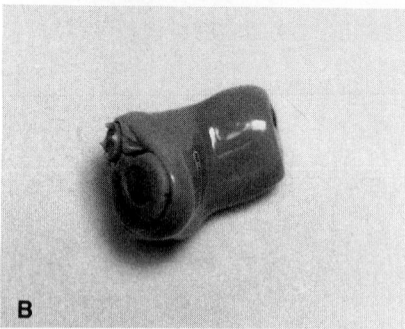

Figure 28–8. Two popular types of hearing aids. **A:** Behind the ear type. **B:** In the ear type.

Types of Hearing Aids

- *Behind-the-ear aid,* the most common type, fits over the ear. An ear mold fits into the ear, and the case, containing the microphone, amplifier, receiver, volume control, batteries, and T/M switch, fits behind the ear.
- *In-the-ear aid,* the most compact, has all of the elements located in the ear mold.
- *Eyeglass aid* involves a hearing aid in one or both temples of a pair of eyeglasses. It functions similarly to the behind-the-ear aid but the components are located in the temples of the glasses.
- *Body-type hearing aid* is used for the most severe hearing losses. The case looks like a pocket-sized transistor radio and can be clipped into a pocket, undergarment, or harness. The case contains the microphone and amplifier and is connected to a receiver, which snaps into an ear mold.

has with it. Care includes careful handling to prevent damage, appropriate use, cleaning of the ear mold, and replacement of dead batteries. Hearing aids are removed and stored before surgery, unless the patient must communicate with operating room personnel before or during surgery.

Although the hearing aid amplifies the sound of voices, it also amplifies background sounds. Patients may continue to have difficulty hearing, especially in a noisy setting. To foster optimal hearing, face the patient, speak slowly and clearly, and rephrase what is said if the patient does not understand. Some hearing-impaired people can lip-read; careful enunciation improves their ability to understand.

Feeding

Patients often have poor appetites because of pain, depression, or medication side effects. The patient may find hospital food unfamiliar or unpalatable. The setting may be uncomfortable, noisy, too warm, or too cool, or there may be unpleasant odors or sights. Other frequent causes of decreased food intake are inability to eat without help due to weakness, fatigue, or paralysis. Assess the patient's feeding ability and the level of support needed for eating; in this way, assistance can be planned and a teaching program can be instituted if appropriate.

Since being fed represents a loss of control, it is important to give the patient some role if possible. This is true for people of all ages. Giving the patient a choice—for instance, the order in which food is eaten—may relieve some of the helpless feelings. Because the process of helping with eating is time-consuming, the patient may feel like a burden. The nurse must avoid reinforcing this belief and should always give the patient ample time to chew and swallow.

Interventions to meet feeding needs are varied. The following are helpful in planning patient care:

- Check chart, Kardex, or diet list to determine whether the patient has limitations on eating (e.g., fasting for laboratory tests or procedures).
- Check each tray for the patient's name and the type of diet. Check any questions with the patient's chart. Verify the patient's name by checking the wristband.
- If pain is a factor limiting food intake or self-feeding ability, time analgesia to permit pain relief at mealtime. If fatigue is a problem, schedule a rest period before eating to enhance appetite and increase independence.
- Help the patient to urinate or defecate if needed to enhance mealtime comfort.
- Enhance the setting. Turn on the lights if needed. Provide good ventilation. Remove room odors and disturbing sights such as soiled dressings.
- Prepare the patient for mealtime by finding dentures

and eyeglasses, brushing teeth, rinsing mouth, and washing hands.
- Help the patient to a comfortable position for eating, usually sitting in bed or a chair. Ensure good body mechanics by positioning the patient high enough in bed to match the bed gatch with the patient's hips. Raise the head of the bed if the patient cannot sit on the side of the bed. A high sitting position is necessary to reduce the danger of choking and aspirating food.
- Clear the overbed table of extraneous items.
- Determine how much help the patient needs (i.e. uncovering containers, removing food from plastic bags, buttering bread, or cutting meat).
- Plan ahead so that patients who need assistance can be helped while their food is still hot. Food that has cooled can be microwaved. Sometimes it is possible to schedule trays for those who require help earlier or later than the others.

See Procedure 33-1 for details on helping a patient to eat.

Adequate swallowing is essential for safe eating. Difficulty swallowing (dysphagia) may occur as a result of disease or trauma to cranial nerves V (trigeminal), IX (glossopharyngeal), or X (vagus). Diseases such as myasthenia gravis and muscular dystrophy that cause muscle weakness may also result in dysphagia. To avoid food aspiration, carefully assess the patient's ability to swallow before feeding. Elicit the gag reflex by placing 1 or 2 ml of sterile water or a small amount of ice chips in the oropharynx, and instruct the patient to swallow. Then place a finger lightly over the larynx to detect upward movement (Larsen, 1981). When there is any doubt as to the patient's ability to swallow, do not try to feed him or her until obtaining an expert opinion.

After a stroke or surgical removal of part of the larynx, the patient may need to relearn how to initiate swallowing (Griffin & Lockhart, 1987). Consulting a speech therapist or an occupational therapist is important in planning a safe rehabilitation program.

Patients who have suffered damage to the left brain have difficulty speaking, reading, writing, and understanding speech. Talking to these patients while they are trying to eat may overwhelm and confuse them, resulting in aspiration of food (Larsen, 1981).

Blind patients can be oriented to the location of food on a plate by referring to the numbers on a clock. They may be used to developing a mental map of the tray by doing a survey with their fingertips; food can be located by gentle probing with a fork. Knowing what the foods are helps a blind person plan how best to eat them. For example, knowing that peas and mashed potatoes are on the plate enables a blind person to eat the peas more easily by pushing them against the mashed potatoes.

Feeding of infants should be relaxed and free of interruptions. Parents or other relatives should feed the child if possible. When giving solid food, position the infant to face the feeder at eye level, and keep the food dish out of reach of exploring hands.

For some patients, hospital food seems strange and unappealing. Special food brought from home or a favorite restaurant may encourage eating.

Many eating aids are available. Plates with guards or lips help the patient get food onto a utensil. Utensil handles can be padded to make them easier to grasp. Cups with spouts help with drinking. Straws may help patients to drink without dribbling.

When the meal is finished, assess the food and fluid intake and record it if indicated. If a calorie count is ordered, record the precise amount of food eaten. Record any pertinent reaction to the meal. Make necessary adjustments in the diet and the care plan.

Toileting

Patients often require assistance with toileting (i.e., help walking to the bathroom or being placed on a bedpan). Needing help with these intimate functions may provoke extreme discomfort for some patients; a kind approach by the nurse helps allay embarrassment. Helping patients to be as independent as possible with toileting is an essential nursing intervention. Most people prize control in this area and benefit greatly from increased self-care. Even if the only independent self-care a patient can manage is to decide when and how elimination will take place, it can help the patient feel more in control.

The following measures can help patients manage self-care of elimination. The nurse can teach these methods and help the patient determine which ones work best.

Increasing fluid intake results in increased urinary output. An intake of 1200 to 1500 ml is recommended, with additional fluid (2000 to 3000 ml) for patients who are immobilized, febrile, or experiencing fluid losses (such as diarrhea). However, fluid limitations are sometimes necessary, as in congestive heart failure and renal impairment; thus, it is important to compare fluid intake and urine output.

Exercise affects micturition by strengthening abdominal and perineal muscles, which enhances voiding and helps to prevent urinary incontinence. For example, Kegel exercises strengthen the muscles of the perineum. These exercises involve contracting the muscles as if trying to stop micturition or by actually practicing stopping the stream of urine while voiding.

Privacy and an opportunity to relax enhances most people's ability to urinate. Worrying about being able to void, especially after surgery or giving birth, may produce tension, so do not pressure patients to void on schedule. The following may help the patient urinate:

- Turn on the bathroom tap.
- Have the patient visualize his or her bathroom at home.
- Warm the bedpan.
- Have the patient assume a comfortable position (standing for men).
- Provide analgesia for pain.
- Pour warm water over the perineum.

See Chapters 37 and 38 for more detail on elimination.

Bedpans. There are two types of bedpans: a *regular bedpan* has a high rim, and a *fracture pan* has a lower rim for patients who cannot raise their buttocks or in whom such movement is contraindicated.

Many patients need help to get on a bedpan. Sitting is the most effective position for passing urine or stool. Some patients can use a bedpan alone if it is left on the bed or covered on a nearby chair; such independence should be encouraged. A trapeze on the bed frame also facilitates moving on and off a bedpan. See Procedure 28-7.

Urinal. A man who is on strict bedrest or who is confined to bed due to weakness or disability may use a **urinal,** a metal or plastic receptacle into which the penis can be placed to facilitate urinating without spilling (see Fig. 37-5). The urinal needs to be emptied frequently into a toilet to prevent spilling and odors. Some men cannot void while sitting or lying in bed; sometimes they can be helped to a standing position long enough to void. Incontinent men may be more comfortable if the urinal is left in place. If this is done, the urinal should be a plastic one, and the scrotum should be padded for protection.

Condom Catheter. A **condom catheter** is a heavy rubber sheath that fits over the penis and is connected to a collection tube and bag. A small bag that can be strapped to the leg may promote self-care for the ambulatory man. Application is outlined and illustrated in Procedure 37-3.

Bedside Commode. As a rule, most patients can progress to the most independent mode of managing elimination that is safe. Many patients on bedrest can tolerate a brief time out of bed to use a bedside **commode,** a portable chair with a toilet seat and a receptacle beneath that can be emptied. In this way, a patient who cannot walk to the bathroom can manage toileting independently. A male patient could stand to urinate and use the commode for a bowel movement. The nurse may need to provide support for these activities by providing water, a washcloth, and a towel for self-cleaning or by performing the cleaning.

Dressing

Dressing and undressing consume a great deal of time and energy, which is why chronically and acutely ill

PROCEDURE 28–7. Using a Bedpan

■ **Purpose**

1. Provide a means for elimination for those patients who are confined to bed or unable to get to the bathroom or bedside commode independently or safely.

■ **Assessment**

• Assess the patient's normal elimination habits and when he or she last voided and/or defecated.

• Assess level of mobility, positioning restrictions, and degree of assistance required.

• Review orders to determine if urine or fecal specimens are needed.

• Identify medications the patient is receiving that would alter the color, consistency, or amount of urine or feces obtained.

■ **Equipment**

1. Clean bedpan or fracture pan (see Fig. 38-6 for two types of bedpans).
2. Toilet tissue.
3. Washcloth, towel, soap.
4. Air freshener (optional).
5. Specimen container (if needed).
6. Cover for bedpan (if toilet for discarding is not in patient's room).
7. Disposable gloves.

■ **Procedure**

Placing the bedpan

1. Wash your hands.
2. Close curtain around bed or shut door.
   Rationale: Provides for privacy and reduces embarrassment.
3. Run warm water over rim of pan; dry with towel.
   Rationale: Warming the pan facilitates patient relaxation and encourages elimination.
   Note: Be careful not to overwarm the pan and burn the patient.
4. Lock siderail up on opposite side of bed from which you will work.
   Rationale: Prevents patient rolling out of bed when turning on and off bedpan.
5. Raise bed to height appropriate for nurse.
   Rationale: Prevents muscle strain and promotes proper body mechanics.
6. For patient who can raise buttocks and assist with procedure:
   a. Fold top linen down on the nurse's side to expose the patient's hips.

Rationale: Exposes the patient minimally to decrease embarrassment and preserve dignity.

b. Have patient flex knees and lift buttocks. Assist patient by placing your hand under sacrum, elbow on mattress, and lifting as a lever.
   Rationale: Patient's body weight is supported by lower legs and feet. Proper body mechanics by nurse prevent muscle strain.

c. Slide rounded smooth rim of regular bedpan under patient. If using a fracture pan, slide narrow flat end under buttocks.
   Rationale: Proper placement prevents spillage and shearing trauma of skin in sacral area.

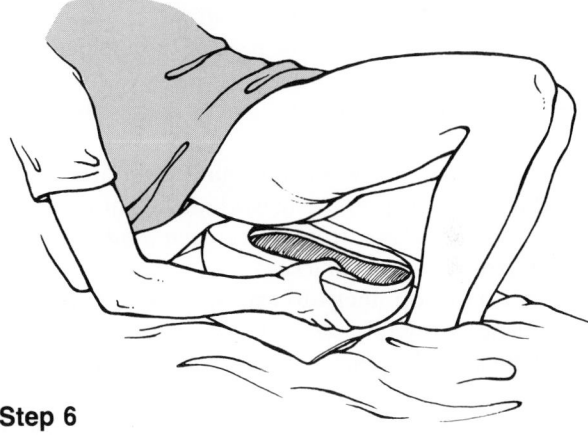

Step 6

7. For patient unable to assist by raising buttocks:
   a. Lower head of bed to flat position.
   b. Fold top bed linens down to expose patient minimally.
   c. Help patient to roll to side-lying position.

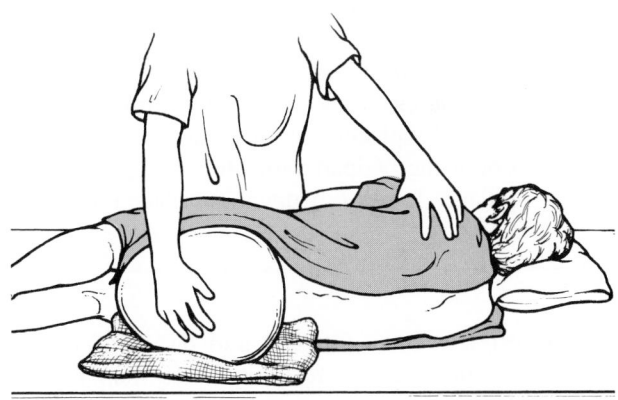

Step 7

(continued)

PROCEDURE 28–7. Using a Bedpan *(continued)*

d. Place bedpan against buttocks and tucked down against mattress. Hold firmly in place and roll patient onto back as bedpan positions under buttocks.
Rationale: Correct placement prevents spillage.

8. Cover patient with linen. Place call bell and toilet paper within reach.
Rationale: Provides for privacy, warmth, independence, and self-dignity.

9. Raise head of bed 30° unless contraindicated.
Rationale: Sitting position reduces discomfort and strain on lower back and facilitates elimination.

10. Lower bed to lowest position. Place siderails up if indicated.
Rationale: Promotes patient safety.

11. Wash your hands. Allow patient to be alone.

Removing the bedpan

12. Answer call bell promptly.

13. Place soap, wet washcloth, and towel at bedside.

14. Raise bed to appropriate working height for nurse.
Rationale: Prevents muscle strain and promotes proper body mechanics.

15. Fold back top linens to expose patient minimally.

16. Put on disposable clean gloves.
Rationale: Prevents contamination of hands with body substances.

17. Assess if patient can wipe perineal area. If not, wipe area with several layers of toilet tissue. If specimen is to be measured or collected, dispose of soiled toilet tissue in separate receptacle, not bedpan.
Note: For female patients, wipe from urethra toward anus to prevent tracking of rectal microorganisms into the urinary meatus. Use as an informal teaching session to reinforce good hygiene practices.

18. For patient who can raise buttocks and assist with procedure:
a. Lower head of bed.
b. Have patient flex knees and lift buttocks. Assist patient by placing one hand under sacrum and supporting bedpan with other hand to prevent spillage. Remove bedpan and place on bedside chair.

c. Offer soap, warm water, washcloth, and towel for patient to wash hands and/or perineal area.
Rationale: Prevents transfer of microorganisms, promotes good hygiene practices, and prevents skin breakdown.

19. For patient unable to assist by raising buttocks:
a. Lower head of bed to flat position.
b. Fold top linen down to expose patient minimally.
c. Help patient to roll off bedpan and onto side. Use one hand to stabilize bedpan during turning to prevent spillage.
d. Wipe anal area with tissue. Wash perineum with soap and warm water. Pat dry.
Rationale: Prevents skin breakdown and excoriation.

20. Assist patient to comfortable position.

21. Cover bedpan and remove from bedside. Obtain specimen if required. Empty and clean bedpan and return it to bedside.
Rationale: Clean pan promptly to minimize spread of offensive odor.

22. Remove and discard gloves. Wash your hands.
Rationale: Reduces spread of microorganisms.

23. Spray air freshener if necessary to control odor, unless contraindicated (patient with respiratory conditions, allergies).
Rationale: Odor is embarrassing to patient and visitors. Self-dignity is preserved by minimizing embarrassment.

■ **Lifespan Considerations**

Child
- A toilet-trained child is reluctant to use a bedpan, as he or she has been taught not to toilet in bed. Use a potty chair at the bedside if possible.

Older Adult
- It is often difficult for the older adult to use a regular bedpan because of limitation of body movement and arthritis. A fracture pan is less difficult and less painful to use.

people often become fatigued and discouraged. The following interventions are designed to help patients relearn dressing skills:

- Schedule dressing or undressing in conjunction with bathing.
- Encourage the patient to use his or her eyeglasses or hearing aid.

- Provide analgesia if needed.
- Organize carefully and allow ample time. Lay clothes out in the order in which they will be needed.
- Choose clothes that are loose and easy to get on and off, with wide sleeves and pant legs and front fasteners. Use Velcro closures when possible. Shoes should have elastic laces or Velcro closures.
- Encourage the patient to help select clothes. Suggest

street clothes rather than nightclothes when appropriate.

- Assess the patient's ability to maintain balance, and put clothes and supplies in easy reach.
- Ensure privacy (within the limits of safety).
- If the patient has visual deficits, tell him or her when you enter and leave the area. If the patient has any sight, place clothing where it can be seen. Remove any unnecessary furniture or other items.
- If the patient has cognitive deficits, develop a routine to lessen confusion. Keep instructions clear and simple, and avoid distractions, which may hinder concentration.
- Teach the use of aids for dressing (e.g., long-handled shoehorn, zipper pull, long-handled reacher, buttonhook). In many institutions, information about the use and availability of such aids can be obtained from the occupational therapist. Help the patient to adapt available equipment to meet specific needs.
- Children over 15 months can participate in dressing by extending their arms and legs when requested. At around 18 months, children can remove socks, mittens, and caps, unzip their clothes, and try to put their shoes on. By 21 months children can pull off their clothes, and at around 24 months they can remove their shoes and help put their clothes on and fasten them.

Care of Unit Environment

The equipment and supplies used by a hospital patient are kept in what is called the patient's *unit*.

Overbed tables, which provide a surface for eating and a work space for nurses, have wheels so they can be maneuvered to fit over the bed or over a chair. Some overbed tables have a mirror and storage space for toilet articles.

Small stands are placed at the side of the bed to provide storage space for personal belongings, a basin for bath water, a small curved basin (emesis basin), supplies for oral care, soap, bedpan, urinal, and toilet paper. A towel bar may be attached to the stand. Closet storage for belongings is usually provided as well. A chair, either a lightly padded straight one or an upholstered armchair, is often provided for the patient or visitors.

In most hospitals, oxygen and suction outlets are installed on the wall above the bed, and often a sphygmomanometer is mounted on the wall with a blood pressure cuff.

The lighting in the unit usually includes diffuse, less intense lighting for general use, a brighter light for patient reading, and an intense light for use during procedures and when visualization is needed for diagnostic purposes.

A call light by which the patient can summon the nurse is attached to the bed. Often, the call light is part of the

sound receiver for the television set as well as the television channel selector. A television and telephone are commonly available, free or for a small fee. Televisions are usually mounted on the wall to facilitate viewing from a Fowler's or flat position. Modern hospitals have individual climate control systems. All these pieces of equipment should be explained to the patient and family at admission.

Beds. Hospitals beds can be moved to a variety of positions, providing comfort for the patient, therapy for some conditions, and proper body mechanics for the nurse. Adjustments in height can usually be made. The high setting permits nurses to perform their tasks without back strain; the low setting permits patients to get in and out of bed easily and safely. Bed position is changed to obtain a specific therapeutic effect. The nurse should be familiar with prescribed bed positions and how to achieve them (see the display). Because bed controls are usually accessible to patients, teaching them how to use the bed enhances independence. Other adjustments that can be made in hospital beds include:

- Elevating the head of the bed to permit eating and other activities
- Simultaneously elevating the head and foot of the bed to prevent sliding toward the foot
- Elevating the foot of the bed when the legs need to be placed above the level of the heart to control swelling
- Tilting the entire bed, with the head of the bed lower than the foot, to enhance circulatory return to the heart

Several kinds of beds are available for patients who

Bed Positions

- Flat position: Mattress is completely flat.
- Fowler's position: The lower part of the bed is raised to the following positions:
  - Low Fowler's position: Head of bed is elevated to semisitting position of 15° to 45°. This position is also called semi-Fowler's position.
  - High Fowler's position: Head and trunk are elevated to 90°. This position is also called simply the Fowler's position.
- Trendelenburg position: The entire bed is tilted with the head downward. This position is not often used because it causes blood pressure to rise, and causes hypotension on return to the supine position.
- Reverse Trendelenburg position: Entire bed is tilted with feet downward.

cannot turn themselves and are at risk for skin break-down (see the display).

Mattresses are usually constructed of inner springs. They give good support and are covered with a water- and soil-resistant material to permit cleaning. Foam-rubber mattresses with an eggcrate configuration can be placed on top of the inner spring mattress for patients who must stay in bed for a long time or who find the mattress uncomfortable. Eggcrate mattresses help relieve pressure on bony prominences, increase comfort, and prevent skin breakdown. Bedboards can be placed under the mattress for added firmness. People with back alignment difficulties may require additional support.

Siderails, a standard part of beds and stretchers, help to prevent accidents caused by patients falling out of bed or getting out of bed by themselves when they are not able to do so safely. They also provide a support for patients to hold while moving in bed and getting up.

Footboards are flat boards of wood or plastic placed at the bottom of the bed at a right angle to the bed. They remove the weight of bedclothes from feet and legs and support the feet to prevent foot drop. Bed cradles can also remove the pressure of bedclothes from the feet and legs. For patients with injured or swollen legs, feet, or toes, removing the pressure of bedclothes may relieve pain and improve circulation.

Poles used for hanging IV containers are located near the bedside in most units. A pole can be inserted into a hole in the bed frame, a free-standing pole can be used, or the containers can be hung from the ceiling.

Bedmaking. A clean, dry, smooth bed enhances the patient's feeling of well-being. Decisions to change linens are made on the basis of patient need and cost, rather than a fixed routine. If the linens are soiled, wet, or stained, they need to be changed. When deciding whether to change linens, however, consider the other needs of the patient and the demands of other patients. For instance, if the patient is tired and weak, it may be better to pad slightly damp or soiled areas and wait until the patient has rested to change the linens. Sometimes straightening and tightening the sheets is adequate. See Procedures 28-8 and 28-9.

Asepsis is important in bedmaking. Drainage on used linens may contain microorganisms that can be transmitted through the air when the linens are shaken, or through contact with the nurse's hands or clothing. Handle linens carefully without shaking them. Avoid touching your clothing, and wash your hands after handling soiled linens. Soiled linens must be put immediately into a linen bag, not on any surfaces of another patient's area. Do not put soiled linens on the floor.

To conserve time and energy, pick up all the necessary linens from the linen supply before beginning. One side of the bed is made as completely as possible before moving to the other side. Raising the bed to a comfortable working height helps prevent back strain.

Specialty Beds for Patients Unable to Turn Themselves

- *Stryker frame:* Facilitates changing position by the use of two mattress sections. The patient lies on the bottom mattress while the top section is secured and the entire frame is manually rotated, turning the patient.
- *Circoelectric bed:* A rotating circular frame that is electrically rotated to turn the patient from head to toe.
- *Rotorest bed:* An electrically driven bed that rocks slowly from side to side. The patient's body is kept in alignment with a series of cushions and straps. The bed can be stopped in any of the positions to facilitate patient care.
- *Clinitron bed:* An airflow mattress that distributes a patient's weight evenly over its surface. It reduces the pressure, shear force, and friction of patient tissues. This device can induce a large amount of perspiration, which cannot be detected in the mattress because of rapid evaporation. Fluid and electrolyte imbalance can develop.

Discharge Planning and Home Care

Patients with self-care deficits need coordinated discharge plans. Self-care deficits limit the ability to function independently, thus contributing significantly to potential inability to cope and to function adequately upon discharge from the hospital. Inability to independently provide for one's hygiene, feeding, grooming, and toileting are key factors necessitating placement in an extended-care facility. When patients with self-care deficits are discharged to their homes, family and community support are often needed to ensure adequate functioning.

The enhancement of self-care skills begins in the hospital with the nurse promoting as much independence in self-care activities as possible. An occupational therapist often helps the patient develop self-care skills, and the nurse can support this learning on a daily basis. The nurse can help the patient anticipate self-care problems at home and plan how to manage them.

The home environment should enhance self-care. In the bathtub or shower, hand grips and nonskid mats can protect against falls. For most patients, getting in and out of the tub poses the greatest problem. Tub seats can be installed so that patients need not lower themselves down into the tub. Hand-held shower appliances also

(Text continues on page 685)

PROCEDURE 28–8. Making an Unoccupied Bed

■ Purpose
1. Provide clean linen and remove sources of skin irritation.
2. Promote comfort.

■ Assessment
- Assess patient's activity level and ability to get out of bed.
- Determine nursing interventions needed in assisting patient out of bed:
  - Vital sign check for orthostatic hypotension.
  - Analgesia.
  - Position precautions (i.e., elevation of body parts).
- Assess patient's potential for excessive perspiration, drainage, or incontinence in determining special linen requirements.

■ Equipment
1. Bottom sheet.
2. Top sheet.
3. Draw sheet.
4. Blanket.
5. Bedspread (changed only if soiled).
6. Mattress pad (changed only if soiled).
7. Pillowcases.
8. Waterproof pads or bath blanket (optional for incontinent or diaphoretic patients).
9. Linen bag.
10. Bedside table or chair.

■ Procedure
1. Wash your hands.
2. Assemble equipment on beside table or chair. Do not place on another patient's bed.
   Rationale: Prevents contamination with microorganisms.
3. Help patient to chair at bedside.
4. Raise bed to comfortable working position.
   Rationale: Promotes good body mechanics and reduces muscle strain to back.
5. Loosen linen on one side of bed. Move to other side of bed and loosen all linen.
6. Remove bedspread and blanket and fold each separately, if they are to be reused. Place over back of chair.
   Rationale: Blanket and bedspread are changed only when soiled at most agencies.
7. Remove pillowcases by grasping seamed end with one hand and pulling pillow out with the other. Place pillows on chair. Discard pillowcases in linen bag.
8. Remove each piece of linen separately by rolling into a ball and discarding into linen bag. Be careful to prevent soiled linen from touching your uniform.
   Rationale: Disposing of linen separately minimizes the chance of nurse's uniform being contaminated by soiled linen. Rolling linen into compact unit prevents microorganisms from shaking off during transfer to linen bag.
9. Slide mattress to head of bed if it has slipped to the foot.
10. Wipe mattress with antiseptic solution if grossly soiled. Dry thoroughly.
11. Working from side of bed where linen is stored, spread mattress pad over mattress and smooth out wrinkles.
    Rationale: Wrinkles in linen irritate the skin, can cause pressure areas, and are uncomfortable.
12. Unfold bottom sheet lengthwise on bed with vertical center crease along center of bed. Unfold top layer toward opposite side of mattress. Pull remaining top sheet over head of mattress, leaving bottom edge of sheet even with mattress edge. Smooth bottom sheet with hand.
    Rationale: If a contour sheet is not used, the bottom sheet is tucked in only at the top of the bed so linen can be changed without undoing the top sheet.
13. Standing near head of bed, tuck the excess sheet under the mattress on your side.

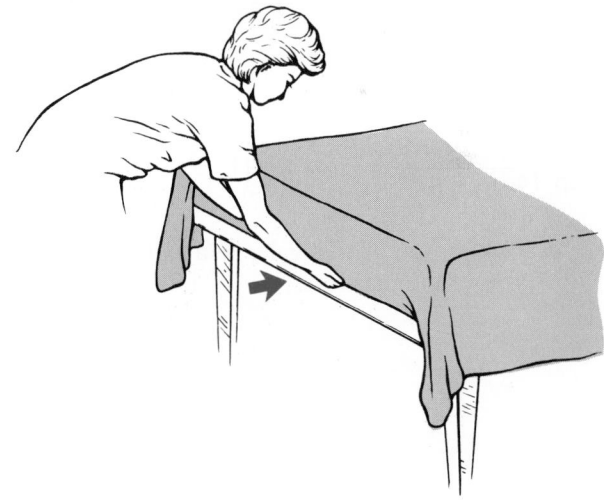

Step 13

14. Miter the corner on your side:
    a. Grasp side edge of sheet about 18 inches down from mattress top.
    b. Lay sheet on top of mattress to form a triangular, flat fold.

(continued)

PROCEDURE 28–8. Making an Unoccupied Bed *(continued)*

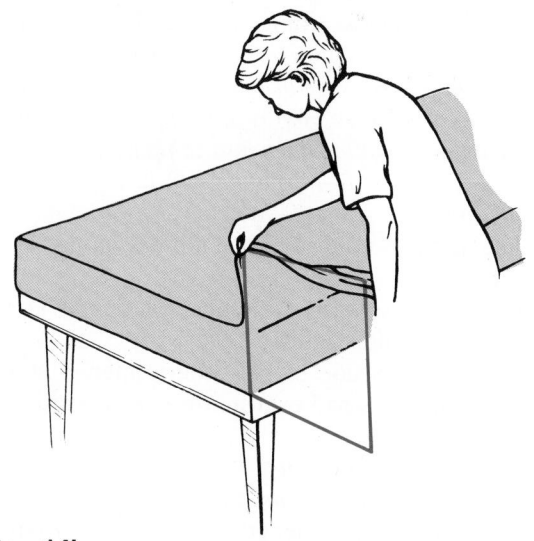

Step 14b

c. Tuck sheet hanging loose below mattress under the mattress, without pulling on the triangular fold.

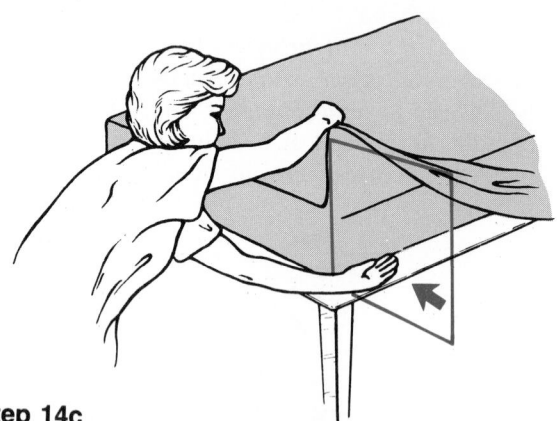

Step 14c

d. Pick up top of triangular fold and place it over side of the mattress.

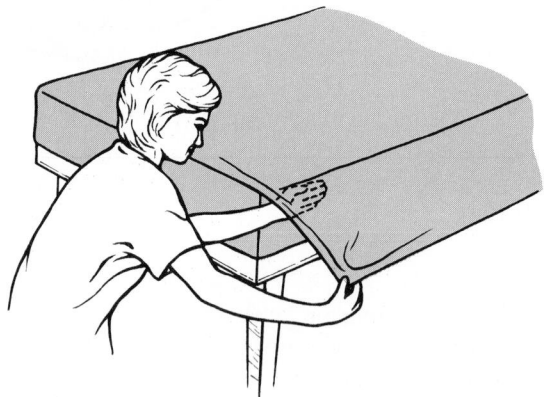

Step 14d

e. Tuck this loose portion of sheet under the mattress.

Rationale: Mitered corners do not loosen easily when patient moves in bed.
Note: If contour sheet is used, fit elastic edges under corner of mattress.

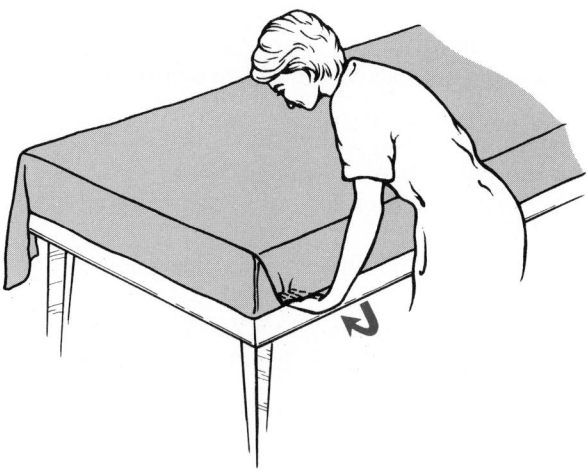

Step 14e

15. Tuck remaining sheet on that side under the mattress.
16. Lay draw sheet (folded in half) on the bed with the center fold at center of bed. Place top edge of draw sheet about 12 to 15 inches from head of bed. Tuck excess draw sheet under mattress.
    Rationale: Draw sheet secures bottom sheet in place to decrease wrinkling.
17. Move to opposite side of bed.
    Rationale: Completing work on one side of bed at a time saves time and decreases energy expenditure.
18. Spread bottom sheet over mattress edge and miter top corner.
19. Tuck excess bottom sheet *tightly* under mattress, pulling gently to smooth out wrinkles.
    Rationale: Taut sheet eliminates wrinkles, which irritate and cause pressure on the skin.
20. Grasp draw sheet, pulling gently. Beginning at middle, tuck draw sheet under mattress firmly. Finish tucking top and bottom.
    Rationale: Tucking middle of draw sheet first prevents wrinkling and poor fit.
21. Return to side of bed where linen is placed.
22. Place top sheet on bed with vertical center fold at center of bed. Unfold sheet with seams facing out and top edge even with top of mattress. Smooth sheet, with excess falling over bottom edge of mattress.
    Rationale: Placing seam side up prevents edges from rubbing and irritating patient's skin.
23. Spread blanket and bedspread evenly over bed.
24. Miter the bottom corner, using all three layers of

(continued)

PROCEDURE 28–8. Making an Unoccupied Bed *(continued)*

linen (sheet, blanket, bedspread). Leave sides un-tucked.

25. Move to opposite side of bed and miter bottom corner, using all three layers of linen.
Rationale: Mitering all three layers together saves time and energy. Mitered corners secure top covers but allow easy access in and out of bed by leaving sides free.

26. Standing at bottom of bed, grasp top covers about 10 inches from bottom of mattress. Loosen linen slightly by pulling on top covers or forming a pleat.
Rationale: Provides additional room for patient's feet for comfort and to prevent pressure on toes.

27. Put clean pillowcases on:
    a. Grasp center of pillowcase, with one hand on seamed end.
    b. Gather case, turning it inside out over the hand holding it.
    c. With same hand, grasp middle of one end of pillow.
    d. Pull case over pillow with free hand.
    e. Adjust case so corners fit over pillow.
    Rationale: This method prevents shaking of pillowcase and linen and distributing microorganisms in room.

28. Place pillows in center at head of bed.

29. Fold top linen back to one side or fanfolded at bottom of bed.

30. Secure call bell within patient's reach and lower bed.
Rationale: Provides for patient safety and makes it easier for patient to return to bed.

31. Arrange the bedside table, nightstand, and personal items within easy reach.

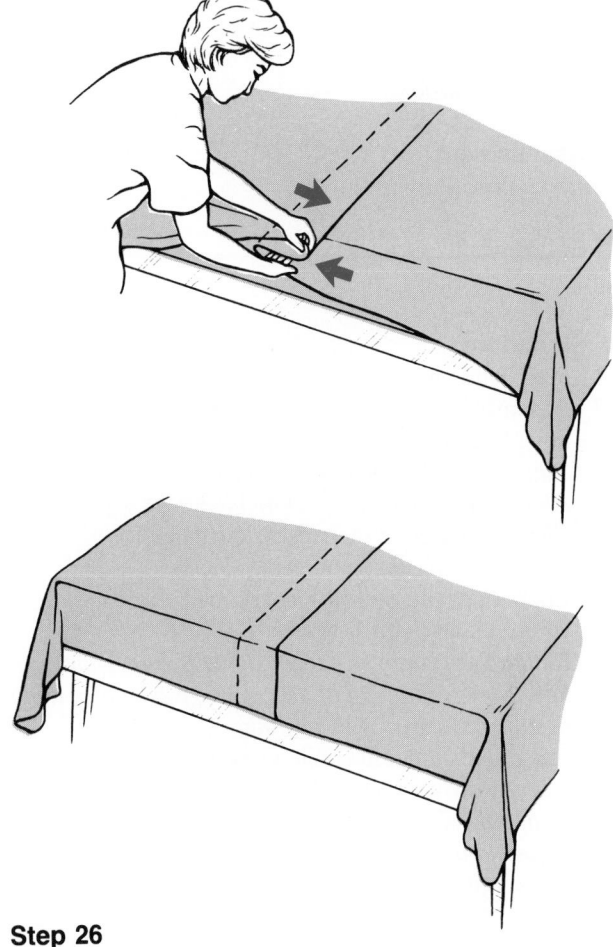

Step 26

32. Discard soiled linen according to agency policy.
33. Wash your hands.

---

can assist with bathing. The hot-water tank thermostat should be set below 120° to avoid burns during bathing.

For the patient who cannot shower or use the bathtub, placing a chair in the bathroom so the patient can wash by the sink may help to conserve energy. Relatives may be available to visit on a weekly basis to supervise or assist with bathing, but often patients are embarrassed to ask relatives or friends to assist with this private, personal activity. If family support is inadequate, home health aides can be used on a routine basis to provide hygiene care for the patient at home.

Independent grooming and dressing should also be assessed and promoted by the nurse before discharge. Many patients do not dress in the hospital and are surprised at how draining this activity can be. Before discharge, patients should be encouraged to practice dressing using energy-conserving measures. The patient should sit as much as possible while dressing and should wear clothes that are easy to get on and off. Sweatsuits

are often ideal for the patient who has difficulty with fine motor skills because they have no buttons or zippers. Slip-on shoes with nonskid soles are easy to put on and help prevent falls. Discuss with the patient the psychological benefits of getting dressed, and work out a plan so that the patient can avoid staying in nightclothes during the day. Often patients need help with laundry. Laundry can be sent to commercial facilities, but this is expensive.

Hair care often provides a morale boost to the homebound patient. Hair should be washed before discharge for patients who might have difficulty with this task. Relatives can take the patient to a local hairdresser for shampoos and hair care, and some beauticians make house calls. Frequently a family member or friend might be encouraged to provide such a service. Applying makeup is important to some women, and lack of coordination or energy can make this activity difficult.

(Text continues on page 688)

PROCEDURE 28–9. Making an Occupied Bed

■ **Purpose**
1. Provide clean linen and remove sources of skin irritation.
2. Promote comfort.

■ **Assessment**
Same as Procedure 28-8.

■ **Equipment**
Same as Procedure 28-8.

■ **Procedure**
1. Wash your hands.
2. Assemble equipment on bedside table or chair. Do not place on another patient's bed.
   Rationale: Placing linen on clean surface prevents contamination with microorganisms.
3. Close room door or bedside curtains.
   Rationale: Maintains patient privacy.
4. Lock siderails up on side of bed opposite from where clean linen is stacked.
   Rationale: Promotes patient safety by preventing patient from rolling out of bed. Also gives patient a bar to grasp to assist with turning.
5. Raise bed to comfortable working position. Lower siderail on your side of bed.
   Rationale: Provides good use of body mechanics to reduce muscle strain on back.
6. Loosen all top linen from foot of bed.
7. Remove bedspread and blanket separately. Without shaking, fold each and place over back of chair if they are to be reused. If they are soiled, hold them away from your uniform and place in linen bag.
   Rationale: Folding linen enables nurse to discard or handle without contaminating uniform. Shaking linen spreads microorganisms through the air.
8. Leave top sheet on patient or cover patient with a bath blanket, then remove and discard top sheet.
   Rationale: Provides warmth and prevents unnecessary body exposure during linen change.
9. Loosen the bottom sheet on your side.
10. Lower head of bed to flat position.
    Note: If patient cannot tolerate flat position, lower head of bed as far as patient can tolerate.
11. With assistance from another worker, grasp mattress lugs and slide mattress to head of bed if it has slipped down.
12. Help patient to roll onto side facing away from you. Patient may grasp siderail to assist. Adjust pillow under head.
    Rationale: Side-lying position provides space for placing clean linen on mattress.

13. Fanfold soiled draw sheet and tuck under buttocks, back, and shoulders. Repeat with soiled bottom sheet and tuck under patient. Do not fanfold mattress pad unless it is soiled.
    Note: Fanfolds under patient should be as tight and smooth as possible to provide space for clean linen and enable patient to eventually roll back over folds.

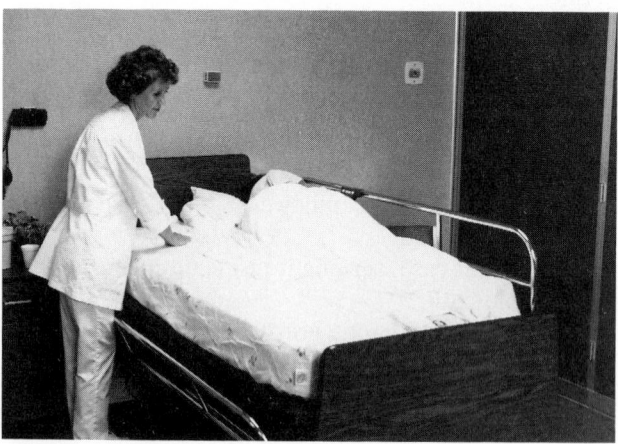

Step 13

14. Place clean bottom sheet on bed. Unfold lengthwise so bottom edge is even with end of mattress and vertical center crease is at center of bed.
15. Bring sheet's bottom edge over mattress sides and fanfold top of sheet toward center of mattress and place next to patient.
16. Tuck top edge of sheet under mattress. Miter top corner on your side (as in Procedure 28-8). Tuck remaining portion of sheet under mattress.
    Note: If a contour sheet is used, fit elastic edges under corner of mattress.
17. Place draw sheet on bed with center fold at center of bed. Position sheet so it will extend from the patient's back to below the buttocks. Fanfold the top edge and place next to patient. Tuck excess under mattress.
    Rationale: Draw sheet is used to reposition patient and absorb excess perspiration.
18. Lock siderails on your side up and move to other side of bed.
    Rationale: Maintains patient safety.
19. Lower siderail. Help patient to roll over folds of linen onto his or her other side.
    Rationale: Exposes other half of bed so soiled linen can be removed and clean linen placed.
20. Move pillow under patient's head.
21. Remove soiled linen by folding into a square or

(continued)

PROCEDURE 28–9. Making an Occupied Bed *(continued)*

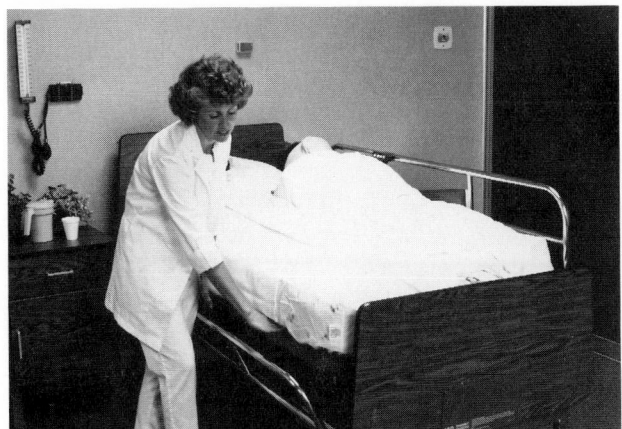

Step 17

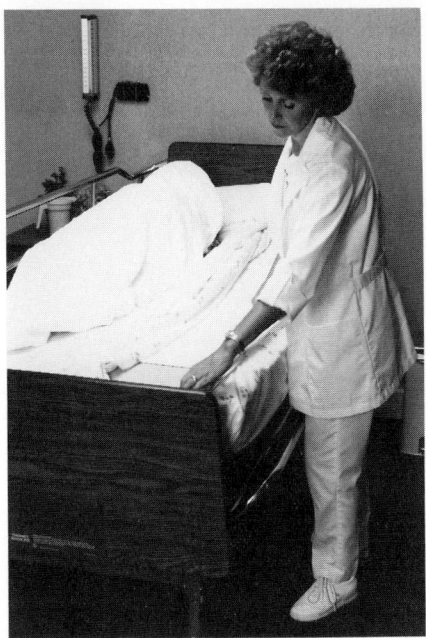

Step 19

cess tightly under mattress. Tuck the middle first, then the top, and finally the bottom.
Rationale: Tucking the center first prevents the draw sheet from pulling sideways, causing a poor fit and wrinkles.

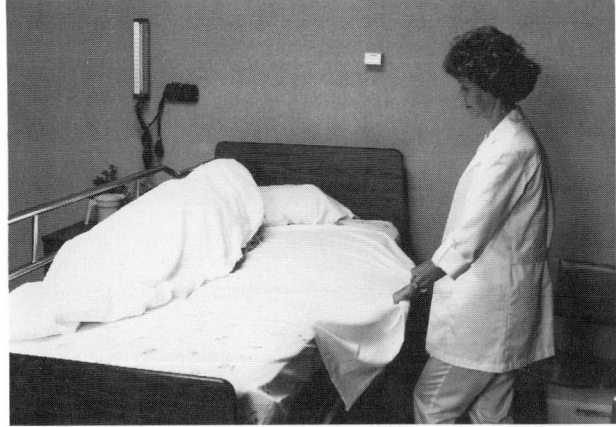

Step 25

26. Help patient to center of bed.
27. Raise siderail if necessary and move to side of bed where remainder of linen is stored.
28. Place top sheet over patient with center crease lengthwise at center of bed with seam side up. Unfold sheet from head to toe.
29. Have patient grasp top edge of clean top sheet. Remove bath blanket or soiled top linen by pulling from beneath clean top sheet. Discard in linen bag.
Rationale: Prevents unnecessary exposure of body parts.

bundle, with soiled side turned in. Place in linen bag.
Rationale: Reduces transmission of microorganisms and prevents patient embarrassment from seeing soiled sheets.
22. Grasp edge of fanfolded bottom sheet.
23. Tuck top of sheet under top of mattress. Miter top corner.
24. Facing bed, pull bottom sheet tight and tuck excess linen under mattress from top to bottom.
Rationale: Maintains a tight fit of the sheet and eliminates wrinkles.
25. Unfold draw sheet by grasping at center. Tuck ex-

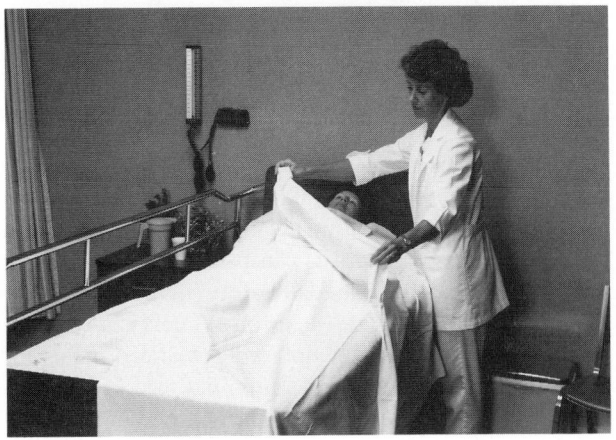

Steps 28 and 29

(continued)

PROCEDURE 28–9. Making an Occupied Bed *(continued)*

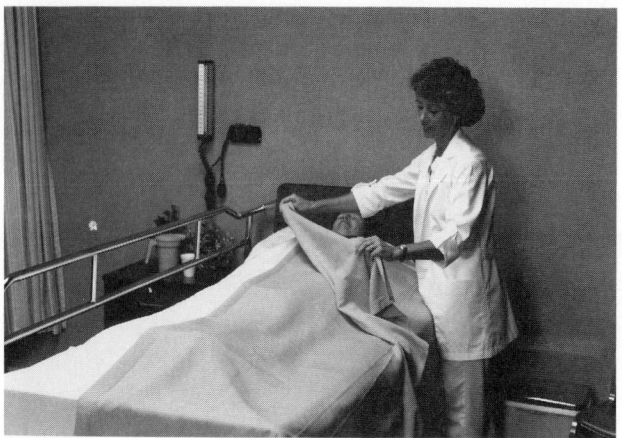

Step 29

30. Complete top covers as described in Procedure 28-8.

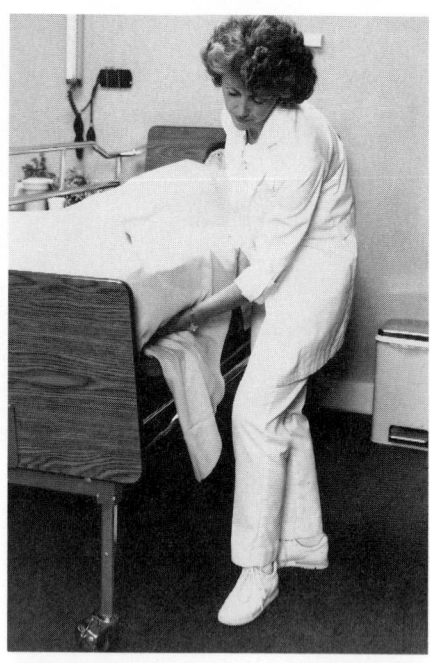

Step 30B

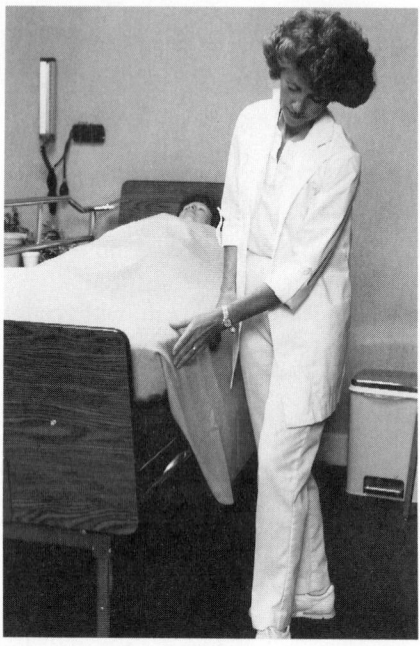

Step 30A

Buying and preparing food can be exhausting, so provide instructions on easy-to-fix, nutritious meals. Frozen foods have improved dramatically in recent years and can be nutritious. Relatives can package single-serving meals so they can be reheated. Safety (i.e., burn prevention) should be stressed. Meals on Wheels is a community service that provides hot, well-balanced meals for the homebound person for a nominal fee. Few supermarkets deliver groceries, but shopping for the homebound person can be done by friends, relatives, or neighborhood young people.

Eating can consume energy. Rest before and after meals should be encouraged. Special utensils can be used by patients with fine motor impairment. Adequate swallowing and chewing is important and should be assessed before discharge.

Self-care deficit in toileting is an important consideration, and home bathroom facilities should be assessed before discharge. If the bathroom is on a different floor from the bedroom, the patient may need a bedside commode or a urinal. If the patient is wheelchair-bound, the bathroom doorway must be wide enough for the wheelchair, and the bathroom must be large enough to permit the patient to transfer from the wheelchair to the toilet.

Patient Teaching: Self-Care and Hygiene

Instruct the patient as follows:

- If you have more energy in the mornings, plan to bathe, shampoo your hair, and put your makeup on then.
- Plan a nap before you eat if eating makes you tired.
- Use the leg bag with your catheter during the day when you're up, but change to the large bag hung down by the side of your bed when you go to bed. This will help the urine drain more effectively.
- Keep a commode (or urinal) downstairs for convenience.
- Include some finger foods such as bread, pieces of fruit, or small sausages at meals.
- Wear your glasses and dentures when eating.
- Use a plate with a suction grip underneath. Push against the plate guard rim while eating.
- Wear loose-fitting clothes if dressing is difficult. Pull-on pants and pullover tops will be handy since you don't need to zip or fasten them. Shoes with Velcro closures or elastic laces are easier. Give yourself plenty of time until you get used to dressing yourself.

Some patients find it difficult to lower themselves onto the toilet and get up again. A high-rise toilet seat can be helpful and is indicated for all patients after hip surgery. Hand grips next to the toilet are also helpful. Patients must be able to wipe themselves and wash their hands after toileting. Prepackaged towelettes can be an easy way to wash hands.

Incontinence can be managed with a Foley catheter or disposable diapers. If a catheter is used, a leg bag can be worn under clothes to promote self-image, and a larger collection bag can be used at night. A condom catheter can also be used with the same urine collection system. Disposable diapers for adults are now widely available, although they are more costly than infant diapers. A more streamlined adult incontinence pad (Depends) is also available.

Patients with self-care deficits and inadequate support may be unable to manage safely at home and may need to be transferred to an extended-care facility or nursing home. When a patient is transferred to another health-care agency, it is important to communicate the level of self-care function to the staff there. Transfer forms usually have a place for the nurse to indicate how independent a patient is in bathing, feeding, grooming, and toileting. Be specific, so that optimum independence can be maintained in the new agency.

EVALUATION

Evaluation of self-care deficit is individualized, based on the outcome criteria developed from the patient goals. Objective and subjective data can be collected from the patient to support successful attainment of patient-centered goals.

Ideally, the patient should exhibit increased independence in bathing, grooming, feeding, and toileting. The patient should be able to state any limitations and should feel comfortable accepting necessary assistance. The patient should demonstrate a positive self-image and satisfaction with accomplishments in self-care despite limitations. The patient should be able to use adaptive devices to facilitate self-care, and self-care should occur without injury.

Examples of outcome criteria are listed here. Some criteria may be important for more than one goal. Specific outcome criteria must be established for each patient.

Goal
Patient will participate as completely as possible in hygiene measures.

Possible Outcome Criteria
- During initial interview, patient states need for assistance to perform hygiene activities that she cannot perform alone.
- After teaching session, patient uses left hand for bathing face, trunk, and arms, as witnessed by nurse.
- Before discharge, patient verbalizes a realistic plan for achieving hygiene measures at home.
- Before discharge, patient expresses enhanced self-esteem.

Goal
Patient will increase level of independence in eating safely.

Possible Outcome Criteria
- By discharge, patient demonstrates using a cup with a built-up handle held with both hands to drink thick liquids.
- Within 4 days, patient uses fingers of either hand to eat finger foods, as witnessed by nurse.
- Before discharge, patient verbalizes a plan for managing eating and drinking at home.

Goal
Patient will participate in dressing self.

Possible Outcome Criteria
- By discharge, patient demonstrates to nurse ability to put on a loose-fitting dress with Velcro fasteners.
- By discharge, patient uses a long-handled reacher to put on slip-on shoes.

Nursing Management Plan
The Patient With Self-Care Deficit

Nursing Diagnosis: Bathing/hygiene self-care deficit related to right-sided weakness manifested by impaired ability to wash most body parts.

Patient Goal: Patient will participate as completely as possible in hygiene measures.

Patient Outcome Criteria

- During initial interview patient states need for assistance to perform hygiene activities that he or she can't perform alone.
- After teaching session, patient uses left hand for bathing face, trunk, and upper extremities, as observed by nurse.
- Before discharge, patient verbalizes a realistic plan for achieving bathing at home.
- Patient expresses enhanced self-esteem before discharge.

Nursing Intervention	Scientific Rationale
1. Assist patient to identify self-care deficits in hygiene.	1. To emphasize ownership of care so that maximum self-participation can occur with maximum self-esteem.
2. Encourage patient to communicate needs and concerns to nursing staff as well as significant others.	2. To reduce the presence of energy-consuming stressors such as isolation and worry.
3. Permit and encourage patient to accept some dependency for as long as it is necessary.	3. A degree of dependence is a necessary part of recovery and rehabilitation for most people.
4. Ensure safety through monitoring and restraining during bathing and hygiene activities.	4. To reduce the possibility of increased injury due to falls.
5. Schedule hygiene self-care 1 hour after breakfast when patient feels rested.	5. Hygiene self-care is a tiring procedure; fatigue can produce confusion.
6. Assist patient to use uneffected hand to wash self, comb hair, and brush teeth within the limits of ability.	6. To enhance independence while providing help and support as needed.
7. Lay out objects for hygiene care in the order to be used and place them on patient's right side on a chair. Don't hurry patient.	7. Gives support, helps to conserve energy. Patient can see objects on the right with visual field split.
8. Provide for the greatest amount of privacy possible.	8. To enhance feeling of dignity and self-worth.
9. Evaluate frequently for indications of fatigue by checking pulse and respiratory rate.	9. Ability to sustain concentrated effort may be limited until endurance is developed.
10. Coordinate self-care rehabilitation with occupational and physical therapy and any other involved health professionals.	10. To ensure that necessary techniques and assistive devices are used in most beneficial manner. Represent patient in negotiations and making arrangements for care.

- During hospitalization, patient expresses a positive approach to solving problems inherent to relearning to dress self.
- Before discharge, patient states plans for dressing self to conserve energy.

Goal

Patient will manage toileting as independently as possible.

Possible Outcome Criteria

- Within 48 hours, patient recognizes and communicates the need to go to the toilet.
- Within 5 days, patient transfers from bed to wheelchair to toilet or from bed to commode with standby assistance.
- Before discharge, patient demonstrates removal and replacement of clothing.
- Before discharge, patient states plan for managing toileting at home.

Key Concepts

- Self-care and hygiene are important factors in promoting health.
- Promoting the highest possible level of self-care independence, beginning at admission, helps reduce the risk that patients will be discharged at a lower level of self-care ability.
- With stress or illness, children and adults often regress to a lower developmental level, permitting them a respite from environmental demands and giving them more energy to deal with the problem at hand.
- Factors affecting self-care are neuromuscular function, energy level, sensory ability, cognition, motivation, sociocultural factors, environmental resources, and age.
- Sudden alterations in functional ability can occur with injury, acute illness, surgery, and pain.
- Chronic illness often poses challenges to independent self-care, since patients must develop coping strategies for functional deficits.
- The ability to maintain independence in self-care is frequently diminished in people who experience a disruptive mental illness. Improved self-care and hygiene often closely follow a return to mental health.
- The nursing assessment provides a specific picture of the self-care deficit to use in planning interventions.
- Although the primary reason for bathing is to enhance cleanliness, there are many other benefits. Warm water and friction enhance circulation, movement provides an opportunity for range of motion, and the experience can be relaxing.
- When providing hygiene care, describe the care measures and obtain permission to proceed. Permission is also needed before cutting hair or shaving facial hair.

References

Bellack, P., & Bamford, P.A. (1884). *Nursing Assessment: A Multidimensional Approach*. Monterey, CA: Wadsworth Health Sciences Division.

Gordon, J. (1987). *Nursing Diagnoses: Process and Application, 2nd ed.* New York: McGraw Hill.

Griffin, C.W (1987). Learning to swallow again. *American Journal of Nursing, 87* (3), 314–317.

Johnston, B.L. (1981). Oxygen consumption and hemodynamic and electrocardiographic responses to bathing in recent postmyocardial infarction patients. *Heart and Lung, 10*(4), 666–671.

Katz, S. (1963). Studies of illness in the aged, the index of ADL's: a standardized measure of biological and psychosocial function. *Journal of the American Medical Society, 185*(12), 914–919.

Katz, S. (1983). Assessing self-maintenance: activities of daily living, mobility, and instrumental activities of daily living. *Journal of the American Geriatric Society, 31*(12), 721–725.

Larsen, G. (1981). Chewing and swallowing. In N. Martin, N.B. Holt, D.J. Hicks (Eds.), *Comprehensive Rehabilitation Nursing*. New York: McGraw Hill.

NANDA (1990). *Taxonomy I revised 1990, with official nursing diagnoses*. St. Louis, MO: North American Nursing Diagnosis Association.

Renn, N. (1989). Oral health and hygiene for the elderly: A shared learning experience. *Home Healthcare Nurse, 7* (3), 37–39.

Sexton, D.L. (1990). *Nursing Care of the Respiratory Patient* (p. 408). Norwalk: Appleton and Lange.

Valentine, A.D. (1988). The case for fluoridation. *Midwife, Health Visitor, and Community Nurse, 24* (5), 158, 160.

Yep, J.O. (1977). Tools for aiding physically disabled individuals increase independence in dressing. *Journal of Rehabilitation, 43* (5), 39–41.

Bibliography

Carpenito. L.J. (1989). *Nursing Diagnosis: Application to Clinical Practice, 3rd ed.* (pp. 374–388). Philadelphia, J.B. Lippincott.

Cleary, M.E. (1985). Aiding the person who is visually impaired from diabetes. *The Diabetes Educator, 10* (4), 12–23.

Dunlap. W.R., & Sands, D.J. (1987). Development of a set of instruments to assess independent living skills. *Journal of Rehabilitation, 53* (1), 58–62.

Goldman, R. (1986). Aging changes in structure and function. In D.L. Carnevali, & M. Patrick (Eds.), *Nursing Management for the Elderly, 2nd ed.* (pp. 82–84). Philadelphia, J.B. Lippincott.

Lorensen, M. (1985). Effects on elderly women's self-care in cases of acute hospitalization as compared with men. *Health Care for Women International, 6* (4), 247–265.

Patrick, M. (1986). Daily living with cognitive deficits and behavior problems. In D.L. Carnevali, & M. Patrick (Eds.). *Nursing Management for the Elderly, 2nd ed.* (pp. 270–283). Philadelphia, J.B. Lippincott.

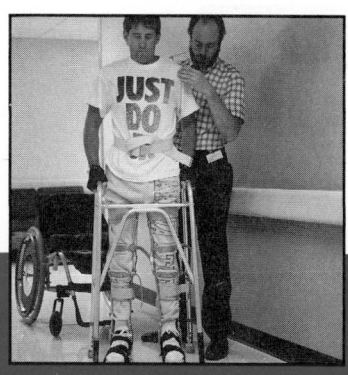

Body Mechanics and Mobility

29

LEARNING OBJECTIVES

Upon completion of this chapter, the student will be able to do the following:

- Describe the roles that bones, muscles, joints, and ligaments play in body movement.
- Discuss normal functions of the musculoskeletal system and characteristics of normal movement.
- Describe normal movement and mobility concerns across the lifespan.
- Identify factors that can affect or alter normal mobility.

- Describe the impact of immobility on each functional health pattern.
- Discuss appropriate objective and subjective data to collect to assess mobility status.
- Identify three NANDA nursing diagnoses for the functional area of mobility.
- Describe nursing interventions to prevent complications to assist the patient with impaired mobility.

KEY TERMS

Active range of motion
Activity intolerance
Aerobic exercise
Anaerobic exercise
Arthroscopy

Atrophy
Body mechanics
Contracture
Flaccidity
Foot drop
Gait
Isometric exercise

Isotonic exercise
Mobility
Passive range of motion
Range of motion
Spasticity

Normal Mobility
  Anatomy of the Musculoskeletal System
    Bones
    Muscles
    Joints
  Normal Physiologic Function
    Alignment and Posture
    Balance
    Coordinated Movement
    Body Mechanics
    Exercise
  Characteristics of Normal Movement
    Full Range of Motion
    Normal Gait
  Factors Affecting Normal Mobility
    Intact Musculoskeletal System
    Nervous System Control
    Circulation and Oxygenation
    Energy
    Lifestyle and Habits
    Coping and Self-Concept
  Lifespan Considerations
Altered Mobility
  Potential for Altered Mobility
    Congenital Problems
    Neuromuscular Deficits
    Musculoskeletal Deficits
    Chronic Health Problems
    Trauma
    Affective Disorders
    Therapeutic Modalities
  Manifestations of Altered Mobility
    Decreased Muscle Strength and Tone
    Lack of Coordination
    Altered Gait
    Falls
    Decreased Joint Flexibility
    Pain on Movement
    Activity Intolerance
  Impact of Immobility on Functional Health
    Health Perception and Health Management
    Activity and Exercise
    Nutrition and Metabolism
    Elimination

    Sleep and Rest
    Cognition and Perception
    Self-Perception and Self-Concept
    Coping and Stress Tolerance
    Roles and Relationships
    Sexuality
  Impact of Altered Mobility on Activities of Daily
    Living
Assessment
  Subjective Data
    Functional Pattern Identification
    Risk Pattern Identification
    Dysfunctional Identification
  Objective Data
    Physical Assessment
    Diagnostic Tests and Procedures
Nursing Diagnoses and Patient Goals
  Impaired Physical Mobility
    Definition
    Defining Characteristics
    Related Factors
  Activity Intolerance
    Definition
    Defining Characteristics
    Related Factors
  High Risk for Disuse Syndrome
    Definition
    Defining Characteristics
    Related Factors
  Related Nursing Diagnoses
  Patient Goals
Implementation
  Nursing Interventions to Promote Health and
    Function
    Physical Fitness Promotion
    Injury Prevention
  Nursing Interventions for Altered Mobility
    Positioning
    Joint Mobility Maintenance
    Ambulation
    Transfers
  Discharge Planning and Home Care
Evaluation
Key Conepts

Mobility, or the ability to move freely within the environment, is fundamental to normal daily functioning. In our highly mobile society, problems affecting mobility are especially significant. Independence is often defined by a person's ability to perform activities of daily living (grooming, dressing, feeding, and elimination), job-related activities, and role-related activities (as a parent or spouse). Limitations in a person's ability to move normally and spontaneously can affect all of these areas.

Changes in mobility also create more subtle effects. Movement is significant in communication. Facial expressions and gestures are significant in nonverbal communication, and talking with someone at eye level promotes equality between those talking. Having to look up at someone from a chair or bed can make a person feel at a psychological disadvantage. Movement is also significant in dispersing negative feelings and tension. Many people find that jogging or participating in athletics helps them to feel healthier and less anxious. Being able to leave uncomfortable or dangerous situations gives most people a feeling of control.

Most people link mobility with health. When patients are confined to bed, they see themselves as sick. Disabilities that affect mobility, such as amputation or a musculoskeletal defect, may impair self-image; the patient may see himself or herself as defective or abnormal.

Like many aspects of health, mobility can be viewed along a continuum, from full mobility to immobility. Full mobility occurs when the person has no physical or psychological factors that limit mobility. Immobility occurs when the person cannot move his or her entire body or a specific body part.

Patients move along this continuum as their abilities change:

- Temporary changes in mobility are often caused by therapeutic treatment, such as traction to repair a fracture.
- Some conditions lead to progressive disability; examples are muscular dystrophy and severe crippling rheumatoid arthritis.
- Permanent changes in mobility occur when physiologic dysfunction that interferes with normal body movement cannot be reversed (i.e., spinal cord injuries that result in paralysis, or cerebral vascular accidents that cause weakness or paralysis on one side of the body).

Rehabilitation is the key to restoring a person with certain disabilities to optimum health, and the nurse plays a significant role in this process.

NORMAL MOBILITY

The musculoskeletal system serves as the supporting framework for the body. It includes the bones and muscles involved in movement and is responsible for the form and shape of the body. The complex activity of movement is coordinated by central and peripheral nerves. Maintaining posture and balance against the force of gravity requires smooth coordination of muscles, joints, and nerves, and a stable center of gravity.

Anatomy of the Musculoskeletal System

The musculoskeletal system is composed of bones, muscles, joints, cartilage, connective tissue, and fibrous tendons. Movement is permitted by flexible connections of bones and muscles at the joints.

Bones

Bones serve as a framework for attachment of muscles, tendons, and ligaments. They facilitate movement, protect vital organs (brain, heart, lungs, liver), store and regulate calcium and phosphate, and form blood cells.

The structure of bones provides for minimum weight and maximum structural strength. Bone tissue is either woven or lamellar. Woven bone is characterized by rapid growth, as in infants, and is generally found where ligaments and tendons insert into the bone of an adult. Lamellar bone is mature bone with highly organized mineralized plates.

Bones can also be classified by shape: long bones (arms, legs); short (tarsals, carpals); flat (cranium); and irregular (vertebral). The components of the long bones are the diaphysis (shaft) and the epiphyses (ends). Most of the bone is covered by periosteum, which contains nerves and blood vessels. The outer portion of long bones is composed of dense, compact bone with a marrow cavity in the center where the blood-forming cells are located.

Muscles

Skeletal muscles are connected to bones at or across joints and are made up of striated, long muscle fibers usually arranged in a parallel alignment. The formation of the striated fibers allows the muscle to contract (shorten) or extend (lengthen) as required by movement. Contraction occurs when the overlapping striated fibers slide toward each other, thereby shortening and increasing the strength of the muscle.

The process of muscle contraction requires a complex mechanical, chemical, and electrical interaction. The contraction is initiated when an action potential (electrical charge) moves down the muscle fiber, releasing large quantities of calcium into the adjacent muscle fibers. Energy for the work of contraction comes from oxidizing fatty acids obtained from the bloodstream. The muscle cells must provide the greatly increased energy needed during exercise since the cardiovascular system alone cannot increase blood flow sufficiently.

Muscles are covered by a layer of connective tissue, which joins with tendon fibers at the end of the muscle fiber where the muscle joins the bone. Muscle fibers are innervated by motor neurons originating from the anterior horn of the spinal cord. All muscle fibers connected to a single motor nerve are called a *motor unit.*

Over a lifetime, the body has only the number of muscle cells with which it was born; however, the work of the muscle determines the size of the muscle cells. When forceful activity is demanded of the muscle, the muscle hypertrophies (the diameter of the muscle increases), causing an increase in the strength of the muscle. Atrophy, the opposite of hypertrophy, causes muscles to decrease in strength and size as a result of disuse. Disuse may be related to lack of exercise, aging, enforced rest, or immobilizing devices.

Joints

Joints are areas where bones meet. The types of joints are fibrous, which do not move (cranial); cartilaginous, with minimal movement (costochondral); and synovial, which are movable (joints of the extremities).

Synovial joints are lined with synovial tissue, which has a rich blood supply and produces synovial fluid. Synovial fluid lubricates the joint, allowing smooth articulation and ease of motion.

Tendons and ligaments connect and support joints. Ligaments stabilize bones in the joints and are more elastic than tendons. Tendons are specialized tissues connecting muscle to bone and are surrounded by synovial-like tissues.

Normal Physiologic Function

Carrying out coordinated movement is a complex process. Even with a framework of bones held together by ligaments and covered with soft tissue and skin, normal function cannot occur without coordinated muscle activity and neurologic integration.

Alignment and Posture

Maintaining upright posture requires proper alignment of the bones, muscles, and joints, and a stable center of gravity (Fig. 29-1). Alignment is achieved when the joints and muscles are not experiencing extremes in

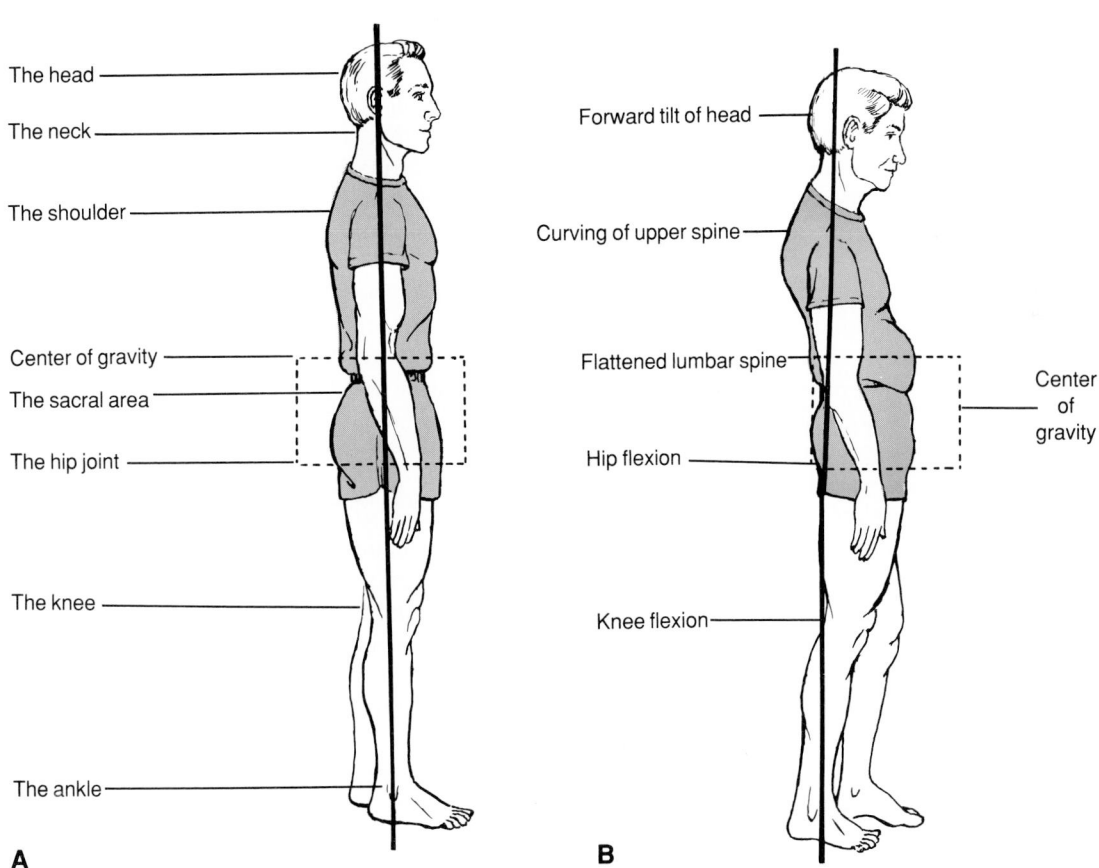

Figure 29–1. Vertical gravity line and posture. **A:** Vertical gravity line and center of gravity. **B:** Postural changes with age.

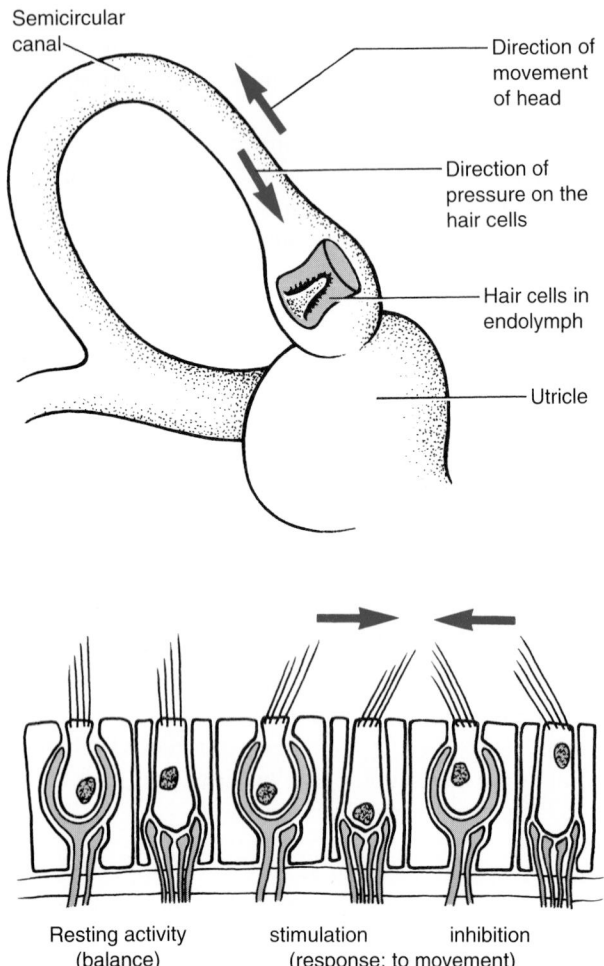

Figure 29–2. Movement of the head stimulates hair cells, transmitting signals to sensory nerve fibers for control of equilibrium and balance.

extension or flexion, or unusual stress, whether lying down, sitting, or standing.

Upright posture and movement require a balanced *center of gravity,* the area where the weight of the body is centered and where the downward forces of gravity are balanced. The usual line of gravity starts at the top of the head and bisects the shoulders, the trunk, the weight-bearing joints, and the base of support; it runs slightly anterior to the sacrum. In the elderly, the lumbar spine tends to flatten and the upper spine and head tend to tilt forward, causing the head to be in front of the usual line of gravity.

Balance

Maintaining balance is a complex function of counteracting gravity and reflexes to maintain posture. The reticular formation provides the nervous energy for supporting the body against gravity by providing most of the intrinsic excitation required for maintaining tone in the exten-

sor muscles. If a person begins to fall to one side, the extensor muscles on that side stiffen while the extensor muscles on the opposite side relax to prevent falling.

Equilibrium is provided largely by the vestibular apparatus of the ear, composed of the cochlear duct, the three semicircular canals, and two large chambers known as the utricle and the saccule (see Fig. 42-2). The function of the cochlear duct is mainly for hearing, not equilibrium. The saccule, utricle, and semicircular canals are vital to maintaining equilibrium and, thus, balance.

The utricle and saccule and the semicircular canals contain tiny hair cells connected to sensory nerve fibers that pass into the vestibular nerve. When the head moves, these hair cells are bent, pulled, or compressed, providing signals to the sensory nerve fibers through the hair cells, transmissions to the appropriate nerve tracts to the brain, and control of equilibrium and balance (Fig. 29-2).

The saccule and utricle provide information about the position of the head relative to the direction of the force of gravity. The three semicircular canals provide a specialized control of equilibrium by signaling the rate of the change. The superior, posterior, and lateral semicircular canals are arranged at right angles to each other, representing all three dimensions of space (Fig. 29-3). When the head suddenly begins to rotate in any direction, the endolymph or fluid within the canals tends to remain stationary while the canals turn. This causes a flow of the fluid in the canals in an opposite direction of the rotation of the head. The fluid flow stimulates the hair cells that signal the sensory nerve fibers.

The information from the semicircular canals serves two purposes. The first is to control the muscles that move the eyes so that when the head moves in any direction, the person can keep the eyes fixed on the point of interest. The second purpose is to control reflex mechanisms for maintaining upright posture and balance (Vander, 1990). Vestibular input for equilibrium comes from vision (vestibulocular input) and from skin and joint receptors (vestibulospinal input).

Coordinated Movement

The cerebellum, cerebral cortex, and basal ganglia are responsible for the control of motor functions such as the mechanisms of alignment, posture, and balance, and for coordinated movement. The cerebellum coordinates the motor activities of movement, the cerebral cortex initiates voluntary motor activity, and the basal ganglia maintains posture. These systems make up the pyramidal and extrapyramidal tracts. The pyramidal tract (the direct corticospinal pathway) initiates transmission of impulses to the spinal cord for voluntary movements. The extrapyramidal tract (the indirect corticospinal pathway) dampens and inhibits impulses to smooth and coordinate skeletal muscle movement.

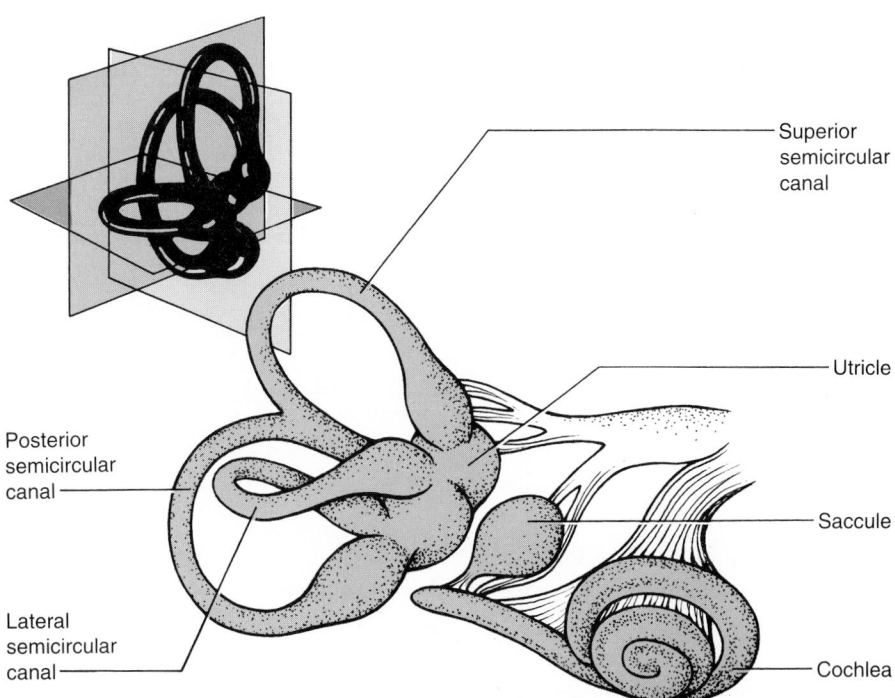

Superior
semicircular
canal

Utricle

Saccule

Cochlea

Posterior
semicircular
canal

Lateral
semicircular
canal

Figure 29–3. The semicircular canals, utricle, and saccule, with illustration of the planes of the canals at right-angle relationships.

The cerebellum has a special role in the control of movement: it controls muscles used in maintaining steady posture and in effecting coordinated, detailed movements. It receives information from both the cortex and subcortical centers on what muscles *should* be doing and compares the input with information from other neurologic sources about what the muscles *are* doing. Based on that comparison, the cerebellum can initiate impulses to correct the discrepancy and smooth the motion (Vander, 1990). The result is that people can have smooth, coordinated movements and can develop fine motor functions, rather than having uncoordinated, arrhythmic movements.

Body Mechanics

Body mechanics can be defined as using alignment, posture, and balance in a coordinated effort to perform activities such as lifting, bending, and moving (Fig. 29-4). Properly performed body mechanics promote safety of the musculoskeletal system and maintain balance without undue strain on muscles. When nurses use their bodies to perform therapies, assist patients with movement, or move equipment, effective body mechanics are required to prevent injury to patient and nurse (see Procedure 29-1).

Components of Body Mechanics. Using effective body mechanics means using gravity advantageously in body alignment, posture, balance, and movement. The center of gravity—where the weight of the body is centered and

where the downward forces of gravity are balanced—tends to be in the area of the pelvis, slightly anterior to the sacrum. Maintaining a balanced center of gravity during movement is essential for alignment, posture, and balance.

Balance is maintained when the spine is kept in vertical alignment, the feet provide a broad base of support, and the body weight is kept close to the center of gravity. When a person lifts or carries a load, that weight be-

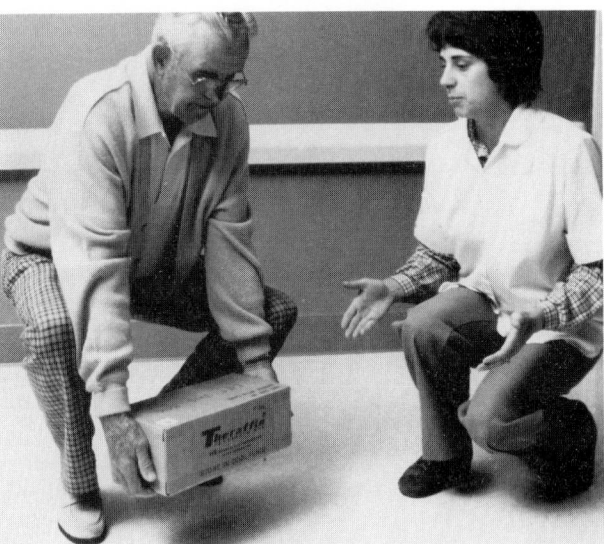

Figure 29–4. The nurse instructs a patient on proper lifting technique to prevent back strain and injury. (Courtesy of Overlake Hospital.)

PROCEDURE 29–1. Using Proper Body Mechanics

■ **Purpose**
1. Prevent injury to the nurse's musculoskeletal system.
2. Prevent injury to the patient during transfer.

■ **Assessment**
• Evaluate weight of patient to be lifted. Arrange for assistance if necessary.
• Assess position and height of patient to be lifted.
• Assess knowledge about body alignment and how to maintain it with position changes.

■ **Procedure**
1. Plan movement before doing it.
   a. Always lock wheels on bed, stretcher, or wheelchair.

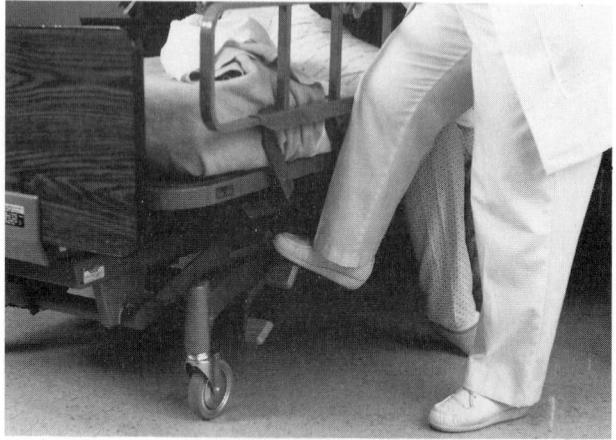

Step 1A

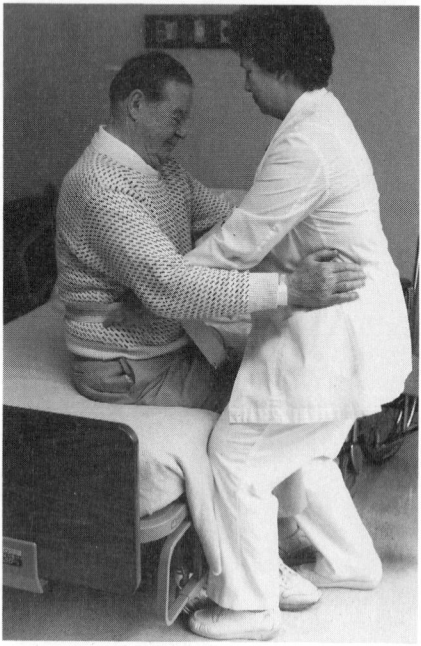

Step 1B

Rationale: Unexpected movements may offset your balance and result in injury to yourself or patient.
   b. Allow patient to assist during transfer.
   Rationale: Helps overcome forces resisting the transfer; encourages patient's sense of independence and provides exercise for patient.
   c. Use mechanical aids (i.e., lifters, slide boards, body mobilizers) or additional personnel to move heavy patients.
   d. Slide, push, or pull patient rather than lifting and carrying when possible.
   Rationale: Your body weight adds power to muscle work. Rocking your own body weight can balance the patient's weight when assisting to a standing position.
   e. Tighten abdominal and gluteal muscles before lifting or moving patient.
   Rationale: Supports the abdomen and stabilizes the pelvis to provide a firm base of support.
   f. Use smooth, rhythmic, coordinated motions.
   Rationale: Smooth motions use less energy and are less likely to cause muscle strain than jerky motions.
   g. If another person is assisting, plan your movements before beginning.
   Rationale: Prevents uncoordinated movements that may result in muscle strain or injury.
2. Begin all movements with proper body alignment and balance.
   a. Face patient to be lifted and pivot your body.
   b. Increase base of support by placing both feet flat on floor, knees slightly bent, with one foot slightly in front of the other or one step apart.
   c. Lower center of gravity toward patient to be transferred.
   Rationale: Maintains body balance, reduces risk of

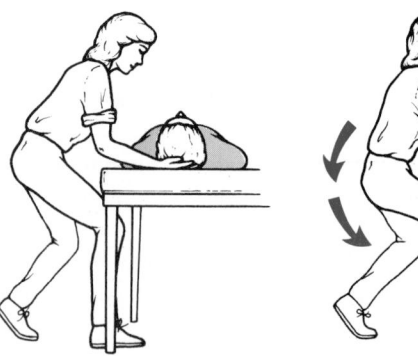

Step 2C

(continued)

PROCEDURE 29–1. Using Proper Body Mechanics *(continued)*

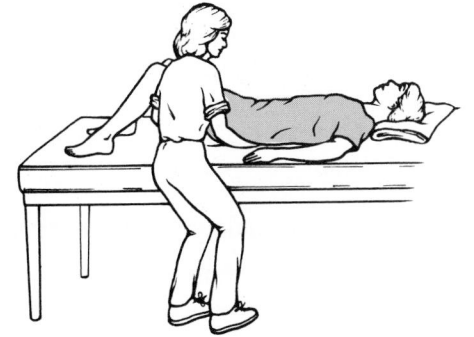

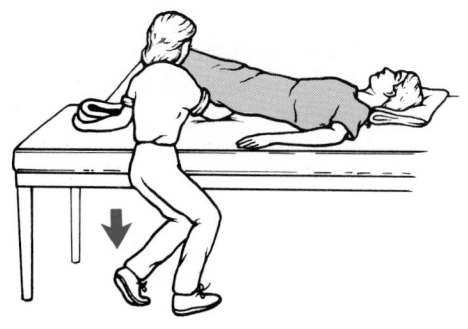

Step 2C

falling, and allows larger muscle groups to work together.

3. Elevate adjustable beds to waist level and lower side-rails to prevent stretching.
4. Carry objects close to body and stand as close as possible to work area.
   Rationale: Maintains the workload near the center of gravity to prevent muscle strain and fatigue caused by hyperextension.

■ **Home-Care Modifications**
• Teach caregivers the above guidelines for body movement.

comes part of the body weight; therefore, it is important to balance that additional weight over the center of gravity.

The larger the base of support, the more stability the person has for changing body position while maintaining alignment, posture, and balance. The weight-bearing joints and skeletal muscles of the legs provide a stable base of support. This base of support can be widened by placing the feet farther apart and flexing the hip and knee joints. These activities lower the center of gravity, making it more stable, and allow flexibility in adjusting position to avoid muscle strain. The base of support must be sufficient so that changes in body position do not cause the center of gravity to fall beyond the edge of the base.

Movement is coordinated by opposing voluntary muscle groups and neuromuscular reflexes. The flexor and extensor muscle groups provide the opposing tensions for movement. When the flexors contract to move a joint, the extensors relax; when the flexors relax, the extensors contract. The flexors of the legs are among the largest and strongest muscles in the body and therefore are used for leverage when using good body mechanics. The neuromuscular reflexes maintain posture by enabling opposing muscle groups to work together in coordinated movement.

Principles of Body Mechanics. Nurses and patients may suffer falls and back injuries as patients are moved from one position or location to another. The more limited the patient's mobility, the greater the need for the nurse to use good body mechanics. Principles of body mechanics that are useful in clinical practice are listed in the display. Some general concepts related to body mechanics are presented here.

The first concept of safe body dynamics is to assess the situation carefully before acting. Planning is crucial. When in doubt, seek assistance before beginning to move a patient. Examine the surroundings for potential obstacles to the desired movement (equipment, cords, tubing, or other items that could trip the nurse or hamper the patient's free movement). Necessary equipment should be placed out of the way of the nurse and patient, usually near the head or foot of the bed. Ventilator tubing, catheters, intravenous (IV) tubing, or wires for cardiac and ventilatory monitoring must be handled by an assistant or positioned to prevent accidental disconnection during the turn or transfer. It helps to use a counting method to coordinate the actions of everyone involved in the movement. Counting "one, two, three" with the position change on "three" helps focus everyone's attention.

The second concept is to use the large muscle groups

Principles of Body Mechanics

Scientific Principles Underlying Body Mechanics

- Less energy is used if all body parts are balanced appropriately.
- The body parts move segmentally and affect balance and function of the musculoskeletal system.
- The larger the base of support, the more stable the body.
- Force can be applied or resisted more effectively when the base of support can be enlarged in the direction of the force.
- Pelvic tilt (contraction of the abdominal and gluteal muscles to stabilize the pelvis) before activity helps protect the lower back from strain and injury.
- Facing the direction of work reduces the chance of injury.
- Less energy is needed to keep an object moving (momentum) than to initiate movement (inertia).
- Moving an object on a level surface requires less effort.
- Reducing friction between the object moved and the surface on which it is moved requires less energy.
- Use of levers reduces energy expenditure.
- Holding an object close to the body requires less energy than farther away.
- Muscle strain can be avoided by using the strong leg muscles when lifting, pushing, and pulling.

- Smooth, continuous movements are easier and safer than sudden, sharp, or uncontrolled movements.
- Using rhythmic movements at a normal rate of speed requires less energy.

Application of Principles of Body Mechanics

- Adjust the height of the work area when possible.
- Assume a starting position that will permit freedom of movement in range, direction, and position.
- Keep body balanced over the base of support with knees relaxed and trunk erect (in relation to the pelvis).
- Bend hips and knees to alter position of body, widening the base of support as needed, for effective leverage and use of energy.
- Face the direction of motion, using muscles of the lower extremities and shifting body weight for lifting, pushing, and pulling actions.
- Hold objects close to the body when lifting.
- Use rhythmic, smooth, and coordinated motions at a reasonable speed.
- Use elbows, hips, and knees as levers when lifting.
- Use mechanical devices when appropriate.
- Remember, holding the breath during a physical activity is an indication of muscle strain and inefficient use of body mechanics.

of the legs, whenever possible, to provide the force for the movement. The back stays straight, the arms maintain a strong grip with elbows slightly flexed, and the hips and knees are bent. Pushing, pulling, or lifting are then accomplished by orienting the torso in the desired direction of movement and straightening the legs. Back injuries that result from moving patients can often be traced to asymmetric use of muscles. Avoid twisting or moving in a diagonal direction.

The third concept is to perform work at the appropriate height for body position. When helping a patient to move in bed, the bed height should be raised to a level close to the nurse's center of gravity, usually between the hips and waist. Often the siderails must be lowered to allow the nurse to bring the patient's weight as close as possible (be careful to prevent an accidental fall from the bed). When moving the patient from the bed to a stretcher, the two surfaces should be at the same height so the patient need not be lifted.

The fourth concept is to use mechanical lifts or assistance whenever needed to facilitate the movement of a patient. In many situations, a lift sheet (also called a turn

or draw sheet) is helpful. This is a sturdy sheet that is positioned under the patient in bed so that it extends from the shoulders to just below the hips. Depending on the patient's weight, two or more nurses (distributed on each side of the bed) can use the lift sheet to move the patient anywhere on the mattress and then to roll the patient onto either side. The key to successful use of the lift sheet is to coordinate the movement of the lifters.

Moving a patient in bed may include turning the patient or moving the patient's position relative to the head of the bed. The patient should be included in the planning for the position change and encouraged to assist whenever possible. Overhead trapezes may provide handholds for patients who wish to assist. Putting the bed in the flat, horizontal position minimizes the muscle work needed to reposition the patient. If the patient cannot assist because of weakness, confusion, or illness, it is better for the patient to cross the arms over the chest than to hold onto the nurse's neck or arms. The nurse can then coordinate and carry out the movement without the risk of unpredictable pulling from the patient.

There are several techniques for transferring a patient

from the bed to a wheelchair, chair, or commode. The choice of technique depends on the patient's ability to assist and cooperate, the nurse's skill, and the number of assistants. The patient should be wearing nonskid footwear and should be assisted symmetrically, preferably by a transfer belt placed snugly around the waist. Explain to the patient the sequence of actions, then use the counting technique to coordinate everyone's efforts. Mechanical lifts are recommended when the patient cannot assist or cooperate, or when the nurse is uncertain about the safety of the transfer.

Exercise

Exercise that makes active use of alignment, posture, balance, and coordinated movement produces many physiologic and psychological benefits. Exercise must be regular and integrated into the person's lifestyle for maximum benefit. Whether a person values and participates in exercise may be influenced by his or her family, culture, job, and health. Recently, exercise has become more popular as people have taken responsibility for decreasing risk factors and leading a healthier life.

Types of Exercise. Exercise may be classified by the source of energy (aerobic or anaerobic) and by the type of muscle tension (isotonic or isometric).

Aerobic exercise requires oxygen to use the energy provided by the metabolic activities of the skeletal muscles. Vigorous, continuous muscle movement (as in walking, running, cycling, cross-country skiing, aerobic dance, or tennis) may be aerobic exercise if the person's heart rate is high enough to promote cardiovascular conditioning.

Anaerobic exercise occurs when the muscle cannot extract enough oxygen from the blood, and anaerobic pathways are used to provide the additional energy for a short time. This type of exercise is useful in endurance training for athletes, primarily.

Isotonic exercise is a dynamic form of exercise in which there is constant muscle tension, muscle contraction, and active movement. Most activities (walking, running, activities of daily living, and range-of-motion exercises) are isotonic.

Isometric exercise is static exercise in which the muscle undergoes tension and contraction but no change in length and no joint movement. Examples of isometric exercise are quadriceps setting to strengthen the quadriceps muscle, maintaining strength in immobilized muscles (casts, traction), and endurance training.

Benefits of Exercise. The human body functions most efficiently when it is used as intended. Exercise provides multiple benefits and affects all areas of function, physiologic and psychosocial. The person who does not exercise regularly is at risk for health problems, just as the immobile patient is at risk for problems related to disuse.

Characteristics of Normal Movement

Full Range of Motion

Range of motion (ROM) is the ability to move all joints through the full extent of function of which they are

---

Terms Describing Joint Motion	
Adduction	Moving a joint or extremity toward the midline of the body
Abduction	Moving a joint or extremity away from the midline of the body
Rotation, internal	Turning a joint or an extremity on its axis toward the body's midline
Rotation, external	Turning a joint or an extremity on its axis away from the body's midline
Flexion	Decreasing the angle between two bones
Extension	Straightening a joint
Hyperextension	Moving a joint past normal extension
Supination	Turning the body or a body part to face upward
Pronation	Turning the body or a body part to face downward
Circumduction	Moving a body part in widening circles
Inversion	Turning the feet inward so toes are pointing toward the midline
Eversion	Turning the feet outward so toes are pointing away from the midline
Opposition	Touching the thumb to each finger

capable. Each joint must be kept actively moving for the joints to maintain mobility, the muscles to maintain strength, and the cardiovascular system to function adequately.

Active range of motion means that the person can initiate and perform exercises in which each joint moves through its complete ROM. The healthy person may complete active ROM as a part of everyday activities and exercise.

Joints move through various planes and ROMs, depending on the type of joint. Table 29-1 shows the types of joints and their ROMs. Terms used to describe and identify movement are listed in the display.

Normal Gait

Walking is the most common form of locomotion. Although most people take the ability to walk for granted, the normal walking gait is a coordinated process requiring equilibrium and balanced posture. To walk efficiently, the person must have strong leg muscles (antigravity support), alternate extension and flexion of the legs (stepping ability), controlled center of gravity for equilibrium, and neuromuscular ability to initiate forward motion (Vander, 1990).

The normal walking gait has two phases:

- The stance phase is composed of three events: heel strike, mid-stance, and push-off.
- The swing phase completes the walking gait with another three events: acceleration, swing-through, and deceleration.

The process of walking is initiated by stepping with a slight forward tilt. The weight of the body is rolled off the ball and toes of one foot and shifted to the heel of the opposite foot and extended leg. In the process, the center of gravity moves from one side to the other and forward at the same time. The body weight is balanced on a narrow base, shifted from side to the other, and supported alternately on one foot and then the other.

Factors Affecting Normal Mobility

Intact Musculoskeletal System

Normal mobility requires adequate muscle strength, bone resiliency and strength, and full ROM of the joints. The integrity of the musculoskeletal system may be affected by anything that interrupts those factors. Muscle strength may be affected by fluid and electrolyte levels, exercise, conditioning, adequate nutrition, or the condition of tendons, ligaments, or soft tissue. With exercise, muscle tone, mass, and strength can be increased, and conditioning of the other musculoskeletal tissues and body organs is enhanced.

The function of the bones and joints depends on the mineral content of bones, which gives them adequate resilience, and by the flexibility of joints and their tendons and ligaments. Adequate intake of calcium, phosphorus, and vitamin B are essential to maintain bone resiliency and an intact skeletal system. Joints must be able to move through their entire ROM so that the body can move freely and maintain mobility.

Nervous System Control

Normal mobility requires the smooth control of movement provided by the nervous system. Motor ability depends on the integrity of the multisynaptic pathways of the afferent and efferent nerves and the central integration provided by the cerebral cortex. Nerve conduction, in turn, needs adequate circulation and an appropriate fluid and electrolyte environment. Balance and stability are the product of equilibrium, which can be affected by some medications (such as those for the common cold), fatigue, or situations that temporarily impair vision and visual input to the vestibular system in the semicircular canals.

Circulation and Oxygenation

The skeletal muscles need adequate amounts of oxygen to function at an optimal level. The lungs must be able to provide oxygen to the hemoglobin while removing carbon dioxide, the by-product of aerobic metabolism in the muscles. For these functions to occur, the lungs and circulatory system must perform dependably.

Factors that can hinder circulation and oxygenation include common minor infections of the upper respiratory system, fatigue, or extremes in temperature. These factors may interfere with adequate intake of oxygen, the heart's ability to increase the rate required by the oxygen demands of the tissue, or the ability to remove the metabolic by-products of muscle activity and metabolism.

Energy

Energy for muscle function is derived from using oxygen and the breakdown products of food to produce muscle contraction. There are two primary types of metabolism: aerobic and anaerobic. Oxidative processes responsible for energy production in aerobic metabolism occur in the mitochondria of cells; water and carbon dioxide are the by-products of this process. Aerobic metabolism is the most efficient form of energy production for long-term activity. In anaerobic metabolism, energy is released from glucose in a process known as glycolysis. This process provides energy when oxygen is inadequate or delayed; lactic acid is the by-product. The depletion of the glycogen stores and the presence of lactic acid produce fatigue in a short time, so this type of metabolism is useful only for short bursts of energy.

TABLE 29–1.

Normal Movement of Body Joints

Location in Body	Type of Joint	Normal Movement
Neck, cervical spine	Pivotal Supine: Cervical	Flexion, extension, lateral flexion, rotation

Supine:

Cervical

Lateral flexion   Rotation   Flexion extension hyperextension

| Shoulder | Ball and socket | Flexion, extension, hyperextension, abduction, adduction, internal rotation, external rotation, circumduction |

Abduction

Adduction   Rotation: outward inward   Flexion extension hyperextension

| Elbow | Hinge joints | |

Supination   Pronation   Flexion   Extension

| Forearm | Pivotal | Supination, pronation |
| Wrist | Condyloid | Flexion, extension, hyperextension, adduction, abduction |

Wrist

Ulnar flexion (adduction)   Radial flexion (abduction)

Flexion   Extension   Hyperextension

| Fingers | Condyloidal Hinge | Flexion, extension, hyperextension, abduction, adduction |

Fingers

Adduction Abduction   Flexion   Extension

| Thumb | Saddle | Flexion, extension, abduction, adduction, apposition   *(continued)* |

TABLE 29-1
(continued)

Location in Body	Type of Joint	Normal Movement
Hip	Ball and socket	Flexion, extension, hyperextension, abduction, adduction, internal rotation, external rotation, circumduction

Abduction
Adduction

Rotation:
outward
inward

Flexion
extension
hyperextension

Knee	Hinge joint	Flexion, extension

Extension

Flexion

Ankle	Hinge joint	Dorsal flexion, plantar flexion

Eversion   Inversion

Dorsiflexion

Plantarflexion

Foot	Gliding	Inversion, eversion
Toes	Condyloid	Flexion, extension, abduction, adduction

Adduction

Abduction

Extension

Flexion

Lifestyle and Habits

The effectiveness of the musculoskeletal system is related to the way in which a person lives. Regular exercise and optimal nutrition are essential to maintain normal mobility and musculoskeletal functioning. If a person has a balanced approach to activity, nutrition, and exercise, mobility will be maintained. The maxim "use it or lose it" is particularly true in regard to the musculoskeletal system: it must be used regularly to maintain function.

Coping and Self-Concept

Activity and the mental state are inextricably linked. Emotional state and self-concept can affect how active a person chooses to be, and physical activity in turn affects the person's self-concept, self-esteem, and ability to cope emotionally. Mobility allows a person to move toward enjoyable experiences, and that reinforces the activity. The feeling of independence that occurs enhances intellectual and sensory stimulation. Consequently, situations that alter the emotional state, such as fatigue, sadness, grief, or depression, may have a direct effect on mobility.

Lifespan Considerations

Newborn and Infant

Movement of the newborn is characterized by random movement and reflex activity. Control over movement occurs progressively during the first year as the neurologic system matures. Development proceeds from proximal to distal parts and in a head-to-toe fashion; babies progress from being able to control their heads, to rolling over, to crawling, to pulling themselves up to a standing position, to standing, and finally to walking. Each successive task requires increasingly coordinated movement. The ages at which these tasks are accomplished vary, but the development always occurs in an orderly progression. Motor activity during the first year characterizes many of the changes that occur in the infant. For this reason, parents often use motor development as a yardstick to evaluate the progress of their infant.

The stepping response can be evoked in newborns by holding them on a solid surface and leaning them slightly forward. The shift in the center of gravity and change in equilibrium initiate the stepping reflex. With maturity, children learn to control and use the same reflex to learn to walk.

Toddler and Preschooler

The ages of 1 to 5 years are marked by refinement of both gross and fine motor skills and by seemingly boundless energy. Fine motor skills generally develop more rapidly in girls than in boys. Young children use their physical abilities to explore their environment and to develop cognitively.

School Age and Adolescent

Physical growth slows between ages 6 and 12. Refinement of gross and fine motor skills continues and is often supported by group activities (e.g., sports, dancing or swimming lessons). Exercise patterns for later life are often determined at this time. Parents should encourage regular physical exercise while avoiding excessive pressure on children to excel. Such expectations can be emotionally and physically damaging for youngsters whose muscles are not fully developed.

Adolescence is a period of rapid physical and sexual development. Teen-agers typically appear gangly and awkward due to rapid growth and variation of growth rates in different body parts. The onset of sexual development and growth varies, causing many adolescents to believe that they are not maturing at a normal rate. Problems with motor function affect body image, which can be especially distressing for the adolescent.

Adult and Older Adult

Life between ages 20 and 40 is usually free from significant physical changes (except pregnancy). As the adult approaches middle age (40 to 60), muscle tone and bone density and mass decrease. Further deterioration in the musculoskeletal system occurs as a person ages. Joints lose elasticity and become less flexible. Bone mass decreases, especially in women with osteoporosis, resulting in more common fractures. Coordination is altered, affecting normal gait. Reaction time is slowed and there is a delayed overall body response to stressors.

With aging, changes in posture and the presence of chronic disorders may affect walking. Flattening of the lumbar spine and changes in the intervertebral discs and vertebral bodies can cause the head and upper spine to tilt forward, resulting in a shift in the center of gravity. Joint degeneration and bone demineralization also affect balance and gait. As a result, the older person often has less extension and swing-through and more side-to-side sway; weight is transferred from the ball of one foot to the ball of the other foot, leading to a wide-based, short-stepped, shuffling gait (Harris, Rodstein, & Still, 1977; Kenshalo, 1979).

The elderly person has more difficulty overcoming inertia and using gravity efficiently. One reason for this is the shift in the center of gravity. In an effort to compensate for the shift, the knees flex slightly for support. The resulting posture is one of a forward-leaning crouch with a widened base.

ALTERED MOBILITY

Potential for Altered Mobility

Normal mobility can be altered by congenital problems, diseases that affect the musculoskeletal or neurologic systems, chronic illness that depletes strength and endurance, trauma, affective disorders, and treatment that requires restrictive devices or voluntary restriction on movement.

Congenital Problems

Congenital problems usually affect normal musculoskeletal or neurologic development. Some, such as congenital hip dysplasia, can be corrected with treatment. Others, such as spina bifida or cerebral palsy, cannot be cured, so treatment is aimed at promoting the greatest degree of functional mobility and preventing complications.

Neuromuscular Deficits

Any disease that impairs the ability of the nervous system to control muscular movement and coordination hinders functional mobility. Often these disorders (such as muscular dystrophy, Parkinson's disease, and multiple sclerosis) are progressive, slowly eroding and destroying the ability to move normally until the person is confined to bed or a wheelchair.

Impairment of the brain or spinal cord also affects normal movement. Central nervous system control can be disrupted by infectious processes (e.g., meningitis), tumors, or cerebral vascular accidents. Treatment can limit or reverse some damage to the central nervous system, but at times dysfunction is permanent and severe.

Musculoskeletal Deficits

Any impairment of the musculoskeletal system can affect joint mobility, skeletal strength, and body movement. Demineralization of the bone, as in osteoporosis or multiple myeloma, increases the risk of fractures. Rheumatoid arthritis, degenerative joint disease (osteoarthritis), and gout limit mobility because movement causes pain. Bone tumors cause pain and can require amputation.

Chronic Health Problems

Chronic health conditions often decrease mobility, because such disorders limit the oxygen and nutrients delivered to the muscles. These substances are important for muscle contraction and movement. Chronic cardiovascular conditions such as congestive heart failure or peripheral vascular disease limit effective blood flow, especially during periods of increased need such as aerobic exercise. Lung disorders decrease the amount of oxygen delivered to all body tissues, including skeletal muscles. Cancer or other conditions that strain nutritional stores deplete the energy necessary for movement.

Trauma

Trauma often results in accidental injury to joints, tendons, ligaments, muscles, or bones. Such damage can be minor, affecting mobility for only a short period of time (e.g., a strain caused by overexerting a muscle, or a sprain caused by twisting a joint). More lengthy disruptions in mobility can occur when joints are dislocated, tendons are torn, or bones are broken. Immobilizing devices are usually used to keep healing body parts in normal alignment.

Severe trauma can also cause extensive damage to the spinal cord or brain. When the spinal cord is severed or severely damaged, paralysis occurs below the level of injury. The term paraplegia is used to describe decreased motor and sensory function to the legs. Quadriplegia is used to describe paralysis of the arms and legs.

Affective Disorders

Severe affective disorders can hinder mobility. Depression and catatonic states result in limited mobility, not because of physical impairments but because the person lacks the desire to move. Fear, especially of pain on movement, may cause people to restrict their movements.

Therapeutic Modalities

Sometimes movement is limited to help treat a medical problem. Restrictive devices such as casts, braces, and splints may be used to immobilize certain areas of the body to promote healing. However, the resulting decreased mobility can have negative consequences.

Bedrest is a common treatment. A patient may be placed on bedrest for the following reasons:

- To promote healing and repair of tissues by decreasing metabolic needs
- To relieve edema
- To decrease pain
- To support a weak, exhausted, or febrile patient.

Bedrest must be psychologically and physically restful. There are various definitions of the extent of bedrest: some physicians permit patients on bedrest to use a bedside commode, others insist on strict confinement to bed.

Manifestations of Altered Mobility

The patient with altered mobility may have a variety of symptoms of varying intensity. Common manifestations are decreased muscle strength and tone, lack of coordination, altered gait, falls, decreased joint flexibility, pain on movement, and decreased ability to tolerate activity.

Decreased Muscle Strength and Tone

Loss of muscle strength and tone is often evident with altered mobility. Normal muscle strength is maintained by frequent contraction of the muscle, which occurs during movement. When movement is limited or abnormal, maximal tension is not applied to muscle groups, decreasing the muscle's ability to contract. This is often accompanied by muscle atrophy; the muscle decreases in size due to disuse.

Decreased strength can be seen when the patient cannot grasp the nurse's hand strongly or can only push weakly with the legs. Weakness may be so severe that the patient's leg muscles cannot support his or her body weight, but at other times decreased strength is less obvious. For example, a patient may be able to extend his or her arms in front of the body, but after a few minutes the arms begin to drift down as the muscles become too fatigued to provide adequate support.

Muscle tone, or the normal resistance to stretch, also decreases with inactivity. Decreased muscle tone is called hypotonicity or **flaccidity.** Decreased tone can cause the muscles to becomes stretched (if they are held in a lengthened position) or contracted (if they are held in a shortened position). Neurologic impairment that results in increased muscle tone, often called **spasticity,** can also affect normal movement.

Lack of Coordination

Lack of coordination occurs when neurologic control and regulation of movement are impaired. This often is the case when trauma or disease affects the cerebellum, which plays an important role in coordinating voluntary muscle movement. Alcohol and certain drugs, such as barbiturates, can also interfere with normal coordinated movement.

Uncoordinated movement appears jerky and uneven and affects the person's ability to move purposefully and efficiently. Many terms are used to describe alterations in coordinated, purposeful movement:

Ataxia is a general term used to describe defective muscle coordination.

A *tremor* is a rhythmic, repetitive movement that can occur at rest or when movement is initiated. A tremor usually interferes with fine motor control, but in the case of Parkinson's disease it can also interfere with coordinated ambulation.

Chorea is spontaneous, brief, involuntary muscle twitching of the limbs or facial muscles; if severe, it can greatly hinder mobility.

Athetosis is movement characterized by slow, irregular, twisting motions.

Dystonia is similar to athetosis but usually involves larger areas of the body.

Altered Gait

Abnormal gait can affect the rhythm, steadiness, or speed of walking.

An *ataxic* gait is characterized by staggering and unsteadiness.

When walking appears stiff and toes appear to catch and drag, the gait is called *spastic*.

Walking with feet wide apart, in a ducklike fashion, is called a *waddling* gait.

A *hemiplegic* gait occurs when one leg is paralyzed or neurologically damaged, so that the leg is dragged or swung around to propel it forward.

A *festinating* gait, typified by walking on the toes as if being pushed, is commonly seen in Parkinson's disease.

Falls

Patients with mobility limitations are likely to experience falls from gait changes, weakness, postural hypotension, or decreased coordination. Falls frequently result in musculoskeletal trauma such as fractures, which can further decrease mobility. Sensory and cognitive changes in the elderly, combined with medication usage, further increase the risk of falls for this age group. Fear of repeated falls may cause some patients to limit their mobility.

Decreased Joint Flexibility

Decreased joint flexibility often occurs with altered mobility because decreased movement causes joints to stiffen. This decreases normal ROM, as fibrosis and fixation of joint structures occur. Muscles atrophy when they do not regularly shorten and lengthen during normal muscle contraction. Initially, decreased flexibility and altered ROM occur in affected joints, but if the joints remain immobilized contractures can occur. A **contracture** is the progressive shortening of a muscle and loss of joint mobility resulting from fibrotic changes in the tissues surrounding the joint.

Pain on Movement

Impaired mobility is often accompanied by pain on movement. Pain can be caused by physical trauma, as in sprains, strains, or torn ligaments. Pain is also commonly associated with degenerative and inflammatory processes. Osteoarthritis (degeneration of the articular surface of weight-bearing joints) and rheumatoid arthritis (an inflammatory disorder that affects joints) cause pain on movement. This pain may cause the patient to avoid movement to decrease discomfort.

Incisional pain decreases the willingness of most patients to ambulate during the postoperative period. Pain caused by inadequate blood flow to the extremities (intermittent claudication) can also severely decrease mobility. Cancer, low back pain, and other disorders that can cause chronic pain often severely limit movement.

Activity Intolerance

Decreased ability to tolerate activity often accompanies impaired mobility. **Activity intolerance** is the state in which the person has inadequate physiologic or psychological energy to endure or complete activity (Carroll-Johnson, 1989). A balance must occur between the activity and the patient's energy. Symptoms associated with activity intolerance are dyspnea, tachycardia, discomfort, weakness, and fatigue.

Commonly, disorders that affect oxygenation, such as respiratory or cardiac problems, decrease a patient's ability to tolerate increases in activity. However, some activity intolerance can be noted in anyone who has been inactive. For example, a 46-year-old man who has been inactive since college will experience activity intolerance if he tries to run two miles. Even short periods of immobility can impair activity tolerance.

Impact of Immobility on Functional Health

Immobility affects all functional health patterns (Table 29-2). Recognizing the possible consequences of immobility allows the nurse to intervene to limit or prevent problems.

Health Perception and Health Management

Immobility often limits the activities and exercise that the patient uses to promote health. When mobility de-

TABLE 29–2.

Comparison of the Effects of Exercise and Immobility on Functional Health Patterns

Functional Health Pattern	Effects of Exercise	Effects of Immobility
Health perception/ health maintenance	Promotes optimal health and well-being	Increases risk of various health problems
	Decreases risk of cardiovascular disease	
Activity/exercise	Strengthens muscles and increases muscle tone	Causes muscle weakness and atrophy, activity intolerance, contractures
	Increases endurance	Decreases range of motion
	Promotes joint mobility	Increases cardiac workload
	Increases cardiac efficiency	Causes orthostatic hypotension
	Decreases resting pulse and blood pressure	Increases risk of thrombus formation
	Improves circulation	Decreases lung expansion
	Increases respiratory rate	Promotes retained secretions
	Increases depth of respirations	Impairs gas exchange
	Improves gas exchange	
Nutritional/metabolic	Increases metabolic rate, appetite, energy	Decreases metabolic rate
	Improves skin tone and turgor	Causes anorexia, negative nitrogen balance, disuse osteoporosis, impaired immunity, skin breakdown and pressure sore development
Elimination	Increases intestinal tone and motility	Decreases intestinal tone and motility
	Increases blood flow to kidneys, promoting optimal excretion of waste products	Causes constipation, urinary stasis
		Increases risk of urinary tract infection, renal calculi
		Decreases bladder tone
Sleep/rest	Improves sleep quality	Decreases sleep quality
Cognitive/perceptual	Increases vitality and well-being	Causes sensory deprivation, confusion, hallucinations, pain and discomfort
Self-perception/ self-concept	Improves appearance, body image, self-concept	Impairs appearance, body image, self-concept
Coping/stress	Reduces stress	Increases stress
		Produces anxiety, anger, depression, powerlessness
Roles and relationships	Fosters relationships if exercise done in groups	Interferes with roles requiring mobility (e.g., going to work, caring for child)
Sexuality	Increases energy available for sexual expression	Can hinder normal sexual expression
	Improves appearance	Immobilizing devices may interfere

creases, the patient is less able to participate in normal activities, including exercise. This decreased level of activity can predispose the patient to a variety of health problems.

Immobility often requires the patient to learn how to manage devices such as casts or splints. The patient with impaired mobility may also need to learn how to use devices such as walkers or canes.

Activity and Exercise

Immobility affects the activity and exercise pattern most significantly. It affects musculoskeletal, cardiovascular, and respiratory function in several ways.

Muscle Atrophy and Weakness. Immobility decreases muscle strength and mass. In a healthy person who has full freedom of movement, muscles keep their size and strength through frequent muscle contractions. Such contractions occur continually with normal activity and movement. Muscle strength and size is proportional to the conditioning the muscle experiences. The athlete who vigorously exercises certain muscles will increase their size and strength, but the sedentary person who exercises infrequently has muscles that are smaller and less capable of work.

Muscle strength and size decrease when immobility limits a person's ability or desire to contract muscles. Reduction in cell size, or **atrophy,** results from the alterations in metabolism that occur during immobility. The body uses a catabolic mode of metabolism in which the body breaks down muscle mass to obtain energy. Changes in strength and mass are substantial and last even after immobility is reversed. Classic experiments by Dietrick and associates (1948) on the effects of immobility on healthy males showed that muscle strength decreased substantially and took 4 to 6 weeks to recover. Leg muscles are affected more by immobilization than other muscles; this is thought to be due to the effects of gravity in maintaining muscle tone. Visual evidence of atrophy can be seen when a cast is removed and the limbs are compared.

Endurance (the ability to tolerate exercise) decreases as the muscle atrophies. This often becomes a vicious cycle. Atrophy experienced by an immobilized patient decreases endurance. This in turn discourages the person from engaging in activity, which contributes to further atrophy.

Contractures and Joint Pain. In the active, mobile person, movement promotes the formation of new connective tissue that is deposited around joints and muscles. This tissue is loose and pliable and remains so as long as normal body movement occurs. But during immobility, stretching of muscles and movement of joints ceases, resulting in the deposition of denser, less pliable fibrotic tissue. Movements involving extension and flexion are most significant in preventing fibrotic changes (Lentz, 1981).

Immobility can cause joints to become fixed and unable to move normally. A contracture (progressive shortening of a muscle and loss of joint mobility) results from fibrotic changes that occur when normal mobility is not maintained. Impaired blood flow to the muscle or joint hastens the formation of contractures. Without appropriate intervention, increasing damage occurs, and a contracture can become irreversible. An irreversible contracture further decreases the person's mobility, since it makes moving the involved muscle difficult or impossible. Contractures also cause disfigurement, which can increase social isolation.

Flexion contractures are most common in immobilized patients. Patients often assume positions of flexion naturally since these positions require less muscle stress and tension to maintain. Also, flexor muscles (those that allow joints to bend) are usually stronger than their extensor counterparts. Common flexor contractures occur at the joints of the elbow, hip, knee, shoulder, wrist, and ankle. **Foot drop** is a contracture in which the foot is fixed in plantar flexion.

Immobility can cause decreased joint stability as a result of decreased tension exerted by ligaments and muscles secondary to loss of muscle tone. Decreased joint stability is thought to be the cause of aches and pains often experienced by immobilized patients. It could also account for the difficulty in ambulation and general stiffness that often follows inactivity and bedrest.

Increased Cardiac Workload. Cardiac workload is increased in the immobilized patient because the heart must work harder when the body is supine than when it is erect. Pooling of blood in the legs usually does not occur in the supine position. With less gravitational pull, blood is redistributed away from the legs toward the trunk. Venous return to the heart is subsequently increased, which means the heart muscle must work harder to pump this increased volume.

Heart rate also increases in the immobilized patient to accommodate the greater amount of blood that must be pumped. Tachycardia is also thought to be due to sympathetic dominance in the inactive person, as with parasympathetic dominance in the active person (Groer & Shekleton, 1989). An important effect of increased heart rate is that the time between contractions is decreased, which shortens the period of myocardial rest and further increases the heart's workload.

Cardiac workload can be taxed even more by use of the *Valsalva maneuver* (forced exhalation against a closed glottis). This maneuver may be used by immobilized patients when they use their arms or upper bodies to move in bed, or when they defecate on a bedpan. During Valsalva, intrathoracic pressure increases, causing the pulse rate and blood flow to the heart to decrease. The subsequent decreases in cardiac output and coronary artery perfusion can be dangerous for the immobilized patient with pre-existing cardiac problems. When breathing is resumed, a large volume of blood is all at once delivered to the heart. This tends to increase pulse rate and to stretch and strain the myocardium.

Orthostatic Hypotension. *Orthostatic hypotension* is the decreased ability to maintain systemic blood pressure when changing from a supine to an upright position. It is commonly seen after a period of immobility. Normally, position changes do not cause systemic blood pressure to drop substantially. This is because arteriolar vasoconstriction prevents large amounts of blood from pooling in the extremities when an upright posture is assumed. Baroreceptors are stimulated when blood flow decreases in the aortic arch and carotid arteries (when, for instance, the person stands up). This in turn triggers increased sympathetic activity, which causes vasoconstriction.

Immobility decreases the effectiveness of this neurovascular reflex. During inactivity, regulatory adjustments are not used and become inactive. It is thought that sympathetic stimulation still occurs in response to standing upright, but peripheral vessels do not respond to this stimulation. Therefore, vasoconstriction does not occur and a drop in blood pressure results.

Another factor that can contribute to orthostatic hypotension is the ineffectiveness of the muscle pump in promoting venous return. This is especially true of muscles atrophied by immobility. As the calf muscles weaken, they are less effective in compressing the veins of the legs and thus are less able to promote venous return. This increases the pooling of blood in the legs and worsens postural hypotension.

Orthostatic hypotension is not apparent during immobilization, but when the patient tries to stand, lightheadedness, dizziness, and increased sympathetic activity (as reflected by an elevated pulse rate and diaphoresis) may occur. Loss of consciousness can occur with severe postural hypotension. A postural drop of more than 10 mmHg in the systolic or diastolic blood pressure or an increase of 10 beats per minute in pulse rate is considered significant (Underhill, et al., 1989).

Thrombus Formation and Embolism. A *thrombus* is a clot composed of platelets, fibrin, and cellular elements of blood that attaches itself to the wall of an artery or vein. A thrombus most commonly originates in the large veins of the legs, due to the relatively low velocity of blood flow there. This is called *deep vein thrombosis.* When the clot breaks away from the vessel wall and enters circulating blood, it is called an *embolus.* Depending on the size of the original thrombus, the clot can lodge in the circulatory system as the diameter of the vessels decreases. This most commonly occurs when the thrombus enters the pulmonary vasculature, where it interferes with blood flow to the lung (a pulmonary embolus). Large pulmonary emboli can cause immediate death, but small thrombi may produce no clinical symptoms.

Normal hemostatic mechanisms regulate the clotting process so that clots normally do not form in veins and arteries. However, the delicate balance in this system can be altered by factors such as venous stasis, hypercoagulability of blood, and trauma or injury to an artery or vein.

Immobility promotes venous stasis. When leg muscles are inactive, venous return to the heart is decreased. Over time, the gravitational effect of the supine position causes the redistribution of body fluids, with a net decrease in venous return (Winslow, 1985). The numerous bifurcations and valves in veins are thought to further promote stasis of blood. This seems to be even more pronounced in the elderly, perhaps explaining in part the increased incidence of thrombus development in the immobilized elderly (Groer & Shekleton, 1989). Poor positioning can cause external pressure on blood vessels, which also contributes to inadequate blood flow and promotes the development of thrombi.

Hypercoagulability of blood is not directly caused by immobility, but often immobilized patients become dehydrated, which can increase blood viscosity. Dehydration may be in part due to the patient's inability to obtain fluids without assistance. It has also been hypothesized that elevated serum calcium levels (a common finding in the immobilized patient) can also affect coagulation.

Trauma to veins or arteries can occur in the immobilized patient secondary to venipunctures or improper positioning. A patient whose immobility is compromised because of trauma is at a higher risk for thrombus formation secondary to vessel injury.

Decreased Lung Expansion. The immobilized patient experiences greater-than-normal resistance to breathing, resulting in underinflation of the lungs and increased work of breathing.

The healthy person keeps the lungs well inflated with practically no effort. In an upright position, the diaphragm can move up and down freely. Airways are kept clear of mucous secretions by an efficient mechanism known as the mucociliary escalator. Periodic sighing and coughing helps to keep even the smallest air sacs (alveoli) open and available for gas exchange. Finally, ordinary activity produces enough carbon dioxide to stimulate a smooth, effective pattern of breathing.

The immobile patient breathes less deeply than normal and with greater effort. The supine patient must overcome two resistances that do not ordinarily work against breathing. First, the diaphragm is prohibited from free movement by the abdominal organs, which shift against it when the patient lies down. To achieve full lung expansion, the patient's diaphragm must push the organs out of the way with each breath. Second, the patient's chest movement is limited by the pressure of the bed against the chest wall. These two factors together result in diminished depth of breathing, or decreased tidal volume. Because the immobilized patient's activity level is less than normal, less carbon dioxide is produced. This results in a lower level of stimulation for breathing, causing further reduction of tidal volume.

Decreased depth of breathing can result in collapse of alveoli, which in turn hinders the exchange of oxygen and carbon dioxide. This condition of alveolar collapse is known as *atelectasis.* In addition to limiting the lungs' ability to exchange gases, atelectasis predisposes the patient to pneumonia. It limits the patient's ability to cough deeply; thus, mucus may become trapped in the lung, providing a rich medium for microbial growth.

Retained Secretions. Secretions of the lung ordinarily perform important protective functions. The liquid part of mucus imparts water vapor to the air entering the respiratory tract. The viscous portion traps bacteria and particulate matter, thus preventing infection or other damage to the sensitive respiratory epithelium. The mucous layer that blankets the airways ordinarily moves steadily upward. The secretions, which contain inhaled debris, are moved into the throat, where they stimulate a cough. Once this occurs, they are expectorated or swallowed.

Immobility can limit the effectiveness of this protective mechanism. Although immobilized patients who have healthy lungs can usually generate sufficient coughs, patients with compromised lung function may be unable to cough out respiratory secretions. As explained above, immobility can inhibit lung expansion, thereby hindering the patient's ability to cough. With an impaired cough mechanism, patients who produce excessive mucus are at risk for secretion retention. The primary dangers of retained secretions are atelectasis secondary to airway blockage, and infection. As airways become obstructed with retained secretions, the alveoli served by them gradually deflate because the oxygen that helps hold them open is absorbed. Since mucus provides a rich, warm growth medium for microorganisms, retained secretions foster bacterial colonies that may eventually cause pneumonia.

Nutrition and Metabolism

The nutritional and metabolic effects of immobility include decreased metabolic rate, anorexia, negative nitrogen balance, disuse osteoporosis, impaired immunity, and increased potential for development of pressure sores.

Decreased Metabolic Rate. The basal metabolic rate is decreased during immobility. The production of many hormones affecting metabolic rate, fluid and electrolyte balance, and the stress response is affected when activity is severely restricted. The amount and pattern of body production of thyroid hormone, adrenocorticotrophic hormone, aldosterone, and insulin are all affected (Rubin, 1988). Metabolism of drugs in the body is also altered.

Negative Nitrogen Balance. In an active person, a balance exists between protein breakdown and protein synthesis. Immobility fosters an elevated rate of protein breakdown, probably due to muscle atrophy. One way to measure this process is to monitor the nitrogen excreted from the body, since nitrogen is excreted as a waste product when protein is broken down by metabolic processes. A negative nitrogen balance occurs when excretion of nitrogen due to protein breakdown exceeds dietary intake. Elevated urinary nitrogen levels are seen in most immobilized patients. The consequence of this state is that the body lacks adequate nitrogen for protein synthesis, resulting in nutritional depletion. This can interfere with wound healing and rebuilding of muscle mass when mobility is resumed.

Immobilized patients often have concomitant factors that further deplete nitrogen balance, such as trauma, burns, surgery, coma, cancer, fever, or infection. Patients with chronic illness or poor nutritional balance before immobilization are at increased risk for negative nitrogen balance.

Anorexia. Anorexia (loss of appetite) is common in immobilized patients. Decreased metabolic rate is accompanied by decreased caloric need. In addition, institutional food, eating in a supine position, environmental factors, and the patient's psychological state can worsen appetite. Stress from hospitalization or from adjustment to alterations in body function can contribute to dyspepsia, gastric stasis, bloating, and distention; all these factors may contribute to anorexia. Regardless of the cause, decreased nutritional intake can impair body function and rehabilitation.

Disuse Osteoporosis. In disuse osteoporosis, bone becomes demineralized secondary to immobility. Bone is a living structure: the bone matrix is in a dynamic state of formation and destruction. Osteoblastic cells are responsible for the proliferation of bone matrix. In contrast, osteoclastic cells destroy bone matrix by absorbing and removing osseous tissue from the bone. Immobility results in an imbalance between osteoblastic and osteoclastic activity, since normal stress and strain imposed on bone via movement is important in osteoblastic processes. In the immobilized patient, osteoblasts continue to lay down bony matrix, but osteoclasts break down bone at a rate faster than osteoblasts build it. The result is a loss of bony matrix. Disuse osteoporosis results in bones that are more porous, brittle, and susceptible to fractures.

Another significant effect of this process is increased serum calcium that must be excreted from the body. Increasing dietary intake of calcium is helpful in preventing disuse osteoporosis only initially (Rubin, 1988). If renal function is insufficient to excrete excess calcium at an adequate rate, calcium may be deposited into the muscles and joints. This can cause discomfort and interfere with normal musculoskeletal function.

Osteoporosis begins soon after loss of mobility occurs. Urinary calcium levels more than double during periods of bedrest (Winslow, 1985). Lengthy immobilization can result in significant bone loss, and return to normal calcium levels may take up to 5 weeks after normal activity is resumed (Rubin, 1988).

Impaired Immunity. The immune system is weakened during immobility. Catabolism of immunoglobulin G doubles, significantly decreasing the normal concentration of circulating antibodies (Rubin, 1988). Leukocytes are less able to engulf and destroy microorganisms. Transport of lymph may be decreased when skeletal muscles are inactive.

Pressure Sores. Pressure sores form when pressure exerted over an area of skin or subcutaneous tissue exceeds the pressure required for adequate blood flow to the area. This causes cells to die because they are not supplied with oxygen and nutrients and because waste products build up. Pressure is usually concentrated on bony prominences but can occur anywhere pressure is great. In the supine position, pressure is greatest over the back of the skull and at the elbows, sacrum, ischial tuberosities, and heels. In the sitting position, the greatest pressure is at the ischial tuberosities and the sacrum.

A compensatory mechanism that responds to this inadequate blood flow is reactive hyperemia. When pressure is removed, blood floods the area in an attempt to prevent tissue necrosis. This mechanism is only effective if it occurs before cellular damage. The critical time period can vary from one person to another.

The normal person can sense pressure buildup and can change position to reduce discomfort, but this is not always possible for the patient with impaired mobility. Patients with neurologic impairment may be incapable of movement or unable to sense the need for position change.

Healing of pressure sores is difficult and slow, especially in the immobilized patient. Pressure sores can prolong immobility and increase the cost and length of hospitalization. See Chapter 34 for more information about pressure sores.

Elimination

Immobility causes alterations in normal elimination patterns, manifested by constipation, urinary stasis, and increased incidence of urinary tract infections and renal calculi.

Constipation. Even in a healthy person, changes in diet, activities, or emotional stress affect normal bowel patterns. In addition to these factors, the immobilized patient experiences additional stressors that interfere with bowel function. Abdominal and perineal muscles can be weakened by muscle atrophy, making it more difficult for the patient to bear down and exert pressure to evacuate stool. As stool descends against the rectum, the stimulus to defecate is felt. In an upright posture, stool descends more quickly into the rectal area, eliciting a strong stimulus. But in the supine position, rectal filling is slow, weakening the stimulus for defecation.

The defecation reflex can also be affected if defecation is postponed when the stimulus to defecate is felt. This happens frequently in the immobilized patient, who may feel embarrassed or may need assistance to use a bedpan. When defecation is delayed, fecal material increases in size and more water is absorbed from the feces, making stool passage even more difficult. Dehydration, common in the immobile patient, can also contribute to constipation. Also, decreased roughage intake because of anorexia adds to the difficulty in stool passage.

This process can lead to fecal impaction (hard stool contained in the rectum that cannot be removed naturally by defecation). With fecal impaction, the patient has a feeling of fullness with a desire to defecate. Often liquid stool seeps around the obstruction formed by the impaction. Fecal impaction can lead to bowel obstruction, so it should be treated promptly with manual removal. Preventive measures should be taken to discourage recurrence.

Urinary Stasis. Normal micturition requires the coordinated interaction of the detrusor muscle of the bladder wall, the perineal muscles, and the internal and external urethral sphincter. As the bladder fills, the sensation of a need to void is transmitted and the internal urethral sphincter relaxes. Control over external sphincters prevents the loss of urine until the perineal muscles are voluntarily relaxed. In the immobilized patient, the signal of the need to void is often not heeded. The patient may not want to bother the nurse by asking for a bedpan. Some patients try to void when they feel the need but have difficulty relaxing the perineal muscles when in the supine position. Delaying micturition causes urine to collect in the bladder. If chronic, this can cause overstretching of the detrusor muscle, which can lead to permanent changes in bladder tone and can have long-term consequences for normal voiding patterns. Prostatic enlargement in the elderly male patient can also interfere with bladder emptying, especially in the supine position.

The supine position promotes the retention of urine. In the upright position, gravity encourages the continual flow of urine from the renal pelvis into the ureter, to eventually be collected in the bladder. When supine, the ureter is above the level of many renal calyces, which means that urine must flow upward against gravity to travel through the ureter.

Urinary retention poses significant problems for the immobilized patient. Stasis of urine contributes to urinary tract infections and renal calculi. When distention is great, patients can experience overflow incontinence. This is embarrassing for the patient and can contribute to skin breakdown.

Urinary Tract Infection. Stagnant urine provides a good medium for bacterial growth. Bladder distention can cause small tears in the delicate bladder mucosa, which contribute to the incidence of urinary tract infection. When the patient experiences distention, catheterization may be necessary to empty the bladder, and any instrumentation of the bladder increases the potential for infection.

Renal Calculi. Stasis of urine and increased serum calcium promotes the formation of renal calculi in the immobilized patient. As serum calcium increases due to loss of calcium from the bones, more of this substance is excreted. This results in an elevation of urinary calcium levels. Calcium can precipitate from solution to form crystals, and stasis of urine encourages the aggregation of crystals into stones. Dehydration, common in the immobilized patient, also increases the incidence of stone formation. Infection caused by some urea-splitting organisms makes the urine more alkaline, which also fosters stone development. Calculi predispose the immobilized patient to increased urinary retention, infection, and hydronephrosis, which can contribute to renal impairment (Patrick, et al., 1991).

Sleep and Rest

Immobility can interfere with normal sleep patterns. Normal activity, especially physical work and aerobic exercise, produces a sense of fatigue that helps the person fall asleep and obtain restful sleep. The immobilized patient may doze frequently during the day, disrupting normal nighttime sleep patterns. The immobilized patient must be awakened frequently to be turned, monitored, or given treatment or medications. Such wakings, especially when numerous, can impair the quality of sleep. The immobilized inpatient must sleep in an unfamiliar, often noisy environment. Stress and health worries can further reduce the amount and quality of sleep.

Cognition and Perception

Immobility reduces the quantity and quality of sensory information available to the patient, since freedom to interact normally with the environment is decreased. This can lead to sensory deprivation. When this occurs, the brain attempts to provide self-stimulation in the form of visual and auditory hallucinations (Rubin, 1988). Initially this may take the form of simple sensory alterations, such as seeing colors or shapes that are not there, or experiencing abnormal sensations such as itching, heat or cold, and involuntary muscle movement. As deprivation continues, more complex abnormal experiences occur, such as hearing voices or seeing people or occurrences that are not real. Symptoms include preoccupation with somatic complaints, difficulty with time perception, difficulty with understanding and following directions, crying, and other emotional outbursts. Confusion is common but reversible if normal sensory input returns.

Pain may occur due to physiologic changes that occur with immobility. Joint stiffness, pneumonia, pressure sores, thrombosis, and emboli can contribute to discomfort for the immobilized patient. The perception of pain may also intensify because focusing on discomfort is more common when diversions are limited.

Self-Perception and Self-Concept

Changes in self-perception and self-concept commonly accompany functional motor impairment or immobility. Immobility contributes to a feeling of powerlessness, since dependence on others is often necessary. Motor impairment can change body image, especially if the impairment results from loss of a body part. Self-concept is altered when patients must depend on devices such as crutches, wheelchairs, or walkers. Problems with coordination can cause embarrassment; patients may worry that they may appear intoxicated. Altered body image can harm self-esteem and lead to lowered self-worth.

Coping and Stress Tolerance

Loss of mobility is not something the patient chooses or desires. With trauma, it occurs suddenly. In some cases it is permanent, requiring the patient to adapt to different functional abilities. Despite supportive social interactions with family and friends, immobilized patients often spend many hours alone and are often bored or lonely. Depression, anger, and anxiety are common.

All of these factors create stress and cause the patient to use coping strategies. How severely the patient is affected depends on his or her perception of the impairment, rather than the specific type or degree of impairment. For example, an elderly man who fractures his hip may think that it marks the loss of his independence. The stress created by the fractured hip for this patient, even though healing is likely, may be greater than that experienced by some patients suffering permanent disability.

Different behavior is exhibited by patients who experience stress due to immobility. Some withdraw, limiting social contact even further. Some complain and become more demanding. The patient who constantly requests assistance may be responding negatively to the stress of immobility.

Roles and Relationships

Immobility affects role function for many people. For children and adolescents, school and social activities are disrupted. For adults, the ability to work is often impaired. This can result in temporary or permanent unemployment with corresponding financial stress. The ability to perform the activities required of a parent or spouse is also disrupted.

Normal family life is affected when any family member experiences immobility. Caring for children may be impossible when a parent is hospitalized or mobility is severely impaired. Arrangements for child care are often difficult to make and stressful for both child and parent. Older children may be better able to care for themselves, but they still require emotional support and guidance from parents. Older children may need to assume more responsibility for tasks normally performed by their parents. When a child is immobilized, this may decrease the quantity and quality of time the parents can spend with other children. This may cause anger and resentment in siblings.

Sexuality

Sexual feelings and activities may be affected by mobility limitations. Lack of privacy, depression, fatigue, and physical limitations can contribute to decreased sexual function. Immobility may impede grooming activities that are often important in maintaining sexual identity. For some patients with long-term motor impairments, such as paraplegics, sexual function may be permanently altered. New methods of sexual expression may need to be learned and valued.

Impact of Altered Mobility on Activities of Daily Living

Impaired mobility severely restricts the patient's ability to perform normal daily activities. Activities of daily living are functions commonly associated with independent functioning, such as eating, performing daily hygiene and grooming, dressing, and toileting. Coordination and muscle strength are necessary to perform these functions. Often the nurse can help the patient learn to function successfully and independently despite physical limitations. This is best done by setting short-term, achievable goals and working with the health-care team (physician, physical therapist, occupational therapist, psychologist, etc.) to develop an appropriate plan. Emotional support is essential.

Difficulty eating is most common among patients with arm involvement (often caused by neuromuscular diseases), or hemiparesis or hemiplegia. Special devices can help the patient grasp a cup or eating utensils. Many patients who lack the coordination to feed themselves also suffer from difficulty swallowing secondary to neurologic impairment; careful nursing supervision is necessary to prevent aspiration of food.

Dressing is often a problem for patients with problems with fine motor skills. Velcro fasteners can be used in place of buttons or zippers. Sweat pants and other loose-fitting clothes are good ideas for the patient who has difficulty dressing.

Since personal hygiene is a private matter for most patients, it is often stressful to have to depend on nursing personnel for this care. Even when patients can perform some hygiene care independently, it can be physically taxing. Sometimes the nurse must do some of the care to prevent overtiring.

Gaining access to toilet facilities is difficult for the patient who cannot move normally. Bedside commodes are often used during hospitalization. Physiologic impairment of bowel or bladder function may occur with some mobility problems involving paralysis. Bowel programs should be instituted to avoid constipation.

Impaired mobility affects other daily activities such as performing housework, driving a car, buying groceries, and paying bills. Social activities may be curtailed, and participating in athletics or exercise programs may be impossible.

ASSESSMENT

To assess the patient's mobility, the nurse must collect subjective and objective information from the patient. Such data help the nurse understand the patient's normal mobility, risk factors for potential alterations in

Nursing Research

Selected Nursing Research Studies

Fitzmaurice, J. B. (1987). Nurses' use of cues in the clinical judgment of activity intolerance. *Classification of Nursing Diagnosis: Proceedings of the Seventh Conference*, pp. 315–323.

Kelly, R. E., et al. (1987). Evaluation of kinetic therapy in the prevention of complications of prolonged bedrest secondary to stroke. *Stroke, 18*, 638–642.

Langemo, D. K., et al. (1990). Explicating the relationship of health measures and self-esteem to exercise practices in adults. *Health Education, 21*(4), 7–11.

MacVicar, M. G., et al. (1989). Effects of aerobic interval training on cancer patients' functional capacity. *Nursing Research, 38*, 348–351.

Videman, T., et al. (1989). Patient handling skill, back injuries and back pain: An intervention study in nursing. *Spine, 14*, 148–156.

Volderi, C., et al. (1990). The relationship of age, sex, and exercise practices to measures of health, lifestyle, and self-esteem. *Applied Nursing Research, 3*(1), 20–26.

Possible Topics for Nursing Inquiry

- What are the risk factors for falls among mobile, noninstitutionalized elderly people?
- What effect do routine exercise programs have on the development of osteoporosis in postmenopausal women?
- What is the psychological impact of routine exercise on depressed terminal cancer patients?
- What impact does extended immobility have on pain perception?
- What impact does posting specific turning schedules at bedside have on compliance?
- What is the impact of bed exercises on reducing perceptual changes associated with prolonged immobility?

mobility, actual impairments in mobility, and management techniques or devices the patient uses to manage impaired mobility.

Subjective Data

Subjective data are initially collected during the nursing interview when the patient enters the facility and at routine intervals as necessary to update information.

Functional Pattern Identification

It is important to determine the patient's normal activity pattern. Ask the patient to describe his or her ability to move normally and perform activities of daily living. A rating scale is often used to document whether the patient is independent, partially dependent, or completely dependent in various activities involving mobility, such as ambulation, toileting, dressing, bathing, and household chores. Ask the patient if there has been any recent change in mobility or activity level. Determine the patient's normal patterns of exercise and leisure activities. If the patient actively engages in aerobic exercise, determine the frequency and appropriateness of the activity.

Assess the patient's satisfaction with his or her current activity level, and note any desire on the patient's part to change the activity pattern. It often helps to ask the patient if any alterations in activity are anticipated after discharge, and how the patient plans to deal with these alterations.

Discuss the patient's lifestyle. Some people enjoy sedentary activities and work at sedentary jobs. Others work at jobs that require vigorous physical exertion and take part in sports and physical activities during their leisure time. People who grew up in a family that valued quiet activities often carry the pattern of inactivity into adulthood.

Risk Pattern Identification

Interviewing the patient can also provide information helpful in identifying risk factors that can contribute to impaired mobility. Document inadequate aerobic activity, which can contribute to an increased risk for chronic disease and deconditioning. Ask if the patient feels weak or fatigued after routine exercise and activity. Ask the patient to describe any distressing symptoms (such as difficulty breathing, pain, or increased heart rate) with activity; document the degree of exercise and the degree of stress. Ask the patient how long the symptoms have occurred and how long they persist after the activity has been discontinued.

Evaluate the patient's risk for falls. Factors that increase this risk are decreased mobility, altered cogni-

tion, the use of alcohol or drugs that impair balance, postural hypotension, and a cluttered environment.

Document current or chronic health problems that may limit mobility or decrease activity tolerance. Common medical conditions important to note are respiratory disease, cardiac disease, anemia, peripheral vascular disease, arthritis, cerebral vascular accidents, multiple sclerosis, Parkinson's disease, brain tumors, head injuries, fractures, spinal cord injuries, and amputations. Evaluate the impact of these problems on mobility.

Dysfunctional Identification

Document any inability of the patient to move normally and with ease. Encourage the patient to explain any problems with mobility or activity tolerance, as well as any adaptations used to promote optimal functioning at home. If the patient reports any limitation in mobility, determine the extent of the problem, when it first occurred, and whether the patient knows the cause. Ask the patient whether the mobility problem has been improving or worsening, and how it affects his or her functional abilities in other areas. Document what the patient can do independently, so that independence within his or her capabilities can be encouraged.

Ask the patient whether he or she uses devices to assist with ambulation (e.g., prostheses, canes, walkers, crutches). If surgery is planned where assistive devices will be used, the patient may be asked to demonstrate skills previously learned.

Perform a comprehensive functional health assessment to determine the impact of decreased mobility on all functional health areas. Note any complications due to limited mobility (e.g., pressure ulcers or renal calculi). To guide the assessment, see Table 29-2, which lists the effects of immobility on functional health patterns.

Discuss with the patient how impaired mobility has affected his or her roles and relationships, self-concept, self-esteem, and body image. Identify family and community support services and evaluate past and present coping abilities.

Objective Data

In addition to collecting subjective information, the nurse uses physical assessment and diagnostic and laboratory tests to help evaluate the patient's mobility.

Physical Assessment

The physical examination is used to collect information about alignment, balance, coordination, gait, joint structure and function, muscle mass, tone, and strength, and activity tolerance. Most often, the nurse uses the technique of inspection to visualize these qualities. When mobility appears normal, more extensive assessment techniques are usually unnecessary, but if mobility is impaired a more detailed assessment may be indicated.

Alignment. Assessing alignment is the first step in determining mobility. First, determine the center of gravity. Proper alignment should be maintained while sitting and standing. When normal alignment is present, an imaginary line can be drawn through the ear lobe, shoulder, hip, femoral trochanter, knee, and front of the ankle. Symmetry of organs and bones should be noted on each side of the body.

Normal spinal alignment is characterized by concave curvature of the cervical spine, convex curvature of the thoracic spine, and concave curvature of the lumbar spine. Extreme curvature of the spine can indicate abnormality. *Scoliosis,* a lateral deviation of the thoracic spine, can be detected by watching the patient bend at the waist from a standing position. *Lordosis,* an abnormal concavity of the lumbar spine, and *kyphosis,* an exaggerated curvature of the thoracic spine, are less common spinal deviations.

Balance. Assess balance by asking the patient to sit or stand, and observe his or her ability to maintain a normal erect posture through postural adjustments. Swaying to one side indicates inability to maintain balance through normal physiologic mechanisms.

Coordination. Watching the patient perform normal activities, including ambulation, allows the nurse to evaluate the coordination of movement. Look for fluid, well-controlled movement. The patient should be able to initiate the desired movement quickly without hesitation. Fine motor skills can be assessed by asking the patient to perform a simple skill such as unbuttoning a shirt or signing papers.

Gait. Observe the patient walk to evaluate **gait,** the character or style of walk. Normal gait should be rhythmic and even, and the stride should be symmetric, with full extension. The head should remain erect and the knees and feet should point forward. Arms should swing alternately with leg movements. The full weight of the body should be easily supported. Observing the patient's shoes to detect patterns of wear can also provide the nurse with information about gait.

Joint Structure and Function. Observation and palpation can detect redness, swelling, or warmth around the joint. Listen for a crunching or grating sound (*crepitus*), which can occur when bones rub against one another during movement because of inadequate protection or lubrication in the joint. Observe the patient's facial expression and nonverbal signs of discomfort during movement. If observation reveals stiffness or guarding during certain body movements, evaluate joint mobility by moving the involved joint through its full ROM (see Table 29-1). When doing this, note the amount of resistance encountered and whether the patient complains of discomfort.

Muscle Mass, Tone, and Strength. Normal muscle mass, tone, and strength can vary greatly from one person to another. Athletes may have bulging, well-defined muscles and great strength and endurance. The elderly may have weak, small muscles with little tone. Increased strength and tone are usually found on the person's dominant side.

Assess muscle strength by evaluating the patient's ability to perform activities of self-care such as feeding, dressing, toileting, and grooming. Strength and coordination can be estimated by observing the ease with which a person can carry out these tasks. Evaluate the strength of specific muscle groups by asking the patient to grip your hand or to use certain muscle groups to push against resistance.

Muscle size in the arms and legs is determined by observation and by comparing measurements. A decrease in circumference in the affected limb usually reflects muscle atrophy from immobility. Atrophy indicates a loss of muscle tone, which decreases endurance.

Postural Blood Pressure. One screening tool to determine if a patient can safely ambulate is monitoring postural blood pressure. See Chapter 19 for instructions on how to measure postural blood pressure. A drop in blood pressure when the patient changes from a supine to a sitting position indicates risk to mobility and ambulation. Complaints of dizziness, lightheadedness, diaphoresis, and tachycardia may accompany orthostatic hypotension and are signs that fainting may occur if ambulation continues.

Risk for Falls. Determine whether independent ambulation is safe. Some facilities list risk factors contributing to falls and ask the nurse to calculate a score to determine those patients at greatest risk. Risk factors include the following:

- Elderly (especially over age 70)
- Visual impairment
- History of previous falls
- History of dizziness, postural hypotension, or syncope
- Cognitive impairments such as confusion
- Use of drugs or alcohol that can impair balance, coordination, or cognitive abilities
- Incontinence.

For more information, see Chapter 25.

Activity Tolerance. In assessing activity tolerance, observe the patient before, during, and after activity to detect abnormal responses. The most common parameters measured are the pulse rate and the respiratory rate. Normally, both increase during activity. Resting vital signs should be within a normal range before activity starts. If the patient begins activity when hypotension, tachycardia, or tachypnea is present, little reserve is available to supply the increased oxygen needed during exercise.

When activity is resumed after bedrest, or when the level of prescribed activity is increased, observe the patient carefully for signs of distress, such as dyspnea, diaphoresis, or dizziness. In high-risk patients such as cardiac or respiratory patients, the nurse may be directed to monitor pulse or respiratory rate during activity, and to discontinue the activity if values are outside the prescribed range. After activity, pulse and respiratory rates should return to pre-activity baseline values within 3 minutes.

Diagnostic Tests and Procedures

Common diagnostic tests used to evaluate musculoskeletal function are radiographic studies and direct visualization of joints. Laboratory values such as hemoglobin and hematocrit may be helpful in assessing activity tolerance.

Radiographic Studies. X-rays are useful in differentiating traumatic injuries such as sprains, dislocations, and fractures. X-rays also help assess the demineralization of bone that occurs in osteoporosis.

Radiographic studies that use injected dye can help evaluate problems with the spine or joints. Defects are revealed through an abnormal pattern of dye distribution in the body part. *Arthrograms* permit visualization of joints and are often used to diagnose tears in ligaments or cartilage. *Myelograms* use radiopaque dye to visualize the spinal canal to detect ruptured vertebral discs or other structural defects.

Arthroscopy. **Arthroscopy** involves examining a joint with a fiberoptic scope to diagnose abnormalities. Minor corrective surgery can also be performed to remove torn cartilage or repair torn ligaments.

Hematologic Studies. Hemoglobin and hematocrit values can be used to evaluate the patient's reserve for activity. Patients with low hemoglobin values have difficulty transporting adequate oxygen to body tissues. Activity expectations may need to be modified for patients with hemoglobin values under 10 g/dL. Low hematocrit values often reflect blood loss or inadequate volume replacement. When patients have low hematocrit values, they are likely to experience postural hypotension and activity intolerance.

NURSING DIAGNOSES AND PATIENT GOALS

NANDA nursing diagnoses that relate to mobility are Impaired Physical Mobility, Activity Intolerance, and High Risk for Disuse Syndrome.

Impaired Physical Mobility

Definition

Impaired physical mobility is a state in which the individual experiences a limitation of ability for independent physical movement (NANDA, 1990).

Defining Characteristics

Inability to purposefully move within the physical environment, including bed mobility, transfer, and ambulation; reluctance to attempt movement; limited range of motion; decreased muscle strength, control, and/or mass; imposed restrictions on movement, including mechanical, medical protocol; impaired coordination (NANDA, 1990).

Related Factors

Intolerance to activity/decreased strength and endurance; pain/discomfort; perceptual/cognitive impairment; neuromuscular impairment; musculoskeletal impairment; depression/severe anxiety (NANDA, 1990).

Activity Intolerance

Definition

Activity intolerance is a state in which an individual has insufficient physiologic or psychological energy to endure or complete required or desired daily activities (NANDA, 1990).

Defining Characteristics

Verbal report of fatigue or weakness (critical); abnormal heart rate or blood pressure response to activity; exertional discomfort or dyspnea; electrocardiographic changes reflecting arrhythmias or ischemia (NANDA, 1990).

Related Factors

Bedrest/immobility; generalized weakness; sedentary lifestyle; imbalance between oxygen supply/demand (NANDA, 1990).

High Risk for Disuse Syndrome

Definition

High risk for disuse syndrome is a state in which an individual is at risk for deterioration of body systems as the result of prescribed or unavoidable musculoskeletal inactivity (NANDA, 1990).

Defining Characteristics

Presence of risk factors such as paralysis; mechanical immobilization; prescribed immobilization; severe pain; altered level of consciousness (NANDA, 1990).

Related Factors

See defining characteristics.

Related Nursing Diagnoses

Lack of normal movement affects all functional health patterns. The patient with a nursing diagnosis of Impaired Physical Activity or Activity Intolerance is often at risk for many other problems. Self-Care Deficits in bathing, grooming, feeding, and toileting are common since these tasks require normal movement and coordination. The disruption of various body systems can result in Altered Skin Integrity, High Risk for Infection, Urinary Retention, Constipation, Altered Nutrition, Impaired Gas Exchange, or Ineffective Airway Clearance. High Risk for Injury is greater since the risk for falls increases if mobility is impaired. Sensory/Perceptual Alterations can occur, and Pain may increase. Altered Sexuality Patterns may be an appropriate diagnosis if spontaneous, normal movement is limited.

Since mobility is linked directly with a person's sense of independence, decreased mobility greatly affects personal feelings. Body Image Disturbance, Self-Esteem Disturbances, Anxiety, and Powerlessness can occur when normal movement is impaired. Altered Role Performance results because some of the responsibilities of a spouse, parent, or employee may require normal movement. Social Isolation and Impaired Verbal Communication can occur when the patient withdraws from social interaction. Ineffective Family or Individual Coping often results from the stress imposed by altered mobility or the need to adjust to permanent disability.

Patient Goals

General goals for the patient with impaired mobility might include:

Patient will increase endurance and tolerance for physical activity.
Patient will actively participate in prescribed therapies to promote optimum healing and restoration of mobility.
Patient will comply with measures to prevent potential complications of immobility.
Patient will maintain optimum functional abilities despite mobility restrictions.

IMPLEMENTATION

Nursing Interventions to Promote Health and Function

Physical Fitness Promotion

Our society has grown more sedentary because machines have reduced the need for physical exertion. Sedentary lifestyles have been implicated in the increased incidence of many diseases. However, physical fitness has recently become more fashionable (Fig. 29-5). Many people jog or participate in exercise programs. Health clubs are available in most communities. Even some companies are beginning to incorporate gymnasiums into their facilities for employees to use. Nonetheless, a relatively small percentage of the population is physically fit.

The nurse is frequently in a position to promote physical fitness. By stressing the importance of exercise for physical and emotional health, the nurse can help prevent mobility problems. Teaching about physical fitness occurs in many areas of nursing. The school nurse can

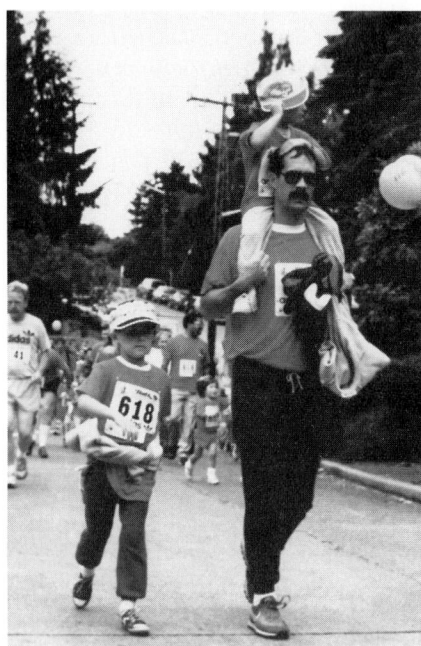

Figure 29–5. Exercise can be a family affair. (Courtesy of University of Washington School of Nursing.)

help young people develop good exercise habits. Physical education should be part of the curriculum in all grades. The school nurse should work with physical education teachers and coaches to promote well-balanced programs. The nurse can teach patients about the value of exercise when they make routine visits to private physicians and clinics. Nurses are often part of the team for weight-reduction programs. Nurses can serve as role models by remaining physically fit.

Exercise programs must be regular to be effective. Aerobic exercise is most beneficial when performed at least three times a week for at least 30 minutes of accelerated heart rate. Exercise tolerance should be increased gradually so as not to place excessive stress on muscles and joints. Pain during exercise is a signal to stop. People may drop out of an exercise program because of soreness if they begin too aggressively.

Exercise programs are part of the rehabilitation process for many patients. Group exercise activities are often planned for patients in extended-care facilities. After a heart attack or cardiac surgery, a specific exercise program is recommended. Exercise is used after a stroke to strengthen affected muscles. Many diabetics use an exercise program to obtain better diabetic control. The patient who has undergone orthopedic surgery is encouraged to exercise certain muscles and joints. The physical therapy staff is often responsible for supervising exercise programs, but the nurse can encourage and reinforce the prescribed therapies.

Injury Prevention

Injuries from accidents commonly cause impaired mobility. The nurse can play a significant role in accident prevention:

- Promoting automobile safety by teaching the importance of using seat belts and proper restraint devices for young children
- Drug and alcohol counseling
- Helping parents provide a safe environment for their children
- Helping to prevent accidents in the workplace.

Specific information on accident prevention is given in Chapter 25.

Nursing Interventions for Altered Mobility

Positioning

Proper positioning is important in preventing complications. A patient with partial mobility can often be taught positioning techniques to be used with or without the nurse's assistance, but immobile patients rely on the nursing staff to reposition them. Helping promote func-

---

Selected Nursing Interventions for Common Altered Mobility Problems

Mobility Assistance

- Turning and positioning
- Transferring
- Assisting with ambulation
- Teaching (preventing falls, ambulation and transfers, using ambulation aids)

Preventing Complications from Immobility

- Range-of-motion exercises
- Leg exercises
- Deep breathing and coughing
- Adequate hydration
- Skin care
- Bowel program

---

tional mobility is an important, independent function of the nurse, who works within mobility restrictions ordered by the physician or physical therapist.

Turning Schedules. According to most reports in the nursing literature, immobile patients should be turned and repositioned every 2 hours, but there is little research to show that this schedule is therapeutic for all

---

Guidelines for Moving Patients

- Assess patients' abilities and limitations.
- Medicate patient to provide optimal pain relief.
- Organize environment and request needed help to ensure safety.
- Explain what you are going to do and how you expect the patient to help.
- Permit patient to do as much as capabilities allow.
- Consider safety precautions (e.g., lock wheels, use transfer belt).
- Use good body mechanics.
- Keep movements smooth and rhythmic.
- Prevent trauma (e.g., friction against skin, pulling joints, grabbing muscles).
- Check patient for proper body alignment and comfort and provide patient with call bell before leaving.

patients. More frequent turning may be needed. Significant factors include the amount of adipose tissue, skeletal structure, underlying pathophysiology, comfort level, skin condition, and level of mobility. Assessing for skin condition and signs of pressure is important in determining the turning schedule. Decreased capillary refill and blanched or reddened areas indicate the need for more frequent turning.

Turning schedules should be incorporated in the care plan and posted at the bedside (Fig. 29-6). This helps ensure consistency of care between different shifts. In extended-care facilities, where many patients require frequent position changes, a specific rotation pattern may be developed to ensure that various positions are used in an orderly fashion.

Positions. Body positions often used in immobile patients are supine, high-Fowler's, semi-Fowler's, prone, side-lying, and Sims' (Table 29-3). Consider the benefits and contraindications of each position when making nursing decisions about positioning (see Procedure 29-2). Unless contraindicated, patients should be moved to a chair twice a day.

Regardless of the specific position, general principles of body mechanics should be used in any position change. Proper body alignment must be maintained, and all body parts must be supported. Pressure, especially over body prominences, should be avoided by adequately padding these areas. Such positioning aids as pillows, splints, footboards, and foam rubber or sheepskin protectors are helpful (Table 29-4).

Organizational skills are required in turning and positioning patients:

- Think through the task before beginning.
- Ensure that all needed equipment is within easy reach.

- Decide whether help from other staff members will be needed, and ensure they are in the room before beginning the position change. If there is a possibility that help may be needed, always request it.
- Explain to the patient exactly what will happen before beginning the position change.
- Enlist the patient's assistance whenever possible, giving instructions and encouragement as necessary.
- When the position change has been completed, ask if the patient is comfortable. Reposition as necessary.
- Tell the patient how long he or she will remain in the position. Provide a call light within easy reach.
- Document position changes and the patient's tolerance of specific positions in the chart.

Logrolling. Logrolling is a technique used for patients who have had surgery or an injury involving the back or spine. To prevent further trauma and injury, the body must be moved as a unit so that the spinal column does not bend or twist. Instruct the patient to keep his or her body as stiff as possible and to avoid any sudden moves during the procedure. A draw sheet can be helpful in logrolling patients smoothly, especially if they are obese. When turning, pillows are placed between the legs; they are left in place if the patient remains in the side-lying position.

Hip Fractures. When turning patients who have had hip surgery, take special care to prevent adduction of the affected hip and leg. Dislocation of the hip can result from movement of the leg toward or past the midline of the body (adduction). To avoid this, abductor pillows should be used. If unavailable, regular pillows should be placed between the legs and an additional staff member should support the affected leg so that it will not fall, even momentarily, during the move.

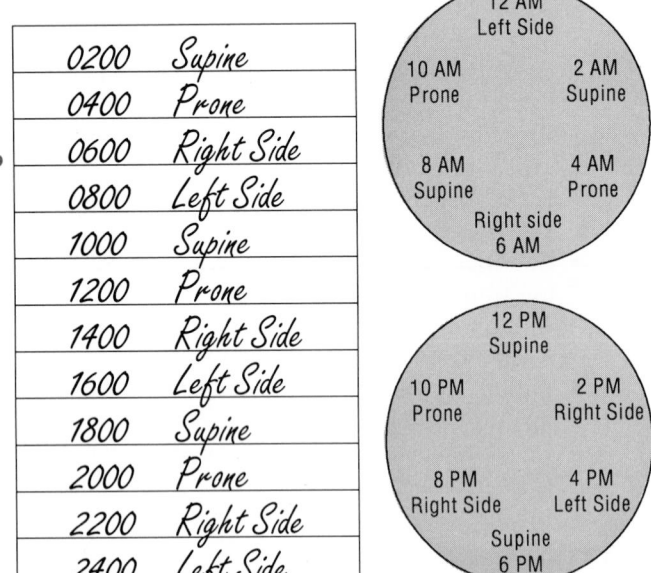

0200	Supine
0400	Prone
0600	Right Side
0800	Left Side
1000	Supine
1200	Prone
1400	Right Side
1600	Left Side
1800	Supine
2000	Prone
2200	Right Side
2400	Left Side

Figure 29–6. Two examples of turning schedules to be posted at the bedside.

TABLE 29–3.

Body Positions for the Immobile Patient

Position	Description	Benefits	Contraindications
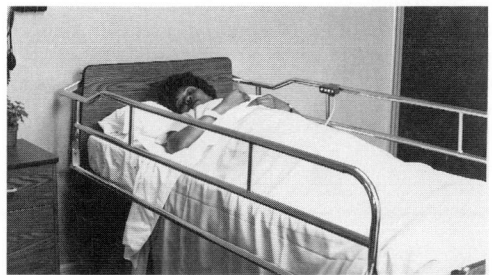 Supine (dorsal recumbent)	Lying on back flat in bed. Pillows may be used under head, knees, and calves to keep heels off mattress.	Alternative position for patients on bedrest; position of choice for patients after spinal surgery and some spinal anesthesia.	Dyspnea, patients at risk for aspiration
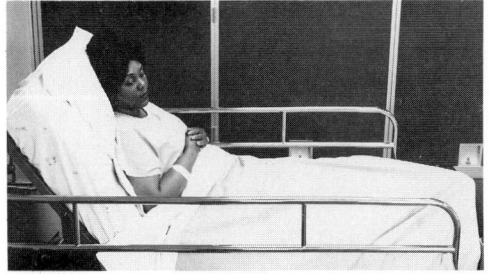 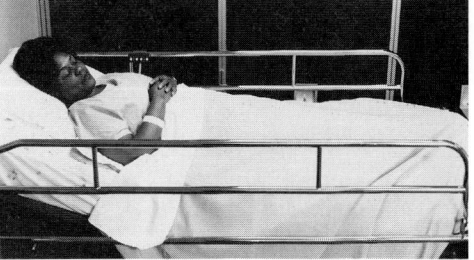 Fowlers' (80° to 90°) Semi-Fowlers' (45°)	Head of bed is raised 45° to 90° and patient is in a sitting position in bed. Small pillows can be used under patient's head and arms, and footboard may be used.	Position of choice for patients with dyspnea from respiratory or cardiac problems, since it improves cardiac output and promotes ventilation. Position is good for eating, talking, watching television, etc.	After spinal or brain surgery
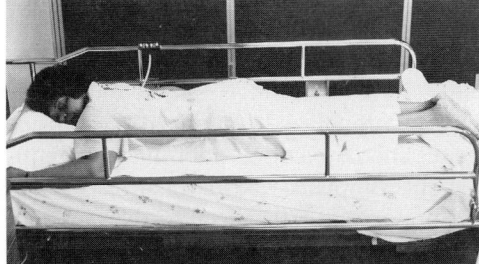 Prone	Lying face-down with head to side and arms over head in flexed position.	Alternative positive for immobilized patient	Abdominal surgery, dyspnea, or other problems of respiratory system or spine
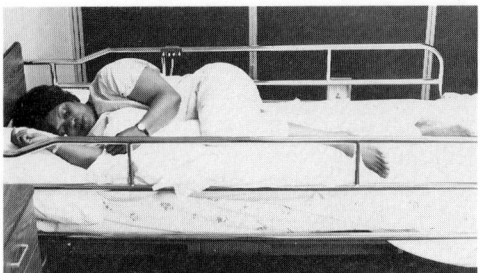 Side-lying (lateral)	Lying on side with most of	Alternative position for im-	Orthopedic surgery, espe-

(continued)

TABLE 29–3.

(continued)

Position	Description	Benefits	Contraindications
	weight distributed to dependent hip and shoulder. Pillows are used to support uppermost leg, arm, and head and are placed behind the back to keep patient on side.	mobilized patient. Relieves pressure from bony prominences on the back. Position of choice for patients with sacral decubitus ulcers.	cially on affected side of hip replacement
Sims' (semiprone)	Lying on side with weight distributed toward anterior ileum, humerus, and clavicle. In this side position, the patient is more prone than in the side-lying position. Legs and arms are flexed and supported with pillows.	Similar to side-lying position	Any spine or orthopedic condition that could be jeopardized by this position

Joint Mobility Maintenance

Each joint's mobility is maintained by normal body movements that exercise the joint within its full ROM. Our daily activities are full of intricate movements that exercise each joint fully. But when mobility is altered, joints stiffen. If this process continues, the joint becomes fixed (a contracture) and movement becomes difficult or impossible. Nursing interventions are aimed at maintaining joint mobility and preventing contractures.

Types of ROM. A patient who can perform ROM unassisted is said to have **active range of motion.** A patient who needs the nurse to perform ROM is said to have **passive range of motion.** Assistive range of motion is when the patient can participate in ROM with assistance. For example, after a cerebral vascular accident the patient may have weakness on one side of the body. With direction, the patient may use the strong muscles on the unaffected side to exercise the weaker muscles on the affected side.

General Principles of ROM Exercises. ROM exercises should be initiated as soon as possible, since changes in affected joints can occur after only 4 days of impaired

mobility. Allow the patient to participate as fully as he or she can. Perform ROM exercises in a systematic order at a designated time each day (most likely during morning care). For high-risk patients, ROM may be indicated more frequently. In some facilities, physical therapists perform ROM for immobilized patients at the bedside.

ROM exercises should be done smoothly and gently. Stop if the patient complains of pain or if resistance is encountered. Support the joint distal to the one being exercised. A physician's order and specific instructions should be obtained to perform ROM for patients with acute arthritis, fractures, torn ligaments, joint dislocation, or acute myocardial infarction. Procedure 29-3 outlines the technique.

Automatic ROM Equipment. Mechanical devices have been developed to provide continuous ROM to a specific joint. Such devices are most commonly used after orthopedic surgery, when such exercise promotes joint mobility and permits rapid rehabilitation. The equipment extends the joint to a prescribed angle for a prescribed period of time, continuously cycling according to parameters set by the physician or physical therapist.

(Text continues on page 726)

PROCEDURE 29–2. Positioning a Patient in Bed

■ Purpose
1. Maintain skin integrity and prevent deformities of the musculoskeletal system.
2. Maintain proper body alignment.
3. Provide comfort.
4. Maintain optimal position for ventilation and lung expansion.

■ Assessment
- Assess patient's body alignment and comfort level in current position.
- Review chart for conditions that influence ability to move or to be positioned (i.e., fractures, paralysis, spinal injury).
- Assess for presence of tubes, lines, incisions, or other equipment that may alter the positioning procedure.
- Assess patient's level of consciousness and ability to understand and follow directions.
- Assess patient's ability to assist with positioning.
- Assess patient's weight and your strength. Determine if additional assistance is needed.

■ Equipment
Pillows.
Draw sheet or turning sheet.
Siderails.

■ Procedure

Moving a patient up in bed (one nurse)
1. Explain procedure and rationale to patient.
   Rationale: Reduces anxiety and increases cooperation.
2. Lower head of bed to flat position and raise level of bed to comfortable working height.
   Rationale: Decreases gravitational pull of upper body and promotes good body mechanics by decreasing back strain.
3. Remove all pillows from under patient. Leave one at head of bed.
   Rationale: Prevents accidental head injury against top of bed frame.
4. Instruct patient to bend legs, put feet flat on bed, and place arm nearest you under your arm and around your shoulder.
5. Place your feet in broad stance with one foot in front of the other. Flex your knees and thighs.
   Rationale: Lowers center of gravity and ensures using large muscle groups of legs.
6. Place one arm under patient's shoulders and one arm under thighs.
   Rationale: Provides support to the heaviest parts of patient's body.

7. Rock back and forth on front and back leg to count of three. On third count, patient pushes with feet as you lift and pull patient up in bed.
   Rationale: Rocking motion helps develop momentum, which provides a smooth lift of patient with minimal use of energy by the nurse.
8. Elevate head of bed and place pillows under head. Raise siderails and lower bed to lowest level.
   Rationale: Provides for patient comfort and safety.

■ Procedure

Moving helpless patient up in bed (two nurses)
1. Explain procedure and rationale to patient.
   Rationale: Reduces anxiety and increases cooperation.
2. Lower head of bed to flat position and raise level of bed to comfortable working height.
   Rationale: Decreases gravitational pull of upper body and decreases back strain.
3. Remove all pillows from under patient. Leave one at head of bed.
   Rationale: Prevents accidental head injury against top of bed frame.
4. One nurse stands on each side of bed with wide base of support and one foot slightly in front of the other.
5. Each nurse rolls up and grasps edges of turn sheet close to patient's shoulders and buttocks.
   Rationale: Turn sheet is used to distribute patient's weight and prevents shearing injury to skin by reducing friction during move.

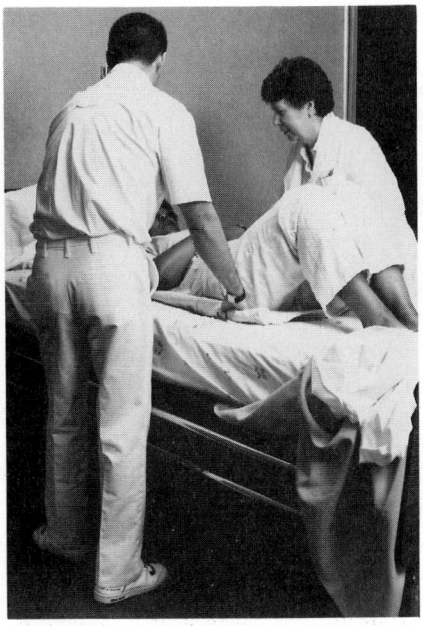

Step 5

(continued)

PROCEDURE 29–2. Positioning a Patient in Bed *(continued)*

6. Flex knees and hips. Tighten abdominal and gluteal muscles.
   Rationale: Prevents back injury by using large muscle groups of legs during transfer.
7. Rock back and forth on front and back leg to count of three. On third count, both nurses shift weight to front leg as they simultaneously lift patient toward head of bed.
   Rationale: Rocking motion develops momentum, which provides a smooth lift of patient with minimal energy use by nurses.
8. Elevate head of bed and place pillows under patient's head. Adjust other positioning pillows as necessary. Put up siderails and lower bed to lowest level.
   Rationale: Provides for patient comfort and safety.

■ **Procedure**

Positioning patient in side-lying position
1. Lower head of bed as flat as patient can tolerate.
   Rationale: Patient turns easier from flat position.
2. Elevate and lock siderail on side patient will face when turned.
   Rationale: Prevents accidental injury from falling out of bed during turn.
3. Place arm that patient will turn toward away from his or her body. Fold other arm across chest.
   Rationale: Facilitates turning by preventing patient from rolling onto bottom arm.
4. Flex patient's knee that will not be next to mattress after turn.

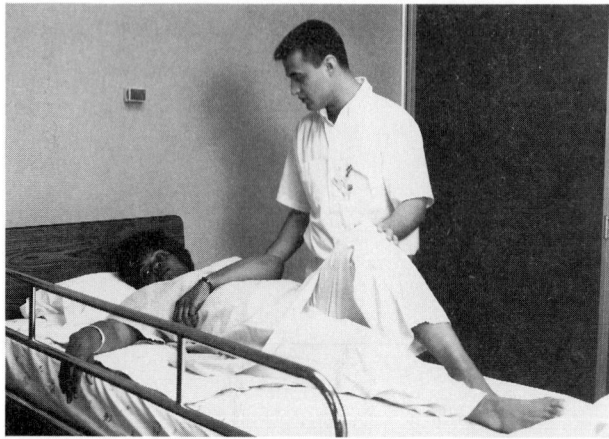

Step 3 and 4

5. Lock siderail. Go around to other side of bed.
6. Assume a broad stance with knees slightly flexed.
   Rationale: Increases balance, lowers center of gravity, and encourages use of large muscle groups during movement.

7. Place one hand on patient's hip and one hand on his or her far shoulder.
   Rationale: Allows you to support heaviest part of patient during turn.
8. Roll patient toward you.

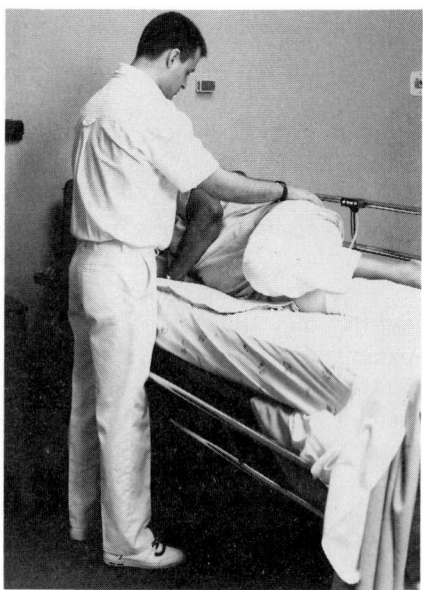

Step 7

9. Align patient properly and place pillow under head.
10. Pull shoulder blade forward and out from under patient. Support upper arm with pillow.
    Rationale: Protects joints from weight and strain. Ventilation may also improve because chest can expand more fully.
11. Fold a pillow lengthwise or roll a towel or bath blanket and tuck behind patient's back.
    Rationale: Provides support to keep patient on his or her side.
12. Place pillow lengthwise between patient's legs from thighs to foot.

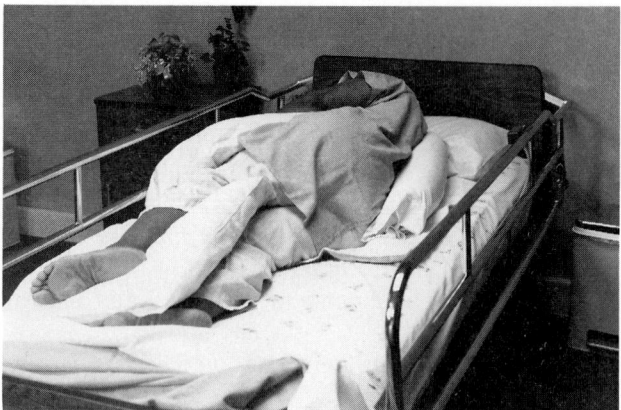

Step 12   *(continued)*

PROCEDURE 29–2. Positioning a Patient in Bed (continued)

Rationale: Maintains leg in alignment and prevents pressure on bony prominences.

■ Procedure

Logrolling

1. Obtain assistance. Two or three nurses are usually required.
2. All nurses stand on same side of bed, with feet apart, one foot slightly ahead of the other. Flex knees and hips.
   Rationale: Increases balance and stability. Ensures use of large muscle groups when turning patient.
3. Place one pillow to support head during and after turn.
   Rationale: Pillow maintains alignment of cervical spine.
4. Place pillows between patient's legs.
   Rationale: Supports the upper leg and prevents adduction during turn.

5. Reach across patient and support head, thorax, trunk, and legs.
6. On count of three, roll patient in one coordinated movement to lateral position.
   Rationale: Maintains alignment of whole body during turn.
7. Support patient in alignment with pillows as described in "Side-lying position."
   Note: Patients with suspected or known spinal injuries should wear cervical collars whenever turning or moving in bed to prevent injury to the spinal cord.

■ Home-Care Modifications

• Caregivers must be taught principles of body alignment and the types of supportive devices used to support and maintain the body in alignment.
• Caregivers need to be aware of devices used to protect bony prominences and prevent pressure sores (i.e., sheepskins, foam mattresses, heel and elbow protectors).

TABLE 29–4.

Positioning Aids

Aid	Purpose	Nursing Considerations
Pillow (feather, foam, or fiber-filled); various sizes	Elevates body part. Supports patient on side. Prevents pressure on skin. Increases comfort by decreasing stress and strain on body parts.	Use pillows small enough to maintain proper body alignment. Assess for allergies to feathers before using.
Bed cradle	Keeps pressure of linen off feet	Position properly over feet.

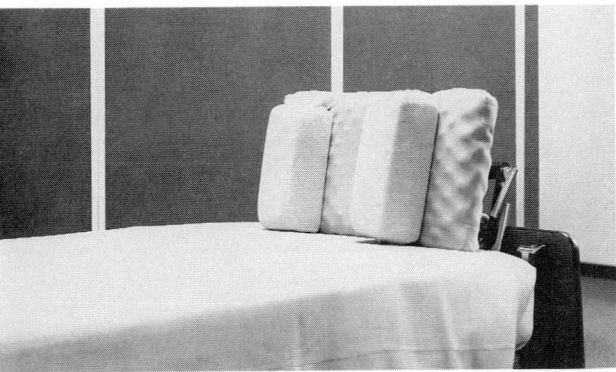

Footboard	Maintains dorsiflexion of the feet, preventing foot drop. If board has antirotation blocks, it can also prevent hip rotation.	Pad board with bath blanket. Position patient's heels over mattress or use heel protectors.
Trochanter roll	Prevents external rotation of legs when in a supine position	Trochanter roll should be placed from patient's iliac crest to mid-thigh. Can be made by rolling bath blanket.

(continued)

TABLE 29–4.

(continued)

Aid	Purpose	Nursing Considerations
Hand roll	Keeps hand in functional position. Prevents finger contractures.	Roll should be large enough to prevent finger flexion and keep thumb in opposition. Rolled washcloth may be used if manufactured hand roll is unavailable.
Hand-wrist splint	Keeps arm and hand in normal functioning position (slight adduction of thumb and dorsiflexion of wrist)	Individually made for each patient. Pad inside of splint. Remove every 4 hours to check for pressure areas.
Heel or elbow protectors (sheepskin or foam)	Reduces mattress pressure on heels or elbows. Helps remove elbow friction when patient moves in bed.	Launder as necessary. Remove every 4 hours to check for pressure areas.
Abduction pillow	Maintains hip abduction after hip surgery	Pad pillow straps. Remove every 4 hours to assess for pressure points. Check pedal pulse to detect interference with circulation.

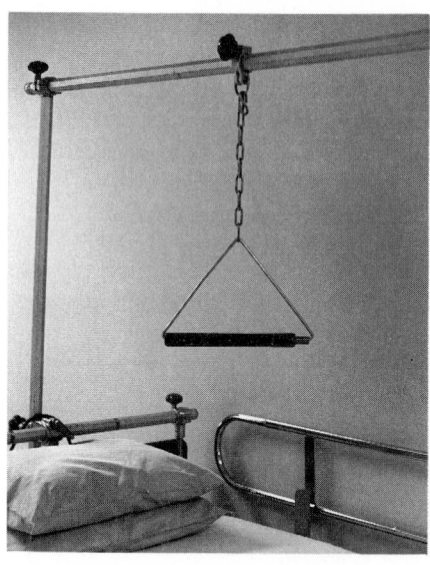

Aid	Purpose	Nursing Considerations
Trapeze bar	Helps patient raise trunk from bed. Allows patient to help in transfers and position changes. Allows patient to strengthen upper arms through exercise.	Teach patient how to use the bar. Avoid hitting your head when you are assisting patient with care.
Siderail	Helps weak patient turn independently. Protects patient from falling out of bed.	Keep in raised position to aid patient mobility and ensure patient safety.
Turn sheet	Helps reposition patient. Can be secured to siderail to support patient in side-lying position.	Position from mid-thorax to below hips. Roll sheet close to patient to obtain better support. Can be made from bath blankets if manufactured models are unavailable.

Ambulation

Early ambulation is significant in reducing complications of immobility. Walking exercises almost all body muscles and promotes joint flexibility. Most surgical patients are permitted to get out of bed and walk on their first postoperative day. Early ambulation significantly reduces the formation of venous clots and atelectasis, thus decreasing respiratory and circulatory complications after surgery. Even a short period of immobility decreases a patient's exercise tolerance, so assistance is often required when walking is resumed. Musculoskeletal or neurologic alterations often require temporary or permanent assistance with ambulation (see Procedure 29-4).

- When transferring a patient to a wheelchair, make sure the wheels are locked to avoid chair movement and possible falls.
- To avoid injury to the caregiver when a patient starts to fall, gently guide the person to the floor rather than attempting to hold the patient up.
- Take postural blood pressures before getting patients up to decrease the chance of falling due to postural hypotension.
- Use ambulation belts when transferring or ambulating patients who are likely to fall.
- Obtain needed help when transferring or ambulating patients; working independently can risk injury to the patient and the caregiver.
- When performing ROM, discontinue movement if the patient complains of pain. Damage could occur if stiff areas are overextended.
- When turning and positioning patients, always keep siderails up if a staff member is not there to prevent falls.
- Make sure all patients who need assistance with mobility have their call lights at all times. Instruct them to call for the nurse if they need to ambulate.
- Keep rooms free of clutter and provide adequate lighting to prevent falls.

Assisting the Patient. Assisting the patient to ambulate safely begins by thoroughly assessing his or her muscle strength and coordination.

First, assist the patient to a sitting position on the side of the bed. Adjust the bed to a high-Fowler's position and help the patient swing his or her legs over the side of the bed. If the patient complains of dizziness, is diaphoretic, or has a postural drop in blood pressure, postpone ambulation. If dangling is well tolerated, ambulation can proceed.

Have the patient wear shoes or slippers with nonskid soles and clear the path of obstacles that might cause the patient to trip. Hallways often have railings the patient can grip. A weak or unstable patient may prefer to push a chair or wheelchair to provide extra support and balance. Encourage the patient to look straight ahead to promote balance and prevent dizziness.

All equipment (IV tubing, Foley catheters, drains) must be attached to a pole. The nurse assisting the patient should not carry equipment, so that his or her hands are free if the patient should fall. The Foley catheter must be kept below bladder level during ambulation.

Watch IV lines carefully. Often the change in position decreases the distance between the bottle and the infusion site. Since gravitational force is decreased, the flow rate can be affected. This usually causes blood to flow up the IV tubing. Unless corrected by readjusting the flow rate, blood will clot at the infusion site and the IV will have to be restarted. Encourage the patient to keep the arm in which the IV is infusing at the side rather than using it to push the IV pole. Nasogastric suction can usually be discontinued while the patient is ambulating and reconnected on return to the room.

While walking, assess the patient for steadiness of gait, diaphoresis, and complaints of fatigue. Pulse and respiratory rate should be monitored before and after ambulation to determine cardiorespiratory response to exercise.

Transfer Belts. Transfer belts (sometimes called safety belts or ambulation belts) should be used if the patient is weak or has problems with coordination. The transfer belt is a canvas belt that can be applied around the waist and tightened over clothing (see Procedure 29-4). The nurse grips the transfer belt as the patient walks so that he or she can provide aid should the patient begin to fall. If the patient becomes dizzy or starts to fall, slowly and gently lower the patient to the floor and call for help (Fig. 29-7). If the patient is at high risk for falls, two nurses may be required to assist with ambulation.

Mechanical Aids. Mechanical devices can help the patient with certain limitations to ambulate safely. Walkers, canes, quad canes, and crutches are helpful in bearing a portion of the patient's weight during ambulation. This helps promote stability and maintain balance. The physical therapist is usually responsible for the initial instruction in the use of these devices, but often the patient requires additional instruction or supervision.

Canes are useful for patients who can bear weight but who need support for balance, or who have decreased strength in one leg. The cane acts as an additional "leg" that provides the patient with three points of support during ambulation. The cane is held in the hand opposite to the weak or injured leg. The affected or weak foot is moved forward with the cane as the weight of the body remains on the stronger extremity (Fig. 29-8). When climbing stairs, the strongest leg advances up the stair first, followed by the cane and the weaker leg. This process is reversed when descending stairs: the cane and the weaker leg are followed by the stronger leg. Instruct the patient to look straight ahead rather than at the feet while walking.

Canes are made of wood or metal and should be about waist high. A variety of canes are available, ranging from a simple straight-leg cane to a three- or four-pronged cane (often called a quad cane).

Walkers are lightweight, tubular metal structures that

PROCEDURE 29–3. Providing Range-of-Motion Exercises

■ Purpose
1. Maintain joint mobility.
2. Improve or maintain muscle strength.
3. Prevent muscle atrophy and contractures.

■ Assessment
- Review medical history to determine specific limitations to joint mobility.
- Assess patient's level of consciousness and physical ability to assist or independently perform range-of-motion exercises.
- Assess for redness, tenderness, pain, swelling, or deformities around joints.

■ Equipment
No special equipment is required except a bed.

■ Procedure
1. Explain procedure and rationale to patient.
   Rationale: Reduces anxiety and encourages cooperation.
2. Position patient on back with head of bed as flat as possible. Elevate bed to comfortable working height.
   Rationale: Promotes proper body mechanics to prevent muscle strain for nurse.
3. Stand on side of bed of joints to be exercised. Uncover only limb to be exerised.
   Rationale: Provides warmth and privacy.
4. Perform exercises slowly and gently, providing support by holding areas proximal and distal to the joint.
   Rationale: Prevents discomfort and muscle spasms from jerky movements.
5. Repeat exercises to each joint five times.
   Note: Discontinue or decrease ROM if patient complains of discomfort or muscle spasm.
6. Neck:
   a. Bring chin to chest.
   b. Bend head toward back.

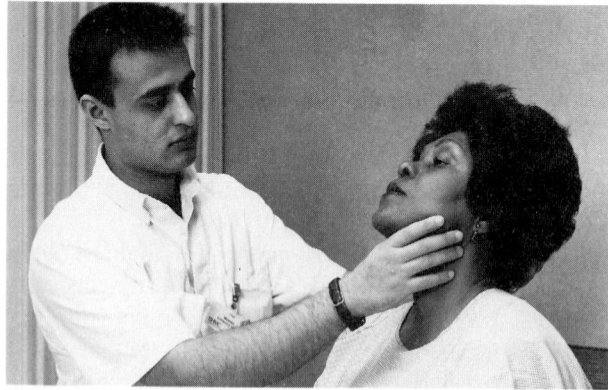

Step 6B

c. Tilt head toward each shoulder.

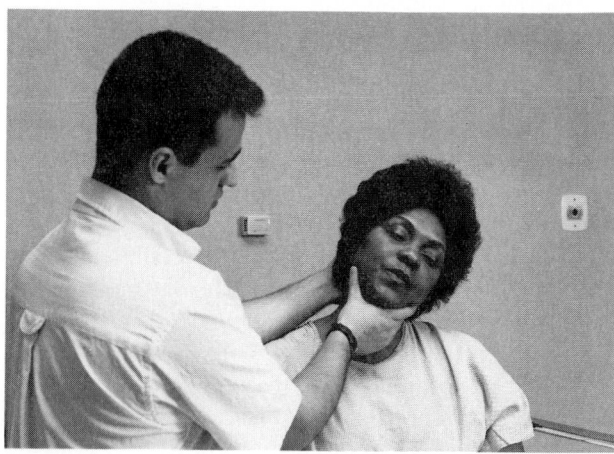

Step 6C

   d. Rotate head in circular motion.
   e. Return to erect position.
7. Shoulder:
   a. Raise arm from side to above head.
   b. Abduct and rotate shoulder by raising arm above head with palm up.
   c. Adduct shoulder by moving arm across body as far as possible.
   d. Rotate shoulder internally and exernally by flexing elbow and moving forearm to touch palm on mattress, then up until back of hand touches mattress.
   e. Move shoulder in a full circle.
8. Elbow:
   a. Bend elbow toward shoulder.

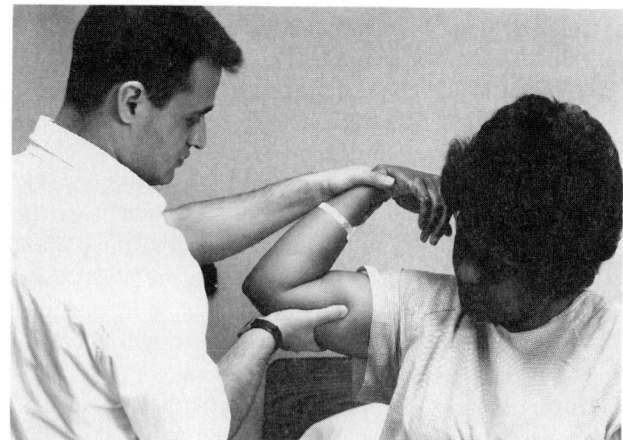

Step 8A

(continued)

PROCEDURE 29–3. Providing Range-of-Motion Exercises *(continued)*

b. Hyperextend elbow as far as possible.

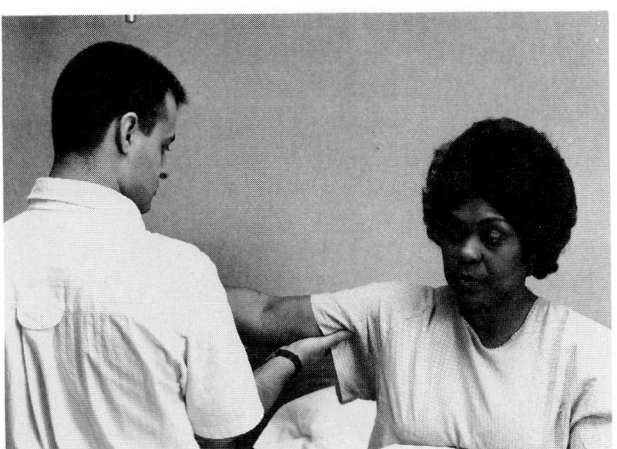

Step 8B

9. Wrist and hand:
   a. Move hand toward inner aspect of forearm.
   b. Bend dorsal surface of hand backwad.
   c. Abduct wrist by bending toward thumb.
   d. Adduct wrist by bending toward fifth finger.
   e. Make a fist, then extend the fingers.
   f. Spread fingers apart, then together.
   g. Move thumb across hand to base of fifth finger.
10. Hip and knee:
    a. Lift leg and bend knee toward chest.
    b. Abduct and adduct leg, moving leg laterally away from body and returning to medial position.
    c. Internally and externally rotate hip by turning leg inward, then outward.
    d. Special care should be taken to support joints of larger limbs.
11. Ankle and foot:
    a. Dorsiflex foot by moving foot so toes point upward.

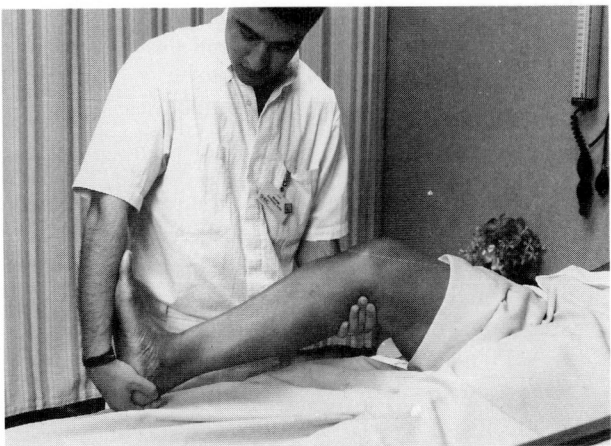

Step 11A

b. Plantarflex by moving foot so toes point downward.
c. Curl toes down, then extend.

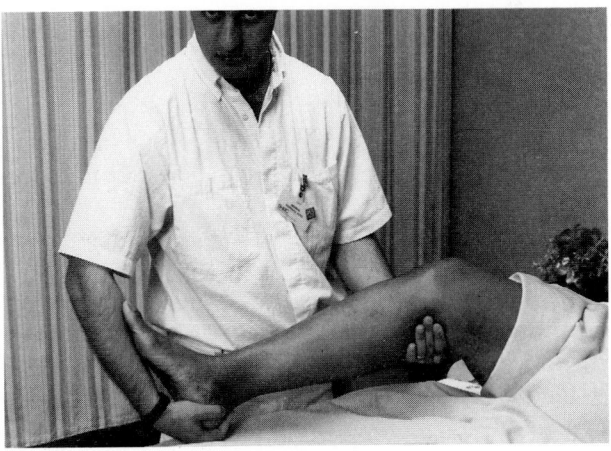

Step 11C

d. Spread toes apart, then bring together.
e. Invert by turning sole of foot medially.
f. Evert by turning sole of foot laterally.
12. Move to other side of bed and repeat exercises.
13. Reposition patient to position of comfort.
14. Document ROM.

provide more support than canes. Walkers have a wide base of support from four rubber-tipped legs. The patient grips the walker, picks it up, and moves it forward. The patient may use a two-point or three-point gait when ambulating with the walker. Clear hallways of any obstructions. Some walkers have wheels and a seat so that if patients become fatigued, they can sit and propel themselves by pushing with their feet.

Crutches allow the patient to walk without weight-bearing. Crutches may be indicated when the patient has a sprain, fracture, or a nonwalking cast. Underarm crutches are most commonly used for these short-term

PROCEDURE 29-4. Assisting with Ambulation

■ Purpose
1. Increase muscle strength and joint mobility.
2. Prevent complications of immobility.
3. Promote self-esteem and independence.

■ Assessment
- Review chart for conditions that impair ambulation (arthritis, fractures, paralysis) and for physician's orders for ambulation or ambulating aids (walkers, canes, crutches).
- Assess comfort level. Medicate as ordered with analgesics. Plan ambulation for time when analgesics have peak action.
- Assess range of motion and muscle strength. Determine if extra assistance is required.
- Obtain baseline vital signs. Obtain orthostatic vital signs if patient has been on prolonged bedrest.

■ Equipment
Ambulation aid (crutches, cane, walker) if required.
Transfer belt (optional).
Robe.
Well-fitting shoes or slippers with nonslip soles.

■ Procedure
1. Explain procedure and rationale for ambulation to patient. Decide together how far and where to ambulate.
   Rationale: Reduces anxiety and facilitates cooperation.
2. Place bed in lowest position.
3. Assist patient to sitting position on side of bed. Assess for dizziness or faintness. Obtain orthostatic vital signs if complaints are present. Allow patient to remain in this position until he or she feels secure.
   Rationale: Minimizes orthostatic hypotension and resulting falls or injury.
4. Help patient don robe and footwear.

■ Procedure

One nurse
1. Wrap transfer belt around patient's waist (optional according to previous assessment).
   Rationale: Provides a firm hold for the nurse to prevent injury to the patient.
2. Assist patient to standing position and assess patient's balance. Return to bed or transfer to chair if very weak or unsteady.
3. Position yourself behind patient while supporting him or her by waist or transfer belt.

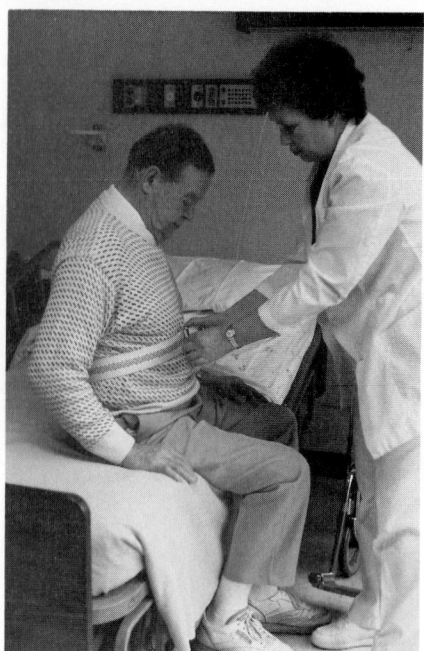

Step 1

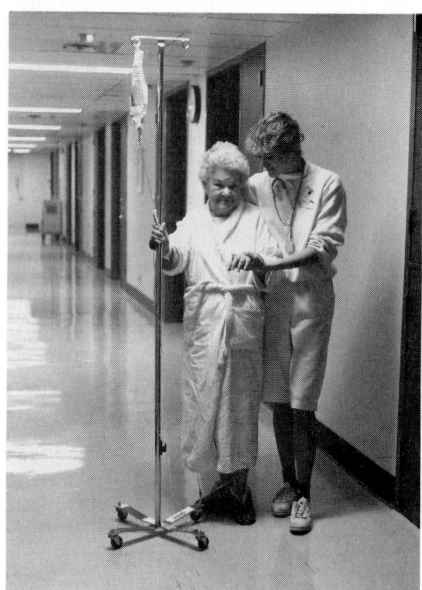

Step 3

Rationale: Allows patient to stand erect and prevents leaning to one side for support from nurse.
4. Take several steps forward with patient, assessing strength and balance.
5. If patient has one-sided weakness, stand on the affected side and provide support by placing arm near-

(continued)

PROCEDURE 29–4. Assisting with Ambulation *(continued)*

est patient around his or her waist. Place other hand around patient's upper arm on affected side.

6. Encourage patient to use good posture and to look ahead, not down at feet.
7. Ambulate for planned distance or time.
8. If patient becomes weak or dizzy, return to bed or assist to chair.
9. If the patient begins to fall, place your feet wide apart with one foot in front. Support the patient by pulling his or her weight backward against your body. Lower gently to floor, protecting head (see Fig. 29-7). *Rationale: Nurse's foot position widens and stabilizes the base of support and enables nurse to support patient's weight with large muscle groups to protect from back strain.*

■ **Procedure**

Two nurses
1. Assist patient to sitting position as described.
2. Assist patient to standing position with one nurse on each side.
3. Each nurse grasps patient's upper arm with the nearest hand and the elbow with the other hand.
   Rationale: Provides firm support by each nurse.
   Note: May use a transfer belt around patient's waist. Each nurse should grasp belt with near hand and elbow with the other hand.
4. Walk with patient using slow, even steps. Assess strength and balance.
   Rationale: Promotes stability of patient.

■ **Procedure**

Using a walker
1. Assist patient to sitting and standing position.
2. Have patient grasp walker handles.

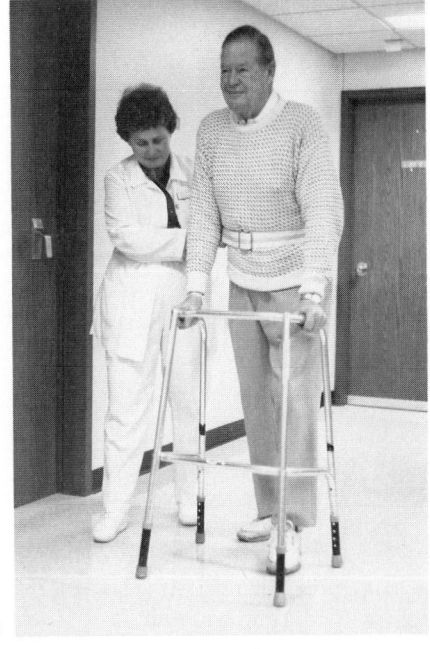

Step 3

3. Patient moves walker ahead 6 to 8 inches, placing all four feet of walker on floor.
4. Patient moves forward to walker.
5. Nurse should walk close behind and slightly to side of patient.
   Rationale: If patient begins to fall, nurse can support him or her and prevent injury.
6. Repeat above sequence until walk is complete.

■ **Home-Care Modifications**
• To provide safety and prevent falls at home, throw rugs and small pieces of furniture should be removed so patient will not trip on them.
• Patient should always wear shoes with nonskid soles.
• The bathroom is a common place for falls and injury. Placing a large rug with a skid-resistant backing on the floor can prevent falls from slipping on wet floors.

purposes. The patient must use the arms to support the body weight, not the shoulders. Using the shoulders can cause skin breakdown at the axilla and nerve damage to the brachial plexus. Underarm crutches must be fitted correctly. There should be 2 inches between the axillae and the top of the crutch when the crutch is placed 2 inches in front of and 6 inches to the side of the foot.

Crutches may also be used to give the support necessary for walking that weak or paralyzed legs cannot provide. For long-term use, Lofstrand crutches, which have metal bands encircling the forearms, are used.

The patient on crutches may use several gaits (see Procedure 29-5):

When the patient can bear partial weight on both feet, the *four-point gait* may be used. The right crutch is placed forward, followed by the left foot, then the left crutch is moved forward, followed by the right foot.

When the patient can bear weight on only one foot, the *three-point gait* is used. Here, both crutches and the weaker leg move forward first, followed by the stronger leg.

The *two-point gait* requires at least partial weight-bearing on each foot, as each crutch moves at the same time as the opposing leg.

The *swing-through gait* is often used by paraplegics, who move both crutches forward, then swing the body

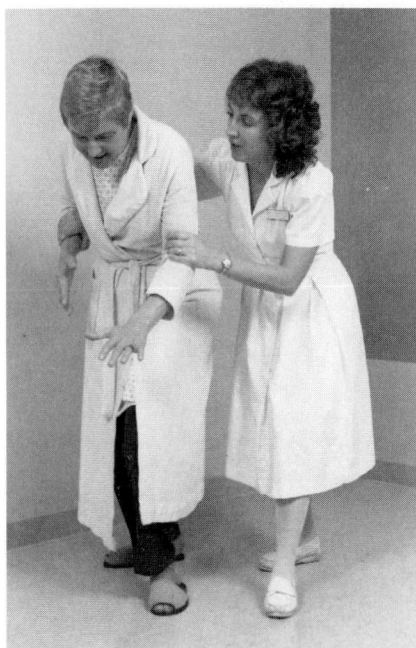
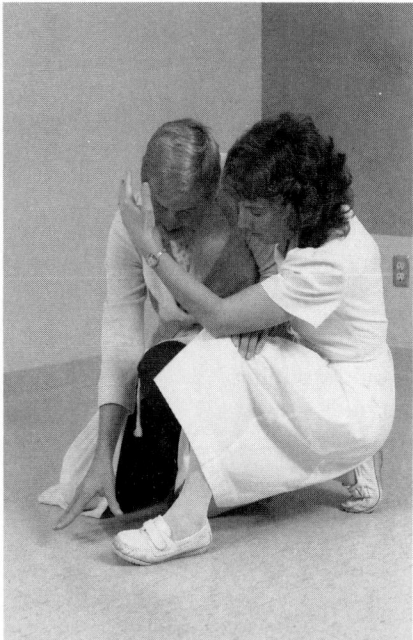
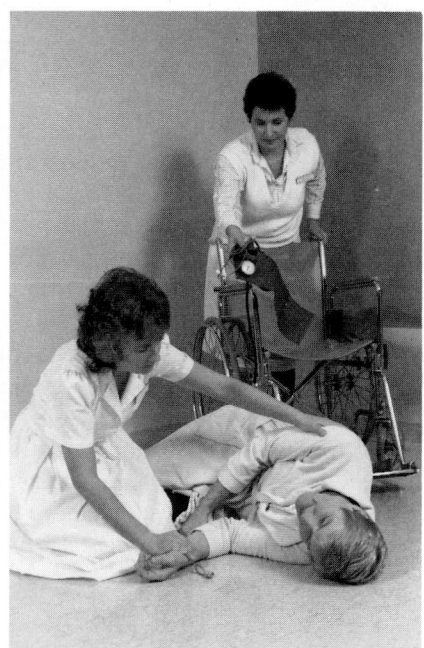

Figure 29–7. Ensure patient safety during a fall by supporting and gently lowering the patient to the ground and then calling for help. Do not try to hold the patient up, as this can result in injury to the nurse.

beyond the crutches to propel themselves forward.

To function independently, the patient on crutches must learn how to rise from a sitting position and climb and descend stairs. This instruction is usually done by a physical therapist. The patient should also be taught to inspect the rubber tips of crutches for wear. Prompt replacement of worn tips can prevent falls.

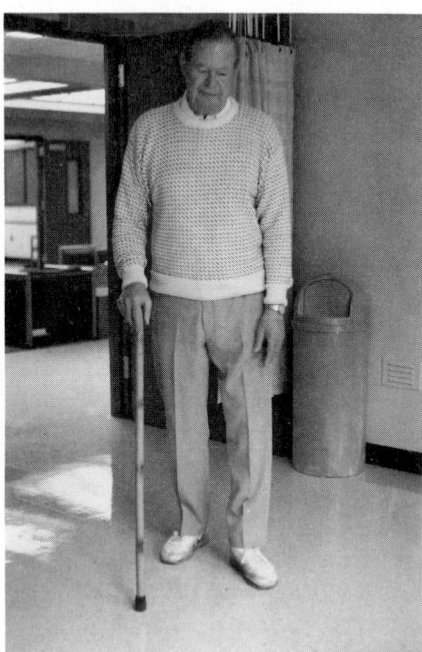

Figure 29–8. Using a cane to ambulate.

Muscle Strengthening to Facilitate Ambulation. Certain muscle groups may need strengthening before some patients can walk. Immobility weakens muscles and can lead to muscle atrophy. Patients on bedrest should be taught to contract their quadriceps, gluteal, and abdominal muscles regularly, since these muscles are important for ambulation. Patients who will use crutches or walkers need to strengthen their arm muscles as well, because increased arm strength will be necessary to support their body weight. *Setting* is a term used to refer to isometric strengthening of muscles. The patient concentrates on one muscle at a time, contracting it for 10 seconds and then permitting it to relax completely. This is repeated a prescribed number of times.

Transfers

Assisted transfers are necessary when the patient is unconscious or extremely weak or has decreased muscle strength or paralysis in the legs. Transfers can involve moving the patient from one flat surface to another, such as from the bed to the stretcher or vice versa (see Procedure 29-6). Another transfer involves moving the patient from the bed to a sitting position, either in a chair or wheelchair (see Procedure 29-7).

Safety is important during transfers. Doing an assessment to identify patient abilities and limitations permits the nurse to individualize the transfer technique and plan for extra help as needed. Use proper body mechanics to prevent injury to patient and nurse. Equipment (transfer belts, transfer boards or sleds, roller

PROCEDURE 29–5. Helping Patients with Crutch Walking

■ Purpose
1. Increase patient's level of activity after musculoskeletal injury.
2. Assist patient to walk safely with crutches using the least amount of energy.

■ Assessment
- Review medical history to determine reason for needing crutches and whether patient is to bear weight on one leg only or can partially bear weight on affected side.
- Assess patient's ability to balance himself or herself.
- Observe for unilateral or unusual weakness.
- Assess muscle strength, especially in legs and arms.
- Determine if patient has past experience with crutch walking.
- Determine appropriate size crutch.

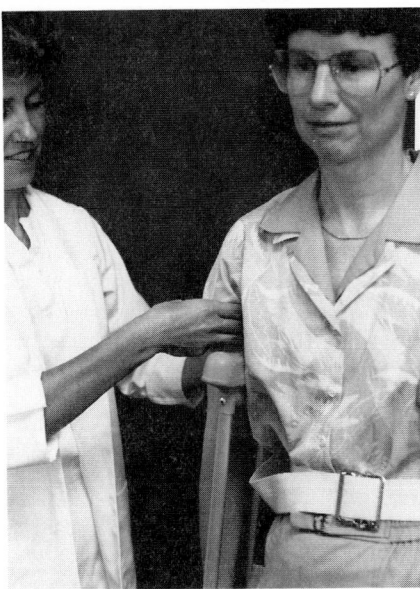

Assessment

■ Equipment
Crutches with suction tips, hand grips, and axillary pads. Shoes with nonskid soles.

■ Procedure

Four-point gait
1. Patient stands erect, face forward in tripod position. Patient places crutch tips 6 inches in front of feet and 6 inches to side of each foot.
   Rationale: This is the position used before crutch walking. It provides a wide base of support so stability and balance are increased.

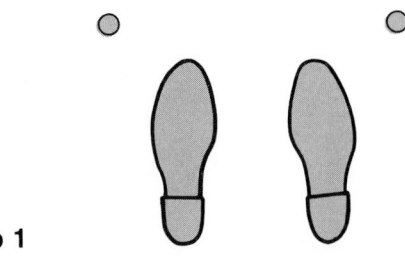

Step 1

2. Patient moves right crutch forward 4 to 6 inches.

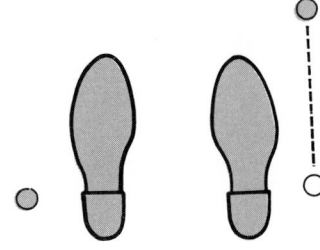

Step 2

3. Patient moves left foot forward to level of right crutch.

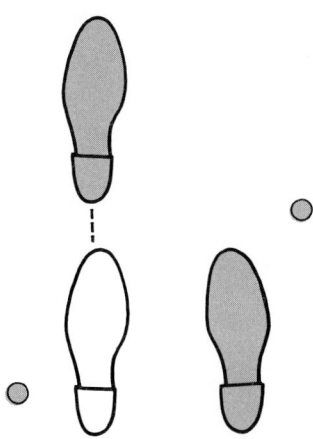

Step 3

4. Patient moves left crutch forward 4 to 6 inches.

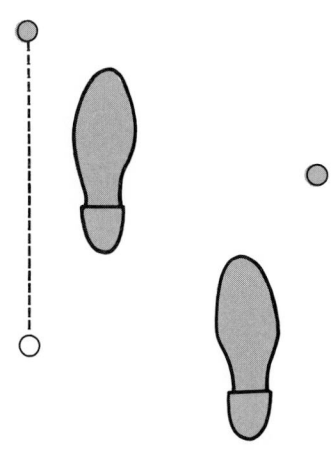

Step 4

(continued)

PROCEDURE 29–5. Helping Patients with Crutch Walking *(continued)*

5. Patient moves right foot forward to level of left crutch.

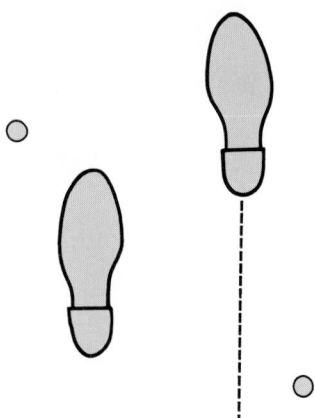

Step 5

6. Repeat sequence.
   Rationale: This gait is the safest and most stable since three points are always on the ground. The crutch and foot positions mimic arm and foot positions during regular walking. The patient must be able to partially bear weight on the affected side to perform this gait.

■ **Procedure**

Three-point gait

1. Beginning in tripod position, patient moves both crutches and affected leg forward.

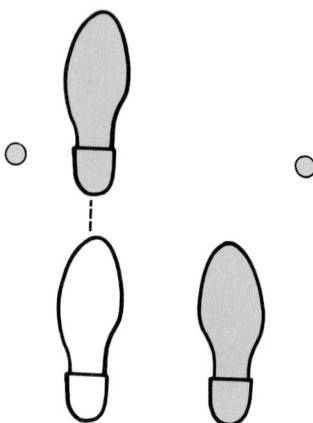

Step 1

2. Patient moves stronger leg forward.
3. Repeat sequence.
   Note: Patient must bear his or her entire weight on the stronger leg to perform this gait.

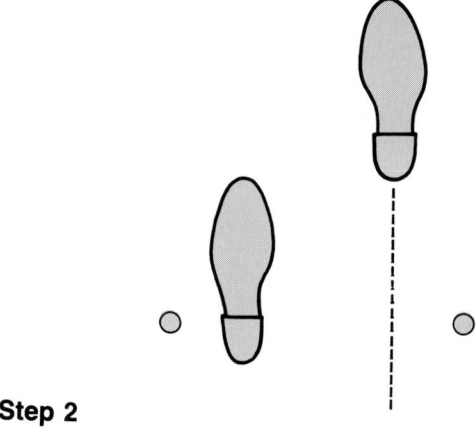

Step 2

■ **Procedure**

Two-point gait

1. Beginning in tripod position, patient moves left crutch and right foot forward.

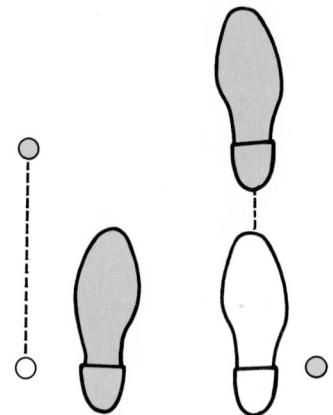

Step 1

2. Patient moves right crutch and left foot forward.

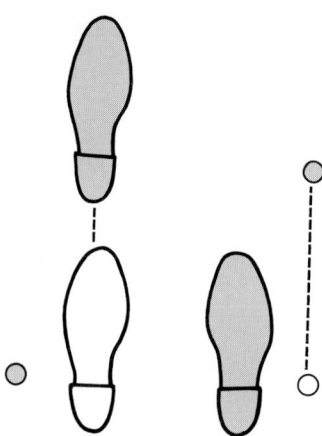

Step 2

3. Repeat sequence.
   Rationale: Crutch and foot movement is similar to arm and leg movement in normal walking. This gait re-

(continued)

quires partial weight-bearing on both feet and is faster than the four-point gait.

■ Procedure

Swinging-to gait

1. Patient forms tripod position and moves both crutches forward.
2. Patient lifts legs and swings to crutches, supporting body weight on crutches.
   Note: Frequently used by patients with paralysis of legs and hips or those wearing weight-supporting braces on their legs.

■ Procedure

Swinging-through gait

1. Patient forms tripod position and moves both crutches forward.
2. Patient lifts legs and swings through and ahead of crutches, supporting weight on crutches.
   Note: Similar to swing-to gait but requires much more strength and coordination.

■ Procedure

Climbing stairs

1. Beginning in tripod position facing stairs, patient transfers body weight to crutches.

2. Patient places unaffected leg on step.
3. Patient transfers body weight to unaffected leg.
4. Patient moves crutches and affected leg to step.
5. Repeat sequence to top of stairs.
   Rationale: The crutches always support the affected leg.

■ Procedure

Descending stairs

1. Patient begins in tripod position facing stairs.
2. Patient transfers body weight to unaffected leg.
3. Patient places crutches onto step and moves affected leg down to stair.
4. Patient transfers body weight to crutches.
5. Patient moves unaffected leg to stair.
6. Repeat sequence to bottom.

■ Lifespan Consideration

- Elderly patients may not have the strength or balance necessary to feel comfortable or safe using crutches. A walker may be preferable.

■ Home-Care Modifications

- The patient using crutches must anticipate problems. If he or she carries books to school or a briefcase to work, a backpack may be a solution until crutches are no longer needed.
- Throw rugs, small pieces of furniture, and toys should be removed from the traffic pattern to provide for safety and ease of walking with crutches.

---

boards, hydraulic lifts) can make transfers easier and safer. Table 29-5 describes common aids.

Two-Person or Three-Person Lifts. Lifts or carries by staff are seldom used in hospitals because they are usually uncomfortable for the patient and pose safety risks for the nurse. However, such carries can be used in emergencies or when the patient being transferred is light. When lifting a patient, place the patient's arms over the chest and have one person available to lift each body area. When moving the patient to another flat surface, one nurse grasps the patient under the head and shoulders, one under the hips, and a third under the thighs and legs. If the patient is being lifted to a chair, one nurse holds the patient under the arms around the chest and the second supports the hips and legs. Synchronize the lift by counting to three. Using proper body mechanics is essential to prevent injury to the lifters.

Hydraulic Lifts. A hydraulic lift is a mechanical device that permits a patient to be transferred from the bed

to a chair (Fig. 29-9). It is used when transferring a patient may pose a safety risk to the patient or the nurse. The lift has a canvas or fabric sling that fits under the patient and hooks into a metal frame. Before using any hydraulic device, read the manufacturer's guidelines for proper operation. The patient may become frightened when lifted away from the bed, so provide verbal support.

Discharge Planning and Home Care

Preparation for discharge and successful home management is an important goal for every patient with mobility problems. This preparation should begin when the patient is admitted and should continue throughout the hospitalization. Waiting until just before the patient is ready to go home is unwise.

Much teaching is aimed at helping the patient learn to use special equipment and to live with any motor limita-

(Text continues on page 740)

PROCEDURE 29–6. Transferring a Patient to a Stretcher

■ **Purpose**

Transfer a patient without injury to nurse or patient.

■ **Assessment**

• Review medical history for conditions that influence or contraindicate ability to move (i.e., fractures, paralysis, spinal injury, generalized muscle weakness, cardiac or respiratory disease that limits exertion).
• Assess patient's range of motion and muscle strength.
• Assess cognitive function or ability to understand and follow directions.
• Assess comfort level. Medicate as ordered with analgesics.
• Assess patient's weight and your strength. Determine if assistance is needed.

■ **Equipment**

Stretcher.
Transfer sled.

■ **Procedure**

1. Explain procedure and rationale to patient.
   Rationale: Reduces anxiety and increases cooperation.
2. Place stretcher parallel to bed.
3. Raise bed to same level as stretcher. Lower siderails. Lock wheels on bed.
4. One or two nurses stand on side of bed without stretcher. Two nurses stand on side of bed with stretcher.
5. Loosen draw sheet on both sides of bed.
   Rationale: Draw sheet assists in transferring patient.
6. Nurses on side without stretcher help patient to roll toward them onto his or her side. May use draw sheet to pull patient onto side or use logrolling technique.
7. Nurses on stretcher side of bed slide sled board under draw sheet and under patient's buttocks and back.

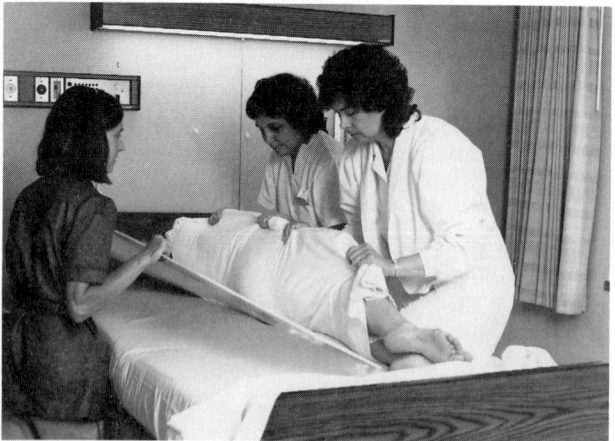

Step 7

8. Roll patient onto sled board into supine position. Place patient's arms across his or her chest.
   Rationale: Prevents injury to arms during transfer.
9. Move stretcher parallel to bed and lock wheels.
10. Nurses on stretcher side of bed assume a broad stance.
    Rationale: Provides a stable base of support.
11. Wrap end of draw sheet over curved end of sled board and slide patient onto stretcher on count of three.
    Rationale: Provides smooth motion for transfer.

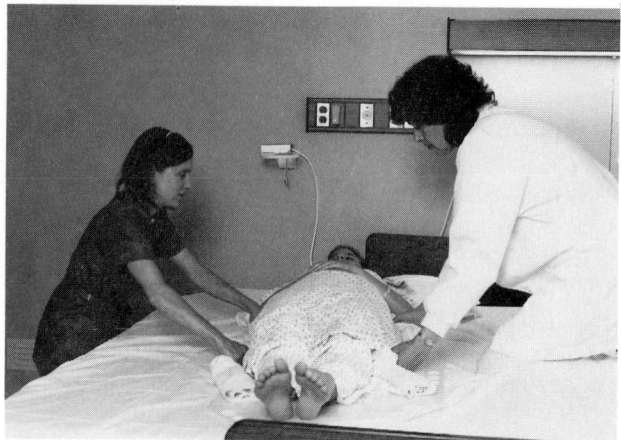

Step 11

12. Lock siderails up on bed side of stretcher and move stretcher away from bed.
    Rationale: Provides for patient's safety.

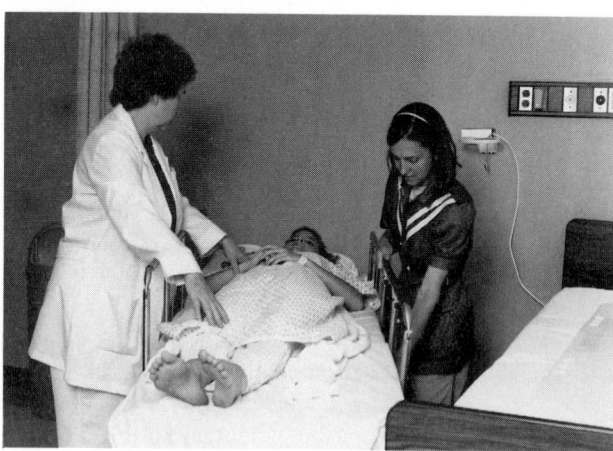

Step 12

13. Roll patient slightly up onto side and pull sled board out from under him or her.
14. Lock other siderails up on stretcher.

(continued)

PROCEDURE 29–6. Transferring a Patient to a Stretcher *(continued)*

---

15. Place cover over patient and lock safety belts across patient's chest and waist. Adjust head of stretcher according to patient limitations.
    Rationale: Provides for comfort, warmth, and safety.

■ **Lifespan Considerations**

Infants and Children
• Infants can be safety moved by one person.

• Children may be moved by one or two people.

Adults
• Depending on level of musculoskeletal function, adults may be able to slide onto a stretcher with minimal assistance.

PROCEDURE 29–7. Transferring a Patient to a Wheelchair

■ **Purpose**
1. Prevent complications of immobility.
2. Promote self-esteem and increase independence.
3. Prevent muscle strain to nurse.

■ **Assessment**
• Assess musculoskeletal function:
  • Joint mobility
  • Paresis or paralysis of extremities
  • Fractures, amputations.
• Assess cognitive function:
  • Ability to understand and follow directions
  • Short-term memory and recognition of physical limitations to movement.
• Assess comfort level. Medicate as ordered with analgesics and plan transfer when pain is relieved.
• Assess baseline vital signs. Assess for history of orthostatic hypotension.
• Review physician's orders for activity level.

■ **Equipment**
Robe.
Slippers or shoes with nonskid soles.
Transfer belt.
Wheelchair.
Restraints (optional as needed).

■ **Procedure**
1. Explain procedure to patient.
   Rationale: Reduces anxiety and gains patient's cooperation.
2. Position wheelchair at 45° angle or parallel to bed. Remove footrests and lock brakes.
   Rationale: Facilitates a smooth, safe transfer from bed to wheelchair.
3. Assist patient to side-lying position, facing the side of bed he or she will sit on.

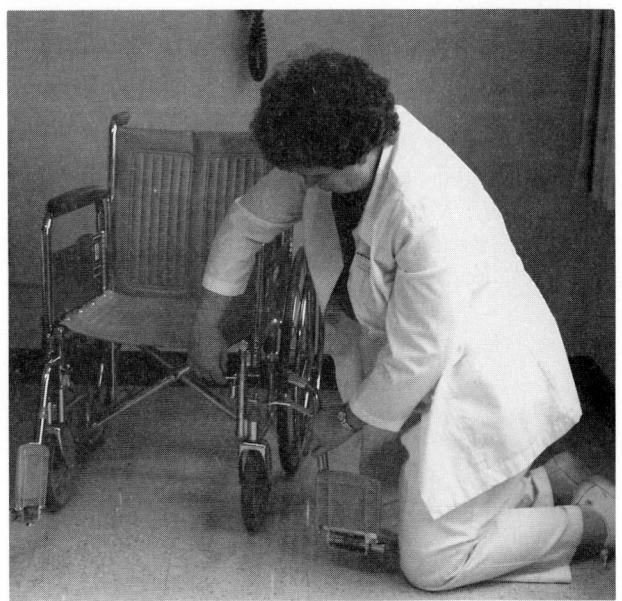

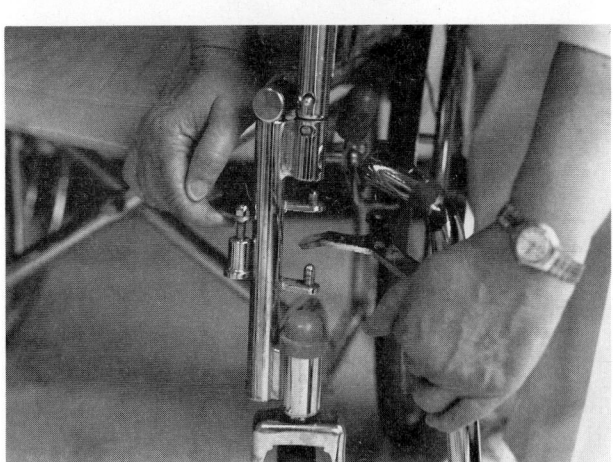

Step 2

(continued)

PROCEDURE 29–7. Transferring a Patient to a Wheelchair *(continued)*

4. Lock bed brakes; lower bed to lowest level and raise head of bed as far as patient can tolerate.
   Rationale: Decreases amount of energy needed to raise patient to sitting position.

5. Lower siderail and stand near patient's hips with foot near head of bed in front of and apart from other foot.
   Rationale: Places nurse's center of gravity near patient's largest weight.

6. Place one arm under patient's shoulders and one arm over patient's thighs.

7. Swing patient's legs over side of bed. At the same time, pivot on your back leg to lift patient's trunk and shoulders.
   Rationale: Gravity lowers patient's legs over bed while nurse transfers weight in the direction of motion.

8. Stand in front of patient and assess for balance and dizziness.
   Rationale: Prevents falls or injury from orthostatic hypotension.

9. Help patient to don robe and nonskid footwear.
   Rationale: Nonskid soles reduce risk of falling.

10. Apply transfer belt if necessary.
    Rationale: Reduces risk of falling during transfer.

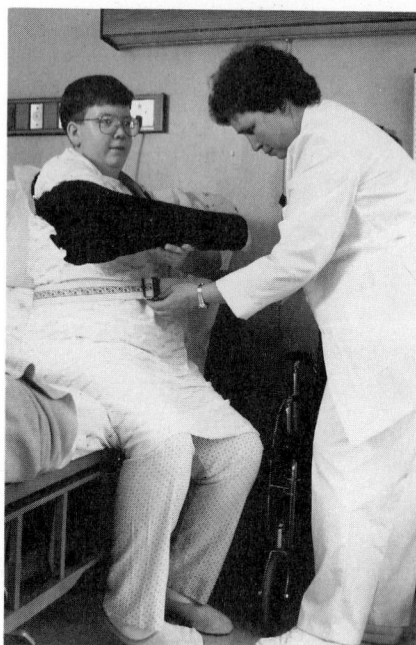

Step 10

11. Spread your feet apart and flex your hips and knees.
    Rationale: Lowers center of gravity and broadens base of support to provide stability and smooth movement using large muscle groups of legs.

12. Put your hands around patient's waist or grasp back of transfer belt.
    Rationale: Provides balance and support.

13. Have patient slide buttocks to edge of bed until feet touch floor.

14. Rock back and forth until patient stands on a count of three.
    Rationale: Rocking motion prevents muscle strain by giving patient's weight momentum and requiring less energy to lift.

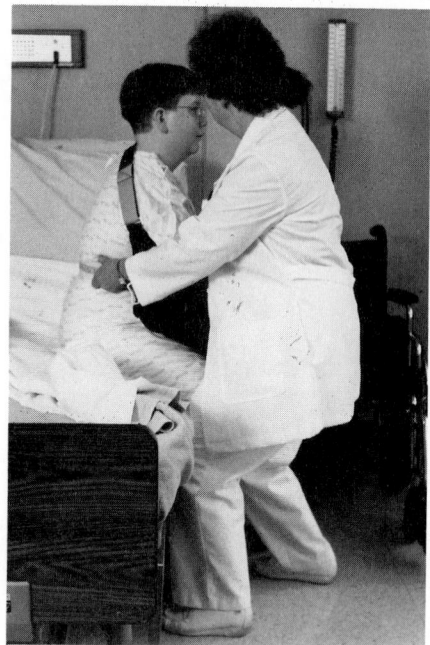

Step 14

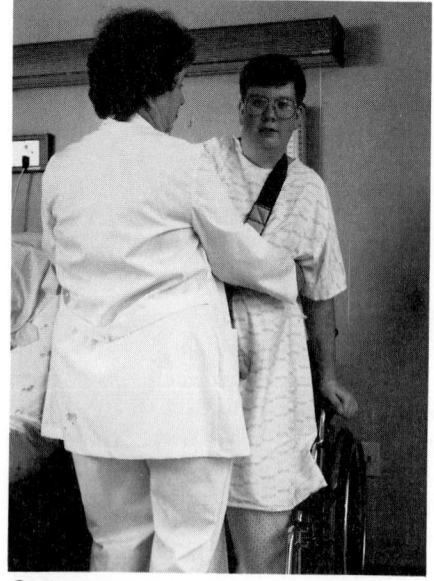

Step 15

(continued)

PROCEDURE 29–7. Transferring a Patient to a Wheelchair *(continued)*

15. Brace your front knee against patient's weak knee as patient stands.
   Rationale: Prevents weak knee from buckling and patient from falling.
16. Pivot on back foot until patient feels wheelchair against back of legs, keeping your knee against the patient's knee.
17. Instruct patient to place hands on chair armrests for support. Flex your knees and hips as you assist patient into chair.
   Rationale: Uses good body mechanics and prevents back injury by supporting weight with large muscle groups.
18. Assess patient's alignment in chair, and secure with restraints as necessary.

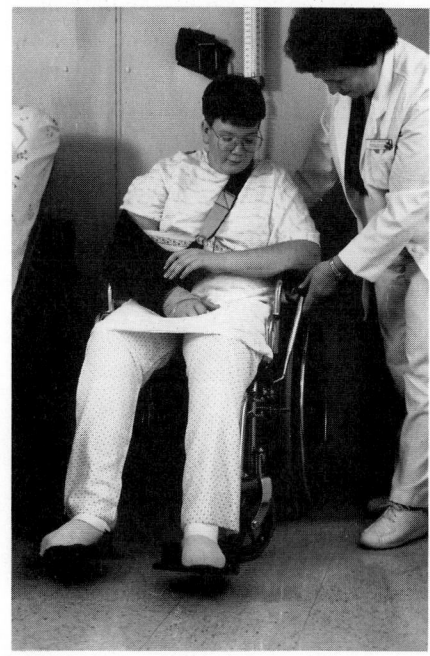

Step 18

TABLE 29–5.

Equipment Assisting Transfers

Device	Purpose	Nursing Considerations
Transfer board or sled	Smooth, flat surface placed under a supine patient to ease the transfer to another flat surface	Use only when transfer surfaces are at the same height. Avoid pinching patient's skin when board is positioned.
Roller board	Also assists with transfers from one flat surface to another. Consists of metal frame covered with longitudinal rollers encased in a fabric covering.	Board is placed in the gap between the bed and the stretcher. Draw sheet is used to slide patient across.
Transfer belt	Used for support during transfers or ambulation, especially for patients who are weak or dizzy or have poor balance	Fasten belt snugly over clothing. Use whenever ambulation may be unsteady.
Hydraulic lift	Used to transfer immobile patients from bed to chair or bathtub. Lift has a canvas sling that fits under patient and hooks into metal frame. Patient can then be elevated and transferred using the hydraulic mechanism.	Reassure patients they will not fall.

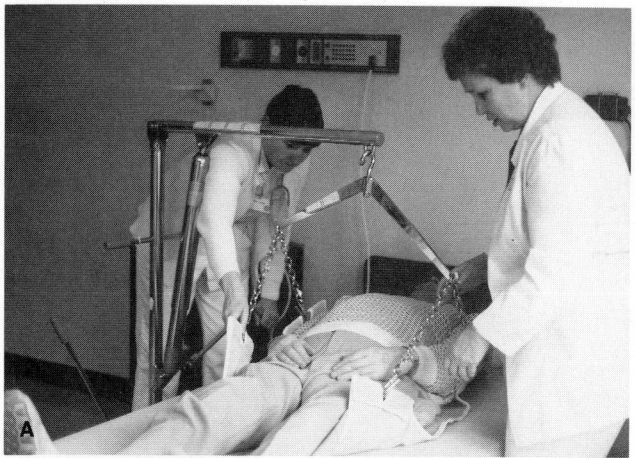
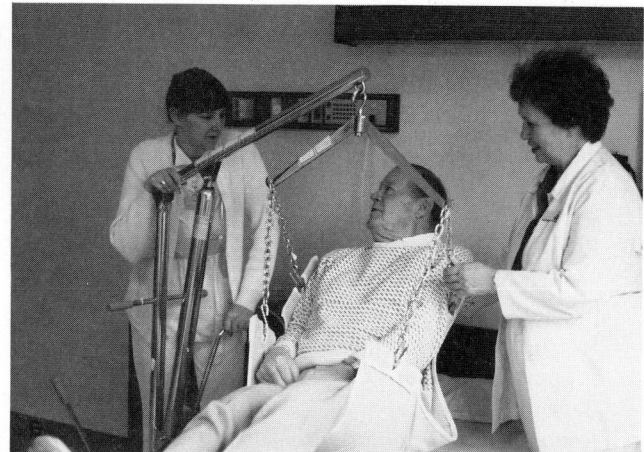
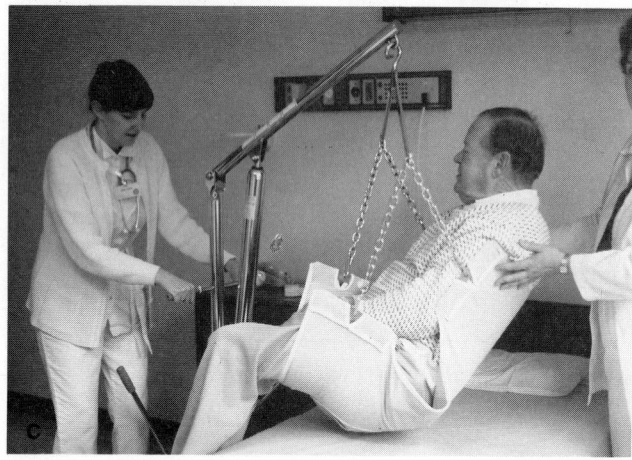
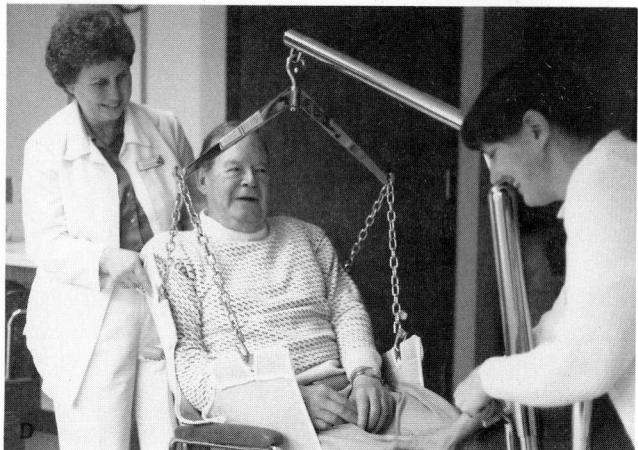

Figure 29–9. Using a hydraulic lift. **A:** Attach fabric sling to frame. **B:** Engage hydraulic system to raise patient from bed. **C:** Move patient to chair. **D:** Lower patient into chair. Sling remains in place and is reattached to frame when patient is moved back into bed.

Patient Teaching

Instruct the patient as follows:

- Practice deep breathing to decrease the potential for respiratory complications during periods of immobility.
- Drink adequate fluids during periods of immobility to prevent urinary stasis and constipation.
- Make sure the back of your legs are in contact with the chair before you sit down.
- Perform leg exercises every hour while in bed to promote circulation and prevent thrombus formation.
- Establish a regular exercise routine with aerobic activities that are enjoyable.
- Start an exercise program gradually and obtain medical clearance as needed.

tions. The patient and family should learn about transfer techniques, ambulation techniques, and the use of special equipment. The physical therapist often does much of this instruction, with reinforcement from the nursing staff. Written instructions are helpful for initial learning and home use.

Before discharge, the nurse may assess the patient's home. Ask about the physical layout of the house, including the number of stairs, the location of bedrooms and bathrooms in relation to living areas, and the ability of the house to accommodate special equipment (e.g., whether a wheelchair can fit through doorways). If disabilities are permanent, reconstruction may be necessary; for example, ramps can be built to permit easy wheelchair access.

Stress the importance of safety to the patient returning home with impaired motor function. Clutter and area rugs should be removed to prevent falls. Plans should be developed for emergencies. Smoke detectors should be installed, and the person's bedroom should be on the ground floor. The local fire department can pro-

Nursing Management Plan
The Patient with Impaired Physical Mobility

Nursing Diagnosis: Impaired physical mobility related to right-leg above-the-knee amputation, as manifested by inability to move purposefully within the environment.

Patient Goal: The patient will move within his or her environment to perform ADLs.

Patient Outcome Criteria

- Patient's hip maintains its flexibility throughout recovery and rehabilitation.
- Patient maintains balance and support by standing on left leg (with help of crutches or walker) one week postoperative.
- Patient demonstrates safe transfer technique (in and out of bed, commode, wheelchair) by one week postop.

Nursing Intervention	Scientific Rationale
1. Keep stump flat and unrotated; do not place pillows under stump.	1. Keeping stump flat prevents contracture.
2. Encourage active ROM exercises every 8 hours.	2. To keep joints flexible.
3. Provide a program of frequent position changes that includes having patient lie prone for 1/2-hour intervals every 8 hours.	3. Frequent position changes enhance mobility and prevent contractures.
4. Do not allow patient to sit up in bed or in a chair for prolonged periods.	4. Sitting up flexes the stump and can cause contractures.
5. Take postural blood pressure measurements before allowing patient to get up.	5. To detect orthostatic hypotension.
6. Encourage patient compliance with physical therapy schedule. Talk to him or her about value of increasing muscle strength in the remaining leg. Note time physical therapy is scheduled and make sure patient has eaten and is medicated (if needed) by that time.	6. Encouraging physical therapy sessions should motivate patient.
7. Remind patient to use abdominal and gluteal muscles to avoid leaning to right side of body when standing.	7. Reminding patient which muscles to use while standing makes it easier for patient to balance.
8. Encourage patient to wear a shoe that provides good support during weight-bearing.	8. Good support is essential for physical recovery and future ambulation.
9. Instruct patient to perform good foot care daily.	9. Foot care is essential since injury to remaining foot greatly reduces mobility and independence.
10. Use trapeze for exercise and preparation for transfer. Attach trapeze above bed. Demonstrate use of trapeze to maneuver in bed and to transfer from bed to chair. Encourage patient to strengthen his or her upper extremities by pulling on trapeze to lift body off bed, then lowering himself or herself slowly.	10. Demonstrating use of equipment increases patient compliance with self-transfers. Using trapeze for exercise should strengthen upper extremity muscles.
11. When patient is in wheelchair, encourage him or her to lift body by pushing down on the arms of the wheelchair.	11. Increases muscle strength in upper extremities. Prevents prolonged pressure and ulcer development.
12. Develop a program of isometric exercises and	12. Isometrics should maintain muscle tone in

(continued)

Nursing Management Plan
The Patient with Impaired Physical Mobility *(continued)*

have patient perform 10 repetitions 3 times a day.

    Lie on back, squeeze cushion between legs.
    Lie on back, spread legs apart against belt buckled around thighs.
    Lie on stomach, lift stump toward ceiling.
    Lie on back, raise stump, then lower stump and hip, pushing down toward bed.

13. Teach transfer from bed to chair using stand–pivot technique.

    Use transfer belt.

    Patient should wear shoe with nonskid sole.
    Verbally walk patient through procedure.

    Praise successful efforts.

right stump and left leg; spelling out exercises helps patient understand the motivation behind them. Using meal time as a reminder to perform exercises should help patient.

13. Patient has good strength in remaining leg and should be able to safely transfer to chair using this technique.
    Enables you to better grip person during transfer.
    Decreases chance of slipping during transfer.
    Provides verbal cuing for movement necessary during transfer.
    Psychological support and praise helpful in motivating patient.

---

vide a decal to be placed on the handicapped person's bedroom window. Arrangements may be made for someone to telephone or check in on the person daily; this is especially important for the elderly, who are at high risk for falls.

Arrangements for special equipment and services should be made before discharge. Sometimes equipment can be rented, or customized equipment may have to be made. Written referrals to home health agencies for nursing care, physical therapy, or other support services should be made. Telephoning such personnel is helpful so that information can be relayed and questions answered before discharge.

Modifications may be necessary when care is transferred to the home setting. When possible, practice should occur in the hospital to simulate the home situation. For example, if a hospital bed will not be available at home, practice transfers in a high-bed position using a board to ease transfer down to the level of the wheelchair. The patient should discuss how he or she will manage such activities as bathing and cooking.

Often much family support is necessary for the patient to manage at home. Family members must feel knowledgeable and comfortable in assuming this responsibility. Relatives must also plan for time away from such responsibilities so that they can recover their strength and enthusiasm. The nurse can give relatives a telephone number or the number of support groups to contact if problems arise.

Great strides have been made in recent years to accommodate people with motor disabilities. Public buildings have wheelchair access, and special facilities can be found in some public restrooms. Some buses and vans are equipped to handle wheelchairs. Equal accessibility to public buildings is a right guaranteed under federal law.

EVALUATION

Measuring outcome criteria helps determine whether the patient has achieved mobility goals. Outcome criteria must be individualized for each patient, but the outcome criteria listed here are examples that may be appropriate.

Goal
Patient will show increased endurance and tolerance for physical activity.

Possible Outcome Criteria
- Within 24 hours, patient states importance of gradually increasing activity or exercise.
- Patient increases amount of exercise or degree of activity daily according to preset parameters.
- With activity or exercise, patient discontinues activity if adverse symptoms (e.g., dyspnea, tachycardia, pain, vertigo) are experienced.

Goal
Patient will actively participate in prescribed therapies to promote optimum healing and restoration of mobility status.

Possible Outcome Criteria

- Patient assists with turning by using trapeze and pushing with legs as instructed during repositioning.
- Patient increases ambulation for a longer period each day.
- Patient demonstrates use of crutches or walker before discharge.
- Patient demonstrates safe transfer technique before discharge.

Goal

Patient will comply with measures to prevent potential complications of immobility.

Possible Outcome Criteria

- Patient practices leg exercises every hour to prevent possible thrombus formation.
- Patient practices deep breathing and coughing every hour to minimize pooling of secretions.
- Patient increases fluid intake to eight glasses of water per day to prevent urinary tract infection and renal calculi.
- Patient performs range of motion daily as instructed to maintain joint flexibility.

Goal

Patient will maintain optimum functional abilities despite mobility restriction.

Possible Outcome Criteria

- Patient performs daily self-care activities involved with bathing, grooming, feeding, or toileting.
- Before discharge, patient demonstrates ability to use ambulation devices safely.
- Before discharge, patient verbalizes realistic plans concerning employment and family responsibiiities.
- Before discharge, patient identifies support groups or people to assist with independent living at home.

Key Concepts

- The normal functions of the musculoskeletal system are proper body alignment, posture, balance, and coordinated movement.
- Proper body mechanics use alignment, balance, and coordinated movement to perform activities such as lifting, bending, and moving in a safe and efficient manner.
- Range of motion is the ability to move a joint through the full extent of its normal movement. Active ROM is when a patient can independently move the joint; passive ROM is when another person must do this for the patient.

- Normal walking gait consists of the stance phase and the swing phase. It requires coordinated effort, balance, and equilibrium.
- Normal mobility requires an intact musculoskeletal system, nervous system control, adequate circulation and oxygenation, adequate energy, appropriate lifestyle values, and a suitable emotional state.
- Symptoms of altered mobility are decreased muscle strength or tone, lack of coordination, altered gait, decreased joint flexibility, pain on movement, and decreased activity tolerance.
- Immobility affects all functional health areas and can contribute to the incidence of many serious complications.
- Nursing assessment includes subjective data collection to determine normal mobility, risk factors for altered mobility, and any current impairments to mobility. Objective data provide information about body alignment, balance, coordination, gait, joint flexibility, muscle tone and strength, and postural blood pressure.
- NANDA nursing diagnoses in the functional area of mobility are Impaired Physical Mobility, Activity Intolerance, and High Risk for Disuse Syndrome.
- Nursing interventions to assist the patient with mobility problems include turning and positioning, providing ROM exercises, transferring, assisting with ambulation, and teaching how to use ambulation aids.
- Patient goals concerning mobility should focus on promoting optimum mobility, increasing endurance and tolerance to exercise, preventing complications from immobility, and adapting to mobility restrictions.

References

Carroll-Johnson, B. (1989). *Classification of Nursing Proceedings of the Eight Conference.* Philadelphia: J. B. Lippincott.
Dietrick, J., et al. (1948). Effects of immobilization upon various metabolic and physiologic functions of normal men. *American Journal of Medicine, 4*(1), 3–36.
Groer, M., & Shekleton, M. (1989). *Basic pathophysiology: A holistic approach* (3rd ed.). St. Louis: C. V. Mosby.
Harris, R., Rodstein, M., & Still, C. N. (1977). Look beyond hurt when an oldster falls. *Patient Care,* October 30, pp. 80–101.
Kenshalo, D. R. (1979) Changes in the vestibular and somasthetic systems as a function of age. In J. M. Ordy & K. Brizzee (Eds.), *Aging: Sensory systems and communication in the elderly,* Vol. 10. New York: Raven.
Lentz, M. (1981). Selected aspects of reconditioning secondary to immobilization. *Nursing Clinics of North America, 16,* 729–737.
NANDA (1990). *Taxonomy I revised 1990, with official nursing diagnoses.* St. Louis, MO: North American Nursing Diagnosis Association.
Patrick, M. L., Woods, S. L., Craven, R. F., et al. (1991). *Medical-surgical nursing: Pathophysiological concepts* (2nd ed.). Philadelphia: J. B. Lippincott.
Rubin, M. (1988). The physiology of bedrest. *American Journal of Nursing, 88*(1), 50–56.
Underhill, S. L., Woods, S. L., Sivarajan, E. S., et al. (1989). *Cardiac nursing* (2nd ed.). Philadelphia: J. B. Lippincott.

Vander, A. J., Sherman, J. H., & Luciano, D. S. (1990). *Human physiology: The mechanisms of body function.* New York: McGraw-Hill.

Winslow, E. H. (1985). Cardiovascular consequences of bedrest. *Heart & Lung, 14,* 236–246.

Bibliography

Byers, P. H. (1985). Effect of exercise on morning stiffness and mobility in patients with rheumatoid arthritis. *Research in Nursing and Health, 8,* 275–281.

Chuman, M. A. (1985). Risk factors associated with ulnar nerve compression in bedridden patients. *Journal of Neurosurgical Nursing, 17,* 338–342.

Curtis, K. A., et al. (1990). Impairment: No barrier to fitness. *Patient Care,* Jan. 15, pp. 130–134.

Fitzmaurice, J. B. (1987). Nurses' use of cues in the clinical judgement of activity intolerance. *Classifications of Nursing Diagnosis: Proceedings of the Seventh Conference,* pp. 315–323.

Holm, K., et al. (1989). Immobility and bone loss in the aging adult. *Critical Care Nursing Quarterly, 12*(1), 46–51.

Kelly, R. E., et al. (1987). Evaluation of kinetic therapy in the prevention of complications of prolonged bedrest secondary to stroke. *Stroke, 18,* 638–642.

Lake, F. R., et al. (1990). Upper-limb and lower-limb exercise training in patients with chronic airflow obstruction. *Chest, 97,* 1077–1082.

Langemo, D. K., et al. (1990). Explicating the relationship of health measures and self-esteem to exercise practices in adults. *Health Education, 21*(4), 7–11.

McGough, C. E. (1988). Introduction to continuous passive motion. *Journal of Burn Care and Rehabilitation, 9,* 494–495.

MacVicar, M. G. et al. (1989). Effects of aerobic interval training on cancer patients' functional capacity. *Nursing Research, 38,* 348–351.

Milde, F. (1988). Impaired physical mobility. *Journal of Gerontologic Nursing, 14*(3), 20–25.

Miers, L. J., et al. (1990). The cardiovascular response to exercise in the patient with congestive heart failure. *Journal of Cardiovascular Nursing, 4*(3), 47–58.

Naso, F., et al. (1990). Endurance training in the elderly nursing home patient. *Archives of Physical Medicine and Rehabilitation, 71,* 241–243.

Olson, E. V. The hazards of immobility. *American Journal of Nursing, 67,* 780–785.

Olson, E. V., et al. (1990). The hazards of immobility. *American Journal of Nursing, 90*(3), 43–48.

Rickert, L. (1989). Benefits of exercise. *Journal of Urologic Nursing, 8,* 758–759.

Sandler, H., & Vernikos, J. (1986). *Inactivity: Physiological effects.* Orlando: Academic Press.

Tyler, M. (1984). The respiratory effects of body positioning and immobilization. *Respiratory Care, 29*(5), 472–483.

Videman, T., et al. (1989). Patient handling skill, back injuries and back pain: An intervention study in nursing. *Spine, 14*(2), 148–156.

Volderi, C., et al. (1990). The relationship of age, sex, gender and exercise practices to measures of health, life-style, and self-esteem. *Applied Nursing Research, 3*(1), 20–26.

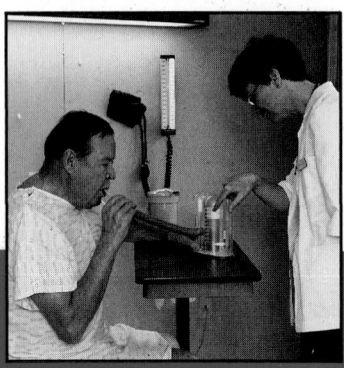

Oxygenation: Respiratory Function

Normal Respiratory Function
  Normal Anatomy of the Respiratory System
  Normal Function of the Respiratory System
    Distribution of Air in the Lungs
    Gas Diffusion
    Gas Transport
    Control of Ventilation
    Defenses of the Respiratory System
  Normal Breathing Pattern
  Factors Affecting Respiratory Function
  Lifespan Considerations
Altered Respiratory Function
  Potential for Altered Function
    Increased Work of Breathing
    Lifestyle Factors
    Environmental Factors
  Manifestations of Altered Respiratory Function
    Cough
    Sputum Production
    Shortness of Breath
    Chest Pain
    Other Signs of Respiratory Dysfunction
  Impact of Respiratory Dysfunction on Activities of
    Daily Living
Assessment
  Subjective Data
    Functional Pattern Identification
    Risk Identification
    Dysfunctional Identification
  Objective Data
    Physical Assessment
    Sputum Assessment
    Diagnostic Tests and Procedures
Nursing Diagnosis and Patient Goals
  Diagnostic Statement: Ineffective Breathing Pattern
    Definition
    Defining Characteristics

    Related Factors
  Diagnostic Statement: Ineffective Airway
    Clearance
    Definition
    Defining Characteristics
    Related Factors
  Diagnostic Statement: Impaired Gas Exchange
    Definition
    Defining Characteristics
    Related Factor
  Related Nursing Diagnoses
  Patient Goals
Implementation
  Nursing Interventions to Promote Health and
    Respiratory Function
    Hydration
    Positioning and Ambulation
    Hyperinflation
    Coughing
    Aerosol Therapy
  Nursing Interventions for Altered Respiratory
    Function
    Oxygen Therapy
    Dyspnea Management
    Altered Breathing Pattern Management
    Chest Physiotherapy
    Suctioning
    Artificial Airways
    Emergency Airway Measures
  Discharge Planning and Home Care
    Infection Control
    Medications
    Home Oxygen Systems
    Energy Conservation
    Fostering Self-Esteem
Evaluation
Key Concepts

The primary function of the respiratory system is breathing, a physiologic function essential to life. By taking in fresh air, the respiratory system continually replenishes the body's supply of oxygen. At the same time, breathing eliminates the waste gas carbon dioxide from the blood.

One of the nurse's responsibilities concerning respiratory function is assessment. The nurse gathers information from the patient, listens to breath sounds with a stethoscope, interprets laboratory tests, and makes important observations to determine the effectiveness of the patient's breathing. Assessment also allows the nurse to identify risk factors that could cause respiratory dysfunction.

The nurse is responsible for promoting normal respiratory function. Two examples are instructing the preoperative patient in deep-breathing techniques and educating the public about the hazards of smoking.

The nurse also performs interventions designed to help the patient with altered respiratory function. From positioning of the debilitated patient to managing sophisticated life-supporting ventilator systems, the nurse plays a vital role in managing the patient with respiratory disease.

Understanding normal respiratory function gives the nurse a solid basis for appreciating the problems of dysfunction. This chapter discusses the process of breathing and its relation to health. Problems concerning breathing and the implications of such problems for the nurse are also presented.

NORMAL RESPIRATORY FUNCTION

Normal Anatomy of the Respiratory System

Breathing delivers air to the lungs, where gas exchange occurs. Before air reaches the lungs, it passes through a series of structures and tubes collectively called the airways (Fig. 30-1).

The upper airway consists of the mouth, nose, and pharynx. The mouth and nose are the normal entryways for air. They are connected by the nasopharynx, which funnels incoming air into the lower portions of the pharynx. Below the pharynx lies the larynx, or voice box. This cartilaginous structure forms the Adam's apple and marks the transition from the upper to the lower airway.

The lower airway consists of the trachea, or windpipe, and its many branches. The average adult trachea is 10 to 12 cm long and 2 to 2.5 cm in diameter. It branches into left and right mainstem bronchi. These branch further into smaller tubes, called lobar bronchi, and again into segmental bronchi. The airways continue to branch in treelike fashion, generating 23 successively smaller (and increasingly numerous) sets of tubes (Des Jardins, 1988).

The smallest of these tubes are the **bronchioles,** which connect the larger conducting airways with the gas-exchange portions of the lungs. This region, known as the lung parenchyma, is made up of millions of tiny air sacs. These sacs, or **alveoli,** are thin-walled epithelial structures that are in contact with a lush capillary network. Oxygen reaching the alveoli crosses the epithelium into the blood, where it is transported to the heart and from there to body tissues.

The tracheobronchial tree and the lungs occupy the thoracic cavity and are the central structures of the respiratory system. They depend on complex, coordinated neuromuscular activity. The lungs can move only pas-

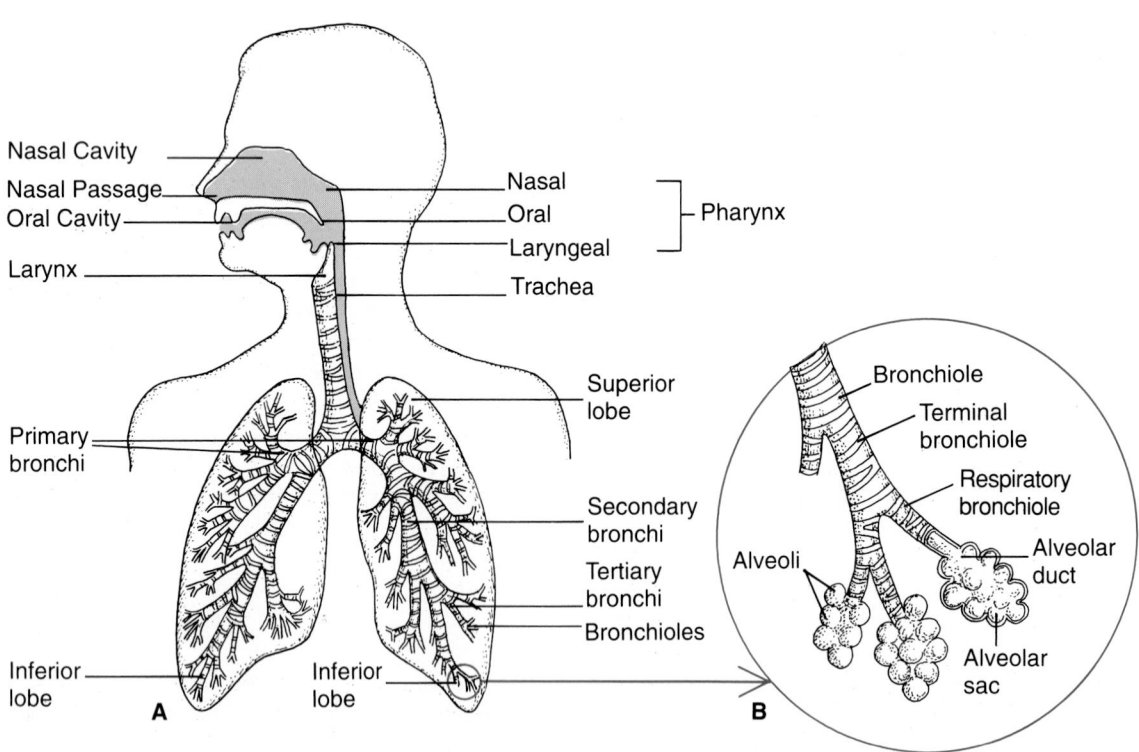

Figure 30–1. Structure of the upper and lower airways. **A:** Airways. **B:** Alveoli.

sively: their stretch comes from muscles such as the diaphragm (which separates the chest from the abdominal cavity) and the intercostal muscles, which lie between the ribs. These muscles receive impulses to contract and relax from the central nervous system, which in turn receives information from specialized nerve centers located in the aorta and carotid arteries.

Normal Function of the Respiratory System

Breathing accomplishes two major tasks: it makes oxygen (O_2) available to the blood, and it allows carbon dioxide (CO_2) to be removed from the blood. Oxygen is carried by the blood through arteries to all cells and tissues, where it is used for metabolism and growth. Without oxygen, cells would die. Carbon dioxide, the waste product that results from the metabolic use of oxygen, continuously enters the blood from the cells. It is carried through the veins to the heart and then to the lungs, where it is excreted. This function of breathing is also vital, since excess carbon dioxide in the blood is toxic to cells.

The respiratory system's function is to ensure that breathing takes place in an efficient and effective manner. When the respiratory system functions properly, breathing is practically effortless; however, chronic and acute respiratory diseases can greatly affect the breathing process. They can cause severe physical discomfort and emotional stress, and may be life-threatening or fatal.

Distribution of Air in the Lungs

Ventilation is the physical act of moving air into and out of the lungs. The term is essentially the same as "breathing." Ventilation allows air to enter the respiratory system so that gas exchange can take place. The mechanical process of ventilation is the result of volume and pressure changes in the chest cavity, or thorax.

When we inspire, the main muscles of ventilation (including the diaphragm and the external intercostal muscles) contract. Their contraction enlarges the volume of the thorax, which causes a decrease in intrathoracic pressure. This in turn causes the lung to be pulled outward with the expanding chest wall. As the lung expands, the pressure within the airways drops. As the airway pressure falls below the atmospheric pressure, air rushes into the lungs.

During exhalation the process reverses. The diaphragm and intercostal muscles relax, causing the thorax to return to its smaller resting size. Pressure in the chest increases, thus allowing air to flow out of the lungs.

Ordinarily, little effort is required to draw air through the conducting airways. The larger airways are held open by cartilage and are large enough for air to flow freely. The smallest conducting tubes of the lower air-

way, the bronchioles, are made primarily of smooth muscle. They remain open by smooth muscle tone and usually provide little resistance to breathing. Because there are millions of bronchioles, they have a collectively large diameter; thus, pulling air through these tiny tubes is easy (Slonim & Hamilton, 1987).

After air finally passes through 20 or more branches of airways, it reaches the respiratory units of the lung parenchyma. Each alveolus that makes up these units is in contact with capillaries of the pulmonary circulation. Because of the large number of alveoli and the near-perfect match of air with blood, the lung parenchyma provides an amazingly large surface area for gas exchange.

Gas Diffusion

Oxygen and carbon dioxide move between the alveoli and the blood by *diffusion,* the movement of molecules from areas of higher concentration to areas of lower concentration. All gases exert pressure against the sides of their containers; thus, carbon dioxide and oxygen exert pressure against the walls of alveoli and blood vessels. Thus we can speak of the partial pressure of oxygen (PO_2) and the partial pressure of carbon dioxide (PCO_2). Gas transfer across the alveolar–pulmonary capillary membrane takes place because of the differences in partial pressures of these two gases.

Air entering the alveoli from the atmosphere contains a relatively large amount of oxygen. Thus, the partial pressure of alveolar oxygen (PaO_2) is relatively high, normally between 80 and 100 mm Hg (Fig. 30-2). By contrast, there is little carbon dioxide in the atmosphere. Because the lungs are the site of excretion for the body's carbon dioxide wastes, the alveoli continually receive a steady stream of carbon dioxide from the blood passing by them. Thus, the partial pressure of alveolar carbon dioxide ($PaCO_2$) is appreciable, but it is considerably lower than the PaO_2. The normal value for $PaCO_2$ is about 40 mm Hg.

Blood entering the pulmonary capillaries has just returned to the heart and lungs after circulating through the body tissues. It is low in oxygen ("deoxygenated") and rich in carbon dioxide. The partial pressure of oxygen of this blood is about 40 mm Hg, the partial pressure of carbon dioxide about 46 mm Hg. As this blood circulates past the alveoli, the difference in partial pressures of these gases between the alveoli and capillary blood allows gas exchange to occur. The partial pressure gradient causes oxygen to diffuse into the blood from the alveoli, and carbon dioxide diffuses out of the blood into the alveoli.

The blood that passes through the pulmonary capillaries enters as oxygen-poor blood from the venous system and leaves as freshly oxygenated arterial blood. After less than a second in the capillary, the partial pressure of oxygen in the new arterial blood (PaO_2) rises

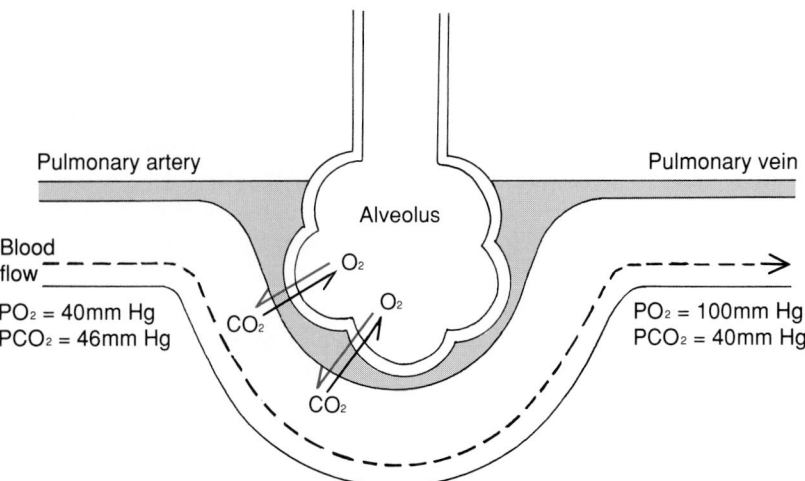

Figure 30–2. Gas exchange in the pulmonary capillary.

to nearly equal that of the alveolus. Carbon dioxide is actually equalized, since the arterial blood leaves the alveoli with a $PaCO_2$ of 40 mm Hg. The arterial blood then flows into the left side of the heart, from which it is pumped into the systemic circulation and carried to the body tissues.

This process of gas exchange follows the same principle when the arterial blood finally is delivered to the body tissues. Metabolism in the tissues uses up oxygen and produces carbon dioxide. Because of metabolic processes, partial pressure of oxygen is lower in the tissues than in the arterial blood. The opposite is true for CO_2. Thus, oxygen diffuses from the blood to the tissues and carbon dioxide from the tissues to the blood, again in response to the difference in partial pressures.

Gas Transport

As oxygen crosses the alveolar–capillary membrane into the blood, it is transported to the tissues in two forms. Small amounts of oxygen are physically dissolved in plasma, but most of the oxygen being carried to the tissues is attached to hemoglobin molecules on red blood cells. Hemoglobin has the unique ability to carry oxygen in its molecular form, rather than as an ion. This is significant because tissues require molecular oxygen for metabolism. Each red blood cell contains many hemoglobin molecules and can carry large amounts of oxygen.

In the healthy person, hemoglobin attracts oxygen like a magnet in the lungs, and releases it to the tissues in response to their need. If blood flow to the tissues is normal, tissue oxygenation can take place.

Carbon dioxide is carried in the blood in several forms. It is transported in a dissolved state, but it also can combine with some amino acids to form carbamino compounds. It can combine with hemoglobin in small amounts, and can be transported as carbonic acid in

small amounts. But the most important transport mechanism for carbon dioxide is in its dissociated form. When chemically combined with water, carbon dioxide dissociates into bicarbonate ions. These ions form the primary component of the bicarbonate buffer system, which plays a major role in acid–base balance within the body (Slonim & Hamilton, 1987).

Control of Ventilation

The process of ventilation is regulated through neural pathways, which are influenced by many factors. Specialized neurons in the brain stem, known collectively as the respiratory centers, generate regular impulses. These impulses are transmitted to the respiratory muscles, causing them to rhythmically contract and relax.

Many neural pathways provide input to the respiratory centers. Stretch receptors in the lung and chest wall limit how far the lungs can expand. These receptors increase the efficiency of breathing by limiting the work the respiratory muscles must do. Peripheral sensory neurons, notably pain and cold receptors, can also provide input to these centers. Finally, although regular rhythmic breathing is primarily an involuntary function, it can be strongly influenced by voluntary thought (Slonim & Hamilton, 1987).

Perhaps the most important influence on the respiratory centers comes from the peripheral and central chemoreceptors. Specialized neural tissue in the aortic arch and carotid arteries (peripheral receptors) and the medulla (central receptors) are sensitive to the blood's chemical content. All of these receptors are sensitive to circulating blood levels of carbon dioxide and hydrogen ions. The peripheral receptors are also stimulated by decreases in PaO_2. These chemoreceptors are linked by neural pathways with the respiratory centers. Information from these specialized tissues greatly influences our pattern of breathing.

Of all the stimuli affecting the chemoreceptors, carbon dioxide plays the primary role in determining the frequency and depth of ventilation. If carbon dioxide levels in the blood increase, the chemoreceptors are stimulated and we breathe more deeply and rapidly. The opposite is also true: our breathing decreases when carbon dioxide levels decrease. Normal breathing is usually regular and smooth, because carbon dioxide levels remain fairly constant. If the blood level of carbon dioxide accumulates or falls appreciably, it ordinarily soon returns to normal by alterations in breathing patterns. The chemoreceptors also increase ventilation if arterial blood pH or PaO_2 falls substantially, but in general the degree of response to these conditions is less than when alterations in $PaCO_2$ occur.

Normally, these mechanisms for changing breathing patterns do not come into play. Only under abnormal or pathologic conditions do these factors affect breathing (Shapiro, Harrison, Kacmarek, & Cane, 1985).

Defenses of the Respiratory System

A major function of the upper airway is to act as an air conditioner. The generous blood flow of the nasal cavity warms inspired air, and its mucosal lining imparts humidity. This moisture and warmth is necessary to maintain the fluid character of the mucus in the lower respiratory tract.

The upper airway also cleans the air we breathe. The nose is a highly effective filter for foreign particles. Dust and irritants are trapped in the hairs lining the nostrils or in the mucus layer of the nasal passages. Incoming air is further purified by the tonsils and adenoids, which are protective lymphoid tissues in the pharynx.

The upper airway protects the lower airway from infection and from injury due to aspiration. The epiglottis acts as a trapdoor, preventing large particles of food or foreign matter from being accidentally aspirated into the lower airway. Below this structure, the vocal cords, false cords, and aryepiglottic folds act as secondary protection against aspiration (Shapiro, et al., 1985).

The conducting tubes of the lower airway further filter and cleanse incoming air. Lining these airways is an epithelial layer containing millions of ciliated cells and mucus-producing glands. This mucous membrane produces a "mucus blanket" that efficiently traps bacteria and microscopic foreign particles. The ciliated cells provide motion to the mucus blanket, allowing it to carry trapped matter upward and out of the respiratory tract. This "mucociliary elevator" protects the airways by constantly sweeping potentially harmful material out of the lungs.

At the alveolar level, specialized scavenger cells called macrophages help decrease the risk of infection by eating bacteria and any minute particles that may have bypassed the mucus blanket.

The lungs and airways are also protected by the sneeze and cough reflexes. Irritants trapped in the nose stimulate sneezing. This helps to expel the trapped material from the nasal passages, thereby decreasing the irritation and helping to prevent infection.

The most important lung defense is a strong and effective cough (Shapiro, et al., 1985). Coughing clears the lower airways much like sneezing helps cleanse the nose. A forceful expulsion of air from the lungs can remove large amounts of germ-laden mucus. This action is vital for keeping the lungs free of infection. Coughing also helps to prevent mucus plugs from forming in airways and to remove plugs that have already formed. In this way, airways are kept open so all areas are available for gas exchange.

Normal Breathing Pattern

Although normal breathing varies depending on age, in general it is smooth, even, and regular. A description of a person's breathing pattern must include information about the rate and depth of breathing, its rhythm, and the effort required to take each breath.

Normal or "quiet" breathing of a person at rest occurs at a rate of 12 to 20 breaths per minute in the older child and adult (Table 30-1). The rate does not vary significantly from one minute to the next unless the person's activity level changes. Usually an awake person breathes slightly faster than one who is asleep.

The rhythm of the normal adult's breathing is steady. All breaths are evenly spaced, with an equal interval between each breath. Exhaling normally takes twice as long as inhaling.

Normally, each breath is about the same size. Despite an occasional sigh or yawn, the chest of a person who is breathing quietly will be seen to rise and fall the same amount from breath to breath. People who use their diaphragms effectively to breathe make their abdomens rise and fall. The average adult moves about a half a liter of air per breath.

Normal breathing is nearly effortless. Little muscular work is required to move air through the lungs. Because of this, quiet breathing is almost unnoticeable; ordinarily no sounds are associated with it.

Factors Affecting Normal Respiratory Function

Respiration, or the exchange of oxygen for carbon dioxide, is highly complex and depends on many factors. Specific physiologic conditions, level of general health, lifestyle, and environment all affect the process. Al-

TABLE 30–1

Respiratory Rates Through the Lifespan

Age Group	Breathing Rate (breaths/minute)
Newborn	30–60
1–5 years	20–30
6–10 years	18–26
10–adult	12–20
Older adult (60 years and older)	16–25

though many factors may contribute to abnormal respiratory function, several others can affect normal breathing in the healthy person.

Body Position. An upright posture allows for the greatest ease of lung expansion. The diaphragm can move up and down most readily when the abdominal organs are not pressed against it. Standing or sitting erect allows gravity to pull the organs down; thus, the diaphragm must push against less resistance. Breathing requires more effort when lying down, because the abdominal contents push against the diaphragm (Slonim & Hamilton, 1987).

Activity and Exercise. Strenuous exercise increases oxygen demand by the body and increases carbon dioxide production. For these reasons, the rate and depth of ventilation increases during exercise. This helps to provide more oxygen to the tissues and to get rid of the extra waste gas.

The cells of the well-conditioned person who exercises strenuously and regularly use oxygen more efficiently than those of the sedentary person. Thus, an athlete normally breathes more slowly and deeply while at rest than someone who is less fit.

Age. The aging process changes all organ systems, including the lungs. They become naturally stiffer with age, and the work needed to stretch them increases. Elderly people, even those without lung disease, usually breathe more shallowly and slightly faster than the young adult.

Pregnancy. During the last trimester of pregnancy, the fetus and amniotic sac grow large enough to displace the diaphragm upward. The mother then breathes faster and more shallowly, even to the point of hyperventilation. During the last few weeks of pregnancy, breathing can become uncomfortable.

Body Weight. A grossly overweight person may experience the same restriction and discomfort in breathing as the pregnant woman. The extra work required to carry extra body weight increases oxygen demands. At the same time, the chest is restricted in its movements (especially in the sitting or supine position), so breathing is more difficult. The very thin person often tends to breathe more rapidly and shallowly than the person of normal body weight.

Environment. All humans are exposed to the same concentration of oxygen: the atmosphere contains about 21% oxygen. Although the concentration of oxygen does not change appreciably, its partial pressure decreases steadily as altitude increases. The partial pressure of oxygen in the atmosphere at 10,000 feet above sea level is only about two-thirds of its partial pressure at sea level. This lower oxygen pressure at higher elevations means that less oxygen is available to the lungs for gas diffusion. Therefore, less oxygen can enter the blood, and tissues receive less oxygen. Thus, even healthy people are likely to experience shortness of breath and activity intolerance at higher elevations.

People's reactions to weather conditions are highly personalized. Some tolerate heat and humidity well; others may complain of difficulty breathing under these conditions. The same is true for cold or dry climates or for sudden changes in weather. People who move to different climates may experience slight changes in breathing patterns until they become acclimated to their new surroundings.

Lifespan Considerations

Like the heart, the lungs perform a lifetime of continual work; however, the structure and function of the respiratory system does undergo normal changes during life.

Newborn and Infant

In the uterus, the fetus's lungs grow rapidly. Branches of airways sprout during the first weeks of pregnancy, and alveoli continue to develop throughout pregnancy. Until the 24th or 25th week of pregnancy, the fetus's lungs do not have enough properly functioning alveoli to make breathing effective (Aloan, 1987). It takes another 10 weeks or more for the fetus to develop fully functional lungs. Surfactant, which decreases surface tension and permits alveolar expansion, is not produced in sufficient quantities until late in pregnancy.

The newborn's first breath requires tremendous physical effort. At birth, the lung is collapsed and the alveoli are filled with amniotic fluid. Although the birth process helps squeeze some of this fluid out of the lungs, it takes several breaths before the alveoli are fully opened.

The newborn breathes rapidly (30 to 60 breaths per minute), and in general larger infants breathe more slowly than smaller ones (Aloan, 1987). The newborn's breathing pattern is characterized by occasional pauses of several seconds between breaths. This periodic breathing is normal during the first 3 months of life, but frequent or prolonged periods of apnea (cessation of breathing of 20 seconds or longer) is abnormal.

Toddler and Preschooler

As the child leaves infancy, the breathing pattern evens out considerably. The respiratory rate of the young child continues to decline. By the child's third birthday, the rate should decrease to around 20 to 30 breaths per minute, and the rhythm is smooth and regular.

During this period, the child must be protected from aspirating foreign objects, which can obstruct his or her small air passages. Providing safe toys and avoiding hard candy or small, hard pieces of food are important to ensure normal respiratory function in this age group.

Child and Adolescent

As the school-age child grows, the rate of respiration steadily slows, until the adult rate of around 12 to 20 breaths per minute is reached. During this period, generally good respiratory health is the rule.

During the teen years, more than 90% of all smokers begin their habit, and thus begin the gradual decline in their lung function. One of the most valuable (and most difficult) functions of the nurse is to educate adolescents about the health risks of smoking.

Adult and Older Adult

Structural and functional changes occur in the lung in the later decades of life. The thoracic wall becomes more rigid and the lungs become less able to stretch. There is no significant decrease in total lung capacity, but dead space ventilation increases. The protective functions of the lung are impaired, as there is decreased ciliary activity and the cough is less propulsive and effective in airway clearance. Finally, gas exchange is affected: normal PaO_2 decreases by 10% to 15% (Carnevali & Patrick, 1986). These respiratory changes contribute to the activity intolerance and increased incidence of respiratory infections in the elderly.

ALTERED RESPIRATORY FUNCTION

Many factors can alter normal respiratory function. Smoking, lack of exercise, poor nutrition, drugs and alcohol, exposure to hazardous fumes or pollutants, cardiopulmonary disorders, developmental abnormalities, restrictive lung movement, airway obstruction, and emotional distress can cause or contribute to illness in general and breathing problems in particular. Conversely, a healthy cardiopulmonary system, clean air, exercise, proper nutrition, and avoiding smoking promote healthy lungs.

Potential for Altered Function

For effective respiration, all parts of the respiratory system must be in good working order. Lungs with narrowed airways or lungs that are stiff and difficult to expand increase the work of breathing. This in turn makes breathing an inefficient, oxygen-robbing activity. Weakened respiratory muscles or dysfunctional pathways between nerves and muscles can also prevent proper ventilation. If an insufficient amount of air enters the lungs with each breath, less oxygen is available to the blood.

The lung must have enough functional alveoli. The respiratory epithelium must be intact and unscarred, so that oxygen and carbon dioxide can pass readily through it. The gas exchange units must also have properly functioning pulmonary capillaries. Enough blood must be flowing through these capillaries so that gas exchange can take place.

Increased Work of Breathing

All bodily functions that require muscle movement involve a certain amount of work. For the healthy person, breathing is practically effortless: the work involved is minimal, and it is normally noticeable only during strenuous exercise. This is because normal lung tissue is stretchy and because the airways are open to allow air to flow through them. Thus, a breath requires little energy to expand the lungs.

In altered respiratory function the amount of work needed for breathing becomes significant, since the amount of oxygen needed for respiratory muscles increases. Although these muscles ordinarily use less than 5% of the oxygen available in the blood, under extreme conditions (when the work of breathing is highest) they may use up to 50% of all the oxygen used by body tissues (Shapiro, et al., 1985). Since a limited supply of oxygen is available in the blood, increased work of breathing can deprive other tissues of needed oxygen. The patient who experiences increased work of breathing is at risk for oxygen deprivation and exhaustion.

There are two general causes of increased work of breathing: restricted lung expansion and airway obstruction.

Restricted Lung Movement. Certain conditions and diseases may cause the lung to stiffen, or may restrict expansion of the chest. This can alter normal respiration in three ways:

Stiffer lungs (or lungs that are not allowed to expand fully) tend to shrivel, and their alveoli collapse. This condition is called **atelectasis.** The amount of space available for gas exchange in the lungs decreases greatly.

Some diseases cause lung tissue to swell and thicken.

Oxygen has greater difficulty in passing through thickened alveolar walls.

Because stiff lungs require more work to expand, the respiratory muscles must consume a disproportionate amount of oxygen.

In all three cases, less oxygen is available to the blood for the tissues.

Actual stiffening of the lung tissues can result from acute or chronic lung injuries. Smoke inhalation, pulmonary fibrosis, respiratory distress syndrome (of the adult or infant), and infections such as pneumonia are examples of disorders that make lung tissues swell and stiffen. They are called *restrictive lung diseases*.

Not all restrictive problems are caused by lung injuries or lung diseases, however. A patient can have perfectly healthy lungs, but if other factors prevent the lungs from expanding completely the same problems with oxygenation occur. Pain from a surgical incision is a common example. The discomfort of stretching the wound's stitches often forces the patient to breathe shallowly; this is why atelectasis is common in postsurgical patients. Other factors that can restrict breathing include severe obesity, chest or abdominal binders, abdominal distension by gas or fluid, medications or anesthesia, injuries to the ribs, musculoskeletal deformities of the chest, and severe weakness or neuromuscular disorders.

Airway Obstruction. Any process that causes the diameter of either the upper or lower conducting airways to decrease results in increased airway resistance. Breathing therefore requires more effort, since air must be drawn through a narrower passageway.

Airways become obstructed in several ways (Fig. 30-3). Their lumens can become plugged by foreign material, mucus, or abnormal growths. Airway obstruction often occurs when small children aspirate objects. Mucus can become so thick and difficult to raise that it obstructs airways. A dehydrated patient or one with chronic bronchitis, cystic fibrosis, or asthma may experience airway obstruction from excessive mucus production. Patients with lung cancer may experience difficulty breathing as tumors obstruct large bronchi.

Altered bronchial smooth muscle tone is also a common cause of airway obstruction. The smallest airways, the bronchioles, are normally held open by smooth muscle tone. When these airways are stimulated by allergy or injury, they can react strongly and may constrict, narrowing their lumens and making breathing difficult. Asthma and chronic obstructive pulmonary disease (COPD) are characterized by **bronchospasm,** or airway smooth muscle hyperreactivity. By contrast, *emphysema* leads to breathing problems because of abnormally low bronchial smooth muscle tone. Years of damage to the bronchiole walls make them floppy and unable to remain open during exhalation. Air becomes trapped in the alveoli, leaving little room for incoming fresh air (Weinberger, 1986).

Airway resistance can also be increased by edema. If the airways become inflamed by irritants or injury, their tissues swell. As the walls of the airways become thicker, they decrease the size of the passage between them. Asthma, bronchitis, and bronchiolitis are examples of conditions in which small airways become inflamed and narrowed. Croup and epiglottitis, most common in young children, obstruct upper airways by swelling the tissues of the throat.

Lifestyle Factors

In addition to obvious pathologic problems, a person's daily activities and habits can also alter normal breathing patterns.

Smoking. Perhaps the most obvious lifestyle choice that can affect respiration is smoking. Smokers are far more predisposed to emphysema, chronic bronchitis, and lung cancer, as well as to heart and cardiovascular

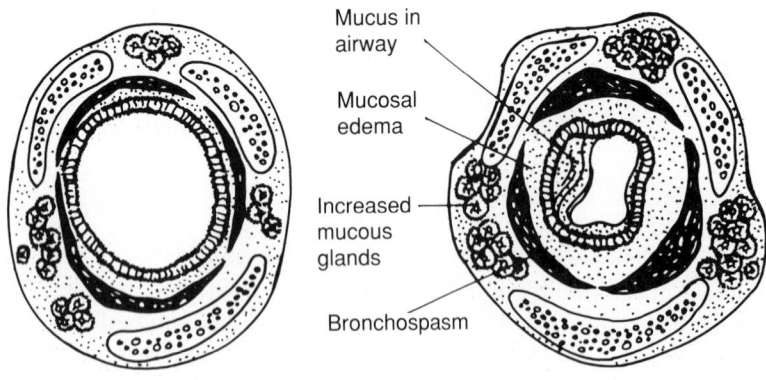

Mucus in airway

Mucosal edema

Increased mucous glands

Bronchospasm

Normal

Asthma

Figure 30–3. Airways can become obstructed by mucus, edema, or bronchospasm.

disease, than are nonsmokers. By producing more mucus and by slowing the mucociliary escalator, smoking promotes airway blockage. It thus provides greater opportunity for bacterial colonization and infection. Whether clinically identifiable lung disease is present or not, smokers usually breathe more rapidly than nonsmokers.

Drugs and Alcohol. Barbiturates, narcotics, and some sedatives (whether legal or illegal) can depress the central nervous system, with a resulting decrease in respiration. Alcohol in large doses can achieve the same effect, but it usually leads to respiratory problems of a different nature. In the chronic alcohol abuser, insufficient nutritional intake results in the body's inability to manufacture hemoglobin and plasma proteins. A drop in hemoglobin decreases the blood's oxygen-carrying ability; fewer plasma proteins can cause fluid to leak into the lungs. Of more immediate concern in the intoxicated person is the danger of vomiting and aspiration of stomach contents into the lungs. Alcohol depresses the reflexes that protect the airways, so if vomiting occurs, stomach contents can easily slip into the trachea, choking the victim. If the victim is revived, aspiration is likely to cause pneumonia.

Nutrition. Without proper diet, plasma proteins and hemoglobin cannot be effectively made by the body. This occurs not only in the alcohol abuser, but also in people who are malnourished from poverty or from eating disorders. In addition, sufficient caloric and protein intake is required for respiratory muscle strength. People with decreased muscle strength work harder at breathing with even slight activity. Adequate fluid intake is necessary to keep secretions thin and easy to expectorate so that airways remain unplugged.

Adequate nutrition is also essential for maintaining a competent immune system. Alcohol abusers and malnourished people are at greater risk for contracting pneumonia and other respiratory infections than are well-fed people.

Stress. The stress of illness can increase oxygen demand and cause increased breathing. In addition, anxiety often causes an increase in the breathing rate. In extreme cases of anxiety the victim hyperventilates and may exhibit symptoms of asthma.

Environmental Factors

The places where we live and work can greatly affect our breathing status. As noted earlier, altitude and climate can affect breathing in people with normal lungs. People with lung disease feel the adverse effects of high elevation or oppressive weather far more acutely than healthy people. Patients with lung disease often need oxygen when traveling in airplanes, since commercial airliners are not pressurized to sea-level conditions (Petty & Nett,

1984). Some asthmatics breathe more easily in warm, dry climates; others may find a damp climate more soothing. People with COPD often find it more difficult to breathe when the weather is hot and humid, since the humidity contributes to the air viscosity. People with COPD or asthma experience more exacerbations of their disease during changes in the weather. Some lung-disease patients benefit from moving to a climate more agreeable to them; others see no difference in their breathing.

In addition to elevation and climate, two other factors can alter normal breathing.

Air Pollution. Industrialized urban areas may have elevated levels of air pollutants. Substances emitted by cars and factories, such as hydrocarbons and oxidants, interfere with oxygenation by directly damaging the lung. Carbon monoxide inhibits the loading of oxygen onto hemoglobin. Because they are respiratory irritants, pollutants cause increased mucus production and may contribute to bronchitis and asthma.

Workers in industrial plants or in certain occupations may be exposed to strong concentrations of specific pollutants and harmful dust. These workers may be prone to develop breathing problems.

Air pollution in the home is also of concern. The role of second-hand smoke (smoke from someone else's cigarette) in the development of childhood breathing disorders such as asthma and respiratory infections is being vigorously investigated.

Pollens and Allergens. Specific substances that cause allergic responses can affect respiration, sometimes severely. The body's attempt to rid itself of substances it perceives as harmful results in the release of chemical mediators that cause an inflammatory response. Substances that trigger such a response are called *allergens*. These are commonly pollens, but dust, foods, or almost any substance can be an allergen. The allergic response precipitates a series of events that leads to tissue damage.

Hay fever is the result of allergies confined to the nose and upper airways. Its dripping nose, itchy eyes, and swollen mucous membranes are annoying and uncomfortable but not life-threatening. When allergic responses take place in the lungs, breathing difficulties are far more severe. Small airways become edematous, more mucus is produced, and inflammatory chemical mediators cause bronchospasm. These are the hallmarks of a common form of asthma. If it is severe and uncontrolled, allergic asthma can be fatal.

Manifestations of Altered Respiratory Function

Cough, sputum production, shortness of breath, and chest pain have been called the cardinal symptoms of

Nursing Research

Selected Nursing Research Studies

Chulay, M., & Graeber, G. (1988). Efficacy of a hyperinflation and hyperoxygenation suctioning intervention. *Heart & Lung, 17*(1), 15–22.

Gift, A., et al. (1986). Psychologic and physiologic factors related to dyspnea in subjects with chronic obstructive pulmonary disease. *Heart & Lung, 15,* 595–601.

Hautman, M. A. (1987). Self-care responses to respiratory illnesses among Vietnamese. *Western Journal of Nursing Research, 9,* 223–243.

Preusser, B., et al. (1988). Effects of preoxygenation on mean arterial pressure, cardiac output, peak airway pressure and postsuctioning hypoxemia. *Heart & Lung, 17,* 290–299.

Rew, L. (1987). Children with asthma. The relationship between behavior and health locus of control. *Western Journal of Nursing Research, 9,* 465–483.

Sexton, D., & Munro, B. (1985). Impact of a husband's chronic illness (COPD) on the spouse's life. *Res in Nurs and Health, 8*(1), 83–90.

Sexton, D., et al. (1988). Living with a chronic illness. The experience of women with COPD. *Western Journal of Nursing Research, 10*(1), 26–39.

Possible Topics for Nursing Inquiry

- What is the rate of compliance with bronchodilator therapy following instructional program?
- What factors contribute to depression among COPD patients?
- How does wearing oxygen supply devices outside the hospital affect the patient's self-image?
- Does intermittent use of oxygen during the day affect quality of sleep at night for the COPD patient?
- After initial instruction, how many patients can effectively use the metered-dose inhaler?
- What is the effect of intermittent versus continuous suction on volume of sputum removed?
- What are effective nursing measures to prevent nasal irritation when receiving oxygen via cannula?

respiratory disease (Cherniack & Cherniack, 1983). When these are present, it is easy to infer that something is wrong with the lungs; however, the spectrum of diseases that can affect the respiratory system is so broad that it is impossible to point to a single group of symptoms that is common to all.

Conversely, some of these symptoms occur so often that they are sometimes taken for granted. It seems that every winter most people develop a cough, often with sputum production. Smokers often dismiss their "smoker's cough" as a normal, expected consequence of smoking. It is common to become short of breath with vigorous exercise, and a "stitch in the side" is familiar to all who have been a bit too vigorous.

When these symptoms are mild and have obvious explanations, it is unlikely that any serious respiratory disorder is present. Signs or symptoms that persist, are not readily explained by immediate circumstances, or are more than mildly noticeable should be examined closely, however.

Cough

A cough is usually a reflex response to irritation in the airways. Smoke is certainly an irritant, and coughing is the natural response to smoke. There is no such thing as a "normal" cough. Any cough, regardless of the obviousness of its origin, is most often an indication that the lungs or airways are being subjected to some form of irritation. A cough's primary function is to help clear offending substances from the airways. A cough also serves as a warning signal: it should alert the cougher to the fact that the airways are being assaulted by possibly harmful stimuli, and that steps should be taken to prevent further irritation.

Coughs can be triggered by a seemingly endless list of chemical or physical substances, or by physical conditions such as hot, dry air. Anything that finds its way into the airway that does not normally belong there can provoke a cough. A cough that accompanies a disease may come from mediators released from inflamed tissues. These mediators, such as histamine, irritate the airways and can trigger a cough.

Not all coughs are pulmonary in origin. The patient with borderline heart failure, for example, often has a chronic cough. Some people may cough for no apparent reason, as a nervous habit.

Since coughs are so prevalent, their value as a diagnostic sign is limited. Many people live with a cough, expressing concern only when it changes in severity or frequency. In contrast, some people may have a serious lung disease and a minimal cough.

Sputum Production

As with a cough, sputum production may be one of the natural consequences of irritation, but it is never really normal. Generally, respiratory mucus, or sputum, is another protective feature of the airways. However, it is normally produced in such small amounts that a cough from a healthy person is dry and nonproductive. Raising mucus with a cough indicates that the lungs are attempting to clear unwanted substances. When a patient coughs productively, it is important to establish the source of the sputum and to assess its color, volume, consistency, and any other noteworthy characteristics.

The lungs may seem to be the obvious source of expectorated sputum, but sometimes coughed-up secretions may originate in the nose or throat. It is necessary to determine whether the patient raises the secretions with a genuine deep cough, or if he or she snorts or "hawks" them out.

Especially frightening can be the coughing up of blood, or hemoptysis. Blood-filled secretions that originate in the lungs may indicate a serious condition, such as lung cancer or tuberculosis. Often, however, bloody secretions originate in the nose. Drainage from the nose or mouth can drip backwards into the throat, staining the mucus of the lower airways. These sources of bleeding should be ruled out before the lungs are considered to be hemorrhaging.

Shortness of Breath

All of us must move a certain amount of air into and out of the lungs every minute to meet the body's metabolic demands. When we cannot breathe sufficiently to meet these requirements, we experience the discomfort of breathlessness. This difficulty in catching the breath is known as **dyspnea.** There are several levels of dyspnea (see display).

The most common cause of dyspnea is the increased work of breathing that occurs with lung disease. Asthmatic or emphysema patients work harder to breathe because their airways are narrower than normal. Patients with pneumonia must work harder at breathing because their lungs do not stretch as readily as normal, and because atelectasis prevents full gas exchange. Very weak patients, or people with neuromuscular diseases such as polio or myasthenia gravis, may experience dyspnea because of weakened respiratory muscles.

There are other causes of dyspnea besides increased work of breathing. High levels of carbon dioxide or low levels of oxygen in the blood may directly cause breathlessness (Slonim & Hamilton, 1987). People with chronic congestive heart failure often experience shortness of breath because of excess fluid in the lungs and low blood oxygen levels. People who become dyspneic during anxiety attacks often have no heart or lung disease.

Shortness of breath is a subjective symptom of lung problems. Some patients who breathe with what appears to be great difficulty may state that their breathing is fine. Others may complain of severe dyspnea even when objective data (such as blood gas values or pulmonary function tests) indicate no apparent problem. The nurse should be ready to investigate all complaints of dyspnea.

Chest Pain

Chest pain can be associated with a wide variety of conditions. Although many common causes of chest pain are nonrespiratory, there are several breathing problems that can lead to it. Diseases characterized by inflammation or infection often cause pain. Inflammatory mediators such as histamine and bradykinin may directly stimulate nerve endings, some of which may be exposed and made hypersensitive by the disease process. This occurs in the airways of the bronchitis patient, who complains of a burning sensation with each cough. Acute bronchitis can make the simple act of breathing painful, because the flow of cooler air across sensitized nerves can cause them to react violently. Mediators may also be responsible for edema formation, which can further contribute to pain. The pressure exerted by swollen tissues on nerves can cause discomfort. Pneumonia patients often experience pain with deep breathing, since each breath increases pressure on pain receptors that are already compressed and irritated by swollen, inflamed lung tissue.

Sometimes chest pain may be the result of cracked ribs or pulled muscles. Patients with severe coughs may actually separate ribs from the cartilage that holds them together. Prolonged or harsh coughing can make the chest muscles sore.

Levels of Dyspnea	
Level I:	patient can walk 1 mile at own pace before experiencing shortness of breath.
Level II:	patient becomes short of breath after walking 100 yards on level ground or climbing a flight of stairs.
Level III:	patient becomes short of breath while talking or performing activities of daily living.
Level IV:	patient is short of breath during periods of no activity.
Orthopnea:	patient is short of breath lying down.

Other Signs of Respiratory Dysfunction

The secondary signs that may appear in a patient with lung disease are less common than the four primary signs, but they are nonetheless important indicators of respiratory problems.

Cyanosis. Cyanosis is a bluish discoloration of the skin caused by a decrease in blood oxygen saturation. Hemoglobin, the major carrier of oxygen in the blood, is bright red when saturated with oxygen. When not carrying oxygen, it becomes deep blue. Sometimes cyanosis is evident in the fingertips on a cold day; this occurs because the blood vessels in the fingers constrict. This is called peripheral cyanosis and is seldom due to respiratory problems.

But when cyanosis can be seen around the face and inside the mouth, a serious problem exists. Since the blood vessels in these areas are not exposed to cold as are the peripheral vessels, the blue color is not caused by vasoconstriction. Rather, this central cyanosis indicates a severe lack of oxygen.

Clubbing. Clubbing is an unusual phenomenon seen in many patients with lung or heart disease. For reasons that are unclear, the tips of the fingers and toes become rounded and enlarged. It is thought that long-term tissue hypoxia causes an alteration of local blood flow in the digits, which in turn affects the tissue growth (Mitchell & Petty, 1989). Clubbing occurs in lung cancer and in lung diseases characterized by pus formation, such as lung abscess.

Engorged Neck Veins. The large jugular veins of the neck may become engorged in some patients with advanced lung disease. Chronic bronchitis, emphysema, pulmonary fibrosis, and occupational lung diseases can lead to congestive heart failure. This may cause blood to back up into the large neck veins. For a more detailed discussion of how this occurs, see Chapter 31.

Abnormal Breath Sounds. The breath sounds heard through a stethoscope can change as a result of lung changes. Wheezes, rumbles (also called rhonchi), and crackles (or rales) are examples of abnormal breath sounds. These will be described further in the section on Functional Assessment.

Impact of Respiratory Dysfunction on Activities of Daily Living

Debilitation caused by lung disease can range from mild to severe. The patient experiences less and less tolerance for activity as the disease progresses. The patient's ability to perform common day-to-day activities may be impaired because of breathlessness or oxygen dependence. Some patients become dyspneic with simple tasks such as shaving, cooking, or talking. The patient with advanced symptoms may be unable to perform these and other activities because of breathlessness.

Meals can pose a problem for the homebound patient. Unless help is available, preparing meals can be exhausting work. Eating is an energy-expending activity, and many people with advanced lung disease cannot eat three large meals daily without feeling severely dyspneic. Knowing this, many of them avoid eating, and this can cause a vicious cycle: the patient has insufficient energy to eat, and without eating weight loss and decreased energy continue. This can contribute to feelings of depression and hopelessness.

Some respiratory patients solve this dilemma by modifying the usual routine of three square meals a day. Instead, they eat several smaller but nutritionally balanced meals. This helps conserve oxygen and prevents the excessive buildup of pressure against the diaphragm caused by larger meals. This regimen provides needed nutrition without causing the breathlessness brought on by a full stomach.

Dressing is also tiring for some respiratory patients. Some may prefer to remain in their bedclothes all day. Whenever dressing is physically possible, the patient should be encouraged to dress daily. This is important for self-esteem and helps keep patients from thinking of themselves as invalids. Garments should be loose-fitting and easy to slip into. Dressing should be done slowly while sitting down.

Getting into and out of a bathtub can exhaust the breathless patient, so showering may be preferred. The patient with a laryngectomy or permanent tracheostomy tube can shower, but should take care to avoid flooding the stoma with water. A washcloth held over the tube prevents this. A shower also imparts humidity to the mucous lining of the airways (Patry-Lahey, 1985).

Toilet concerns of the respiratory patient are important to consider. Constipation can cause abdominal distension, thereby limiting diaphragm movement. Extra straining can also tire the patient and cause shortness of breath. Prescribed stool softeners and good hydration can help to prevent constipation.

Mobility within the home can be a problem for the patient with extreme dyspnea. Use of prescribed oxygen during periods of daily in-home activity is helpful in building up tolerance to exertion. Frequent rest is needed.

Mobility outside the home can also present special problems for the patient with poor respiratory function. Public transport may be available but may be several blocks from the patient's home. Thus, the patient may have to rely on taxis or a private car. If the patient uses oxygen and wants to fly, advance arrangements must be made with the airline. The patient who is a marginal candidate for oxygen therapy may find a greater need for it on an airplane or at a high elevation (Petty & Nett, 1984).

Respiratory patients are often less communicative than other patients. This may be because of depression and feelings of isolation. They may also be less talkative because the act of speaking can cause shortness of breath. It is difficult to inhale while speaking, so the dyspneic patient typically speaks in short, terse sentences. This may make respiratory patients appear crabby and unpleasant, but in fact they are merely attempting to conserve their energy.

ASSESSMENT

The basis for appropriate nursing interventions is a thorough respiratory assessment. Information from the assessment enables the nurse to identify potential or actual nursing diagnoses and to individualize nursing care. If relevant data is missed or goes unreported by the nurse, the respiratory patient's condition may worsen or may even become life-threatening.

Although it is essential to gather facts from the patient, the person who is severely short of breath may be unable to respond fully to a battery of questions. The hypoxic patient may respond with confused answers, and forcing the dyspneic patient to speak can worsen shortness of breath. The nurse must be sensitive to the patient's ability to answer questions and should understand that sometimes it is appropriate to ask as few questions as possible.

Subjective Data

Relevant subjective information to be gathered by the nurse includes data to help identify the patient's functional breathing pattern. The nurse must also identify factors that show the patient to be at risk for respiratory dysfunction. Finally, the nurse must be alert to the presence of breathing problems in the patient. The nursing history is the starting point for getting this information.

Functional Pattern Identification

Unlike eating, sleeping, or elimination patterns, normal breathing is usually nondescript. Unless a person has experienced breathing problems previously, he or she is likely to have taken no notice of the normal breathing pattern. Few people can provide specific information about how often or how deeply they breathe. The nurse is generally safe in assuming that the patient with no previous history of lung disorders breathes normally.

The normal breathing pattern of the person with chronic respiratory problems may differ greatly from that of the healthy person, however. For example, the patient with chronic asthma may ordinarily breathe with a slight wheeze. Although this would be considered uncomfortable and abnormal by most people, the asthmatic may have grown to tolerate it. Indeed, because asthmatics know from past experience how difficult breathing can be, they may regard the slight wheeze as normal, and consider only a severe wheeze as abnormal.

Similarly, the patient with COPD may grow to accept as normal shortness of breath after walking two city blocks. Only if exercise tolerance decreases below this standard might the patient begin to consider that something is wrong.

These examples show that the nurse must be careful in eliciting information about normal breathing patterns. Patients who indicate that their breathing is ordinarily fine or unremarkable may have adjusted to a baseline breathing pattern that is abnormal for most people. The nurse can identify the normal functional breathing pattern by asking relevant questions about cough, dyspnea, sputum production, and discomfort associated with breathing. Although these symptoms are normally assessed with regard to the patient's complaints, they also may give some insight into the normal breathing pattern.

The nurse should establish whether a cough is ordinarily present, for example, and if so, at what time of the day it usually occurs. The patient may deny being usually short of breath unless the nurse can specify degrees of dyspnea to which he or she can relate. The nurse can ask how far the patient can walk before needing to rest ("A mile; a city block; a flight of stairs; 20 feet?"). The patient can be asked how much sputum he or she usually coughs up ("A teaspoon; a tablespoon; a half cup?") and about its color.

Many other questions are listed in the display. Family members and people close to the patient may be helpful in providing supportive information.

Risk Identification

Causes of the patient's breathing problem may be rooted in long-term habits, occupational exposure, or past illnesses. The nursing history must include information about the risk factors that can lead to respiratory dysfunction.

Information about smoking habits is most important for giving insight into the patient's condition. The duration and extent of cigarette smoking is sometimes expressed in terms of "pack-years": 1 pack-year is equal to smoking one pack of cigarettes a day for a year. A person who has smoked two packs a day for 40 years would thus be said to have an 80 pack-year smoking history. Chronic bronchitis, emphysema, and lung cancer are directly related to smoking and are more likely to occur in patients with long histories of heavy smoking.

Other lifestyle factors can also affect lung health. The patient who has lived in poverty and is malnourished, for example, is more at risk for infections such as tuberculosis. This and other respiratory infections are also more common in alcohol abusers. These people are likely to have problems fighting infection because of self-

---

Initial Respiratory Assessment Questions

- Describe your cough.
- Does the cough produce sputum? If so, how much?
- Does the cough occur at any particular time of day, or under any particular circumstances? Is it constant, or intermittent?
- What is the color and consistency of the sputum? Is it thick or thin? Is it difficult to raise? Is there any odor or bad taste to the sputum? Has there been any blood in the sputum?
- When do you become short of breath? How much activity can you tolerate before you become dyspneic? How severe is the dyspnea?
- Do you have pain associated with breathing? Where is the pain located? How can it be described? Is it continuous, does it occur only on inspiration, or during coughing, or at other noticeable times?

---

neglect and the lowered effectiveness of their immune systems.

A respiratory patient's work history may be relevant to understanding breathing problems. Many occupations involve exposure to fumes or dust such as silicon and asbestos, which are toxic to lung tissue. Agricultural workers are exposed to organic dusts such as molds that can cause infections and asthma-like symptoms.

Family and personal history can also contribute to a thorough evaluation. Cystic fibrosis is genetically transmitted, as is a type of emphysema that develops in early adulthood. The patient with asthma often recalls a childhood with allergies and eczema. A history of poor dental hygiene may explain a patient's bronchiectasis or lung abscess.

Dysfunctional Identification

The nurse needs to determine whether the patient has come to the hospital with a completely new breathing problem, or whether help is being sought because of a change in a chronic respiratory condition. Because acute breathing trouble is frightening, people with no history of previous respiratory difficulties usually seek medical help quickly when they find they are having trouble breathing. This may also be true for most patients with chronic lung disease. Since many such patients are taught by their physicians to recognize and treat certain changes in breathing status, however, some may wait longer than others before seeking medical and nursing help. Sometimes infections or other problems worsen their already poor breathing sufficiently to motivate

them to seek extra medical care. In either case, a full description of the symptoms that have led the patient to seek care can help clarify the cause of the immediate breathing problem.

When gathering information about the onset and duration of the recent breathing problem, the nurse should determine whether the problem is continuous or intermittent. If the problem seems to be continuous, perhaps some new exposure has triggered a hypersensitivity reaction, such as new carpeting or a new pet. The patient may have contracted an infection that has progressed or has remained subacute. If the problem comes and goes, the nurse should ask whether the patient can identify the circumstances that bring on the difficulty. Perhaps the patient's breathing worsens at certain times of the day, or when the patient engages in certain activities.

The nurse should also assess cough, dyspnea, sputum production, and discomfort or pain. Relevant questions are listed in the display.

Breathing problems are accompanied by a variety of emotions. Acute episodes of dyspnea bring anxiety and fear. Panic occurs when the patient feels severely dyspneic. The discomfort caused by difficult breathing can make the patient worry that breathing may stop altogether. Some patients become verbal and express their panic in words, but others become quiet and withdrawn. The nurse must recognize that either response may accompany breathlessness. Regardless of the reaction, the patient needs reassurance that the breathing complaint is being taken seriously.

Since panic exacerbates the dyspnea attack, the nurse must quickly assess both the physical and psychological components of the dyspnea. Generally, the degree of panic exhibited by the patient is proportional to the degree of dyspnea. Although some patients may experience more fear than others when dyspnea strikes, decreasing patient anxiety helps bring the breathing problem under control. A calm demeanor on the nurse's part is important to help decrease the patient's anxiety.

Patients with chronic respiratory problems may experience self-consciousness and embarrassment because of their dysfunction. Because breathlessness may interfere with the ability to communicate, the chronic respiratory patient may feel isolated and appear aloof. This can contribute to frustration and irritability, and may end in depression caused by continued illness and loss of independence.

The nurse can assess these feelings by asking appropriate questions and by observing the patient. Observations made by the patient's family and friends and other members of the health-care team are invaluable in helping the nurse determine how the patient is adjusting to the illness.

Decreased self-sufficiency can cause stress in the patient's support system. The spouse, family, or significant others may need to assume a greater role in the patient's care after discharge. The nurse must assess the understanding and abilities of the patient and those who will assist the patient at home. If the nurse determines that inadequate support is available, referrals to appropriate community resources are necessary.

Objective Data

A complete assessment of respiratory status can be a lengthy and involved process. In addition to the subjective information obtained through the nursing history, objective, measurable data must be gathered. This information includes observations made by the nurse, information gained by hands-on examination of the chest, and laboratory data.

Physical Assessment

The primary techniques used in physical assessment are inspection, palpation, percussion, and auscultation. Sputum is visually examined.

Inspection. An essential observation is the rate and pattern of respiration. The respiratory rate is significant because a steady amount of air must enter and leave the lungs every minute to ensure proper blood levels of oxygen and carbon dioxide. Breathing too slowly causes too little oxygen or too much carbon dioxide in the blood. Conversely, breathing too quickly causes excessive elimination of carbon dioxide, which causes dizziness and possibly respiratory alkalosis. Rapid breathing also indicates excessive work of breathing. If breathing work becomes too great, the patient may become exhausted and stop breathing altogether.

The pattern of breathing is also important. Normal respirations should be smooth and regular. Except in the newborn, uneven or irregular breathing can mean airway obstruction, or it can signal neurologic or muscle problems. As noted earlier, babies breathe rapidly and often have regular brief periods of apnea between groups of breaths. This is abnormal only when the apnea periods are frequent or last more than 10 or 15 seconds (Aloan, 1987).

To accurately assess the resting patient's respiratory rate, the nurse should count the number of times the chest rises and falls during a 30-second period and multiply that number by two. The patient should be unaware of the nurse's observation, since he or she may become self-conscious and alter the breathing pattern. During normal rounds to check vital signs, the nurse can assess respirations immediately after assessing the patient's pulse. The nurse can take the patient's pulse for 30 seconds, and while still holding the patient's wrist, count the respiratory rate for the next 30 seconds. The patient will believe that the nurse is still counting the pulse. If

silence is maintained during this period, an accurate count can be made.

The patient's breathing pattern also includes the depth of respiration, the rhythm, and the effort required to breathe. The chest should move noticeably with each breath. Overly shallow or deep breaths are abnormal and should be documented. The actual volume of air moved with each breath can be measured by a respirometer, but this is usually necessary only for the critically ill patient. All breaths should be roughly equal in size.

Breaths should also be evenly spaced. The nurse should note also the relative length of inspiration and exhalation. Normally, inspiration takes about half as long as exhalation. Prolonged inspiration, especially with high-pitched noises, indicates obstruction of the upper airways, as in croup or epiglottitis. An abnormally long exhalation indicates air trapping in the lower airways, as in asthma or emphysema.

The nurse can describe the patient's breathing effort by noting obvious use of shoulder or neck muscles. The patient with COPD often sits in a forward-leaning position, using these so-called accessory muscles to help enlarge the chest cavity and make room for more air. This indicates shortness of breath, and may be seen in patients without COPD as well. Other obvious signs of dyspnea should be noted, such as gasping, audible wheezing, or panting respirations. In the infant, flaring of the nostrils and retractions of the ribs during inspiration are notable signs of air hunger and extraordinary work of breathing.

In addition to describing the breathing pattern, the nurse should observe the patient's color. Cyanosis around the lips and under the tongue indicates serious hypoxemia.

Finally, the nurse inspects the chest to detect obvious chest deformities, wounds, or masses. The overall shape of the chest is important but less obvious. Over time the COPD patient's chest becomes hyperinflated because of an inability to fully exhale. This gives it the characteristic barrel shape seen in so many of these patients. A severe asthma attack can also cause air trapping and temporary hyperinflation of the chest.

Palpation. The hands are used to assess abnormalities such as swelling or tenderness. Palpation is also used to determine the extent and pattern of thoracic expansion and to note the position of the trachea. Abnormal chest wall vibrations transmitted through inflamed or fluid-filled lung tissues may be detected by palpation.

Percussion. Tapping on different areas of the chest with the fingertips produces characteristic sounds. Percussion can be used to distinguish air-filled portions of the lung from those that are fluid-filled or consolidated. It also allows the nurse to identify the borders of the diaphragm and to compare both sides of the chest. A keen ear and experience with pulmonary assessment are needed to interpret correctly the various alterations in pitch, intensity, duration, and quality of percussion notes.

For more information on palpation and percussion in the physical examination of the chest, consult a text on respiratory care nursing or general physical assessment.

Auscultation. Listening to breath sounds with a stethoscope provides vital information for evaluating the patient's respiratory status.

The most important reason for listening to the chest is to determine whether air is moving through all areas of the lung. When auscultating with a sensitive stethoscope, the nurse should be able to hear air moving in all lung fields. Breath sounds should be equally loud on both sides of the chest.

Absent or distant-sounding breath sounds in any area of the lung can indicate airway obstruction, or can mean that fluid or air is in the pleural space. A "quiet chest" in an asthmatic who is experiencing severe shortness of breath may indicate poor ventilation. It is regarded as a grave sign of impending respiratory failure.

The quality of breath sounds can also be assessed by auscultation. Normal breathing should make soft rustling sounds, like a breeze blowing gently through leaves on trees. Only inspiratory sounds should be noticeable, with expiration being quiet.

The nurse must also be familiar with common abnormal breath sounds. *Rales or crackles* are heard on inspiration and indicate the presence of fluid in the lungs. These sounds are often heard in patients with obstructive diseases or pneumonia. When they are coarse and loud and occur with severe dyspnea, rales may be a telling sign of congestive heart failure and pulmonary edema.

Rhonchi or rumbles are low-pitched sounds caused by air flowing past large plugs of mucus. They are common in patients with chronic bronchitis and asthma, or in any disorder in which an excess of mucous secretions are produced. Often rhonchi clear with a strong cough. If the patient has a weak cough and cannot clear the secretions, coarse rhonchi can indicate the need for airway suctioning.

Wheezes have been described as high-pitched, musical sounds. They are most often heard during exhalation. Wheezing is caused when air is forced through narrowed airways, as in asthma or emphysema. Coughing does not usually make the wheeze disappear. In many cases, bronchodilators are required to open the patient's airways and ease breathing. Inspiratory wheezes can be heard when the upper airways are swollen and edematous. The most severe type of inspiratory wheeze is called stridor, heard most commonly in children with croup or epiglottitis. If upper airway obstruction becomes too severe, an artificial airway (such as an endotracheal tube or a tracheostomy) must be used to ensure an open passage for breathing.

Sputum Assessment

If the patient is coughing up sputum, it should be inspected. Normal respiratory secretions are clear or white. Normal sputum has no odor and is of medium consistency. Sputum that is thick and sticky is usually difficult to expectorate. It may indicate that the patient is poorly hydrated. Sputum produced by asthma patients is stringy, like thickened egg white. The patient with pulmonary edema has frothy, pinkish secretions.

Sputum that is yellow or greenish or has a putrid or musty odor usually indicates infection. When infection is suspected, a sputum sample should be collected in a sterile container and sent to the laboratory for examination.

Blood-streaked mucus indicates airway inflammation, and although it can be alarming it is not often serious. It commonly occurs during harsh coughing episodes in patients with bronchitis. Frankly bloody mucus is a sign of continual bleeding somewhere in the airways, and should be thoroughly investigated.

Diagnostic Tests and Procedures

The most commonly used tests for assessing respiratory status are chest X-ray, pulmonary function tests, sputum culture, and arterial blood gas analysis. More specialized tests include bronchoscopy, lung scans, pulmonary angiography, skin testing for allergies in asthma, and skin tests for tuberculosis.

Chest X-ray. The chest x-ray is widely used to identify pathologic changes in the lung and chest that may explain the patient's breathing problems. From a chest x-ray the radiologist can detect abnormal fluid or air in the pleural space. The x-ray can also show whether portions of the lungs are consolidated (as in pneumonia) or airless (as in atelectasis). Tumors are often first detected by routine x-rays. The chest x-ray can also be used to determine the position of catheters and tubes and to monitor a patient's response to therapy.

Pulmonary Function Tests. Specialized breathing tests measure lung volumes and flow rates of air through the airways. These tests are performed with a spirometer, and the resulting depiction of the lung volumes and flows is called a spirogram. When measured correctly, lung volumes and flow rates can indicate the presence of disease. Restrictive lung disease is identified by less-than-expected lung volumes. Obstructive diseases, which are characterized by air trapping and narrowed airways, can also be detected by tests that measure airflow. More specialized pulmonary function tests can give information on lung diffusion abilities, the ability of the lungs to stretch, and the volume of lung actually being used for gas exchange.

Sputum Culture. The patient who has a productive cough, is febrile, and may otherwise show signs of infection should have a sample of sputum evaluated by the laboratory. A Gram stain can be done to determine quickly whether an infection is present. Information about the specific bacteria causing the infection and the best antibiotic to use against it can be gained from a sputum culture and sensitivity. Although this test yields precise information, it takes 2 to 3 days for the results. A Gram stain can be done immediately.

Arterial Blood Gases. These blood tests are regarded as the most reliable indicator of oxygenation and ventilation. Blood flowing through the arteries has just passed through the lungs, where it has undergone the process of exchanging carbon dioxide for oxygen. Since it has yet to circulate past the tissues, arterial blood contains the most oxygen and the least carbon dioxide of any blood in the body.

Tissues rely on arterial blood for nutrients such as glucose, minerals, and electrolytes. The arterial blood also contains the body's oxygen supply. The PaO_2 is a good indicator of how much oxygen is available to tissues. When the PaO_2 is lower than normal, tissues may experience **hypoxia.** This is dangerous to all tissues and organs but can be especially damaging to the heart and the brain, where it can result in a myocardial infarction or a cerebrovascular accident. Although the normal value for PaO_2 declines with age, an abnormally low PaO_2 is a sure sign of lung disease. The more severe the lung impairment is, the lower the PaO_2 (see display).

Arterial blood gases give important information about oxygenation and the lungs' ability to ventilate. The $PaCO_2$ of arterial blood shows how effective the lungs are at removing this waste product. Too much or too little CO_2 can alter the acid–base balance of the blood, adversely affect heart function, alter the drive to breathe, and impair the ability of the tissues to use oxygen.

The $PaCO_2$ stays nearly constant in the person with healthy lungs. A $PaCO_2$ lower than 35 mm Hg indicates **hyperventilation,** or breathing in excess of metabolic needs. This can occur voluntarily in healthy people; it can also occur in healthy but hysterical people. Hyperventilation can also happen during an asthma attack, or in some patients with head injuries.

A $PaCO_2$ above 45 mm Hg indicates **hypoventilation.** This means that the patient is not breathing sufficiently to rinse the blood of the carbon dioxide waste produced by the tissues. This condition usually occurs only in patients with severe obstructive airway disease such as COPD, or in patients whose respiratory drive has been diminished by narcotics, barbiturates, or trauma.

An arterial blood sample also provides information about the blood's acidity or alkalinity. Biochemical processes that are essential to all cell life require a close balance of the blood's acids and bases. The pH is a

---

Levels of Hypoxemia

Mild: PaO_2 of 60–80 mm Hg
Moderate: PaO_2 of 40–60 mm Hg
Severe: PaO_2 of less than 40 mm Hg

Note: PaO_2 naturally declines with age. For every year over 60, subtract 1 mm Hg from the normal range. For example, a man of 70 would be expected to have a PaO_2 of 70–90 mm Hg.

Also, the newborn infant is normally hypoxemic during the first 12–24 hours of life. A PaO_2 of 80–100 mm Hg is achieved after this time.

Adapted from Shapiro, B., Harrison, R., Kacmarek, R., & Cane, R. (1985). *Clinical applications of respiratory care* (3rd Ed.). Chicago: Year Book Medical Publishers.

---

measure of the acid–base balance of the blood. Normally, arterial blood is slightly alkaline with a value of 7.40. If the arterial pH is below 7.35, the person is said to be acidotic. A pH above 7.45 indicates the person is alkalotic (Table 30-2).

Acid–base imbalances are caused by either respiratory or metabolic problems. Ordinarily, breathing too rapidly depletes carbon dioxide (the primary blood acid), and respiratory alkalosis results. Conversely, hypoventilation allows carbon dioxide to build up, resulting in respiratory acidosis.

A number of conditions can cause metabolic acidosis or alkalosis. When a diabetic patient has insufficient insulin, for example, excessive amounts of acid are produced because of inefficient glucose metabolism. Severe diarrhea can cause rapid loss of bicarbonate, a major base, from the gastrointestinal system. Both of these result in metabolic acidosis. In contrast, vomiting or excessive removal of stomach acids via nasogastric suction may cause an imbalance resulting in a relative excess of base. The same can occur with overuse of antacids. Both of these can lead to metabolic alkalosis. For a more detailed discussion of acid–base balance, refer to Chapter 32.

Bronchoscopy. Bronchoscopy allows the physician to directly visualize the airways. A flexible fiber-optic tube connected to a viewing screen is inserted through the

TABLE 30–2
Normal Arterial Blood Gas Values

PaO_2:	80–100 mm Hg
$PaCO_2$:	35–45 mm Hg
pH:	7.35–7.45
HCO_3-:	22–26 mEq/L
Base excess:	±2

patient's nose. The scope is directed into the trachea and bronchi by a hand-held control. The bronchoscope can be used to collect sterile sputum specimens or tissue samples for laboratory examination, or to withdraw large sputum plugs or aspirated objects that have obstructed the airways.

Lung Scan and Angiography. Lung scans and angiography are used to determine the pattern of blood flow and ventilation in the lung. They are often used to establish the presence and extent of pulmonary embolism. They involve the use of radiopaque substances and x-rays.

Skin Tests. Skin tests are done for two purposes. One type of skin testing involves injecting small amounts of substances ("antigens") under the skin to determine the cause of allergies. Small skin eruptions indicate sensitivity to the injected antigen. Since asthma is often caused by allergy, skin testing can help identify the source of the attacks. The physician can then attempt to desensitize the patient by gradually increasing his or her exposure to the antigen, allowing the immune system to slowly adjust to the presence of the allergy-causing substance.

Another type of skin test is used to establish whether a patient has been exposed to specific infections. The most common test of this type is the PPD (purified protein derivative) test for tuberculosis. In this test a small amount of serum containing a derivative of tuberculosis bacteria is injected into the skin. If the patient has been exposed to the disease, the injection site becomes swollen within about 48 hours. Although a positive PPD test does not necessarily indicate the presence of active tuberculosis, the result should be called to the attention of the physician, and further investigation should be undertaken.

NURSING DIAGNOSES AND PATIENT GOALS

People with respiratory dysfunction display many problems and have the potential to develop many others. Patient assessment data substantiate a potential or actual nursing diagnosis. There are nursing diagnoses that relate specifically to alterations in respiratory function. Primary NANDA nursing diagnoses included in this category are Ineffective Breathing Pattern, Ineffective Airway Clearance, and Impaired Gas Exchange.

Diagnostic Statement: Ineffective Breathing Pattern

Definition

Ineffective breathing pattern is the state in which an individual's inhalation and/or exhalation pattern does not enable adequate pulmonary inflation or emptying (NANDA, 1990).

Defining Characteristics

Dyspnea; shortness of breath; tachypnea; fremitus; abnormal arterial blood gas values; cyanosis; cough; nasal flaring; respiratory depth changes; assumption of three-point position; pursed-lip breathing or prolonged expiratory phase; increased anteroposterior diameter; use of accessory muscles; and altered chest excursion (NANDA, 1990).

Related Factors

Neuromuscular impairment; pain, musculoskeletal impairment; perception or cognitive impairment; anxiety; decreased energy and fatigue (NANDA, 1990).

Diagnostic Statement: Ineffective Airway Clearance

Definition

Ineffective airway clearance is the state in which an individual is unable to clear secretions or obstructions from the respiratory tract to maintain airway patency (NANDA, 1990).

Defining Characteristics

Abnormal breath sounds (rales [crackles], rhonchi [wheezes]); changes in rate or depth of respiration; tachypnea; effective or ineffective cough, with or without sputum; cyanosis; dyspnea (NANDA, 1990).

Related Factors

Decreased energy and fatigue; tracheobronchial infection, obstruction, secretion; perceptual or cognitive impairment; trauma (NANDA, 1990).

Diagnostic Statement: Impaired Gas Exchange

Definition

Impaired gas exchange is the state in which an individual experiences a decreased passage of oxygen and/or carbon dioxide between the alveoli of the lungs and the vascular system (NANDA, 1990).

Defining Characteristics

Confusion; somnolence; restlessness; irritability; inability to move secretions; hypercapnea; hypoxia (NANDA, 1990).

Related Factor

Ventilation perfusion imbalance (NANDA, 1990).

Related Nursing Diagnoses

Other nursing diagnoses are common for people with respiratory dysfunction. These include High Risk for Infection, Altered Nutrition: Less Than Body Requirements, Pain, and Sleep Pattern Disturbance. Breathing difficulties and respiratory disease also affect the patient's ability to carry out activities of daily living. Possible nursing diagnoses related to this include High Risk for Activity Intolerance or Self-Care Deficit. Anxiety, Self-Esteem Disturbance, and Ineffective Individual or Family Coping are examples of possible psychosocial nursing diagnoses. Knowledge Deficit regarding treatment plan, and Impaired Adjustment are also potential nursing diagnoses for many patients with respiratory dysfunction.

Patient Goals

The following general areas should be included in the formulation of patient goals:

Patient will demonstrate knowledge regarding prevention of respiratory dysfunction.
Patient's tissues will have adequate oxygenation.
Patient will mobilize pulmonary secretions.
Patient will effectively cope with changes in self-concept and lifestyle.

Patient goals differ substantially depending on the prognosis. For the healthy person, the goals will probably be to prevent respiratory problems and to learn good pulmonary hygiene. For the patient with an acute problem, the goal will be to recover from the respiratory problem without any residual respiratory complications. Goals for the chronic respiratory patient focus on the patient's ability to live within limitations imposed by the disease, and to accept changes in lifestyle and self-concept. For the terminal respiratory patient, goals should be to maintain adequate comfort and to accept impending death.

IMPLEMENTATION

The nurse plays a central role in educating patients with respiratory dysfunction, as well as preventing and treating this problem. Interventions are aimed at restoring, maintaining, and promoting respiratory health. The selection of appropriate nursing interventions is based on assessment, the resultant nursing diagnoses, and patient goals (see display).

Nursing Interventions to Promote Health and Respiratory Function

The nurse can become involved in hospital or community activities that promote healthy lungs. In the hospital, the nurse is a credible teacher who can offer facts about the dangers of smoking. This can also be done in the community, in schools, and at community-sponsored health fairs. The American Lung Association sponsors activities in many areas to call attention to pulmonary health. "Better Breather" clubs provide a social and educational outlet for those with chronic breathing problems. Meetings of these groups combine pot-luck dinners with informal, instructional talks by nurses, physicians, and therapists.

The nurse can also actively campaign for local and regional legislation designed to control air pollution. Asbestos removal from schools and public buildings, indoor air pollution, and auto emissions controls are

---

Selected Nursing Interventions for Selected Respiratory Dysfunctions

Airway maintenance

- Positioning
- Hydration
- Humidification (e.g., nebulizers or humidifiers)
- Coughing
- Increased mobility
- Chest physiotherapy
- Postural drainage
- Suctioning
- Airway care

Inadequate gas exchange

- Positioning for optimum lung expansion
- Deep breathing
- Pursed-lip breathing
- Incentive spirometry
- Oxygen administration (via cannula, mask, Venturi mask, rebreathing mask)
- Bronchodilator therapy
- Ventilators

Ineffective breathing pattern

- Verbal cues regarding respiratory rate or depth
- Judicious use of pain medication
- Anxiety management

Patient Teaching

Instruct the patient as follows:

- Learn to breathe correctly. Using the diaphragm helps the patient with chronic lung disease to increase breathing efficiency. Breathe with your abdomen: push out with inspiration, and exhale by pulling your abdomen in.
- Use pursed-lip breathing to exhale more fully. To do this, almost close your lips, forming a small circle, and exhale slowly against the lips, as if you are whistling.
- If you are taking prescribed medications for your breathing, do not use over-the-counter medications without the advice of your physician. Undesirable interactions can occur.
- Use bronchodilators according to the prescribed schedule. Exceeding the prescribed dose can cause serious side effects, such as heart irregularities and seizures.
- To help keep secretions thin and easy to cough up, drink at least 6 glasses of water each day.
- Notify your physician if your breathing becomes more difficult, your sputum increases in amount or changes color, or you have an elevated temperature. These signs may indicate respiratory infection.
- When using oxygen at home, instruct friends and family members not to smoke. Keep oxygen away from open flames and space heaters.

---

examples of issues that are unresolved in many states. Nurses can join or form political organizations in favor of candidates who support clean-air legislation.

Nurses in industry promote respiratory health by teaching workers how to avoid or minimize harmful exposures to fumes or dust. This may include instruction in the proper use of filtration-type respirators. The nurse may also help workers to recognize early symptoms of respiratory problems.

The nurse can use a number of therapies to promote respiratory function. Airway maintenance measures are used to improve airway clearance. Important interventions to keep airways open include adequate hydration, positioning and ambulation, aerosol therapy, coughing, chest physiotherapy, management of artificial airways, and suctioning. Hyperinflation techniques (such as deep breathing, incentive spirometry, and intermittent positive pressure breathing) can help improve the patient's breathing pattern. Oxygen therapy is used to promote gas exchange.

Hydration

Proper hydration is vital for many functions, including maintaining electrolyte balance, removing waste products from the blood, and regulating temperature. Insufficient fluid can adversely affect these and other functions, not the least of which is secretion mobilization. Inadequate hydration causes respiratory mucus to become thick and difficult to cough up. Sticky, tenacious sputum that coats the linings of the respiratory tract can cause breathing difficulties for any patient. For the patient with lung disease, extra mucus in the airways makes already difficult breathing even worse.

Mucus that remains stuck to the airways acts as a germ trap. Normally this is a protective function of mucus, but only when the mucus can be easily removed by coughing. When mucus is hard to expectorate, the bacteria caught in it have a chance to multiply and cause pneumonia.

Other problems caused by dried, sticky mucus can include excessive coughing and absorption atelectasis. When extra mucus builds up in the airways and becomes thick, it becomes an irritant and causes a cough. Ideally, the mucus can be expelled with a cough. However, thick mucus is difficult to raise, and the persistent cough it can create may be nonproductive. This can deprive the coughing patient of sleep. It can cause pain in surgical patients and can cause the weakened patient to become dyspneic.

The nurse can help maintain the mobility of mucus by encouraging fluids in all patients who are at risk for dried secretions. Unless the patient is severely restricted in the amount of fluid allowed, water and juices should be encouraged and taken frequently to keep the sputum thinned. Milk should be avoided since it tends to thicken secretions. Patients can set an intake goal and independently keep track of their fluid intake. For patients who are weak or need assistance in obtaining fluids, the nurse should offer fluids regularly. Patients whose oral intake is restricted may require additional aerosol therapy to ensure secretion fluidity.

Positioning and Ambulation

Ambulation and the ability to frequently change position are two natural means for keeping the lungs open and clear of secretions. Movement helps shift respiratory mucus in the airways. This is beneficial because the mucus moves into areas of the airways where it can generate a cough, and thus can be expelled easily. This keeps mucus from pooling and minimizes the risk of bacterial colonization and infection.

Mucus tends to pool in the lungs of people who cannot or will not move around. Bedridden patients, patients in pain (such as those who have undergone surgery), and patients who cannot tolerate exercise (because of heart or lung disease) have limited mobility and thus are prone to secretion retention. The patient with an artificial airway and the patient whose cough is otherwise impaired are also inclined to have mucus pooling.

To assist these patients in the removal of secretions, the nurse should see that they frequently change position. Simply moving the patient from one side to another or assisting with ambulation when possible helps the natural clearance mechanisms of the lung. For the severely debilitated patient, frequent positioning also aids circulation and prevents skin breakdown.

Ambulation is difficult for some respiratory patients because of dyspnea with exertion. Whenever possible, each patient must be helped to increase exercise tolerance by encouraging independence. Additional benefits of increased exercise tolerance include extra strength for effective coughing and decreased oxygen consumption (Ries, 1987). Portable oxygen may be needed during periods of ambulation.

Hyperinflation

Several techniques are available to prevent and counteract atelectasis. Shallow breathing or an ineffective cough can lead to atelectasis, mucus plugging, hypoxemia, and pneumonia (Shapiro, et al., 1985). Hyperinflation of the lungs can expand alveoli and promote an effective cough, thereby decreasing the risk of atelectasis.

Deep Breathing. Deep breathing is essential for the prevention of pulmonary complications in the hospitalized patient. Pain, lung disease, muscle weakness, or neurologic impairment can hinder a patient's ability to breathe deeply. A major task of the nurse is to coach and encourage the patient in deep-breathing techniques.

Deep breathing is useful for any patient with limited activity, but is perhaps most useful for the postoperative patient. There are no contraindications to deep breathing: anyone can do it at practically any time. Although patients with incisional pain or broken ribs may find it uncomfortable to inhale deeply, it causes no harm. A deep breath can open alveoli that have collapsed as a result of shallow breathing. It also stimulates the specialized cells of the alveoli that are responsible for surfactant production (Slonim & Hamilton, 1987). A deep breath also strengthens the cough and aids in the movement of mucus in the tracheobronchial tree.

The nurse should instruct the patient to deep-breathe by inhaling slowly through the nose. Holding the breath for 2 or 3 seconds at the peak of inspiration allows the air to distribute optimally throughout the airways. A relaxed passive exhalation through the mouth is recommended for most patients. (See Procedure 30-1, Teaching Coughing and Deep-Breathing Exercises.)

Pursed-Lip Breathing. Pursed-lip breathing is a special measure to be used by selected patients along with deep breathing. Patients with obstructive lung diseases such as COPD or asthma should be taught this technique to aid in the release of trapped air from obstructed airways.

To perform pursed-lip breathing, the patient inhales deeply, holds the breath for a moment, then exhales slowly through lips that are held almost closed. By pushing the air against the small orifice made by the pursed lips, pressure is created back through the airways. This back-pressure effect pushes the airways open throughout exhalation. This allows more air to escape during exhalation and helps to prevent air trapping.

Incentive Spirometry. Deep breathing can be performed by almost anyone, but some patients need assistance. Numerous devices have been developed to help patients deep-breathe, but the most widely used one is the incentive spirometer. It operates on the principle that spontaneous sustained maximal inspiration is most beneficial to the lungs and has virtually no adverse effects. Its simplicity, minimal cost, and effectiveness have made incentive spirometry one of the most commonly prescribed therapies.

The incentive spirometer measures roughly the patient's inspired volume and offers the "incentive" of measuring progress. Models vary greatly, but all offer the patient some observable indicator of how deep a breath has been taken. Volume-oriented incentive spirometers require the patient to inspire deeply from a bellows. To use these models, the patient inhales steadily and deeply, causing the bellows to deflate and rise as air is evacuated from the bellows. The objective is to motivate the patient to inspire more deeply each time the device is used. Because volume is indicated on the device, the patient can see how much is inspired with each breath. The patient and nurse can set realistic goals for each breathing session, and the patient can work independently toward achieving each goal.

Flow-oriented incentive spirometers use "floating" ping-pong balls or similar objects to indicate patient effort (Fig. 30-4). Inspiration must be quick and deep. The subatmospheric pressure caused by the deep inspiration raises the balls, and the objective is to keep the balls floating for as long as possible. The balls float as long as inspiratory flow is sustained and the chamber is evacuated of air. Although volume is not accurately measured with these devices, they are popular because they are inexpensive and just as effective as the volume-oriented devices, and patients enjoy the challenge of making the balls float as if by magic. As with volume-oriented spirometers, the nurse and patient can establish goals for each breathing session.

Regardless of the type of equipment used, the purpose of incentive spirometry is to motivate the patient to take responsibility for the success or failure of deep-breathing therapy. When properly performed, incentive spirometry can give all the benefits of deep breathing. A reasonable schedule for this therapy is eight to ten breaths

PROCEDURE 30–1. Teaching Coughing and Deep-Breathing Exercises

■ **Purpose**

1. Facilitate respiratory functioning by increasing lung expansion and oxygenation.
2. Encourage expectoration of mucus and secretions that accumulate in the airways after general anesthesia and immobility.

■ **Assessment**

- Assess patient's risk factors for developing respiratory complications (i.e., general anesthesia, history of pulmonary disease or smoking, chest wall trauma, cold or respiratory infection within past week).
- Assess quality, rate, depth of respiration.
- Auscultate breath sounds.
- Inspect placement of incision and evaluate whether it interferes with chest expansion.
- Evaluate patient's physical ability to cooperate and perform pulmonary exercises:
  - level of consciousness
  - language or communication barriers
  - ability to assume Fowler's position
  - expression of pain (medicate as ordered)

■ **Equipment**

Pillows for positioning and to splint incision

■ **Procedure**

Deep Breathing

1. Assist patient to Fowler's or sitting position.
   Rationale: Upright position allows increased diaphragmatic excursion secondary to downward shift of internal organs from gravity.
2. Have patient place hands palm down, with middle fingers touching, along lower border of rib cage.
   Rationale: Allows patient to feel movement of chest and abdomen during deep breathing.
3. Ask patient to inhale slowly through the nose, feeling middle fingers separate. Hold breath for 2 or 3 seconds.
   Rationale: Inhaling through nose allows air to be filtered, warmed, and humidified. Holding breath allows lungs to fully expand.

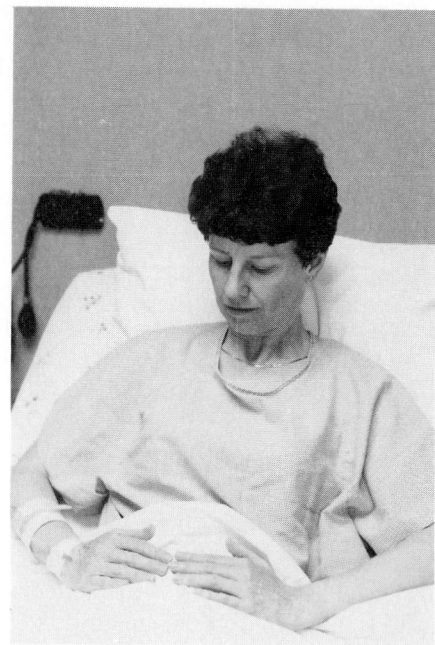

Step 2

4. Have patient exhale slowly through mouth. Repeat 3 to 5 times.
   Rationale: Slow expulsion of air frequently initiates the coughing reflex, which facilitates expectoration of mucus.

■ **Procedure**

Controlled Coughing

1. If voluntary coughing does not occur, have patient take a deep breath, hold for 3 seconds, and cough deeply 2 or 3 times. Nurse should stand to the patient's side to ensure the cough is not directed at him or her.
   Note: Patient must cough deeply, not just clear the throat.
   Rationale: Several consecutive coughs are more effective than one single cough at moving mucus up the respiratory tree.
2. If the patient has an abdominal or chest incision that will be painful during coughing, instruct the patient to hold a pillow firmly over the incision (splinting) when coughing.

(continued)

PROCEDURE 30–1. Teaching Coughing and Deep-Breathing Exercises *continued*

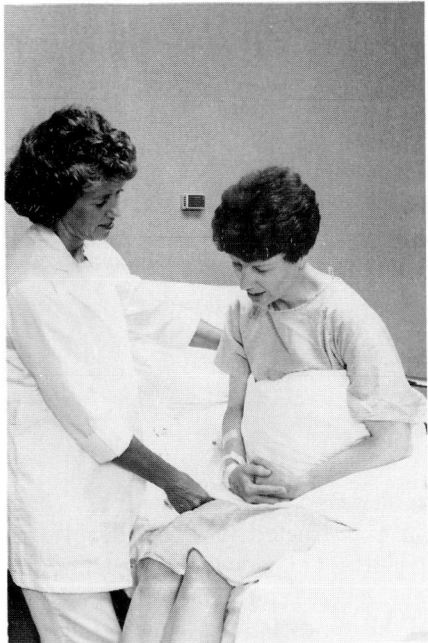

Step 2

Rationale: Coughing uses abdominal and accessory respiratory muscles, which may have been cut during surgery. Splinting supports the incision and surrounding tissues and reduces pain during coughing.

3. Instruct, reinforce, and supervise deep-breathing and coughing exercises every 2 to 3 hours post-operatively.
4. Document procedure.

■ **Lifespan Considerations**

Infants and Children

• Infants cannot cooperate with coughing and deep-breathing exercises, but crying is thought to hyperinflate the lungs.
• Young children learn through games and imitation. A preoperative game of "Simon Says" is one way to teach them lung exercises: "Simon says touch your nose," "Simon says stick out your tongue," "Simon says take a deep breath," "Simon says cough."

hourly during waking hours. Care should be taken to perform the exercises slowly, to avoid hyperventilation. (See Procedure 30-2, Promoting Breathing with the Incentive Spirometer.)

Intermittent Positive Pressure Breathing. When patients are unable or unwilling to breathe deeply, either on their own or with an incentive spirometer, intermittent positive pressure breathing (IPPB) provides an alternative hyperinflation therapy. This treatment uses a mechanical ventilator to provide a pressurized breath on inspiration. The machine pushes air into the lungs much like a bicycle pump fills a tire. As the lungs fill, pressure builds throughout the patient circuit and cycles the ventilator off. After each positive pressure breath, the patient exhales passively.

When assisting with IPPB, the nurse should have the patient sit up or lie in semi-Fowler's position. Pressure and flow controls should be set to deliver enough air to fill the lungs but not to make the patient uncomfortable. The patient inspires from the mouthpiece of the ventilator tubing, triggering the machine to deliver a breath. The lungs are allowed to fill passively, and exhalation takes place when the chest has expanded fully. The patient must keep air from leaking through the nose or from around the mouthpiece and must not breathe too fast. The nurse should allow regular rest periods and should assess the patient regularly for adverse effects.

It is difficult to teach some patients to use IPPB correctly. The equipment is expensive, and specially trained personnel are needed to provide and monitor therapy. Complications include hyperventilation, spread of infection, air swallowing with resultant gastric distension, danger of causing or worsening a pneumothorax, and the possibility of increasing air trapping in patients with obstructive diseases. In addition, IPPB is no more effective at providing a deep breath for most people than is spontaneous deep breathing or incentive spirometry (Burton, Hodgkin, & Ward, 1991).

Coughing

No single measure is more effective for maintaining secretion control than a strong cough. The patient who produces excessive secretions breathes more easily and more comfortably if the secretions can be expectorated. Sputum retention causes increased work of breathing and may contribute to atelectasis and hypoxemia.

A cough is the sudden movement of air behind secretions that pushes the secretions forward. To establish the forward push, the air must exert sufficient pressure against the mucus. Usually this is accomplished by having the patient inspire deeply and then close the glottis. As the patient begins to exhale before the glottis opens, pressure builds in the airways. When the glottis suddenly opens, the quick release of pressure generates rapid airflow, which pushes the mucus up and out.

For many patients, a strong cough is difficult or impossible. Postoperative or trauma patients in pain may be unable or unwilling to cough deeply. Patients with severe

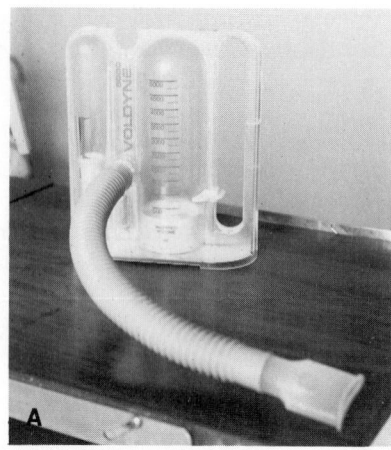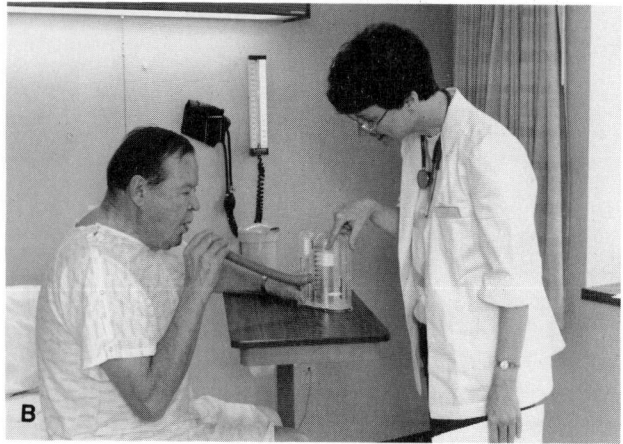

Figure 30–4. Incentive spirometers. **A:** Flow-directed incentive spirometer. **B:** Patient using incentive spirometer.

COPD may be unable to quickly release air from their lungs, and thus cannot generate an effective cough. Some patients are simply too weak to cough, and others may not understand how to produce an effective cough. Finally, a patient with a tracheostomy or endotracheal tube cannot cough with optimal efficiency, since the glottis cannot close.

The nurse must be an effective coach to elicit a proper cough. Many patients need encouragement and assistance, and all patients should be told clearly the rationale for coughing. Different types of coughs should be used by different patients.

Deep Cough. The postoperative patient who does not have lung disease should be taught to cough deeply, to mobilize secretions and to open alveoli that may have collapsed after anesthesia. The deep cough can cause pain around the incisional area in patients who have had abdominal or thoracic surgery. To help control the pain, the nurse can show the patient how to support the incisional area with a pillow. The patient uses the pillow as a splint to keep the incision immobilized during the cough. By holding the pillow tightly during a deep cough, the patient can minimize discomfort. In patients with severe incisional discomfort, it may be wise to schedule coughing sessions after pain medications have been administered.

Stacked Cough. Some patients find it painful to cough despite premedication. For them, a stacked cough may be less uncomfortable and almost as effective. Stacked coughing is the release of several short blasts of air instead of one deep cough. This type of cough prevents excessive stretching of stitches and also decreases the airway collapse that may come with deep coughing.

Low-Flow (Huff) Cough. A third type of cough is called low-flow or "huff" coughing. This method of

clearing the airways is most effective for COPD patients. The patient is instructed to inhale deeply. Instead of closing the glottis and allowing a large amount of pressure to build, the patient then "huffs" the air out. The low airflow this type of cough generates helps prevent airway collapse while still propelling mucus upward in the bronchi. A similar method of coughing can be used for patients with tracheostomies.

Quad Cough. Some patients with neuromuscular disease and those who are quadriplegic may need direct assistance in generating an effective cough. For these patients, the quad cough technique is useful. The patient takes a deep breath, or the nurse provides a deep breath with a resuscitation bag. The deep breath is held for a moment. With hands placed just below the patient's ribcage, the nurse forces the patient to exhale rapidly by quickly pushing in and upward. The resultant rush of air can act as a cough by helping to propel mucus up and out of the airways.

Aerosol Therapy

An aerosol is a suspension of microscopic liquid particles in air. Aerosol therapy may be given for any of the following reasons:

- To add humidity to certain oxygen delivery systems.
- To hydrate thick sputum.
- To relax bronchioles constricted by bronchospasm.
- To administer anti-inflammatory drugs or asthma prevention drugs.
- To deliver antibiotics to the lungs to fight infection.

Sputum that is dried and thickened is difficult to raise, even with the most powerful cough. Despite adequate hydration, a patient's sputum may become dry, requiring aerosol therapy. A large-volume nebulizer or an

---

■ **Purpose**
1. Improve pulmonary ventilation and oxygenation.
2. Loosen respiratory secretions.
3. Prevent or treat atelectasis by expanding collapsed alveoli.

■ **Assessment**
• Identify patients at risk for atelectasis.
• Complete respiratory assessment (i.e., history of smoking, breath sounds, respiratory rate and rhythm, sputum production.
• Review physician's orders for incentive spirometry.

■ **Equipment**
Incentive spirometer (flow-oriented or volume-oriented)
Note: Type of incentive spirometer is usually determined by equipment available through respiratory therapy.
Mouthpiece (if not already connected to spirometer)
Nose clip (optional)

■ **Procedure**
1. Wash your hands.
   Rationale: Reduces transfer of microorganisms.

2. Assist patient to high Fowler's or sitting position.
   Rationale: Facilitates optimal lung expansion.
3. Instruct patient in procedure:
   a. Seal lips tightly around mouthpiece.
      Rationale: Prevents leakage of air around mouthpiece.
   b. Inhale slowly and deeply through mouth. Hold breath for 2 or 3 seconds.
      Rationale: Maintains maximal inflation of alveoli.
      Note: Patient can see his or her progress by watching the balls elevate or lights go on, depending on type of equipment used.
   c. Exhale slowly around mouthpiece.
   d. Breathe normally for several breaths.
4. Repeat procedure 5 to 10 times every 1 to 2 hours, per physician's orders.
5. Wash your hands.

■ **Lifespan Considerations**
Note: Patients who are too young to follow directions, are cognitively impaired or malnourished, or lack necessary motor skills are likely to be unsuccessful at using incentive spirometry.

---

ultrasonic nebulizer can deliver a thick mist continuously to the airways. The water is absorbed into the mucus blanket, loosening it and facilitating its removal. The watery mist is also soothing to inflamed airways. Heating the water before aerosolization can increase the amount of water vapor carried in the aerosol.

This treatment is provided through an aerosol mask, or via a tracheostomy collar or "T-piece" for patients with artificial airways. Often oxygen is used to power the nebulizer, in which case the patient receives additional oxygen therapy. The nurse should periodically check these nebulizers to ensure that they are filled with sterile water, are screwed together tightly, and are not too hot.

Aerosols can work efficiently to loosen dried secretions. Patients with distant but relatively clear breath sounds may develop coarse rumbles after aerosol therapy. This is a sign that the treatment has successfully moistened thick mucus. Once the secretions are loosened, they must be coughed out or removed by suctioning.

Hand-Held Nebulizers. Bronchodilator drugs are powerful medications that are best delivered by means of small-volume hand-held nebulizers. Most of these agents can reverse bronchospasm quickly. They can also cause the heart to work much harder and make the patient feel generally nervous. These medications are

packaged in a wide variety of dosages, so the nurse should carefully check the ordered dose against the available unit-dose packages. Some patients are particularly susceptible to the side effects of these medications, so all patients should be closely monitored for signs such as increased pulse rate, agitation, and restlessness.

The hand-held nebulizer can be operated by means of a compressor or by oxygen at 4 to 5 liters per minute (LPM). The patient should inhale deeply and hold the breath for a moment. This allows the aerosol to deposit in the distant portions of the lungs and to open the airways more effectively. This should be repeated at a slow breathing rate until the medication is gone from the nebulizer. Some of the more widely used aerosolized bronchodilators are isoetharine (Bronkosol), metaproterenol (Alupent), terbutaline (Brethine, Bricanyl), and albuterol (Proventil, Ventolin).

Other types of medications can also be delivered by small-volume nebulizers. Cromolyn sodium (Intal) can be given only by inhalation. It may be aerosolized as a liquid, or it may be inhaled as a powder via a device called a Spinhaler. This medication is used to prevent asthma attacks. Antibiotics may also be delivered by aerosol. This is usually done only if the patient has a particularly stubborn lung infection. Aerosolized corticosteroids such as beclomethasone (Vanceril, Beclo-

TABLE 30–3

Common Medications for Patients with Respiratory Conditions

Agent	How Provided	Clinical Notes
Bronchodilators		
Isoetharine (Bronkosol) Metaproterenol (Alupent) Terbutaline (Brethine, Bricanyl) Albuterol (Ventolin, Proventil)	Metered-dose inhalers (MDI), unit dose packs, solution for administration via hand-held nebulizer or IPPB; some solutions for injection	1. Used to treat wheezing from asthma, COPD 2. May cause nervousness and tremors 3. May cause tachycardia. Note heart rate before and after treatment. 4. Aerosol chamber (or "spacer") improves dispersal of medication.
Theophylline (Theo-Dur, Slo-bid, aminophylline, many others)	Oral via tabs and liquids; injectable IV solution is aminophylline	1. Same as 1–3 above 2. Side effects include nausea, headache, agitation. 3. Toxic effects may include cardiac arrhythmias and seizures. 4. Blood levels should be monitored, kept at 10–20 µg/dL 5. Wide variety of available preparations; use extra caution in administration.
Anti-inflammatory agents		
Beclomethasone (Beclovent, Vanceril) Flunisolide (AeroBid) Triamcinolone (Azmacort)	Metered-dose inhaler	1. These agents are locally acting steroids. They decrease inflammation in asthma and COPD. 2. These agents are not effective in acute dyspnea attacks. 3. Patient should rinse mouth after use.

Safety Alert

- Do not smoke or use heat-generating devices nearby when oxygen is in use. Oxygen accelerates combustion and a fire may result.
- Handle oxygen cylinders with care. Damage to the tank or its valve can result in an explosion.
- Closely monitor oxygen administration and be sure the prescribed concentration or liter flow rate is not exceeded. Hypoventilation, oxygen toxicity, and eye damage may occur if selected patients are given too much oxygen.
- When suctioning a patient, hyperinflate and pre-oxygenate with 100% oxygen before each attempt. This will help prevent atelectasis and hypoxemia.
- Limit each suctioning attempt to 15 seconds to minimize the risk of trauma and hypoxemia.
- Monitor patients receiving theophylline preparations closely for toxic effects such as nausea, tachycardia, and nervous agitation. This bronchodilator can cause cardiac arrhythmias and seizures in excessive doses.

vent) and triamcinolone (Azmacort) are being used more frequently to fight lung inflammation and to avoid the negative systemic effects that accompany long-term oral use of steroids. Table 30-3 lists common respiratory medications.

Metered-Dose Inhalers. Gas-powered, cartridge-type nebulizers called metered-dose inhalers (MDIs) provide a premeasured dose of aerosolized medication to the patient with each breath. The MDI usually contains a bronchodilator or steroid. MDIs are ordinarily self-administered by the patient, but the nurse is often responsible for instructing the patient in their use. An aerosol chamber that attaches to the MDI can help the patient increase the MDI's efficiency. Figure 30-5 shows an MDI.

Nursing Interventions for Altered Respiratory Function

Oxygen Therapy

Some patients need oxygen therapy to maintain adequate arterial blood oxygen levels. Lung disease, cardiovascular problems, blood disorders such as anemia, and extraordinary metabolic demands of healing tissues can

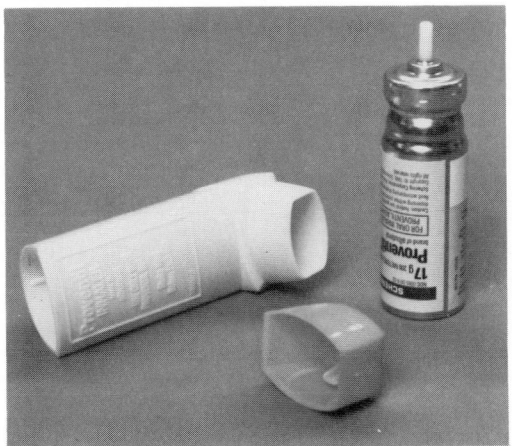

Figure 30–5. Metered-dose inhaler.

limit the body's oxygen supply. By providing these patients with supplemental oxygen, their PaO_2 can usually be brought within reasonable limits.

Oxygen therapy is used primarily to reverse **hypoxemia** (low blood oxygen levels). This action can help to accomplish three fundamental goals (Shapiro, 1985):

- Improved tissue oxygenation.
- Decreased work of breathing in dyspneic patients.
- Decreased work of the heart in patients with cardiac disease.

First, increasing the amount of oxygen available to the patient's lungs increases the amount of oxygen available to the blood. This makes more oxygen available for the vital organs.

Second, the hypoxemic patient must often work harder at breathing to maintain adequate blood oxygen levels. As a result, the respiratory muscles use a disproportionate amount of oxygen just to maintain the process of breathing. By replacing the oxygen taken by the overworked muscles, the patient can use less effort to breathe.

Third, hypoxemia normally causes the heart to beat faster. This is a compensatory mechanism: by increasing the amount of blood flow to tissues, the heart can make up for a decreased amount of oxygen in the blood. By reversing the hypoxemia that causes this increased heart rate, myocardial work can be decreased.

Administration of Oxygen. For the average patient with lung disease, oxygen therapy can help eliminate dyspnea and thereby improve comfort. For the critically ill patient, meticulous oxygen therapy can be life-saving.

Because oxygen is a drug, a prescription is required for its use. The fact that it is so commonly and sometimes casually prescribed may give the nurse the impression that oxygen is harmless. Improperly administered it can be worthless at best, however, and it can be dangerous. The nurse must understand how various oxygen delivery systems work and must learn how to operate them safely.

Once oxygen therapy has been started, the patient's blood gases should be monitored regularly. An alternative to arterial blood gas analysis is pulse oximetry. The oximeter is noninvasive and convenient for measuring the degree to which hemoglobin is saturated with oxygen. It attaches to the patient's ear lobe or finger and can provide a continuous display of the percentage of hemoglobin saturation.

Oxygen is prescribed either in terms of flow (expressed in liters per minute [L/min]) or percent (often expressed as fraction of inspired oxygen, or FIO_2). A general rule for safe oxygen therapy is to use the lowest level of oxygen possible to achieve an acceptable PaO_2 or percent saturation. This level of oxygen should be used only as long as necessary. Oxygen should normally be used continuously until the patient can maintain a satisfactory PaO_2 or percent saturation without it.

Because oxygen is drying, oxygen therapy is usually delivered using humidification. A humidifier is attached to the flow meter (Fig. 30-6), and the oxygen tubing is attached to the humidifier.

Oxygen Delivery Systems. Various pieces of equipment have been designed to provide oxygen in a wide range of flows and percentages. The device best suited for the patient's needs is determined first by its capability and second by patient comfort (Table 30-4). Common oxygen devices are shown in Figure 30-7.

The amount of supplemental oxygen the patient needs must be established. The aim of oxygen therapy in most cases should be to maintain the patient's PaO_2 above 60 mm Hg, or the oxygen saturation of hemoglobin above 90%. It is rarely necessary to keep the PaO_2 higher than 90 or 100 mm Hg.

Most patients require relatively low concentrations of oxygen to correct hypoxemia. If a small amount of addi-

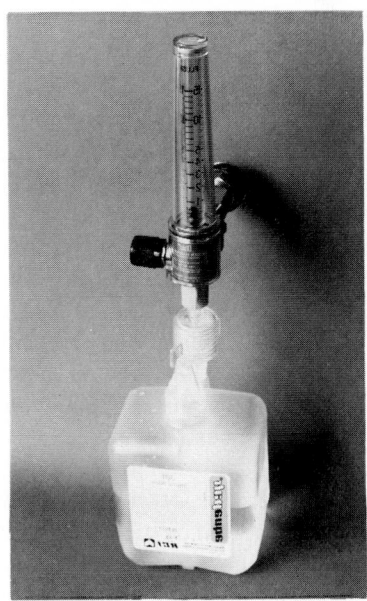

Figure 30–6. Flow meter.

TABLE 30–4

Oxygen Therapy Equipment

Device	Oxygen Capability	Nursing Considerations
Cannula (nasal prongs)	22%–44% when operated at 1–6 L/min	1. "Rule of 4" gives an approximation of concentration: for each L/min of oxygen, concentration of O_2 delivered increases by 4% (e.g., 1 L/min yields 22%, 2 L/min yields 26%, etc.) 2. Maximum flow should be no more than 6 L/min to avoid mucosal drying. 3. Generally most convenient and comfortable O_2 device
Venturi mask	24%–50% when L/min run at 3–8 L/min as specified on side of mask	1. Precise delivery system 2. Noisy; like all masks it may cause claustrophobia.
Simple mask	40%–60% when run at 6–10 L/min	1. Most common midrange O_2 device 2. Not usually desirable for COPD patient because of potential for excessive oxygenation
Reservoir mask	90% and up when run at 10–15 L/min	1. Used for critically ill patients 2. Use sufficient flow to keep reservoir bag inflated.
Incubator	22%–40% and up	1. Frequent analysis required 2. Very imprecise delivery in O_2 ranges above 30%
Oxyhood	22%–90% and up	1. Precise O_2 delivery for infants 2. O_2 must be prewarmed and humidified.

tional oxygen is needed to maintain the PaO_2 over 60 mm Hg, a cannula or low-percentage Venturi-type mask can be used. If the patient requires a moderate amount of oxygen, a simple mask is preferable. When a high concentration of oxygen is needed, a reservoir-type mask is required.

Nasal Cannula. The nasal cannula is the most commonly used oxygen delivery system. Also called nasal prongs, this device can provide oxygen concentrations between approximately 22% and 44%. The cannula is widely used because of its comfort. It is well tolerated by most patients because it allows for good mobility, it is quiet, and unlike a mask it seldom causes feelings of claustrophobia.

The cannula is worn with both prongs inserted into the nostrils. The prongs must be kept snugly in place. The oxygen flow-meter should be set according to the physician's order, between 1 and 6 L/min. More than 6 L/min can dry the patient's nasal passages, and they may become sore and bleed. If the patient's nasal passages are patent, the cannula delivers oxygen whether the patient breathes through the mouth or nose.

The cannula is a satisfactory oxygen system for the patient who requires a low but not necessarily precise concentration of oxygen. The actual percentage of oxygen delivered by the cannula per breath varies depending on the patient's breathing pattern. A deep breath causes more room air to mix with the oxygen coming from the cannula than does a shallow breath. This results in greater dilution of the oxygen, so a lower concentration is delivered. The same is true if the patient breathes rapidly: a lower concentration of oxygen is provided at a given flow rate than if the patient breathes slowly. Although most patients' breathing patterns are regular, the cannula can deliver only an estimated concentration of

oxygen. It has the potential for inconsistency. (See Procedure 30-3, Administering Oxygen by Nasal Cannula or Mask.)

Venturi-Type Mask. A Venturi-type mask can be used if precise, low-concentration oxygen delivery is required. These masks allow air to mix with the incoming oxygen in specific ratios. For each liter of oxygen used to power the mask, several liters of air are pulled into the mask. This results in a consistent dilution of the oxygen, and a high total flow of oxygen-enriched air to the patient. Because of the high total flow into the mask, the patient's breathing pattern does not affect the concentration of oxygen.

Some Venturi-type masks can deliver only one specific percentage of oxygen (usually 24%, 28%, 35%, or 40%). Other masks may be adjusted to provide several different concentrations of oxygen through the same mask. Some models can provide up to 50% oxygen, although the consistency of oxygen delivery at this setting may not be guaranteed.

The disadvantages of these masks is that they are noisy and may contribute to feelings of confinement or claustrophobia. For these reasons some patients may not keep them on continually, and their precision will be lost.

Oxygen Catheters. About 15 years ago, nasal oxygen catheters were commonly used to deliver lower oxygen concentrations. They are almost never used now because a cannula is just as effective, more covenient, and less invasive.

Transtracheal catheters (Figs. 30-8, 30-9) are being implanted with increasing frequency. These catheters (12 Fr or smaller) are inserted through the patient's neck into the trachea. They are attached to a portable "walker" oxygen system. They are provided to select patients who can care for the device.

Their disadvantage is the invasiveness of the procedure used to insert them. Many people are frightened by the prospect of having a hole in their throats. But they have several advantages: they are extremely efficient in delivering oxygen, and they are almost unnoticeable. Patients who require 2 L/min of oxygen via cannula can use as little as 0.5 L/min with the catheter. There is no waste of oxygen as there is with the cannula, since all the oxygen coming through the catheter directly enters the lungs. Catheters are less obvious than a cannula: they are small and easy to hide under a scarf or collar. This minimizes the self-consciousness commonly felt by the respiratory patient and bolsters the patient's self-confidence.

Simple Oxygen Mask. A simple oxygen mask is the easiest way to deliver between 40% and 65% oxygen. The mask fits over the mouth and nose and is held in place with an elastic strap. The mask should be operated with no less than 5 L/min; lower flows are insufficient to flush out the patient's exhaled air. A rate of 5 or 6 L/min is likely to provide a concentration of about 40% to 45% oxygen. Up to 12 L/min may be needed to deliver 60% to 65% oxygen. As with the cannula, the actual percentage of oxygen received by the patient varies depending on the breathing pattern.

Reservoir Mask. A reservoir mask is a simple mask with a bag attached. Between breaths, oxygen collects in the bag. This makes a larger volume of oxygen available to the patient for each breath. These masks therefore can provide higher oxygen concentrations: when run on 10 to 15 L/min, reservoir masks can deliver up to 90% oxygen. These masks are used primarily by the critically ill patient.

Large-Volume Pneumatic Nebulizers. Large-volume pneumatic nebulizers may be used to deliver oxygen along with continuous aerosol therapy. These aerosol generators can deliver supplemental oxygen in varying concentrations. Oxygen can be given through an aerosol mask or, if the patient has a tracheostomy, through a special tracheostomy mask or a T-piece.

Continuous Positive Airway Pressure. Continuous positive airway pressure is another method of oxygen delivery. This form of therapy was previously limited to infants with respiratory distress syndrome, but has found popularity as a treatment for adult disorders such as

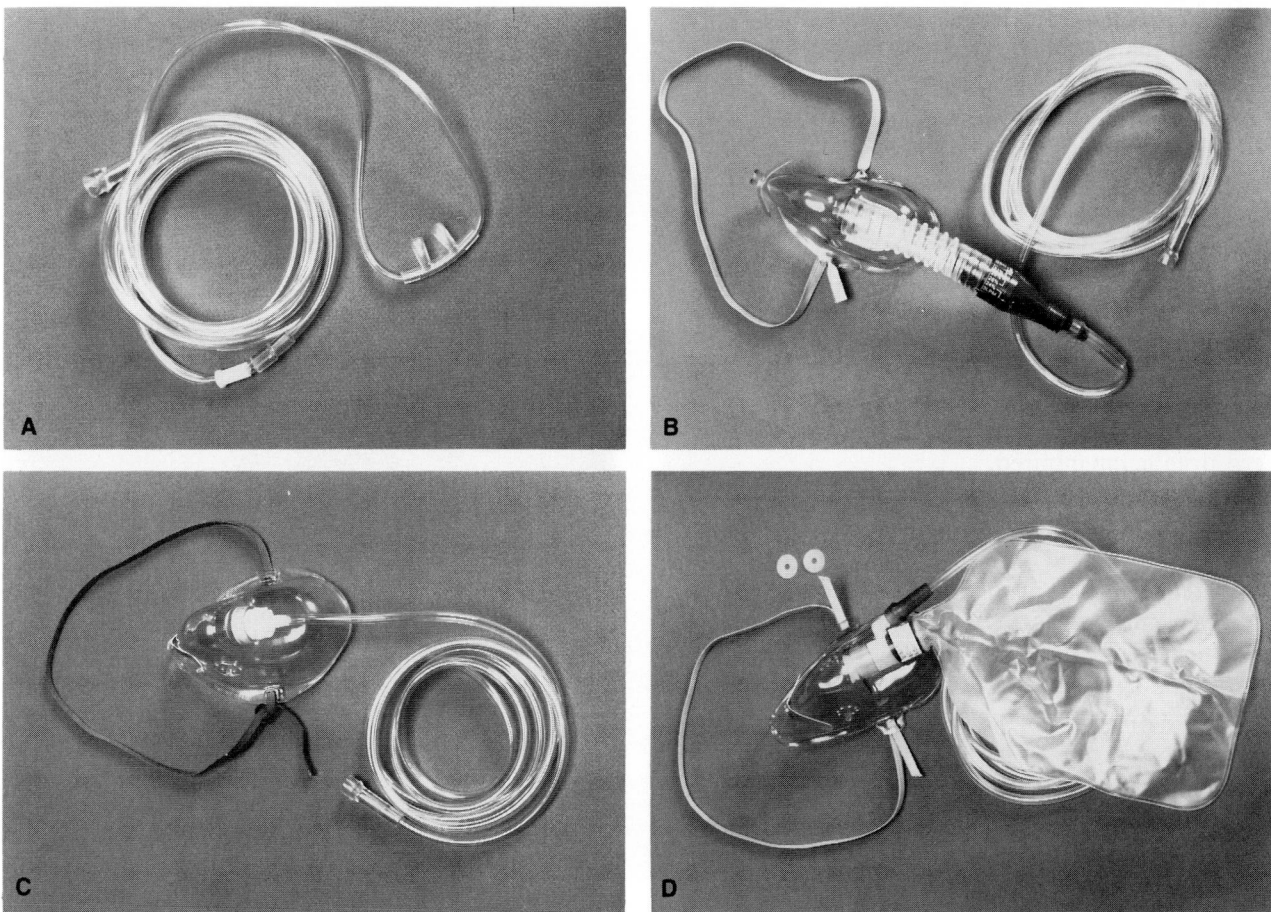

Figure 30–7. Common oxygen delivery devices. **A:** Cannula. **B:** Venturi-type mask. **C:** Simple oxygen mask. **D:** Reservoir mask.

PROCEDURE 30–3. Administering Oxygen by Nasal Cannula or Mask

■ **Purpose**

Deliver low to moderate levels of oxygen to relieve hypoxia.

■ **Assessment**

- Assess respiratory status (i.e., breath sounds, respiratory rate and depth, presence of sputum, arterial blood gases if available, past medical history).
  Note: For patients with chronic obstructive pulmonary disease (COPD), hypoxemia is often the stimulus to breathe since they chronically have high blood levels of carbon dioxide. If additional oxygen is needed, a low-flow system is essential to maintain slight hypoxemia so breathing is stimulated.
- Assess for clinical signs and symptoms of hypoxia: anxiety, decreased level of consciousness, inability to concentrate, fatigue, dizziness, cardiac arrhythmias, pallor or cyanosis, dyspnea.
- Review chart for physician's order for oxygen to include method of delivery, flow rate, duration of therapy.

■ **Equipment**

Appropriate oxygen delivery system:
  Nasal cannula and tubing (O_2 concentrations: 22%–44%)
  Simple oxygen mask (O_2 concentrations: 40%–60%)
  Partial rebreather mask–low-flow system (O_2 concentrations: 50%–70%)
    Reservoir bag allows patient to rebreathe a portion of exhaled air.
    Bag must not totally deflate during inspiration, or O_2 flow rate should be increased.
  Nonrebreather mask
    Delivers the highest O_2 concentrations possible without mechanical ventilation (80%–90%).
    One-way valve prevents room air or exhaled air from being inspired.
  Venturi mask
    Delivers O_2 concentrations accurate within 1% (24%–50%).
    Frequently used with COPD patients.
Oxygen source
Flow meter
"No smoking" sign
Humidifier and distilled water (optional)

■ **Procedure**

1. Wash your hands.
2. Explain procedure to patient. If using cannula, encourage patient to breathe through nose.
3. Assist patient to semi- or high-Fowler's position, if tolerated.
   Rationale: Facilitates optimal lung expansion.

4. Attach humidifier flow meter. Attach oxygen to humidifier nozzle, particularly if using a high O_2 flow.
   Rationale: O_2 in high concentrations can be drying to the mucosa.

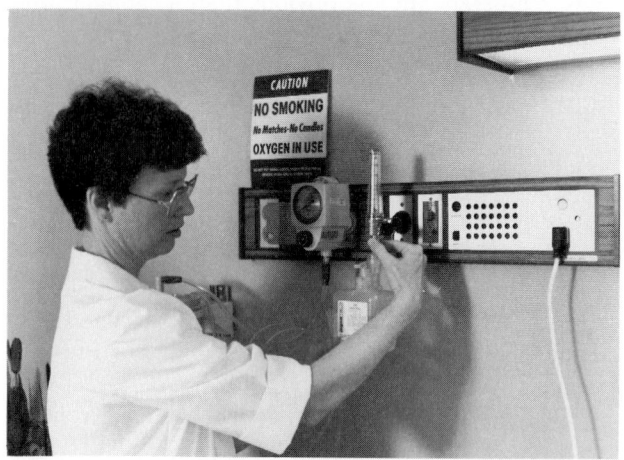

Step 4

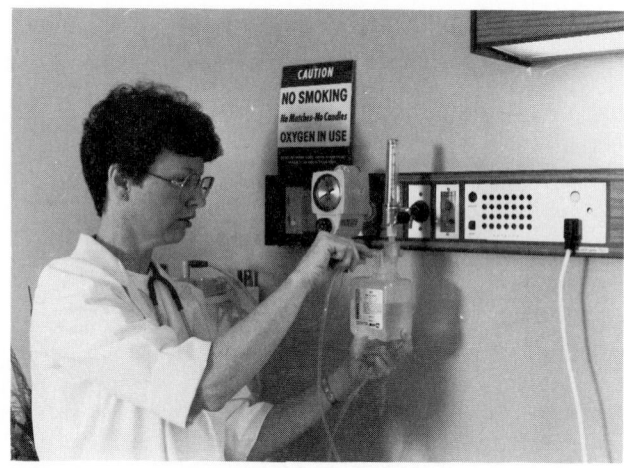

Step 4B

5. Turn on the oxygen at the prescribed rate. Check that oxygen is flowing through tubing.
6. Cannula.
   a. Place cannula prongs into nares.
   b. Wrap tubing over and behind ears.
   c. Adjust plastic slide under chin until cannula fits snugly.
7. Mask.
   a. Place mask on face, applying from the nose and over the chin.
   b. Adjust the metal rim over the nose and contour the mask to the face.

(continued)

PROCEDURE 30–3. Administering Oxygen by Nasal Cannula or Mask *continued*

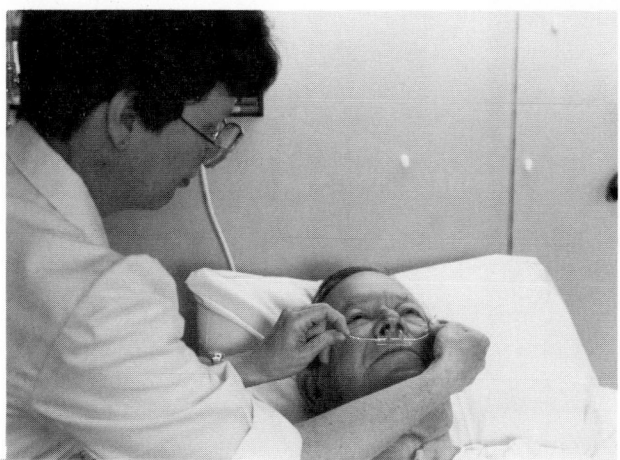

Step 6

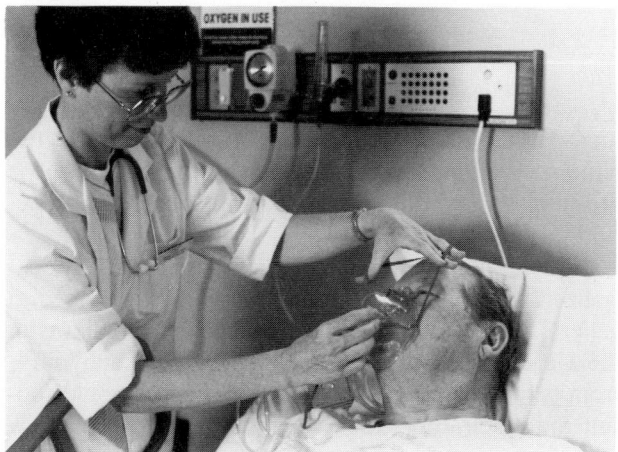

Step 7

Rationale: When the mask fits the face properly, little oxygen escapes.

  c. Adjust elastic band around head so mask fits snugly.
    Rationale: Patient is more likely to comply with therapy if equipment fits comfortably.

8. Assess for proper functioning of equipment and observe patient's initial response to therapy.

9. Monitor continuous therapy by assessing for pressure areas on the skin and nares every 2 hours and rechecking flow rate every 4 to 8 hours.
10. Document procedure and observations.

■ Lifespan Considerations

Infants and Children

- Isolettes (incubators) and tents are used for administering oxygen and humidity to infants and newborns. It is difficult to maintain high concentrations of oxygen in an isolette or tent, but it is nonintrusive and non-irritating.
- Plan nursing care so tent or isolette is entered as little as possible to prevent oxygen levels from dropping.
- Children frightened by the oxygen tent may feel more secure with their favorite toy or blanket.

■ Home Care Modifications

- In-home oxygen supply is delivered by cylinders, liquid oxygen, or oxygen concentrators. Portable oxygen systems are available to increase independence and social activities.
- Equipment vendor and home-care nurse should instruct patient on how to use oxygen equipment and how often the equipment must be filled.
- The patient should be informed about using an oxygen vendor whose services include:
  - Trained personnel to instruct the patient in use and maintenance of the equipment.
  - 24-hour emergency service.
  - Monthly follow-up visits for equipment maintenance and patient instruction.
  - Vendor insurance billing.
- Needing oxygen at home can be a psychological trauma for the patient. Patients should be encouraged to share their fears and concerns. A local support group of other patients using home oxygen may help patients to discuss their feelings.

sleep apnea and postoperative atelectasis. Oxygen is delivered under pressure to the patient through a tightly fitted mask, or through a special set of nasal prongs. The pressure helps to open alveoli, providing more space for the oxygen to diffuse.

Pediatric Oxygen Delivery Systems. Pediatric oxygen delivery systems include incubators and oxygen hoods. An incubator is an enclosed unit designed for environmental control. The incubator is used in newborn nurs-

eries to provide precise control of temperature, to deliver humidity, and to isolate the infant. It can also be used to deliver oxygen. The incubator's oxygen inlet accepts from 1 to 12 L/min of oxygen. Although it is can achieve higher concentrations, the incubator should be used to deliver no more than 30% to 35% oxygen. The accuracy of delivery varies greatly each time the incubator is opened; the unreliability is increased at higher concentrations.

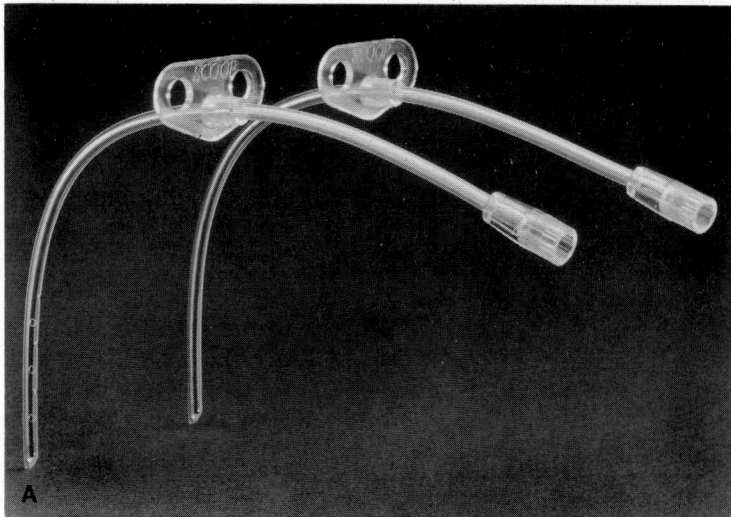
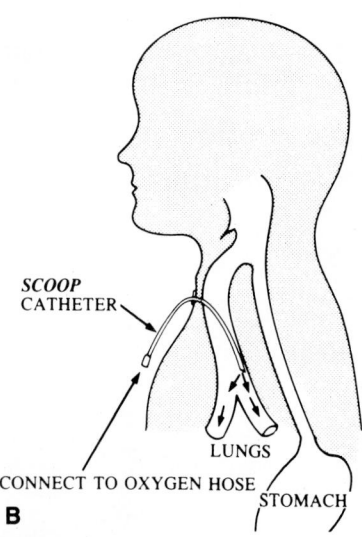

Figure 30–8. The SCOOP transtracheal catheter delivers oxygen directly to the lungs. **A:** Catheter. **B:** Placement of the catheter. The transtracheal catheter is surgically implanted on an outpatient basis and causes very little discomfort. (Courtesy of Transtracheal Systems, Englewood, CO)

For more precise control of oxygen delivery to infants, a hood should be used. This plastic chamber fits around the baby's head. The oxygen should be warmed, humidified, preblended to the prescribed percentage, and analyzed before it enters the hood. A flow of at least 7 L/min is needed to keep the hood from filling with the baby's exhaled air. The temperature of the incoming oxygen must be about 95°F to prevent chilling the infant. The concentration of oxygen that can be delivered through a hood ranges from 22% to almost 100%.

Oxygen Tents. Oxygen tents were once widely used for all patients who needed oxygen, but their use is now limited. They are infrequently used for the small child who refuses to wear a mask or cannula. They also are used as a "mist tent" for children with croup. Like the incubator, the tent is inefficient in its delivery of oxygen. Unless it is tucked tightly under the mattress, the tent leaks oxygen and the oxygen percentage inside fluctuates. Tents must be kept cool: modern units have a self-cooling feature, but older tents must be cooled manually by adding ice. The nurse must ensure that the tent is cool and securely tucked in and that the crib rails are up.

Ventilators. Ventilators are mechanical devices used to assist the breathing of patients who cannot maintain satisfactory oxygenation and ventilation with spontaneous breathing. Until recently, these machines were used only in the intensive care unit. Lately, however, more ventilator patients are being cared for on general medical-surgical and rehabilitation units. Patients are even being discharged with ventilators to their homes.

A positive-pressure ventilator delivers oxygen under pressure to the patient who cannot breathe effectively. These machines range from simple pressure-limited devices to microprocessor-driven volume-limited ventila-

tors. They can be used to control every aspect of the patient's breathing, or merely to assist the patient who is too weak to maintain effective ventilation for long periods.

Most ventilators require frequent monitoring by specialized personnel. If a ventilator patient is assigned to general floor care, the nurse must become familiar with the alarm system of each machine. Alarms may differ from one machine to another, so the nurse should consult the respiratory care practitioner each time a new ventilator patient arrives on the unit.

More information on negative-pressure ventilators follows in the home care and rehabilitation section of this chapter. For additional information on intensive ventilator care, consult texts on respiratory therapy or critical care nursing.

Safety Considerations. Oxygen is generally safe when used properly, but certain precautions must be observed. As with all drugs, there is the potential for causing harm with misuse.

When oxygen therapy starts, the nurse should inform the patient of the importance of wearing the oxygen device. A "no smoking" sign must be posted in the patient's room, and this warning must be strictly enforced. Although oxygen is not flammable, it greatly accelerates combustion and could cause a fire from a small spark.

The flow of oxygen should be checked often to ensure that the prescribed amount is being delivered. If a humidifier or nebulizer is being used, the nurse must ensure that these are attached properly. A leak can prevent the patient from receiving the full flow of oxygen.

Blood gases, color, respiratory rate, and breathing

POSTURAL DRAINAGE POSITIONS

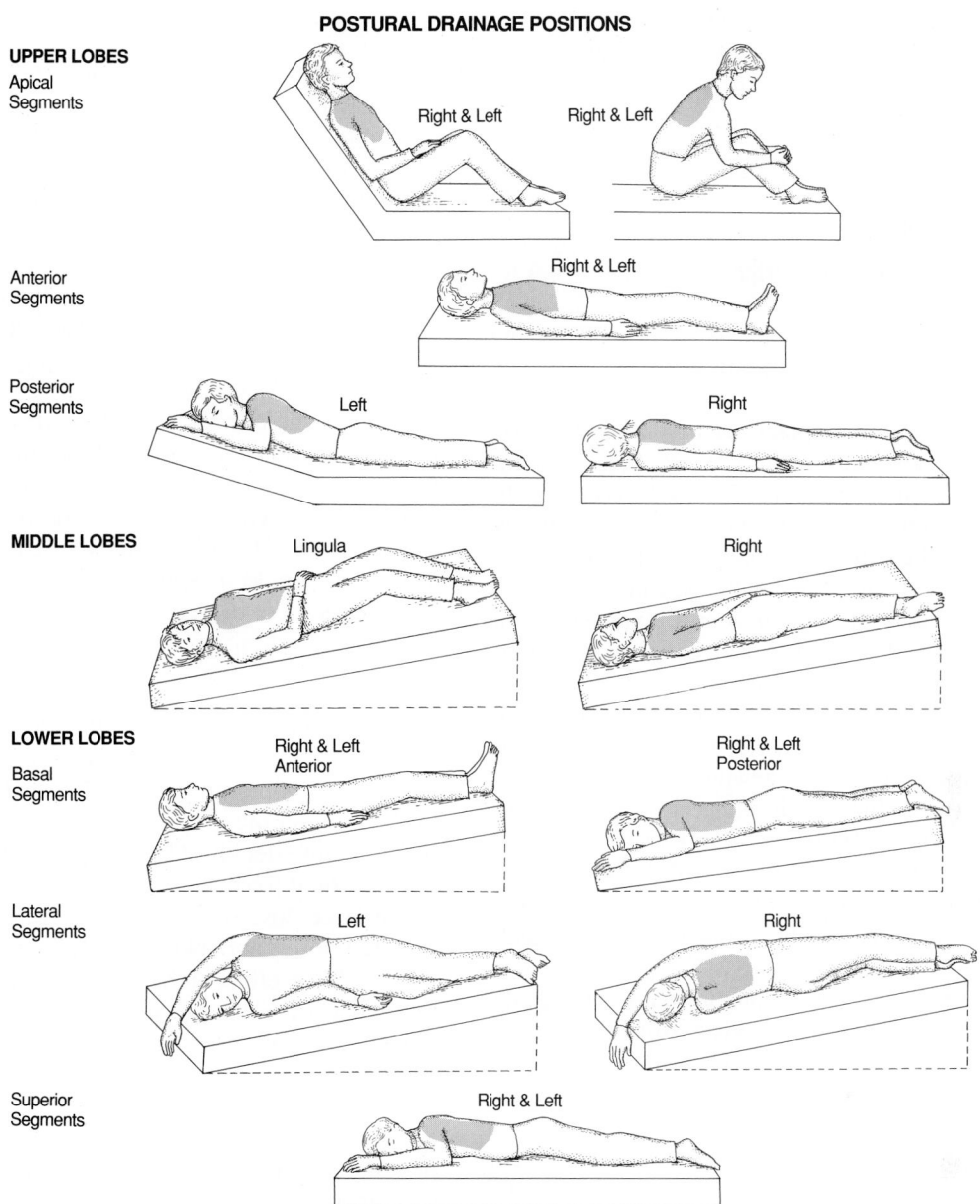

Figure 30–9.   Various postural drainage positions are used to mobilize secretions from specific lobes and segments of the lungs.

effort are general indicators of the success of oxygen therapy. The patient's status should be assessed regularly to determine the need for continuation or adjustment of therapy.

In addition to the fire hazard posed by its use, oxygen can be dangerous in several other ways.

First, infants exposed to even relatively low concentrations of oxygen can develop severe eye damage called retrolental fibroplasia. This disorder can result in blindness, and although it is more common in premature babies, it can affect any newborn. For this reason, meticulous monitoring of all newborns receiving oxygen therapy is essential.

Second, high concentrations of oxygen are toxic to lung tissue. Severely ill patients who require intense oxygen therapy for extended periods of time may actu-

ally suffer lung damage as a result. Although this is not usually a concern for the average patient on a nasal cannula, oxygen toxicity is a danger for the long-term intensive care respiratory patient.

Third, oxygen can cause hypoventilation in certain patients with chronic lung disease. Some of these patients breathe primarily as a response to hypoxemia. If they receive too much oxygen, their PaO_2 rises excessively and their drive to breathe can disappear. This can cause hypoventilation, which could lead to respiratory arrest. Although this is rare, patients who should be most closely watched for this are the COPD patient, the child or adult in advanced stages of cystic fibrosis, and the infant with bronchopulmonary dysplasia.

Oxygen in high concentrations can also cause atelectasis, which can actually hinder gas exchange and may encourage the development of pneumonia. Finally, a patient may develop a psychological dependence on oxygen. This can be expensive and at the least poses an unneeded fire hazard.

Dyspnea Management

Dyspnea is one of the most frightening experiences for the patient. As each breath becomes more difficult, anxiety rises. This worsens the dyspnea, and a vicious cycle is established. The nurse must therefore treat two aspects of dyspnea: the physical and the psychological.

When the patient complains of dyspnea, the nurse must quickly determine its general cause. Most often the episode is brought on by exertion. A brief walk down the hall, a physical therapy session, a shower, or perhaps just a walk across the room can precipitate dyspnea in the compromised patient. When exertion causes dyspnea, the nurse must make the patient comfortable in a resting position. Usually the patient is most comfortable sitting, since this keeps the diaphragm unrestricted. If oxygen is ordered on an as-needed basis, it should be worn and the prescribed flow rate administered. The nurse should focus the patient's efforts on slowing the breathing rate. The patient should breathe through the nose if possible, using the diaphragm for inspiration. Pursed-lip breathing is appropriate for asthma and COPD patients. The nurse must not rush the patient: with gentle encouragement and reassurance, the breathing rate will gradually decrease and the dyspnea will pass.

Next to exertion, the most common cause of dyspnea is anxiety or emotional upset. Visits from loved ones, upsetting telephone conversations, or worry over home affairs or finances may cause the patient to breathe faster and less efficiently. This can progress to dyspnea. The nursing treatment is the same as for exertional dyspnea. The nurse may need to spend a few moments with the patient, as an empathetic listener. Some patients may have standing orders for diazepam or another mild anxiety-controlling medication to be administered during periods of anxiety. These must be used cautiously, since some of these agents have the potential for decreasing the patient's respiratory drive.

Dyspnea not brought on by obvious exertion or anxiety may be due to organic problems such as infection, pulmonary embolism, bronchospasm, or a worsening of the patient's underlying condition. The nurse must assess the situation fully and refer the problem to the physician as necessary.

In all cases of dyspnea, the nurse must try to establish the immediate cause and extent of dyspnea. Comfort measures are always appropriate, as is oxygen when a standing order is available. Many institutions have policies allowing nurses to begin oxygen therapy for the dyspneic patient while a physician's order is sought. When these measures do not decrease dyspnea in a short period of time, the physician should be notified.

Altered Breathing Pattern Management

Hyperventilation Management. Hyperventilation occurs when the patient breathes in excess of metabolic demands. It is identified by a $PaCO_2$ below normal (below 35 to 45 mm Hg), rapid breathing, and symptoms such as dizziness and tingling sensations. The subjective complaint of dyspnea may or may not be present. Nursing efforts should be directed at decreasing patient anxiety and getting the patient to breathe at a slower rate.

If this cannot be done by simple encouragement, a paper bag can be prescribed by the physician for use as a rebreathing device. The nurse has the patient breathe in and out of the bag for several breaths. This allows the patient's carbon dioxide to collect in the bag. By rebreathing the exhaled gas, the patient can restore the arterial level of carbon dioxide to normal. This naturally slows the rate of breathing, and the dizziness and tingling sensations should disappear. As with dyspnea, a complete assessment of hyperventilation is needed, and referral to the physician may be required.

Hypoventilation Management. Inadequate ability to remove carbon dioxide from the blood is hypoventilation. The hypoventilating patient is often groggy and most often is breathing slowly. Depending on the cause of the hypoventilation, the nurse must have the patient breathe more deeply. The heavily sedated patient, such as the patient fresh from surgery or the patient who has had a large dose of analgesic medication, needs to be watched closely and told to take deep breaths frequently. Gradually the effect of the medication will diminish, and breathing will return to normal. But until it does, the nurse must stay close by and continually tell the patient to breathe.

When chronic lung disease causes hypoventilation, the nurse must be aware of the patient's need for secretion removal or for bronchodilators and other pharmacologic agents. By providing these therapies as prescribed, the nurse can help the patient maintain clear airways, thereby minimizing the risk of hypoventilation. COPD patients benefit from pursed-lip breathing, since a more complete exhalation helps eliminate carbon dioxide.

If hypoventilation cannot be reversed by these measures, more aggressive therapy (such as intubation and mechanical ventilation) may be needed. Because hypoventilation is potentially serious, all cases should be brought to the attention of the physician.

Chest Physiotherapy

One method for improving airway clearance is chest physiotherapy. It is a mainstay of treatment for many patients with cystic fibrosis, bronchiectasis, lung abscess, COPD, and pneumonia. This therapy is based on the fact that mucus can be knocked or shaken from the walls of the airways and helped to drain from the lungs.

The primary techniques of this method of secretion mobilization are percussion, vibration, and postural drainage. Any of these physiotherapy techniques can be used alone, but they are most effective when used together. The patient's ability to tolerate these procedures may limit the vigor with which they are applied, so positioning and clapping techniques may need to be modified.

Percussion. Percussion produces a wave of energy that is transmitted through the chest wall to the mucus-coated bronchial tubes. The chest is struck rhythmically with cupped hands over the area where secretions are located. Care must be taken to avoid striking over the spine or kidneys, on female breasts, or on incisions or broken ribs. Gas-powered or electric chest percussors are also available.

Vibration. Vibration works in much the same manner as percussion. In this technique, the nurse's hands are used like a gentle jackhammer. They are placed on the patient's chest and are rapidly and vigorously shaken during the patient's exhalation. This technique may help dislodge secretions and stimulate a cough.

Postural Drainage. Postural drainage uses gravity to assist in the movement of secretions. The patient is placed in various positions to facilitate the flow of mucus from different segments of the lung. By placing a mucus-filled portion of the lung higher than the rest of the lung segments, the mucus in that portion is given a downhill course on which to slide. The mucus thus enters larger airways and is then more easily removed by cough or suctioning.

Not all postural drainage positions are well tolerated by all patients. The Trendelenburg (head-down) position can increase shortness of breath in the COPD patient because the abdominal organs put pressure on the diaphragm. The head-down position can increase intracranial pressure and should be used cautiously for patients with head injuries. It can also be stressful for patients with cardiac problems.

Suctioning

Patients who cannot cough effectively to remove their secretions are at risk for pneumonia, atelectasis, and even asphyxiation from choking on mucus. To prevent this, the nurse may have to suction their airways (Fuchs, 1984).

Suctioning or mechanical aspiration of the airways involves inserting a catheter through the nose, mouth, or tracheal tube. The catheter is attached to a portable or wall unit suction device. Secretions are removed in much the same manner as dirt is drawn up by a vacuum cleaner. See Procedure 30-4 for a step-by-step guide to oropharyngeal and nasopharyngeal suctioning.

Some patients with large amounts of oral secretions may benefit from mouth suctioning. A "tonsil tip" (Yankauer) suction catheter can be used to evacuate excess saliva and thick mucus from the back of the throat.

Risks. Patients with deep bronchial secretions may require deep endobronchial suctioning. Properly performed, suctioning can greatly improve airflow in the lungs and thus promote oxygenation. However, the procedure carries several risks. It can cause temporary hypoxia, since oxygen along with mucus is extracted from the airways. For this reason it is essential to provide the patient with 100% oxygen before each suctioning attempt. Also for this reason, each suction attempt should never take longer than 15 seconds.

Suction should be applied intermittently to help decrease grabbing of the trachea's delicate mucosal lining by the catheter. Only as much suction as necessary to remove secretions should be used. Usually the suction regulator should be set between 80 and 120 mm Hg for larger children and adults, and 60 to 80 mm Hg for infants. (See Procedure 30-5, Suctioning Nasotracheal Secretions).

In addition to causing hypoxia, suctioning can cause cardiac arrhythmias, hypotension, and atelectasis. Because suctioning can stimulate a gag reflex, vomiting (with the potential for aspiration) is possible. Thus, this procedure requires the utmost caution.

Suctioning can greatly relieve the dyspnea that accompanies excessive secretions, but for nearly all patients it is frightening and unpleasant. The nurse should be prepared to offer a great deal of reassurance.

Artificial Airways

An artificial airway is a device that provides a more direct route to the lungs than the natural airway. Oropharyngeal airways, nasopharyngeal airways ("nasal trumpets"), endotracheal tubes, and tracheostomy tubes are examples of artificial airways.

Oral or Nasal Airways. These airways are used to bypass upper airway obstructions or to facilitate secretion removal (Fig. 30-10). Oral airways are simple to insert but are poorly tolerated by all but the comatose patient. The noncomatose patient is likely to gag on an oral airway, so a nasal trumpet is preferable. These airways should be well lubricated with water-soluble gel before they are inserted.

Endotracheal Tubes. An endotracheal tube is a plastic tube inserted through the nose or mouth into the trachea. These airways are used to ventilate a patient during surgery or when mechanical ventilation is necessary.

Tracheostomy. The **tracheostomy** is an artificial airway in which a plastic tube is surgically inserted just below the larynx into the trachea, bypassing the mouth and upper airway. The surgical procedure that establishes the artificial airway is called a tracheotomy; the resultant airway is a tracheostomy. This procedure is most often done as a temporary measure. Unlike a per-

(Text continues on page 785)

PROCEDURE 30–4. Suctioning Oropharyngeal and Nasopharyngeal Areas

■ **Purpose**
1. Remove excess oral and nasal secretions to maintain patent upper airway.
2. Prevent aspiration of blood or vomitus.
3. Collect sputum or secretions for diagnostic testing.

■ **Assessment**
• Assess respiratory system:
  Note rate, depth, rhythm of respirations.
  Note noisy, wet, or snory respirations.
  Auscultate breath sounds.
• Assess patient's ability to cough. Note amount and character of sputum.
• Assess vital signs. Compare to baseline vital signs. Note an elevation in temperature.
• Assess level of consciousness and ability to protect airway (i.e., presence of cough reflex). Note any drainage from mouth.

■ **Equipment**
Portable or wall suction apparatus with tubing and reservoir
Sterile suction kit containing:
  Appropriate-sized catheter: infants, #5 to #8 Fr; children, #8 to #10 Fr; adults, #12 to #18 Fr
  Pair of gloves
  Container for saline to flush and lubricate catheter
Sterile NaCl (may be provided in kit)
Water-resistant disposal bag
Facial tissues
Towel (optional)

■ **Procedure**
1. Wash your hands.
   Rationale: Prevents transmission of microorganisms.
2. Explain procedure and purpose to patient.
   Rationale: Reduces anxiety and encourages cooperation with procedure.
3. a. Position the conscious patient with an intact gag reflex in a semi-Fowler's position.
      Rationale: Helps prevent aspiration of secretions.
   b. Position the unconscious patient in a side-lying position facing you.
      Rationale: Facilitates drainage of secretions by gravity and prevents aspiration.
4. Turn suction device on and adjust pressure: infants and children, 50 to 75 mm Hg; adults, 100 to 120 mm Hg.
   Rationale: Excessive negative pressure traumatizes mucosa and can induce hypoxia.
5. Open and prepare sterile suction catheter kit.
   a. Unfold sterile cup, touching only the outside. Place on bedside table.

b. Pour approximately 100 ml sterile NaCl into cup.
c. Put on sterile gloves.

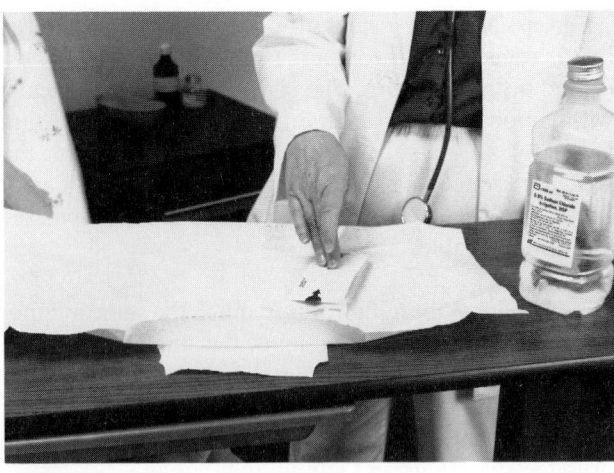
Step 5A

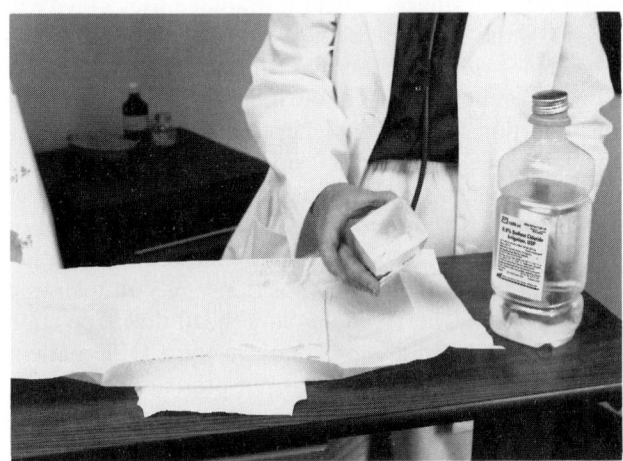
Step 5A

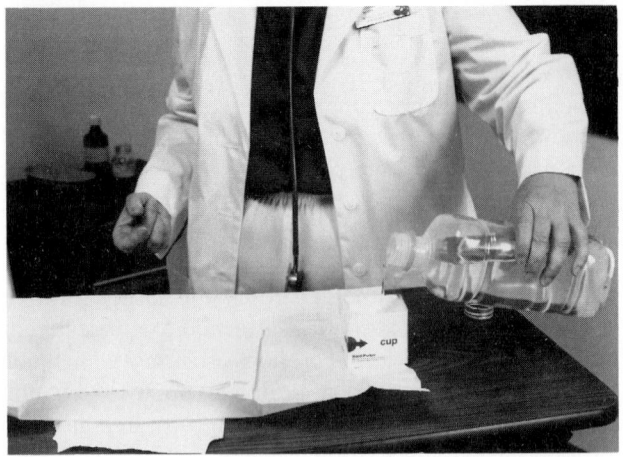
Step 5B

(continued)

PROCEDURE 30–4. Suctioning Oropharyngeal and Nasopharyngeal Areas *continued*

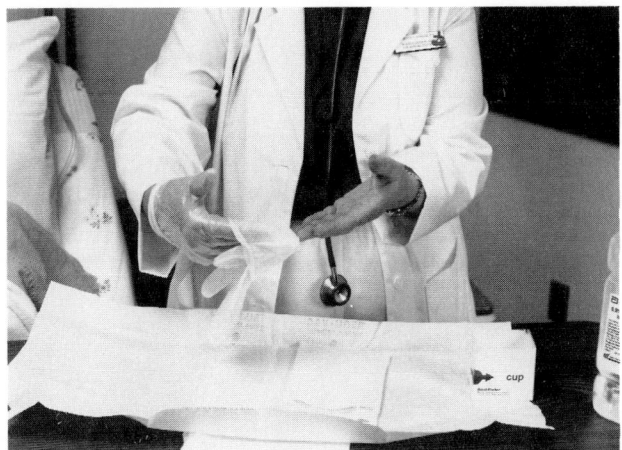

Step 5C

> *Note:* If kit provides only one glove, place on dominant hand. Dominant hand will remain sterile. A clean disposable glove may be used on nondominant hand and is used to protect yourself from mucous membrane and sputum exposure.

6. Pick up catheter with dominant hand. Pick up connecting tubing with nondominant hand. Attach catheter to tubing without contaminating sterile hand.

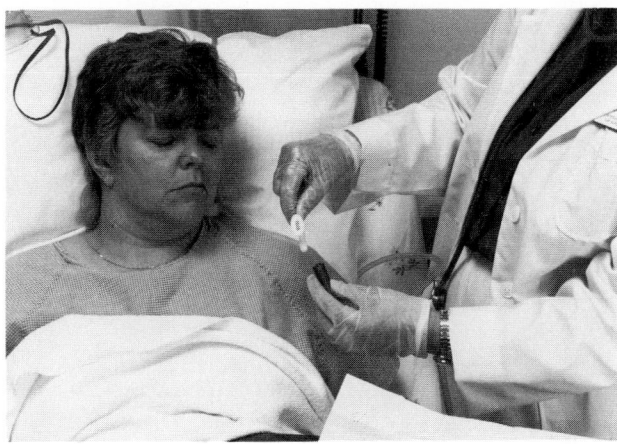

Step 6

7. Place catheter end into cup of NaCl. Test functioning of equipment by applying thumb from nondominant hand over open port to create suction.
   Rationale: Lubricates catheter for easier insertion and ensures proper functioning of suction equipment.

8. If patient is using an oxygen delivery system, remove with nondominant hand.

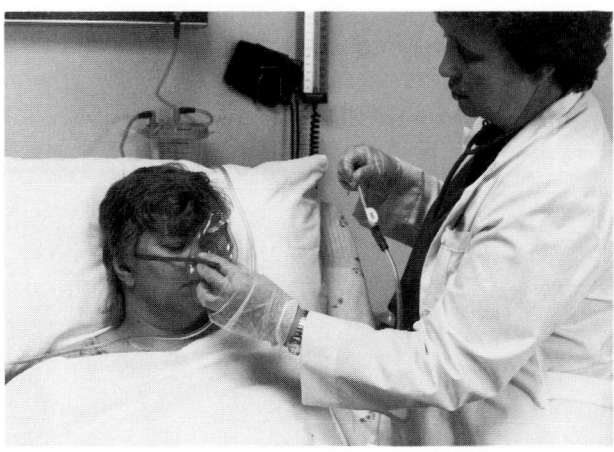

Step 8

9. Without applying suction, insert catheter gently into nostril, directing slightly downward. If one nostril is not patent, do not force, but try the other nare. Advance catheter into pharynx.
   Rationale: Not applying suction and gentle insertion prevent trauma to mucosa.

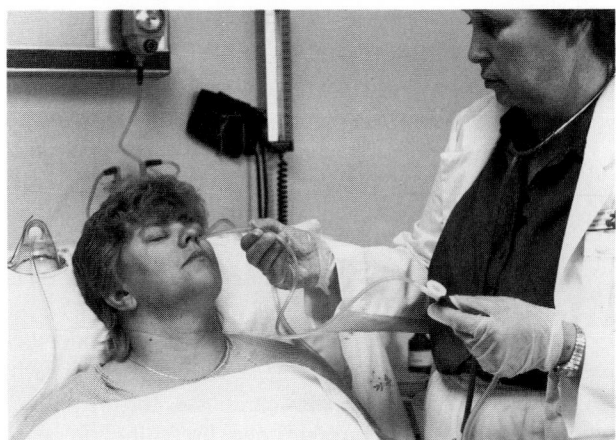

Step 9

10. Apply suction by placing thumb of nondominant hand over open port. Rotate the catheter with your dominant hand as you withdraw the catheter. This should take 5 to 10 seconds.
    Rationale: Rotation of catheter prevents trauma to mucous membrane from prolonged suctioning of one area. Limiting the suction time to 10 seconds or less prevents hypoxia.

(continued)

PROCEDURE 30–4. Suctioning Oropharyngeal and Nasopharyngeal Areas *continued*

11. If patient is using supplemental oxygen, replace for several minutes between subsequent suction passes. *Note:* If patient is not using supplemental oxygen, allow 1 to 2 minutes for ventilation between subsequent passes. Encourage deep breathing.
Rationale: Prolonged suctioning can induce hypoxia.

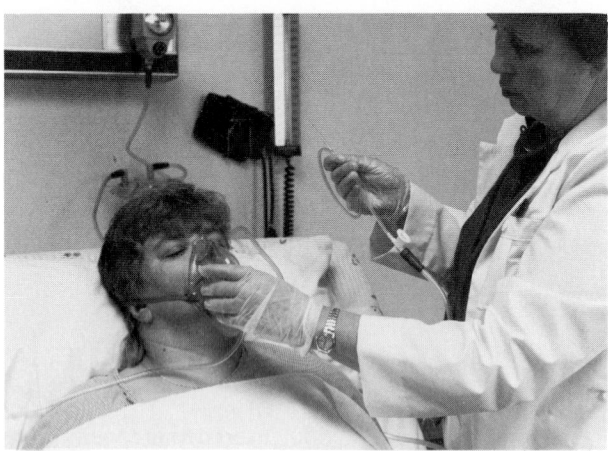

Step 11

12. Rinse catheter thoroughly with NaCl.
Rationale: Clears secretions from catheter.
13. Repeat steps 9 to 12 until nasopharynx is clear.
14. Without applying suction, insert the catheter gently along one side of the mouth. Advance to the oropharynx.
Rationale: Oropharynx is suctioned after nasopharynx because the nose is considered cleaner than the mouth. Directing the catheter along the side of the mouth prevents stimulation of the gag reflex.
15. Apply suction for 5 to 10 seconds as you rotate and withdraw catheter.
Rationale: Rotation of the catheter prevents trauma to the mucous membrane.
Note: Be sure to remove secretions that pool beneath the tongue and in the vestibule of the mouth.
16. Allow 1 to 2 minutes between passes for the patient to ventilate. Encourage deep breathing. Replace oxygen if applicable.
17. Repeat steps 14 and 15 as necessary to clear oropharynx.
18. Rinse catheter and tubing by suctioning NaCl through.
19. Remove gloves by holding catheter with dominant hand and pulling glove off inside out. Catheter will remain coiled inside the glove. Pull other glove off inside out. Dispose of in trash receptacle.

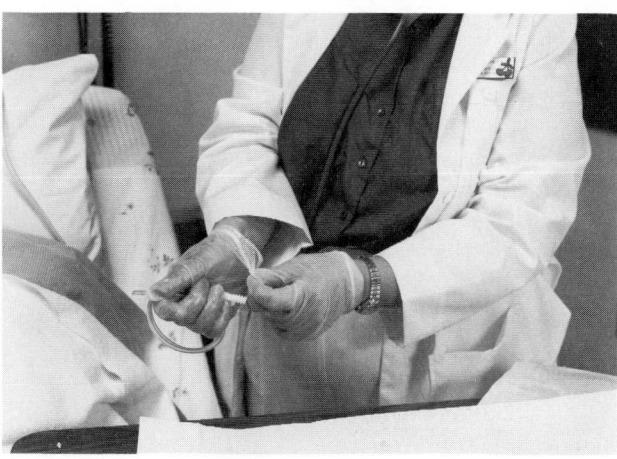

Step 19

Rationale: Patient secretions are contained inside gloves to reduce transmission of microorganisms.
20. Turn off suction device.
21. Assist patient to comfortable position. Offer assistance with oral and nasal hygiene. Replace oxygen mask if used.
Rationale: Accumulated respiratory secretions irritate the mucous membranes and are unpleasant for the patient.

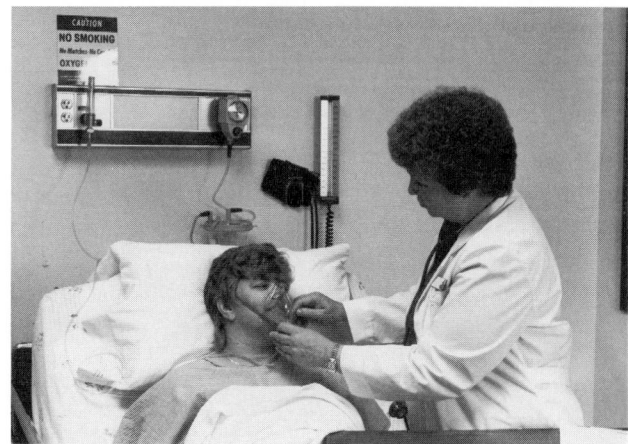

Step 21

22. Dispose of disposable supplies.
23. Wash your hands.
24. Ensure that sterile suction kit is available at head of bed.
Rationale: Provides immediate access to suction equipment when needed.
25. Document procedure and observations.

(continued)

PROCEDURE 30–4. Suctioning Oropharyngeal and Nasopharyngeal Areas *continued*

■ Lifespan Considerations

Infants and Children
- Infants and young children have airways that are easily occluded by a small amount of secretions. The nasal airway is smaller in diameter, the epiglottis is higher, and the tongue is proportionately larger.
- A bulb syringe is often used to aspirate secretions from an infant's nasal and oral cavities. This is a clean rather than a sterile procedure because the pharynx is not entered.

■ Home Care Modifications
- Patients may need to be taught to suction their secretions if they have difficulty coughing them up. Main-taining adequate hydration thins secretions and facilitates their removal.
- The type and number of microorganisms available to contaminate the respiratory system are different at home than in the acute-care setting. The patient or caregiver may be taught to use plain paper cups for suctioning, not a sterile basin. The cups should be kept in a sealable package. A clean cup is removed from the bottom of the package for each suctioning effort. The package should be resealed between uses.
- Suction catheters can be clean, not sterile. They should be washed in soapy water, rinsed well, and soaked in a vinegar-and-water solution.
- To decrease expenses, saline solution can be made by boiling water and adding salt.

---

manent laryngectomy, in which the entire larynx is removed, a tracheotomy leaves the structure of the airway intact.

Indications. Indications for tracheostomy placement are varied. A patient may require this procedure to bypass a severe or recurrent upper airway obstruction. The patient who regularly aspirates food or stomach contents may need a tracheostomy to protect the airway. A few patients may need this type of airway to help with secretion control, since a tracheostomy provides a readily accessible route for suctioning. Finally, the patient who requires long-term mechanical ventilation may be tracheotomized to provide the safest and most stable artificial airway available. Many tracheotomized patients on the general nursing unit are former patients of the intensive care unit, or have had head and neck surgery (Hoffman & Maszkiewicz, 1987).

Risks. Risks of a tracheostomy are numerous. Immediately after surgery, bleeding of the tracheostomy site is common. Dressings need to be changed frequently during this period. The nurse must also assess the extent of blood loss and be prepared to call the surgeon if bleeding is excessive.

Meticulous care of the stoma is necessary to keep it free from infection. Since the tracheostomy bypasses the defenses of the upper airway, the patient is at risk for pneumonia. Thus, sterile technique should be used when cleaning the tracheostomy site and when suctioning the patient.

Often patients who are tracheotomized have marginal breathing ability. It is this type of patient who must be protected most diligently against plugging of the tube. Dried secretions can completely occlude the tube, creating a respiratory emergency. For this reason tracheostomy patients must be well hydrated, and the air they breathe must be completely humidified by a nebulizer or high-output humidifier.

A tracheostomy also poses communication problems. Because the vocal cords are above the level of the tracheostomy tube, the patient cannot speak. A tablet and pencil can save a great deal of frustration. Specialized tracheostomy tubes, such as the Pitt Speaking Tube or Communi-Trach, allow the patient to speak in short sentences. The Olympic Trach-Talk can be attached to a standard tracheostomy tube, making speech possible. Tracheostomy buttons are used to temporarily plug the tracheostomy so that the patient's ability to breathe through the natural airway can be assessed. When these are in place, the patient can once again speak.

Such devices are more effective for some patients than for others. They are appropriate for use only by the patient with strong spontaneous respirations. The nurse must scrupulously follow the directions for each of these specialized devices, because unless they are used properly they are unlikely to work. Also, if improperly applied they may cause complete airway blockage.

Body image is a potential problem for these patients. The tracheotomized patient may feel embarrassed or inadequate because of the stoma. The patient may perceive the stoma as ugly and disfiguring and may be embarrassed by its messy, bubbling secretions. Feelings of defeat and depression may result from the inability to perform such a basic function as breathing without assistance. The patient is also likely to feel fear and anxiety about the inability to speak.

The nurse can be supportive and help to allay these fears. When the tracheostomy is temporary, the nurse can reassure the patient that the ability to communicate will return. Knowing that the incision will heal completely may help the patient to better accept the temporary disfigurement.

PROCEDURE 30–5. Suctioning Nasotracheal Secretions

■ Purpose
1. Remove secretions and maintain patency of lower airway.
2. Stimulate a cough reflex to assist patient in clearing secretions.

■ Assessment
Assess respiratory system:
  Note rate, depth, rhythm of respirations.
  Note noisy, wet, or snory respirations.
  Auscultate breath sounds.
Assess patient's ability to cough. Note amount and character of sputum.
Assess vital signs. Compare to baseline vital signs. Note an elevation in temperature.
Assess level of consciousness and ability to protect airway (i.e., presence of cough reflex). Note any drainage from mouth.

■ Equipment
Portable or wall suction apparatus with tubing and reservoir
Sterile suction kit containing:
  Appropriate-sized catheter: infants #5 to #8 Fr; children, #8 to #10 Fr; adults, #12 to #18 Fr
  Pair of gloves
  Container for saline to flush and lubricate catheter
Sterile NaCl (may be provided in kit)
Water-resistant disposal bag
Facial tissues
Towel (optional)
Oxygen source with mask or manual resuscitator

■ Procedure
1. Wash your hands.
   Rationale: Prevents transmission of microorganisms.
2. Explain procedure and purpose to patient.
   Rationale: Reduces anxiety and encourages cooperation with procedure.
3. a. Position the conscious patient with an intact gag reflex in a semi- or high-Fowler's position.
      Rationale: Helps prevent aspiration of secretions.
   b. Position the unconscious patient in a side-lying position facing you.
      Rationale: Facilitates drainage of secretions by gravity and prevents aspiration.
4. Turn suction device on and adjust pressure: infants and children, 50 to 75 mm Hg; adults, 100 to 120 mm Hg.
   Rationale: Excessive negative pressure traumatizes mucosa and can induce hypoxia.
5. In accordance with agency policy and physician's orders, place oxygen mask or resuscitator bag over patient's nose and mouth. Have patient take several deep breaths.
   Rationale: Counteracts the hypoxic side effects associated with tracheal suctioning.
6. Open and prepare sterile suction catheter kit while patient deep-breathes.
   a. Unfold sterile cup, touching only the outside. Place on bedside table.
   b. Pour approximately 100 ml sterile NaCl into cup.
   c. Put on sterile gloves.
      Note: If kit provides only one glove, place on dominant hand. Put clean disposable glove on nondominant hand to protect yourself from mucous membrane and sputum exposure.
7. Pick up catheter with dominant hand and attach to suction tubing without contaminating sterile hand.
8. Place catheter end into NaCl. Test functioning of equipment by applying thumb from nondominant hand over open port to create suction.
   Rationale: Lubricates catheter for easier insertion and ensures proper functioning of suction equipment.
9. Remove oxygen delivery device with nondominant hand.
10. Without applying suction, gently insert catheter into nares using slight downward slant, or alongside and through mouth.
11. Advance catheter into trachea during inspiratory phase of respiratory cycle. In adults, insert catheter 20 to 24 cm; adolescents, 14 to 20 cm; children and infants, 8 to 14 cm.
    Note: Patient will usually cough when catheter is in trachea.
    Rationale: Epiglottis is open during inspiration and facilitates movement of catheter into trachea.
    Note: If resistance is felt when catheter is inserted the recommended distance, the tip is probably on the carina. Pull the catheter back 1 cm before applying suction to prevent mucosal trauma.
12. Apply suction by placing thumb of nondominant hand over open port. Rotate the catheter with your dominant hand as you withdraw the catheter. This should take about 5 to 10 seconds.
    Rationale: Rotation of catheter prevents trauma to mucous membrane from prolonged suction in one spot. Limiting the suction time to 10 seconds or less prevents hypoxia.
13. Replace supplemental oxygen. Encourage deep breathing and coughing. Allow several minutes of ventilation between suction passes.
    Note: Monitor for alterations in cardiopulmonary status (bronchospasm, hypoxia, cardiac arrhythmias).

(continued)

14. Rinse catheter with saline until clear.
15. Repeat steps 10 to 14 until trachea is clear of secretions.
16. Perform nasopharyngeal or oral pharyngeal suctioning to clear secretions from the upper airway.
17. Remove gloves by holding catheter with dominant hand and pulling glove off inside out. Catheter will remain coiled inside the glove. Pull other glove off inside out. Dispose of in trash receptacle.
    Rationale: Patient secretions are contained inside gloves to reduce transmission of microorganisms.
18. Turn off suction device.
19. Assist patient to comfortable position. Offer assistance with oral and nasal hygiene.
20. Dispose of disposable supplies.
21. Wash your hands.
22. Ensure that new sterile suction kit is available at head of bed.
    Rationale: Provides immediate access to suction equipment when needed.
23. Document procedure and observations.

■ Lifespan Considerations

Infants and Children

- Infants and young children have airways that are easily occluded by a small amount of secretions. The nasal airway is smaller in diameter, the epiglottis is higher, and the tongue is proportionately larger.
- A bulb syringe is often used to aspirate secretions from an infant's nasal and oral cavities. This is a clean rather than a sterile procedure because the pharynx is not entered.

■ Home Care Modifications

- Patients may need to be taught to suction their secretions if they have difficulty coughing them up. Maintaining adequate hydration thins secretions and facilitates their removal.
- The type and number of microorganisms available to contaminate the respiratory system are different at home than in the acute-care setting. The patient or caregiver may be taught to use plain paper cups for suctioning, not a sterile basin. The cups should be kept in a sealable package. A clean cup is removed from the bottom of the package for each suctioning effort. The package should be resealed between uses.
- Suction catheters can be clean, not sterile. They should be washed in soapy water, rinsed well, and soaked in a vinegar-and-water solution.
- To decrease expenses, saline solution can be made by boiling water and adding salt.

Tracheostomy Care. Tracheostomy care is necessary to minimize the risk of infection and to ensure that crusted secretions do not plug the tube, and for general cleanliness. The nurse must clean around the incision site and clean the inner cannula of the tube. This should be done with sterile water or normal saline solution. A small brush is used to scrub the lumen of the inner cannula, and cotton-tipped applicators are useful for cleaning the stoma. If there are encrusted secretions on the skin, a dilute solution of hydrogen peroxide can be used to loosen them. Peroxide also is useful for clearing mucus from the inner cannula. This solution must be thoroughly rinsed away with sterile water.

The nurse should also change any stoma dressings. Commercially made tracheostomy dressings are available, or gauze may be folded to size. Dressings cut with scissors should not be used because threads from the gauze can cause an inflammatory reaction at the stoma. If the patient has large amounts of secretions, tracheostomy dressings should be changed as often as necessary. If the tracheostomy produces few secretions, the dressing may need changing only once or twice a day. Well-established dry tracheostomies may require no dressing (Carroll, 1986).

The tapes used to fasten the tracheostomy in place usually need replacement once or twice a day. Great care must be taken during this portion of the procedure, since the unsecured tracheostomy tube can be easily coughed out. Because the patient who coughs out the tracheostomy tube may no longer have a patent airway, it is the policy of many institutions to have two nurses change tracheostomy tapes. One nurse should hold the tube in place while the other threads the tapes through the

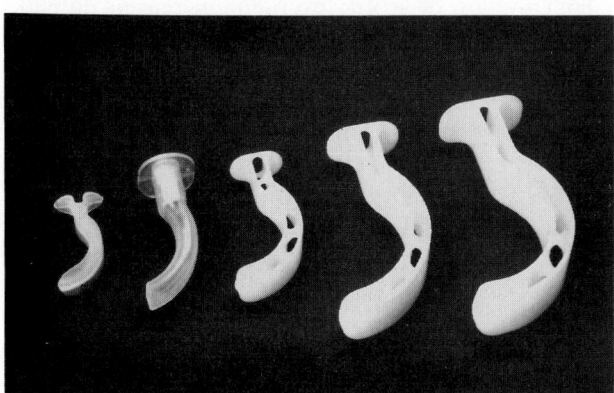

Figure 30–10.   Oral airways.

flange and secures them. Unless Velcro fasteners are used, the tapes should be tied securely with a square knot. See Procedure 30-6 for detailed instructions on tracheostomy care.

Emergency Airway Measures

Soft-tissue obstruction usually means that the tongue has fallen backwards and blocked the airway. Obstruction by the tongue can interfere with oxygenation and can cause carbon dioxide retention. This is particularly a problem for the neurologically impaired patient, such as the stroke victim, or the comatose patient. This form of obstruction is identified by a loud snoring sound. It is easily remedied by positioning the patient on one side or the other. If this is undesirable or impractical, an oral or nasal airway may be needed.

Airway obstruction requires immediate attention to prevent catastrophe. The choking victim cannot breathe, and the airway must be cleared to prevent a cardiorespiratory arrest. When the nurse first discovers the choking victim, he or she should stay with the victim and shout for help. The nurse must take immediate action to clear the obstruction. The person first arriving to help will be ready to alert the CPR team if necessary, and to offer other immediate support.

Heimlich Maneuver. The Heimlich maneuver is recommended by the American Heart Association for the treatment of foreign body obstruction in adults and children (AHA, 1986). In this procedure, abdominal thrusts are used to generate high pressures that can dislodge an aspirated obstruction. After establishing that the choking victim cannot cough or speak, the nurse must act quickly. The nurse must stand behind the victim, and wrap his or her arms around the victim's waist. With one fist against the abdomen and the other grasping the opposite wrist, the nurse squeezes rapidly and tightly, using an upward thrusting motion. This must be repeated until the obstruction is successfully dislodged, or until the victim loses consciousness. (See Procedure 30-7, Managing an Obstructed Airway.)

If unconsciousness occurs, the victim is laid in a supine position. The nurse should sweep the victim's mouth with the fingers in an attempt to pull out any obstruction. If no obstruction is obvious, the nurse must try to ventilate the victim with a manual resuscitator or with mouth-to-mouth breathing. This is followed by abdominal thrusts, and the sequence is repeated until it is successful.

The Heimlich maneuver or its modified technique is not recommended for pregnant women or for infants. Chest thrusts should be used for these choking victims.

Discharge Planning and Home Care

Some patients are discharged from the hospital with orders to receive home respiratory therapy such as hand-held aerosol treatments, chest physiotherapy, oxygen, or ventilator care. How much and what kind of home therapy the patient receives depends on many factors, including the patient's age, ability to learn procedures, family support, degree of impairment, and motivation. The nurse is often the one to assess these characteristics for the purpose of making recommendations to the physician. Often the nurse is also responsible for much of the teaching for home care.

Infection Control

The procedures of home respiratory care differ somewhat from those in the hospital. A home patient may use disposable items for longer than the time allowed for in-hospital use. Pieces of equipment normally considered disposable after 2 or 3 days in the hospital, such as cannulas or small-volume nebulizers, are likely to be used for much longer in the home. Hospital procedures performed under sterile conditions, such as tracheostomy care and suctioning, may be done using clean technique at home.

These differences are due in part to cost considerations and limited facilities at home for sterilization. They are usually justified by the fact that the patient is exposed to fewer dangerous foreign microorganisms at home than in the hospital.

Because these differences in procedures can foster germ growth, one of the most important aspects of home nursing care of the respiratory patient is infection control. The patient must be taught effective cleaning of all equipment. To assess compliance, the nurse should secure an order for periodic culturing of equipment.

The nurse must ensure that the patient clearly understands the importance of infection control, since potentially lethal pneumonia may result from respiratory infection. The patient should have yearly flu vaccinations and during flu season should avoid crowds. The COPD patient should be encouraged to discuss pneumonia immunization with the physician.

The patient should know the signs of impending infection: increased sputum production, change of sputum color to yellow or green, fever, and increasing difficulty in raising sputum. If the patient has a standing order for antibiotics, it is appropriate to begin taking the medication when these signs appear. If relief is not obtained within a day or two, contact the physician. Appreciable amounts of blood in the sputum, a severe increase in shortness of breath, or any other severe symptoms should be referred immediately to the physician.

Medications

Home use of respiratory medications can be simplified by prepackaged unit-dose medications, but these are

(Text continues on page 792)

PROCEDURE 30–6. Providing Tracheostomy Care

■ Purpose
1. Maintain airway patency by removing encrustations.
2. Prevent infections of the tracheal site.
3. Promote cleanliness and prevent skin breakdown at stoma site.

■ Assessment
- Assess for excess peristomal secretions, excess intra-tracheal secretions, or soiled tracheostomy dressing and ties.
- Assess respiratory status: breath sounds, respiratory rate, skin color, labored breathing, flared nares or sternal retractions, arterial blood gases.
- Identify factors that influence tracheostomy care:
  Inadequate nutritional status predisposes patient to infection, poor healing, and weak cough reflex.
  Respiratory infection: pulmonary secretions increase in amount. Note color, amount, and odor.
  Fluid status: inadequate hydration increases tenaciousness of secretions. Patient may have difficulty coughing thick secretions up.
  Humidity: tracheostomy collars deliver humidified air to prevent dry, cracked membranes and thickened secretions.
- Identify type of tracheostomy tube used and if inner cannula is present.
- Assess patient's ability to understand and perform independent tracheostomy care.

■ Equipment
Sterile tracheostomy care kit containing:
  Two basins
  Small brush or pipe cleaners
  4″ × 4″ gauze
  Commercially available tracheostomy dressing
  Twill tape or trach ties
Hydrogen peroxide
Normal saline
Sterile gloves
Scissors
Tracheostomy suction supplies

■ Procedure
1. Wash your hands and don gloves.
   Rationale: Reduces transmission of microorganisms.
2. Explain procedure to patient. Place in semi- to high-Fowler's position.
3. Suction tracheostomy tube. Before discarding gloves, remove soiled tracheostomy dressing, and discard with catheter inside glove.
   Note: Follow procedure 31-5, Suctioning Nasotracheal Secretions, but insert catheter through

tracheostomy tube and advance about 10 to 12 cm in an adult.
   Rationale: Removing secretion maintains a patent airway while doing tracheostomy cleaning.
4. Replace oxygen or humidification source and encourage patient to deep-breathe as you prepare sterile supplies.
5. Open sterile tracheostomy kit. Pour normal saline into one basin, hydrogen peroxide into the second. Open several sterile cotton-tipped applicators and one sterile precut tracheostomy dressing and place on sterile field. If kit does not contain twill tape, cut two 15″ ties and set aside.
   Rationale: Preparing equipment allows for smooth, organized performance of tracheostomy care.
6. Don sterile gloves. Maintain sterility of dominant hand throughout procedure.
   Rationale: Prevents transmission of microorganisms to trachea.

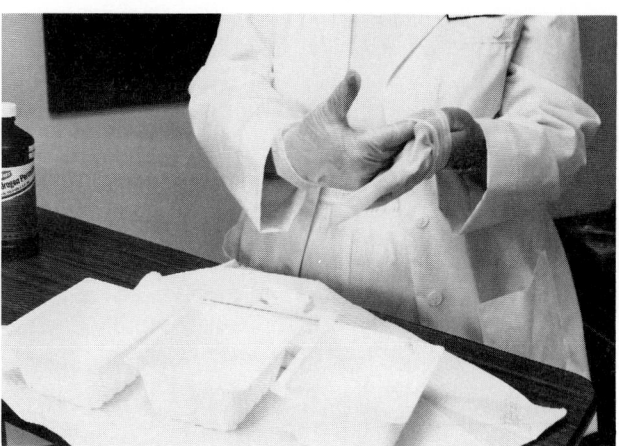

Step 6

7. Remove oxygen or humidity source.
   Note: For tracheostomy tube with inner cannula, complete steps 8 to 25. For tracheostomy tube without inner cannula or plugged with a button, complete steps 13 to 25.
8. Unlock inner cannula by turning counterclockwise. Remove inner cannula and place in basin with hydrogen peroxide.
   Rationale: Loosens and removes secretions from inner cannula.
9. Replace oxygen source over or near outer cannula.
   Rationale: Maintain constant supply of oxygen to prevent respiratory or cardiac distress.
   Note: Not all patients require a constant oxygen supply during tracheostomy care.

(continued)

PROCEDURE 30–6. Providing Tracheostomy Care *continued*

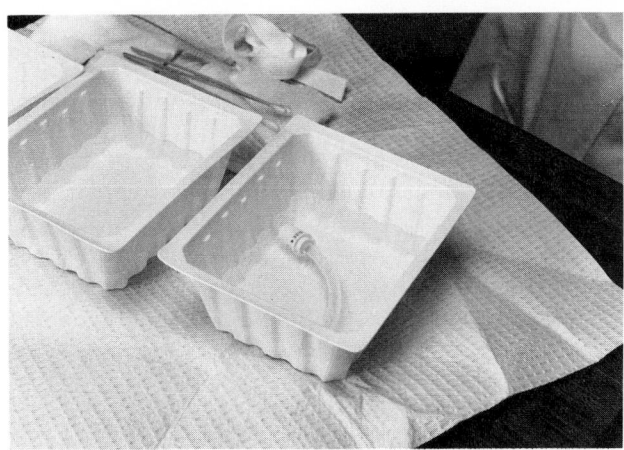

Step 8

10. Clean lumen and sides of inner cannula using pipe cleaners or sterile brush.
    Rationale: Mechanical force and friction are needed to remove thick or dried secretions.

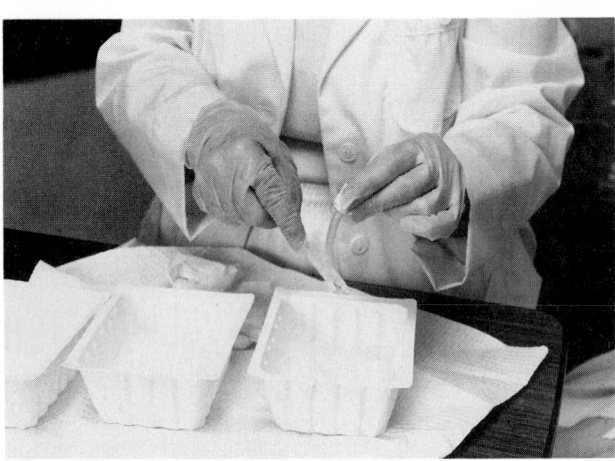

Step 10

11. Rinse inner cannula thoroughly by agitating in normal saline for several seconds.
    Rationale: Removes secretions and water from cannula. Also provides lubrication to each insertion.
12. Remove oxygen source and replace inner cannula into outer cannula. "Lock" by turning clockwise until the two blue dots align. Replace oxygen or humidity source.
    Rationale: Reestablishes oxygen to a secured inner cannula.

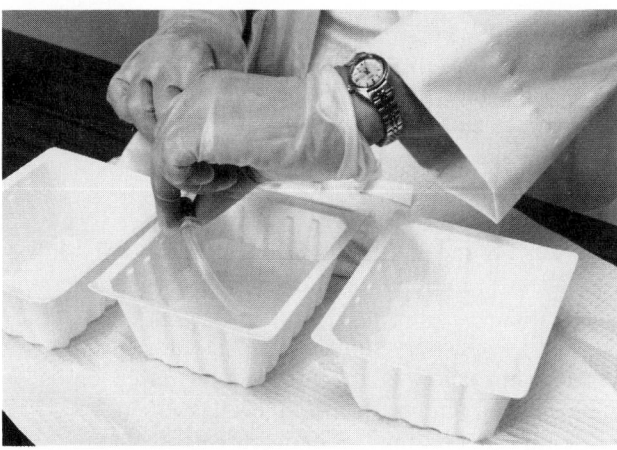

Step 11

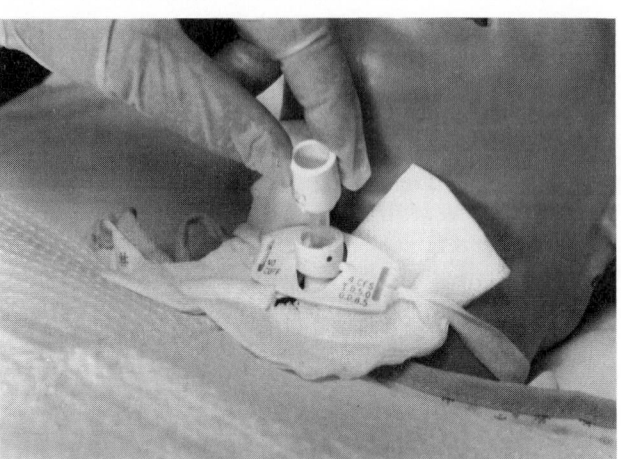

Step 12

13. Clean stoma under faceplate with circular motion using hydrogen peroxide-soaked cotton applicators. Cleanse dried secretions from all exposed outer cannula surfaces.

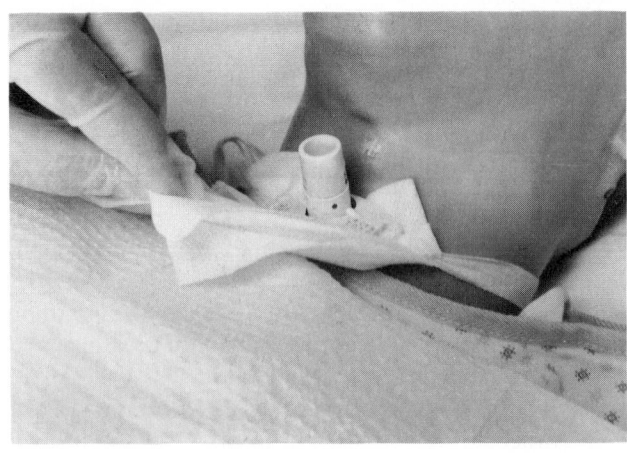

Step 13

(continued)

PROCEDURE 30–6. Providing Tracheostomy Care *continued*

14. Remove foaming secretions using normal saline-soaked cotton-tipped applicators.
    Rationale: Hydrogen peroxide can be irritating to the skin.
15. Pat moist surfaces dry with 4″×4″ gauze.
    Rationale: Moist surfaces support growth of microorganisms and skin excoriation.
16. Place dry, sterile, precut tracheostomy dressing around tracheostomy stoma and under faceplate. Do not use cut 4″×4″ gauze.
    Rationale: Frayed cotton fibers could be aspirated into the trachea.
17. If tracheostomy ties are to be changed, have an assistant don a sterile glove and hold the tracheostomy tube in place.
    Rationale: Prevents accidental displacement of the tracheostomy tube if the patient moves or coughs when the ties are not secure.
18. Cut a ½″ slit approximately 1″ from one end of both clean tracheostomy ties. This is easily done by folding back on itself 1″ of the tie and cutting a small slit in the middle.
19. Remove and discard soiled tracheostomy ties.
20. Thread the slit end of one clean tie through the one eyelet of the faceplate. Thread the other end of the tie through the slit and pull it taut against the faceplate.
    Rationale: Secures the ties to the faceplate without using knots.

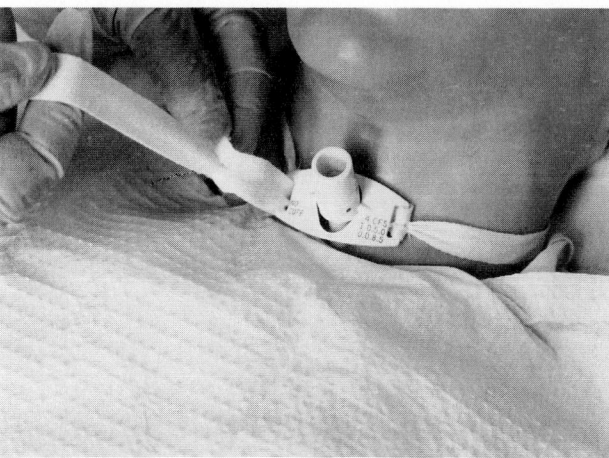

Step 20B

Rationale: Ties must be taut enough to prevent accidental dislodging of tracheostomy tube, but loose enough not to cause choking or pressure on the jugular veins. Ties at side of neck are more comfortable for the patient.

23. Remove gloves and discard disposable equipment. Label, date, and store reusable supplies.
    Note: Opened normal saline is considered sterile for 24 hours.
24. Assist patient to comfortable position and offer oral hygiene.
25. Wash your hands.
26. Document procedure and observations.

■ Lifespan Considerations

Infants and Children
- Additional assistants may be necessary during tracheostomy care to prevent active children from dislodging or expelling their tracheostomy tubes.
- Parents may be encouraged to participate with the procedure in an effort to comfort the child and promote patient teaching.

■ Home Care Modifications
- The patient or caregiver must be taught:
    That handwashing is the most important step before touching the tracheostomy.
    The function of each part of the tracheostomy tube.
    To remove, change, and replace the inner cannula. It is recommended that the inner cannula be cleaned two or three times a day.
    To cleanse the tracheostomy stoma.
    To suction tracheal secretions.
    To assess for symptoms of infection (i.e., increased

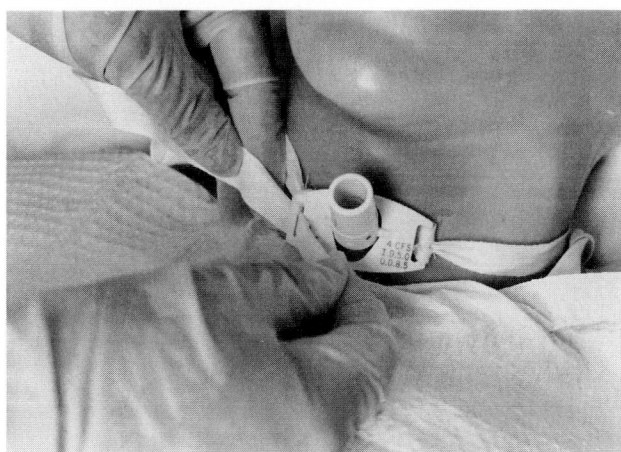

Step 20A

21. Repeat step 20 with the second tie.
22. Bring both ties together at one side of the patient's neck. Assess that ties are only tight enough to allow one finger between tie and neck. Use two square knots to secure the ties. Trim excess tie length.
    Note: Assess tautness of tracheostomy ties frequently in patients whose neck may swell from trauma or surgery.

(continued)

temperature, increased amount of secretions, change in color or odor of secretions).
• A vaporizer may be used in the home to replace moisture into the air.
• The patient may wear a scarf or 4″×4″ over the tracheostomy if the air is dusty.
• Home care may be a clean rather than sterile procedure:
    Plain single-use paper cups may be used for soaking the inner cannula.

Tap water may be used to rinse secretions from the inner cannula.
    Gloves need not be worn, but thorough handwashing is imperative.
• A list of needed supplies and equipment and the names of medical supply houses is useful.
• Names and telephone numbers of health-care professionals who are available for emergencies or advice 24 hours a day should be readily available.

---

more expensive than stock bottles of medications. Dosage measurement, if the patient can learn to do it, may be more cost effective.

The patient should be taught to recognize side effects of medications and to understand why they are dangerous. The dangers of taking medications more frequently than ordered should also be stressed. If the medications provide no relief, the patient should be taught to call the physician.

Home Oxygen Systems

The equipment used by lung patients at home also differs from hospital equipment. At home the patient can receive oxygen from high-pressure cylinders, liquid gas systems, or electrically powered concentrators. Compressed oxygen from high-pressure tanks is best for the patient who requires only occasional oxygen. Liquid oxygen systems allow the patient to leave home. Portable "walkers" can be filled from a stationary unit at home. The walkers are small enough to be carried or wheeled in a small cart, but they can hold up to several hours' worth of oxygen (Fig. 30-11). A concentrator is a device that chemically separates oxygen from room air. It is an excellent choice for the patient who requires continuous oxygen in low concentrations.

Home ventilators also are different from those found in the intensive care unit. Wrap-around pulmonary-aid belts only assist patients with breathing and are not the best choice for those who cannot breathe. For these patients, or for those with severe weakness at night, a negative-pressure ventilator (for example, an iron lung or chest cuirass) is more appropriate.

The companies that rent these items or supply the oxygen should be well established and reliable. They should be able to provide service 24 hours every day. The patient should have the telephone numbers of the suppliers and must be able to get service whenever necessary. Reputable suppliers often hire respiratory thera-

pists to routinely visit the patient at home and to assess respiratory status and equipment function. Coordination between these services and community health nursing services should be arranged.

Energy Conservation

Activities of daily living can be seriously affected by respiratory dysfunction, but with slight modifications they can be performed by most patients. Energy conservation and the motivation to be independent are keys to success. Performing activities of daily living does wonders for the patient's self-esteem and self-confidence.

The nurse should base suggestions for modifying activ-

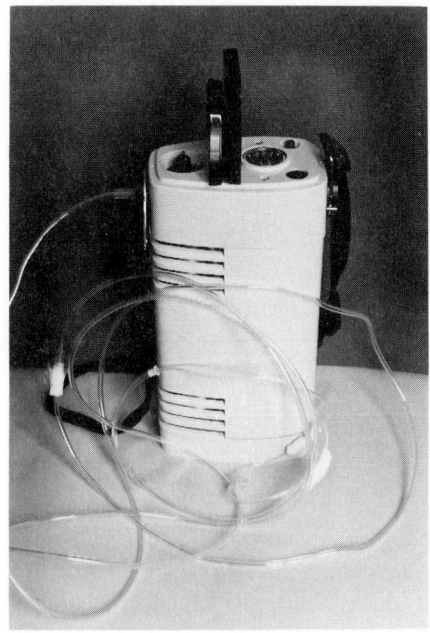

Figure 30–11. Portable oxygen walker.

PROCEDURE 30–7. Managing an Obstructed Airway (Heimlich Maneuver)

■ **Purpose**
Remove a foreign body from obstructing the airway in order to prevent anoxia and cardiopulmonary arrest.

■ **Assessment**
• Identify disorders that put patients at greater risk for airway obstruction:
    Cerebral vascular accident with hemiparesis
    Amyotrophic lateral sclerosis
    Seizure disorders
    Tumors of neck or esophagus
    Decreased level of consciousness
    Heavy narcotic or sedative use
    Alcohol intoxication
    Diminished or absent cough and gag reflex
• Assess patients for signs and symptoms of airway obstruction.
    Symptoms *not needing* immediate intervention:
      Ability to speak
      Ability to breathe in and out
      Ability to cough
      Stable vital signs
      Note: Stay with the patient and allow him or her to cough to clear airway.
    Symptoms *needing* immediate intervention:
      Universal distress signal for complete airway obstruction
      Irregular, slow, shallow breathing
      Apnea
      High-pitched wheezing
      Inability to cough forcibly or at all
      Inability to speak
      Vomitus in mouth or on face
      Loose, free-floating dentures
      Cyanosis
      Abnormal pulse (irregular, rapid, or slow)
• Determine which variation of the Heimlich maneuver (chest thrusts, finger sweep) to use.

■ **Equipment**
No equipment is mandatory; suction equipment and emergency cart are useful if in hospital setting.

■ **Procedure**

    Conscious Adult (Heimlich maneuver)
1. The patient will be standing or sitting.
2. Stand behind the patient.
3. Wrap your arms around patient's waist.

4. Make a fist with one hand. Place thumb side of fist against patient's abdomen, above the navel but below the xiphoid process.

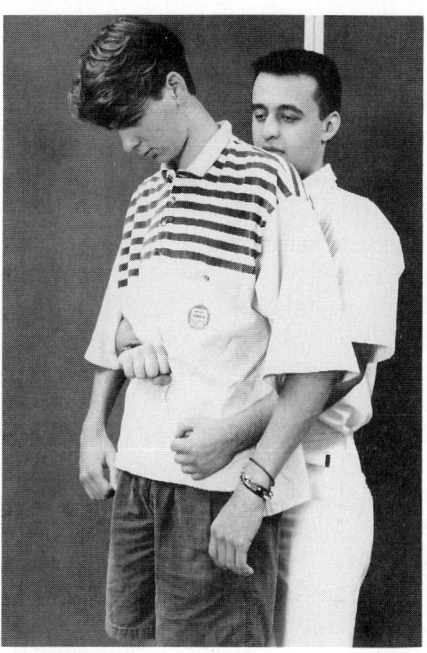

Step 4

5. Grasp fist with other hand.

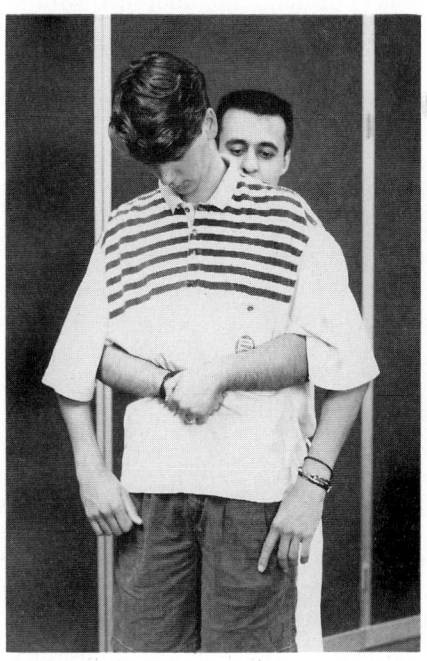

Step 5

(continued)

PROCEDURE 30–7. Managing an Obstructed Airway (Heimlich Maneuver) *continued*

6. Press fist into abdomen with a quick upward thrust. *Rationale: Increases intrathoracic pressure and creates an artificial cough, which forces air and foreign objects out of the airway.*
7. Repeat distinct separate thrusts until foreign body is expelled or patient becomes unconscious.

■ **Procedure**

Unconscious patient (Heimlich maneuver, abdominal thrust)
1. Patient will be lying on the ground.
2. Turn patient on back and call for help.
3. Finger sweep.
   a. Use tongue-jaw lift to open mouth. *Rationale: Draws tongue away from back of throat to relieve obstruction or visualize foreign body.*
   b. Insert index finger inside cheek and sweep to base of tongue. Use a hooking motion if possible to dislodge and remove the foreign body. *Note: Finger sweeps are avoided in infants and children, since the foreign body can easily be pushed further into the airway. Remove only if clearly visible and easily reached.*
4. Straddle patient's thighs or kneel to the side of thighs.
5. Place heel of one hand on epigastric area, midline above the navel but below the xiphoid process.
6. Place second hand on top of first hand.
7. Press heel of hand into abdomen with a quick upward thrust. *Rationale: Increases intrathoracic pressure and creates an artificial cough to force air and foreign body out of airway. Note: Be careful to thrust in the midline to prevent injury to the liver or spleen.*
8. Repeat abdominal thrusts 6 to 10 times.
9. If airway is still obstructed, attempt to ventilate using mouth-to-mouth respiration and head tilt-chin lift.
10. Repeat steps 5 to 8 until successful.

■ **Lifespan Considerations**

■ **Procedure**

Infants Under 1 Year of Age (Back Blows and Chest Thrusts)
1. Straddle infant over your arm with head lower than trunk.
2. Support head by holding jaw firmly in your hand.
3. Rest your forearm on your thigh and deliver four back blows with the heel of your hand between the infant's scapula.
4. Place free hand on infant's back and support neck while turning to supine position.
5. Place two fingers over sternum in same location as for external chest compression (one fingerwidth below nipple line).
6. Administer four chest thrusts.
7. Repeat steps 1 to 6 until airway is not obstructed.

■ **Procedure**

Children Over 1 Year of Age
1. Perform Heimlich maneuver with child standing, sitting, or lying as for adult, but more gently.
2. Rescuer may need to kneel behind child or have child stand on a table.
3. Prevent foreign body airway obstruction in infants and children by teaching parents or caregivers to:
   a. Restrict children from walking, running, or playing with food or foreign objects in their mouths.
   b. Keep small objects (i.e., marbles, beads, beans, thumb tacks) away from children under 3 years of age.
   c. Avoid feeding popcorn and peanuts to children under 3 years of age, and cut other foods into small pieces.
4. Parents and caregivers should be instructed in the management of foreign body airway obstruction.

■ **Procedure**

Pregnant women or very obese adults (chest thrusts)
1. Stand behind patient.
2. Bring your arms under patient's armpits and around chest.
3. Make a fist and place thumb side against *middle* of sternum.
4. Grasp fist with other hand and deliver a quick backward thrust.
5. Repeat thrusts until airway is cleared.
6. Chest thrusts may be performed with patient supine and hands positioned with heel over lower half of sternum (as for cardiac compression). Administer separate downward thrusts until airway is clear.

■ **Prevention**
- Cut food into small pieces. Chew thoroughly, especially if wearing dentures.
- Avoid laughing and talking while swallowing and chewing.
- Avoid excessive alcohol before and during meals.

ities of daily living on a thorough assessment of the extent to which each activity has been affected by respiratory dysfunction. For instance:

If meal preparation is a problem, the nurse may be able to provide a referral to a "Meals on Wheels" program.
Sponge baths may be a practical alternative to tub bathing if mobility is impaired.
An elevated toilet seat may help decrease the work needed to rise from the toilet.

Patients must never be encouraged to exceed their abilities, but they should be encouraged to work gradually toward increasing exercise tolerance. Helping the patient to set realistic goals is of utmost importance. Conversely, goals should provide enough challenge to allow the patient to feel the endeavor is worthwhile. The nurse must praise small accomplishments, since progress at building endurance is often slow.

Fostering Self-Esteem

Like most of us, the person with lung disease wants to be an independent, contributing member of society. The patient must feel self-reliant, not like a burden to others. The ability to get around independently and to do meaningful work can help foster these feelings. These activities are also essential to avoid the debilitating effects of depression.

Work is often a source of satisfaction and self-esteem. The diagnosis of pulmonary disease does not mean the person is automatically unable to work. On the contrary, if the patient derives satisfaction from a job, it is important for him or her to continue working as long as possible. Frequent illness can make it difficult for the severely dyspneic patient to hold a demanding job. Although it is not always feasible for the patient's employer to offer flexibility of scheduling, this option should be explored. The nurse can help the patient by offering encouragement, by discussing possible work options, and by acting as a resource. The nurse can further identify patients who might benefit from discussions with the occupational therapist.

Respiratory disease can severely inhibit sexual desire and the ability to perform. Shortness of breath and its resultant fatigue can be responsible for the loss of this function. Often, however, newly developed sexual problems in these patients may be based on the *fear* that the disease will prevent satisfactory performance. This fear, along with perhaps depression and lowered self-esteem, can bring about a self-fulfilling prophecy: the patient who expects sexual problems to develop will almost certainly be right.

Recognition by the patient of these limitations should not mean resignation to a less-than-full life. Sexual difficulties may be common among respiratory patients, but they can be surmounted (Petty & Nett, 1984). The nurse

can suggest using prescribed bronchodilators before sexual relations. This helps some patients maintain good breathing throughout sexual activity. The nurse can inform the patient that passive positions save energy. Perhaps most important, the nurse must stress the importance of open communication between the patient and his or her partner.

The nurse can help further by offering suggestions for activities outside of the home. Social outlets can help the patient to cope with the day-to-day frustrations of lung disease. The American Lung Association sponsors classes and support groups for people with respiratory disease. These groups may meet in or out of the hospital. Often staff nurses, physicians, or therapists are guest speakers at such gatherings. Rehabilitation programs are more structured activities organized at the hospital. Their purpose is to increase the patient's ability to function with lung disease. Such programs may provide breathing retraining, exercise, and diet and occupational counseling.

EVALUATION

The nurse works with the patient to develop goals. Outcome criteria are specific observable indicators that can measure goal attainment. For each general goal, outcome criteria are suggested, but it is important to individualize outcome criteria depending on the patient's current status.

Goal
Patient will demonstrate knowledge regarding prevention of respiratory dysfunction.

Possible Outcome Criteria
- After teaching session, patient demonstrates deep-breathing and coughing techniques.
- After teaching session, patient discusses the physiologic effects of smoking.
- After teaching session, patient lists signs of respiratory infection and knows when to call the physician.
- After teaching session, patient describes, for any medication administered for respiratory problems, the name of the drug, dose to be taken, action of the medication, side effects of the medication, and any special considerations for administration.
- After teaching session, patient demonstrates pursed-lip breathing.
- Patient joins and regularly attends meetings of a stop-smoking program for 6 months.

Goal
Patient's body tissues will have adequate oxygenation.

Nursing Management Plan
The Patient with Ineffective Airway Clearance

Nursing Diagnosis: Ineffective airway clearance related to tracheobronchial infection as manifested by weak cough, adventitious breath sounds, and copious green sputum production.

Patient Goal: Patient will mobilize pulmonary secretions.

Patient Outcome Criteria

- After teaching session, patient demonstrates proper coughing techniques.
- Patient drinks at least six glasses of water per day while in hospital.
- Patient demonstrates correct self-suctioning technique before discharge.

Nursing Intervention	Scientific Rationale

1. Provide and teach the patient the importance of adequate hydration.
    Encourage fluids (2000 to 3000 mL per 24 hours).
       Intake and output.
       Avoid milk and milk products.
       Ultrasonic nebulizer treatment.
	1. Adequate hydration thins secretions, which prevents mucus from plugging airways.
	
	To help evaluate hydration status of patient.
	Milk products tend to thicken secretions.
	To moisten and aid mobility of respiratory secretions.

2. Position and encourage to cough to promote mobilization of secretions.
    Deep breathing every 2 hours.
    Huff coughing.
    Assume sitting position if possible.
	2. To open alveoli and prevent further atelectasis.
	To prevent airway collapse.
	To permit deep inspiration and forceful abdominal contractions necessary for coughing.

3. Administer analgesic before cough session if pain limits coughing effectiveness.	3. If patient fears pain he or she hesitates to breathe deeply and cough effectively.

4. Provide or teach patient tracheal suctioning if he or she is unable to remove secretions with effective coughing.
    Hyperoxygenate with 100% O_2 before and after suctioning procedure.
    Suction for no longer than 15 seconds per suctioning attempt.
    Provide opportunities for patient to practice and demonstrate suctioning technique if self-suctioning is necessary.
	4. A weak, nonproductive cough causes secretions to be retained in airways and interfere with gas exchange.
	To prevent hypoxemia, which can occur during the suctioning procedure.
	Longer periods of suction can contribute to tissue trauma and hypoxemia.
	Suctioning is a complex motor skill that requires practice for skill acquisition and comfort.

5. Provide or teach postural chest physiotherapy as ordered by doctor. Have patient or family members demonstrate when comfortable with skill mastery.	5. To allow secretions to drain from major airways using the force of gravity.

Possible Outcome Criteria
- By discharge, patient demonstrates arterial blood gases within baseline values.
- By discharge, patient maintains a respiratory rate of normal depth and rhythm between 12 and 20 breaths per minute (values may be adjusted for patients with chronic respiratory problems).

- By discharge, patient reports improved comfort with breathing.
- By discharge, patient reports improved activity tolerance.

Goal
Patient will mobilize pulmonary secretions.

Possible Outcome Criteria

- After teaching session, patient demonstrates proper coughing technique.
- By discharge, lungs are clear on auscultation.
- Patient drinks at least six glasses of water a day while in the hospital.
- Patient demonstrates correct self-suctioning technique before discharge.

Goal

Patient will effectively cope with changes in self-concept and lifestyle.

Possible Outcome Criteria

- Within 6 months of diagnosis, patient verbalizes how the respiratory condition has caused changes in lifestyle.
- Within a week of diagnosis, patient verbalizes support people to provide emotional strength.
- By end of teaching session, patient lists community agencies and services that he or she plans to use.
- Before discharge, patient demonstrates oxygen-conserving measures such as sitting while dressing and planning rest periods.
- Before discharge, patient demonstrates the safe use of home oxygen equipment.
- Before discharge, patient verbalizes sexual positions requiring less oxygen expenditure.

Key Concepts

- The primary functions of breathing are the delivery of oxygen to the blood, the removal of carbon dioxide from the blood, and maintenance of acid–base balance.
- Breathing is normally almost effortless, but the work required for breathing increases tremendously when the airways are obstructed by inflammation, bronchospasm, or excessive mucous secretions.
- Deep breathing and coughing are two of the most important measures for preventing postoperative pulmonary complications.
- Adequate hydration is essential to keep respiratory secretions moist and easily coughed up from the respiratory tract.
- Patients with COPD must not receive too much oxygen, since it can cause hypoventilation. They normally require only 2 to 3 L/min through a nasal cannula or 28% through a Venturi mask.
- Smoking is the single most important factor affecting pulmonary health.
- Common manifestations of respiratory dysfunction are cough, dyspnea, chest pain, and sputum production.
- The most common respiratory conditions the nurse encounters are asthma, COPD, pulmonary embolism, and pneumonia.
- Major nursing interventions for the respiratory patient are measures to promote airway patency, improve the distribution of air in the lungs, and to promote oxygenation.
- Airway maintenance interventions include hydration, positioning, coughing, chest physiotherapy, suctioning, and management of artificial airways.
- Hyperinflation techniques, such as deep breathing, incentive spirometry, and intermittent positive pressure breathing, help prevent atelectasis and promote a strong cough.
- Oxygen therapy raises the amount of oxygen in the lungs, thereby making more oxygen available to the blood and tissues.
- A cannula or Venturi mask provides a relatively low concentration (less than 40%) of oxygen. Medium (40% to 60%) concentrations of oxygen are provided by simple masks. Reservoir-type masks deliver high oxygen concentrations (above 60%).
- Dyspnea, excessive mucous secretions, dried secretions, hyperventilation, and hypoventilation are common nursing problems of the hospitalized respiratory patient.
- Discharge planning must be individualized for the respiratory patient. Ability to perform activities of daily living and manage home procedures must be considered carefully before discharge.

References

Aloan, C. A. (1987). *Respiratory care of the newborn: A clinical manual.* Philadelphia: J. B. Lippincott.

American Heart Association (1986). Standards and guidelines for cardiopulmonary resuscitation and emergency cardiac care. *Journal of the American Medical Association, 255,* 2972.

Burton, G., Hodgkin, J., & Ward, J. (1991). *Respiratory care* (3rd ed.). Philadelphia: J. B. Lippincott.

Carnevali, D., & Patrick, M. (1986). *Nursing management for the elderly* (2nd ed.). Philadelphia: J. B. Lippincott.

Carroll, P. (1986). Artificial airways, real risks. *Nursing '86, 16*(8), 56–59.

Cherniack, R., & Cherniack, L. (1983). *Respiration in health and disease* (3rd ed.). Philadelphia: W. B. Saunders.

DesJardins, T. (1988). *Cardiopulmonary anatomy and physiology: Essentials for respiratory care.* Albany, NY: Delmar Publishers Inc.

Fuchs, P. (1984). Streamlining your suctioning techniques, part 1: Nasotracheal suctioning. *Nursing '84, 14*(5), 55–61.

Hoffman, L., & Maszkiewicz, R. (1987). Airway management for the critically ill. *American Journal of Nursing, 87,* 39–54.

Mitchell, R., & Petty, T. (1989). *Synopsis of clinical pulmonary disease* (4th ed.). St. Louis: C. V. Mosby.

NANDA (1990). *Taxonomy I revised 1990, with official nursing diagnoses.* St. Louis, MO: North American Nursing Association.

Patry-Lahey, R. (1985). Helping a laryngectomy patient go home. *Nursing '85, 15*(3), 63–65.

Petty, T., & Nett, L. (1984). *Enjoying life with emphysema.* Philadelphia: Lea & Febiger.

Ries, A. (1987). Pulmonary rehabilitation. *Resp Management, 17*(2), 39–44.

Shapiro, B., Harrison, R., Kacmarek, R., & Cane, R. (1985). *Clinical application of respiratory care* (3rd ed.). Chicago: Year Book Medical Publishers.

Slonim, N., & Hamilton, L. (1987). *Respiratory physiology* (5th ed.). St. Louis: C. V. Mosby.

Weinberger, S. (1986). *Principles of pulmonary medicine.* Philadelphia: W. B. Saunders.

Bibliography

Ahrens, T., & Rutherford, K. (1987). The new pulmonary math. *American Journal of Nursing, 87,* 337–340.

Ariagno, R., & Glotzbach, S. (1987). Home monitoring of high-risk infants. *Chest, 91,* 898–899.

Barnes, P. (1987). Using anticholinergics to best advantage. *Journal of Respiratory Disease, 8*(5), 84–95.

Barnes, T. (1988). *Respiratory care practice.* Chicago: Year Book Medical Publishers.

Bergbom-Engberg, I., et al. (1989). Assessment of patients' experience of discomfort during respiratory therapy. *Critical Care Medicine, 17,* 1068–1072.

Buschiazzo, L. (1986). What's new in CPR? *Nursing '86, 16*(1), 34–37.

Callaghan, T. (1986). Bronchial hygiene in cystic fibrosis. *Respiratory Therapy, 16*(4), 13–16.

Callahan, M. (1985). A prudent pulmonary rehabilitation program. *American Journal of Nursing, 85,* 1368–1369.

Carlson, K. (1989). Assessing a child's chest. *RN, 52*(11), 26–32.

Daily, D. (1987). Home oxygen therapy for infants with bronchopulmonary dysplasia: Growth and development. *Respiratory Management, 17*(3), 13–20.

Dean, N., Costello, E., Duffy, S., & Flynn, S. (1987). The role of ketotifen in preventive therapy for asthma. *Respiartory Management, 17*(3), 40–43.

Dennison, R. (1986). Cardiopulmonary assessment: How to do it better in 15 easy steps. *Nursing '86, 16*(4), 34–40.

Eggland, E. (1987). Teaching the ABC's of COPD. *Nursing '87, 17*(1), 60–64.

Falck, S. (1985). Chronic ventilator patients: Alternatives to hospital care. *Respiratory Therapy, 15*(1), 27–35.

Garcia, M. K. (1989). Asthma: Old problems and new strategies. *Sch Nurs, 5*(3), 25–32.

Garrity, E., & Gross, N. (1987). Prompt management for status asthmaticus. *Journal of Respiratory Disease, 8*(5), 21–32.

Geisman, L. K. (1989). Advances in weaning from mechanical ventilator. *Critical Care Nursing of North America, 1,* 697–705.

Geller, R., & Fisher, J. (1987). The role of symptomatic treatment for the common cold. *Journal of Respiratory Disease, 8*(1), 20–34.

Gregg, B. L. (1989). Inspiratory muscle training with a weighted incentive spirometer in subjects with chronic airway obstruction. *Respir Care, 34,* 860–867.

Griffin, C., & Lockhart, J. (1987). Learning to swallow again. *Am J Nurs, 87,* 314–317.

Hahn, K. (1987). Slow teaching the COPD patient. *Nursing '87, 17*(4), 34–42.

Herman, J. (1987). New oxygen delivery systems: Gaining patient compliance. *Resp Management, 17*(3), 30–39.

Holland, W. (1987). International workshop on the etiology of asthma. *Chest, 91*(supplement).

Jenne, J. (Ed.). (1987). Rationale for the use of theophylline in COPD: Bronchodilation and beyond. *Chest, 92*(supplement).

Lapidov, M. (1989). Respiratory distress revisited. *Neonate Netw, 8*(3), 9–14.

Libby, L. (1986). Cystic fibrosis and genetics. *Resp Therapy, 16*(3), 13–16.

Lieberman, J. (1985). Cystic fibrosis: Concepts in pharmacologic treatment. *Resp Therapy, 15*(2), 35–43.

Lindell, K. O., et al. (1990). Breaking bronchospasm's grip with metered-dose inhalers. *Am J Nurs, 90*(3), 34–41.

Lough, M., Doershuk, C., & Stern, R. (1985). *Pediatric respiratory therapy* (3rd ed.). Chicago: Year Book Medical Publishers.

Mayo, J., & Hamner, J. (1987). A nurse's guide to mechanical ventilation. *RN, 50*(8), 18–24.

McCorkle, R., et al. (1989). A randomized clinical trial of home nursing care for lung cancer patients. *Cancer, 64,* 1375–1382.

McFadden, E. (1987). Cromolyn: First-line therapy for chronic asthma? *J Resp Disease, 8*(1), 39–48.

Mischler, E., Felice, M., Fitzpatrick, S., Yankaskas, J., & Knowles, M. (1987). Managing lung disease in adult cystic fibrosis patients. *J Resp Disease, 8*(2), 23–33.

Mischler, E., Felice, M., Fitzpatrick, S., Yankaskas, J., & Knowles, M. (1987). Cystic fibrosis in adults: The nonrespiratory aspects. *J Resp Disease, 8*(3), 89–102.

Moody, L. E. (1990). Measurement of psychophysiologic response variables in chronic bronchitis and emphysema. *Appl Nurs Res, 3*(1), 36–38.

O'Ryan, J. (1987). An overview of mechanical ventilation in the home. *Resp Management, 17*(2), 27–36.

Peck, G. H. (1989). RCPs develop expertise in smoking intervention. *AARC Times, 13*(10), 73–78.

Petty, T. (1985). Definitive criteria for prescribing home oxygen systems. *Resp Therapy, 15*(2). 13–21.

Petty, T. (1987). Drug strategies for airflow obstruction. *Am J Nurs, 87,* 180–184.

Petty, T. (1987). New developments in home oxygen therapy. *Resp Management, 17*(3), 24–29.

Rau, J. (1989). *Respiratory care pharmacology* (3rd ed.). Chicago: Year Book Medical Publishers.

Robinet, K., Holmes, E., & Hartnett, J. (1987). Facing down the fear of ventilator patients. *RN, 50*(8), 14–16.

Romanski, S. (1986). Interpreting arterial blood gases in four easy steps. *Nursing '86, 16*(9), 58–64.

Senn, S., et al. Efficacy of a pulsed oxygen delivery device during exercise in patients with chronic respiratory disease. *Chest, 96,* 467–472.

Shapiro, B., Harrison, R., & Walton, J. (1989). *Clinical application of blood gases* (4th ed.). Chicago: Year Book Medical Publishers.

Snider, D. (1987). Tuberculosis in children: Time for short-course chemotherapy. *J Resp Disease, 8*(4), 70–80.

Soffer, A. (Ed.). (1987). Neurohumoral mechanisms in obstructive airway disease: The role of inhaled anticholinergic agents. *Chest, 91*(supplement).

Summer, S., & Grau, P. (1986). An update on BCLS standards. *Nursing '86, 16*(11), 48–49.

Taylor, D. (1985). Clinical applications: Assessing breath sounds. *Nursing '85, 15*(3), 60–62.

Transtracheal oxygen: The nose knows the difference. (1987). *Am J Nurs, 87,* 421–422.

Walsh, T. (1987). Helping patients cope with terminal COPD or lung cancer. *J Resp Disease, 8*(3), 23–34.

Weisman, S. W. (1989). Understanding transtracheal oxygen. *Nursing, 19*(12), 43–47.

Wesmiller, S. W., et al. (1989). Interpreting your patient's oxygenation status. *Orthop Nurs, 8*(6), 56–60.

West, J. (1985). *Respiratory physiology: The essentials* (2nd ed.). Baltimore: Williams & Wilkins.

White, K., & Perez, P. (1986). Your ventilator patient can go home again. *Nursing '86, 16*(12), 54–56.

Wilkins, R., Sheldon, R., & Krider, S. (1985). *Clinical assessment in respiratory care.* St. Louis: C. V. Mosby.

Wimsatt, R. (1985). Unlocking the mysteries behind the chest wall. *Nursing '85, 15*(11), 58–63.

Zwillich, C. (1986). Asthma therapy: An update. *Resp Therapy, 16*(2), 13–17.

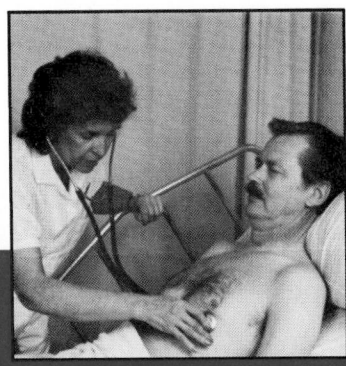

Oxygenation: Cardiac Function and Tissue Perfusion

LEARNING OBJECTIVES

Upon completion of this chapter, the student will be able to do the following:

- Describe the cardiovascular system.
- Discuss factors that contribute to normal cardiac output and tissue perfusion.
- Describe the consequences of altered cardiovascular function and their causes.
- Understand how altered cardiovascular function can impact normal activities.
- Discuss cardiovascular changes that occur during the lifespan.

- Perform a basic nursing assessment of cardiovascular function.
- Identify common procedures and diagnostic tests used in the evaluation of the cardiovascular patient.
- State relevant nursing diagnoses for the patient with cardiovascular dysfunction.
- Discuss several nursing measures directed at promoting and restoring cardiovascular function.

KEY TERMS

Angina
Aneurysm
Arrhythmia
Arteriosclerosis
Contractility

Diastole
Infarction
Ischemia
Myocardium
Perfusion

Stenosis
Systole
Thrombus
Transient ischemic attack (TIA)

Normal Cardiovascular Function
  Anatomy of the Cardiovascular System
    The Heart
    The Blood Vessels
    The Cardiovascular System
  Normal Function of the Heart and Blood Vessels
    Heart
    Blood Vessels
  Normal Cardiovascular Functional Pattern
    Heart Rate
    Blood Pressure
    Skin Temperature and Color
    Other Indicators
  Factors Affecting Normal Cardiovascular Function
    Age
    Activity and Exercise
    Gender
    Body Position
    Temperature
    Coping and Stress Tolerance
    Lifestyle and Habits
  Lifespan Considerations
Altered Cardiovascular Function
  Potential for Altered Cardiovascular Function
    Decreased Pumping Ability of the Heart
    Altered Blood Flow
    Altered Blood Composition
    Risk Factors
  Manifestations of Altered Cardiovascular Function
    Changes in Vital Signs
    Ischemia
    Edema and Thrombus Formation
    Organ Dysfunction and Failure
  Impact of Cardiovascular Dysfunction on Activities
    of Daily Living
Assessment
  Subjective Data
    Functional Pattern Identification

    Risk Identification
    Dysfunctional Identification
  Objective Data
    Physical Assessment
    Diagnostic Tests and Procedures
Nursing Diagnoses and Patient Goals
  Diagnostic Statement: Altered Tissue Perfusion
    (Renal, Cerebral, Cardiopulmonary,
    Gastrointestinal, Peripheral)
    Definition
    Defining Characteristics
    Related Factors
  Diagnostic Statement: Decreased Cardiac Output
    Definition
    Defining Characteristics
    Related Factors
  Diagnostic Statement: Activity Intolerance
    Definition
    Defining Characteristics
    Related Factors
  Related Nursing Diagnoses
  Patient Goals
Implementation
  Nursing Interventions to Promote Health and
    Function
  Nursing Interventions for Altered Cardiovascular
    Function
    Patient Teaching
    Promotion of Venous Return
    Edema Reduction
    Positioning
    Pain Management
    Energy Conservation
    Rehabilitation
    Cardiopulmonary Resuscitation
Evaluation
Key Concepts

Throughout a person's life, the heart and the blood vessels work together as the main components of the cardiovascular system. The primary function of this system is to transport oxygen and nutrients to the tissues, and to deliver the end-products of tissue metabolism to appropriate organs for their excretion.

The proper function of every organ and tissue depends on the efficiency and the effectiveness of the cardiovascular system. A healthy heart is essential to provide an adequate flow of blood into the blood vessels. The blood vessels distribute the blood and precisely regulate the amount of blood made available to every tissue of the body. Thus, the cardiovascular system ensures that a constant supply of blood is circulated to the body organs 24 hours each day. The fact that this takes place over a span of 70 or more years attests to the remarkable durability of this system.

This chapter focuses on the vital role played by the cardiovascular system in the maintenance of overall health. Dynamics of normal circulation are discussed, and the role of the nurse in supporting cardiovascular health is examined.

NORMAL CARDIOVASCULAR FUNCTION

Anatomy of the Cardiovascular System

The Heart

The heart is a hollow, muscular organ that acts as a powerful pump. Its job is to keep blood moving throughout the body. Because blood contains the nutrients and oxygen that are essential for life, the heart is responsible for providing all tissues with a constant supply of fresh, life-sustaining nutrition.

Heart Tissues. The heart consists of three layers. The innermost layer of the heart, the endocardium, is made of endothelial cells and connective tissue. The thick muscular middle layer is called the **myocardium.** The outer layer of the heart, or epicardium, is made of epithelial cells. This last layer becomes the pericardium, which is a thin-walled sac that surrounds the heart and attaches it to the diaphragm, the large arteries and veins, and the sternal wall of the thorax.

The bulk of the heart is muscle. Similar to both striated (skeletal) and smooth muscle, cardiac muscle is recognized as unique because of its automaticity (Landau, 1986b). The heart is capable of beating without external neural stimuli. Its rhythmicity is created by its own automatic electrical conduction system. This system consists of small tissue focal points and pathways that generate and conduct electrical impulses.

Several structures make up the heart's conduction system. The sinoatrial (SA) node is located on the posterior wall of the right atrium, just below the vena cava entry into this chamber. The atrioventricular (AV) node is found in the lower part of the right atrium. The AV node connects to the bundle of His, which branches right and left and spreads along the ventricle walls. These branches terminate in a network of nervelike Purkinje fibers, which spread throughout the ventricular myocardium.

Heart Structure. The heart is a hollow organ, with dividing walls that form four chambers. It is divided into left and right halves by a strong muscular wall, or septum. These halves are further divided crosswise by a

"fibrous skeleton" of connective tissue. The upper chambers are called the atria, and the lower chambers are called the ventricles.

The muscle in the left side of the heart is much thicker than that in the right. This reflects the fact that the left heart must generate higher pressures than the right (Halpenny & Bond, 1989). The left side of the heart must pump blood to all tissues of the body; the right side of the heart serves only the low resistance pulmonary system of the lungs.

Valves. Valves separate the atria from the ventricles. Attached to rings of connective tissue, the valves are fibrous structures that open and close in response to pressure differences between chambers. Each of these AV valves appears as flaps or leaflets that fold together to form a tight seal between chambers. The tricuspid valve separates the right atrium from the right ventricle; the mitral valve separates the left atrium and left ventricle.

Valves also separate the ventricles from the large blood vessels they fill. These valves are called semilunar valves, because of the half-moon shape of their leaflets.

Coronary Circulation. The coronary circulation provides the heart tissue with oxygenated blood. A pair of main coronary arteries, each with multiple branches, delivers fresh blood to all layers of the heart. One artery serves the right side of the heart; the other serves the left. The blood used by the heart is emptied into the coronary sinus, which drains into the right atrium.

The Blood Vessels

The heart empties its contents into an interconnected network of arteries, capillaries, and veins. These are collectively called blood vessels. These vessels range in size from microscopic to over an inch in diameter. Arteries convey blood away from the heart; veins carry blood from the tissues back to the heart. They are linked together by smaller vessels called capillaries.

Arteries. Arteries are relatively thick-walled, muscular vessels. This gives them strength and elasticity, which allows them to withstand the high pressure of blood being constantly forced into them by the heart. The largest artery, the aorta, arises from the left ventricle of the heart. Like a tree trunk that divides into limbs, smaller branches, and twigs, the aorta branches into successively smaller and more numerous channels. Major arteries of the head, limbs, and vital organs branch from the aorta. From each of these major arteries, many smaller arteries arise, carrying blood to every tissue of the body. The smallest arteries, called arterioles, connect to the capillaries and regulate the flow of blood into them.

Capillaries. These near-microscopic vessels run through all the body's tissues. Capillaries in the skin, muscles, and other tissues of the body are narrow channels with few branches; those in the lungs are multi-channeled. The thin endothelial walls of all capillaries are variably permeable, which allows for the exchange of nutrients and waste products between the blood and tissues.

Veins. After blood has passed through capillaries, it drains into the veins. Veins are less muscular than arteries, and therefore more distensible. Because of their distensibility, veins can stretch to accommodate relatively large volumes of blood. The treelike branching of the venous system is similar to that of the arteries, but in reverse. At their junction with capillaries, veins are small. These empty into successively larger veins, finally ending in the vena cavae. This major vessel has a superior branch, which drains blood from the head and upper limbs. The inferior vena cava collects blood from the abdominal organs and lower limbs. Together they return deoxygenated blood (or blood that has given up oxygen to the tissues) from the systemic circulation to the right atrium of the heart.

The Cardiovascular System

The heart and blood vessels comprise the cardiovascular system. It is a closed circuit, with all of its many branches ultimately beginning and ending at the heart. This system has two major portions: the pulmonary circulation and the systemic circulation (Fig. 31-1).

Pulmonary Circulation. This series of vessels carries blood through the gas exchange portions of the lungs. Deoxygenated blood from the vena cavae is pumped from the right atrium to the right ventricle. From the right ventricle the blood is ejected into the pulmonary artery. This vessel follows the branching of the tracheobronchial tree in the lungs and ends in a lush network of capillaries covering all 300 million alveoli (air sacs). These multichanneled pulmonary capillaries bring the blood into contact with air, where it can absorb oxygen and release carbon dioxide. The pulmonary capillaries empty their oxygen-enriched blood into tiny venules. In turn, the venules empty into successively larger veins, finally ending in one of four large pulmonary veins. These veins empty passively into the left atrium of the heart.

Systemic Circulation. Virtually all tissues of the body are nourished by the systemic circulation. It provides all tissues with "fresh," oxygenated blood, and collects and removes tissue waste products. Circulation begins with the left atrium, which receives oxygenated blood from the pulmonary veins. From the left atrium the oxygenated blood is pumped into the left ventricle, and from there into the aorta. The oxygenated blood is dispersed through the many branches of the arterial system, finally passing through tissue capillaries. Here tissues absorb oxygen and nutrients from the fresh blood in exchange

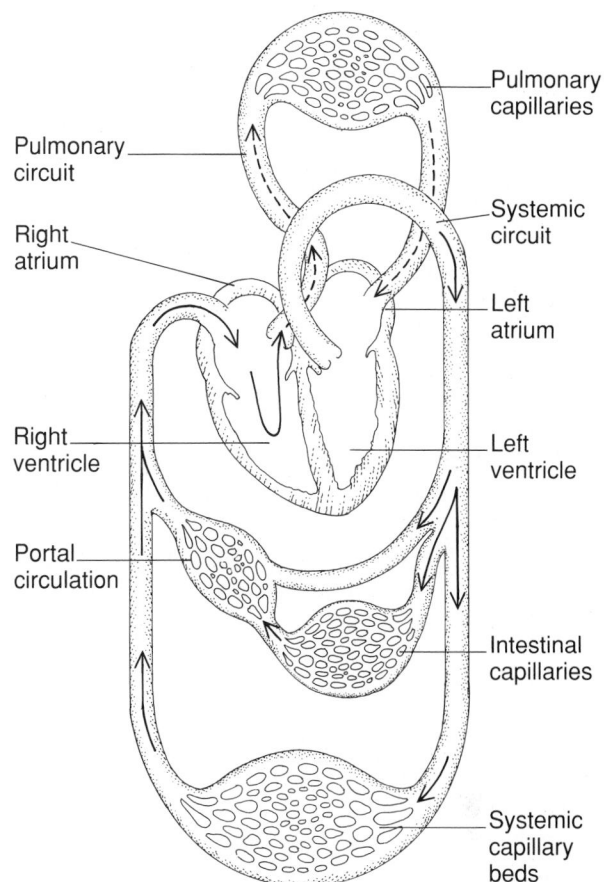

Figure 31-1. Schematic representation of the pulmonary and systemic circulation.

for their waste products. The deoxygenated blood enters the veins and returns to the right atrium by way of the vena cavae. Then the blood is pumped from the atrium into the right ventricle, and the cycle begins once again.

Normal Function of the Heart and Blood Vessels

The normal heartbeat is a repetitive cycle of rhythmic contraction and relaxation. With each contraction, during the period called **systole,** blood is ejected from the atria into the ventricles, and from the ventricles into the arteries. Between contractions, in the period called **diastole,** the heart muscle relaxes and its chambers fill with blood. Throughout the cycle, blood continually flows past the body's tissues, exchanging vital nutrients for their wastes.

The cardiac cycle begins with the generation of a small electrical impulse within the heart. This impulse is translated into mechanical activity, which results in muscle contraction and pumping motion.

Heart

The effectiveness of the heart as a pump depends on several factors. Three of the most important factors are its ability to generate and conduct electrical impulses, its ability to fill and empty properly, and the strength with which it can contract.

Impulse Conduction. Whereas contraction and relaxation of most muscles are controlled by the nervous system, the heart has its own inherent, automatic ability to control its activity (Fig. 31-2). Impulses that stimulate contraction normally originate in specialized cells near the top of the right atrium. In these cells (known as the sinoatrial [SA] node), small but significant chemical changes regularly occur. Concentrations of ions such as potassium, sodium, and calcium inside and surrounding the SA node fluctuate suddenly and rapidly. This rapid ionic fluctuation causes a change in the electric potential of the cells, known as depolarization. This generates a small electrical impulse. Because the SA node establishes impulses that determine the rate at which the heart beats, it is often called the pacemaker of the heart.

This tiny electrical impulse is significant because it travels from one myocardial cell to the next, causing similar ionic changes in the heart muscle. This wave of depolarization leads to muscle contraction. After the impulse has passed over the cells, their ionic concentrations return to previous levels (repolarization), and the muscle relaxes.

From the SA node, the electrical impulse travels over the surface of the atria. This causes smooth and uniform atrial contraction. When the impulse reaches the lower portion of the atria, it is delayed briefly before it continues into the ventricles. This delay is important because it allows time for the atria to contract fully. Thus, the atria can empty their contents into the ventricles before the lower chambers contract.

Leaving the atria, the impulse is channeled through the AV node, the bundle of His, and into its right and left branches. It finally enters the many Purkinje fibers that extend throughout the ventricular muscle. As the impulse spreads, the ventricular myocardial cells contract.

This entire sequence of electrical events takes less than a second. It occurs 60 to 100 times during each minute of life.

Blood Flow Through the Heart. The electrical impulse generates an orderly, sequential contraction. The coordinated contraction of all muscle fibers is essential for maximum cardiac pumping power. Proper valve function is another essential element for effective pumping.

The valves act as doorways between the atria and ventricles, and between the ventricles and their major arteries. They allow blood to flow in one direction only, maximizing efficiency and preventing the backflow of blood. This unidirectional action of the valves allows the heart chambers to develop high pumping pressures. This is necessary to ensure that blood is ejected with sufficient force to reach the farthest tissues of the body.

Between heartbeats, the heart is at rest. During this time, the atria fill passively, receiving blood from the vena cavae (on the right side of the heart) and the pulmonary veins (on the left). When the atrial muscle cells contract, pressure builds within the atrial chambers. The pressure forces the atrioventricular valves to open, and the blood is pushed into the ventricle below each atrium.

As the ventricles fill, the spreading electrical impulse causes a similar mechanical action in the ventricles. The ventricular muscle cells begin to contract, squeezing the volume of blood inside the chambers. This squeeze gen-

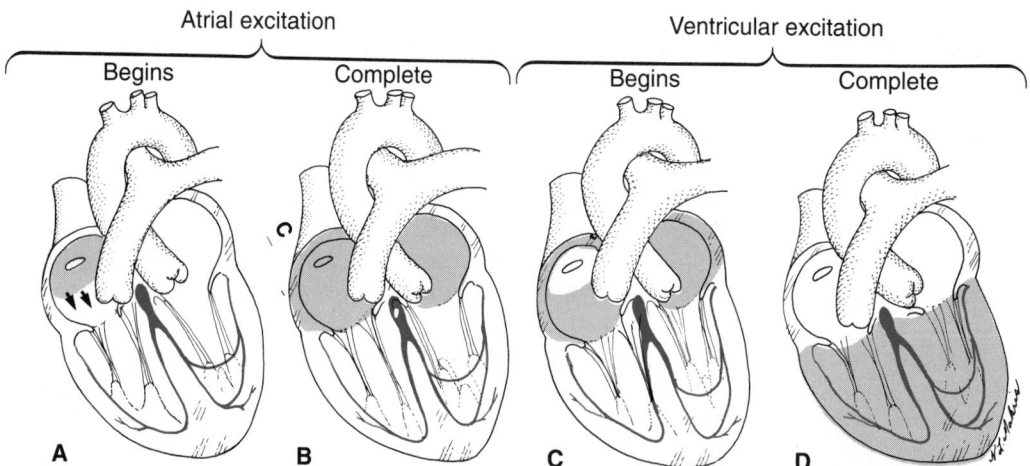

Figure 31–2. Conduction system of the heart. **(A)** Impulse originates at sinoatrial node and **(B)** spreads across atria to atrioventricular node. **(C)** Brief delay allows ventricles to fill before impulse spreads through bundle of His, its branches, and **(D)** Purkinje fibers.

erates pressure. The rising pressure within the ventricles forces the atrioventricular valves to close. As the pressure in each ventricle rises, the valves to the pulmonary artery and the aorta are eventually forced open. The blood from the right ventricle is ejected into the pulmonary circulation for gas exchange, and the blood from the left ventricle enters the systemic circulation.

Cardiac Output. The amount of blood pumped by the heart each minute is referred to as cardiac output. In the normal resting adult, cardiac output is approximately 5 to 6 L/min. This is equal to the total amount of blood contained within the circulatory system (Landau, 1986b). The healthy person is able to increase cardiac output to several times this amount in response to changing metabolic demands.

Cardiac output is a function of two factors, heart rate and stroke volume. Heart rate is simply the number of times the heart beats each minute. Stroke volume refers to the amount of blood ejected by the heart with each beat. An increase or decrease in either of these factors may change cardiac output.

Heart rate is primarily determined by the heart's pacemaker, the SA node. This tissue receives information constantly from the autonomic nervous system, however. The parasympathetic branch of this system slows heart rate; the sympathetic branch increases it. Increased metabolic activity (such as vigorous exercise) produces cardiac stimulating metabolites; it also stimulates the sympathetic nervous system. Thus, cardiac output increases under these conditions to meet the extra demands of the tissues.

Stroke volume depends on three factors. First, the amount of blood that enters the heart determines how much can be pumped out. Healthy heart muscle is usually able to stretch to accommodate the volume of blood returning to it. Second, stroke volume also depends on the natural strength of the heart muscle, or its **contractility.** Like any muscle, the healthy, well-exercised heart is a stronger and more efficient heart, so it is able to eject a larger volume of blood with each beat. Finally, stroke volume depends on the resistance to blood flow offered by the circulatory system (Laurent-Bopp, 1986). Normally, the heart generates much higher pressures than the pressure within the vascular system. Thus, the heart can eject its contents, making room for more blood to fill it.

Blood Vessels

The intricate tubing network that makes up the vascular system is more than a passive recipient of the heart's contents. Arteries, capillaries, and veins are dynamic structures whose proper function is essential for complete health.

Distribution of Blood Flow. As the heart ejects blood, the thick, muscular walls of the arteries stretch slightly,

then rebound. The relative stiffness and elasticity of the arteries allow the blood to maintain its forceful forward momentum. This is important to maintain blood pressure and to ensure that the blood has enough force to reach the tissues.

The smallest arteries are called arterioles. These tiny vessels are able to increase or decrease their caliber to meet local tissue needs. Consider the example of a person who is jogging. The jogger's active leg muscles require more oxygen and nutrients than do the digestive tract organs. Metabolites from the working leg muscles, rapid depletion of the local muscle oxygen supply, and the autonomic nervous system cause the arterioles serving the leg muscles to dilate. By opening wider, the vessels allow more blood to flow into the legs to meet the tissue needs. At the same time, arterioles within the digestive tract may actually constrict, limiting the amount of blood entering the digestive tract. In this manner, the body is able to direct blood flow to where it is needed most. Thus, the arterioles are the primary regulators of blood flow, and they play a key role in the moment-to-moment regulation of blood pressure.

By the time blood enters the capillaries, its pressure and velocity have decreased greatly. The slower flow rate of blood through the capillaries is necessary to allow sufficient time for tissues to extract oxygen and nutrients. The slow flow also allows the tissues adequate time to deposit their wastes into the blood so they can be removed.

The veins collect blood from all the capillaries. Blood flows slowly in the veins; the initial force of the heartbeat is greatly diminished by the time the blood has passed through the capillaries. In addition, venous blood must overcome gravity in the upright person. Backward flow of the venous blood could be a problem were it not for one-way valves in the veins. Skeletal muscles, particularly those of the legs, squeeze the veins, pushing blood forward and opening the valves. As the muscles relax, the valves of the veins snap shut, preventing backflow (Fig. 31-3).

Veins are stretchy, compliant vessels. This characteristic allows them to expand to accommodate large volumes of blood. As much as 75% of the total blood volume can be in the venous system at one time (Halpenny & Bond, 1989).

Tissue Perfusion. To maintain life, all living cells of the body must have a constant supply of oxygen and nutrients. These substances are delivered by the blood through the cardiovascular system. The flow of blood through the tissues of the body is called tissue **perfusion.**

Individual cells and tissues receive oxygen, glucose, and various ions through the walls of capillaries. Their thin endothelial walls are permeable to most small molecules. In the arterial end of the capillary, the forward force of the blood helps to push fluid and soluble particles out of the vessel. This fluid surrounds the cells, and nutrients are exchanged for wastes. Oxygen and other molecules enter the cells primarily by diffusion, moving from an area where they are highly concentrated (the fluid) to an area of lower concentration (the cell). Metabolites such as carbon dioxide diffuse from the cell into the fluid, also in response to a concentration difference.

At the venous end of the capillary, tissue pressure forces some of the fluid back into the vessel. The remaining fluid is pulled into the capillary by large protein molecules in the plasma. This spongelike action of the plasma proteins is called oncotic pressure.

The vital organs require continuous perfusion for their optimal function. The kidneys must receive a steady flow of blood to effectively filter and cleanse the blood. An adequate blood pressure is needed to keep the renal arteries patent and to ensure continuous blood flow and urine production.

The brain relies on a sophisticated network of neural receptors to guarantee a near constant level of perfusion. These receptors, located in the major arteries leading to the brain, are sensitive to variations in blood pressure. When pressure increases, the receptors cause arterial constriction. This reflex action protects the brain's delicate capillaries from possible injury caused by a sudden rise in pressure. If blood pressure drops, the arteries dilate, thus ensuring a consistent flow of blood through the brain despite a possible momentary decrease elsewhere.

The coronary arteries that nourish the heart tissue are perfused primarily during the resting portion of the cardiac cycle, or diastole. With their openings just above the aortic valve, the coronary arteries can receive blood only when the valve is closed. When systole ends, some of the

blood ejected by the left ventricle falls back against the valve. This closes the valve and allows blood to enter the coronaries. Adequate coronary perfusion depends, to a great extent, on adequate cardiac output. Within the normal range of heart rate, there is usually sufficient time for the coronary arteries to fill completely.

Perfusion of the pulmonary vascular system is similar to perfusion of other body tissues. Here, however, the diffusion gradients for oxygen and carbon dioxide are reversed. The air in the lung contains a high concentration of oxygen and a low concentration of carbon dioxide. The blood that enters the pulmonary system is deoxygenated and rich in carbon dioxide: it has given up its oxygen to the tissues in exchange for carbon dioxide before reaching the lungs. For this reason, as blood passes through the pulmonary capillaries it is able to absorb oxygen and rid its excess carbon dioxide.

Normal Cardiovascular Functional Pattern

Heart rate, blood pressure, skin temperature and color, and the absence of pain with exertion all help to identify normal cardiovascular function. Urine output and sensorium are also indicators of normal perfusion and cardiac output.

Heart Rate

The number of times the heart beats each minute is termed the heart rate. This is reflected by the pulse, which is determined by palpating over an artery, or by listening over the heart with a stethoscope.

In the healthy adult, the heart beats rhythmically, with an equal time interval between each beat. Also, every beat is normally the same strength or intensity as all other beats.

Normal heart rate in the adult is around 70 beats/min, although this value can vary greatly from one person to another. Resting heart rate in the person who exercises regularly is usually lower than in the person who does not. For this reason, the range for normal heart rate is from 60 (or lower) to 100 beats/min.

Exertion normally increases heart rate. The heart beats faster to meet the additional metabolic demands of hard-working muscles. It continues to do so for a short while after the exertion has stopped. Both the level and the duration of heart rate increase depend on the level of exertion and the conditioning of the person. The well-conditioned person experiences a smaller and shorter increase in heart rate with exertion than the person who does not exercise regularly (Hammond, 1985).

Heart rate varies considerably throughout the lifespan of the person. In general, heart rate is highest in the newborn, and it decreases steadily through early and middle adulthood. The person who is free of cardiovascular and lung disease generally maintains a stable

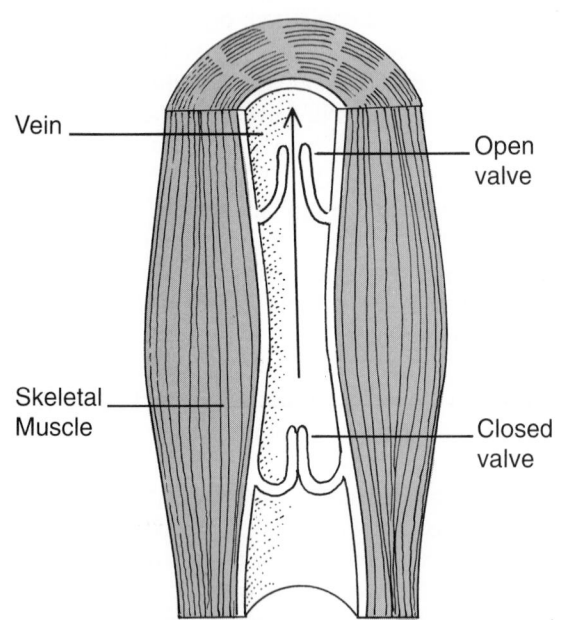

Figure 31–3. The skeletal muscle pump. Contraction of skeletal muscle compresses vein, raising venous pressure and pushing blood toward heart.

Vein

Open valve

Skeletal Muscle

Closed valve

pulse well into old age. (See the section entitled "Lifespan Considerations" for a more specific discussion of heart rate and age.)

Blood Pressure

The force with which the blood is pushed through the arterial system is called blood pressure. Like heart rate, blood pressure varies with age. (See the section entitled "Lifespan Considerations" for further discussion.)

Normal blood pressure ranges from 120/70 (in the healthy young adult) to 150/85 in the healthy elderly adult. Women tend to have slightly lower average blood pressure than men (National Heart, Lung & Blood Institute, 1984).

Blood pressure varies throughout the day, being generally highest during late afternoon. Body position affects normal blood pressure only slightly. The blood pressure of an upright person is a few points lower than when it is measured in the same person who is lying down. Finally, physical exertion causes minimal changes in diastolic blood pressure, but systolic pressure can rise by as much as 60 to 80 mm Hg (Rowell, 1986).

Skin Temperature and Color

Skin temperature is a rough indicator of cardiovascular function. The person with good circulatory status is warm, with a fairly uniform skin temperature over all parts of the body. Cool ambient temperatures may cause local constriction of blood vessels in exposed skin, such as the hands, face, or ears. Under such conditions, these areas are cool to the touch. Warm outside temperatures do not raise skin temperature appreciably, however, because the sweating mechanism helps to cool the body. Skin temperature increases somewhat with strenuous exercise. In this situation, blood vessels open to release excess body heat.

Skin color is also reflective of circulatory status. It can roughly indicate the level of blood oxygenation, as well as adequacy of local blood flow. Because skin color varies so greatly among individuals, it is difficult to apply general norms. Regardless of external skin color, however, the mucous membranes of all people are generally deep pink in color. These areas include the inner linings of the lips and mouth and the inner lining of the eyelids.

Other Indicators

Absence of Pain. Neither normal activity nor strenuous exercise should cause pain. Discomfort, shortness of breath, even the familiar "stitch in the side" may be expected outcomes of severe exercise, but these activities do not cause chest pain in the healthy person.

Urine Output. At rest, the kidneys receive approximately 20% of the total cardiac output (Halpenny &

Bond, 1989). They filter the blood continually, making urine in the process. Urine output is a direct reflection of renal blood flow. Adequate kidney perfusion is indicated by a normal volume of urine output.

Sensorium. The brain must receive adequate blood flow for it to perform its many functions. Appropriate speech and cognitive function indicate that the brain is well perfused. Normal cognitive functions, such as problem-solving and recognition of familiar faces and situations also indicate normal perfusion.

Factors Affecting Normal Cardiovascular Function

Heart rate, blood pressure, and the other indicators of cardiovascular function can vary from one person to another. They can also fluctuate normally within the same person. Several factors are responsible for this variance.

Age

The rapid metabolic rate of the newborn demands tremendous blood flow to developing tissues. Thus, the heart rate is considerably faster in the infant than in the older child whose growth rate has slowed. The heart rate of the adult whose bodily growth has almost stopped is slower still. Only in old age, when the vascular system has naturally narrowed and stiffened somewhat, does the heart rate again increase slightly.

This same loss of elasticity of the blood vessels is also responsible for an increased blood pressure in the elderly (Craven, 1989). The heart must pump the blood with greater force to move it through the narrowed network of vessels. In turn, the additional effort required of the heart forces it to beat faster to meet its own metabolic demands.

Activity and Exercise

Increased metabolic requirements of exercising muscles force the heart to beat faster. The contraction and relaxation of muscles against veins increase return of blood to the heart; consequently, cardiac output increases.

The increase in metabolism raises the temperature of the muscle. Increased muscle temperature, in turn, causes vascular dilation, which increases local blood flow. Locally acting vasoactive mediators and the muscles' rapid depletion of their oxygen supply may also cause local vasodilation.

Exercise may also protect the cardiovascular system. There is evidence that regular vigorous exercise helps to control serum levels of cholesterol, a major factor in the onset of atherosclerosis (Cowan, 1983).

Gender

Heart rate and blood pressure vary slightly between the sexes. The average man has a slower pulse, but higher blood pressure, than the average postpubescent woman. In women, blood pressure may increase slightly after menopause, probably as a result of hormonal changes.

Body Position

Because blood is a fluid, it is affected by gravity. It tends to pool in the lower, gravity-dependent areas of the body. In the standing person, blood must overcome gravity to reach the heart. The heart must work slightly harder to force blood through the system because venous blood must be forced upward.

In contrast, in the supine person the blood vessels are on the same level as the heart. In this case gravity promotes venous return to the heart. For this reason stroke volume is generally greater when a person is lying down than when the same person is standing. In the healthy person the supine position usually causes a drop in systolic blood pressure with a slight rise in diastolic blood pressure. A slight decrease in heart rate also occurs.

Temperature

A primary function of the autonomic nervous system is to maintain a consistent body temperature. The body absorbs heat when the outside temperature is warm, and it generates heat from its own metabolic processes. This heat must be removed from the body because the vital organs function well only within a narrow temperature range.

One mechanism for shedding extra heat from the body is vasodilation (the increase in diameter of a vessel due to the relaxatuion of the vessel's smooth muscle). When body temperature begins to rise, the autonomic system signals the peripheral arterioles to open wide. This allows blood to flow freely into capillaries near the body's surface. The excess heat radiates from the blood to the surrounding air. Sweating enhances the heat removal process, causing further opening of blood vessels and (through evaporation) additional heat loss (Brengleman, 1983).

The opposite occurs when temperatures are cold. Peripheral arterioles constrict, thereby limiting blood flow to the extremities and to the body surface. In this way, heat loss from the body's core is minimized.

Coping and Stress Tolerance

The autonomic nervous system may also cause momentary increases in blood pressure and heart rate when fear, pain, or anxiety is experienced. Stimulation of the adrenal gland to release epinephrine can prolong this effect. When these emotions are extreme, the opposite can occur, with a resultant drop in blood pressure.

Much has been written about personality types and their predisposition toward heart disease (Haynes, Feinleib, & Kannel, 1980; Jenkins, 1982; Rosenman, 1974; Rosenman, et al., 1970). For many years, the hardstriving, competitive, highly assertive person with the type A personality was believed to suffer an appreciably higher incidence of heart attacks than the easygoing, relaxed, more cooperatively oriented type B person. Recent studies have raised questions about the validity of this belief, speculating instead that the competitive nature of the type A personality may actually offer protection against heart attacks (Shekelle, et al., 1985). More research is needed to study this further.

Lifestyle and Habits

Smoking increases heart rate, blood pressure, and peripheral vascular resistance. Many over-the-counter and prescription medications, including those for noncardiovascular problems, can affect heart rate, blood pressure, or local blood flow. Drinkers of caffeinated coffee and cola usually have higher heart rates and blood pressures than those who drink decaffeinated beverages.

Finally, the effects of alcohol on the cardiovascular system have been studied and documented for many years. Unfortunately, many studies concerning alcohol's effects show conflicting or inconclusive results. It has been established that alcohol increases cardiac output at rest. Alcohol may also cause arrhythmias and contribute to or cause hypertension (Altman, 1989). The effects of light and moderate alcohol consumption are a source of great controversy. Recent studies reached opposing conclusions concerning mortality and morbidity from cardiovascular disease among light to moderate drinkers.

Lifespan Considerations

Although the functions of cardiac output and tissue perfusion remain unchanged throughout life, age-related changes in hemodynamics do occur.

Newborn and Infant

The newborn's heart rate is normally 130 to 160 beats/min. It is commonly irregular in its rhythm. A heart rate of less than 100 in a newborn is cause for alarm. As the infant matures, the heart rate becomes more rhythmic and slower, but it can easily increase during activity or when the infant cries.

Blood pressure is lowest during the newborn period. The newborn's systolic pressure is low, usually in the mid-40s. By 1 month of age, average systolic pressure is 80 to 90 mm Hg, with diastolic pressure ranging from the mid-40s to 60 mm Hg. By 1 year of age, the average blood pressure is around 96/65 mm Hg (National Heart, Lung & Blood Institute, 1984).

Toddler and Preschooler

The heart rate slows somewhat as the infant becomes a toddler. Steady activity, however, is likely to keep it high throughout the daytime hours. By the end of this period, the heart rate has decreased to a resting rate of around 100 beats/min.

Blood pressure varies slightly within this age group but generally remains within the 95 to 100/65 mm Hg range.

School Age and Adolescent

As the heart grows in size, its rate continues to decline. Blood pressure changes are gradual and slight during this period. At any given age during this time, boys generally have slightly higher blood pressure and lower heart rate than girls. By the age of 17, both heart rate and blood pressure have stabilized at the adult values of 60 to 80 and 120/70, respectively.

Adult and Older Adult

By the time the person reaches adulthood, age-related changes have already occurred within the cardiovascular system. As maturing continues, these changes may lead to decreased activity tolerance and decreased endurance. Along with natural "wear and tear," diet, stress, smoking, and several other lifestyle factors may have contributed to the processes of calcification, fatty degeneration, and diminished elasticity of the blood vessels. This is likely to account for the gradual and expected rise in blood pressure as the adult grows older. Because of the added work this places on the heart, the heart rate is often slightly higher in the older adult.

Most people notice few serious vascular changes related to aging. Many older adults display minor signs of decreased tissue perfusion, such as dry skin or nailbed changes. In some older adults, a decrease in oxygen supply to the extremities or to organs such as the brain or kidney may produce activity or behavioral changes.

Diseases leading to problems with tissue perfusion are uncommon in early adulthood. As chronic disorders develop or worsen, however, the potential for the development of peripheral vascular disease increases. Thus, peripheral vascular disease and its resultant perfusion problems increase in frequency with age (Craven, 1989). Disorders such as diabetes mellitus, chronic hypertension, kidney disease, or problems with lipid metabolism cause peripheral vascular disease in the aged.

Although coronary heart disease (CHD) is not considered part of the normal aging process, it has traditionally affected older adults more frequently than younger. There is growing evidence that lifestyle changes have led to lower death rates from CHD over the past several years, with the greatest reduction in deaths occurring among younger middle-aged adults. This finding implies that CHD development is indirectly related to age, inso-far as duration of exposure to CHD risk factors is longer in the aged (Gillum, et al., 1984; Pell & Fayerweather, 1985).

ALTERED CARDIOVASCULAR FUNCTION

For years cardiovascular disease has ranked as America's number one cause of death and debilitation. Worldwide, its incidence has grown steadily as modernization has spread. It is a contributing factor in untold numbers of cases of debilitating and disabling conditions.

Because of the complexity of the cardiovascular system, the potential for alteration in function is great. A host of factors can adversely affect cardiovascular function. Lifestyle choices, such as nutritional status, exercise, and smoking, along with trauma and pathologic conditions, can contribute greatly to problems of the heart and blood vessels.

Potential for Altered Cardiovascular Function

Tissue oxygenation requires that all portions of the cardiovascular system work properly. Alterations in the conduction system, improper opening or closing of the valves, or damage to cardiac muscle fibers can diminish the effective pumping ability of the heart. Changes in the blood vessels and in the blood can also create the potential for altered function.

Decreased Pumping Ability of the Heart

A healthy heart is able to create tremendous pressure and eject blood through the arteries to the lungs and body tissues. To do so, electrical impulses must proceed through its fibers in an orderly manner. The valves must open and close at precisely the correct moment, and the cardiac muscle must have sufficient strength to overcome resistance of the blood vessels.

Conduction Problems. Proper function of the conduction system ensures the orderly contraction of myocardial muscle fibers. This results in a coordinated, concerted pumping action, with all muscle fibers operating as a unit. If the conduction system is damaged or if it malfunctions, the electrical impulses it generates do not spread sequentially through the muscle. Thus, the fibers that normally contract together may do so out of sequence or may contract independently of each other. This discordant fiber contraction affects the inherent rhythm of the heart and may consequently impair its ability to pump effectively.

An **arrhythmia** is an abnormality in heart rhythm, commonly caused by disturbances in the conduction system. Arrhythmias are diagnosed by electrocardiography (ECG or EKG). Arrhythmias range from minor, clinically insignificant abnormalities to life-threatening conditions. Arrhythmias may be caused by damage to the heart muscle, diminished coronary blood flow, decreased blood oxygen levels, medications, alterations in serum electrolytes (such as potassium or calcium), stress (from exercise, fever, or emotional stress), or overstretching of the heart muscle (Woods, 1989).

Valve Dysfunction. The four valves of the heart must be able to open fully and close tightly to guarantee forward blood flow. Any of the heart's valves may be damaged by inflammation, infection, or trauma, or they may be congenitally malformed. The most common cause of acquired valve damage is rheumatic fever.

Generally, valve damage results in **stenosis** (narrowing). This condition can limit stroke volume and force the heart to work much harder than normal to maintain an adequate cardiac output. Over time the heart becomes less able to maintain normal cardiac output and heart failure occurs. For example, if the mitral valve becomes stenotic, the left atrium may not be able to empty its entire contents into the left ventricle. This causes a backup of blood in the atrium, which in turn results in a backup of blood into the pulmonary circulation. Eventually, this can cause heart failure.

Muscle Damage. A competent heart contracts with sufficient force to generate enough pressure to pump blood into all areas of the body. It must do this with each beat, approximately 70 times per minute, during every minute of life. To maintain normal rhythm, the heart requires a constant supply of oxygen and nutrients. If blood flow decreases through the coronary arteries, the active muscle becomes hypoxic. Unless blood flow is restored, portions of the heart muscle can die. This is called a myocardial **infarction,** or heart attack. The person who survives a heart attack may have areas in the heart muscle where the damaged muscle tissue is replaced by scar tissue.

A second cause of cardiac muscle damage or weakening is severe overwork of the heart. The normal heart responds to extra work by enlarging. Eventually, excessive demands stretch the heart to its limits. It finally weakens and fails. Increased vascular resistance (often caused by **arteriosclerosis,** or hardening of the arteries), excessive blood volume, and alterations in blood viscosity are common contributing factors in the development of heart failure.

Finally, the heart muscle can be damaged by infection, inflammatory or infiltrating metabolic disease, nutritional deficiencies, trauma, and drug abuse (Laurent-Bopp, 1986).

Altered Blood Flow

Blood vessels bring lifegiving nourishment to all organs and tissue of the body. They also control the amount of blood entering (and, therefore, leaving) the heart. Consequently, conditions that affect the arteries and veins can alter both tissue perfusion and cardiac output.

Arterial Dysfunction. Conditions that affect the structure of the arteries disrupt their normal function. Arteries can become occluded, or they can dilate abnormally because of **aneurysms** (weakened areas of arterial walls).

Atherosclerosis is by far the most common cause of arterial occlusion. This condition is characterized by fatty deterioration of the arterial smooth muscle walls. Over time, the lumen of the arteries narrows as their walls absorb increasing amounts of circulating fat particles, or lipids. Affected vessels also become stiff and fibrinous, and eventually may close completely. The resultant change in the walls of the vessel is called *plaque* formation (Fig. 31-4). This degenerative process occurs gradually, over a period of years. It is more common in certain susceptible people and is associated with a wide range of lifestyle factors. High blood pressure, high serum lipid levels, and cigarette smoking are the most important of these (Cowan, 1989). Atherosclerosis is the primary cause of peripheral vascular disease (PVD) and CHD, and is the most common disorder of the cardiovascular system. It seriously compounds the problems of hypertension (described below) and is the single most important factor in the vast majority of strokes and heart attacks.

Other important causes of arterial occlusion include infection, inflammation, or trauma to the arteries. Arteries can also experience increased smooth muscle tone as a result of increased sympathetic nervous system stimulation. Finally, arteries can be occluded by edema (swollen tissues) and thrombi (blood clots).

Capillary Dysfunction. As passive structures, capillaries are mainly affected by the arteries, veins, and surrounding tissues. Capillaries can become occluded by pressure from surrounding tissue. This can happen when tissues are swollen by edema, bruising, or tumors.

Capillaries can become leaky and can cause or contribute to tissue edema. Increased blood pressure or venous congestion can excessively stretch the walls of the capillaries, allowing fluid to leak out. Clogged lymphatic channels are unable to reabsorb normal capillary fluid, so the fluid can build up in the tissues as edema. Toxins, trauma, and inflammation can increase capillary permeability, thereby promoting fluid leakage. Finally, capillaries can leak if plasma proteins are deficient, because these substances are responsible for exerting the osmotic pressure that retains fluid in the blood vessels.

Venous Pooling. Decreased venous blood flow can aggravate hypertension and cause ischemia. Unless blood is kept moving steadily through the veins, tissue edema or clot formation may occur. Causes of venous

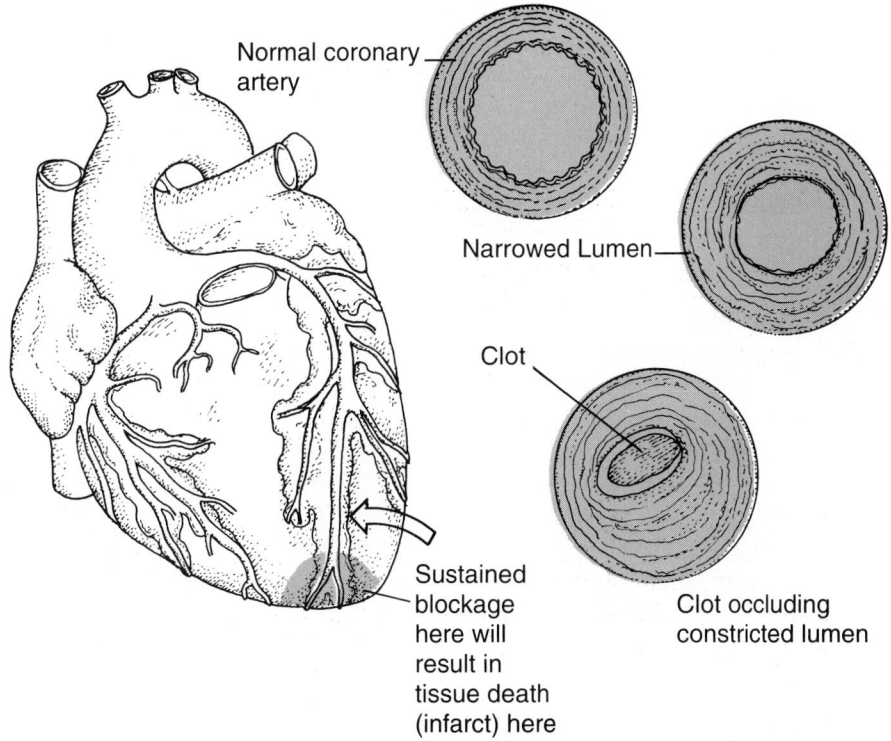

Figure 31-4.   Atherosclerotic plaque: a buildup of fat, cholesterol, fibrin, cellular waste products, and calcium on the endothelial lining of an artery.

pooling include right heart failure and ineffective venous valves.

If the right side of the heart is weakened by disease, or if the pulmonary vasculature is highly resistant, the heart may be unable to pump effectively. Blood collects in the vena cavae faster than the heart can pump it into the pulmonary system. As the heart falls further behind in its pumping efficiency, the returning blood backs up. Blood flow slows as the larger and then the smaller veins become engorged with pooled blood.

Venous valve incompetency can be caused by trauma or by vein inflammation (phlebitis). More often, however, gravity and muscle inactivity are responsible for valve dysfunction and venous pooling. In the upright person, gravity hinders venous return, thereby promoting the gradual collection of blood in the veins of the lower leg. A person who must stand or sit for long periods (or who is immobile, such as the patient confined to bed) does not have the benefit of regular muscle compression against the veins. As more blood collects in the leg veins, the veins can become dilated and distorted varicosities (Fitzgerald, et al., 1984). The valves become so overstretched that their edges cannot approximate, so blood moves backward as well as forward through the incompetent valves.

An additional effect of venous pooling is increased myocardial work. Because stroke volume depends on how much blood enters the heart, venous pooling limits venous return. To maintain normal output, the heart must beat faster. This added work is compounded by the fact that increased venous pressure causes increased vascular resistance. Thus, the heart must increase its efforts to push against the pooled blood.

Finally, in some cases venous pooling is caused by edema and thrombi. More often, edema and thrombi are potential consequences of venous pooling. These serious problems are discussed in the next section.

Altered Blood Composition

The blood carries essential nutrients to the cells, but it can do this effectively only if the composition of the blood is normal and if there is a sufficient volume of blood to fill the cardiovascular system. Alterations in the red blood cells or plasma, or changes in circulating blood volume or consistency can affect cardiovascular function.

Altered Red Blood Cells.   The red blood cells are responsible for delivering oxygen, which is carried on the hemoglobin portion of the cell. An insufficient number of cells (as in anemia) or damage to the hemoglobin molecules results in tissue hypoxia. Whereas hypoxia affects all tissues, the brain and heart are particularly sensitive to oxygen deprivation. Hypoxia causes brain damage and cardiac arrhythmias leading to possible cardiac arrest.

Altered Plasma Composition. The liquid portion of the blood carries glucose, electrolytes, and trace minerals and nutrients to the cells. Changes in the normal levels of any of these substances, or in pH, can cause alterations in cardiovascular function. For example, slight changes in serum potassium levels can cause serious arrhythmias. Increased sodium intake can cause an increase in blood volume, which increases cardiac work. An acidotic blood pH can decrease the ability of hemoglobin to carry oxygen.

Altered Blood Volume. To function optimally, the cardiovascular system must contain a relatively constant blood volume. Dehydration or hemorrhage causes a decrease in circulating volume. Because tissue perfusion depends on a sufficient volume of circulating blood, any decrease in volume can lead to tissue hypoxia. This occurs in the condition commonly called shock.

Excessive blood volume can occur in victims of congestive heart failure, kidney failure, and mismanagement of intravenous (IV) fluid therapy. Excess blood volume causes increased blood pressure. The heart must work harder than normal to pump the additional blood through the vascular system. The additional blood volume and pressure also overload capillaries, causing edema. In the peripheral tissues, overloading causes swelling and decreased perfusion. If fluid overload occurs in the lung, pulmonary edema fills the air sacs and causes asphyxiation and possibly death.

Altered Blood Viscosity. The thickness (or viscosity) of the blood is generally consistent. Anemia or excessive fluid in the blood not only affects cardiovascular function in the aforementioned ways, these conditions also increase cardiac work through a secondary mechanism. Thinner, less viscous blood flows more quickly than normal blood flows through the vessels. Increased blood flow increases venous return to the heart. This usually forces the heart to pump faster to empty itself.

The opposite condition, called polycythemia, results in thicker, more viscous blood. Polycythemic blood flows more slowly through the vessels. To pump this thicker blood through the system, the heart must work harder than usual.

Risk Factors

Many factors contribute to the development of cardiovascular problems. Adequate knowledge of these risk factors and the impact they have on cardiovascular health can encourage lifestyle changes that help to prevent cardiovascular dysfunction. See the accompanying list of uncontrollable, controllable, and contributory risk factors for cardiovascular disease.

Smoking. Smoking has been called the most important single modifiable risk factor for cardiovascular disease (Surgeon General, 1979). Smoking increases the

---

Coronary Heart Disease Risk Factors

Uncontrollable Risk Factors

Gender—risk increases for all men, risk increases for women after menopause
Family history of heart disease
Age—risk increases with age
Diabetes mellitus

Controllable Risk Factors

Cigarette smoking
High blood pressure
Hyperlipoproteinemia (high blood lipids; results from excessive intake of cholesterol and saturated fats)
Sedentary lifestyle
Stress
Obesity

Contributing Factors

Lack of exercise
Oral contraceptives
Excessive alcohol intake

---

heart rate, increases blood pressure, constricts arterioles, and may cause irregular cardiac rhythm. It enhances the process of atherosclerosis and is the major cause of peripheral vascular disease. Smoking also limits the oxygen-carrying capacity of the blood by displacing oxygen with carbon monoxide.

Nutrition. The relationship between dietary factors and cardiovascular problems is complex, but a diet high in saturated fats and cholesterol has been shown to be strongly associated with atherosclerotic lesions. Cholesterol is the primary component of the plaque (fatty lesion) that gradually occludes arteries. This leads to peripheral vascular disease and hypertension, which greatly increase the chance of myocardial infarction (MI) from coronary artery disease or stroke from cerebral vascular disease. A diet high in triglycerides (found primarily in alcoholic beverages and in foods rich in refined carbohydrates) may also be related to cardiovascular disease (Goe, 1989).

The role of salt in foods has received close scrutiny. Because sodium is hydrophilic, a diet high in salt content can increase blood volume and thereby increase cardiac work. This can seriously aggravate chronic hypertension or congestive heart failure. Convenience foods and preserved foods often contain a large amount of sodium. A diet that includes many such foods may increase the susceptible person's risk for cardiovascular problems.

Body Size and Body Fat. Being overweight places excessive demands on the cardiovascular system. The extra adipose tissue must be supplied with blood to meet its metabolic requirements. The extra cells are served by literally miles of blood vessels. To perform the additional work of pumping blood to these tissues, the heart may become enlarged. Blood pressure increases, but perfusion may decrease. Obesity has also been associated with elevated blood levels of cholesterol and triglycerides, and with increased risk of heart disease (Hubert, et al., 1983).

Exercise. A sedentary lifestyle leads to an increased risk for cardiovascular disease (Rigotti, Thomas, & Leaf, 1983). Just as regular exercise strengthens leg and arm muscles, it also makes the heart stronger and improves its pumping efficiency. Increased blood circulation also helps prevent the formation of thrombi and atherosclerotic plaques by decreasing platelet stickiness and serum cholesterol (Underhill & Stephen, 1989). Thus, the well-conditioned person has a lower risk of heart or circulatory problems than the person who does not exercise regularly.

Cardiovascular problems may be related to the patient's job. Occupations that require the worker to stand or sit for long periods promote venous pooling and predispose the person to varicose veins and possible hypercoagulation problems. A sudden change from a sedentary occupation to a physically demanding job may aggravate cardiovascular problems.

Medical and Family History. Some cardiovascular problems may result from current or previous medical conditions. Diabetes mellitus is often accompanied by serious circulatory changes. Rheumatic fever can be responsible for damage to the heart valves. Clinical evidence of valve damage may not be evident until years after the rheumatic fever has disappeared. In addition to rheumatic fever, recent systemic infections, particularly those that have gone untreated or have responded poorly to antibiotic therapy, may increase the patient's risk for endocarditis.

Trauma can also be responsible for cardiovascular problems. Severe trauma may cause direct damage to vascular beds. Vessel trauma coupled with edema can result in diminished blood flow to the injured area. Recent long bone fractures can cause emboli.

High blood pressure is an important risk factor for stroke, MI, and dissection (bursting) of aneurysms. Reports of previous or ongoing treatment for hypertension may provide the explanation for current symptoms.

Although it is clear that many cardiovascular problems have no hereditary basis, it is possible that genetics may play a role in certain disorders. For example, some patients may report that an unusually high number of close relatives have suffered strokes or heart attacks. Hypertension is also known to be more prevalent in some families than in others. Thus, a positive family history for cardiovascular disease must be considered carefully.

Medications and Drug Use. Prescription or over-the-counter drugs may affect cardiac output or blood pressure. Asthma preparations and some cold remedies may substantially increase heart rate. Diuretics (either prescribed or so-called natural diuretics from health products stores) can decrease blood volume and can alter electrolyte balance. This can cause potentially dangerous changes in heart rhythm. Birth control pills significantly enhance the process of blood clot formation and increase the risk of embolism.

The use of illicit drugs can have serious cardiovascular complications. IV use of any drug provides an entry for bacteria into the bloodstream and puts the user at high risk for bacterial endocarditis. Impurities in the injected drug can cause cardiac inflammation and may form the nucleus of an embolism. Repeated IV injections can also result in phlebitis and eventual destruction of the vessel.

Cocaine use has been increasingly associated with sudden cardiac arrest. Overdoses of opiates (such as heroin or morphine) can cause severe hypotension. They may also induce pulmonary edema.

Patients who take illegal drugs often deny that they use them. Nonetheless, because these drugs have such an impact on the cardiovascular system, it is important to ask about them in the patient interview.

Stress. Stress is often mentioned as a cause of high blood pressure, angina, and MI. Its precise role in the development or progression of these disorders has not been established, but its association with cardiovascular disease is well known. People with preexistent cardiac problems who encounter extraordinary or protracted periods of business, family, or personal stress may be at added risk for exacerbations of these problems.

Manifestations of Altered Cardiovascular Function

There are many ways in which cardiovascular function is altered, with a wide range of manifestations. Vital signs are typically affected. When cardiovascular changes cause tissue ischemia, common indicators of inadequate tissue perfusion include pain and changes in the skin and sensorium. Edema and **thrombus** (clot) formation are manifestations as well as causes of alterations in blood flow. Finally, organ dysfunction and possible failure are important manifestations of altered cardiovascular status.

Changes in Vital Signs

Changes in cardiovascular status are reflected by changes in blood pressure, pulse character and rate, and respiratory rate.

Nursing Research

Selected Nursing Research Studies

Bauer, W., & Dracup, K. (1987). Physiological effects of back massage in patients with acute myocardial infarction. *Focus on Critical Care, 14*(6), 42–46.

Gilliss, C., & Rankin, S. (1988). Social and sexual activity after cardiac surgery: A report of the first six months. *Progress in Cardiovascular Nursing, 3*(3), 93–97.

Johnson Fletcher, B., Lloyd, M. S., & Fletcher, G. (1988). Outpatient rehabilitative training in patients with cardiovascular disease: Emphasis on training method. *Heart and Lung, 17*(2), 199–205.

Karlik, B. & Yarcheski, A. (1987). Learning needs of cardiac patients: A partial replication study. *Heart and Lung, 16*(5): 544–551.

Keeling, A. (1988). Health promotion in coronary care and step-down units: Focus on the family—linking research to practice. *Heart and Lung, 17*(1), 28–34.

Possible Topics for Nursing Inquiry

- Impact of the application of antiembolitic stockings on heart rate and blood pressure of the person wearing the hose.
- Accuracy of dosage measurement of nitroglycerine ointment using scale papers provided.
- Does upper body extremity effort cause increased incidence of angina compared to similar energy output from lower extremities?
- Assessment of cardiovascular health of children who consistently eat diets low in vegetables and fruit.
- Effectiveness of using clinical simulation to decrease new graduate's anxiety regarding code management.

Blood Pressure. Blood pressure may fluctuate with changes in cardiac output and tissue perfusion. Decreased circulating volume or increased venous pooling may be indicated by orthostatic hypotension. This condition is present when there is a drop of more than 15 mm Hg after assumption of an upright position (Underhill & Stephen, 1989). Abnormally low blood pressure (below 100/60 mm Hg) accompanied by other indicators of diminished oxygenation is a serious sign of decreased cardiac output.

High blood pressure, formerly called hypertension, is undoubtedly the most common manifestation of altered blood flow, affecting 30% of the adult population (Joint National Committee of 1984, 1985). It is the most common risk factor for cardiovascular disease in developed and developing countries (Sollek & Lee, 1989). A complex phenomenon, high blood pressure contributes to the morbidity and mortality of millions of people annually.

High blood pressure is nearly always caused by narrowing of the arteries. To maintain a normal, constant cardiac output, the heart must work harder to force blood through the narrowed vessels. High blood pressure also promotes atherosclerosis, which further increases blood pressure.

The underlying cause of high blood pressure is unknown in as many as 95% of all cases (Cunningham, 1986). Several theories explaining elevated blood pressure have been offered, but no single explanation is prevalent. Researchers have postulated that primary high blood pressure is caused by an increased level of circulating vasoactive substances or by increased sympathetic nervous system activity. Increased blood pressure may be caused by changes in sodium excretion or by changes in arterial smooth muscle contractility caused by changes in calcium absorption (Caris, 1985).

High blood pressure can affect anyone, but it occurs most often in those with a positive family history, in men, and in the aged. Urban dwellers, particularly blacks, are most susceptible. Important modifiable risk factors include smoking, sodium intake, high serum lipids, weight control, and stress.

High blood pressure is unique in that it is both a manifestation of cardiovascular dysfunction and, in turn, a cause of further dysfunction. For this reason, it is considered both a sign of disease and a disease in its own right. As a disease, it is extremely dangerous because of its potential for severe tissue and organ damage.

Pulse Character. Diminished or absent pulses may indicate inadequate blood flow to an area. Although the pulse normally becomes fainter as the distance from the heart increases, absence of pulse usually indicates vessel occlusion. Complete vessel occlusion is most often associated with other signs, such as skin changes and pain. In some people, the most distal peripheral pulses (the dorsalis pedis and posterior tibial) may not be palpable but may be confirmed with the use of a Doppler instrument (Hudson, 1983).

Pulse Rate. The heart rate increases in response to increased oxygen demand. It decreases at rest when oxygen demands are low. A heart rate of 100 beats/min at rest may indicate problems with cardiac output if known contributing factors (such as fever, pain, medications, or anxiety) are absent. An increase in heart rate greater than 20 beats/min during mild activity (such as walking or moving to the commode) may indicate that decreased cardiac output is contributing to activity intolerance. Conversely, heart rate that does not increase with exercise may indicate the heart is unable to adjust to changing oxygen demands (King & Sivarajan-Froelicher, 1989).

Respiration. Respiratory rate and effort often increase in the person with cardiovascular dysfunction. Decreased cardiac output or diminished tissue blood flow limits the amount of oxygen available to the tissues. As activity increases and tissues demand more oxygen, respiration increases to supplement blood oxygenation. Shortness of breath can occur in the person with heart or circulatory problems with even slight activity, because the cardiovascular system is unable to meet the added oxygen demand. In extreme cases, the person may experience shortness of breath at rest or when lying down. Finally, a hacking cough is a common manifestation of heart failure.

Ischemia

Decreased tissue perfusion causes tissue hypoxia because less oxygen is available for metabolism. The tissue also experiences starvation because less blood flow brings fewer nutrients. Finally, tissue that is underperfused undergoes slow poisoning because its metabolic wastes are not fully removed by the bloodstream. This condition of inadequate perfusion, along with its consequences, is called **ischemia.**

No living tissue can function without adequate blood flow. Subnormal tissue perfusion causes suboptimal tissue function. Although ischemia is better tolerated by some tissues than others, it is never desirable. The manifestations of ischemia include pain, changes in skin and sensorium, and organ dysfunction.

Pain. Pain occurs commonly with ischemia when tissues are deprived of oxygen. The exact mechanism by which this occurs is not fully understood, but it has been hypothesized that peripheral nerve endings may be stimulated by pressure caused by cellular edema, or the nerves may release chemical pain mediators as a response to their own hypoxia (Solack, 1982). Reversal of hypoxia by restoring blood flow eliminates the pain if the tissue is still viable. Pain that is not lessened by rest or by measures to improve blood flow and oxygenation may signal tissue infarction.

Angina. **Angina** is chest pain associated with decreased coronary blood flow. Most often it occurs with exertion. Cold temperatures, heavy meals, smoking, and emotions have also been known to precipitate episodes of angina (Underhill & Stephen, 1989). It usually subsides within 10 minutes; relief is hastened by rest or medication. It has been described as a crushing, oppressive pressure. Angina spreads across the chest and may radiate peripherally to the arms, neck, and jaw. In se-

vere cases of coronary heart disease, angina can occur even at rest.

Intermittent Claudication. Intermittent claudication is limb pain caused by poor blood flow. Most often this refers to cramps, numbness, and aching in the legs after even mild activity. The usual cause is atherosclerosis or arterial spasm. Extra activity increases muscle oxygen demand, and the narrowed vessels are unable to supply sufficient blood to meet the additional demand. As with angina, rest decreases the pain because decreased muscle activity requires less oxygen. With rest, the muscle has lowered oxygen requirements, so the limited blood flow delivered by the narrowed vessels is once again sufficient to meet its needs.

Changes in Skin Color, Temperature, and Character. Alterations in cardiac output and tissue perfusion can become apparent by changes in the skin.

Skin color varies widely, so changes in color may not be evident in all people. In light-skinned people, however, sudden constriction of peripheral blood vessels (caused by fear, low cardiac output, or trauma) causes blanching of the skin. Patients experiencing these circumstances appear "ashen." Chronically decreased tissue perfusion or anemia causes pallor.

Rubor is a bluish-red skin coloration caused by hyperemia, or increased blood flow. Temporary increases in skin perfusion cause flushing, as is evident during fever or times of embarrassment (Pfister & Bruno, 1986).

Cyanosis occurs when hemoglobin is not carrying an adequate amount of oxygen, resulting in a bluish appearance. Peripheral cyanosis (of the fingers, toes, and ear lobes) occurs when blood flow is restricted. Cold weather is a common cause of transient peripheral cyanosis and usually is not clinically significant. In contrast, central cyanosis is a serious sign of decreased oxygenation. It appears around the lips and tissues of the oral cavity.

Skin temperature rises with increased blood flow to the skin; vascular constriction or poor perfusion cools the skin. If the sympathetic nervous system has caused the constriction (e.g., in shock), sweat glands may become activated and the patient feels clammy to the touch.

Skin character changes occur with alterations in perfusion. Chronically poor perfusion may result in loss of hair in the affected area, thickened nails, and shiny, dry skin indicative of inadequate tissue nutrition. Some people with chronic heart disease also have clubbed fingers and toes.

Poor perfusion causes tissue malnutrition. This leaves the cells weak, edematous, and unable to withstand normal wear and tear. Skin lesions, dermatitis, and ulcerations can develop readily in patients with compromised skin perfusion. Chronically limited arterial flow to an area can cause skin breakdown, with possible tissue necrosis and gangrene. Decubitus ulcers are common examples of this condition.

Changes in Sensorium. The brain is extremely sensitive to any alterations in normal blood flow. When cerebral blood supply diminishes even slightly, changes in sensorium occur. Most commonly, the patient is restless and anxious. Confusion, fatigue, listlessness, and slurring of speech may occur with a prolonged decrease in cerebral blood flow, as in shock. Chronic brain ischemia limits cognitive function.

When the blood supply to the brain is acutely diminished or completely interrupted, dizziness and loss of consciousness may occur. This occurs when the vessels to the brain are blocked or when cardiac output is abnormally low. A **transient ischemic attack (TIA)** is a temporary decrease in blood flow to the brain, with brief disturbances in speech, vision, and mobility; confusion; and numbness felt on one half of the body. TIAs are important warning signs of possibly impending strokes (Osborne, 1986).

Complete lack of blood flow to specific areas of the brain causes tissue infarction, resulting in a cerebrovascular accident (CVA, or "stroke"). Depending on the areas affected, speech, cognition, or motor function can be severely disrupted. Massive strokes can be fatal or can reduce a person to a comatose state.

Edema and Thrombus Formation

Edema. An excess of fluid collected in the interstitium is called edema. Often it is the result of venous pooling caused by heart failure or incompetent venous valves. Increased venous blood volume leads to increased venous pressure. This additional pressure becomes extra resistance for blood flowing through the capillaries. The capillaries become engorged, stretching the epithelium and eventually allowing fluid to leak from the overstretched vessel. This extravascular fluid collects in the surrounding tissue.

The resultant edema can cause pain by compressing local nerves. More importantly, swollen tissues compress capillaries and smaller arteries, limiting blood flow and causing ischemia.

In addition to venous pooling, edema can be caused by hypervolemia, decreased levels of plasma proteins, and increased capillary permeability (Bates, 1987).

Thrombus Formation. Inappropriate blood clot formation is another potential consequence of venous pooling. Blood clotting factors can be activated when blood flow is slowed, especially if veins have been damaged. Polycythemia, infection, pregnancy, and oral contraceptives greatly heighten the risk of clot formation (Gregerson & Wild, 1989).

A thrombus can steadily increase in size until it occupies the entire lumen of the vein. This halts blood flow because the clot becomes a barrier to incoming arterial blood. Wherever a clot blocks a vessel, ischemia, infarction, and tissue necrosis can occur.

A clot may also break loose and travel toward the heart. It may be pumped into the pulmonary circulation, where it continues to travel until the continually narrowing vasculature stops its progress. The clot becomes wedged in a branch of the pulmonary artery and shuts off blood flow to the affected portion of the lung. This *pulmonary embolism* disrupts gas exchange; if large enough, it can cause death.

Thrombi can form in any blood vessel, but they are particularly likely to form in the deep veins of the legs. The surgical patient, the immobile patient, and those with added risk for clot formation are the most susceptible to thrombus formation.

Organ Dysfunction and Failure

The vital organs require consistent, normal cardiac output and perfusion for optimal function. High blood pressure or ischemia can have serious consequences.

Brain. The effects of ischemia on the brain have been noted above. High blood pressure can cause a cerebrovascular accident where excessive pressure can burst delicate vessels.

Heart and Major Arteries. Coronary ischemia causes angina, which can severely limit activity, and should serve as warning of immediate danger to the heart. High blood pressure forces the heart to work harder than normal, causing cardiac enlargement, which can lead to eventual heart failure. Because it promotes atherosclerosis, high blood pressure contributes to coronary artery disease. These effects greatly increase the risk of MI. Finally, high blood pressure can enlarge aneurysms. If pressure is sufficient, aneurysms may burst and cause severe hemorrhage.

Kidneys. High blood pressure can damage the delicate capillaries that form the glomeruli in the kidney. Renal ischemia limits the kidneys' ability to filter the blood. Either condition can eventually cause irreversible kidney failure. This is manifested as fluid and electrolyte imbalances, decreased urine production, disorders of acid–base balance, and the accumulation of toxic metabolites in the blood. These sequelae, in turn, cause all other organs and tissues in the body to function poorly. In addition, renal ischemia stimulates the release of hormones that contribute to high blood pressure.

Other Organs. High blood pressure can damage delicate capillaries of the eye, leading to visual disturbances and possible blindness. The bowel is subject to necrosis from ischemia. Liver failure can occur as a result of right heart failure, because passive congestion of blood causes pressure within the liver to build. In this situation, the liver is unable to produce clotting factors, metabolize medications, and assist with protein and carbohydrate metabolism. These conditions can lead to abnormal bleeding, medication toxicities, and nutritional deficits.

Impact of Cardiovascular Dysfunction on Activities of Daily Living

The functional range of activities for the patient with cardiovascular problems varies widely. Some patients are severely disabled by their disease; others may experience little change in their activity levels. The ability to perform activities of daily living (ADLs) is determined by the extent to which the disease has affected oxygen delivery to tissues. Because all activity increases tissue oxygen demands, severe ischemia greatly limits activity. Conversely, minor alterations in blood flow or cardiac output have less effect on ADLs.

The hospitalized cardiac patient is often restricted from any form of activity for a day or two after an uncomplicated MI. The patient is assisted to the commode and helped with the bath. Patients are usually allowed to brush their own teeth and wash their own faces, provided they have sufficient energy. Once the patient has been allowed to ambulate in the room, showers may be permitted. If the patient is weak, the shower can be taken while sitting in a chair.

Patients with an MI complicated by heart failure, shock, or other conditions return to normal activities at a slower rate. The nurse must carefully chronicle the patient's progress in performing ADLs to assist the physician in deciding how and when to increase the patient's activity level.

The patient may continue to experience fatigue after discharge. The time needed to return to work, to normal social interaction, and to normal sexual activity varies but is ordinarily within 6 to 8 weeks of discharge.

The patient with peripheral vascular disease performs ADLs in accordance with the degree of pain caused by the problem. Patients with leg cramping and pain may require help ambulating. Time needed for walking from place to place must include adequate time for rest. Those patients who have limited perfusion of their hands experience a decrease in strength, and simple tasks such as opening jars and using eating utensils may become more difficult.

The patient who has had a stroke can initially have great difficulty in accomplishing ADLs. Ability to perform them as the condition improves varies greatly depending on the extent of brain damage caused by the stroke.

Any patient who has limited activity tolerance probably needs help with those normal tasks that require extensive movement or effort. In some communities, service groups are available to help with shopping, meal preparation, housekeeping, or transportation.

ASSESSMENT

To formulate accurate nursing diagnoses and to establish appropriate interventions, the nurse must conduct an assessment of the patient's cardiovascular status. This includes the gathering of subjective data, most of which comes from the health history. Objective data may include information gained through a physical examination of the patient, as well as data from laboratory and diagnostic tests.

The extent and timeliness of this assessment vary depending on the immediate condition of the patient. All patients must be assessed thoroughly and methodically, but this is easier to accomplish in patients with stable or chronic cardiovascular conditions. Acutely ill patients who are experiencing severe chest pain or other symptoms of MI must be assessed rapidly and on a moment-to-moment basis. In such cases, intervention is begun immediately, and evaluation is ongoing. Only after the patient is stabilized can a thorough assessment be conducted.

The method of assessment described here focuses on the patient with stable cardiovascular problems. For a discussion of emergency assessment of the critically ill cardiac patient, consult texts on cardiovascular or critical care nursing.

Subjective Data

Information obtained by the nurse often provides the basis for intervention. Conversely, essential interventions may never become part of the patient's care plan if relevant data are not reported. The gathering of subjective data through the nursing history is usually the first step in the assessment process.

The nursing history helps the nurse identify patterns of normal cardiovascular function. To use the nursing history to its fullest advantage, the nurse must be aware of factors that may place the patient at risk for cardiovascular problems. Finally, the nurse must be able to use information from the nursing history (as well as from objective data sources) to identify basic patterns of cardiovascular dysfunction, so that appropriate intervention can be initiated.

Functional Pattern Identification

Like breathing, normal cardiovascular function is taken for granted; as a continuous process, the regularity of the system becomes virtually unnoticeable. Unlike other natural functions, we take notice of pulse and perfusion only when something goes wrong. Unless the patient experiences symptoms of dysfunction, it is difficult to identify the normal functional pattern of the patient from subjective data. For this reason, the nursing history is much more helpful in pinpointing cardiovascular dysfunction.

The nurse can gain information about the patient's normal functional pattern by assessing activity tolerance. The ability to perform a normal range of daily activities and to tolerate a reasonable level of physical exertion is strongly indicative of good cardiovascular health. Most people experience no chest pain or other remarkable discomfort while at rest or while engaged in moderate activity. Practically everyone is aware that strenuous work or exercise causes the heart to beat faster and more forcefully. Because this is recognized as normal, few people would call these changes "pain" or "discomfort." Consequently, complaints of chest pain with activity always warrant a full investigation.

The nurse assesses activity tolerance by first determining whether the patient experiences pain, discomfort, or any other symptom during periods of physical activity. The majority of people who report no pain or activity restriction are usually free of significant cardiovascular disease. Unfortunately, the reported absence of pain or activity restriction with vigorous exercise does not guarantee freedom from cardiovascular problems. In most cases, however, it is a highly positive indicator of good cardiovascular health. Along with objective indicators such as pulse and blood pressure, reports of normal activity tolerance allow the nurse to understand the patient's functional pattern.

People with cardiovascular problems often experience discomfort, pain, or other symptoms at a lower level of activity than the healthy person. This usually leads to self-imposed restriction of activities as the person adjusts to the condition. For this reason, the cardiovascular patient's "normal" pattern may be different from that of the healthy patient. (Because activity restriction is not normal, assessment of activity intolerance is discussed in the section entitled "Dysfunctional Identification.")

Risk Identification

Many factors contribute to the development of cardiovascular problems. Direct observations and the nursing history can be instrumental in identifying those factors. The nurse should seek information concerning any factors that would increase the risk for cardiovascular dysfunction.

The nurse should question the patient concerning past cardiovascular conditions, such as a previous MI, stroke, or circulatory difficulties. It is also important to determine any functional deficits that resulted from these conditions and the management program the patient is using. Increased risk can also be assessed by asking the patient if any close family members have had cardiovascular problems.

The nurse should determine the extent of the patient's smoking. The number of packs of cigarettes smoked daily and the number of years smoked (pack/year history) are important measures of the patient's total exposure to smoking.

Dietary intake of saturated fats, cholesterol, and sodium should be assessed. Patients can be asked directly about cooking habits and dietary patterns, but many people are unaware of the fat, cholesterol, and sodium content of specific foods. It may help to ask the patient to describe a normal day's intake and ask for an estimate of specific high-risk foods (e.g., how many eggs do you eat per week?). Despite an increased emphasis on health, much of the prepackaged supermarket food and food sold in "fast food" restaurants contains an extremely high percentage of fat and sodium. Because many people regularly eat these convenience foods, the nurse should investigate the patient's eating habits with this in mind.

Activity and exercise patterns should also be assessed to determine increased risk for cardiovascular dysfunction. Questions such as, "How often do you exercise each week, and what type of activities do you enjoy?" may be helpful. Assess how much of the patient's work day is comprised of sedentary activity.

Information concerning any medications the patient is taking is important to obtain. Many medications have side-effects that can have an impact on cardiovascular function. If the medication is specifically for a cardiovascular condition, the nurse should assess the length of time the medication has been taken, the dose, the patient's knowledge of the medication, and any side-effects the patient may have experienced. The use of recreational drugs, especially IV drug abuse or cocaine use, should also be determined.

Dysfunctional Identification

The nurse identifies cardiovascular dysfunction by assessing symptoms and signs. The patient (or a family member or significant other) can often provide information important in the diagnosis and treatment of the problem.

Finding out why the patient has sought medical care is the first step in determining the nature of the patient's health complaint. The patient should be allowed to explain in his or her own words without interruption. After the initial explanation, the nurse should seek specific clarification concerning the problem.

Pain is the most common reason for people with cardiovascular dysfunction to seek medical and nursing aid. The nurse should determine the specific nature of the pain: its location, its intensity, and the circumstances that cause it. See the display listing questions to ask the patient who is experiencing chest pain.

Activity restriction is an important subjective measure of cardiovascular dysfunction. The nurse must establish the level of activity associated with the onset of pain or discomfort. Some relevant questions to determine activity restriction include: do the symptoms occur only during strenuous exercise, such as running or playing basketball? Do they occur with walking at a normal pace? If so, how far can the patient walk before the symptoms begin? Does quiet household activity bring on the symptoms? Does the patient experience the symptoms during periods of rest? Are there any other circumstances, such as weather or emotional stress, that also tend to cause or exaggerate the problem? Do the symptoms appear at particular times of the day?

Other complaints must be thoroughly examined. A nocturnal cough or dyspnea, dizziness, "blackouts," swelling of hands or ankles, and changes in skin color or sensation may also indicate cardiovascular dysfunction. The nurse must gather as much specific information concerning these symptoms as possible. This information forms the basis for physical examination and further diagnostic investigation.

Objective Data

Physical Assessment

Physical examination of the patient is helpful to assess cardiovascular status, as well as to detect actual or potential alterations in cardiovascular function.

Inspection. Observing the patient's general behavior and appearance yields significant information about tissue perfusion and cardiac output. Because the brain is extremely sensitive to any decrease in blood flow, assessment of sensorium and level of consciousness provides clues about cerebral perfusion. Decreased cardiac output, vascular disease, or both can change cognitive and perceptual function.

Sensorium is often the first indicator of perfusion to be assessed because it is readily apparent in the nurse's first interactions with the patient. People with normal cerebral perfusion usually speak in a normal cadence, answer questions quickly and appropriately, and are oriented to person, place, and time. They are also able to follow directions. The nurse should note slowness of speech or other overt difficulties with speaking. Inappropriate responses to questions or statements, confusion, apathy, decreased understanding, disorientation, restlessness, or anxiety are all possible signs of decreased cerebral perfusion.

Level of consciousness is indicated by patient arousability. The well-perfused patient is easily aroused; one who requires much stimulation to respond may have diminished cerebral blood flow.

Appearance of the patient also provides information about circulatory status. Because skin color can roughly indicate blood flow adequacy, the person should be examined for both central and peripheral cyanosis. In light-skinned patients, pallor or blanched skin should be noted as evidence of possible ischemia or anemia. Localized skin discolorations, such as bruises, redness, or mottling, are also to be noted. The presence of dependent edema (in the hands, sacrum, or ankles) indicates possible circulatory problems. Neck veins should be relatively flat; engorgement of these veins implies inefficient right heart pumping.

The legs and arms are inspected for changes in hair distribution, shiny skin color, ulcerations, edema, and venous distention. Any varicosities are noted. Toenails and fingernails should be smooth; ridged and thickened, hornlike nails indicate decreased peripheral perfusion. Digits are normally round in shape, but exaggeratedly rounded, "clubbed" fingertips are associated with oxygenation problems, either from lung disease or from cardiovascular disease.

Palpation. The well perfused patient is warm and dry to the touch. Although cool extremities are normal in many people, chronically cold fingers and toes often indicate poor circulation.

Capillary refill time also reflects peripheral tissue perfusion and cardiac output. This is determined by pressing a nailbed until it blanches (Fig. 31-5). Pressure is released, and the time it takes for the nail to return to its original color is noted. This "capillary refill time" is ordinarily less than 3 seconds. A longer refill time indicates narrowing of the blood vessel serving the digit, decreased circulating blood volume, or otherwise decreased cardiac output.

Edema is also palpated, and its extent is noted (Fig. 31-6). Edema has traditionally been described in terms of a scale ranging from zero (no edema present) to four (severe, pitting edema). This scale offers a subjective but moderately useful means for indicating the amount of edema present.

More accurate means of measuring edema include serial measurements of affected extremities or abdominal girth (for ascites). Daily weight assessment can also indicate the extent of edema present. A weight gain of 10 lb (indicative of 5 L of extracellular fluid volume) precedes visible edema in most patients (Underhill & Stephen, 1989).

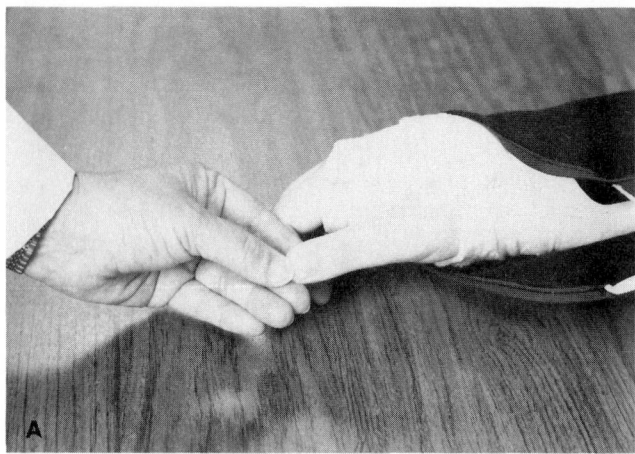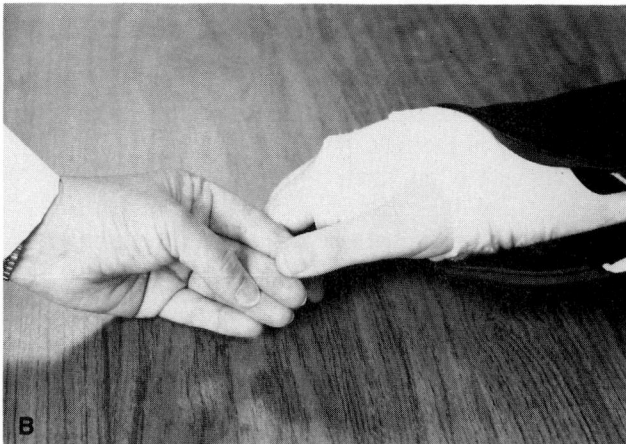

Figure 31–5. Test for capillary refill. Pressure is applied to nail bed **(A)**, then released **(B)**. Time for nail to regain color is noted.

Homan's sign is assessed by experienced practitioners to determine the possibility of deep vein phlebitis. This test is performed by bending the patient's foot upward toward the leg (dorsiflexion). When performed properly, pain or tenderness in the calf is suggestive of vein inflammation.

Pulse is palpated for quality and rate. Regularity of rhythm, pulse intensity, and the number of beats per minute are noted. Peripheral circulation is assessed, with the nurse checking femoral, popliteal (behind the knee), and dorsalis pedis (ankle) pulses for equal intensity in both legs.

Auscultation. A stethoscope is used to determine blood pressure, to count the apical pulse, and to identify normal and abnormal heart sounds.

Blood pressure is assessed to establish the presence of hypotension, high blood pressure, positional differ-

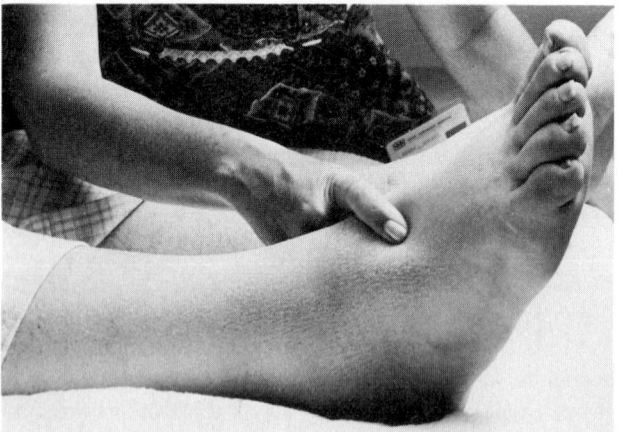

Figure 31–6. Pitting edema. An impression of the finger remains after pressure is released.

ences, and to quantitate blood flow into a limb. (For a detailed discussion of pulse and blood pressure assessment, see Chap. 19.)

Apical pulse is determined by auscultation to establish its rate and character. This is a simple yet essential measurement for the complete assessment of the patient who has a pulse that is difficult to palpate. It is also necessary to auscultate the apical pulse when administering certain medications, notably cardiac glycosides such as digoxin.

Normal heart sounds, murmurs, or other adventitious sounds are also audible by stethoscope. Interpretation of these sounds takes a considerable amount of practice and a strong understanding of their underlying physiology (see Chap. 18).

Diagnostic Tests and Procedures

The most common tests and procedures are described briefly here. For a more detailed discussion of diagnostic tests and procedures, consult Chapter 20 or a text on cardiovascular nursing. Table 31-1 lists selected tests and diagnostic procedures used to assess cardiovascular function.

Laboratory Studies. Several laboratory tests yield useful information concerning cardiovascular function. These tests range from basic blood assessment to highly sophisticated assays.

The complete blood count (CBC) provides information on white blood cells, platelets, and sedimentation rate. In addition, the CBC determines the number of red blood cells, hemoglobin, and hematocrit. These latter measures are important indicators of the oxygen-carrying capability of the blood.

Cardiac enzymes are proteins that are liberated from cells when tissue damage occurs. Serum levels of cre-

TABLE 31–1

Selected Tests and Procedures Used to Assess Cardiovascular Function

Test/Procedure	Purpose
Complete blood count	Yields information on platelets, presence or absence of infection, oxygen-carrying capacity; to diagnose anemias, nutritional deficiencies, and selected metabolic disorders
Blood chemistry tests	Determine serum electrolytes, lipids; also creatinine and BUN to assess kidney function
Serum enzymes	Rule out or confirm myocardial infarction (MI)
EKG	Identify arrhythmias, determine types and extent of heart damage from MI
Stress EKG (treadmill)	Identify cardiac abnormalities not evident on resting EKG
Echocardiography	Measure heart size and thickness; observe valve function; measure cardiac output
Heart catheterization	Measure pressure within heart chambers to determine heart strength, valve competency, cardiac output, and fluid volume status
Angiography	Outlines bloodflow through vessels to identify blockages, aneurysms

atine kinase (CK) and lactic dehydrogenase (LD) are measured to confirm a suspected MI.

Kidney function studies can indicate problems with perfusion. Blood urea nitrogen (BUN) and creatinine may be elevated in patients with hypoperfusion of the kidneys.

Serum electrolytes directly affect cardiovascular function. Deviations from normal levels can adversely affect cardiovascular function. Arrhythmias result from potassium imbalances. Sodium increases lead to extra fluid volume and increased cardiac work. Levels of these electrolytes are affected by diuretics and other drugs that affect cardiac function. They are also altered by changes in kidney function, acid–base status, and fluid balance.

Blood lipids include cholesterol and triglycerides. Lipids, linked to proteins known as lipoproteins, are also measured. Elevated blood levels of the low-density variety of lipoproteins (LDLs) are strongly associated with peripheral vascular disease and coronary artery disease. Conversely, high-density lipoproteins (HDLs) have been associated with a reduced risk for cardiovascular diseases. Although this test does not confirm or rule out the presence of cardiovascular disease, it is considered a useful screening tool for identifying those who are at risk (Report of NCEP, 1988).

Diagnostic Procedures. A variety of invasive and noninvasive procedures have been devised to study the cardiovascular system. Some are simple and require relatively basic skills and equipment. Others can be conducted only with the most technologically advanced facilities.

Diagnostic procedures yield information about cardiac function or blood flow. Tests relating to the heart include those that measure its electrical conductivity (such as electrocardiography and exercise testing) and those that measure its size and mechanical ability (such as echocardiography and cardiac catheterization). Angiography and hemodynamic monitoring are used to provide precise information concerning blood flow.

Electrocardiography records electrical impulse conduction of the heart in the resting patient. Electrodes are placed on specific areas of the patient's limbs and chest. The electrodes are connected to a highly sensitive voltmeter, which controls a delicate pen. As the electrodes detect electrical impulses, the pen scribes a tracing on a moving strip of paper. The various deflections of the ECG tracing correspond to the individual events of the cardiac conduction cycle (Fig. 31-7).

Electrodes are placed on several areas of the limbs and chest to provide several "views" of cardiac impulses. Many views (called "leads") are needed to differentiate among the various conditions that can affect the heart, because abnormalities may not appear in all leads. Single-lead ECGs are useful for continuous monitoring of a patient, but the standard 12-lead ECG is needed for a thorough evaluation of the heart's electrical conductivity. When properly interpreted, the ECG can detect myocardial damage, cardiac ischemia, alterations from normal heart rhythm, changes in heart position or size, or problems within the conduction system.

Exercise testing can assess a person's response to cardiovascular stress. In some people, problems of cardiac ischemia may not be detectable with a conventional resting ECG because these problems may occur only during periods of activity.

The test involves the use of a treadmill, a "moving sidewalk" with adjustable speed and slope. The subject

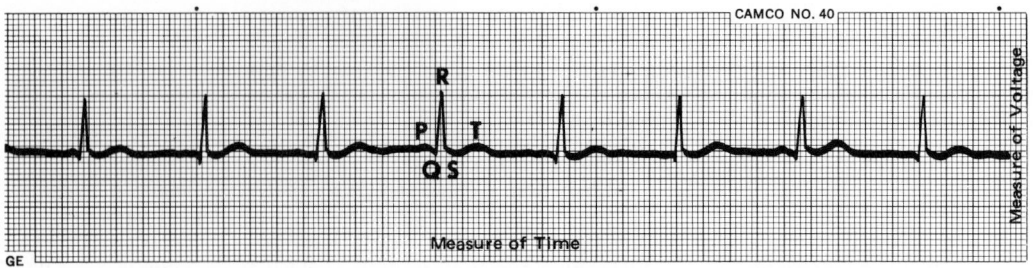

Figure 31–7. An electrocardiogram provides valuable information about the heart's ability to conduct impulses.

begins walking at a normal pace on the treadmill. The ECG and blood pressure are monitored continually while the speed and slope of the treadmill are gradually increased. The test usually lasts about 15 minutes, unless it is terminated because of ECG or blood pressure changes, or by the patient's fatigue, pain, or shortness of breath. Exercise testing allows practitioners to determine with some precision the degree of the person's functional ability.

Echocardiography uses ultrasonic waves to diagnose structural defects of the heart. This technique evolved from the use of marine sonar equipment, in which sound is bounced off structures, forming identifiable patterns. A penlike probe sends high-frequency sound waves through the chest wall. The waves produce "echoes" as they bounce off the heart, and the echo pattern is recorded. Using these patterns, cardiologists can obtain an accurate view of the heart without performing potentially dangerous invasive procedures such as catheterization. Myocardial muscle thickness and motion, structure and motion of the valves, the size of the chambers, and the presence of fluid around the heart can be detected with echocardiography.

Catheterization of the heart and large vessels is used to determine precise information concerning valve function and cardiac muscle strength. Various types of catheters can be inserted through a vein or artery and directed (under fluoroscopy) into the chambers of the heart. The catheter is able to measure the pressure generated within each of the chambers and to establish how efficiently the heart is pumping.

Some types of cardiac catheters can also be used to measure cardiac output and pressures within the pulmonary vascular system. Because they furnish information about vascular pressures, indwelling catheters are valuable tools in fluid and blood pressure management. Pulmonary artery and central venous pressure (CVP) catheters are used for this purpose.

Arterial catheters allow the nurse to monitor arterial blood pressure closely and to draw blood for evaluation of oxygenation and acid–base status. Arterial catheters, as well as other indwelling vascular catheters, are used only where constant monitoring is possible, usually in an intensive care setting.

Blood flow studies determine the patency and shape of blood vessels, as well as the direction and volume of blood flow through them. The simplest and least expensive test of this type is Doppler examination.

Doppler instruments enhance the turbulent sounds made by blood as it circulates through the heart or vessels. Using ultrasound technology, the Doppler instrument produces a graphic representation of the course of blood flow. Arterial blood flow can be detected in an extremity with this instrument, making it especially valuable in the assessment of the vascular surgical patient.

More involved (and more invasive) are tests that use contrast media or radioactive tracers. Angiography uses a radiopaque dye to outline blood vessels and to confirm or rule out vessel blockage. This technique is also used to detect aneurysms. Radionuclide examinations use radioactive substances to detect MI and decreased myocardial blood flow.

The chest x-ray can establish the size and shape of the heart and aorta, and detect pulmonary congestion or edema. It is also used to confirm correct placement of indwelling heart catheters and pacemakers.

NURSING DIAGNOSES AND PATIENT GOALS

Appropriate nursing diagnoses concerning the patient's response to altered cardiovascular function are based on accurate interpretation of assessment data. The nurse should be familiar with NANDA nursing diagnoses that pertain to the cardiovascular function. The two primary NANDA nursing diagnoses that specifically address problems of cardiovascular function are Altered Tissue Perfusion and Decreased Cardiac Output. Activity Intolerance is also a significant problem for many patients with cardiovascular dysfunction, although Activity Intolerance is not exclusively a cardiovascular problem.

Diagnostic Statement:
Altered Tissue Perfusion (Renal, Cerebral,
Cardiopulmonary, Gastrointestinal,
Peripheral)*

Definition

Altered tissue perfusion is the state in which an individual experiences a decrease in nutrition and oxygenation at the cellular level due to a deficit in capillary blood supply (NANDA, 1990).

Defining Characteristics

Table 31-2 lists defining characteristics with chances of characteristics in diagnoses, as outlined by NANDA.

Related Factors

Interruption of arterial blood flow; interruption of venous blood flow; exchange problems; hypovolemia; hypervolemia (NANDA, 1990).

Diagnostic Statement:
Decreased Cardiac Output

Definition

Decreased cardiac output is a state in which the blood pumped by an individual's heart is sufficiently reduced that it is inadequate to meet the needs of the body's tissues (NANDA, 1990).

Defining Characteristics

Variations in blood pressure readings; arrhythmias; fatigue; jugular vein distention; color changes, skin and mucous membranes; oliguria; decreased peripheral pulses; cold clammy skin; rales; dyspnea, orthopnea; restlessness.

Change in mental status; shortness of breath; syncope; vertigo; edema; cough; frothy sputum; gallop heart rhythm; weakness (NANDA, 1990).

Related Factors

As yet, not developed by NANDA.

Diagnostic Statement: Activity Intolerance

Definition

Decreased activity intolerance is a state in which an

* The subcomponents cerebral, renal, and gastrointestinal require further work.

individual has insufficient physiologic or psychological energy to endure or complete required or desired daily activities (NANDA, 1990).

Defining Characteristics

Verbal report of fatigue or weakness (critical); abnormal heart rate or blood pressure response to activity; exertional discomfort or dyspnea; electrocardiographic changes reflecting arrhythmias or ischemia (NANDA, 1990).

Related Factors

Bedrest/immobility; generalized weakness; sedentary lifestyle; imbalance between oxygen supply/demand (NANDA, 1990).

Related Nursing Diagnoses

Other nursing diagnoses are common for people with cardiovascular dysfunction. These include: Fluid Volume Excess; High Risk for Infection; Altered Nutrition: Less Than Body Requirements; Pain; and Sleep Pattern Disturbance. Circulatory problems and heart disease also affect the patient's ability to carry out activities of daily living. Possible nursing diagnoses related to this include Activity Intolerance or Self-Care Deficit. Anxiety and Ineffective Individual or Family Coping are examples of possible psychosocial nursing diagnoses.

Patient Goals

Type of condition and patient health status determine patient goals. In general, the following are appropriate goals for the cardiovascular patient:

- Patient will demonstrate adequate knowledge concerning cardiovascular dysfunction prevention or care.
- Patient will maintain adequate cardiac output.
- Patient will demonstrate adequate tissue perfusion with adequate oxygenation of body tissue.
- Patient will cope effectively with resulting changes in self-concept and lifestyle.

Specific goals for the healthy person focus on prevention of cardiovascular problems by increased awareness of risk factors associated with cardiovascular dysfunction. Goals pertinent to the patient admitted with an acute problem focus on recovery from the cardiovascular problem without residual complications. Realistic goals for the chronic cardiovascular patient focus on helping

TABLE 31–2
Defining Characteristics for Altered Tissue Perfusion

	Chances That Characteristics Will Be Present In Given Diagnosis	Estimated Sensitivities and Specificities. Chances That Characteristic Cannot Be Explained By Any Other Diagnosis
Skin temperature, cold extremities	High	Low
Skin color		
Dependent blue or purple	Moderate	Low
Pale on elevation; color does not return on lowering of leg*	High	High
Diminished arterial pulsations*	High	High
Skin quality: shining	High	Low
Lack of lanugo	High	Moderate
Round scars covered with atrophied skin		
Gangrene	Low	High
Slow-growing, dry, brittle nails	High	Moderate
Claudication	Moderate	High
Blood pressure changes in extremities		
Bruits	Moderate	Moderate
Slow healing of lesions	High	Low

*Highly specific and sensitive for diagnosis.
Adapted from NANDA (1990). *Taxonomy I revised 1990, with official nursing diagnoses.* St. Louis, MO: North American Nursing Diagnosis Association.

the patient to live within limitations imposed by the disease, and to improve acceptance of changes in lifestyle and self-concept. Goals for the terminal cardiovascular patient should revolve around the maintenance of adequate comfort and acceptance of impending death.

IMPLEMENTATION

The assessment process forms the basis for establishing nursing diagnoses, which in turn help the nurse determine appropriate patient goals. Therapeutic nursing action and its implementation are based on patient goals.

The nurse helps to educate patients and the public in the prevention of cardiovascular problems. Further effort is aimed at educating patients with perfusion problems in ways to manage their conditions. Nursing interventions and clinical therapeutics relating to cardiovascular function are directed at promoting optimal cardiac output and tissue perfusion. Prevention of potential complications of diminished tissue blood flow and the management of specific cardiovascular health problems are also objectives of nursing implementation. The next section discusses how the nurse promotes cardiovascular health. The following section presents selected nursing actions and nursing skills relevant to the cardiovascular patient.

Patient Teaching

Instruct the patient as follows:

- Restrict fat, cholesterol, and sodium in your diet to promote cardiovascular health.
- If you have chronic angina, take nitroglycerin before activities requiring exertion.
- If you take digoxin, monitor your pulse and notify your doctor if the pulse rate falls below 60 (unless instructed otherwise), and/or you are experiencing irregularities of rhythm, nausea, weakness, or visual changes; these symptoms may indicate digoxin toxicity.
- If you have poor peripheral circulation, examine your feet daily for redness or signs of skin breakdown. Poor circulation decreases sensation and increases the time it takes for sores to heal.
- Do not cross your legs or wear constricting clothing because impaired circulation can occur.
- If you experience ischemia (angina or intermittent claudication), alternate periods of activity with periods of rest to lessen pain.
- Apply antiembolic stockings before getting out of bed in the morning to prevent dependent edema and to make application easier.

Nursing Interventions to Promote Health and Function

The primary prevention of cardiovascular disease starts with an understanding of its causal factors. The nurse can be instrumental in promoting cardiovascular health by instructing people and groups on the dangers posed by the many risk factors associated with cardiovascular disease. Presenting information concerning risk factors in a nonsensational, objective manner can help consumers decide on appropriate behavior modification measures.

The nurse can help patients who are seeking to modify their risk for cardiovascular disease by being knowledgeable about (and taking part in) local support groups and classes that focus on this goal. The recent proliferation of self-help programs, fitness clubs, and aggressively advertised diets has provided the consumer with many choices. The nurse should be able to offer guidance in program selection and to help the patient identify (and avoid) programs that promise overly simplistic or unrealistic means to cardiovascular health.

The patient may need to be made aware of appropriate supervised physical activity programs. If the patient has a known medical problem or is over 35 years of age, the nurse should recommend a complete physical examination before the patient starts an exercise regimen. Various classes or support groups may be available to help the patient alter unhealthful lifestyle habits. Diet management, smoking cessation, and stress management programs are often sponsored by the hospital or other local agencies. Nurses may be instrumental in developing and implementing such programs in the private workplace. The goal of these programs is the promotion of cardiovascular health.

Nursing Interventions for Altered Cardiovascular Function

Patient Teaching

The patient with cardiovascular disorders should be taught to recognize warning signs of decreased cardiac output or decreased perfusion. Signs and symptoms that indicate the need for medical help are listed in the display. The nurse should be certain the patient is aware of the importance of infection prevention. The patient should also be instructed in how to promote blood flow and to reduce edema, how to promote skin integrity, and how to avoid fatigue.

The cardiovascular patient often must take numerous medications. The quality of teaching done by the nurse can determine the degree of patient compliance with the medication regimen. Cardiovascular drugs are complex and may be confusing to the patient. Therefore, it is

---

Selected Nursing Interventions for Cardiac Problems

Activity Intolerance

- Monitor pulse, respiratory rate, and subjective feelings during activity.
- Space activities.
- Permit rest periods before activity.
- Limit activity 1 hour after meals.
- Teach energy conservation measures.

Edema

- Instruct patient to avoid constricting garments.
- Instruct patient to elevate edematous area.
- Instruct patient to avoid dependent positioning.
- Teach patient about fluid- or sodium-restricted diet.
- Apply antiembolism stockings.

Pain (due to inadequate oxygen supply)

- Instruct patient to stop activity when pain occurs.
- Administer nitroglycerine or vasodilators as ordered.
- Pace activities within patient's limits.
- Instruct patient to avoid cold temperature and smoking.
- Instruct patient to report unrelieved pain to appropriate health-care professional.

---

beneficial to include the patient's spouse or significant other in discussions concerning medications. The nurse should explain clearly the reasons for taking prescribed medications. The explanation, "This is for your heart" is inadequate because the patient may have several prescribed heart medications. Simple yet accurate descriptions of each medication's action help the patient appreciate and remember the importance of complying with the medication regimen. The nurse should also stress the importance of taking medications as ordered. The patient must be warned against missing doses or stopping a medication without consulting the physician. The nurse must be certain the patient understands how and when to take medications, whether any foods or other substances should be avoided (to prevent interactions), and what side-effects to expect. The patient should also be taught to recognize signs of overdose or toxicity, and when to contact the physician.

Instruct the patient as follows:

Call Your Doctor When You Experience

- Any sign of infection—redness, swelling, pain and tenderness.
- Unusual insomnia or extreme, prolonged fatigue after physical exercise.
- Angina pain that does not subside with rest or after three nitroglycerin tablets taken 5 min apart (for patients who have documented chronic angina).
- Sudden confusion or incoordination.
- Unusual fatigue.
- Prolonged depression.

Call An Ambulance (911, If Available) When You Experience

- New, sustained pressure or pain in the chest, arms, neck, or jaw (if this is not a normal occurrence).
- Rapid, irregular, or unusually slow heart beat (if this is abnormal).
- Dizziness or fainting.
- Severe pain and loss of normal color in an extremity (which is not due to exposure to cold).

Reasons for other medical therapies should also be explained thoroughly. The patient's usual lifestyle and culture should be taken into consideration when schedules for treatments and medications are planned. Flexibility should be allowed where possible.

In addition to patient teaching, the nurse promotes cardiovascular function by employing various therapeutic interventions. Measures described below are valuable for optimizing tissue perfusion and maintaining cardiac output. Because adequate cardiac output is essential for the maintenance of tissue perfusion, some basic nursing measures help to accomplish both of these goals.

Promotion of Venous Return

Venous stasis in the patient with limited mobility may result in edema and embolization. The nurse helps to reduce the risk of dangerous clot formation by taking measures to improve the return of blood to the heart. Leg exercises, antiembolic stockings, and avoidance of constriction help to prevent venous stasis.

Leg Exercises. Leg exercises improve circulation and prevent venous stasis. Leg exercises are commonly taught to preoperative patients to prevent postoperative circulatory complications. These simple exercises are helpful for any patient with impaired mobility, especially those patients on bedrest.

Leg exercises alternately contract and relax the quadriceps and gastrocnemius muscles of the lower extremity. Contraction of these muscles helps promote the flow of blood back to the heart. Three separate leg movements can be encouraged (Fig. 31-8). First, have the patient perform *calf pumping* exercises, which involve alternate dorsiflexion and plantar flexion of the feet. Second, have the patient bend one knee, sliding the foot up as far as possible along the mattress and back again. Repeat this process with the other leg. Finally, have the patient alternately raise and lower each straight leg off the mattress as far as comfort allows.

Leg exercises should be begun as soon as the patient returns from surgery or whenever the patient is immobile. Exercises should be performed at least once every 1 to 2 hours while the patient is awake. If the patient is not able to perform leg exercises independently because of decreased strength or neurologic impairment, it is important for the nurse to assist with passive leg exercises, encouraging as much patient participation as possible.

Antiembolic Stockings. Immobility deprives the bedridden patient of the circulatory benefit of muscular contraction against the veins. Venous engorgement can be offset in these patients by the use of antiembolic stockings.

Antiembolic stockings are made of strong elastic material. When correctly fitted and applied, they exert gentle pressure against the legs. The stockings promote venous return in much the same manner as the leg muscles, using continuous instead of intermittent pressure.

To do their job effectively, antiembolic stockings must fit properly. Stockings that are too large for the patient cannot provide sufficient vein compression; stockings that are too tight can shut off blood flow to the legs. Guidelines for proper measurement and size selection of antiembolic stockings are available from the manufacturer and should be followed instead of estimating stocking size by the height or weight of the person. Wrinkles or poorly made seams can lead to pressure sores on the skin. The nurse must inspect the patient's legs and feet regularly to ensure that circulation is not impeded by the stockings. Antiembolic stockings are usually removed once during every 8-hour period for 30 minutes. When in place, the toes should remain warm, and there should be no obvious constriction or excoriation caused by the stockings.

The elastic stocking is best applied with the stocking inside out to the heel. The toes are placed in the stocking, and each side is pulled onto the foot as far as possible. The stocking is first pulled past the midpoint of the heel, and the fabric beyond the toes is pulled over the foot. The fabric is pulled over the ankle and pulled up the calf to the point of measurement, without allowing it to

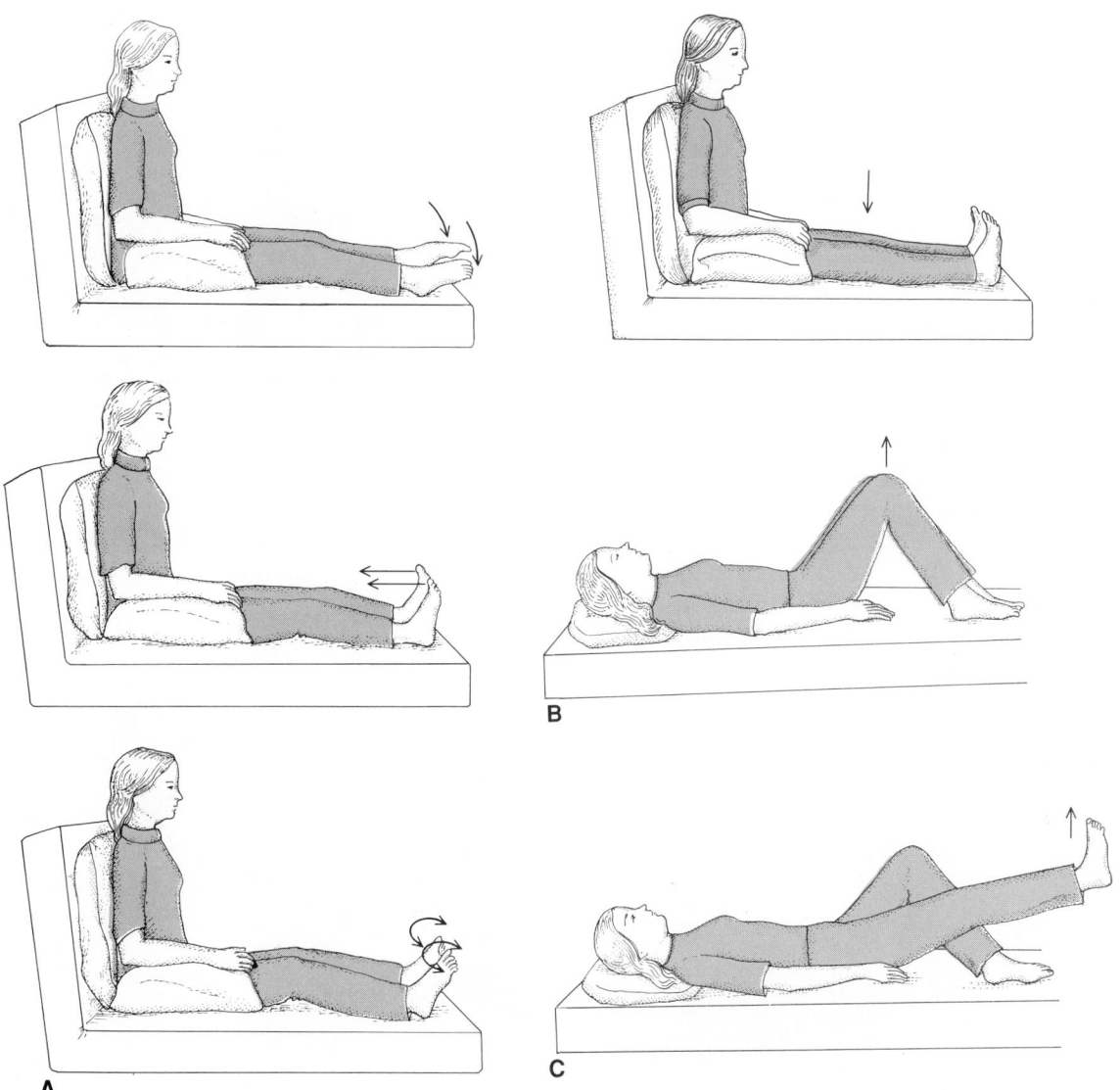

Figure 31–8.   Leg exercises to improve circulation.   **(A)** Calf pumping exercises: dorsiflexion and plantarflexion. Point toes of both feet toward foot of the bed; relax; pull toes toward the chin; relax; make circles with both ankles, one direction and then the other; repeat three times; relax.   **(B)** Knee flexion and extension. With knees flexed and feet flat on the bed, slide feet forward as far as possible and back to flexed position.   **(C)** Raising and lowering leg. Raise and lower each straight leg alternatively while the other leg is flexed. Raise as far as comfort allows without straining.

roll at the top. Final adjustments include adjusting the heel as necessary and slightly pulling the fabric away from the toes to minimize pressure. The stockings should be applied in the morning, before the patient has gotten out of bed. This allows them to be fitted while the patient's legs are least edematous (see Procedure 31-1).

Avoiding Constriction.   Both immobilized and active patients must be warned against venous constriction. Any article of clothing that exerts excessive pressure on the calves or thighs may constrict the veins. This diminishes venous return and promotes the formation of clots and varicosities. The use of garters or the practice of wearing stockings knotted above the knee should be

discouraged. Socks with tight elastic bands around the tops and short-legged pants with tight elastic or belted bottoms should be avoided.

In addition to garments, orthopedic casts made of plaster or other materials can tighten and restrict blood flow. Warm fingers or toes indicate sufficient blood flow, but cool extremities, numbness or tingling, and limited capillary refill may indicate a need for altering the cast or recasting.

The nurse should point out that crossing the legs creates pressure points against veins. This activity should be avoided. Patients who must sit for extended periods (such as at work) should be careful not to create venous constriction by sitting too far back in chairs. The back of the calves should not rest against the edge of the chair

---

PROCEDURE 31-1. Applying Antiembolic Stockings

■ Purpose
1. Supplement the action of muscle contraction and aid venous return from the lower extremities.

■ Assessment
- Identify patients at high risk for deep vein thrombosis (e.g., long-term bedrest or cardiovascular disease).
- Obtain physician order.

■ Equipment
Stockings (available in knee-high or thigh-high lengths). Measure length (heel to groin) and width (calf and thigh) of patient's leg before ordering.
Baby powder or talcum powder

■ Procedure
1. Position patient in supine position for one half hour before applying stockings.
   Rationale: Veins should not be distended with blood when stockings are applied.
2. Provide privacy for patient.
3. Gather material from length of stocking down to the toe.
   Rationale: Makes application easier.

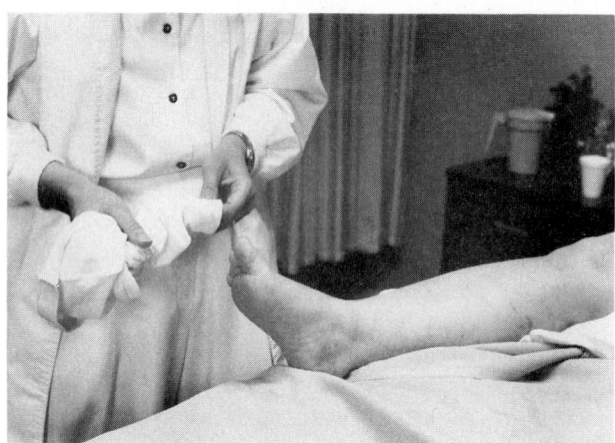

Step 3

4. Ease the stocking over the patient's toe and heel and adjust to fit snugly.
   Rationale: Wrinkles impede circulation.
5. Gently pull the stocking over the leg removing all wrinkles.
   Rationale: Irregularities in fit may cause pressure areas.
   Hint: Baby powder or talc lightly sprinkled over the foot and leg may make stocking application easier.

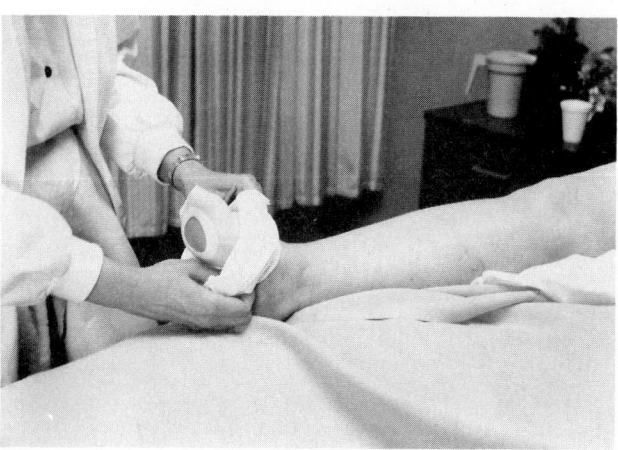

Step 4

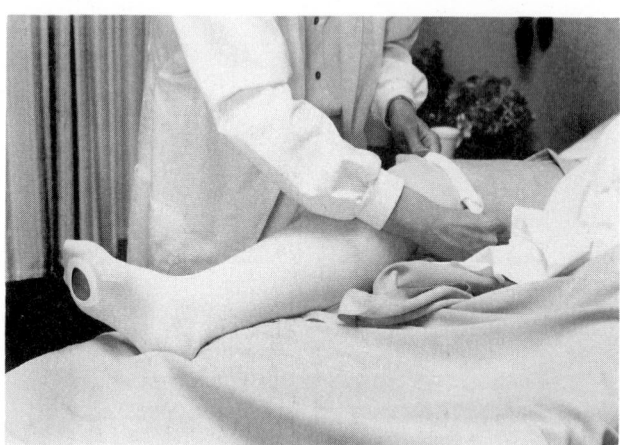

Step 5

6. Assess toes for circulation and warmth. Check area at the top of the stocking for binding.
   Rationale: Constriction and rolling down of stockings during wear is a result of poor fit and can impede circulation and cause thrombosis.
7. Antiembolic stockings should be removed at least twice daily.
   Rationale: Enables skin to be washed and assessed for edema or irritation.

■ Lifespan Considerations

Children
- Antiembolic stockings are infrequently used in children.

(continued)

PROCEDURE 31–1. Applying Antiembolic Stockings (continued)

■ **Special Considerations**

The Obese Patient
- Proper fitting of antiembolic stockings is difficult with the obese patient, requiring special attention for areas of constriction and binding.
- Elastic (Ace) bandages may be an alternative to provide antiembolic protection in patients from whom

correct fit is impossible with standard stocking sizes.

■ **Home Care Modifications**
- Patients need to be instructed to remove stockings regularly for skin inspection and cleansing.
- Be sure patients understand that commercial support stockings *are not* a substitute for medical antiembolic stockings.

---

because this compresses the veins. These people also should be taught to flex their leg muscles periodically, and to stand and walk frequently to encourage venous return.

Edema Reduction

Peripheral edema can impede blood flow to the tissues. It is also unsightly and is often uncomfortable or painful for the patient. Control of edema is an important nursing priority.

Elevation of Limbs. One of the simplest measures for reducing edema is to elevate affected limbs. This allows gravity to assist venous return to the heart and helps to decrease venous pressure. This reduces the leakage of fluid from vessels and promotes its reabsorption. Vessels can reopen, and perfusion is improved.

Care must be taken to avoid causing venous constriction when elevating edematous limbs. Legs should be fully supported when elevated, and there must be no pressure points. The leg should not be lifted so high that a constriction occurs at the groin. The knee gatch on the hospital bed should not be used because this restricts venous flow behind the knee.

Diet Teaching. The patient with fluid retention problems usually benefits from a low-sodium diet. Because sodium molecules attract water, limiting salt intake helps to control edema. The nurse can help the patient develop an awareness of the importance of salt and sodium restriction.

Limited use of table salt is a logical first step in a sodium-restricted diet, but the patient must also be made aware of "hidden" sodium content. The patient should learn to look for sodium content on the labels of beverages, health products, and over-the-counter medicines (especially antacids), as well as in foods. The patient should avoid highly processed convenience foods. Vinegar, spices, and herbs can be used as a replacement for salt in cooking. Finally, the patient should be encouraged to discuss possible salt substitutes with the physician.

Fluid Restriction. Patients who have fluid-volume excess must restrict fluid intake until balance is restored. Intake and output are monitored carefully to assess fluid status. An intake that is more than 2 L (2000 mL) greater than output suggests fluid retention.

The patient should also be weighed daily, preferably at the same time and ideally before breakfast. Weight should not vary by more than 1 kg (2 lb) per day.

Positioning

Body position affects cardiac work and tissue perfusion. The heart works harder in the supine person than in the upright person (Winslow, 1985). Lying flat promotes venous return. Because all vessels are at the same level of the heart, gravity's effect on the blood is minimized. Blood can flow more freely into the vena cavae. The increased volume of blood entering the atria increases stroke volume.

For the patient with compromised cardiac status, such as the patient with an MI or heart failure, lying supine can be uncomfortable and can increase the work of the heart. A semi-Fowler's position for these patients reduces their cardiac work by limiting venous return.

Conversely, the patient who is in shock should not be placed in the semi-Fowler's position. Without sufficient blood to fill the vascular space, the shock victim requires improved cardiac output. Trendelenburg's position, with the foot of the patient's bed elevated and the head down, enhances venous return and temporarily improves blood flow to the brain. Within a minute or two, pressure-sensitive baroreceptors in the carotid arteries are stimulated. These receptors signal the brain to constrict the arteries as a protective measure against excessive pressure within the cranium. For this reason, the shock victim should be placed in Trendelenburg's position for only a few minutes. After this time, the patient should be lowered to a supine position. During this period, the victim must also receive specific treatment for the cause of the shock to ensure restoration of perfusion to all vital organs.

On a smaller scale, positioning can be used to improve perfusion to selected underperfused areas. Arterial flow is enhanced by gravity. Allowing ischemic hands or feet to hang in dependent positions may improve perfusion; however this is contraindicated in the edematous patient.

Pain Management

Some cardiovascular patients experience infrequent, relatively slight pain; others have constant debilitating pain. Helping these patients to manage their pain is an essential nursing skill.

Chest Pain. Complaints of chest pain must never be ignored. It has many causes, but unless proven otherwise chest pain in the cardiac patient must be assumed to be a serious sign of cardiac hypoxia. Although the patient may want to attribute some chest pains to anxiety or excitement, these are unlikely causes. People with normal coronary arteries do not experience chest pain with anxiety or excitement.

When acute chest pain is evident, the patient should stop all activity and should rest. The patient should sit comfortably; lying flat inhibits full chest expansion and limits gas exchange in the lung, so this position should be avoided. Oxygen should be started as ordered.

Sublingual nitroglycerin should be administered if it has been ordered for chest pain. Blood pressure should be assessed 5 minutes after this medication has been given, because nitroglycerin is a vasodilator and blood pressure may fall. If the pain is not relieved after repeat doses of nitroglycerin, the physician should be notified.

The patient should rest after an episode of pain. The nurse should document the duration, activity during onset, and vital signs during the episode, and should report this information to the physician.

Patients with chronic angina can be helped primarily by assistance with activity management. They should be taught to monitor their pulse rates and to pace activities to prevent increases of greater than 20 beats/min above the baseline rate. Activities should be done on an empty stomach whenever possible to avoid acute angina. Because blood is diverted to the gut after eating, less oxygen is available to the muscles, including the heart. For this reason, the nurse should not schedule procedures or activities such as bathing or walking right after meals. If sublingual nitroglycerin is ordered, the patient should take a dose before performing an activity that has previously produced pain.

Claudication and Peripheral Ischemic Pain. These categories of pain from peripheral vascular disorders are not life-threatening, but the discomfort they produce can be crippling. Pain may be precipitated by cold surroundings, by cigarette smoking, or by activities that exceed individual tolerance. Nursing measures to prevent such pain are directed at enhancing oxygen delivery to tissues by improving blood flow or by decreasing oxygen demand.

Heat helps relieve peripheral vascular pain. Warm, moist heat applied to the extremities promotes vasodilation, thereby improving circulation to the tissues. This is accomplished through the use of warm compresses or by soaking the hands or feet in a basin of warm water. A warm pad may be wrapped around a limb.

Chronically impaired perfusion of extremities can cause impaired perception of the sensation of heat. For this reason, the patient with vascular disease is prone to burns. The nurse must exercise great care to avoid excessively hot soaks or compresses. Their temperature should not exceed 95° to 100°F (35° to 38°C). When a heating pad is used, it should be covered with a towel or pillowcase and not allowed to come into direct contact with the skin.

Energy Conservation

Closely related to pain management is energy conservation. Pain can occur when the patient exceeds normal activity tolerance. Effective conservation of energy can promote activity tolerance and, thus, can help to prevent pain.

Repeated movement of the upper arms should be avoided by newly diagnosed patients with MI. This movement increases the metabolic demands of the arm muscles. The heart is forced to pump harder for the blood to overcome gravity.

The patient should be warned against Valsalva's maneuver, which occurs during grunting. Air in the chest pushes against a closed glottis, raising intrathoracic pressure. This can suddenly increase blood pressure while simultaneously hindering venous return. Activities involving lifting or pushing heavy objects, and straining during bowel movements often involve Valsalva's maneuver. The patient with an acute MI should be instructed to avoid the stress this places on the heart by consciously maintaining a steady breathing pattern during such activities.

The most important energy conservation measure for the cardiovascular patient is rest. Regular rest periods should be provided. The patient should rest undisturbed for an hour after meals. Rest should be encouraged before and after activities such as bathing, or when lengthy treatments are scheduled.

Activities should be spaced to avoid fatigue. Periods of work should alternate with rest or lighter activity. During activities, the patient should sit whenever possible to avoid cardiovascular strain. When activities or tasks require the gathering of several materials, good planning is essential to eliminate unnecessary and inefficient wasted effort. The patient should immediately stop any activity that produces fatigue, breathlessness, pressure, or pain.

Rehabilitation

For most patients, cardiovascular problems need not permanently prevent them from enjoying a normal lifestyle. The purpose of rehabilitation is to help the cardiovascular patient restore or improve lost function.

The success of rehabilitation efforts varies greatly from one person to another. Its effectiveness depends on the acuity and the extent of the patient's condition. Of great importance, too, is the patient's motivation, as well as the enthusiasm and skill of health-care workers. In some cases, successful rehabilitation means regaining and perhaps improving on previous function. In other cases, rehabilitation means that the person manages some of the activities and demands of daily living without incurring excessive pain and discomfort.

Central to the concept of rehabilitation is the premise that patients with cardiovascular disorders should return to as active and productive a life as possible. This goal depends on physical endurance, which is improved by graded physical activity. Thus, although rest is an essential part of the management of cardiovascular problems, activity also must play a part.

Promotion of activity tolerance starts after the medical problem has been identified and treated. Next, a functional assessment of the patient is conducted. Only after the patient's physical, mental, and emotional readiness for rehabilitative measures has been thoroughly assessed can appropriate measures be implemented.

Gradual rehabilitation of the hospitalized patient usually can begin with simple in-bed activity. Examples of nonstrenuous exercises include rotation and dorsiflexion of the ankles, and working the feet against a footboard. Self-care activities, such as shaving, washing, eating, or brushing the teeth, should be encouraged. These activities help prevent deconditioning by maintaining joint mobility and by preserving some muscle tone. They may also help to maintain the patient's spirits by forcing the realization that their condition has not rendered them helpless.

As the patient progresses to ambulation, accurate assessment is essential to prevent the patient from attempting to do more than he or she is ready to do. The nurse must observe the patient closely for subjective signs of pain. The cardiac patient should be monitored by telemetry, which records the patient's electrocardiogram while he or she is walking. Changes in blood pressure, mentation, or color, or patient complaints of lightheadedness or weakness are indications that the exercise is too strenuous. The patient should sit and rest immediately. Breathlessness or increased heart rate lasting for more than 10 minutes after exercise indicates a need to go slower in the rehabilitation effort. Nocturnal insomnia or daytime fatigue may also mean that the previous day's exercise has been too strenuous.

Activity can be increased daily on the basis of the patient's tolerance or by exercise prescription. The New York Heart Association Functional Classification Index is often used to classify cardiac patients according to their functional capacity (Table 31-3). Management of activity can be based on this information.

Exercise should be part of a continuing rehabilitation program after the patient's discharge from the hospital. The nurse should teach the patient about safe exercise practices at home. Warm-up exercises prevent sudden demands on the heart; cooling down exercises help prevent pooling of blood in the legs. Exercise should not be performed in extremes of weather, nor should it be performed within an hour of meals. Isometric exercises should be avoided because they involve the Valsalva's maneuver.

The patient should also be instructed to recognize untoward symptoms of overexertion, such as palpitations or fluttering in the chest, racing pulse, pain, and pressure. The nurse should instruct the patient how to take the pulse using the carotid or radial sites. The patient should stop activity if the pulse rate exceeds the specific target zone prescribed by the physician. If the pulse lowers with activity, if it becomes irregular, or if the heart rate does not return to its resting level within 10 minutes after exercise, the patient should contact the physician (Lindskog, et al., 1983).

Patience is essential for both the patient and the nurse: neither should try to hurry the rehabilitation process. Exercise must be graduated, with more strenuous activities being added to the regimen only as patient tolerance

TABLE 31–3
Functional and Therapeutic Classification of Patients with Diseases of the Heart

Functional Classification	Therapeutic Classification
Class I Patients with cardiac disease but without resulting limitations of physical activity. Ordinary physical activity does not cause undue fatigue, palpitation, dyspnea, or anginal pain.	**Class A** Patients with cardiac disease whose physical activity need not be restricted in any way.
Class II Patients with cardiac disease resulting in slight limitation of physical activity. They are comfortable at rest. Ordinary physical activity results in fatigue, palpitation, dyspnea, or anginal pain.	**Class B** Patients with cardiac disease whose ordinary physical activity need not be restricted, but should be advised against severe or competitive efforts.
Class III Patients with cardiac disease resulting in marked limitation of physical activity. They are comfortable at rest. Less than ordinary physical activity causes fatigue, palpitation, dyspnea, or anginal pain.	**Class C** Patients with cardiac disease whose ordinary physical activity should be moderately restricted, and whose more strenuous efforts should be discontinued.
Class IV Patients with cardiac disease resulting in inability to carry on any physical activity without discomfort. Symptoms of cardiac insufficiency or of the anginal syndrome may be present even at rest. If any physical activity is undertaken, discomfort is increased.	**Class D** Patients with cardiac disease whose ordinary physical activity should be markedly restricted. **Class E** Patients with cardiac disease who should be at complete rest, confined to bed or chair.

From New York State Heart Association. (1964).

allows. The patient must be warned against the attitude: "If this much exercise is good, twice as much will cure me in half the time." Exercise can provide several valuable physiologic and psychological benefits to the patient with cardiovascular disease, but it is not a cure-all. Exercise is only one facet of a multipronged approach to regaining health. Adherence to prescribed medical therapies, reduction of stress, and modification of lifestyle risk factors are vital parts of any successful rehabilitation program.

Cardiopulmonary Resuscitation

Cardiac arrest is the most serious emergency that can occur in the hospital. When a patient's heart stops, acute hypoxia begins to destroy all tissues. Unless oxygenation is restored quickly, the victim will die. Cardiopulmonary resuscitation (CPR) is a means of artificially supporting circulation and oxygenation until the victim's heart begins beating on its own.

CPR is a systematic approach to life support that has been revised and refined over the years. In 1986, the American Heart Association and the American Red Cross established a single set of protocols for managing cardiac arrest. Basic CPR is outlined in Procedure 31-2.

Most hospitals require practically all personnel to be trained in basic cardiac life support (BCLS). The ability to maintain a cardiac arrest victim's breathing and circulation with basic CPR skills is essential to the success of all resuscitation efforts. No matter how much sophisticated equipment is available or how knowledgeable the nurse is about resuscitation drugs, the victim will only survive if basic CPR is performed properly. All nurses should master CPR and update their skills regularly. The Red Cross and other agencies offer classes for BCLS certification. These courses can be completed in a day, often through the hospital.

(Text continues on page 836)

PROCEDURE 31–2. Administering Cardiopulmonary Resuscitation (CPR)*

■ Purpose
1. Restore cardiopulmonary functioning.
2. Prevent irreversible brain damage from anoxia.

■ Assessment
- Determine that the patient is unconscious. Shake the patient and shout at him or her to confirm unconsciousness rather than being asleep, intoxicated, or hearing impaired.
- Assess for presence of respirations.
- Assess carotid artery for pulse.
  Note: Presence of pulse *and* respiration contraindicates initiation of cardiopulmonary resuscitation (CPR).

■ Equipment
A hard surface: Patient may be placed on floor, ground, or use a backboard.

No additional equipment is necessary but in the hospital setting, an emergency (crash) cart with defibrillator and cardiac monitoring should be brought to the bedside by additional personnel A crash cart usually contains:

  Airway equipment
  Suction equipment
  Intravenous equipment
  Laboratory tubes and syringes
  Prepackaged medications for advanced life support

■ Procedure

One Rescuer—Adult Patient
1. Assess to determine responsiveness. Shake gently.
   Rationale: Determine need for resuscitation.
2. Call for help.

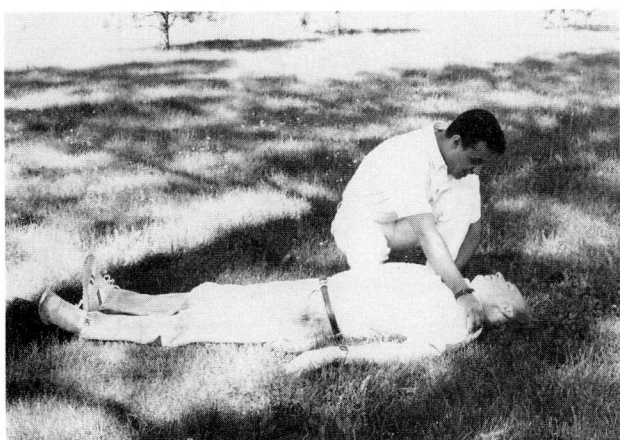

Step 1

3. Turn patient onto back while supporting head and neck. Place a cardiac board under the back or place patient on the floor.
   Rationale: A firm surface is needed for adequate compression of the heart between the sternum.
4. Open the airway using a head tilt/chin lift.
   Note: Use modified jaw thrust if a neck injury is suspected.

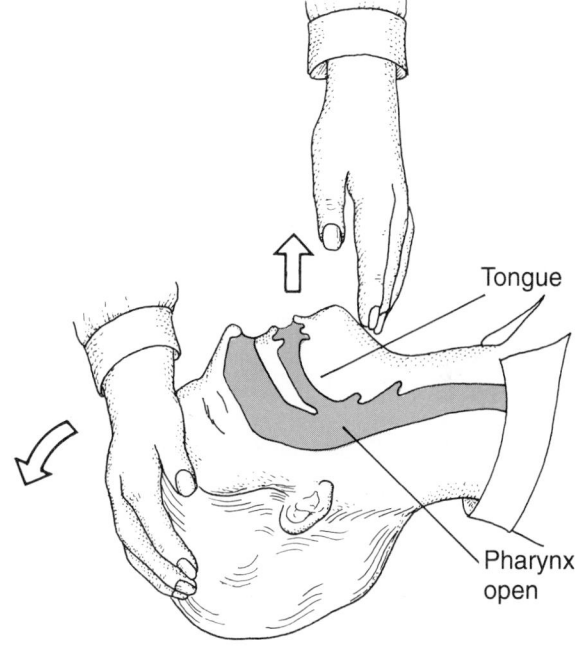

Tongue

Pharynx open

Step 4

5. Place your ear over patient's mouth, and observe the chest for rising with respiration. *Listen, look,* and *feel* for breathing for 3 to 5 seconds.
6. Pinch the patient's nostrils with thumb and index finger of hand holding the forehead.
   Rationale: Pinching the nostrils prevents air from escaping.
7. Take a deep breath and place your mouth around the patient's mouth with a tight seal.
   Note: If patient wears dentures, they should remain in place to enable an airtight seal.
8. Ventilate two full breaths. Each breath should take 1 to 1.5 seconds to deliver. Pause between breaths to allow for lung deflation and to take another deep breath.
9. Assess for carotid pulse for 5 seconds on the side next to which you are kneeling. Maintain head tilt with the other hand.
10. *If patient is pulseless:* Call for help.

(continued)

PROCEDURE 31–2. Administering Cardiopulmonary Resuscitation (CPR)* *(continued)*

11. With hand nearest patient's legs, place middle and index fingers on lower ridge of near ribs and move fingers up along ribs to the costal-sternal notch (in center of lower chest).

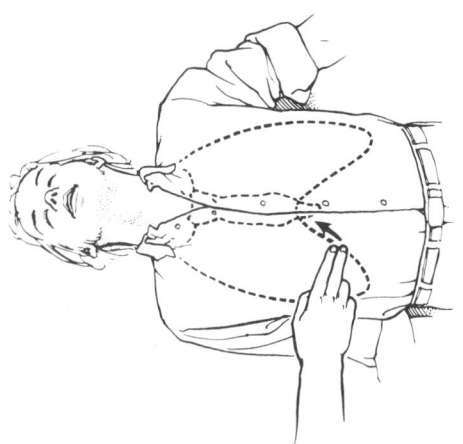

Step 11

12. Place middle finger on this notch and the index finger next to the middle finger on the lower end of the notch.

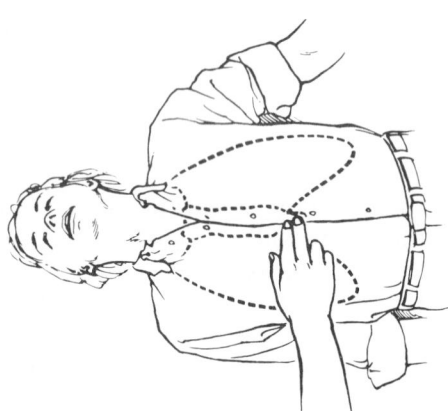

Step 12

13. Place heel of other hand along the lower half of the sternum, next to the index finger.
Rationale: Careful attention to hand placement during cardiac compression prevents fractured ribs and organ trauma.

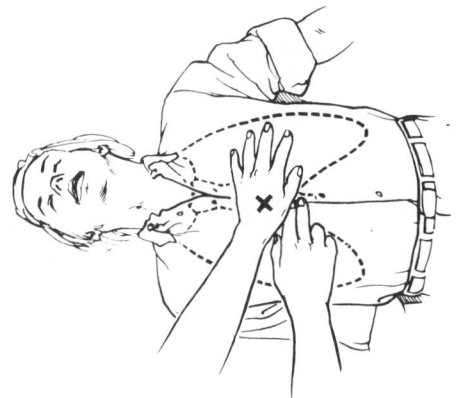

Step 13

14. Remove first hand from the notch and place heel of that hand parallel over the hand on the chest. Interlock fingers, keeping them off patient's chest.
15. Keeping your hands on sternum, extend your arms, locking the elbows, with your shoulders directly over the patient's chest.
Rationale: Weight of your upper body and strength of both arms are needed for adequate cardiac compression. Placing your shoulders over patient's chest provides additional muscle power and prevents hands from slipping off sternum and breaking ribs.
16. Press down on chest, depressing sternum 1.5 to 2 in.
Rationale: Compresses the heart between sternum and vertebrae to pump blood out of heart.

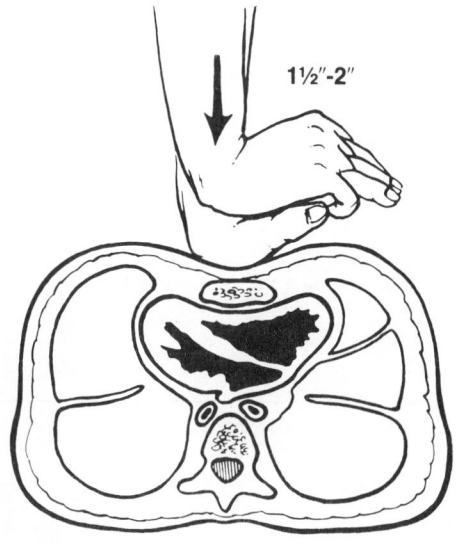

1½"–2"

Step 16

(continued)

PROCEDURE 31–2. Administering Cardiopulmonary Resuscitation (CPR)* *(continued)*

17. Completely release compression while maintaining your hand position. Repeat in a smooth rhythm 80 to 100 times/min.
    Note: Saying the mnemonic "one and two and . . . fifteen" may help maintain the rhythm.
    Rationale: Pressure on the sternum must be released between compressions to allow the heart to fill with blood. Leave your hands in position on the chest to prevent internal injury from malposition of the hands.

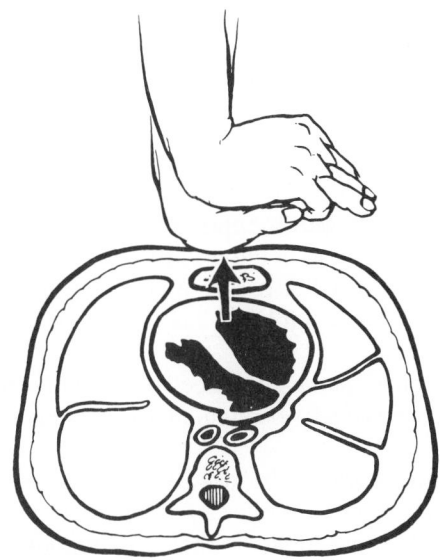

Step 17

18. Ventilate with 2 full breaths after every 15 chest compressions.
19. Repeat 4 cycles of 15 chest compressions and 2 ventilations.
20. Reassess for carotid pulse. If patient is pulseless, continue CPR. Reassess for carotid pulse every few minutes.
    Note: Never interrupt CPR for longer than 7 seconds.

■ **Procedure**

Two Rescuers—Adult Patient

1. When second rescuer arrives, the first rescuer stops CPR after completing two ventilations and assesses for a carotid pulse for 5 seconds.
2. The second rescuer moves into the chest compression position.
3. If pulselessness continues, the first rescuer states "no pulse" and delivers one ventilation.
4. The second rescuer begins chest compression while counting out loud, "one and two and three and four

and five and." The compression rate is 80 to 100/min.
5. The first rescuer gives one full ventilation after every five chest compressions. The first rescuer also assesses carotid pulse during chest compressions to evaluate effectiveness.

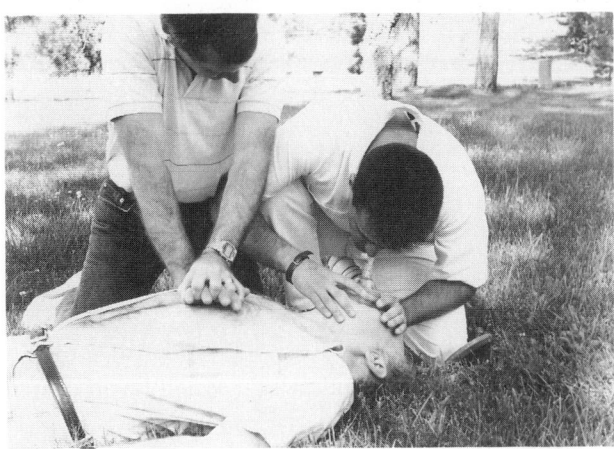

Steps 4 and 5

6. If second rescuer wishes to change positions he or she states, "Change, one and two and three and four and five and."
7. The first rescuer delivers the ventilation then moves into the chest compression position.
8. The second rescuer moves to the ventilator position and assesses for a carotid pulse for 5 seconds. If pulseless, resume CPR.
   Note: Do not interrupt CPR for more than 7 seconds.

■ **Procedure**

One Rescuer CPR—Infant and Child

1. Assess unresponsiveness.
2. Call for help.
3. Place child on hard surface.
4. Open the airway using head tilt/chin lift. Avoid overextension of head in infants.
   Rationale: Overextension of the head is thought to collapse the trachea in infants, causing an airway obstruction.
5. Place your ear over child's mouth and observe chest for rise.
   Listen, look, and *feel* for breathing.
   Note: If airway obstruction from food or foreign object is suspected, perform Heimlich maneuver.
6. If breathlessness is determined, seal mouth and nose and ventilate twice (1 to 1.5 seconds for each breath). Observe for chest rise.
   Note: Infants and small children may require the

(continued)

PROCEDURE 31–2. Administering Cardiopulmonary Resuscitation (CPR)* *(continued)*

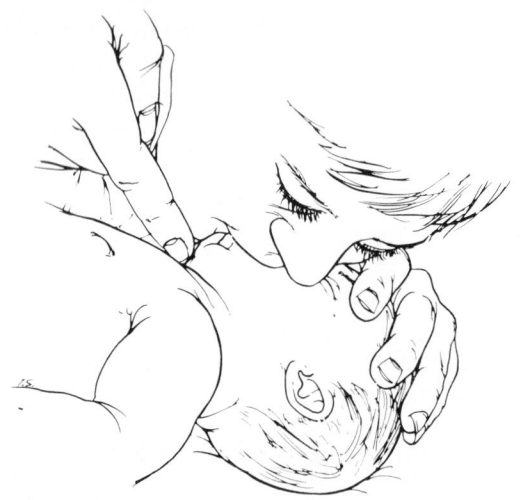

Step 6

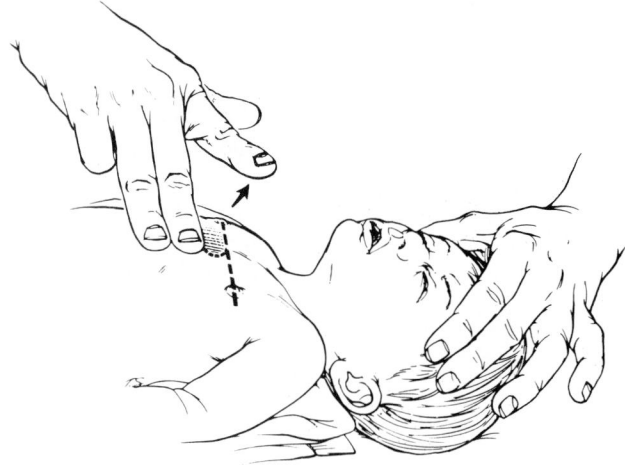

Step 8

rescuer to place mouth over the mouth and nose to establish an airtight seal.

7. Assess pulselessness by palpating for carotid artery on near side in children over 1 year of age. In infants less than 1 year, assess brachial pulse for 5 seconds. *Rationale: Infants less than 1 year have short, chubby necks, which make it difficult to assess the carotid pulse.*

8. Begin chest compression if pulseless.
   a. For infant up to 1 year:
      1) Visualize an imaginary line between the infant's nipples.
      2) Place your index finger on the sternum just below this imaginary line.
      3) Place your middle and fourth finger on sternum next to index finger. This is the location for cardiac compression.
   b. For child 1 to 8 years of age:
      1) Placement of hand on sternum is the same as for adult CPR. Use one hand to compress sternum 1½ inches 80 to 100 times/min.
      2) Continue chest compressions and ventilate at the rate of one breath to five compressions.
      3) Continue CPR as for an adult.

■ **Home-Care Modifications**

• Public education in the performance of CPR must be emphasized. CPR is a complex skill, and efforts to decrease the complexity for lay people must be addressed.

  Emphasis should be placed on teaching one-rescuer CPR because two-rescuer CPR is rarely used by lay rescuers.

  Courses should be developed to allow people to concentrate on an area of Basic Life Support that most closely applies to their life situation. For example, families of patients with heart disease may learn one-rescuer CPR of adults, while parents may learn only infant/child resuscitation and Heimlich maneuvers.

• Nonphysicians who initiate CPR should continue resuscitation efforts until:

  Spontaneous circulation and ventilation are effectively restored.

  Another competent person is available to continue CPR.

  A physician or physician-directed team assumes responsibility.

  The rescuer is physically exhausted and unable to continue CPR.

*All figures from the American Heart Association (1987). *Heartsaver manual; A student handbook for cardiopulmonary resuscitation and first aid for choking. American Heart Association. Pamphlet No. 70-1002 (CP). Dallas: American Heart Association.*

Advanced cardiac life support (ACLS) requires extensive training and rigorous testing. People certified in ACLS are trained in ECG interpretation and advanced airway management. They are qualified to administer cardioactive drugs or electrical shock (defibrillation) as needed.

Hospital resuscitation is often referred to as a "code" (e.g., different institutions announce cardiac arrests as

"Code 199," or "Code Blue"). The "code" team consists of physicians, nurses, pharmacists, and respiratory therapists. All members of the code team should be certified in ACLS.

The nurse is most often the first person to discover a cardiac arrest victim in the hospital. Knowing what to do before and after help arrives increases the chances for the victim's survival. Along with the techniques of CPR, the nurse must be proficient in handling many duties at the scene of a cardiac arrest. The following discussion focuses on some of the important nursing aspects of hospital CPR efforts. (Specific cardiac arrest protocols are established by each hospital and are usually published in the nursing procedure manual. It is the responsibility of each nurse to be familiar with these protocols.)

Initial Management. A multitude of responsibilities accompany the discovery of a cardiac arrest victim. After quickly establishing that an arrest has occurred, the nurse must shout for help and press the emergency button at the head of the bed (if available). At the same time, the hospital telephone operator must be alerted. The nurse must dial the emergency number and announce to the operator, "There is a cardiac arrest on (floor or wing), room (number)." The operator can summon help using the hospital paging system.

The nurse's first calls for help should bring other nurses to the victim's room. They bring the emergency supplies ("crash cart") while the discoverer begins preparations for CPR. Whether or not assistance comes immediately, *the discovering nurse must stay with the victim* and continue to call for help until it arrives.

If the patient has been sitting upright, the bed must be lowered to a flat position. The overbed table should be moved away from the bed for easy access to the patient. The nurse should remove the pillow from under the patient's head. If the bed is elevated to stretcher level, it should be lowered. All of these adjustments must be made as quickly as possible, and CPR must be initiated immediately. Other nurses can move the furniture from around the bed to make room for the crash cart, defibrillator, and ECG machine.

The Code Team. Management of a cardiac arrest usually requires no fewer than four people. The first team member is responsible for establishing and managing the patient's airway. This is often a nurse anesthetist, anesthesiologist, or respiratory therapist. The second performs chest compressions to maintain circulation. The third team member establishes IV lines and administers medications. The fourth member maintains an accurate record of medications and interventions and can help by fetching needed supplies. Team members may switch roles during the resuscitation effort and take turns at compressions, because this is especially fatiguing.

After Resuscitation Begins. Once the code team has taken charge, the nurse who discovered the victim should remain with the team to provide essential information. The circumstances under which the victim was found, the patient's pre-arrest status, primary diagnoses, recent medications, and recent laboratory data are relevant. The nurse may also be needed to assist with procedures. The person in charge assigns specific duties to members of the code team. Those who are not actively participating in the resuscitation efforts are asked to leave the room.

Consideration of privacy is important. If the room is shared by another patient, the roommate should be moved elsewhere if possible. If this is not practical, the curtain should be drawn, and a nurse should stay with the second patient. This patient may be anxious; his or her questions should be answered honestly.

Finally, one of the most difficult tasks for the nurse is in dealing with the sorrow and fears of the victim's loved ones. These people need support during and after the resuscitation. The nurse provides honest information but should not speculate on the patient's condition. Questions concerning the patient's immediate condition should be answered only by those who are absolutely certain of it.

EVALUATION

Patients with cardiovascular dysfunction show widely variable rates of progress. For this reason, specific goals for these patients must be individualized. Together, the nurse and the patient can establish realistic goals with appropriate outcome criteria for measuring goal attainment.

General goals for all patients with cardiovascular dysfunction include:

Goal
Patient will demonstrate adequate knowledge concerning cardiovascular dysfunction prevention or care.

Possible Outcome Criteria
By the end of the teaching session
- Patient demonstrates an understanding of cardiovascular risk factors by reciting those that apply to him or her and discussing their physiologic effects.
- Patient describes a specific plan and timetable for modifying his or her cardiovascular risk factors.
- Patient states the following for any medication administered for cardiovascular problems: name of the drug, dose to be taken, action of the medication, side-effects of the medication, and any special considerations for administration.
- Patient describes the rationale(s) for prescribed therapies.
- Patient lists and describes signs or symptoms that warrant calling the physician.

Goal
Patient will maintain adequate cardiac output.

Possible Outcome Criteria
During hospitalization, patient's
- Heart rate has regular rhythm and remains between 60

Nursing Management Plan
The Patient with Activity Intolerance

Nursing Diagnosis: Activity intolerance related to an imbalance between oxygen supply and demand manifested by verbal reports of fatigue or weakness; abnormal heart rate or blood pressure response to activity; exertional discomfort or dyspnea.

Patient Goal: Patient will balance activity with physical limitations.

Patient Outcome Criteria

- Patient's heart rate has regular rhythm and remains between 60 and 100 beats per minute at rest. (Values may require adjustment for patients with chronic cardiovascular or pulmonary problems.)
- Patient's heart rate rises in proportion to level of activity and does not exceed prescribed maximum limits.
- Patient's blood pressure remains within normal limits for the person's age group; fluctuations with position are minimal.

Nursing Intervention	Scientific Rationale
1. Limit activity 1 hour after meals.	1. Blood flow is directed to digestive tract to aid digestion, increases workload on the heart.
2. Plan heavy activities (e.g., morning hygiene, ambulation) to alternate with rest period of 1 to 2 hours.	2. Careful scheduling allows for uninterrupted rest period. Spacing activity conserves energy and avoid activity intolerance.
3. Offer prescribed nitroglycerine before activity or when pain develops with activity.	3. Nitrates redistribute blood flow to coronary vessels, increasing blood supply to the myocardium and decreasing ischemic pain or increasing activity tolerance.
4. Monitor pulse, blood pressure and respiratory rate before, during, and after activity.	4. Sudden changes in vital signs indicate activity intolerance and provide a parameter for scheduling activity.
5. Gradually increase activity within physician's activity order.	5. Gradual increase in activity level helps patient build endurance and better tolerate increased activity.

Patient Goal: Patient will effectively cope with necessary lifestyle and activity changes.

Patient Outcome Criteria

- Patient demonstrates energy-conserving measures, evidenced by sitting while dressing and planning rest periods during hospital stay.
- Patient discusses realistic plans concerning return to work and other normal activities by end of hospital stay.

Nursing Intervention	Scientific Rationale
1. With patient, establish a plan for day's activity schedule.	1. Offering opportunity to plan activity periods increases patient's feeling of control.
2. Educate patient regarding signs of activity tolerance, e.g., shortness of breath, increased heart rate.	2. Knowledge of symptoms of activity intolerance helps patient identify activity tolerance and manage own activity level.
3. Encourage goal-setting for future activity periods (i.e., "Next time, what would you hope to be able to do for yourself?").	3. Permits patient to become goal directed and in greater control of situation. Communicates confidence that progress will occur.
4. Explore with the patient inventive ideas to conserve energy (e.g., doing tasks from a chair rather than standing; sitting in shower).	4. Conservation of energy increases energy available for other more important activities and increases independence.

and 100 beats/min at rest. (Values may require adjustment for patients with chronic cardiovascular or pulmonary problems.)

- Heart rate rises in proportion to level of activity and does not exceed prescribed maximum limits.
- Blood pressure remains within normal limits for the person's age group; fluctuations with position are minimal.

Goal

Patient will demonstrate adequate tissue perfusion with adequate oxygenation of body tissue.

Possible Outcome Criteria

Within 48 hours of initiation of nursing interventions

- Patient reports absence of severe ischemic pain and presence of improved comfort.
- Patient demonstrates improved color and temperature of extremities.
- Patient demonstrates improved activity tolerance by experiencing decreasing pain with ambulation.
- Patient is oriented to person, place, and time.

Goal

Patient will effectively cope with changes in self-concept and lifestyle.

Possible Outcome Criteria

By Discharge

- Patient verbalizes how his or her cardiovascular condition has caused life changes.
- Patient identifies support people from whom emotional strength can be derived.
- Patient demonstrates energy conservation measures, evidenced by sitting while dressing and planning rest periods.
- Patient discusses realistic plans concerning return to work and other normal activities.

Key Concepts

- Good cardiovascular function depends on a healthy heart to pump blood, an adequate blood volume, and healthy blood vessels to distribute blood to tissues.
- Tissue perfusion, or the flow of blood through the tissues of the body, is essential for cell viability. Tissue perfusion depends on adequate functioning of the cardiovascular system to supply body tissues with oxygen and to remove waste products.
- Normal cardiovascular function usually produces a pulse rate between 60 and 100 beats/min, a blood pressure between 100/60 and 150/85, and an absence of pain on exertion.
- Normal cardiovascular function is affected by age,

gender, exercise, body position, temperature, stress, smoking, and the ingestion of drugs or alcohol.

- Age-related changes in hemodynamics do occur throughout a person's life.
- Altered cardiovascular function can occur when the heart is less effective as a pump (e.g., arrhythmias, muscle damage, valve dysfunction), when the blood vessels are not able to deliver blood adequately to the tissues (atherosclerosis, vein problems, clots, or emboli), or when abnormalities occur within the blood (anemia, low blood volume).
- Modifiable cardiovascular risk factors include smoking, high cholesterol, obesity, lack of exercise, hypertension, stress, and the abuse of IV drugs.
- Manifestations of altered cardiovascular function include: changes in vital signs, ischemic pain, changes in the color or temperature of the skin, changes in sensorium, edema, organ system failure
- Cardiovascular dysfunction can have a great impact on a person's ability to perform activities of daily living and may necessitate lifestyle changes.
- Assessment of cardiovascular function includes gathering subjective data (interviewing) and objective data (physical assessment and laboratory and diagnostic information) to differentiate normal and dysfunction cardiovascular status as well as identifying people at risk for cardiovascular dysfunction.
- Primary NANDA nursing diagnoses for the patient with cardiovascular dysfunction include Altered Tissue Perfusion, Altered Cardiac Output, and Activity Intolerance.
- The nurse is instrumental is promoting optimum cardiovascular health by teaching risk modification for the general public.
- Nursing measures that can help maximize cardiovascular health and prevent complications include improving venous return, minimizing edema, teaching energy conservation, and helping the patient to manage ischemic pain.
- Cardiac arrest is a medical emergency for which cardiopulmonary resuscitation must be quickly and effectively performed to prevent morbidity and mortality.
- Patient goals and outcome criteria should be individualized for the patient with cardiovascular dysfunction including: prevention of dysfunction through adequate patient knowledge, maintenance of adequate cardiac output, maintenance of adequate tissue perfusion, and adequate coping with changes in self-concept and lifestyle.

References

Altman, G. (1989). Alcohol and drug abuse. In S. L. Underhill, S. L. Woods, E. S. Sivarajan Froelicher, & C. J. Halpenny (Eds.). *Cardiac nursing* (2nd ed.; pp. 1000–1007). Philadelphia: J. B. Lippincott.

Bates, B. (1987). *A guide to physical examination* (4th ed.). Philadelphia: J. B. Lippincott.

Caris, T. N. (1985). *A clinical guide to hypertension.* Littleton, MA: P. S. G. Publishing.

Carpenito, L. J. (1987). *Nursing diagnosis: Application to nursing practice* (2nd ed.). Philadelphia: J. B. Lippincott.

Cowan, G. O. (1983). Influence of exercise on high-density lipoproteins. Symposium. *American Journal of Cardiology, 52*(4), 13b–16b.

Cowan, M. J. (1989). Pathogenesis of atherosclerosis. In S. L. Underhill, S. L. Woods, E. S. Sivarajan Froelicher, & C. J. Halpenny (Eds.). *Cardiac nursing* (2nd ed.; pp. 184–193). Philadelphia: J. B. Lippincott.

Craven, R. F. (1989). Physiologic adaptations with aging. In S. L. Underhill, S. L. Woods, E. S. Sivarajan Froelicher, & C. J. Halpenny (Eds.). *Cardiac nursing* (2nd ed.; pp. 170–175). Philadelphia: J. B. Lippincott.

Cunningham, S. L. (1986). Hypertension. In M. L. Patrick, S. L. Woods, R. F. Craven, J. S. Rokosky, & P. M. Bruno (Eds.). *Medical-surgical nursing. Pathophysiological concepts* (pp. 603–621). Philadelphia: J. B. Lippincott.

Fitzgerald, F. T., Graor, R., Lofgren, E. P., et al. (1984). When the complaint is varicose veins. *Patient Care, 18,* 22–54.

Gillum, R. F., Folsom, A. R., & Blackburn, H. (1984). Decline in coronary heart disease mortality. *American Journal of Medicine, 76*(6), 1055–1065.

Goe, M. R. (1989). Hyperlipoproteinemia. In S. L. Underhill, S. L. Woods, E. S. Sivarajan Froelicher, & C. J. Halpenny (Eds.). *Cardiac nursing* (2nd ed.; pp. 858–867). Philadelphia: J. B. Lippincott.

Gregerson, L. A., & Wild, L. R. (1989). Abnormalities of coagulation: Bleeding and clotting. In S. L. Underhill, S. L. Woods, E. S. Sivarajan Froelicher, & C. J. Halpenny (Eds.). *Cardiac nursing* (2nd ed.; pp. 944–956). Philadelphia: J. B. Lippincott.

Halpenny, C. J., & Bond, E. F. (1989). Cardiac anatomy. In S. L. Underhill, S. L. Woods, E. S. Sivarajan Froelicher, & C. J. Halpenny (Eds.). *Cardiac nursing* (2nd ed.; pp. 11–26). Philadelphia: J. B. Lippincott.

Haynes, S. G., Feinleib, M., & Kannel, W. B. (1980). The relationship of psychosocial factors to coronary heart disease in the Framingham Study. III. Eight-year incidence of coronary heart disease. *American Journal of Epidemiology, 111*(1), 37–58.

Hubert, H. B., Feinleib, M., McNamara, P. M., et al. (1983). Obesity as an independent risk factor for cardiovascular disease: A 26-year follow-up of participants in the Framingham heart study. *Circulation, 6*(5), 968–976.

Hudson, B. (1983). Doppler ultrasound stethoscope. *Nursing '83, 14*(5), 55–57.

Jenkins, C. D. (1982). Psychosocial risk factors for coronary heart disease. *Acta Medica Scandinavica (Suppl), 660,* 123–136.

Joint National Committee of 1984. (1985). Hypertension prevalence and the status of awareness, treatment, and control in the United States: Final report of the subcommittee on definition and prevalence. *Hypertension, 7*(3), 457–468.

King, S. C., & Sivarajan Froelicher, E. S. (1989). Cardiac rehabilitation: Activity and exercise program. In S. L. Underhill, S. L. Woods, E. S. Sivarajan Froelicher, & C. J. Halpenny (Eds.). *Cardiac nursing* (2nd ed.; pp. 739–756). Philadelphia: J. B. Lippincott.

Landau, B. R. (1986a). Review of anatomy and physiology—Blood vessels and lymphatics. In M. L. Patrick, S. L. Wood, R. F. Craven, J. S. Rokosky, & P. M. Bruno (Eds.). *Medical-surgical nursing. Pathophysiological concepts* (pp. 585–592). Philadelphia: J. B. Lippincott.

Landau, B. R. (1986b). Review of anatomy and physiology—The heart. In M. L. Patrick, S. L. Woods, R. F. Craven, J. S. Rokosky, & P. M. Bruno (Eds.). *Medical-surgical nursing. Pathophysiological concepts* (pp. 463–469). Philadelphia: J. B. Lippincott.

Laurent-Bopp, D. (1986). Cardiomyopathy and infectious and inflammatory cardiac disorders. In M. L. Patrick, S. L. Woods, R. F. Craven, J. S. Rokosky, & P. M. Bruno (Eds.). *Medical-surgical nursing. Pathophysiological concepts* (pp. 585–592). Philadelphia: J. B. Lippincott.

Laurent-Bopp, D. (1989). Pathophysiology of heart failure. In S. L. Underhill, S. L. Woods, E. S. Sivarajan Froelicher, & C. J.

Halpenny (Eds.). *Cardiac nursing* (2nd ed.; pp. 220–227). Philadelphia: J. B. Lippincott.

Lindskog, B., Kempf, T. M., Newton, K., Silvarajan, E., & Coppel, D. (1983). Teaching outline: Cardiac education classes. Seattle: American Heart Association, Washington Affiliate.

NANDA (1990). *Taxonomy I revised 1990, with official nursing diagnoses.* St. Louis, MO: North American Nursing Diagnosis Association.

National Heart, Lung, and Blood Institute. (1984). The 1984 report of the Joint National Committee on Detection, Evaluation, and Treatment of High Blood Pressure. USDHHS (PHS), NIH. Reprinted in *Archives of Internal Medicine, 144,* 1045.

Osborne, P. A. (1986). Cerebrovascular accidents. In M. L. Patrick, S. L. Woods, R. F. Craven, J. S. Rokosky, & P. M. Bruno (Eds.). *Medical-surgical nursing. Pathophysiological concepts* (pp. 887–920). Philadelphia: J. B. Lippincott.

Pell, S., & Fayerweather, W. E. (1985). Trends in the incidence of myocardial infarction and in associated mortality and morbidity in a large employed population, 1957–1983. *New England Journal of Medicine, 312*(16), 1005–1011.

Pfister, S., & Bruno, P. M. (1986). Assessment of integument function. In M. L. Patrick, S. L. Woods, R. F. Craven, J. S. Rokosky, & P. M. Bruno (Eds.). *Medical-surgical nursing. Pathophysiological concepts* (pp. 1378–1384). Philadelphia: J. B. Lippincott.

Report of the National Cholesterol Education Program expert panel on detection, evaluation, and treatment of high blood cholesterol in adults. (1988). Reprinted in *Archives of Internal Medicine, 148,* 36–69.

Rigotti, N. A., Thomas, G. S., & Leaf, A. (1983). Exercise and coronary heart disease. *Annual Review of Medicine, 34,* 391–412.

Rosenman, R. H. (1974). The role of behavior patterns and neurogenic factors in the pathogenesis of coronary heart disease. In R. S. Eliot (Ed.) *Stress and the heart* (pp. 123–141). Mt. Kisco: Futura.

Rosenman, R. H., Friedman, M., Strauss, R., et al. (1970). Coronary heart disease in the Western Collaborative Study Group: A follow-up experience of 4½ years. *Journal of Chronic Diseases, 23,* 173–190.

Rowell, L. B. (1986). Human circulation regulation during physical stress (pp. 213–406). New York: Oxford University Press.

Shekelle, R. B., Hulley, S. B., Neaton, J. D., et al. (1985). The MRFIT behavior pattern study. II. Type A behavior and the incidence of coronary heart disease. *American Journal of Epidemiology, 122*(4), 559–570.

Sollek, M. V., & Lee, K. A. (1989). High blood pressure. In S. L. Underhill, S. L. Woods, E. S. Sivarajan Froelicher, & C. J. Halpenny (Eds.). *Cardiac nursing* (2nd ed.; pp. 814–857). Philadelphia: J. B. Lippincott.

Surgeon General. (1979). The health consequences of smoking: Cardiovascular disease. USDHHS (PHS) publication #84–50204.

Underhill, S. L., & Stephen, S. A. (1989). Coronary heart disease risk factors. In S. L. Underhill, S. L. Woods, E. S. Sivarajan Froelicher, & C. J. Halpenny (Eds.). *Cardiac nursing* (2nd ed.; pp. 194–206). Philadelphia: J. B. Lippincott.

Woods, S. L. (1989). Electrocardiography, vectorcardiography, and polarcardiography. In S. L. Underhill, S. L. Woods, E. S. Sivarajan Froelicher, & C. J. Halpenny (Eds.). *Cardiac nursing* (2nd ed.; pp. 309–348). Philadelphia: J. B. Lippincott.

Bibliography

Bauer, W., & Dracup, K. (1987). Physiological effects of back massage in patients with acute myocardial infarction. *Focus on Critical Care, 14*(6), 42–46.

Brenglemann, G. L. (1983). Circulatory adjustments to exercise and heat stress. *Annual Review of Physiology, 45,* 191–212.

Dunklee, J. E. (1984). Protocol: Congestive heart failure. *Nurse Practitioner, 9*(9), 15–21.

Ellstrom, K., & Bella, L. D. (1990). Understanding your role during a code. *Nursing '90, 20*(5), 36–44.

Fahey, V. A. (1984). Deep vein thrombosis. *Nursing '84, 14*(3), 34–41.

Feldstein, A. (1986). Detect phlebitis and infiltration before they harm your patient. *Nursing '86, 16,* 44–47.

Fletcher, B. J., Lloyd, A., & Fletcher, G. F. (1988). Outpatient rehabilitative training in patients with cardiovascular disease: Emphasis on training method. *Heart and Lung, 17*(2), 199–205.

Fletcher, G. F. (1984). Long-term exercise in coronary artery disease and other chronic disease states. *Heart and Lung, 13,* 28–46.

Gilliss, C. L., & Rankin, S. H. (1988). Social and sexual activity after cardiac surgery: A report of the first six months. *Progress in Cardiovascular Nursing, 3*(3), 93–97.

Grundy, S. M. (1983). Can modification of risk factors reduce coronary heart disease? In S. H. Rahimtoola (Ed.), *Controversies in coronary heart disease.* Philadelphia: F. A. Davis.

Grundy, S. M., Greenland, P., Herd, A., et al. (1987). Cardiovascular and risk factor evaluation of healthy American adults. *Circulation, 75*(6), 1340a–1362a.

Halpenny, C. J. (1989). The systemic circulation. In S. L. Underhill, S. L. Woods, E. S. Sivarajan Froelicher, & C. J. Halpenny (Eds.), *Cardiac nursing* (2nd ed.; pp. 62–79). Philadelphia: J. B. Lippincott.

Halpenny, C. J. (1989). Regulation of cardiac output and blood pressure. In S. L. Underhill, S. L. Woods, E. S. Sivarajan Froelicher, & C. J. Halpenny (Eds.), *Cardiac nursing* (2nd ed.; pp. 86–107). Philadelphia: J. B. Lippincott.

Hammond, H. K., & Froelicher, V. F. (1985). Normal and abnormal heart rate responses to exercise. *Progress in Cardiovascular Diseases, 27*(4), 271–296.

Johnson Fletcher, B., Lloyd, M. S., & Fletcher, G. (1988). Outpatient rehabilitative training in patients with cardiovascular disease: Emphasis on training method. *Heart and Lung, 17*(2), 199–205.

Jones, S., & Bagg, A. M. (1988). Lead drugs for cardiac arrest. *Nursing '88, 18*(1), 34–41.

Kannell, W. B., Doyle, J. T., Ostfield, A. M., et al. (1984). Optimal resources for primary prevention of atherosclerotic diseases. *Circulation, 70,* 157a–205a.

Karlik, B., & Yarcheski, A. (1987). Learning needs of cardiac patients: A partial replication study. *Heart and Lung, 16*(5), 544–551.

Keeling, A. (1988). Health promotion in coronary care and step-down units: Focus on the family—Linking research to practice. *Heart and Lung, 17*(1), 28–34.

Larson, E., Lunche, S., & Tran, J. T. (1984). Correlates of IV phlebitis. *National Intravenous Therapy Association, 7,* 203–205.

Miracle, V. A., & Allnutt, D. R. (1990). Using a manual resuscitator correctly. *Nursing '90, 20*(5), 49–51.

Patrick, M. L., Woods, S. L., Craven, R. F., Rokosky, J. S., & Bruno, P. M. (Eds.). (1986). *Medical-surgical nursing. Pathophysiological concepts.* Philadelphia: J. B. Lippincott.

Peterson, F. Y. (1983). Assessing peripheral vascular disease at the bedside. *American Journal of Nursing, 83,* 1549–1551.

Report of the Subcommittee on Definition and Prevalence of the Joint National Committee on Detection, Evaluation, and Treatment of High Blood Pressure. (1985). Hypertension prevalence and the status of awareness, treatment, and control in the United States. Approved by the National High Blood Pressure Education Committee.

Solack, S. D. (1989). Pathophysiology of myocardial ischemia and infarction. In S. L. Underhill, S. L. Woods, E. S. Sivarajan Froelicher, & C. J. Halpenny (Eds.). *Cardiac nursing* (2nd ed.; pp. 207–219). Philadelphia: J. B. Lippincott.

Standards and guidelines for cardiopulmonary resuscitation and emergency cardiac care. (1986). *Journal of the American Medical Association, 255*(7), 2841–3044.

Underhill, S. L. (1989). History taking and physical examination of the patient with cardiovascular disease. In S. L. Underhill, S. L. Woods, E. S. Sivarajan Froelicher, & C. J. Halpenny (Eds.), *Cardiac nursing* (2nd ed.; pp. 242–274). Philadelphia: J. B. Lippincott.

Underhill, S. L., Woods, S. L., Sivarajan Froelicher, E. S., & Halpenny, C. J. (Eds.). (1989). *Cardiac nursing* (2nd ed.). Philadelphia: J. B. Lippincott.

Willens, J. S., & Copel, L. C. (1989). Performing CPR on adults. *Nursing '89, 19*(1), 34–43.

Winslow, E. H. (1985). Cardiovascular consequences of bed rest. *Heart and Lung, 14,* 236–244.

Wright, C. (1984). Managing stable angina pectoris: Nitroglycerin, beta blockers, and risk factor reduction, *Nurse Practitioner, 9*(2), 54–62.

UNIT VIII
Nutrition and Metabolism

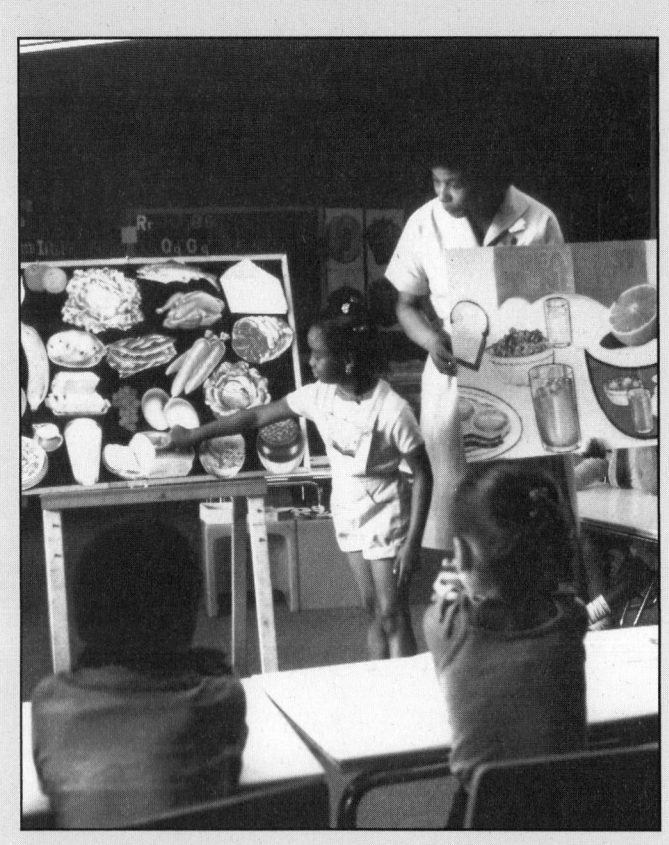

CHAPTERS

32 Fluid, Electrolyte, and Acid–Base Balance

33 Nutrition

34 Skin Integrity and Wound Healing

35 The Body's Defenses Against Infection

36 Thermoregulation

Assessing for nutritional and metabolic needs and intervening to meet those needs encompass a wide range of nursing activities. Using the nursing process as a framework, Unit VIII explores the many facets of nutrition and metabolism. These areas of human function include not only the intake and use of food and fluids, but also such indicators of nutritional and metabolic status as skin and tissue integrity, immune system function, and body temperature regulation.

The first two chapters in this unit discuss the concepts and nursing care associated with the intake of food and fluids and acid–base and fluid and electrolyte balance in the body. Meeting nutritional needs and maintaining the chemical balance within the body require accurate assessments and nursing diagnoses that result in effective nursing interventions. Every patient encounter reveals a patient need for nursing care since these areas of function require that the nurse emphasize health promotion as well as health restoration or support. The next three chapters in this unit explore concepts and nursing care pertinent to situations that indicate the status of nutritional and metabolic function: skin integrity and wound healing, the body's defenses against infection, and thermoregulation.

This unit discusses concepts, principles, and nursing care issues relevant for every patient. In addition to emphasizing nursing interventions to promote health and function, each chapter features assessments and holistic interventions for high risk situations as well as nursing care needs for patients with altered function.

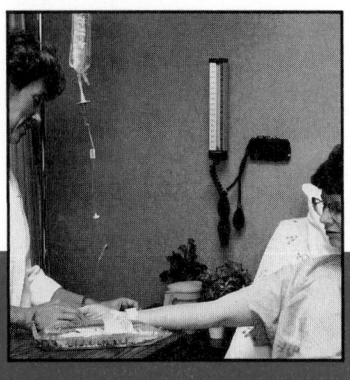

Fluid, Electrolyte, and Acid–Base Balance

LEARNING OBJECTIVES

Upon completion of this chapter, the student will be able to do the following:

- Describe physiologic factors that affect fluid, electrolyte, and acid–base homeostasis.
- Describe common alterations in fluid, electrolyte, and acid–base balance.
- Recognize the impact of age changes on fluid and electrolyte status.
- Describe assessment parameters for the patient with potential and/or actual fluid and electrolyte imbalance.
- Identify appropriate NANDA nursing diagnoses for patients with fluid imbalance.
- Implement appropriate patient teaching to prevent or manage fluid and electrolyte imbalance.
- Describe appropriate nursing interventions concerning intravenous therapy and blood transfusions.

KEY TERMS

Acid	Electrolyte	Hypotonic
Active Transport	Filtration	Infiltration
Anion	Fluid Volume	Ion
Base (or Alkali)	Deficit	Isotonic
Buffer	Fluid Volume	Osmosis
Cation	Excess	Osmotic Pressure
Diffusion	Hypertonic	

32

Normal Fluid and Electrolyte Balance
  Fluid Compartments
  Total Body Water
  Electrolytes
    Sodium
    Potassium
    Calcium
    Magnesium
  Fluid and Electrolyte Distribution
    Processes of Fluid and Electrolyte Movement
    Pressures Affecting Fluid and Electrolyte
      Movement
  Factors Affecting Fluid and Electrolyte Balance
    Fluid Intake
    Food Intake
    Fluid Output
    Hormonal Control
  Lifespan Considerations
Normal Acid–Base Balance
  Acids, Bases, and pH
  Acids and Bases in the Blood
  Factors Affecting Acid–Base Balance
    Respiratory Buffering
    Renal Buffering
Altered Fluid, Electrolyte, and Acid–Base Balance
  Altered States of Fluid, Electrolyte, or Acid–Base
    Balance
    Fluid Imbalance
    Electrolyte Imbalance
    Acid–Base Imbalance
  Potential for Altered Fluid, Electrolyte and Acid–
    Base Balance
    Inadequate Oral Intake
    Excessive Loss
    Stress
    Chronic Illness
    Surgery
    Pregnancy
  Manifestations of Fluid, Electrolyte, or Acid–Base
    Imbalances

Imbalance of Intake and Output
Changes in Mental Status
Changes in Vital Signs
Abnormal Tissue Hydration
Abnormal Muscle Tone or Sensation
  Impact of Fluid, Electrolyte, or Acid–Base
    Imbalance on Activities of Daily Living
Assessment
  Subjective Data
    Functional Pattern Identification
    Risk Identification
    Dysfunctional Identification
  Objective Data
    Physical Assessment
    Laboratory and Diagnostic Tests
Nursing Diagnoses and Patient Goals
  Diagnostic Statement: Fluid Volume Deficit
    Definition
    Defining Characteristics
    Related Factors
  Diagnostic Statement: Fluid Volume Excess
    Definition
    Defining Characteristics
    Related Factors
  Related Nursing Diagnoses
  Patient Goals
Implementation
  Nursing Interventions to Promote Health and
    Function
  Nursing Interventions for Altered Fluid and
    Electrolyte Status
    Oral Fluids
    Electrolyte Replacement
    Intravenous Therapy
    Blood Transfusions
  Discharge Planning and Home Care
Evaluation
Key Concepts

Health and normal body functioning depends on fluid, electrolyte, and acid–base balance. Fluids surrounding the cells of the body are important in the transportation of oxygen, nutrients, and other chemicals essential for sustaining cell viability. They also facilitate waste removal and ensure that cells are capable of carrying on specialized cell functions. Fluids are also essential for the maintenance of adequate blood volume. Optimal cell function depends on the volume and composition of body fluids being maintained within a narrow, normal range.

The balance of fluid and electrolytes within the body is delicate and depends on many complex physiologic mechanisms. Simple activities of daily life, such as excessive exercise, skipping meals, or sunbathing, might upset the precise balance of fluids and electrolytes if the body were not capable of making fine adjustments. Healthy adults and children compensate for such potential hazards; for example, on a hot summer day most people will increase their fluid intake due to thirst.

Minor illness, such as vomiting and diarrhea, or surgery can temporarily disrupt fluid and electrolyte homeostasis despite general good health. For example, sustained vomiting and diarrhea may require hospitalization so that intravenous therapy can be instituted. Chronic diseases such as congestive heart failure, kidney impairment, or liver dysfunction seriously disrupt the body's ability to maintain fluid and electrolyte balance. People with such medical problems are in constant danger of serious disruptions of fluid or electrolyte status, the results of which could be life-threatening.

The nurse plays a vital role in promoting normal fluid and electrolyte balance, and in preventing serious, life-threatening imbalances. Patient teaching regarding the importance of adequate fluid intake and the treatment of common problems such as fever, vomiting, and diarrhea can prevent many potential fluid and electrolyte imbalances. Nursing assessment of fluid and electrolyte balance is essential in detecting imbalances early so that appropriate interventions can be begun promptly. Interventions such as promoting fluid intake, assisting with eating, monitoring intravenous infusions, and administering medications can all help to promote fluid and electrolyte balance.

NORMAL FLUID AND ELECTROLYTE BALANCE

Body fluid is composed primarily of water and chemical compounds called electrolytes. Fluid balance refers to the relative constancy of the distribution of water in the two major fluid compartments of the body. Fluid imbalance refers to an increase or decrease in water within these fluid compartments.

Fluid Compartments

The two fluid compartments within the body are the intracellular fluid compartment (ICF) and the extracellular fluid compartment (ECF) (Fig. 32-1). As the names imply, the intracellular fluid consists of all the fluid contained within the body's cells; the extracellular fluid consists of all the fluid outside the cells. The extracellular fluid is further divided into the intravascular fluid, which consists of plasma, and interstitial fluid, which is the fluid between the cells. Adults have about two thirds of their total fluid within the intracellular compartment and one third in the extracellular compartment (Vander, Sherman, & Luciano, 1985). Body fluids in infants are more evenly distributed, with approximately one half of their body fluid in the intracellular and one half in the extracellular compartment (Goldberger, 1986).

Total Body Water

The total body water comprises from 45% to 85% of the body weight. The variation of body water depends on body fat, sex, and age. Fat contains proportionately less water than does muscle (Cunningham, 1989). Therefore, obese individuals contain relatively less water than lean individuals. Water accounts for 46% to 52% of the body weight in adult women and 52% to 60% of the body weight in adult men. The lower water content in women is due to the greater amount of adipose tissue (Metheny, 1987). Infants have a greater proportion of body water than adults (Whaley & Wong, 1989). Percentage of total body fluid in relation to age and sex is illustrated in Table 32-1.

Electrolytes

Electrolytes are chemical compounds that dissociate in solution into separate particles. These particles carry an electrical charge and are known as **ions.** Positively charged ions are referred to as **cations,** and ions that have a negative charge are referred to as **anions** (Metheny, 1987). Important cations include sodium (Na^+), potassium (K^+), calcium (Ca^{++}), and magnesium (Mg^{++}). Chloride (Cl^-), phosphate (HPO_4^-), sulfate (SO_4^-), and bicarbonate (HCO_3^-) are common anions. Concentration of electrolytes differ in the intracellular and extracellular fluid compartments. The most common electrolytes in the extracellular fluid are sodium and chloride, whereas potassium and phosphate are found in greatest concentration in the intracellular fluid.

Electrolytes are measured in terms of their combining power, or the ability of cations to combine with anions, rather than by their absolute weight in solution. The milliequivalent is used as the measure of this chemical activity. The amount of electrolytes in a solution is most commonly expressed in terms of milliequivalents per liter (mEq/L). For example, 1 mEq of Mg^{++} will combine with 2 mEq of Cl^-.

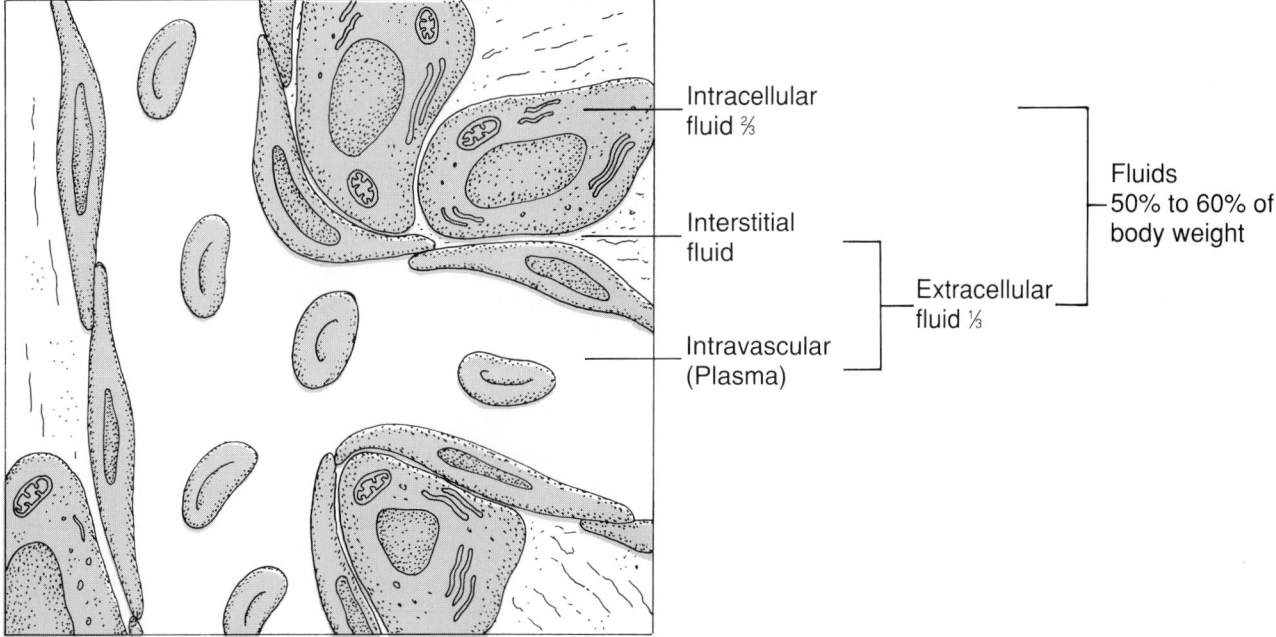

Figure 32–1.   Fluid compartments, showing intracellular fluid, extracellular fluid (which contains intravascular and interstitial fluid), and plasma. Total body fluid is 50% to 60% of body weight.

An analogy may help to illustrate this concept. The hostess who is planning a dinner party would be more concerned over the number of men and the number of women to invite, rather than the total weight of women compared to the total weight of the men. An equal number of each sex will help to ensure a successful party, whereas the total weight of each group has little significance.

Electrolyte balance refers to the relative consistency of the distribution of electrolytes in the serum. Electrolyte imbalance refers to the increase or decrease of the concentration of ions within the serum. Because of the dynamic nature of fluids and electrolytes, changes in serum electrolyte concentrations are indicative of cellular electrolyte changes. The concentration of electrolytes can be determined in the cell as well as in the serum. However, the determination of the electrolyte concentration within the cell requires special techniques. Therefore, the health-care worker must rely on changes in the serum as reflective of electrolyte imbalance. Normal serum electrolyte ranges for the adult are given in Table 32-2. Normal values may vary slightly between laboratories. It is important to look at trends rather than make a diagnosis based on a single laboratory value.

Sodium

Sodium is the most abundant cation in the extracellular fluid. Normal serum levels of sodium are between 135 and 145 mEq/L (Barta, 1987). Serum levels of sodium within these limits are necessary for proper body functioning. Sodium is responsible for the osmotic pressure of extracellular fluid and is also a factor in the transmis-

sion of nerve impulses and in muscle contraction. Sodium also joins with bicarbonate to help maintain proper acid–base balance within the body.

Serum sodium depends on a balance of dietary intake and renal excretion. Sodium is commonly found in table salt (sodium chloride). Other food sources include dairy products, meat, eggs, and certain vegetables; food processing also tends to add salt in the preserving process. The kidneys excrete excess sodium from the body. Aldosterone, an adrenal hormone, helps to regulate this process.

Potassium

Normal potassium levels are essential for proper cardiac, neural, and muscle function and contractility (Fischbach,

TABLE 32–1

Variations in Total Body Fluid According to Age and Sex

Age	Total Body Fluid (% Body Weight)
Premature infant	85%
Newborn (full-term)	70%–80%
Twelve months	64%
Puberty to 39 years old	Male: 60%
	Female: 52%
40 to 60 years	Male: 55%
	Female: 47%
Over 60 years	Male: 52%
	Female: 46%

From Metheny, N. (1987). *Fluid and electrolyte balance: Nursing considerations* (p. 5). Philadelphia: J. B. Lippincott.

TABLE 32-2

Normal Serum Electrolyte Values

Electrolyte	Serum Value
Cations	
Sodium (Na$^+$)	135–145 mEq/L
Potassium (K$^+$)	3.5–5.0 mEq/L
Calcium (Ca^{++})	4.3–5.3 mEq/L
	(8.5–10.5 mg/dL)
Magnesium (Mg^{++})	1.5–2.5 mEq/L
	(1.8–3.0 mg/dL)
Anions	
Chloride (Cl$^-$)	95–108 mEq/L
Bicarbonate (HCO$_3^-$)	22–26 mEq/L
Phosphorus (PO$_4^-$)	1.7–2.6 mEq/L
	(2.5–4.5 mg/dL)

Normal value ranges may vary slightly from laboratory to laboratory.

1988). Potassium also plays an important role in cellular functions such as protein and glycogen synthesis (Porth, 1990). Normal serum potassium ranges are between 3.5 and 5.0 mEq/L (Schwartz, 1987).

There are two major hormonal controls of the extracellular concentration of potassium: insulin and aldosterone. Insulin, a pancreatic hormone, promotes the transfer of potassium from the extracellular fluid into the intracellular fluid of skeletal muscle and liver. Aldosterone enhances renal excretion of potassium. An increase in serum potassium stimulates the release of aldosterone to lower the concentration of the ion. Conversely, a decrease in serum potassium inhibits the release of aldosterone to reduce excretion of the ion.

The body needs approximately 40 to 80 mEq of potassium per day, which is met by dietary intake (Corbett, 1987). The kidneys play the major role in the maintenance of potassium balance, varying excretion with daily intake. Any excessive amount of potassium is also excreted from the body via the stool and in perspiration.

Calcium

The normal serum calcium levels are between 8.5 mg/dL and 10.5 mg/dL (or 4.3 to 5.3 mEq/L) (Byrne et al., 1986). Approximately 99% of the calcium within the body is located within the skeletal system and teeth. The remainder is located in the serum. Calcium is present in the blood primarily in two forms, the ionized form and the albumin-bound form. Approximately 50% of the serum calcium is ionized, with the remainder bound to proteins, mainly albumin. Since a large portion of the calcium is bound to albumin, it is important to correlate serum calcium levels with the serum albumin levels when evaluating laboratory data.

Calcium is indispensable for healthy functioning. The cell membrane structure depends on calcium, as it pro-

motes cell adhesiveness. Calcium is also important in wound healing, proper synaptic transmission in nervous tissue, proper membrane excitability, and in providing the structure for teeth and bones. The contractility of muscle tissue also depends on a normal level of calcium. Calcium is essential for blood clotting and also is critical in metabolic reactions involved in the production of energy (glycolysis).

There are many good dietary sources for calcium. Dairy products such as milk, cheese, and yogurt are excellent sources. Sardines, whole grains, and leafy green vegetables also contribute calcium.

Magnesium

The normal serum magnesium level is 1.5 to 2.5 mEq/L (1.8 to 3.0 mg/dL) (Byrne, et al., 1986). Seventy percent of magnesium is distributed in the bones, and 30% within the soft tissue and body fluids. Like potassium, magnesium is primarily an intracellular ion, with only 1% in extracellular fluid.

Less is known about the function of magnesium than other cations. It is important in regulating neuromuscular function and cardiac activity (Metheny, 1987).

Magnesium is supplied in the diet. Good sources of magnesium include green leafy vegetables, legumes, citrus fruit, peanut butter, and chocolate. The kidney helps to regulate magnesium levels by reabsorbing the ion when the serum level is low and excreting the ion when the serum level is high.

Fluid and Electrolyte Distribution

The membranes of individual cells, the vascular capillary walls, and the lymphatic capillary walls create a semipermeable membrane that separates fluid compartments. Movement between compartments is constant and necessary for cell viability. Water and some electrolytes move easily across this membrane, but larger molecules such as proteins are less able to move across capillary walls. The mechanisms by which fluid movement occurs include osmosis and filtration. Electrolytes and other dissolved particles move by means of diffusion, filtration, and active transport. These mechanisms respond to fluid pressures, which include hydrostatic pressure and oncotic pressure.

Processes of Fluid and Electrolyte Movement

Diffusion. Diffusion is the process of molecules moving from an area of higher concentration to an area of lower concentration. Molecules are in constant motion; if a highly concentrated substance is placed in one side of a container of fluid, the molecules will bombard each other until they are equally distributed in the solution.

Diffusion is an important process in maintaining electrochemical neutrality. Electrochemical neutrality is a state in which the numbers of anions and cations are balanced within each fluid compartment. Since oppositely charged particles attract, electrochemical neutrality is normal within compartments. If any compartment contains an excess of cations, then an identical number of anions must diffuse into the compartment so that the charge is balanced. The same is true if an excess of anions is present: a sufficient number of cations will diffuse into the compartment to balance the electrical charge and ensure electrochemical neutrality.

Osmosis. **Osmosis** refers to the movement of a fluid through a semipermeable membrane. A semipermeable membrane allows some substances to travel through but not others. Osmosis can occur if a semipermeable membrane separating two fluid compartments is permeable to water, and if one compartment contains a greater concentration of a dissolved substance than the other compartment. Water passes through the membrane to the area of greater concentration of the dissolved substance. The net effect of osmosis is to equalize solution concentrations on both sides of the membrane. The principle to remember is, given a semipermeable membrane, water always moves in the direction of greater concentration of dissolved particles (Fig. 32-2).

Active Transport. At times, substances must move across the semipermeable membrane from an area of less concentration to an area of greater concentration. **Active transport** is the process by which this is accomplished. Energy must be available and used to move substances against a concentration gradient. Enzymes facilitate this process.

A specific carrier substance binds with each specific substance that is to be transported against the concentration gradient. The carrier and the combined substance then move through the semipermeable membrane, after which they once again separate. This process can be inhibited by decreasing the temperature of the cell, decreasing the supply of glucose and nutrients available to the cell, or by exposing the cell to toxins.

The process of active transport can be illustrated by the functioning of the sodium–potassium pump in the body. A high concentration of sodium ions is present in extracellular fluid (135 to 145 mEq/L), whereas a low concentration of sodium is present in the intracellular fluid (10 mEq/L) (Barta, 1987). Diffusion of sodium ions across the cell membrane into the cell is facilitated by this concentration gradient. If left unchecked, intracellular sodium would continue to rise and extracellular sodium would continue to fall. The sodium–potassium pump prevents this from happening by actively transporting sodium out of the cell. The difference in concentration of sodium and potassium in intracellular and extracellular compartments is essential for the initiation of action potentials; nerve impulse propagation and muscle contraction depends on this process.

Filtration. **Filtration** involves the transfer of water and dissolved substances through a permeable membrane from a region of high pressure to a region of low pressure. Hydrostatic pressure, or the pressure exerted by fluid against the walls of its container, promotes outflow of fluid from capillaries. Filtration occurs within the glomerular capillaries of the kidney and also at a tissue level to promote fluid and electrolyte balance.

Pressures Affecting Fluid and Electrolyte Movement

Fluid pressures are significant in determining fluid movement between intracellular and extracellular fluid compartments. The most significant pressures involved in fluid movement are osmotic pressure and hydrostatic pressure.

Osmotic Pressure. **Osmotic pressure,** the force of attraction for water by undissolved particles, helps to keep fluid within vessels and prevents a net flow outward. Osmotic

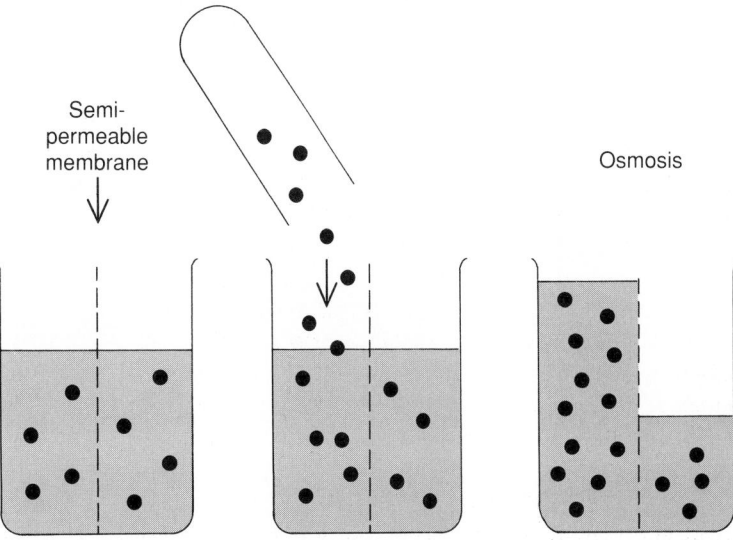

Figure 32–2. Osmosis. Water will always cross a semipermeable membrane in the direction of greater concentration of dissolved particles.

pressure depends on the osmolarity of the solution. Osmolarity refers to the proportion of dissolved particles (solute) in a fluid. Osmolality refers to the concentration of dissolved substances on the basis of weight-to-weight rather than weight-to-volume. These terms are often used interchangeably. Osmolarity is expressed in milliosmols per liter (mOsm/L), whereas osmolality is expressed in milliosmols per kilogram (mOsm/kg).

The normal osmolality of blood plasma is 280 to 300 mOsm/kg (Heitkemper & Bond, 1988). Plasma proteins contribute to the osmotic pressure because they are hydrophilic, which means they attract water. Another term for the osmotic pressure that is produced by plasma proteins is colloid oncotic pressure.

Fluids can differ in osmolarity depending on the concentration of their solutes (Fig. 32-3). A solution that has the same osmotic pressure or osmolarity as blood plasma is called isoosmotic or **isotonic.** When an isotonic solution enters the circulation, there is no net movement of water across the membrane, so cells retain their normal size. A hypoosmotic or **hypotonic** solution has a concentration of solute that is less than blood plasma. When a hypotonic solution (such as water) surrounds a cell, water will cross the membrane into the cell, causing it to swell. The opposite is true for a hyperosmotic or **hypertonic** solution. In a hypertonic solution, the concentration of solute is greater than blood plasma. When a hypertonic solution such as 3% sodium chloride is infused, water will leave the cell, causing the cell to decrease in size.

Hydrostatic Pressure. Hydrostatic pressure promotes filtration of fluid from the vessels into the interstitial compartment. Factors that affect hydrostatic pressure include the arterial blood pressure within vessels, the force with which the heart pumps blood, the rate of blood flow, and venous pressure.

Filtration Pressure. Hydrostatic pressure minus osmotic pressure equals the filtration pressure. To illustrate what happens as blood circulates through the capillary bed, the filtration pressure needs to be examined. In the arteriole the net hydrostatic pressure of the blood is around 32 mm Hg, and the osmotic pressure is 22 mm Hg. The filtration pressure of the arteriole is the difference between them, or +10 mm Hg. Since this is a positive pressure, it supports filtration out of the vessel into the interstitial fluid. In a similar manner, the filtration pressure of the venule can be calculated. The hydrostatic pressure is 12 mm Hg, while the osmotic pressure remains the same at 22 mm Hg. The filtration pressure is the difference, which is −10 mm Hg. Since this is not a positive pressure, filtration from the venule will not occur and the osmotic pressure will pull fluid back into the vessel (Fig. 32-4).

This process of fluid leaking out of the arterioles, only to be reabsorbed in the venules, is continuous. It is also the manner by which the body is able to transport oxygen and other nutrients to the cells and remove waste products. In the healthy person, this process is balanced so that almost all filtered fluid is returned to the vascular space. The lymph system functions to return excess fluid or protein from the interstitial space into the circulation. If the hydrostatic pressure is greatly increased or the osmotic pressure is greatly reduced, some of the filtered fluid may remain in the interstitial space; this is referred to as edema. Damage to lymph drainage can also produce edema.

Factors Affecting Fluid and Electrolyte Balance

In the healthy person, homeostasis demands a balanced fluid and electrolyte status. Normally, the amount of fluids and electrolytes lost from the body is replenished through adequate intake. Hormonal controls and adequate kidney function regulate this process; Table 32-3 gives a summary of typical intake and output for a 24-hour period.

Fluid Intake

Daily intake of water enters the body via the oral route. About two-thirds of ingested water is in the form of drink-

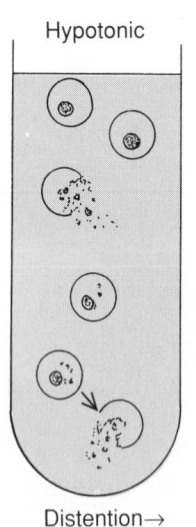

Distention→
lysis

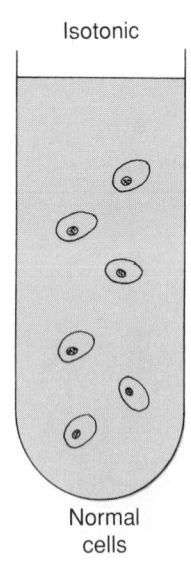

Normal
cells

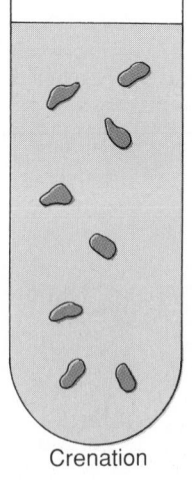

Crenation

Figure 32-3. Hypotonic, isotonic, and hypertonic solutions. In an isotonic solution, cells maintain normal size by effective fluid balance. Cells absorb water from less concentrated (hypotonic) solutions and lose fluid when the surrounding solution is more concentrated (hypertonic).

ing water or beverages containing water; the remainder is through food. Also, a small amount of water is produced by the body through the process of oxidation of hydrogen during food metabolism. An average daily intake for an adult is 1300 mL of water (about six glasses). An additional 1000 mL of water is obtained through foods, especially fruits and vegetables, which are about 80% to 90% water. Only 300 mL of water is obtained through food oxidation (Metheny, 1987).

The thirst mechanism helps to regulate fluid intake. The thirst center is located in the hypothalamus and is stimulated by an increase in plasma osmolarity or a decrease in blood volume. Psychologic factors or a dry mouth may also stimulate the thirst center. Adequate intake of fluids will satisfy thirst if blood volume is restored and osmolarity returns to normal.

Food Intake

In addition to food providing approximately one third of the body's fluid needs, food provides the body with electrolytes. Calcium is abundant in dairy products. Sodium is found in salt, processed meat and food, bread products, and dairy products. Bananas, melons, oranges, apricots, broccoli, raisins, and dates are all good sources of potassium. A well balanced diet usually replaces any necessary electrolytes.

Fluid Output

Water can be lost from the body in four ways: through the kidneys as urine, through the skin as perspiration, through the lungs as insensible water loss, and through the gastrointestinal tract in stool or in vomit.

The kidney is the main organ regulating fluid balance. Glomerular filtration and tubular reabsorption permit the kidneys to conserve or excrete water and electrolytes as necessary to maintain homeostasis. These processes are controlled through the hormonal regulation of antidiuretic hormone and aldosterone, which will be discussed in depth in the following section. Normal urine output for 24 hours is approximately 1500 mL. Loss of fluid through the gastrointestinal system in the form of feces is usually minimal (approximately 200 mL) (Metheny 1987).

Loss of fluid through the skin in the form of perspiration accounts for an average daily loss of 100 to 200 mL of fluid. In addition to perspiration, insensible fluid loss through the skin amounts to about 300 to 400 mL per day. Insensible water loss occurs when water molecules move from an area of higher concentration (the body) to an area of lower concentration (the atmosphere). This differs from perspiration, during which sweat glands actively expel water through the skin.

The final route for fluid loss is via the lungs during respiration. Exhalation not only contains carbon dioxide but also water vapor. The loss of water through respiration is approximately 300 mL per day (Metheny, 1987).

Hormonal Control

Two hormones, aldosterone and antidiuretic hormone, fine-tune the delicate fluid balance in the body. They permit the body to make adjustments so that urine output or urine concentration can change as necessary to maintain fluid and electrolyte balance.

Antidiuretic Hormone. Antidiuretic hormone (ADH) is produced in the supraoptic and paraventricular nuclei of the hypothalamus. From these nuclei, ADH passes down along axons into the posterior lobe of the pituitary, where it is stored. With appropriate stimulation, it is released into the systemic circulation. Antidiuretic hormone maintains the osmolarity of the blood within normal limits by adjusting the amount of water excreted in

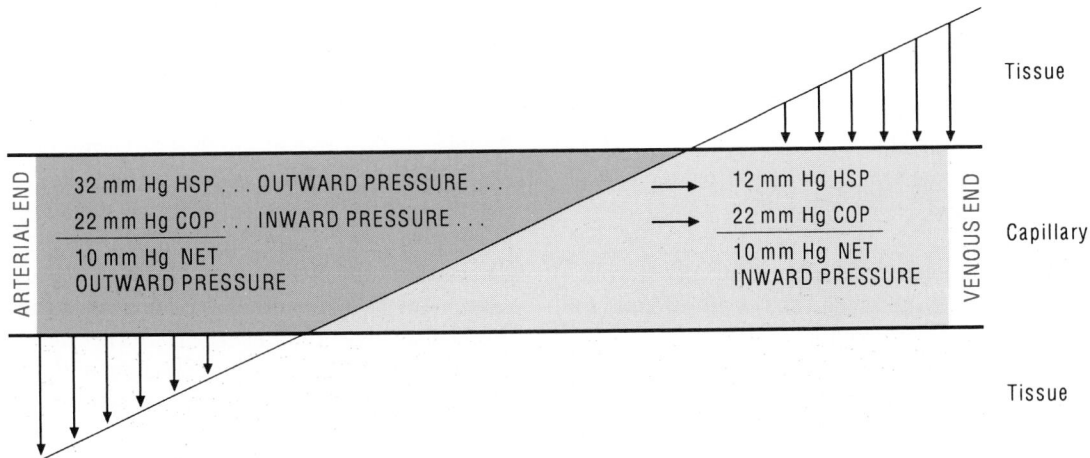

Figure 32–4. Filtration pressure in a capillary. In the arterial end of a capillary, fluid is pushed out into the tissues; in the venous end, fluid is absorbed back into the circulation.

TABLE 32–3
Typical 24-Hour Intake and Output

Intake		Output	
Oral fluids	1300 mL	Urine	1500 mL
Fluid in food	1000 mL	Feces	200 mL
Oxidation of food	300 mL	Perspiration	100–200 mL
Total	2600 mL	Insensible loss	
		Skin	300–400 mL
		Respiration	300 mL
		Total	2400–2600 mL

the urine. The hormone acts on the distal tubules and collecting tubules in the kidney, making them more permeable to water (Vander, et al., 1985). This promotes reabsorption and serves to conserve water in the body.

The two major factors that control the release of ADH are changes in plasma volume and changes in plasma osmolarity. An increase in plasma volume, such as occurs with an increase in water intake, will cause the following to occur: the hypothalamic cells receive input from the vascular baroreceptors, particularly those located in the left atrium. The increase in blood volume subsequently increases the arterial blood pressure, which in turn stimulates the baroreceptors. The baroreceptor stimulation sends impulses to the hypothalamus to inhibit the production and release of ADH. This increases urine production and decreases excess circulating volume. This process is reversed when plasma volume is decreased, such as occurs in shock. The subsequent release of ADH causes an increase in tubular permeability to water and subsequently water reabsorption, which increases blood volume.

Changes in osmolarity of the serum also affect the production of ADH. Cells known as osmoreceptors, which are located in the hypothalamus, detect changes in serum osmolarity. An increase in serum osmolarity stimulates the production of ADH in the hypothalamus and the release of ADH from the posterior pituitary. Antidiuretic hormone acts to decrease urine production by promoting reabsorption of fluid into the circulating blood. When this occurs, the serum osmolarity decreases. This causes the stimulation of osmoreceptors to cease, which stops production and release of ADH. Since the antidiuretic effect is no longer present, urine production increases.

Aldosterone–Angiotensin System. The aldosterone-angiotensin system is the second major hormonal control of fluid and electrolyte balance. It is most significant in regulating extracellular fluid volume balance.

As blood flow decreases to the kidney, renin is released. Renin is an enzyme produced and secreted by special cells in the kidney. Renin splits angiotensinogen into angiotensin I. A converting enzyme in the lung converts angiotensin I into angiotensin II as blood flows

through the lungs. Angiotensin II is a potent stimulator of aldosterone.

Aldosterone is a hormone produced by the adrenal cortex; it regulates sodium reabsorption in the distal tubules and collecting ducts of the kidney. Sodium and water reabsorption help to maintain circulating blood volume and blood pressure.

Parathyroid Hormone. Parathyroid hormone (PTH) helps to regulate calcium and phosphate balance in the body. The presence of PTH causes serum calcium levels to increase by increasing bone, gut, and renal reabsorption of calcium. Usually, there is a reciprocal relationship between calcium and phosphorus levels. Parathyroid hormone increases serum calcium levels but decreases serum phosphate levels, and, conversely, decreased secretion of PTH will lower serum calcium levels and increase serum phosphate concentration.

Lifespan Considerations

Age is a significant factor in fluid and electrolyte balance. The very young and the elderly are more likely to experience fluid or electrolyte imbalances. An understanding of age-related differences is important for the nurse in order to prevent, identify, and treat fluid and electrolyte problems.

Newborn and Infant

Proportionally, the infant has a larger percentage of weight (70% to 80%) as water than the adult (60%) (Metheny, 1987). Preterm infants have an even greater amount of body water, up to 90% (Metheny 1987). A greater amount of the water is within the extracellular compartment in the infant as compared to the adult. The infant also has a greater surface area in relation to weight than the adult. Hence, a large volume of fluid can be lost through the skin. Fluid requirements vary according to age, as do normal urine outputs. Generally the infant has greater fluid requirements and greater fluid losses. The kidneys of the infant are immature, lacking the ability to fully concentrate urine. Metabolic rate is high in the infant, as is the respiratory rate, both of which contribute to increased insensible loss of fluid.

Fluid loss can occur very rapidly in this age group. Parents need to be taught how potentially serious vomiting or diarrhea can be for the infant, and the importance of contacting their health-care provider if these symptoms persist.

Toddler and Preschooler

Approximately 62% of the toddler's weight is water. Fluid requirements vary but are generally 1000 to 1200 mL for a 24-hour period. Urine output increases from approximately 500 to 700 mL per day at age 2 to 600 to 850 mL per day at age 5. Water loss via the skin, respiration, urine, and stools is greater for the young child than for the adult.

Child and Adolescent

The ratio of total body water to total body weight decreases throughout the child and adolescent period. By the time the child is 12 years old, the percentage of body water to body weight is approximately the same as in the adult.

Children of this age group often drink soda or sugared beverages to supply their fluid needs. Water and other more nutritious fluids such as milk should be encouraged. Children and adolescents should be cautioned against the potential dangers of excessive exercise without adequate fluid replacement, especially in hot weather. Balanced dietary intake is important in promoting normal electrolyte balance. Dietary intake is often erratic in the adolescent. Fad diets or purging to lose weight, which have become increasingly frequent among adolescent girls, can cause severe fluid and electrolyte imbalances.

Adult and Older Adult

Water accounts for 45% to 50% of the body weight in adult women and 55% to 60% of the body weight in adult men. The lower water content in women is due to greater amounts of adipose tissue. In middle age, there tends to be an increase in adipose tissue, thus accounting for a continual decrease in total body fluids after the age of 40. After the age of 25, there is a decline in the number of nephrons in the kidney. By the time an individual is 85 years old, there is 30% to 40% fewer functioning nephrons. Consequently, the kidney has less ability to concentrate urine and conserve body fluids.

Adults most often develop fluid and electrolyte imbalances after an acute illness or elective surgery. Older adults commonly experience alterations in fluid and electrolyte status secondary to chronic illness such as renal failure or heart failure. Diuretics, commonly given to treat congestive heart failure, can cause hyper-

natremia or hypokalemia. Excessive use of laxatives can reduce gastrointestinal absorption of potassium, promoting hypokalemia and fluid loss. Some elderly restrict their fluid intake to prevent urinating in the middle of the night. Although calcium levels are often normal in the elderly, calcium leaves the bones of the body, predisposing the person to fractures when falls occur.

NORMAL ACID–BASE BALANCE

For the body's cells to operate with maximum efficiency, they need oxygen, nutrients, electrolytes, a controlled temperature, and an otherwise predictably stable environment. An important component of cellular environment is the hydrogen ion concentration ($[H^+]$). Too much or too little of this ion can dangerously alter cell metabolism.

The healthy body has mechanisms that closely control the amount of H^+ in the blood. The maintenance of this substance within a narrow concentration range is called acid–base balance. Such vital functions as nerve conduction, hormonal activity, and cardiac electrophysiology depend on a stable acid–base environment. Because significant deviations from normal blood $[H^+]$ may be life-threatening, the nurse must have a thorough understanding of the processes of acid–base balance.

Acids, Bases, and pH

Any substance that can donate free H^+ ions to a solution is called an **acid.** By contrast, any substance that can decrease H^+ in a solution is a **base** (also called an **alkali**).

An example of a strong acid is hydrochloric acid, which is found in the stomach. When it enters into solution, it breaks down (or dissociates) almost completely into hydrogen and chloride ions. A small amount of a strong acid in water can generate a large number of free H^+ ions.

Sodium hydroxide (lye) is one example of a strong base. In solution, it binds with some of the H^+ provided by water, greatly reducing the number of free H^+ ions. Weak acids and bases act much the same as strong acids and bases, but they cause only limited changes in $[H^+]$. A solution that contains more acid than base is described as acidic, whereas solutions containing relatively more base are termed basic (or alkaline).

The number of H^+ ions in any solution is indicated indirectly by means of the pH scale. This numeric scale describes the degree of acidity or alkalinity of solutions. The pH scale ranges from 1 to 14, with 7 representing a neutral solution that is neither acidic nor alkaline. Acidic solutions are indicated by the low end of the scale. Weak acids have a pH only slightly below 7, whereas the strongest acids have the lowest pH values. Similarly, bases have pH values above 7, with higher pH values indicating increasingly strong bases.

Acids and Bases in the Blood

The body's extracellular fluids have an average pH of between 7.35 and 7.45 (Saari, 1986). This relatively stable pH is the result of a balance between the body's naturally occurring acidic and alkaline compounds.

The most important acid in the body is carbonic acid. The waste substance carbon dioxide is produced each moment by cells as they use oxygen to metabolize glucose. By itself, carbon dioxide could be considered a neutral compound, but as it enters the blood, it combines chemically with water to form carbonic acid. This weak, unstable acid dissociates to H^+ and HCO_3- (bicarbonate) ions:

$$H_2O + CO_2 \langle = = =\rangle H_2CO_3 \langle = = =\rangle H^+ + HCO_3^-$$

Bicarbonate ion is the body's most important base. Although other acids and bases are found in the blood, it is the balance between carbonic acid (and the hydrogen it provides) and bicarbonate ions which is primarily responsible for maintenance of normal blood pH.

Factors Affecting Acid–Base Balance

The balance between blood acids and bases is closely regulated. The concentration of HCO_3^- in the blood is normally 20 times greater than that of carbonic acid. The 20-to-1 ratio of base to acid is the key to normal acid–base balance (Saari, 1986).

As long as this ratio remains stable, blood pH will remain within its normal range. If the usual concentration of one of these substances should change, the body adjusts the concentration of the other proportionally in an effort to maintain the 20:1 base-to-acid ratio. This adjustment process is called compensation, and it is accomplished through buffering mechanisms.

Buffers are substances that help prevent large changes in pH by absorbing or releasing H^+ ions. Thus, when the blood has an excess of acid, successful buffering prevents a large drop in pH despite the influx of extra H^+ ions into the blood. In such cases, buffers combine with the additional H^+ ions released by the acid, minimizing the potentially damaging effect of extra free H^+ ions in the blood. Similarly, a deficit of blood acid can result in a serious increase in pH. Successful buffering will cause extra H^+ ions to be released into the blood, so the 20:1 ratio of base to acid can be regained.

The body relies on several buffer mechanisms. The plasma proteins, such as albumin and globins, along with hemoglobin in the red blood cell, have limited capacities for regulating H^+ ion concentration. Compounds such

as phosphate and ammonia assist in the removal of H^+ ions to the urine, and thus play a part in acid–base balance.

The most important buffering mechanism in the body involves the respiratory and renal systems. Moment-to-moment maintenance of acid–base status is handled by the lungs, because they can react almost instantly to minute changes in blood pH. The kidneys are responsible for regulating gradual or long-term changes in acid–base balance. They are slower than the lungs to react to changes, but their effect is usually more powerful. Failure of either system can lead to life-threatening illness.

Respiratory Buffering

The lungs are directly responsible for controlling the amount of carbon dioxide in the blood. Carbon dioxide can change rapidly from a liquid to a gas state. It dissolves into the blood from the tissues and, in its liquid state, is carried primarily as carbonic acid, bicarbonate, and hydrogen ions. When this blood reaches the lungs, these substances recombine into carbon dioxide, which then quickly diffuses from the blood into the lung and is exhaled. The lungs normally maintain carbon dioxide levels in the arterial blood ($PaCO_2$) of between 35 and 45 mm Hg (Corbett, 1987).

When large amounts of carbon dioxide are being produced by the tissues, the lungs normally respond with an increase in the rate and depth of ventilation. This increases the rate at which this acid is excreted and prevents any significant change in pH. The respiratory system reacts in an opposite manner if carbon dioxide production decreases. Since breathing is also needed to supply oxygen to the blood as well as to regulate carbon dioxide, however, people are able to decrease ventilation only to a limited extent.

Renal Buffering

The kidneys play a major role in the regulation of acid–base status. By manipulating the rate of excretion or retention of H^+ and HCO_3- ions, they greatly influence the maintenance of the normal base-to-acid ratio.

Gradual increases in the blood acids are buffered in two ways by the kidneys. They will increase excretion of H^+ ions into the urine and return HCO_3- ions to the blood. Additional serum bicarbonate is thus made available to absorb more free H^+ ions, and normal pH can be reestablished.

The kidneys balance a gradual loss of blood acid (or excess of blood base) by increasing retention of H^+ ions and increasing the excretion of HCO_3- ions into the urine. Thus, any rise in pH is prevented as the relative concentration of bases and acids is kept in the correct ratio.

The response of the kidneys to acid–base imbalance is generally long-lasting; however, it can take as long as 2 days before the kidneys' response is complete. For this reason, the kidneys are less effective than the lungs in handling sudden changes in acid–base status. Table 32-4 gives normal values for arterial blood gases.

ALTERED FLUID, ELECTROLYTE, AND ACID–BASE BALANCE

Altered States of Fluid, Electrolyte, or Acid–Base Balance

Disruptions in homeostasis can affect fluid balance, electrolyte balance, or acid–base balance. Fluid imbalances include fluid volume deficit and fluid volume excess. Imbalances of sodium, potassium, calcium, and magnesium can involve either too much or too little of any of these electrolytes in the blood. Acid–base imbalances encompass the problems of respiratory acidosis, respiratory alkalosis, metabolic acidosis, and metabolic alkalosis.

Frequently, more than one imbalance occurs at a time. For simplicity, each imbalance will be discussed separately. Refer to a medical–surgical nursing text for more information on complex problems of fluid and electrolyte imbalance.

Fluid Imbalance

A state of fluid imbalance can occur if there is too much or too little fluid in any of the fluid compartments. **Fluid volume deficit** (FVD) is the term used to describe a deficiency of fluid, while **fluid volume excess** (FVE) is the term used to describe too much fluid.

Fluid Volume Deficit. Fluid volume deficit involves the loss of extracellular fluid containing equal proportions of solute (which is primarily sodium) and water. This loss of isotonic fluid causes a decrease in the volume of the extracellular fluid compartment. Initially there is no shift of fluid, but with acute or prolonged loss of isotonic fluid, fluid can shift from the intracellular compartment into the extracellular compartment. Other common terms that are used for FVD include hypovolemia, saline deficit, and isotonic dehydration. Fluid volume deficit can occur because of inadequate intake or abnormal losses such as vomiting or diarrhea.

A special type of FVD known as "third spacing" occurs when fluid leaves the intravascular volume and is trapped in another area of the body (Metheny, 1987). A "third space" is any area where fluid accumulates and is physiologically unavailable to return to its appropriate compartment. For example, third space fluid in the peritoneal cavity is known as ascites.

Symptoms of a FVD include postural hypotension, weak, rapid pulse, weight loss (except in third spacing), dry mucous membranes, thirst, poor skin turgor, de-

creased urine output, and slow-filling peripheral veins. Serum sodium values often remain within normal limits since isotonic fluid loss has occurred. Treatment of FVD includes either oral or intravenous replacement of sodium and water. The patient must be protected from injury that could occur secondary to postural hypotension.

Fluid Volume Excess. Fluid volume excess involves an increase of extracellular fluid comprised of approximately equal proportions of sodium and water. Increases in saline volume often occur with cardiac failure, renal failure, or liver disease. When excess fluid cannot be eliminated, hydrostatic pressure forces it into the interstitial space, where it is observable as edema. A significant increase in extracellular volume has to occur before edema is visible.

Rapid weight gain (greater than 0.5 kg per day) is the most significant symptom indicating FVE. A weight gain of 1 kg reflects retention of 1 liter of saline. Increased blood pressure, bounding pulse, fullness of neck veins, and decreased urine output may also accompany FVE. Excess extracellular volume can leak into the lungs, causing pulmonary edema, indicated by dyspnea and abnormal breath sounds (rales). As with FVD, serum sodium values may be within normal limits.

Medical management of FVE involves a sodium-restricted diet and the administration of diuretics. The underlying pathology is identified and treated. Fluid restriction may be necessary.

Electrolyte Imbalance

Electrolyte balance is significant for maintaining normal physiologic function. Too much or too little sodium, potassium, calcium, or magnesium in the blood can cause serious disruptions in homeostasis and, when severe, prove life-threatening.

Sodium Imbalance. Hypernatremia is the term signifying excess serum sodium concentration (above 145 mEq/L), whereas hyponatremia indicates a subnormal sodium concentration in the blood (less than 135 mEq/L). Sodium imbalance involves changes in serum osmolarity and thus causes shifts of fluid between intracellular and extracellular fluid compartments.

Hypernatremia. Hypernatremia involves an increase in serum osmolarity. It can be caused by a decrease in water relative to sodium, or by an increase in sodium relative to water. As serum sodium increases, water is drawn from the intracellular compartment, causing cellular shrinking. As fluid is pulled from the cells of the brain, confusion, agitation, and finally convulsions may result. Other symptoms include dry mucous membranes, decreased urine output, a serum sodium above 145 mEq/L, and a serum osmolarity above 300 mOs/kg. Other terms used for hypernatremia include water defi-

TABLE 32–4
Normal Arterial Blood Gas Values

Abbreviation	Normal Range	Definition
pH	7.35–7.45	Reflects the hydrogen ion concentration of arterial blood Acidosis: <7.35 Alkalosis: >7.45
$PaCO_2$	35–45 mm Hg	Reflects partial pressure of carbon dioxide in arterial blood Hypocapnia: low partial pressure of carbon dioxide in arterial blood, <35 mm Hg Hypercapnia: high partial pressure of carbon dioxide in arterial blood, >45 mm Hg
PaO_2	80–100 mm Hg	Partial pressure of O_2 in arterial blood
HCO_3^-	22–26 mEq/L	Amount of bicarbonate in arterial blood

cit, hypertonic dehydration, and hyperosmolarity.

Hyponatremia. Hyponatremia involves a decrease in serum osmolarity, due to loss of sodium relative to water, or to an increase in water relative to sodium. As serum osmolarity falls below 280 mOs/L, water leaves the vascular space and enters the cells of the body, causing cellular swelling. This can result in central nervous system disruption, causing lethargy, headache, and confusion, possibly progressing to convulsions or coma. Nausea, vomiting, and an elevated blood pressure can also accompany hyponatremia. Other terms used for hyponatremia include hypotonic disorder, water excess, and hypoosmolarity.

Potassium Imbalance. An excess of serum potassium (above 5.0 mEq/L) is known as hyperkalemia, and a deficit of serum potassium (below 3.5 mEq/L) is known as hypokalemia.

Hyperkalemia. Hyperkalemia most often accompanies kidney failure, since renal impairment prevents the proper excretion of excess potassium. Hyperkalemia has also been associated with cellular damage, which causes potassium to diffuse from the cell into the extracellular fluid; with insulin deficiency, which decreases the amount of potassium moved into the cell, and with adrenal deficiency, due to decreased production of aldosterone. Sudden infusions of large amounts of potassium intravenously can also cause hyperkalemia (Lowery & Ash, 1988).

An increase in the serum potassium concentration leads to an increased responsiveness of the cell membranes to stimuli, which can be seen in changes in skeletal, smooth, and cardiac muscle. Anxiety, irritability, gastrointestinal hyperactivity (diarrhea and intestinal cramping), and cardiac arrhythmias (irregular heart rate or rhythm) may be present. If serum potassium is elevated (above 8 mEq/L), responsiveness of the cell membranes to stimuli is decreased. Symptoms similar to those of hypokalemia then appear.

Medical treatment for hyperkalemia includes renal dialysis, diuretics, or ion-exchange resins to help lower potassium levels. Insulin and glucose or bicarbonate infusions may be used to move potassium into the cell. The underlying cause for the hyperkalemia should be detected and treated.

Hypokalemia. Hypokalemia occurs with abnormal loss of potassium and inadequate replacement, or a redistribution from extracellular to intracellular stores (Stein, 1988). A reduction in serum potassium concentration leads to a decreased responsiveness of cellular membranes to stimuli. The resulting lack of responsiveness to stimuli leads to characteristic skeletal, smooth, renal, and cardiac manifestations. Symptoms usually appear when serum potassium is below 3 mEq/L. Muscle weakness and fatigue are common. Muscle weakness begins in the lower extremities, and moves up the trunk to the upper extremities. In severe cases of hypokalemia, the muscles of respiration are affected. A decreased responsiveness of the smooth muscle in the gastrointestinal area can produce abdominal distention, nausea, vomiting, constipation, and paralytic ileus. Because the effectiveness of ADH depends on an adequate serum level of potassium, increased urination frequently accompanies hypokalemia. The decreased ability to concentrate urine may also result in increased thirst. Arrhythmias occur in the presence of hypokalemia. Low serum potassium levels may suppress insulin release, thus elevating blood glucose level.

Hypokalemia is corrected by increasing the intake of potassium by encouraging potassium-rich foods in the diet, administering oral potassium supplements, or, in severe cases, administering potassium intravenously. The underlying cause for potassium loss should be identified and preventive teaching implemented.

Calcium Imbalance. Hypercalcemia is an elevated serum calcium and occurs when serum calcium rises above 10.5 mg/dL (5.3 mEq/L). Hypocalcemia refers to a low

Selected Nursing Research Studies

Gaspar, P. M. (1988). What determines how much patients drink. *Geriatric Nursing, 9,* 221–224.

Josephson, A., et al. (1987). The relationship between intravenous fluid contamination and the frequency of tubing replacement. *CINA Journal, 3*(2), 17–18, 20–21.

Leibovici, L. (1989). Daily change of an antiseptic dressing does not prevent infusion phlebitis: A controlled trial. *American Journal of Infection Control, 17*(1), 23–25.

McKee, J. M., et al. (1989). Complications of intravenous therapy: A randomized prospective study. *Journal of Intravenous Nursing, 12,* 288–295.

Popovsky, M. A., & Ilstrup, D. M. (1986). Randomized clinical trial of transparent polyurethane IV dressings. *NITA, 9,* 107–110.

Shearer, J. (1987). Normal saline flush versus dilute heparin flush: A study of peripheral intermittent IV devices. *Journ NITA, 10,* 425–427.

Possible Topics for Nursing Inquiry

- What are the criteria and incidence a staff nurse uses for irrigating an intravenous line?
- What is the cost benefit of using heparin verses saline to flush heparin locks?
- What is the age-related incidence of phlebitis versus infiltration with the use of angiocatheters?
- What are the perceptions of thirst with intake of liquids of different temperatures?
- How is the anxiety of people needing a blood transfusion affected before and after education regarding HIV screening of blood?
- During how many nurse–patient interactions is the patient on "push fluids" offered liquid to drink?
- What is the comparison of selected fruit juices on a person's perception of thirst?

serum calcium level and occurs when the serum calcium concentration falls below 8.5 mg/dL (4.3 mEq/L).

Hypercalcemia. Hypercalcemia occurs with excessive intake of vitamin D, excessive intake of milk or alkaline "antacids," hyperparathyroidism, immobilization, and reduced renal function. The presence of various types of malignancies can also cause hypercalcemia.

Hypercalcemia causes decreased neuromuscular excitability, which can result in various symptoms. Muscle weakness, lack of coordination, confusion, lethargy, impaired memory, gastrointestinal problems such as nausea, vomiting, and constipation, pruritis, kidney stones, and bone pain are symptoms that can occur in the person with high serum calcium levels.

Hypocalcemia. Hypocalcemia is associated with parathyroid deficiency, vitamin D deficiency, and renal disease. Some malignancies, pancreatitis, various treatments such as massive blood transfusion, and the abuse of laxatives or enemas can decrease serum calcium levels.

A reduction in calcium in the serum can cause spontaneous discharge of both sensory and motor fibers of the peripheral nervous system. This produces the following symptoms in the patient: mild hypocalcemia begins with paresthesia, which is a tingling in the hands, fingers, feet, or around the mouth. Tetany is manifested by grimacing, muscle twitching, cramping, hyperactive reflexes, and severe flexion of the wrist and ankle joints. Both can develop as the serum calcium falls lower. If untreated, laryngospasm, seizures, and cardiac arrest can cause death.

Oral calcium supplements should be given in mild cases of hypocalcemia. In more severe cases, intravenous (IV) calcium must be given slowly. Rapid IV replacement of calcium can result in cardiac arrhythmias. Seizure precautions may be necessary.

Magnesium Imbalance. Hypermagnesemia occurs when the serum concentration of magnesium is more than than 2.5 mEq/L (3.0 mg/dL), whereas hypomagnesemia occurs when the serum concentration of magnesium is less than 1.5 mEq/L (1.8 mg/dL).

Hypermagnesemia. Hypermagnesemia can occur in renal failure, diabetic ketoacidosis, or when magnesium sulfate is given in therapy (Metheny, 1987). It also can occur with the use of magnesium-based laxatives (Cunningham, 1989). High serum magnesium levels depress muscular irritability, which can cause hypotension, weakness, depressed reflexes, paralysis, bradycardia, respiratory failure, and cardiac arrest.

Hypomagnesemia. Hypomagnesemia can be due to impaired intake, impaired intestinal absorption, and excessive urinary excretion secondary to diuretics and chronic alcoholism. Hypomagnesemia causes neuromuscular irritability, which can be seen in tremors, cramps, difficulty swallowing, and cardiovascular changes

Acid–Base Imbalance

A consistent arterial pH of between 7.35 and 7.45 is necessary for efficient cellular metabolism. When pH of arterial blood falls below this range, acidosis is said to be present. Alkalosis occurs if pH is greater than 7.45. Acidosis and alkalosis can be categorized as either respiratory or metabolic, depending on the primary cause. Acid–base imbalances can be either acute or chronic, reflecting the effectiveness of the body's compensatory mechanisms. Disturbances in acid–base balance can severely alter blood oxygen transport, neurologic function, and cardiac rhythmicity.

Acidosis. Respiratory acidosis is present when low pH is caused by hypoventilation. Metabolic acidosis occurs when the kidneys are unable to retain enough bicarbonate ion to buffer free hydrogen ions in the blood (Mathewson, 1987).

Respiratory Acidosis. Respiratory acidosis is indicated by a subnormal pH accompanied by an elevated level of carbon dioxide ($PaCO_2$ greater than 45 mm Hg.) The lungs normally maintain blood concentrations of this metabolic waste product within a narrow range. When breathing ability is compromised, by lung diseases such as asthma or emphysema, or by depressed neural or muscular function (such as with narcotic overdose, head trauma, or polio), carbon dioxide accumulates in the blood. As this acid increases, free hydrogen ion is released, causing pH to drop.

Over time, the kidneys may be able to compensate for this excessive build-up of acid. They increase excretion of H^+ ion into the urine and return HCO_3^- to the blood. In this way normal pH can be reestablished.

Metabolic Acidosis. Metabolic acidosis is characterized by low pH and decreased plasma HCO_3^- level (below 22 mEq/L). It occurs with loss of bicarbonate from severe diarrhea, or with accumulation of atypical acids (such as ketoacids, caused by diabetes, or lactic acids, caused by oxygen deprivation) (Romanski, 1986).

The respiratory system attempts to compensate for these conditions by increasing ventilation. The lungs cannot directly decrease the concentration of these atypical acids in the blood, nor can they alter the amount of available bicarbonate. By increasing the rate of excretion of carbonic acid, however, the lungs can help to balance the abnormal pH.

Alkalosis. Respiratory alkalosis is caused by hyperventilation. Metabolic alkalosis occurs when there is excessive loss of body acids, or with unusual intake of alkaline substances (Romanski, 1986).

Respiratory Alkalosis. Respiratory alkalosis is present when a high pH is accompanied by decreased blood carbon dioxide levels (below 35 mm Hg). Hyperventilation (caused most commonly by anxiety and asthma) increases removal of carbon dioxide from the blood. This leads to a relative excess of blood base, with a resultant increase in pH. To compensate, the kidneys attempt to increase excretion of HCO_3^- into the urine. By reducing the normal level of this base, the normal ratio of blood bases to acids is reestablished, and pH thus returns toward normal.

Metabolic Alkalosis. Metabolic alkalosis is usually caused by vomiting or vigorous nasogastric suction (Corbett, 1987). Occasionally, endocrine disorders or the ingestion of large amounts of antacids can also bring about metabolic alkalosis. The loss of stomach acid, or an excessive amount of base in the stomach, will cause H^+ shifts in the blood, and pH will increase.

Compensation for this disorder is limited. The respiratory system is able to decrease breathing to some extent in an attempt to allow blood carbon dioxide to rise. The retention of this acid helps to balance the loss of the other acids. Breathing can only be slowed slightly before oxygenation is threatened, however, so this compensatory mechanism is only partially effective.

Potential for Altered Fluid, Electrolyte, and Acid–Base Balance

Many factors can increase the risk for fluid, electrolyte, or acid–base imbalance, including inadequate oral intake, excessive loss of fluid or electrolytes, stress, chronic illness, and surgery.

Inadequate Oral Intake

Many factors can affect the ability to achieve adequate fluid intake. Fluids and food have to be readily accessible. The elderly may be unable to get out to shop for or prepare a well-balanced diet, thus decreasing their intake of needed electrolytes and fluid. People in bed may be too weak to reach for and drink fluids and too fatigued to consume entire meals.

Psychologic factors such as depression or confusion may also contribute to decreased oral intake. Some people may purposely limit oral intake to lose weight or decrease the number of times they must void. Often, lack of knowledge regarding the consequences of these actions contributes to such behavior.

Physiologic factors such as nausea often limit oral intake. The inability to swallow, such as after a stroke, or discomfort while swallowing, such as with a sore throat, can also contribute to inadequate oral intake.

Excessive Loss

Fluid and electrolyte problems can occur when an individual experiences abnormal loss of fluid or electrolytes. This commonly occurs in vomiting, diarrhea, diaphoresis, or increased urine output secondary to the administration of diuretics.

Vomiting depletes the body of fluid and electrolytes. As hydrochloric acid is lost from the stomach, hydrogen ions and chloride ions are depleted, leading to a metabolic alkalosis. If vomiting contains alkaline duodenal fluid along with stomach contents, no significant shift in acid–base balance may occur. Gastric contents are also high in potassium and sodium, and prolonged vomiting can deplete these electrolytes. Vomiting compounds fluid and electrolyte problems because the ability to maintain adequate intake usually is also affected.

Diarrhea depletes the body of both fluid and electrolytes. Intestinal secretions contain much bicarbonate; thus most diarrhea causes a metabolic acidosis. Intestinal contents are also rich in sodium and potassium, and diarrhea can deplete both of these electrolytes. Often, fluids are withheld from the patient with diarrhea, since oral intake increases intestinal peristalsis, which in turn aggravates the diarrhea.

Diaphoresis, or excessive sweating, can increase the loss of fluid and electrolytes. Sweat is a hypertonic fluid containing sodium, potassium, and chloride. Diaphoresis can occur with increased physical activity, fever, or exposure to elevated environmental temperatures. Fluid containing sodium (e.g., tomato juice or broth) should be used to replace both fluid and electrolytes that are lost when diaphoresis occurs.

Diuretics can be prescribed to promote the excretion of sodium and water from the body. Usually, diuretics are ordered for patients with chronic heart, renal, or liver problems. At times, the medications may remove too much fluid or sodium from the body, resulting in a fluid or sodium deficit. Many diuretics (e.g., thiazides) also promote the excretion of potassium from the body, increasing the risk for potassium depletion. Frequently, patients receiving such diuretics are given potassium supplements to prevent electrolyte imbalance.

Stress

Stress affects fluid and electrolyte balance. Stress can be caused by many factors, such as physical trauma, anxiety, and pain. When stress occurs, aldosterone production is increased, causing retention of sodium and water. Stress also increases ADH production, resulting in decreased urine production. Both of these mechanisms tend to increase circulating volume, which can contribute to fluid overload in high-risk people.

Chronic Illness

Many chronic medical problems adversely affect a person's ability to maintain normal fluid, electrolyte, and acid–base homeostasis. Chronic renal problems, chronic heart problems, and chronic respiratory problems are significant. Other problems such as liver disorders, cancer, and diabetes mellitus also can significantly affect fluid and electrolyte balance.

Renal Failure. As the kidneys become less able to function properly due to disease, there is an abnormal build-up of sodium, chloride, potassium, and fluid in the body. The kidneys are less able to control precisely the selective removal of excess electrolytes, so toxic levels may build up in the body. Since the body normally produces more acid wastes than alkaline wastes, metabolic acidosis occurs when the kidneys fail to function. Hyperkalemia and hypocalcemia are often present.

Cardiac Failure. As the heart fails to work effectively to pump and circulate blood, fluid collects in both the lungs and the rest of the body. Fluid volume excess is complicated by the fact that, as the heart pumps less effectively, decreased blood reaches and perfuses the kidneys, thus increasing fluid retention. Systemic and pulmonary edema can occur in heart failure.

Respiratory Failure. Chronic respiratory problems affect acid–base balance. Chronic destruction of alveoli limits the lungs' functional ability to remove excess hydrogen ion from the body. The pH of the blood falls and respiratory acidosis occurs.

Surgery

Many preoperative and postoperative factors influence the surgical patient's fluid and electrolyte status. Preoperatively, the patient is kept *non per os* (NPO; nothing by mouth) and may receive numerous enemas. During surgery, increased insensible water loss occurs as the internal body structures are exposed to air. Blood loss, often significant, can occur during surgical procedures. Potassium levels frequently fall after surgery due to cellular trauma and inadequate intake. As cells are destroyed, potassium is released from inside the cell, which will cause a temporary increase in serum potassium. As this potassium is excreted in the urine, serum potassium can become depleted and supplemental potassium may be necessary. Frequently, the postoperative patient is NPO or on a restricted diet for a period of time. Drainage from nasogastric tubes or surgical drains increases the potential for loss of fluids and electrolytes. Emotional stress, pain, nausea, and vomiting are common postoperatively and can contribute to fluid and electrolyte imbalance.

Pregnancy

Physiologic changes occur during pregnancy that can alter fluid, electrolyte, and acid–base status. Fluid retention and edema occur frequently, although the exact mechanism underlying this is not completely understood (Metheny, 1987). Aldosterone production increases during pregnancy. There is an overall increase in blood volume as well as total body fluid volume. Alteration in acid–base balance also occurs. Hyperventilation is caused by higher progesterone levels and results in alkalosis as the $PaCO_2$ decreases.

Manifestations of Fluid, Electrolyte, or Acid–Base Imbalances

Although each specific fluid, electrolyte, or acid–base imbalance has specific symptoms, general groups of symptoms frequently accompany states of imbalance, namely, a significant difference between intake and output, a change in the mental status of the patient, a change in the vital signs of the patient, abnormal tissue hydration, and abnormal muscle tone. The degree of the imbalance and the suddenness with which it occurs will determine the severity of symptoms. In evaluating manifestations, it is important to see if all data support the same conclusion. The nurse should suspect fluid, electrolyte, or acid–base imbalance for any patient who presents the following clinical symptoms.

Imbalance of Intake and Output

Intake and output should be approximately equal for a 24-hour period. When output is significantly greater or significantly less than intake, the nurse should suspect a fluid balance problem. Before arriving at any conclusions, the nurse should make certain that the intake and output record is accurate, since mistakes in such records are common. Normally, urine output is around 1500 mL per 24-hour period, but a wide range of individual variation is considered normal, depending on many factors. A decrease in this amount can occur in fluid volume deficit, and an increase or decrease in this amount in fluid volume excess.

In evaluating trends in intake and output, it is important to consider at least the last 48 hours. For some patients with chronic health problems, it may be important to consider data over a longer period of time. The nurse should look for a pattern of imbalance between intake and output (e.g., over the last 5 days the patient's urine output has decreased when the oral intake has remained approximately the same).

Changes in Mental Status

Subtle changes in a person's ability to understand and relate to his or her environment are some of the earliest indications that a fluid or electrolyte imbalance is present. When changes are detected in the normal cognitive–perceptual functioning of an individual, fluid and electrolyte imbalance must be suspected.

Level of consciousness (LOC) is the state of awareness and arousal of an individual. Changes in LOC can occur with changes in serum osmolality or changes in serum sodium. At first, changes are minor and may not be picked up unless the nurse knows the patient well. The patient may simply feel fatigued, restless, or apprehensive. Confusion can occur as the imbalances become more severe. Changes in LOC can vary from excessive excitability to lethargy. Lethargy can progress to coma

and, eventually, death. The abruptness of the onset of the imbalance will increase the severity of symptoms.

Changes in Vital Signs

Most states of fluid, electrolyte, or acid–base imbalance are accompanied by a change in the patient's vital signs. The nurse should observe for changes from baseline vital sign readings in the patient.

Respiratory Rate and Depth. Deep, labored respirations may occur to compensate for metabolic acidosis, whereas shallow respirations may be present in alkalosis. Fluid volume excess can cause fluid to leak within the lungs and thus impede oxygenation. Dyspnea may indicate that this has occurred. Lung auscultation can detect rales, a subtle sign of fluid excess, prior to frank dyspnea.

Heart Rate and Rhythm. The quality of the pulse depends in part on the amount of circulating volume. In volume excess the pulse is strong, full, and bounding. In volume deficits the pulse is usually weak, thready, and increased in rate. Irregular heart rhythms are common in electrolyte imbalances involving potassium and magnesium.

Blood Pressure. Increased blood pressure may occur with fluid volume excesses. A corresponding decrease in blood pressure occurs in fluid volume deficits. A more sensitive way to assess a volume deficit is to determine the affect that position change has on blood pressure. The blood pressure and pulse is first measured in the supine position, then measured again after 2 minutes in a sitting position, and finally 2 minutes later, standing. Normally, within 2 minutes, the body can adjust to changes in position, and blood pressure and pulse rate should return close to baseline. A drop of greater than 15 mm Hg in systolic pressure or a 10 mm Hg drop in diastolic pressure with an increase in pulse rate is significant, and frequently means the patient is volume depleted (Underhill, 1989). Postural blood pressure readings are a significant assessment tool for the nurse and should be employed routinely for all patients at risk for volume depletion (e.g., postoperatively).

Abnormal Tissue Hydration

When fluid imbalance occurs, tissues can retain excess fluid, appearing edematous, or lose fluid, appearing dry and shriveled. Tissue hydration can be noted in the mouth, where the mucous membranes and tongue can appear dry and may have ridges due to lack of moisture. Tissue turgor, or the ability of the skin to return to normal position immediately after being pinched, is affected by fluid imbalance. Poor tissue turgor occurs in fluid deficit or when elasticity is lost from the skin during normal aging.

Edema, or the presence of fluid in the interstitial space, is not observable, in most patients, until 5 L of fluid has been retained (Underhill, 1989). Edema is most noticeable in dependent areas of the body (e.g., the legs when walking, the back and sacral area when supine in bed). When edema is severe, an indentation can be left when a finger is pressed into the edematous tissue; this is known as pitting edema.

Abnormal Muscle Tone or Sensation

Changes in muscle tone and muscle irritability frequently accompany fluid, electrolyte, and acid–base imbalances. Excessive neuromuscular stimulation can be seen in increasing irritability, muscle weakness, twitching, or cramping. Patients with electrolyte imbalance often experience tingling and other paresthesias. The nurse should also observe patients for seizure activity, which can occur in severe imbalances.

Impact of Fluid, Electrolyte, or Acid–Base Imbalance on Activities of Daily Living

The ability of the patient with a fluid, electrolyte, or acid–base imbalance to perform common activities of daily living may be impaired. For the patient who has an IV line, eating may be difficult because the dominant hand may be immobilized or he or she cannot use both hands in cutting meat, buttering bread, and so forth. The nurse needs to anticipate these problems and make sure necessary assistance is provided.

The patient with fluid, electrolyte, or acid–base imbalance may tire easily. For these patients, activities should be limited, with frequent rest periods provided during energy-consuming activities. For example, a patient who is responsible for his or her own bath and is fatigued can conserve energy by bathing parts of the body at different intervals with established rest periods. Bathing in a tub may be too strenuous, so a bed bath may be a preferred alternative. Dressing may be exhausting; consequently, the patient may prefer to remain in bedclothes all day. Garments should be loose-fitting and easy to slip on and off. Patients with IVs have difficulty dressing, especially in placing the garments over the affected extremity, and may need assistance so that the IV will not be inadvertently dislodged.

Confusion may occur in the patient with a fluid, electrolyte, or acid–base imbalance. The nurse needs to make sure that safety precautions are implemented. These may include restricting the patient to bed, orienting the patient to person, place, and time, keeping the side rails up, and generally assisting the patient with activities of daily living that cannot be safely performed independently.

Mobility can become a problem for patients with fluid, electrolyte, and acid–base imbalances. Stand-by assistance may be necessary. When patients assume an upright posture, it is important to wait until dizziness subsides before beginning ambulation. Postural blood pressure should be assessed on high-risk individuals. Aids such as ambulation belts, walkers, and canes can assist the patient to ambulate more safely.

ASSESSMENT

Gathering data concerning the fluid and electrolyte status of an individual is important to determine potential problems and actual disturbances. Subjective and objective data are obtained in the nursing assessment through the nursing history, the physical assessment, and through evaluating information obtained from laboratory and diagnostic tests.

Subjective Data

The collection of subjective information helps the nurse identify the normal pattern of fluid and electrolyte status for the patient, any risk factors that may predispose the patient to fluid and electrolyte imbalance, and any actual dysfunctions that are present.

Functional Pattern Identification

The nurse usually begins the assessment of a patient's fluid and electrolyte status by obtaining or reviewing his or her history. In this process, the nurse gains an understanding of normal fluid status for the person and any factors that may predispose the person to imbalance.

The nurse should question the patient regarding normal functional patterns of intake and output and any recent changes that have occurred. Special diet restrictions such as sodium-restricted diets or the use of salt substitutes should be noted. Reported increased thirst or a decreased fluid intake are also significant. The amount and pattern of urine output should also be assessed, along with any changes.

Risk Identification

The collection of subjective data can also help the nurse identify risk factors that could contribute to dysfunction. The nurse should elicit information concerning recent acute illness. Vomiting or diarrhea is especially important to document, as well as the presence of a fever or diaphoresis. The severity and duration of these problems should be noted.

Certain chronic diseases also predispose a person to fluid and electrolyte imbalance. The patient should be questioned about the presence of the following: renal failure, congestive heart failure, respiratory dysfunction, diabetes mellitus, diabetes insipidus, Addison's disease, Cushing's disease, or thyroid disease. If any of these are present, the patient should be questioned regarding his or her individualized management plan and any complications that have occurred.

The nurse should also question the patient regarding intake of any prescription or nonprescription medications. Various medications, such as insulin, diuretics, steroids, laxatives, and antacids can contribute to fluid and electrolyte disturbances. The use of vitamins and calcium supplements should also be noted.

Finally, the nurse should assess spiritual or sociocultural factors that may affect fluid and electrolyte balance. Religious beliefs, such as the Jehovah's Witness's refusal to receive blood products, could increase the potential for fluid deficit problems if a patient hemorrhages after surgery. A fixed income or the lack of transportation could prevent a person from getting medicine or food to comply with medical treatment.

Dysfunctional Identification

The nurse can use the subjective data he or she collects to help identify actual fluid and electrolyte problems. Actual fluid and electrolyte imbalances are most likely to cause altered cognitive functioning or imbalances of intake and output. The patient can provide information regarding significant differences from their normal patterns of intake or output. It is helpful to validate subjective data with objective information gained through the physical assessment and the evaluation of laboratory test results before an actual diagnosis is made.

Objective Data

In addition to gathering subjective data, the nurse also collects objective data concerning the patient's fluid and electrolyte status through physical assessment of the patient and reviewing laboratory tests results.

Physical Assessment

Objective data are obtained from all functional health patterns. Physical assessment data can be collected by assessing intake and output, body weight, vital signs, skin for turgor and hydration, edema, and fullness of neck and hand veins. More invasive assessment techniques include monitoring central venous pressure and pulmonary artery pressure.

Monitoring Intake and Output. Intake and output is an important assessment to help evaluate fluid and electrolyte status. The physician may order intake and output assessment (I & O) on a patient after surgery or when evaluation of medical problems such as congestive heart failure is necessary. Often it is the nurse who decides when it is important to monitor a patient's intake

and output. Guidelines that the nurse can use include when fluid intake or urinary output is less than normal, when abnormal losses are occurring such as from a surgical drain or vomiting, when intravenous therapy is being administered, when the patient has medical problems that affect fluid or electrolyte status, and when the patient is not physiologically stable, such as after surgery or trauma.

Intake measurements include oral and parenteral fluids. Oral fluids include any liquids ingested or any foods that will become liquid at room temperature. Jello, sherbert, popsicles, and ice cream are types of solid foods that should be included in intake and output. Puréed food is not considered fluid intake. Other oral intake includes feedings delivered via any tube that enters the body (e.g., a nasogastric tube going into the stomach through the nose; a jejunostomy tube entering the jejunum through the abdomen; or a gastrostomy tube entering the stomach through the abdomen). Parenteral intake includes any intravenous fluids, intravenous medications, and any blood products administered.

Output measurements include urine, liquid stool, vomit, drainage from a wound or operative site (e.g., chest tube, hemovac drain), and drainage from a nasogastric tube. Diaphoresis or drainage on a dressing cannot be precisely measured, but if they are excessive their presence can be noted without an exact value for output.

Intake and output is recorded on a graphic sheet, which is individualized for each agency. Most forms permit the nurse to list the intake and output and obtain subtotals for each shift and a total for the entire 24-hour period (see the display). Some agencies also have worksheets that can be posted on the patient's door or on the bathroom door to alert all staff that the patient is on I & O. The cubic centimeter (cc) or milliliter (mL) is the standard of measurement, rather than household measures such as cups or ounces. One cubic centimeter is equal to 1 mL, and there is approximately 30 mL in a fluid ounce.

Intake measurements are often obtained by knowing the standard measurements of containers. Often, what is normal for the agency will be printed on the I & O sheet as a handy reference for the nurse. For example, when a milk carton contains 240 mL and the patient drinks half of the milk, 120 mL is recorded on the I & O sheet. It is important to include all intake. Sips of water taken during the day can add up to significant intake, as can oral medications, such as antacids, that are given frequently. Ice chips should be recorded as approximately half their volume.

Urine output is measured every time the patient voids. Toilet paper should be kept separate from the urine to obtain accurate measurement. If the patient voids in a bedpan or a commode, the urine is transferred into a calibrated container so that a measurement can be obtained. If the patient is able to get up to the toilet, a measuring device (sometimes called a hat) is placed

Intake and Output Documentation Form

BED	DATE

INTAKE			OUT PUT					
TIME	PO/NG	AMOUNT	TIME	URINE	STOOL	EMESIS/GASTRIC	OTHER	OTHER
N I G H T								
NIGHT TOTAL ▶			NIGHT TOTAL					
D A Y								
DAY TOTAL ▶			DAY TOTAL					
E V E N I N G								
EVENING TOTAL ▶			EVENING TOTAL					

PT. I.D.

between the toilet seat and the toilet to collect the urine (Fig. 32-5). If a voiding cannot be measured, it is usually indicated on the I & O record (e.g., 320 mL plus incontinent × 1). If a patient has a Foley catheter, the collection bag is usually emptied and the urine is measured at the end of each shift unless the bag becomes full sooner.

Other drainage is also usually emptied and measured at the end of each shift.

In addition to measuring and recording intake and output, the nurse evaluates patterns and values that are outside the normal range. Intake and output should be roughly equal, as seen in Table 32-3. For an adult the

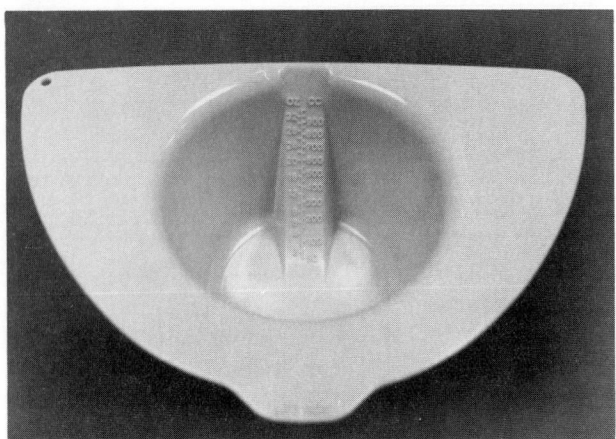

Figure 32–5. Urinary "hat" for measuring urine.

urinary output is usually 40 to 80 mL per hour, or approximately 1500 mL per day. Typically, the intake of fluid is 1300 mL per day. The reason there is a difference in intake and output is that water is also ingested in food. When a person has significant other losses (e.g., vomiting, diarrhea), it may also affect urinary output. Urine values less than 30 mL per hour are significant. If large discrepancies occur between intake and output, it is important to ascertain the accuracy of the data collected. Since many people may be responsible for recording I & O, some intake or output could inadvertently have not been recorded.

Body Weight. Assessing weight provides data concerning fluid balance. Rapid changes in weight are indicative of body fluid changes. Each kilogram of weight lost or gained equals approximately 1 L of fluid. A rapid loss of 2% of total body weight indicates a mild fluid deficit, whereas a rapid loss of 8% or more indicates a severe fluid deficit (Metheny, 1987).

Daily weights are often ordered for patients who are at risk for fluid problems. Weights should be measured at the same time of day (preferably in the morning before breakfast), with the patient wearing the same clothing, using the same scale, to ensure accuracy. If a patient is too ill or weak to stand to be weighed, a bedscale weight can be obtained. A bedscale is a portable scale on wheels onto which the patient can be transferred and weighed.

Often the nurse uses data from intake and output and daily weight together to assess for fluid imbalance. A decreasing output in conjunction with an increasing weight would indicate the patient is retaining fluid. A sudden weight loss with low urine output may indicate fluid volume deficit.

Integumentary Assessment. Changes in the skin and mucous membranes can indicate fluid imbalance. The general appearance of the skin is important to note.

Flushed, dry skin may signal a fluid volume deficit. Lack of tearing or perspiration is also important to note. Since the composition of the eyes is primarily water, eyes that appear sunken and feel soft to the touch indicate a fluid deficit.

A lack of moisture of the mucous membranes of the mouth may indicate a water or sodium imbalance. Dry mucous membranes can also be caused by mouth breathing. If lack of moisture is detected when a finger is inserted between the cheek and gum, this is probably due to a fluid or electrolyte imbalance. Deep furrows or ridges in the tongue can also occur in fluid deficits.

Decreased skin turgor can accompany volume deficits. Turgor refers to the elastic quality of the skin. When the skin is pinched and released, it should immediately return to its normal position. Skin turgor can be assessed by pinching the skin over the sternum, inner aspects of the thighs, and forearm. If the skin flattens slowly after a pinch, there is poor skin turgor. It should be noted that poor skin turgor is common in older individuals due to changes in the elasticity of their skin (Fig. 32-6).

Edema, or the excessive accumulation of interstitial fluid, can also be detected on examining the skin. This collection of interstitial fluid can occur in various parts of the body, such as around the eyes, around the sacrum, in the extremities, or other dependent parts of the body. Before edema is apparent, 5 to 10 pounds of excessive body fluid must be present. Edema is best assessed by pressing a finger over tissues. Edema is measured by the use of + signs, ranging from + (1+) to + + + + (4+). One + indicates edema that is just perceptible (2 mm); + + and + + + indicate moderate edema (4 to 6 mm); and + + + + indicates severe edema (8 mm or more). Pitting edema occurs when an indentation remains in the skin (often for 15 to 30 seconds) after a finger presses into edematous tissue. Pitting edema is not apparent until there is approximately a 10% increase in body weight. Edema may also be evaluated by measuring the circumference of body parts (e.g., leg or abdomen). If the circumference is measured at the same location with the same technique, an increase in circumference would indicate increased fluid in the interstitial space. Accumulation of fluid in the abdominal cavity (ascites) is often evaluated in this manner.

Vital Signs. Vital signs are important parameters to monitor and detect potential fluid, electrolyte, and acid–base imbalance. Variations in vital signs have been discussed under "Manifestations of Fluid, Electrolyte, and Acid–Base Balance."

Neck Veins. Distention of neck veins accompanies fluid overload. The jugular veins are visible in the neck. Changes in jugular vein distention can indicate alterations in fluid volume. To assess jugular vein distention, the nurse should place the patient in a sitting position with the head elevated to a 30- to 45-degree angle. The neck should be straight in alignment with the body. With the patient in this position, the distention within the jugular vein should not extend more than 2 cm above the sternal angle (angle of Louis). An increase in fluid volume may be indicated by distention of the neck veins from the top portion of the sternum to the angle of the jaw.

Hand Veins. Assessment of peripheral veins, such as those in the hand, may also be helpful in evaluating a patient's fluid status. To assess hand veins, the nurse should elevate the patient's hands for about 3 to 5 seconds. Normally, the veins empty and appear flattened. The hands should then be placed in a dependent position. Normally, the veins become distended within 3 to 5 seconds. If the veins take longer than 5 seconds to fill when in the dependent position, this may indicate a fluid volume deficit. If the veins take longer than 5 seconds to empty when elevated, this may indicate a fluid volume excess.

Central Venous Pressure. Central venous pressure is a more accurate method of evaluating fluid status than visually inspecting distention within veins of the body. The central venous pressure is the pressure of the right atrium or vena cava. The normal pressure is approximately 4 to 11 cm of water. An increase in the pressure may indicate an excessive amount of fluid volume, as seen in congestive heart failure. A decrease in pressure may indicate a deficiency of fluid volume.

Pulmonary Artery Pressure. Evaluating pulmonary artery pressure (PAP) is a more precise method of evaluating fluid status than central venous pressure monitoring. Pulmonary artery pressure is measured by using a catheter placed through the right heart into the pulmonary artery. Normal pulmonary artery pressure is

$$\frac{20 \text{ to } 30 \text{ mm Hg}}{8 \text{ to } 15 \text{ mm Hg}}$$

Low PAP readings correspond to volume deficits, and elevated PAP readings correspond to fluid excess. Monitoring pulmonary artery pressures is an invasive procedure and needs to be limited to critical care situations.

Bowel Assessment. Bowel elimination is also important to consider in detecting fluid and electrolyte imbalances. Fluid volume deficits often are accompanied with hard, dry stool as the body attempts to conserve needed fluid. Since diarrhea predisposes an individual to fluid and electrolyte disorders, any diarrhea should be evaluated carefully. Bowel tones should be assessed and hypoactive or hyperactive bowel sounds noted. Hyperactive bowel sounds or the presence of diarrhea can occur with a sodium deficit or a potassium excess. Abdominal distention, hypoactive bowel tones, or a paralytic ileus, can accompany a potassium deficit.

Laboratory and Diagnostic Tests

The nurse uses laboratory data to assist in the early identification and the continuous monitoring of fluid and electrolyte imbalances. Trends revealed in laboratory data are more significant than any single value. The nurse should be familiar with serum electrolyte values, hematocrit, serum or urine osmolality, urine specific gravity, and arterial blood gases. Information from these laboratory tests can help the nurse individualize his or her plan of care.

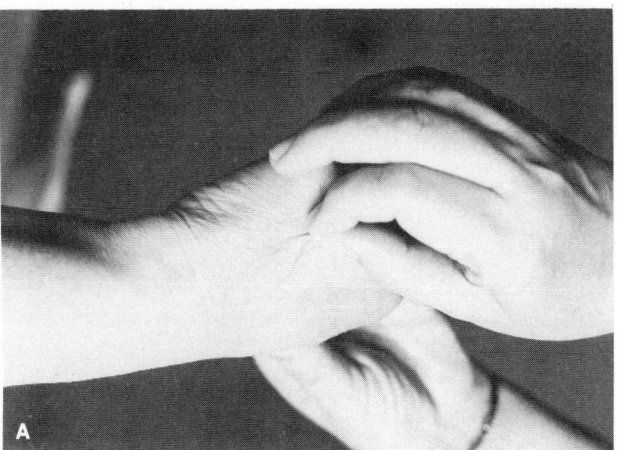 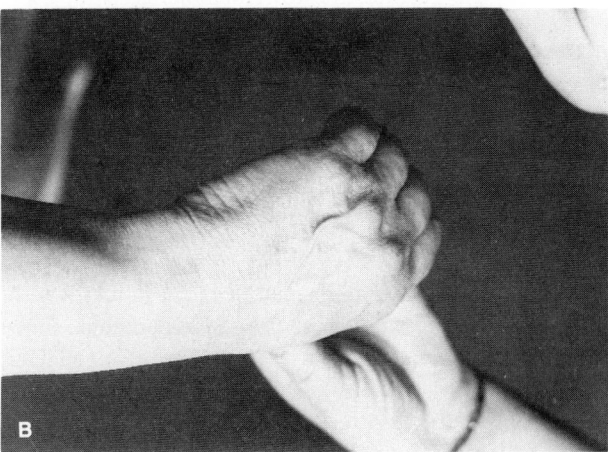

Figure 32–6. Assessing for skin turgor. Normally, when the skin is pinched it will return immediately to its natural state. When there is fluid loss, however, the skin is not elastic and does not return to normal as quickly.

Serum Electrolytes. Monitoring serum electrolyte values permits the nurse to evaluate trends and assess whether electrolyte imbalances are improving or getting worse. Electrolytes are usually obtained and evaluated in groups rather than singularly. Two standardized groupings are common. A profile including serum calcium, carbon dioxide, chloride, phosphate, magnesium, potassium, and sodium may be ordered to help screen electrolyte abnormalities. A more comprehensive profile that also includes other blood components such as glucose, blood urea nitrogen, creatinine, and protein (total, albumin globulin [A/G] ratio) can be helpful in evaluating the total fluid and electrolyte status. Normal reference values for each blood chemistry are found in Appendix B. Since venous blood samples are used to measure the quantity of electrolytes, serum electrolyte values reflect amounts within extracellular fluid.

Serum Osmolality. Serum osmolality can be obtained with a venous blood sample. Normal osmolality is 280 to 300 mOs/kg. Serum osmolality is decreased in water excess and elevated in water deficit.

The nurse may double the serum sodium to obtain a rough approximation of serum osmolarity. If necessary, the nurse is able to more accurately calculate serum osmolality by using the following formula: $2 \times$ plasma sodium concentration + blood glucose divided by 18. Although urea contributes to the absolute value of the serum osmolality, it is not used in the calculation because it is permeable to cell membranes and will not act to hold water within either compartment.

Urine Osmolality. Urine osmolality measures the solute concentration of the urine. Increasing the amount of nitrogenous wastes such as urea, creatinine, and uric acid will elevate the urinary osmolarity. The circulating amount of ADH will affect urine osmolality. Normal urine osmolality ranges from 50 to 1200 mOsm/kg, with an average being 550 mOsm/kg. The more concentrated the urine, the greater the urine osmolality.

Specific Gravity. Specific gravity measures the weight of a substance compared to an equal part of water. The specific gravity of water is 1.000. With normal fluid intake, urine specific gravity is usually 1.010 to 1.020. A higher specific gravity is obtained when the urine is concentrated, whereas a lower specific gravity is obtained when the urine is dilute.

Hematocrit. Hematocrit measures the percentage of whole blood that is composed of red blood cells. Since the hematocrit evaluates the relationship between RBCs and plasma, an increase or decrease in either red blood cells or plasma will affect the hematocrit. Loss of red blood cells, as occurs in hemorrhage, will lower hematocrit, whereas conditions that increase red blood cell production, such as polycythemia, will increase hematocrit. Alteration in fluid balance can also alter hema-

tocrit. Fluid deficit will increase hematocrit, whereas fluid excess will decrease hematocrit.

Arterial Blood Gases. Arterial blood gases measure the pH, the partial pressure of carbon dioxide ($PaCO_2$), the partial pressure of oxygen (PaO_2), the bicarbonate (HCO_3^-), and the oxygen saturation of hemoglobin (O_2 sat) found in arterial blood. Arterial blood gases are used to evaluate the acid–base balance in the body and adequate pulmonary function. A pH below 7.35 indicates acidosis, whereas a pH greater than 7.45 indicates alkalosis. Normal ranges for other blood gas values are given in Table 32-4.

NURSING DIAGNOSES AND PATIENT GOALS

Using information gathered in the assessment, the nurse is able to identify actual or potential fluid and electrolyte problems. Two nursing diagnoses related to fluid and electrolyte disturbances have been accepted by NANDA, namely, Fluid Volume Deficit and Fluid Volume Excess. Fluid Volume Excess or Fluid Volume Deficit can be actual or potential nursing diagnoses. Fluid and electrolyte imbalance can also cause other related potential or actual problems for the patient.

Diagnostic Statement: Fluid Volume Deficit

Definition

Fluid volume deficit is the state in which an individual experiences vascular, cellular, or intracellular dehydration (NANDA, 1990).

Defining Characteristics

Change in urine output; change in urine concentration; sudden weight loss; decreased venous filling; hemoconcentration; change in serum sodium.

Hypotension; thirst; increased pulse rate; decreased skin turgor; decreased pulse volume/pressure; change in mental state; increased body temperature; dry skin; dry mucous membranes; weakness (NANDA, 1990).

Related Factors

Active fluid volume loss; failure of regulatory mechanisms (NANDA, 1990).

Diagnostic Statement: Fluid Volume Excess

Definition

Fluid volume excess is the state in which an individual experiences increased fluid retention and edema (NANDA, 1990).

Defining Characteristics

Edema; effusion; anasarca (generalized, massive edema); weight gain; shortness of breath; orthopnea; intake greater than output; S/3 heart sound; pulmonary congestion (chest x-ray); abnormal breath sounds, rales (crackles); change in respiratory pattern; change in mental status; decreased hemoglobin and hematocrit; blood pressure changes; central venous pressure changes; pulmonary artery pressure changes; jugular vein distention; positive hepatojugular reflux (distention of the jugular vein induced by pressure over the liver); oliguria; specific gravity changes; azotemia (presence of urea or other waste products of nitrogen metabolism in the blood); altered electrolytes; restlessness and anxiety (NANDA, 1990).

Related Factors

Compromised regulatory mechanism; excess fluid intake; excess sodium intake (NANDA, 1990).

Related Nursing Diagnoses

Many other nursing diagnoses can be present in patients with fluid and electrolyte imbalances. Related nursing diagnoses can be actual or potential, and early identification permits the nurse to intervene successfully. Self-Care Deficit or Activity Intolerance can occur if fatigue, weakness, or muscular irritability are present. High Risk for for Injury can occur if electrolyte or fluid imbalances cause postural hypotension, loss of consciousness, or impaired cognition. Impaired Skin Integrity is frequently associated with edema, and either constipation or diarrhea is often associated with fluid or electrolyte imbalances. Knowledge Deficit or Noncompliance can occur when new treatment regimes are instituted without adequate patient teaching.

Patient Goals

The nurse and patient work together to set realistic, individualized goals. Patient goals should include:

The patient will reestablish normal fluid and electrolyte balance.
The patient will demonstrate knowledge regarding how to promote future fluid and electrolyte balance.
The patient will have an absence of complications from fluid or electrolyte imbalance.

The nurse and patient can work together to determine specific outcome criteria to individualize the plan of care. Short-term goals, such as the patient will increase fluid intake to 2000 mL per 24 hours, may be easy to reach within a short period of time. Other goals may involve changes in long-established dietary patterns, which may take much longer to achieve.

IMPLEMENTATION

Nursing intervention is important in preventing and promoting adequate fluid and electrolyte balance, as well as in treating imbalances as they occur. Patient teaching, assisting with fluid and dietary intake, and monitoring and managing intravenous infusion of fluids or blood are all important nursing interventions to promote optimal fluid and electrolyte balance.

Nursing Interventions to Promote Health and Function

Teaching people in the community, or people seeking assistance within the health-care system, is an important nursing role to prevent fluid and electrolyte problems from occurring. Nurses can help people understand how fluid and electrolyte imbalances occur and how they can be prevented.

Teaching can occur in a variety of settings and for all age groups. The nurse who interacts with new parents should stress fluid needs of the newborn, how quickly serious problems can develop if the infant should develop vomiting, diarrhea, or a fever, and symptoms that warrant contacting a physician. Follow-up teaching can occur as the child grows, explaining normal fluid requirements and dietary patterns. When the child is ill, the nurse can explain measures to help the parents adequately hydrate the child. Balanced electrolyte solutions are available commercially. Ice pops and other frozen treats may be helpful in encouraging fluid intake in the reluctant child.

The school nurse can reinforce teaching in health classes. Often school-age children are involved in sports activities. Encouraging adequate fluid intake after strenuous exercise is important. The dangers of fad diets and eating disorders should be discussed, especially among adolescents.

Nurses who work in industry should be aware of working conditions that could affect fluid and electrolyte balance. When employees must work in hot, humid environments performing strenuous exercise, periodic breaks should be scheduled so that adequate fluid replacement is possible. The nurse may be influential in supporting policies and legislation to ensure such practices.

Health teaching is especially important among the elderly. Classes can be offered in senior citizen centers or community agencies to reinforce good diet and fluid requirements. Often older individuals are taking medications, such as diuretics, that can affect fluid and electrolyte balance. Teaching is important to ensure patient compliance and help prevent any problems that can occur with treatment. Patients can be taught to detect signs of fluid and electrolyte imbalance such as rapid weight gain or loss, swelling, changes in normal urine output, muscle weakness, or abnormal skin sensation, and they can be given guidelines for when to notify a physician.

Nursing Interventions for Altered Fluid and Electrolyte Status

Planned nursing interventions are important in promoting optimum fluid and electrolyte balance. The nurse must individualize his or her approach for specific patients, considering their current condition.

Oral Fluids

Depending on the patient's current status, oral fluids may need to be regulated. The nurse may determine this from his or her own nursing assessment and nursing diagnosis. If the nurse has identified a potential or actual fluid volume deficit, he or she will want to institute a plan to increase oral fluid intake, whereas if the nursing diagnosis is potential or actual fluid volume excess, the nurse will want to curtail oral intake. The physician may also order that fluids be restricted or encouraged.

Increasing Oral Fluids. "Force fluids" or "push fluids" are general terms used to designate that increased fluid intake is required. Individual goals should be set for each patient, depending on the current fluid status. To help ensure patient compliance, it should be explained why the increased fluid intake is desirable, and the patient should help set individual goals for fluid intake. Patient teaching and goal-setting may include the family if the patient is unable or reluctant to drink fluids independently. The nurse should encourage the family members to offer sips of water continually during their visit and record how much the patient was able to drink on the I & O sheet.

Fluids should always be kept within the patient's reach. Bedside water pitchers should be changed frequently so that the water is cold and fresh. If the patient is unable to drink independently, the nurse should offer fluids and encouragement for drinking during every patient interaction. Some patients may verbally refuse fluids, but when the straw or glass is placed in their mouth and encouragement given they may decide to drink. Providing fluids that the patient especially likes may increase fluid intake. It is important to consider any dietary restrictions when providing patients with additional fluids. For example, a diabetic patient should have only sugar-free soft drinks, and a patient on a potassium-restricted diet should not be offered fluids high in potassium, such as orange juice. When making dietary choices, the nurse can encourages foods that have a high fluid content such as custards, soups, and ice creams.

When a specific fluid order is given (e.g., increase fluids to 2000 mL per 24 hours), the nurse should plan how much should be consumed in each shift. The bulk of fluids is usually consumed during the daytime and early evening hours. Large amounts of fluids taken close to bedtime may necessitate getting up to the bathroom during the night, consequently interrupting sleep.

Adequate fluid replacement is also necessary for patients who are receiving tube feedings. Frequently, these patients need additional water to prevent fluid volume deficits. They are often people who cannot independently drink when they are thirsty, or even notify the nurse of their thirst. For this reason, the nurse should assess carefully the fluid needs of patients receiving tube feedings, and fluids should be administered as needed.

Restricting Oral Fluids. Oral fluids may need to be restricted when fluid volume excess is present or when certain medical conditions occur, such as congestive heart failure or renal failure. Assisting the patient to comply with limited fluid intake despite thirst can be a challenge for the nurse.

Patient Teaching

- Drink plenty of fluids. At least six glasses of water should be encouraged.
- If you exercise vigorously, replenish both fluids and electrolytes with solutions such as Gator Ade.
- Increase fluid intake if you are experiencing increased loss of fluids through diarrhea, fever, or vomiting.
- Infants are especially susceptible to rapid and serious problems with fluid and electrolyte balance. Diarrhea and vomiting that is severe or lasts for more than 24 hours, should be reported to the physician.
- If you are on diuretics (except potassium-sparing diuretics), eat a banana a day or take potassium supplements as ordered by your physician.
- Follow the list of foods you should eat or should avoid for your specific electrolyte imbalance.
- Call the nurse if the IV site begins to hurt, or starts to swell, or if the bottle is almost empty.
- If you are ambulating with an IV, do not push the pole with the affected arm. Blood may back up the tubing if there is not enough distance between the infusion site and the IV bottle.
- If you are receiving a blood transfusion, notify the nurse if you feel hot, have chills, ache or develop a headache, develop a rash, have difficulty breathing, or develop low back pain.

The physician's orders for fluid restriction will include the number of milliliters of fluid to be taken per 24 hours. Most fluid restrictions include all fluids ingested. When a free water restriction is ordered, only free water is restricted, since other fluids, such as tomato juice or milk, contain sodium and would not contribute further to a sodium deficit.

The nurse and patient plan how to best allocate the allotted fluid during a 24-hour period. Some patients prefer to drink fluids with their meals, whereas others prefer to save fluids for between meals. Most fluids are designated for day and evening shifts, with usually about 100 mL left over for nights in case the patient should have to take medication or want a drink. Ice chips may be helpful for people on fluid restriction. Ice melts to one half its volume and should be noted as such on the intake and output record. Water pitchers may be removed from the room and water offered in small cups to avoid the temptation of drinking too much at one time. Diversional activities may also help the patient focus less on the thirst he or she is experiencing. Television may not be a good diversional activity since viewing many advertisements that promote various beverages may stimulate thirst.

To minimize thirst for patients on fluid restrictions, salty or very sweet fluids should be avoided. Gum and hard candy may temporarily relieve thirst by drawing fluid into the oral cavity because the sugar content increases oral tonicity. Fifteen to 30 minutes later, oral membranes may be even drier than before. To avoid this rebound effect, try to encourage sugar-free candy and gum. Dry foods such as crackers and bread may also increase the patient's feeling of thirst. Thirst may be decreased by allowing the patient to rinse his or her mouth frequently. A sip of water is taken, swished around the oral cavity, and then spit out before it is swallowed. Mouth washes containing alcohol should be avoided since they have a drying effect. Frequent oral care is necessary for anyone on a fluid restriction. Lips can be moistened with a water-soluble gel to prevent drying and cracking.

Electrolyte Replacement

From the nursing assessment, the nurse can identify those patients at risk for electrolyte deficit or excess. The nurse can help to promote optimum electrolyte balance by teaching the patient about which foods should be restricted or encouraged, and administering oral or intravenous electrolyte supplements.

Diet Teaching. Once the nurse has identified the potential for an electrolyte imbalance, a diet teaching plan can be individualized. The patient should be provided with a list of foods high in the identified electrolyte and given some guidelines for the amount to be consumed each day (Table 32–5). For example, for the patient who

has recently been ordered a thiazide (potassium-depleting) diuretic, the nurse may indicate that it is important to eat at least one banana or one other potassium-rich food each day.

Electrolyte Supplements. When normal dietary intake is not sufficient, electrolyte supplements can be administered orally or intravenously. The intravenous administration is usually reserved for severe electrolyte imbalances or when the patient is unable to take anything orally. Liquid oral potassium supplements are very foul-tasting and should be mixed with juice to promote compliance. Intravenous preparations of potassium must be administered carefully. Concentrated infusion could cause damage to the veins or cause rebound hyperkalemia, which is potentially dangerous.

Intravenous Therapy

Intravenous therapy is frequently used with hospitalized patients to prevent or treat fluid and electrolyte imbalances. The nurse is responsible for initiating, monitoring, and discontinuing the intravenous infusion. The type and amount of IV fluid and electrolyte replacement is ordered by the physician.

Purpose of Intravenous Therapy. Intravenous therapy is initiated for a variety of reasons, including: to provide the patient with fluids when adequate fluid in-

TABLE 32–5
Selected Dietary Sources for Electrolytes

Electrolyte	Dietary Source
Sodium (Na^+)	Salt (sodium chloride), monosodium glutamate (MSG), soy sauce, dairy products (milk, cheese), processed food (luncheon meats, bacon), snack foods (peanuts, chips, pretzels), boullion, canned or packaged soup, pickles, olives, sauerkraut, tomato juice
Potassium (K^+)	Fruits (banana, cantaloupe, apricots, peaches, dates, raisins), vegetables (avocado, navy beans, potatoes, squash, carrots, cauliflower), orange juice, tomato juice
Calcium (Ca^{++})	Dairy products (milk, cheese, yogurt, ice cream), dark green vegetables (broccoli, spinach, greens), sardines, salmon, oysters, tofu
Magnesium (MG^{++})	Nuts and peanut butter, egg yolk, milk, whole grain cereals, bananas, citrus fruit, dark green vegetables, legumes, seafood

take cannot be obtained through oral intake; to provide the patient with electrolytes to maintain normal electrolyte balance; to provide the patient with glucose to use as an energy source; to provide an access route to administer medications intravenously; to provide a venous access to administer blood products; and to provide a venous access so that treatment can be administered promptly if an emergency situation should occur.

Types of Intravenous Solutions. Intravenous solutions can be isotonic, hypotonic, or hypertonic depending on the tonicity of the fluid. Specific patient fluid and electrolyte needs will determine which solution is ordered.

Isotonic fluids are solutions that have the same osmotic pressure as that found within the cell. Isotonic fluids are used to expand the intravascular compartment and thus increase circulating volume. Because these solutions do not alter serum osmolarity, interstitial and intracellular compartments remain unchanged. An isotonic solution would be helpful for hypotension caused by hypovolemia. Examples of an isotonic solution include normal saline (0.9% NaCl) and lactate Ringers.

Hypotonic fluids are solutions that have less osmotic pressure than the cell. When a hypotonic solution is infused, it lowers serum osmolarity, causing body fluids to shift out of the blood vessels and into the cells and interstitial space. For this reason, hypotonic fluids are administered when a patient needs cellular hydration. Half normal saline (0.45 NaCl) is an example of a hypotonic solution. Five percent dextrose in water, although an isotonic solution before administration, quickly becomes a hypotonic solution once in the body, as the dextrose is quickly metabolized, leaving only the water.

Hypertonic fluids are solutions that have greater osmotic pressure than the cell. When a hypertonic solution is infused, it raises serum osmolarity, pulling fluid from the cells and the interstitial tissues into the vascular space. Hypertonic solutions are often administered to the postoperative patient to maintain circulating volume and prevent edema. Examples of hypertonic solutions include 5% dextrose in normal saline, 5% dextrose in half normal saline, and 5% dextrose in lactate Ringers.

Equipment for Intravenous Infusion. A variety of equipment is available to provide intravenous therapy to patients. Brands may vary slightly among different manufacturers. Intravenous set-ups contain the following: an access device that gains entry to a vein; a bag or bottle containing the IV solution; and tubing that connects the IV bag with the access device (Fig. 32-7). Intravenous equipment is sterile, and sterility is maintained during use to prevent potentially life-threatening infection.

Access devices most commonly used for peripheral intravenous therapy include butterfly needles and over-the-needle catheters (angiocatheters) (Fig. 32-8). Butterfly needles are short, beveled needles with plastic flaps; they often are used for short-term therapy or when

therapy is given to a child or infant. Butterfly needles are also referred to as scalp vein needles. Angiocatheters are plastic catheters that are placed over metal stylets. The metal stylet is used to pierce the skin and enter the vein, after which the plastic catheter is threaded into the vein and the metal stylet is removed. Both types of devices come in a variety of sizes. The lumen size is measured in gauges, the most common adult sizes being 22, 20, and 18. As the numbers increase the lumen size decreases; thus a 22-gauge needle is smaller in diameter than an 18-gauge needle.

Intravenous therapy is sometimes administered through large, central veins of the body, most commonly the subclavian. When central access is necessary, an inside-the-needle catheter (intracatheter) may be used (see Fig. 32-8). In these devices the plastic catheter is inserted through the needle, the needle is pulled back, encased in a plastic sleeve, and fastened outside the infusion site. When intravenous therapy is needed over a long period of time, a more permanent type of silicone catheter can be used. Hickman or Broviac are two common brand names of these catheters. The catheters are approximately 90 cm in length and contain a Dacron cuff. They are tunneled through subcutaneous tissue and placed into the subclavian vein (Fig. 32-9). Eventually, fibrous tissue grows around the Dacron cuff, which stabilizes it in place, decreases infection rates, and permits usage as a long-term venous access route.

Containers for IV fluid include glass bottles and plastic bags. Plastic bags have become increasingly popular over the last 10 years because they require less room for storage and eliminate the potential dangers of breakage. Plastic bags collapse as they empty and therefore require no vent to equalize pressure. The amount of fluid remaining in the bag may be difficult to measure accurately, however, because of the semirigid nature of the bag. One other disadvantage of plastic bags is that certain drugs (e.g,. insulin) bind with the plastic, making IV administration of these drugs with plastic bags difficult.

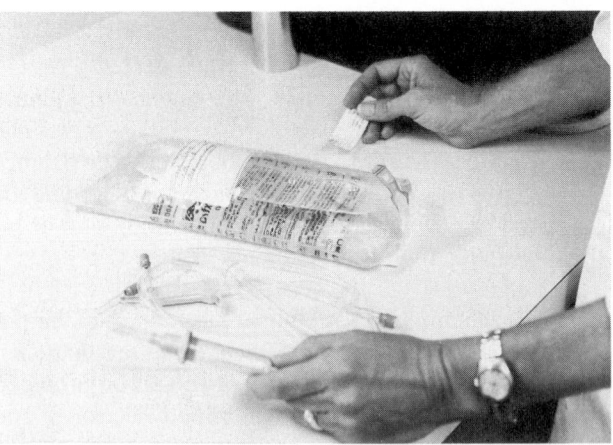

Figure 32–7. Intravenous bag and tubing.

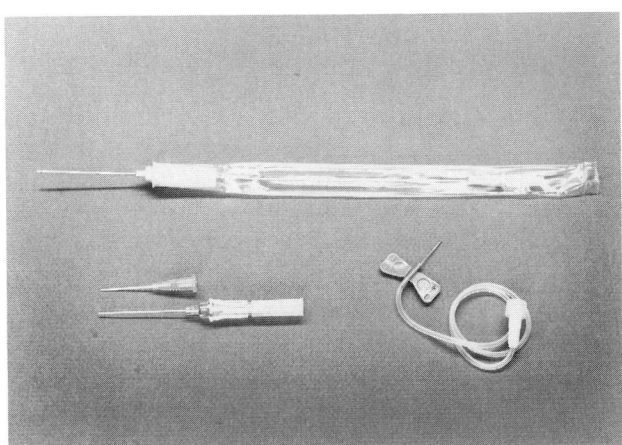

Figure 32–8. Intravenous access devices: butterfly (bottom right), angiocatheter (bottom left), and intracatheter (top).

Both bottles and bags come in a variety of sizes. Usually 1000-mL containers are used for normal hydration purposes. Smaller bags (e.g., 500 mL) may be used for children or when fluid is infusing at a very slow rate. Smaller containers (50, 100, or 250 mL) are often used to dilute and dispense medications.

Intravenous tubing connects the IV bag or bottle to the access device (Fig. 32-10). Normally, IV tubing includes the following features:

The spike, which permits the tubing to access the IV container.

The filter, which traps any particles and prevents their entry into the patient's blood stream.

The drip chamber, which allows the nurse to visualize and count the drops of IV fluid as they enter the system.

Roller or slide clamps, which permit regulation of flow rate.

Injection sites or ports, which permit the administration of medications, blood products, or other IVs.

Tubing.

A needle adaptor for connection to the needle or angiocatheter.

In addition to these features, a vent must also be included in the tubing when an unvented bottle system is used.

Individual manufacturers produce tubing with different drip rates. Two general classification of tubing are Macrodrip and Minidrip (Fig. 32-11). Macrodrip tubing delivers 10, 15, or 20 drops per mL, depending on the manufacturer. Minidrip tubing delivers 60 drops per mL. Macrodrip tubing is generally used for adult patients, especially when large volume replacement may be required (e.g., during surgery). Minidrip tubing is used for infants, children, or when fluids are infused slowly.

Venipuncture. Venipuncture is the technique that permits access to a vein so that a needle or catheter can be inserted. Venipuncture is a sterile procedure since the integrity of the skin is broken. In most hospitals, it is the nurse who is responsible for starting intravenous therapy in this manner. In some agencies, a special IV team is responsible for all IV starts, and, in some cases, general IV maintenance. The IV team is usually composed of nurses with training and much experience with veni-

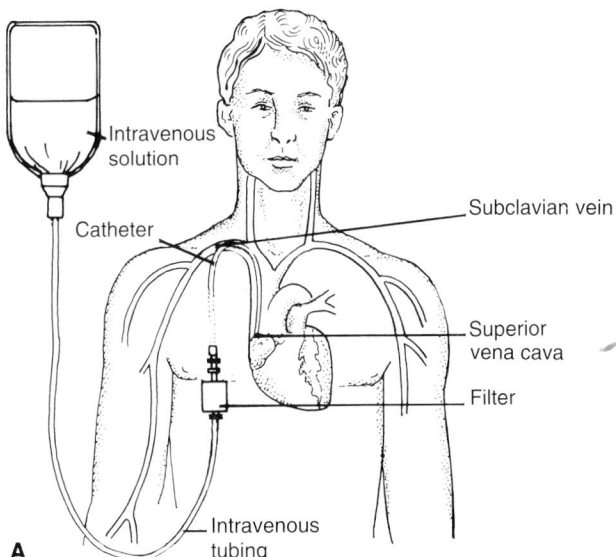

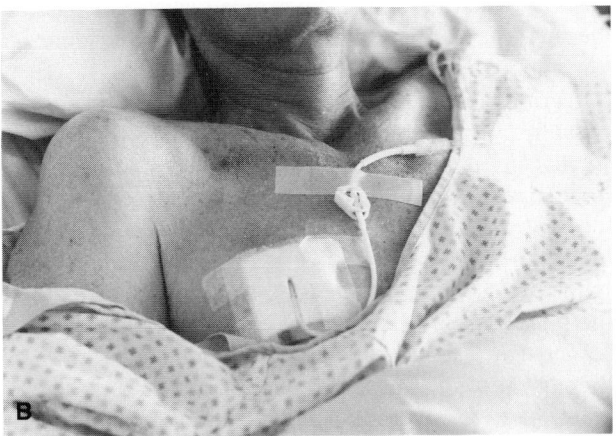

Figure 32–9. Central line catheter. **A:** Placement of catheter into subclavian vein. **B:** Patient with Hickman line in place.

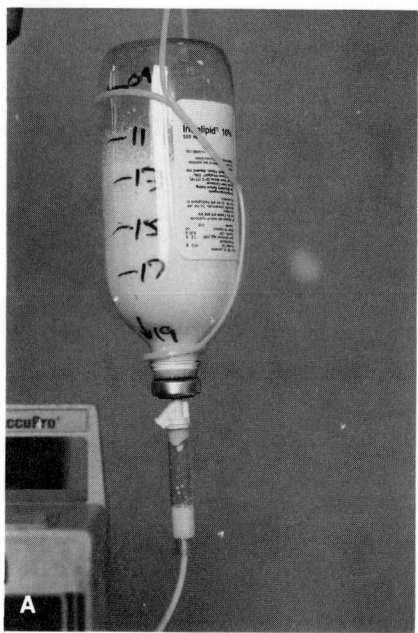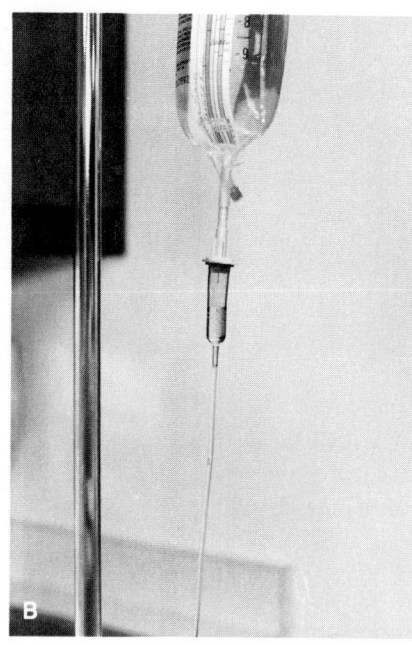

Figure 32–10. Intravenous tubing. **A:** Vented tubing. **B:** Unvented tubing.

puncture. In hospitals that do not employ IV teams, nurses are usually certified in venipuncture technique. Only physicians insert central venous catheters.

In the adult, the veins of the hand and forearm are commonly used for intravenous infusion. When the basilic or cephalic vein is used, the ulna and radius act as natural splints, which allows the patient greater freedom of movement. Any vein selected should be free of sclerosis, pain, or hematomas. Whenever possible, larger veins are used. The distal portion of the vein is punctured first, leaving the more proximal sites for later venipunctures. Because infants and young children have very small veins, scalp veins in the temporal region are often used. Veins located directly over movable joints should be avoided because their use increases the possibility that the IV will dislodge and infiltrate. Veins of the lower extremities should be avoided whenever possible because they limit mobility and increase the incidence of thrombophlebitis.

Various techniques are employed to help locate and visualize veins before venipuncture. First, the nurse visually inspects the patient's veins, avoiding any areas that appear bruised or sclerosed. A tourniquet is placed on the extremity to distend the vein with blood. This will make the vein more visible and permit the needle to puncture the vein more easily. Additional tips that can help fill veins are to lower the extremity below the level of the heart, to ask the patient to open and close his or her fist several times, to tap lightly over the selected vein, or to use warm soaks for 5 minutes before venipuncture to vasodilate the selected vessel.

Adequate site preparation is necessary to avoid infection. Hair around the site may be clipped. Shaving is avoided because small microscopic nicks or abrasions can provide entry for microorganisms. The site is prepared with 70% alcohol or a povidine–iodine (Betadine) solution. Povidine–iodine is a better bactericide, but some people are allergic to it. Gloves should be worn by the nurse during this procedure because contamination with the patient's blood is a possibility.

All equipment should be assembled prior to attempting venipuncture. Tape is cut and all equipment placed within reach. To insert the needle, stretch the skin taut over the vein with the thumb and index finger. Hold the needle with the bevel up and enter the skin at a 45-degree angle. As the skin is pierced, decrease the angle of the needle to 30 degrees. This will permit entry into the vein at an angle and decrease the likelihood of accidentally puncturing the opposite vein wall. Insert the needle one-half inch into the vein. A blood return will ensure access to the vein. When using an angiocatheter, the plastic catheter must be threaded into the vein. When placement of the needle or catheter in the vein is assured, attach the tubing and release the tourniquet. Loop the tubing and anchor well, using tape and a transparent dressing, over the infusion site. Adjust the infusion according to the prescribed rate.

Monitoring Intravenous Infusions. The nurse is responsible for monitoring intravenous infusion to ensure that the fluid infuses at the proper rate and that complications of intravenous therapy are detected promptly. (See Procedure 32-1, Monitoring an Intravenous Infusion.)

Calculating flow rate is the first step in ensuring the proper infusion of IV fluids. After the administration set

PROCEDURE 32–1. Monitoring an Intravenous Infusion

■ Purpose
1. Provide a dependable, patent route for infusion of intravenous therapy.
2. Protect the patient from introduction of air or microorganisms into the vascular system.

■ Assessment
- Review patient's chart for diagnosis and medical plan for intravenous therapy.
- Assess patient's treatment schedule to identify times for drug administrations and laboratory sampling.
- Assess patient for clinical signs of fluid or electrolyte imbalances.

■ Equipment
May need:
   3 mL sterile syringe.
   Heparinized NaCl.
   Sterile NaCl.
   Alcohol or Betadine wipe (according to hospital policy).
   Clean, disposable gloves.
   Dressing supplies.

■ Procedure
1. Compare intravenous fluid currently infusing with the ordered solution.
   Rationale: Ensures prompt recognition and correction of errors.
2. Inspect the rate of flow at least every hour. Check actual flow rate for 15 seconds and compare with prescribed rate of flow (see Fig. 32-12). If the infusion is ahead of schedule, slow it so the infusion will complete at the planned time. If infusion is behind schedule, review hospital policy before increasing flow rate. Many agencies require a physician's order to increase the rate of flow.
   Rationale: Intravenous therapies that are not on schedule can be detrimental to the patient. Fluids that are infused too rapidly may cause circulatory overload with resultant pulmonary edema and cardiac failure. Fluids that are behind schedule deliver insufficient fluids and nutrients.
3. Inspect the system for leakage and, if present, locate the source. Tighten all connections within the system. If leak is still present, slow IV flow rate to keep vein open and replace tubing with sterile set.
   Rationale: Intravenous therapy is a sterile procedure. A break or leak in the tubing allows microorganisms to enter and contaminate the entire system.
4. Inspect the tubing for kinks or blockages. The tubing should be loosely coiled and placed on the bed.

Rationale: Blockages in the tubing impede the flow of solution and the patient may not receive the necessary fluids and nutrients.
5. Observe the fluid level in the drip chamber. If it is less than half full, squeeze the chamber gently to allow more fluid in.
   Rationale: If the fluid level in the drip chamber is too low, turbulence from the fluid dripping into the chamber may create air bubbles that may enter the tubing.
6. Inspect the infusion site for infiltration. This occurs when the needle becomes dislodged from the vein and intravenous fluid flows into the interstitial tissue. The signs of infiltration are: decreased rate of flow, swelling, pallor, coolness, and discomfort at or above the needle insertion site. If present, the IV site must be changed. If a large amount of fluid infiltrated, elevate the arm above the heart on several pillows.
   Rationale: Prompt detection is important to promote patient comfort and permit early treatment. Elevation facilitates venous and lymphatic drainage.
7. Inspect arm above the insertion site for phlebitis, inflammation of the vein. This may occur as a result of trauma or chemical irritation secondary to intravenous additives or solution pH. The signs of phlebitis include: redness, swelling, warmth and pain along the vein above the IV insertion site. If present, the IV must be discontinued and restarted in another area.
8. Inspect the insertion site for bleeding.
9. Monitoring intravenous therapy is a nursing responsibility but if the patient is able to comply, teach him or her to contact the nurse if:
   - The flow rate changes suddenly.
   - The fluid container is almost empty.
   - Blood is in the tubing.
   - The site becomes uncomfortable.
10. Chart any findings indicating complications of intravenous therapy (e.g., infiltration).

■ Lifespan Considerations

Infants and Children
- Children change position frequently and their tubing can easily become kinked or disconnected. Taping all connections and protecting the insertion site with a medicine cup and rigid arm board may prolong the efficacy of the IV.

Additional
- Armboards and soft wrist restraints or mitt restraints may be used to protect the IV site in any

(continued)

PROCEDURE 32-1. Monitoring an Intravenous Infusion *continued*

patient, regardless of age, who is at risk for purposefully disrupting the intravenous system.

■ Home Care Modifications
- Patient or caregiver must be taught to:
  - Inspect the insertion site at least four times daily through the transparent dressing.
  - Assess for infiltration, phlebitis, or obvious dis-

lodged catheter. If any of these situations occur, caregiver should clamp the IV tubing, remove the catheter, and call the nurse.
- Observe flow rate for sluggishness or lack of dripping. Should this occur, caregiver should open roller clamp and look for kinked tubing. If problem continues, contact health-care provider.

---

is selected or known, the drip rate of the infusion can be calculated from the physician's order using the following formula:

$$\text{Drops/minute} = \frac{\text{Total volume infused} \times \text{drop factor}}{\text{Total time for infusion in minutes}}$$

The size of the drop that the administration set creates is known as the drop factor, which can be found on the packaging of the administration set. This factor may change with different manufacturers, since macrotubing can deliver 10, 15, or 20 drops per mL. To calculate the drip rate of an IV that is to infuse 1000 mL in 8 hours using tubing that has a drip factor of 10, the nurse would use the above formula, obtaining a rate of 20 to 21 drops per minute:

$$\text{Drops/minute} = \frac{1000 \times 10}{8 \text{ hr} \times 60} = \frac{10000}{480} = 21 \text{ drops/min}$$

Manual regulation of the infusion can be done once the IV drip rate has been calculated. The roller clamp is used to adjust the rate of flow. The nurse usually counts the drops as they fall into the drip chamber for 15 seconds. This number is multiplied by 4 to determine the drip rate for a full minute. The nurse then uses the roller clamp to adjust the flow rate until it corresponds with the prescribed rate of flow (Fig. 32-12).

A time strip, which can be made from adhesive tape or purchased commercially, can also help ensure accurate infusion of IV fluids. The time strip is placed along the IV bag or bottle next to the calibrated numbers that indicate the volume remaining in the container. The strip is marked in hourly increments, indicating where the fluid level will be at specific times. This device permits the nurse, at a glance, to assess when the IV is getting behind or ahead of schedule (Fig. 32-13). It is important that the nurse check IV infusions every hour to ensure proper infusion of fluid.

An IV pump or controller may be used to regulate accurately the infusion rate. This is especially useful if

Macro IV tubing

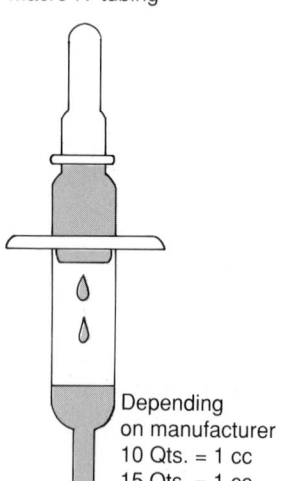

Depending on manufacturer
10 Qts. = 1 cc
15 Qts. = 1 cc
20 Qts. = 1 cc

A

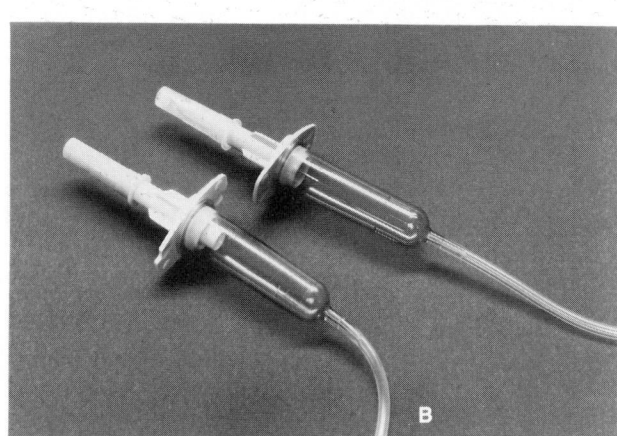

B

Micro IV tubing

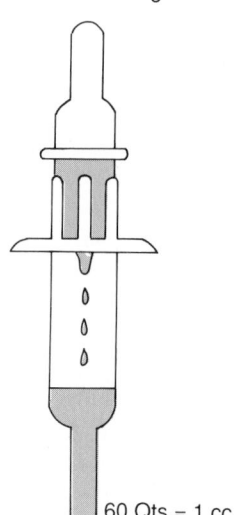

60 Qts.= 1 cc

Figure 32-11.   Microdrip IV tubing (60 drops per mL). Microdrip IV tubing (10, 15, 20 drops per mL).

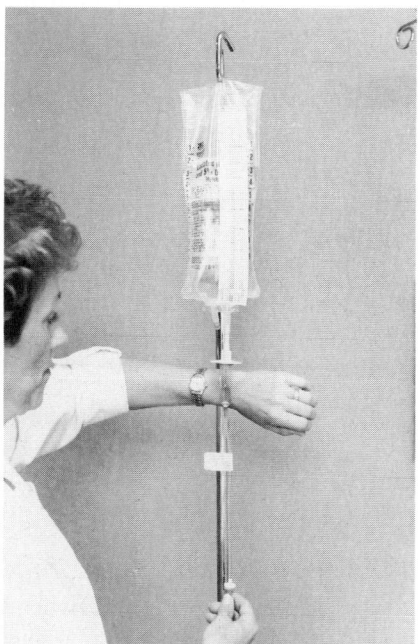

Figure 32–12.   Manual regulation of IV drip rate.

fluid administration must be watched very carefully, such as when infusing fluid to an infant or administering certain medications. A pump uses positive pressure to deliver the prescribed volume of fluid, whereas a controller depends on gravity to maintain a precise flow rate (Fig. 32-14).

The pump regulates the flow by volume, whereas the controller senses the drops infusing. Most newer models of pumps and controllers can be electronically programmed. The nurse enters the amount of fluid that is hung (e.g., 1000 mL) and the rate at which it is to infuse in cubic centimeters per hour. The machine displays how many cubic centimeters have infused and how many are remaining in the IV container at any given time.

Most regulating devices have alarms that indicate when fluid cannot be delivered at the prescribed rate for any reason (e.g., the bottle is empty, the tubing is kinked, air is in the line, or the vein is clogged). Infiltration will not necessarily trigger the alarm. The nurse can troubleshoot to identify the cause of the problem and correct it to ensure proper infusion of fluids. Since many different types and models of these devices are used, it is important that the nurse become knowledgeable and read specific operating guidelines for any machine that is used. Alarms must not be turned off until the underlying problem has been discovered.

Factors Affecting the Infusion Rate. Careful assessment of the intravenous infusion is necessary routinely after the IV is adjusted because many factors other than drip factor can affect the rate of infusion. Such factors as the height of the IV bottle, the position of the extremity, the position of the catheter within the vein, the patency

of the catheter, a constriction or kink in the tubing, and clogged air vents can affect the flow rate of an intravenous infusion.

Height of the IV bottle will affect the rate of infusion since IV infusions are affected by gravity. As the height of the bottle from the infusion site is increased, the gravitational force will be greater and the fluid will flow in faster. Conversely, as the distance between the bottle and IV site decreases, the fluid will infuse more slowly. This often can be seen when the patient gets up and walks in the hall, pushing his or her IV pole with the hand in which the IV is flowing; the drip rate slows and often stops altogether, and blood may flow back into the tubing. The nurse must watch for this and temporarily speed up the IV so that the infusion is not disrupted. After ambulation, the rate should be reregulated if necessary to prevent improper infusion of fluids.

The position of the extremity can also affect the infusion of fluid. As the extremity is elevated, the fluid will infuse more slowly. Also, bending the extremity at the wrist or the elbow, or leaning on the arm can slow the rate of infusion. Patients should be cautioned not to raise their arm over their head or sleep on the side where the IV is infusing.

Constriction or kinking of IV tubing can also contribute to altered flow rates. Tubing can become kinked if it is placed inadvertently under the patient. Tubing can also be obstructed if tape is applied too tightly, or if edema develops when the tape interferes with venous blood return in the extremity.

The position of the needle within the vein can also affect the rate of flow. Sometimes position changes can cause the needle bevel to rest against a vein wall; this is known as a positional IV. Care must be taken to frequently monitor an IV that appears to be positional. When the

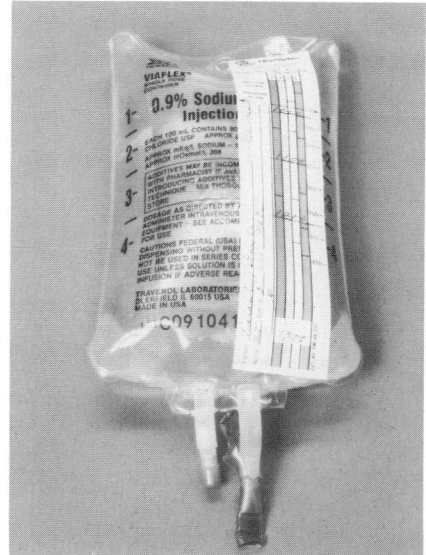

Figure 32–13.   IV time strip.

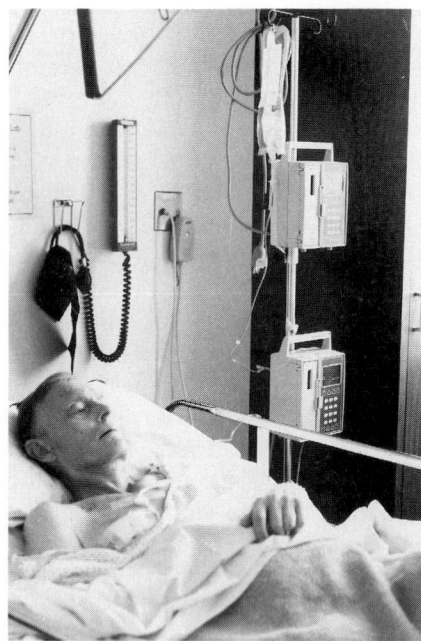

Figure 32–14. McGraw IV infusion pump.

IV slows down, the nurse should increase the rate, but if the patient moves again and the bevel becomes free of the vein wall, the rate of infusion will once again increase. Armboards are somewhat helpful in immobilizing joint movement and decreasing the chance of needle movement.

Patency of the catheter is also important to ensure proper infusion of fluids. A blood clot can form at the end of the catheter and stop the infusion. If the clot does not completely obstruct the lumen of the catheter, the flow rate may slow and become sluggish. Whenever flow of fluids is interrupted for any reason (e.g., bending at a joint, kinking of tubing, etc.), clotting can occur. This is often a problem when IVs are infusing very slowly to keep the vein open (TKO or KVO). When a KVO rate is ordered, the nurse often can periodically speed up the flow rate to flush the catheter and prevent clot formation (Metheny, 1987). If the flow has stopped completely, the catheter should never be irrigated since this pushes the clot into the circulation, which can cause an embolus or systemic infection. Some institutions support a policy of separating the tubing from the catheter and aspirating the clot with a syringe.

Clogged air vents can also slow the rate of IV flow. If the air vent on a solution bottle or volume control chamber should become clogged, fluid cannot leave the system because air is unable to enter to replace it. Changing the tubing may be necessary to correct this problem.

Changing IV Bottles and Tubing. The nurse is responsible for changing the IV bag or bottle as needed and changing IV tubing according to agency policy. The IV bag or bottle is changed when the previous container is empty, when there is a change in IV orders, or when the

IV container has been hanging for more than 24 hours.

All IV bag and tubing changes must be done under strict aseptic technique to prevent infection. Most agencies have policies that indicate the frequency and protocol for these procedures. (See Procedure 32-2, Changing Intravenous Solution and Tubing.)

Intravenous Site Care. Agency policies also specify expectations for site care. Semipermeable dressings are frequently used to cover the IV site. The nature of these dressings permits continual viewing of the site so that assessment can be made frequently (Fig. 32-15). These dressings also reduce the frequency of dressing changes and the incidence of infection. Some agencies still prefer gauze dressing for IV site care. Whenever site care is performed, the nurse must take extra care not to dislodge the catheter.

Complications of Intravenous Therapy. An important nursing responsibility is monitoring the patient for possible complications of intravenous therapy. The most significant complications of intravenous therapy include infiltration, phlebitis, infection, air embolism, and fluid overload.

Infiltration occurs when fluid enters the subcutaneous tissues. This can occur if the needle or catheter slips out of the vein or if intravenous fluid leaks from the vein into subcutaneous tissue. When infiltration occurs, the patient may complain of pain and have swelling around the infusion site, which usually becomes cool to the touch. When infiltration has occurred, the IV usually infuses more slowly because of the increased pressure within the subcutaneous tissues. Absence of blood return into the tubing as the IV bag is lowered below the level of the infusion supports the possibility that infiltration may have occurred. Absence of a blood return is not diagnostic, since some angiocatheters do not readily permit the back flow of blood, and the location of the bevel of the needle may also make back flow difficult. Nursing intervention when infiltration occurs is to discontinue the IV and restart it in a new location. Elevation and application of a warm soak may help reduce edema. The nurse should also consider prevention measures, such as stabilizing the joint with an armboard and making sure the needle or catheter is adequately secured.

Phlebitis refers to an inflammation of a vein. If a blood clot accompanies the inflammation, it is referred to as a thrombophlebitis. Factors that contribute to the development of a phlebitis include increased length of time the catheter is in a vein, infusion of irritating substances such as potassium chloride or antibiotics, and using small veins or veins of the lower extremities where blood flow is relatively sluggish. Clinical manifestations of phlebitis include complaints of discomfort and a vein that appears red and feels warm and hard (almost cordlike) when palpated. The IV will be sluggish, especially if a clot is

PROCEDURE 32-2. Changing Intravenous Solution and Tubing

■ Purpose
1. Maintain sterility of intravenous system.
2. Continue ordered therapeutic regimen.

■ Assessment
- Determine if intravenous catheter needs to be restarted in a new site.
  - It is recommended that periphral IV sites should be changed every 72 hours. Review the policy of your agency.
  - Inspect IV site for signs of infiltration, sluggish flow, or phlebitis.
- Determine what time next solution container is due. Prepare next solution 1 hour before it is due. Plan to change container when less than 50 mL remains.
- Review physician's orders for current intravenous fluid orders.
- Check label on currently infusing solution and tubing for the date and time they were hung.
  - IV solutions are not considered sterile if they are open longer than 24 hours.
  - It is recommended that IV tubing be changed every 48 hours to ensure sterility of system. Review the policy of your agency.
- Inspect intravenous system to determine type of tubing required. Many different administration sets are available. Some infusion pumps use specially designed cassette tubing. Review the policy of your agency.

■ Equipment
Sterile container of ordered amount and type of solution.

An appropriate sterile tubing administration set.

Adhesive tape or pre-marked strips for labeling and timing solution container and tubing.

Tape for securing tubing.

Clean, disposable gloves (for tubing change).

Dressing material and antiseptic solution if IV site dressing is to be changed. Follow agency procedure.

■ Procedure

Changing Solution Container
1. Wash hands.
2. Compare solution with physician orders.
3. Label solution container with patient's name, solution type, additives, date, and time hung. Time label side of container. Record solution change.
4. Prepare container for spiking:
   a. If solution is in a plastic bag, remove plastic cover from entry nipple. Maintain sterility of nipple end.

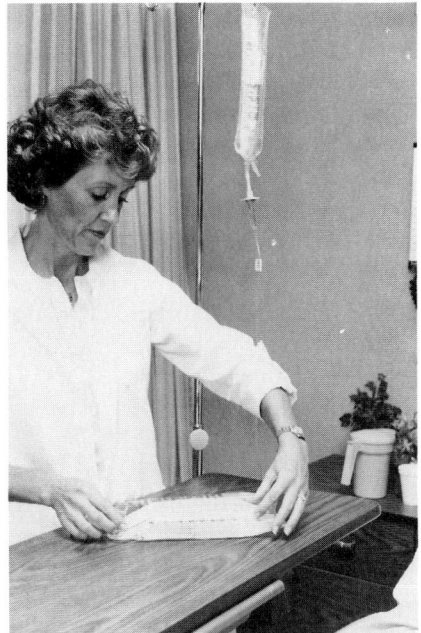

Step 3

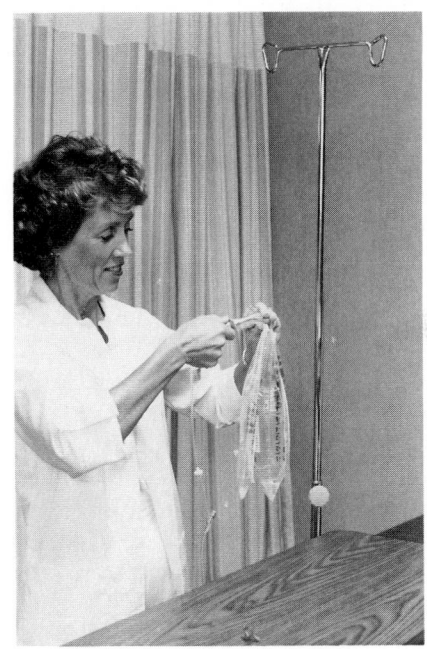

Step 6

   b. If solution is in a bottle, remove metal cap, metal disk, and rubber disk. Maintain sterility of bottle top.

Rationale: Prevents transmission of microorganisms into container when spike is inserted.

(continued)

PROCEDURE 32-2. Changing Intravenous Solution and Tubing *continued*

5. Close the clamp on the existing tubing.
   Rationale: Prevents fluid in drip chamber from emptying and air entering tubing during changing procedure.

6. Take old solution container from IV pole, invert it.
   Rationale: Brings work to eye level and prevents fluid remaining in container from emptying onto floor when tubing is removed.

7. Remove spike from used container, maintaining its sterility. Spike new intravenous container with firm push/twist motion.

8. Hang new container on IV pole.
   Rationale: Allows gravity to augment fluid filling drip chamber.

9. Inspect tubing for air bubbles and assess that drip chamber is one-half full of solution.
   Rationale: Reduces risk of air embolism.

10. Adjust clamp to regulate flow rate, according to orders.
    Rationale: Deliver IV fluids as ordered to restore fluid balance.

■ **Procedure**

Changing Solution and Tubing

1. Follow first three steps of *Changing Solution Container* only.

2. Open new tubing package, keeping protective covers on spike and catheter adapter.
   Rationale: Maintain sterility of new tubing set.

3. Adjust roller clamp on new tubing to fully closed position.
   Rationale: Prevents fluid spillage when new solution container is attached.

4. Prepare new solution container as directed in *Changing Solution Container.*

5. Remove protective cover from spike, maintaining sterility, and spike into new solution container.

6. Hang container and "prime" drip chamber by squeezing gently, allowing to fill one-half full.
   Rationale: Prevents air bubbles from entering tubing with the solution.

7. Remove protective cap from catheter adapter and adjust roller clamp to flush tubing with fluid. Replace protective cap.
   Rationale: Removes air from tubing to protect patient from risk of air embolus. Protective cap maintains sterility of system.

8. Adjust roller clamp on old tubing to fully close.
   Rationale: Prevents fluid leakage when tubing is disconnected.

9. Don clean, disposable gloves.
   Rationale: Protects nurse from transfer of microorganisms if blood inadvertently gets on hands.

10. Hold catheter hub with fingers of one hand (may use hemostat). With other hand, disconnect tubing using gentle twisting motion.
    Note: The dressing may have to be removed.
    Rationale: Holding catheter hub firmly maintains needle position in the vein.

11. Grasp new tubing, remove protective catheter cap, and insert tightly into needle hub, while continuing to stabilize catheter hub with other hand.

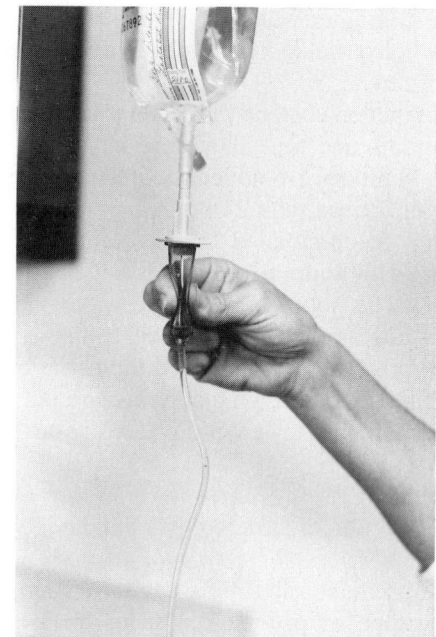

Step 6

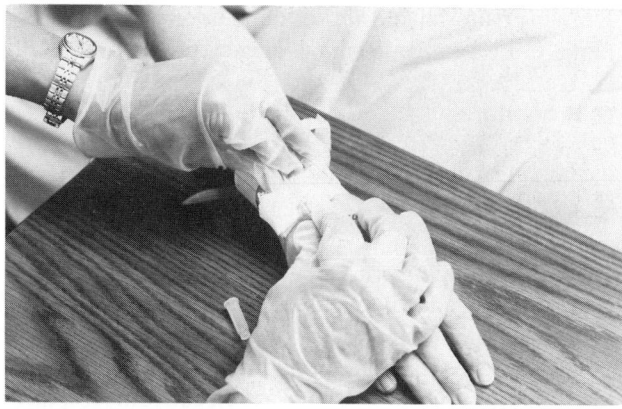

Step 11

(continued)

PROCEDURE 32–2. Changing Intravenous Solution and Tubing *continued*

12. Adjust roller clamp to start solution flowing according to physician's order.
13. Discard gloves.
14. Secure tubing with tape.
    Rationale: Prevents pulling on catheter hub and accidental dislodging of catheter in the vein.
15. If dressing was removed, apply new dressing to IV site according to agency policy.
16. Label new tubing with date and time and your initials.
17. Label solution container with patient's name, solution type, additives, date and time hung. Time label side of container. Record solution and tubing change.
    Rationale: Facilitates monitoring by other staff members.

■ **Lifespan Considerations**

Infants and Children
- Infants and children are at risk for circulatory overload if intravenous fluids are accidentally infused too rapidly. IV solutions are available in 250 and 500 mL containers to guard against such accidents. Volume control administration sets are also available to allow only a preset amount of fluid to be infused. All children under 2 years of age should have this type of safety device during intravenous therapy.

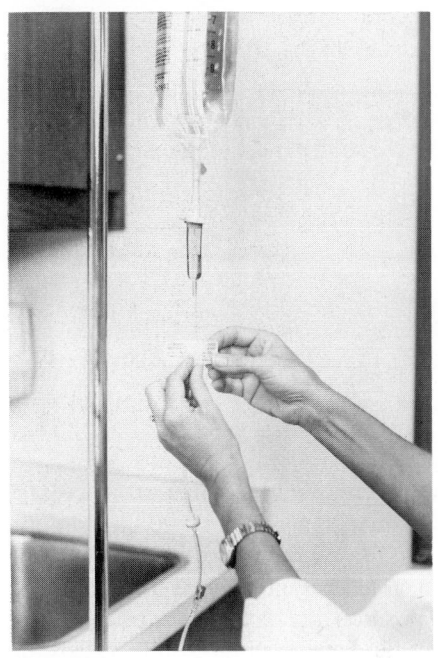

Step 16

---

present. The IV should not be irrigated since irrigation could push the clot into the systemic circulation, thus contributing to systemic infection. Nursing interventions for phlebitis include discontinuing the IV and restarting it in a different site, and the application of a warm compress to decrease inflammation. Phlebitis can be reduced if large veins are used for venipuncture, needles are used rather than catheters, irritating substances are diluted properly and infused slowly, and IV sites are changed per agency protocol (the Centers for Disease Control recommends every 72 hours) (Metheny, 1987).

Infection can occur systemically or at the IV infusion site. The longer an IV is in one site, the greater the chance for infection, thus IV sites often are routinely changed according to guidelines given in agency policies (e.g., every 72 hours). Signs and symptoms of infection can be local (redness, warmth, or purulent drainage at the site) or systemic (fever, chills, general discomfort). If infection is suspected, the physician should be notified. The discontinuation and restarting of the IV, as well as the culturing of the IV catheter, may be ordered.

Air embolism refers to air entering the blood system and moving in the vessel. Air emboli are more common when central veins or infusion pumps are used. A significant amount of air (usually over 5 mL) must enter the peripheral venous circulation before it poses a significant health risk for the patient. Smaller amounts of air are significant when a central venous catheter is used for intravenous therapy. A few bubbles entering the system are not harmful, but may worry the patient. When large amounts of air enter the system, the patient may become hypotensive, tachycardic, cyanotic, and actually lose consciousness. Treatment for air embolism includes placing the patient on the left side with head down. This will allow the air to rise into the right ventricle and allow blood to pass into the lungs.

Fluid overload may occur if the patient receives intravenous fluid too rapidly. The elderly, especially those with poor cardiac function, and the very young are prone to fluid overload. Fluid overload can occur if the nurse tries to "catch up" when the IV infusion gets behind. The patient may complain of headache, have neck vein

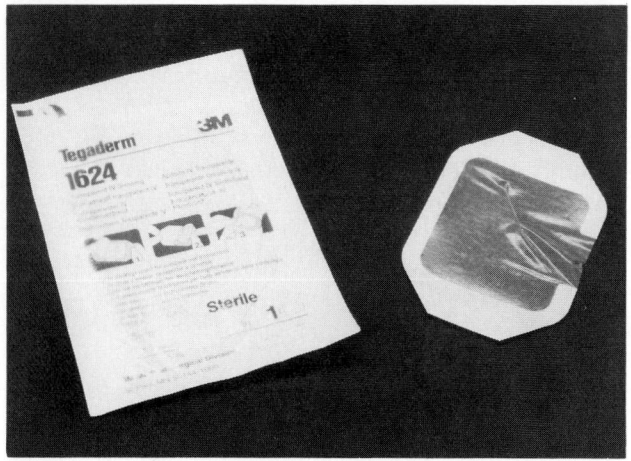
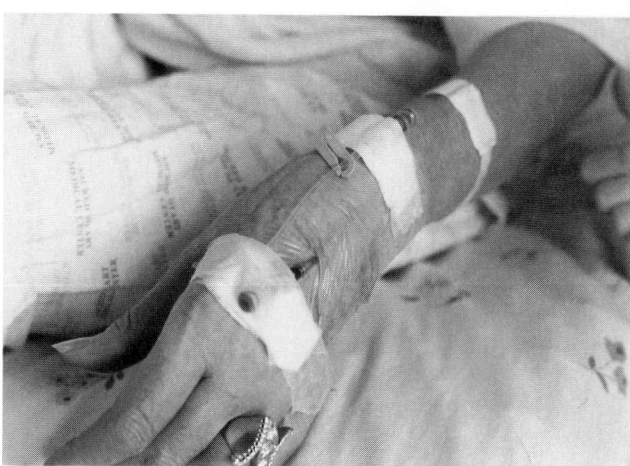

Figure 32–15. Tegaderm dressing for IV site.

distention, increased blood pressure, increased respiratory rate, and dyspnea. The nurse should slow down the IV to a KVO rate (30 to 50 cc per hour) and contact the physician. The patient should be placed in a semi-Fowler's position and oxygen may be administered. Prevention of fluid overload is possible by careful monitoring of all IVs and placing high-risk patients on controllers or pumps.

Discontinuing an Intravenous Infusion. An infusion is discontinued when all ordered fluids have infused or when complications develop. Before discontinuing an infusion, it is important to don disposable gloves, since contact with blood can occur. The flow of fluid is stopped by moving the roller clamp to the off position. Tape is carefully removed, while supporting the catheter. A gauze pad is placed over the venipuncture site as the catheter is withdrawn, and then pressure is applied over the site. A band-aid can be applied if necessary. It is important to document the amount of fluid infused, the time the infusion was discontinued, any complications of therapy that occurred, and any nursing measures taken (such as application of a warm compress).

Blood Transfusions

Blood transfusion refers to the introduction of whole blood or blood components (packed red cells, plasma, platelets) directly into a patient's circulatory system. Transfusions are given primarily to restore circulating blood volume, restore coagulation factor deficiencies, improve oxygen-carrying capacity of the blood, and increase white blood cells to decrease the chance of infection.

Blood Components. The patient does not always need all components of whole blood, so certain blood compo-

nents can be selectively transfused depending on the unique needs of the patient. Common blood products for transfusion include whole blood, packed red cells, white blood cells, platelets, plasma, albumin, and cryoprecipitate. The nurse should become knowledgeable regarding the indications and nursing considerations for each product.

Whole blood contains all blood components and is usually transfused to people who need both blood cells and volume replacement, such as after significant blood loss. A unit of whole blood is approximately 500 mL.

Packed red cells contain a concentration of red cells with most plasma removed. A unit of packed cells is approximately 250 mL. Packed red cells provide the same oxygen-carrying capacity, without the volume, as whole blood. They are especially useful in the treatment of chronic anemia. Problems of fluid overload and electrolyte imbalances can be avoided since packed cells contain less volume and less sodium and potassium. To prevent an allergic response, the packed red cells can be washed to remove most antibodies from the cell.

White blood cells, or granulocytes, can be administered to patients with low or abnormal white blood cell count. Infusion of white cells is helpful in assisting in fighting infection. They are frequently given to cancer patients who have low white cell counts due to chemotherapy or the effects of the cancer.

Platelets may be administered in fresh blood, platelet concentrates, and platelet-rich plasma. The major function of platelets is to initiate blood clotting and hemostasis.

Whole plasma is the fluid component of the blood in which the corpuscles are suspended. Plasma consists of organic and inorganic substances dissolved in water. Whole plasma can be used to correct hypovolemia due to selective loss of plasma, such as occurs in extensive burns. Electrolyte solutions and albumin often replace the need for plasma infusions.

Albumin is a plasma protein contained within the plasma. It is used as a volume expander, because fluid is pulled back into the vasculature due to the oncotic force the protein exerts. Another advantage of albumin is that it, unlike whole plasma, carries no risk of hepatitis transmission.

Cryoprecipitate is a plasma fraction rich in fibrinogen and blood clotting factor VIII. Cryoprecipitate is concentrated from many units of blood and administered to hemophiliacs, who are predisposed to bleeding problems because genetically they lack factor VIII.

Blood Compatibility. To safely administer blood, it is important that the donor blood be compatible with the blood of the patient. To ensure this, the blood of both the patient and the donor is tested to determine ABO and Rh compatibility. Blood typing refers to testing the person's blood type, and crossmatching is the process of assuring that it is compatible with the donor blood.

ABO blood groups can be determined by testing for antigens on the erythrocyte. The population can be divided into four ABO blood groups, types A, B, AB, and O. The erythrocytes of a person in group A have the A antigen, group B the B antigen, group AB both A and B antigens, and group O has neither A nor B antigens. In addition to antigens, each blood group also contains naturally occurring antibodies (agglutinins) in the serum. Group A has anti-B antibodies, Group B has anti-A antibodies, Group AB has no A or B antibodies, and Group O has anti-A and anti-B antibodies in the serum. Anti-A antibodies destroy A antigens and anti-B antibodies destroy B antigens, which results in red cell destruction, known as hemolysis. Type O blood is often referred to as the universal donor, since it has neither A nor B antigens and it can safely be given to people with other blood types. Likewise, AB blood is often referred to as the universal recipient, because the lack of antibodies enables accepting transfusions from other blood types.

Rh factor is also important to determine before transfusion to prevent blood incompatibility. Five antigens in the Rh system, the most important of which is D, are located on the surface of the erythrocyte. The presence of D antigen determines that a person is Rh positive (85% of whites), whereas the lack of this antigen designates an individual as Rh negative (15% of whites). Antibodies against Rh factor do not occur naturally. Such antibodies only form when Rh-negative blood is exposed to Rh-positive cells. After antibodies form, it is only on subsequent exposure to Rh-positive blood that a reaction (agglutination) occurs in which there is hemolysis of cells. Rh factor is especially important in obstetrics. If an Rh-negative mother carries an Rh-positive fetus, antibodies can form in the mother's blood. If the mother should become pregnant again with an Rh-positive fetus, Rh agglutinogens can enter the circulation of the fetus and cause a hemolytic reaction. RhoGam, a commercial name for antibodies directed against Rh factor, is given to the mother after the first miscarriage, abortion, or pregnancy to prevent future problems.

Selection of Blood Donors. Nurses are frequently responsible for screening prospective blood donors and overseeing the process of blood collection. The nurse is responsible for ensuring the safety of both the blood donor and the recipient of the blood donation. To do this, the nurse interviews the prospective donor to rule out any history of hepatitis or recent hepatitis exposure, recent infectious exposure, syphilis or malaria, recent immunizations, recent reception of any blood product transfusion, and exposure to the HIV virus, (or risky behaviors such as IV drug abuse or homosexual or bisexual activities). To ensure safety of our blood supply, screening for these factors is important to identify and prevent high-risk people from donating. To protect the blood donor, people are not permitted to donate if they are pregnant, anemic, do not fall within weight restrictions, have abnormal blood pressure, or have donated whole blood within the last 56 days.

Blood is tested for antibodies to the HIV virus and hepatitis B. At this time there is no way to test blood for non-A, non-B hepatitis, and transmission of this form of hepatitis can occur with blood transfusions. The chance of contracting AIDS through blood transfusions has been significantly reduced since the development and implementation of testing all blood for antibodies to the HIV virus. It is important to recognize that the blood donor is not at risk for acquiring any infectious disease, including AIDS, since all blood procurement is done under strict aseptic conditions.

Transfusion Technique. To administer any blood product, the nurse must understand correct technique for administration and be aware of the complications that can occur. The procedure for administering a blood transfusion is given in Procedure 32-3. Important considerations when infusing blood products include proper identification of the patient and the blood, using a large enough access device (usually 18-gauge or larger) to avoid damage to the blood cells as they infuse, and using only compatible IV solutions of normal saline to prevent cell hemolysis. The nurse also frequently assesses the patient for signs of a transfusion reaction.

Complications of Blood Transfusion. The administration of blood or blood products involves a number of risks. The nurse should monitor the patient carefully for any untoward effects. The major risks include febrile reaction, circulatory overload, septic reaction, allergic reaction, and acute hemolytic reaction.

Febrile reaction to blood products can occur due to hypersensitivity of the recipient to the donor's blood cells. In this reaction, the patient develops a fever and chills, and complains of headache and malaise. Sometimes an antipyretic, such as aspirin, is ordered before blood administration to prevent a febrile reaction. If symptoms occur after the infusion has been started, the infusion should be stopped and the IV kept open with normal saline. The physician should be notified and vital signs monitored.

Allergic reactions can also occur when blood products are administered. This complication may occur because the patient has a sensitivity to the plasma protein from the donor's blood. Symptoms of an allergic reaction include flushing, urticaria (hives), wheezing, and a rash with itching. Once again, the infusion must be stopped, the IV kept open with normal saline, and the physician notified. An antihistamine may be ordered to decrease the severity of the reaction and make the patient more comfortable. If hives are the only manifestation, the physician may elect to continue the infusion at a slower rate. The nurse must then monitor the patient carefully for manifestations of a more severe reaction that could cause respiratory difficulty.

Hemolytic reactions are the most serious of the acute complications of blood transfusions, and can be life-threatening. A hemolytic reaction occurs when the donor's blood is incompatible with the recipient's blood. This can occur if the wrong blood is mistakenly administered to a patient. Hemolysis, or destruction of red cells, occurs when the antibodies in the recipient's blood quickly react to the donor's blood cells. Symptoms are immediate and include facial flushing, fever, chills, headache, low back pain, tachycardia, dyspnea, hypotension, and blood in the urine. Prompt intervention is essential to decrease mortality in hemolytic reactions. Vital signs should always be monitored before starting the infusion and during the first 5 minutes, when the blood is infused slowly. If the nurse suspects a hemolytic reaction, the blood administration should be stopped and the IV kept open with normal saline. The physician will order drugs to treat the hypotension and have the patient monitored closely. Blood from both the donor and recipient will be tested to assess whether a hemolytic reaction has occurred. A urine specimen is also collected to determine if renal involvement is present.

Circulatory overload can occur when blood products are infused too quickly or too much volume is infused. Circulatory overload is more likely to occur in the very young or in the elderly with poor cardiac function. Symptoms of circulatory overload include increased venous pressure, distended neck veins, dyspnea, coughing, and abnormal breath sounds. Circulatory overload can be prevented by infusing packed cells rather than whole blood for high-risk patients, and carefully monitoring the infusion rate of blood products. If the nurse suspects circulatory overload, he or she should slow the infusion of blood, position the patient in an upright position with feet dependent, and notify the physician.

Selected Nursing Interventions for Common Fluid and Electrolyte Problems

Fluid Volume Deficit

- Increase oral fluids
- Increase food with high fluid content
- Intravenous therapy
- Limit fluid losses by treating vomiting or diarrhea

Fluid Volume Excess

- Limit fluid intake
- Limit dietary sodium intake
- Administer diuretics as ordered by the physician
- Carefully monitor any IV infusion or blood transfusion to prevent rapid infusion of fluid

PROCEDURE 32-3. Administering a Blood Transfusion

■ **Purpose**

Replace blood volume or blood components lost through trauma, surgery, or a disease process.

■ **Assessment**

- Review physician's order for transfusion.
- Review chart for pertinent, baseline laboratory values (i.e., CBC, platelets).
- Review chart for previous transfusion history, noting if patient has ever had a transfusion reaction.
- Inspect patient's current IV for patency and intactness. Assess that IV catheter is an 18- or 19-gauge angiocatheter, which will facilitate transfusion flow and prevent hemolysis of red blood cells. Restart if necessary.

■ **Equipment**

Packaged blood component from blood bank according to agency protocol.
250 mL IV container of sterile 0.9 normal saline.
Blood administration set with filter.
Blood warmer and pressure bag (optional) may be used if infusing large volumes of blood rapidly.
Alcohol swabs and tape.

■ **Procedure**

1. Explain procedure to patient. Have patient sign consent form if required by hospital policy.
2. Obtain patient's vital signs to include temperature. *Rationale: Provides baseline, pretransfusion vital signs to compare against vital signs taken during and after transfusion.*
3. With another RN at the patient's bedside, verify the blood product *and* the patient's identity by comparing the laboratory blood record with:

   a. The patient's name and identification number both verbally and against patient's wrist band.
   b. The blood unit number on the blood bag label.
   c. The blood group and RH type on the blood bag label.

   Also verify the type of blood component and the expiration date noted on the blood label. Document verification by both RN signatures on transfusion record.
   Rationale: Strict adherence to verification prior to blood administration greatly reduces the risk of infusing the wrong blood type.
4. Wash your hands.
5. Open Y-type blood administration set and clamp both rollers completely.
   Rationale: Prevents spilling and wastage of blood.
6. Spike 0.9 NaCl container. Prime drip chamber and tubing with saline.
7. Spike blood or blood component unit with second spike. Keep roller clamp shut.
8. Remove primary IV tubing from catheter hub and cover end with sterile protector.
   Rationale: Ensures sterility of IV so it can be reconnected following transfusion.
9. Attach blood administration tubing to catheter hub and secure with tape.
10. Close clamp to 0.9 NaCl container. Open clamp to

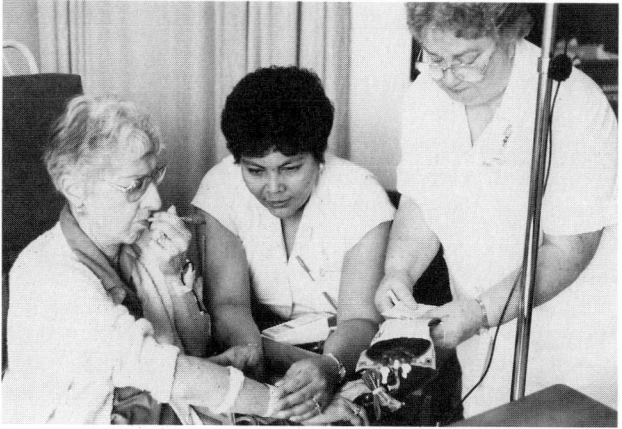

Step 3

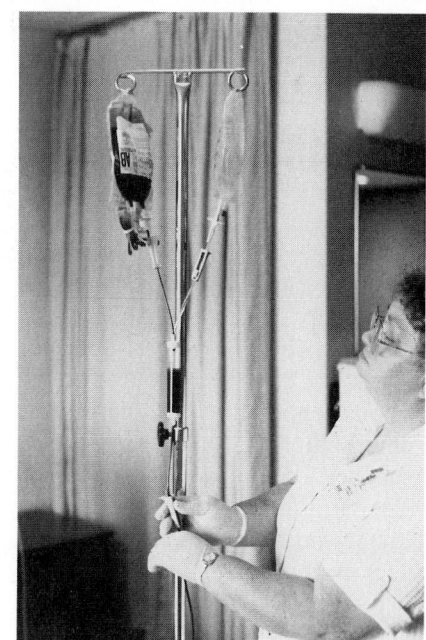

Step 10

(continued)

blood product. Open roller clamp below drip chamber and begin transfusion.

11. Infuse blood slowly for first 15 minutes (10 drops per minute).

12. Monitor and document vital signs every 5 minutes during first 15 minutes, assessing for chilling, back pain, headache, nausea or vomiting, tachycardia, hypotension, tachypnea, or skin rash.

    Rationale: Most blood reactions occur within first 15 to 20 minutes of transfusion. Altered vital signs or other adverse reactions are early indications of a transfusion reaction. Infusing blood slowly during this period limits the amount of blood the patient receives if there is a reaction.

    Note: If any adverse reactions occur, close clamp to blood, open clamp to 0.9 NaCl, and notify physician immediately. Follow agency policy for laboratory notification and obtaining blood and urine specimens.

13. If no adverse reactions occur after 15 minutes, regulate clamp to increase infusion according to physician's orders. Monitor vital signs hourly until transfusion is complete.

14. When blood transfusion is complete, clamp roller to blood and open roller to 0.9 NaCl. Infuse until tubing is clear.

    Rationale: Prevents wastage of blood product and prevents hemolysis of cells from noncompatible IV solutions.

15. Obtain and document post-transfusion vital signs.

16. If second blood component unit is to be transfused, slow 0.9 NaCl to keep vein open until next unit is available. Follow verification procedure and vital sign monitoring for each unit.

17. If transfusion orders are complete, disconnect the blood administration tubing from the catheter hub. Reconnect the primary intravenous solution and tubing and adjust to desired rate.

18. Wash hands and document procedure.

■ **Lifespan Considerations**

Infants and Children
- Many blood banks have "pedi-packs" of blood available in 50 and 100 mL sizes for infusing to children.
- Follow agency protocol for administering blood and blood components to children.

Older Adult
- If the patient has cardiac failure, careful assessment to prevent fluid overload is necessary. Packed red blood cells are frequently infused to limit the volume being infused. The infusion of 0.9 NaCl may be limited to the minimum needed to irrigate the tubing. The infusion time may be increased to decrease the load on the heart.

Septic reactions to blood administration can also occur if the blood products have been contaminated with bacteria. The patient will likely have a rapid onset of fever and chills, and perhaps vomiting, diarrhea, and hypotension. The transfusion should be stopped and the physician notified. Septic reactions can be minimized if blood products are kept refrigerated until used and infused in less than 4 hours. The longer blood products remain at room temperature, the more likely bacteria will grow and multiply.

For all complications of blood therapy, the role of the nurse is essential in prompt detection of untoward effects. The nurse can also identify high-risk patients so that treatment can be individualized to prevent complications.

Discharge Planning and Home Care

Many patients continue treatment for fluid and electrolyte imbalances in the home. It is fairly common for the patient to have intravenous therapy in the home setting; consequently, the patient and family members must be taught proper management of the fluids and how to use the equipment to regulate flow rate. Also, it is important to teach the patient and the family about potential complications of intravenous therapy. The patient should be given the name and telephone number of the supply company, and have a plan for what to do if equipment malfunctions or problems with intravenous therapy develop. To develop hypothetical problems that could occur and ask the patient what could be done is a good method of evaluating problem-solving abilities and skills.

Fluid and electrolyte imbalances may necessitate dietary changes. Certain restrictions may be enforced or certain foods may need to be encouraged. Lists of such foods should be given to the patient and a plan worked out as to who will do the shopping and prepare the meals. These tasks may prove tiring for those who are weak from fluid or electrolyte imbalances.

Patients with fluid and electrolyte imbalances may

Nursing Management Plan
The Patient With Fluid Volume Deficit

Nursing Diagnosis: Fluid volume deficit related to inadequate oral intake as manifested by concentrated urine, change in urine output, dry mucous membranes, postural hypotension, and change in serum sodium.

Patient Goal: Patient will reestablish normal fluid and electrolyte balance.

Patient Outcome Criteria

- Patient maintains equal intake/output within ±300 mL per 24 hours.

Nursing Intervention	Scientific Rationale
1. Monitor intake and output.	1. Observation of trends in intake and output provides essential data regarding patient's fluid and electrolyte status and guides interventions. Intake should approximately equal output but observing for trends and significant increases or decrease is more important than specific numbers.
2. Monitor serum electrolytes, serum osmolality, specific gravity, and hematocrit.	2. To provide essential data regarding patient status and guide interventions. (Common abnormal laboratory values in fluid volume deficit include increased Hct, increased serum sodium, increased serum osmolality, increased specific gravity.)
3. Increase oral fluid intake to at least 2000 mL per 24 hours or as ordered by physician.	3. Increased intake of fluids (and high fluid-content foods) helps correct fluid volume deficit and maintain adequate hydration.
4. Monitor IV fluid therapy as prescribed.	4. To provide fluids when adequate intake cannot be obtained by oral intake alone. Monitoring ensures infusion at prescribed rate and allows early detection of complications.
5. Assess fluid preferences.	5. Patient more likely to increase fluid intake with fluids that are appealing.
6. Ensure optimal access to preferred fluids and assist as needed.	6. Availability and assistance necessary to ensure increased fluid intake.
7. Give positive reinforcement or verbal cuing as necessary.	7. To increase compliance for patients who may be forgetful or disinterested.

Patient Goal: Patient will demonstrate knowledge regarding how to promote fluid and electrolyte balance.

Patient Outcome Criteria

- Patient verbalizes the importance of drinking eight glasses of water per day by the end of the teaching session.
- Patient lists foods that are high in sodium and verbalizes needed modifications in diet by discharge.
- Patient maintains a daily record of weight for next month.
- Patient verbalizes a plan to cope with temporary problems of diarrhea or vomiting by discharge.

Nursing Intervention	Scientific Rationale
1. Assess reason for inadequate fluid intake before admission.	1. Many possible reasons for inadequate intake, e.g., increased need secondary to diarrhea, depression, desire to decrease voidings, and

(continued)

---

inability to access and prepare food. Important to understand reason to individualize plan for care and prevention.

2. Teach patient or family about the significance (e.g., rehospitalization, potential for confusion and injury) and prevention (e.g., daily fluid requirement, method for recording intake) of fluid volume deficit.

2. Increased knowledge leads to increased compliance and more successful outcomes.

3. Provide a list of symptoms of or conditions that increase risk for fluid volume deficit (e.g., diarrhea) that require contact with a physician.

3. May result in earlier treatment. Written material may be referred to in the future to help ensure compliance.

---

have various medications prescribed. The medication, purpose, dosage, frequency, precautions, and potential side effects and complications should be emphasized. If the patient has a prescription for a medication (e.g., diuretics), it is important to explain the manifestations of the potential electrolyte imbalance and methods of circumventing the problem. For example, for the patient taking diuretics that enhance excretion of potassium, it is necessary to emphasize the importance of potassium replacement by taking ordered supplements or making necessary dietary changes (e.g., eating a banana a day).

Because fluid and electrolyte imbalances may cause poor coordination, weakness, confusion, and altered gait, the nurse should emphasize the need for a safe home environment. Such teaching may include assistance with ambulation or suggestions for safety features in the home (night lights, hand railings next to the tub or toilet, removing throw rugs).

Explaining to the patient before discharge the symptoms that need to be relayed to the physician is an important part of discharge teaching. For example, some physicians may want to be informed if the patient gains more than 5 pounds, or has vomiting or diarrhea that lasts for more than 1 day. All patient teaching is beneficial in preventing future occurrences of fluid and electrolyte imbalances.

EVALUATION

The nurse uses specific outcome criteria to measure the attainment of patient goals. If outcome criteria have not been achieved, the nurse can revise his or her plan of care or set more realistic goals. The process of evaluation and revision of care is dynamic and continual.

Outcome criteria should be individualized for the patient. Possible outcome criteria are given as a guide.

Goal
The patient will reestablish normal fluid and electrolyte balance.

Possible Outcome Criteria
- The patient maintains equal intake/output within + or − 300 mL per 24 hours.
- By discharge, the patient demonstrates weight within 2 kg of baseline weight (give specific amount of weight to be lost or gained).
- The patient does not experience sudden changes in weight (increasing or decreasing more than 1 kg per day).
- By discharge, the patient reestablishes electrolyte values within normal limits.
- The patient experiences a decrease in postural blood pressure.
- By discharge, the patient verbalizes that he or she does not have excessive thirst.
- By discharge, the patient has an absence of edema.
- By discharge, the patient has absence of concentrated urine.

Goal
The patient will demonstrate knowledge regarding how to promote fluid and electrolyte balance.

Possible Outcome Criteria
- By the conclusion of the teaching session, the patient verbalizes the importance of drinking eight glasses of water per day.
- By the conclusion of the teaching session, the patient lists foods that are high in sodium and verbalizes needed modifications in diet.
- The patient maintains a daily record of weight for next month.
- The patient notifies the physician of any significant weight gain, as evidenced on daily record.

- By the conclusion of the teaching session, the patient verbalizes a plan to cope with temporary problems of diarrhea or vomiting.
- By the conclusion of the teaching session, the patient lists foods high in potassium.
- The patient complies with physician's recommendations by taking oral potassium supplements at each dosage scheduled.

Goal

The patient will have an absence of complications from fluid or electrolyte imbalance.

Possible Outcome Criteria

- The patient stands and walks without falling during hospital stay.
- The skin remains intact despite edema until edema is reduced.
- The patient has an absence of infiltration or phlebitis during hospital stay.

Evaluation is important to ensure that the goals of promoting optimum fluid and electrolyte balance, preventing complications of fluid and electrolyte imbalance, and increasing the patient's knowledge to prevent fluid and electrolyte imbalance, are achieved. Modification of the plan of care, or more realistic outcome criteria, may be necessary if goal attainment has not occurred.

Key Concepts

- Homeostasis of body fluids, electrolytes, and pH is necessary for cellular function and the maintenance of health.
- Homeostasis is maintained by processes such as diffusion, osmosis, active transport, and filtration that facilitate fluid or electrolyte movement.
- Intracellular fluid refers to the fluid within the cells of the body, whereas extracellular fluid refers to the intravascular fluid and the interstitial fluid.
- Cations are positively charged electrolytes (sodium, potassium, calcium, and magnesium), and anions are negatively charged electrolytes (chloride, phosphate, sulfate, and bicarbonate). Balance between anions and cations is a dynamic process necessary to maintain neutrality.
- Hormonal control (ADH, aldosterone, parathyroid hormone) and buffering mechanisms (respiratory and renal) help to maintain fluid, electrolyte, and acid–base balance.
- States of altered fluid balance include fluid volume excess or fluid volume deficit.
- States of electrolyte imbalance include hypernatremia, hyponatremia, hyperkalemia, hypokalemia, hypercalcemia, hypocalcemia, hypermagnesemia, and hypomagnesemia.
- States of altered acid–base balance include respiratory acidosis, metabolic acidosis, respiratory alkalosis, and metabolic alkalosis.
- Inadequate intake; excessive loss through vomiting, diarrhea, diaphoresis, or diuretics; stress; chronic illness such as renal failure, cardiac failure, or respiratory failure; surgery; or pregnancy can increase the potential for altered fluid, electrolyte, and acid–base balance.
- Age-related, developmental changes can affect fluid, electrolyte, and acid–base balance.
- Alterations in normal fluid, electrolyte, or acid–base balance are manifested by imbalances in intake and output, changes in mental status, changes in vital signs, abnormal states of tissue hydration, or abnormal neuromuscular status.
- Alterations in fluid and electrolyte status can affect functional abilities as a person becomes weak, fatigued, or confused.
- Intake and output, weight, edema, tissue turgor, neck vein and hand vein engorgement, and vital signs are all important objective data to collect to identify actual problems in fluid and electrolyte status.
- Laboratory data, such as serum electrolytes, serum osmolality, urine specific gravity, hematocrit, and arterial blood gases, also provide important information for identifying potential disruption in fluid and electrolyte status.
- Accepted NANDA diagnoses include Fluid Volume Excess and Fluid Volume Deficit.
- Important nursing interventions include preventive health teaching; regulating oral fluids; assisting with electrolyte replacement; and initiating, regulating, and monitoring intravenous therapy and monitoring blood transfusions.
- Height of the bottle, position of the extremity, position of the catheter in the vein, and patency of the catheter and tubing are all factors that can affect the infusion rate.
- Potential complications of IV therapy include infiltration, phlebitis, infection, air embolism, and fluid overload.
- Blood transfusions are administered to restore circulating volume, to improve oxygen-carrying capacity of the blood, to restore coagulation factors, and to increase white blood cell count to decrease the risk of infection.
- To prevent serious adverse reactions from blood administration, careful screening and matching of donor and recipient blood is necessary.
- Possible goals for the patient with fluid and electrolyte disturbances include restoration of normal fluid and electrolyte balance, promotion of balance through adequate knowledge, and avoidance of potential complications.

References

Barta, M. A. (1987). Correcting electrolyte imbalances. *RN, 50*(2), 30–33.

Byrne, J., Saxton, D., & Pelilcan, P. (1986). *Laboratory tests: Implications for nursing care* (2nd ed.). Menlo Park, CA: Addison-Wesley.

Corbett, J. V. (1987). *Laboratory tests and diagnostic procedures with nursing diagnoses* (2nd ed.). Norwalk, CT: Appleton & Lange.

Cunningham, S. L. (1989). The physiology of body fluids. In H. D. Patton & A. F. Fuchs, et al. (Eds.), *Textbook of physiology* (21st ed.). Philadelphia: W. B. Saunders.

Fischbach, F. (1988). *A manual of laboratory diagnostic tests* (3rd ed.). Philadelphia: J. B. Lippincott.

Goldberger, E. A. (1986). *Primer of water, electrolyte and acid base symptoms* (7th ed.). Philadelphia: Lea & Febiger.

Heitkemper, M., & Bond, E. (1988). Fluid and electrolytes: Assessment and interventions. *Journal of Enterstomal Therapy, 15*(1), 18–23.

Lowery, S. J., & Ash, S. R. (1988). Diminishing the risk of IV potassium chloride. *Nursing 88, 18*(6), 64.

Mathewson, M. K. (1987). Thyroid disorders. *Critical Care Nursing, 7*(1), 74–85.

Metheny, N. (1987). *Fluid and electrolyte balance: Nursing considerations*. Philadelphia: J. B. Lippincott.

NANDA (1990). *Taxonomy I revised 1990, with official nursing diagnoses*. St. Louis, MO: North American Nursing Diagnosis Association.

Porth, C. M. (1990). *Pathophysiology: Concepts of altered health states* (3rd ed.). Philadelphia: J. B. Lippincott.

Romanski, S. O. (1986). Interpreting ABG's in four easy steps. *Nursing 86, 16*(9), 58–63.

Saari, M. (1986). Innovations and excellence: Arterial acid–base balance and arterial blood gases. *Perioperative Nursing Quarterly, 2*(2), 52–62.

Schwartz, M. W. (1987). Potassium imbalances. *American Journal of Nursing, 87*, 1292–1298.

Underhill, S., Woods, S., Sivarajan-Froelicher, E., & Halpenny, J. (1989). *Cardiac nursing* (2nd ed.). Philadelphia: J. B. Lippincott.

Vander, A., Sherman, J., & Luciano, D. (1985). *Human physiology: The mechanisms of body function* (4th ed.). New York: McGraw Hill.

Whaley, L. F., & Wong, D. L. (1989). *Essential of pediatric nursing*. St. Louis: C. V. Mosby.

Bibliography

Calloway, C. (1987). When the problem involves magnesium, calcium or phosphate. *RN, 50*(5), 30–35.

Carpenito, L. (1989). *Nursing diagnosis: Application to clinical practice* (3rd ed.). Philadelphia: J. B. Lippincott.

DeRubertis, F. R. (1984). Hypercalcemia and hypocalcemia. *Topics in Emergency Medicine, 5*(4), 64–78.

Epstein, Y., et al. (1985). Fluid balance in hot climates: Sweating, water intake and prevention of dehydration. *Public Health Review, 13*(1/2), 115–137.

Ehlinger-Sherman, J. (1989). IV therapy that clicks. *Nursing 89, 19*(5), 50–51.

Feldstein, A. (1986). Detect phlebitis and infiltration before they harm your patient. *Nursing 86, 16*(1), 44–47.

Finberg, L. (1984). Oral electrolyte/glucose solutions. *Journal of Pediatrics, 105*, 939–940.

Gasparis, L. (1989). IV solutions: Which one is right for your patient? *Nursing 89, 19*(4), 62–64.

Girard, N. J., Morgan, R. G., & Orr, M. D. (1988). Autologous salvage of blood. *AORN Journal, 47*(2), 492–503.

Greenburg, A. (1984). Common emergencies of acid–base balance. *Topics in Emergency Medicine, 5*(4), 1–6.

Gurevich, I. (1986). Are IV in-line filters worth the price? *Nursing 1986, 16*(7), 42–43.

Guyton, A. (1986). *Textbook of medical physiology*. Philadelphia: W. B. Saunders.

Hakki, A., et al. (1986). A simple formula for monitoring parenteral infusion. *Critical Care Nursing, 6*(3), 57–62.

Irwin, M. (1987). Encourage oral intake—Yes, but how? *American Journal of Nursing, 87*(1) 100–106.

Keating, S., & Kelman, G. (1988). *Home health care nursing: Concepts and practice*. Philadelphia: J. B. Lippincott.

Kokko, J. P., & Tannen, R. L. (1986). *Fluid and electrolytes*. Philadelphia: W. B. Saunders.

Landier, W. C., et al. (1987). How to administer blood components to children. *Maternal Care Nursing, 12*(3), 178–184.

Mascaro, J. (1986). Managing IV therapy in the home. *Nursing 86, 16*(5), 50–51.

Masiak, M., Naylor, M., & Hayman, L. (1985). *Fluid and electrolytes through the life cycle*. Norwalk, CT: Appleton-Century-Crofts.

McFadden, E., & Zaloga, G. (1983). Calcium regulation. *Critical Care Quarterly, 6*, 313–315.

Mintz, P., et al. (1988). The latest protocols for blood transfusions. *Nursing 88, 18*(10), 34–41.

Nelson, R., & Miller, H. (1986). Keeping air out of IV lines. *Nursing 86, 16*(3), 57–59.

Rose, B. (1984). *Clinical physiology of acid–base and electrolyte disorders* (2nd ed.). New York: McGraw Hill.

Peck, N. (1985). Perfecting your IV therapy techniques. *Nursing 85, 15*(5), 38–43.

Stein, J. H. (1988). Hypokalemia: Common and uncommon causes. *Hospital Practice, 23*(3), 55–64.

Stuhler-Schlag, M. K. (1982). Pre and postoperative fluids and electrolytes. *Today's OR Nurse, 4*(7):11–15, 66–67.

Swearington, P., Sommers, M., & Miller, K. (1988). *Manual of critical care*. St. Louis: C. V. Mosby.

Walpert, N. (1990). An orderly look at calcium metabolism disorders. *Nursing 90, 20*(7), 60–64.

Witek Janusek, L. (1990). Metabolic acidosis: Pathophysiology, signs, symptoms. *Nursing 90, 20*(7), 52–53.

Wendorff Burrows, C. Take a step toward making better IV needle selections. *Nursing 84, 14*(12), 32–33.

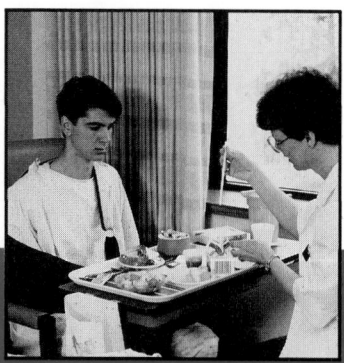

Nutrition

LEARNING OBJECTIVES

Upon completion of this chapter, the student will be able to do the following:

- List essential nutrients and give examples of good dietary sources for each.
- Describe normal digestion, absorption, and metabolism of carbohydrates, fats, and proteins.
- List factors that can affect normal dietary patterns.
- Discuss nutritional considerations across the lifespan.
- Describe manifestations of altered nutrition.
- Describe nursing interventions to promote optimal nutrition and health.
- Discuss nursing responsibilities for interventions used to treat altered nutritional states (e.g., therapeutic diets, tube feedings, total parenteral nutrition).

KEY TERMS

Calorie (kilocalorie)
Carbohydrates
Complete protein
Fats
Fiber
Glycogenesis
Incomplete protein

Monosaccharides
Negative nitrogen balance
Nutrients
Partially complete proteins

Polysaccharides
Positive nitrogen balance
Protein
Vitamins

Normal Nutritional Function
  Anatomy of the Digestive System
  Normal Physiologic Function of Nutrients
    Carbohydrates
    Protein
    Fat
    Vitamins
    Minerals
    Water
  Normal Physiologic Function of the Digestive
    System
    Digestion
    Absorption
    Metabolism
    Excretion
  Characteristics of Normal Nutrition
    Ideal Body Weight
    Physical Status
    Normal Laboratory Values
  Normal Nutritional Functional Pattern
    Basic Four Food Groups
    Recommended Dietary Allowances
    U.S. Recommended Daily Allowances
    World Nutrient Guides
    Nutrient Density
    Dietary Guidelines for Americans
    Energy Balance
  Factors Affecting Normal Nutrition
    Physical Factors
    Lifestyle and Habits
    Culture and Religion
    Economic Resources
    Gender
    Pregnancy and Lactation
  Lifespan Considerations
Altered Nutritional Function
  Potential for Altered Nutritional Function
    Inadequate Intake of Nutrients
    Excess Intake of Nutrients
    Inability to Use Ingested Nutrients
    Increased Metabolic Demand
    Surgery
    Cancer and Cancer Treatment
    Alcohol and Drug Abuse
    Psychological State
  Manifestations of Altered Nutrition
    Overweight
    Obesity
    Underweight

    Recent Significant Weight Gain or Loss
    Decreased Energy
    Altered Bowel Patterns
    Altered Skin, Teeth, Hair, and Mucous
      Membranes
Assessment
  Subjective Data
    Functional Pattern Identification
    Risk Identification
    Dysfunctional Identification
  Objective Data
    Physical Assessment
    Diagnostic Tests and Procedures
Nursing Diagnoses and Patient Goals
  Altered Nutrition: Less than Body Requirements
    Definition
    Defining Characteristics
    Related Factors
  Altered Nutrition: More than Body Requirements
    Definition
    Defining Characteristics
    Related Factors
  Altered Nutrition: High Risk for More than Body
    Requirements
    Definition
    Defining Characteristics
    Related Factors
  Impaired Swallowing
    Definition
    Defining Characteristics
    Related Factors
  Related Nursing Diagnoses
  Patient Goals
Implementation
  Nursing Interventions to Promote Health and
    Function
    Community Nutrition Programs
    Patient Teaching
    Optimal Intake Promotion
  Nursing Interventions for Altered Function
    Withholding Food
    Special Diets
    Nutritional Supplements
    Enteral Tube Feedings
    Peripheral Parenteral Nutrition
    Total Parenteral Nutrition
  Discharge Planning and Home Care
Evaluation
Key Concepts

As part of a holistic approach to good health, a nutritionally adequate diet is vital for promoting normal growth and development and preventing deficiency states. Optimal nutrition is essential to maintain health and prevent disease. An adequate diet is necessary to maintain bodily functions, to promote healing, to maintain healthy tissues, to maintain body temperature, and to build resistance to infection.

Nutrients are biochemical substances obtained from ingested food and fluids. Carbohydrates, proteins, and fats are nutrients that supply the body with energy. Vitamins, minerals, and water do not supply energy but are important in regulating body processes. Essential nutrients cannot be synthesized by the body in adequate amounts and therefore must be provided through the diet. Dietary intake of nonessential nutrients is not required, since these nutrients can be synthesized in adequate amounts by the body or are not required for body functioning.

Nurses are in a key position to assess, monitor, and promote good nutrition, both in health-care institutions and in the community. In a variety of settings (e.g., health fairs, classes in schools and community centers, and interactions with families during health screening) they can teach principles of normal nutrition. Nurses also screen for altered nutritional states to detect obesity, malnutrition, or anorexia. Nutritional assessment is also important for any preoperative patient. Nurses teach patients how to adapt to dietary restrictions when special diets are necessary. Nurses are also responsible for monitoring nutritional therapies, such as enteral tube feedings or total parenteral nutrition, that may be necessary to maintain optimal nutrition in patients with significant impairments.

NORMAL NUTRITIONAL FUNCTION

The body uses nutrients to build and maintain body tissues, to furnish energy, and to regulate body processes (Eschleman, 1991). Cell makeup is constantly changing. Nutrients are needed to supply building materials, whether calcium for teeth and bones or fat for padding and support of vital organs. Each cell requires energy to fulfill its task, whether it be maintenance or something as obvious as walking. Chemicals in the form of nutrients act and react to regulate body processes, whether it is as basic a process as breathing or as circumstantial as wound healing. Water, which makes up one half to two thirds of adult weight, is an important regulator in body processes.

In a complex series of processes, the body breaks down the ingested nutrients into a form that can be absorbed and used. Metabolism is the process by which energy from nutrients can be used by the cells or stored for later use. Anabolic processes build up substances and body tissues; catabolic processes break down substances and

or body stores. These reserves are called on when the person is not eating, as in a serious illness, or when there is an increased need for nutrients, as in pregnancy.

Energy obtained from food is measured in the form of a large calorie or kilocalories (abbreviated calories or cal) or in Canada kilojoules (KJ). The large **calorie** is the amount of heat required to raise one kilogram of water 1°C.

Anatomy of the Digestive System

The digestive system consists of the organs of the gastrointestinal (GI) tract through which food enters, travels, and exits the body (mouth, pharynx, esophagus, stomach, small intestine, large intestine) and accessory organs that play a role in the process of digestion (tongue, salivary glands, teeth, liver, pancreas, and gallbladder) (see Fig. 38-1).

The mouth is lined with mucous membrane. The tongue is composed of skeletal muscle and is covered with mucous membrane. The papillae, which are the elevations on the tongue, contain the taste buds. The salivary glands are the sublingual (in the anterior part of the mouth under the tongue), the submandibular (in the posterior part of the floor of the mouth), and the parotid (near the temporomandibular joint). The salivary glands secrete saliva, which contains the salivary enzymes involved in mastication. Mastication includes chewing, the resultant reduction of size of food particles, and the mixing of food with saliva.

The pharynx extends from the base of the skull to the esophagus and is composed of muscle lined with mucous membrane. Food and air pass through this organ before reaching the appropriate outlet (the esophagus for food and the bronchi for air). The epiglottis closes off the airway during swallowing. The esophagus extends from the pharynx to the stomach and transports food from the mouth to the stomach. It is a long, collapsible tube composed of muscular walls lined with mucous membrane.

The stomach lies in the left upper portion of the abdominal cavity. It is connected to the esophagus at the upper end and to the duodenum at the lower end. The stomach varies in size according to body size, sex, and distention. The stomach is lined with mucous membrane and has a muscle layer and an outer fibroserous layer.

The small intestine lies in the abdominal cavity and measures about an inch in diameter and 20 feet in length. It has a mucous lining, two muscle layers, and an outer visceral peritoneal layer. The small intestine consists of the duodenum, the jejunum, and the ileum.

The large intestine, located at the lower end of the GI tract, is about 2 to 3 inches in diameter and 6 feet long. It has a mucous lining, a muscle layer, and an outer visceral peritoneal layer. The large intestine consists of the cecum, the colon (ascending, transverse, descending, and sigmoid), and the rectum (see Fig 38-2).

The accessory organs of digestion are located outside the GI system, but their secretions are conveyed there by ducts. The liver, the largest gland in the body, lies in the right upper quadrant of the abdominal cavity. Bile produced in the liver is transported through the hepatic duct and the cystic duct to the gallbladder, where it is stored and concentrated. The common bile duct transports bile to the duodenum, where it participates in digestion. The pancreas is located behind the stomach and lies in the curvature of the duodenum. Pancreatic enzymes are transported to the duodenum through the pancreatic ducts.

Normal Physiologic Function of Nutrients

Nutrients, or food containing elements for normal body functioning, are divided into six categories: carbohydrates, protein, fat, vitamins, minerals, and water. Energy is provided by the metabolism of carbohydrates, fat, and protein. Water is essential to maintain normal fluid balance and to promote normal digestion, absorption, and metabolism of food. Vitamins and minerals are organic and inorganic compounds important for normal body processes.

Carbohydrates

Carbohydrates are simple sugars (**monosaccharides**) and complex sugars (**polysaccharides**). They are composed of carbon, hydrogen, and oxygen. The polysaccharides are hydrolyzed into simple sugars during digestion by acid hydrolysis and digestive enzymes. Sugars, syrups, molasses, honey, fruit, and milk are excellent sources of simple carbohydrates. Complex carbohydrates are contained in bread, cereal, potatoes, rice, pasta, crackers, flour products, and legumes.

The main function of carbohydrates is to provide energy. Each gram of oxidized carbohydrate yields about 4 kcal. Carbohydrates are also important in oxidizing fats in normal fat metabolism; promoting desirable bacterial growth in the GI tract, which is vital to the synthesis of B-complex vitamins; producing the carbon component in the synthesis of nonessential amino acids; and producing other essential body acids and compounds.

Polysaccharides not digested in the GI tract are one of the main components of dietary fiber. Dietary **fiber** is a minimal source of energy but plays an essential role in stimulating peristalsis and maintaining normal bowel elimination. Another noteworthy characteristic of carbohydrates is their protein-sparing action. Protein sparing is when the body uses carbohydrates rather than protein as a source of energy, thus sparing protein for the vital function of tissue building.

The circulation of blood supplies glucose to the cells as a source of energy and for the production of vital substances. The blood glucose level is maintained within relatively narrow limits (about 80 to 110 mg/dL). In the fasting state, the blood glucose level is about 60 to 80 mg/dL, but shortly after a meal the level can rise to 140 to 160 mg/dL (Patrick, et al., 1991). *Hyperglycemia,* a condition in which the blood glucose level is higher than normal due to inadequate production or use of insulin, occurs in diabetes mellitus. *Hypoglycemia,* a condition in which the blood glucose level is lower than normal, can be symptomatic of liver or pancreatic abnormalities.

Protein

Proteins are vital to growth, development, and the normal functioning of nearly all body systems. They are the major constituents of most living cells and body fluids, including bones, skin, teeth, muscle, hair, blood, and serum. **Proteins** are organic compounds composed of polymers of amino acids connected by peptide bonds. They contain carbon, hydrogen, oxygen, and nitrogen. Depending on the specific amino acids they are composed of, proteins may also contain phosphorus, iron, sulfur, or copper. These proteins are synthesized by the body for specific functions, including: hemoglobin for carrying oxygen to tissues, insulin for blood glucose regulation, and albumin for regulating osmotic pressure in the blood. These functions generally cannot be performed by another body protein.

The main functions of proteins include growth, regulation of body functions and processes, replacement of cellular proteins, and as a source of energy. Protein catabolism supplies 4 kcal per gram. Protein also plays an important role in regulatory functions and in the body's immune system. Catalytic enzymes derived from proteins function in the regulation of digestion, absorption, metabolism, and catabolism.

Proteins can be classified as complete, partially complete, or incomplete:

Complete proteins contain sufficient amounts of the essential amino acids to maintain body tissues and to promote body growth. Essential amino acids must be supplied by the diet since they cannot be synthesized by the body at a rate sufficient to meet the body's needs. Nonessential amino acids can be synthesized by the body from available sources. An adequate diet contains a good supply of both essential and nonessential amino acids. Good sources of complete protein are meat, fish, poultry, milk, cheese, and eggs.

Partially complete proteins contain sufficient amounts of amino acids to maintain life but do not promote growth.

Incomplete proteins do not contain sufficient amounts of amino acids to maintain life, to build tissue, or to promote growth. By themselves, incomplete proteins are not compatible with maintaining life. Sources of incomplete protein are dried peas and beans, peanut butter, seeds, fruits and vegetables, bread, cereal, rice, and pasta.

A person's protein requirement depends on his or her state of health, age, size, state of nutrition, stress level, activity level, and other factors. One measure of the protein requirement is a person's state of nitrogen balance. Nitrogen equilibrium, the normal state for a healthy adult, exists when the amount of nitrogen taken in equals the amount of nitrogen excreted. A state of **positive nitrogen balance** exists when the intake of nitrogen is greater than the amount excreted. This situation exists when new tissues are being synthesized as in recovery from illness, athletic training, pregnancy, and childhood growth. A **negative nitrogen balance** exists when the excretion of nitrogen exceeds the intake. This is an undesirable condition that may exist when a disease is causing excessive tissue breakdown or when the diet is inadequate in protein, calories, or both.

Fat

Fats, also called lipids, include neutral fats, oils, fatty acids, cholesterol, and phospholipids. **Fats** are organic substances composed of carbon, hydrogen, and oxygen. They are a significant component of the American diet.

Fat is a component of all body cells and makes up approximately 20% of the body weight of healthy, nonobese people. Fat performs many important functions in the human body, including cellular transport, insulation, protection of vital organs in the form of padding, provision of energy, energy storage of adipose tissue, vitamin absorption, and carrying fat-soluble vitamins (e.g., vitamins A, D, E, and K).

The energy value of fats is significant, supplying 9 kcal per gram of oxidized fat. This is more than twice as much energy per gram than is provided from oxidation of an equal amount of protein or carbohydrate. Fats also have a significant satiety value: they give us a feeling of fullness because they remain in the stomach longer than carbohydrates or protein.

Fats are classified as saturated or unsaturated, based on chemical differences. Saturated fats have two hydrogen atoms attached to each of the carbon atoms in the carbon atom chain. An unsaturated fat has a single hydrogen atom missing from each of two side-by-side carbon atoms and thus, a double bond will be formed between the two carbon atoms. This difference is significant in terms of the physical characteristics of the fats, including such factors as melting point, hardness, and the ability to form an emulsion.

Most sources of fats contain a combination of saturated and unsaturated fatty acids. Sources of animal fats, especially beef and lamb, generally contain a higher percentage of saturated fatty acids and are harder than vegetable sources of fatty acids. Coconut oil, palm oil, and palm kernel oil are also highly saturated. Chicken fat contains a significantly higher percentage of unsaturated fatty acids and is measurably softer than beef or lamb fat. Fish and vegetable sources are classified as unsaturated, as they contain a higher percentage of unsaturated fatty acids and are also generally softer than animal fats.

Vitamins

Vitamins are organic compounds that are essential to the body in small quantities for growth, development, maintenance, and reproduction (Table 33-1). They do not supply energy, but they assist in the use of energy nutrients. Most vitamins (except vitamins D and K) cannot be synthesized by the body and must therefore be supplied by the diet. Recommended daily allowances (RDAs) specify the intake of vitamins needed to supply normal daily requirements. Vitamins are present in small quantities in food and can be destroyed by exposure to light, air, and heat, and during food preparation. Because of this, fresh foods are usually the best source of vitamins. Some foods, such as fortified milk or cereals, have extra vitamins added.

Vitamins are classified as fat-soluble or water-soluble. Fat-soluble vitamins (A, D, E, K) are absorbed with fat into the circulation. A deficiency of fat-soluble vitamins can occur when fat digestion or absorption is altered. Excess fat-soluble vitamins are stored in the liver or adipose tissue; thus, excessive intake of vitamins A and D can cause toxicity.

The water-soluble vitamins are vitamin C and the B-complex vitamins. Water-soluble vitamins are not stored in the body, although some body tissues can hold limited amounts. Adequate daily intake of water-soluble vitamins is recommended to prevent deficiencies. When the intake of water-soluble vitamins exceeds the amount absorbed by the tissues, the excess is excreted in the urine.

Fat-Soluble Vitamins
Vitamin A. Vitamin A is important in:

- Maintenance of normal vision, especially in dim light
- Maintenance of healthy epithelium
- Promotion of normal skeletal and tooth development
- Promotion of normal cellular proliferation.

The effects of a vitamin A deficiency are significant, and in many countries vitamin A deficiency is the most prevalent vitamin deficiency. Signs of vitamin A deficiency are:

- Night blindness
- Epithelial changes such as keratinization (progressive degeneration of the cells that may lead to infections in the eyes, ears, or nasal passages)

TABLE 33–1

Summary of Vitamins

Vitamin	Function	Deficiency	Sources
Fat-Soluble Vitamins			

A
(retinol;
  precursor:
  carotenes)
	Formation of visual purple and visual violet; normal growth of epithelial tissue, and visual violet; especially skin and mucous membranes; normal bone and tooth structure	Night and glare blindness; deterioration of epithelial tissue leading to decreased resistance to infection; dry, scaly skin; eye changes; xerophthalmia leading to blindness	Liver; whole milk and foods containing milk fat, such as butter, cream, cheese; margarine; as carotene in dark green leafy vegetables and some fruits

D (calciferol)	Promotion of absorption of calcium and phosphorus; normal use of these minerals in skeleton and soft tissue	Faulty bone and tooth development; rickets; osteomalacia	Fortified milk; direct exposure of skin to sunlight; fish liver oils
E (tocopherols)	Antioxidation—protection of substances that oxidize readily, such as essential fatty acids; thus, prevention of damage to cell membranes	Destruction of red blood cells (hemolysis); deficiency is rare	Vegetable oils and shortening; margarine; green leafy vegetables; whole grains, legumes, nuts
K (menadione)	Normal blood clotting	Prolonged clotting time; hemorrhagic disease in newborns	Synthesis by intestinal bacteria; green leafy vegetables
Water-Soluble Vitamins			
Ascorbic Acid (vitamin C)	Collagen formation: strong blood vessels, healthy skin, healthy gums, wound healing; formation of red blood cells; absorption of iron, conversion of folacin to its active form	Adult acne; easy bruising; poor wound healing; swan-neck; hair deformity; sore gums; hemorrhages around bones; scurvy	Citrus fruit; broccoli; strawberries, cantaloupe; guava, mango, papaya; peppers; tomatoes; greens; potatoes
Thiamine (B$_1$)	Energy metabolism; synthesis of DNA, RNA	Poor appetite; fatigue; constipation; neuritis of legs; beriberi: wasting, paralysis of legs, heart failure, mental confusion	Meats, especially pork; wheat germ; whole-grain and enriched bread; legumes; peanuts, peanut butter, nuts
Riboflavin (B$_2$)	Energy metabolism; protein metabolism; essential for functioning of B$_6$ and niacin	Eye irritation; cheilosis; glossitis; seborrheic dermatitis.	Milk; organ meats; meat, fish, eggs; green leafy vegetables; enriched breads and cereals
Niacin (precursor: tryptophan)	Energy metabolism; production of fatty acids, cholesterol, steroid hormones	Fatigue; poor appetite; weakness; anxiety; pellagra; diarrhea, dermatitis, deteriorated mental state	Liver, meat, fish, poultry; peanuts; legumes; whole-grain and enriched breads and cereals; sources of tryptophan; complete protein foods
Pyridoxine (B$_6$)	Amino acid metabolism involving protein synthesis; synthesis of regulatory substances such as serotonin; niacin production; hemoglobin synthesis	Anemia; dermatitis; irritability; convulsions	Liver, kidney; chicken; fish; pork; eggs; whole-grain cereals; legumes
Folacin (folic acid)	Protein metabolism: synthesis of DNA and RNA, red blood cell formation	Macrocytic anemia	Green leafy vegetables; liver, kidney, meats, fish; nuts; legumes; whole grains; bacterial synthesis

(continued)

TABLE 33–1

(continued)

Vitamin	Function	Deficiency	Sources
Cobalamin (B_{12})	Protein metabolism: synthesis of DNA, production of red blood cells; healthy nervous system: carbohydrate metabolism, myelin formation (Intrinsic factor of gastric secretions is required for absorption)	Pernicious anemia: macrocytic anemia, sore mouth, poor appetite, poor coordination in walking, mental disturbances	Found only in animal products: meat, fish, poultry, eggs, milk, cheese; bacterial synthesis
Pantothenic Acid	Energy metabolism; synthesis of amino acids, fatty acids, cholesterol, steroid hormones, hemoglobin	Unlikely unless part of a deficiency of all B vitamins Associated with "burning feet" syndrome	Organ meats; salmon; eggs; broccoli; mushrooms; pork; whole grains; legumes (by bacterial synthesis)
Biotin	Protein, fat, and carbohydrate metabolism	Hair loss; dermatitis. Deficiency rare; can be induced by aviden, a protein in raw egg white.	Liver, egg yolk, soy flour, cereal Bacterial synthesis

From Eschleman, M. M. (1991). *Introductory nutrition and diet therapy,* 2nd ed. (pp. 202–203). Philadelphia: J. B. Lippincott.

- Follicular hyperkeratosis (skin changes leading to rough, dry, and scaly skin)
- Dryness of the eyes (xerophthalmia)
- Inadequate tooth and bone development.

The RDA of vitamin A for adult men is 1000 RE (or 5000 IU [international units]) and for adult women 800 RE (or 4000 IU), with more needed for pregnant or lactating women (Eschleman, 1991). Vitamin A is stored in the liver and excessive intake can be toxic. Excellent sources of vitamin A are dark-green leafy vegetables, yellow fruits and vegetables, fish oils, liver, whole milk and whole-milk cheeses, fortified low-fat milk and cheeses, and egg yolk.

Vitamin D. Vitamin D is synthesized in the skin by ultraviolet light activity, in the liver, and in the kidney. Vitamin D is important in:

- Intestinal absorption of calcium
- Mobilization of calcium and phosphorus from bone
- Renal reabsorption of calcium.

These effects increase the blood levels of calcium and phosphorus, allowing for normal mineralization of bone and cartilage and for the maintenance of calcium in extracellular fluid for normal muscle contraction.

A deficiency in vitamin D intake is significant because it leads to an inadequate absorption of calcium and phosphorus and to a deficiency of mineralization in bones and teeth. The bones become soft and cannot bear weight, resulting in skeletal deformities. Signs of vitamin D deficiency are:

- Rickets in children (soft, fragile bones and skeletal deformities)

- Poor dental health
- Tetany (low serum calcium resulting in muscle twitching and convulsions)
- Osteomalacia (soft bones and a tendency toward spontaneous fractures secondary to a vitamin D and calcium deficiency).

The RDA of vitamin D for adults is 5 µg and 10 µg for pregnant or lactating women (Robinson & Weighley, 1984). Excellent sources of vitamin D are fish oils, fortified milk, and sunlight exposure. Excessive amounts can be toxic.

Vitamin E. The physiologic effects of vitamin E are not well understood. The major function is thought to be its role as an antioxidant, in which it assists in maintaining the integrity of cellular membranes and in protecting vitamin A from oxidation.

Vitamin E deficiency is rare, but signs of severe deficiency are increased hemolysis of red blood cells, poor reflexes and impaired neuromuscular functioning, and anemia.

The RDA of vitamin E for adult men is 10 mg α-TE and for adult women 8 mg α-TE (more for pregnant or lactating women) (Eschleman, 1991). Excellent sources are vegetable oils, green leafy vegetables, nuts, and legumes. Vitamin E is not stored in the body to any appreciable extent, and toxicity is rare.

Vitamin K. An adequate intake of vitamin K is necessary for the formation of prothrombin and other clotting factors. The major physiologic effect of vitamin K appears to be its role in blood coagulation.

Vitamin K deficiencies are manifested in two ways: an increased tendency to hemorrhage (prolonged clotting time) and hemorrhagic disease of the newborn. This disease of the newborn is most likely to occur in premature or anoxic infants.

RDAs for vitamin K were set for the first time in 1989 (Eschleman, 1991). The RDA for adult men is 80 µg/day and for adult women 65 µg/day. It is thought that about half of the body's requirement of vitamin K is synthesized by bacteria in the lower intestinal tract. The major sources are green leafy vegetables, liver, and intestinal synthesis. Vitamin K is not stored in the body to an appreciable extent. Large amounts can be toxic.

Water-Soluble Vitamins

B-Complex Vitamins. Each B-complex vitamin has its own function and RDA.

Vitamin B_1 (thiamine) functions in carbohydrate metabolism, and adequate thiamine intake will result in healthy nerve functioning and normal appetite and digestion. Deficiency symptoms are poor appetite, apathy and mental depression, fatigue, constipation, edema, cardiac failure, and neuritis. The disease associated with inadequate thiamine intake is beriberi. Acute beriberi adversely affects the cardiac, nervous, and GI systems. Death can result from cardiac failure. The RDA of thiamine is 1.4 mg for men and 1.0 mg for women, with additional amounts recommended for pregnant or lactating women (Robinson & Weighley, 1984). Excellent sources are whole-grain breads and cereals, green vegetables, milk, meat, fish, and poultry.

Vitamin B_2 (riboflavin) functions in protein and carbohydrate metabolism and contributes to healthy skin and normal vision. Deficiency symptoms are cheilosis (cracking and fissures at the corners of the mouth), dermatitis, and increased vascularization of the cornea and other vision irregularities. The RDA of riboflavin is 1.6 mg for men and 1.2 mg for women, with additional amounts recommended for pregnant or lactating women (Robinson & Weighley, 1984). Excellent sources are milk, eggs, green leafy vegetables, and organ meats.

Vitamin B_3 (niacin) is involved in glycogen metabolism, tissue regeneration, and fat synthesis. The niacin deficiency disease is pellagra; its symptoms are fatigue, headache, loss of appetite and weight loss, abdominal pain, diarrhea, dermatitis, and neurologic deterioration. The RDA of niacin is 18 mg for men and 13 mg for women, with additional amounts recommended for pregnant or lactating women (Robinson & Weighley, 1984). Excellent sources are meat, fish, poultry, and whole grains.

Vitamin B_{12} (cyanocobalamin) functions in the formation of mature red blood cells and in the synthesis of DNA and RNA. It requires intrinsic factor for absorption. A vitamin B_{12} deficiency leads to pernicious anemia, other forms of anemia, and neurologic deterioration. The RDA of vitamin B_{12} is 3 µg for adults, with additional amounts recommended for pregnant or lactating women (Robinson & Weighley, 1984). This vitamin is found only in animal foods (meats, fish, poultry, milk, and eggs).

Other important B vitamins are vitamin B_6, pantothenic acid, and biotin. Deficiencies are rare.

Vitamin C. Vitamin C is important in:

- Protection against infection
- Adequate wound healing
- Collagen formation
- Iron absorption
- Metabolism of several important amino acids.

Vitamin C also acts as an antioxidant and thus protects vitamins A and E from excessive oxidation.

Signs of vitamin C deficiency are:

- Inadequate formation of collagen (poor wound healing), increased susceptibility to infection, retardation of growth and development, joint pain, anemia
- Scurvy (now rare, but formerly common among sailors whose diets lacked fresh fruits and vegetables, particularly citrus fruits). Symptoms of scurvy are joint pain, leg swelling, fever, infections, irritability, bone degeneration, tooth and gum degeneration, and anemia.

The RDA for vitamin C is 60 mg for adults and 80 to 100 mg for pregnant or lactating women (Robinson & Weighley, 1984). Excellent sources of vitamin C are citrus fruits, strawberries, melons, broccoli, fresh tomatoes, and green leafy vegetables. Little vitamin C is stored in the body, so a daily supply is needed. Although megadoses (30 to 100 times the recommended allowances) of vitamin C have not been proven toxic, excessive doses are not advised due to the possibility of kidney-stone formation and GI disturbances.

Minerals

Minerals are inorganic substances found in nearly all body tissues and fluids. When plant or animal tissue is burned, what remains is ash or mineral matter. Minerals function in the building of body tissues and in the regulation of body metabolism. There are over 25 known minerals in the adult body, but only the most notable are described here or in Table 33-2.

Calcium. Nearly all the calcium in the body is found in the bones and teeth. The bones provide the framework for the body and serve as a storage area for calcium to keep the plasma concentration of calcium relatively constant. Calcium is also important in:

- Conversion of prothrombin to thrombin, and other steps of the coagulation process
- Nerve impulse transmission, by participating in the formation of acetylcholine
- Regulation of materials in and out of cells
- Contraction and relaxation of muscles, most notably the heart muscle.

TABLE 33–2

Summary of Minerals

Mineral	Function	Deficiency	Sources
Calcium	Bone and tooth formation; blood clotting; cell permeability; nerve stimulation; muscle contraction; enzyme activation	Stunted growth; rickets; osteomalacia; osteoporosis (porous bones); tetany (low serum calcium)	Milk; hard cheese; salmon and small fish eaten with bones; some dark green vegetables; legumes (tofu)
Iron	Hemoglobin and myoglobin formation; cellular enzymes	Anemia	Liver, lean meats; legumes, dried fruits, green leafy vegetables; whole grain and fortified cereals
Sodium	Osmotic pressure; water balance; acid–base balance; nerve stimulation; muscle contraction; cell permeability	Rare: nausea; vomiting; giddiness; exhaustion; cramps	Table salt, salted foods, MSG and other sodium additives; milk; meat, fish, poultry, eggs
Potassium	Osmotic pressure; water balance; acid–base balance; nerve stimulation; muscle contraction; synthesis of protein; glycogen formation	Nausea; vomiting; muscular weakness; rapid heart beat; heart failure	Widely distributed in food: meats, fish, poultry; whole grains; fruits, vegetables, legumes
Iodine	Synthesis of thyroid hormones that regulate basal metabolic rate	Goiter; cretinism, if deficiency is severe	Iodized salt; seafood; food grown near the sea
Fluoride	Resists dental decay	Tooth decay in young children	Fluoridated water (1 part per million)
Phosphorus	Bone and tooth formation; energy metabolism—component of ATP and ADP; protein synthesis—component of DNA and RNA; fat transport; acid–base balance; enzyme formation	Stunted growth; rickets (due to excessive excretion rather than to dietary deficiency)	Distributed widely in foods: milk; meats, poultry, fish, eggs; cheese; nuts; legumes; whole grains; processed foods
Magnesium	Component of bones and teeth; activates many enzymes, including those involved in energy metabolism; nerve stimulation; muscle contraction	Seen in alcoholism or renal disease: tremors leading to convulsive seizures	Green leafy vegetables; nuts; whole grains; meat; milk; seafood
Selenium	Antioxidant—prevents oxidative damage to body tissue	Keshan disease; damage to heart muscle	Fish, meat, breads and cereals
Zinc	Constituent of many enzyme systems, including those involved in protein digestion and synthesis, carbon dioxide transport, and vitamin A use	Delayed wound healing; impaired taste sensitivity. Severe deficiency (rare in US): retarded growth and sexual development; dwarfism	Oysters, herring; meat, liver, fish; milk; whole grains; nuts; legumes

From Eschelman, M. M. (1991). *Introductory nutrition and diet therapy,* 2nd ed. (p. 170). Philadelphia: J. B. Lippincott.

The absorption of calcium takes place mainly from the duodenum by active transport. Calcium is also passively diffused across the intestinal mucosa from the jejunum and the ileum. The amount of calcium absorbed is mainly determined by the body's need. About 30% to 40% of the calcium in the diet is absorbed in the healthy adult. Growing children and teen-agers and pregnant and lactating women absorb a greater percentage of their dietary calcium because of the increased need. Some of the calcium ingested forms insoluble salts, which cannot be absorbed.

Absorption of calcium is assisted by adequate amounts of vitamin D, parathyroid hormone, ascorbic acid, lactose, several other amino acids, and physical activity. Calcium absorption can be decreased by inadequate amounts of vitamin D, insufficient exposure to sunlight, decreased amounts of ascorbic acid, decreased physical activity, and emotional stress. Other factors, such as a high consumption of dietary fiber and excessive phosphorus intake, are thought to impair the absorption of calcium. These factors are still being researched.

The effects of calcium deficiency can be profound:

Rickets, a disease of infants and children caused by inadequate calcium and vitamin D, involves the inadequate deposition of calcium and phosphorus in the bone. Symptoms include soft bones, enlarged joints, enlarged skull secondary to delayed closure of the cranial fontanels, bowed legs, and spinal and chest deformities.
Osteomalacia, the adult form of rickets, results from an inadequate intake of calcium, phosphorus, and vitamin

D. The mineral content of the bone is reduced but the bone stays the same size.

Osteoporosis involves a reduction in bone mass. It is mainly seen in women over age 50 who have had a chronically insufficient intake of calcium. Other factors contributing to the development of osteoporosis may include decreased estrogens, heredity, smoking, race, and decreased physical activity. Symptoms vary in severity and may include reduced bone mass, leading to poor posture; increased fragility of bones, leading to an increase in bone fractures; and delayed healing of fractured bones. Malabsorption syndromes can lead to problems in calcium absorption and osteoporosis can develop.

Interestingly, low dietary intake of calcium has also been associated with hypertension; research is continuing (Robinson, 1986).

The RDA for calcium is 800 mg for adults, with additional amounts recommended for teen-agers and pregnant or lactating women (Robinson & Weighley, 1984). Excellent sources are yogurt, milk (whole, skim, buttermilk), and hard cheese. Other sources are ice cream, cottage cheese, salmon, clams, oysters, collards, mustard and turnip greens, and tofu.

Iron. Most of the iron in the body is found in hemoglobin, the red-pigmented iron-containing protein. Hemoglobin carries oxygen from the lungs to the tissues and helps transport carbon dioxide to the lungs. Iron is also found in the body's myoglobin, an iron–protein compound in the muscle that serves as an oxygen storage system for the muscles.

Iron deficiencies may manifest themselves in iron-deficiency anemia. This form of anemia is not uncommon, especially in infants and menstruating women. In an anemia, circulating hemoglobin is reduced and the blood cannot provide for the oxygen needs of the tissues. Iron-deficiency anemia may result from a diet chronically deficient in iron. Other factors that may lead to iron-deficiency anemia are blood loss, chronic disease, pregnancy and lactation, diarrhea, and other nutritional deficiencies (protein and calorie). Symptoms of iron-deficiency anemia are excessive fatigue, lethargy, and poor resistance to infection. Since obtaining sufficient iron to combat anemia by dietary measures alone is impractical, recommended treatment includes taking iron salts (ferrous sulfate or gluconate) along with a well-balanced diet.

The RDA of iron for the adult man is 10 mg and for the adult woman 18 mg, with additional amounts recommended for pregnant or lactating women (Robinson & Weighley, 1984). Good sources of iron are meat (especially liver), fish, and poultry. Other fairly good sources are eggs, bread, enriched cereals, and leafy vegetables.

Sodium. Sodium is found primarily in the extracellular fluid in the body and helps maintain the body's fluid and acid–base balance. RDAs for sodium intake have not been set. The average diet contains more sodium than the body requires, and sodium deficiencies (except in rare circumstances) have not been identified. Many people would benefit from eating less sodium, and sodium restriction is important for people with heart disease, hypertension, edema, renal disorders, liver disease, congestive heart failure, and toxemias of pregnancy. Sodium is present in many foods, including salt, salt compounds, milk, meat, poultry, fish, eggs, and processed foods.

Potassium. Potassium is found primarily in the intracellular fluid of the body and functions in fluid balance, in protein synthesis, and in the regulation of muscle contraction. RDAs have not been set, and deficiencies have not been identified, except in cases of severe vomiting and diarrhea and diabetic acidosis. Potassium restriction is indicated for patients with renal impairment and renal failure. Potassium is present in many foods, including protein-rich foods, bread, cereal, fruits, and vegetables.

Iodine. Although considered a trace element, iodine is an important mineral. The primary location of iodine in the body is the thyroid gland. The major function of iodine is as a component of the thyroid hormones, thyroxine and triiodothyronine. These hormones help regulate energy metabolism, nervous and muscle cell functioning, and mental and physical growth.

A chronic deficiency of iodine can lead to endemic goiter. The major initial symptom is an enlarged thyroid gland. This condition is especially significant in pregnant women because it can lead to physical and mental retardation in the fetus. In its severe form, this condition in the infant is known as *cretinism*. Cretinism is rare in the United States but remains a problem in certain areas of Central and South America, Africa, and Asia. Characteristics of cretinism are muscle flabbiness, weakness, dry skin, thick lips, skeletal retardation, and severe mental retardation. Thyroid hormone given early to infants can be of some value, but certain physical and mental deficiencies are irreversible. Everyone, especially pregnant women, should eat a diet sufficient in iodine.

The RDA of iodine for adult men and women is 150 μg, with additional amounts recommended for pregnant or lactating women (Robinson & Weighley, 1984). Good sources of iodine are salt-water fish, shellfish, and iodized salt. A half-teaspoon of iodized salt contains nearly 200 μg of iodine.

Fluorine. Fluorine is found primarily in the bones and teeth. It functions to maintain bone structure and to reduce tooth decay by strengthening tooth enamel. There is no RDA, but the estimated safe intake level is 1.5 to 4.0 mg per day for adults (Robinson & Weighley, 1984). Fluorine is found in the diet, the water, and the soil in generally safe and adequate amounts. Many areas in the United States have added fluoride, a fluorine compound, to the water in amounts equivalent to the normal soil concentration (1 part fluoride per 1 million parts water or soil).

Water

Water is necessary to maintain normal cell function. Water is obtained by drinking fluid and eating foods with a high water content (fresh fruits and vegetables) and by the oxidation of food. Thirst signals the need for water and encourages a person to drink. Fluid balance is covered in Chapter 32.

Normal Physiologic Function of the Digestive System

The digestive system performs the vital function of converting the foods we eat into substances that can be absorbed and used by the cells of the body. This conversion involves the processes of digestion, absorption, metabolism, and excretion.

Digestion

Digestion is the process by which foods are broken down and used by the body for growth, development, healing, and prevention of disease. Digestion includes the mechanical and chemical processes necessary to convert the food into a physically absorbable state.

The mechanical process of digestion consists of the following events:

1. Mastication takes place in the mouth. Food particles are reduced in size and mixed with enzymes in saliva.
2. Deglutition (swallowing) begins in the mouth and continues in the pharynx and the esophagus.
3. Churning movements and peristalsis move the ingested material through the stomach and into the duodenum.
4. In the small intestine, the ingested material is further churned and mixed with digestive enzymes, and comes in contact with the intestinal mucosa to allow for absorption.
5. Peristalsis moves the ingested material into the large intestine.
6. Further churning, peristalsis, and absorption help move the ingested mass along the full length of the large intestine, where it is stored until evacuation from the body occurs.

The chemical processes of digestion change the composition of ingested material. Only carbohydrates, fats, and proteins must be chemically reduced for absorption.

Carbohydrate Digestion. Carbohydrate digestion involves the hydrolysis of polysaccharides (with the exception of cellulose and other fibers) into disaccharides by the amylase enzymes found in saliva and pancreatic juices. Hydrolysis is a chemical process between a compound and water that results in the division of the compound into simpler components. A polysaccharide is a carbohydrate compound containing three or more saccharide groups, a disaccharide contains two saccharide groups, and a monosaccharide contains only one saccharide group. Disaccharides are further hydrolyzed into monosaccharides by the enzymes sucrase, maltase, and lactase secreted by the intestines.

Fat Digestion. Fat digestion is accomplished by emulsification of fats, facilitated by bile. Emulsification involves the breaking down of fats into smaller fat droplets and the dispersion of these droplets into solution. The pancreatic enzyme lipase hydrolyzes the small fat droplets into fatty acids and glycerol.

Protein Digestion. Protein digestion involves the hydrolysis of the larger protein compounds into amino acids. This is done by the protease enzymes, which include pepsin from the gastric fluid, trypsin and other proteases from the pancreatic fluid, and peptidases from the intestinal fluid.

Absorption

Absorption is the process by which the digested protein, fats, and carbohydrates as well as vitamins, minerals, and water are actively and passively transported through the intestinal mucosa into the blood or lymphatic circulation. The proteins, as amino acids, and the digested carbohydrates and simple sugars, in the form of monosaccharides, are absorbed into the bloodstream through the intestinal capillaries. The fats, in the form of glycerol and fatty acids, are absorbed into the lymphatic system through the lymphatic capillaries in the intestinal villi. Some finely emulsified neutral fats are absorbed undigested into the capillaries.

Metabolism

After the ingested food is digested and absorbed, it is ready to be metabolized. *Metabolism* is the complex chemical process that occurs in the cells to allow for energy use and for cellular growth and repair. Metabolism involves both catabolic and anabolic processes: catabolic processes break down complex substances into simpler substances (e.g., tissue breakdown) and anabolic processes convert simple substances into more complex ones (e.g., tissue repair).

Carbohydrate Metabolism. Short-term glucose excesses are changed into glycogen in the presence of insulin by the liver cells. This is an anabolic process called **glycogenesis.** Glycogen is stored in the liver and skeletal muscles until needed and is then converted back into glucose by a catabolic process called glycogenolysis.

Longer-term storage of glucose in the presence of insulin takes the form of fat deposits (adipose tissue). When the amount of glucose entering the cells is not enough to meet cellular demands, gluconeogenesis (the formation of glucose from protein and fat in the liver) occurs. This catabolic process yields 4.1 kcal of energy per gram of oxidized carbohydrate (Luke, 1984).

Fat Metabolism. Fats are converted to adipose tissue and stored in the body's fat deposits. Stored fat deposits make up the body's largest reserve energy source. The catabolism of fats involves the hydrolysis of fat into glycerol and fatty acids. The fatty acids are then converted by a series of chemical reactions known as ketogenesis into ketone bodies. Next, in the tissue cells, ketones are converted via the citric acid cycle into energy, carbon dioxide, and water. Glycerol is converted by gluconeogenesis into glucose. Fats are a more concentrated source of energy than carbohydrates, yielding 9 kcal of energy per gram of catabolized fat.

Protein Metabolism. Protein anabolism plays the important role of tissue-building, antibody production, blood cell replacement, and tissue repair. Temporary excesses of protein are stored in the liver and in skeletal muscle. Protein catabolism involves the hydrolysis of cellular proteins into amino acids in the tissue cell. It also involves the deamination process of amino acids, in which an amino group is split off from an amino acid to form ammonia and keto acid. This process takes place in the liver cell to form glucose and urea.

Excretion

The excretory organs (kidneys, sweat glands, skin, lungs, and intestines) remove waste products from the body. Water, toxins, salts, and nitrogen wastes are excreted through the skin and sweat glands. Carbon dioxide and water are excreted through the lungs. Digestive and metabolic wastes are excreted through the intestines and the rectum.

Characteristics of Normal Nutrition

Normal nutrition involves a balanced intake of food to meet the energy requirements necessary for organ function, body movement, and work. Adequate food intake also provides raw materials for the production of enzymes and the production of cells necessary for growth, replacement of tissues, and tissue repair. See the display for the characteristics of a well-nourished person.

Ideal Body Weight

Normal nutritional intake usually results in body weight appropriate for a person's height and frame. Ideal body weight (IBW) is the estimated weight optimal for body

---

> **Characteristics of a Well-Nourished Person**
>
> - Normal weight and height for age, body build, and developmental stage
> - Adequate appetite
> - Active, alert, and able to maintain adequate attention span
> - Firm, healthy skin and mucous membranes
> - Erect posture, with straight arms and legs
> - Well-developed muscles without excess body fat
> - Normal schedule of tooth eruption and healthy teeth and gums
> - Normal urinary and bowel elimination patterns
> - Normal sleep patterns
> - Normal hemoglobin, hematocrit, and serum protein levels
> - Absence of diet-related abnormalities

---

functioning and health. Ranges for IBW according to height and body frame are listed in standardized tables (see Appendix D). Sometimes such information can be misleading, since it does not always reflect accurately the amount of body fat present. For example, a body builder may be heavier than the IBW listed but may have a less-than-average amount of body fat.

A rule of thumb for estimating IBW is that a 5-foot-tall woman should weigh about 100 pounds; 5 pounds should be added for each additional inch. The IBW for a 5-foot-tall man is 105 pounds, to which 6 pounds should be added for each additional inch.

Physical Status

Normal nutrition is apparent in the normal appearance of many parts of the body. The patient's general appearance should reflect alertness and responsiveness. The skin should have normal tone and good turgor. The mouth, gums, and lips should appear moist and pink and should be free from lesions. Hair and nails should appear healthy. Bones should hold the body erect, and muscles should maintain good tone. Normal reflexes should be apparent. The abdomen should appear flat and undistended.

Normal Laboratory Values

Laboratory values are usually within normal ranges in healthy people. Normal hematocrit and hemoglobin values reflect adequate iron stores and hydration status. Plasma protein values such as serum albumin reflect adequate protein intake.

Normal Nutritional Functional Pattern

Normal diets vary widely among people. The following guidelines can help each person to make good dietary choices and evaluate the adequacy of his or her diet.

Basic Four Food Groups

The basic four food groups, as recommended by the U.S. Department of Agriculture, provide a general guide for planning nutritious, appetizing meals. The four groups are the fruit and vegetable group, the bread and cereal group, the meat group, and the milk group. Fats, sugars, and alcohol are included in a fifth group. Guidelines suggest an appropriate daily number of servings from each group (Fig. 33-1). Food selected according to these guidelines provides approximately 1200 kilocalories daily.

Fruit and Vegetable Group. The fruit and vegetable group includes cooked and uncooked parts of plants, including roots, bulbs, flowers, stems, and leaves. Four or more daily servings are recommended. One serving of an uncooked fruit or vegetable is roughly equal to one medium-sized fruit or vegetable (e.g., one apple, one orange, one potato). A serving of a cooked fruit or vegetable is about a half-cup.

Since this group provides a major source of vitamin A, vitamin C, and fiber, it is recommended that the four servings include:

- One serving of a significant source of vitamin C (e.g., citrus fruits, strawberries, melon, spinach, broccoli, or green peppers)
- One serving of a dark-green or yellow vegetable for vitamin A (e.g., squash, pumpkin, carrots, spinach, broccoli, asparagus, or beet greens)
- One serving of a significant source of fiber (e.g., uncooked and unpeeled fruits and vegetables).

In addition to vitamin A and vitamin C, the fruit and vegetable group is also a fair to good source of calcium, iron, potassium, and all the B vitamins except B_{12}. As a group, these foods have a high water content and are generally low in calories, protein, and fat. Fruits and vegetables are free from cholesterol. The carbohydrate content varies depending on the type of vegetable or fruit and the method of processing and preservation.

Bread and Cereal Group. The bread and cereal group is an important food source in many countries. Rice, wheat, and corn are staples in the diets of people worldwide. This group includes whole grains, breads, cereals, rice, noodles, pasta, and products made with enriched flour and cereal. Four daily servings are recommended; one serving is about a half-cup of a cooked product (pasta, rice, or cereal), one slice of bread, or one ounce of uncooked cereal.

Breads and cereals are good sources of thiamine, iron, niacin, and riboflavin. Many breads and cereals are enriched, especially those processed and sold in the United States. Enrichment with vitamins and minerals adds to their nutritive value. Whole grains are also excellent sources of zinc, copper, B vitamins, and vitamin E. As a group, these foods are a good source of carbohydrates, calories, and incomplete proteins and are low in fat.

Meat Group. Two servings from the meat group are recommended daily; a serving is 2 or 3 ounces of the edible part of meat, fish, or poultry. This group also includes eggs, dry beans or peas, lentils, soybeans, nuts, seeds, and peanut butter. One ounce of meat is roughly equal to one egg, a half-cup of dry beans or peas, or 2 tablespoons of peanut butter.

The meat group is an excellent source of protein and is also a good source of several vitamins and minerals, including vitamin A, phosphorus, magnesium, iron, and the B vitamins. Some shellfish are a good source of calcium, and salt-water fish are a good source of iodine. This group can contain a large amount of fat, depending on the cut of the meat, the type of meat, and the method of processing and preparation. Animal food can contain a significantly larger amount of cholesterol and saturated fat, but fish is generally lower in cholesterol. Egg yolks in particular contain a large amount of cholesterol.

Milk Group. The milk group is an important source of nutrition for all people, but is especially important for infants, children, and pregnant or lactating women. This group includes milk, ice cream, ice milk, yogurt, and cheese. The recommended number of daily servings depends on the person's physiologic needs, age, and developmental level. Children under 12 need two or three servings; teen-agers need four servings; adults need two or three servings; pregnant women need three or four servings; and lactating women need four servings. One serving equals a cup (8 ounces) of milk, 1.5 cups of ice cream, or about 1.3 ounces of cheese.

Milk is an excellent source of calcium, phosphorus, and riboflavin. It is also fairly rich in sodium, potassium, magnesium, vitamin A, thiamine, vitamin B_6, vitamin B_{12}, niacin, and vitamin D. Milk is an excellent source of protein. There is little iron in milk. The fat content of milk depends on the type of product. In recent years, many people have started drinking low-fat milk and eating low-fat cheese to decrease their fat intake.

The nutritional characteristics of cheese are similar to those of milk, depending on the type of cheese. One noteworthy difference (which could be important for people with a lactase deficiency) is that cheese contains only a trace amount of lactose.

Fats, Sugars, and Alcohol Group. The foods in this group—for example, sugar, jelly, jam, shortening, butter, margarine, salad dressings, soft drinks, and alcoholic beverages—add flavor, variety, and interest to our

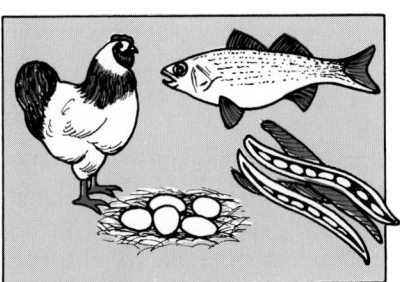

Meat, poultry, fish, and beans group
(2 servings)

½ serving is:
1 to 1½ ounces lean, boneless, cooked
   meat, poultry, or fish
1 egg
½ to ¾ cup cooked dry beans, peas, lentils,
   or soybeans
2 tablespoons peanut butter

Poultry and fish preferred over red meats.

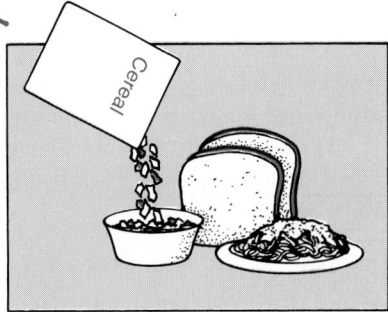

Bread and cereal group (4 servings)

1 serving is:
1 slice bread
½ to ¾ cup cooked cereal or pasta
1 ounce ready-to-eat cereal

Choose whole-grain products.

Daily Meal Planning

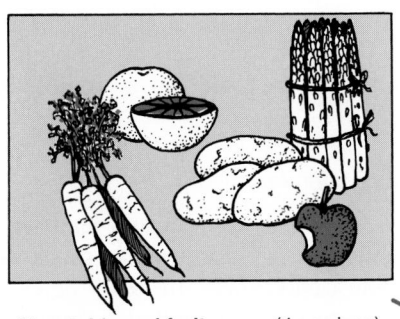

Vegetable and fruit group (4 servings)

1 serving is:
½ cup   an orange
a small salad   ½ grapefruit
a medium-sized potato

Use citrus fruit, melon, berries, or tomatoes
daily and a dark-green or dark-yellow
vegetable frequently. Eat unpeeled fruits
and vegetables.

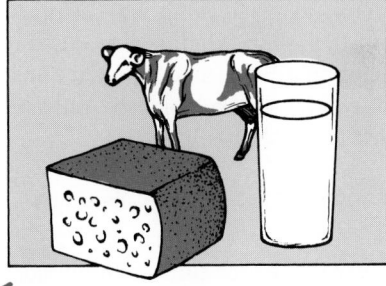

Milk and cheese group (2 to 4 servings)

Servings:
Adults   2
Children under 9 years old   2-3
Children 9 to 12 years old
   and pregnant women   3
Teens and nursing mothers   4

1 serving is:
1 cup milk or yogurt
1⅓ ounces cheddar or swiss cheese
1½ cups ice cream or ice milk
2 cups cottage cheese

Skim, nonfat, and low-fat milk and milk
products provide calcium and keep fat
intake down.

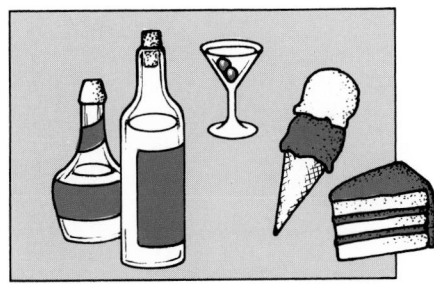

Fats, sweets, and alcohol group
Use sparingly.

Figure 33–1.   Basic four food groups permit nutritional daily meal planning.

meals. There is no recommended number of daily servings, and these foods should be restricted by people who want to lose weight. It is important to minimize the intake of sugar and fats, especially saturated fats. Foods in this group add to the energy value of our diets but generally add little nutritive value. One noteworthy exception is fortified margarine, a fair source of vitamin A and vitamin E.

Recommended Dietary Allowances

The Food and Nutrition Board of the National Academy of Sciences has developed recommended dietary allowances for kilocalories, protein, and certain vitamins and minerals (see Appendix D). These values are recommendations for healthy people and do not take into consideration factors that may significantly increase metabolic demands (e.g., exercise or hypermetabolic states). Since nutritional requirements vary with age, sex, pregnancy, and lactation, separate values are given for each category. Recommended levels are set to include about 98% of the people in the group, so a recommended dietary allowance may be more than a specific person in the group may need at a particular time. A common mistake is to think the "D" in RDA stands for "daily" rather than "dietary," necessitating consistent daily recommended intake for each nutrient. It is sufficient to average intake for each nutrient over 1 week (Wardlaw & Insel, 1990).

U.S. Recommended Daily Allowances

The Food and Drug Administration has established standards derived from the recommended dietary allowances known as U.S. **Recommended Daily Allowances (RDAs).** Four categories are used: infants less than 1 year, toddlers 1 to 4 years, children over 4 and

adults, and pregnant and lactating women. The RDAs usually use the highest nutrient recommendation in each category. Nutrition labels on food packages usually give the percentage of RDAs provided in one serving.

World Nutrient Guides

Many countries have developed nutrition guides similar to the RDAs. Canada's Department of National Health and Welfare developed Recommended Nutritional Intakes. Great Britain also developed a nutrition guide. The World Health Organization, together with the United Nations Food and Agriculture Organization, developed a nutritional guide similar to the RDA for worldwide use. Factors within each country and the opinions of scientists vary, explaining the slight differences in recommendations. Table 33-3 compares different nutrition guides.

Nutrient Density

The concept of *nutrient density* can be used to evaluate the nutritional quality of foods. Foods that provide more nutrient value than kilocalories are nutrient dense. Foods with low nutrient density (e.g., sugar or alcohol) provide energy but often lack essential nutrients. Foods that are nutrient dense are preferred to promote optimal nutrition.

Dietary Guidelines for Americans

Because many Americans overeat and lead sedentary lives, there has been a significant rise in cardiovascular problems, diabetes, and cancer. In 1977, the U.S. Senate Select Committee on Nutrition and Human Needs prepared dietary goals in an effort to reverse the trend (see the display).

TABLE 33–3

Comparison of Dietary Standards

Classification	Kcal	Protein (grams)	Calcium (mg)	Iron (mg)	Vitamin A (RE)	Thiamine (mg)	Riboflavin (mg)	Vitamin C (mg)
United States								
Female (63 kg, 1.63 m)	2200	50	800	15	800	1.1	1.3	60
Male (79 kg, 1.76 m)	2900	63	800	10	1000	1.5	1.7	60
United Kingdom								
Female	2150–2500	54–62	500	12	750	0.9–1.0	1.3	30
Male	2500–3350	63–84	500	10	750	1.0–1.3	1.6	30
Canada								
Female (55.8 kg)	2100	41	700	14	800	0.9	1.1	45
Male (71.1 kg)	3000	57	800	8	1000	1.2	1.5	60
FAO/WHO								
Female	2300	39	400–500	18	750	0.9	1.3	30
Male	3200	46	400–500	10	750	1.2	1.8	30

Figures are based on 1980 for the United States and United Kingdom, 1983 for Canada, and 1974 for WHO.
From Shils, M. E., & Young, U. R. (1988). *Modern nutrition in health and disease* (7th ed.). Philadelphia: Lea & Febiger.

United States Dietary Goals

1. To avoid overweight, consume only as much energy (calories) as is expended; if overweight, decrease energy intake and increase energy expenditure.

2. Increase the consumption of complex carbohydrates and "naturally occurring" sugars from about 28% of energy intake to about 48% of energy intake.

3. Reduce the consumption of refined and processed sugars by about 45% to account for about 10% of total energy intake.

4. Reduce overall fat consumption from approximately 40% to about 30% of energy intake.

5. Reduce saturated fat consumption to account for about 10% of total energy intake; balance that with polyunsaturated and monounsaturated fats, which should account for about 10% of energy intake each.

6. Reduce cholesterol consumption to about 300 mg a day.

7. Limit the intake of sodium by reducing the intake of salt to about 5 g a day.

Suggested Changes in Food Selection and Preparation

1. Increase consumption of fruits and vegetables and whole grains.

2. Decrease consumption of refined and other processed sugars and foods high in such sugars.

3. Decrease consumption of foods high in total fat, and partially replace saturated fats, whether obtained from animal or vegetable sources, with polyunsaturated fats.

4. Decrease consumption of animal fat, and choose meats, poultry, and fish that will reduce saturated fat intake.

5. Except for young children, substitute low-fat and non-fat milk for whole milk, and low-fat dairy products for high-fat dairy products.

6. Decrease consumption of butterfat, eggs, and other high-cholesterol sources. Some consideration should be given to easing the cholesterol goal for premenopausal women, young children, and the elderly in order to obtain the nutritional benefits of eggs in the diet.

7. Decrease consumption of salt and foods high in salt content.

U.S. Senate Select Committee on Nutrition and Human Needs. (1990). *Dietary goals for the United States* (3rd ed.).

Energy Balance

Adjusting dietary patterns to maintain a balance between caloric intake and energy expenditure is important to provide optimal nutrition. *Basal metabolism* is the amount of energy required to carry out involuntary activities at rest (such as breathing, circulating blood, or maintaining body temperature). Men usually have a higher basal metabolic rate (BMR) than women due to a proportionally greater muscle mass. Other factors, such as growth, infection, fever, stress, and extreme environmental temperatures, can increase BMR. Decreased BMR can be due to aging, prolonged fasting, and sleeping. Increased physical exercise creates caloric demands above basal requirements.

To maintain body weight, dietary intake of calories must equal caloric expenditures. When caloric intake is greater than energy expended, weight gain occurs, as energy is stored in body fat. When caloric intake is less than energy expended, weight loss occurs, as body stores of energy are depleted. For an average person, a daily deficit of 500 calories (3500 calories per week) will result in the loss of one pound a week.

Caloric requirements can be calculated by estimating how much energy is required for basal activities and adding the calories needed for voluntary muscular activity. The display shows one method of calculating kilocalorie energy output for BMR and voluntary muscular activity.

Factors Affecting Normal Nutrition

Factors affecting a person's nutritional status are many and varied.

Physical Factors. Healthy body functioning is important to promote digestion and absorption of food. Healthy teeth and gums or well-fitting dentures are important for chewing, which is necessary to break up food particles to facilitate digestion. The GI system must function well to promote optimal use of ingested nutrients. Hormone production of insulin and pancreatic digestive enzymes also is important for food use.

Physical factors can affect a person's ability to buy, transport, cook, and eat food. Physical mobility and energy is necessary for shopping, cooking, and eating. When a person cannot complete such tasks due to physical limitations, assistance may be necessary to ensure adequate nutrition.

Lifestyle and Habits. Eating patterns are highly individualized and greatly determined by personal preference. Food preferences and eating habits are often set during childhood and may be handed down from one generation to the next. Some families are adventurous and love trying new recipes; other families derive security from having certain meals, prepared in exactly the

Shortcut for Estimating Energy Output: Basal Metabolism

Use the factor 1.0 kcalorie per kilogram of body weight per hour for men or 0.9 for women. The following is an example for a 150-pound man.

1. Change pounds to kilograms:

$$\frac{150 \text{ lb}}{2.2 \text{ lb}} \times 1.0 \text{ kg} = 68 \text{ kg}$$

2. Multiply weight in kilograms by the BMR factor:

$$68 \text{ kg} \times 1 \text{ kcal/kg/hr} = 68 \text{ kcal/hr}$$

3. Multiply the kcalories used in 1 hour by the hours in a day:

$$68 \text{ kcal/hr} \times 24 \text{ hr/day} = 1632 \text{ kcal/day}$$

Energy for BMR equals 1632 kcalories per day.

Shortcut for Estimating Energy Output: Voluntary Muscular Activity

The figures we use are crude approximations based on the amount of muscular work a person typically performs in a day. To select the one appropriate for you, remember to think in terms of the amount of *muscular* work performed. Don't confuse being *busy* with being *active*.

- For sedentary (mostly sitting) activity (a typist), add 50% of the BMR.
- For light activity (a teacher), add 60%.
- For heavy work (a roofer), add 100% or more.

If the man we used in the previous example were a typist, we would estimate the energy he needed for physical activities by multiplying his BMR kcalories per day by 50%.

$$1632 \text{ kcal/day} \times 50\% = 816 \text{ kcal/day}$$

His energy need for activities equals 816 kcalories per day.

From Cataldo, C., Nyenhuis, J., & Whitney, E. (1987). *Nutritional and diet therapy: Principles and practice* (2nd ed.). St. Paul: West Publishing Co., pp. 90, 91.

same way, over and over. If a child is raised in a family that eats throughout the day, rather than having three distinct meals, this pattern will seem normal and will probably influence his or her eating patterns throughout life. The amount and type of food eaten is also determined by early experience. If a child is given large servings and rewarded with desserts, overeating may become a problem later in life. The atmosphere created at mealtime also subtly affects our feelings about food and eating.

Peer pressure and sex-role stereotypes can affect eating patterns. Adolescents survive for years on hamburgers, french fries, pizza, and soda. A man may be less likely to order a quiche or salad for lunch than a woman; likewise, a woman may feel less comfortable eating a big steak sandwich.

Food fads can also affect dietary patterns. Some foods can be linked with beliefs about health that are not grounded in scientific fact. For instance, bran was recently extolled as a source of dietary fiber, although the importance of dietary fiber has been well known. Popular literature touted bran as a cure-all for many common ills, even as a way of preventing cancer. Many people started eating large amounts of bran due to exaggerated claims about its value.

A single professional person who works long hours may not have enough time to shop for and cook food. Likewise, a family with two working parents may find themselves eating out due to lack of time and energy to shop and cook. Single retired people may find that although they have the time to cook, they have limited motivation to cook and eat meals alone. People who lead active lives with strenuous physical exertion may need more frequent meals and more calories to meet their minimal nutritional requirements. On the other hand, sedentary people who spend hours in front of the TV may gain weight from decreased physical activity and increased snacking.

Culture and Religion. Culture plays a significant role in the type of food we eat and our feelings about diet and nutrition. Ethnic origin provides for great diversity and creativity in food preparation. Staple products may vary among different cultural groups; for example, Asians may eat rice with most meals and people of Italian descent may prefer pasta. Spices and methods of cooking also vary from culture to culture.

Some religions dictate when or if certain foods can be eaten, and how food is to be prepared. An example of this is the Jewish dietary law, which restricts (among other things) the eating of dairy and meat products at the same time. Most religions have special foods that are traditional for specific religious observances.

Economic Resources. Dietary adequacy is related to a person's finances. Money is needed to buy and transport food and to obtain and maintain the equipment needed to cook and store food safely. The lower a person's economic level, the less likely it is that his or her diet is nutritionally adequate. Low-income areas often have fewer grocery stores, with less selection and often with higher prices. Low-income people may not have the transportation to shop outside of their own neighborhoods. Affluent people can stock up when items are on sale, stretching their food budget; poor people cannot do so.

Low-income families often must sacrifice their food budget to leave enough money for other bills. The result may be less expensive meals that are low in protein and high in starch. Sources of protein such as meat and dairy products are usually expensive and require refrigeration.

Gender. Nutritional requirements vary slightly between men and women. Men usually need more calories and protein to maintain a larger muscle mass. Women have proportionally more adipose tissue and need fewer calories to maintain body weight. To prevent anemia, women need more dietary iron to offset losses from menstruation.

Pregnancy and Lactation. The pregnant woman's diet should include a substantial increase in calories, protein, calcium, folic acid, and iron. Often a prenatal multivitamin and mineral supplement is prescribed. The pregnant woman should gain weight throughout her pregnancy as prescribed and monitored by her health-care professional. Pregnant women at particular risk for nutritional deficiencies are adolescents, underweight women, obese women, women with chronic nutritional problems, women who smoke or ingest alcohol or drugs, low-income women, and women with chronic illnesses such as diabetes or anemia.

The lactating (nursing) woman also has special needs. Minor deficiencies in the lactating woman's diet are more likely to influence her nutritional state than the nutritional quality of her milk. Major deficiencies in the woman's diet may result in a decrease in the nutritional quality and quantity of her milk. Lactating women need to increase their intake of calcium, protein, and calories. These increases are important because the quality and quantity of breast milk produced directly affects the adequacy of the breastfeeding infant's diet.

Lifespan Considerations

Although people vary widely in their nutritional needs throughout the lifespan, there are certain characteristics people have in common at different ages.

Newborn and Infant

Adequate nutrition during infancy is vitally important because the infant's growth and development is more rapid during the first year of life than at any other time. Birth weight usually doubles within the first 4 to 6 months and triples by 12 months. The newborn needs more calories per pound of body weight because the BMR is so high. The infant's growth and development is also influenced by genetic characteristics and the quality of prenatal nutrition and care.

Milk, from the breast or bottle, is the food of choice for the newborn. Breastfeeding should occur as soon after birth as possible. For the first 3 days after birth, the mother's breasts produce colostrum, a thin, watery fluid. Breast milk, which contains about 20 calories per ounce, is produced after the third day. Weight gain may be less rapid in the breastfed infant. Feedings are usually frequent (e.g., every 2 to 3 hours) since breast milk is easily digested. Breast milk gives the infant immunity against some bacteria and viruses, decreases the production of bacteria in the intestine, decreases the incidence of allergies, and provides a well-balanced, ideal source of nutrition. The breastfeeding mother should avoid taking drugs, since small amounts can be transferred to the breast milk and ingested by the infant.

Formula is a safe and nutritious substitute for mothers who prefer not to breastfeed or cannot do so. Iron-fortified commercial formulas should be used until at least 6 months of age. Most formulas are modified cow's milk, which has been heat-treated to aid digestion. Soy formulas and predigested formulas are also available.

Foods (juices, fruits, vegetables, and iron-fortified cereal) are gradually added to the infant's diet to provide additional nutrition and to begin to accustom the infant to foods of different textures, flavors, and consistencies. The age at which these foods are introduced varies according to the infant's need, the practices of the health-care provider, and the influence of the infant's culture and environment. Juices are often added at about 1 month, cereal, fruits and vegetables, and egg yolk at about 4 to 6 months. When teeth begin to erupt at about 6 months, crackers and teething biscuits are often added. New foods should be introduced one at a time, so that the offending food can be identified if allergies develop. In the second half of the first year, motor development has improved so that the infant can begin to sit up, eat finger foods, and drink from a cup.

Toddler and Preschooler

Adequate nutritional intake is important between the ages of 1 and 5 years because this is a period of physical growth and development. Variations between toddlers necessitate some differences in their diets. During this period, the growth rate begins to decline and the appetite also decreases as less food is needed to meet normal metabolic demands. The child's appetite may be erratic. Teeth continue to erupt into the second and sometimes the third year. Muscle mass and bone density increase. This requires adequate protein, calcium, and phosphorous in the diet. Energy levels remain high, requiring adequate caloric intake.

Independence in feeding greatly increases during this period, as the child increases coordination and ability to use eating utensils. Many children can feed themselves by age 2. Mental abilities and language development are also increasing, so the child is better able to communicate food likes and dislikes. Values and attitudes about eating develop during this period. It is important not to use food to punish, reward, bribe, or convey love. Some children may become picky eaters, especially when not eating gains them attention from their parents.

Maintaining adequate dietary habits for toddlers and preschoolers is important because good habits are established at an early age. The most common dietary deficiency in this age group is iron deficiency, which leads to iron-deficiency anemia. A diet that includes iron-rich foods is indicated, and iron supplements may also be necessary. Vitamins A and C also may be deficient in the diets of toddlers and preschoolers, so it is important to ensure that foods rich in these vitamins are eaten. Active children in this age group benefit from nutritious between-meal snacks.

Child and Adolescent

Growth evens out during childhood and adolescence, but there is great variation in the growth rates of individual children. The digestive system matures and permanent teeth erupt. Children can eat larger meals less frequently, requiring fewer calories per unit of body weight. Adolescence is a period of rapid growth and sexual maturation.

A diet that includes the recommended allowances of protein, carbohydrates, vitamins, and minerals for the individual age group, physical status, and developmental level is necessary for optimal health. Nutritional deficiencies most likely to occur during childhood and adolescence are iron, calcium, vitamin A, and vitamin C (Luke, 1984). It is important to provide adequate amounts of these vitamins and minerals in the diet. Health problems that respond well to nutritional intervention during this age include dental caries, anemia, and obesity.

The school-lunch program can play a vital role in providing nutritionally balanced, low-cost meals. Some schools also have a breakfast program and a snack program. These programs are usually available either free or at a reduced cost for needy children. In addition to providing a substantial part of the daily nutritional needs of children, these programs make a valuable contribution in terms of nutrition education and developing good nutritional habits.

Social pressure and emotional stress can have adverse effects on the young person's efforts to maintain a nutritionally adequate diet. Peers may dictate dietary choices. Fewer meals may be eaten at home; fast food, soda, and candy are often favorites, despite their low nutritional density. Smoking, drinking, and substance abuse can also affect nutritional status.

The child or teenager may experience an unbalanced pattern of activity or rest. Increased participation in sports requires additional caloric intake. Weight gain is common during the preadolescent period, as the body prepares for rapid growth. If the child leads a sedentary life and eats a high-calorie diet, weight gain can be excessive and can contribute to obesity. On the other hand, weight consciousness, especially among adolescent girls, can lead to fad diets, anorexia nervosa, and bulimia.

Adult and Older Adult

Growth stops and metabolism declines during adulthood, so fewer calories are required. Weight gain is common, especially if physical activity is limited. Calcium deficiency and osteoporosis can be a concern for adults, especially postmenopausal women. Adults should maintain a calcium intake of 800 to 1200 mg per day throughout adulthood. Adequate intake of calcium is especially important before age 30, when peak bone mass is being attained (Robinson & Weigley, 1984).

Inadequate nutritional intake during this time may be due to increased daily demands that decrease the time and energy available for buying, cooking, and eating food. Dietary patterns can be affected when both parents in a family work. Some adults lack adequate resources or knowledge about good nutrition. Pregnancy and lactation, as discussed above, greatly alter nutritional requirements.

Physiologic changes occur in later years that have a major impact on nutrition. Metabolic rate continues to decline. Even though the need for calories decreases, the need for iron and vitamins remains high. The diets of many elderly people are deficient in calories, calcium, vitamins A, C, D, B-complex, folate, thiamine, and riboflavin (Blumberg, 1986). Adequate fiber intake is necessary to prevent constipation, a common problem of the older adult. The senses of taste and smell diminish, which can affect enjoyment of eating and cause decreased intake of food. Digestion is affected by a change in the contents of bile and pancreatic secretions, decreased peristalsis, and decreased blood flow to the GI tract. Periodontal disease and ill-fitting dentures can make chewing difficult and painful.

For older adults, socioeconomic factors can also contribute to inadequate nutrition. Getting to and from stores and carrying groceries can be problems for the older person with a mobility impairment. Older adults may have trouble using cooking appliances because of failing eyesight and arthritis, or because of the complexity of modern appliances. Selecting economical, nutritious foods can be difficult for the older shopper because of the wide variety of products available.

Social isolation, which can occur due to chronic illness or depression, can also hinder nutrition. Those who have lost many of their friends and live far from their relatives may become lonely and depressed, which can make cooking and eating more difficult.

Several community resources have been developed to help older adults continue living at home by combating the problems of inadequate nutrition, social isolation, poverty, and inadequate transportation. Programs for home-delivered meals, such as Meals on Wheels, provide nutritious, low-cost meals for older people who have difficulty preparing their own food. This program is able to remain low in cost partly because of a volunteer staff. Food stamps and food banks are also useful in helping older adults and needy people to achieve a more nutritious diet.

Another excellent resource for older adults is a local senior center, which can provide meals, health screening and medication assistance, transportation assistance, dietary counseling, recreational activities, and assistance and referral for economic and legal problems.

ALTERED NUTRITIONAL FUNCTION

The body constantly undergoes renewal. If proper nutrition is not provided, body tissues will not be adequately maintained, energy will not be adequate for activities, and normal body processes will suffer.

Potential for Altered Nutritional Function

Inadequate intake of essential nutrients (protein, carbohydrates, fats, vitamins, minerals, or water) can impair nutritional status. Problems associated with excessive intake have emerged only recently and are primarily limited to developed countries in which food is plentiful and lifestyles are more sedentary.

Despite adequate intake, some people experience altered nutritional status because of inadequate digestion and absorption of nutrients. Medical conditions causing inflammation or obstruction of the GI tract decrease nutrient use. Inadequate production of hormones or enzymes can also affect digestion and absorption. A person who cannot use ingested nutrients may decrease his or her food intake due to anorexia, nausea, bloating, or vomiting.

Inadequate Intake of Nutrients

Inability to Acquire and Prepare Food. People who are unable to purchase, transport, and prepare food will often suffer from inadequate intake unless other people or agencies can be found to fulfill this need. In Third World countries, starvation is common due to drought and famine (Fig. 33-2). Starvation or malnutrition can also occur in developed nations when people lack the resources to obtain adequate food. People who are weak or disabled by chronic disease have difficulty shopping and cooking. A confused or disoriented person may not remember to eat or may be unable to organize the complex tasks of buying and cooking food independently.

Inadequate Knowledge. Some people may not eat a healthful, balanced diet because they lack information about nutrition. A person is likely to eat only what tastes good or is convenient if he or she does not know or care that such an eating pattern can be unhealthy. The consequences of poor nutrition are not immediately observable, so the motivation to change bad eating patterns may not be strong.

Swallowing Impairment. People who have difficulty swallowing may be unable to ingest enough nutrients to meet daily requirements. Swallowing impairment can occur when the gag reflex is absent due to neurologic

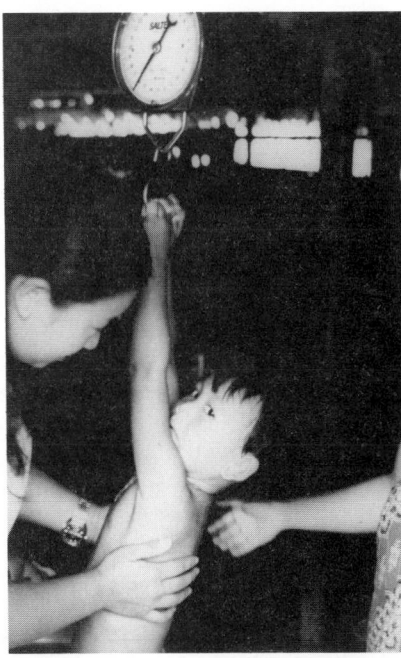

Figure 33–2. Nurses conduct a malnutrition survey in a refugee camp, Khao I Dang, Thailand. (Photo courtesy Marjorie A. Muecke.)

dysfunction (such as a cerebral vascular accident) or muscle weakness. Obstruction of the oropharyngeal cavity secondary to a tumor or edema can also impair swallowing.

Discomfort During or After Eating. When a person experiences discomfort during or after eating, he or she may decrease food intake. A sore throat, a tonsillectomy, a mouth lesion, or ill-fitting dentures can cause pain during eating.

Anorexia. Anorexia, or loss of appetite, can occur for a variety of reasons. Depression, GI dysfunction, infectious illness, and the side effects of many medications can cause anorexia and the resultant decrease in food intake.

Nausea and Vomiting. Nausea, or the unpleasant feeling that vomiting is imminent, frequently precedes vomiting. Nausea and vomiting can interfere with normal food intake. They may be due to motion sickness, viral or bacterial infections of the GI tract, gallbladder disease, general anesthesia, disruption of inner-ear function, side effects of various medications, and pregnancy. Some people may feel nauseated or vomit from unpleasant smells or sights.

Excess Intake of Nutrients

Calories. Caloric intake in excess of daily energy requirements results in storage of energy in the form of increased adipose tissue. As the percentage of stored fat increases, a person becomes overweight or obese. Excess weight increases the stress on body organs and predisposes the person to chronic health problems such as diabetes mellitus or hypertension. Excessive caloric intake does not ensure an adequate intake of essential nutrients; the obese person may be malnourished due to a lack of essential vitamins or nutrients.

Fats. Americans have a higher percentage of fat in their diets than do people in many other countries: studies have shown that fat makes up about 40% of the calories in the American diet (Robinson & Weigley, 1986). An excess intake of fat has been related to obesity, an increased risk of coronary artery disease (especially increased intake of saturated fats), and several forms of cancer, including breast, colon, and uterine cancer. Dietary modifications can lower fat and cholesterol intake (see the display).

Inability to Use Ingested Nutrients

Inflammation of the Gastrointestinal Tract. Inflammation of the lining of the gastrointestinal tract causes discomfort and interferes with the absorption of nutrients.

Esophagitis, an inflammation of the esophagus, can be caused by burns, poisons, infections, or chronic vomiting. This causes discomfort and impairs swallowing.

Gastritis is characterized by inflammation of the mucosal layer of the stomach, which can proceed to ulceration if untreated. Mucosal cells of the stomach can atrophy and become unable to absorb Vitamin B12, leading to pernicious anemia (Lewis, 1986).

Cholecystitis is an inflammation of the gallbladder, usually caused by the presence of gallstones. The presence of inflammation and stones causes pain after the ingestion of a meal high in fat, since the gallbladder spasms as it attempts to release bile to assist with fat digestion.

Inflammatory bowel disease (e.g., Crohn's disease, or ulcerative colitis) greatly affects absorption of nutrients

---

Suggested Dietary Modifications to Reduce Fat and Cholesterol

- Use low-fat or skim milk instead of whole milk.
- Reduce intake of ice cream, using ice milk or yogurt instead.
- Increase use of low-fat cheese, and limit intake of cheese high in fat.
- Use lean meats and trim all observable fat; avoid frying.
- Eat more fish and chicken; avoid red meat.
- Avoid shellfish (e.g., shrimp, lobster).
- Avoid organ meats (e.g., liver).
- Limit use of eggs, especially yolks.
- Use soft margarine and polyunsaturated cooking oils; avoid butter, lard, and solid shortenings.

---

and water from the intestine. the intestinal inflammation greatly increases the movement of nutrients through the gastrointestinal tract, resulting in severe diarrhea. Treatment frequently requires resection of large inflamed areas of the intestine, permanently altering absorption in the area.

Obstruction of the Gastrointestinal Tract. Any obstruction caused by scar tissue, benign or cancerous growths, or structural abnormalities can alter normal nutritional status. Esophageal obstruction can severely limit intake or restrict oral intake to fluids. A hiatal hernia is a protrusion of the stomach upward into the mediastinal cavity, causing esophageal reflux, or the backflow of stomach contents into the esophagus, resulting in heartburn. Intestinal obstruction usually necessitates withholding all oral intake until the obstruction has resolved or has been surgically corrected.

Malabsorption of Nutrients. Malabsorption syndromes can be caused by the inability to tolerate certain foods. An allergic reaction to gluten, which is found in wheat, rye, oats, and barley, can affect absorption. Gluten causes mucosal villi to atrophy, decreasing their absorptive abilities. Lactose intolerance occurs when there is a deficiency of lactase, a digestive enzyme that breaks down the sugar commonly found in milk.

A decrease in pancreatic enzyme production occurs in some pancreatic disorders, resulting in altered digestion of fats and protein. In cystic fibrosis, an inherited disorder, excessive mucus production plugs pancreatic ducts, leading to altered protein and fat digestion.

Malabsorption can also occur secondary to surgical intervention. Gastric or intestinal resection removes large areas of the GI tract normally involved in absorption of nutrients. Decreased blood flow to the GI tract can also decrease the rate of nutrient absorption.

Diabetes Mellitus. Diabetes mellitus is a chronic condition in which insufficient amounts of insulin are produced or the body cannot effectively use circulating insulin. Insulin is a hormone essential for proper metabolism of fats and carbohydrates. When adequate insulin is unavailable, the transfer of glucose into the cell is impaired and the glucose level of the blood rises. Thus, the available energy source cannot be used by the body.

Increased Metabolic Demand

Certain conditions increase the body's nutritional requirements, potentially contributing to altered nutritional status. They include:

- Periods of rapid growth (infancy, adolescence, or pregnancy)
- Conditions that increase the basal metabolic rate (fever, exercise, or hyperthyroidism)
- Stress (from emotional distress, fear, surgery, or illness)

• Cancer (greatly increases the metabolic rate, which can result in rapid weight loss despite normal food intake).

Surgery

Surgery greatly increases the risk for nutritional deficits. Studies by Shirreff noted weight and serum albumin loss for all subjects studied after surgery (Shirreff, 1990). Increased metabolic demands due to the stress of surgery and wound healing, along with inadequate postoperative intake, compound nutritional deficits. Many surgical patients are nutritionally depleted at the time of the operation due to chronic illness or GI problems.

Cancer and Cancer Treatment

Cancer greatly increases metabolic demands of the body, and cancer cells compete with normal cells for nutrients. Cancer patients often experience anorexia, nausea, vomiting, and depression, all of which can decrease food consumption. Radiation or chemotherapy can also alter normal nutrition because loss of appetite, nausea, and vomiting are commonly associated with such treatments. Mouth lesions known as stomatitis often occur with cancer therapy, causing pain and difficulty with chewing. Chemotherapy and radiation cause fatigue, decreasing the amount of energy available for cooking and eating.

Alcohol and Drug Abuse

Excessive, chronic ingestion of alcohol can impair nutrition. Normal eating may be greatly affected when excessive alcohol intake occurs, impairing the necessary intake of calories and nutrients. Money normally spent on food may be used to buy alcohol. Deficiency of B vitamins (thiamine, folate, niacin, and B_6) is common because they are necessary to metabolize alcohol. Alcohol's toxic effect on the intestinal mucosa can impair the normal absorption of nutrients. Chronic alcohol use can also cause irreversible changes to the cells of the liver, affecting the liver's role in metabolic pathways.

Drug abuse also can affect nutrition. Addiction to heroin or cocaine can decrease the user's desire for food, as preoccupation with buying drugs disrupts normal daily routines. Other drugs, such as amphetamines and barbiturates, can cause an increase or decrease in food intake.

Psychological State

A person's psychological state can affect his or her desire to eat. Anxiety causes some people to increase their food intake; others eat less when they feel anxious. Depression often decreases the person's appetite and depletes the energy available for cooking and eating. Some people may willingly alter eating patterns to help achieve weight loss. Rather than changing eating patterns, rapid weight loss is often obtained through crash diets. **Anorexia nervosa** is an eating disorder in which the person refuses to eat due to a fear of becoming overweight, even in the presence of normal or less than ideal body weight.

Manifestations of Altered Nutrition

Indications of altered nutrition are overweight, obesity, underweight, recent significant weight loss or gain, decreased energy levels, altered bowel patterns, and altered appearance of the skin, hair, teeth, and mucous membranes (Table 33-4). If the patient's weight varies significantly from IBW, a nutrition problem is likely.

Overweight

A person is said to be overweight if his or her body weight exceeds IBW by 1% to 20%. The National Center for Health Statistics estimates that over 20 million American adults (or just under 20% of the adult population) are overweight (Robinson, 1986). A person gains weight when he or she takes in more calories than the body needs.

TABLE 33-4

Signs of Poor Nutrition and Possible Nutrient Deficiency

Signs	Possible Lacking Nutrient
Hair: thin, coarse, lacking luster, breaks easily	Protein
Skin: excessive bruising, bleeding	Vitamin K
Skin: pressure sores, poor wound healing	Vitamin C and protein
Gums: swollen, bleeding	Vitamin C
Muscles: wasting	Protein
Lack of growth	Protein, calories
Skeletal: poor posture, painful joints, bowed legs, increase in bone fractures	Calcium, vitamin D, vitamin C, protein
Mental: confusion, motor weakness	Thiamine: niacin, B complex

Obesity

A person is said to be obese if he or she is more than 20% over IBW. Morbid obesity is obesity that can interfere with normal functioning, such as mobility or breathing. Excess calories do not ensure adequate nutritional intake, so the obese patient may be undernourished in many important nutrients.

Underweight

A person is said to be underweight if he or she is 1% to 20% less than IBW. This occurs when caloric intake is insufficient to meet the body's nutritional requirements.

Recent Significant Weight Gain or Loss

Minor fluctuations in weight occur on a day-to-day basis due to fluid losses and gains, but changing weight patterns over weeks or months may indicate altered nutrition. A significant weight gain can occur when a person eats more than the body needs for energy expenditure. This can happen when a person becomes less active or when the intake of food is increased due to stress or boredom. Significant weight loss, especially when intake has remained constant, can indicate hypermetabolic states such as cancer or hyperthyroidism, or an inability to use ingested nutrients.

Decreased Energy

Nutrition provides the body with energy to perform normal cellular processes and carry out normal movement and activities. When nutritional deficits occur, adequate energy may be unavailable. Fatigue or activity intolerance are common manifestations of altered nutrition. The patient may complain of feeling tired or weak.

Altered Bowel Patterns

Inadequate dietary intake may affect bowel function and regularity. Constipation can occur when fiber or fluid intake is inadequate. Diarrhea can occur when large quantities of fresh fruits are eaten. With food intolerance (e.g., lactase deficiency) or malabsorption syndrome, GI distress occurs. When a patient's bowel regularity changes, nutritional deficits must be ruled out as a causative factor.

Altered Skin, Teeth, Hair, and Mucous Membranes

Skin, nails, hair, and mucous membranes are rapidly growing tissues that continuously require adequate nutrition for growth. Protein is especially important in this process. Vitamin deficiencies are also often manifested by altered development and growth of skin, teeth, hair, and mucous membranes. When protein is lacking, hair may become thin and lack luster and can break easily. Skin heals slowly and may appear thin and fragile when nutrition is inadequate. Mucous membranes may develop sores and bleed easily. Teeth and gums are more prone to disease.

ASSESSMENT

Subjective Data

In a nutritional assessment, the nurse determines the person's nutritional health. Information is collected by interviewing the patient about normal dietary patterns and preferences, risk factors that may contribute to nutritional alterations, and actual nutritional deficits.

Functional Pattern Identification

The nurse asks questions to determine the patient's normal eating patterns and food preferences. Ask the patient to describe his or her appetite as good, fair, or poor, and whether eating and mealtime is usually a pleasant experience.

Asking the patient to describe food and fluid intake on a typical day gives the nurse a sense of what is normal for the patient. Two surveying methods can be used, the 24-hour recall or the food diary. The 24-hour recall asks the person to recall and record the type, quality, and method of preparation of all food eaten within a 24-hour period. In the food diary, the person keeps a log of the amount, time, and manner of preparation for all food consumed within a specific period of time. This time period can vary, but is often 3 days to 1 week; this permits the evaluation to be affected less by "one-time-only" dietary indiscretions. Both surveying methods are subject to recall and recording errors.

Ask about food likes and dislikes, normal timing of meals, and routine snacks. Determine whether the patient follows a special diet for any reason, has food allergies, or limits the intake of certain foods. Discuss cultural or religious dietary concerns. For some patients, it may be important to inquire how stress affects eating patterns. Some people under stress limit their food intake, but others increase the amount and frequency of food consumption.

Ask who in the family is responsible for shopping and cooking, or whether such responsibilities are shared by more than one family member. Also ask about the use of prepackaged prepared food, and the number of times per week that the patient eats out.

Risk Identification

The nutritional assessment helps to identify patients at risk for nutritional deficits. Discuss the patient's knowledge and values about nutrition; questions such as, "Do you feel your diet helps promote health?" and "What (if any) changes in your diet do you feel might be beneficial?" are appropriate. If the patient is on a specific diet, asking which foods are important to include or avoid can help assess the patient's understanding of the dietary restrictions.

Identify the presence of anorexia, chewing problems, sore mouth, dysphagia, nausea and vomiting, and when present the length of time food intake has been affected. Note any chronic or acute health problems affecting the GI tract (e.g., ulcers, gallbladder disease, inflammatory bowel disease). Document any chronic health conditions (e.g., diabetes mellitus, cancer, renal disease, heart disease, lung disease) and assess their effect on appetite and food intake. Note any condition that impairs swallowing (e.g., a neurologic impairment) and outline specific deficits.

Assessing socioeconomic factors is also important to determine possible nutritional deficits. Does the patient have money and transportation to buy nutritious food? Are there safe storage and adequate cooking facilities? Does the patient or caretaker have the energy to shop for and prepare meals?

Also assess drug intake. Document excessive alcohol intake, as well as the use of illicit drugs such as cocaine and heroin. Note the use of prescription medications such as insulin, antacids, chemotherapeutic agents, and steroids, as well as over-the-counter preparations, and assess for any impact on nutrition.

Dysfunctional Identification

Nutrition can be impaired if the patient cannot buy and prepare food, if the patient is unwilling or unable to eat, if the patient's intake is excessive, or if the patient cannot use ingested nutrients. Assessing such dysfunctions is often done by asking questions to determine normal patterns or nutritional risk.

Nutritional alterations can be identified if the patient's weight is significantly greater than or less than IBW. Reports of significant recent weight loss without altered diet indicate an inability to meet normal nutritional requirements. A dietary intake that supplies significantly less than recommended dietary allowances also helps to identify a deficit. Signs and symptoms such as fatigue, muscle wasting, and obesity show nutritional dysfunction.

Objective Data

Objective data are gathered by general observations, anthropometric measurements, calorie counts, mouth examination, and swallowing evaluation. Laboratory and diagnostic tests can provide data to evaluate nutritional status and the functional ability of the GI system.

Physical Assessment

General Observations. General observation of the patient provides important information on nutritional status. An adequately nourished person should appear robust, vital, and energetic and should have erect posture. Skin, hair, and nails should appear healthy. See the first display in this chapter and compare it to Table 33-4.

Anthropometric Measurements. Anthropometric measurements include height and weight, skinfold measurements, and arm circumference measurements (Fig. 33-3). Skinfold and arm circumference measurements are not commonly performed on the hospitalized patient, but may be used for nutritional screening.

Height and weight are measured and compared to a table of standard measurements grouped by age, sex, and body frame (see Appendix D). Small, medium, or

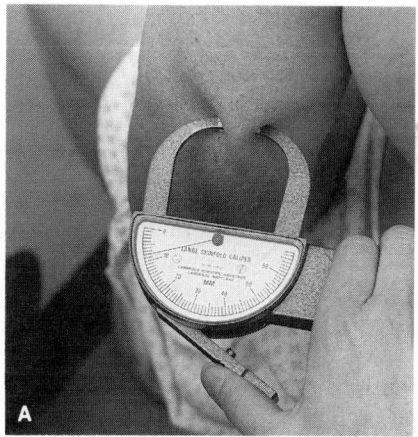

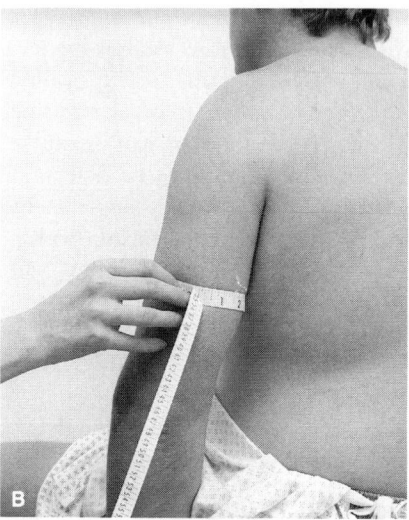

Figure 33-3. Anthropometric measurements. **A:** Calipers are used to measure triceps skin fold. **B:** A tape measure is used to measure the upper arm. Values are compared to standards to detect increased body fat.

large body frame can be estimated by measuring wrist circumference. Also, ask what the person thinks his or her IBW is; this may vary from standardized tables.

Skinfold measurements are used to help determine fat stores in the body. The triceps skinfold and the subscapular skinfold are most commonly used. Using a caliper, the fold of skin, which includes the subcutaneous tissue but not the underlying muscle, is measured. Measurements are compared to a table of standards grouped by age and sex to detect excess fat.

Arm circumference measurements are taken of the upper arm to provide information about the muscle mass. Since muscles serve as the major protein stores, measuring arm circumference helps evaluate protein status. Again, measurements are compared to a table of standards.

Calorie Count. When inadequate intake is suspected, a calorie count can be done. The nurse records exactly how many cubic centimeters or bites of food have been ingested. This information is used by the dietitian to calculate the calories and to evaluate whether the caloric intake is adequate for the patient's needs.

Mouth Inspection. The nurse observes the condition of the teeth, gums, and mucous membranes. Mucous membranes should be moist and adequate saliva present. Caries, excessive plaque, and gingivitis are noted. If dentures are present, proper fit and condition are evaluated. Lesions of the oral cavity (canker sores, stomatitis, *Candida* infections) should be detected and treated promptly, since discomfort associated with such lesions can alter food intake.

Swallowing Evaluation. A swallowing evaluation is necessary when potential difficulty in swallowing is suspected. Often the patient is referred to a speech therapist for a swallowing evaluation, but the nurse may need to evaluate swallowing abilities to determine whether feeding is safe. A swallowing evaluation includes assessment of motor function of the facial, oral, and tongue muscles, cough reflex, swallowing reflex, and gag reflex (DiIorio & Price, 1990).

Motor function is assessed by observing the face, jaw, and tongue for symmetry and strength during normal movements. Asking the patient to cough will permit evaluation of the briskness and strength of the cough reflex, which is necessary to clear aspirated food from the airway. Ability to swallow is evaluated by placing the index finger and thumb on the patient's laryngeal protuberance and asking the patient to swallow. As the patient with an intact swallowing reflex swallows, the nurse will feel the larynx elevate.

Finally, the gag reflex is evaluated by stroking the patient's right or left pharyngeal wall with a tongue blade.

Diagnostic Tests and Procedures

Biochemical data can be used to confirm a diagnosis, help determine what type of dietary modification will be necessary, or help identify specific nutritional deficiencies before clinical signs are apparent. Evaluating blood and urine is most useful in analyzing a patient's nutritional state. The most common laboratory data used are hemoglobin, serum albumin, serum transferrin, and total lymphocyte count. Anergy testing can be done to identify severe nutritional deficits.

Hemoglobin. A hemoglobin count measures the blood's oxygen- and iron-carrying capacity. A decreased hemoglobin value indicates decreased iron intake or decreased iron reserves, which often is present in anemia.

Serum Albumin. Serum albumin accounts for over half of the body's total serum protein. Serum albumin values reflect protein intake or absorption. Values of less than 3.5 g/dL indicate nutritional deficits.

Serum Transferrin. Transferrin, a blood protein that binds with iron and is important in its transport, is considered a sensitive indicator of protein deficiency. Transferrin, which is synthesized in the liver, increases when iron stores are low and decreases when iron stores are high. Changes in protein intake or visceral protein stores are more rapidly reflected in serum transferrin levels than in serum albumin levels.

Creatinine Excretion. The rate of creatinine formation is proportional to total muscle mass. Creatinine is released during skeletal muscle metabolism and is excreted from the body via the kidneys. Creatinine excretion is usually measured by collecting and measuring creatinine in all voided urine during a 24-hour period. As muscles atrophy during malnutrition, creatinine excretion decreases.

Immunocompetence Testing. Immunity is affected by nutritional status. In severe nutritional depletion, the patient may be unable to mount an immune response (anergy). Commonly this is seen as the lymphocyte count decreases with protein depletion. Skin testing may also be performed to evaluate the impact of nutritional deficits on immune function. Antigen skin tests (e.g., tuberculosis, *Candida,* mumps) may be given to evaluate the patient's response to antigens to which he or she has already been sensitized. If no skin response is observed after 48 hours, anergy is said to be present (Curtas, et al., 1989). Anergy indicates the need for aggressive nutritional support.

NURSING DIAGNOSIS AND PATIENT GOALS

Assessment of the patient allows the nurse to identify strengths, nutritional risk factors, and altered nutritional states. Four accepted NANDA nursing diagnoses have been identified for the area of nutrition: Altered Nutrition: Less Than Body Requirements; Altered Nutrition: Greater Than Body Requirements; Altered Nutrition: High Risk For More Than Body Requirements; and Impaired Swallowing.

Altered Nutrition: Less than Body Requirements

Definition

The state in which an individual experiences an intake of nutrients insufficient to meet metabolic needs (NANDA, 1990).

Defining Characteristics

Loss of weight with adequate food intake; body weight 20% or more under ideal; reported food intake less than recommended daily allowance; weakness of muscles required for swallowing or mastication; reported or evidence of lack of food; aversion to eating; reported altered taste sensation; satiety immediately after ingesting food; abdominal pain with or without pathology; sore, inflamed buccal cavity; capillary fragility; abdominal cramping; diarrhea and/or steatorrhea; hyperactive bowel sounds; lack of interest in food; perceived inability to ingest food; pale conjunctiva and mucous membranes; poor muscle tone; excessive loss of hair; lack of information, misinformation; misconceptions (NANDA, 1990).

Related Factors

Inability to ingest or digest food or absorb nutrients due to biologic, psychological, or economic factors (NANDA, 1990).

Altered Nutrition: More than Body Requirements

Definition

The state in which an individual experiences an intake of nutrients that exceeds metabolic needs (NANDA, 1990).

Defining Characteristics

Weight 10% to 20% over ideal for height and frame; triceps skinfold greater than 15 mm in men, 25 mm in women; sedentary activity level; reported or observed dysfunctional eating pattern: pairing food with other activities, concentrating food intake at end of day, eating in response to external cues such as time of day or social situation, eating in response to internal cues other than hunger (e.g., anxiety) (NANDA, 1990).

Related Factors

Excessive intake in relation to metabolic need (NANDA, 1990).

Altered Nutrition: High Risk for More than Body Requirements

Definition

The state in which an individual is at risk of experiencing an intake of nutrients that exceeds metabolic needs (NANDA, 1990).

Defining Characteristics

Presence of risk factors such as reported or observed obesity in one or both parents; rapid transition across growth percentiles in infants or children; reported use of solid food as major food source before 5 months of age; observed use of food as reward or comfort measure; reported or observed higher baseline weight at beginning of each pregnancy; dysfunctional eating patterns: pairing food with other activities, concentrating food intake at end of day, eating in response to external cues such as time of day or social situation, eating in response to internal cues other than hunger (e.g., anxiety) (NANDA, 1990).

Related Factors

Excessive intake in relation to metabolic need (NANDA, 1990).

Impaired Swallowing

Definition

The state in which an individual has decreased ability to voluntarily pass fluids and/or solids from the mouth to the stomach (NANDA, 1990).

Defining Characteristics

Major. Observed evidence of difficulty in swallowing (e.g., stasis of food in oral cavity, coughing/choking).

Minor. Evidence of aspiration (NANDA, 1990).

Related Factors

Neuromuscular impairment (e.g., decreased or absent gag reflex, decreased strength or excursion of muscles involved in mastication, perceptual impairment, facial paralysis); mechanical obstruction (e.g., edema, tracheostomy tube, tumor); fatigue; limited awareness; reddened, irritated oropharyngeal cavity (NANDA, 1990).

Related Nursing Diagnoses

Altered nutritional status affects many functional areas and can contribute to many other nursing problems. Alterations in normal elimination patterns (Diarrhea, Constipation) can occur due to nutritional deficits or the inability to use ingested nutrients. Decreased nutritional status greatly increases the risk for infection and delays wound healing. Skin breakdown (Impaired Skin Integrity, Impaired Tissue Integrity) is also more common in the poorly nourished person. Fluid status alterations (Fluid Volume Deficit) can occur in severe malnutrition. Altered nutritional status often results in fatigue, since the energy supply to the cells of the body is inadequate. When this occurs, or when morbid obesity is present, the patient may develop Activity Intolerance or Self-Care Deficit. If these conditions are extreme, such limitations can affect the person's ability to independently manage in the home setting (Impaired Home Maintenance Management).

Knowledge Deficit often occurs in patients who are placed on new diets (e.g., diabetic or heart patients) or new nutritional therapies (e.g., hyperalimentation or tube feedings). Noncompliance with diet orders or dietary restrictions can occur.

Altered nutritional status frequently affects appearance as body weight is gained or lost. Extreme alterations in body weight can lead to Body Image Disturbance and Self-Esteem Disturbance and may lead to Social Isolation.

Patient Goals

Patient goals for nutrition include ensuring adequate nutritional intake and understanding and complying with dietary modifications. Suggested goals include:

- Patient will use a nutritionally sound dietary intake to meet body requirements and promote health.

- Patient will maintain dietary intake adequate to meet energy expenditures of the body.
- Patient will demonstrate adequate knowledge to adhere to dietary prescription or therapies to promote health.

IMPLEMENTATION

Nursing Interventions to Promote Health and Function

In collaboration with the health-care team, the nurse is responsible for promoting optimal nutrition through health teaching. Nutritional counseling can occur in the community or hospital. Promoting optimal nutrition by providing assistance and creating an atmosphere that encourages eating is also an important nursing role.

Community Nutrition Programs

Governmental programs have been developed for people who need dietary enhancement and nutrition education. Nurses are actively involved in providing education and care through such programs. Community-based programs include:

- Senior center services
- Home-delivered meals
- Food stamps
- Missions and shelters
- WIC, a nutrition and health-care program for pregnant women, new mothers, infants, and children
- Child-care centers
- School lunch programs
- The M & I Program (maternal and infant nutritional supplementation and health care).

In addition to providing food for high-risk groups, many of these services also provide nutrition education and counseling. The Nutrition Education and Training (NET) program has been developed to help public schools incorporate nutrition education in their curricula.

Community resources also include the nutritional services of public health nurses, nutritionists, home health caregivers, and welfare agency workers. The services these people provide—education, assistance with meal planning and food buying, consultation, nutrition referrals, and research—are significant to the community's nutritional health.

International agencies promote health and nutritional adequacy on a worldwide level. These programs include the United Nations Food and Agriculture Organization (FAO), the World Health Organization (WHO), and the United Nations Children's Fund (UNICEF).

Patient Teaching

Nurses are active in a variety of settings to promote good nutrition. In addition to nutrition teaching in community-based programs, teaching can occur in a variety of settings, such as health fairs, schools, prenatal classes, health screening visits, and at home (Fig. 33-4). The goal of such education is to encourage good nutrition by increasing the person's understanding of the importance of a healthy diet. The nurse in these settings can refer high-risk people to appropriate private and community resources.

Patient teaching about nutrition also occurs in the hospital. When hospitalized, some patients are receptive to nutrition teaching. Statements can be directed at actions the patient can take currently (for example, "While your incision is healing, it's important to eat enough protein."). Informal diet instruction can occur when helping patients make menu selections. The nurse can praise good food choices, emphasizing the importance each food plays in staying healthy. Gentle encouragement can be given to improve diet selections (for example, "Have you ever tried 1% milk rather than 2% milk? Many people don't notice the difference, and it's a good way to reduce the fat intake in your diet.").

Patients often question the nurse about nutrition or ask for suggestions for altering diets. For example, an overweight patient may ask the nurse's opinion of a new diet recommended by a friend. It is important to provide the person with accurate factual information, encouragement, praise, and referral to appropriate resources.

Optimal Intake Promotion

Hospitalization often affects eating, and the nurse plays a role in encouraging optimal nutrition for patients. Provide an environment that facilitates enjoyment of food.

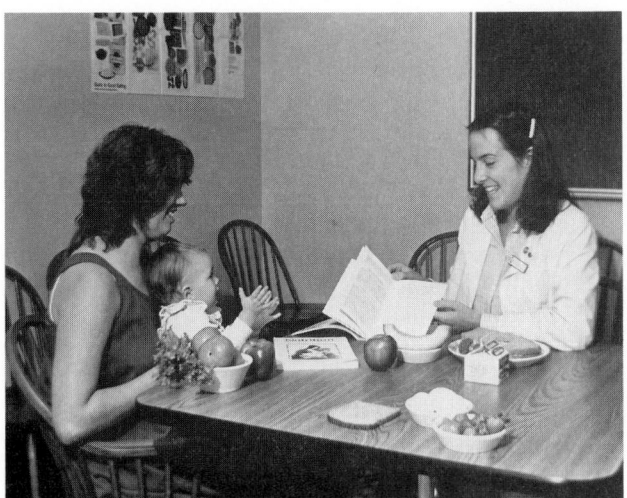

Figure 33–4. Teaching in the home setting to help a mother plan nutritious meals for her family. (Courtesy of Overlake Hospital Medical Center.)

Patient Teaching

Instruct the patient as follows:

- Eat a well-balanced diet from the four food groups.
- Develop regular eating patterns.
- Obtain recommended daily allowances of vitamins and minerals to promote health and prevent deficiencies.
- Make sure your diet has enough fiber by eating fresh fruits and vegetables and whole-grain cereals.
- Avoid excess calorie intake and refined sugar.
- Limit fat intake by using low-fat milk, reducing the intake of whole-fat cheese and ice cream, and eating chicken and fish rather than red meat.
- Limit sodium intake by decreasing the amount of salt used. Avoid processed or preserved foods.
- Learn proper storage and food preparation techniques to avoid bacterial contamination and possible foodborne infections.

The room should be clean, well ventilated, and free from strong odors. The atmosphere should be relaxing. Avoid interruptions such as treatments and procedures during mealtime. Oral care before eating promotes comfort. Medications to control nausea and pain should be timed so that optimal relief is achieved at mealtimes.

Food should be served in an appetizing manner and at the right temperature. Many hospital units have microwave ovens to rewarm cooled food. Food preferences should be considered, and the food should be arranged attractively. Small servings are preferable since they do not overwhelm the patient. Family members should be encouraged to bring favorite foods from home, as long as such food is permitted on the patient's diet.

Having pleasant company while eating can improve eating for some patients, but conversation should not distract the patient. Verbal cues and encouragement during eating provided by staff or relatives may be necessary for the confused or reluctant patient.

It is important to get patients out of bed and sitting in a chair for meals. This position facilitates chewing and swallowing and prevents reflux of stomach contents after eating. Assist patients who need help cutting food, opening packages, or eating; see Procedure 33-1.

Nursing Interventions for Altered Function

Nursing responsibility for the patient with altered nutrition includes providing special diets and nutritional supplements, and monitoring nutritional therapies such as

---

PROCEDURE 33–1. Assisting an Adult with Feeding

■ Purpose
1. Maintain nutritional status.
2. Provide a time for socialization.

■ Assessment
- Assess patient's physical and emotional ability to feed self (i.e., motor function, coordination, level of consciousness, vision, interest, depression).
- Assess eating habits and food preferences. Cultural and religious beliefs may eliminate food from the diet.
- Review history for food allergies.
- Assess ability of GI tract to absorb and digest oral nutrition (i.e., presence of bowel sounds, regular bowel movements, history of GI disorders, Crohn's disease, duodenal ulcers, pancreatitis, cholecystitis, ulcerative colitis).
- Review physician's orders for type of diet.

■ Equipment
Personal hygiene supplies for patient to wash hands.
Glasses, if necessary.
Special devices (splints, prostheses, spoons, cups).
Meal tray.
Oral hygiene equipment.

■ Procedure
1. Prepare patient's environment for meal:
   a. Remove urinals, bedpans, dressings, trash.
   b. Ventilate or aerate room for unpleasant odors.
   c. Clean overbed table.
      Rationale: Clean, uncluttered environment enhances appetite.
2. Prepare patient for meal:
   a. Help patient to urinate or defecate.
   b. Help patient to wash face and hands.
   c. Assist with oral hygiene.
   d. Help patient to apply dentures, glasses, or special appliances.
   e. Assist to upright position in bed or chair.
      Rationale: Promotes comfort and optimal physical condition to stimulate appetite and ingest meal.
3. Wash your hands before touching meal tray.
   Rationale: Prevents transfer of microorganisms.
4. Check patient's tray against diet order.
   Rationale: Prevents giving wrong diet to patient.
5. Place tray on overbed table and move in front of patient.
6. Prepare tray. Open cartons, remove lids, season food, cut food into bite-size pieces.
   Rationale: Patients with impaired physical or cogni-

tive function may be unable to prepare food for eating.
7. Place a napkin or towel under patient's chin.
8. If patient can feed self, the nurse may leave at this point. Return after 10 to 15 minutes to determine if patient is tolerating diet.
   Rationale: Enhances feelings of independence and positive self-esteem.
   Note: Do not leave patients with overly hot liquids or food unless they are fully independent with feeding.
   Rationale: Decreased sensation or lack of motor coordination could result in burns from hot foods or liquid.
9. If patient needs help to eat, sit in chair facing patient. If patient must remain in bed, nurse may stand.
   Rationale: Conveys an unhurried, social impression.

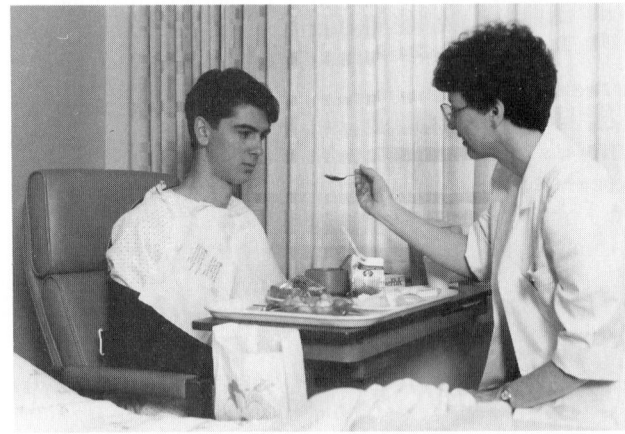
Step 9A

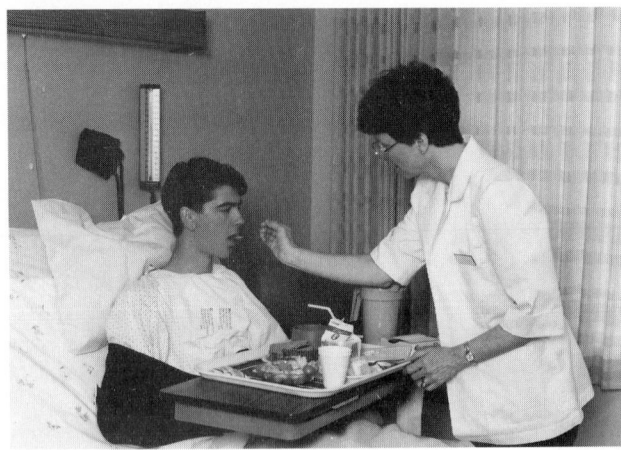
Step 9B

(continued)

PROCEDURE 33–1. Assisting an Adult with Feeding *(continued)*

10. Allow patient to choose the order he or she would like to eat. If patient is visually impaired, identify the food on the tray.
11. Warn patient if food is hot or cold.
12. Allow enough time between bites for adequate chewing and swallowing.
    Rationale: Avoids feeling of rushing through the meal.
13. Offer liquids as requested or between bites. Use a straw or special drinking cup if available.
    Rationale: Assists swallowing.
14. Provide conversation during meal. Choose topic of interest to patient. Reorient to current events or use meal as an opportunity to educate on nutrition or discharge plans.
    Note: Do not talk to patients who are relearning swallowing techniques; they need to concentrate.
15. Help patient to wash hands and face, and perform oral hygiene after meal.
16. Assist to comfortable position and allow rest period.
    Note: If at risk for aspiration, leave head of bed elevated for 30 minutes after eating.
17. Record fluids and amount of meal consumed, if ordered.
18. Remove and dispose of tray.
19. Wash your hands.

■ **Lifespan Considerations**

Infant
- Infants do not usually need food other than breast milk or formula until 4 to 6 months of age. Strained or blended foods may be introduced at that time.
- At 6 months of age, infants are interested in self-feeding with a spoon or teething crackers.

Toddler
- Toddlers are often very independent and insist on feeding themselves.
- Appropriate "finger foods" include meatballs, hard-boiled eggs, cooked carrots, peas, fruit slices (without skins), cheese pieces, dry cereal, crackers.

Preschool
- This is a period of slow growth, so a decrease in appetite can be expected.
- Using foods in color games and allowing the child to help with food preparation (stirring gelatin and pudding, peeling oranges, washing vegetables) stimulate the child's interest and teach good eating habits.

Adolescent
- Ages 10 to 11 (girls) and 12 to 13 (boys) are a period of rapid growth. Larger consumption of nutrients and calories are needed.
- Girls beginning menstruation need increased iron in their diets.

Older Adult
- Elderly patients may have diminished appetites from loss of taste and smell and decreased number of taste buds.
- Many older adults wear dentures. Poorly fitting dentures can impair their ability and desire to eat properly.
- Fewer calories are usually needed in this age group because of decreased activity and slowing metabolism.

■ **Home Care Modifications**
- Loneliness and poverty may decrease a patient's ability or interest in eating balanced meals at home.
- Federal programs such as food stamps and Supplemental Security Income can increase the food-buying power for patients at home.
- In 1972, a federally funded nutrition program for the elderly was instituted that provides low-cost, nutritious meals served in community settings. These programs also provide socialization for the lonely elderly.
- Meals on Wheels is available in many communities to deliver nutritious meals to patients in their homes.

---

total parenteral nutrition and tube feedings. Patient teaching is important in each of these therapies.

Withholding Food

The term *NPO* or nothing by mouth (Latin, *non per os*) is used when patients cannot ingest food or fluids orally. Withholding food may be indicated to:

- Rest the GI tract to promote healing

- Clear the GI tract of contents before surgery or diagnostic procedures
- Prevent aspiration during surgery or in high-risk patients
- Give normal intestinal motility time to return during the postoperative period
- Treat severe vomiting or diarrhea
- Treat medical problems such as bowel obstruction or acute inflammation of the GI tract.

Well-nourished patients can tolerate lack of food for

Selected Nursing Interventions for Common Nutritional Problems

Less Nutrition Than Body Requires

- Encourage and cue verbally to eat
- Provide high-protein and high-caloric snacks
- Give dietary supplements
- Use enteral tube feedings
- Use peripheral parenteral nutrition
- Use total parenteral nutrition

More Nutrition Than Body Requires

- Explain low caloric diets
- Identify and encourage healthy eating habits and patterns
- Give encouragement and positive reinforcement
- Refer for behavior modification techniques
- Encourage increased activity and regular exercise
- Refer to support groups and appropriate agencies for weight reduction

Impaired Swallowing

- Provide rest period before meals
- Position patient upright in chair or high-Fowler's position in bed with neck slightly flexed
- Thicken liquids
- Provide small bites and check for pocketing of food
- Provide simple, short verbal cues to "chew," "swallow," etc.
- Keep stimuli to a minimum to prevent distractions
- Provide enough time and appear unrushed
- Initiate appropriate referrals as needed

---

a few days, but fluids must be provided to prevent fluid and electrolyte disturbances. Some patients find it difficult to be unable to eat. Nursing measures to promote comfort during this period include:

Provide frequent oral hygiene.
Give ice chips, hard candy, and gum or mouth rinses if permitted.
Avoid exposure to people eating or advertisements for food.

If the NPO period is longer than a few days, alternate forms of nutritional support may be necessary.

Special Diets

Dietary intake must often be altered to promote healing and restore health. Objectives of dietary treatment may be to increase or decrease weight, to allow an organ to rest, to remedy nutritional deficits, to promote healing, and to provide nutrients the body can metabolize.

When a patient can eat any food, the diet is referred to as general, regular, or house. A regular diet is well balanced and supplies the metabolic requirements of a sedentary person (about 2000 calories per day). Menus allow the patient to select from a wide variety of choices, but all offerings are nutritionally planned to supply recommended daily allowances. Special requests or preferences (such as vegetarian or kosher diets) and food allergies should be reported to the dietary department when the patient is admitted.

It may be necessary to modify the diet's texture, consistency, calories, or other nutrients if the patient has had surgery or has a medical condition that requires an altered diet. Modifications of consistency are clear liquid, full liquid, soft, mechanical soft, and bland.

Clear Liquid. This diet includes only liquids that lack residue, such as juices without pulp (e.g., apple, cranberry), tea, gelatin, soda pop, and clear broth. It is used as a first diet postoperatively, before some diagnostic tests, and after an acute episode of vomiting or diarrhea.

Full Liquid. A full liquid diet includes all fluids and foods that become liquid at room temperature (ice cream, sherbet). This diet may be ordered postoperatively after a clear liquid diet has been well tolerated, or for patients who cannot chew food adequately.

Soft. Soft diets include soft foods and those with reduced fiber content, which require less energy for digestion. Soft diets are appropriate for the person who has difficulty chewing, or who has no teeth. *Mechanical soft* diets are further chopped or puréed. Soft diets may also be used for the postoperative patient as the diet progresses from full liquid.

Bland. Bland diets eliminate chemical irritation (from highly seasoned foods), mechanical irritation (from food high in fiber), and thermal irritation (from foods that are very hot or cold). Caffeine and alcohol are also limited to prevent chemical irritation.

Diet as Tolerated. Diet as tolerated (DAT) is ordered when the patient's ability to tolerate certain foods may change, such as during the postoperative period or after GI distress. The nurse orders the diet based on the patient's appetite and ability to eat. For example, on the first postoperative day, a patient may be given a clear liquid diet. If no nausea occurs, normal intestinal motility has returned, and the patient feels like eating, the diet may be advanced to a regular diet.

TABLE 33–5
Dietary Modifications for Diseases

Disease	Modification
Renal disease	Restrict intake of sodium, potassium, and protein.
Liver disease (cirrhosis)	Restrict intake of sodium; increase intake of protein.
Congestive heart failure	Restrict intake of sodium and calories.
Coronary artery disease	Restrict intake of sodium, calories, and fats (saturated fats and cholesterol).
Burns	Increase intake of calories, protein, vitamin C, and the B-complex vitamins.
Respiratory (emphysema)	A soft, high-calorie, high-protein diet is recommended.
Tuberculosis	Increase intake of protein, calories, calcium, and vitamin A.
Hypertension	Restrict sodium intake; lose weight, if appropriate.

Restrictive Diets. Diets may be ordered to fulfill a special requirement of the patient with chronic disease or altered metabolism. For example, the patient with cardiac problems may need to limit sodium and cholesterol, the obese patient may need calorie restriction, and the diabetic patient may follow a prescribed American Diabetes Association diet. Examples of such dietary modifications for different diseases are given in Table 33-5. It is important to be aware of any such dietary restrictions, since any food or fluid given must fit the restrictions.

When a patient is placed on a restrictive diet, it is important to provide teaching to promote necessary dietary changes. The dietitian may do initial diet teaching, and the nurse reinforces such teaching. Written materials are available to assist in patient teaching. Changes in long-established eating patterns are difficult for many patients to make, and goals must be realistic and individualized for each patient.

Nutritional Supplements

Nutritional supplements may be added to the prescribed diet to provide necessary nutrients, especially during periods of increased metabolic demand. Supplements can take the form of protein-rich formulas or vitamins and minerals. Protein supplements, such as Ensure, can be requested by the nurse or ordered by the physician. These supplements are typically milkshake-type drinks given between meals three or four times a day to increase calorie and protein intake. Malnourished patients or patients with excessive metabolic demand from trauma, fever, infection, surgery, or cancer benefit from such therapy.

Enteral Tube Feedings

Enteral nutrition is the direct delivery of nutrients into the GI system. Tube feedings are nutritionally balanced commercial formulas that are given through a tube di-

rectly into the esophagus, stomach, jejunum, or duodenum. Access to the GI system can be achieved by inserting a tube through the nose into the stomach or intestine.

If long-term tube feedings are likely, a surgical procedure is performed to create an opening directly into the stomach or intestines through which feedings can be directly administered. A *gastrostomy* is an opening into the stomach. A newer procedure for gastrostomy placement involves endoscopic percutaneous insertion of a

---

Safety Alert

- Keep hot liquids away from toddlers or confused patients who may accidentally spill them.
- When ability to swallow is questionable, never give oral food or fluids until a complete evaluation is done.
- Sit patients upright when eating to minimize the chance of accidental aspiration.
- Use caution when using microwaves to reheat food. Burns can result from steam when containers are opened or if portions of the food become very hot.
- Always check proper tube placement before beginning tube feedings to prevent accidental aspiration of feedings.
- Dilute infant formulas or tube feedings according to manufacturer's specifications to avoid administering highly osmotic solutions, which could cause significant fluid and electrolyte imbalances.
- Be familiar with the Heimlich maneuver, and use it to dislodge aspirated food particles if the patient cannot independently clear airway.

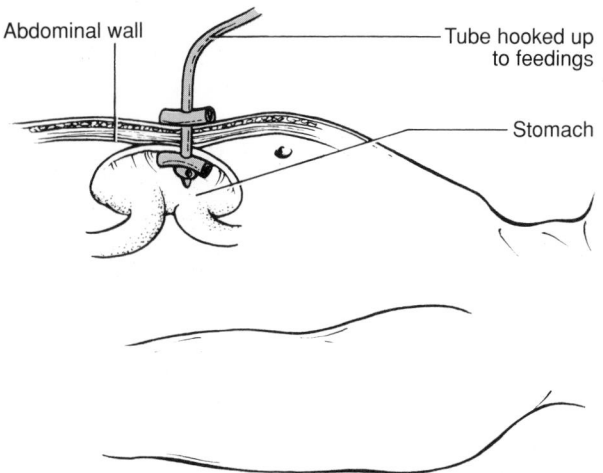

Figure 33–5. Percutaneous endoscopic gastrostomy (PEG) permits placement of a tube in the stomach for feedings. Mushroom catheter prevents dislodgement.

mushroom catheter into the stomach (Fig. 33-5). Known as *percutaneous endoscopic gastrostomy* (PEG), this procedure is safer and less expensive since it does not require a general anesthetic and can often be done on an outpatient basis (Starkey, et al., 1988). Because GI motility is not decreased by surgery or anesthesia in this procedure, feedings can start immediately. An opening into the jejunum (*jejunostomy*) is often used when aspiration has been a problem (Eisenberg, 1989). A *gastrostomy/jejunostomy* tube can be inserted if decompression is necessary along with feeding. A double-lumen tube allows feeding to enter the jejunum while the other lumen drains the stomach (Eisenberg, 1989).

Indications. Tube feedings are used to provide nutrition to patients who cannot swallow or who have an esophageal obstruction. Obstruction can occur secondary to edema from head or neck surgery or trauma (e.g., swallowing caustic substances or inhaling smoke). Tube feedings are also indicated when the patient's decreased level of consciousness prevents safe eating. Tube feedings can be used as adjunctive therapy for patients who can eat but who cannot consume adequate nutrients to meet nutritional demands of the body (e.g., cancer patients). Premature infants who have an inadequate sucking reflex or lack strength to feed can also be fed through gavage. Tube feedings are appropriate only when the patient can absorb nutrients from the GI tract (Fig. 33-6).

Types of Tubes. The type of tube used to deliver enteral feedings depends on where and how the feeding is delivered. A nasogastric tube, such as a Levin tube, can be used for short-term tube feedings. Because such tubes are relatively rigid and have a large diameter compared to the nasal passage, discomfort and mucosal breakdown is common with prolonged therapy. More flexible, small-

bore tubes have been developed when long-term feeding is indicated but a surgical opening in the GI tract is undesirable. These tubes vary in size from 6 to 12 French and are composed of polyurethane, silicon, or polyvinyl chloride. Most have weighted distal tips and are placed using a stylet. The tubes are radiopaque so that tube placement can be confirmed by x-ray. Nasogastric tubes are attached to the nose with tape.

Tubes that are surgically placed in the stomach or intestines are usually larger in diameter and made of plastic or rubber. Initially they are sutured in place to prevent leakage and avoid dislodgement. Aseptic care of the incision is important until healing has occurred. The tube can be clamped off between feedings. When the incision has healed, the tube can be removed and reinserted when feeding is required.

Enteral Formulas. Enteral feedings consist of nutritionally balanced formulas that contain proteins, carbohydrates, and fats. Many brands are commercially available; they vary in relative proportions of nutrients and calories, osmolality, and ease of digestibility and absorption. Most formulas can be stored unrefrigerated until opened, but then should be refrigerated to limit microbial growth.

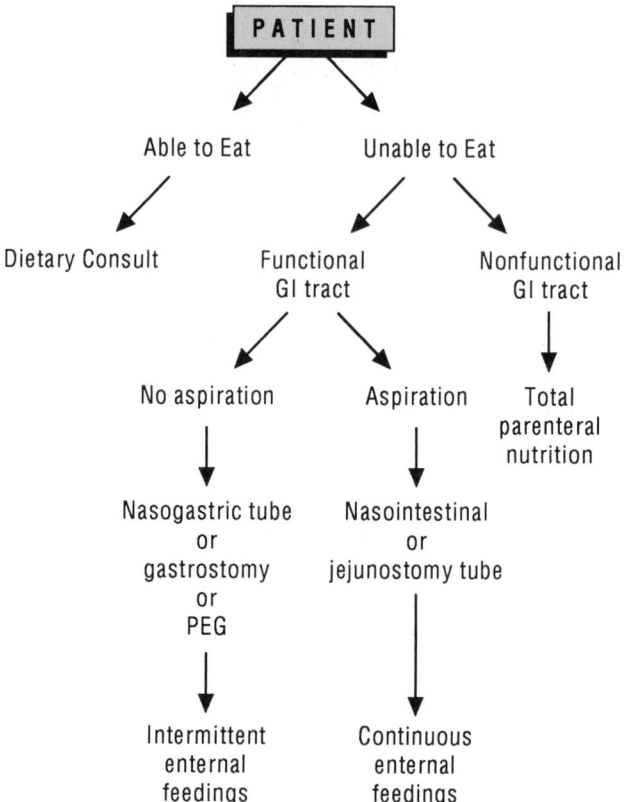

Figure 33–6. Indications for selection of different types of nutritional support. (Modified from Eisenberg, P. (1989). Enteral nutrition: Indications, formulas, and delivery techniques. *Nursing Clinics of North America* 24(2), 326.)

Continuous Versus Intermittent Feedings. Enteral feedings may be given on an intermittent or continuous basis (see Procedure 33-2). The physician orders the rate of infusion and the formula to be used. Continuous feedings are permitted to flow in at the prescribed rate using a gravitational drip method, or they are monitored by an infusion pump. For the patient who is eating, feedings may be ordered to infuse continuously during the night and are discontinued a few hours before breakfast in hopes of stimulating the appetite.

Intermittent feedings are given at specific intervals, usually corresponding to mealtimes. Intermittent feedings should be given slowly over a 15-minute period, either using a syringe or by gravity flow.

Hazards and Complications. Nursing responsibilities for the patient receiving tube feedings include prevention and assessment of complications such as nausea, vomiting, aspiration, fluid and electrolyte imbalance, diarrhea, intestinal cramping, occlusion of the tube, and hyperglycemia.

Nausea and vomiting usually occur when the feeding is administered at a rate faster than the formula can be absorbed. To assess for this, check the residual volume left in the stomach after feedings or at periodic intervals if tube feedings are continuous. If residuals are greater than 100 mL, the feeding should be stopped or the rate decreased, since aspiration is likely if vomiting occurs (Eisenberg, 1989).

Aspiration can also be minimized by checking proper placement of the tube before feedings are initiated and at frequent intervals, and by keeping patients in Fowler's position at all times when feedings are infusing and for 30 minutes after an intermittent feeding. Blue food coloring can be added to the formula of patients at risk for aspiration. If blue-tinged respiratory secretions are produced, aspiration has probably occurred.

Diarrhea, intestinal cramping, and fluid loss are related to the high osmolality of the formulas used. Diluting the concentration by adding water or giving the patient adequate free water may prevent severe osmotic fluid shifts. Slow administration of room-temperature feedings helps limit GI intolerance.

Feeding tubes, especially those with small-bore lumens, clog easily. Take care to avoid tube occlusion even for a short period of time. Clogging can be prevented by frequent flushing of the tube with water, especially after giving medications.

Hyperglycemia may occur in patients who cannot produce enough insulin to deal with the carbohydrate load in the formula. For diabetic patients and any high-risk person, blood glucose monitoring permits careful regulation of increased insulin need.

Peripheral Parenteral Nutrition

Intravenous therapy provides the patient with fluid and electrolytes, but only a limited amount of nutrients and calories (e.g., 170 kcals in 1000 mL 5% dextrose in water). Intravenous therapy does not meet a patient's basal nutritional needs; this causes catabolism of nutrient stores in the body. When nutritional support is needed for a short period of time, or when invasive procedures to deliver more concentrated nutritional support intravenously are not feasible, peripheral parenteral nutrition (PPN) may be an option. PPN infuses isotonic lipids into peripheral vessels to meet caloric requirements. Such infusions can deliver nearly 2000 kcals per day (Worthington & Wagner, 1989). The increased incidence of phlebitis with PPN limits the frequency with which this therapy is used (Worthington & Wagner, 1989). PPN is more appropriately used to prevent malnutrition than to correct nutritional deficits.

Total Parenteral Nutrition

Total parenteral nutrition (TPN), also known as hyperalimentation, is the administration of hypertonic solutions containing dextrose, proteins, vitamins, and minerals into the venous circulation. With the addition of lipid emulsions, a nutritionally complete diet can be delivered intravenously. See Procedure 33-3.

Indications. Since TPN requires more invasive procedures, it is usually used when tube feedings are ineffective or contraindicated. TPN is indicated in conditions that interfere with absorption of nutrients from the GI tract, when diarrhea or vomiting is persistent and does not respond to treatment, and when complete bowel rest is necessary to promote healing. TPN is initiated when parenteral nutrition will be needed for more than 5 days (Worthington & Wagner, 1989).

Venous Access. Because it is a highly osmotic solution, TPN must be infused in central vessels. Irritation and sclerosing of the vein, as well as sudden fluid shifts, are less likely when the hypertonic solutions are mixed adequately with blood. Common vessels used for central catheter insertion are the subclavian and jugular veins. Nonsurgical insertion can occur when a standard central venous line is inserted into a vessel and advanced to the appropriate place. When TPN is anticipated for an extended period, a more permanent catheter (e.g., Hickman, Broviac) may be surgically placed (Fig. 33-7).

TPN Solution. All TPN solutions contain essential nutrients including protein, carbohydrates, electrolytes, vitamins, water, and trace elements. The proportion of each ingredient is individualized based on the patient's need. The carbohydrate source is often a 50% dextrose solution, and protein is provided as synthetic crystalline amino acids. The patient's caloric need is carefully assessed to provide the number of calories needed for anabolism. Electrolytes, vitamins, and trace elements are added based on laboratory assays.

(Text continues on page 929)

PROCEDURE 33–2. Administering Nutrition via Nasogastric or Gastrostomy Tube

■ Purpose

1. Provide enteral nutrition in patients who cannot swallow or who have an esophageal obstruction.
2. Provide nutrition to comatose or semiconscious patients.
3. Provide additional nutrients for patients who cannot orally consume total caloric requirements.

■ Assessment

- Assess patient's nutritional status and identify need for tube feedings:
  - Impaired swallowing
  - Decreased level of consciousness
  - Head, neck, or facial surgery or trauma
  - Extraordinary caloric requirements.
- Review chart for food allergies and physican's order as to type, amount, rate, route, and frequency of feeding.
- Assess patient's GI system:
  - Observe and palpate for distention; tenderness.
  - Auscultate bowel sounds.
  - Determine time of last bowel movement.
  - Assess for presence of existing feeding tube.

■ Equipment

Formula.
Blue food coloring (optional).
Disposable gavage bag and tubing.
60-cc catheter tip irrigation syringe.
Infusion pump (optional).
Water.
Measuring container.

■ Procedure

1. Wash your hands.
2. Close room door or curtains around bed.
   Rationale: Provides for privacy and decreases embarrassment.
3. Explain procedure to patient.
4. Help patient to high-Fowler's position by elevating head of bed at least 60° or assisting to a chair. If high-Fowler's position is contraindicated, help patient to a right side-lying position with head slightly elevated.
   Rationale: Positions prevent aspiration of formula into lungs and facilitate flow of feeding into intestine.
5. Confirm placement of tube in stomach:
   a. Attach 60-mL irrigation syringe to tube and inject 10 mL of air while auscultating over epigastrium.
   Rationale: Air can be heard entering stomach.
   Note: Auscultation of air is not always a reliable index of tube placement when a small-bore feeding tube is used.

   b. Aspirate all stomach contents and measure for residual.
   Rationale: Presence of gastric fluid confirms tube placement in the stomach. Gastric residuals are checked to evaluate if gastric emptying is adequate.

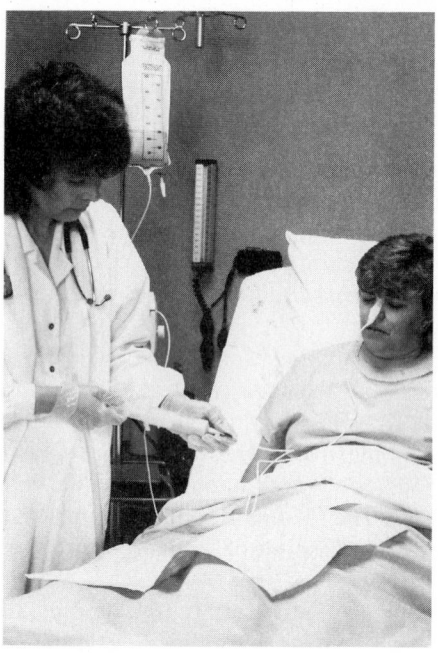

Step 5B

   c. If 100-mL or more than half of the last feeding is aspirated, contact the physician before proceeding with tube feeding. The feeding is usually held.
   d. Reinstill the aspirated gastric contents through the tube and into the stomach.
   Rationale: Gastric content is rich in electrolytes. Electrolyte imbalance could occur if residuals are discarded.
6. Prepare correct amount and strength of formula. Formula should be room temperature. Add several drops of food coloring (optional).
   Rationale: Strength and amount of formula is gradually increased to prevent diarrhea and gastric intolerance. Formula should be at room temperature because it will not be warmed or cooled by the oral and esophageal mucosa as occurs in normal swallowing. Cold formula can cause abdominal cramping and discomfort; hot formula can burn the stomach. Food coloring is frequently used when tube-feeding patients are at risk for aspiration. If formula is aspirated, nasotracheal suction reveals bluish secretions. Check agency policy.

(continued)

PROCEDURE 33–2. Administering Nutrition via Nasogastric or Gastrostomy Tube *(continued)*

■ **Procedure**

Bolus or Intermittent Feeding

1. Remove plunger from irrigation syringe. Clamp gastric tubing and attach syringe. If using gavage bag, attach tubing to gastric tube.
Rationale: Clamping tubing prevents air from entering stomach and prevents stomach contents from leaking out.
2. Fill syringe or gavage bag with formula.
3. Allow feeding to flow in slowly (10 to 15 min.). If using syringe, raise or lower syringe to adjust flow rate by gravity. Refill syringe as needed without disconnecting, avoiding air spaces in tubing. If gavage bag is used, hang bag on IV pole and adjust flow rate with clamp on tubing.
Rationale: Feedings given too rapidly cause nausea, vomiting, flatus, and abdominal cramps.
4. Clamp tubing just as feeding is completing. Rinse tube with 30 to 60 mL tap water. Do not allow air to enter tubing.
Rationale: Clamping tubing prevents air from entering stomach to reduce bloating or cramps. Rinsing with water clears the gastric tube to prevent blockage and bacterial growth.
5. Clamp gastric tube and disconnect from syringe or gavage bag.
6. Have patient remain in high-Fowler's or elevated side-lying position for 30 to 60 minutes after feeding.

■ **Procedure**

Continuous Feeding

1. Connect gavage tubing to gastric tube.
2. Hang gavage bag on IV pole.
3. Pour in desired amount of formula.
Note: Usually hang amount of formula to infuse in 3 hours. Check agency policy.
4. Connect tubing to infusion pump and set rate.
Rationale: Prevents feeding from infusing too rapidly, which may result in vomiting and cramps.
5. Patients on continuous feedings should have gastric residuals checked every 4 to 6 hours, according to agency policy. Then flush tubing with 30 to 60 mL water.
Rationale: Assesses for adequate absorption of feeding and verifies correct placement of tube.
6. Have patient remain in high-Fowler's or in slightly elevated right side-lying position.
7. Wash any reusable equipment with soap and water. Change equipment every 24 hours or according to agency policy.

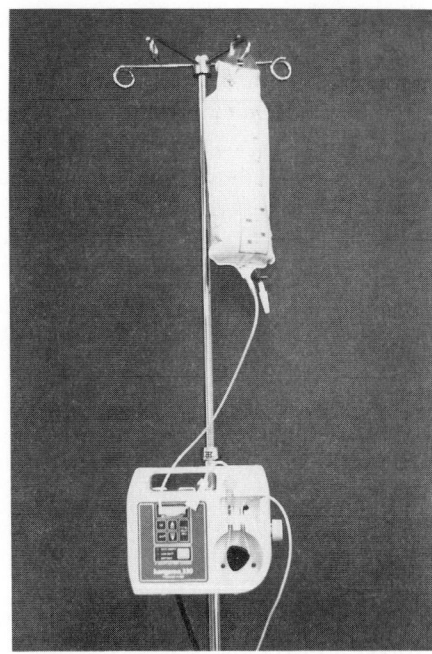

Step 4

8. Wash hands.
9. Document appropriately.

■ **Lifespan Considerations**

Infants and Children

• Intermittent feeding and reinsertion of nasogastric feeding tube at each feeding is recommended in children. There is significant risk of stomach perforation, nasal airway obstruction, and ulceration and irritation of the mucous membrane if a feeding tube is left in continuously.

■ **Home Care Modifications**

• Patients are encouraged to participate in the preparation and procedure of tube feeding if possible to increase their feelings of independence and self-esteem.
• Patient or caregiver must be educated in correct technique and rationales as stated above.
• Feedings can be provided from commercially prepared formulas or home-blended foods. Formulas may be thinned with juice, milk, or water.
• Caregiver must be taught proper storage of extra formula:
  • Commercially prepared formulas should be sealed and stored in refrigerator once the can is open. Use within 24 hours.
  • Home-blended feedings should be tightly sealed, dated, and refrigerated. Use within 24 hours after preparation.

(continued)

PROCEDURE 33–2. Administering Nutrition via Nasogastric or Gastrostomy Tube *(continued)*

- Tube-fed patients may feel isolated or may have altered self-esteem and body image from the loss of sensory and social stimulation associated with eating. Feedings can be scheduled with family mealtimes.
- If medically permitted, the patient can consume some favorite foods orally. If swallowing is contraindicated,

it may be possible for the patient to chew and taste a few favorite foods, then spit them out.
- Followup and consultation with a home health nurse often allows patients and caregivers to arrange creative solutions to problems or concerns that arise.

PROCEDURE 33–3. Administering Total Parenteral Nutrition (TPN)

■ Purpose

1. Provide parenteral nutritional support to malnourished patients.
2. Provide parenteral nutritional support to patients requiring bypass of the GI tract for prolonged periods.
3. Provide parenteral nutritional support to patients who have excessive metabolic needs due to trauma, cancer, or hypermetabolic states.

■ Assessment

- Assess nutritional needs of patient.
- Check pattern of weight loss or gain, and intake and output balance.
- Check physician's order for TPN, noting additives and rate of infusion.
- Compare bottle of TPN against physician's order to ensure that it is correct.
- Assess patient's knowledge of TPN and need for patient teaching.

■ Equipment

Total parenteral nutrition solution (usually prepared by pharmacy).
Appropriate IV tubing with filter.
Infusion control pump.
TPN dressing kit as per hospital protocol (usually contains transparent dressing, acetone swabs, Betadine swabs).
Sterile gloves and mask.
Blood glucose monitoring equipment.

■ Procedure

Monitoring TPN therapy

1. Schedule and assist patient with chest x-ray after central catheter insertion.
   Rationale: Documents that catheter is in correct position and whether pneumothorax occurred during insertion.

2. Confirm correct solution is running at ordered rate. Check expiration date of solution. Use infusion controller to monitor and regulate flow rate.
   Note: Solutions with more than 10% dextrose must be infused directly into the subclavian or internal jugular vein to rapidly dilute the solution and prevent thrombophlebitis. Constant flow rate helps prevent hyperglycemia and electrolyte imbalances.

3. Inspect tubing and catheter connection for leaks or kinks. Tape all connections. Change tubing every 24 hours according to hospital policy.
   Rationale: Leaks prevent patient from receiving prescribed volume of solution and are a potential entry site for bacteria. Kinks in tubing can obstruct flow of solution and result in clotting of catheter. Taping connections prevents accidental disconnection.

4. Inspect insertion site for infiltration, thrombophlebitis, or drainage. If present, notify physician.
   Note: The physician may order the catheter to be removed. If infection is suspected, catheter tip may be placed in sterile specimen cup and sent to laboratory for culture.

5. Monitor vital signs, including temperature, every 4 hours.
   Rationale: Elevated temperature may indicate catheter-related sepsis.

6. Assess for symptoms of air embolism (i.e., decreased level of consciousness, tachycardia, dyspnea, anxiety, "feeling of impending doom," chest pain, cyanosis, hypotension).
   Note: If suspected, lay patient on left side with head in Trendelenburg position.
   Rationale: Lying on left side may prevent air from flowing into the pulmonary veins. Lying in Trendelenburg position increases intrathoracic pressure, which decreases the amount of blood pulled into the vena cava during inhalation.

7. Use the TPN line *only* for TPN. Do not use the line for any other reason.

(continued)

Rationale: Minimizes breaks in integrity of line to prevent infection.

8. Test urine every 6 hours for specific gravity and ketones.
9. Perform test for glucose every 6 hours. Notify physician if abnormal.
   Rationale: Hyperglycemia may be an indication that patient needs insulin to help metabolize glucose or may be an early indication of sepsis.
10. Monitor laboratory tests of electrolytes, BUN, glucose, as ordered, and report abnormal findings.
11. Maintain accurate record of intake and output to monitor fluid balance.
12. Weigh patient daily and record.
13. Inspect dressing once a shift for drainage and intactness. Change whenever loose or moist and at least every 48 hours.

■ Procedure

Changing TPN Tubing and Dressing
1. Wash your hands.
   Rationale: Reduces transmission of microorganisms.
2. Cross-check new hyperalimentation solutions with physician's order. Check expiration date.
   Note: TPN must be used within 24 hours of preparation.
3. Attach sterile tubing and filter to new parenteral hyperalimentation solutions. Prime tubing as you would a conventional IV.
4. Place patient in supine position.
   Rationale: Position decreases pressure in vena cava to reduce risk of air embolism when catheter is disconnected.
5. Don a mask. Instruct patient to turn head facing opposite direction of insertion site, and not to cough or talk during dressing change.
   Note: Place mask on patient if he or she cannot cooperate.
   Rationale: Protects insertion site and catheter from microorganisms from the nurse or patient's nose and mouth.
6. Don gloves.
   Rationale: Protects nurse from patient's secretions.
7. Remove old dressing and discard.
8. Inspect insertion site for redness, drainage, swelling.
9. Remove gloves.
10. Wash your hands.
11. Open sterile supplies and place on bedside table.
12. Put on sterile gloves.
13. Cleanse insertion site with gauze soaked in 10%

acetone. Wipe in circular motion, moving from the insertion site outward.
Rationale: Acetone removes old adhesive tape and defats the skin.
Note: Keep acetone from contacting catheter, because it could break down the plastic.

14. Cleanse site with same circular motion for 2 minutes using povidone-iodine solution (Betadine). Allow to air dry.
    Rationale: Betadine has antimicrobial properties to reduce the number of microorganisms at the catheter insetion site.
15. Cleanse connection of catheter and tubing with Betadine.
16. Hospital policy may dictate cleansing Betadine off skin with alcohol.
17. Apply Betadine ointment to insertion site.
    Rationale: Provides long-term antimicrobial action.
18. Loosen tubing at catheter hub.
19. Ask patient to hold breath and bear down (Valsalva) while you quickly disconnect old tubing and attach new tubing to catheter hub.
    Rationale: The Valsalva maneuver increases pressure on large veins in chest and reduces chance of air embolism when catheter is open.
20. Tape all connections.
    Rationale: Prevents accidental disconnection of tubing.
21. Place transparent, semipermeable dressing over insertion site. Optional: Paint skin margins with tincture of benzoin before placing dressing to ensure a tighter seal.
    Rationale: Transparent dressing is preferred so insertion site can be easily assessed without disrupting or manipulating dressing.
22. Loop and tape tubing next to dressing.
23. Label dressing and tubing with date and your name.
24. Adjust flow rate per physician's order.
25. Discard used solution and tubing. Remove gloves. Document amount infused on intake and output record.

■ Procedure

Administering Intralipids
1. Check solution against physician's order. Inspect solution for separation of emulsion into layers or for froth. Do not use if present.
   Rationale: Solution is spoiled.
2. Wash your hands.
3. Attach intralipid tubing to bottle. Prime tubing as for a conventional IV.

(continued)

PROCEDURE 33–3. Administering Total Parenteral Nutrition (TPN) *(continued)*

Rationale: Intralipid tubing has no in-line filter that would cause separation of the emulsion.

4. Place 19- or 21-gauge 1-inch needle on distal end of tubing.
5. Identity patient.
6. Identity Y-port on hyperalimentation tubing (below in-line filter).
7. Cleanse Y-port with antiseptic swab. Allow to dry. Insert needle into port. Secure with tape.
    Note: Intralipids can be infused into a peripheral IV.
8. Adjust flow rate to infuse at 1.0 mL/min for adults and 0.1 mL/min for children. Infuse at this rate for 30 minutes while you monitor the patient and vital signs every 10 minutes.
    Note: If any adverse reactions occur, stop infusion and notify physician.
9. If no adverse reactions occur, adjust flow rate:
    a. Adults: 500 mL intralipid over 4 to 6 hours.
    b. Children: up to 1 gm/kg over 4 hours.

■ **Lifespan Considerations**

Infants and Children

• TPN solutions for children generally start with a 10% dextrose solution, increased to 25% dextrose. Exogenous insulin is usually not needed, as a child's pancreas adapts easily to higher glucose levels. TPN solutions also usually contain higher concentrations of calcium, phosphorus, magnesium, and vitamins.

• Children are usually more active than adults and require frequent assessment of the tubing to prevent disconnections or obstruction during ambulation or play.

• Instruct parents on preventing accidental disconnection or obstruction of tubing.

• Soft restraints may be necessary to prevent the child from pulling out the catheter. Provide play therapy, books, and stimulation to distract the child.

■ **Home Care Modifications**

• The health-care team must determine that the patient or a guardian is responsible and able to be present during therapy.

• Identify and consult with a home health nurse who can be available 24 hours a day to troubleshoot complications.

• A long-term infusion device such as a Hickman or Groshung catheter should be in place before the patient's discharge.

• The patient or caregiver must be taught how to initiate, monitor, and maintain an IV catheter and infusion according to the above protocol.

• The patient usually is weighed daily. Intake and output are recorded. Blood values are monitored at least every other week.

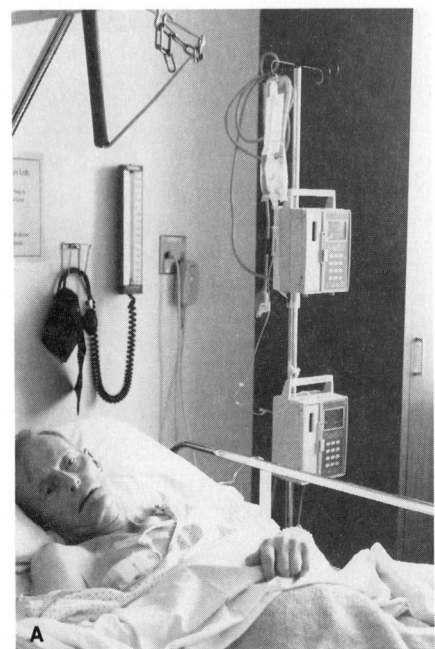
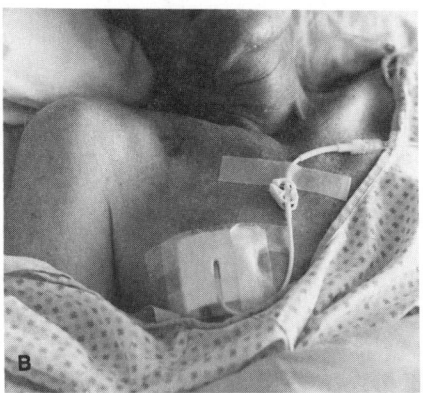

Figure 33–7. **A:** Malnourished patient receiving TPN through a central venous catheter. **B:** Enlargement of **A** showing catheter.

To supply all necessary nutrients, fat in the form of 10% or 20% lipid emulsions is often given with TPN. These isotonic solutions, which look like milk, are compatible with TPN and can be infused intravenously (Fig. 33-8). Recently, a system known as Total Nutrient Admixture (TNA), which mixes lipid emulsions with amino acid and dextrose solutions, has become available in the United States. This permits all necessary nutrients to be given in a single bottle, decreasing expense and possible infection risk (Worthington & Wagner, 1989).

Continuous Versus Cycling Infusions. Often, TPN is given continuously and monitored via an infusion pump to prevent inadvertent sudden infusion. Cycling, or the interruption of infusion for a period of time, is routinely used for patients receiving home therapy. It permits increased freedom, as nutrition is delivered only at night. When instituting cyclic infusions, rates should be increased gradually, so as not to cause sudden fluid shifts or hyperglycemia.

Complications. Many potentially serious complications, such as pneumothorax, air embolism, infection, fluid overload, and hyperglycemia, are associated with TPN.

Pneumothorax can occur if the lung is punctured during insertion of the central venous line. Symptoms of pneumothorax are chest or shoulder pain, sudden shortness of breath, tachycardia, and absence of breath sounds on the affected side.

Air embolism, or the introduction of air into the vascular system, can occur when the catheter is introduced or if air is introduced into the intravenous line at any time. Having the patient perform the Valsalva maneuver when the line is inserted or whenever the system is disconnected reduces the risk of air embolism. Tubing should be connected with Luer locks to prevent accidental separation, and the patient should take care not to pull on or dislodge tubing when moving.

Infection is a potentially serious complication of TPN. TPN is a glucose-rich solution that can support microbial growth. Use strict aseptic technique during insertion of the catheter, dressing changes, and tubing and bottle changes. Agency protocol determines the frequency and technique to be used for routine care of the site and tubing. Avoid piggybacking into the TPN line. Frequently assess the insertion site. Inflammation at the site and fever usually necessitates catheter removal. The catheter tip should be cultured after removal.

Fluid overload can occur if the osmotic solution is infused too quickly, drawing fluid into the circulatory system. This risk is especially high for patients who have a history of congestive heart failure and cannot tolerate rapid fluid shifts. TPN infusion should always be regulated by a pump or controller to avoid sudden infusion of fluid. Monitor daily weights and intake and output.

Hyperglycemia, or elevated blood glucose, can occur when insufficient insulin is produced to handle the glucose load provided by TPN. Blood glucose levels are monitored and insulin coverage may be necessary. The TPN infusion is usually started gradually and tapered off gradually to avoid sudden shifts in glucose.

Discharge Planning and Home Care

Nutrition is an important consideration in planning for discharge and independent management at home. All patients should be counseled on desirable food intake

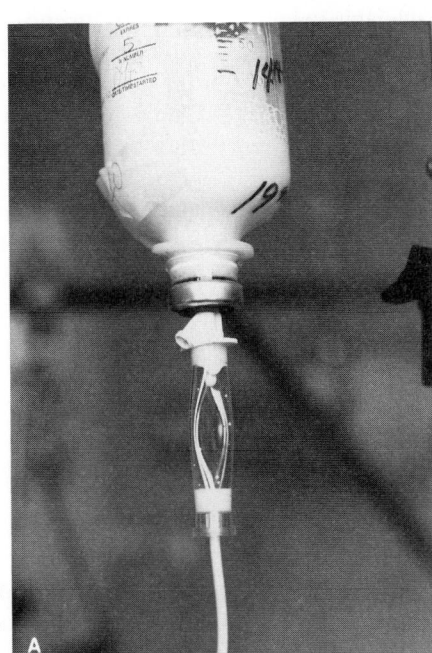
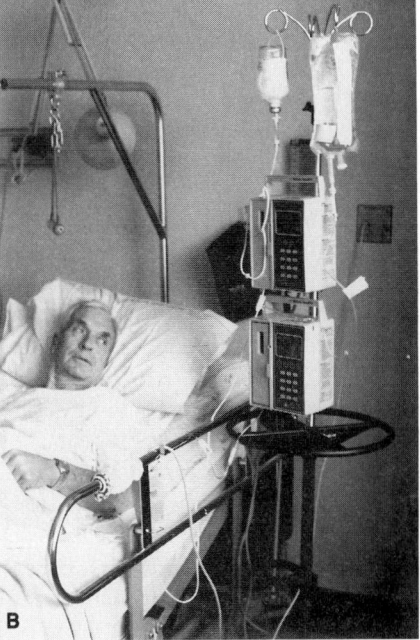

Figure 33–8. **A:** Lipid emulsion for intravenous administration. **B:** TPN and lipids infusing together.

Nursing Research

Selected Nursing Research Studies

Bowman, M., et al. (1989). Effect of tube feeding osmolality on serum sodium levels. *Critical Care Nursing, 9*(1), 22–28.

Eisenberg, P., et al. (1989). Nasoenteral feeding tube properties and the ability to withdraw fluid via a syringe. *Applied Nursing Research, 2,* 168–172.

Johnson, M. L., et al. (1990). Dietary practices, nutrition knowledge and attitudes of coronary heart disease patients. *Health Values, 14*(1), 3–8.

Perez, S., & Brant, K. (1989). Enteral feeding contamination: Comparison of diluents and feeding bag usage. *Journal of Parenteral and Enteral Nutrition, 13,* 306–308.

Petrosino, B. M., et al. (1989). Implications of selected problems with nasoenteral tube feedings. *Critical Care Nursing Quarterly, 12*(3), 1–18.

Prendergast, J. M., et al. (1989). Clinical validation of a nutritional risk index. *Journal of Community Health, 14,* 125–135.

Schols, A., et al. (1989). Inventory of nutritional status in patients with COPD. *Chest, 96,* 247–249.

Possible Topics for Nursing Inquiry

- What is the effect of prompted cueing on nutritional intake in nursing home patients?
- What is the relationship of preoperative albumin levels on postoperative wound healing and incidence of wound infection?
- How does nurse followup teaching affect compliance with a low-sodium diet?
- What is the impact of continuous versus intermittent tube feedings on the sensation of hunger and desire to eat?
- How does the length of hospital stay compare for nutritionally adequate patients versus patients with nutritional deficits undergoing coronary bypass surgery?
- What are the nutritional risk factors for low-birth-weight infants during the first year of life?

---

after discharge. For example, the surgical patient should be told to eat enough protein to promote wound healing. Assess whether the patient can buy, prepare, and eat food; often patients may need assistance with shopping or cooking. Family and friends are often available to help for a short period of time. If adequate supports are unavailable, community agencies such as Meals on Wheels may be necessary.

Patients with chronic health problems often pose greater nutritional challenges. Many local and national agencies, such as the American Cancer Society, American Heart Association, and American Diabetes Association, publish pamphlets that provide dietary guidance and realistic suggestions. For patients who are malnourished or at high risk for nutritional deficits, a referral to community health agencies may be necessary.

When new restrictive diets are ordered for patients, teaching should be started as soon as possible so that appropriate reinforcement can be given before discharge. A dietitian may begin the teaching. When possible, patients should receive written materials that outline which foods to include and exclude from the diet. The nurse can help patients to determine how best to incorporate the dietary changes into their lives.

Nutritional support technologies, such as tube feedings or TPN, are now often managed at home. In many agencies, it is the nurse who teaches the patient how to administer such therapies at home. Teaching should begin early in the hospitalization, by explaining TPN or tube feedings as they are performed. Before discharge, the patient should be able to demonstrate necessary administration techniques and to solve problems that may occur. When possible, family members or caregivers should be included in teaching sessions. Arrangements for equipment and supplies should be made before discharge, and the name of the vendor should be provided to the patient.

EVALUATION

Goal
Patient will use a nutritionally sound dietary intake to meet body requirements and promote health.

Possible Outcome Criteria
- Within 24 hours, patient describes a diet providing the recommended dietary allowances for self as indicated by age, sex, and physiologic state.

Nursing Management Plan
The Patient with Altered Nutrition

Nursing Diagnosis: Altered nutrition: less than body requirements, as manifested by being underweight, having a low hematocrit, and having an inadequate intake of calcium, iron, protein, vitamin A, and vitamin C.

Patient Goal: Patient will construct a diet that meets the RDA standards, is psychologically satisfying, can be readily understood, and is relatively easy to prepare or obtain.

Patient Outcome Criteria
- Patient obtains correct, useful information in which she expresses confidence.
- Patient describes the basic function of nutrients.
- Patient uses a diet that contains adequate amounts of all nutrients to meet the RDA standards.
- Patient reports satisfaction with the diet and an increased energy level.
- Patient increases weight within the normal range for height, age, and sex.

Nursing Intervention	Scientific Rationale
1. Assess patient lab values (hematocrit, hemoglobin, serum albumin) and physical parameters (height, weight, skin-fold measurements).	1. To detect deviations from baseline and deviations from normal standards so that measures can be taken to correct deficiencies.
2. Assess the patient's ability to obtain food.	2. To detect possible problems to minimize or prevent financial or physical limitations from contributing to an inadequate diet.
3. Assess the patient's motivational level and ability to learn and follow the new diet prescription.	3. To detect potential problems to prevent motivational or learning difficulties from interfering with obtaining a nutritionally adequate diet.
4. Instruct the patient in the new diet prescription and assess understanding (increased intake of protein, calcium, iron, vitamins A and C, and calories).	4. To provide an improved intake of nutrients, especially those that had been determined to be low.
5. Provide the patient with written information on the basic functions of the major nutrients; discuss this information with the patient and assess understanding.	5. To provide the patient with basic information for personal use; written format assists the patient in retaining the information.
6. Answer patient's questions; discuss areas of concern futher; provide the patient with additional reference material as necessary.	6. To assist the patient toward increased knowledge; to relieve uncertainties; to improve knowledge of self-care activities.
7. Assess the patient's family history of diabetes and the patient's predisposing characteristics toward the possible development of diabetes.	7. To establish a baseline of information so that potential problems can be prevented or detected early and treated promptly.

- Within 3 days, patient verbalizes use of proper daily food selection from the basic four food groups.
- Patient uses healthful diet by limiting the intake of saturated fats, refined sugar, calories, and sodium, as witnessed by the nurse at 5 meals during next 5 days.
- By discharge, patient's skin and nails demonstrate absence of clinical signs of nutrition deficiency or excess.
- During hospitalization patient's blood glucose, albumin, etc. remain within normal limits as shown in laboratory tests.

Goal
Patient will maintain dietary intake adequate to meet energy expenditures of body.

Possible Outcome Criteria
- Within 24 hours, patient describes dietary changes necessary to meet adequate caloric intake during current period of increased demand (e.g., pregnancy, lactation, adolescence, trauma, or surgery).
- Patient works toward maintaining ideal body weight by exercising daily during next week.

- For 1 month, patient uses nutritional supplements (e.g., protein supplement, vitamins) during periods of increased demand.

Goal

Patient will demonstrate adequate knowledge to adhere to dietary prescription or therapies to promote health.

Possible Outcome Criteria

- After teaching session patient lists foods to avoid on special diet (e.g., low-sodium, low-fat).
- Before discharge patient describes how to alter lifestyle (eating in restaurants, preparing food) to comply with dietary restrictions.
- Before discharge, patient discusses realistic use of family and community support groups to ensure adequate nutrition after discharge.
- Before discharge, patient or caregiver demonstrates how to administer hyperalimentation or tube feedings.

Key Concepts

- Adequate nutritional intake is important to maintain body functions, promote healing, maintain healthy tissues, maintain body temperature, and build resistance to infection.
- Essential nutrients are carbohydrates, protein, fat, vitamins, minerals, and water.
- Complex physiologic processes, including digestion, absorption, and metabolism, permit the body to break down food so that it can be used by the body as energy.
- Great variations exist in dietary intake among different people, but guidelines such as food groups, recommended daily allowances, and caloric requirements can be useful in evaluating adequate intake.
- Many factors affect normal eating patterns.
- The potential for impaired nutrition exists when the patient's intake is inadequate or excessive, when the patient cannot use ingested nutrients, or when there is increased metabolic demand or an altered psychological state.
- Manifestations of altered nutrition include body weight that is above or below ideal, a recent significant weight gain or loss, decreased energy, altered bowel patterns, and altered skin, teeth, hair, or mucous membranes.
- Nutritional needs vary across the lifespan.
- The health assessment includes collecting subjective data on normal eating patterns, risk factors for nutritional deficits, and identification of altered nutrition.
- Anthropometric measurements (height and weight, skinfold measurements, and arm circumference), calorie counts, and swallowing evaluation can provide objective data to help assess a patient's nutritional state.
- NANDA nursing diagnoses in the functional area of nutrition are Altered Nutrition: Less than Body Requirements, Altered Nutrition: Greater than Body Requirements, and Impaired Swallowing.
- Nursing interventions to promote optimal nutrition include patient teaching, measures to encourage eating, and community-based nutrition programs.
- Therapeutic diets are used to promote health, manage disease, or encourage healing.
- Nutritional support can be given through dietary supplements, enteral tube feedings, or total parenteral nutrition.
- Patient teaching and discharge planning are important to promote optimal nutrition at home.

References

Blumberg, J. B. (1986). Nutritional requirements for the healthy elderly. *Contemporary Nutrition, 11*(6),.

Curtas, S., Chapman, G., & Megurd, M. (1989). Evaluation of nutritional status. *Nursing Clinics of North America, 24,* 301–311.

DiIorio, C., & Price, M. E. (1990). Swallowing: An assessment and practice guide. *American Journal of Nursing, 90*(7), 38–46.

Eisenberg, P. (1989). Enteral nutrition: Indications, formulas, and delivery techniques. *Nursing Clinics of North America, 24,* 315–337.

Eschleman, M. M. (1991). *Introductory nutrition and diet therapy* (2nd ed.). Philadelphia: J. B. Lippincott.

Lewis, C. M. (1986). *Nutrition and nutritional therapy in nursing.* Norwalk, CT: Appleton-Century-Crofts.

Luke, B. (1984). *Principles of nutrition and diet therapy.* Boston: Little, Brown & Co.

NANDA (1990). *Taxonomy I revised 1990, with official nursing diagnoses.* St. Louis, MO: North American Diagnosis Association.

Patrick, M., Woods, S., Craven, R. et al. (1991). *Medical-surgical nursing: A pathophysiological approach* (2nd ed.). Philadelphia: J. B. Lippincott.

Robinson, C., & Weigley, E. (1984). *Basic nutrition and diet therapy.* New York: Macmillan.

Robinson, C. et al. (1986). Normal and therapeutic nutrition. New York: Macmillan.

Shirreff, A. (1990). Preoperative nutritional assessment. *Nursing Times, 86*(8), 69–72.

Starkey, et al. (1988). Percutaneous endoscopic gastrostomy (PEG). *American Journal of Nursing, 88,* 42–45.

Wardlaw, G., & Insel, P. (1990). *Perspectives in nutrition.* St. Louis: Times Mirror/Mosby.

Worthington, P., & Wagner, B. (1989). Total parenteral nutrition: Advances in Nutritional Support. *Nursing Clinics of North America, 24,* 355–369.

Bibliography

Anderson, B. (1986). Tube feeding: Is diarrhea inevitable? *American Journal of Nursing, 86,* 704–706.

Berger, R., et al. (1989). Nutritional support in the critical care setting, part 2. *Chest, 96,* 372–380.

Bowman, M., et al. (1989). Effect of tube feeding osmolality on serum sodium levels. *Critical Care Nursing, 9*(1), 22–28.

Cataldo, C., Nyenhuis, J., & Whitney, E. (1989). *Nutrition & diet therapy: Principles and practice* (2nd ed.). St. Paul: West.

Chernoff, R. (1990). Physiologic aging and nutritional status. *Nutrition in Clinical Practice, 5*(1), 8–13.

Collinsworth, R., et al. (1989). Nutritional assessment of the elderly. *Journal of Gerontologic Nursing, 15*(12), 17–39.

D'Agostino, N. (1989). Managing nutrition problems in advanced cancer. *American Journal of Nursing, 89,* 50–56.

Eisenberg, P., et al. (1989). Nasoenteral feeding: Tube properties and the ability to withdraw fluid via a syringe. *Applied Nursing Research, 2,* 168–172.

Finn, S. C. (1989). Applying new technology to nutritional assessment. *Caring, 8*(10), 18–22.

Gavan, C., et al. (1988). Explication of Neuman's model: A holistic systems approach to nutrition for health promotion in the life process. *Holistic Nurse Practitioner, 3*(1), 26–38.

Heitkemper, M., et al. (1989). Nursing research opportunities in enteral nutrition. *Nursing Clinics of North America, 24,* 415–426.

Johnson, M. L., et al. (1990). Dietary practices, nutrition knowledge, and attitudes of coronary heart disease patients. *Health Values, 14*(1), 3–8.

Marcuard, S. P., et al. (1989). Clearing obstructed feeding tubes. *Journal of Parenteral Nutrition, 13*(1), 81–83.

Murphy, J. (1990). Tube feeding problems and solutions. *Advanced Clinical Care, 5*(2), 7–11.

Perez, S., & Brant, K. (1989). Enteral feeding contamination: Comparison of diluents and feeding bag usage. *Journal of Parenteral and Enteral Nutrition, 13,* 306–308.

Petrosino, B. M., et al. (1989). Implications of selected problems with nasoenteral tube feedings. *Critical Care Nursing Quarterly, 12*(3), 1–18.

Prendergast, J. M., et al. (1989). Clinical validation of a nutritional risk index. *Journal of Community Health, 14*(3), 125–135.

Sandall, M. J., et al. (1989). The impact of diagnostic-related groups/prospective payment systems on nutritional needs in home health and extended-care facilities. *Journal of the American Dietetic Association, 89,* 1444–1447.

Schols, A., et al. (1989). Inventory of nutritional status in patients with COPD. *Chest, 96,* 247–249.

Seller, B. (1989). Strengthening nutrition care in hospitals. *Nutrition in Clinical Practice, 4*(4), 123–124.

Sultemeier, A. (1988). An innovative approach to teaching prenatal nutrition. *Journal of Community Health Nursing, 5*(4), 247–254.

Walden, R. (1989). The relationship of dietary supplemental calcium intake to bone loss and osteoporosis. *Journal of the American Dietetic Association, 89,* 397–400.

Whitney, E., Cataldo, C., & Rolfes, S. (1987). *Understanding normal and clinical nutrition* (2nd ed.). St. Paul: West.

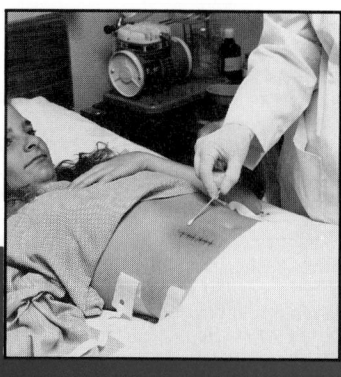

Skin Integrity and Wound Healing

LEARNING OBJECTIVES

Upon completion of this chapter, the student will be able to do the following:

- Discuss factors that affect normal integumentary function.
- Identify manifestations of altered integumentary function.
- Describe normal wound healing and factors that affect it.

- Discuss nursing assessment of skin integrity and wound healing.
- Discuss nursing interventions to prevent pressure sores or altered skin integrity.
- Explain scientific principles in wound management and in the application of heat and cold to promote wound healing.

KEY TERMS

Abrasion	Evisceration	Pruritus
Approximate	Fistula	Puncture wound
Debridement	First intention	Sanguineous
Decubitus ulcer	Granulation tissue	Second intention
Dehiscence	Hematoma	Serosanguineous
Dermatitis	Integument	Serous
Dermis	Laceration	Subcutaneous layer
Epidermis	Macerated	Suppuration
Eschar	Pressure sore	Wound healing

34

Normal Integumentary Function
Anatomy
  Skin Layers
  Skin Appendages
Normal Physiologic Function
  Protection
  Thermoregulation
  Fluid and Electrolyte Balance
  Vitamin D Synthesis
  Regeneration
Characteristics of Normal Skin
  Color
  Temperature
  Moisture
  Texture and Thickness
  Odor
Normal Integumentary Functional Pattern
Factors Affecting Normal Integumentary Function
  Circulation
  Nutrition
  Lifestyle and Habits
  Knowledge
  Condition of the Epidermis
Lifespan Considerations
Altered Integumentary Function
Potential for Altered Integumentary Function
  Allergic Reactions
  Infections
  Abnormal Growth Rate Disorders
  Wounds
  Stasis Dermatitis
  Pressure Sores
  Burns
Manifestations of Altered Integumentary Function
  Pruritis
  Rash
  Lesions
Wound Healing in Altered Integumentary Function
  Phases of Wound Healing
  Types of Wound Healing
  Factors Affecting Wound Healing

Complications of Wound Healing
Impact of Integumentary Dysfunction on Activities
  of Daily Living
Assessment
Subjective Data
  Functional Pattern Identification
  Risk Identification
  Dysfunctional Identification
Objective Data
  Physical Examination
  Diagnostic Tests and Procedures
Nursing Diagnoses and Patient Goals
Diagnostic Statement: Impaired Skin Integrity
  Definition
  Defining Characteristics
  Related Factors
Diagnostic Statement: Impaired Tissue Integrity
  Definition
  Defining Characteristics
  Related Factors
Related Nursing Diagnoses
Patient Goals
Implementation
Nursing Interventions to Promote Health and
    Integumentary Function
  Patient Teaching
  Pressure-Sore Prevention
Nursing Interventions for Altered Integumentary
    Function
  Pruritus Relief
  First Aid for Minor Wounds
  First Aid for Minor Burns
  Dressings
  Wound Support
  Drainage Management
  Wound Debridement, Irrigation, and Packing
  Local Application of Heat and Cold
  Emotional Support
Discharge Planning and Home Care
Evaluation
Key Concepts

Skin, also called **integument,** is the external covering of the body and is the body's largest organ. It helps protect the body and has sensory and regulatory functions. Disruptions in normal skin integrity can interfere with important skin functions.

A **wound** is a break in skin integrity. Accidental wounds can occur when the skin is exposed to extremes in temperature, caustic chemicals, excessive pressure, trauma, or radiation. Wounds may also occur if surgical intervention is necessary to treat various health problems. Regardless of the cause of the wound, the body responds to any injury with a complex restorative process called **wound healing.**

The nurse has a significant role in preventing impaired skin integrity and promoting optimal healing when disruptions in the skin or underlying structures occur. The nurse teaches patients how to avoid accidental injury, provides first-aid measures for traumatic skin injuries, manages wound care for lesions or surgical incisions, and prevents pressure sores in high-risk patients.

NORMAL INTEGUMENTARY FUNCTION

Anatomy

The skin, a vital organ, is part of the integumentary system. Various skin appendages are also included in this system.

Skin Layers

The skin has three layers: epidermis, dermis, and subcutaneous layer (Fig. 34-1).

The **epidermis** is the outer layer of skin. It is avascular and relies on the dermis for its nutrition. The epidermis specializes to form the hair, nails, and glandular structures. The epidermis is composed of five layers of stratified squamous epithelium. The thin, outermost layer of the epidermis (the stratum corneum) is continuously shed in a process called desquamation. The major cell of the epidermis, the keratinocyte, produces keratin, the primary material in the shed layer of cells. Basal layers of the epidermis contain melanocytes, which produce *melanin,* the brown substance that colors the skin.

The **dermis** underlies the epidermis and makes up the bulk of the skin. It is composed of tough connective tissue and is well vascularized. Lymphatic vessels and nerve tissues are also found in the dermis. This dermal matrix supports and nourishes the constantly changing epidermis.

The **subcutaneous layer** underlies the dermis. It consists primarily of fat and connective tissues that support other layers of the skin.

Skin Appendages

The skin appendages (hair, nails, eccrine sweat glands, apocrine sweat glands, and sebaceous glands) are formed by invagination of the epidermis into the under-

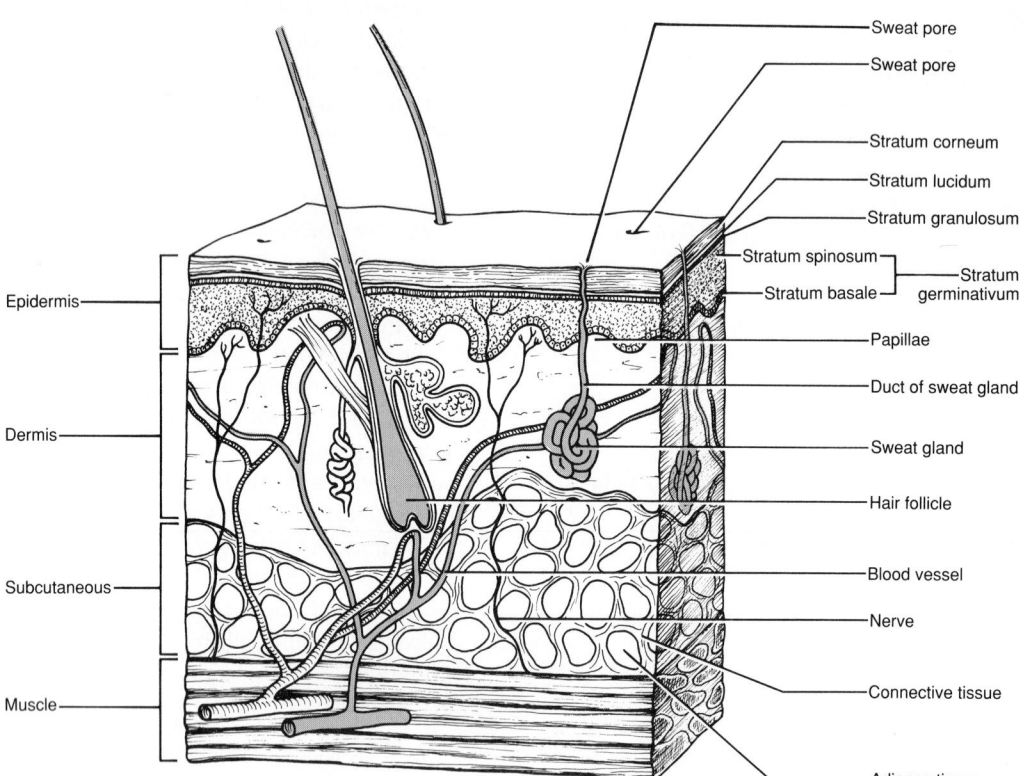

Figure 34–1. Cross-section of skin showing the three layers: epidermis, dermis, and subcutaneous layer.

lying dermis. Hair is dead keratin that is formed at about 3 mm per day. Nails are dead keratin plates produced by epidermal cells. Hair and nails have no nerve endings or blood supply. The eccrine and apocrine glands are sweat glands: eccrine glands, which are widely distributed throughout the skin, help transport sweat to the outer skin surface, and apocrine sweat glands are found primarily in the axilla and the genital area. The apocrine duct empties into the hair follicle. Sweat produced by apocrine glands contributes to a characteristic body odor when the secretions are decomposed by bacteria. **Sebaceous glands** secrete sebum, which lubricates the outer layer of skin.

Normal Physiologic Function

The skin has several functions: protective, regulatory, and regenerative.

Protection

Intact skin protects the body from physical and chemical injury. Infection is less likely when intact skin provides a barrier to microorganisms. Lymphocytes, leukocytes, and mast cells surround small blood vessels within the skin to protect the body from foreign invasion. Melanin protects the skin from the sun's ultraviolet rays.

Thermoregulation

The skin's regulatory functions include thermoregulation, fluid and electrolyte balance, and vitamin D synthesis. Heat loss through the skin is controlled by dilation or constriction of blood vessels; this regulates the loss or retention of heat as needed by the body and helps the body adjust to external changes of temperature.

Fluid and Electrolyte Balance

Continual fluid and electrolyte loss would occur if skin did not provide an external covering for the body. Fluid and electrolyte loss can be increased by profuse sweating (through eccrine glands in the skin) if the body temperature needs to be lowered. Sebum produced by the sebaceous glands helps to conserve heat by preventing evaporation of moisture from the skin.

Vitamin D Synthesis

From the sun's ultraviolet rays, the skin synthesizes vitamin D, which is necessary for efficient absorption of calcium and phosphorus.

The skin also has a sensory function. Within the skin are located nerve receptors for touch, pain, temperature, and pressure. Integrating such data from the environment is important in maintaining homeostasis.

Regeneration

Regeneration is a normal function of the skin. The outer part of the epidermis is constantly sloughing off cells and replacing them; the normal turnover rate is 14 to 20 days. Humans cannot regenerate limbs, but the functional cells of the kidney, liver, and pancreas have regenerative capacities, as do the epithelial cells of the skin and those lining the gastrointestinal tract.

Characteristics of Normal Skin

Characteristics of normal skin include color, temperature, moisture, texture, thickness, turgor, and odor.

Color

Normal skin tones vary among races depending on the production and accumulation of melanin in the skin. The greater the accumulation of melanin, the darker the skin tone. In races with darker skins, melanocytes produce more melanin when the skin is exposed to sunlight; skin tones can range from tan to dark brown or black. The skin color of lighter-pigmented races also varies, ranging from ivory to pink. Areas of hyperpigmentation, such as freckles, normally occur in light-skinned people. Some races have yellow or olive undertones to their skin color. In all people, sun-exposed areas, such as the face or arms, can be darker.

Temperature

Skin is normally warm, but peripheral areas, such as the feet or hands, may be cool if vasoconstriction in the skin has occurred.

Moisture

Normally the skin is dry to the touch, but moisture can accumulate in folds of the skin. Moisture can be felt on the skin if the person is in a warm climate or has recently exercised. Anxiety can increase the moisture normally detected in the axilla or palms of the hands.

Texture and Thickness

The texture of unexposed skin is smooth, but areas exposed to friction (such as the soles of the feet or the palms of the hands) may become rough. Sun exposure can also make skin less smooth.

Skin thickness varies depending on the body location. The skin on the soles of the feet may be a quarter-inch thick, but the skin covering the eyelids may be only one-fiftieth of an inch thick.

Normal skin has good elasticity and rapidly returns to its normal shape when pinched between the thumb and forefinger. As a person ages, skin turgor normally decreases. Skin turgor can also be affected by other factors such as loss of fluid.

Odor

Skin is usually free from odor, but a pungent aroma is normal with perspiration, especially in the axilla and groin.

Normal Integumentary Functional Pattern

In addition to its physiologic functions of protection, regulation, and regeneration, the skin also plays an important role in developing self-concept because it provides the basis for personal appearance. The skin, hair, and nails are often decorated and provide a basis for cultural sexual differences.

The skin is also a means of communication between people. Nurses have developed Therapeutic Touch, a process of healing by a particular kind of touch. Muscles under the skin allow facial expression, another form of communication. Smiling, winking, blinking, frowning, and sneering are forms of facial expression that communicate.

Factors Affecting Normal Integumentary Function

Normal skin viability depends on blood flow, nutrient supply, personal hygiene, knowledge, and the integrity of the epidermis. Age-related changes can also affect normal integumentary status.

Circulation

Adequate blood flow to the skin is necessary for healthy, viable tissues. Adequate skin perfusion requires four factors:

The heart must be able to pump adequately.
The volume of circulating blood must be sufficient.
Arteries and veins must be patent and functioning well.
Local capillary pressure must be higher than external pressure.

Nutrition

A well-balanced diet promotes healthy skin. With a deficiency of protein or calories, hair becomes dull and dry and may fall out, and skin becomes dry and flaky. Adequate intake of vitamins A, B_6, C, and K, niacin, and riboflavin is important to prevent abnormal skin changes. Adequate intake of iron, copper, and zinc is important to prevent abnormal pigmentation and changes in nails and hair.

Lifestyle and Habits

Lack of cleanliness can hinder skin health, because washing removes debris, bacteria, and sweat from the skin and keeps pores open and unclogged. Hygiene practices vary widely among different people and different cultures.

Knowledge

The patient's understanding of skin care and hygiene is an important factor in maintaining skin integrity. The need for cleaning the body is the first step. Skin care is especially important in the heat and direct sunlight of the summer and the cold, chapping winds of the winter. Ill patients should know the importance of frequent turning in bed. Parents should be taught how to care for their newborn's skin. Cognitive changes could affect safety when using items such as heating pads, stoves, hot pans, frozen items, and hot and cold water.

Condition of the Epidermis

To maintain its protective function against invading microorganisms, the epidermis should be free from any breaks. The natural moisture of skin should be maintained, since abnormal drying can cause microscopic cracks in the skin.

Lifespan Considerations

Skin changes during the lifespan, with the greatest variations occurring in the very young and the elderly.

Newborn and Infant

The neonate's skin is thinner and more sensitive than that of the older infant. Superficial blood vessels are so prominent that they give the newborn's skin a characteristic red color. Only the sebaceous glands are active during early infancy. **Milia** are sebaceous retention cysts that can be seen as white, opalescent spots around the chin and nose. They appear during the first few weeks of life and disappear spontaneously. Fine hair called **lanugo** covers the newborn's body. It is lost during the first weeks of life and replaced by hair of a different color and texture. Infants characteristically have long, thin fingernails and toenails that often scratch their delicate skin.

The infant's skin is susceptible to blistering, chafing, and rashes related to friction or irritation. Exposure to a warm, humid environment can lead to prickly heat, and frequent bathing can cause dryness, leading to other skin problems. Contact dermatitis and bacterial infections can occur from exposure to soiled diapers.

Other common skin disorders of infancy are diaper rash and eczema. Diaper rash can be avoided by keeping the infant clean and dry and by avoiding rubber pants, disposable diapers, or detergents to which the baby is sensitive. Eczema may be an allergic response to foods, soaps, or other stimuli, so new foods should be introduced one at a time into the infant's diet.

During the first year of life, the proportion of subcutaneous fat increases. Raw areas called *intertrigo* may develop in obese youngsters as skin rubs against skin. The proportion of subcutaneous fat decreases in the second year of life, and intertrigo is less common.

Toddler and Preschooler

After the first year of life, the normal child shows little changes in the skin until puberty. As motor skills develop, children are more prone to accidents, which can cause lacerations or abrasions. Falls increase as the child learns new skills (walking, running, jumping) but does not yet have adequate motor coordination. Despite the risk of injury, it is important to give children the freedom to develop their skills.

Toddlers and preschoolers are also susceptible to burns. Hot liquids should be kept out of their reach, and they should be kept away from heaters, barbecue grills, stoves, and fires. Electric outlets should be capped with protective covers to prevent accidental electrical burns.

Today, more children attend day-care centers or nursery schools, increasing the risk of contracting communicable diseases. The poor hygiene practices of most young children compound the problems of disease transmission in this age group.

Child and Adolescent

The skin remains stable until adolescence. Skin integrity is most affected by communicable illnesses in this age group. Impetigo and head lice can also occur; such problems cause embarrassment for the child and family and require absence from school. Older children are more aware of their bodies and are concerned when rashes or scars affect their appearance. The nurse can identify rashes in children and institute measures to avoid the spread of infectious diseases that impair skin integrity. The nurse can also provide emotional support for both parents and children, so the child is better able to cope with the stress and discomfort of skin disruptions.

During adolescence, pubic, axillary, and other body hair appears. The most common disorder of adolescence is acne vulgaris. As the sebaceous glands enlarge at puberty, the production of sebum increases. Acne lesions result from the plugging of pilosebaceous glands. Lesions form primarily on the face and neck and to a lesser extent on the back, chest, and shoulders. Because adolescence is a time when physical appearance is important to self-concept, severe acne can be emotionally disturbing to the adolescent.

Adolescents engage in many leisure activities that involve sun exposure (e.g., swimming, outdoor sports, sunbathing). Because excessive sun exposure has been linked to skin cancer, they should be taught to protect their skin by using effective sunscreen products.

Adult and Older Adult

Skin changes occur as part of the normal aging process. As skin ages, it generally becomes thinner because dermal and subcutaneous mass is lost. Because sebaceous and sweat glands are less active, dry skin is more common as a person ages. Wrinkling and poor skin turgor result from the loss of elastic fibers and collagen changes in the dermal connective tissue. Because circulation to the skin is reduced, healing is slower. Skin breakdown occurs more easily and tissue repair takes longer. There is less hair and nail growth. The nails may become thickened and brittle, and hair may lose its pigment and turn gray. **Pruritus** (itching) commonly occurs in the elderly, due mainly to dry, scaling skin.

There is also a marked increase in the size and number of benign skin growths in the elderly, which can affect the person's appearance and self-concept. *Skin tags* are loose flaps of skin that occur mainly around the neck, eyelids, and axillary areas. *Keratoses* are horny growths that are slow-growing proliferations of the keratinizing cells of the epidermis. *Senile lentigines,* also called age or liver spots, are pigmentation changes that occur on sun-exposed areas. Although many skin changes are benign, older people should have regular skin examinations because the incidence of malignant skin problems increases with age.

ALTERED INTEGUMENTARY FUNCTION

Potential for Altered Integumentary Function

Allergies, infections, growth disorders, accidental and surgical wounds, burns, and pressure sores can significantly impair skin integrity. Any impairment in skin integrity is likely to alter normal function.

Allergic Reactions

Allergic reactions and skin inflammation are responses to injury mediated by histamine release. The reactions may be caused by external or internal irritants. The irritants may be chemical in nature (shampoo, skin creams, detergents, cosmetics, clothing, plants such as poison ivy or poison oak), or the reaction may be caused by mechanical means (for example, rubbing against an irritant such as wool). Berries, shellfish, chocolate, sulfur, and penicillin may cause skin reactions. **Dermatitis** is an inflammation of the skin. Chronic dermatitis can be characterized by changes to the epidermis characterized by thickening, scaling, and increased pigmentation.

Infections

Skin infections can be bacterial, viral, or fungal. Streptococcal and staphylococcal organisms are responsible for most bacterial infections. Impetigo, which usually is caused by beta-hemolytic streptococci, is the most common bacterial skin infection.

Herpesvirus infection is the most common viral cause of skin disruption. Common locations are the lips, face, mouth, and genitals. Many communicable childhood illnesses of viral origin cause rashes. Pruritus often accompanies these rashes and may lead to secondary infection.

Fungal infections can infect nonhairy skin (tinea corporis), the scalp (tinea capitis), the genitofemoral region (tinea cruris or "jock itch"), nails (tinea unguis), and most commonly the feet (tinea pedis or "athlete's foot"). Candidal (formerly called monilial) fungal infections often occur when normal body flora is disrupted secondary to antibiotic therapy or immunosuppression.

Abnormal Growth Rate Disorders

When the skin is produced at an abnormal rate by malignant or nonmalignant processes, normal integrity can be disrupted.

Psoriasis is a nonmalignant, chronic disorder that greatly increases the rate of skin production: the normal epidermal turnover rate of 14 to 20 days is accelerated to 3 to 4 days. The elbows, knees, scalp, and soles of the feet are common sites for psoriasis. Periods of remission are followed by exacerbations, which can be triggered by stress, infection, or environmental factors.

Benign or malignant *neoplasms* can also affect skin integrity. Most benign neoplasms result from viral infections or normal aging, but most malignant lesions result from prolonged exposure to solar radiation.

Wounds

Although regeneration is a normal function of skin, any trauma to the skin—such as a wound—creates a risk for altered skin function. Wounds can be divided into broad categories of accidental and surgical (Table 34-1).

Accidental Wounds. Common accidental wounds are abrasions, lacerations, and puncture wounds: An **abrasion** is caused when skin rubs against a hard surface. Friction scrapes away the epithelial layer of skin, exposing the epidermal or dermal layer. Falls onto hands, elbows, or knees cause most abrasions. A **laceration** is an open wound or cut. Most lacerations affect only the upper layers of skin and subcutaneous tissue underneath, but permanent damage may occur if there is injury to internal structures such as muscles, tendons, blood vessels, or nerves. Accidents involving automobiles, machinery, or knives may result in lacerations. A **puncture wound** is made when tissue is penetrated by

TABLE 34-1
Types of Wounds

Wound	Description
Broad Categories	
Accidental	Unintentional injury such as knife, gunshot, burn; jagged edges; bleeding; unsterile
Surgical	Planned therapy such as surgical incision, needle introduction; clean edges; controlled bleeding; controlled surgical asepsis
Skin Integrity	
Open	Break in skin or mucous membranes; may bleed with tissue damage; infection risk
Closed	No break in skin integrity, but soft-tissue damage present; may have internal injury and bleeding
Descriptors	
Abrasion	Wound involving friction of skin; superficial; dermatologic procedure for scar-tissue removal
Puncture	Intentional or unintentional penetrating trauma; made by sharp instrument that penetrates skin and underlying tissue
Laceration	Ragged wound edges with torn tissues; object may be contaminated; infection risk
Contusion	Closed wound; bleeding in underlying tissues caused by blunt blow; bruise
Cleanliness/Contamination	
Clean	Closed surgical wound that did not enter gastrointestinal, respiratory, or genitourinary systems; low infection risk
Clean/contaminated	Wound entering gastrointestinal, respiratory, or genitourinary systems; infection risk
Contaminated	Open, traumatic wound; surgical wound with break in asepsis; high infection risk
Infected	Wound site with pathogens present; signs of infection

a sharp, pointed instrument. Damage to underlying structures or gross contamination with debris and pathogens may result. Nails, pins, tacks, and other sharp objects are common causes.

Surgical Wounds. Surgical wounds vary from simple and superficial (such as a thyroidectomy incision) to deep and contaminated (such as an abdominal incision done for septic peritonitis). They may be divided into several categories (see Table 34-1).

- Superficial or deep (penetrating a cavity, joint space, or muscle group)
- Clean or contaminated (through contaminated skin or viscera)
- Open (incision is left open to encourage drainage and minimize sepsis) or closed.

The severity of the wound determines the time for healing, the degree of pain, the probability of wound complications, and the presence of any tubes, drains, or suction devices.

Ostomies are surgical openings in the abdominal wall that allow part of the intestine to open onto the skin. Many medical conditions, such as cancer of the intestine or urinary bladder or an inflammatory bowel disease, may require an ostomy. Because the skin surrounding the opening (stoma) may be continuously exposed to feces, urine, or intestinal secretions, skin irritation may occur. Erythematous rashes, excoriations, and areas of painful raw skin may develop as a result of drainage and poor skin care at the ostomy site.

Stasis Dermatitis

Stasis dermatitis is caused by impairment of venous return secondary to varicose veins. Pooling of blood leads to edema, vasodilation, and plasma extravasation, all of which result in dermatitis. If untreated, stasis dermatitis may progress to a frank ulcer.

Pressure Sores

Pressure sores, sometimes called **decubitus ulcers** or bedsores, result when capillary blood flow to the skin is impeded. These ulcers occur primarily as the result of unequal distribution of pressure over certain parts of the body. Because of decreased blood flow, the supply of nutrients and oxygen to the skin and underlying tissues is impaired. This causes cells to die and decompose and an ulcer to form. If pressure is not relieved and treatment instituted, damage may spread and involve the fascia, muscle, and bone. Infection and sepsis commonly occur.

Sometimes underlying tissue can be compressed and necrosis may occur deep below the skin surface.

Ulcer Staging. Pressure sores are classified according to their stage of development (Fig. 34-2):

A Stage I ulcer involves inflammation and reddening of the skin. Any breakdown present during this stage involves only the epidermis. Usually Stage I ulcers are reversible if pressure is relieved.

A Stage II ulcer appears as a shallow crater or skin blister. It involves the dermis and can penetrate to the subcutaneous fat layer. This ulcer is swollen and painful and requires a number of weeks to heal once pressure is relieved.

A Stage III ulcer involves destruction of the subcutaneous tissue layer and capillary beds. The ulcer is not painful but may have foul-smelling yellow or green drainage. Stage III ulcers can require months to heal.

A Stage IV ulcer involves extensive damage to underlying structures and may extend to the bone. On the skin surface the sore may appear small, but beneath the skin deep tunnels extend away from the opening. They often are necrotic and have foul-smelling drainage. At its edges the ulcer may develop a leathery black crust (**eschar**), which may eventually cover the ulcer. Infectious complications, such as osteomyelitis, are common. Months or years can elapse before a Stage IV ulcer heals.

Risk Factors. Factors causing ulcer formation include increased pressure and decreased tissue tolerance. The conceptual model shown in Figure 34-3 was developed by Braden and Bergstrom (1987) to illustrate the complex etiology of pressure-sore development.

Pressure can be increased by decreased mobility, decreased activity, and decreased sensory/perceptual ability. Extrinsic factors that decrease tissue tolerance and increase the likelihood of pressure-sore development are moisture, friction, and shearing force. Other contributing factors are malnutrition, age, or low arteriolar pres-

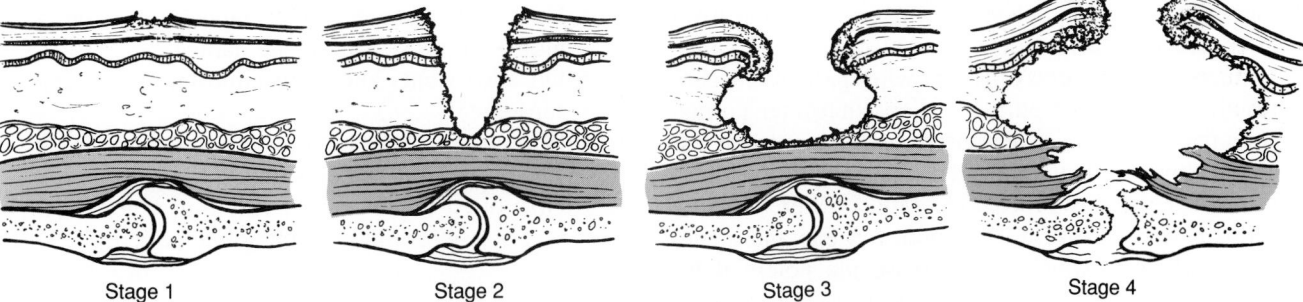

| Stage 1 | Stage 2 | Stage 3 | Stage 4 |

Figure 34–2. Staging of pressure sores. Stage I, redness and inflammation of the epidermis. Stage II, shallow crater or blister that usually involves the dermis. Stage III, full-thickness skin loss exposing subcutaneous tissue. Stage IV, extensive damage to underlying structures, including muscle and bone.

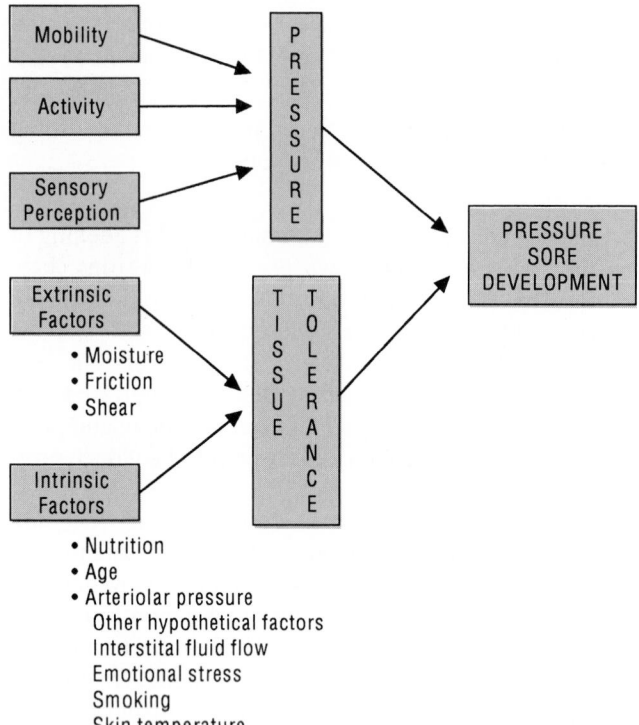

Figure 34–3. A conceptual schema by Braden and Bergstrom outlining the cause of pressure sores.

sure. Often it is the relationship between risk factors that ultimately causes a pressure sore to develop.

When unevenly distributed, *pressure* can exceed normal capillary pressure (32 mm Hg). The greater the pressure and the longer its duration, the more likely it is that a pressure sore will develop. Any rigid object (such as a bed or chair) puts pressure on the skin. When the patient is sitting or lying, gravity increases the pressure exerted over bony prominences; this pressure is increased when the patient is obese. Normally, a person unconsciously shifts his or her body weight to prevent the occlusion of capillaries due to increased pressure. Everyone has had the experience of numbness or a prickly sensation in an area of the body to which blood flow was impeded due to pressure. But people who cannot sense increased pressure or cannot independently reposition themselves (e.g., paraplegic or comatose patients) are at increased risk for the development of pressure sores.

Altered mental status can occur when patients are confused, comatose, or on medications that alter normal cognitive processes. When this occurs, patients are less aware of pressure buildup and may not reposition themselves as needed to prevent ulceration. Altered mental status may also contribute to poor hygiene and inadequate self-care, which can increase the potential for ulcer formation.

Moisture can predispose skin to breakdown. Skin that is continually bathed in moisture softens, increasing its susceptibility to trauma and infection. Skin continually exposed to moisture becomes **macerated.** Incontinence

Nursing Research

Selected Nursing Research Articles

Bergstrom, N., et al. (1987). A clinical trial of the Braden scale for predicting pressure-sore risk. *Nursing Clinics of North America, 22,* 417–428.

Copeland-Fields, L., & Hoshiko, B. (1989). Clinical validation of Braden and Bergstrom's conceptual schema of pressure sores risk factors. *Rehabilitation Nursing, 14*(5), 257–260.

Dai, T., & Catanzaro, M. (1987). Health beliefs and compliance with a skin-care regimen. *Rehabilitation Nursing, 12*(1), 13–16.

HoldenLund, C. (1988). Effects of guided imagery on surgical stress and wound healing. *Res Nurs Health, 11,* 235–244.

Jacobs, M. A. (1989). Comparison of capillary blood flow using a regular hospital bed mattress, ROHO mattress, and a medicus bed. *Rehabilitation Nursing, 14,* 270–272.

LaMantia, J., et al. (1987). A program design to reduce chronic readmission for pressure sores. *Rehabilitation Nursing, 12*(1), 22–25.

Whitney, J. D. (1989). Physiologic effects of tissue oxygenation on wound healing. *Heart Lung, 18,* 466–474.

Possible Topics for Nursing Research

- What is the effect on wound healing of listening to music during dressing changes?
- What is the effect of dry verus moist cold therapies for pruritus relief?
- What is the incidence of pressure-ulcer development in immobile patients with hemoglobin values less than 9 g/100 ml?
- What effect does hourly wheelchair tilting have on capillary blood flow and pressure-sore development?
- How effective are various tape-removal techniques on preventing tissue damage?
- Do adolescents know the importance of using sunscreen?
- What is the correlation between albumin levels and postoperative dehiscence?
- How often is the prone position used for pressure-sore prevention in immobile patients?

often causes the patient to lie in urine or feces. Diaphoresis or inadequate drying after hygiene, especially in skin folds, can also increase moisture.

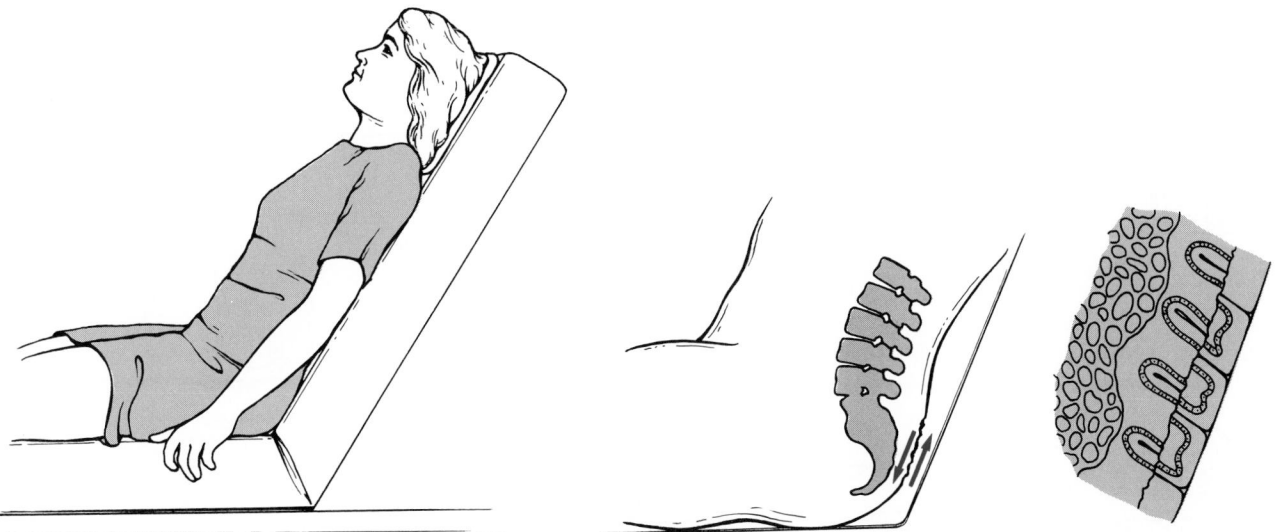

Figure 34–4.   Shearing force contributes to pressure-sore development when opposing forces cause capillaries to stretch and tear as the patient slides down in bed.

Friction occurs when two surfaces rub together. When skin rubs against a firm surface such as bedclothes or the hands of a caregiver, small abrasions can occur, increasing the possibility of ulcer formation. Adequate lubrication of the skin and care when handling, moving, and washing patients limits the negative effect of friction.

Shearing force occurs when tissue layers move on each other, causing the stretching of blood vessels passing through subcutaneous tissue (Fig. 34-4). Most commonly this occurs when the patient slides down in bed or is pulled up in bed. The patient's skin remains relatively immobile since friction anchors it to the sheets, but deeper structures such as fascia move with the patient, as they are attached to bone. In the process, capillaries in the underlying tissue are stretched and often torn, increasing the risk of ulcer formation.

Altered nutritional status increases the risk of pressure-sore development because inadequately nourished cells are more easily damaged. In nutritionally depleted patients, capillaries become more fragile, and as they break, blood flow to the skin can be impaired. Severely malnourished patients experience weight loss, decreased subcutaneous tissue, and decreased muscle mass. This limits the amount of padding between skin and underlying bone, aggravating the effects of pressure over bony prominences.

Common Locations. Pressure sores most commonly develop over bony prominences, where body weight is distributed over a small area with inadequate padding (Fig. 34-5). When supine, the greatest points of pressure are the back of the skull, the elbows, the sacrum and coccyx, and the heels. When sitting, the greatest points of pressure are the ischial tuberosities and the sacrum.

Burns

A burn involves damage to tissues as the result of exposure to excessive heat, electricity, caustic chemicals, or radiation. Burns range from minor injuries such as a simple sunburn to major insults that cause significant life disruptions. The degree of damage depends on the type of burn, its extent and depth, and the patient's preburn state of health.

Partial-thickness burns may be superficial or moderate to deep. A superficial partial-thickness burn (first degree; epidermal) is pinkish or red with no blistering; a mild sunburn is a good example. Moderate to deep partial-thickness burns (second degree; dermal or deep dermal) may be pink, red, pale ivory, or light yellow-brown. They are usually moist with blisters. Exposure to steam may cause this type of burn.

A full-thickness burn (third degree) may vary from brown or black to cherry red or pearly white. Thrombosed vessels and blisters or bullae may be present. The full-thickness burn appears dry and leathery. Sometimes when extensive damage is done to fascia, muscle, or bone, the injury is called a fourth-degree burn.

Thermal burns, the most common type, are caused by contact with a variety of heat sources, including flames, hot liquids, hot surfaces, and steam. Chemical burns are caused by contact with noxious substances. The amount of tissue damaged as a result of chemical injury depends on the concentration of the chemical and the length of exposure. The severity of an electrical burn depends on the type and voltage of the current, the pathway the current takes through the body, and the duration of contact. Radiation burns occur when a person is accidentally exposed to radiation or when radiation is used as a form of therapy. If intense enough, radiation can kill cells through ionization.

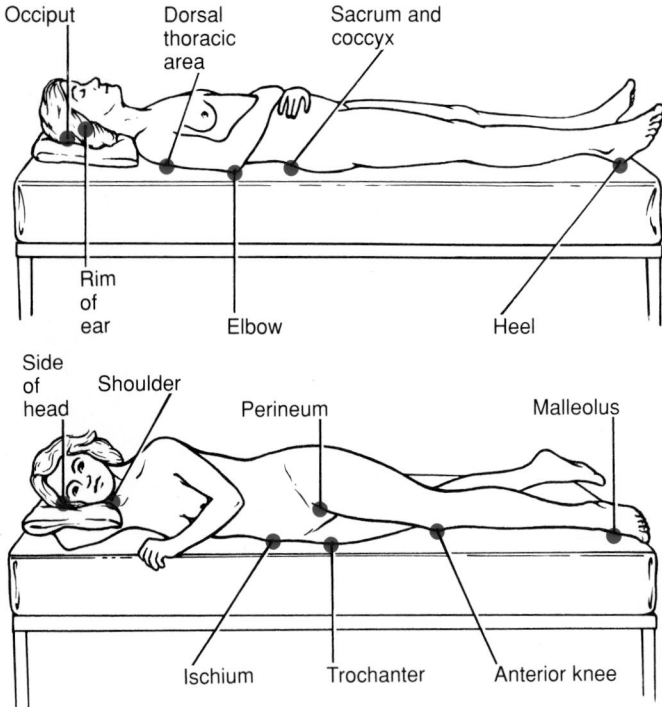

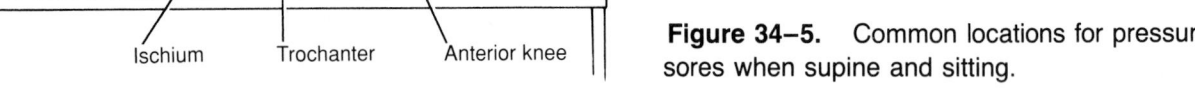

Figure 34–5. Common locations for pressure sores when supine and sitting.

Manifestations of Altered Integumentary Function

Disruption in normal skin integrity can manifest as breaks in the skin, rash, lesions, or pruritus; often more than one of these symptoms may occur.

Any break in the epidermal layer of the skin signifies that altered skin integrity is present. Often the disruption to the epidermis is evident, but it may be smaller and less obvious; microscopic breaks in the skin may manifest as redness due to inflammation.

Pruritus

Pruritus, or itching, is a common symptom associated with several skin and systemic problems. Conditions that cause itching may be dermatologic, environmental, systemic, or psychological. Pruritus is often the cause of secondary lesions, since scratching breaks skin surfaces. Common causes of pruritus include:

- Infestation by mites or lice
- Inflammatory reactions due to irritants or allergens
- Skin diseases of rapid cell proliferation, such as psoriasis
- Sunburn
- Overdrying of the skin
- Diabetes mellitus
- Liver or renal disease.

The itching sensation arises from a particular pattern of sensory impulses as the result of multiple-fiber stimulation. Various external stimuli decrease the threshold to itching. Chemical mediators such as histamine, serotonin, and kinins have also been implicated in itching.

Rash

Many conditions, such as excessive heat, communicable disease, allergy, or emotional distress, can cause a *rash,* a general term used for a temporary skin eruption. A rash is described according to its characteristics. A macular rash is level with the skin surface; a papular rash involves solid elevations above the skin surface. A generalized rash covers most areas of the body; a localized rash is limited to specific areas. Pruritus may accompany a rash.

Lesions

A *lesion* involves the loss of normal tissue, in terms of either structure or function. Lesions may vary in size from a fraction of a millimeter to many centimeters in diameter.

Various terms are used to describe different lesions. A *wheal,* which normally occurs from insect bites or allergic skin reactions, is an elevated, irregularly shaped area of cutaneous edema. *Urticaria,* more commonly called hives, is a linear wheal that forms in response to capillary dilatation and passive transudation of plasma. Vesicles, bullae, and pustules are superficial elevations of skin formed by fluid. A *vesicle* is less than 1 cm in diameter and is filled with serous fluid. A *bulla* is a vesicle greater than 1 cm in diameter. A *pustule* is filled with pus rather than serous fluid.

Eczema, which is a symptom rather than a disease, is an acute or chronic inflammatory condition in which erythema, papules, vesicles, scales, crusts, or scabs appear alone or together. It is a severe form of atopic dermatitis.

Lesions can also be classified by shape, arrangement, and distribution. Primary lesions arise in previously normal skin, and secondary lesions may develop from primary lesions. Examples of secondary lesions include scales, crusts, and fissures. In the acute form of dermatitis, vesicles develop, the vesicles burst and ooze, and crusts form. See Table 34-2 for a description of primary and secondary lesions.

Wound Healing in Altered Integumentary Function

when the skin is wounded, a type of healing by replacement occurs. The nature of this healing process is essentially the same for all wounds, but the timeframe for healing depends on the location of the wound, its depth and extent, the regenerative capacity of the injured cells, and the overall state of the patient's health.

Phases of Wound Healing

The three phases in first-intention wound healing are the defensive phase, the reconstructive phase, and the maturation phase. The entire healing process may take from a few weeks to years.

Defensive Phase. In the defensive phase, also known as the inflammatory or exudative phase, the body responds to the wound by setting up defenses against further invasion. Its combined forces of hemostasis, inflammation, and cell migration are important to control bleeding, seal the wound, protect the tissues from bacterial contamination, remove the debris resulting from cell injury, and provide a scaffolding for later deposition of collagen fibers (Bruno, 1979). This stage begins at the time of inury and lasts about 4 to 6 days.

Hemostasis, the process to stop bleeding, is the first step in the defensive phase. It occurs as the result of vasoconstriction of the injured vessels, platelet aggregation and clot formation, and deposition of fibrin, which forms a matrix for cellular repair.

To understand this process, it may help to visualize the chain of events that occurs after a simple paper cut. First, blood flows rapidly to the gash. For the next 5 to 10 minutes, there is localized vasoconstriction with clot formation that prevents further hemorrhage. This also serves to cement the wound edges, reducing further entry of organisms into the wound. The scab, consisting of clots and dead tissue, provides excellent protection. Beneath the scab, epithelial cells begin to migrate, and as they meet they close the wound edges.

The *inflammatory response* is the next event in the defensive phase. Unlike vasoconstriction, which is characterized by hemostasis, increased blood flow to the injured area characterizes the inflammatory stage. The venules dilate, capillaries open, and there is an increased vascular permeability to plasma. Symptoms at this stage may include pain, redness, swelling, and warmth, as

fluids containing plasma proteins, water, and electrolytes enter the wound around the clot.

The final event in the defensive stage is *cell migration*. White blood cells (neutrophils and monocytes) are the first cells to migrate into the wound, arriving about 6 hours after the injury. Their purpose is to phagocytize (engulf) bacteria, necrotic tissue, and other cellular debris to prepare the site for reconstruction.

Reconstructive Phase. The reconstructive or proliferative phase begins on the third or fourth day. In this phase, which lasts about 2 weeks, the fibroblasts multiply and form a latticework for migrating cells. The epithelial cells also proliferate and form buds containing tiny capillaries that nourish new granulation tissue. The synthesis of collagen is the major event in this stage. A gain in tensile strength is seen, but only 35% to 59% of wound strength is reached by the end of the month.

Maturation Phase. The maturation or remodeling phase, which completes the healing process, begins about 3 weeks after the injury and may last up to 2 years. The number of fibroblasts decreases, collagen synthesis stabilizes, and collagen fibrils become increasingly organized, resulting in greater tensile strength of the wound. The tissue generally reaches maximum strength in 10 to 12 weeks, but even after complete healing only 70% to 80% of the original strength can be expected.

Types of Wound Healing

Wounds heal differently depending on whether or not tissue loss has occurred. The types of wound healing are classified as first, second, and third intention (Fig. 34-6).

Healing by First Intention. Wounds with minimal tissue loss, such as clean surgical incisions or shallow sutured wounds, heal by **first intention**. The edges of the wound **approximate** (approach each other) rapidly, granulation tissue is not visible, and scarring is generally minimal. Infection risk is lower when a wound heals by first intention.

Healing by Second Intention. Wounds with tissue loss, such as deep lacerations, burns, and decubitus ulcers, have edges that do not readily approximate. They heal by **second intention**: the open wound gradually fills with soft pinkish-red buds that bleed easily (**granulation tissue**). Eventually, epithelial cells grow over these granulations, completing the cycle. Scarring is more prevalent, and because the wound remains open for a longer time, there is an increased risk of infection.

Healing by Third Intention. Healing by third intention occurs when a wound is closed at a later stage, after the wound surfaces have already started to granulate. This may happen when a deep wound is not sutured

TABLE 34–2.

Skin Lesions

Primary Skin Lesions

Primary skin lesions are original lesions arising from previously normal skin. Secondary lesions can originate from primary lesions.

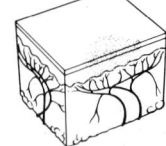
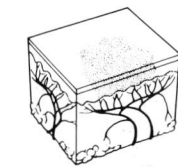

Macule, Patch

Macule

Patch

- *Macule:* <1 cm, circumscribed border
- *Patch:* >1 cm, may have irregular border
- Flat, nonpalpable skin color change (color may be brown, white, tan, purple, red)

Examples:

Freckles, flat moles, petechia, rubella, vitiligo, port wine stains, ecchymosis

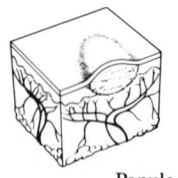

Papule, Plaque

Papule

Plaque

- *Papule:* <0.5 cm
- *Plaque:* >0.5 cm
- Elevated, palpable, solid mass
- Circumscribed border
- Plaque may be coalesced papules with flat top

Examples:

Papules: Elevated nevi, warts, lichen planus
Plaques: Psoriasis, actinic keratosis

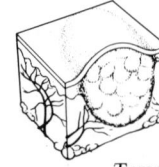

Nodule, Tumor

Tumor

- *Nodule:* 0.5–2 cm
- *Tumor:* >1–2 cm
- Elevated, palpable, solid mass
- Extends deeper into the dermis than a papule
- Nodules circumscribed
- Tumors do not always have sharp borders

Examples:

Nodules: Lipoma, squamous cell carcinoma, poorly absorbed injection, dermatofibroma
Tumors: Larger lipoma, carcinoma

Secondary Skin Lesions

Secondary skin lesions result from changes in primary lesions.

Erosion

- Loss of superficial epidermis
- Does not extend to dermis
- Depressed, moist area

Examples:

Ruptures vesicles, scratch marks

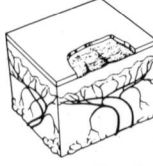

Erosion

Vesicle, Bulla

Bulla

Vesicle

- *Vesicle:* <0.5 cm
- *Bulla:* >0.5 cm
- Circumscribed, elevated, palpable mass containing serous fluid

Examples:

Vesicles: Herpes simplex/zoster, chickenpox, poison ivy, second-degree burn (blister)
Bulla: Pemphigus, contact dermatitis, large burn blisters, poison ivy, bullous impetigo

Wheal

Wheal

- Elevated mass with transient borders
- Often irregular
- Size, color varies
- Caused by movement of serous fluid into the dermis
- Does not contain free fluid in a cavity as, for example, a vesicle

Examples:

Urticaria (hives), insect bites

Pustule

- Pus-filled vesicle or bulla

Examples:

Pustule

Acne, impetigo, furuncles, carbuncles

Cyst

- Encapsulated fluid-filled or semisolid mass
- In the subcutaneous tissue or dermis

Examples:

Sebaceous cyst, epidermoid cyst

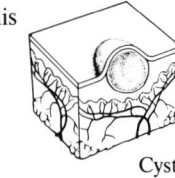

Cyst

Scar (Cicatrix)

- Skin mark left after healing of a wound or lesion
- Represents replacement by connective tissue of the injured tissue
- Young scars: red or purple
- Mature scars: white or glistening

Example:

Healed wound or surgical incision

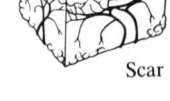

Scar

(*continued*)

TABLE 34–2
(continued)

Ulcer

- Skin loss extending past epidermis
- Necrotic tissue loss
- Bleeding and scarring possible

Examples:

Stasis ulcer of venous insufficiency, decubitus ulcer

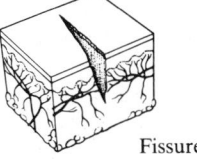
Ulcer

Fissure

- Linear crack in the skin
- May extend to dermis

Examples:

Chapped lips or hands, athlete's foot

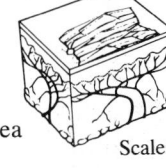
Fissure

Scales

- Flakes secondary to desquamated, dead epithelium
- Flakes may adhere to skin surface
- Color varies (silvery, white)
- Texture varies (thick, fine)

Examples:

Dandruff, psoriasis, dry skin, pityriasis rosea

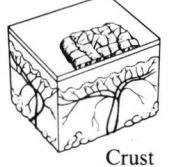
Scales

Crust

- Dried residue of serum, blood or pus on skin surface
- Large adherent crust is a scab

Examples:

Residue left after vesicle rupture: impetigo, herpes, eczema

Crust

Keloid

- Hypertrophied scar tissue
- Secondary to excessive collagen formation during healing
- Elevated, irregular, red
- Greater incidence in blacks

Example:

Keloid of ear piercing or surgical incision

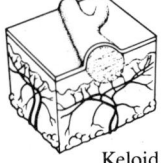
Keloid

Atrophy

- Thin, dry, transparent appearance of epidermis
- Loss of surface markings
- Secondary to loss of collagen and elastin
- Underlying vessels may be visible

Examples:

Aged skin, arterial insufficiency

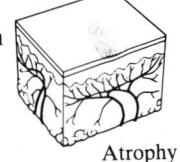
Atrophy

Lichenification

- Thickening and roughening of the skin
- Accentuated skin markings
- May be secondary to repeated rubbing, irritation, scratching

Example:

Contact dermatitis

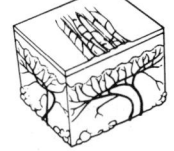
Lichenification

immediately. It can also occur when a wound is purposely left open until there is no sign of infection; this is known as delayed primary closure. When a wound heals by third intention, a deeper and wider scar is common.

Factors Affecting Wound Healing

Many variables exist that either promote or inhibit wound healing. Systematic factors such as nutrition, circulation, oxygenation, and immune cellular function can affect wound healing. Individual factors including age, obesity, smoking history, and drug therapy can also affect the rate of wound healing. Finally, local factors such as the nature of the injury, the presence of infection, and the local wound environment play a part in either enhancing or retarding the wound healing process.

Systemic Factors

Nutrition. Sound nutrition is essential for optimal wound healing. Nutritional deficiencies retard wound healing by prolonging the exudative phase and by inhibiting collagen synthesis. Nutritional requirements increase with stresses such as surgery, large open wounds, burns, and infections. Septic patients, burn patients, and surgical patients (especially those with major abdominal surgery) are susceptible to protein deficiency. Patients with protein deficiencies are most likely to develop wound infections because they have decreased leukocytic functions (such as phagocytosis and immunogenesis).

Protein and vitamins A and C are especially important in healing wounds. Carbohydrates and fats also play key roles in wound healing. Glucose is needed for the increased energy requirements of cells (especially leukocytes and fibroblasts), and fats are essential because they are the building blocks for the cell membranes being formed.

Many vitamins and minerals are important in wound healing:

Vitamin A promotes epithelialization and enhances collagen synthesis and cross-linking.

The vitamin B complex serves as a cofactor of enzyme systems.

Vitamin C (ascorbic acid) has been shown to be essential for collagen production; with decreased amounts of

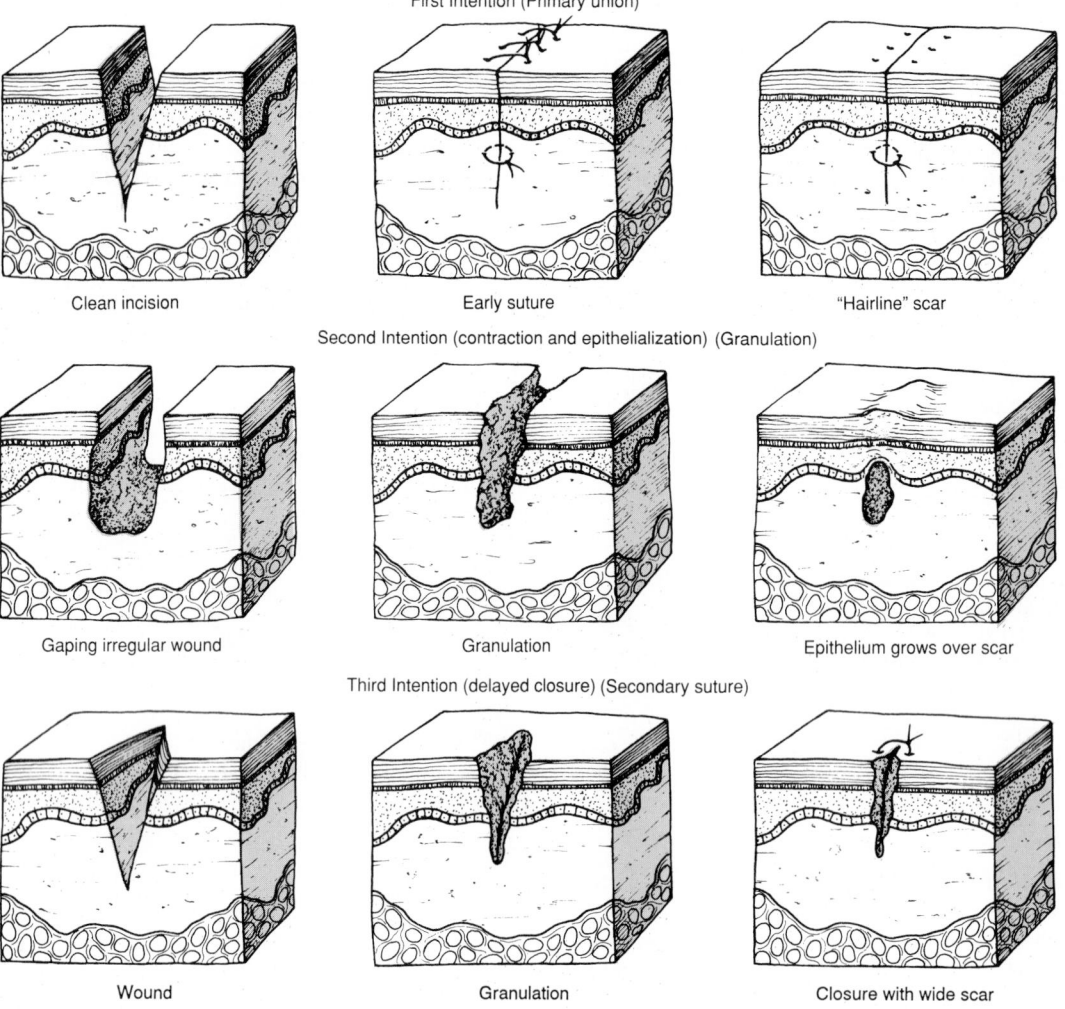

First Intention (Primary union)

Clean incision   Early suture   "Hairline" scar

Second Intention (contraction and epithelialization) (Granulation)

Gaping irregular wound   Granulation   Epithelium grows over scar

Third Intention (delayed closure) (Secondary suture)

Wound   Granulation   Closure with wide scar

Figure 34–6. Wound healing by first, second, and third intention.

vitamin C, the tensile strength of the wound decreases. Ascorbic acid also enhances capillary formation and decreases capillary fragility. It provides a defense to infection by playing a role in the immune response.

Vitamin K is essential in the synthesis of prothrombin, which is important in coagulation.

Minerals such as iron, zinc, and copper are involved in collagen synthesis.

Circulation and Oxygenation. Circulation to the involved wound and oxygenation of the tissues greatly influence wound healing. Wound healing slows whenever there is reduced local blood flow, which is why venous stasis ulcers, and decubitus ulcers are so notoriously hard to heal. Decreased arterial oxygen tension alters both collagen synthesis and formation of epithelial cells (Whitney, 1989). When hemoglobin levels are reduced by more than 15%, such as in severe anemia, oxygenation is reduced and tissue repair is altered. Anemia may combine with preexisting states such as diabetes or arteriosclerosis to further impair blood flow and therefore retard wound healing.

Immune Cellular Function. Drugs and therapies can affect immune cellular function and, therefore, wound healing. Immunosuppressive drugs such as corticosteroids, which may be given to prevent organ rejection in transplant patients, also depress the natural defenses against infection and mask the inflammatory response. Immunosuppressive agents usually also suppress protein synthesis, wound contraction, and epithelialization (Flynn & Rovee, 1982).

Cancer patients are often at risk for delayed wound healing and infection. Some patients have deficient or defective circulating antibodies. Chemotherapy and radiation treatments often retard wound repair. Chemotherapeutic agents such as 5-fluorouracil inhibit fibroblast replication and collagen synthesis, whereas vincristine suppresses antibody production. Radiation therapy negatively affects fibroblastic activity.

Individual Factors

Age. Changes that are part of the normal aging process can hinder wound healing. Circulation slows slightly, compromising oxygen delivery to the wound. Changes occur in the clotting process, and the inflammatory response and phagocytosis are impaired, increasing the risk of infection. Fibroblastic activity and collagen synthesis decrease with age, so cell growth and differentiation and reconstruction are slower. Because the scar tissue produced is less pliable, there is a greater risk that the body part will have a functional problem. Impaired healing may result from associated factors such as poor nutrition, which is more common in the elderly population, rather than as a direct result of the aging process.

Obesity. Wound healing may be retarded in obese patients. Because adipose tissue is relatively avascular, it provides only a weak defense against microbial invasion and impairs delivery of nutrients to the wound. Obese patients are at increased risk for complications and are often advised to lose weight before elective surgery. In general, surgery on an obese person takes longer, and suturing adipose tissue can be difficult. The potential for dehiscence and evisceration and subsequent infection is also greater in the obese patient.

Smoking. Physiologic changes occur in smokers that hinder wound healing. Functional hemoglobin levels decrease, impairing oxygen release to the tissues. Long-time smokers have an increased number of platelets, and the platelets are more adhesive. This hypercoagulability leads to the formation of thrombi, which may block small vessels. Oxygen delivery to the tissues may ultimately be compromised, which causes delayed wound healing.

Drugs. A number of drugs, in addition to those that directly affect the immune response, affect wound healing. Oral anticoagulants, given to decrease potential thrombus formation, increase the potential for bleeding into the wound. Even over-the-counter drugs, such as aspirin, decrease platelet aggregation and prolongs bleeding time. Antibiotics may be prescribed preoperatively for certain operative procedures that carry a high risk for postoperative infection. This prophylaxis is generally given for only a short time, because when antibiotics are used for a long time the risk of infection can increase and wound healing can be delayed.

Stress. Physical and emotional stress triggers the release of catecholamines; they cause blood vessels to constrict, decreasing blood flow to the wound. Stress can be caused by trauma, pain, and hospitalization. Recent research studies indicate increased wound healing when relaxation and guided imagery are used to reduce stress (HoldenLund, 1988).

Local Factors

Nature of the Injury. Usually, a surgical incision made using strict aseptic technique heals faster than, for instance, a deep wound embedded with gravel from a bicycle accident. The deeper the wound and the more extensive the tissue loss, the longer the wound will take to heal. Even the shape of the wound has an effect: the greater the irregularity, the more prolonged the wound healing process. If trauma has caused hematomas (blood clots) to form, this can also impede healing.

Presence of Infection. Infection hampers wound healing. When debris is not fully debrided or cleansed from a wound, infection is common. Infection may be introduced in the hospital by inadequate handwashing and poor dressing-change techniques. Infection may result from a surgical procedure, especially when a contaminated area such as the gastrointestinal or genitourinary tract is the operative site.

Local Wound Environment. Many factors in the local wound environment affect healing. The pH should be between 7.0 and 7.6; it can be altered by drainage, which may need to be contained or siphoned away for proper healing.

Tension or stress on the wound is also a factor in healing. Undue stress can be caused by improper handling of the wound during surgery or any activity that puts tension on the wound during the early postoperative period (e.g., applying a dressing or binder incorrectly, stress during movement). Vomiting, coughing without splinting, and abdominal distention can cause tension on an abdominal incision, potentially interfering with wound healing.

Complications of Wound Healing

Inadequate or delayed wound healing can cause a number of complications: hemorrhage, hematoma formation, infection, dehiscence, evisceration, and fistula formation. Such complications can lead to increased mortality and morbidity, and at best delay recovery.

Hemorrhage. After the initial trauma, bleeding is expected, but within several minutes hemostasis occurs as part of the first phase of wound healing. However, when large blood vessels are severed or the patient has poor clotting ability, bleeding may continue. Hemorrhage may also occur later in the postoperative period if a suture slips, a clot dislodges, erosion through a blood vessel occurs, or abnormal stress is applied to the incisional area.

Hemorrhage may occur internally or externally. External bleeding is obvious: bloody drainage, more than what is normally expected, is visible from the wound. Dressings may become saturated with blood, and gravity may even pool blood under the patient. Internal bleeding is less observable and may be indicated by swelling of the affected area, an abnormal amount of bloody drainage from a catheter or drain, an increase in pain, or abnormal vital signs.

Hematomas. A **hematoma,** a localized collection of blood, appears as a swelling or mass underneath the skin surface and often has a bluish color. Small hematomas are readily absorbed into the systemic circulation as debris from the wound, but larger hematomas may take weeks to reabsorb, creating dead space and dead cells that inhibit healing. A large hematoma near a major artery or vein is especially dangerous, since local pressure exerted by the hematoma can disrupt blood flow.

Large hematomas may require evacuation or surgical removal to promote optimal wound healing.

Infection. A break in skin integrity, whether due to a surgical incision or accidental trauma, gives microorganisms a portal for entry into the body. Bacterial contamination of the wound can result in infection if the patient's defenses are inadequate. The incidence of wound infection depends on the following:

- Local factors: contamination, degree of closure, presence of foreign bodies
- Treatment factors: length of hospital stay, length of surgery, surgical closure
- Host factors: patient's age, nutritional status, chronic health problems.

Symptoms of an infected wound are purulent drainage, an inflamed incisional area, fever, and an elevated white blood cell count. Wound infections greatly increase the cost of medical care and can substantially lengthen recovery time. See Chapter 35 for detailed information on wound infection.

Dehiscence and Evisceration. Dehiscence is a total or partial disruption in wound edges (Fig. 34-7). As wound edges separate, an increase in drainage usually occurs. Dehiscence most commonly occurs before collagen formation is complete in high-risk patients (3 to 14 days after injury). Obesity, poor nutritional status, and increased stress on the incisional area through abdominal distention or trauma increase the risk of dehiscence. Patients often report feeling that their incision has "given way" after activities such as coughing or vomiting that increase pressure on the incision. Dehiscence may also occur when sutures or staples are removed before the wound has healed adequately.

Evisceration. Evisceration is the protrusion of viscera through a wound opening (Fig. 34-3). Evisceration can follow dehiscence if the opening has not been reclosed and is large enough to allow internal organs to protrude. Evisceration often occurs when dehiscence occurs suddenly and is extensive. When evisceration occurs, reassure the patient, cover the area with sterile saline dressings, and notify the surgeon immediately. Do not try to push viscera back into the abdomen. The patient usually must return to surgery for wound closure. Infection is more likely when dehiscence and evisceration have occurred, and often antibiotics are given.

Fistula. A fistula is an abnormal tubelike passageway that forms between two organs or from one organ to the outside of the body. Fistula tracts are usually the result of poor wound healing after tissue injury from surgery or vaginal delivery. Normal wound healing promotes tissue layer closure, thus preventing abnormal communication

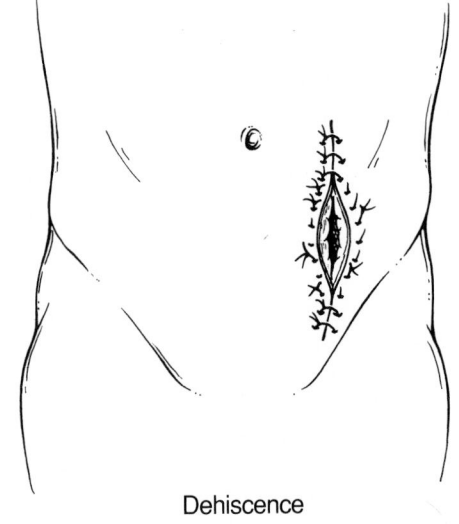

Dehiscence

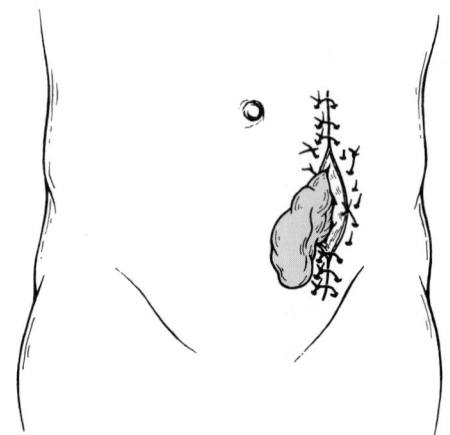

Evisceration

Figure 34–7. Dehiscence is the disruption of wound edges: Evisceration is the protrusion of viscera through that wound opening.

between organs of the body. The name of the fistula designates the site of the abnormal communication; for example, a rectovaginal fistula is an abnormal opening between the rectum and the vagina that permits feces to enter the vagina.

When a fistula opens onto the outside skin surface, drainage (especially gastric or intestinal) may contribute to skin breakdown. Small fistulas may heal under optimal conditions, but surgical intervention may be needed for larger fistulas that do not heal with conservative treatment.

Impact of Integumentary Dysfunction on Activities of Daily Living

Altered skin integrity can change a patient's lifestyle and ability to perform activities of daily living (ADLs). Patients with a diminished sense of touch may have difficulty buttoning clothes or grooming themselves. Large draining wounds may limit the patient's mobility and sap the energy necessary for ADLs. Systemic responses to skin alterations such as fever and malaise may also lower the patient's activity tolerance.

Some skin conditions may require the patient to be confined at home, or the patient may choose isolation because of changes in body image and lowered self-esteem. This is especially true if the skin impairment is highly visible, such as on the face. Resulting feelings of anxiety or depression may alter the patient's ability and motivation to perform ADLs.

Elderly patients may be particularly hampered in performing ADLs because they often have other chronic health problems that may aggravate the problems created by their skin alterations. Tissue repair and healing may take longer in the elderly, so these patients may need wound care for longer periods of time. Elderly patients often have fewer family members or significant others to assist with skin treatments or dressings and to help with hygiene or nutritional needs.

ASSESSMENT

A systematic assessment of skin integrity and wound healing is essential. It provides data to identify potential or actual problems and allows the nurse to develop an individualized care plan. Subjective and objective data are collected during the first encounter with the patient, and ongoing assessment is done to detect changes in skin integrity or wound-healing status.

Subjective Data

Interviewing the patient allows the nurse to gather data about the patient's normal skin status, the history of skin problems, and the presence of risk factors that can increase the potential for altered skin integrity or wound healing. Subjective data also gives the nurse detailed information on the development of actual skin or wound problems and how the patient has managed them.

Functional Pattern Identification

When interviewing the patient, the nurse should ask what the patient's skin, hair, and nails are normally like. Reports of excessively dry or oily skin should be noted. Questions about normal skin-care practices and individual preferences help the nurse to individualize care; often patients bring with them skin-care products, creams, and lotions to maintain their skin in its normal state. The nurse should assess what self-care activities the patient can independently perform. If the patient has been unable to care for his or her hair or nails, arrangements for such care can be made.

If the patient manages a chronic skin or wound condition, the nurse should document specific management techniques. For the ostomy patient, the nurse notes what type of equipment is used to keep the skin around the stoma free from irritation and breakdown. For the patient with a wound, the nurse gathers information about normal wound-management practices.

Risk Identification

In the interview, the nurse can identify patients at risk for problems with skin integrity or delayed wound healing.

Obtain an allergy history, with a description of the allergic response (including dermatologic symptoms) and identification of the allergen. For patients with a positive allergy history, specific foods, medications, or products (e.g., soaps or tape) should be noted on the patient's record. When a patient reports numerous allergies, take care to avoid new products that may cause an allergic response.

Obtain a history of past skin conditions. Ask what factors triggered the problem, whether the condition was seasonal or aggravated by stress, and how the patient handled the problem (e.g., home remedies, over-the-counter preparations). Question the patient about a family history of skin problems, since some dermatologic problems (e.g., eczema, psoriasis) commonly run in families.

Document any recent exposure to factors that can cause skin trauma, rash, or lesions. Note any contact with family members or others with infectious illnesses (e.g., measles, chickenpox, scabies, lice). Travel to foreign countries or activities such as hiking or camping can expose the patient to parasites or poisonous plants. Exposure to caustic chemicals, excessive heat, or radiation may also be important in identifying the risk for skin alterations.

When a patient is admitted for surgery, it is important to assess risk factors that may delay wound healing, such as malnutrition, impaired circulation, immunosuppression, obesity, smoking, diabetes mellitus, infection, and stress. Assess the amount and quality of incisional pain postoperatively by asking the patient to describe and quantify the pain. Observe the patient for nonverbal cues such as grimacing or splinting that often occur with pain. Movement and activity commonly increase incisional pain, but a sudden unexplained increase may indicate wound complications such as infection or dehiscence.

It is also important to determine the risk for pressure-ulcer formation. A patient who cannot move independently or will be immobilized is at increased risk. Diabetics with neuropathy or patients with paralysis are at increased risk due to impaired sensation. The risk for ulcer development is increased if the patient is malnourished, is incontinent of urine or feces, is obese or very thin, or has altered cognitive functioning.

The Braden Scale for Predicting Pressure-Sore Risk (Bergstrom, et al., 1987) helps quantify pressure ulcer risk. Risk factor categories, which include sensory–perception, skin moisture, activity, mobility, friction and shear, and nutritional status, are used to evaluate potential risk for pressure sore development (see Fig. 34-5). A study of the Braden scale validated 9 of the 13 physiologic factors, but recommended that psychosocial factors such as noncompliance, family dynamics, or socioeconomic factors be included as well (Copeland-Fields & Hoshiko, 1989).

Dysfunctional Identification

Ask the patient if any skin problems (rash, sores, or breaks in the skin) are present. If they are, ask how long the condition has been present, what it looked like when it first appeared, if and how it spread, and any associated symptoms. Ask if any treatments have been used, including home remedies and over-the-counter preparations.

If an accident has resulted in a wound, burn, or other injury, evaluate the nature of the events leading to the trauma. Note any contamination of the area with dirt or debris. Ask parents about their child's injuries, and if they give vague or suspicious explanations, a follow-up evaluation should be done to determine if child abuse has occurred. For all accidental wounds, even minor ones, ask about the status of the patient's tetanus immunization, and update it if necessary.

Interview questions can also help assess the impact a skin condition or wound has on ADLs. Such conditions can affect self-concept, causing the patient to withdraw from social interaction. Watching the patient's nonverbal cues helps the nurse assess the psychological impact of the skin impairment.

Objective Data

Objective information obtained during the physical examination can identify actual problems in skin integrity or wound healing. Inspection and palpation help the nurse to collect objective data about skin integrity and wound status. Laboratory and diagnostic tests may be done to confirm a diagnosis of cancer or the presence of infection.

Physical Examination

Inspection of the Skin. A general inspection of the skin is followed by a more detailed examination of any abnormalities noted. Examine the skin for color, vascularity, turgor and mobility, texture, and the presence or absence of lesions. A good source of light is essential. Compare for symmetry in contralateral areas throughout the examination.

Skin color varies from one person to another, from one part of the body to another, and according to race. Some pigment variations are normal. Pigment changes also normally occur during pregnancy. Other changes in skin color may be evidence of systemic disease. Cyanosis (bluish discoloration) in nailbeds may be due to vasoconstriction, although cyanosis in the mouth or conjunctiva may indicate hypoxemia secondary to heart or lung dysfunction. The yellow hue of jaundice may indicate liver or biliary disease.

Skin texture refers to the palpable and visible surface structure, its fineness or coarseness, and whether it is scaly, crusted, or macerated. Skin may appear thick and tough, or thin and friable. Experienced nurses can sometimes predict, based on skin appearance, which patients are more likely to suffer skin breakdown.

When any skin abnormality is present, note its shape, pattern, distribution, and color. Note whether the abnormality is localized or generalized and whether distribution is symmetric. Lesions can occur in clusters, circles, or lines, or their placement may be irregular. Measure the size of the lesion so that changes in size can be detected.

Also examine the patient's hair and nails. Inspect the hair for distribution, quantity, and quality. Absence of hair growth on lower extremities can indicate decreased peripheral blood flow. Thinning and brittle nails may be caused by nutritional deficits or impaired circulation. Nail clubbing (Fig. 18-7), a change in the angle of the fingernail and nail base, is associated with chronic respiratory and cardiac dysfunction. Capillary refill time is illustrated in Figure 31-5.

Inspection of the Wound. Inspection permits the nurse to evaluate wound healing and detect possible wound complications. Appraise the general appearance of the wound, type and amount of drainage, functioning of drainage systems, amount and characteristics of incisional pain, and signs of wound complications, such as infection.

General Appearance. Note the size and shape of the wound and compare it with previous notations in the chart. Size is usually estimated in millimeters or the size of common coins. In some situations where wound healing is watched carefully, size and shape may be measured daily with concentric circle overlays.

Surgical incisions are usually closed with sutures, staples, or clips so the skin edges are well approximated to promote healing. Initially the incision may appear slightly swollen or red, due to normal inflammation. Usually within a week of surgery, the wound edges heal together and swelling subsides. When staples have been in for a prolonged period, they may rise and show signs of inflammation where they enter the skin.

When wound edges are not well approximated and healing does not occur by first intention, healing occurs by granulation. Initially the area appears red, as capillary beds proliferate from which connective tissue will eventually develop. As healing occurs, epithelium grows over these capillary beds and the wound decreases in size. This shrinkage in wound size can be observed.

Color Code to Classify Wounds. The three-color concept of wound classification developed by Marion Laboratories (see Table 34-3) helps the nurse to assess wound healing and identify an appropriate plan of treatment (Cuzzell, 1988). The wound is classified by color (red, yellow, or black) rather than the depth of tissue destruction. For a red wound, the goal of treatment is to protect the area so that healing can occur. When the wound is yellow, the goal of treatment is cleansing to remove nonviable tissue and purulent drainage. Black wounds need to be debrided to remove necrotic tissue or eschar so that wound healing can occur. As wounds change color, treatment plans are changed accordingly.

Drainage Systems. Drainage devices are placed in the wound when the surgeon anticipates a large amount of fluid accumulation, which inhibits wound healing. Closed drainage systems consist of a drain attached to a portable or external suction source. Open drainage systems, such as a Penrose drain, drain directly from the wound and are associated with a higher rate of wound infection.

A *Penrose drain* is a hollow, flat rubber tube placed directly into the incision or into a stab wound in the incisional area (see Fig. 34-15). It allows fluid to drain via capillary action into absorbent dressings. Penrose drains may be advanced or shortened to drain different areas.

A *Hemovac* is placed into vascular areas where bloody drainage is expected after surgery. Suction is maintained by compressing a springlike device (see Procedure 34-3, Step 7). When inspecting a Hemovac drain, expect bloody drainage and ensure that the Hemovac remains in the compressed state. Suction can be interrupted if leaks are present in the system or if the Hemovac has filled with drainage.

A *Jackson-Pratt* or grenade drain permits drainage to collect in a bulblike device, which can be compressed to create gentle suction (see Fig. 34-14). Suction is lost when the bulb is expanded either from too much drainage or a leak in the system.

Inspect the drainage system to ensure patency and function. Drains may or may not be sutured in place, so take care not to inadvertently remove them during inspection.

Wound Drainage. The type and amount of drainage varies depending on the type and location of surgery. Note the amount, color, consistency, and odor of any drainage. Terms commonly used to describe wound drainage are:

Serous drainage is clear, watery, and plasmalike.
Sanguineous drainage is bloody, as from a fresh wound.

Serosanguineous drainage is pale and thin and contains plasma and red cells.
Purulent drainage contains white cells and microorganisms and occurs when infection is present. It is thick and opaque and can vary from pale yellow to green or tan, depending on the offending organism.

In closed systems, the amount of drainage can be accurately monitored since the drainage is measured every 8 hours. The greatest amount of drainage is expected in the early postoperative period. The amount tapers off as edema subsides and fluid is removed from the site. Most surgeons remove drains when drainage is minimal. An unexpected increase in drainage is important to note, since it can precede wound complications such as dehiscence. A change in the character of drainage is also important to observe and report, especially if there is a sudden increase in bloody drainage or if drainage become purulent.

Assessing the amount of drainage is more difficult when a closed drainage system is not used. The nurse can help to quantify the amount of drainage by noting the number of dressings that were saturated and the number of times the dressing required changing. When the dressing is not being changed, drainage is sometimes circled on the dressing and marked with a date and time.

Inspection for Infection. Observe for symptoms that may indicate infection in the wound, such as pain, redness, swelling, and purulent drainage. Systemic signs include fever and an elevated white blood count. Wound infection can occur a few days after surgery if mass contamination has occurred, but often such infections do not become apparent until later in the postoperative period. See Chapter 35 for a detailed discussion of wound infections.

Palpation. Palpation can be used along with inspection to gather objective data about wound status or skin integrity. Use gloves when palpating skin surfaces to avoid exposure to infectious agents; sterile gloves are needed if the skin is not intact or if a drain is present. Palpation is helpful in assessing raised surfaces of the skin and the skin texture and temperature. When wound infection is suspected, gently palpate the incisional area to detect swelling or hardness.

Diagnostic Tests and Procedures

Laboratory and diagnostic tests may be performed to confirm the cause of a skin or wound abnormality. Most commonly, a culture and sensitivity is done to identify infectious organisms that can cause a skin lesion or infect a wound. See Chapter 35 for more information on wound cultures. A biopsy is sometimes performed to rule out malignant causes of skin abnormalities.

NURSING DIAGNOSES AND PATIENT GOALS

Impaired Skin Integrity and Impaired Tissue Integrity are NANDA diagnoses used to identify problems with skin breakdown and healing. Impaired Skin Integrity is used to identify potential problems or actual problems that involve only the epidermal or dermal layer. Impaired Tissue Integrity is used when the damage involves more than the dermis; often connective tissue, muscles, and nerves are involved.

Diagnostic Statement: Impaired Skin Integrity

Definition

A state in which the individual's skin is adversely altered (NANDA, 1990)

Defining Characteristics

Disruption of skin surface, destruction of skin layers, invasion of body structures (NANDA, 1990).

Related Factors

External (Environmental). Hyperthermia or hypothermia; chemical substance; mechanical factors (shearing forces, pressure, restraint); radiation; physical immobilization; humidity.

Internal (Somatic). Medication; altered nutritional state (obesity, emaciation); altered metabolic state; altered circulation; altered sensation; altered pigmentation; skeletal prominence; developmental factors; immunologic deficit; alterations in turgor (change in elasticity) (NANDA, 1990).

Diagnostic Statement: Impaired Tissue Integrity

Definition

A state in which an individual experiences damage to mucous membrane, corneal, integumentary, or subcutaneous tissue (NANDA, 1990).

Defining Characteristics

Major. Damaged or destroyed tissue (cornea, mucous membrane, integumentary, or subcutaneous) (NANDA, 1990).

Related Factors

Altered circulation; nutritional deficit/excess; fluid deficit/excess; knowledge deficit; impaired physical mobility; irritants, chemical (including body excretions, secretions, medications); thermal (temperature extremes); mechanical (pressure, shear, friction); radiation (including therapeutic radiation) (NANDA, 1990).

Related Nursing Diagnoses

A patient with impaired skin or tissue integrity is at risk for other problems. Any break in the skin increases the risk for infection. When impairment involves large surface areas, such as with extensive burns, Ineffective Thermoregulation or Fluid Volume Deficit may occur. Healing of impaired skin or tissues requires increased nutritional resources and may result in Altered Nutrition. When tissue or skin impairment is severe, it may limit the patient's mobility and self-care abilities. Knowledge Deficit may be present if the patient must learn complex management protocols.

Psychological effects of impaired skin or tissue integrity are important to consider. Altered self-concept, body image, and self-esteem commonly accompany skin impairments, especially if the impairment is highly visible. When severe, this can cause Anxiety, Ineffective Individual Coping, or Social Isolation.

Patient Goals

Patient-centered goals for skin and tissue integrity involve preventing damage and promoting optimal healing of damaged tissues.

The patient's skin will remain intact without areas of local inflammation.
The patient's skin will demonstrate evidence of healing of existing lesions.
The patient will demonstrate increased knowledge of skin care.
The patient/family will comply with the treatment plan to promote wound healing and skin integrity.

IMPLEMENTATION

Nursing interventions are aimed at promoting optimal skin integrity, preventing skin or tissue damage, and treating impaired skin to promote optimal wound healing and skin function.

Nursing Interventions to Promote Health and Integumentary Function

Nursing care plays an important role in preventing skin alterations. Optimal skin integrity is maintained by promoting adequate oxygen, nutrients, water, and waste removal for the skin and mucous membranes.

There are several basic principles of skin care (see the display). One of the most important involves maintaining intact skin since it is the body's first line of defense against trauma and infections. Measures to prevent irritation or injury are imperative. Skin breakdown can be prevented by avoiding mechanical irritation from rubbing or friction. Remove tape carefully and pat patients dry to avoid traumatizing delicate skin. To minimize chemical irritation, use mild soaps, plain water, or products containing emollients. Very young, elderly, emaciated, or obese patients may have particularly sensitive skin that is more prone to chemical irritation.

Maintaining adequate hydration of the skin also contributes to healthy skin function. Because very dry skin is susceptible to breakdown, avoid drying agents such as alcohol and use lotions or creams with lanolin. Patients with dry skin should be bathed only once or twice a week. However, skin that is exposed to excessive moisture for prolonged periods of time can lead to bacterial growth and irritation. Patients who are incontinent of urine or stool or who perspire excessively need prompt, thorough, frequent washing and drying. Areas where skin lies in folds (e.g., under the breasts, in the gluteal folds) can collect moisture and need special attention. A gauze pad or a light dusting of powder may help prevent moisture buildup.

Adequate nutrition is essential for normal skin integrity. Adequately nourished cells can better resist injury and disease, so a diet with appropriate vitamins, minerals, and protein is essential. A patient who has poor absorption of nutrients, excessive losses of protein, or

inadequate food and fluid intake may need additional nutritional support (high-protein supplements, total parenteral nutrition) to prevent skin breakdown and ensure healing.

Adequate circulation is also needed to maintain cell life. Inadequate blood flow to the skin results in ischemia and tissue breakdown. Keeping patients warm prevents vasoconstriction. Treating underlying cardiac or circulatory problems helps ensure adequate blood flow to the skin. Getting adequate exercise and avoiding constrictive clothing can help ensure optimal blood flow. Frequent turning and repositioning can avoid localized obstruction of blood flow due to increased pressure.

Patient Teaching

Hygiene teaching is important to maintain skin integrity. Because patients with impaired sensation are less able to sense injury to the skin, they should be taught to inspect skin surfaces (especially the feet) routinely for signs of breakdown. When wearing new shoes, they should take care to avoid blisters and irritation. Since temperature discrimination is also affected, hot-water heaters should be turned down to avoid accidental burns.

Hygiene teaching is also important for the parents of a newborn. Teaching should include how to prevent skin trauma (for example, clipping fingernails short and putting mittens on the child when scratching is anticipated). Reassure parents about normal skin changes or congeni-

---

Principles of Skin Care

- Intact skin is the body's first line of defense against trauma and infection.
- Breakdown of the skin's integrity must be prevented.
- Skin must be adequately hydrated.
- The body's cells must be adequately nourished.
- Adequate circulation is needed to maintain cells.
- Skin hygiene is necessary.
- Skin sensitivity varies among people and according to their health status.

Patient Teaching

Instruct the patient as follows:

- If you have decreased skin sensations, inspect your skin carefully and take actions to prevent skin injury resulting from trauma or burns.
- Reduce your risk of skin cancer by avoiding overexposure to the sun and using effective sunscreen products.
- Report any change in size, shape, color, or healing activity of lesions to your health-care provider.
- Reduce skin irritation by regular applications of lotion and moisturizers, especially if you are an older adult.
- Install smoke detectors and learn to use fire extinguishers, and routinely practice what to do should fire break out.
- Keep dry any areas that hold moisture (e.g., under the breasts, between fat folds, between the legs) to prevent maceration of skin.

tal lesions of the skin. Parental bonding with the infant can be hindered if the parents view the infant as deformed or scarred.

Education about accident prevention is important. Many automobile accidents can be avoided by careful driving, adhering to speed limits, and using seat belts or air bags. Bicycle injuries can be prevented or limited by observing safety rules and wearing helmets. Smoke detectors should be installed to prevent serious burns. See Chapter 25 for more information on safety.

Pressure-Sore Prevention

Preventing pressure ulcers begins with accurate assessment of at-risk patients and appropriate prevention and treatment measures (see display). Comprehensive teaching programs have been effective in preventing

readmissions for pressure sores (LaMantia, et al., 1987). Frequent turning and positioning, keeping the skin clean and dry, improving nutritional status, and avoiding friction and shearing force all help prevent pressure sores.

Pressure buildup can be decreased by using support surfaces such as foam, air-filled, flotation, or alternating-air mattresses. Surfaces are usually used on beds, but some can be adapted for wheelchair use.

Foam surfaces are available in various shapes and depths; an eggcrate mattress is an example (Fig. 34-8). The thicker and denser the foam, the greater the pressure protection provided. These surfaces are inexpensive and lightweight, but are difficult to clean (especially if soiled with urine or stool) and are not very durable. Often these surfaces are used for high-risk patients who are immobilized temporarily (e.g., postoperatively).

Air-filled surfaces are similar to the air mattresses used for camping or for floating in swimming pools. Bladders are pumped full of air, preventing the body from touching the bed surface. The inflation level should be checked daily by placing a hand between the bed and the mattress to see if body prominences can be felt. An inadequately inflated mattress loses its protective value. Air-filled mattresses are easy to clean, lightweight, and durable, but must be protected from punctures.

Flotation surfaces are filled with water, gel, or a combination of materials to provide good pressure distribution. As with air-filled mattresses, they must be monitored frequently; the manufacturer provides specific guidelines. These surfaces are durable and soilproof but expensive. Gel-filled devices can solidify at cold temperatures.

Alternating-air surfaces contain air cells that are alternately inflated and deflated to avoid pressure buildup. These devices malfunction frequently, and repairs are costly. Studies have not demonstrated any advantage over less-costly surfaces (Daechsel & Conine, 1985).

Pressure-Sore Prevention

Relieve Pressure

- Change position frequently, alternating supine, side-lying, and prone.
- Support surfaces to decrease capillary pressure.
- Pad bony prominences.
- Raise seat from wheelchair.
- Tilt wheelchair back to relieve pressure from gravity.

Avoid Shearing Force and Friction

- Avoid semi-Fowler's position.
- Use trapeze bar.
- Use turning sheet to pull patient up in bed.
- Use heel and elbow protectors.

Keep Skin Clean and Dry

- Pat dry carefully after bathing.
- Clean skin carefully after every incontinent episode.
- Use appropriate drainage-collection measures.

Provide Optimal Nutrition

- Encourage high-protein foods.
- Encourage foods high in vitamin C.
- Keep hemoglobin and albumin levels within normal limits.
- Encourage adequate caloric intake.

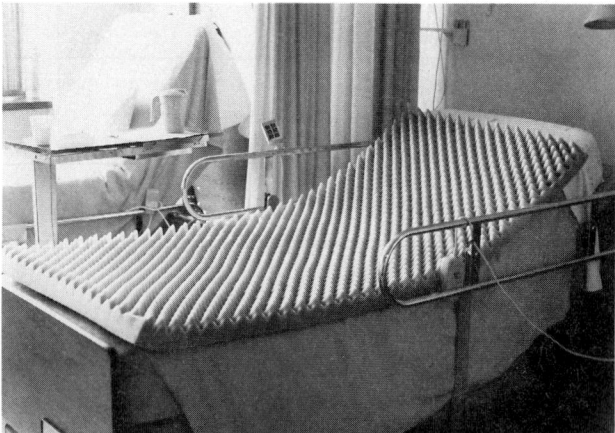

Figure 34–8. An eggcrate mattress prevents pressure sores by distributing body weight equally.

Nursing Interventions for Altered Integumentary Function

Wound care is planned by the members of the health-care team, and nursing interventions are significant for promoting optimal wound healing and skin integrity. Nursing interventions to encourage independence, reinforce patient accomplishments, and teach the patient and family to achieve optimal self-care are important. Depending on the type of wound the nurse may want to protect the area to promote optimum regeneration of tissue (red wound), cleanse the area to treat or prevent infection (yellow wound) and debride the area to remove debris which impairs wound healing (black wound). Refer to Table 34-3 for a summary of wound care according to the color concept method. Heat and cold can also be used as therapeutic modalities to promote healing.

Pruritus Relief

Pruritus often accompanies skin problems. Nursing management is aimed at relieving the situations that cause pruritus, decreasing the associated discomfort, and preventing additional trauma to the skin.

Pruritus is often caused by excessive drying of the skin, especially in elderly patients. Lotions and moisturizing creams should be applied regularly to promote rehydration of dried areas. Bathing should be limited; if soap is used, it should be thoroughly rinsed from the skin, and specific brands that increase irritation should not be used. Oil may be added to the bath water, but care should be taken since oil increases the slipperiness of the

---

TABLE 34-3

Color Classification of Wounds

Color	Goal	Possible Treatment
Red	Protection	Telfa, semipermeable (film) dressings; moist compresses
Yellow	Cleansing	Wet-to-dry dressings; irrigation; semipermeable (film) dressings; occlusive dressings
Black	Debridement	Hydrotherapy, chemical debridement, surgical debridement, occlusive dressings

---

tub and may contribute to falls. Using tepid, not hot, water and gently patting the skin dry also decrease skin irritation.

Explaining the importance of not scratching may increase compliance for adults, but cautions rarely work for young children. Keeping children's fingernails cut short and having them wear cotton gloves may decrease skin trauma. In severe cases elbow restraints may be needed. Diversional activities and guided imagery may also help focus the patient's attention away from unpleasant sensations.

Cool baths and moist cool compresses promote vasoconstriction and provide relief. Baking soda or oatmeal baths are soothing. Medications may be ordered by the physician and used on a PRN basis. Antihistamines and sedatives, although commonly used, have systemic side effects. Topical medications such as corticosteroids or antibiotics can decrease inflammation or treat infection. A paste made from baking soda and water can also be applied to decrease itching.

First Aid for Minor Wounds

Basic principles in caring for minor accidental wounds are to promote hemostasis, cleanse the wound, and protect it from further injury.

Bleeding can be controlled by putting direct pressure on the wound or by elevating the affected part. Initial bleeding may help remove dirt and contaminants from the wound.

Cleansing the wound removes potential sources of infection. Try to remove foreign materials such as dirt or cinders unless the wound is extensive or the patient complains of excessive pain. For most minor wounds, running water as an irrigating solution and mild soap as a cleansing agent is recommended.

After bleeding has subsided and the area has been cleansed, the wound is protected with a sterile or clean dressing. Small cuts may be left open to the air. Extensive wounds may require a bulky dressing applied with pressure to minimize movement.

The wound should be assessed for potential complications, and any patient with a wound that requires more extensive treatment should be referred to the appropri-

---

Selected Nursing Interventions for Common Skin Integrity Problems

Primary Wound Healing

- Apply dressings (permeable or semipermeable).
- Promote drainage:
    Ensure patency of open and closed drainage systems.
    Recharge closed drainage systems.
    Advance drains.
- Support the wound with Steristrips or butterflies, sutures and staples, bandages, and binders.
- Apply heat to local site.

Secondary or Tertiary Wound Healing

- Apply dressings (semipermeable or occlusive).
- Debride, irrigate, or pack wound as needed.
- Apply heat to local site.

ate health-care agency. Signs of infection usually take up to 24 hours to develop. Exudate, fever, or severe redness and swelling indicate that the wound needs a physician's attention. When excessive bleeding occurs, sutures are usually necessary to ensure healing by primary intention.

First Aid for Minor Burns

The type of burn dictates the appropriate first-aid measures. In all cases, it is important to halt the burning process and prevent further damage.

With a thermal burn, the heat source must first be removed. If someone is on fire, immediate action should be to "stop, drop, and roll." After the heat source has been removed, the burned area should be flushed with copious amounts of cool water. If done quickly, this action halts the burning process by speeding heat dissipation, and it relieves pain. The patient's clothing and jewelry in the affected area should be removed, since clothing and metal can retain heat. If clothing sticks to the burned area, cut around it rather than pulling, which may traumatize underlying burned tissues (Smith & Savinski-Bozinko, 1989). Ointments and home remedies should be avoided because they can complicate burn healing.

Treatment of chemical burns is similar to that of thermal burns. The first step is to remove the patient's clothing and flush the burned area with water, which dilutes the chemical and halts the burning process. To be most effective, the irrigation should be at low pressure but should last at least 20 minutes (Smith & Savinski-Bozinko, 1989). If a large area has been exposed, placing the patient in a shower may be the easiest way to flush the burned area. Brush powdered chemicals off the area before irrigating. Avoid splashing any of the irritant, since even dilute exposure to some chemicals can result in burns or irritation of mucous membranes. Some chemicals (e.g., alkali powders) may react with water to produce heat, so industrial nurses should be knowledgeable about the chemicals used in their workplaces.

Before treating an electrical burn, the victim must be freed from the electrical source. If the person is still in contact with the electrical current, it must be turned off at its source. If you must separate the victim from energized current, make sure you are well grounded and use nonconductive equipment such as a lineman's glove, polydacron rope, or dry wood. After removing the victim from the current, if the injury site or clothing are smoldering, douse them with water to dissipate the heat. Cardiopulmonary resuscitation may be necessary, since ventricular fibrillation or cardiac arrest often occurs with electrical burns. After stabilizing a victim of an electrical burn, contact the power company and describe any malfunction or problem that led to the burn. The company will conduct a safety inspection of the electrical system.

Dressings

A *dressing* is a protective covering placed over a wound. Dressings are used for the following reasons:

- To absorb drainage
- To prevent contamination
- To prevent mechanical injury to the wound
- To help maintain pressure so that excessive bleeding is avoided
- To immobilize the wound so that further trauma does not occur
- To provide psychological and aesthetic comfort for the patient.

The type of dressing used depends on the type of wound, location, status, and personal preference.

Types of Dressings. Dressings are of three general types: permeable, semipermeable, and occlusive (Table 34-4).

Permeable dressings allow air to reach the wound so it can dry. Absorbent gauze, whether in small squares (2×2's or 4×4's), large rectangles (Surgipads, abdominal pads, ABDs), or rolls (Kerlix), is selected based on the size and location of the wound and the amount of drainage. Most products are available in presterilized packages.

Telfa is a type of gauze that has a nonadherent coating on one surface, which prevents it from sticking to the wound. Granulating tissue is not disrupted when a Telfa dressing is removed. Some gauze dressings are impregnated with petroleum jelly to keep the wound moist and prevent destruction of new, sensitive tissue.

Semipermeable dressings, such as Op-site or Tegaderm, provide a transparent covering that permits oxygen to reach the wound but prevents contamination by microorganisms. A layer of fluid collects under the dressing, providing a moist environment for wound healing. The nurse can see through the dressing to inspect the wound without changing the dressing. Semipermeable dressings are often left in place for a week, which prevents the destruction of newly formed tissues from frequent dressing removal.

Occlusive dressings, such as Duoderm, Restore, or Tegasorb, are not transparent and are impermeable to oxygen. The inner surface of these hydrocolloid dressings interacts with the wound exudate, forming a hydrated gel over the wound. When debridement and autolysis is needed, these dressings may be changed every few days, but when granulation is present the dressing may be left in place for 7 days. When these dressings are removed, the gel may be thick, yellow, and malodorous, but this does not indicate infection if the wound appears clean when the gel is removed (Conforti, 1989).

Methods of Securing Dressings. Tape, Montgomery straps, bandages, or binders can hold a dressing in place.

Tape is the most commonly used securing device. Adhesive tape is not often used on the skin: it holds securely, but

TABLE 34–4

Types of Dressings

Type	Description	Examples	Purpose	Uses
Permeable	Absorbent gauze	2 × 2's, 4 × 4's, ABDs	Allows air to dry the wound; absorbs wound drainage	Dry incisions, wet-to-dry dressings, incisions with Penrose drain and drainage
Semipermeable	Transparent, self-adhering film	Op-site, Tegaderm	Allows oxygen to reach the wound and provides a moist environment for wound healing; permits easy inspection	Covers incision or IV site, skin abrasions, Stage I or Stage II (with minimal drainage) pressure sores, partial-thickness burns
Occlusive	Hydrocolloid and hydrogel products	Duoderm, Restore, Vigilon	Does not allow oxygen to reach the wound; liquefies necrotic debris; exudate absorbers absorb drainage	Draining or necrotic wounds (e.g., Stage III pressure sores); partial-thickness burns

removal can be painful. If adhesive tape must be used, hair should be clipped before application and a tape-remover solution used when the tape is gently pulled from the skin. Nonallergenic paper or plastic tape is preferred for dressings that adhere to the skin. Microfoam tape is a pliable, foamlike tape used for compression or pressure dressings.

Montgomery straps or ties, used when dressings require frequent changing, are commercially prepared strips of nonallergenic tape (Fig. 34-9). Ties are inserted through the holes at one end. Montgomery straps help prevent skin breakdown because they eliminate the need to remove tape with every dressing change. Changing the Montgomery straps is required only when they become loose or soiled.

Bandages and *binders* can also be used to hold gauze dressings in place. Specific information on different types of bandages and binders is given later in this chapter.

Agents Used to Clean Wounds. If left in place, wound exudate provides a warm, moist environment that fosters microbial growth. Sterile saline (0.9% NaCl) is the most common solution used to clean wounds. Povidone–iodine (Betadine) may be used if an antiseptic is needed. Hydrogen peroxide, an oxidizing agent, may be used at half-strength if wound debridement and cleansing is desired. All cleansing agents should be sterile.

Dressing Changes. The type of dressing used and the frequency of dressing changes are determined by wound status. Sometimes the physician may order the type of dressing and the frequency of dressing changes, but at other times the nurse determines what type of dressing will best promote healing. In many hospitals, one nurse specializes in skin and wound care and can advise nurses

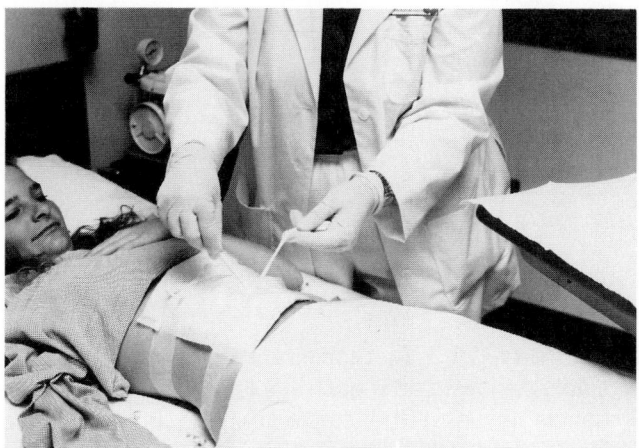
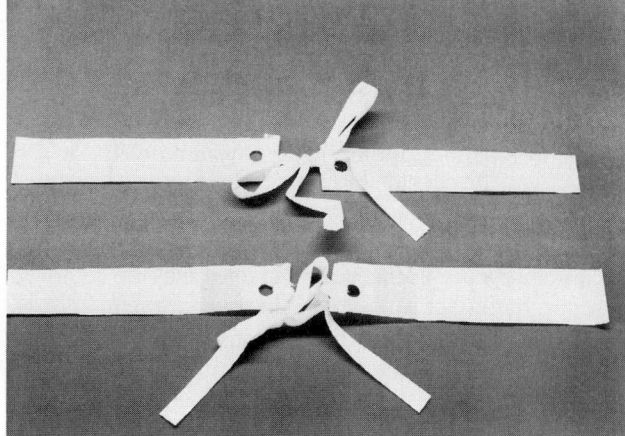

Figure 34–9.   Montgomery straps or ties are used to prevent skin breakdown from frequent tape removal when dressings need to be changed often.

and physicians about the best management approach for a specific wound.

Procedures for changing a dry sterile dressing and applying wet-to-dry dressings are given in Procedures 34-1 and 34-2.

Wound Support

Supporting the wound area and preventing stress and tension on the incision helps promote healing.

Butterflies and Steristrips. Butterflies and Steristrips are applied to wounds to approximate wound edges and promote healing. A butterfly is a type of adhesive strip shaped like a butterfly. One edge is adhered to the skin and the other edge is pulled until wound approximation is achieved; then the other adhesive side is adhered to the skin. On small wounds, a butterfly may eliminate the need for sutures. Steristrips are commercially prepared adhesive strips used for the same purpose. They come in different widths. Tincture of benzoin may be sprayed on the skin before application to help them stick longer.

Sutures and Staples. In a surgical incision, the support is provided by using sutures, surgical staples, or surgical clips to hold the incision together until healing occurs. The type of material used for wound closure affects wound healing.

Suture, the material used to sew an incision together, can be absorbable (e.g., catgut or chromic) or nonabsorbable (e.g., nylon, silk, or polypropylene). The type of suture used depends on the size and location of the wound, how strong the suture material needs to be, the desired cosmetic effect, and the surgeon's preference. Generally, the least amount of suture and the smallest size of suture results in optimal wound closure.

Skin staples are made of stainless steel and are minimally reactive to the body as a foreign substance. Often when skin staples are used, absorbable sutures are used to close viscera and underlying tissue layers. Staples decrease the risk of infection and reduce tissue handling because they allow faster wound closure. Larger stainless-steel clips may also be used to approximate wound edges.

Sutures, staples, or clips are inspected when the dressing is changed or routinely if a transparent dressing is used. The physician determines how long they must remain in place. Sutures are usually removed 7 to 10 days after surgery, if wound edges are well approximated and healing appears normal. Skin staples may be removed sooner, but larger retention sutures may remain in place for a longer time. Sometimes the physician orders the removal of every other staple or suture, to ensure that adequate healing has occurred and to avoid dehiscence. Most surgical patients also have absorbable sutures in place holding deeper layers of tissue or fascia together.

Staples are removed with a staple remover (Fig. 34-10A). It is inserted under each staple and the handle is compressed. The pressure causes the staple to bend in the middle, and the edges pop out of the skin. The patient may experience minor discomfort as the staples are removed. Steristrips are usually applied after the staples are removed to support the wound until healing is more complete.

Sutures are removed with a forceps and scissors. The suture is cut close to the skin, and the forceps is used to remove the suture (Fig. 34-10B). Care must be taken to avoid pulling the visible portion of the suture through underlying tissue, since this can contaminate the incisional area and contribute to an infection. Sutures may be intermittent or continuous, and the nurse must discern the suturing technique before removing the sutures. As with staples, Steristrips are often applied after suture removal.

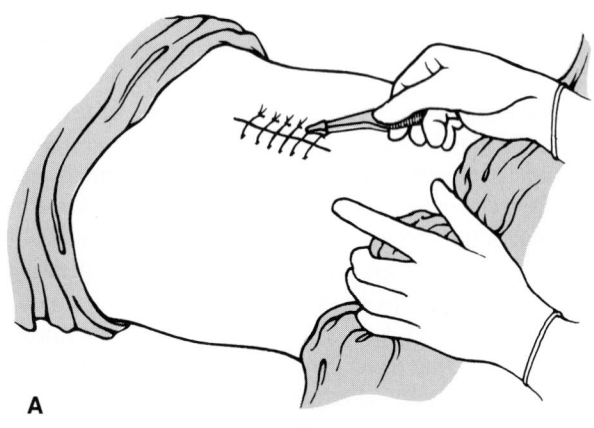

A

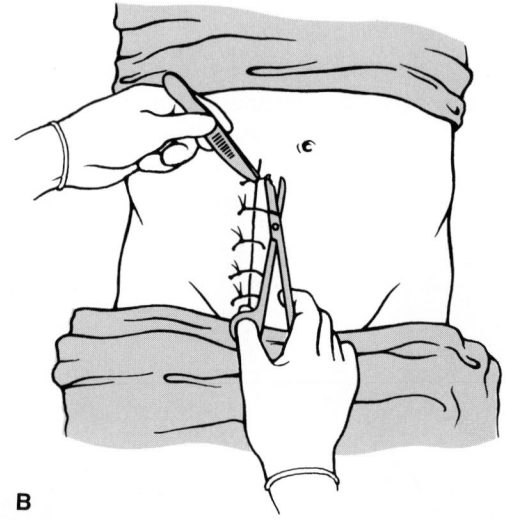

B

Figure 34–10. **A.** Staples are removed by inserting a staple remover under each staple and compressing the handle, causing the staple to bend in the middle. **B.** To remove a suture, cut close to the skin and use forceps to pull through, taking care to avoid pulling the visible part of the suture through underlying tissue.

PROCEDURE 34–1. Changing a Dry Sterile Dressing

■ **Purpose**

1. Protect wound from trauma and external contamination.
2. Provide opportunity to assess the wound.
3. Provide a dry environment for wound healing.

■ **Assessment**

- Assess location and degree of pain. Medicate if necessary.
- Assess for presence of generalized symptoms of infection (i.e., elevated temperature, leukocytosis, diaphoresis).
- Assess dressing for drainage. Observe bedclothes and linen for drainage.
- Review medical history and identify factors that may contibute to delayed wound healing (i.e., poor nutritional status, age, obesity, immunosuppressive therapy, disorders such as anemia or diabetes mellitus).
- Assess patient's ability to cooperate during procedure. Arrange for assistant if necessary to ensure patient's safety during procedure.
- Note patient allergies to tape or dressing materials.

■ **Equipment**

Clean gloves, sterile gloves.
Sterile, prepackaged dressing(s).
Sterile towel.
Clean, flat work surface.
Tape (micropore or paper).
Montgomery straps (optional).
Disposable suture-removal set for scissors and forceps (optional).
Cleansing solution as ordered, applicator.
Plastic bag.

■ **Procedure**

1. Close patient's door or close curtains around bed. Explain procedure to patient.
2. Position patient comfortably. Expose only wound area.
   Rationale: Provides safety, privacy, and comfort.
3. Wash your hands.
   Rationale: Handwashing helps prevent spread of microorganisms.
4. Make a cuff on top of plastic bag and place within easy reach of dressing table.
   Rationale: Cuff allows contaminated dressing to be easily contained without contaminating outside of bag.
5. Put on clean disposable gloves.
   Rationale: Gloves protect nurse from becoming contaminated by wound drainage.

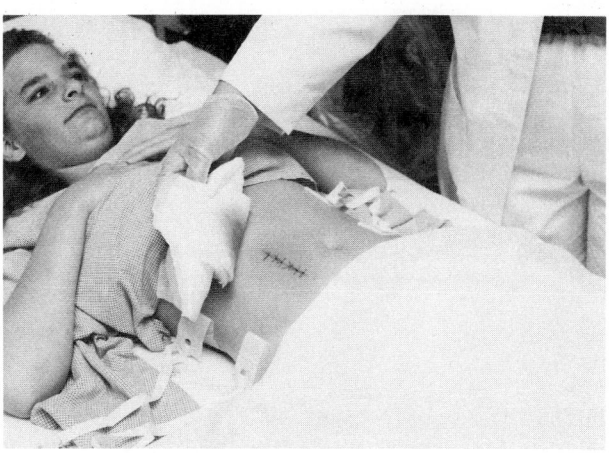

Step 6

6. Remove dressing from wound and discard into plastic bag.
   Note: If dressing adheres to wound, pour a small amount of sterile saline on the wound to loosen the dressing, to prevent disruption of healing tissue.
7. Dispose of gloves. Wash your hands.
   Rationale: Gloves are contaminated. Handwashing helps prevent spread of microorganisms.
8. Set up sterile supplies. Open sterile towel and hold it by the edges. Place it on a clean, flat surface without contaminating the center of the towel. Open dressing package(s) by peeling paper down to expose dressing. Let it fall onto the sterile field. Open

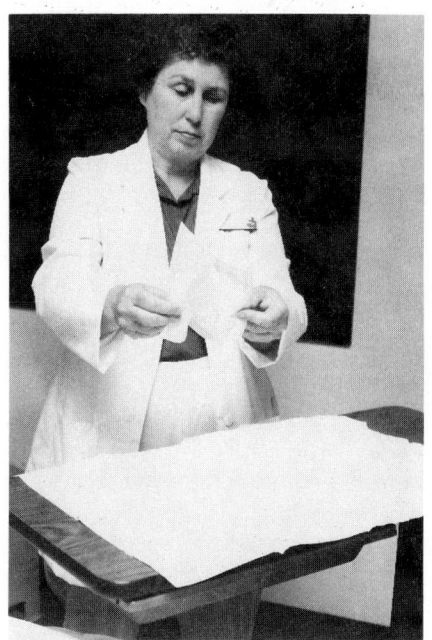

Step 8A

(continued)

PROCEDURE 34–1. Changing a Dry Sterile Dressing (continued)

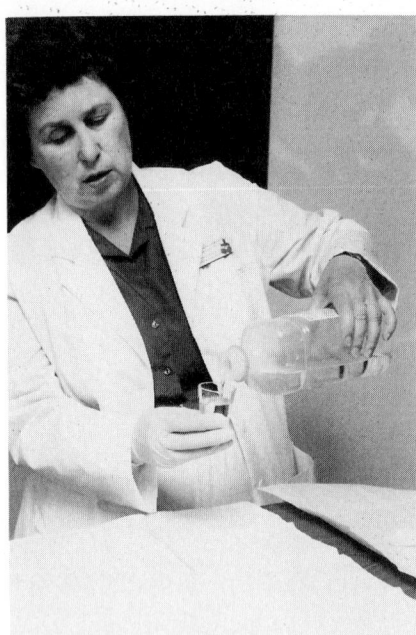

Step 8B

cleansing solution container and applicator packages. Set them at the side of the sterile field.
Rationale: Setting up sterile supplies after removing and discarding the soiled dressing allows the nurse to assess what dressing material is needed and to make changes if necessary without charging the patient for unneeded supplies.
Optional: Instead of using the sterile towel as a sterile field, the nurse may open the dressing packages and suture set carefully, allowing the inside of the packaging material to serve as the sterile field.
9. Don sterile gloves. Grasp applicators at nonabsorbent end and dip them into the cleansing solution.

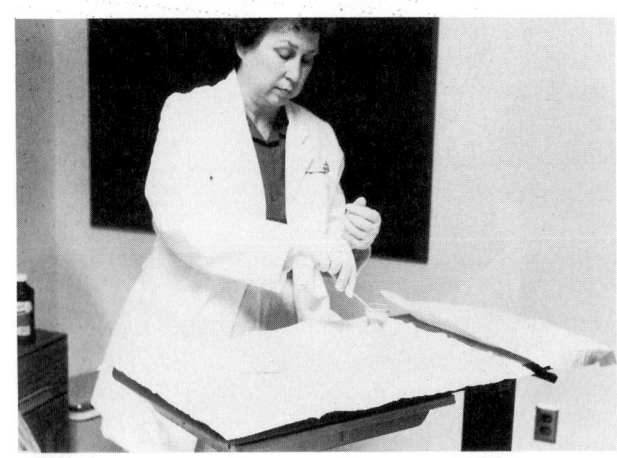

Step 9

10. Clean drainage from the wound with strokes moving from the top toward the bottom of the wound, or from the outside toward the center. Use each applicator once and discard it. Do not place it back into the cleansing solution.
Rationale: Cleansing from the least contaminated toward the most contaminated areas prevents spreading microorganisms throughout the wound. Using applicators only once prevents the transfer of microbes into the cleansing solution container.

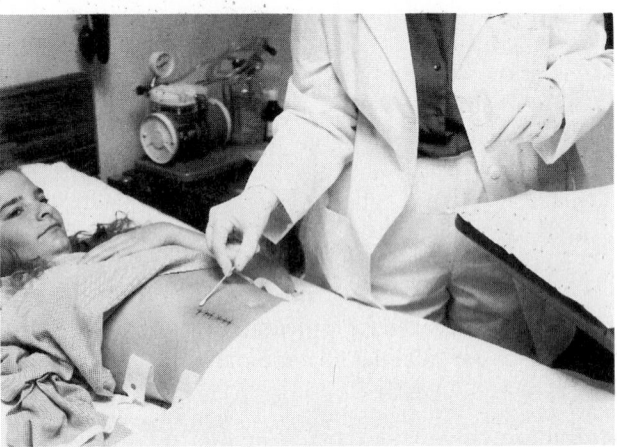

Step 10

11. Dry the wound with gauze held by forceps.
Rationale: Microorganisms grow well in dark, moist environments.
12. Inspect the incision for bleeding, inflammation, drainage, and healing. Note any areas of dehiscence (opening or gaping of wound edges).
Rationale: Inadequate healing or complications must be noted and treated immediately.
13. Apply sterile dressings one at a time over the wound.

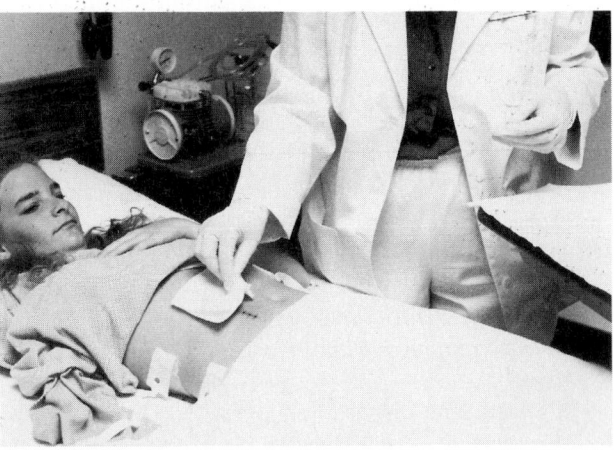

Step 13A

(continued)

PROCEDURE 34–1. Changing a Dry Sterile Dressing (continued)

Rationale: Prevents introduction of microorganisms into the wound.

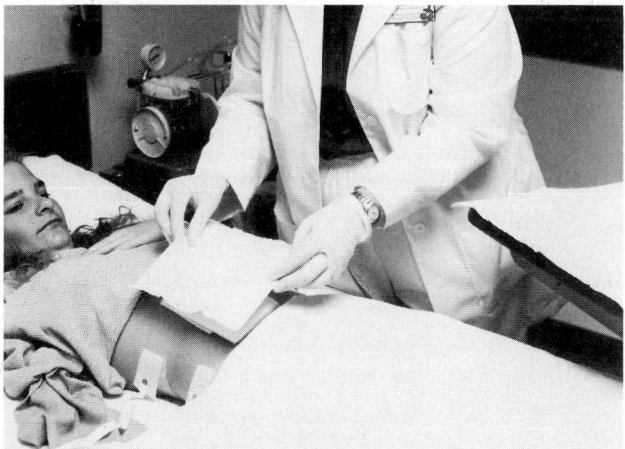

Step 13B

14. Secure the dressing with tape or Montgomery straps.

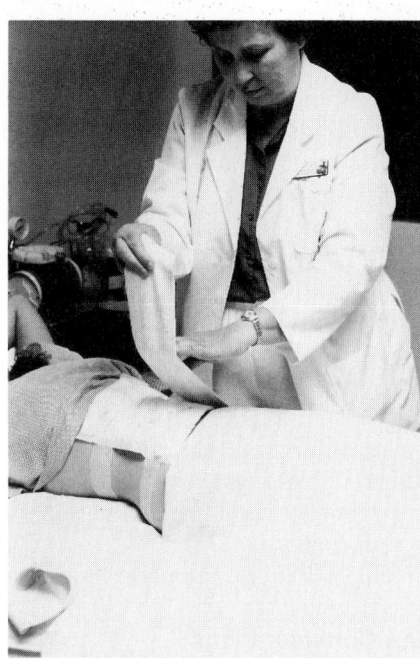

Step 14

15. Wash your hands.
    Rationale: Prevents spread of microorganisms.
16. Document procedure and observations.

■ Lifespan Considerations

Children

• Young children need to be reminded not to touch the incision when their dressing is removed. An assistant may be needed to prevent the child from moving and contaminating the wound or the sterile field.
• Preschool and young school-age children may feel that the part of their body covered by a dressing is not there. It reassures them to set the body part. Allow them to see their incision if they are interested.
• If the child is not toilet-trained and the dressing becomes wet with urine or feces, change the dressing. Consider using wide plastic tape over the dressing to keep it dry.

Older Adult

• As skin ages, it loses its elasticity and becomes more sensitive. Adhesive tape may tear the skin. Paper tape or Montgomery straps are more protective.

■ Home Care Modifications

When a patient needs to change dressings at home instruct him or her:

• That handwashing before and after the dressing change is the most important aspect of maintaining asepsis. For some dressings gloving is not required.
• Where to buy and how to open and use dressings.
• How to clean the wound and which antiseptic to use.
• Signs of infection that indicate the need to call the nurse or physician.

Bandages. **Bandages** are used to support the wound area, secure dressings or splints, apply pressure as necessary to promote hemostasis or minimize edema, and immobilize an area. They are available in various sizes and in materials such as gauze, Kling (a gauze that stretches and molds to the body), elasticized material (e.g., Ace bandage), muslin, or flannel. Gauze bandages are inexpensive and practical for wrapping areas of the body such as the fingers, hands, feet, arms, and legs. Elasticized material is used when pressure is required to promote hemostasis or decrease edema.

For ease in application, bandages usually come in

PROCEDURE 34–2. Applying Wet-to-Dry Dressings

■ Purpose
1. Debride the wound.
2. Promote healing.
3. Protect the wound from contamination and mechanical trauma.

■ Assessment
- Review the physician's orders for type and strength of solution to be used and frequency of dressing changes.
- Assess location and size of wound to determine needed dressing supplies.
- Assess patient's level of comfort. Give analgesics as needed before wound care.
- Review nursing notes for previous wound description and for presence of generalized symptoms of infection (i.e., elevated temperature, leukocytosis).

■ Equipment
Clean disposable gloves.
Sterile gloves.
Sterile dressing instrument set (forceps, scissors).
Sterile thin-mesh gauze dressing.
Sterile gauze dressings.
Extra sterile gauze dressings or ABD pads.
Sterile basin.
Prescribed sterile solution.
Sterile saline.
Tape or ties.
Waterproof disposal bag.
Sterile cotton-tipped applicators (optional).
Sterile drape (optional for sterile field).

■ Procedure
1. Prepare patient and remove dressing according to steps 1–5 of Procedure 34-1.
   Note: Forceps may be used to remove a soiled dressing. If dressing adheres to underlying tissues, do not moisten it. Gently remove the dressing while assessing patient's discomfort level.
   Rationale: Dressing removal is intended to debride exudate and necrotic tissue from the wound. Moistening the dressing impairs the debridement process.

2. Observe dressings for amount and characteristics of drainage.
3. Observe wound for eschar (thick layer of dead cells and dried plasma), granulation tissue (reddish capillary loops that bleed easily), or epithelial skin buds.
   Rationale: Assessment of wound for healing.
4. Prepare sterile supplies. Open sterile instruments, sterile basin, solution, and dressings.
5. Place fine-mesh gauze into basin and pour the ordered solution over mesh to saturate.
   Rationale: Gauze touching the wound surface must be thoroughly moistened to increase its absorptive ability.
   Note: If the wound is very large, warm the ordered solution to body temperature to prevent excessive loss of body heat.
6. Don sterile gloves.
   Rationale: Prevents contamination of wound or supplies with microorganisms. Protects nurse from contamination from body fluids.
7. Cleanse wound with antiseptic solution as prescribed or with normal saline, moving from least to most contaminated areas.
   Rationale: Assists cleansing of debris from wound.
8. Gently pack moistened gauze into the wound. If wound is deep, use forceps or cotton-tipped applicators to press gauze into all wound surfaces.
   Rationale: Moist gauze absorbs drainage and adheres to necrotic debris as it dries.
9. Apply several dry, sterile 4 × 4's over the wet gauze.
   Rationale: Absorbs excess moisture from under dressings.
10. Place ABD pad over dry 4 × 4's.
    Rationale: Protects wound from contamination.
11. Dispose of sterile gloves.
12. Secure dressings with tape, Kerlix gauze (for circumferential dressings), or Montgomery ties.
13. Assist patient to a comfortable position.
14. Wash your hands.
15. Document procedure and observations.

■ Lifespan Considerations and Home Care Modifications
See Procedure 34-1.

---

rolls. One hand is used to hold the free end of the bandage in place until it is anchored, while the other hand slowly unrolls the needed length of bandage as it is smoothly applied to the area.

Bandages may be applied using different techniques, depending on the site (Fig. 34-11):

Circular turns anchor bandages in place by overlapping the previous bandage turn completely.
Spiral turns are used to cover cylindrical body parts such as the wrist or arm, ascending the body part by overlapping the previous turn by one-half or two-thirds the width of the bandage.

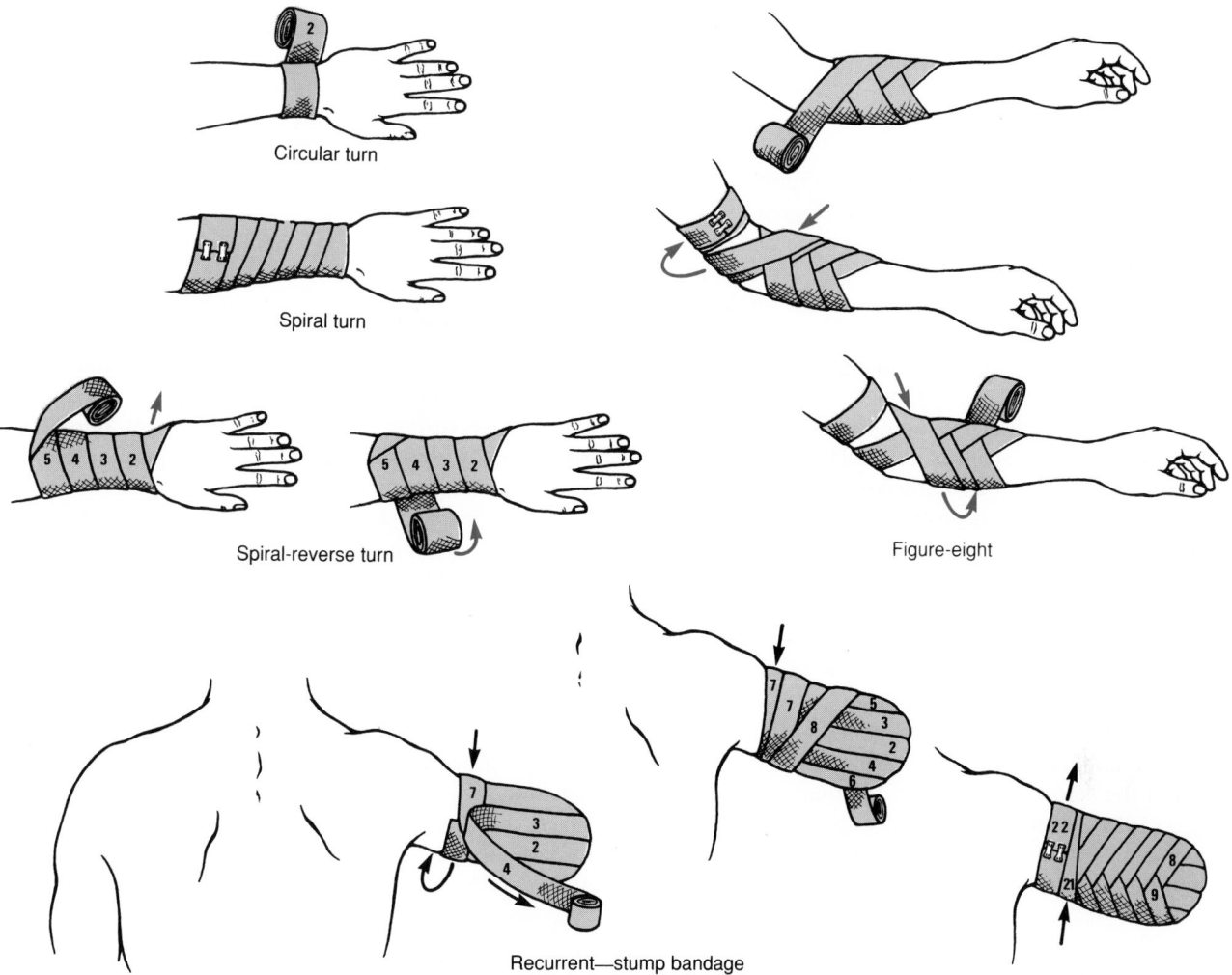

Circular turn

Spiral turn

Spiral-reverse turn

Figure-eight

Recurrent—stump bandage

Figure 34-11.   Techniques for bandage application.

Spiral reverse turns, useful when bandaging the leg, thigh, or forearm, require a twist that reverses the bandaging direction halfway through each turn.

Figure-eight turns consist of overlapping, alternating ascending and descending oblique turns that resemble a figure eight. This technique is especially useful when bandaging a joint.

Recurrent or stump bandaging is used for the head, digits, or amputated limbs. The bandage is anchored with a few circular turns, then turned back over itself, repeating until the distal end of the body part is covered. Once the end is covered, the bandage is anchored by using figure-eight and circular turns.

To promote healing and prevent discomfort, a bandage must be applied correctly. Bandages should be applied snugly, but never so tightly that circulation is impeded or pain occurs. Even tension should be exerted as the bandage is applied. Uneven overlapping of turns or exposed skin should be avoided to prevent undue pressure on tissues. When possible, bandages should be applied with the body part in its normal position. When bandaging an extremity, start bandaging at the distal end

to decrease the chance of edema or circulatory impairment. Soiled bandages should be changed, since bandages can harbor organisms that can cause infection. Friction between skin surfaces can be prevented by padding susceptible areas with gauze or cotton. Bandages are fastened in place with tape, metal clips, or safety pins. Knots, ties, or pins should be located away from the skin to avoid creating areas of localized pressure.

Frequent assessment of body parts distal from the bandage site (e.g., fingers, toes) is important to detect impaired circulation promptly. Cyanosis, pallor, coolness, numbness, tingling, swelling, or absent or diminished pulses are signs that circulation may be decreased. Many bandages are routinely removed so that the area can be inspected and areas of pressure avoided. If a bandage was applied by a physician or during surgery, the nurse may need an order before removing or adjusting it.

Binders.   **Binders** are used to support a specific body part or to hold dressings in place. The use of Velcro in binders has increased their ease of application and comfort. Velcro fasteners permit individualized adjustments and securely fasten the binder in place, while permitting quick and easy release. Binders come in different shapes and sizes depending on the area for use. The binders most commonly used for support are abdominal binders, T-binders, and slings (Fig. 34-12).

An *abdominal binder* is used to support the torso, especially after abdominal surgery (Fig. 34-13). It is usually a straight piece of elastic fabric, 15 to 20 cm wide and long enough to go around the torso. Newer versions have Velcro fasteners; previously, cloth binders were fastened with pins.

A *many-tailed* or *scultetus binder* once was commonly used to support the abdomen, but it is used infrequently today. This binder is a rectangular piece of cloth with a fringe of 5-cm-wide strips of cloth. The rectangular section is placed under the supine patient's lower back and the tails are firmly criss-crossed, starting from the hip. When the last tail is in place, it is fastened with a safety pin or tucked under other tails to prevent slipping.

A *T-binder* is used to secure dressings after surgery on the perineal or rectal area. T-binders are made of cloth and are shaped like the letter T. The top of the T fits around the patient's waist, and the tail is brought between the legs until it can be fastened at the waist. The male T-binder is split so that the tail of the T can easily fit around the scrotum and penis. Padding against tender areas of the perineum may be necessary. Wound drainage may be frequent, and the T-binder must be changed when it becomes soiled.

A *sling* is used to support the arm, usually after trauma or injury. Commercially manufactured slings use Velcro for fastening and adjustments. If a commercial sling is unavailable, a triangular piece of cloth can be placed under the bent arm and folded as necessary to create a proper support. The sling is tied to the side of the neck so that the knot does not press against the cervical vertebrae.

Drainage Management

A large amount of wound drainage can inhibit wound healing and impair skin integrity around the wound. Nurses are responsible for promoting optimal wound drainage by ensuring that drainage systems function properly and by advancing or removing drains as ordered by the physician. Nurses also protect skin from irritation by changing dressings frequently when caustic drainage is present.

Drains must be patent to remove drainage from the wound effectively. Patients should be prevented from lying on drainage systems because this can kink or compress the drain, thereby obstructing drainage flow. Some drains are sutured in place, but others are not, so care must be taken not to remove a drain accidentally. When the patient ambulates, the drainage system is pinned to the patient's gown; this avoids placing excessive tension on the drainage system and incisional area, especially when the system is full of drainage. Preventing tension on the drainage system also decreases patient discomfort.

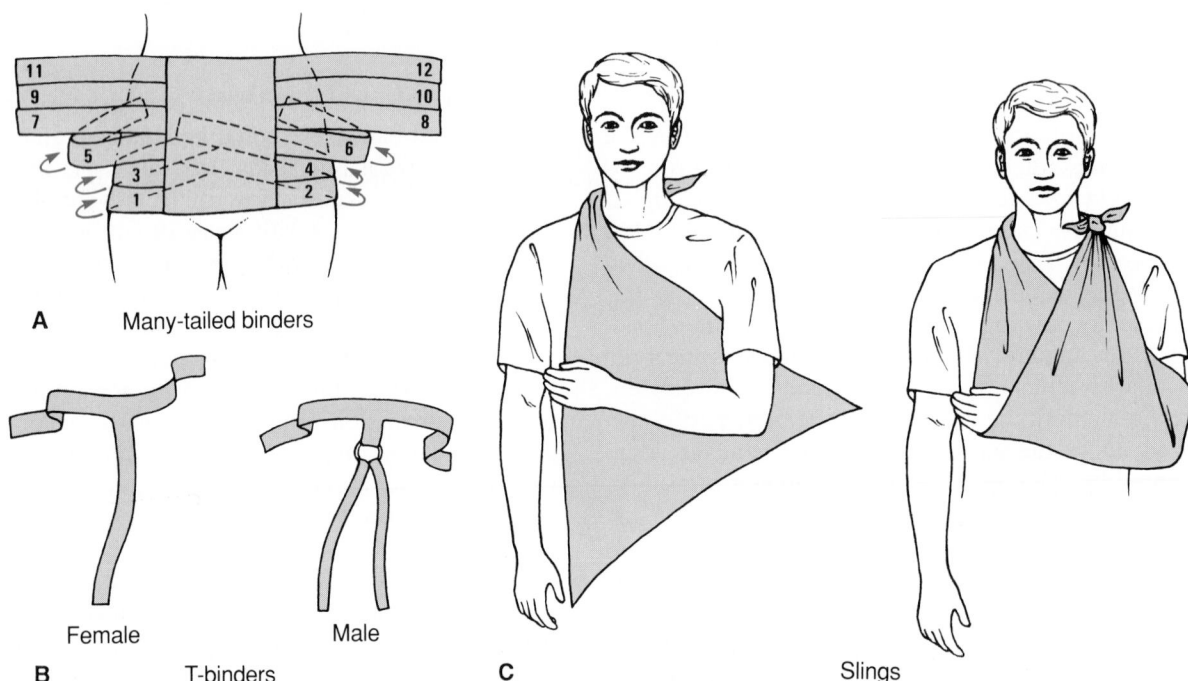

A Many-tailed binders

Female   Male

B T-binders

C Slings

Figure 34–12. Binder application. **A.** Many-tailed. Criss-cross tails starting at the hip. **B.** T-binder. Bring tail or tails through the legs and attach at the waist. **C.** Sling. Fold a triangular cloth and tie it at the side of the neck to prevent vertebral pressure.

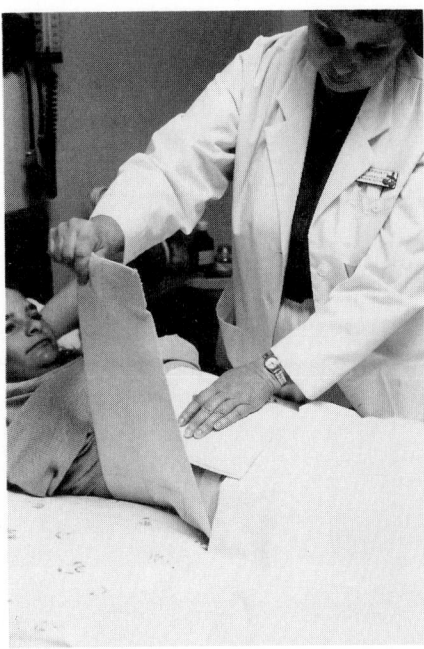

Figure 34–13.   Abdominal binder. Pull tight and fasten Velcro.

Closed Drainage Systems. Appropriate suction permits drainage to be evacuated from the wound. If the drain is attached to external suction, check that the prescribed amount of suction is registered on the suction source. When the attachment tube is disconnected, suction should be apparent.

When closed drainage systems (such as the Hemovac or Jackson-Pratt) are used, suction is usually maintained by compression of a spring or bulb. Refer to Procedure 34-3. Specific instructions accompany drainage systems and should be consulted before handling. When most drainage systems expand fully, gentle suction is no longer available to assist drainage flow. This can occur if there is a leak in the system or if the collection container is full of drainage. *Recharging* (reactivating the suction) is done by opening the appropriate port, emptying drainage if necessary, and compressing the spring or bulb while closing the port (Fig. 34-14) The nurse should wear gloves during this procedure since contact with drainage can occur. Routinely, drainage is emptied and measured at the end of each shift and the drainage system is recharged. If the system stays compressed for only a short time, it usually indicates a leak in the system, and external system pieces may need to be exchanged.

Advancing and Removing Drains. In many hospitals, nurses are responsible for advancing or removing drains, as ordered by the physician. Usually drains are advanced or removed when little drainage is being discharged. Advancing a drain allows evacuation of drainage from different areas of a wound without the need for more than one drainage tube.

To advance or shorten a drain, any sutures holding the drain in place must first be removed. Sterility must be maintained, so sterile forceps or sterile gloves are used as the drain is advanced. When shortening a Penrose drain, a sterile safety pin is attached to the end of the drain (Fig. 34-15). This helps to prevent inadvertent loss of the drain back into the wound. Any excess part of the drain is cut off with scissors. Advancing some drains can cause the patient discomfort. This can be minimized by asking the patient to breathe deeply as the drain is pulled and by premedicating the patient. After drain advancement or removal, increased drainage can be expected for a short time.

Wound Debridement, Irrigation, and Packing

When wounds are healing by second intention, debridement, packing, and irrigation may be necessary to promote wound healing.

Debridement. **Debridement** is the removal of foreign material or dead tissue from a wound to discourage the growth of microorganisms and to promote wound healing. Surgical debridement is performed by a physician in the operating room or at the bedside. Foreign matter

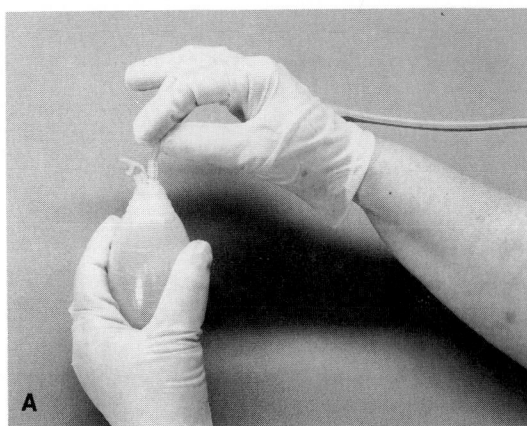

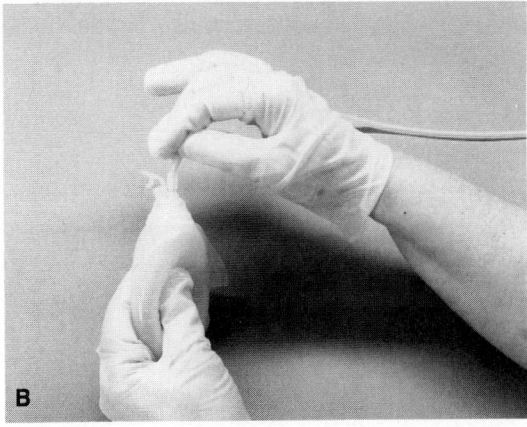

Figure 34–14.   Recharging a Jackson-Pratt drainage system. Also see Procedure 34–3, Step 7.

PROCEDURE 34–3. Maintaining a Portable (Hemovac) Wound Suction

■ **Purpose**

1. Facilitate healing by removing drainage from the incisional area where granulating tissue is forming.

■ **Assessment**

• Assess patient for generalized signs of infection (i.e., elevated temperature).
• Assess drainage for amount, color, clarity, and odor.
• Assess the patient for inflammation or discomfort around the drain.

■ **Equipment**

Clean disposable gloves.
Calibrated drainage receptacle.

■ **Procedure**

1. Explain procedure, assist patient to a comfortable position, pull curtains or close door.
2. Wash your hands. Don clean disposable gloves.
   Rationale: Prevents transfer of microorganisms.
3. Expose Hemovac tubing and container while keeping patient draped.
   Rationale: Provides for privacy and warmth.
4. Examine tubing and container for patency and suction seal.
   Note: If the system's seal is broken, the Hemovac reservoir will be expanded and not compressed.
5. Open the drainage plug (it is labeled).
6. Pour drainage into a calibrated receptacle without contaminating the drainage spout.
   Rationale: Prevents transfer of microorganisms to the wound.
7. Reestablish suction by placing reservoir on a firm, flat surface. With drainage plug open, compress the unit and reinsert drainage plug.
   Rationale: Establishes a closed drainage system with suction.

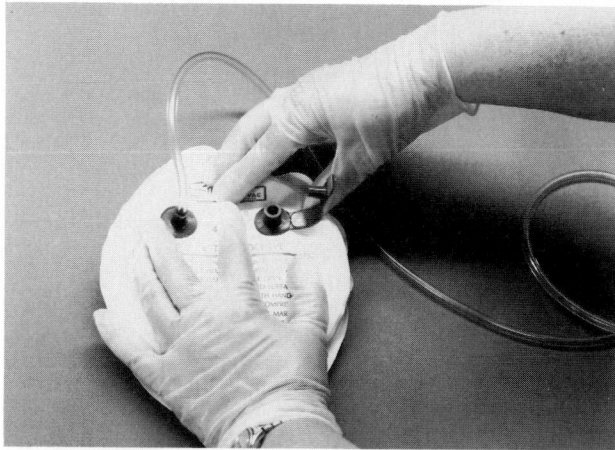
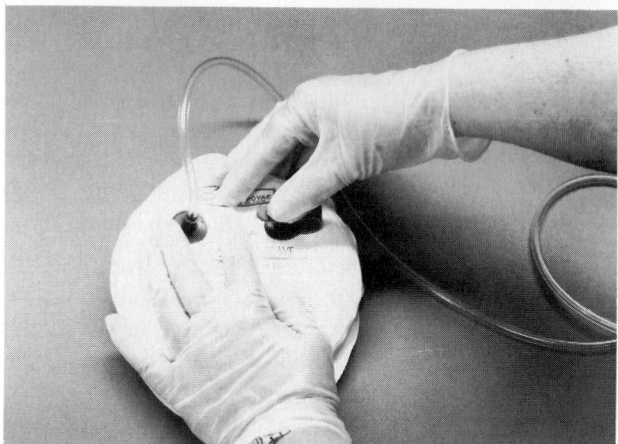

Step 7

8. Remove and discard gloves.
9. Return patient to a comfortable postion.
10. Measure drainage and record amount, color, and any other pertinent information.

---

may be cut from the wound or flushed with saline or hydrogen peroxide (H_2O_2). Hydrogen peroxide oxidizes protein, which causes the foaming that occurs when hydrogen peroxide comes in contact with dead tissue. Hydrogen peroxide should always be diluted to half strength before use, since at full strength it can irritate tissues and can cause serious side effects, especially if used in deep, semiclosed wounds (Bassam & Dudai, 1982).

Wet-to-dry dressings may be ordered to help debride a wound. Moist dressings are applied to a wound and permitted to dry before they are removed. The dried dressings adhere to foreign matter and dead tissue, which are then pulled away from the wound as the dressing is removed.

Wet-to-dry dressings are usually changed every 4 to 8 hours, depending on how long it takes the premoistened gauze pads to dry (see Procedure 34-2).

Irrigation. **Irrigation** involves flushing a wound with a solution to clean out exudate or debris. Irrigation is most commonly used when the open wound is infected or deep. Various sterile solutions such as normal saline, hydrogen peroxide, povidone–iodine, or antibiotic solutions can be used. A large Asepto (cone-shaped) syringe or a catheter is used to direct the fluid over the appropriate area, and a basin is used to collect fluid as it flows from the wound. Since splashing may occur, goggles and

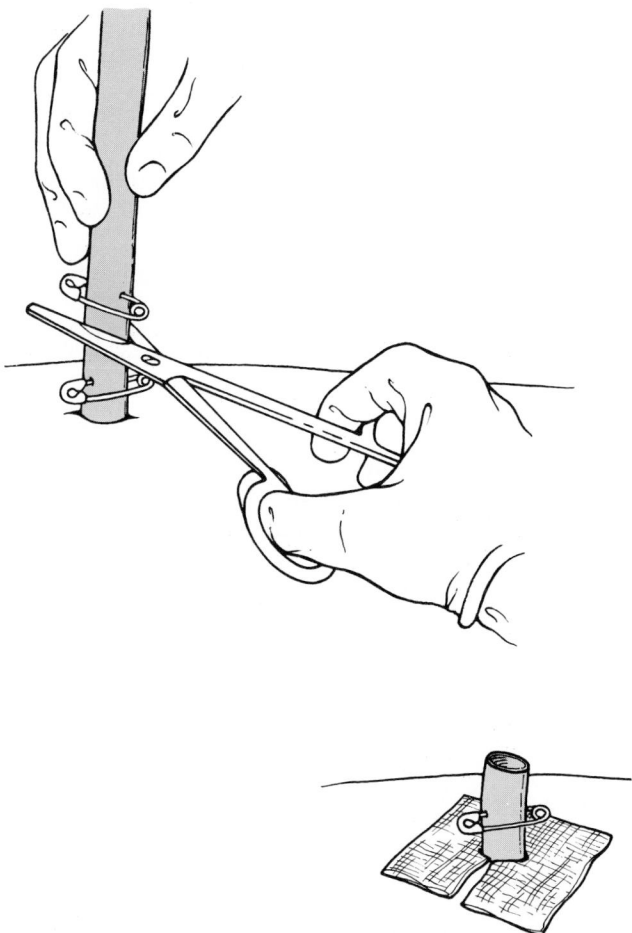

Figure 34–15. To advance a Penrose drain, don sterile gloves and remove any sutures. With sterile forceps, carefully advance the drain the appropriate length and attach a second sterile safety pin to prevent inadvertent loss back into the wound. Cut between the pins. Place a gauze square around the drain to absorb drainage and protect skin integrity.

protective barriers should be used to prevent contamination. Procedure 34-4 describes how to irrigate a wound.

Packing. Sterile packing can be inserted into an infected wound or an open wound that has the potential for infection. Packing prevents the wound from closing prematurely, which could lead to microorganism growth and abscess formation. Packing is commercially prepared in long, thin strips. Usually plain gauze packing is used, but gauze impregnated with iodophor, petrolatum, or povidone–iodine is also available. A sterile cotton applicator is used to insert packing into the wound as deeply as possible until the wound is fully packed.

Packing may also be used after surgery on areas of the body that are hard to suture (e.g., vagina, nasal septum) to apply pressure and prevent blood loss from small capillaries. When packing has been inserted during surgery, this should be noted on the patient's record so that it is not accidentally removed when the dressing is changed. Pressure packing is usually left in place for 2 or 3 days and then removed by the surgeon or by the nurse with a physician's order, so that it does not become a reservoir for the growth of microorganisms.

Local Application of Heat and Cold

Heat and cold can be used as therapeutic interventions to promote healing (Table 34-5).

Cold therapies are usually used early in wound management to control hemorrhage, edema, and pain. Cold is used to control local bleeding because it causes vasoconstriction, which decreases blood flow to the area. Cold helps control swelling by reducing the permeability of capillary walls and the escape of extracellular fluids.

Heat therapies are used to increase blood flow, resolve inflammation, improve healing of soft tissues, and relieve muscular pain and stiffness. Local heat causes vasodilation, increasing the supply of oxygen, nutrients, leukocytes, and antibodies to the tissues. The increased blood flow also promotes removal of metabolic wastes and dissipation of heat. Heat increases the local cellular metabolic processes, which in turn increases the demand for more oxygen. As a result of this activity, increased healing of soft tissues occurs. The inflammatory process is also accelerated when heat is applied because heat reduces the viscosity of blood. This allows leukocytes and antibodies to reach the infected area more quickly.

Safety Alert

- Monitor patients with decreased sensation to skin surfaces closely when using heating pads or hot water. Thermal burns may result from impaired temperature perception.
- Never use the high setting on heating pads or other heating units. During use, inspect the skin frequently for signs of thermal damage.
- Move and position the immobile patient carefully to prevent injury to the skin as a result of shearing force.
- Monitor postoperative wounds carefully and prevent undue stress to the wound by supporting the wound during coughing or vomiting.
- Monitor toddlers and preschoolers around hot liquids, cigarettes, heaters, barbecue grills, and stoves to prevent thermal burns.

PROCEDURE 34–4. Irrigating a Wound

■ **Purpose**
1. Cleanse the wound.
2. Instill medication into the wound.
3. Promote wound healing.

■ **Assessment**
• Review physician's orders for type and strength of solution to be used for irrigation.
• Assess location and size of wound to determine needed dressing supplies.
• Assess patient's comfort level. Give analgesics as needed before wound care.
• Assess for symptoms of anxiety.
• Review chart for presence of generalized symptoms of infection (i.e., elevated temperature, leukocytosis).

■ **Equipment**
Sterile dressing instrument set and dressing materials as in Procedure 34-2.
Sterile gloves.
Sterile basin.
Mask, goggles, and gown may be indicated to protect nurse's eyes, mouth, and uniform from splatter.
Clean basin to collect contaminated irrigating solution.
Prescribed irrigating solution warmed to body temperature.
Sterile irrigating solution.
Sterile Robinson catheter (optional for deep wounds).
Waterproof disposal bag.
Waterproof underpad.

■ **Procedure**
1. Close door or curtains around bed. Explain procedure to patient.
2. Position patient comfortably to allow irrigating solution to flow by gravity across the wound and into a collection basin.
   Rationale: Solution must flow from least contaminated to most contaminated area. Gravity directs the flow.
3. Expose only the wound area. Place waterproof pad under patient.
   Rationale: Protects linen from spill of irrigating solution.
4. Wash your hands.
   Rationale: Prevents transfer of microorganisms.
5. Don mask, goggles, and gown if needed.
   Rationale: To prevent contamination of nurse's mucous membranes and uniform if splatter from wound irrigation is anticipated.

6. Remove dressing and inspect wound. See steps 1–4 of Procedure 34-2.
7. Pour warmed irrigating solution into sterile basin.
   Rationale: Warmed solution is more comfortable for patient.
8. Open irrigating syringe and place into basin with solution.
9. Place second basin at distal end of wound to catch contaminated irrigating solution.
10. Don sterile gloves.
    Rationale: Maintains surgical asepsis.
11. Fill irrigating syringe with solution. Holding syringe tip about an inch above the wound, gently flush all areas of the wound. Continue flushing until solution draining into basin is clear.
    Rationale: Holding syringe tip above tissue prevents trauma to granulation tissue. Irrigating until clear ensures that all debris and exudate are removed.

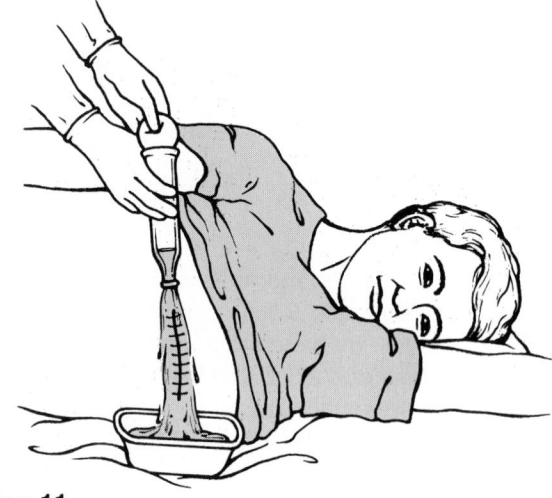

Step 11

12. If the wound is deep, attach a Robinson catheter to filled syringe with irrigating solution. Gently insert catheter into wound and flush until returning solution is clear.
    Rationale: Catheter introduces solution deeper into wound.
    Note: When refilling irrigation syringe with solution, disconnect catheter, fill syringe, and reconnect catheter. This prevents contaminating the basin of solution with microorganisms from the catheter.
13. Dry wound edges and surrounding skin with dry gauze dressings.
    Rationale: Excess moisture on skin promotes growth of microorganisms and skin breakdown.

(continued)

PROCEDURE 34–4. Irrigating a Wound *(continued)*

---

14. Apply sterile dressing.
    Rationale: Provides protective barrier over wound.
15. Remove and discard gloves.
16. Secure dressing with tape or Montgomery straps.
17. Assist patient to a comfortable position.
18. Dispose of equipment.
    Note: Retain remaining bottle of sterile solution for future irrigations. Mark date and time of opening on bottle for reference. Dispose of according to agency policy.
19. Wash your hands.
20. Document procedure and observations.

■ **Lifespan Considerations and Home Care Modifications**
Refer to Procedure 34-1.

Heat increases **suppuration** by allowing pus to consolidate in infected areas. Heat also promotes muscular relaxation and relieves muscular tension and spasms and joint stiffness. A disadvantage of local heat is that increased capillary permeability can increase edema formation.

Safety Considerations. Patient safety is an important consideration when using heat or cold, because they can damage tissues or alter thermoregulation. Table 34-6 lists precautions for the safe use of heat and cold.

The duration of application is important. Maximum vasodilation or vasoconstriction usually occurs in 30 min-

TABLE 34–5

Uses for Heat and Cold

Effect	Physiologic Mechanism	Selected Uses
Heat Application		
Promotes healing and suppuration (consolidation of pus)	Vasodilation leads to increased blood flow, thus increasing oxygen and nutrients to the area and promoting removal of waste products	Surgical wounds, infected wounds, hemorrhoids, episiotomies
Decreases inflammation by accelerating inflammatory process	Increases capillary wall permeability, increases leukocyte and antibody flow to area, promotes action of phagocytes	Phlebitis, IV infiltration
Decreases musculoskeletal discomfort	Increases sensory nerve conduction, promotes muscle relaxation, decreases viscosity of synovial fluid	Low back pain, menstrual cramps, contractures, arthritis, muscle spasms
Cold Application		
Controls bleeding	Vasoconstriction decreases blood flow, which in turn decreases metabolic tissue demands as well as the supply of oxygen and nutrients	Fractures, trauma, superficial lacerations, puncture wounds
Decreases edema	Decreases capillary permeability, vasoconstriction	Sprains, muscle strains, sports injuries
Relieves pain	Decreases nerve conduction velocity, induces numbness or paresthesia	Arthritis, trauma, musculoskeletal injuries

utes, and prolonged application may result in burns or freezing. Very young or elderly patients have a decreased ability to tolerate heat and cold and are more likely to suffer adverse effects. Impaired circulation, impaired sensation, or impaired cognitive abilities also increase the incidence of injury. Body areas where heat or cold therapy is used can be more or less sensitive, depending on the sensitivity and thickness of skin. Impaired skin integrity increases the chance that heat or cold application could damage tissues.

Extensive exposure to heat or cold can have systemic as well as local effects. Unexpected adverse effects can occur, especially in high-risk patients such as the very young or elderly. Refer to Chapter 36 for more details.

Cold Packs and Ice Bags. Cold packs and ice bags are used to deliver local dry cold. Commercial cold packs contain an alcohol-based solution that is released inside the bag when it is squeezed or kneaded, creating a cold temperature. The outer covering is soft and pliable, so it can be molded to fit the contours of the body and applied directly to the skin surface. These packs cannot be refrozen. Procedure 34-5 decsribes how to apply a cold pack.

Ice bags come in a variety of sizes and can be used to control localized bleeding, reduce swelling, and reduce pain. Ice bags are made of rubber and have screw-on caps for filling. Some ice bags do not use ice but instead contain a solution that must be frozen; they must be refrozen after each use. Before applying an ice bag, a cloth cover should be applied over the rubber surface to avoid irritating the skin and to maintain medical asepsis.

Cold Compresses. Cold compresses are used to relieve swelling and inflammation. Gauze pads are moistened with chilled saline or water and applied to the appropriate area. If applied to an open wound, sterility must be maintained. Compresses easily conform to the contour of the intended area and can soften exudate. Because cold compresses quickly warm to the temperature of the patient's skin, frequent changing is needed. If left on the wound for a prolonged period, maceration can occur.

Warm Compresses. Warm compresses are generally applied to open wounds to improve circulation and promote suppuration. If an open wound is involved, surgical asepsis principles must be followed, but medical asepsis is sufficient if the compress is applied to intact skin. Compresses mold easily to body contours. Commercially packaged sterile compresses are available that must be heated under an infrared lamp before opening and application. If commercially prepared compresses are unavailable, solution can be warmed and applied to

TABLE 34–6

Precautions for the Safe Use of Heat and Cold

Assessment Factor	Rationale
Acute sudden pain that may indicate abscessed tooth or appendicitis	Application of heat may cause rupture, with systemic spread of infection.
Broken skin or deep open wounds	Subcutaneous and visceral tissues are more sensitive to temperature extremes. Fewer pain and temperature receptors are available to warn of possible tissue damage.
Circulatory impairment (peripheral vascular disease, diabetes)	Cold application vasoconstricts, thus decreasing circulation to the already compromised area. Heat is not dissipated well from the area, making tissue damage more likely.
Sensory deficits (cerebral vascular accident, paraplegia, quadriplegia)	Alterations in nerve conduction limit the sensation of temperature or pain, thus increasing the likelihood of tissue damage.
Mental status impairment (confusion, decreased level of consiousness)	Decreased reliability of reporting pain and altered sensation increases the possibility of tissue damage.
Age extremes	Very young childen have immature thermoregulation, cannot communicate pain or discomfort specifically, and cannot alter their environment. Elderly have reduced sensation to pain and often have another impairment (circulatory, sensory, etc.) that compounds the risk. Heat should not be applied to the abdomen of a pregnant women because fetal growth could be affected.
Metallic implants (pacemakers, total joint replacements)	Metal is a good conductor of heat, thus increasing the potential for burns since the implant cannot be readily removed.

PROCEDURE 34–5. Applying a Cold Pack

■ Purpose
1. Promote capillary vasoconstriction to prevent or decrease edema of traumatized tissue, to control bleeding, or to reduce pain.

■ Assessment
- Identify the purpose for cold therapy.
- Examine the condition of the affected skin or injury.
- Assess sensitivity of affected area to temperature and touch to determine if patient has impaired sensation to cold.
- Determine baseline level of pain.
- Obtain baseline vital signs and assess patient's ability to tolerate cold therapy. (See Lifespan Considerations below).
- Review physician's order for frequency and duration of therapy.
- Assess patient's understanding of procedure.

■ Equipment
Ice bag, collar, and ice or commercially prepared ice pack.
Pillowcase or bath towel.

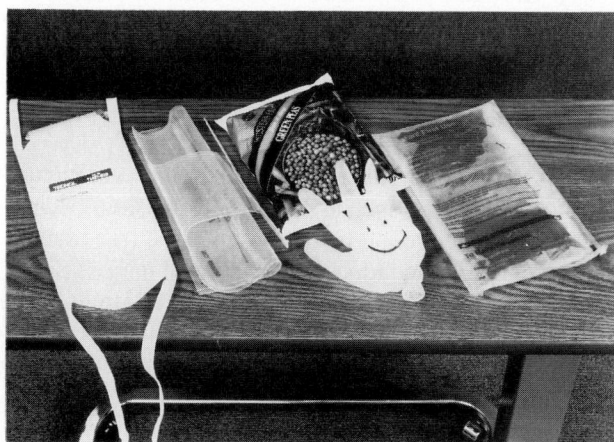

Equipment

■ Procedure
1. Prepare ice pack. Fill bag or collar two-thirds full with crushed ice. Expel excess air from bag and secure cap. Commercial pack must be squeezed or kneaded.
   Rationale: Excess air in ice bag acts as insulation and interferes with cold conduction. Squeezing commercial pack releases alcohol-based solution to activate cold.
2. Place towel or pillowcase over cold pack.
   Rationale: Direct contact of ice pack to skin can cause destruction of skin cells from intense vasoconstriction.

Note: Some commercial packs have an outer insulating wrap and can be applied directly to skin.
3. Close bed curtains or room door.
4. Assist patient to a comfortable position and expose only area to be treated.
   Rationale: Maintains patient privacy and comfort.
5. Apply prepared ice pack to area to be treated. Secure with tape or ties if necessary. Cover patient.
6. Monitor condition of skin after 5 minutes.
   Rationale: Skin should be slightly pale and cool to touch. Cold therapy is too intense if skin surface is blue or mottled.
7. Remove pad after 30 minutes and observe condition of treated skin.
   Rationale: Maximum effect of cold therapy is achieved in 30 to 60 minutes. After 60 minutes, a secondary vasodilation will occur. Wait 1 hour before reapplying.
8. Assist patient to a comfortable position and dispose of ice or commercial pack.
   Rationale: Plastic ice collars and bags are reusable if not soiled. Commercial ice packs cannot be frozen for reuse.

■ Lifespan Considerations

Infants
- Infants lose body heat readily. Ice packs are generally contraindicated because of the potential for loss of core body heat. Cold therapy may be used cautiously on limited areas (i.e., an extremity).

Toddlers and Children
- Increased cooperation and compliance can be achieved if the child thinks of the ice pack as a friendly object. A plastic glove or ice bag with a face marked on it changes it from a treatment to a friend.

Older Adults
- Patients with atherosclerosis may have decreased blood supply to a body part. If cold is applied to an area with decreased circulation, treatment-induced vasoconstriction may causes tissue damage.
- Patients with cardiovascular or pulmonary disease are at risk for fluid overload if cold is applied on a large area or extremity. Cold-induced vasoconstriction shifts blood into the central circulation and may cause heart failure or pulmonary edema. Be alert to the patient's overall circulatory status before applying cold.

Home Care Modifications
- Ice packs are frequently ordered for home use. Assess the patient's or significant other's knowledge of the procedure and safety measures. Educate as necessary.

gauze pads. Avoid using temperatures that might cause burns.

The heat of a warm compress dissipates quickly, but heat can be retained longer by applying a layer of plastic over the compress. If a constant warm temperature is desired, the nurse can apply a heating mechanism over the compress (e.g., an aquathermia pad), but because moisture conducts heat the temperature of the heating mechanism must be low.

Warm Soaks. Warm soaks involve immersing a body part in a warm liquid (usually water) to promote relaxation, improve circulation, soften wound exudate, or debride a wound. They can also be used to apply a medicated solution. Warm soaks usually take about 20 minutes, and the solution may need to be changed since cooling may occur. Sterility should be maintained for open wounds.

Sitz Baths. A sitz bath provides moist heat to the pelvic and perineal area. A sitz bath is used after rectal or perineal surgery or after vaginal delivery to decrease inflammation and discomfort.

The patient sits in a special tub or in a basin that fits onto the toilet seat, so the legs and feet remain out of the water. Using a bathtub does not serve the same purpose, since immersing the entire body in warm water nullifies the effect of local heat applied to the pelvic area. The patient's feet and upper torso should remain covered to prevent chilling. The sitz bath is filled with warm water (105°F to 110°F or 40°C to 43°C). A plastic bag with attached tubing is filled with warm water and inserted into the portable sitz bath, where it slowly replenishes warm water during the procedure. Sitz baths usually last for about 20 minutes.

Because heat is being applied to a large area of the body, vasodilation can occur, causing the patient to feel lightheaded and faint. If this occurs, the nurse should assess the patient for a rapid pulse, pale facial color, or complaints of nausea. If these signs and symptoms are present, the sitz bath should be discontinued.

Paraffin Baths. Paraffin baths, a mixture of heated paraffin wax and mineral oil, are used for arthritic patients with painful joints. The treatment is usually given by a physical therapist.

Hot Packs. Dry local heat can be applied with hot-water bottles or K-packs. Hot-water bottles are similar to ice bags, but they are filled two-thirds full with hot water (125°F or 52°C for the normal adult; 110°F or 43°C for a young child or debilitated adult). Make sure the temperature of the water will not burn the patient. Place a cloth covering over the rubber container to avoid irritation to the skin and to maintain medical asepsis. The water should remain warm for 20 to 45 minutes, depending on its initial temperature. Hot-water bottles are used infrequently in hospitals but are common in the home setting.

K-packs or commercial hot packs are disposable, commercially prepared packages that produce specified amounts of heat when squeezed or kneaded. They cannot be reused.

Heating Pads. Although often used at home, heating pads are seldom used in hospitals because of the increased risk of burns. A thermostat controls the amount of heat the unit delivers, and when used in hospitals the unit is often adjusted so that it can operate only on the low setting. When a heating pad is used, the patient should be advised not to lie on the unit or operate it near moisture, since this increases the chance of a burn. A heating pad should not be applied to the skin for longer than 20 to 30 minutes at any one time.

Aquathermia Pads. An aquathermia (water flow) pad is a popular heat-producing device used for treating muscle sprains and mild inflammation. This unit consists of a waterproof pad through which water circulates; the temperature of the circulating water can be controlled. The unit is filled two-thirds full of water and should be checked periodically for evaporation. If significant evaporation occurs, the unit must be refilled.

The waterproof pad should not be in direct contact with the patient's skin. It is usually covered with a pillowcase or towel. The pad is positioned over the intended area and left there for 20 to 30 minutes. The patient should not lie on the pad, as pressure prevents normal distribution of the circulating water. Procedure 34-6 describes how to use aquathermia pads.

Heat Lamps. Heat lamps are used to increase circulation to small areas, such as episiotomy incisions or pressure sores. The area to be treated must be free of moisture, which could conduct heat. The heat lamp is placed an appropriate distance away from the treatment area (at least 45 cm), and low-wattage bulbs (40 to 60 watts) are used. The treatment lasts about 20 minutes. During treatment, the patient's skin should be assessed periodically to ensure that no burn occurs.

Heat Cradles. Heat cradles also deliver radiant heat, but they cover a much larger surface area. The cradle contains a row of small (25-watt) bulbs along the top of a dome-shaped device. The bedsheets can be placed over the metal frame to protect the patient's privacy and to prevent cooling from air currents. The patient should be assessed several times during the treatment, because cutaneous vasodilation can occur.

Emotional Support

Skin conditions may cause low self-esteem and altered body image, especially if there is disfigurement or the altered skin function is evident on the face. The patient

PROCEDURE 34–6. Applying Aquathermia Pads

■ Purpose
1. Provide warm dry heat at a constant temperature.
2. Increase circulation and promote healing in localized areas.
3. Reduce edema and inflammation in localized areas.
4. Relieve the discomfort of muscle spasms of sprain.

■ Assessment
- Observe condition of skin area to be covered with aquathermia pad.
- Determine baseline level of discomfort or degree of restricted range of motion, if treatment is for muscle spasms or strain.
- Assess sensitivity in affected area to temperature and touch to determine impaired patient sensation to heat extremes.
- Obtain baseline vital signs.
- Review physician's order for frequency and duration of therapy.
  Note: Temperature is usually determined by hospital policy.
- Assess equipment for fraying of electric cords.
- Assess patient's understanding of procedure.

■ Equipment
Aquathermia unit.
Distilled water.
Pillowcase or bath towel.
Paper tape.

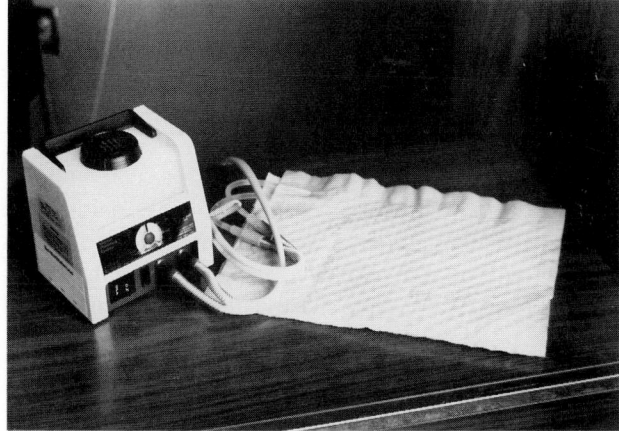

Equipment

■ Procedure
1. Close bed curtains or door.
   Rationale: Provides privacy for patient.

2. Assist patient to a comfortable position and expose area to be treated.
   Note: Patient should never lie directly on heating pad.
   Rationale: Lying on top of heating pad prevents heat from dispersing, increasing the risk of burns.
3. Place aquathermia reservoir on bedside stand. Adjust temperature to below 105°F. Plug into electrical outlet. Turn unit on and observe water level in unit. Refill with distilled water as necessary.
   Rationale: Distilled water has no minerals that could precipitate and damage the unit. Running the unit without water could also damage it.
4. Cover the heating pad with a pillowcase or wrap the treatment area with a towel.
   Rationale: Placing rubber directly against the skin does not allow absorption of perspiration and can cause maceration of the skin.
5. Place pad on affected area and secure with tape if necessary.
   Note: Do not use safety pins; they could puncture the pad and cause a leak.
6. Five minutes after application, monitor skin for erythema.
   Rationale: Prevents a burn or adverse reaction.
7. Remove pad after 20 to 30 minutes and store until next treatment.
   Rationale: Maximum effect of heat application is achieved in 20 to 30 minutes. Capillary vasoconstriction, which counters the healing process, occurs as a secondary effect after 60 minutes of heat application.
8. Wait 1 hour before reapplying.
9. Observe treatment area. Question patient to determine comfort level and assess for improved range of motion, if used on an extremity.
   Rationale: Heat applications stimulate large-diameter sensory nerves and block pain impulses by smaller nerve fibers.
10. Assist patient to a comfortable position.
11. Document procedure.

■ Lifespan Considerations

Infants and Children
- Children under 12 years of age should not be left unsupervised with an electric heating unit because they may accidently burn themselves by turning the gauges on the unit or repositioning themselves on top of the unit.
- Children may not complain of a heat sensation until the treated area is burned.

(continued)

Older Adults
- Elderly patients may have decreased sensitivity to heat, so use extreme care to monitor equipment temperature and prevent burns.
- Elderly patients with decreased subcutaneous fat stores have loss of insulating ability and may complain of discomfort at temperatures that are comfortable to the nurse.

Special Considerations
- Comatose or paralyzed patients have impaired senses. Heating pads are contraindicated because of the increased risk of burns.

- Any patient with decreased sensation (i.e., diabetic neuropathy) must be closely monitored during treatment because of the increased risk of burns.
- Patients receiving analgesics, sedatives, or hypnotics may have altered sensory perceptions and are at increased risk for burns during treatment.

■ **Home Care Modifications**
- Heating pads are often ordered for use at home. Assess patient's or significant other's knowledge of procedure and safety measures. Educate as necessary.

---

may choose isolation over appearing in public. Getting the patient to express feelings about perceived or actual disfigurement is the first step in facing the problem. The nurse, with the patient, can identify appropriate diversional activities. Support people can help the patient work through the isolation. Referrals to appropriate community resources can also be made to help avoid isolation.

Discharge Planning and Home Care

Most skin and wound disorders can be successfully managed at home with appropriate assistance from healthcare personnel. Areas for the nurse to assess include:

- Environmental safety and cleanliness
- Access to needed supplies
- Patient's knowledge of self-care or treatment and ability to perform self-care
- Dietary needs
- Support systems.

A supportive home environment is one that has the human and physical resources needed by the patient. Patients who cannot manage self-care or who have complicated dressing changes or new ostomies are at high risk for potential problems with home management. Such patients may need a referral to community resources.

Pressure-sore prevention is important for all immobile patients who are cared for at home. Caregivers should be taught the importance of frequent turning and proper positioning, proper patient hygiene, and adequate nutrition, in addition to any prescribed dressings or treatments. Support mattresses or beds can be bought or rented for home use to assist with pressure-sore prevention.

Patients who need clean or sterile dressings must demonstrate before discharge the knowledge and ability to

perform wound care. Written instructions that include information on where to buy necessary supplies and equipment should be given at discharge. The family should be involved in wound management instruction. Patients and family members should be taught how to detect infection, including how to monitor the patient's temperature. Family members' acceptance of the skin impairment and their willingness to assist with care boosts the patient's self-esteem.

For some patients, shopping and cooking can be difficult. Family members, neighbors, or agencies such as Meals on Wheels can provide nutritious meals. A clean home environment is necessary to prevent infection. Family members or outside agencies may need to assist with cleaning and laundry. Families of children with lice or scabies need information on extermination and laundering techniques.

EVALUATION

The evaluation of patient-centered goals determines whether outcome criteria have been met. Outcome criteria should be individualized for each patient and revised as necessary. Below are listed patient goals and possible outcome criteria concerning prevention of tissue damage and promotion of optimal wound healing.

Goal
Patient's skin will remain intact without areas of local inflammation.

Possible Outcome Criteria
- Patient has no skin lesions or pressure sores during hospital stay.
- During hospitalization patient develops no redness or abrasions of skin.
- Before discharge, patient has moist skin without excessive drying or flaking.

Nursing Management Plan
The Patient with Impaired Skin Integrity

Nursing Diagnosis: Impaired skin integrity related to pressure, friction, and immobility manifested by quarter-sized, second-stage sacral pressure sore
Patient Goal: Patient/family will comply with regime to prevent and treat pressure sores
Patient Outcome Criteria

- Patient discusses pressure sores with nurse during hospital stay.
- Patient describes five contributing factors to pressure sore development before discharge.
- Patient inspects skin daily during hospital stay.
- Before discharge patient demonstrates interventions to effectively relieve pressure sores.

Nursing Intervention	Scientific Rationale
1. Teach the patient and family what pressure sores are; use photos	1. Knowledge is important in developing values to maintain preventive health practices
2. Discuss factors that can increase incidence of pressure sore formation	2. Specific knowledge allows patient to develop specific interventions that help prevent pressure sores
3. Teach patient to inspect all skin areas daily and to use a mirror for hard to visualize areas	3. To detect any evidence of skin abnormality promptly
4. Elicit patient preference for equipment (e.g., support surfaces), skin treatment, turning schedules	4. Active involvement of patient in individualizing prevention plan helps ensure compliance

Patient Goal: Patient's skin will demonstrate evidence of healing of existing lesions.
Patient Outcome Criteria

- By discharge, patient demonstrates increased granulation tissues in healing wound.
- During hospitalization, patient demonstrates absence of redness, swelling, and purulent drainage.

Nursing Intervention	Scientific Rationale
1. Reposition q 2 hours, increase frequency of positioning if redness or blanching does not disappear	1. Repositioning relieves pressure, which can occlude capillary bloodflow leading to tissue damage and ulcer formation
2. Do not allow patient to lie on healing pressure sore. Turn right to left, left to right, right to prone	2. Delicate healing tissues are more susceptible to trauma and impaired blood flow; pressure delays healing
3. Use pillows to position and support boney and high-risk areas for pressure sores	3. Padding decreases pressure and friction, which can increase pressure sore development
4. Get up in chair at least 30 minutes twice a day	4. Improves overall circulation and relieves pressure from ulcer area
5. Communicate turning schedule on wall at patient's bedside	5. Communication of specific times and positions helps promote compliance with turning schedule
6. Avoid high-Fowler or semi-Fowler position while in bed	6. Increases shearing force, which impairs circulation as patient slides down in bed
7. Use turning sheet when moving patient up in bed	7. Decreases shearing force and friction from bed when moving patient
8. Apply appropriate mattress (e.g., alternating air) to bed	8. Decreases chance of occlusion of capillary blood flow, which can increase pressure sore development and delay healing

(continued)

Nursing Management Plan
The Patient with Impaired Skin Integrity (continued)

Nursing Intervention	Scientific Rationale
9. Massage skin areas around the pressure sore and other boney areas	9. Improves circulation to areas that are at risk for breaking down
10. Keep skin clean and dry, especially after episodes of incontinence	10. Moisture promotes maceration of tissues and delays healing
11. Apply semipermeable dressing to pressure sore; change every 7 days unless barrier is broken. Inspect every shift	11. Permits easy visualization of area and permits oxygen to reach ulcer, yet provides a seal to promote healing and prevent infection
12. Encourage protein and vitamin rich diet; assess dietary intake and assist with menu choices	12. Adequate nutrition is necessary for wound healing

Goal

Patient's skin will show evidence of healing of existing lesions.

Possible Outcome Criteria

• Within 24 hours, wound edges are well approximated.
• Within 48 hours, healing wound has increased granulation tissues.
• By discharge, wound has no redness, swelling, or purulent drainage.

Goal

Patient will show increased knowledge of skin care.

Possible Outcome Criteria

• After teaching session, patient verbalizes interventions that can prevent pressure-ulcer formation.
• By discharge, patient identifies causes of mechanical or chemical tissue destruction.
• By discharge, patient demonstrates routine skin care to prevent excessive drying or abrasions.
• Before discharge, patient discusses signs of wound and skin infection and when to contact a health-care provider.
• Before discharge, patient discusses effective use of heat or cold therapies to prevent skin injury.

Goal

Patient/family will comply with treatment plan to promote wound healing and skin integrity.

Possible Outcome Criteria

• After teaching session, patient states important measures to promote skin integrity and wound healing.
• Patient maintains adequate nutritional intake, as witnessed by nurse during hospital stay.

• By discharge, patient/family demonstrate wound care and dressing change.
• Before discharge, patient/family demonstrate proper use of special equipment needed to promote skin integrity.

Key Concepts

■ The health of skin depends on adequate blood flow, adequate nutrition, intact epidermis, proper hygiene.
■ Skin's normal physiologic functions are protection, thermoregulation, maintenance of fluid and electrolyte balances, vitamin D synthesis, sense of touch, and regeneration (wound healing).
■ The very young and the very old are most susceptible to skin disruption.
■ Potential for alterations in skin function include allergic reactions, infections, abnormal growth rate, wounds, pressure sores, and burns.
■ Altered skin integrity may be manifested by pruritus, rash, lesions, and inadequate wound healing.
■ Understanding the types of wound healing (first, second, or third intention) is vital for proper wound assessment and management.
■ Hemorrhage, infection, dehiscence, evisceration, and fistula formation are potential complications of wounds.
■ Factors affecting wound healing include oxygenation and nutrient supply, immune cellular function, age, obesity, smoking, drug intake, stress, nature of the injury, wound infection, and environment.
■ In the nursing assessment, data are collected about normal skin status, risk for skin impairment, and identification of altered skin integrity.

- Planned nursing interventions are important to prevent pressure-sore development and trauma to skin.
- Permeable, semipermeable, and occlusive dressings are used to promote wound healing.
- Wound support can be provided by sutures, staples, clips, Steristrips, bandages, and binders.
- Effective management of drainage systems (ensuring patency, recharging, and advancing drains) promotes optimum wound healing.
- Local application of heat and cold can decrease inflammation, improve healing, and reduce pain.
- Discharge planning and home care are important for long-range promotion and maintenance of skin integrity.

References

Bassam, M., & Dudai, S. (1982). Near-fatal systemic oxygen embolism due to wound irrigation with hydrogen peroxide. *Postgraduate Medical Journal, 58,* 448.

Bergstrom, N., Demuth, P. J., & Braden, B. J. (1987). The Braden scale for predicting pressure-sore risk. *Nursing Research, 36*(4), 205–210.

Braden, B. J., & Bergstrom, N. (1987). A conceptual schema for the study of etiology of pressure sores. *Rehabilitation Nursing, 12*(1), 8–12.

Bruno, P. (1979). The nature of wound healing. *Nursing Clinics of North America, 14,* 667–682.

Conforti, C. (1989). Pressure sores: Dressed for successful healing. *Nursing '89, 19*(3), 58–61.

Copeland-Fields, L., & Hoshiko, B. (1989). Clinical validation of Braden and Bergstrom's conceptual schema of pressure-sore risk factors. *Rehabilitation Nursing, 14*(5), 257–260.

Cuzzell, J. (1988). The new RYB color code. *American Journal of Nursing, 88,* 1342–1346.

Daechsel, D., & Conine, T. A. (1985). Special mattresses: Effectiveness in preventing decubitus ulcers in chronic neurological patients. *Archives of Physical Medicine and Rehabilitation, 66,* 246–248.

Flynn, M., & Rovee, D. T. (1982). Promoting wound healing. *American Journal of Nursing, 82,* 1543–1558.

HoldenLund, C. (1988). Effects of guided imagery on surgical stress and wound healing. *Research in Nursing and Health, 11,* 235–244.

LaMantia, J., et al. (1987). A program designed to reduce chronic readmission for pressure sores. *Rehabilitation Nursing, 12*(1), 22–25.

NANDA (1990). *Taxonomy I revised 1990, with official nursing diagnoses.* St. Louis, MO: North American Nursing Diagnosis Association.

Smith, G., & Savinski-Bozinko, G. (1989). Giving emergency care for burns. *Nursing '89, 19*(9), 55–62.

Whitney, J. D. (1989). Physiologic effects of tissue oxygenation on wound healing. *Heart & Lung, 18,* 466–474.

Bibliography

Bayley, E., & Smith, G. (1987). The three degrees of burn care. *Nursing '87, 17*(3), 34–43.

Cuzzell, J., & Stotts, N. (1990). Wound care: Trial and error yields to knowledge. *American Journal of Nursing, 90*(10), 53–64.

Fay, M. (1987). Drainage systems: Their role in wound dressings. *AORN Journal, 46,* 442.

Jackson, D. S., et al. (1988). Current concepts in wound healing: Research and theory. *Journal of Enterostomal Therapy, 15,* 33.

Hotter, A. (1982). Physiologic aspects and clinical implications of wound healing. *Heart & Lung, 11,* 522–531.

Lingner, C., Rolstad, B., Wetherill, K., et al. (1984). Clinical trial of a moisture vapor-permeable dressing on superficial pressure sores. *Journal of Enterostomal Therapy, 11,* 147–149.

Makleburst, J., Mondoux, L., & Sieggreen, M. (1986). Pressure relief characteristics of various support surfaces used in prevention and treatment of pressure ulcers. *Journal of Enterostomal Therapy, 13,* 85–89.

Neuberger, G., & Reckling, J. (1985). A new look at wound care. *Nursing '85, 15*(2), 34–42.

Norton, D. (1989). Calculating the risks: Reflections on the Norton scale. *Decubitus, 2,* 24–31.

Oleske, D., et al. (1986). A randomized clinical trial of two dressing methods for the treatment of low-grade pressure ulcers. *Journal of Enterostomal Therapy, 13,* 90–98.

Rosequist, C., & Shepp, P. (1987). The nutrition factor. *American Journal of Nursing, 87,* 45–47.

Sebern, M. (1987). Home-team strategies for treating pressure sores. *Nursing '87, 17,* 50–53.

Trelease, C. (1986). A cost-effective approach for promoting skin healing. *Nursing Economics, 4,* 265–266.

Young, M. E. (1988). Malnutrition and wound healing. *Heart & Lung, 17,* 60.

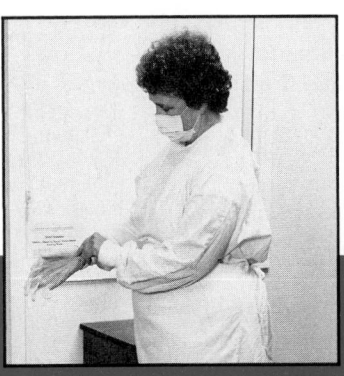

The Body's Defenses Against Infection

35

Normal Resistance to Infection
Characteristics of Normal Resistance to Infection
Nonspecific Natural Defenses
Specific Acquired Defenses
Factors Affecting Normal Resistance to Infection
Cognition and Perception
Intact Skin and Mucous Membranes
Personal Hygiene
Nutrition
Environment
Immunization
Lifespan Considerations
Altered Resistance to Infection
Potential for Infection
Presence of Infectious Agents
Type of Infection
Hospitalization
Compromised Host
Manifestations of Infection
Nonspecific Symptoms
Fever
Increased Pulse and Respiratory Rate
Inflammatory Symptoms
Pain
Purulent Drainage
Enlarged Lymph Nodes
Rash
Gastrointestinal Symptoms

Impact of Infection on Activities of Daily Living
Assessment
Subjective Data
Functional Pattern Identification
Risk Identification
Dysfunctional Identification
Objective Data
Physical Assessment
Diagnostic Tests and Procedures
Nursing Diagnoses and Patient Goals
Diagnostic Statement: High Risk for Infection
Definition
Defining Characteristics
Related Nursing Diagnoses
Patient Goals
Implementation
Nursing Interventions to Promote Health and
Function
Infection Prevention Among the General Public
*Infection Prevention Within the Health-Care
System*
Nursing Interventions for Altered Function
Host Defenses Enhancement
Antimicrobial Therapy
Prevention of Infection Spread
Discharge Planning and Home Care
Evaluation
Key Concepts

Infectious diseases have changed history by wiping out large numbers of people, stopping industrial growth, causing migrations, and altering social structures. Infection continues to have a significant impact today. For instance, childhood diseases interrupt development by interfering with school and play, and lifelong physical or mental deficits may result. Sexually transmitted diseases such as herpes, gonorrhea, and AIDS have spread rapidly in the past two decades because of changing sexual practices and increased travel, and now have enormous social consequences.

Infectious diseases are responsible for more health-care contacts than any other reason. Infections consume billions of dollars in health-care costs and are a major cause of absenteeism from work and school. They are a common cause of death in Third World countries and cause significant morbidity and mortality in the developed world.

For infection to occur, an uninterrupted chain of conditions must be present that allows microorganisms to grow, reproduce, be passed from place to place, and to enter a susceptible host. This "chain of infection" is described in detail in Chapter 22. When the chain of infection remains intact, people must rely on their bodily defenses to fight disease-causing microorganisms.

NORMAL RESISTANCE
TO INFECTION

Humans are bathed in a sea of microorganisms called **normal flora.** Their presence in or on the body is normal and is usually **symbiotic,** meaning that there is no harm to either organism. These organisms live on the skin, in the nasopharynx, in the gastrointestinal tract, and on other body surfaces.

Infection is the result of an interaction between an agent that can alter the normal functioning of the body and a host that provides an environment for the agent's replication and growth. Microorganisms that can cause disease are called **pathogens.**

Characteristics of Normal
Resistance to Infection

The body's defenses against infection can be divided into two major groups:

Nonspecific natural barriers include the skin and the mucous membranes covering the gastrointestinal, respiratory, and urinary tracts.

Specific acquired defenses occur in response to a particular organism and are mobilized to fight that specific invader.

The types of human defenses against infection are outlined in Table 35-1.

Nonspecific Natural Defenses

A person's general health (including nutritional status, lifestyle, and stress level) is an important factor in determining his or her resistance, along with age, sex, and place of residence.

Racial origin also plays an important role. A population's exposure to an infectious agent over generations can lead to increased resistance to that microorganism. For instance, measles was carried by European explorers to the New World, causing the deaths of millions of

TABLE 35–1
Human Defenses Against Infection

Defense	Examples
Nonspecific Natural Defenses	
Individual factors	Heredity
	Good hygiene practices
	Nutritional balance
	Immunization history
Anatomic barriers	Skin
	Mucous membranes
Mechanical removal of microorganisms	Gastrointestinal motility
	Ciliary action in the respiratory tract
	Cleansing effect of the flow of urine
	Expulsive effect of coughing and sneezing
	Lavaging effects of tears and saliva
	Shedding of uterine lining in menstruation
	Flow of organ secretions through ducts (i.e., bile)
Chemical factors*	Acidity of gastric secretion
	Acidity of vaginal secretions
	Acidity of fatty acids of the skin
	Lysozyme enzymes in tears, nasal secretions, urine, and saliva
	Hormones secreted by the adrenal cortex and pancreas
Local tissue factors	Indigenous microflora (competition)
	Tissue surface receptor (occupancy)
White blood cell function	Inflammation
	Fever
	Phagocytosis
Acquired Specific Resistance†	Immune response
	Cellular immunity (T-lymphocytes elaborate killer cells and helper cells)
	Humoral immunity (B-lymphocytes produce antibodies to specific microorganisms)
	Memory of the organisms produces lasting immunity

* Factors that retard growth and provide less favorable media for growth.
†Resistance may be required naturally if the person has had the infectious disease or has been immunized.

inhabitants of North and South America. Today, African Americans who have the genetic disease of sickle-cell anemia do not contract malaria, presumably because the shape of the cell makes it difficult for the parasite to enter. Because malaria kills more than a million people a year, this is an important form of immunity, but it carries its own consequences as a disease. Many ethnic groups have developed cultural habits that act as a barrier to the spread of infection, and scientists are sorting out the differences between customs and genes.

Mechanical and Chemical Barriers. Intact skin and mucous membranes that cover body cavities are the most important barriers to infection. Infection is rare if these barriers remain intact. The physical barriers of the skin and mucous membranes are aided by their chemical composition, and some barriers also have specialized cells. Normal flora that grows on healthy tissues uses the local nutrients, thus inhibiting the colonization and growth of pathogens by depleting the supply of food and oxygen. Mechanical forces, such as tears, saliva, and urine, wash bacteria from surfaces as they flow through ducts and tracts. Peristalsis increases the mechanical cleansing of organ walls. **Interferon** is a nonspecific chemical inhibitor secreted by body cells in response to invasion by viruses.

White Blood Cells. The phagocytes and inflammatory response make up the second line of defense to microbial invasion. *Phagocytes,* cells that can ingest microbes, are the white blood cells found in the blood and certain tissues. There are two types of white blood cells (also called leukocytes):

• Polymorphonuclear cells, which contain granules of digestive enzymes (granulocytes)
• Mononuclear cells, which are either monocytes or lymphocytes (also called agranulocytes because they lack digestive enzymes).

Table 35-2 lists the actions of various white cells. Appendix B also includes a table of differential white blood cell counts.

Inflammatory Response. Inflammation is a nonspecific response to tissue injury that may be caused by microbial invasion or mechanical, chemical, or heat injury. The purpose of inflammation is to limit the extent

TABLE 35–2

White Blood Cell Functions in Infection

Cells	Action
Neutrophils	Phagocytes. They ingest and break down foreign particles, particularly bacteria and parasites. They are also an important link in the generation of fever to combat the proliferation of microorganisms.
Eosinophils	Allergic reaction. They increase in response to allergic and parasitic conditions when there is an antibody–antibody response.
Basophils	Unknown. They contain heparin and histamine in their granules, which may be important in preventing blood clotting during an inflammatory response.
T-lymphocytes	Synthesis of immunoglobins. Effective in destroying bacteria, viruses, and cancer cells, they recognize antigens and stimulate B-lymphocytes and macrophages. Three types have been identified: helper cells, which stimulate other leukocytes; killer T-cells, which recognize and destroy virus-infected cells; and suppressor cells, which tell the other cells to stop fighting after the antigenic substance is cleared. They produce cellular immunity.
B-lymphocytes	Synthesis of antibodies. Important in the immune response, they are stimulated by the T-cells to divide and produce the plasma cells, which then produce specific antibodies to the antigen. The memory of the antigen is carried on memory cells that produce lasting immunity to the specific microorganism. They produce humoral immunity.
Macrophages	Scavenger cells. They dispose of cellular debris. Their numbers increase in the late stage of acute infections and during chronic infections. Levels also rise in response to viral, bacterial, and parasitic infections. They are considered important in activating the lymphocytes and are found in the reticuloendothelial system (RES).

of the injury. Blood vessels dilate and plasma flows out of the capillaries into the irritated tissue. White blood cells migrate into the area; neutrophils are usually first, followed by the clean-up crew of monocytes. The area then begins to show the four signs of inflammation:

- Redness from blood accumulation in the dilated capillaries
- Warmth from the heat of the blood
- Swelling from the accumulation of fluid
- Pain from pressure or injury to the local nerves.

The area is red, warm, swollen, and tender. It is inflamed but not necessarily infected. The inflammatory response is discussed further in Chapter 34.

Inflammation and phagocytosis work together to contain microorganisms. If they are successful, a collection of dead leukocytes, digested bacteria, dead tissue cells, and plasma may form into the material called *pus*.

Fever. Elevated body temperature also aids in the battle against infection. The hypothalamus raises the body's thermostat in response to pyrogens, and cell metabolism increases. Pyrogens are released by phagocytic cells (granulocytes, monocytes, and macrophages) after being stimulated by microorganisms or endotoxins (Wertz, 1991).

Research has shown that fever (defined as a body temperature above 101°F or 38.2°C) helps combat infection by interrupting viral replication and slowing the rate of bacterial growth. Fever is also reported to increase the mobility of leukocytes and to enhance their ability to phagocytize microorganisms. Also, the effects of endotoxins are shortened with elevated temperatures.

Thus, fever is thought to have a beneficial effect on the outcome of an infection if other body systems are not compromised. If fever is too high or is prolonged, the patient may become severely debilitated or suffer convulsions.

Specific Acquired Defenses

Another important barrier to the spread of infectious organisms is the specific response of acquired defenses that develop immunity. **Antigens** are usually foreign particles, such as microbes that enter the host, but they may be a person's own cells in some autoimmune diseases. The specific response to an antigen takes place at two sites: in the blood (humoral immunity) and in the cells of the lymphatic system (cellular immunity).

The immune system response is stimulated when the antigens enter the lymphatic and circulatory systems. The antigens are phagocytized by macrophages, monocytes, or neutrophils, and the microbe is digested. Portions of the microbe are antigenic determinants, particles that stay with the phagocyte and are carried to the lymphoid tissue in the lymph nodes or the spleen. The phagocyte, usually a macrophage, presents this processed antigen to the lymphocytes, which then work to produce immunity.

There are two types of lymphocytes: T-lymphocytes and B-lymphocytes. Both originate from stem cells in the bone marrow and differentiate to become the lymphopoietic cells. Some of them pass through the thymus gland in the chest and are modified to form the thymus-dependent lymphocytes or T-lymphocytes (also known as T-cells). The others are modified by unknown mechanisms and become B-lymphocytes. There are several subgroups of lymphocytic cells, and much research is being done on their functions (see Table 35-2).

Immune System. The immune system, if properly functioning, can produce resistance to a recurrence of a disease. Immunity to a specific pathogen usually follows an active infection, which may or may not be symptomatic. Other forms of immunity can be produced to prevent a specific disease from occurring.

The immune system conveys lasting resistance to infection by forming a "memory" of the antigen within the body. T-lymphocytes and B-lymphocytes, the building blocks of the immune system, accumulate in lymph nodes along lymphatic vessels and are exposed to all antigens except those that enter the bloodstream directly. These lymphocyte cells are heavily concentrated in the tonsils and spleen, which are important tissues in children and young adults.

Cellular Immunity. Cellular immunity, principally composed of T-lymphocyte activity, is stimulated by fungi, protozoa, some viruses, and bacteria. After the T-lymphocytes are stimulated, they enter the circulation from the lymphoid tissues and seek the site of the microbe. At the site, the lymphocytes produce proteins called lymphokines that draw more phagocytes to the area, keep them there to fight the invader, and increase their killing power. Lymphokines disappear after the antigen has been eliminated, but some of the T-cells remain in the tissues and keep a memory of the antigen. Memory T-lymphocytes are reactivated rapidly if the same antigen reappears.

Humoral Immunity. Humoral immunity takes place in the bloodstream. B-lymphocytes produce humoral immunity by producing antibodies that convey specific resistance to many viral infections. B-lymphocytes are stimulated by the antigenic determinants contained within the macrophages and produce plasma cells. The plasma cells then produce antibodies that are released into the bloodstream from the lymphoid tissue. Antibodies, also called immunoglobulins, circulate in the bloodstream and interact there with the antigens they encounter; this gives rise to the term humoral, or blood, immunity.

Antibodies are formed in response to substances found in bacterial cell walls, toxins, microbial enzymes, viruses, and other individual allergens. They can make the bacteria more susceptible to phagocytosis or help in bacterial cell lysis. Antibodies formed in response to a virus neutralize the virus, act as antitoxins, or cause the microbes to clump together or precipitate. Others simply make it easier for microbes to be ingested by phagocytes. Memory B-lymphocytes remain in lymphoid tissue, where they can become reactivated if the pathogen reappears.

The complement system, a series of proteins found in the bloodstream, also aids in the antigen–antibody reaction. The complement system enhances phagocytosis of microbes, helps in lysis of bacterial cell walls, and encourages the inflammatory response.

Active Immunity. Active immunity is produced when the immune system is stimulated, either naturally or artificially, to produce antibodies (Fig. 35-1) Natural immunity follows the course of an infection: the patient experiences a disease and produces a good response to the antigen. Active immunity can also be produced by vaccination (the injection of weakened or killed organisms into a person, stimulating antibody production and producing an artificially acquired active immunity).

Passive Immunity. Passive immunity can be conveyed by two means. Antibodies can pass from the mother via the placenta to the fetus, or through breast milk to the newborn. Also, antibodies from a person or animal that has had the disease can be taken from the blood and given to a person for temporary passive protection (Fig. 35-1). Passive immunity, which provides only temporary protection, is given in the form of immune globulins or antitoxins when there is not enough time for the person to acquire active immunization, or when a vaccine does not exist for the disease.

Relative Versus Absolute Immunity. Immunity to a specific pathogen may be absolute (such as that generated to measles) or relative (when susceptibility to infection persists but the symptoms are usually less severe, such as

those seen in respiratory viral infections). The immune response protects the person early in an infectious process only if the person has been previously exposed to the invading organism. An initial response takes 2 to 4 weeks to be effective against a previously unknown antigen. To produce these reactions, the patient must be well nourished and must have a competent immune system.

Factors Affecting Normal Resistance to Infection

A person's ability to resist infection is affected by his or her knowledge, hygiene, nutrition, environment, and immunization status.

Cognition and Perception

Children should be taught the values of cleanliness, sanitation, and infection control at an early age, because understanding infection, its dangers, and its prevention play an important part in our ability to defend ourselves against infection. For instance, people responsible for cooking must learn how to handle food safely and how to wash their hands properly.

Intact Skin and Mucous Membranes

Intact epithelial surfaces of the skin and mucous membranes stop microbial invasion. Epithelial surfaces include the skin; the linings of the oral, anal, vaginal, gastrointestinal, respiratory, and urinary tracts; the conjunctiva; and the lining of the external ear. Few pathogens can penetrate these intact anatomic boundaries.

Secretions and mechanical functions help to remove organisms that are deposited and colonized on these

Figure 35–1. Establishing immunity to disease. **A.** Naturally acquired active immunity occurs when a person is exposed to antigens (may have symptoms of the disease or be symptomatic). **B.** Naturally acquired passive immunity occurs when antibodies from the mother are transferred to the fetus. **C.** Artificially acquired active immunity occurs when inoculation of toxoid or vaccine is administered. **D.** Artificially acquired passive immunity occurs when antibodies from another person or animal are injected. Adapted from Alcamo, I. E. (1987). *Fundamentals of microbiology.* Menlo Park, CA: Benjamin/Cummings Publishing Company.

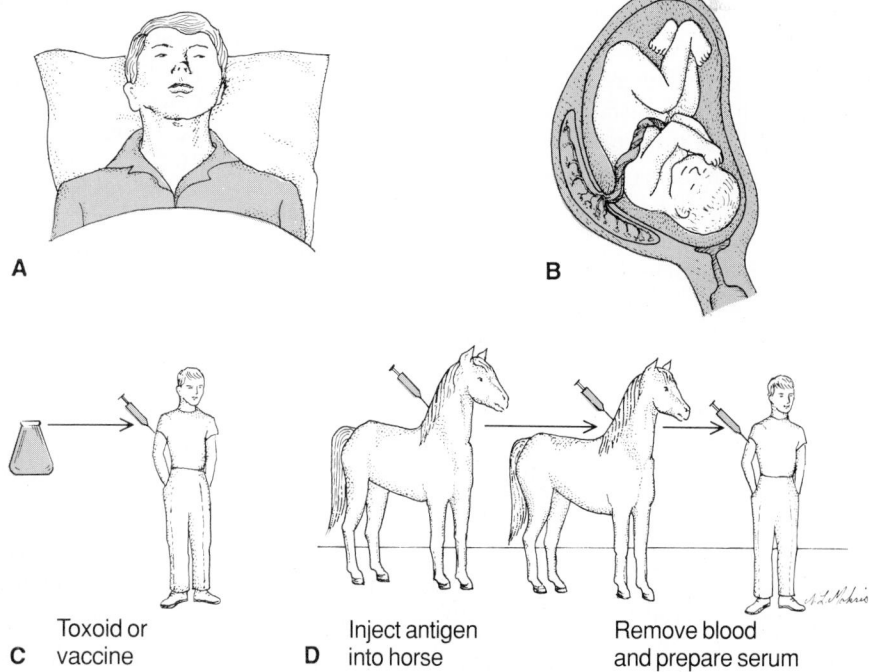

A

B

C   Toxoid or vaccine

D   Inject antigen into horse

Remove blood and prepare serum

surfaces. For organisms to invade tissues, they must first attach to the surface, and this attachment is impeded by the local pH, mobility of the surface, flow of mucus, beating of cilia, washing of the surface by fluids, and renewal of surface cells by desquamation.

Personal Hygiene

Routine personal grooming fosters normal host defenses against infection. Normal cleansing of the skin is important in removing transient microorganisms and decreasing colonization. Handwashing is the most significant way to decrease the spread of microorganisms. Hygiene also helps to lubricate skin surfaces and to maintain an intact epidermis. Routine oral care removes debris and plaque, which attract microorganisms to the mouth. Routine washing of clothes and accessories also decreases the number of microorganisms on the body.

Nutrition

Adequate nutrition is essential for normal host defense against infection. The body's ability to synthesize antibodies, which are proteins, becomes ineffective if protein stores are depleted. Adequate energy, supplied by the breakdown of ingested food, is necessary to mount an effective attack against invading organisms.

Environment

Environmental factors influencing resistance to infection include sanitation, climate, and population density.

Adequate treatment of water and waste products is essential to prevent the spread of infection. Governmental agencies supervise and control the treatment of human waste. Communities ensure that garbage is collected and sewage is chemically treated before it enters the water system. Adequate sanitation reduces the number of microorganisms.

Warm, moist climates provide a good environment for the growth of organisms or vectors (e.g., mosquitoes or ticks) that can transmit disease. Cold temperatures increase the amount of time most people spend indoors, which is why the incidence of colds and viruses rises during the winter.

Densely populated areas increase the transmission of infection. Avoiding overcrowding, both in the community and in each household, can decrease the risk of infection.

Immunization

Vaccines are made of inactivated viruses or bacterial cells that cannot multiply in the body, or weakened (attenuated) organisms that multiply slowly in the body but do not cause symptoms. Some produce lifelong immunity, but most bacterial vaccines (with the exception of the pertussis vaccine) last only a few months. Vaccinations against bacterial diseases are given when there is an outbreak of the disease or when a person travels to an area where the disease is endemic.

Toxoids, also called antitoxins and immune globulins, stimulate immunity to toxins produced by bacteria or viruses. They convey temporary artificial passive immunity. Diphtheria and tetanus produce active immunity that is long-lasting, but revaccination is required throughout the lifespan. Toxoids are produced from the serum of humans and animals that have been exposed to viral or bacterial toxins and have produced antitoxins.

Lifespan Considerations

The type of infections that a person is exposed to and vulnerable to depend on that person's physical integrity and activities. The very young and the very old have high rates of infection because their defense mechanisms against infections are lowered.

Newborn and Infant

The immune system does not become fully operational until about 6 months of age. Before then, the infant's resistance to infection comes from the antibodies passed via the placenta and breast milk. Neonates have difficulty localizing infections (preventing the spread of organisms from the site of contact). Their phagocytes have difficulty trapping microbes, and they do not produce enough antibodies. Viral diseases such as chickenpox or herpes simplex, acquired from the birth canal or from infected siblings, can cause severe disseminated disease.

Neonates have immature thermoregulatory mechanisms and do not become febrile. Instead, they manifest infections more subtly: they become lethargic or restless, or stop feeding. After 2 to 4 months of age, infants begin producing antibodies, and by 6 months their lymphocytes are fully operational if they have had adequate nutrition (Alcamo, 1986; Chusid, 1984; Donowitz, 1987).

Toddler and Preschooler

Preschool children need supervision to prevent infections. They are exposed to many pathogens as they increase their mobility, and they have poor personal hygiene. Toddlers often play in dirt, they are incontinent of urine and feces, and they put things in their mouths. Although they are developing mature immune systems, they have not been exposed to pathogens to give them immunity. By age 3 to 4 years, the immune system has matured to a level similar to that of adults in producing antibodies. Childhood vaccinations are timed to take advantage of this developing immunocompetence.

Children who live in low socioeconomic conditions with poor hygiene are exposed to viruses in their food and water. When these viral diseases occur in children, they are often milder than in adults. Children may develop lifelong immunity from some of these viral infections, but diseases caused by bacteria, such as salmonella and shigella, do not produce immunity and may recur frequently.

The most common infections in early childhood are respiratory tract infections. Because children's eustachian tubes are shorter and straighter than those of adults, middle-ear infections (otitis media) are common as bacteria pass to the ear canal from the nasopharynx. Children may suffer many colds each year, but by age 5 or 6 years their immune system and body defenses have matured to a level where the infections are more localized. The common communicable diseases are transmitted as children play with others.

Preventing infections in early childhood requires:

• Adult supervision of play activities
• Good hygienic care of the child and his or her food
• Adequate vaccinations
• Early treatment to prevent spread or preventable complications
• Isolation from infected people (Alcamo, 1986; Ford-Jones, 1987; Fox, 1981).

Child and Adolescent

Communicable diseases are most prevalent as children enter school and organized play activities, and they are most common during the winter, when children stay indoors. Children are also exposed to skin diseases such as impetigo (from staphylococcal infections), roundworm infestations, and lice (from sharing combs, clothes, and sports equipment). There is a high incidence of streptococcal infections in children ages 6 to 12 years, resulting in pharyngitis, tonsillitis, and scarlet fever (which may have rheumatic and renal complications).

Accidents are common in this age group, resulting in abrasions, lacerations, and fractures. Although most accidents from play and sports are relatively minor, they carry an infection risk.

Sexually transmitted diseases such as infectious mononucleosis, chlamydia, herpes simplex, syphilis, gonorrhea, and AIDS are on the rise in adolescents. Young adults who contract them run an increased risk of serious consequences; for instance, pelvic inflammatory disease in young women is a major cause of ectopic pregnancy and infertility, and inflammation and infection of the urethra and testes can lead to sterility in men. The immune system should be fully mature by adolescence but may be compromised by malnutrition or acquired deficiencies (Farley, 1991; Halverson & Graham, 1991).

Adult and Older Adult

Immunity to many diseases is established by adulthood. Adults have fewer respiratory tract infections but more chronic lung diseases, which can increase infection risk. Sexually transmitted diseases continue to be a major problem in this age group, depending on the person's lifestyle.

Accidents, both industrial and recreational, have infectious complications. Many deaths from motor-vehicle accidents are caused by infections that cause the failure of organ systems.

Infections in a pregnant woman can be transmitted across the placenta to the fetus. A minor or subclinical infection can be passed to the fetus, who may suffer either minor consequences, major congenital anomalies, or death.

As people age, the effects of their lifestyles begin to affect their ability to resist infection. The thymus begins to shrink in late adolescence and continues to diminish into middle age, leading to a decline in cell-mediated and humoral immunity. Cardiovascular disease, cancer, diabetes, obesity or malnutrition, alcoholism, anxiety, depression, and stress have all been shown to decrease defense mechanisms against infection. The medications and treatments used to combat these diseases may also decrease immune system function. Adults with chronic diseases require more frequent hospitalization, putting them at risk for **nosocomial infections** (infections acquired while receiving health care).

With the increase in air travel and the development of global economic ties, people are traveling more and living in foreign countries where they may be exposed to infectious diseases that are not endogenous to their native area. They may then take these infectious organisms home, contributing to the spread of infection. Because they have their initial exposure as adults, the symptoms and complications of the disease may be severe (Wertz, 1991).

The skin of elderly people becomes thinner and drier. It loses elasticity and fat and receives less circulation, leading to an increased susceptibility to injury and infection. Bedridden patients are more susceptible to the development of infected decubitus ulcers.

There are changes in other defense mechanisms with aging. The pH of body secretions changes, peristalsis slows, and the endogenous flora changes with age and medications. The cough and gag reflexes of elderly patients may be impaired after a stroke or from medications that cloud their thinking. Loose-fitting dentures and impaired swallowing mechanisms may lead to aspiration, which can contribute to respiratory infection.

Elderly adults may have problems with urinary retention, which leads to bacterial growth in stagnant urine and decreased cleansing of the urethra by a brisk stream of urine. Ascending infections also occur, especially in the bedridden adult. Incapacitated adults may be incontinent of urine and feces, causing excoriation of the skin in the perineal and sacral regions and further contributing to infections. If they are confused or agitated, elderly patients may carry microorganisms from these areas to their nose or mouth if they are not given adequate help with hygiene.

The immune systems of elderly patients may be impaired. White blood cell counts do not always rise in response to infections, and phagocytosis is ineffective. There is a decreased inflammatory response, and body temperature may not be elevated in response to an infection. The ability to wall off and limit the spread of infection is decreased. There is a decreased cellular immune response, and old infections such as tuberculosis may be reactivated. Both nonspecific and specific responses to microbial invasion are diminished.

As a cause of death in the elderly, infections are exceeded only by cancer and myocardial infarction; urinary tract and respiratory tract infections are the most common and the most lethal. Infections use up energy necessary for other body processes. The elderly have twice the incidence of influenza as young adults, and the mortality rate is higher. They are also vulnerable to postoperative infections, particularly when the chest or abdomen is the operative site.

Increasing numbers of elderly people in the United States live in nursing homes. They are at increased risk for infection for a variety of reasons: their chronic diseases may predispose them to infection, they may be housed in crowded rooms with other infected patients, they may have invasive devices such as Foley catheters, and they may be unable to take adequate nutrition by mouth. The inability to care for their own hygienic needs, coupled with the inadequate staffing in many long-term care facilities, increases infection risk. Additional exposure to infection may come from visitors with active respiratory infections or caregivers who fail to wash their hands before and after care (Craven, 1991; Fox, 1984; Garibaldi & Nurse, 1986; Gross & Levine, 1987).

ALTERED RESISTANCE TO INFECTION

Potential for Infection

Infection transmission can occur because of the virulence of the infectious agent or because of alterations in normal host defense mechanisms. Often, the combination of many factors leads to an infection.

Presence of Infectious Agents

The type and number of microorganisms and their virulence, pathogenicity, and invasiveness determine whether an infection occurs. **Virulence** means the vigor with which

the organism grows and multiplies, *pathogenicity* is its ability to cause harm, and *invasiveness* involves its ability to penetrate tissues. Large numbers of organisms that are virulent, pathogenic, and invasive are most likely to cause infection.

The **incidence** of infection can be represented by this equation:

$$\text{Infection} = \frac{\text{Bacteria} \times \text{Virulence}}{\text{Host defenses}}$$

In the past, only a few organisms were thought to be pathogenic, but that idea is changing as we recognize that almost any microorganism can cause disease, given the right conditions for entry and growth in the body. Even normal flora can cause disease under the right circumstances. Such organisms are *opportunistic*: although normally not considered pathogens, they take advantage of being in the right place at the right time and cause infection.

Bacteria, viruses, fungi, and parasites are pathogenic organisms. Common infectious diseases caused by bacteria and viruses are listed in Table 35-3.

Bacteria. Bacteria are simple, single-celled organisms with no membrane-bound internal organelles. Reproduction is by simple fission. The group of organisms called bacteria contains thousands of species, but only a few hundred of them cause human disease. They are what most people think of when they say "germs."

Gram-positive bacteria such as staphylococci are commonly found in wound infections and food poisoning; streptococci contribute to skin, wound, and respiratory infections. Gram-negative rods, normally found as normal flora of the bowel, are often associated with hospital-acquired infections started by self-contamination of the patient. They are also the most common cause of urinary tract infections.

Anaerobes, or organisms requiring reduced oxygen tension for growth, are often associated with serious infections. They are often seen in infections in which a mixture of organisms are present (polymicrobial infections). Anaerobes are part of the normal flora of the mouth, intestines, and female genital tract.

Toxins liberated by bacteria include exotoxins and endotoxins. Exotoxins of gram-positive bacteria are diffusible and cause tissue injury. Exotoxins are liberated by bacteria that cause tetanus, diphtheria, botulism, cholera, and staphylococcal food poisoning. Gram-negative bacteria usually contain toxic substances in their cell wall; these are released on cell lysis and are called endotoxins. Endotoxins are particularly potent poisons when they gain access to the bloodstream.

Viruses. Viruses are particles of nucleic acid and protein, often covered with membranes. They replicate in living cells and cause a number of diseases. Their replication process is unique. A virus invades a living cell many times its size, uses the cell's metabolism, and produces copies of itself while either destroying the cell or changing the cell's genetic makeup. The virus cannot reproduce independently, but in the cell it is efficient and deadly to the larger organism.

Viruses cause AIDS, chickenpox, colds, cold sores, encephalitis, hepatitis, herpes, influenza, measles, mononucleosis, mumps, polio, rabies, shingles, pneumonia, and many other diseases. They have been associated with some cancers and leukemias and with many autoimmune diseases, including multiple sclerosis, rheumatoid arthritis, and diabetes. They cause disease in humans and in every other organism (including bacteria) and are a constant threat to livestock and agriculture. Some viruses, such as herpes simplex, may remain latent in the cell for long periods, then start replicating and manifesting symptoms in response to illness or stress.

Fungi. Only a few fungal infections cause disease in humans, but fungi can be deadly if they disseminate through the body tissues. Unicellular fungi, called yeasts, that cause disease in humans are often normal flora of the skin and mucous membranes. They do not injure the host until defenses are lowered (for instance, *Candida* in the mouth of infants [thrush] or in cancer or AIDS patients) or until antibiotics have destroyed normal bacterial flora. Infestations of yeast by inhalation of spores can cause coccidioidomycosis or histoplasmosis lung infections. The most common yeast infections affect the skin, hair, and nails, such as athlete's foot, ringworm, and groin itch.

Parasites. Parasites that infect humans are either protozoa, helminths, or arthropods. Parasitic infections are associated with poor socioeconomic conditions with inadequate sanitation measures for water and sewage. When public-health measures do not control these organisms, disease is prevalent.

Protozoal infections are common in underdeveloped countries and probably cause more suffering worldwide than any other group of diseases. Trichomoniasis, a sexually transmitted disease, is the one common protozoal disease in the United States and causes 2.5 million infections annually (Alcamo, 1986). Other diseases include African sleeping sickness, malaria, and giardiasis. Pneumocystosis, a disease of the alveolar sacs, is increasing in frequency in immunosuppressed cancer patients and in patients with AIDS.

Helminths are flatworms and roundworms. Some invade the tissues; others live in the gastrointestinal tract or blood. When infected pork is insufficiently cooked, trichinae pass to human muscles, causing trichinosis. Pinworms are found worldwide and are one of the most common parasites in humans. Roundworms are also passed among humans and are common. Flatworms are best known from reports of intestinal tapeworms. Another form, flukes, may enter the human bloodstream.

Arthropods include mites, ticks, fleas, lice, and fly larvae. The arthropods cause a skin irritation from the toxins they introduce when they bite humans. The dermatitis they cause is often further complicated by bacterial superinfections. They also serve as vectors for some protozoal infections and for dreaded bacterial infections such as bubonic plague (Alcamo, 1986; Flower, 1987).

Type of Infection

Colonization is the introduction of microorganisms onto a body surface where they grow and multiply but do not invade the body or cause an immune response or symptoms (Wertz, 1991). The host, if ill or in a vulnerable state, may become ill and get an infection. There is a difference between being infected and becoming ill. Illness results when the agent gains the upper hand and there is a change from the normal state of health. When an obvious complex of symptoms occurs, the infection is called a clinical disease. When the body successfully resists being overwhelmed by the infection, it is called subclinical. There may be few symptoms and the host may be unaware of the exposure, but antigens form that can be recovered from the person's blood.

Infection is described as primary when it occurs in an otherwise healthy person or secondary when it develops in a weakened patient.

Community Acquired. Infections that are acquired in the course of everyday living are called community acquired. They include the communicable diseases of childhood, which are called contagious because the infectious agent is easily passed between hosts. However, infections may also be noncommunicable. These are single-event infections, such as tetanus, which occurs when *Clostridium* spores enter tissues from a puncture wound. The agent is acquired from the environment, but it is not easily transmitted to another host.

Nosocomial Infections. Infections that are acquired while receiving health care are called nosocomial infections. The patient is exposed to and starts incubating the infection while receiving care in a hospital, extended-care facility, outpatient clinic, surgical facility, or mental institution. Depending on the length of the incubation period, the patient may not manifest signs and symptoms of the infection until after discharge. Acute-care hospitals pose a high risk of infection to vulnerable people. This is because of their concentration of ill people who are having procedures that invade their skin and mucous membrane barriers and who are receiving drugs or other therapies that alter their defenses. There is a high concentration of pathogens in the hospital because of the nature of the ill patients. Infections that are not easily transmitted in the community may be easily transmitted

(Text continues on page 994)

TABLE 35–3
Common Infectious Diseases

Infection	Agent	Transmission	Symptoms	Possible Complications	Prevention
General Infections					
Common cold	Rhinovirus	Respiratory droplet	Sneezing, nasal and sinus stuffiness, nasopharyngeal irritation, watery eyes, chills, malaise	Pneumonia, otitis media	Avoid direct contact with infected individuals. Keep body defenses strong through good nutrition, exercise.
Influenza	Virus	Respiratory droplet	Coldlike symptoms, fever, body stiffness and discomfort; gastrointestinal symptoms of vomiting and diarrhea with some strains of flu	Pneumonia	Avoid direct contact. Keep body defenses strong. Flu virus vaccines are available.
Childhood Infections					
Measles (rubeola)	Virus	Respiratory droplet or secretions or direct contact	Fever, malaise, anorexia, photophobia, coryza, cough, Koplik spots on lateral surface of the mouth followed a few days later by a red rash	Encephalitis	Measles vaccine is available. Avoid contact with infected individuals if not immuned. Wear a mask if contact with an infected person is necessary.
German measles (rubella)	Virus	Respiratory droplet or body secretions (urine, blood, feces). Can cross placenta to fetus during pregnancy.	Malaise, headache, swollen lymph glands, anorexia, low-grade fever, and runny nose followed by maculopapular rash	Severe retardation and birth defects if contracted in utero	Obtain rubella vaccine. Avoid contact with infected people if not immuned. Wear mask if contact with infected person is necessary.
Mumps	Virus	Respiratory droplet or contact with saliva	Malaise, muscle aches, headache, anorexia, swollen and tended parotid glands, fever	Encephalitis, arthritis, deafness, sterility in adult males	Obtain mumps vaccine. Avoid contact with infected people if not immuned. Mask may help decrease infection.
Chickenpox	Varicella-zoster virus	Respiratory droplet, contact with lesions before they have scabbed over	Fever, malaise, anorexia, rash characterized by macules, papules, and vesicles that crust over; pruritus secondary to rash	Secondary skin infections due to scratching	No vaccine is available. Isolate infected person until lesions are scabbed over or disappear.
Scarlet fever	Streptococcal bacteria	Respiratory droplet or direct contact	Sore throat, bright red tongue, high fever, nausea, vomiting, rash	Rheumatic fever, glomerulonephritis, renal failure	Avoid direct contact with infected people. Isolate the patient until 24 hours after antibiotic treatment.

Pertussis (whooping cough)	Gram-negative bacillus (*Bordetella pertussis*)	Respiratory droplet	Cold symptoms that progress to a severe cough that includes a "whoop" as the glottis closes during deep inspiration. Vomiting, epistaxis and hemorrhaging can occur from severe coughing bouts.		Pertussis vaccine is available. Isolate the patient from nonimmune people and use a mask during acute infectious stage.

Neurologic Infections

Encephalitis	Enterovirus, arbovirus, or as a sequela of measles, rubella, chickenpox, or influenza	Respiratory droplet or direct contact with gastrointestinal secretions	Fever, vomiting, aching head, neck, and back muscles, drowsiness, convulsions, paralysis, coma	Brain damage	Vaccinations are available for measles, rubella, and influenza.
Meningitis	Gram-negative bacteria or virus	Respiratory droplet, spread to meninges through the bloodstream	Fever, anorexia, intense headache, intolerance to light and sound, delirium, convulsions, coma	Shock, respiratory distress, brain damage	
Polio	Virus	Ingestion of contaminated food and water	Nausea, vomiting, cramps, paralysis of arms, legs and body; if nerve supply is affected, impaired swallowing and breathing	Permanent paralysis	Salk or oral Sabin vaccination is available. Take enteric precautions for infected patients.

Sexually Transmitted Diseases

Syphilis	Spirochete *Treponema pallidum*	Sexual contact, mother to fetus via placenta, blood transfusion if donor is in early stage of disease and undiagnosed	Primary stage: genital lesion, enlarged lymph nodes. Secondary stage (6 weeks later): lesions of skin and mucous membrane, with generalized symptoms of headache and fever	Tertiary stage: central nervous system and cardiovascular damage, paralysis, psychosis	Public should be educated on safe sex practices. Screen blood donors. Do serologic testing before and during pregnancy. Avoid contact with body secretions from infected patients.
Gonorrhea	Gonococcus *Neisseria gonorrhoeae*	Sexual contact; mother to fetus during delivery	Yellow mucopurulent discharge of the genital area, painful or frequent urination, pain in the genital area; may be asymptomatic	Sterility, cystitis, arthritis, endocarditis	Public should be educated on safe sex practices. Mother should be tested before delivery. Newborn's eyes should be treated with silver nitrate. All contacts should be treated with antibiotics.
Genital herpes	Virus Herpes simplex type 2	Sexual contact; mother to fetus during vaginal delivery	Genital soreness, pruritus, and erythema. Vesicles appear that usually last for about 10 days, during which time transmission of virus is likely		Public should be educated on safe sex practices. Sexual contact should be avoided when lesions are present. Infected mothers should have a cesarean delivery.

(continued)

TABLE 35–3
Continued

Infection	Agent	Transmission	Symptoms	Possible Complications	Prevention
Chlamydia	Bacteria *Chlamydia trachomatis*	Sexual contact; mother to fetus during vaginal delivery	Mucopurulent genital discharge, genital pain, dysuria	Sterility	Public should be educated on safe sex practices. Sexual contact should be avoided when lesions are present. Infected mothers should have a cesarean delivery.
Acquired immune deficiency syndrome (AIDS)	Human immuno-deficiency virus (HIV)	Sexual contact; exposure to blood or blood products; mother to fetus	Active phase: rash, cough, malaise, night sweats, lymphadenopathy Asymptomatic phase: no symptoms but test is positive for HIV antigens AIDS-related complex (ARC): lymphadenopathy, diarrhea, oral candidiasis, weight loss, fatigue, skin rash, recurrent infections, fever AIDS: rare infections such as Pneumocystis carinii pneumonia or rare cancers such as Kaposi's sarcoma or B-cell lymphomas	Neurologic impairment	Public should be educated on safe sex practices, especially high-risk groups. Blood or blood products used for transfusion should be carefully screened. IV drug abusers should not share needles. Universal precautions should be used consistently in all health-care settings. Institute measures to avoid needlesticks among health-care workers.

Blood-Borne Infections

Infection	Agent	Transmission	Symptoms	Possible Complications	Prevention
AIDS (see above)					
Hepatitis A	Hepatitis A virus (HAV)	Contaminated water or food or fecal–oral contamination	Malaise, anorexia, nausea, vomiting, fever, headache, abdominal pain, jaundice, enlarged liver	Hepatic damage or failure, encephalopathy	Public should be educated on good sanitation and personal hygiene, especially after using the toilet and before handling food. Food handlers and day-care workers should be educated and monitored. Enteric precautions should be taken with all infected individuals. Immunoglobulin may be given to travelers visiting endemic areas.
Hepatitis B	Hepatitis B virus (HBV)	Transfusion with infected blood or blood products (less common with other body fluid contact), punctures with HBV-contaminated sharps, mother to fetus in utero	Malaise, anorexia, nausea, vomiting, fever, headache, abdominal pain, jaundice, enlarged liver	Hepatic damage or failure, encephalopathy	Hepatitis B vaccine is recommended for high-risk individuals who often come in contact with blood. If exposed, immune globulin may be given. Screen blood donors. Avoid needlesticks. Use universal precautions.

Food- or Water-Borne

Disease	Causative agent	Mode of transmission	Signs and symptoms	Complications	Prevention
Typhoid fever	Bacteria *Salmonella typhi*	Contaminated water or food, contact with urine or feces of a carrier	Headache, weakness, fever, rash, abdominal tenderness, diarrhea, decreased level of consciousness (stupor, delirium, coma)	Intestinal hemorrhage or perforation	Water sanitation and waste disposal should be regulated and flies should be controlled. Vaccinations should be given in regions with contaminated water supply. Good handwashing after using the toilet should be encouraged. Use enteric precautions for infected patients. Milk and dairy products should be pasteurized.
Salmonella	Bacteria (various species of *Salmonella*)	Contaminated food, especially inadequate refrigeration or sanitation; improperly cooked meat	Vomiting, diarrhea, abdominal cramps, fever	Dehydration, shock due to fluid volume deficit	Food, especially eggs and poultry, should be properly handled, refrigerated, and cooked.
Shigella	Bacteria *Shigella*	Contaminated water or food; crowded environments such as jails or institutions	Vomiting, diarrhea, abdominal cramps, fever	Dehydration possibly leading to shock	Food should be properly stored and prepared.

Accident-Related

Disease	Causative agent	Mode of transmission	Signs and symptoms	Complications	Prevention
Tetanus (lockjaw)	Bacteria *Clostridium tetani*	Puncture wound from needle, nail, dog bite, or gunshot wound	Increased neuromuscular tone and irritability, twitching, convulsions	Respiratory arrest and death	Keep immunization current; after accident booster dose or tetanus may be given to stimulate recall. If prolonged time has elapsed since booster, combination of antitoxins (tetanus immune globin) and tetanus and diphtheria toxoids is given.

in the hospital. This leads to the increased danger that patients may be colonized by microorganisms that are not their normal flora and may become ill from them (Alcamo, 1986; Centers for Disease Control, 1984; Ford-Jones, 1987; Weinstein, 1986).

Local Versus Systemic Infections. An infection may be localized to a single area of the body, or may disseminate to deeper organs. When it spreads to other body systems, the infection is called *systemic.* If bacteria spread through the bloodstream, the term *bacteremia* is used. Another term, *septicemia,* is often used as a synonym, but it more accurately refers to the presence of microorganisms (or their toxic products) in the bloodstream that are disrupting normal body functions. Streptococcal or staphylococcal blood infections were formerly called "blood poisoning."

Acute Versus Chronic Infections. An infection may be acute or chronic depending on the severity and duration of symptoms. An acute infection usually develops rapidly, causes symptoms, comes to a climax, and then fades fairly quickly. A chronic infection, on the other hand, can linger: symptoms usually develop more slowly, and convalescence may take months. An acute infection can become chronic when the body cannot rid itself of the organism.

Hospitalization

About 5% to 6% of all hospitalized patients acquire a nosocomial infection (Castle & Ajemian, 1987). The vast majority of these infections involve the urinary tract, surgical or traumatic wounds, the respiratory tract, or bacteremias in association with intravascular lines. The incidence of these infections is shown in Figure 35-2.

Risk for Urinary Tract Infections. The incidence of urinary tract infections in hospitalized patients is directly related to instrumentation. The most common causes of urinary tract infections are continuous indwelling Foley catheters and diagnostic or therapeutic procedures that traumatize the urethral mucosa or introduce organisms into the bladder.

Catheter-associated infections result from a lack of strict aseptic technique during insertion, a break in the closed drainage system, an ascending infection by organisms from the perineum of a patient with fecal incontinence, and direct contamination from a caregiver's hands. The display lists factors contributing to the incidence of urinary tract infection. See Chapter 37 for detailed information on preventing and treating urinary tract infections.

Risk for Wound Infections. Contributing to the significant problem of wound infections in hospitals are:

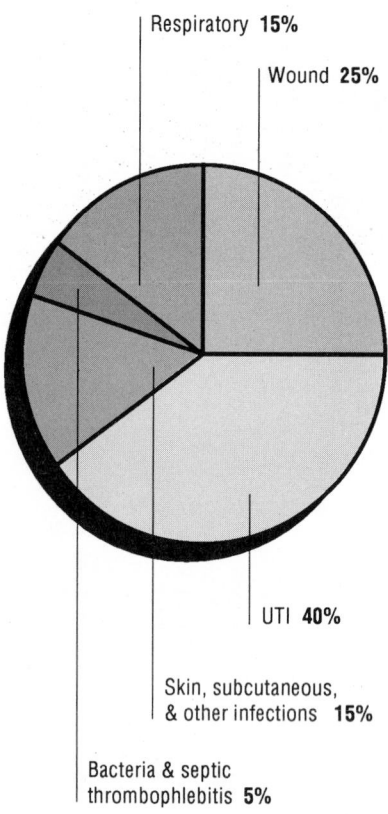

Figure 35–2.   Rates of common hospital-acquired infections. (From Centers for Disease Control (1984). National nosocomial infection surveillance.

- More complicated, longer surgical procedures
- The increase in the number of older patients with chronic diseases who are having surgery
- New surgical procedures in which foreign materials (such as heart valves, joints, vessels, or orthopedic hardware) are implanted
- The increase in the number of organ transplant recipients who require immunosuppressive agents
- The increased use of diagnostic or treatment modalities that expose patients to bacteria or suppress their normal host resistance.

Three factors contribute to the incidence of wound infection: local tissue factors in the wound, treatment factors, and host factors (see the display). Figure 35-3 shows the relationship between the number of preoperative days and increasing rates of infection in clean wounds. The longer the patient is in the hospital, the more likely it is that he or she will suffer an infectious complication (Cruse, 1986).

Infections that appear during the first 48 hours after surgery are usually the result of massive contamination and are due either to streptococcal infections or clostridial infections (which present as gas gangrene). Staphylococcal infections generally do not appear until

Factors Predisposing to Urinary Tract Infection

Factors That Increase Contamination of Urethral Area

- Fecal incontinence
- Atrophic changes (senile vaginitis)
- Hospital environment

Factors That Facilitate Ascent of Organisms up Urethra

- Catheterization
- Surgery
- Sexual intercourse
- Pelvic relaxation with aging
- Urethral incompetence (incontinence)
- Diapering incontinent patients

Factors That Reduce Flow of Urine

- Outflow obstruction (urethral stricture, prostatic hypertrophy, fecal impaction)
- Neurogenic bladder
- Inadequate fluid intake (dehydration)

Factors That Promote Bacterial Colonization

- Foreign body (tumor, calculi)
- Aging (epithelial cell changes, reduced mucus production, waning immunity)

From Fox, R. A., & Horan, M. A. (1984). Genitourinary infection. In R. A. Fox (Ed.), *Immunology and infection in the elderly* (p. 115). Edinburgh: Churchill-Livingstone.

Factors Contributing to Wound Infection Development

Local Factors

- Degree of contamination of the wound
- Virulence of contaminating organisms
- Adequacy of local blood supply
- Amount of necrotic or injured tissue in the wound
- Degree of closure of the wound
- Presence of dead spaces, hematomas, and seromas
- Presence and type of foreign bodies
- Location of the wound
- Mechanism of injury

Treatment Factors

- Length of hospital stay
- Time, type, and thoroughness of treatment
- Duration of operative procedure(s)
- Timeliness and appropriateness of antibiotic administration
- Appropriate surgical closure
- Surgical technique
- Appropriateness of wound dressing
- Nutritional support
- Adequacy of oxygenation and tissue perfusion
- Use of invasive devices for monitoring, drainage, and fluid or nutritional support
- Adequate treatment of coexisting infections

Host Factors

- Age
- General immunologic competence
- Chronic health problems
- Preoperative nutritional status
- Obesity
- Remote infections
- Extent of injury (multiple wounds or extensive surgery)

after the third postoperative day, and polymicrobial infections until after the fourth day. See Table 35-4.

Risk for Respiratory Tract Infections. Most hospital-acquired respiratory infections are caused by Gram-negative organisms that often are the antibiotic-resistant flora of the institution. These are often polymicrobial infections.

Many factors can predispose the hospitalized patient to respiratory tract infections, including factors that:

- Increase secretion production
- Decrease chest wall movement
- Inhibit secretion clearance
- Depress the respiratory drive
- Increase the risk of microbial colonization.

Refer to the display for factors that predispose the patient to respiratory infections.

Smoking, atelectasis, chronic lung disease, obesity, alcoholism, and malnutrition contribute to the development of respiratory infections. Compromised host defenses lead to increased rates of infection and increased morbidity and mortality. See Chapter 30 for specific

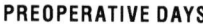

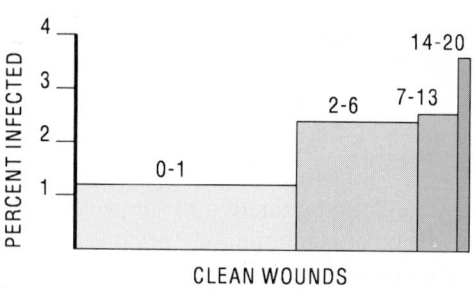

Figure 35–3. Relationship of length of hospital stay to wound infection. The longer the patient is in the hospital before surgery, the more susceptible he or she is to wound infection. From Cruse, P. (1986) Surgical infection: Incisional wounds. In J V. Bennett and P. S. Brachman (Eds.), *Hospital infections* (2nd ed., p. 427). Boston: Little, Brown & Co.

information on preventing and treating respiratory infections.

Risk for Bacteremias. Bacteremias are caused by microorganisms that enter the bloodstream from infected wounds or contaminated devices. The most common cause of bacteremias are contaminated intravascular catheters and monitoring devices. When microorganisms enter and proliferate in the bloodstream, serious infections can occur, including cellulitis, septicemia, endocarditis, and distal infections in the lung, liver, and spleen (Messner & Gorse, 1987).

Risk for Bone and Joint Infections. Bone infection, or osteomyelitis, is a serious type of infection that is difficult to treat. Normal bone has an excellent blood supply, but because of its rigid structure, once pus forms inside the periosteum, increased pressure develops that can occlude the bone's blood supply. This produces areas of infected, devitalized bone. Ligaments and tendons have poor blood supplies and do not resist infection well. Joints contain avascular cartilage and menisci, and because of the inadequate blood supply, antibiotics cannot reach the infecting organism in bactericidal concentrations.

Bone and joint infections are associated with orthopedic injury or surgery, peripheral vascular disease, decubitus ulcers, infected puncture wounds, or long-term use of intravenous therapy that causes bacteremia.

Compromised Host

A few infections occur as a direct result of the virulence of the agent of infection or its by-products, but most infections occur as a result of decreased host defenses. Before an infectious process becomes a disease, there must be a breakdown or impairment of the physical and chemical barriers to bacterial colonization, the inflammatory and febrile response, and the response of the white blood cells, including those involved in immunity. Unfortunately, this occurs frequently in a person's life.

Decreased resistance to infection may be due to age, pre-existing diseases, medical therapy, malnutrition, or stress. The body's anatomic barriers may be broken by many conditions. The display lists many host factors that can alter resistance to infection.

Breaks in Skin and Mucous Membranes. Breaks in skin and mucous membranes predispose a person to infection. Both natural and therapeutic processes can alter intact epithelial surfaces.

Skin in infants and elderly people is thin and more easily broken or penetrated by microorganisms. Some medications, such as steroids, cause thinning of the skin and add to the potential for breakdown.

Surgical intervention and many diagnostic procedures break normal skin integrity, greatly increasing the possibility of infection. Therapeutic procedures invade every epithelial surface. Nasogastric tubes, urinary catheters, suction catheters, and rectal thermometers can cause surface abrasions and obstruct the natural flow of cleansing fluids.

TABLE 35–4

Clinical Onset of Wound Infection

Postoperative Day*	Responsible Pathogen	Presents As
1–2	B-hemolytic streptococcus, *Clostridium* sp.	Cellulitis with or without deep or central gangrene: gas gangrene
3–4	*Staphylococcus aureus*	Wound abscess with halo cellulitis
5–6	Aerobic Gram-negative bacilli plus various anaerobes	Wound abscess with or without synergistic gangrene centrally
7–8	Aerobic Gram-negative bacilli alone	Wound abscess

*The interaction between the pathogen and the host determines when the infection becomes apparent.

Factors Predisposing to Pulmonary Infections

Factors That Increase Secretion Production

- Smoking
- Intubation
- Chemical irritation (air pollution, allergies, inhalation anesthetics, aspiration of gastric contents, impaired cough or swallowing mechanisms)

Factors That Decrease Chest Wall Movement

- Pain (chest or abdominal injuries or incisions)
- Obesity
- Abdominal distention
- Tight casts or bandages
- Age
- Skeletal deformities (traumatic or congenital [e.g., scoliosis])

Factors That Inhibit Secretion Clearance

- Dry, tenacious secretions
- Dehydration
- Chronic lung disease
- Decreased diaphragmatic movement (neurologic deficits, paralysis, muscle weakness)

Factors That Depress the Respiratory Center (Hypoventilation)

- Sedatives
- Narcotics
- Altered levels of consciousness (resulting from trauma or cerebrovascular events)
- Acid–base imbalance

Factors That Increase the Risk of Microbial Colonization

- Extended hospital stay
- Residence in long-term care facility
- Endotracheal intubation
- Tracheostomy
- Suprainfection after long-term use of antibiotics
- Malnutrition
- Primary or acquired immune deficiency
- Contaminated respiratory equipment
- Steroids
- Immunosuppressive therapy
- Poor personal hygiene practices

Factors That Alter Resistance to Infection

Patient Conditions

- Diabetes mellitus
- Advanced malignancy
- Obesity
- Malnutrition or nutritional deficiencies
- Uremia
- Burns
- Trauma
- Leukemia
- Premature birth
- Advanced age
- Drug and alcohol abuse
- Chronic pulmonary disease
- Cardiovascular disease
- Peripheral vascular disease
- Obstructive stones in gallbladder and ureteral ducts
- Immune deficiency diseases
- Immobility
- Cigarette smoking

Therapeutic Procedures

- Intravascular lines
- Indwelling urinary catheters
- Extensive surgical procedures
- Implantation of prosthetic devices
- Hyperalimentation
- Endotracheal and tracheostomy tubes
- Feeding tubes
- Radiation

Drugs

- Steroids
- Cancer therapy
- Inappropriate or prolonged use of antibotics
- Antimetabolites

Invasive Devices. Any invasive device that enters the body provides a portal of entry for microorganisms, thus increasing the chance for infection. Invasive devices are often used to treat illness, especially in hospitals. Tubes through the skin and body orifices provide microorganisms with direct access to internal organs and the bloodstream. Intravascular lines are inserted to give medications and fluids or to serve as monitoring devices. Urinary catheters or tubes placed in the gastrointestinal tract for decompression or feeding also increase infection risk. Surgical drains placed postoperatively to promote adequate wound drainage provide an access route for microorganisms into the wound.

Stasis of Body Fluids. Stagnant secretions in the body provide a warm, moist environment that fosters bacterial growth. Normal defense mechanisms prevent stasis of body fluids, but these can be altered for a variety of reasons. Tubes inserted into the trachea or drugs that cause sedation may bypass or suppress the normal cough and sneezing clearance of respiratory secretions. Smokers inhibit normal nasopharyngeal ciliary action by inhaling toxic chemicals in cigarette smoke. Tumors or other obstructions in ducts of exocrine glands obstruct the flow of normal secretions, providing a media rich for microbial growth. Decreased fluid intake, immobility, and urinary tract obstruction foster urinary stasis, increasing the risk of urinary tract infection.

Inadequate Nutrition. Malnutrition depresses almost every normal defensive response to infection. Neutrophil and macrophage function is defective, blood levels of complement are low, and both cellular and humoral immune reactions are diminished. When infection occurs, cellular metabolism increases as the body tries to fight it. Because increased metabolism requires increased calories and protein, inadequate protein stores decrease the body's ability to manufacture antibodies and white blood cells. A vicious cycle occurs, with increased nutritional needs and decreased body reserves. Residents of Third World countries experience this cycle of malnutrition and infection many times during their lives. Malnutrition may also occur if the patient cannot eat because of anorexia or indwelling tubes in the gastrointestinal tract, and the body cannibalizes its own muscle mass.

Stress. Stress increases greatly when a patient is ill or hospitalized. Surgery or trauma are emotionally and physically stressful. Physical or emotional stress causes the body to release cortisol, which can increase the risk of infection. Cortisol increases the level of serum glucose, a good medium for bacterial growth. The metabolic rate is increased, depleting energy stores necessary for tissue healing and the production of antibodies. Extreme continuous stress causes exhaustion, which limits a person's ability to resist infection.

Humoral Immune Dysfunction. The immune system's ability to finish the killing process by producing memory cells and antibodies can be impaired in several ways. Immunodeficiency may be congenital or acquired. Diseases affecting immunocompetence include AIDS, alcoholism, the presence of pre-existing infection, burns, cancer, the absence or removal of the spleen in children, bone marrow depression from radiation or chemotherapy, chemical poisoning, and malnutrition.

Coexisting Medical Problems. Cancer, especially if it affects bone marrow production of leukocytes, increases the risk of infection. Cancers such as leukemia may accelerate the rate of leukocyte production, but the cells are immature and ineffective in fighting infection. Treatment of many forms of cancer by chemotherapy or radiation may cause bone marrow suppression, affecting the body's ability to resist infection.

Some diseases affect the factors that attract neutrophils and wandering macrophages to the site of infection. This attraction, called chemotaxis, is decreased in diabetes mellitus, cirrhosis, and uremia. Patients with burns have impaired neutrophils that do not ingest and destroy microorganisms efficiently. Because neutrophils release mediators of inflammation, impairment of their number and effectiveness has a profound effect on host defenses.

Medical problems that affect the circulation of blood and nutrients can impair host defenses. Cardiovascular conditions, such as peripheral vascular disease and congestive heart failure, can limit the body's ability to supply leukocytes and antibodies to the site of an infection, thus decreasing the infection-fighting potential.

Inflammatory disorders can also increase the risk of infection. The inflammatory response normally helps destroy and contain microbes to prevent systemic infection. However, inflammation can be destructive if it causes loss of vascular control and if the tissue exudate is extensive enough to provide a media for microbial growth.

Drug Therapy. Drug therapy can cause defects in the host's response to infection. Steroids, chemotherapy, antimetabolites, and the inappropriate or prolonged use of antibiotics can all increase the risk of infection.

Opportunistic infection (sometimes referred to as superinfection) can occur with antibiotic therapy. If the course of antibiotic administration is prolonged or if an incorrect antibiotic is chosen, bacterial growth may be stimulated as normal flora in the gut, mouth, and skin is destroyed. These opportunistic organisms take advantage of the bad luck of the normal flora, leading to serious infections in the host.

Manifestations of Infection

The way an infection becomes apparent varies depending on the infectious agent, the host, and the organ system involved. Nonspecific symptoms may precede overt clinical signs.

Nonspecific Symptoms

The human body has a variety of internal sensors that signal when something is wrong. Often this inner sense is the first warning of an impending infection. These early warnings include malaise (a general sense of feeling not completely well), listlessness, inability to concentrate, uneasiness, light-headedness, weakness, muscle or joint discomfort, headache, and anorexia. As the person becomes more ill, the symptoms change from subjective, vague complaints to objective findings.

Fever

Fever is a common manifestation of infection and should be considered a sign of infection until other causes are ruled out (Hoeprich & Boggs, 1983). Fever is the response of the thermoregulatory center in the hypothalamus to circulating pyrogens. These pyrogens are released when phagocytic cells (granulocytes, monocytes, and macrophages) are stimulated by microorganisms or endotoxins (Wertz, 1991). Very young children tend to produce high fevers (up to 105°F or 40°C) in the presence of infection, but elderly people may not show a fever or may produce only a low-grade fever when infection is present.

Figure 35-4 shows common causes of fever during the postoperative period. During the first postoperative day, an elevated temperature is most likely caused by the physiologic stress of surgery, atelectasis, or a wound infected with *Clostridia* or streptococci. Pneumonia is most likely to cause a fever during the first to fifth postoperative day, urinary tract infection on the second to eighth postoperative day, and wound infection from the third to eleventh postoperative day. Deep operative infection or infected prosthetic devices may be detected when fever develops weeks or months after surgery.

Increased Pulse and Respiratory Rate

Infection increases the body's metabolic rate, which increases the heart rate. The pulse may become bounding. The rate and depth of respiration also increase as the body tries to get rid of excess waste products produced during increased metabolism.

Inflammatory Symptoms

Infection stimulates the inflammatory response to promote leukocyte migration to the area. The inflammatory response is discussed in detail in Chapter 34. As inflammation occurs, the area appears red, swollen, and warm.

Pain

Most infections cause discomfort. Pain can occur when inflammation causes swelling within an enclosed area, or

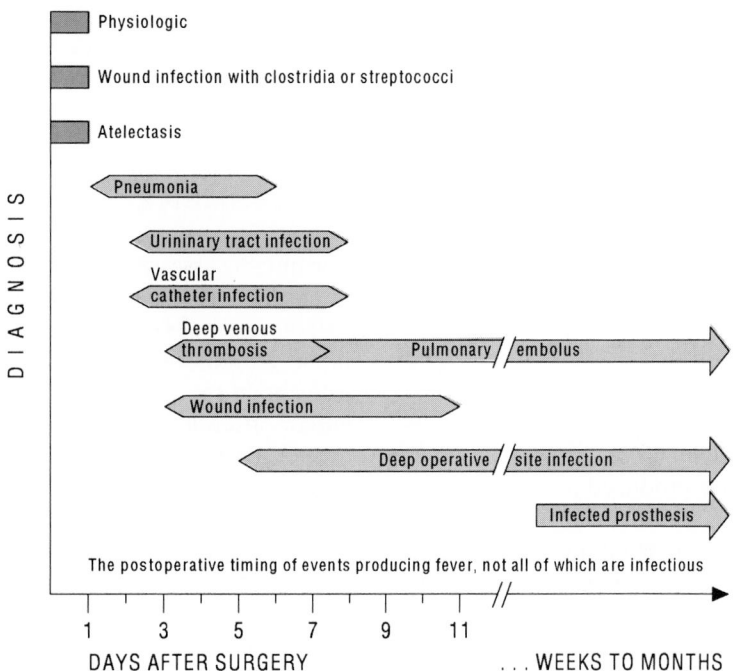

Figure 35–4.   Common causes of fever according to days after surgery. From Bohnen, J. M. & Meakins, J.L. (1985). Postoperative infection. In L. A. Mandell & E. D. Ralph (eds.), *Essentials of infectious disease* (p. 356). Boston: Blackwell.

when normal function is impeded. Examples of pain caused by infection include the following:

- Pleuritic pain when breathing, with a respiratory infection
- Burning on voiding, with a urinary tract infection
- Pain on swallowing, with a streptococcal throat infection.

Purulent Drainage

As white blood cells migrate to the infection, **purulent** (containing pus) drainage may be observed. Because of the increased numbers of white cells, body fluids such as urine or sputum may become cloudy or whitish-yellow. Purulent drainage is usually thicker than normal and often foul-smelling.

Enlarged Lymph Nodes

During an infection, the lymph nodes that drain an infected area may become enlarged and easily palpable ("swollen glands"). As the swelling increases, the nodes may also become tender. During inflammation, the lymphatic capillaries dilate as excess interstitial fluid, proteins, and invading microorganisms enter the lymphatic system. The swelling shows that lymphocytes and macrophages in the lymph node are fighting the infection and trying to limit its spread.

Rash

A rash may accompany many conditions. It often occurs with primary infections of the skin (e.g., impetigo) but may accompany some generalized infectious diseases. The diagnosis of many communicable childhood diseases is made on the specific characteristics of the rash. Many rashes cause pruritus, and scratching may disrupt the skin's integrity, which can result in secondary skin infections.

Gastrointestinal Symptoms

Acute gastrointestinal inflammation can be caused by viruses, bacteria, and toxins produced by certain bacteria and parasites. Anorexia, nausea, and vomiting often occur when the stomach lining is inflamed; diarrhea is more common when the small or large intestine is inflamed.

"Traveler's diarrhea" may occur when tourists drink water and eat uncooked food that contains endemic bacteria or parasites. Travelers have little previous exposure to these microorganisms, so they have limited antibodies to fight the infectious agent.

Impact of Infection on Activities of Daily Living

Depending on the severity and duration of the infection, the patient's normal daily activities may be affected. The patient may experience pain or other physical discomfort, may be separated from his or her peers, and may be disfigured or have a long-term disability. The community suffers from the patient's loss of economic contribution and inability to participate in church, political, or charitable activities.

All age groups are affected by the consequences of infection. Infants may fail to meet their nutritional needs for growth and development. Toddlers may experience delays in developmental task attainment, such as walking or talking, and may suffer separation anxiety if they require hospitalization. School-age children miss the opportunity to participate in school projects and may fall behind in schoolwork. Adolescents and young adults may miss social or athletic events. Parents may stay home from work or pay for someone to watch the sick child (if such a person can be found). Wage-earners may lose their salary if they do not have sick time as an employee benefit, and may be forced to pay for medical care if they do not have medical insurance.

An infection saps the energy needed for normal daily activities. The infected patient may not have enough energy for normal grooming. Sexual and social relations can be hindered due to fatigue. If the infection is located in a joint or requires bedrest, mobility is affected. Pain and the need for antibiotics during the night can disrupt normal sleep patterns. Food intake can be affected by decreased appetite, the inability to buy or cook food, or the vomiting and diarrhea that may accompany infection or antibiotic therapy.

ASSESSMENT

The nursing assessment includes gathering data from the nursing history, physical examination, and laboratory and diagnostic tests. As part of the nursing history, the nurse should observe for signs of infection and should ask about the patient's infection risk factors, paying careful attention to cues given by the patient or caregiver. The nurse collects information from the patient and secondary sources such as the family, school or employee health-care providers, and friends or co-workers. Diagnostic studies and laboratory data are also an important source of information used to identify or rule out infection.

The nurse must use all five senses to pick up cues indicating the presence of infection. For instance, the smell of drainage may be a subtle sign of infection, or changes in taste in the nurse's mouth can signal a room harboring an infection.

Subjective Data

Subjective data is collected from the patient to help the nurse determine normal patterns, the risk for infection, and the history of specific infections.

Functional Pattern Identification

The nurse is interested in the patient's normal defense system against illness. The nurse should ask the patient or caregiver about measures normally taken to avoid illness, including questions about the patient's normal pattern of rest and exercise, nutrition, use of vitamins and folk remedies, and understanding of germ exposure. The nurse should obtain a history of immunizations and determine whether they are complete and current. A description of the patient's usual experience of illness, including childhood diseases, allows the nurse to determine if the pattern is normal.

Risk Identification

The nurse should closely screen the patient for infection risk and should document any recent exposure to infectious illness. Sometimes this means asking questions such as, "Has anyone in your immediate family recently been infected with (specify disease)?" School records and community documentation of infectious disease outbreaks should be considered in evaluating each patient for risk. Questions about the patient's general health (such as normal sleep and exercise patterns, nutritional history, use of drugs, cigarettes, or alcohol, and sexual practices) should be included. Any chronic health conditions, such as heart disease, lung disease, or diabetes, and their treatment should be explored. It is important to determine whether the patient has been treated with chemotherapy or radiation, since such treatment often increases the risk of infection by suppressing the immune system. A medication history should also be taken, focusing on immunosuppressive drugs such as steroids and the current or previous use of antibiotics (see the display).

Dysfunctional Identification

If an infection was one of the reasons the patient sought medical assistance, the nurse's questions should elicit more specific information:

- How long has the infection been present?
- What symptoms first occurred?
- Was the occurrence of the infection associated with any change in routine?
- How does the infection affect the patient's ability to perform activities of daily living?

Health Interview Questions

Ask about immunization history, history of exposure to communicable diseases, and any recent acute infections.

Ask about chronic diseases that have been complicated by infections, and the usual method of treatment. Ask about the signs and symptoms the patient has experienced and the medications the patient has used.

Learn what medications or medical therapy the patient is receiving (e.g., antibiotics, steroids, immunosuppression drugs, chemotherapy, or radiation therapy).

Ask about the patient's usual diet, and assess its nutritional adequacy.

Ask about the patient's patterns of sleep, exercise, and recreation to determine health beliefs and lifestyle factors that may contribute to the risk of infection.

Elicit a history of nausea, vomiting, diarrhea, anorexia, general malaise, muscle aches, or headaches.

If an infection was not one of the reasons the patient sought advice, but the patient displays symptoms of infection anyway, further questioning is indicated:

- Is there any pain, redness, swelling, or abnormal drainage? When did it start? How long has it lasted? What is its intensity?
- Has the patient suffered nausea, vomiting, diarrhea, malaise, or general aches and pains (symptoms that accompany many viral infections)?

See the display for symptoms of common infections.

Information about the patient's present level of functioning in each of the health patterns should be obtained when infection is present. The nursing history (as opposed to the medical history) focuses on how the infection has affected the patient's ability to function normally and to carry out usual activities and routines.

Objective Data

Physical Assessment

The nurse performs a physical assessment to provide more information on the presence of infection and how it has affected the patient's functional ability.

Common Manifestions of Infection

Wound Infection

- Redness
- Swelling
- Pain
- Localized heat
- Fever
- Purulent or malodorous drainage
- Bruising around incision or induration of area around wound

Urinary Tract Infection

- Urgency
- Increased frequency of urination
- Burning with urination (dysuria)
- Cloudy, bloody, or malodorous urine (pyuria, hematuria)
- Fever
- Frank pain

Respiratory Disease

- Nasal congestion or discharge
- Productive cough
- Fever, increased pulse and respiratory rate
- Sore throat
- Painful breathing (pleuritic chest pain)
- Difficulty in breathing (dyspnea)

Gastroenteritis

- Severe abdominal cramping and nausea after eating
- More than usual number of stools and/or loose watery or bloody stools

General Inspection. The nurse gets a general impression of the patient when they first meet. The nurse can see whether the patient is comfortable or in obvious pain. Signs of fatigue can be detected in the patient's posture and in how he or she moves. Abnormal skin color and the presence of rashes or lesions is often apparent, and swelling and signs of inflammation can also be detected.

Vital Signs. Vital signs are frequently monitored in hospitals (often every 4 hours) to detect the presence of infection or to monitor its progress. The accuracy of such assessment is important in determining the presence of infection. In a patient with an infection, the nurse often finds an elevated temperature (often above 101°F), an elevated pulse rate, and an increased respiratory rate.

When evaluating the significance of vital signs that differ from baseline values, the nurse must consider other factors that could be responsible. It is helpful to look at the pattern of changes in vital signs. A consistently elevated and rising temperature is significant. Often the physician obtains cultures and begins to look for the source of a possible infection when the temperature rises above 101°F. It is important to remember that some people, such as elderly and immunosuppressed patients, may not show a fever when infection is present.

Auscultation of Breath Sounds. Auscultating breath sounds can help detect respiratory infections. Pneumonia can alter normal breath sounds, producing rales, rhonchi, and wheezes. Atelectasis, which can predispose a patient to respiratory infection, is noted by diminished breath sounds.

Auscultation of Bowel Sounds. Auscultating bowel sounds can help detect increased intestinal peristalsis. Increased peristalsis often accompanies microbial irritation of the gut, which can cause diarrhea.

Palpation of Lymph Nodes. Lymph nodes can enlarge and become tender due to localized and systemic infection. Gentle palpation using the tips of the middle three fingers can detect any enlargement in lymph nodes. Normally, cervical lymph nodes are less than 1 cm in diameter and are soft and mobile. The nurse should note any tenderness during palpation.

Diagnostic Tests and Procedures

Because clinical signs sometimes provide insufficient evidence to identify a pathogen, diagnostic procedures are used to detect and identify the source of an infection. Laboratory analysis and culturing of body fluids and x-rays and other imaging methods are used to locate the source of infection. Antibiotic sensitivities and therapeutic drug monitoring are used to identify optimal drug therapy.

Common studies included in an initial infection work-up are:

- A complete blood count (CBC), including hemoglobin (Hbg), hematocrit (Hct), and white blood cell (WBC) count
- Urinalysis
- Erythrocyte sedimentation rate (ESR or sed rate).

When infection is highly suspected, the physician may also order a series of WBC counts with differentials and body fluid cultures and sensitivities.

White Blood Cell Count. The number of WBCs, or leukocytes, rises in response to infection, tissue necrosis, stress, and neoplastic changes in bone marrow. A rise in circulating WBCs to above the normal adult range of 5000 to 10,000 cells per cubic millimeter is called **leukocytosis.** Infectious processes may become evident by examining the WBCs and differentiating the cell types. By examining the types of WBCs, a diagnosis can be confirmed and progress can be followed. The cells are counted and the cell types are reported as a percentage of the total number (see Appendix B).

Neutrophils normally compose about 50% to 70% of all WBCs. Their numbers increase during infection, but there is also an increase in the number of immature cells, called a leftward shift in the granulocytic differential count. This shift is considered a strong indication of bacterial infection. As the body responds to infection, it releases stored leukocytes from the bone marrow and increases its production of new cells to combat the infection. As the infectious process continues, the warrior cells do not have time to mature fully before they are released into the circulation; thus the leftward shift is seen in the differential count. When the proportion of neutrophils increases, the patient's resistance is good and the body is considered to be fighting the infection well. The greater the leftward shift, the more worrisome the infection appears.

Some patients, such as those who are malnourished, elderly, immunosuppressed, or on steroids, cannot produce more WBCs in response to an infection. In these cases, the absence of an increase in total WBCs or a lack of clarity on the differential does not rule out infection.

A specimen of 5 to 10 mL of blood is sent to the laboratory in a vacuum tube with a solution to prevent clotting. Results from the laboratory are reported in both absolute numbers and the relative percentage of subtypes of WBCs. Abnormal results should be reported to the physician.

Urinalysis. The urine is routinely examined to check for kidney and endocrine function and to identify the presence of urinary tract infection. Urinalysis provides information about the color, pH, specific gravity, and presence of protein, glucose, and ketones in the urine. Microscopic examinations search for casts, red and white blood cells, epithelial cells, and bacteria. Changes in color, concentration, or odor of the urine may indicate an infectious process. Alkaline urine (pH above 8) may indicate bacteriuria. High levels of glucose and protein may indicate systemic or urinary tract infection. Red or white blood cells or their cellular casts may also indicate infection, but may be caused by noninfectious inflammatory conditions. Large numbers of white cells usually indicate a urinary tract infection. A clean-catch or midstream urine specimen is requested if more than four WBCs are found or if bacteria are seen on the slide made from the urine sample. See Chapter 37 for more information on collecting urine samples. Abnormal results should be reported to the physician so that treatment can be started.

Erythrocyte Sedimentation Rate. The ESR measures the rate at which red blood cells settle in unclotted blood in millimeters per hour. The result is elevated both in acute noninfectious inflammatory conditions and in infectious processes. Collagen disease, tissue necrosis, malignancies, and stress can also increase the rate of sedimentation. This test is most commonly used to provide a crude estimate of a disease process and of the response to therapy. Because it is affected by drugs and other factors, all medications the patient is taking should be brought to the laboratory's attention.

Culture and Sensitivity. Cultures are obtained from body fluids to isolate the source of unknown fevers and to identify the microorganism causing the signs of clinical infection. Culture specimens are obtained from blood, sputum, stool, throat or wound exudate, and urine as well as spinal, joint, pleural, and other body cavity fluids. Most specimens are obtained using sterile swabs with a solid or liquid medium, a sterile container with a lid, or a sterile syringe with a sterile bottle of medium to receive the specimen.

Specimens are sent to the laboratory for Gram stain and **culture and sensitivity** results. Properly prepared Gram stains provide information as soon as the slide smears are prepared and give broad classifications of the microorganisms. This information may be used to order antibiotic therapy while waiting for specific culture results. Four reagents are used on the slide smears of the cultured material. Microorganisms retain one of two dyes depending on whether they are Gram-positive or Gram-negative. Information on the report also indicates the shape of the organisms (such as rods or cocci). Results of Gram stains can be obtained from the laboratory in less than 30 minutes; it usually takes 24 to 36 hours to grow good cultures and 48 hours to obtain growth and sensitivity results.

Sensitivity testing of microorganisms to antibiotics is a benefit of obtaining good culture specimens. After microorganisms are grown in culture media, different concentrations of antibiotics are added to a known quantity of the inoculum to test their ability to inhibit growth or to kill the organism. The laboratory reports the names of the organisms present and whether they are sensitive or resistant to specific antibiotics. The drugs are then tested for their range of effectiveness against the pathogen.

The accuracy of laboratory analysis for all cultures is only as good as the specimen provided. Factors affecting the results of the analysis include:

• Contamination of the specimen
• Delay in sending the specimen (which increases the

growth of contaminating organisms and causes deterioration of the constituents to be examined)
- Use of inappropriate containers and culture media
- Failure to identify the source of the specimen
- Failure to tell the laboratory about current patient medications (e.g., antibiotics) that may affect the analysis.

The nurse can elicit the patient's cooperation by explaining why the specimen is being obtained. Specimens should be taken before starting medications that could alter the results. They should be labeled with the time, date, and site of collection and should be immediately delivered to the laboratory. When cultures are being obtained, aseptic technique should be used and gloves should be worn by the caregiver to avoid potential transmission of pathogens.

Many hospitals allow nurses to culture suspicious exudates from tubes or wounds as a matter of policy. Because the cost of processing a specimen is often not covered by insurance without a physician's order, however, a written order should be obtained to decrease the financial burden on the patient.

Blood cultures are ordered when there is a high degree of suspicion that an infectious process is occurring. Blood cultures are usually obtained from two separate venipuncture sites. Because indwelling intravascular lines may be contaminated with surface pathogens or seeded by microorganisms that are localized to the catheter tip, blood is not usually drawn for culture from previously inserted lines. The ideal specimen is drawn just before or during the rise in temperature, since the pathogens are usually circulating in high concentrations at that time.

Obtaining a blood culture requires a set of culture bottles, a sterile syringe, two sterile needles, skin preparation equipment, and a tourniquet. The skin is cleansed according to the institution's procedure; usually a combination preparation of povidone–iodine (Betadine) and alcohol is recommended. The tops of the culture bottles are cleansed and allowed to dry. Gloves are worn while the sterile needle and syringe are used to aspirate blood. The needle is then usually changed before inoculating the culture media into special vacuum bottles. After ensuring hemostasis at the puncture site, the nurse removes the gloves and washes his or her hands before transporting the specimen to the laboratory.

Sputum cultures are obtained in a fever work-up when the patient has a productive cough. Since infections may be located in either the upper or lower respiratory tract, a good culture specimen should contain little saliva; saliva and postnasal drip secretions contaminate the specimen. Sputum should ideally be obtained in the morning, before the patient eats. It should be collected in a sterile container with a lid and should be transported to the laboratory as soon as it is obtained (unless it is a 24-hour specimen, which usually is placed in a special fixative).

Occasionally a patient cannot cooperate with sputum specimen collection, or a specimen must be obtained from a patient who is endotracheally intubated. A specimen is then obtained via suctioning with a sterile suction catheter via the nasotracheal or endotracheal route. The physician may also elect to insert a small catheter through a needle inserted into the trachea and aspirate secretions transtracheally. Specimens can also be obtained through bronchoscopy. Again, specimens should be immediately transported to the laboratory.

Throat cultures are obtained with a sterile cotton swab that is touched to the back of the throat as the patient says "aaahh." This should be done as quickly as possible, since it may trigger the gag reflex. Maintaining sterility, the swab is placed into a culture medium and transported to the laboratory.

Wound cultures are taken when signs of local inflammation or purulent discharge from the wound are noted. Suitable culture media or kits are obtained from the hospital supply service. Fresh exudate should be used for culture specimens. After removing the dressing, any crusted drainage should be gently wiped away with sterile gauze before swabbing the area. The specimen should be obtained from deep in the wound if possible; swabs from the skin are usually of no value.

Body cavity fluid cultures are obtained using aseptic technique when there is an indication of inflammation in the area. Spinal taps, joint aspirations, and pleural cavities are commonly cultured for microorganisms based on clinical observations and a high index of suspicion for an infectious process. Special kits are available from the hospital supply service, and sterile technique is always used. The nurse assists the physician in obtaining these specimens by ordering supplies, positioning and draping the patient, and ensuring rapid transport of the specimens to the laboratory.

Stool cultures may be ordered to rule out infectious causation of diarrhea. Cultures are usually necessary to examine the stool for leukocytes and to identify enteric pathogens of bacterial or fungal origin. Parasites, another common cause of diarrhea, lay eggs in the gastrointestinal tract that can be detected on examination. When a patient is being screened for parasitic infection, stool specimens are collected daily for 3 days. Moving organisms can easily be detected in fresh specimens.

Stool specimens should be collected in a sterile bedpan and transferred to a sterile container with a sterile tongue blade. On the laboratory form the nurse should identify the test required, should note if the patient has been out of the country, and should specify the organism to be screened for. Stool specimens can be affected by urine, toilet paper, soap, disinfectants, antibiotics, antacids, barium, laxatives, enemas, and cool temperatures.

Serology Tests. Serology tests are sometimes done as part of a fever work-up. Early in the course of the infection, an acute-phase blood specimen is collected. If the cause of the infection is not determined by the third week, a convalescent-phase specimen is obtained, and both specimens are examined simultaneously for a change in antibody titer. The laboratory needs to know the clinical signs and symptoms of the patient and the patient's immunization history. By comparing antigen–antibody reactions of the two specimens, a diagnosis can be made.

Therapeutic Drug Monitoring. Drug monitoring is used to test the concentration of a drug in body tissues. Drugs have both beneficial and adverse effects on body tissues: the goal is to give the right drug, in the right amount, at the right intervals, to avoid adverse reactions. Drugs are cleared from the body by the liver and kidneys after being metabolized by various organs. The clearance of a drug may depend on the patient's clinical status and the functional state of the liver and kidneys. Serum plasma levels of some drugs can be measured and their dosage changed depending on the results of laboratory analysis. Blood levels of antibiotics are tested to avoid possible toxic effects such as renal damage (nephrotoxicity) and eighth cranial nerve damage (ototoxicity).

The timing of specimen collection is of critical importance in drug monitoring. For the laboratory and physician to interpret the plasma drug level, they must know when the last dose of antibiotic was given and when the specimen was obtained. The highest level of drug concentration (peak level) should occur shortly after the drug is given, and the lowest level (trough level) should occur after the antibiotic has been metabolized. The goal of therapy is to keep the peaks from being too high and the troughs from being too low. Specimens must be labeled as to whether they are being analyzed as a peak or trough specimen. Depending on the test results, the amount of the antibiotic and the frequency of dosing may be adjusted to match the patient's rate of metabolism and drug clearance.

Diagnostic Imaging. Rapid advances are being made in the ability to visualize internal organs and to evaluate them for infection. Chest x-rays are used to diagnose pneumonia, lung abscesses, and tuberculosis. Endoscopic procedures are used to visualize the respiratory and gastrointestinal tract and to obtain specimens for microbiologic testing.

Computed axial tomography (CAT or CT) is used to obtain multidimensional images of the body, which are interpreted by computer to construct images of internal structures. By visualizing the differences in densities of organs, and organ deformity, the study can help locate abscesses or other areas of infection. The study can be done with contrast media, which enhances visualization of normal versus abnormal tissue.

Magnetic resonance imaging (MRI) is expected to be used with increasing frequency to detect infection of the nervous system. The procedure uses opaque contrast materials, injected intravenously, that have affinities for concentrations of white blood cells in abscesses or other areas of infection.

After these tests, the nurse must monitor vital signs and, when contrast material is used, observe for any signs of allergic reaction.

NURSING DIAGNOSES AND PATIENT GOALS

Nursing diagnoses are used to identify dysfunctional health patterns that predispose the patient to disruption of daily activities. Infection can affect many functional areas, including psychosocial and physiologic functioning. Dysfunctional health patterns are identified from subjective data collected during the patient interview and objective data collected during the physical examination.

Nursing assessment can also identify health patterns conducive to the patient's well-being. Once identified, these strengths should be positively reinforced with verbal recognition and incorporated into the care plan.

Diagnostic Statement: High Risk for Infection

Definition

High risk for infection is the state in which an individual is at increased risk for being invaded by pathogenic organisms (NANDA, 1990).

Defining Characteristics

Presence of risk factors such as inadequate primary defenses (broken skin, traumatized tissue, decrease in ciliary action, stasis of body fluids, change in pH secretions, altered peristalsis); inadequate secondary defenses (decreased hemoglobin, leukopenia, suppressed inflammatory response) and immunosuppression; inadequate acquired immunity; tissue destruction and increased environmental exposure; chronic disease; invasive procedures; malnutrition; pharmaceutical agents; trauma; rupture of amniotic membranes; insufficient knowledge to avoid exposure to pathogens (NANDA, 1990).

Related Nursing Diagnoses

People at risk for infections, as well as those who are infected, often present with other common nursing diagnoses. Knowledge Deficit is often present; for instance, inadequate knowledge of hygiene or infection control measures can contribute to increased incidence of infection. The presence of an infection may require the patient to learn skills to treat the infection (for example, changing a dressing using sterile technique).

Impaired Home Maintenance Management can be diagnosed when a patient does not have the knowledge, skill, or support to cope with his or her situation at home.

Pain is another common nursing diagnosis associated with infection. The inflammation that accompanies infection causes discomfort, and discomfort also occurs secondary to the fever that accompanies many infections. Sleep Pattern Disturbance can occur if discomfort is great.

Depending on the infection's location, the function of various body systems can be affected. Impaired Physical Mobility can occur if the infection is in an extremity or bedrest is needed to treat the infection. Altered Urinary Elimination can occur with a urinary tract infection. Bowel Incontinence can occur if the infection results in diarrhea or if the patient experiences diarrhea as a side effect of antibiotic therapy. Impaired Gas Exchange is common with lung infections.

Finally, Impaired Skin Integrity can occur secondary to the rashes that accompany many infections or due to impaired healing of surgical incisions in the presence of an infection.

Nursing diagnoses also involve psychosocial aspects of functioning. Self-Esteem Disturbance can result when a person assumes the sick role or adjusts to a changing body image. Anxiety and Ineffective Individual Coping can occur when patients and their families are faced with severe infection. Altered Role Performance may be a consequence when an infection limits a person's ability to work, go to school, or carry out normal family responsibilities. Sexual Dysfunction can occur because of lowered energy reserves or as a direct consequence of a sexually transmitted disease.

Patient Goals

Patient goals are aimed at preventing the occurrence of infections and minimizing the complications of infections that are already present. Patient goals related to infection include:

Patient or caregiver will demonstrate adequate knowledge to recognize and report signs of infection.
Patient or caregiver will use good health practices to prevent occurrence and spread of infection.
Patient will comply with treatment regimens to help cure infection and prevent possible complications.

IMPLEMENTATION

The perception of health and health management is influenced by the patient's developmental level, cultural and religious beliefs, social interactions, and biologic

framework (Gordon, 1987). Nursing interventions and therapeutic regimens that fail to consider this interaction of biology, behavior, and beliefs fail to achieve their highest goals.

The potential for infection is a set of risk factors that depends on the patient's behavior and situation. Identifying patterns of behavior that prevent infection is as important as identifying factors that cause infection in the patient.

Nursing interventions are directed at the following:

- Controlling the spread of infection
- Reducing or eliminating the adverse effects of infection on functional abilities
- Supporting normal defense mechanisms and behaviors that prevent infection
- Detecting behaviors that increase the potential for infection
- Providing education to modify the negative behaviors.

Nursing Interventions to Promote Health and Function

Patient teaching is important in preventing infection. Nurses collaborate with many other disciplines and public agencies to teach preventive health practices, monitor the incidence of infection, and treat infection.

Infection Prevention Among the General Public

Preventing the spread of microorganisms must take place at four levels:

- The person and family or other living group
- The community
- The nation
- The world.

Nurses can work at all these levels to plan, implement, and evaluate health practices.

Protection from infection starts with people and their household cohabitants. People protect themselves and their families by using good hygiene practices, maintaining household cleanliness, eating a well-balanced diet, and exercising regularly. They enhance their protection by getting recommended vaccinations against communicable diseases associated with childhood or with foreign travel.

But even the best individual regimen is incomplete without community infection control programs. Local agencies regulate the quality of drinking water and food served in public places by setting standards and monitoring practices. They also regulate the disposal of sewage and control solid-waste disposal. Many communities and states have passed laws forbidding unimmunized children from attending school. Some bar children with

Nursing Research

Selected Nursing Research Articles

Cools, H. J. M., et al. (1988). Infection control in a skilled nursing facility: A six-year survey. *J Hosp Infect, 12*(2), 117–124.

Lopey, J., et al. (1988). Infection control in day-care centers: Present and future needs. *Am J Infect Control, 16*(1), 26–29.

Maki, D. G., et al. (1988). Evaluation of dressing regimens for prevention of infection with peripheral intravenous catheters. *CINA J, 4*(4), 9.

Reid, E. (1988). Breast milk banks and HIV. *Midwife Health Visit Community Nurse, 24*(7), 287.

Ribner, B. S., et al. (1989). Outbreak of multiply resistant *Staphylococcus aureus* in a pediatric intensive care unit after consolidation with a surgical intensive care unit. *Am J Infect Control, 17*(5), 258–263.

Road, L. L., et al. (1989). The importance of nosocomial transmission of measles in the propagation of a community outbreak. *Infect Control Hosp Epidemiol, 10*(4), 161–166.

Sadousky, D. A., et al. (1988). Use of nonsterile gloves for routine noninvasive procedures in thermally injured patients. *J Burn Care Rehabil, 9,* 613–615.

Spence, M. R., et al. (1990). Hepatitis B: Perceptions, knowledge, and vaccine acceptance among registered nurses in high-risk occupations in a university hospital. *Infect Control Hosp Epidemiol, 11*(3), 129–133.

Possible Topics for Nursing Inquiry

- How reliable is fever as a symptom of infection in patients over 65?
- How successful in reducing the incidence of infection is a teaching program encouraging preschool workers to provide proper hygiene after preschoolers' toileting?
- What is the incidence of nonvaccinated children in community shelters for the homeless?
- What is the incidence of bacteremia when alcohol versus Betadine is used to clean IV ports before injection?
- How successful are current blood bank standards in preventing HIV-contaminated blood from reaching the public?
- What is the patient's or public's perception of blood supply safety?
- Does admission the morning of surgery decrease the rate of postoperative infection?

active infections from the classroom. Community or regional health authorities gather statistics on the incidence of infectious diseases in their communities. They decide which diseases pose a hazard to the community's well-being and must be reported to their agency.

Some countries have public-health agencies that gather statistics from the regional reports and compile them for yearly comparisons. They govern the quality of air, water, food, and wastes that cross state, regional, or international boundaries, and set standards for reduction of pollutants and microorganisms. They bar people with designated acute infections from immigrating into the country, and prohibit the return of native citizens without proof of immunizations against diseases endemic in the areas to which they have traveled.

Several international health organizations gather statistics from national groups and have formed commissions for the education of health-care providers. These organizations establish priorities for infection control and make recommendations about immunizations for international travel. International commissions also pro-

vide supplies and personnel for some immunization programs (Fig. 35-5).

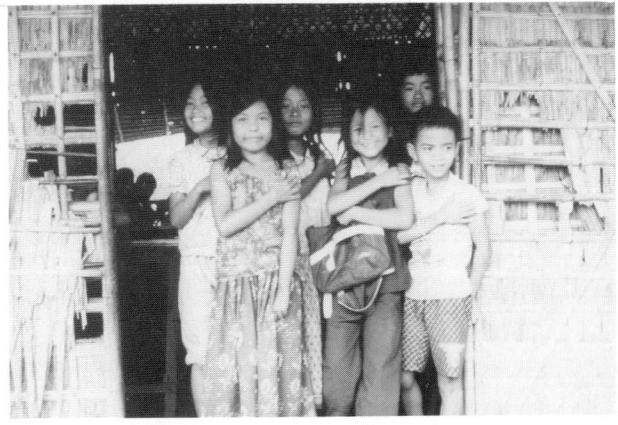

Figure 35–5. Refugee camp schoolchildren posing after receiving their immunizations at Khao I. Dan, Thailand. (Courtesy of Sherry Riddick.)

Immunization Programs. Nurses participate in establishing programs for people and groups to receive immunizations. They help to identify outbreaks of infectious disease in communities, give vaccinations, establish record-keeping mechanisms, and counsel people about precautions and possible complications of immunization. Nurses work in clinics, schools, and industry to teach about immunizations.

Immunizations may be given by injection, oral solutions, or nasal sprays. To avoid multiple injections, they are given in combination with each other (when the compounds are stable and there is minimal danger of overwhelming the immune system). Booster injections of some vaccines are given throughout the lifespan to stimulate the memory cells of the immune system (Table 35-5).

Because of frequent changes caused by new information, new immunization guidelines must be obtained yearly. This information is available from the Advisory Committee on Immunization Practices of the U.S. Public Health Service and from the Committee on Infectious Diseases of the American Academy of Pediatrics. Similar committees exist in Canada and the World Health Organization.

Immunization records should be maintained by parents during childhood and given to the children as they leave home. Physicians need to record this information and make patients aware of any unusual reaction they may have had. Commonly, excellent vaccination records are kept through the first years of school, but then the parent or child neglects to update the record. This information may be needed if questions arise about whether immunizations are current (especially tetanus, after an accidental injury).

Contraindications to vaccinations include immunodeficiency states, allergy to eggs, or previous allergic reactions. Live vaccines should not be given during pregnancy, during acute debilitating disease, or during periods of severe malnutrition.

Infection Prevention Within the Health-Care System

Controlling infection in the health-care system is a major function of the nursing staff. Infection control is essential in clinics, physicians' offices, outpatient departments, outpatient surgical centers, private laboratories, and in both acute and long-term care facilities. Infection control is most highly regulated and scrutinized in hospitals. It will be interesting to see if the trend toward short stays and outpatient care decreases the incidence of major infectious complications. Current standards of infection

---

TABLE 35–5

Recommended Schedule for Immunization of Healthy Infants and Children*

Recommended Age[†]	Immunizations[‡]	Comments
2 months	DTP, HbCV,[§] OPV	DTP and OPV can be initiated as early as 4 weeks after birth in areas of high endemicity or during epidemics
4 months	DTP, HbCV,[§] OPV	2-month interval (minimum of 6 weeks) desired for OPV to avoid interference from previous dose
6 months	DTP, HbCV,[§]	Third dose of OPV is not indicated in the U.S. but is desirable in other geographic areas where polio is endemic
15 months	MMR,[‖] HbCV[¶]	Tuberculin testing may be done at the same visit
15–18 months	DTP,[**,††] OPV[‡‡]	See footnotes
4–6 years	DTP,[§§] OPV	At or before school entry
11–12 years	MMR	At entry to middle school or junior high school unless second dose given previously
14–16 years	Td	Repeat every 10 years throughout life

* For all products used, consult manufacturer's package insert for instructions for storage, handling, dosage, and administration. Biologics prepared by different manufacturers may vary, and package inserts of the same manufacturer may change from time to time. Therefore, the physician should be aware of the contents of the current package insert.

† These recommended ages should not be construed as absolute. For example, 2 months can be 6 to 10 weeks. However, MMR usually should not be given to children younger than 12 months. (If measles vaccination is indicated, monovalent measles vaccine is recommended, and MMR should be given subsequently, at 15 months.)

‡ DTP, diphtheria and tetanus toxoids with pertussis vaccine; HbCV, *Haemophilus* b conjugate vaccine; OPV, oral poliovirus vaccine containing attenuated poliovirus types 1, 2, and 3; MMR, live measles, mumps, and rubella viruses in a combined vaccine; Td, adult tetanus toxoid (full dose) and diphtheria toxoid (reduced dose) for adult use.

§ As of October 1990, only one HbCV is approved for use in children younger than 15 months.

‖ May be given at 12 months of age in areas with recurrent measles transmission.

¶ Any licensed *Haemophilus* b conjugate vaccine may be given.

** Should be given 6 to 12 months after the third dose.

†† May be given simultaneously with MMR at 15 months.

‡‡ May be given simultaneously with MMR and HbCV at 15 months or at any time between 12 and 24 months; priority should be given to administering MMR at the recommended age.

§§ Can be given up to the seventh birthday.

Reprinted with permission from *Report of the Committee on Infectious Diseases.* Copyright © 1991, American Academy of Pediatrics.

control are based on recommendations by the Joint Commission on Accreditation of Healthcare Organizations (JCAHO) and local health departments, some of which do not cover nontraditional health-care settings.

Infection Control Committees. To qualify for JCAHO approval, a hospital must have an infection control program responsible for controlling, investigating, reporting, and preventing infections in the facility. A committee of hospital employees and physicians is usually formed to evaluate practices designed to prevent hospital-associated infections. Committee membership varies depending on the institution, but all major medical services should be represented, as well as representatives of nursing, housekeeping, the laboratory, pharmacy, central services, and the operating room.

One member of the committee is designated to coordinate its work. Most institutions have one person, usually a nurse, who is employed to implement the infection control program and to collate the data that is generated. The position has various titles; practitioners are often called hospital epidemiologists. Large hospitals may have several people in the epidemiology department.

Nursing Interventions for Altered Function

When an infection becomes established, nursing measures are directed toward helping the patient combat the illness and preventing the spread of the infection to others.

Host Defenses Enhancement

Because nothing is more important in controlling infection than maintaining the natural barriers to infection, nurses devote a great deal of time to supporting these defenses. Enhancing host defenses is both preventive and supportive therapy.

Decrease of Transient Microorganisms. Decreasing the number of microorganisms present on body surfaces can help prevent and fight infection. Handwashing is the most significant measure to decrease the transient growth of microorganisms. Patients should be encouraged to wash their hands after using the toilet, before eating, and after contact with articles likely to be contaminated. Regular bathing, shampooing, and general grooming are important in keeping body surfaces clean. In some instances, such as before a surgical procedure, antimicrobial soap may be used to further impede microbial growth.

Daily brushing and flossing of teeth remove microorganisms that collect in the oral cavity. Regular dental check-ups are important so that plaque and tartar, which provide good foci for bacterial growth, can be removed from the teeth.

Special eye care must be given to patients who have an impaired blink reflex or cannot tear. Regular cleansing of the eye and the instillation of artificial tears help prevent eye infections.

Intact Skin and Mucous Membranes. Intact skin and mucous membranes provide a physical barrier against the invasion of possible pathogens. Adequate hydration and lubricants or creams can prevent excessive drying. A water-soluble lubricant can be applied to the nares or lips to prevent cracking. Avoiding trauma that could impair skin integrity is important. Harsh chemicals, excessive heat, or friction can abrade skin and should be avoided.

For bedridden patients, establishing regular turning schedules and massaging bony prominences decrease the chance of skin breakdown and possible infection. Specialized equipment such as kinetic beds or special mattresses may be used for high-risk patients.

Rest and Relaxation. Adequate rest and freedom from stress are important in fighting and preventing infection. Sleep disturbances can occur when patients must be awakened at night for antibiotic therapy. If this is necessary, other activities (such as vital signs and dressing changes) should be scheduled to coincide with antibiotic administration. The environment should be kept quiet and comfortable to induce sleep. Naps during the day may be indicated. Activities that promote relaxation and reduce stress should be encouraged.

Nutrition. Patients with infections require high-calorie, high-protein diets with adequate vitamins to promote healing and to manufacture the components of the immune system. Fever increases the metabolic needs of body tissues. Loss of nutrients from vomiting, diarrhea, and wound drainage often necessitates supplemental feedings, such as between-meal snacks. Hyperalimentation may be necessary if the patient cannot consume adequate nutrition orally. Providing frequent, small meals that the patient likes and can manage increases the chances of meeting nutritional goals. Giving oral hygiene before and after meals enhances patient enjoyment and decreases the chances for opportunistic infection of the mouth. As always, it is important to avoid any food with questionable methods of preparation or refrigeration.

Hydration. Infection often causes large fluid losses from sweating, vomiting, diarrhea, or excessive wound drainage. Adequate hydration is important to prevent drying and cracking of the skin and mucous membranes. The nurse should encourage adequate fluid intake to preserve intravascular volume and to maintain adequate urinary output. Decreased urine volume increases urinary stasis and the risk of urinary tract infection. If the patient cannot drink, intravenous fluid administration may be necessary.

Ambulation and Positioning. Regular periods of aerobic exercise should be encouraged if possible. If mobility is limited, the nurse should encourage as much activity as the patient can tolerate without excessive fatigue. Ambulation that does not exceed the activity tolerance of a compromised respiratory system or infected joints promotes circulation, facilitates chest wall excursion, promotes digestion, and decreases stasis of bodily fluids.

When ambulation is impossible, patients may require assistance with turning and positioning. Patients should be assisted in turning every 2 hours while awake and every 2 to 4 hours while sleeping. Ambulation resumes as soon as the patient's condition permits. Extremities may need to be elevated to facilitate drainage when infection is present.

Pulmonary Toilet. Encouraging patients to cough, deep-breathe, blow their noses, and move promotes clearance of respiratory secretions, which may become infected if allowed to pool in the lower respiratory tract. Retained secretions prevent adequate gas exchange at the alveolar membranes and reduce the amount of oxygen available to the tissues to combat infection, heal injured tissues, and meet metabolic needs. Secondary infections are commonly associated with impaired respiratory tract function.

Patients should be taught to cover their mouths when they cough or sneeze to prevent droplet transmission of microorganisms. When blowing the nose, one nostril should always remain open to prevent secretions from becoming forced into the ear canal. Youngsters should be taught not to pick their noses, since infected organisms can easily be transmitted to other parts of the body and other people. Everyone should be taught to dispose properly of tissues and respiratory secretions. See Chapter 30 for detailed information on pulmonary hygiene and care.

Comfort Measures. Manifestations of infection such as aches and pains, feelings of lethargy or malaise, fever, chills, nausea and vomiting, and itching cause generalized discomfort that is most often managed by relieving the symptoms. In general, comfort measures are aimed at relieving debilitating symptoms to conserve the patient's energy for healing and fighting infection.

Aches and pains are treated with mild analgesics or narcotics, based on their impact on rest, sleep, and ambulation. Feelings of malaise may be relieved with warm broth, a cool cloth to the head, warm blankets, and rest. Fevers may be treated, if prolonged or excessive, with tepid sponge baths, antipyretics, or cooling blankets. Shaking chills can be relieved by warm blankets and warm fluids, but may require intravenous meperidine if prolonged. Nausea and vomiting may be relieved by removing objects with objectionable odors from the patient's room, offering carbonated beverages, providing a darkened, quiet room, or in more severe cases by withholding oral intake and giving antiemetics. Itching may be treated with moist cool cloths, calamine lotion, pastes made from baking soda, or prescribed antihistamines (e.g., diphenhydramine).

Antimicrobial Therapy

Antimicrobial agents are used to combat the growth and replication of microorganisms. Giving these drugs and monitoring therapy is a collaborative function of nurses, physicians, pharmacists, and laboratory technicians.

Antibiotics should be given based on the presumed antibiotic sensitivity of the infecting species. A culture and sensitivity is obtained to determine appropriate antibiotic therapy. Antibiotics should not be used routinely in all infections. Several species of organisms have mutated over the years since antibiotics were introduced, and now are resistant to all but a few toxic drugs.

It is important to remember what antibiotics can and cannot do. They do not cure the patient: at best they slow the growth of or kill the organism, which is necessary for recovery from infection. They control the size of the microbial population with which the patient's immune system must contend. Antibiotics "buy time" during which the patient's own immune system can be mobilized. Eliminating the microbes may prevent further injury, but a return to normalcy depends on the body's healing capacity (Alcamo, 1986).

Antibiotics as a group have a wide range of safety but they can produce severe allergic reactions and toxic effects. Patients should be asked about allergies and the drugs they currently use so that incompatibilities can be detected. Renal and hepatic failure, interactions with other drugs, the patient's underlying disease, and extremes of age predispose the patient to adverse reactions. Both the very young and the very old have impaired renal clearance of drugs, and their dosage should be adjusted accordingly. Monitoring blood levels of antibiotics is one method of ensuring safety and optimal effectiveness; see the section above on therapeutic drug monitoring.

Antibiotics may eradicate the endogenous flora of the skin and mucous membranes of the mouth, gastrointestinal tract, and vaginal tract. This flora normally protects the host's mucous membranes, and when it is eliminated, opportunistic organisms may invade the tissues. Opportunistic infection is a secondary infection that often occurs when normal flora is destroyed by antibodies, immunosuppression, or cancer treatment. Opportunistic infection are more common when antimicrobials are given in large doses, when several antimicrobials are given concurrently, or when broad-spectrum antibiotics are used. Often such infection appears 4 to 5 days after antimicrobial therapy is begun.

Prevention of Infection Spread

When caring for a patient with an infection, it is important to perform nursing interventions that prevent the spread of infection to others.

Handwashing and Sterile Technique. Handwashing and sterile technique are two significant factors in pre-venting the occurrence and transmission of infection in health-care settings (Fig. 35-6). Hands should be washed before and after contacts that have the potential for transmission of infectious materials, either from or to the caregiver. Even with the new emphasis on gloving for contact with body fluids, nothing is more effective than good handwashing in preventing the transmission of infectious organisms. Although experts say that proper handwashing can reduce nosocomial infection rates by 50%, several studies have demonstrated that it is the least common infection control measure in hospitals (Castle & Ajemian, 1987). See Chapter 22 for specific information on handwashing.

Sterile technique (surgical asepsis) is used when:

- A body cavity is entered with an object that may damage the mucous membranes
- The intravascular compartment is entered
- A surgical procedure is performed
- Any procedure is performed on an immunosuppressed patient.

Examples of these procedures include inserting intravenous or urinary catheters, giving injections, irrigating drainage devices, and changing surgical dressings.

Isolation. Often the nurse is the first person to identify symptoms indicating infection and to institute precautions for the transmission of infection. Various isolation systems are discussed in Chapter 22. Isolation procedures are a matter of hospital policy, but current Centers for Disease Control recommendations emphas-

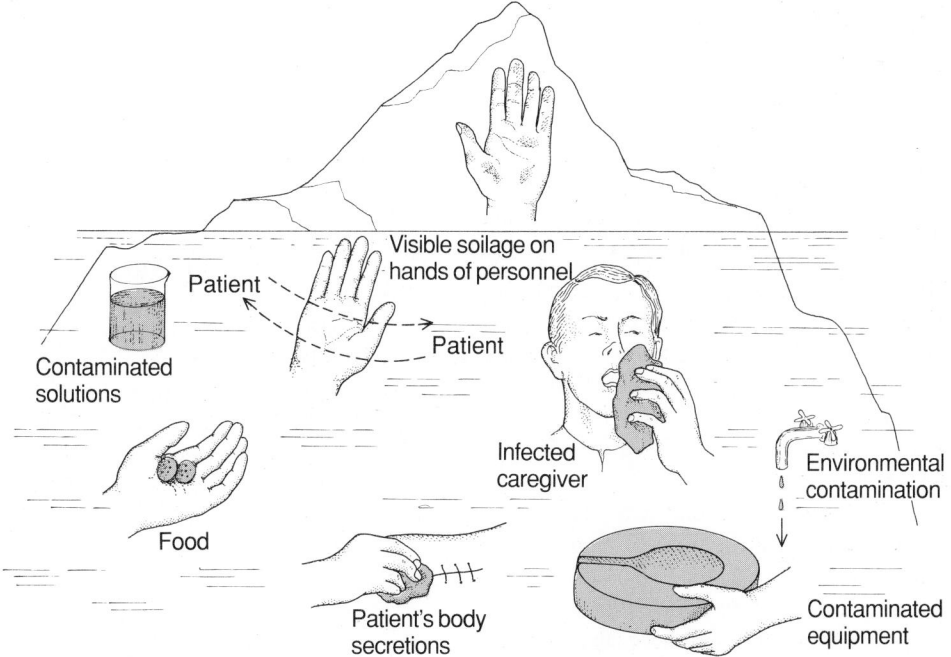

Figure 35–6. Contamination iceberg. Visible soilage on the hands of personnel is only the tip of the iceberg. The risk for carrying infection is greater but many times is hidden.

ize the need to treat blood and other body fluids from all patients as potentially hazardous. This approach is known as universal precautions. Gloves should be worn for all contact with body fluids. Gowns, gloves, masks, and goggles should be worn when there is a danger of splashing body fluids into the face, eyes, or clothing of the caregiver. Specific precautions, such as a private room with negative airflow, should be taken for airborne transmission.

Secretion Disposal. Patients and their families should be instructed about proper methods for disposing of body secretions such as sputum, feces, urine, and wound drainage. The nurse should provide the patient with tissues to cover the nose and mouth while coughing and sneezing, and disposal bags should be within convenient reach. Full bags should be emptied and replaced. Family members should be taught that diapers soiled by infants or adults should be rinsed in the toilet before placing them in covered trash containers or sending them to the laundry service. Dressings used for containing wound drainage should be placed in disposable, moistureproof bags and removed from the patient-care area. Hand-washing is essential for patients and health-care workers when any contact with body secretions occurs.

Discharge Planning and Home Care

Home-care management may be as simple as caring for a patient with influenza or as complex as managing home care for a terminal cancer patient recovering from extensive surgery. Whether the care is short- or long-term, avoiding infectious complications and supporting the family is important in maintaining functional abilities (see the display).

Safety Alert

- Wash your hands! The most common cause of transmission of microorganisms in the hospital is contact with unwashed hands.
- Adhere strictly to aseptic technique when indicated.
- Keep your immunizations up to date. Communicable diseases can be serious or fatal.
- Avoid any contact with body fluids with bare hands. Use gloves to prevent the transmission of infections.
- Institute preventive measures to ensure that skin and mucous membranes remain intact. Disruptions in the epithelial layer greatly increase the risk of infection.

Issues in Home Management

Barriers to Home Management of Infection

The patient or caregiver may:

- Lack knowledge
- Lack financial resources
- Perceive the behavior needed as unacceptable or uncomfortable
- Lack technical skill
- Experience depression or anger that impedes his or her incentive to practice healthy behaviors or deliver care
- Have religious or sociocultural beliefs and behaviors that oppose the recommendations of the health-care provider.

Interventions to Facilitate Positive Outcomes

Meet Educational Needs
- Assess level of knowledge of disease and preventive behavior (rest, exercise, nutrition, mode of transmission of the disease, use of medications, aseptic technique)
- Provide simple written instructions.

Meet Needs for Supplies and Equipment
- Insurance coverage evaluation
- Referral to social services
- Referral to volunteer organizations
- Instruction in use of generic brands of medications.

Meet Needs for Support in Alteration of Lifestyle
- Emphasize the positive aspects of increase in well-being.
- Set realistic goals with the patient and significant others.
- Modify the care plan to avoid conflict with religious beliefs or cultural practices by incorporating those behaviors that do not cause adverse effects.
- Enlist the support of other members of the family and social or religious group.

Provide a Supportive Social Network
- Give appropriate referrals to groups and agencies.
- Identify health-care providers who will provide assistance.
- Counsel family members or significant others.

There is a trend toward keeping all but the most seriously ill patients at home for the delivery of health care. When this is impossible, patients often receive necessary care in inpatient facilities and return to their homes for recuperation. Many patients are discharged from acute-care facilities with indwelling devices that increase the risk for infection. Many institutions now employ nurses and social workers whose sole function is to arrange for continuity of care in the home. Some hospitals even have their own home-health agencies or have contracts with others.

The nurse must assess the caregiver's knowledge level and health-care beliefs and practices. The home must be evaluated to help the family arrange for convenient care delivery. Caregivers must be involved in the planning and should choose solutions that are acceptable to them. They need assistance in buying or renting equipment and in obtaining supplies and medications. A daily record-keeping system must be created to record information about vital signs, medications, treatments, and food and fluid intake. There should be a place on the record where caregivers can note questions to ask the health-care professional.

Roles may change in the family as a result of the

Nursing Management Plan
The Patient at Risk for Infection

Nursing Diagnosis: High risk for infection related to delayed wound healing, immunosuppressive treatment for cancer of the bowel, and age manifested by insufficient knowledge of wound healing and infection.

Patient Goal: Patient/family will demonstrate knowledge about methods of preventing and detecting infection.

Patient Outcome Criteria

- Patient/family member describes methods to avoid infection and dispose of contaminated articles by second day.
- Patient/family member verbalizes signs and symptoms of infection by third day.
- Patient/family member demonstrates acceptable technique in applying a dressing by discharge.
- By discharge, patient/family member describes food and fluid that will meet nutritional needs.

Nursing Intervention	Scientific Rationale
1. Begin instruction of wound care as early in the course of recovery as possible. Include family member.	1. To prepare patient in wound management before discharge.
2. Review principles of good handwashing before wound care.	2. Handwashing is the single most important mechanism in stopping the transmission of pathogenic organisms.
3. Demonstrate the technique for dressing change (see Procedure 34-1). Allow time for practice and a return demonstration.	3. Technical skills are better acquired if they are observed and practiced.
4. Demonstrate removal of old dressing, including how to discard in moisture-proof bag.	4. Proper waste disposal is important in preventing the spread of microorganisms.
5. Review the causes of wound contamination.	5. Better understanding aids patient compliance.
6. Discuss activites that may cause trauma to the wound and how to avoid them.	6. Trauma can prevent wound healing and increase the chance of infection.
7. Review signs and symptoms of infection, encouraging patient and family to ask questions.	7. Early detection and treatment of infection decreases incidence of serious complications.
8. Instruct patient in the importance of well-balanced diet high in protein calories. Discuss sources of vitamin C and vitamin supplements.	8. Wound healing requires protein and calories for building new cells. The immune system depends on protein and calories to produce antibodies.
9. Provide the patient with written instruction concerning how to change the dressing and when to call their physician.	9. Instructions given in the hospital may be forgotten when at home. Written instructions provide a handy reference.

illness. The caregiver assumes more responsibility, and the newly dependent patient may find that his or her self-concept is altered. Family members must be counseled about these changes and helped to express feelings about the role transitions. Support systems should be arranged for the caregiver so that he or she has the freedom to accomplish desired goals. Support systems can also help ensure that the caregiver can get adequate rest and avoid emotional or physical exhaustion.

The caregiver must be taught how to evaluate vital signs, give medications, and observe for signs of toxicity. Basic aseptic practices should be taught to the patient and family members. The importance of handwashing and proper disposal of contaminated supplies must be stressed. The caregiver may require instruction in basic hygiene measures such as bathing, toileting, and oral care. Instruction in sterile technique is necessary for applying dressings, managing intravenous devices and medications, and caring for urinary catheters.

The caregiver should be taught to wear rubber gloves when caring for the patient with a known infection. Lightweight rubber gloves, the kind commonly used for dishwashing and household cleaning, are suitable for the home care of patients with diarrhea or wound infections. These gloves can be washed with mild soap and water and reused after drying. They must be kept separate from those used in food preparation or dishwashing.

EVALUATION

The success of a program to avoid or contain infection requires cooperation between the patient and the health-care team. Excellent communication is required and high levels of trust must be established. People must assume responsibility for their own behavior and health-care practices, and the health-care system must educate the public and scrutinize its own infection prevention practices. Health-care workers must be diligent in practicing infection control.

The optimal outcome of efforts to control infection (which is not always attainable) is freedom from the signs and symptoms of infection. Some outcome criteria for goals involving infection include:

Goal
Patient will demonstrate adequate knowledge to recognize and report signs of infection.

Possible Outcome Criteria
- Before discharge, patient or caregiver lists four signs of infection.
- Before discharge, patient or caregiver verbalizes indications that would require contacting a health-care professional.
- Before discharge, patient or caregiver demonstrates accurate monitoring of body temperature.

Goal
Patient will use good health practices to prevent the occurrence and spread of infection.

Possible Outcome Criteria
- Patient or caregiver demonstrates good handwashing technique after the teaching session.
- Before discharge, patient or caregiver verbalizes proper methods of infection control to be used at home.
- By discharge, patient verbalizes selected strategies to minimize the risk of infection.

Goal
Patient will comply with treatment regimens to help cure infection and prevent possible complications.

Possible Outcome Criteria
- Patient keeps the next three appointments with health-care providers.
- Patient uses recommended aseptic practices for dressing changes or invasive devices as a return demonstration at the next teaching session.
- Patient takes prescribed medications to treat or prevent infections, as reported to the nurse at the next appointment.

Key Concepts

- Microorganisms are everywhere but usually do not cause harm.
- The body has an elaborate system of barriers to invasion by microorganisms.
- Infections are responsible for more visits to health-care facilities than any other reason.
- Advances in medical technology are often the means of transmission for infection.
- Infection requires an uninterrupted chain of events; if any link in the chain is broken, infection cannot occur.
- Although a few infections are caused by the microorganism's ability to cause disease almost every time it comes in contact with a human, most infections are caused by a breakdown of host defenses.
- Nosocomial infections are infections acquired during the course of health-care delivery.
- Infections may be acute or chronic.
- Host defenses are specific and nonspecific.
- The four signs of inflammation are redness, warmth, swelling, and tenderness.
- Fever is an important mechanism in fighting infection, but it consumes a great deal of metabolic energy.
- T-lymphocytes and B-lymphocytes form memory cells that can be reactivated on reexposure to an antigen. This is the basis of lasting immunity.

■ Production of cellular immunity and antibodies takes 2 to 4 weeks after the first exposure to an organism.

■ Immunizations are given to children and adults depending on the maturity of the patient's immune system and the activities the age group participates in.

■ Because communicable childhood diseases may have severe complications, all children should be immunized.

■ Very young and very old people have decreased resistance to infection. Both nonspecific and specific barriers to infection are affected.

■ A communicable disease is caused by an agent that is easily transmitted among hosts.

■ The inflammatory response helps control the spread of infection, but if it goes on too long it can harm the patient.

■ The most common complications of surgery are infections. The most common hospital infections are urinary tract infections, wound infections, respiratory tract infections, and bacteremias from intravascular line insertion.

■ A compromised host is a person whose natural barriers to infection have been decreased by medical therapy, a chronic condition, or an inadequate immune system.

■ Laboratory analysis is necessary to identify the specific organism or group of organisms causing an infection.

■ Preventing infection is an individual, community, national, and international responsibility.

■ Increasing numbers of patients are being treated at home for chronic conditions or rehabilitation, and many of them have several risk factors for infection. Nurses must assume the responsibility for teaching these patients or their caregivers how to avoid infection.

References

Alcamo, I. E. (1986). *Fundamentals of microbiology.* Reading, MA: Addison-Wesley.

Bohnen, J. M., & Meakins, J. L. (1985). Postoperative infection. In L. A. Mandell & E. D. Ralph (Eds.), *Essentials of infectious diseases* (pp. 353–370). Boston: Blackwell.

Castle, M., & Ajemian, E. (1987). *Hospital infection control: Principles and practice* (3rd ed.). New York: John Wiley & Sons.

Centers for Disease Control. (1984). *National nosocomial infection surveillance.* CDC Surveillance Summaries 33(2SS).

Chusid, M. J. (1984). Special pediatric infectious disease problems. In M. W. Rytel & W. J. Mogabgab (Eds.), *Clinical manual of infectious disease* (pp. 215–239). Chicago: Year Book Medical Publishers.

Craven, R. F., Patrick, M. L., & Bruno, P. M. (1986). Changes with Aging. In M. Patrick, S. L. Woods, R. Craven, et al. (Eds.), *Medical-surgical nursing: Pathophysiological concepts.* Philadelphia: J. B. Lippincott.

Cruse, P. (1986). Surgical infection: Incisional wounds. In J. V. Bennett & P. S. Bachman (Eds.), *Hospital infections* (2nd ed., pp. 423–436). Boston: Little, Brown & Co.

Donowitz, L. G. (1987). Infection in the newborn. In R. P. Wenzel (ed.), *Prevention and control of nosocomial infections* (pp. 481–493). Baltimore: Williams & Wilkins.

Farley, M. P. (1991). Multiple trauma. In M. Patrick, S. L. Woods, R. Craven, et al. (Eds.), *Medical-surgical nursing: Pathophysiological concepts* (pp. 1576–1601). Philadelphia: J. B. Lippincott.

Flower, J. (1987). The other side of AIDS. *Healthcare Forum, 30*(6), 33–36.

Ford-Jones, E. L. (1987). The special problems of nosocomial infection in the pediatric patient. In R. P. Wenzel (Ed.), *Prevention and control of nosocomial infections* (pp. 494–540). Baltimore: Williams & Wilkins.

Fox, J. P. (1981). Epidemiology of infectious diseases. In R. D. Feigin & J. D. Cherry (Eds.), *Textbook of pediatric infectious diseases* (pp. 4–69). Philadelphia: W. B. Saunders.

Fox, R. A. (1984). The effect of aging on the immune response. In R. A. Fox (Ed.), *Immunology and infection in the elderly* (pp. 289–309). Edinburgh: Churchill-Livingstone.

Garibaldi, R. A., & Nurse, B. (1986). Infections in the elderly. *American Journal of Medicine, 81*(suppl 1A), 53–58.

Gordon, M. (1987). *Nursing diagnosis: Process and application* (2nd ed.). New York: McGraw-Hill.

Gross, P. A., & Levine, J. F. (1987). Infections in the elderly. In R. P. Wenzel (Ed.), *Prevention and control of nosocomial infections* (pp. 541–559). Baltimore: Williams & Wilkins.

Halverson, S. G., & Graham, S. K. (1991). Infections and inflammatory disorders affecting reproductive function. In M. Patrick, S. L. Woods, R. Craven, et al. (Eds.), *Medical-surgical nursing: Pathophysiological concepts* (pp. 1499–1523). Philadelphia: J. B. Lippincott.

Hoeprich, P. D., & Boggs, D. R. (1983). Manifestations of infectious diseases. In R. D. Hoeprich (Ed.), *Infectious diseases* (pp. 85–98). Philadelphia: Harper & Row.

Messner, R. L., & Gorse, G. J. (1987). Nursing management of peripheral intravenous sites. *Focus on Critical Care, 14*(2), 25–33.

NANDA (1990). *Taxonomy I revised 1990, with official nursing diagnoses.* St. Louis, MO: North American Nursing Diagnosis Association.

Weinstein, R. A. (1986). Multiply resistant strains: Epidemiology and control. In J. V. Bennett & P. S. Bachman (Eds.), *Hospital infections* (2nd ed., pp. 151–169). Boston: Little, Brown & Co.

Wertz, M. J. (1991). Infection. In M. Patrick, S. L. Woods, R. Craven, et al. (Eds.), *Medical-surgical nursing: Pathophysiological concepts.* Philadelphia: J. B. Lippincott.

Bibliography

Benenson, A. S. (1981). *Control of communicable diseases in man* (13th ed.). Washington, DC: American Public Health Association.

Burke, I. F. (1978). *The infection-prone hospital patient.* Boston: Little, Brown & Co.

Carnevali, D. L. (1983). *Nursing care planning: Diagnosis and management* (3rd ed.). Philadelphia: J. B. Lippincott.

Jaroff, L. (1988, May 23). Stop that germ. *Time Magazine*, pp. 56–64.

Joint Commission on Accreditation of Hospitals. (1986). *A guide to JCAH nursing services standards.* Chicago: Author.

Kee, J. L. (1987). *Laboratory and diagnostic tests with nursing implications* (2nd ed.). Norwalk, CN: Appleton & Lange.

Koepke, J. A., & Koepke, J. F. (1987). *Guide to clinical laboratory diagnosis* (3rd ed.). Norwalk, CN: Appleton & Lange.

McFarland, M.B., & Grant, M. M. (1988). *Nursing implications of laboratory tests* (2nd ed.). New York: John Wiley & Sons.

Seedor, M. W. (1979). *Introduction to asepsis: A programmed unit for nurses* (3rd ed.). New York: Teachers College Press.

Smith, W. (1987). *Respiratory and infectious disease: A profile of health and disease in America.* New York: Facts on File Publications.

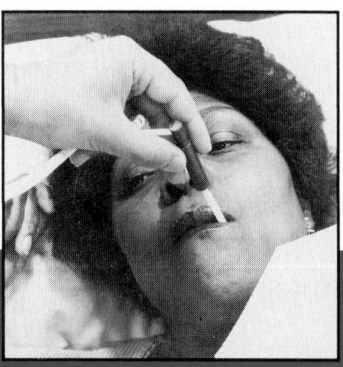

Thermoregulation

LEARNING OBJECTIVES

Upon completion of this chapter, the student will be able to do the following:

- Describe how heat is produced in the body.
- Describe how the body reduces core temperature.
- Describe the effects of various factors on the body's thermoregulation.
- Discuss lifespan considerations for temperature regulation.
- Identify risk factors that predispose to altered body temperature.
- Describe manifestations of altered body temperature.

- Discuss appropriate assessment parameters concerning thermoregulation.
- List four NANDA nursing diagnoses concerning potential or actual altered body temperature.
- Discuss the importance of patient teaching in prevention and treatment of altered thermoregulation.
- Understand appropriate nursing interventions for fever management.

KEY TERMS

Antipyretic
Basal body temperature
Basal metabolic rate

Core temperature
Febrile
Fever
Hyperthermia
Hyperpyrexia

Hypothermia
Insensible evaporation
Metabolism
Surface temperature

36

Normal Thermoregulation
  Heat Production
    Basal Metabolic Rate
    Exercise or Muscle Activity
    Thyroid Hormones
    Sympathetic Nervous System
  Heat Loss
    Radiation
    Conduction
    Convection
    Evaporation
  Normal Pattern of Body Temperature
  Factors Affecting Normal Body Temperature
    Physiologic Processes
    Behavioral Responses
  Lifespan Considerations
Altered Thermoregulation
  Potential for Altered Thermoregulation
    Environmental Extremes
    Altered Thermoregulatory Mechanisms
    Exercise
    Altered Cognitive States
    Stress
    Altered Nutrition
  Manifestations of Altered Thermoregulation
    Pyrexia or Fever
    Heat Exhaustion
    Heat Cramps
    Heat Stroke
    Hypothermia
    Frostbite
  Impact of Altered Temperature on Activities of
    Daily Living
Assessment
  Subjective Data

    Functional Pattern Identification
    Risk Identification
    Dysfunctional Identification
  Objective Data
    Assessment of Body Temperature
    Inspection
Nursing Diagnoses and Patient Goals
  Diagnostic Statement: High Risk for Altered Body
    Temperature
    Definition
    Risk Factors
  Diagnostic Statement: Hypothermia
    Definition
    Defining Characteristics
    Related Factors
  Diagnostic Statement: Hyperthermia
    Definition
    Defining Characteristics
    Related Factors
  Diagnostic Statement: Ineffective Thermoregulation
    Definition
    Defining Characteristics
    Related Factors
  Related Nursing Diagnoses
  Patient Goals
Implementation
  Nursing Interventions to Promote Health
  Nursing Interventions for Altered
    Thermoregulation
    Fever Management
    Nursing Management of Hyperthermia
    Nursing Management of Hypothermia
  Discharge Planning and Home Health Care
Evaluation
Key Concepts

NORMAL THERMOREGULATION

A person's body temperature is a sensitive indicator of the presence of physiologic changes occurring in the body. These changes can be the result of a disease process, a traumatic injury, or a therapeutic intervention. Because of the sensitive nature of a person's body temperature, monitoring the patient's temperature is one of the common routine procedures performed on any person entering the health-care system.

The nurse is often the person to screen patients using temperature monitoring, identifying deviations in temperature and reporting significant findings to the physician so that appropriate therapy can be instituted. Although the skill itself is readily learned, the physiology underlying thermoregulation is complex. For nurses to competently provide care for patients with normal or abnormal temperature states, it is important that the nurse possess a sound understanding of the physiologic processes involved in temperature regulation.

Core temperature, or the temperature of the interior body tissues, remains almost constant (within +/− 0.6°C [1°F]) in a healthy state. In contrast, a person's **surface temperature,** or the temperature of the skin and tissue immediately underlying the skin, rises and falls according to the temperature of the surrounding environment (Guyton, 1986). Core temperature is the product of the precise balance between heat production and heat loss. Figure 36-1 illustrates behavioral and physiologic factors involved in the production and loss of heat from the body.

Heat Production

Heat is produced continually in the body as a by-product of the chemical reactions taking place in all of the cells of the body. The collective process of chemical reactions occurring in the cells, with the by-product of heat production, is known as **metabolism.** The rate of heat production is directly determined by a person's metabolic rate. Factors such as level of activity, age, hormones, psychologic well-being, nutritional status, body temperature, and environmental temperature can increase or decrease the metabolic rate, however, and consequently, the amount of heat produced. In a resting state, most of the body heat is produced in the body core, which includes the trunk, viscera, and brain. During a

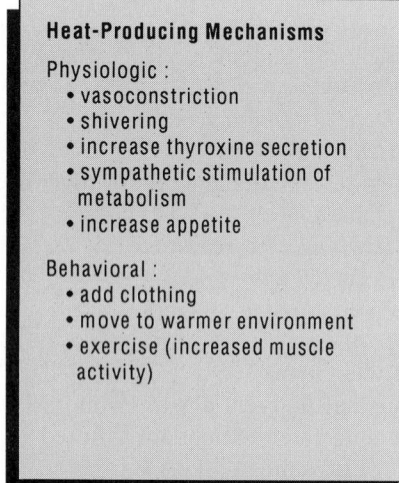

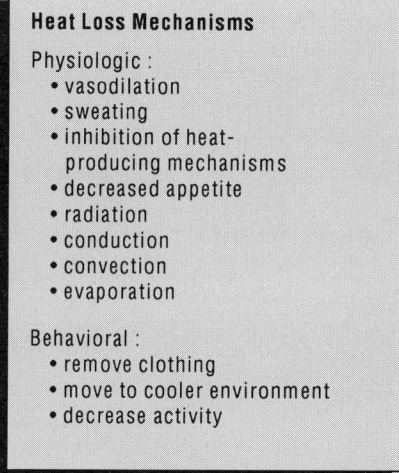

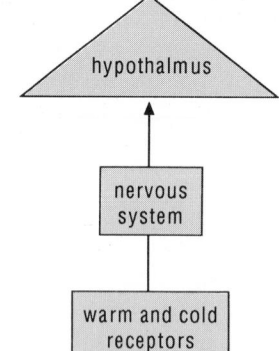

Figure 36–1. Body temperature: the balance between heat production and heat loss.

working state, most of the heat is produced in the musculature. The process of thermoregulation maintains a fairly constant core temperature regardless of where the heat is being produced.

Basal Metabolic Rate

The **basal metabolic rate** (BMR) is the amount of energy used by the body during absolute rest in an awake state (so-called basal conditions). To measure the BMR, the person is placed in basal conditions, as outlined in the display. The rate of oxygen used by the body under these conditions is measured with a metabolator. Then the metabolic rate is calculated in terms of kilocalories per square meter of body surface (kcal/m^2). The BMR is normally expressed as a percentage above or below the normal mean value (Vick, 1984).

The BMR varies with age and sex. A young child has a metabolic rate almost twice that of an adult because of the growth process that is occurring in children (Guyton, 1986). After 2 years of age, a girl's BMR is about 5% to 10% less than a boy's of the same age and size. The greatest difference of BMRs (18% to 27%) between the sexes occurs during adolescence (Vick, 1984). The BMR rate decreases rapidly from birth to about 20 years, and then declines more gradually.

Temperature, both external and internal, affects the BMR. People living in a tropical climate will probably have a lower BMR than people living in a temperate

---

Basal Conditions for Measuring BMR

- No food consumption for 12 hours because digestion of food increases the metabolic rate.
- A restful night of sleep because rest reduces the activities of the sympathetic nervous system and other metabolic excitants to their minimum level.
- No strenuous exercise after waking; rest in a reclining position for 30 minutes before the test. This is most important because of the profound effect exercise has on metabolism.
- Individual must be in a comfortable position and have as little psychologic stimulation as possible in order to reduce the degree of sympathetic activity.
- Environmental temperature should be between 20°C to 26.6°C (68°F to 80°F). Temperatures lower than this range increase sympathetic nervous activity, and higher temperatures cause discomfort and sweating.

From Guyton, A. C. (1986). *Textbook of medical physiology* (7th ed.) (p. 847). Philadelphia: W. B. Saunders.

---

zone, and their BMRs will be more closely related to their body weight than to their surface area. An increased body temperature, which speeds up the metabolic process, causes the BMR to rise approximately 14% for each degree Celsius of fever (7% per degree Fahrenheit) (Ganong, 1989).

Exercise or Muscle Activity

Exercise or muscle activity has profound effects on a person's metabolic rate, particularly if the person participates in some form of strenuous activity. Maximal muscle exercise can increase the body's overall heat production by about 50 times the normal amount for a few seconds, and in well-trained athletes, heat production can be increased by about 20 times the normal amount for a sustained period (Guyton 1986).

Thyroid Hormones

The thyroid hormones thyroxine and triiodothyronine also have a profound effect on the rate of body metabolism. These hormones increase the metabolic rate in most cells of the body, except the cells in the brain, testes, spleen, and retina. Thyroxine has a slow, prolonged effect on the metabolic process, whereas the actions of triiodothyronine occur about four times as rapidly as thyroxine (Guyton, 1986). To maintain a normal basal metabolic rate, the precise amount of thyroid hormone must be released at the appropriate time. This controlling function is regulated by the thyroid-stimulating hormone (TSH), which is secreted by the anterior pituitary gland.

People who have excessive levels of thyroid hormones (hyperthyroidism) have a higher metabolic rate and a temperature chronically elevated by as much as 0.5°C (1°F). The converse is true for people with low thyroid hormone levels (hypothyroidism) (Ganong, 1989).

Sympathetic Nervous System

Stimulation of the sympathetic nervous system, with the release of norepinephrine and epinephrine, increases the metabolic process within many cells. In the newborn child, the sympathetic stimulation of the mitochondria in a certain type of fat tissue called brown adipose tissue (BAT), which is located in the infant's interscapular region, increases the metabolic rate of the BAT, resulting in an increase in the rate of heat production by as much as 100% (Guyton 1986). This marked increase in metabolism and subsequent heat production is referred to as nonshivering thermogenesis (Vander, Sherman, & Lucinno, 1985). The magnitude of the effect of BAT thermogenesis in adults is questionable, and it is currently being investigated by numerous researchers (Baker, et al., 1984; Glick, 1987).

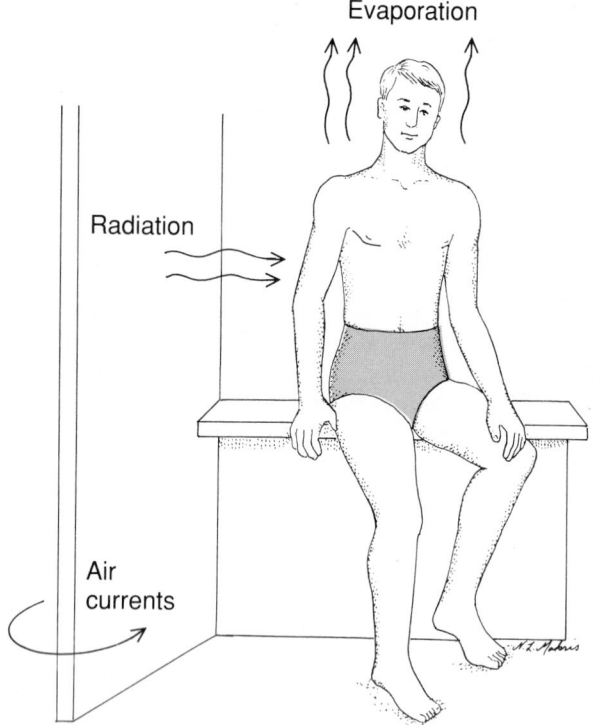

Evaporation

Radiation

Air
currents

Figure 36–2. Heat is lost by four processes: radiation, conduction, convection, and evaporation. Adapted from Guyton, A. C. (1986). *Textbook of medical physiology* (7th ed.), (p. 850). Philadelphia: W. B. Saunders.

Heat Loss

Just as heat is continuously being produced by the body, it is also continuously being lost. Heat is lost from the body by four processes: radiation, conduction, convection, and evaporation. Figure 36-2 depicts heat loss by each of these four processes. An understanding of these processes enables the nurse to control the amount of heat lost from the body.

Radiation

All objects that are not at absolute zero temperature radiate heat in the form of infrared heat rays. Heat loss in this manner is based on the principle that objects facing each other are always radiating heat toward one another. If the temperature of the body is greater than the environment, then a greater quantity of heat is radiated to the environment than to the body, and vice versa. A nude person in a room of normal temperature loses about 60% of their total body heat via radiation (Guyton, 1986). The nurse must consider heat lost by radiation when implementing procedures that expose the patient's skin surface to the environmental temperature (e.g., preparing the patient for a surgical procedure

in the cool operating room; adjusting the room temperature to compensate for heat loss during a bath; caring for a neonate in an isolette).

The amount of heat lost by radiation can be reduced by covering the body with closely woven fabrics. Dark-colored clothing absorbs more solar rays than light-colored fabrics. The same is true for dark skin tones compared with light ones.

Conduction

Conduction of heat is the transfer of heat from one object to another through direct contact. When a person grasps an empty metal container, heat will be conducted readily from the hand to the container, but within a few minutes the temperature of the container equals that of the hand, and thereafter the container actually acts as an insulator to prevent further heat loss from the hand. The body only loses minute amounts of heat via conduction to other objects.

The body does lose considerable amounts of heat to the air through conduction, however. If the air immediately adjacent to the skin is cooler, then the heat from the body will warm the air. Once the air next to the skin equals the temperature of the skin, there is no further loss of heat from the skin surface. Wearing several layers of clothing allows layers of warmed air to be created, thus insulating the body and helping to keep it warm. If the clothing becomes wet, its effectiveness as an insulator is lost because the conductivity of water increases the rate of heat transmission as much as 20-fold or more (Guyton, 1986).

The body also loses heat to water by conduction. Since water can absorb more heat than air, the body cannot form a zone of insulation around the body to reduce heat loss. The rate of heat loss from the skin can be quite high when there is immersion in water that is cooler than body temperature. Water used to bathe patients should be slightly above body temperature, unless the patient has an elevated temperature, called **febrile.** For febrile patients, the water should be warm but below body temperature, so the water will absorb heat from the patient.

Heat is also conducted from the internal organs of the body to the surface of the skin by the flow of blood. The skin and subcutaneous tissues, particularly the fat, act as heat insulators for the body. Fat conducts heat only one third as readily as other tissues. Women tend to have a thicker layer of subcutaneous fat than men. This insulating property of the skin and subcutaneous tissues plays an important role in maintaining a consistent core temperature.

A person can gain heat from the environment if it is warmer than their skin surface. This is not a source of heat production, and normally has little effect on the thermoregulation process; however, it can be a threat to the person if the temperature is extremely hot and the body is not able keep the core temperature within a normal range.

Convection

For heat to be lost from the body by convection, it must be conducted from the body to the air and then carried away by air currents. Normally, a warm layer of air exists adjacent to the skin surface. As the air becomes heated, it rises and passes into the cooler air mass. If the skin surface is in contact with air currents, the process of convection is increased. If during this process the temperature of the skin surface is cooled to equal the temperature of the air, then rate of heat loss cannot increase. Instead the rate at which heat can be conducted from the core of the body to the skin is the factor that then determines the rapidity of heat loss.

Heat loss by convection can be increased by opening windows or by forcing the exchange of air by placing a fan in a room. Activity such as walking or running also increases the amount of heat lost by convection.

If a person is exposed to an extremely cold environment, whether it is air or water, the environment is capable of carrying away essentially all of the heat that can reach the skin from the body core (Guyton, 1986).

Evaporation

Approximately 0.6 kcal of heat is lost for every gram of water that evaporates from the body (Mountcastle, 1980). Water is continuously being lost through evaporation from the skin and lungs at a rate of about 600 mL per day (Guyton 1986). This is referred to as **insensible evaporation,** and it cannot be controlled for purposes of temperature regulation because it results from continual diffusion of water molecules through the skin and respiratory tract mucosa, regardless of body temperature.

When the temperature of the surroundings becomes greater than the temperature of the skin surface, the only means by which the body can rid itself of heat is by the process of evaporation. In a very hot, humid environment, evaporation of water from the body is reduced because the surrounding air is already saturated, thus posing a potential health risk for some people, such as the elderly.

Normal Pattern of Body Temperature

The normal oral temperature of a healthy adult is considered to be 37°C (98.6°F); however, this is an average value. Each person has a unique circadian thermal rhythm that may be slightly higher or lower than 37°C. Table 36-1 outlines the normal temperature ranges for people throughout the lifespan.

The body has several repetitious patterns, one of which is the circadian thermal rhythm, which occurs in a 24-hour cycle. Studies have identified 5 PM to 7 PM (1700 to 1900 hours) as the peak of the daily cycle, when body temperature is likely to be elevated (Samples, et al., 1985). The time when body temperature is lowest occurs in the early morning.

Normal monthly fluctuations in body temperature occur in women because of hormonal factors. Progesterone, a female hormone secreted by the ovaries, is believed to have a thermogenic effect that causes the core temperature of many women to be elevated by 0.6°C (1°F) in the last half of their menstrual cycle (Shaver, 1991). This rise in temperature occurs at ovulation. By measuring oral body temperature every morning before rising (basal conditions), a woman can determine when ovulation has occurred. This early morning body temperature measurement is known as the **basal body temperature,** and provides the basis for the rhythm method of birth control.

Various parts of the body will normally have different temperature readings. The rectal temperature is considered to be the most representative of core body temperature, as this site varies least with environmental changes. Oral temperature is considered to be 0.6°C (1°F) lower than the rectal temperature (Guyton, 1986), and it is affected by many factors, including the ingestion of hot or cold fluids, gum-chewing, smoking, exercise, and mouth breathing (Carpenito, 1989). The reason for the higher rectal temperature is that the mouth is constantly being cooled by evaporation. The axillary temperature is considered to be 0.6°C (1°F) lower than the oral temperature. Variations in temperature readings can occur within a particular site. For example, the posterior sublingual pocket of the mouth has been found to be significantly higher than the area under the front of the tongue (Erickson, 1980).

TABLE 36–1
Normal Temperature Ranges

Age	Site	Degrees Celsius	Degrees Fahrenheit
Newborn	Axilla	35.5–37.5	96–99.5
6 months	Axilla	37.5	99.5
5 years	Oral	37	98.6
13 years	Oral	36.6	97.8
Adult	Oral	37	98.6
>70 years	Oral	36	96.9

Factors Affecting Normal Body Temperature

Body temperature is determined by the delicate balance that occurs between heat production and heat loss, as shown in Figure 36-1. Normal body temperature depends mainly on physiologic processes, and, to a lesser extent, on behavioral responses.

Physiologic Processes

The integrated functioning of many body systems is required to maintain the body temperature within a normal range. The hypothalamus, nervous system, circulatory system, shivering mechanism, and sweat glands interdependently play a significant role in thermoregulation. The skin plays an important role for both systemic and local temperature regulation.

The Hypothalamus. The hypothalamus, often considered the body's thermostat, is able to maintain the internal temperature of the body within half a degree of the normal average range (Guyton, 1986). The preoptic area, located in the most anterior portion of the hypothalamus, contains thermosensitive neurons that directly respond to the temperature of the blood. When these neurons detect that the temperature of the blood is too warm, signals radiate to the "heat-loss center" located in the anterior portion of the hypothalamus. This anterior center is composed mainly of parasympathetic nerves that, when stimulated automatically, initiate mechanisms to decrease body heat. If cold is detected, signals are sent to the "heat-promoting center" located in the posterior portion of the hypothalamus. This center operates mainly through the sympathetic nervous system, which stimulates mechanisms to produce body heat.

The Nervous System. The nervous system acts as the communicating mechanism to assist the hypothalamus in maintaining body temperature within the critical temperature level, which is referred to as "set point." While the heat center in the preoptic area of the hypothalamus is mainly responsible for detecting heat, the detection of cold relies mainly on the cold receptors of the skin. To a lesser extent, the cold receptors in the spinal cord and abdominal organs also serve this purpose (Guyton, 1986). Temperature sensors receive information about the temperature of the internal or external environment and transmit this information to the hypothalamus along neural pathways. Once the signals have been reached by the heat-sensitive neurons in the hypothalamus, messages are then sent to initiate heat-producing or heat-reducing mechanisms.

The Circulatory System. The circulatory system functions as a transportation mechanism responsible for carrying heat from the body core, where heat is produced, to the body surface. Once heat arrives at the body surface, it can be transferred to the air via radiation, conduction, convection, and evaporation. When the hypothalamus sends out messages to cool the core temperature, the blood vessels dilate, increasing the blood flow to the skin surfaces. Conversely, vasoconstriction occurs when the body needs to conserve heat. The degree of vasoconstriction is controlled by the sympathetic nervous system. In the most exposed parts of the body, such as the hands, feet, and ears, the blood is supplied directly from the arterioles to the veins. This allows for tremendous variation in the rate of blood flow. In such areas, the rate of blood flow can be almost zero, or it can increase to 30% of the cardiac output (Guyton, 1986).

The Skin. The skin plays a major role in thermoregulation. The skin contains mainly cold (and some warmth) receptors, which send signals to the hypothalamus. When the skin is chilled over the entire body, immediate reflex effects are initiated to increase the body temperature. First, a strong reflex causes shivering, which produces heat. Concurrently, vasoconstriction of the blood vessels occurs and the sweating process is inhibited. When only a portion of the body is affected by a temperature change (e.g., when a person places one hand in warm water), local skin reflexes occur. These reactions are caused both by the local effects of temperature changes directly on the blood vessels and sweat glands, and by local cord reflexes conducted from the skin receptors to the spinal cord and back to the same skin area. The intensity of such a reaction is monitored by the hypothalamus to prevent excessive heat exchange from locally cooled or heated areas of the body (Guyton, 1986).

The skin also contains numerous blood vessels that transport heat from the core of the body to the skin surface, where heat loss mechanisms disperse the heat to the air. In addition, the skin acts as an insulator. Fat tissues within the subcutaneous layer of the skin help to keep heat inside the body.

The Shivering Mechanism. The shivering mechanism is an involuntary motor activity that increases body temperature through increased heat production. Shivering is controlled by a center located in the dorsomedial portion of the posterior hypothalamus. This center is extremely sensitive and becomes activated when the body temperature falls a fraction of a degree below the set point. When this center receives cold signals from the skin and spinal cord, it transmits impulses through bilateral tracts down the brain stem into the lateral columns of the spinal cord, and then to the anterior motor neurons. These nonrhythmic impulses increase the tone of the skeletal muscles. Once the muscle tone reaches a critical level, shivering probably results from feedback oscillation of the muscle spindle stretch reflex mechanism. To help maintain normal body temperature, heat production can rise as high as four to five times normal during maximum shivering.

The Sweat Glands. Sweat glands located beneath the dermal layer of the skin secrete a watery solution containing high concentrations of sodium and chloride. This secretion passes through tiny ducts onto the skin surface. Once on the surface of the skin, it evaporates, thus cooling the surface of the skin. As the skin cools, the blood flowing near the surface of the skin is also cooled. The preoptic area of the anterior hypothalamus initiates the sweating process via impulses transmitted in the autonomic pathways to the spinal cord, and then through the sympathetic outflow to the skin everywhere on the body.

Behavioral Responses

Humans can also help regulate body temperature through behavioral responses. A person must be alert and physically able to successfully manipulate the environment to use behavioral responses to assist with temperature control. To increase body temperature, a person can put on more clothes, raise the temperature of the room, or increase physical activity. To decrease body temperature, a person can remove clothing, increase convection currents by sitting near a fan or breeze, or move to a cooler environment.

Lifespan Considerations

The very young and the elderly are at high risk when any deviation from normal body temperature occurs. Understanding the developmental considerations in thermoregulatory mechanisms will help the nurse prevent and treat altered temperature states.

Newborn and Infant

The premature infant is neurologically underdeveloped, with limited capability for thermoregulation. Low birth weight significantly decreases the amount of body fat available to act as insulation. Premature infants have temperature receptors on their face in the trigeminal area. When stimulated (e.g., when cool air currents blow over the face), the infant will start to burn brown fat, increasing metabolic rate and oxygen consumption, even if the rest of the body is warm (Schreiner & Kisling, 1982). This can result in respiratory distress, apnea, and metabolic acidosis, leading to significant physiologic problems for the infant. The premature infant is placed in an incubator, so that the temperature of the environment can be carefully regulated.

All infants are at risk for alterations in temperature regulation because of a number of factors. A large sur-

face area, as compared to weight, creates problems in maintaining the heat infants produce. In addition, the very young do not have the capacity to increase their body temperature by shivering, reduce their temperature by sweating, or make behavioral adjustments in their environment (Dodman, 1987). During the first year of life, the immune system is immature, so infants are prime candidates for infection, which in turn produces fevers.

The infant depends totally on parents or other caregivers to assist with temperature regulation by maintaining a constant, comfortable environmental temperature. Parents frequently must be taught not to overdress a newborn. Many parents must also be taught how to take an axillary temperature for their newborn.

Toddler and Preschooler

As the child enters the second year of life, thermoregulation is more stable, although not fully mature. Weight gain during the first year has added fat to help insulate the body from heat loss.

A common neurologic disorder associated with fever that affects a small portion of young children is febrile convulsions. Most febrile convulsions occur after 6 months of age, with increasing frequency until 18 months. They are unusual after 5 years of age (Whaley & Wong, 1989). The cause of the convulsions is unknown, but they occur during a temperature rise rather than after prolonged elevation. Convulsions can be frightening for parents. The nurse frequently assumes the role of teacher, helping parents become knowledgeable on how to treat fever or convulsions in their young children.

Child and Adolescent

As children grow and develop, their sweat glands and shivering mechanism become more functional. By the time the child reaches puberty, these two temperature-regulating mechanisms are fully functional.

Childhood illnesses continue to cause fever in the school-age child and adolescent. Adolescents begin to take part in many activities, such as hiking and sports, that may expose them to extremes in environmental temperature. Sports that require excessive exertion in warm temperatures (e.g., running laps in football practice) should be done with caution. If youngsters participate in skiing or hiking, they should be informed on how to dress properly to avoid exposure. Swimming lessons should include information on how to protect oneself from hypothermia if accidental exposure to cold water is possible.

Adult and Older Adult

The thermoregulating system of the adult is fully operational to maintain core body temperature. Unless adults are exposed to some form of trauma (e.g., head injury, accidental hypothermia) or disease process (e.g., skin disorders that disrupt the ability to sweat; tumors involving the hypothalamus; breakdown in the immune system) that impedes the functioning of their regulatory system, their bodies can cope with minor deviations in normal temperature range.

The normal temperature range decreases as people reach old age. Research has documented mean oral temperature of the elderly adult as 36.2°C (97.2°F) (Kurtz, 1982). This implies that the elderly have less heat to lose. Also, their BMR has decreased, they often have less body fat to act as an insulator, they are less active, and can be poorly nourished. The elderly are particularly sensitive to extremes in the environmental temperature because of the decreased functioning of their thermoregulatory system. The older population has been found to have an increased body temperature threshold before sweating begins, as well as a decreased sweating rate (Yurick, Spier, Robb, & Ebert, 1989). The elderly may also live in poorly ventilated apartments and have inadequate resources for heating or cooling their homes. Cognitive changes may make the older person less mentally capable of making appropriate behavioral responses, especially if drugs such as hypnotics or alcohol are used. The elderly have a much higher mortality rate associated with abnormal temperature states than do infants. Perhaps this higher mortality rate occurs because the elderly are not given the same degree of protection and nurturing as infants.

ALTERED THERMOREGULATION

Despite finely tuned physiologic mechanisms for temperature control, situations can occur that overwhelm the body's homeostatic mechanisms and result in abnormal body temperature. Abnormal body temperature can be slight, such as with low-grade fever with a cold, or life-threatening, as in severe cases of hypothermia or hyperthermia. Knowledge of factors that can alter normal body temperature is important for the nurse in preventing and treating alterations in thermoregulation.

Potential for Altered Thermoregulation

Extremes in environmental temperature, altered thermoregulatory mechanisms, infection, strenuous exercise, and stress can cause deviations from normal body temperature.

Environmental Extremes

The person's environment may influence the temperature of the body. Exposure to very warm temperatures for an extended period of time can lead to hyperthermia.

Hyperthermia is a state in which the core temperature is higher than the acceptably normal range for the person. Humans are capable of surviving extremes of environmental temperature, provided precautions are taken to avoid injury. The extremes of heat a person can safely tolerate depend on the moisture content of the air. If the air is dry and there are air currents present to allow evaporation, a person may tolerate a temperature of 65.5°C (150°F) for several hours; however, if moisture is present in the air and the environmental temperature is high, the process of evaporation is impeded, and the person can only tolerate a temperature of 34.4°C (94°F). If a person has existing health problems (such as heart disease), or if they are required to do physical work, even moderately elevated temperatures may be difficult to tolerate.

A period of acclimatization occurs when a person is suddenly exposed to very warm temperatures. At first, physical work is difficult and the person may actually feel weak and ill. Over a period of a few days, sweat mechanisms become more effective in cooling the body. As acclimatization occurs, sweat composition changes to contain less sodium (Vander, Sherman, & Luciano, 1985); this decreases the likelihood that fluid and electrolyte imbalance will occur.

Exposure to temperatures that are well below freezing present local and systemic problems, because such extremely low temperatures can result in freezing of the skin's surface, as well as lowering the body core temperature. When the core temperature of the body falls below 34.4°C (94°F), the ability of the hypothalamus to regulate body temperature is impaired.

Altered Thermoregulatory Mechanisms

Any condition that interferes with normal mechanisms of thermoregulation can contribute to altered body temperature.

Nervous System Impairment. Tumors or trauma to the brain or spinal cord interfere with nervous system control over temperature regulation. If the spinal cord is severed in the neck above the sympathetic outflow from the cord, as in the quadriplegic patient, the hypothalamus can no longer control the degree of vasoconstriction or sweating anywhere in the body. Local temperature reflexes originating in the skin, spinal cord, and intra-abdominal receptors can still function, but their effectiveness is limited. A person with this sort of disability must rely on behavioral responses or environmental control for temperature regulation.

Malignant Hyperthermia. Malignant hyperthermia is an inherited condition in which normal thermoregulatory mechanisms can be disrupted by the administration of certain anesthetic agents. Following the administration of halothane, succinylcholine, or lidocaine, the regulatory mechanisms of the hypothalamus are suppressed. The patient may experience tachycardia, arrhythmias, muscle rigidity (especially of the jaw), and extremely elevated body temperature. Temperature of the body increases very rapidly due to a hypermetabolic state. The patient's body temperature may reach 44°C to 46°C (111°F to 131°F) (McConnell, 1987). Excessive body temperature can cause irreversible cell injury, especially to brain cells. Survival depends on early recognition of the symptoms of malignant hyperthermia and immediate treatment to lower body temperature. Since this is an inherited problem, all people undergoing surgery should be questioned concerning any family member experiencing any adverse reactions to the administration of anesthetic agents.

Circulatory Impairment. Circulatory problems can impede normal temperature regulation. Patients with peripheral vascular disease or neuropathy (decreased blood flow to the nerves) are not able to constrict or dilate blood vessels to control heat loss from the body. Treatment with medications, such as antihypertensive agents, can also interfere with vasoconstriction as a regulatory mechanism.

Skin Impairment. Damage to large areas of skin can impede the body's ability to regulate body temperature. Severe burns can cause a hypermetabolic state that increases body temperature. In severely burned patients, above-normal body temperature is often present for a few weeks until the core temperature can be readjusted. Damage to the microcirculation of the skin decreases the patient's ability to retain body heat. For this reason, it is important to control the environment of the patient with severe burns to prevent significant drops in body temperature.

Endogenous Pyrogens. Infection caused by bacteria, viruses, fungi, and other microbes elevates normal body temperature. These agents cause the host to produce specific proteins called endogenous pyrogens (EP). Endogenous pyrogens are released from immunologically active phagocytic cells. Some tumor cells are also capable of producing EP (Shaver, 1982).

Endogenous pyrogens are transported to the brain, where they alter the firing rate of the temperature-sensitive neurons located in the preoptic area of the hypothalamus. As a result, the set point is increased, causing the thermoregulatory center to sense the existence of a lower-than-desired temperature. This causes the thermoregulatory center to initiate heat-conserving and heat-producing mechanisms, such as shivering, until the core temperature reaches the new set point (Guyton, 1986).

It usually takes the body several hours to reach the higher set point. During this period, the person experiences chills and feels cold, even though the body temperature may be elevated. The skin surface feels cold and the person shivers. Once the higher temperature is reached, the person feels neither hot nor cold.

When the factor causing the release of EP is removed, the hypothalamic thermostat is set at a lower, often normal rate. This triggers the preoptic area to initiate heat-loss mechanisms. When this happens, the person will experience intense sweating and sudden development of hot skin because of vasodilation. This sudden change is known as the "crisis," and often heralds the return to normal body temperature.

Exercise

An increase in muscle activity causes increased metabolic rate and an increase in body heat production. Exercise causes the body temperature to vary according to the strenuousness of the activity. Very strenuous exercise, such as long-distance running, can raise the rectal temperature to 40°C (104°F) in healthy people (Guyton, 1986). If the person is already febrile, then exercise can cause the temperature to rise even higher.

Conversely, inactivity can decrease normal heat production. A paralyzed person who is in a very cool environment cannot use body movement to effectively increase body temperature. This increases the likelihood that hypothermia can occur.

Altered Cognitive States

To employ behavioral responses to alter body temperature, a person must be cognitively alert and able to interpret environmental stimuli. The confused patient may be unaware that the ambient temperature of his or her surroundings is abnormal, and therefore may not dress appropriately or regulate environmental temperature.

Medications and drugs that impair cognitive states can also affect temperature regulation. Narcotics, sedatives, and alcohol decrease levels of consciousness and sensation, thus decreasing the recognition of (and behavioral responses to) abnormal temperature.

Stress

Physical and emotional stress can cause the body temperature to rise because of the hormonal and neural stimulation concurrent with a state of stress. Usually such fluctuations in body temperature are minor.

Altered Nutrition

People who are severely nutritionally depleted lack normal body fat to act as an insulator against heat loss. Lack of appetite and inability to eat decrease heat produced through the metabolism of food.

Manifestations of Altered Thermoregulation

Alterations causing above-normal body temperature are evidenced by fever, heat cramps, heat exhaustion, and heat stroke. Below-normal body temperature can be seen in hypothermia or frostbite.

Nursing Research

Selected Nursing Research Studies

Durham, M. L., Swanson, B., & Paulford, N. (1986). Effects of tachypnea on oral temperature estimation: A replication. *Nursing Research, 35,* 211–214.

Morgan, S. P. (1990). A comparison of three methods of managing fever in the neurological patient. *Journal of Neuroscience Nursing, 22*(1), 19–24.

Mravinac, C. M., Dracup, K. & Clochesy, J. M. (1989). Urinary bladder and rectal temperature monitoring during clinical hypothermia. *Nursing Research, 38,* 73–76.

Stephens, D., Beak, R., & Boyce, P., et al. (1989). The effect of heated oxygen on body temperature: A pilot study. *Journal of Post-Anesthesia Nursing, 4,* 75–87.

Wehmer, M. A., & Baldwin, B. J. (1986). Inadvertent hypothermia: Clinical nursing research. *AORN Journal, 44,* 788, 790, 792–793.

White, H. E., Thurston, N. E., Blackmore, K. A., Green, S. E., Hannah, K. J. (1987). Body temperature in the elderly surgical patient. *Research in Nursing and Health, 10,* 317–321.

Wirtz, B. J. (1987). Effects of air and water mattresses on thermoregulation. *Journal of Gerontolological Nursing, 13*(5), 13–17.

Possible Topics for Nursing Inquiry

- How effective are tepid sponge baths in reducing core body temperature?
- Are normal circadian thermal patterns influenced by dietary intake?
- What is the effect of a routine exercise program on core body temperature in people over age 65?
- What is the effect on core body temperature, in the newborn, of wearing a knit cap during the first 24 hours after delivery?
- What is the effect on body temperature of giving cool versus warm fluids to a patient with a fever?

Pyrexia or Fever

Pyrexia or **fever** can be defined as a regulated state in which the body's core temperature rises above the normal level for that person during rest. A low-grade fever is a temperature slightly elevated to approximately 37.1°C to 38.2°C or 98.8°F to 100.6° F. A temperature elevation above 38.2°C is considered a high-grade fever, and temperature elevations above 40.5°C (104.9°F) are referred to as **hyperpyrexia.**

Fever is viewed as an adaptive state, if it is kept within acceptable limits (Shaver, 1982). Although the adaptive value of fever is not fully understood, research has provided evidence of some body mechanisms that are influenced by fever in ways deemed beneficial. The growth of some species of bacteria is inhibited by the high temperatures associated with fever. Higher body temperatures increase the mobility of leukocytes, thus enhancing their rate of phagocytosis. Fever inhibits the bacteria's ability to use iron, a key nutrient necessary for their survival (Shaver, 1982). Also, the higher rates of chemical reactions that occur during a fever may allow cells to repair damage more quickly (Guyton, 1987).

Types of Fever. There are four common types of fever, which differ according to the pattern each one establishes (Table 36-2).

A sustained fever is a rise in body temperature that remains consistently elevated with little fluctuation.

An intermittent fever rises or "spikes" at some point during a 24-hour period. This "spiking" usually occurs late in the afternoon or evening. An intermittent fever alternates between elevated and normal levels on a day-to-day basis.

A remittent fever occurs when the temperature is always elevated, but the amount of elevation may fluctuate. This could occur when a patient has a temperature of 38°C to 38.5°C for most of the day, but which rises to 40°C in the late afternoon.

A relapsing fever is characterized by an elevated temperature lasting for several days, alternating with several days of normal temperature.

Phases of Febrile Episode. A febrile episode has three distinct phases, the chill phase, the fever phase, and the flush phase or crisis. Each phase exhibits unique symptoms.

During the chill phase, the body's heat-producing mechanisms are attempting to increase the core body temperature. The patient will experience a feeling of being cold and may shiver. The appearance of goose flesh, which is caused by the contraction of the arrector pili muscles in an attempt to trap air around body hairs, may be evident. The patient's skin will appear pale and cool due to vasoconstriction.

The fever phase occurs when the fever has reached the new, higher set point. The patient's skin feels warm to the touch and appears flushed because of vasodilation.

TABLE 36-2

Differences in Types of Fevers

Type of Fever	Fever Pattern
Sustained fever	Rise in temperature above normal that remains consistently high with little fluctuation
Intermittent fever	Rises or spikes at some point during 24-hour period; usually late afternoon or evening
Remittent fever	Rise in temperature that is always elevated, but amount of elevation fluctuates
Relapsing fever	Elevated temperature lasting for several days, alternating with several days of normal temperature

During this phase of the fever, the patient feels neither hot nor cold. The patient may experience thirst if fluid volume deficit has occurred. The patient may complain of general malaise, weakness, and aching muscles, which are due to the increased rate of protein catabolism. In addition, the patient may be either drowsy or restless. An unchecked fever can cause the patient to become delirious and suffer from convulsions because of the irritation to nerve cells in the brain.

The flush or crisis phase is the third phase in a febrile episode. During this phase, the patient experiences profuse diaphoresis, decreased shivering, and possible fluid volume deficit. The patient's skin will appear flushed and warm to the touch because of vasodilation.

Heat Exhaustion

Heat exhaustion (or heat prostration) occurs from exercising in the heat. Exercising in warm temperatures results in the loss of large amounts of fluid through sweating, especially if fluid replacement does not occur. Body temperature may be only slightly elevated or even below normal, but the loss of fluids causes significant circulatory problems. The patient will experience tachycardia, dyspnea, and hypotension. The skin will be pale and feel cold and clammy. To treat heat exhaustion, the person should lie in a dorsal recumbent position and drink salty fluids. To prevent further episodes, people can ingest sodium (salt tablets) before exercise and drink balanced electrolyte solutions during exercise.

Heat Cramps

Heat cramps are painful, intermittent spasms of the skeletal muscles brought about by vigorous exercise and profuse sweating, which disturbs the body's sodium balance. When people experience these cramps, they should cease their activity and replace depleted sodium with sodium tablets or fluids high in sodium content (e.g., tomato juice).

Heat Stroke

Heat stroke occurs when the body temperature rises beyond a critical temperature to a higher range of 41.1°C to 42.2°C (106°F to 108°F) (Guyton, 1986). This rise in body temperature is precipitated by exposure to high environmental temperatures and resulting excessive sweating. Consequently, as the hypothalamus becomes excessively heated, its heat-regulating ability becomes depressed and sweating diminishes. Thus, a high body temperature will perpetuate itself unless checked by external temperature-reducing interventions.

The person experiences dizziness, abdominal distress, and delirium, which will lead to unconsciousness if the temperature is not reduced. These symptoms are probably the result of circulatory shock brought on by the excessive loss of fluid and electrolytes. Hyperpyrexia, an excessively high body temperature, can cause damage to the body tissues, particularly to the brain cells, in a matter of minutes.

Elderly people, particularly those who are in the lower socioeconomic group, are more prone to heat stroke during environmental heat waves. This can be attributed to poor ventilation and preexisting health problems, such as poor nutrition, and respiratory and cardiac diseases. Also, the sweat mechanism is less efficient in the elderly, limiting their ability to safely cope with high environmental temperatures.

Hypothermia

Hypothermia is a state in which the core body temperature is lower than an acceptably normal range for a given person. This condition can be artificially induced for therapeutic reasons, or it can result from unintentional exposure to extremely cold environmental temperatures.

When the core temperature of the body falls below 33°C (92°F), thermoregulation is impaired. A vicious cycle begins: low body temperature causes the metabolic rate to decrease, which decreases the amount of heat produced by the body. Insufficient heat is available to return the body temperature to a normal range, which in turn slows the metabolic rate even more. If this cycle continues uninterrupted, death will occur when the core temperature reaches about 24°C (75°F) (Guyton, 1987).

Induced (Artificial) Hypothermia. Induced, or artificial, hypothermia is the deliberate lowering of the core temperature to a range of 30°C to 32°C (86°F to 89.6°F) (Rafalowski, 1987). This hypothermic state is induced by administering drugs that depress the hypothalamic thermostat, or by encasing the patient in a cooling blanket, which gradually decreases the core temperature. A person can remain in this state of suspended animation for days or several weeks without damage to body tissues (Guyton, 1986).

Induced hypothermia is used during cardiac surgery to decrease the metabolic rate, thus preserving the function of vital organs. It also reduces blood loss, due to the vasoconstrictive effect of the hypothermia. It may also be used as a treatment for patients who are hyper-pyrexic, in whom the core temperature is above 40°C (104°F). Hypothermia is also induced to prevent or re-duce intracranial pressure in neurosurgical patients.

Accidental Hypothermia. Accidental hypothermia occurs when a person is unintentionally exposed to a cold environment that causes the core temperature to be reduced below an acceptable normal temperature. The severity of hypothermia depends on the age and health status of the person and the length of time he or she is exposed to the cold environment.

Hypothermia causes body functions to be depressed and impairs the function of the hypothalamus. Conse-quently, heat-producing mechanisms are diminished, so the person becomes even colder. When a person feels cold, they become drowsy, which reduces the body's ability to produce heat through muscle activity. Eventu-ally the person becomes comatose and death will ensue.

Frostbite

Frostbite occurs when the skin is exposed to extremely cold temperatures, freezing its surface. The most suscep-tible areas of the body to frostbite are the digits of the hands and feet, the earlobes, and the tip of the nose. Careless application of ice packs can also result in freez-ing the skin surface. If the frozen area is bathed imme-diately in warm water, not exceeding 43.3°C (110°F) in temperature, it can be thawed without permanent dam-age. Otherwise, prolonged freezing impairs the circula-tory network in the affected area, resulting in permanent tissue damage. Gangrene can develop in the damaged tissue, and amputation of the frostbitten area may be necessary.

Impact of Altered Temperature on Activities of Daily Living

Altered temperature states have differing effects on how well a person can perform normal daily activities. The warmer environment causes the person to be lethargic and to have less energy to perform normal daily activ-ities. Appetite tends to decrease, with a consequent decrease in the amount of food eaten. At the same time, thirst increases, increasing normal fluid intake. For peo-ple with preexisting health problems such as a cardiac condition, a respiratory condition, or obesity, increased environmental temperatures prove more taxing. In-volvement in daily activities, especially those involving physical exertion, will be uncomfortable and will place

them at risk for developing conditions associated with hyperthermia.

People living in warm environmental temperatures must dress with light-weight, loose-fitting clothing to allow air currents to circulate close to their skin and promote cooling. Bathing is usually more frequent to promote comfort and prevent body odor. For people unable independently to take care of their own hygiene needs, this can prove difficult.

Cold environmental temperatures pose problems of a different sort. People are at risk for developing hypo-thermia if they do not take appropriate measures when exposed to cold environmental conditions. People living in these environments must wear several layers of densely woven fabrics to trap layers of air, providing insulation from cold outdoor temperatures. They must either stay indoors more or protect their skin surfaces from freezing when they venture outdoors. Outdoor physical exercise may be limited in periods of extreme cold.

Economic burdens may be great for those living in extreme environmental climates. Monthly heating or air-conditioning bills may severely stress the person's finances, especially if that person is living on a fixed income. Some jobs may be dangerous when tempera-tures are extremely hot or extremely cold. The welder who must work in a shop that is not air-conditioned may be at risk for heat stroke. Likewise, the ski instructor who must work when extremely cold conditions persist, may develop hypothermia or frostbite. Sometimes work is cancelled when weather conditions prove dangerous, thus economically affecting the worker.

ASSESSMENT

When collecting data about a patient's temperature sta-tus, the nurse is gathering data for purposes of screening, to determine if a problem exists, or for monitoring an existing problem. Objective and subjective data are im-portant to elicit from the patient.

Subjective Data

Interviewing the patient helps the nurse to understand the patient's normal body temperature range, isolate any risk factors that may predispose the patient to alter-ations in body temperature, and identify actual altered temperature states.

Functional Pattern Identification

When questioned about normal body temperature, some patients may be able to tell the nurse their normal temperature range. More likely, the patient will describe his or her temperature as normal or elevated. If a temperature elevation has been present, people often monitor their temperature and can provide the specific temperature measurements they have obtained.

Patients can also provide information about whether they generally feel cold or warm, the temperature they keep their thermostat set at, and how many blankets they use at night. This information about what is normal for the patient will help the nurse to adjust the environment to promote comfort whenever possible.

Risk Identification

The patient history helps elicit information identifying risk factors the patient may have for abnormal temperature states. Any past occurrence of hyperthermia or hypothermia should be documented. Metabolic problems, such as cancer or endocrine imbalances, can alter metabolic rate and should be noted. A systems review should detect problems in circulation, neurologic status, and skin integrity, since all can affect normal thermoregulatory mechanisms. Chronic illnesses such as cardiac problems, respiratory disease, or obesity should be considered as risk factors for altered temperature status. The medication history should be assessed for the use of drugs that affect vascular tone or level of consciousness, since these drugs increase the risk for altered temperature status.

Risk identification should also include environmental and situational data. The type of home the patient lives in and the adequacy of heating and air conditioning should be ascertained. Information concerning the job or leisure activities of the patient should be explored, especially noting if these activities take place outdoors in climates with temperature extremes, or if they involve strenuous physical exertion.

If the patient is scheduled for a surgical procedure that involves the administration of anesthetic agents, the nurse should inquire if there is a history of malignant hyperthermia in the family. If the patient reports that any family member had difficulty or died suddenly during surgery or in the immediate postoperative period, the anesthesiologist should be notified.

Dysfunctional Identification

If the nurse obtains a temperature reading outside the range of normal, or if the patient verbalizes having an abnormal body temperature, additional information should be collected to help determine the cause of the temperature abnormality. If the temperature is elevated, the nurse should seek information to determine how long the patient has been aware of the elevated temperature, whether the patient has experienced any chills or diaphoresis, and whether the patient feels hot or cold. Questions can be directed to better understand whether the fever has established any pattern (intermit-

tent, remittent, relapsing), what the patient thinks is the cause of the fever, and how the patient has been treating the fever. The nurse should also consider other factors that can cause elevated temperature, such as strenuous activity, ingestion of hot liquids, ovulation, degree of hydration, environmental temperature, and anxiety.

If the temperature is lower than normal for the patient's age, the nurse may suspect the patient is suffering from hypothermia. The nurse will need to validate this hypothesis by determining the mentation of the patient, the patient's feelings of warmth or cold, the nutritional status of the patient, the patient's previous activity level, the socioeconomic class of the patient, and medications the patient has been taking. The nurse should inquire as to what the patient thinks caused the hypothermia. In addition, the nurse should consider other factors that may cause low body temperature, such as a low environmental temperature, ingestion of cold liquids before measuring the temperature, or other factors that could have caused an inaccurate reading.

Objective Data

Objective data collection should include accurate measurement of body temperature, and observation of physical signs and symptoms that may be indicative of temperature abnormality or fluctuation.

Assessment of Body Temperature

Measuring the body temperature is a way of assessing the function of the thermoregulatory system. This is accomplished by measuring the core body temperature at various locations of the body. The temperature varies throughout the body, and no single value is "the" body temperature. The most common site for measuring the temperature is the oral cavity, specifically the posterior sublingual pocket located at the base of the tongue. For specific information on how to accurately determine body temperature at various body sites, refer to Chapter 19.

One study recommends that the optimal time to measure body temperature to screen for fever is once a day at 6 PM (1800 hours). This recommendation is based on the influence of the circadian thermal rhythm on a person's body temperature (Samples, et al., 1985).

Other vital signs should be monitored along with temperature to evaluate whether changes in other vital signs correspond appropriately with the diagnosed alteration of body temperature.

Inspection

Areas of the body should be inspected for signs of alterations in body temperature. The skin should be observed for color, temperature, moisture, and the presence of piloerection (goose flesh) or shivering. The nurse should note whether color and temperature changes are localized or occur over most of the body. General observations should include the patient's level of consciousness, body weight, and the state of nutrition and hydration.

NURSING DIAGNOSES AND PATIENT GOALS

Subjective and objective data assist the nurse in identifying actual and potential problems of altered body temperature. NANDA has identified four accepted nursing diagnoses involving temperature alteration: High Risk for Altered Body Temperature, Hypothermia, Hyperthermia, and Ineffective Thermoregulation.

Diagnostic Statement: High Risk for Altered Body Temperature

Definition

High risk for altered body temperature is the state in which an individual is at risk for failure to maintain body temperature within a normal range (NANDA, 1990).

Risk Factors

Extremes of age; extremes of weight; exposure to cold/cool or warm/hot environments; dehydration; inactivity or vigorous activity; medications causing vasoconstriction/vasodilation; altered metabolic rate; sedation; inappropriate clothing for environmental temperature; illness or trauma affecting temperature regulation (NANDA, 1990).

Diagnostic Statement: Hypothermia

Definition

Hypothermia is the state in which an individual's body temperature is reduced below normal range (NANDA, 1990).

Defining Characteristics

Major. Reduction in body temperature below normal range; shivering (mild); cool skin; pallor (moderate) (NANDA, 1990).

Minor. Slow capillary refill; tachycardia; cyanotic nailbeds; hypertension; piloerection (NANDA, 1990).

Related Factors

Exposure to cool or cold environment; illness or trauma; damage to hypothalamus; inability or decreased ability

to shiver; malnutrition; inadequate clothing; consumption of alcohol; medications causing vasodilation; evaporation from skin in cool environment; decreased metabolic rate; inactivity; aging (NANDA, 1990).

Diagnostic Statement: Hyperthermia

Definition

Hyperthermia is a state in which an individual's body temperature is elevated above his or her normal range (NANDA, 1990).

Defining Characteristics

Major. Increase in body temperature above normal range (NANDA, 1990).

Minor. Flushed skin, warm to the touch; increased respiratory rate; tachycardia; seizures/convulsions (NANDA, 1990).

Related Factors

Exposure to hot environment; vigorous activity; medications/anesthesia; inappropriate clothing; increased metabolic rate; illness or trauma; dehydration; inability or decreased ability to perspire (NANDA, 1990).

Diagnostic Statement: Ineffective Thermoregulation

Definition

Ineffective thermoregulation is the state in which an individual's temperature fluctuates between hypothermia and hyperthermia (NANDA, 1990).

Defining Characteristics

Fluctuations in body temperature above or below the normal range. See also major and minor characteristics present in hypothermia and hyperthermia (NANDA, 1990).

Related Factors

Trauma or illness; immaturity; aging; fluctuating environmental temperature (NANDA, 1990).

Related Nursing Diagnoses

People with altered body temperature are at risk for other problems. Those with hyperthermia may experience Fluid Volume Deficit, Activity Intolerance, High

Risk for Injury, and Altered Nutrition: Less than Body Requirements. Hypothermia may cause Pain, Altered Tissue Perfusion, and Impaired Skin Integrity.

Patient Goals

Patient goals are individualized for each patient who is at risk for developing, or who has, actual problems in maintaining normal body temperature. Goals should focus around the following:

Patient will maintain body temperature within normal range.
Patient will identify factors that can precipitate alterations in body temperature.
Patient will verbalize strategies to prevent and treat deviations from normal body temperature.

IMPLEMENTATION

Nursing interventions are focused on preventing problems of thermoregulation, assisting regulation of temperature when alteration has occurred, and educating the patient to manage and prevent problems of thermoregulation.

Nursing Interventions to Promote Health

The nurse's role is ideal for teaching people how to avoid potential problems with thermoregulation, and what to

---

Nursing Interventions for Alterations in Thermoregulation

Hypothermia

- Increase environmental temperature
- Apply layers of clothing or blankets
- Keep clothing dry
- Increase physical activity
- Increase intake of food and warm fluids

Hyperthermia

- Decrease environmental temperature
- Increase air movement (e.g., fans)
- Remove clothing
- Sponge skin with cool water
- Replenish fluids
- Decrease physical activity

Patient Teaching: Thermoregulation

Instruct the patient as follows:

- To properly obtain your oral temperature, place the thermometer in the posterior sublingual pocket, which is right under the tongue. Smoking, drinking, chewing gum, and exercise can affect accuracy of the temperature reading obtained.
- Wear light, loosely woven fabrics that are light in color to keep cool in hot weather. Drink extra fluid when weather is very hot.
- To prevent hypothermia, dress in several layers of clothing (wool is an especially good insulator), making sure to keep your head warm and all clothing dry.
- If you are elderly, you are less able to tolerate extremes in temperature.
- If you elderly, you are less likely to have a fever during an infectious episode, and may normally run subnormal temperatures.

---

do if such problems should occur. Teaching can occur in many settings, as well as in social interactions with the general public.

The nurse can be a credible teacher for the parents of a newborn. Instruction about thermoregulation is imperative for parents of the premature infant. Explanations should include a discussion of the immaturity of the infant's ability to regulate temperature. The nurse should instruct the parents to protect the newborn from temperature extremes (e.g., to avoid chilling during the bath, to avoid overdressing the infant). The nurse should also explain how to monitor axillary temperature and when to contact the physician regarding a fever.

The public should have a good knowledge of hypothermia and hyperthermia. Proper dress for different weather conditions is important. Keeping the head covered to prevent excessive loss of heat is also important, since 40% of body heat can be lost through the head. When weather conditions are extreme, ways to cope with severe hot or cold weather should be emphasized. This is especially important for the elderly, or those with chronic illnesses such as respiratory or cardiac disease. Community resources to help people pay for high heating or cooling bills, or to install insulation to make their homes more energy-efficient, may be available for those on a fixed income. The nurse can refer people to such community services.

The nurse can speak to community groups, such as the Boy Scouts or Girl Scouts, to explain the effects of temperature extremes and how to avoid thermoregulation problems. Health classes, which are frequently taught by the school nurse, also offer an excellent opportunity to instruct youngsters on such problems. Senior citizen centers also welcome instruction on how problems of thermoregulation can be avoided in the elderly.

People indulging in strenuous exercise, especially in hot weather, should be taught to replenish fluids and recognize signs of hyperthermia. The school nurse is an excellent authority for seeing that athletic events and practices are conducted safely, so that children are not exposed to heat stroke.

Nursing Interventions for Altered Thermoregulation

In a variety of clinical settings, the nurse must treat patients with altered body temperature. Interventions for fever management, hyperthermia, and hypothermia are important therapies the nurse uses to help patients regain normal body temperature when an imbalance has occurred.

Fever Management

The management of a fever varies according to the phase of the fever and the signs or symptoms the patient is experiencing (see the display).

Management During Chill Phase. Nursing interventions during the chill phase will focus on patient comfort. Blankets or extra clothing can be provided to help the patient feel warmer. The patient should be given adequate nourishment and fluids to meet the body's needs due to increased metabolic rate. The patient with a preexisting respiratory or cardiovascular problem may require activity restriction or supplemental oxygen to meet the demands of the increased metabolic rate. The nurse should monitor the patient's vital signs frequently

---

Guidelines for Care of a Febrile Patient

During the Chill Phase

Patient Can Experience
Feeling cold
Shivering
Paleness of skin
Skin cool to touch
Appearance of "gooseflesh"
Increase in body temperature

Nursing Interventions
Apply extra blankets
Increase fluid intake
Restrict activity
Supplement oxygen if patient has preexisting cardiac or respiratory problem

During Fever Phase

Patient Can Experience
Feeling neither hot nor cold
Dry oral mucosa
Thirst
Possible dehydration
General malaise, weakness, aching muscles
Drowsiness or restlessness
Possible convulsions
The possibility of becoming comatose

Nursing Interventions
Cover with light, warm clothing to avoid chilling patient
Encourage fluids (cool)
Restrict iron from diet if necessary
Rest
Apply lubricant to dried lips and nasal muscosa
Use tepid sponging if temperature becomes very high
Increase air circulation to encourage cooling
Implement safety precautions to protect patient if restless, delirious, or convulsions occur

Flush Phase

Patient Can Experience
Profuse sweating
Decreased shivering
Possible dehydration
Flushed skin
Skin warm to touch

Nursing Interventions
Use tepid sponging, avoid chilling patient
Encourage oral fluids (cool)
Restrict activity
Cover with light clothing or bed linens

to detect any deviations from the normal range and determine the effect of the fever on other body systems.

Management During Fever Phase. Once the fever has reached the new higher set point, nursing interventions will continue to focus on patient comfort and adequate patient hydration. The patient should be covered with adequate clothing to prevent shivering. Frequently, mouth care is important, since lips and mucous membranes may become dried out because of dehydration. Cool oral fluid should be encouraged, preferably fluids high in protein to cope with the increased rate of metabolism. Food or fluids high in iron should be avoided, since bacteria need good iron supplies to survive (Shaver, 1982). The patient should be encouraged to rest.

As the temperature approaches 40°C (104°F), the patient may be given a tepid sponge bath to promote cooling by evaporation and conduction. To further promote heat loss, the temperature of the environment can be cooled and the circulation of the air increased by the use of fans.

If the patient becomes restless, delirious, or convulses, then patient safety becomes an additional concern for the nurse. Padded siderails may be indicated to prevent the patient from falling out of bed or becoming injured if the siderail is struck. The patient should be monitored closely if convulsions are anticipated, and safety precautions should be instituted to prevent injury.

Management During Flush Phase. Nursing intervention during the flush phase continues to focus on patient comfort and hydration. The patient should be covered with a minimal amount of light clothing to prevent conservation of heat. Cool, tepid sponging and increased air circulation assist the patient's cooling mechanisms to reduce the core temperature. The diaphoretic patient's clothing and bed linens must be changed frequently to prevent skin breakdown and provide patient comfort. The nurse should assist the patient to maintain adequate hydration by encouraging cool liquids. Physical activity should be limited to prevent heat production.

Antipyretics. Drugs such as aspirin, acetaminophen, and aminopyrine are called **antipyretics** because they lower the setting of the hypothalamic thermostat so that the temperature of the body falls. Antipyretics may be used to reduce the temperature when the fever becomes a threat to the patient's well-being. Aminopyrine, which decreases the normal body temperature, may be used by physicians to induce a hypothermic condition.

Antipyretics should be used judiciously in children and the elderly because of their body size and metabolic function. The use of antipyretics has been questioned in routine fever treatment, since higher body temperatures may help support body defenses to fight infection (Cunha, 1985).

Aspirin is effective in lowering an elevated temperature, but will not reduce the temperature to a lower than normal range. Aspirin promotes heat loss by dilating blood vessels and fostering diaphoresis, but does not affect heat production in the body. Often, people take aspirin mainly to reduce the aches and discomforts associated with fever. Aspirin should not be given to children with flulike illnesses because it has been associated with Reye's syndrome, a potentially fatal condition involving liver damage and encephalopathy (Reeves-Swift, 1990).

When a nurse administers an antipyretic to a febrile patient, the patient's temperature should be taken immediately before the medication is given and approximately 1 hour later to determine if the medication has had the desired effect.

Tepid Baths. Tepid baths or sponging are administered to febrile patients when their temperature reaches a seriously elevated level. These should be administered to the patient when his or her temperature is consistently high, not during the chill phase of a fever. Tepid water is used to avoid the chilling effects of cool water. This procedure may be either soothing or uncomfortable for the patient, depending on the patient's skin temperature. Tepid baths or sponging are intended to artificially replace the body's sweating mechanism by cooling the surface of the skin, thereby cooling the blood being delivered to the body core. Also, this procedure allows cooling to occur by the process of evaporation. The nurse must be cautious to avoid chilling the patient, which will trigger the shivering mechanism. Before administering a tepid sponge bath, the nurse should measure the patient's temperature, and it should be measured 30 minutes after the procedure to determine the effectiveness of the intervention.

A study by Neuman (1985) suggests that sponging febrile children should be abandoned as a method of reducing elevated body temperature caused by an infectious process. Research has demonstrated that the administration of antipyretics without sponging is just as effective as combining the two procedures (Neuman, 1985). Alcohol sponging is not recommended because rapid evaporation increases the risk of shivering, and the fumes can be noxious.

Hypothermia Blankets. These special blankets can be used to reduce the temperature of the hyperpyrexic patient. The blanket consists of rubber or vinyl coils through which distilled water or alcohol is pumped. The temperature of the fluid can be programmed by a control device similar to a thermostat. When cooling is desired, the blanket is usually set slightly lower than normal body temperature (e.g., 35°C or 96°F). A rectal probe is inserted into the patient to constantly monitor core body temperature, so that excessive cooling does not occur. During use of the hypothermia blanket, the

Safety Alert

- Protect infants from extremes in temperature.
- Avoid chilling during bathing.
- Do not permit children under 2 years of age in a hot tub.
- Monitor the temperature via rectal probe when a hypothermia blanket is used, so that core body temperature will not drop too low.
- After hypothermia, rewarm the patient slowly to prevent massive vasodilation and possible shock.
- Do not administer aspirin to children with flulike illness as an antipyretic, since its administration has been linked with potentially lethal Reye's syndrome.
- Provide prompt treatment for heat stroke; it is a medical emergency that must be promptly treated to prevent cellular damage.

administration of medication may be necessary to block the shivering mechanism.

Nursing Management of Hyperthermia

Many conditions other than fever that involve sustained elevation of core body temperature above the normal range require therapeutic intervention. Based on a sound understanding of thermoregulation, the nurse should focus care on decreasing heat production and increasing heat loss from the body. The environment should be cool and the circulation of air increased by the use of fans. Fluid intake should be encouraged and physical activity should be limited.

When a patient experiences heat stroke, immediate measures must be instituted to prevent cellular damage and possible mortality. Application of ice packs to the head, axilla, and groin, where there are abundant blood vessels close to the skin surface, assists in quickly lowering core body temperature. Spraying or sponging the affected person with water establishes an artificial sweating mechanism and allow heat loss by means of evaporation. If conscious, the person should be encouraged to take oral fluids. Transfer to a medical facility, where the patient can be closely monitored, is often necessary for anyone suffering from heat stroke. A hypothermia blanket, medications, and intravenous fluids may be needed to stabilize the patient.

Nursing Management of Hypothermia

When treating hypothermia, the nurse should use measures to promote heat production and limit heat loss from the body. The environment should be warm, with layers of clothing applied to trap air in between layers to act as insulation. In severe cases of hypothermia, more aggressive rewarming by immersion into warm fluids or using external heat sources may be necessary. Warming should occur gradually to prevent massive vasodilation, which can lead to shock.

If frostbite is present, the affected area should be bathed in water not exceeding 43.3°C (110°F) to prevent permanent damage (Guyton, 1986). The area should not be rubbed or bumped, since frozen skin can be easily damaged.

Discharge Planning and Home Care

The nurse is in an ideal position to teach patients how to care for themselves and others when they have an alteration in thermoregulation. People of all ages need to know how to prevent hyperthermic conditions, such as heat cramps and heat stroke, and hypothermic conditions, such as hypothermia and frostbite. Patients need information on how to treat these conditions at home and when to seek professional help.

Fever is a condition involving altered body temperature that is commonly treated in the home. The nurse needs to provide information concerning the different stages of fever and the appropriate care during each phase. Information about caregiving should include aspects related to nutrition, fluid balance, activity, heat reduction techniques, and nonprescription medications. Teaching may be required as to how to measure temperature at various body sites with equipment purchased at the local drug store. Information needs to be given regarding when professional advice should be sought for the febrile person.

Parents of newborn infants need to know about the importance of maintaining a consistent environmental temperature. Types of clothing appropriate for the newborn should be discussed, as well as how to keep the infant cool in hot weather.

The elderly need to know that the aging process creates changes in their perception of temperature as well as in their ability to cope with environmental changes. Changes in lifestyle and control of the environment should be discussed to prevent alterations in body temperature.

Some patients may need to be counseled regarding home heating and cooling. Air-conditioning units may be important for those people with chronic health problems who live in very hot areas. Heating systems should be safe and efficient. Houses should be well insulated to promote comfort and to decrease the cost of heating or cooling. Furnace filters should be changed frequently to prevent excessive dust in the environment. Space heaters should be used with caution and positioned away from flammable items. Kerosene heaters should be well vented to prevent carbon monoxide poisoning. Community agencies are available to assess individual heating systems, and in some cases to help financially with the high cost of heating or cooling for those who cannot afford to pay.

EVALUATION

Evaluation is an ongoing part of the nursing process. As a nurse completes an intervention, the patient must be reassessed to determine if the intervention was effective in helping to achieve the desired goal. This reassessment or evaluation process is accomplished by comparing the actual patient outcomes to the outcome criteria established for each patient goal.

Patient goals and outcome criteria need to be individualized for each patient with potential or actual problems with thermoregulation. Examples of appropriate goals and outcome criteria for selected patients might be:

Goal
Patient will maintain body temperature within normal range.

Nursing Management Plan
The Patient with Ineffective Thermoregulation

Nursing Diagnosis: Ineffective thermoregulation related to the aging process, as evidenced by low body temperature.
Patient Goal: Patient will maintain body temperature within normal range.
Patient Outcome Criteria

- Patient maintains body temperature within $\pm 1°$ of normal body temperature for next 48 hours.
- Patient expresses comfort related to heat or cold for next 48 hours.

Nursing Intervention	Scientific Rationale
1. Monitor oral temperature daily at 6 PM.	1. Temperature should be assessed using the same site to ensure consistency. The oral site is accurate and easy to use. 6 PM is when the temperature is highest because of the circadian thermal rhythm, and taking the measurement at the same time also ensures consistency.
2. Encourage patient to walk for 20 minutes daily.	2. Exercise increases the metabolic rate, which produces heat.
3. Increase temperature of the environment (room).	3. To prevent heat lost to the environment by radiation and conduction.
4. Encourage patient to wear layers of tightly woven clothing.	4. Layers of clothing trap the air between the layers and provide insulation, thus reducing heat loss.

Patient Goal: Patient will identify factors that can precipitate altered body temperature.
Patient Outcome Criteria

- By end of teaching session, patient verbalizes three risk factors for developing hypothermia.
- At next appointment, patient identifies factors within his or her lifestyle that could contribute to altered body temperature.

Nursing Intervention	Scientific Rationale
1. Encourage patient to eat a well-balanced diet.	1. Eating properly prevents loss of fat. Fat is needed to help insulate the body and reduce heat loss.
2. Teach the patient about interventions to prevent hypothermia.	2. If the patient understands the ways to prevent hypothermia, he or she is more likely to comply.

Possible Outcome Criteria

During the period of hospitalization

• Patient maintains body temperature within 1 degree of normal body temperature.

• Patient does not complain of feeling uncomfortably cold or warm.

Goal

Patient will identify factors that can precipitate altered body temperature.

Possible Outcome Criteria

By the end of the teaching session

• Patient verbalizes three risk factors for developing hypothermia.

• Patient verbalizes three risk factors for developing hyperthermia.

• Patient identifies factors within his or her lifestyle that could contribute to altered body temperature.

Goal

Patient will verbalize strategies to prevent and treat deviations from normal body temperature.

Possible Outcome Criteria

By discharge

• Patient describes three ways to alter the environment to prevent personal altered body temperature.

• Patient discusses how to monitor temperature and how to manage fever at home.

• Patient identifies when a health-care provider should be consulted in the occurrence of altered body temperature.

Key Concepts

■ Heat is continuously being produced in the body as a by-product of the chemical reactions taking place in all body cells.

■ Body temperature is the delicate balance between heat produced and heat lost.

■ Heat production in the body is influenced by the person's basal metabolic rate, their thyroid hormone level, stimulation of their sympathetic nervous system, as well as their level of muscle activity.

■ Heat is lost from the body by means of radiation, conduction, convection, and evaporation.

■ The hypothalamus, nervous system, circulatory system, shivering mechanism, and sweat glands interdependently play significant roles in the thermoregulation of the entire body.

■ Human beings are capable of behavioral responses that allow them to make adjustments (e.g., remove or

add clothing, adjust the temperature of a room) to aid in the regulation of their body temperature.

■ The normal temperature range decreases slightly as the individual ages.

■ When assessing body temperature, the nurse must consider the effects that age, hormones, exercise, and stress have on the person's thermoregulating mechanism.

■ A person's core temperature fluctuates according to his or her circadian thermal rhythm. In addition, a woman's menstrual cycle influences her core temperature.

■ A person's body temperature is a sensitive indicator of the presence of physiologic changes occurring in his or her body.

■ Death generally occurs when the core body temperature reaches 44°C to 45°C (112°F to 114°F), or when the core temperature drops below 24°C (75°F).

■ Fever is viewed as an adaptive state if it is kept within acceptable limits.

■ Three common types of fevers are intermittent, remittent, and relapsing fevers.

■ In the care of a febrile patient, the nursing interventions should focus on each phase of the patient's fever.

■ The nurse should recognize the early symptoms of malignant hyperthermia, heat cramps, heat exhaustion, and heat stroke, and implement appropriate independent and collaborative interventions.

■ Hypothermia, in a controlled environment, may be used as a therapeutic intervention.

■ The very young, the elderly, and the infirm are at risk when any deviations in their body temperature occurs.

■ The nurse collects data about a patient's temperature status for purposes of screening, to determine if a nursing problem exists, or for monitoring an existing nursing problem.

■ The nurse assesses the patient's temperature by indirect measurement, using a mechanical device, and by palpating the patient's skin to detect variation in surface temperature.

■ The nurse must determine which is the most appropriate site for measuring a patient's temperature.

■ The nurse is in an ideal position to teach people how to care for themselves, or others, when they have a minor febrile condition, or to teach people about other factors influencing thermoregulation.

■ Nursing diagnoses related to thermoregulation include High Risk for Alterted Body Temperature, Hypothermia, Hyperthermia, and Ineffective Thermoregulation.

References

Baker, N., Cerone, S. B., Gaze, N., & Knapp, T. (1984). The effect of type of thermometer and length of time inserted on oral temperature measurement of afibrile subjects. *Nursing Research, 33,* 109–111.

Carpenito, L. J. (1989). *Nursing diagnoses: Application to clinical practice* (3rd ed.). Philadelphia: J. B. Lippincott.

Cunha, B. A. (1985). Significance of fever in the compromised host. *Nursing Clinics of North America, 20,* 163–169.

Dodman, N. (1987). Newborn temperature control. *Neonatal Network, 5*(6), 19–23.

Erickson, R. (1980). Oral temperature differences in relation to thermometer and technique. *Nursing Research, 29,* 157–164.

Ganong, W. F. (1989). *Review of medical physiology* (14th ed.). Los Altos, CA: Lange Medical Publications.

Glick, Z. (1987). Brown fat thermogenesis after single meals—hormonal and dietary influences. *International Journal of Obesity, 2*(2), 43.

Guyton, A. C. (1986). *Textbook of medical physiology* (7th ed.). Philadelphia: W. B. Saunders.

Guyton, A. C. (1987). *Physiology of the human body* (7th ed.). Philadelphia: W. B. Saunders.

Kurtz, K. J. (1982). Hypothermia in the elderly: The cold facts. *Geriatrics, 37,* 85.

McConnell, E. A. (1987). *Clinical considerations in perioperative nursing* (pp. 372–387). Philadelphia: J. B. Lippincott.

Mountcastle, V. B. (1980). *Medical physiology* (14th ed.). St. Louis: C. V. Mosby.

NANDA (1990). *Taxonomy I revised 1990, with official nursing diagnoses.* St. Louis, MO: North American Nursing Diagnosis Association.

Neuman, J. (1985). Evaluation of sponging to reduce body temperature in febrile children. *Canadian Medical Association Journal, 132,* 641–642.

Rafalowski, M. M. (1987). Relationship of core temperature at time of blanket removal to subsequent core temperatures in patients immediately after coronary artery bypass. *Heart and Lung, 16,* 9–13.

Reeves-Swift, R. (1990). Rational management of a child's acute fever. *American Journal of Maternal Child Nursing, 15*(2), 82–85.

Samples, J. F., VanCott, M. L., Long, C., King, I. M., & Kersenbrock, A. (1985). Circadian rhythms: Basis for screening fever. *Nursing Research, 34,* 377–379.

Schreiner, R., & Kisling, J. (1982). *Practical neonatal respiratory care.* New York: Raven Press.

Shaver, J. (1982). The basic mechanisms of fever: Considerations for therapy. *Nurse Practitioner, 10,* 15–19.

Shaver, J. (1991). Assessment of reproductive function. In Patrick, M. L., et al. (Eds.), *Medical–surgical nursing: Pathophysiological concepts.* (2nd ed., pp. 1904–1913). Philadelphia: J. B. Lippincott.

Vander, A., Sherman, J., & Luciano, D. (1985). *Human physiology: The mechanisms of body function* (4th ed.). New York: McGraw Hill.

Vick, R. L. (1984). *Contemporary medical physiology.* Menlo Park: Addison-Wesley.

Whaley, L. F., & Wong, D. L. (1989). *Essentials of pediatric nursing* (3rd ed.). St. Louis: C. V. Mosby.

Yurick, A. G., Spier, B. E., Robb, S. S., & Ebert, N. J. (1989). *The aged person and the nursing process* (3rd ed.). Norwalk, CT: Appleton-Century-Crofts.

Bibliography

Carroll, S. M. (1989). Nursing diagnosis: Hypothermia. *Classification of Nursing Diagnoses: Proceedings of the 8th Conference,* 425–428.

Doyle, M. A. (1987). Whole body hyperthermia: Making things too hot for cancer. *RN, 50*(8), 39–40.

Durham, M. L., Swanson, B., & Paulford, N. (1986). Effects of tachypnea on oral temperature estimation: A replication. *Nursing Research, 35,* 211–214.

Enright, T., & Hill, M. G. (1989). Treatment of fever. *Focus on Critical Care, 16*(2), 96–102.

Erbstoesser, M. (1989). Care of the patient with malignant hyperthermia. *Journal of Postanesthesia Nursing, 4,* 71–74.

Johnson, S. E. (1989). Alteration in temperature regulation: Hypothermia. *Classification of Nursing Diagnoses: Proceedings of the 8th Conference,* 378–380.

Litwack, K. (1988). Practical points in the management of hypothermia. *Journal of Postanesthesia Nursing, 3,* 339–341.

Lydon, J., McDonald-Lynch, A., Marshall, I., & Villanueva, W. (1989). Patient teaching about hyperthermia. *Oncology Nursing Forum, 16,* 855–860.

Michal, D. M. (1989). Management of hypothermia in the multitrauma patient. *Journal of Emergency Nursing, 15,* 416–421.

Morgan, S. P. (1990). A comparison of three methods of managing fever in the neurological patient. *Journal of Neuroscience Nursing, 22*(1), 19–24.

Mravinac, C. M., Dracup, K., & Clochesy, J. M. (1989). Urinary bladder and rectal temperature monitoring during clinical hypothermia. *Nursing Research, 38,* 73–76.

Stephens, D., Beak, R., Boyce, P., et al. (1989). The effect of heated oxygen on body temperature: A pilot study. *Journal of Postanesthesia Nursing, 4,* 75–78.

Wehmer, M. A., & Baldwin, B. J. (1986). Inadvertent hypothermia: Clinical nursing research. *AORN Journal, 44,* 788, 790, 792–3.

White, H. E., Thurston, N. E., Blackmore, K. A., Green, S. E., & Hannah, K. J. (1987). Body temperature in the elderly surgical patient. *Research in Nursing and Health, 10,* 317–321.

Wirtz, B. J. (1987). Effects of air and water mattresses on thermoregulation. *Journal of Gerontological Nursing, 13*(5), 13–17.

U N I T IX
Elimination

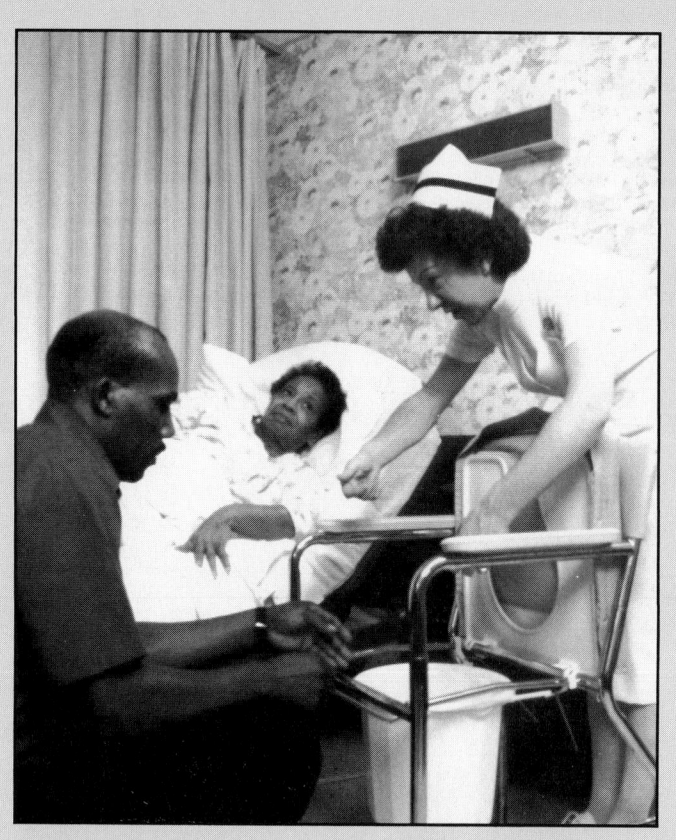

CHAPTERS

37 Urinary Elimination

38 Bowel Elimination

Elimination of body wastes is a universal human need. It is also an area of concern for most patients in a health care facility and at home, when self-care becomes the focus. Unit IX explores the human functions of urinary and bowel elimination.

Each chapter considers the concepts and principles related to normal function. The nursing process serves as a framework to present the knowledge base necessary to assess function and either plan and intervene to promote health and function or intervene for altered function. The assessment discussion focuses on uncovering the normal pattern of elimination for each patient, including the assistance of any devices, such as laxatives, to control elimination. Each chapter emphasizes patient teaching to promote normal elimination and considers all forms of elimination, including those that require devices, such as ostomy bags.

Elimination is a concern for every patient regardless of the problem for which they need nursing care. This unit is applicable to every patient the nurse encounters.

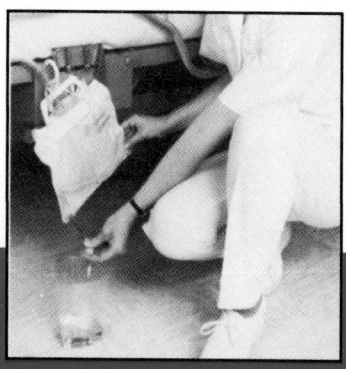

Urinary Elimination

LEARNING OBJECTIVES

Upon completion of this chapter, the student will be able to do the following:

- Describe the normal structure and function of the urinary system.
- Understand the process of micturition.
- List several factors that influence urinary elimination.
- List and describe alterations in normal voiding patterns.
- Describe factors that can alter normal urinary function.
- Recognize age-related differences in urinary elimination.
- Discuss nursing assessment of urinary function.
- Identify nursing diagnoses related to urinary elimination.
- Describe nursing interventions to promote normal urinary elimination.

KEY TERMS

Anuria
Condom Catheter
Detrusor
Diuresis
Dysuria
Enuresis

Frequency
Hematuria
Incontinence
Indwelling Catheter
Micturition
Oliguria

Polyuria
Pyuria
Residual Urine
Retention
Urgency

37

Normal Urinary Function
  Anatomy of the Urinary Tract
    Kidneys
    Ureters
    Bladder
    Urethra
  Normal Function of the Urinary System
    Urine Formation
    Process of Urination
  Characteristics of Normal Urine
  Normal Pattern of Urinary Elimination
  Factors Affecting Normal Urinary Elimination
  Lifespan Considerations
Altered Urinary Function
  Potential for Altered Urinary Function
    Obstruction of Urine Flow
    Infections of the Urinary Tract
    Hypotension
    Neurologic Injury
    Decreased Muscle Tone
    Pregnancy
    Surgery
    Medications
    Urinary Diversion
  Manifestations of Altered Urinary Function
    Dysuria
    Polyuria
    Oliguria
    Urgency
    Frequency
    Nocturia
    Hematuria
    Pyuria
    Urinary Retention
    Incontinence
    Enuresis
  Impact of Urinary Dysfunction on Activities of
    Daily Living
Assessment
  Subjective Data
    Functional Pattern Identification
    Risk Identification
    Dysfunctional Identification
  Objective Data
    Assessment of Urine

    Assessment of Urinary Retention
    Physical Assessment
    Diagnostic Tests and Procedures
Nursing Diagnoses and Patient Goals
  Diagnostic Statement: Stress Incontinence
    Definition
    Defining Characteristics
    Related Factors
  Diagnostic Statement: Urge Incontinence
    Definition
    Defining Characteristics
    Related Factors
  Diagnostic Statement: Reflex Incontinence
    Definition
    Defining Characteristics
    Related Factors
  Diagnostic Statement: Functional Incontinence
    Definition
    Defining Characteristics
    Related Factors
  Diagnostic Statement: Total Incontinence
    Definition
    Defining Characteristics
    Related Factors
  Diagnostic Statement: Urinary Retention
    Definition
    Defining Characteristics
    Related Factors
  Related Nursing Diagnoses
  Patient Goals
Implementation
  Nursing Interventions to Promote Health and
    Urinary Function
    Patient Teaching
    Urinary Collection Devices
  Nursing Interventions for Altered Function
    Bladder Training
    External Catheters and Protective Pants
    Urinary Catheterization
    Bladder Credé
    Urinary Diversion
    Renal Dialysis
  Discharge Planning and Home Care
Evaluation
Key Concepts

The elimination of fluid waste is an essential function of the human body. Failure of the urinary system to function properly can result in serious, possibly life-threatening conditions. Less serious urinary dysfunction, although not life-threatening, can be embarrassing and debilitating for the person.

The nurse is instrumental in promoting optimal urinary function and preventing urinary complications for all patients. The nurse individualizes teaching and specific interventions to help patients of all ages deal with problems of incontinence, urinary retention, and prevention of urinary tract infection. An understanding of anatomy and physiology of the urinary system, and of the factors that can affect normal and abnormal functioning of urinary elimination, are important for the nurse in individualizing patient care.

NORMAL URINARY FUNCTION

Normal urinary function depends on the normal anatomy and physiology of the kidneys, ureters, urinary bladder, and urethra. Many factors can affect normal urine production and elimination of urine from the body.

Anatomy of the Urinary Tract

Structures within the urinary tract include the kidneys, where the urine is formed; the ureters, which connect the kidneys with the bladder; the bladder, which stores urine; and the urethra, which permits the urine to exit from the body (Fig. 37-1).

Kidneys

The two kidneys are located on the posterior abdominal wall, in front of and on either side of the vertebral column. They lie approximately between the twelfth thoracic and third lumbar vertebrae. Each kidney is enclosed by a fibrous capsule and supported by a mass of adipose tissue.

The functional unit of the kidney is called a nephron (Fig. 37-2). Each kidney has over 1,000,000 nephrons, and each nephron is capable of forming urine. The nephron consists of the glomerulus, Bowman's capsule, proximal convoluted tubules, loop of Henle, the distal tubule, and the collecting duct. The glomerulus is a network of blood vessels, surrounded by Bowman's capsule, where the formation of urine begins. The tubules, loop of Henle, and collecting ducts are passageways that permit the urine to flow to the bladder. More importantly, they selectively reabsorb or secrete substances from the urine so that fluid and electrolyte balance is maintained.

Ureters

The ureters are narrow (1.25 cm), smooth muscle tubes that serve as passageways for urine to flow from the

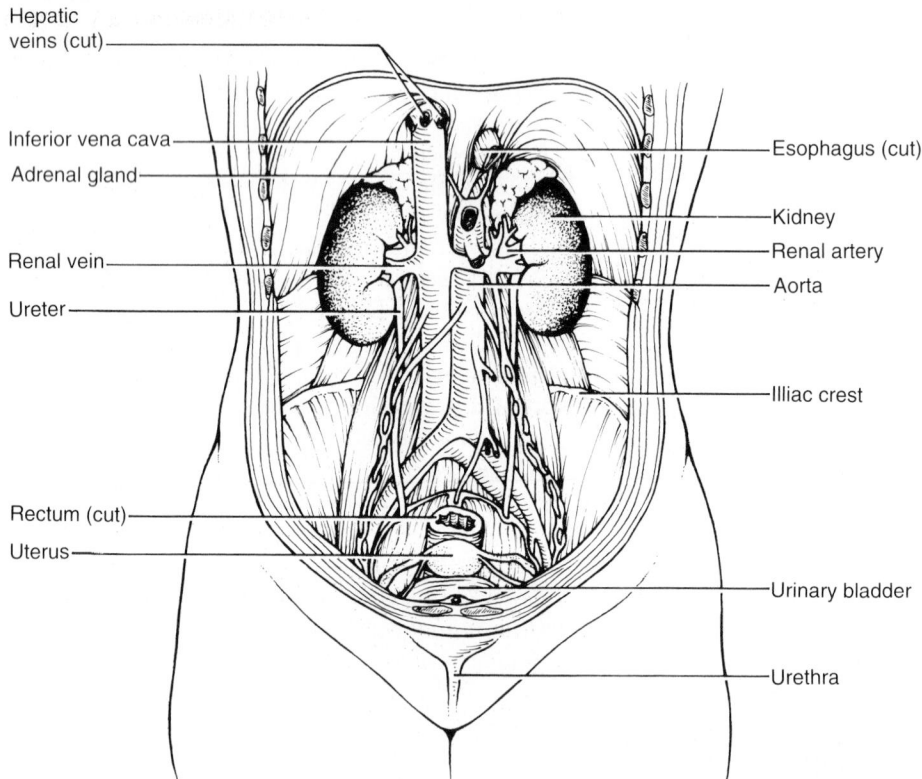

Hepatic
veins (cut)

Inferior vena cava

Adrenal gland

Renal vein

Ureter

Rectum (cut)

Uterus

Esophagus (cut)

Kidney

Renal artery

Aorta

Illiac crest

Urinary bladder

Urethra

Figure 37–1. Anatomic structures of the urinary tract.

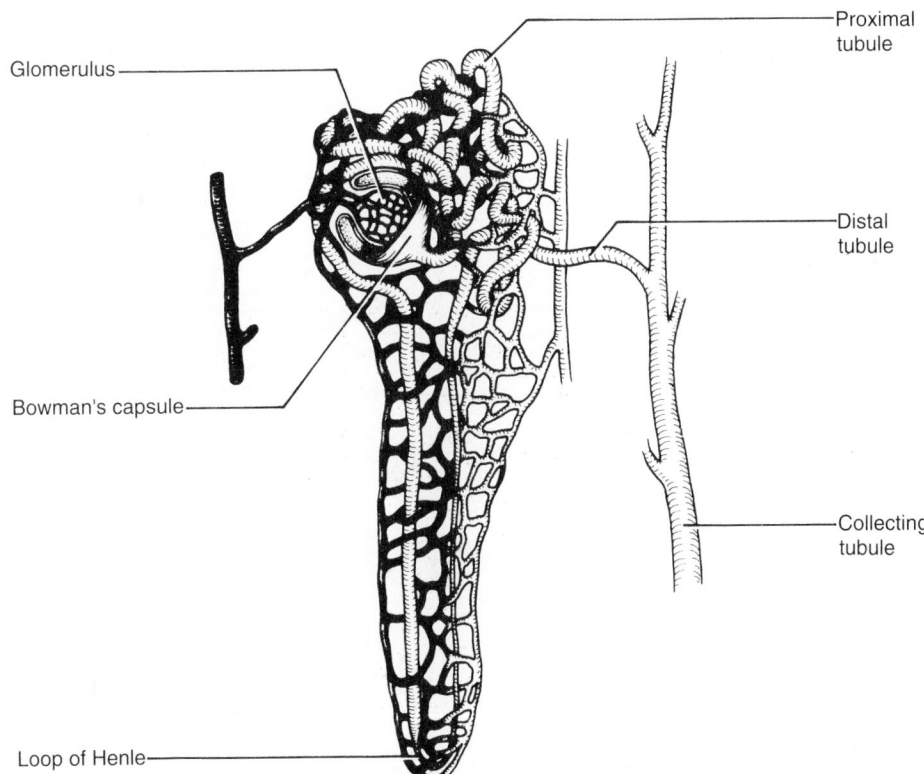

Figure 37–2. The nephron: the functional unit of the kidney.

kidneys to the bladder. The ureters have a peristaltic movement that propels the urine toward the direction of the bladder. The frequency of the peristaltic movement ranges from once every 10 seconds to once every 2 to 3 minutes (Guyton, 1986). A flap of mucous membrane, which acts as a valve, covers the juncture between the ureters and the bladder. Under normal conditions, this prevents reflux of urine up through the ureter into the kidney.

Bladder

The bladder is the storage compartment for urine. It is a hollow, smooth muscle that lies behind the symphysis pubis when empty (Fig. 37-3). In the woman, the bladder is located in front of the uterus and the vagina. In the man, the bladder is located in front of the rectum and above the prostate gland.

The body of the bladder is composed of three layers of smooth muscle. The inner and outer layers are longitudinal, whereas the middle layer is circular. Collectively, these three layers are called the **detrusor** muscle. The bladder is hollow when empty, but is capable of expansion to hold a considerable amount of urine.

The lower portion of the bladder, approximately 2 to 3 cm long, is called the bladder neck or internal urinary sphincter. Autonomic nervous innervation affects smooth muscle control of the internal sphincter. Sympathetic impulses cause the sphincter to contract, keeping the urine in the bladder. Parasympathetic nerve stimulation results in contraction of the detrusor muscle and

relaxation of the internal sphincter; this causes urination to occur.

Urethra

The urethra is the exit passageway for urine from the bladder. In women the urethra is short, about 3 to 5 cm (1 to 2 in), a factor that increases the opportunity for the entrance of bacteria into the urinary system. In men, the urethra is longer, about 20 cm (8 in), and serves to transport semen as well as urine.

The external sphincter is located in the urethra. The external sphincter is a band of skeletal muscle that surrounds a section of the urethra and permits voluntary control of urination. The external sphincter is usually contracted to keep the urethra closed and prevent constant emptying of urine from the bladder. When the external sphincter relaxes, urine can flow out from the bladder.

Normal Function of the Urinary System

The elimination of fluid waste from the body is the function of the urinary system. Small amounts of fluid waste are excreted by the gastrointestinal, respiratory, and integumentary systems, but the great majority of fluid waste is excreted through the renal system. The process of fluid waste elimination can be divided into two parts, urine formation, and excretion of urine from the body.

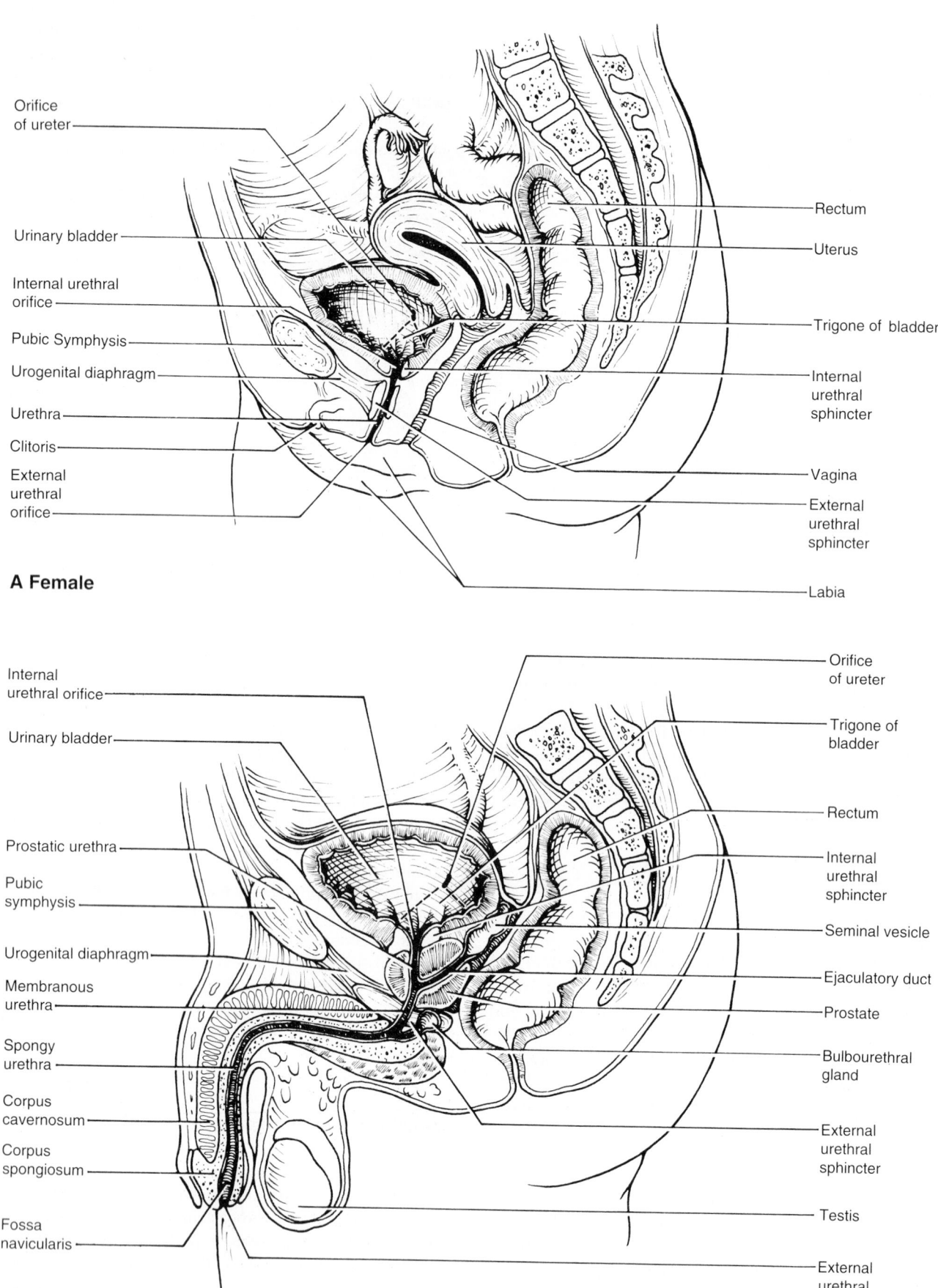

Orifice of ureter

Urinary bladder

Internal urethral orifice

Pubic Symphysis

Urogenital diaphragm

Urethra

Clitoris

External urethral orifice

Rectum

Uterus

Trigone of bladder

Internal urethral sphincter

Vagina

External urethral sphincter

Labia

A Female

Internal urethral orifice

Urinary bladder

Prostatic urethra

Pubic symphysis

Urogenital diaphragm

Membranous urethra

Spongy urethra

Corpus cavernosum

Corpus spongiosum

Fossa navicularis

Orifice of ureter

Trigone of bladder

Rectum

Internal urethral sphincter

Seminal vesicle

Ejaculatory duct

Prostate

Bulbourethral gland

External urethral sphincter

Testis

External urethral orifice

B Male

Figure 37–3. Genitourinary tract showing the location of the urinary bladder and urethra: **A:** Female. **B:** Male.

Urine Formation

The major function of the kidney is regulation of volume and composition of the extracellular fluid (ECF) of the body. It does this by selectively retaining wanted water and other substances, and excreting unwanted water and other substances in a fluid waste called urine. Urine formation occurs by the processes of filtration, reabsorption, and secretion.

Filtration. The process of filtration begins at the glomerulus. The renal arteries bring blood to the kidneys; the smaller branches of these arteries bring blood to the glomerulus of each nephron. The capillaries of the glomerulus are porous, and as the blood passes through the glomerular capillaries, some of the constituents of the blood are actually filtered out. The red blood cells and the proteins are too large to be filtered, and remain in the capillary, but most of the remaining plasma constituents can be filtered. The fluid that is filtered out of the glomerulus into the Bowman's capsule is called the glomerular filtrate.

Reabsorption. The glomerular filtrate then enters the second segment of the nephron, the tubule. The tubule actively and passively reabsorbs substances that the body wants to retain. These substances include varying amounts of water and electrolytes (Na^+, K^+, Cl^-, and HCO_3^-), and all of the glucose and amino acids. Reabsorption occurs mostly in the proximal convoluted tubule, but also in the distal and collecting tubules (Patrick, et al., 1991). Almost 99% of the glomerular filtrate is reabsorbed by the tubules. Only 1% of the glomerular filtrate remains unabsorbed by the tubules, to form the fluid waste called urine (Brunner & Suddarth, 1988).

Secretion. In addition to reabsorbing substances, the tubules secrete some substances to rid them from the body. Varying amounts of H^+ ions and K^+ ions are secreted, as well as ammonia, creatinine, uric acid, and some other metabolites (Patrick, et al., 1991). Urine then consists of the 1% of unreabsorbed glomerular filtrate plus some secreted substances. By forming urine, the kidney successfully accomplishes its major role of regulating the volume and composition of the ECF.

Process of Urination

Several words are used to describe the process of excreting urine from the body, including urination, voiding, and **micturition.** In adults, the emptying of the bladder usually occurs when the bladder is stretched or distended by about 250 to 400 mL of urine. Smaller amounts of urine trigger bladder emptying in children. When the volume of urine in the bladder reaches the range of 250 to 400 mL, the pressure of that amount stretches the detrusor sufficiently to begin to force the bladder neck to open. This sensation of stretch in the detrusor is transmitted to sacral segments of the spinal cord; reflex motor action is transmitted back to the detrusor muscle to cause it to contract. The detrusor contraction causes even more stretch and pressure, and it is usually at this point that the person perceives a full bladder and the need to urinate. This reaction of bladder stretch, leading to bladder contraction and the perceived need to void is called the micturition reflex. The micturition reflex is an involuntary spinal cord reflex.

In children under the age of 3, the micturition reflex leads to spontaneous urination. Beyond age 3, however, most people have learned to postpone urination until the time and place is more socially acceptable; this is because the act of urination is ultimately controlled by higher nerve centers in the brain. The person can consciously decide to postpone voiding by keeping the external sphincter, a skeletal muscle, contracted in a closed position. This effectively keeps urine from being released, even in the presence of the micturition reflex. When the person decides the time and place is right for voiding, the external sphincter can consciously be relaxed, permitting urine to flow from the bladder. The emptying of the bladder also involves the contraction of abdominal muscles and the relaxation of pelvic floor muscles. The amount of urine emptied is usually in the range of 250 to 400 mL per void. All but 5 to 10 mL of urine is typically emptied from the bladder (Guyton, 1986).

Characteristics of Normal Urine

Common characteristics of urine include amount, color, clarity, and odor. Many factors can produce normal variations among different people, or even variations at different times for the same person.

Volume. The average amount of urine per void for an adult is approximately 250 to 400 mL. Urinary output can vary greatly, depending on intake and other fluid losses. A catheterized patient should drain a minimum of 30 mL of urine per hour. Urine output less than 30 mL per hour can indicate inadequate blood flow to the kidneys.

Color. The color of urine ranges from a light yellow, to a darker yellow, to a dark yellow–brown, called amber. The patient's state of hydration alters the color. Urine may be almost colorless if it is very dilute secondary to a high fluid intake. Urine may be dark amber or orange–brown if it is very concentrated secondary to a decreased fluid intake. Medications may also alter the color of urine. The urine may appear dark reddish-brown or streaked with blood if a woman is menstruating.

Clarity. Urine is normally transparent. Freshly voided urine should appear clear without sediment.

Urine draining from a retention catheter should appear clear and without sediment in the tubing, but may contain occasional mucus shreds. Urine that has been sitting unemptied in a urinal or collecting device for an hour or more may normally appear cloudy secondary to separation or settling of urinary constituents.

Odor. The odor of freshly voided urine is typically described as aromatic. Generally, the more dilute the urine, the fainter the odor, and the more concentrated the urine, the stronger the odor. Urine that has been sitting unemptied for a long period of time may have a strong ammonia odor. Medications and certain foods may alter the odor of urine. A strong, offensive odor is not normally present in urine free of infection.

Normal Pattern of Urinary Elimination

Many people have a routine pattern associated with urinary elimination. Most people void four to six times a day. Typically, people void soon after getting out of bed in the morning. Many people tend to void within an hour after mealtime and once again before bedtime. Variations in the pattern of fluid intake have a direct effect on the routine pattern of voiding.

The total amount of urine voided during a 24-hour period usually ranges from 1200 to 1500 mL. Each void should contain a minimum of approximately 200 mL and a maximum of 500 mL.

Factors Affecting Normal Urinary Elimination

Many factors can affect normal urinary elimination. Fluid intake, loss of body fluid, dietary intake, body position, and psychologic factors all can affect normal urinary patterns.

Fluid Intake. The amount of fluid ingested by a person is the most influential factor in determining urine output. If all other factors are held constant, a complementary relationship exists between fluid intake and urine output. If a person increases the volume of fluid intake there will be an associated increase in the volume of urine output. Conversely, a decrease in fluid intake will cause a corresponding decrease in urine output. This relationship is hormonally controlled.

Several hormones, the most important of which is antidiuretic hormone (ADH), play significant roles in the reabsorption of water in the tubules of the nephron. The name "antidiuretic" implies its function, which is to prevent **diuresis,** or the excretion of water. Antidiuretic hormone is secreted by the hypothalamus and released by the posterior pituitary in the brain. Increased plasma osmolarity stimulates the release of ADH (this is discussed in detail in Chapter 32). When ADH is present,

the distal tubule of the nephron becomes more permeable to water. The release of ADH causes more water to be reabsorbed by the kidney, thus producing a more concentrated urine. When fluid intake is increased, ADH release is suppressed. In the absence of ADH, the renal tubules become relatively impermeable to water, and little water is reabsorbed. This produces increased volume of dilute urine.

Not only does the amount of fluid intake have an effect on the amount of urine produced, but it also influences the frequency of urination. If fluid intake is greatly increased, frequency of voiding increases because the bladder fills more quickly. Conversely, if fluid intake is low, voiding frequency decreases.

Loss of Body Fluid. When a person loses a great deal of body fluid, the kidneys increase reabsorption of water from the glomerular filtrate to maintain the proper osmolarity of the extracellular fluid. This saving of water to regulate the concentration of solutes in the ECF results in decreased urine output. Increased loss of body fluids can occur with vomiting, diarrhea, excessive diaphoresis secondary to fever or exercise, excessive wound drainage, extensive burns, or blood loss from trauma or surgery.

Nutrition. Diet may affect urinary elimination. If the diet contains a high percentage of foods that have a high water content (e.g., fresh fruits and vegetables), urine volume will be greater than if these foods are ingested on a limited basis. If large quantities of salty foods are ingested without increasing water intake, urine output will decrease and be more concentrated.

Alcohol or foods containing caffeine (such as coffee, tea, cola, and chocolate) also affect urinary output. Alcohol and caffeine both contain a diuretic and increase urine output.

Body Position. Body position plays an important role in the ability to completely empty the bladder with each voiding. The typical body position for urinary elimination in men is the upright standing position. Some men find it difficult to fully empty their bladder into a urinal while lying flat in bed. Commonly, this alters the voiding pattern so that voiding is more frequent, with less volume. The normal position for voiding in women is the sitting position. If a woman must use a bedpan while flat in bed, she may also be unable to completely empty her bladder.

Psychological Factors. Since the release of urine from the bladder is ultimately under voluntary conscious control, the process of voiding can be influenced by anything that causes one to think about voiding. If another person talks about the need to void, one may also feel the urge to void. If one reads a chapter about urinary elimination, one may need a bathroom break before finishing. If one hears running water, the need to void may be intensified. Pouring warm water over a patient's inner thigh or perineal area may stimulate voiding; giving a patient a cold bedpan may temporarily prevent voiding.

Stress or anxiety can have an effect on urinary elimination. In a stressful or anxious situation, a person can experience a strong urge to urinate. Stress can also cause the reverse problem of urinary retention. A person's muscles become so tense that relaxation of the perineal muscles does not occur, thus inhibiting voiding.

Privacy for voiding is an important psychologic factor to consider. Many people are unable to relax their perineal muscles if they feel they have inadequate privacy. Women, in particular, have been culturally trained to require more privacy for voiding. Women's public restrooms always have private stalls for elimination, whereas men's public restrooms have open rows of receptacles for urinary elimination. People have varying requirements of privacy for voiding.

Lifespan Considerations

Newborn and Infant

The kidneys of the fetus begin functioning and the fetus voids urine in utero from about the third month after conception. The newborn, therefore, may have urine in his or her bladder at birth and should be able to void within the first 24 hours after birth. The first voiding may be of slightly pink-tinged urine. The pinkish color is due to an accumulation of uric acid crystals. It is important to note the first voiding after birth to verify that urine formation and elimination are adequate. The kidneys at birth are still not fully developed; Bowman's capsule and the tubules are still refining their respective filtering and reabsorption abilities. It is likely that the newborn will void small amounts (15 to 30 mL, up to 30 to 40 times a day) of a dilute, light yellow-colored urine. As the infant grows, he or she is able to void in slightly larger amounts at slightly less frequent intervals. The color of the urine remains pale yellow throughout infancy. The total amount of urine voided in a 24-hour period depends on total fluid intake and fluid losses from other sources. The average urine output for the newborn or infant is about 500 to 600 mL in 24 hours. Table 37-1 gives the normal ranges of daily urine output during the lifespan.

TABLE 37–1

Normal Ranges for Daily Urine Output During Lifespan

Age (years)	Output (mL)
Newborn–2	500–600
2–5	500–800
5–8	600–1200
8–14	1000–1500
14 and over	1500

An infant has no voluntary control of urinary elimination. The sacral spinal cord segments innervating the bladder are not yet mature. The bladder will empty in reflex fashion after a degree of bladder stretch has occurred.

Serious alterations in urinary elimination may be caused by congenital malformations of the urinary tract or the central nervous system. Urinary tract infections, which are more common in the female infant than the male infant, can also cause disruption of normal urinary function.

Toddler and Preschooler

It is during toddlerhood and the preschool years that a child usually achieves voluntary urinary continence. During this time, a child becomes physiologically and psychologically capable of this task. Sometime between 12 to 18 months, the myelinization of the sacral spinal segments that control the bladder becomes complete, and a child can then perceive bladder fullness. A good indicator of the maturation of the spinal cord is when a toddler can walk independently.

Even though a toddler can perceive bladder fullness by age 18 months, he or she may not choose to voluntarily hold the urine in the bladder and delay voiding. Sometime between 2.5 to 3 years, most children can perceive a full bladder *and* voluntarily delay voiding. Children also need a sufficient vocabulary to communicate the need to urinate, easy access to toilet facilities, and sufficient fine motor control to loosen or remove necessary clothing. In the American culture, most parents sense their child's readiness to begin toilet training at age 2.5 to 3 years. They notice that the child is voiding less frequently (longer periods of diaper dryness) and is able to acknowledge in words that he or she does feel bladder fullness. Sometimes toddlers need to experience some outdoor play time without a diaper to visually see what happens when they experience bladder fullness followed by urethral relaxation and bladder emptying. They begin to understand cognitively the relationship between bladder fullness and voluntary bladder emptying, and are ready for toilet training. Children in the American culture usually achieve daytime urinary continence by age 3; boys may take longer to achieve daytime continence. Nighttime continence may not occur until age 4 or 5.

Child and Adolescent

School-age children have achieved both daytime and nighttime urinary continence. These children and adolescents are approaching the urinary elimination habits of adults; they void straw-colored urine six to seven times a day. The amount of urine output is greatly influenced by the amount of oral fluid intake. See Table 37-1 for the average ranges of urine output in a 24-hour period. A small percentage of school-age children continue to experience involuntary urinary incontinence, which is termed enuresis. Parents often seek advice from healthcare providers when nocturnal enuresis occurs past age 7. Specific nursing interventions for the management of nocturnal enuresis are discussed later in this chapter.

Adult and Older Adult

By the time a person has reached adulthood, he or she has developed a urinary elimination pattern that is normal or typical for him or her. A typical pattern of urinary elimination in a healthy adult is the painless voiding of approximately 250 to 400 mL clear, yellow urine with an aromatic odor about four to five times per day. Normal or expected deviations from this pattern occur with an increase or decrease in fluid intake.

In late middle age, men may experience altered urinary elimination related to prostatic hypertrophy, and women may experience altered urinary elimination related to weakened perineal muscles (cystocele or rectocele).

As a result of cardiovascular changes that occur with aging, there is usually decreased blood perfusion to the kidneys in the elderly. This decreased arterial flow to the renal arteries is a gradual change that results from decreased cardiac muscle strength, which reduces cardiac output to the periphery, and a decrease in the elasticity of the peripheral blood vessels. Over time, due to decreased arterial perfusion, there is a progressive decrease in kidney function; the kidneys become a less effective regulator of the body's extracellular fluid. The ureters, bladder, and urethra lose some muscle tone with aging. The bladder becomes less able to hold large amounts of urine (decreased bladder capacity), and the elderly person may experience an urgency to empty the bladder more frequently of smaller amounts of urine. The urge to void may be sensed when the limit of bladder is at capacity, which diminishes the ability to voluntarily delay voiding (Turner & Plymat, 1987). Uninhibited bladder contractions can further increase the sense of urgency. These factors place the elderly at risk for incontinence. Nocturia is a frequent complaint in the elderly, and urinary retention is also more common in the elderly. This predisposes the elderly to urinary tract infections. Women may experience stress incontinence as they age, related to weakened perineal muscles. Older men eventually experience urinary hesitancy and difficulty starting the urinary stream, related to prostatic hypertrophy.

ALTERED URINARY FUNCTION

Potential for Altered Urinary Function

Many factors can predispose a person to disruption of normal patterns of urinary elimination (see the display).

Factors Associated with Altered Urinary Elimination

Obstruction of urine flow
  Renal calculi
  Prostatic enlargement
  Tumors
  Structural abnormalities
Infection
Hypotension
Neurologic injury
  Spinal cord injury
  Cerebral vascular accident (stroke)
  Brain tumor
Decreased muscle tone
  Aging
  Multiple pregnancies
  Obesity
Medications
Surgery
  Anesthesia
  Edema
  Immobility
Pregnancy
Urinary diversions

Obstruction of urine flow, urinary tract infections, hypotension, neurologic injury, medications, surgery, pregnancy, and urinary diversion all affect urinary function.

Obstruction of Urine Flow

Obstruction of the normal flow of urine can lead to problems in urinary elimination, and, when severe, can cause kidney damage. Urinary obstruction can be caused by structural abnormalities within the urinary tract, urinary tumors or other tumors that press against the urinary tract, renal stones, or prostatic enlargement. Obstruction can also occur when a patient has a catheter or tubes in place to drain urine, and they become plugged or kinked.

One of the complications of obstruction within the urinary system is hydronephrosis. Hydronephrosis is the distention of the kidney pelvis with urine secondary to the increased resistance caused by obstruction to normal urine flow. Unrelieved hydronephrosis can cause renal cell atrophy and necrosis, which can cause permanent kidney damage.

Urinary stasis also occurs secondary to urinary obstruction. The stagnant urine proximal to the obstruction provides a good growth medium for microorganisms, and thus fosters the development of urinary tract infections.

Infections of the Urinary Tract

Urinary tract infections (UTIs) are usually caused by microorganisms normally found in the gastrointestinal tract. The microorganisms commonly responsible for UTIs are of the enterobacteriaceae species, including *Escherichia coli, Klebsiella,* and *Proteus* (Conti & Eutropius, 1987). These microorganisms typically gain access to the urinary system via the urethral meatus. Hence, the most common UTIs are infections of the urethra (urethritis) or bladder (cystitis). Urethritis and cystitis are classified as lower urinary tract infections, whereas infections of the ureters (ureteritis) and the kidney pelvis or tubule system are classified as upper urinary tract infections. Upper urinary tract infections occur less frequently, but are more serious, since kidney damage and renal failure may result.

Normally the urinary tract is sterile, except at the urethral meatus. In the healthy person, bacteria tend to be flushed away during the act of voiding. Infection occurs when microorganisms from the surrounding perineal skin or anal opening find their way to the urinary meatus and ascend the urethra. Women are more susceptible to lower urinary tract infections because of the short length of the female urethra and the proximity of the vagina and anus to the urinary meatus. Men are less susceptible to lower urinary tract infections because of the longer length of the male urethra, and also due to the antibacterial properties of prostatic secretions (Conti & Eutropius, 1987).

Other factors that can increase the incidence of UTIs include incorrect wiping of the anal area after a bowel movement, sexual intercourse, which can bring perineal microorganisms into closer contact with the urinary meatus, and any procedure that places an object in the urethra or bladder for diagnostic or therapeutic reasons. The longer a catheter remains in the bladder, the greater the chance of nosocomial infection (Cox, 1988).

Infections of the urinary tract can disrupt the normal pattern of urinary elimination in a number of ways. Voiding becomes painful and more frequent. The person with a UTI often experiences urgency, a subjective feeling of being unable to voluntarily delay the urge to void. Urine becomes abnormal, containing pus (pyuria) and blood (hematuria). Ultimately, if the infection ascends to the kidney, renal damage can occur and possibly result in renal failure.

Hypotension

It is important to maintain adequate blood perfusion to the kidneys to ensure urine formation. When arterial blood pressure drops too low, the renal arteries do not have enough pressure to cause glomerular filtration. Inadequate circulating volume or inability of the heart to pump adequately can decrease blood flow to the kidneys. Decreased circulating volume can occur after surgery, trauma, or when the patient has severe loss of fluids, such as from diarrhea or vomiting. When urine output drops below 30 mL per hour for 2 consecutive hours, decreased perfusion of blood to the kidneys and other vital organs must be suspected.

Neurologic Injury

Neurologic injury, such as occurs after a stroke or spinal cord injury, can cause disruption in normal patterns of urinary elimination. Injury (by trauma, hemorrhage, or tumor) to the frontal lobes of the brain, which control the voluntary nature of voiding, can lead to incontinence. This type of incontinence is called uninhibited neurogenic bladder (Patrick, et al., 1991).

The micturition reflex occurs at the sacral level of the spinal cord. If the spinal cord is injured at the sacral level or above, the person will experience a change in control of urinary elimination. A person may experience reflex voiding, which results in incontinence. This occurs because as soon as the bladder is stretched to a certain degree, a reflex contraction of the bladder occurs, resulting in loss of urine. This condition is called reflex neurogenic bladder If the reflex arc itself is injured, the bladder may fill without the bladder stretch contraction mechanism working, resulting in urinary retention. This condition is called autonomous neurogenic bladder.

Decreased Muscle Tone

Weakened abdominal and perineal muscles can impair bladder contraction and control of the external urinary sphincter. Abdominal and perineal muscles can become weak due to obesity, multiple pregnancies, stretching during childbirth, menopausal atrophy due to decreased estrogen, and chronic constipation. A cystocele is the protrusion or herniation of the bladder into the vaginal canal; it produces symptoms of stress incontinence, frequency, dribbling, and an inability to completely empty the bladder.

Continuous bladder drainage with a catheter can also cause decreased bladder tone. Continuous bladder drainage prevents the bladder from ever getting full; thus, stretch of the bladder musculature is limited, promoting bladder atrophy. After the removal of a catheter, some patients experience dribbling and difficulty with urinary control. This is usually temporary, lasting until bladder tone returns.

Pregnancy

Pregnancy can cause an alteration in urinary elimination. The increasing size and weight of the growing uterus can exert pressure on the bladder, a common cause of frequency in pregnant women. Compression of the bladder by the uterus may also lead to obstruction of urinary flow and incomplete emptying of the bladder. During the early postpartum period, a woman is also prone to altered urinary function. Trauma from vaginal delivery causes swelling in the perineal area, which can obstruct the flow of urine.

Surgery

Postoperative patients should be able to void within 10 hours after surgery. Some patients have difficulty voiding postoperatively for a number of reasons. Often, postoperative patients are volume-depleted due to limited fluid intake and loss of blood and fluid during surgery. The stress of surgery triggers the release of ADH, which decreases urinary output. During the immediate postoperative period, patients often are unable to get up and use the bathroom. Using a bedpan or urinal in a supine position often impedes normal urinary patterns.

Surgery involving the urinary system, intestines, or reproductive organs predisposes a patient to urinary retention. Trauma to tissues can cause edema, which can potentially obstruct the flow of urine. The use of a retention catheter is indicated after any surgery on the urinary tract.

Anesthesia can also affect urinary elimination. Anesthetic agents slow the glomerular filtration rate, reducing urinary output. People receiving a spinal or regional block during surgery are at increased risk for postoperative urinary problems, as these agents impair the sensory and motor impulses that control micturition. Until the anesthesia has worn off, the patient will be unable to perceive bladder fullness and will not be able to initiate voiding. This can cause urinary retention.

Medications

Medications can be given therapeutically to affect urinary elimination, and medications administered for other reasons can have side effects that influence normal urinary patterns. Some medications also change the color of urine.

Medications classified as diuretics have as their intended effect an increase in urine output. They accomplish this by affecting the reabsorption of sodium and water in the tubules of the nephron. Commonly used diuretics include chlorathiazide, hydrochlorathiazide, furosemide, spironolactone, and triamterene. People with edema or a propensity to develop edema are candidates for diuretic therapy. Cholinergic medications (e.g., urecholine) may be given to promote voiding, since they stimulate contraction of the detrusor muscle.

Side effects of medications used to treat other health problems can adversely affect urinary elimination. The risk of urinary retention is increased with medications having anticholinergic effects. Belladonna alkaloids, phenothiazines, tricyclic antidepressants, and antihistamines are examples of such drugs. Narcotics can decrease glomerular filtration rate and decrease the sensation of bladder fullness.

Some medications can change the color of urine. For example, pyridium causes the urine to turn bright orange, and amitriptyline turns urine blue–green.

Urinary Diversion

A urinary diversion is a surgical procedure in which the normal pathway of urine elimination is altered. The ureters are rerouted from a diseased or damaged urinary system to a new outlet, called a stoma, created by the surgeon on the patient's abdomen. The diversion may be permanent, as with cancerous conditions that require removal of the bladder (cystectomy). In other conditions, such as trauma or severe chronic urinary tract infections, the diversion may be temporary to promote healing.

Urinary diversions alter normal urinary elimination, as the person no longer has control over voiding. Although the person is able to engage in all normal activities, adjustment to the urinary diversion and learning to manage it may take some time.

Four types of urinary diversions are the ileal conduit (or ileal loop), the Kock pouch diversion, the ureterostomy, and the vesicostomy (Fig. 37-4).

Ileal Conduit. The procedure known as an ileal conduit or ileal loop involves removing a small segment of the ileum and then reattaching the two portions of the intestine that have been severed. One end of the removed section is sutured closed to form a conduit for urine collection and passage; the other end is brought out through the abdominal wall to form a stoma. The stoma usually protrudes 0.5 to 0.75 inch above the abdominal skin. The ureters are then implanted into the conduit so that urine flows from the kidneys into the conduit (through the ureters), and out through the stoma. The patient is fitted with and uses a stoma appliance to collect urine. The ileal conduit is the most common type of urinary diversion.

Kock Pouch Diversion. The Kock pouch diversion is similar to the ileal conduit except that it requires no external appliance to collect urine. Instead, a pouch is formed by taking a 60- to 70-cm segment of ileum, which will hold urine inside the body. The urine is prevented from leaking out of the pouch through the stoma by an outlet nipple valve, which is created using intussuscepted portions of the ileal segment (the tissue is folded back against itself in such a way that the path of fluid is obstructed). Reflux of urine from the pouch back into the ureters is prevented with a similar inlet nipple valve. Urine is removed from the internal pouch on a scheduled basis, usually four to six times a day, by inserting a catheter through the stoma, through the outlet valve, and into the pouch.

Ureterostomy. The ureterostomy urinary diversion has the ureters diverted from their normal attachment in

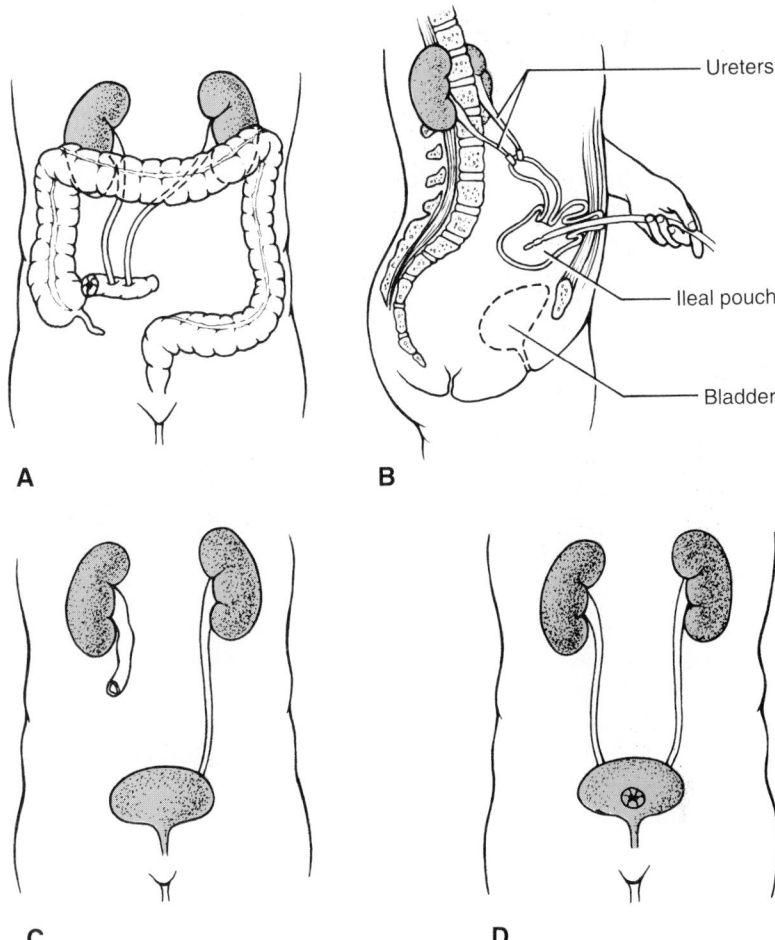

Figure 37–4. Urinary diversions: **A:** Ileal conduit. **B:** Kock Pouch. **C:** Ureterostomy. **D:** Vesicostomy.

the bladder to the patient's abdominal wall or flank. Like the ileal conduit, a stoma is created, one or two depending on whether or not one ureter has been connected to the other before being brought to the body's surface. Urine drains continuously from the ureters out through the stoma, which necessitates the use of an appliance to collect urine.

Vesicostomy. The vesicostomy urinary diversion involves suturing closed the neck of the bladder, bringing forward the anterior wall of the bladder to the abdomen, and then forming a tube and stoma from a portion of the anterior bladder wall. Urine drains continuously from a portion of the bladder through the exit tube and stoma, so a urinary diversion appliance must be worn. A continent vesicostomy is similar to the Kock pouch diversion, however, in that it can be created by forming an outlet nipple valve from intussuscepted portions of the anterior wall. The patient is routinely catheterized or performs self-catheterization to remove urine.

Manifestations of Altered Urinary Function

Disruption of normal patterns of urinary elimination can be seen in the following signs and symptoms: dysuria, polyuria, oliguria, urgency, frequency, hematuria, urinary retention, incontinence, and enuresis. The nurse plays a significant role in detecting abnormal patterns of urinary elimination, as well as in preventing such problems. The nurse also assists the patient in coping with irreversible dysfunctional patterns.

Dysuria

Dysuria means painful voiding. Pain is often associated with urinary tract infections and is felt as a burning sensation during urination. Any bladder inflammation or trauma, or inflammation of the urethra can cause dysuria. Dysuria may occur temporarily after sexual activity, and is often associated with sexually transmitted disease in both men and women. Some medications can cause dysuria. Painful voiding should be referred to a physician, since there are many causes of dysuria.

Polyuria

Polyuria is the formation and excretion of excessive amounts of urine in the absence of a concurrent increase in fluid intake. Urine output of greater than 2500 to 3000 mL in 24 hours is considered polyuria. Untreated diabetes insipidus and diabetes mellitus can greatly increase urine output. Ingestion of diuretics, caffeine, and alcohol also results in polyuria.

Oliguria

Oliguria is the formation and excretion of decreased amounts of urine, or urinary output less than 500 mL in 24 hours. A severe decrease in fluid intake, or any disease state or injury that leads to an excessive loss of body fluids, can cause oliguria. For example, excessive vomiting, diarrhea, diaphoresis, burns, or bleeding can decrease urine output. Persons with renal disease may be oliguric. As the kidney approaches complete failure as a functioning organ, the person may become anuric. **Anuria** is the formation and excretion of less than 100 mL of urine in 24 hours.

Urgency

Most adults can delay emptying the bladder until it contains 250 to 400 mL of urine. **Urgency** describes the subjective feeling of being unable to voluntarily delay the urge to void. Urgency implies a strong micturition reflex due to inflammation or irritation of the bladder, incompetent urethral sphincter, weak perineal muscle control, or psychologic stress.

Frequency

Voiding at frequent intervals is known as **frequency.** This occurs when a person voids more frequently than the normal pattern, without a significant increase in fluid intake. Each void usually contains less than 250 mL of urine. Frequency not associated with increased fluid intake can be related to other factors, such as urinary tract infections or pressure on the bladder from pregnancy. Frequency and urgency often occur together.

Nocturia

Voiding during normal sleeping hours is called nocturia. If a person voids before going to bed, it should be possible to sleep for 7 to 8 hours without feeling a strong micturition reflex. Ingestion of large amounts of fluids before bed, especially those containing alcohol or caffeine, may promote nocturia. People with medical conditions such as congestive heart failure may also experience nocturia. When lying supine, edema decreases as fluid enters the circulation. This increases blood flow to the kidneys and thus increases glomerular filtration and urine output.

Hematuria

Hematuria indicates blood in the urine; it can be gross (visible on visual examination), or occult (not visible on visual examination). Occult blood may change the color of urine from normal clear yellow or amber to a cloudy or hazy yellow or amber. As the number of red blood cells increases, the urine may become bright red in color. Pathologic causes of hematuria include urinary tract infections, urinary tract tumors, renal calculi, poisoning, and trauma to the urinary mucosa. Hematuria is expected and temporary after urinary tract or prostatic surgery.

Pyuria

Pyuria means the urine contains pus, which is the accumulation of the end-products of an inflammatory response. These end-products include microorganisms and white blood cells. Pus gives urine a cloudy color and, often, a strong, unpleasant odor. Pyuria occurs in the presence of any urinary tract infection.

Urinary Retention

Urinary **retention** is the inability to empty the bladder of urine. In urinary retention, the person is either unable to perceive the growing bladder fullness, or is unable to relax the bladder neck and external urethral sphincter to allow passage of urine from the body. Since the kidneys continue to form urine, the volume within the bladder grows, until, in extreme cases, the bladder can hold up to 2000 to 3000 mL of urine.

Urinary retention often involves the inability to void within 8 to 10 hours of the last voiding. The absence of voiding may be followed by suprapubic discomfort, and a feeling of fullness and restlessness. The person may or may not perceive a strong urge to void. Bladder distention of more than 600 mL can often be palpated in the suprapubic area of the abdomen. Urinary retention is distinguished from oliguria by the presence of bladder distention.

Urinary retention with overflow is the loss of small amounts of urine from an overdistended bladder. As the bladder becomes overdistended with urine, it no longer responds to bladder stretch as a stimulus to initiate detrusor contraction and voiding. The bladder can maintain only a certain degree of overdistention before excess urine is eliminated in small amounts at frequent intervals. The small amounts of urine that are voided are known as "overflow."

Complications of urinary retention include the loss of bladder tone secondary to the excessive stretch of the detrusor muscle fibers. Even after the primary retention is relieved, it may take a period of weeks for the bladder/ stretch–bladder/emptying response to return to normal. The accumulation of urine in the bladder also leads to stasis of urine, which predisposes the person to urinary tract infection and calculus development. Bladder distention can also lead to hydronephrosis as the urine backs up into the ureters and kidney.

Persons at risk for developing urinary retention include those with neurologic impairment, such as spinal cord injury or brain lesions. Postoperative patients often are afflicted with temporary urinary retention until edema subsides and spinal anesthesia wears off. After vaginal delivery of a baby, swelling of the urinary meatus is a common occurrence that may cause a temporary obstruction to the outflow of urine.

Incontinence

Urinary **incontinence** is the involuntary loss of urine from the bladder. Five types of urinary incontinence are identified by patterns of uncontrolled voiding and related causative factors. The five classifications are stress, urge, reflex, functional, and total incontinence.

Stress Incontinence. The sudden, involuntary loss of small amounts (less than 50 mL) of urine that accompanies a sudden increase in intra-abdominal pressure is called stress incontinence. Examples of activities that increase intra-abdominal pressure are coughing, sneezing, laughing, lifting, and jumping.

Factors associated with stress incontinence include a weakening of the pelvic floor muscles, high intra-abdominal pressure, damage to the bladder neck, or side effects of medications. The pelvic floor muscles can be weakened by the stretching that occurs during childbirth. Women who have experienced a long and difficult labor and delivery or who have experienced multiple childbirths are most likely to have weakened pelvic muscles. Estrogen is necessary to maintain the normal tone of reproductive organs and associated musculature; therefore, postmenopausal women who have decreased estrogen levels may suffer from stress incontinence (Turner & Plymat, 1988). Obesity or pregnancy can cause high intra-abdominal pressure. Obese, postmenopausal women who have had multiple pregnancies are most likely to develop stress incontinence. Another cause of stress incontinence is direct trauma, which may occur due to a fractured pelvis or during genitourinary surgery.

Urge Incontinence. The involuntary loss of urine after a strong feeling of the need to urinate is termed urge incontinence. The person with urge incontinence is unable to simultaneously perceive a full bladder and hold urine until the bathroom is reached. Urge incontinence is often accompanied by frequency, dysuria, and nocturia.

Factors associated with urge incontinence include urinary tract infections, the use of diuretics, the consumption of fluids containing caffeine or alcohol, or an increase in fluid intake. An overdistended bladder can precipitate urge incontinence. Some patients experience urge incontinence for a short period of time after an indwelling catheter has been removed. They have become accustomed to an empty bladder, and need time to accommodate the usual degree of bladder distention.

Reflex Incontinence. An involuntary loss of urine that occurs at somewhat predictable intervals when a specific bladder volume is reached is called reflex incontinence. The person is unable to sense bladder fullness due to neurologic impairment, and the bladder simply empties when a certain degree of bladder stretch has been reached. Bladder emptying occurs at the sacral reflex level, because the connection to the cerebrum allowing voluntary inhibition of voiding is impaired. Reflex incontinence is seen in the patient with neurologic impairment, such as spinal cord lesion, cerebrovascular accident, or brain tumor.

Functional Incontinence. Functional incontinence involves the inability or unwillingness of a person with normal bladder and sphincter control to reach the bathroom in time to void. Environmental barriers, disorientation, or physical limitations can contribute. The amount of urine that is lost is typically large.

Many factors can interfere with the ability to reach the toilet in time. A poorly lit, cluttered room may obstruct easy access to the bathroom. Raised siderails or a call bell that is out of reach can contribute to functional incontinence in the hospitalized patient. Sensory or cognitive factors are also associated with functional incontinence, as confusion, disorientation, and sedatives or side effects of medications can impair cognitive functioning. Motor deficits, such as impaired gait and loss of fine motor control needed to release necessary clothing, can also contribute.

Total Incontinence. The continuous, involuntary, unpredictable loss of urine from a nondistended bladder is termed total incontinence. The designation is sometimes used when the observed incontinence does not fit any other incontinence category and does not respond to usual incontinence treatment methods.

Factors associated with total incontinence include a specific neurologic lesion in the brain or spinal cord, traumatic or surgical injury to the genitourinary area or spinal cord, or a congenital malformation within the urinary tract or spinal cord.

Enuresis

Enuresis is involuntary voiding with no underlying pathophysiologic origin, after the age that bladder control is usually achieved. By the time most children are 4 or 5 years old, they can control urinary elimination during both the day and night. Enuresis beyond the age of 5 is typically nocturnal. Nocturnal enuresis is called bedwetting by most parents. Involuntary voiding during sleep can occur during naps during the day but is more frequent during longer periods of sleep at night.

Factors associated with nocturnal enuresis include small bladder capacity, sound sleeping, stress and anxiety at home or school, urinary tract infections, and family history of nocturnal enuresis.

Impact of Urinary Dysfunction on Activities of Daily Living

The elimination of fluid wastes from the body is an important function of daily living. The inability to do this properly has serious psychologic and social implications. Incontinence can lead to social isolation, since many people fear that bladder incontinence will prove embarrassing in social situations (National Institutes of Health, 1988). Sometimes this limits trips outside the home or limits social encounters to only close friends, who will understand if incontinence should occur. The loss of control over this basic body function can create feelings of anxiety or fear, whether in the 8-year-old with enuresis, or the 80-year-old who has developed a bladder control problem (Yu, 1987).

Alterations in urinary elimination may place an extra financial burden on the person who has to purchase protective pants and special garments. Frequent trips to the physician and required medications can add to the financial burden. Frequently, extra energy and time must be spent washing clothing and bedding. Clothing should be chosen that is easy to get on and off and does not require dry cleaning. Some people may need to choose styles that will hide protective pants.

Incontinence and enuresis can disrupt sleep, as one has to get up and change clothes, wash, and then try to get back to sleep. If it is a child who is experiencing nocturnal enuresis, sleep is usually also disrupted for the parent who gets up to help the child with these tasks. The lack of sleep can cause tension and irritability, which in turn increases the stress that is felt due to altered patterns of urinary elimination.

Adequate hygiene is important for people with alterations in urinary function. Adequate bathing after incontinence will decrease odor and prevent skin breakdown. Adequate washing may be difficult for the elderly, those who are cognitively impaired, or the child who has to get to school on time.

Frequent uncontrolled incontinence in the elderly often contributes to the family's decision to seek institutional care. For many people, a move to an extended care facility drastically affects independence in the tasks of daily living. As the percentage of the aged population increases, the impact on society at large is considerable.

ASSESSMENT

Functional assessment allows the nurse to collect subjective and objective data regarding normal urinary status

and risk factors that can contribute to urinary dysfunction, and to identify dysfunctional urinary patterns. The nurse can collect such information by asking direct questions, watching for subtle nonverbal cues, performing physical assessment, and evaluating information gathered in diagnostic and laboratory tests.

Subjective Data

The collection of subjective information from the patient (or other significant person) about urinary status usually begins with obtaining a detailed history. The nurse should ensure patient privacy, and be sensitive to feelings of embarrassment the patient may experience during the discussion of urinary function.

Functional Pattern Identification

It is often easier for the patient to describe alterations in urinary elimination pattern than to describe normal urinary elimination. Normal patterns of elimination can be affected by many factors in daily living, so that some people have difficulty recognizing their own normal pattern within daily variation.

Specific questions regarding when the last voiding occurred, how many times per day urination usually occurs, whether each void contains a small, medium, or large amount of urine, and whether the patient often wakes during the night to void, helps the nurse identify normal patterns of urinary elimination. The nurse may have to clarify the term "urinating" by using other words the patient may be more familiar with, such as voiding, peeing, passing water, or "going potty". The data the nurse gathers from such questions can then be analyzed to evaluate whether the patient's typical pattern falls within expected parameters of the healthy child or adult.

Risk Identification

A nursing history also allows the nurse to identify factors that could potentially alter urinary elimination. Information should be elicited concerning previous renal or urinary tract problems, such as kidney failure, renal calculi, or urinary tract infections. If one of these conditions is present, the nurse should obtain a history of the condition and how it was treated and resolved. The nurse should question the patient about any previous genitourinary surgery, such as prostatic surgery or repair of a cystocele. Other acute or chronic medical problems, such as congestive heart failure or neurologic injury, should be evaluated in terms of their impact on normal patterns of urinary function.

Data should be elicited about recent changes in daily routine concerning exercise, food, or fluid intake. A significant change in oral intake or the consumption of beverages containing alcohol or caffeine should be noted. Medications that can alter urinary output or function, such as diuretics or anticholinergics, should also be indicated.

Motor or cognitive dysfunction that could impede successfully getting to a bathroom should be evaluated. Visual impairment or communication difficulties could also affect the ability to reach the bathroom in a timely manner in a new environmental setting. The general ability to understand and follow directions should be assessed so that teaching can be individualized for the patient.

Dysfunctional Identification

The collection of subjective data can also help the nurse identify dysfunctional patterns of urinary elimination. An open-ended question such as, "Have you noticed any problems with your urinating lately?" is often a good way to begin. If the patient responds by indicating no urinary difficulties, clarify the meaning of his or her response by asking more specific questions, such as:

Do you have any pain or burning with urination?
Have you noticed any pink or reddish color in your urine?
Do you feel you are able to empty your bladder completely every time you urinate?
Do you accidentally lose any urine when you sneeze or cough?
Do you have any difficulty stopping or starting your urinary stream?

Such questions are useful because alterations in normal urinary function often occur gradually and are perceived as normal by the patient. For example, the elderly man may have had difficulty starting his urinary stream for the past 10 years due to prostatic enlargement, and does not view this as a urinary problem.

Abnormal patterns of voiding such as polyuria, oliguria, or anuria are important to document, as well as hematuria, dysuria, frequency, or urgency. When present, the nurse should question the patient as to the length of time the problem has persisted, and when it first began.

If the patient does indicate a chronic problem with urinary function, such as stress incontinence or a urinary diversion, the nurse should question the patient regarding individual management of the problem. At this time the nurse can also ask the patient how he or she would like things handled during hospitalization. For example, the woman who manages her stress incontinence by wearing sanitary napkins at home may want to continue doing so while hospitalized for an acute appendectomy.

When a problem in urinary elimination is identified, the nurse should assess the patient's support system. Because urinary elimination problems are often stressful, the support of family and friends is often helpful and necessary for the patient. The nurse can use subjective data to evaluate how the patient and family members are coping with problems in urinary function.

Objective Data

Objective data can be collected by visually examining the urine, and by physical assessment of the lower abdomen and perineal area. Information from diagnostic and laboratory tests can also help the nurse evaluate the urinary status of the patient.

Assessment of Urine

Assessment of urine is best done when the patient does not void directly into the toilet, but rather into a urine collection device (urinal for men; bedpan for women), or when a retention catheter is in place. When assessment of the urine is important, the nurse may have to request that the patient void into one of these devices. A "hat" is a device that can be placed in between the toilet and the toilet seat to catch urine (see Fig. 32-5). Using a hat permits the patient to void normally in the toilet, but still allows for visual inspection or measurement of urine.

Assessment of urine includes visual inspection for color, clarity, the presence of blood or mucus, and noting the odor of the urine. (Refer to the normal characteristics of urine that have already been discussed in this chapter.) The amount of urine should be assessed for each void, as should the total urine output over a 24-hour period. The 24-hour output can be compared to the intake, and any significant difference noted. Trends of increasing or decreasing output should be evaluated.

Assessment of Urinary Retention

To assess a patient for urinary retention, the nurse should examine the patient's voiding pattern. If the patient's intake and output (I & O) are being monitored, a written record of the time and amount of each void is maintained. When examining this flowsheet, the nurse can determine the pattern of voiding and the balance of overall intake and output. Within a 24-hour period, the intake and output is usually within 200 to 300 mL. The absence of voiding during any 8-hour period or the frequent voiding of small amounts of urine (50 to 100 mL) per void suggest urinary retention or urinary retention with overflow voiding.

When a patient's I & O is not being monitored, it is important to obtain subjective information regarding urinary elimination at least once every 8 hours. Question the patient as to whether voiding has occurred and whether any difficulty in voiding was experienced. Risk factors, such as anticholinergic medications, surgery, vaginal delivery, or prostatic hypertrophy should be considered. Physical assessment of the lower abdomen is indicated for any patient in whom urinary retention is suspected.

Physical Assessment

Inspection. Inspection of the lower abdomen and perineum is one of the most helpful parts of the physical assessment in evaluating urinary function. The nurse inspects the patient's lower abdomen when the patient's history or recent voiding pattern indicates that urinary retention is a potential urinary alteration. When the patient is lying in a supine position, a bulge in the central lower abdomen just above the symphysis pubis can be noted if the bladder is distended. When the bladder contains less than 500 mL, no bulge will be present. When the bladder holds more than 700 mL, the bulge may be observed extending in the direction of the umbilicus. It may not be easy to observe a distended bladder in an obese person.

It is not necessary to inspect the patient's perineal area routinely, unless the patient complains of severe dysuria and the presence of purulent drainage. When there are no specific complaints, the nurse can examine the urinary meatus when performing perineal hygiene for the patient unable to meet his or her own hygiene needs. The nurse should always inspect the urinary meatus when inserting or removing a urinary catheter. If healthy, the skin surrounding the urinary meatus is nonreddened, moist, and without discharge. Smegma, an accumulation of white, odorous secretions from sebaceous glands found under the labia minora in women and under the foreskin in men, is normal, and is not discharge from the urinary meatus. Abnormal findings on inspection of the perineum are reddened, inflamed skin surrounding the urinary meatus, and purulent discharge.

Percussion. Percussion of the lower abdomen follows inspection to determine the presence of a distended bladder. Percussion should begin at the umbilicus and proceed downward toward the symphysis pubis. If the bladder is empty or contains less than 150 mL of fluid, a hollow note will be heard, the normal sound expected over the abdomen. Percussion over a distended bladder will produce a duller sound. Urine, being liquid, is denser than the mixture of air and fluid in the small intestines, and therefore produces a duller sound. The closer the dull sound is to the umbilicus, the greater the degree of bladder distention. Percussion is the most reliable element of the physical assessment in evaluating the degree of bladder distention.

Palpation. Palpation is the final component of physical assessment of the lower abdomen to assess for bladder distention. As with percussion, palpation should start at the level of the umbilicus and move in a downward direction toward the symphysis pubis. The finger-tips of both hands should be used to palpate deeply in an attempt to feel the top edge of the bladder. When the bladder contains more than 150 mL of urine, the edge of the bladder will feel smooth and rounded. The top edge of the distended bladder should be at the same level of the abdomen where percussion changed from a hollow to a dull sound. Even though palpation of the bladder must be deep to feel the edge of the bladder, it should be done gently. Palpation may cause discomfort and stimulate voiding.

Table 37-2 gives a comparison of normal and abnormal findings during physical assessment of the lower abdomen.

Diagnostic Tests and Procedures

The nurse is responsible for collecting urine specimens for laboratory examination. Some urine tests are performed by the nurse, while others require that the urine be sent to a laboratory for more sophisticated examination. The nurse is also involved in preparing the patient for diagnostic procedures that help identify pathologic urinary conditions. The nurse is responsible for patient teaching and preparation before such procedures, as well as assisting with procedures and providing the patient with postprocedure care.

Collection of Urine Specimens. The nurse is responsible for collecting urine specimens for a number of different types of tests. Different tests require different collection procedures. The urine collected can be a random urine specimen, a clean catch, or midstream specimen, a 24-hour urine specimen, or urine withdrawn from an indwelling urinary catheter. Special considerations may be required during collection of urine from an infant or small child. Guidelines for these procedures are given in Procedure 37-1, "Collecting Urine Specimens."

Random Specimen. Random urine specimen collection is used when sterile urine is not required. The clean specimen can be collected in a urinal, bedpan, hat, or directly into a specimen cup. The urine should not be

---

TABLE 37–2

Comparison of Normal and Abnormal Findings on Physical Examination of Lower Abdomen for Bladder Distention

Normal	Abnormal
Inspection	
No distention	Bulging above symphysis pubis
Percussion	
Hollow	Dull
Palpation	
Bladder not palpable	Smooth, round edge of bladder

PROCEDURE 37–1. Collecting Urine Specimens

■ Purpose
1. Obtain a noncontaminated urine specimen for routine or diagnostic studies that include culture and sensitivity tests.

■ Assessment
- Determine patient's ability to understand directions and to obtain specimen independently.
- Identify purpose for obtaining specimen to guide selection of best method for obtaining specimen.
- If collecting specimen from indwelling urinary system, assess tubing for sampling port.

■ Equipment
Disposable gloves.
Container, label.
For collecting sterile urine specimen from an indwelling catheter: Betadine swab, 10-mL syringe with 23 to 25 gauge needle, sterile specimen container.
For collecting midstream urine specimen: cleansing solution, towel, specimen container.
For collecting a specimen from child without urinary control: cleansing solution, towel, pediatric urine collection bag, diaper.

■ Procedure

Collecting Sterile Specimen from an Indwelling Catheter
1. Explain procedure to patient.
2. Wash hands. Put on disposable gloves.
   Rationale: Prevents transmission of microorganisms.
3. Position patient so that catheter is accessible.
4. Cleanse the aspiration port of the drainage tubing with Betadine swab.
   Rationale: Prevents microorganisms from entering the drainage tubing.

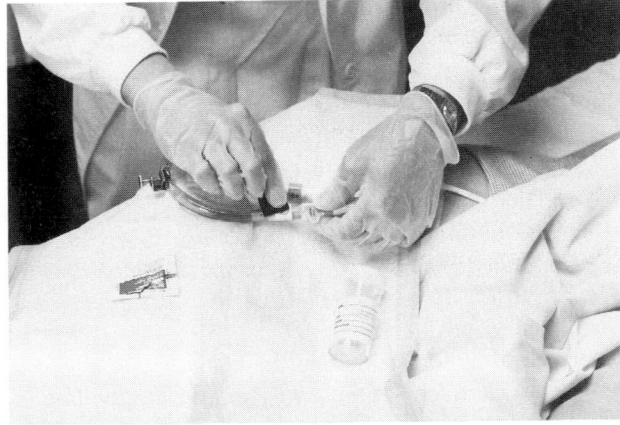

Step 4

5. Allow urine to collect in tubing by clamping or bending tubing (2 mL of urine is sufficient for a culture and sensitivity specimen).
   Rationale: Fresh urine is needed for accurate test results.
6. Insert needle into aspiration port. Draw urine sample into syringe by gentle aspiration. Remove needle.

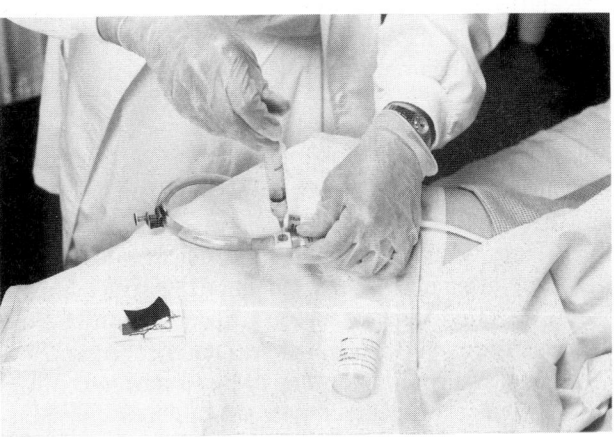

Step 6

7. Transfer urine from syringe into a sterile specimen container.
   Note: Hospital policy may allow specimen to be transported to laboratory in syringe with sterile cap on syringe in place of needle.
8. Label the container. Date and time laboratory requisition.
   Rationale: Incorrect identification of specimen could cause diagnostic or therapeutic error.
9. Send specimen to laboratory within 15 minutes or place in specimen refrigerator.
   Note: If specimen is for microbiology testing, it must be sent immediately and not refrigerated.
   Rationale: Microorganisms grow quickly in urine, especially at room temperature. Refrigeration retards bacterial growth.
10. Dispose of all contaminated supplies. Wash hands.
11. Document procedure and observations.

■ Procedure

Collecting Midstream Urine Specimen for a Woman
1. Instruct patient how to cleanse urinary meatus and obtain urine specimen.
2. Wash hands.
3. Separate labia minora and cleanse perineum with cleansing agent Betadine swab, starting in front of

(continued)

PROCEDURE 37–1. Collecting Urine Specimens *(continued)*

the urethral meatus and moving swab toward the rectum.
Rationale: Prevents spread of microorganisms from the rectum to the urinary meatus.

4. Begin to urinate while continuing to hold labia apart. Allow first urine to flow into toilet.
Rationale: Washes microorganisms and cellular debris out of meatus.

5. Hold specimen container under the urine stream and collect sample.

6. Remove specimen container, release hand from labia, seal container tightly, and finish voiding.

■ **Procedure**

Collecting Midstream Urine Specimen for a Man

1. Wash hands.

2. Cleanse end of penis with cleansing agent Betadine swab. If man is not circumcised, instruct him to retract foreskin to expose urinary meatus before cleansing and throughout specimen collection.

3. Begin to urinate, allowing urine to flow into toilet.
Rationale: Washes microorganisms and secretions from urethra before collecting specimen.

4. Pass specimen container into urine stream and collect sample.

5. Remove container, seal tightly, and finish voiding.

6. Follow steps 7 to 10 above.

7. The nurse should put on disposable gloves to receive specimen container from patients. Clean and rinse outer surface of container with disinfectant.
Rationale: Prevents transfer of microorganisms to other health-care workers from possible urine spillage outside containers.

8. Label the container. Date and time laboratory requisition.
Rationale: Incorrect identification of specimen could cause diagnostic or therapeutic error.

9. Send specimen to laboratory within 15 minutes or place in specimen refrigerator.
Note: If specimen is for microbiology testing, it must be sent immediately and not refrigerated.
Rationale: Microorganisms grow quickly in urine, especially at room temperature. Refrigeration retards bacterial growth.

10. Dispose of all contaminated supplies. Wash hands.

■ **Procedure**

Collecting a Specimen from a Child Without Urinary Control

1. If parents are present, explain procedure to them.

2. Position child gently on back. Put on disposable gloves. Remove diaper.

3. Clean perineal–genital area gently with soap and water, followed by Betadine antiseptic.

4. For a girl: Separate labia and cleanse from front of urethral meatus toward the rectum. Rinse with sterile water and dry with cotton balls.
Rationale: Cleansing removes lotions, powders, fecal matter, as well as decreases the numbers of microorganisms present on the skin. Drying the area thoroughly facilitates adhesion of the urine collection bag.

5. For a boy: Cleanse the penis and scrotum. If boy is not circumcised, retract foreskin and cleanse. Rinse with sterile water and dry with gauze or cotton balls.
Rationale: Same as for a girl.

6. Remove paper backing from adhesive of collection bag.

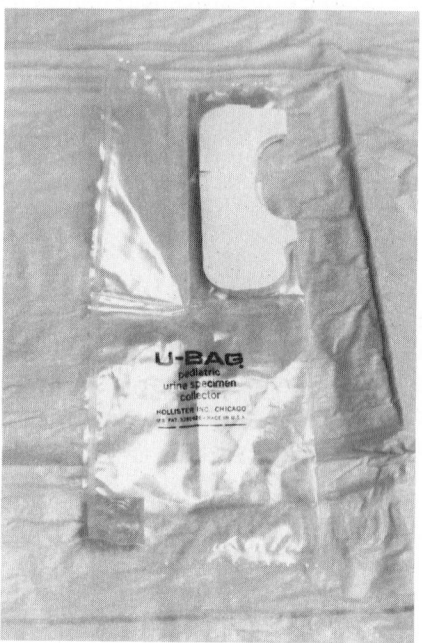

Step 6

7. Spread the child's legs widely apart.
Rationale: Separates and flattens skin folds to increase adhesion of bag and decrease chances of leaking.

8. Apply collection bag over child's perineum, covering penis and scrotum on boy, and urinary meatus and vagina of girl. Press adhesive to secure, starting at the perineum and working outward.
Rationale: Securing adhesive from the center toward the outside decreases wrinkling and subsequent leaking of urine.

9. Place a diaper on the child loosely.
Rationale: Helps to hold the urine collection bag in place.

(continued)

PROCEDURE 37–1. Collecting Urine Specimens *(continued)*

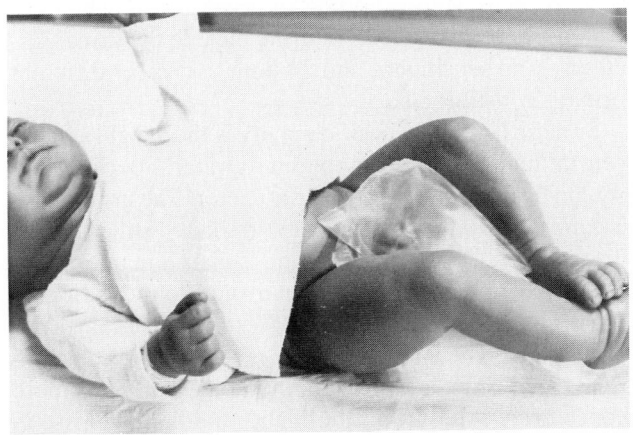

Step 8

10. Remove gloves, wash hands.
11. Check the collector for urine every 15 minutes.
    Note: Parents can check child for urine specimen.

12. When urine specimen is obtained, glove again, and gently remove collection bag from the skin and empty urine into specimen container.
13. Tighten lid and cleanse outside of container if contaminated with urine.
    Rationale: Cleansing the outside of container prevents spread of microorganisms.
14. Label the container. Date and time laboratory requisition.
    Rationale: Incorrect identification of specimen could cause diagnostic or therapeutic error.
15. Send specimen to laboratory within 15 minutes or place in specimen refrigerator.
    Note: If specime is for microbiology testing, it *must* be sent *immediately* and not refrigerated.
    Rationale: Microorganisms grow quickly in urine, especially at room temperature. Refrigeration retards bacterial growth.
16. Dispose of all contaminated supplies. Wash hands.
17. Document that specimen was collected and sent.

contaminated with feces or toilet paper. If a woman is menstruating, this should be noted on the specimen. The specimen should be properly labeled and promptly sent to the laboratory, or used for a test to be made at the bedside.

Clean-Catch or Midstream Specimen. A clean-catch or midstream-voided specimen is used when a specimen relatively free of microorganisms is required. A sterile specimen cup or sterile bedpan or urinal is used to collect the urine specimen. The urinary meatus should be cleansed of the organisms normally found on the skin surrounding the meatus. Women need to be instructed to clean the perineal area well with soap and water or a disinfectant before voiding. Cotton balls with soap or disinfectant should be used only once, wiping from front to back to avoid contamination from the anus. This cleansing is usually repeated three times with different cotton balls. Men should clean the end of the penis in a circular motion starting at the tip. The patient is then asked to void a small amount of urine into the toilet, stop the urinary flow, and then void midstream urine into the specimen container. Obtaining a midstream urine specimen decreases the chance that the sample will be contaminated with microorganisms from the perineal skin or vaginal secretions. The sample is not acceptable if contaminated with stool, vaginal secretions, or menstrual blood.

The container should be properly labeled and immediately transported to the laboratory. If the specimen cannot be taken to the laboratory immediately, it must be refrigerated. Changes in the urine begin to occur within an hour if it is left unrefrigerated. Multiplying bacteria may split urea, which produces a more alkaline urine.

24-Hour Specimen. A 24-hour urine specimen is required to accurately measure kidney excretion of certain substances. The nurse is responsible for explaining the procedure to the patient and for taking steps to ensure that *all* urine is saved. Inadvertent discarding of even a small amount of urine invalidates the test results, necessitating that collection of urine be started all over again. A sign over the patient's bed and on the bathroom door helps alert all hospital personnel and family members that all urine must be saved. A large container for urine collection is usually provided by the laboratory. A preservative may be added to this container to prevent the breakdown of certain urinary constituents.

Often a 24-hour sample is started early in the morning after the patient's first void. The nurse should instruct the patient to void until the bladder is completely empty. This voided urine should be discarded and the time noted as the beginning of the 24-hour period during which all urine must be saved. The patient may void into any clean urinary container (bedpan, hat, urinal), but care must be taken to avoid contamination with stool or toilet paper. All urine is then emptied into the 24-hour collection container, taking care not to splash, since the added preservative can be caustic. The large container should be refrigerated or placed in a bucket of ice during the 24 hours of collection. At the end of the 24 hours, the patient should be asked to empty his or her bladder, and this urine is added to the collection container. The container is then labeled and sent to the laboratory.

Specimen from Catheter. Obtaining a specimen from a catheter may be necessary when the patient is unable to void or already has a catheter in place. Urine collected in this manner is sterile. When obtaining urine from a catheter, it is important to maintain strict asepsis at all times to prevent entry of microorganisms into the bladder.

When catheterization is necessary to obtain urine, an in-and-out catheterization is performed. This means the catheter is left in place only long enough to obtain the specimen (see Procedure 37-4). The sterile urine is permitted to flow into the specimen container, and then the container is properly labeled and sent to the laboratory.

When the patient already has a retention catheter in place, the specimen is obtained by using a syringe to draw urine from a self-sealing port in the catheter (Procedure 37-1). The specimen port of the catheter is cleansed with alcohol. A small-gauge needle (e.g., 23 or 25 gauge) is inserted into the port and the necessary amount of urine is withdrawn into the syringe. Once the urine is obtained, it is usually transferred to a specimen container, labeled, and sent to the laboratory. It may be necessary to clamp the catheter tubing just below the specimen port for 20 to 30 minutes with a rubber band to allow enough urine to collect in the tubing so that a specimen can be obtained. This is especially true if more than a few cubic centimeters of urine are needed in the specimen.

Urine should not be collected from the catheter drainage bag. This urine is not considered sterile, since the collection system has been opened to drain urine at different intervals. Also, as the urine sits for long periods of time in the drainage bag, growth of bacteria can occur.

Collecting Urine from Children. Collecting urine from infants and children may necessitate special attention if the child has not yet achieved control of voiding. Catheterization is often difficult, and not recommended because of the small meatal opening and the trauma to the young child. Plastic collection devices are a more acceptable method of collecting urine from an infant or young child. Clear plastic bags with adhesive material can be attached over the child's urethral meatus (Procedure 37-1). The child's perineal area is washed and dried thoroughly before application of the bag over the perineum. Bags should be applied according the manufacturer's instructions, and care taken to avoid trauma to the delicate meatus of the young child.

Collecting specimens from children who have achieved bladder control may also be challenging. Often children find it difficult to start their stream on command. Drinking a glass of water, running a faucet, and permitting the parent to help the child obtain the urine specimen may increase the chances of success.

Urine Tests. Common tests that are routinely performed on urine by the nurse include specific gravity, pH determination, and assessing for the presence of glucose, protein, ketone bodies, or occult blood. The most common laboratory tests of urine include the urinalysis, culture and sensitivity, and 24-hour assays for different urinary constituents.

Specific Gravity. Specific gravity is the weight or concentration of urine as compared to water. Specific gravity can be measured using a urinometer. The urinometer is calibrated to float at the 1.000 mark in distilled water. To test for specific gravity, urine is placed in a test tube and the urinometer is gently spun and allowed to float in the urine (see Procedure 37-2, "Testing Specific Gravity of Urine"). The specific gravity is read where the meniscus of the urine hits the urinometer marking. The more concentrated the urine, the higher the float will rise in the urine, and the higher the specific gravity reading. Normal specific gravity of urine is 1.010 to 1.025 g/mL. A low specific gravity usually occurs because of overhydration or a pathologic condition that affects the kidneys' ability to concentrate urine. A high specific gravity occurs because of fluid volume deficit.

Reagent Strips. Reagent strips (or dipsticks) are available to measure the amount of certain substances such as glucose, protein, or ketones in the urine. Such strips can also be used to determine urinary pH or the presence of occult blood. The instructions for proper use of the various reagent strips are clearly printed on the container and should be followed precisely to ensure accurate results. The procedure usually involves dipping the reagent strip into the urine sample and comparing any color changes to the color chart provided on the container. Timing is crucial for the accurate interpretation of results for some tests, such as testing for glucose or ketones. Assessment of the urine by reagent strips is ordered by the physician when he or she wants to closely monitor certain parameters on high-risk patients (e.g., assessing pregnant women for protein in their urine), or to continually monitor the urine status for each voiding. The nurse may independently decide to use reagent strips when necessary for comprehensive assessment of high-risk patients.

Urinalysis. Urinalysis is one of the most common screening tests performed on urine. A urinalysis provides data about the color, turbidity, pH, and specific gravity of the urine, as well as indicating the presence of protein, glucose, ketones, red blood cells, white blood cells, bacteria, and casts in the urine. The collection of a urine specimen for urinalysis is routine for all hospitalized patients. The test can be performed on any random specimen of 20 to 30 mL of urine. Although the specimen can be collected at any time during the day, the first voided morning specimen is preferred. The first urine voided in the morning is ordinarily more concentrated, since the patient is usually without fluids during

PROCEDURE 37–2. Testing Specific Gravity of Urine

■ Purpose

1. Evaluate the extent to which the urine is being concentrated in the kidney.
2. Monitor the patient's hydration status in response to therapies such as intravenous fluids and drugs (mannitol, antidiuretic hormone).

■ Assessment

- Assess patient's ability to collect urine specimen. Determine alternate methods of specimen collection, if necessary.
- Assess related clinical signs/symptoms of hydration status:
  - Intake and output records.
  - Vital signs.
  - Serum electrolytes.
  - Skin turgor, mucous membranes.
  - In infants, position of fontanel.

■ Equipment

Urinometer (hydrometer).
Glass cylinder.
20 ml freshly obtained urine.
Clean, disposable gloves.

■ Procedure

1. Wash hands, put on clean, disposable gloves.
   Rationale: Protects against microorganisms being transferred from urine specimen to nurse's hands.
2. Pour urine into glass cylinder until it is one-half to three-quarters full.
   Rationale: Urometer will not float unless glass cylinder is at least one-half full.
3. Place urometer into the cylinder. Gently spin stem of urometer.
   Rationale: Prevents the urometer from adhering to the side of the cylinder.
4. Place cylinder on flat surface at eye level. When twirling stops, read where the urine level meets the calibrated urometer at the base of the meniscus.
   Rationale: The concentration of dissolved solutes in the urine affects the depth at which the urometer floats.
5. Discard urine, wash equipment with soap and water, allow to air dry. Discard gloves. Document findings.
   Rationale: Prevents growth of microorganisms in equipment in between uses.

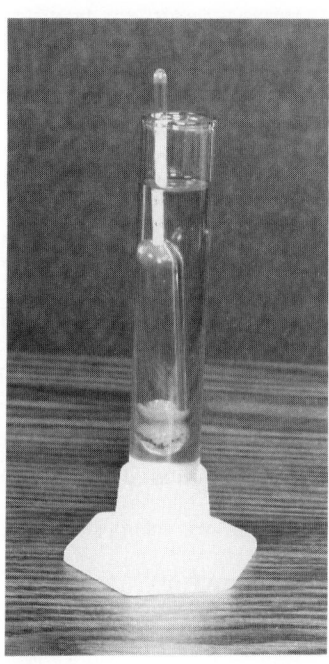

Step 4A

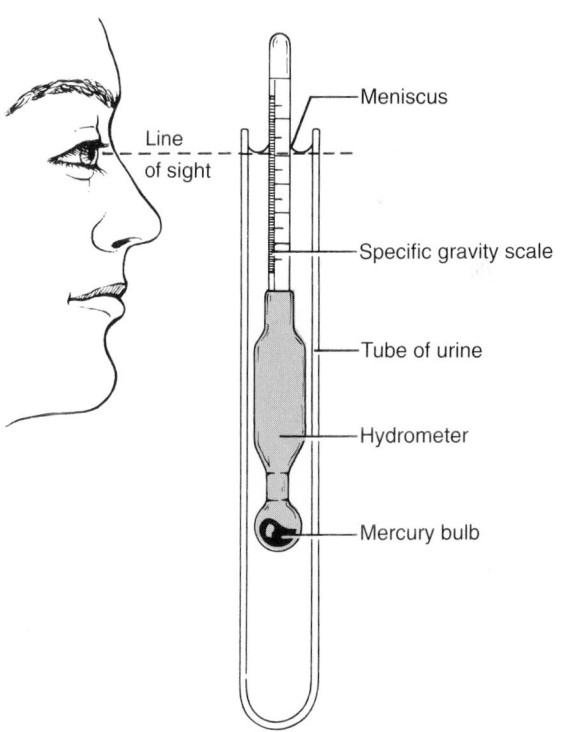

Step 4B

the night. The influence of diet and activity is minimized. All these factors make the first voided specimen more likely to reveal any abnormalities that are present. Table 37-3 presents a concise summary of the parameters tested in a urinalysis, the range of acceptable normal values, and the clinical significance of abnormal values.

Urine Culture and Sensitivity. Culture and sensitivity tests can be performed on the urine to identify any microorganism causing a urinary tract infection, and to identify those antibiotics that can effectively kill the organism. The culture allows the bacteria to grow and multiply over a period of at least 48 hours. After 24 hours of growth, the laboratory is able to make a preliminary identification of the organism. Another 24 to 48 hours may be necessary to conduct the definitive analytic tests that identify the exact microorganism responsible for the infection. After identification of the organism, the laboratory can test to see which antibiotics inhibit growth of the organism. If an antibiotic inhibits bacterial growth, the bacteria is said to be sensitive to the antibiotic. If the antibiotic does not inhibit bacterial growth, the organism is considered resistant. The purpose of performing a culture and sensitivity is to ensure effective antibiotic therapy in the treatment of urinary tract infections.

24-Hour Specimens. Twenty-four-hour urine specimens may be used to measure kidney excretion of certain substances. Some substances excreted by the kidney are not excreted at the same rate throughout the day. A single random specimen may give incomplete, inaccurate results about these urinary solutes. Some of these substances include total urine protein, creatinine, urobilinogen, uric acid, electrolytes, and hormones. To evaluate accurately the presence and amount of these substances, all urine excreted by a patient during a 24-hour period is collected and sent to the laboratory for examination.

Blood Test. Small samples of blood can be analyzed in the laboratory to screen for kidney disease. Two of the more commonly performed tests are blood urea nitrogen (BUN) and serum creatinine.

Blood urea nitrogen measures the amount of urea nitrogen in the blood. Urea, the major nitrogenous end waste product of metabolism, is formed in the liver. Urea is carried in the bloodstream from the liver to the kidneys for excretion. When the kidney is diseased, it is unable to adequately excrete urea and urea begins to accumulate in the blood causing the BUN to rise. Normal BUN is 8 to 25 mg/100 mL. Since other factors, such as high dietary intake of protein, fluid deficit, infection, gout, or excessive breakdown of protein stores can also elevate BUN, it is not a highly sensitive indicator of impaired renal function.

Serum creatinine is a more sensitive indicator of renal function. Creatinine is the waste product formed from the breakdown of skeletal muscle tissue; its formation is not influenced by diet or other factors. As creatinine is formed, it is carried in the bloodstream to the kidneys for

TABLE 37–3

Urinalysis Parameters

Parameter	Normal Values	Clinical Significance of Variations
Color	Light yellow–amber	Almost colorless: ↑ fluid intake; Dark color: ↓ fluid intake; Pink, red, dark brown: red blood cells in urine; Pink, orange, red, brown, blue–green: medications or foods
Turbidity	Clear	Hazy; cloudy, smoky: urine specimen allowed to stand at room temperature; red blood cells, white blood cells, bacteria, mucus threads: mucosal irritation secondary to indwelling catheter
pH	Normal: 6 Range: 4.6–8	<6: Diet high in meat or some fruits (cranberries); metabolic acidosis (diabetes mellitus, starvation); respiratory acidosis (emphysema) >6: Diet high in vegetables and citrus fruits; urinary tract infections; metabolic alkalosis (vomiting, prolonged diuretic therapy); respiratory alkalosis (hyperventilation)
Specific gravity	Range: 1.015–1.025	<1.015: ↑ Fluid intake, diuretic therapy, diabetes insipidus, renal diseases >1.025: ↓ Fluid intake; ↑ fluid loss (vomiting, diarrhea, fever); ↑ ADH secretion (trauma, stress)
Protein	None–trace	Present in: severe stress, renal disease, pre-eclampsia of pregnancy
Glucose	None	Present in: diabetes mellitus
Ketones	None	Present in: diabetes, ketoacidosis, starvation
Microscopic examination: High-Power Field		
Red blood cells	0–3	>3: Urinary tract infection, bleeding, urinary tract trauma, anticoagulant therapy
White blood cells	0–5	>5: Urinary tract infection
Bacteria/yeast	None–few	Few: contamination from perineal skin Many: urinary tract infection
Casts (precipitation or clumping of protein substances)		
	None–occasional	Many: possible renal diseases

filtration and excretion. Damage to a large number of nephrons prevents efficient excretion of creatinine and causes the build-up of creatinine in the blood. An elevated serum creatinine is indicative of impaired renal function. When the BUN and serum creatinine are both elevated, it is a reliable indicator of kidney dysfunction.

Creatinine clearance is a combination blood and urine test that measures the rate at which creatinine is cleared from the blood by the kidneys. Creatinine is excreted in the urine by the process of glomerular filtration. Creatinine is not secreted by the kidney tubule, nor is it reabsorbed anywhere in the kidney tubule. Therefore, its excretion is an accurate measure of glomerular filtrating ability of the kidney. To compute the creatinine clearance, a measurement of the creatinine level in the blood, the creatinine level in the urine, and the amount of urine produced in a set period of time (usually 24 hours) is needed. A decreased creatinine clearance value indicates renal impairment.

Diagnostic Procedures.   The physician can order many diagnostic urologic procedures to better understand the functioning of the patient's urinary system, and to identify any abnormalities. The nurse prepares the patient physically and psychologically for these tests, monitors the patient during and after the procedure, and uses the information obtained to individualize the plan of care for the patient.

X-ray Examination.   X-ray examination can provide helpful information concerning the status of the urinary tract. The two most commonly performed x-ray examinations for this purpose are the flatplate of the abdomen to visualize the kidneys, ureters, and bladder (KUB), and the intravenous pyelogram (IVP).

The plain abdominal x-ray that visualizes the kidneys, ureters, and bladder is helpful in detecting malformations in the size or shape of the kidneys, ureters, or bladder, and to detect the presence of any stones that could obstruct the flow of urine. This x-ray procedure is painless and requires no special care before or after the procedure.

An intravenous pyelogram (IVP) is an x-ray that visualizes the urinary system by the use of a radiopaque (contrast) dye. The dye is injected intravenously and x-rays are taken at set intervals. This permits visualization of the dye as it is excreted by the kidneys, emptied into the ureters, and finally deposited in the bladder. An x-ray is also taken immediately after the patient voids to check if the bladder is completely emptying. The procedure takes about 1 hour to complete. Special preparations before the procedure include clear liquids or a light meal the evening before the test; nothing by mouth after midnight (although sometimes clear fluids are permitted); and enemas and laxatives to clear the colon of feces, since fecal contents can interfere with visualization. The nurse should also check for any history of allergy to iodine (x-ray dye) before beginning preparation for the test.

Several other tests are helpful in visualizing the urinary system and detecting abnormalities of the kidney or bladder (Table 37-4). They include computerized axial tomography (CT) scan, magnetic resonance imaging (MRI), renal scan, and abdominal ultrasound. During these procedures, various types of energy are directed over the abdomen. Computer technology converts the information into visual pictures of the kidney. Patient preparation varies with each test. There may be some discomfort associated with maintaining body position during the procedure, but the procedures themselves are not painful.

Cystoscopy.   Cystoscopy involves the insertion of a tube into the bladder for the purpose of direct visualization. A cystoscope is a flexible tube that can be inserted into the urethra and guided into the bladder. A light at the end of the cystoscope allows the physician to look for abnormalities such as tumors, stones, or structural problems. Specialized instruments can be passed through the cystoscope to remove small stones or to take tissue biopsies. Radiopaque dye may be injected for subsequent kidney x-rays; this is known as a retrograde pyelogram. The patient needs to sign a consent form before the cystoscopy. After the procedure, the nurse needs to

TABLE 37-4

Diagnostic Procedures to Assess Kidney Function

Test	Technology	Image Produced
Computerized axial tomography	X-ray machine rotates 180° around abdomen	Three-dimensional cross-section of kidney
Magnetic resonance imaging	Large magnet and radio waves	Visual display on computer screen
Renal scan	IV infusion of radio-nuclide; subsequent reading of radio-activity of target organ (kidney)	Two-dimensional picture of kidney
Ultrasound	Sound waves	Visual display on computer screen

assess for hematuria, urinary retention, dysuria or bladder spasms, and any signs or symptoms of urinary tract infection. A retention catheter may be left in place for a short period of time after the cystoscopy.

Urodynamic Studies. Urodynamic studies are used to detect abnormalities in bladder function or voiding. These procedures measure pressure (from the bladder, urethra, and within the abdomen), urinary flow, and striated muscle activity. The names of these procedures and the dynamics of urination tested are listed in Table 37-5. These procedures require no special preparation before testing. Urodynamic studies generally are not painful, but the patient may experience some intermittent discomfort during the procedure.

Noninvasive Urine Volume Monitoring. Noninvasive urine volume monitoring is a new technique that can be performed at the bedside by the nurse. A new portable ultrasound device has been developed to measure the volume of urine contained within the bladder. This noninvasive technique allows the nurse to evaluate the amount of urine in the bladder if he or she suspects urinary retention. It may also be helpful in measuring post-void residual urine, thus avoiding the necessity of in-and-out catheterization.

A probe is attached to a machine that contains a screen capable of visualizing the bladder with ultrasound. Lubricating jelly is placed on the lower abdomen, and the probe is moved until a clear outline of the bladder is present on the screen. Two separate readings are taken, from which the machine computes the volume of urine (Fritz, 1989).

NURSING DIAGNOSES AND PATIENT GOALS

Accepted NANDA nursing diagnoses involving alterations in urinary elimination include urinary retention and five types of urinary incontinence: stress, urge, reflex, functional, and total. The nurse uses data from the assessment of urinary elimination to determine the presence or risk any of these disruptions in normal urinary elimination patterns.

TABLE 37-5
Diagnostic Procedures to Assess Bladder Function

Test	Purpose
Uroflowmetry	Measures characteristics of voided urine stream: peak and average flow rates.
Cystometrogram	Measures bladder pressure during bladder filling and during voiding.
Electromyogram	Measures activity of the striated muscles in the perineum.
Urethral Pressure Profile	Evaluates smooth muscle activity of urethra.

Diagnostic Statement: Stress Incontinence

Definition

Stress incontinence is the state in which an individual experiences a loss of urine of less than 50 mL occurring with increased abdominal pressure (NANDA 1990).

Defining Characteristics

Major. Reported or observed dribbling with increased abdominal pressure.

Minor. Urinary urgency; urinary frequency (more often than every 2 hours) (NANDA, 1990).

Related Factors

Degenerative changes in pelvic muscles and structural supports associated with increased age; high intra-abdominal pressure (e.g., obesity, gravid uterus); incompetent bladder outlet; overdistention between voidings; weak pelvic muscles and structural supports (NANDA, 1990).

Diagnostic Statement: Urge Incontinence

Definition

Urge incontinence is the state in which an individual experiences involuntary passage of urine occurring soon after a strong sense of urgency to void (NANDA, 1990).

Defining Characteristics

Major. Urinary urgency; frequency (voiding more often than every 2 hours); bladder contracture/spasm.

Minor. Nocturia (more than twice per night); voiding in small amounts (less than 100 mL) or in large amounts (more than 550 mL); inability to reach toilet in time (NANDA, 1990).

Related Factors

Decreased bladder capacity (e.g., history of pelvic inflammatory disease, abdominal surgeries, indwelling urinary catheter); irritation of bladder stretch receptors causing spasm (e.g., bladder infection); alcohol; caffeine; increased fluids; increased urine concentration; overdistention of bladder (NANDA, 1990).

Diagnostic Statement: Reflex Incontinence

Definition

Reflex incontinence is the state in which an individual experiences an involuntary loss of urine, occurring at somewhat predictable intervals when a specific bladder volume is reached (NANDA, 1990).

Defining Characteristics

Major. No awareness of bladder filling; no urge to void or feelings of bladder fullness; uninhibited bladder contraction/spasm at regular intervals (NANDA, 1990).

Related Factors

Neurologic impairment (e.g., spinal cord lesion that interferes with conduction of cerebral messages above the level of the reflex arc) (NANDA, 1990).

Diagnostic Statement: Functional Incontinence

Definition

Functional incontinence is the state in which an individual experiences an involuntary, unpredictable passage of urine (NANDA, 1990).

Defining Characteristics

Major. Urge to void or bladder contractions sufficiently strong to result in loss of urine before reaching an appropriate receptacle (NANDA, 1990).

Related Factors

Altered environment; sensory, cognitive, or mobility deficits (NANDA, 1990).

Diagnostic Statement: Total Incontinence

Definition

Total incontinence is the state in which an individual experiences a continuous and unpredictable loss of urine (NANDA, 1990).

Defining Characteristics

Major. Constant flow of urine occurs at unpredictable times without distention or uninhibited bladder contractions/spasm; unsuccessful incontinence-refractory treatments; nocturia.

Minor. Lack of perineal or bladder filling awareness; unawareness of incontinence (NANDA, 1990).

Related Factors

Neuropathy preventing transmission of reflex indicating bladder fullness; neurologic dysfunction causing triggering of micturition at unpredictable times; independent contraction of detrusor reflex due to surgery; trauma or disease affecting spinal cord nerves; anatomic (fistula) (NANDA, 1990).

Diagnostic Statement: Urinary Retention

Definition

Urinary retention is the state in which an individual experiences incomplete emptying of the bladder (NANDA, 1990).

Defining Characteristics

Major. Bladder distention; small, frequent voiding or absence of urine output.

Minor. Sensation of bladder fullness; dribbling; residual urine; dysuria; overflow incontinence (NANDA, 1990).

Related Factors

High urethral pressure caused by weak detrusor; inhibition of reflex arc; strong sphincter; blockage (NANDA, 1990).

Related Nursing Diagnoses

The patient with urinary dysfunction can experience many other problems. Individual nursing diagnoses are supported from data collected in the nursing assessment. The patient with Altered Urinary Elimination can experience Impaired Skin Integrity and Fluid Volume Deficit. Psychologic stress due to problems with urinary elimination can result in Anxiety or Ineffective Individual Coping. Sleep Pattern Disturbance and Sexual Dysfunction can also result. Knowledge Deficit is also common in the patient with urinary dysfunction, since new treatment regimens will have to be learned to prevent or cope with problems with urination.

Patient Goals

Goals for the patient with urinary dysfunction should be individualized depending on patient assessment. General patient goals should encompass the following:

Patient will strengthen or maintain adequate perineal muscle control.
Patient will reestablish control over voiding.
Patient will verbalize understanding of procedures necessary to promote optimal urinary function.

IMPLEMENTATION

The nurse plays a significant role in preventing and managing urinary dysfunction. Patient teaching can inform the general population as well as each individual patient how urinary problems can be prevented. The nurse also implements specific measures to promote optimum urinary elimination, such as comfort measures, catheterization, administering medications, and caring for the patient with a urinary diversion or one who is undergoing renal dialysis. Individual management plans are developed for people with special urinary problems such as urinary retention, incontinence, or enuresis.

Nursing Interventions to Promote Health and Urinary Function

Patient Teaching

Patient teaching is important in promoting optimum health and urinary function. All patients should be taught the importance of adequate fluid intake, how to avoid urinary tract infections, and measures to maintain adequate perineal muscle tone.

Fluid Intake Promotion. Educating people regarding the importance of adequate fluid intake is a significant nursing intervention. Normally, an adult should drink between six to eight glasses or about 1500 to 2000 mL of fluid per day. Fluid intake may have to increase proportionally with any excessive loss of body fluid.

Fluid intake should be spaced throughout the waking hours to prevent transitory dehydration. Fluid intake may be restricted before bed to avoid waking during the night. Water is a preferred fluid, since excessive intake of caffeine, glucose, or sodium can alter urinary elimination.

Adequate fluid intake serves two functions: adequate urine production will flush microorganisms out of the urinary system, thus decreasing the chance of infection or obstruction from stones; and producing large amounts of urine will help to distend and stretch the detrusor muscle, preventing atrophy. For these reasons, adequate fluid intake is helpful in preventing urinary tract infection and maintaining bladder tone.

Urinary Tract Infection Prevention. In addition to maintaining adequate fluid intake, other measures can prevent urinary tract infection. Adequate perineal hygiene is important in preventing contaminating microorganisms of the anus or vagina from entering the urethra. Women should be instructed at an early age to always wipe from front to back after urinary or fecal elimination. Voiding immediately after sexual intercourse also helps to prevent bacteria from entering the woman's urinary tract. Adequate perineal care is impor-

tant during the postpartum period and during menstruation. Men and women, including all health-care workers, should be reminded of the importance of washing hands carefully with soap and water whenever the perineal area or body fluids are touched.

The nurse can also teach the signs and symptoms of urinary tract infections, namely fever, flank pain, dysuria, frequency, urgency, pyuria, or hematuria. Teaching is especially important after any instrumentation of the bladder. Some people may be embarrassed to contact their physician about urinary problems, so the importance of prompt treatment for potential urinary tract infections should be stressed.

Optimum Muscle Tone Promotion. Loss of perineal and abdominal muscle tone can contribute to urinary retention and incontinence. Promoting regular exercise of these structures can prevent loss of tone. Kegel exercises involve tightening of the perineal and anal muscles. This should be done several times per hour, and incorporated into activities of daily living so that life-long habits can be formed. Kegel exercises are discussed in Chapter 48. Another muscle strengthening exercise involves having the patient voluntarily stop and start the stream of urine when voiding. Exercise instruction is especially important during the postpartum period. Patient teaching concerning weight reduction for the obese person is also helpful in improving muscle tone.

Urinary Collection Devices

Illness and hospitalization can disrupt a person's usual routine of urinary elimination. Unfamiliar and sometimes uncomfortable medical procedures, loss of privacy, strange surroundings, and anxiety concerning medical diagnosis and/or prognosis are just a few of the factors that may disrupt usual urinary elimination habits. In addition to promoting an adequate fluid intake, there are a number of comfort measures that the nurse can employ to promote urinary elimination and to assist the patient in maintaining his or her usual elimination habits:

- Provide a private setting for voiding.
- Allow adequate, unhurried, and uninterrupted time for voiding.
- If nursing assistance is needed for voiding, assess the patient's usual voiding times (such as when awakening, before meals, and at bedtime), offer assistance at those times in particular, and be available for assistance at in-between times.
- Promote relief of physical discomfort and anxiety-producing situations. These may increase muscle tension and inhibit the relaxation needed for urination. Provide medications for pain as ordered, and emotional support and reassurance.
- Aid the patient in assuming a comfortable and, if at all

possible, physiologic position for voiding. This is a sitting or squatting position for women and a standing position for men.

- If the patient has difficulty starting to urinate, it may be helpful for the nurse to provide sensory stimuli that act either by promoting relaxation or by the concept of suggestion. These stimuli include pouring warm water over the perineum, running water from the faucet, having the patient relax in a warm bath, placing the patient's hands in warm water, stroking the inner thighs, providing music or reading material, and offering a beverage.

Urinary collection devices to promote normal urinary elimination are the toilet, bedside commode, urinal, and bedpan.

Toilet. For patients who are ambulatory, the typical procedure for urinary elimination involves walking to and from the bathroom and using the toilet for voiding, with assistance provided by the nurse as necessary. For some patients who have difficulty sitting down on and arising from a conventional-height toilet, a raised or elevated toilet seat can be attached, so that the patient has a decreased distance to lower and raise himself or herself. Based on previous assessment, necessary comfort measures should be provided for the patient using the bathroom, and opportunity given after voiding for the patient to wash his or her hands. This may be a good time to instruct the patient about hygiene techniques, such as the importance for the woman to wipe the perineum from front to back after voiding.

Bedside Commode. If the patient is unable to ambulate as far as the bathroom, but can transfer out of bed to a chair, then a commode may be the device of choice for urinary elimination. A commode is a straight-backed armchair, frequently with locking wheels, with a toilet-like seat and receptacle for urine and feces. Some commodes are made with their own receptacles; others have a place for attaching a conventional bedpan. Many commodes have a flat seat covering the toilet seat, so that it may also be used as a chair. Before assisting the patient to the commode, the nurse must assess whether or not the patient can safely transfer independently and, if not, just how much support he or she needs. If the patient is at risk for falling, it may be necessary for the nurse to remain with the patient or to stand just beyond the privacy curtains while he or she urinates. Other comfort measures must be provided as needed, and the patient should be provided with a means of handwashing after voiding.

Urinal. When a male patient is confined to bed, he may use a urinal as a convenient collection device for urine (Fig. 37-5). Although urinals are made in a number of designs, and some urinals are designed specif-

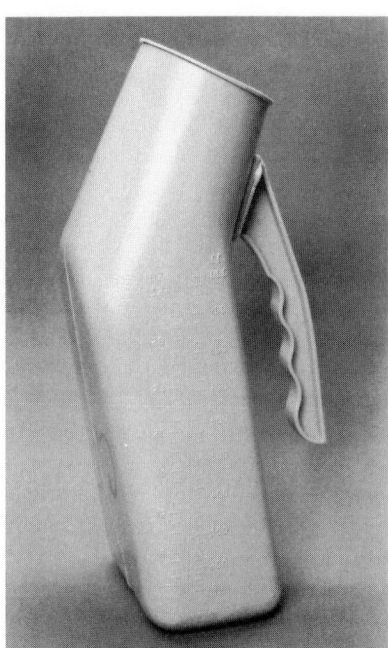

Figure 37–5.   A urinal may be used by the male when the patient cannot walk to the bathroom.

ically for women, it is typically the man who uses the urinal. Assisting the patient to stand at the bedside when voiding while using the urinal is physiologically advantageous. Sometimes, however, this is contraindicated, and consequently the patient is positioned in bed in as close to an upright position as feasible. In most instances the patient is able to place and hold the urinal himself. If he is unable to do so, then the nurse may need to hold the urinal in place while the patient urinates, or place the urinal and then leave the patient alone for a few moments. When the patient has completed voiding into the urinal, he will typically place it on the overbed table or hang it on the siderail of his bed. To avoid having the urinal bumped or knocked and the contents spilled, and to avoid any embarrassment that may be caused by having the patient's urine clearly visible at the bedside, it is important that the nurse remember to empty and rinse the urinal in a timely manner. Once again, it is also important for the nurse to provide comfort measures as needed and a means of handwashing after voiding.

Bedpan. For female patients confined to bed, the bedpan is the collection device frequently used for urinary elimination. Typically, the male patient uses the urinal for urine elimination and the bedpan for bowel elimination, and the female patient uses the bedpan for both. Two types of bedpans are commonly available (Fig. 37-6): the first, known as a regular bedpan, is rounded somewhat like a toilet seat and has a higher back; the second type, called a fracture pan, is smaller and more flat. Fracture pans are used primarily for patients who have physical limitations or have difficulty lifting their

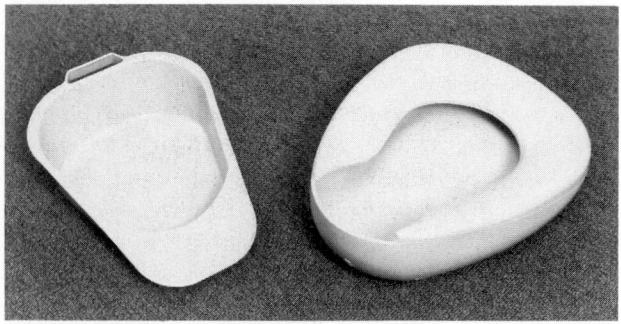

Figure 37–6. Two types of bedpans: fracture pan (left); regular pan (right).

buttocks onto the bedpan. Fracture pans are also used for patients whose medical complications contraindicate lifting onto a regular bedpan.

Some patients who are confined to bed can independently use the bedpan for urinary elimination. The bedpan should be kept within easy reach, along with toilet paper or other means of cleansing the perineum after urination. The nurse may need only to assure privacy, to empty and cleanse the bedpan in a timely manner, return the bedpan to the patient, and provide supplies for hand-washing.

For many patients confined to bed, however, more assistance by the nurse is required. Having to use a bedpan for urine elimination may be an embarrassing, uncomfortable, and tiring procedure. Some patients may say that they feel it requires less energy to get up to use a commode than to get onto and off a bedpan. The positioning may be awkward, particularly if the patient is unable to sit erect. It may feel as if she is sitting in a precarious position on top of the bedpan. In addition, complete emptying of the bladder may be inhibited when the patient must attempt to urinate in a more recumbent position. This incomplete bladder emptying may lead to urinary retention and other problems discussed throughout this chapter.

Measures to promote urinary elimination for patients who must use a bedpan for urination include many of the previously noted comfort measures. Privacy must be ensured and the patient placed in a comfortable, physiologic position for voiding if at all possible. Often it is helpful for the nurse to elevate the head of the patient's bed to a Fowler's position and to place a small supportive pillow or rolled towel under the small of the back. It may also be helpful to have the patient flex her knees and hips to provide as close to a normal position for voiding as possible. Warming the bedpan under running tap water just before placing it frequently helps to promote relaxation and avoid the muscle-contracting sensation of bare skin on cold metal or plastic. The nurse may find it helpful to place a small amount of talc or cornstarch on the seat of the bedpan to facilitate sliding the bedpan under the patient and removing it after voiding. It may also be a prudent measure to place extra absorbent pads under the patient and bedpan during the procedure to prevent soiling of the bed linen if the bedpan tips when being removed. For specific guidelines about assisting a patient onto and off of a bedpan, refer to that specific section in Chapter 28.

In timing or scheduling the use of the bedpan, toilet, urinal, or commode, the nurse must assess each patient as to the amount of assistance required. Some patients are capable of monitoring their own elimination needs and will request assistance as necessary. For other patients, however, this is not the case. Some patients may feel the need to urinate but have difficulty communicating that need, or have awareness of the need to urinate and be able to communicate that need, but have difficulty using the collection devices independently. Others may have difficulty controlling urinary elimination, and may need assistance in planning and implementing a regular schedule of times for urinary elimination, frequently at 2-hour intervals. No matter what the difficulty, however, it is important for the nurse to approach the patient in a calm, matter-of-fact manner and to provide appropriate comfort measures as necessary for promotion of optimal urinary elimination.

Nursing Interventions for Altered Function

The nurse can use many therapeutic nursing interventions to assist the patient with altered urinary function. External catheters, protective pants, or indwelling catheters can be used for incontinent patients if bladder training in unsuccessful.

**Selected Nursing Interventions
for Common Urinary Problems**

Urinary Retention

- Verbal prompting
- Physiologic positioning for voiding
- Running water
- Bladder credé
- Intermittent or in-and-out catheterization

Urinary Incontinence

- Bladder training
  Regulating fluid intake
  Voiding schedule
  Abdominal and perineal muscle
    strengthening
- External and indwelling catheters
- Protective pants

Bladder Training

Bladder training is the major independent nursing intervention used to treat urinary incontinence. Bladder training involves regulation of fluid intake, establishment of a regular voiding schedule, and a program of abdominal and perineal muscle-strengthening exercises.

Sufficient fluid intake is important for the success of a bladder training program. The bladder requires at least 200 mL volume to initiate the micturition reflex. A fluid intake of at least 2000 mL daily is recommended to provide sufficient hydration to allow the normal bladder stretch–contraction reflex to occur. The nurse and the patient together should decide on the daily fluid volume goal. Most fluids should be taken during daytime hours, decreasing intake of fluids as bedtime approaches. Fluids with a diuretic effect such as coffee, tea, cola, or alcohol are best avoided during bladder retraining.

Establishing and maintaining a voiding schedule is the most challenging aspect of bladder training. Several options are available, and if one is unsuccessful another may be tried.

* Traditional bladder retraining starts with scheduled voidings. The patient is asked to void at scheduled times (usually every 2 hours) and suppress the urge to void before the scheduled time. The time interval is gradually increased to every 4 hours.
* Habit retraining schedules the patient's voiding in an attempt to gradually approximate the patient's usual voiding pattern.
* Timed voiding is the continuous use of an unchanged fixed voiding schedule (usually every 2 hours).
* Prompted voiding involves the use of regular checks to see if the patient perceives the urge to void. Sometimes just the reminder or suggestion of the need to void is sufficient stimulus to initiate voiding. Prompted voiding can prevent incontinence when there is difficulty perceiving bladder fullness.

It is important that the patient and all nurses responsible for the patient's care be aware of the method of bladder retraining and the schedule. The success of bladder retraining depends on consistency over time, as the bladder is being retrained to response to normal micturition reflex. Refer to the Nursing Management Plan for an example of a bladder retraining schedule.

Muscle strengthening exercises are the third part of a bladder retraining program. Kegel exercises to strengthen the pubococcygeal muscles and exercises such as sit-ups to strengthen the abdominal muscles are helpful in promoting optimum urinary control.

External Catheters and Protective Pants

For some patients, use of urinary collection devices such as the urinal, bedpan, or commode, may not be satisfactory because of an inability to control voiding. These may be elderly patients with some form of cognitive dysfunction, unconscious patients, or others with extreme weakness. Patients who are unable to control urination will need assistance with urine collection. They will also need frequent cleansing or bathing to remove odors and to maintain clean, dry, and intact tissues in the perineal area.

Condom (Texas) Catheter. A device called an external catheter (or **condom catheter,** "Texas" catheter) is sometimes used for male patients unable to control voiding. External catheters have a much lower risk of urinary tract infection than indwelling catheters. The external catheter is comprised of a condom that is placed on the penis and attached to tubing which inserts into a closed collection bag. The collection bag may be similar to the type used for indwelling catheters or, for patients who are more mobile, it may be a bag that attaches securely to the leg. When applying or removing an external catheter, it is important to carefully follow the specific directions of the manufacturer or agency policy. For general guidelines on applying and removing an external catheter, see Procedure 37-3, "Applying a Condom Catheter." The external catheter should be removed daily to cleanse the penis and surrounding tissues, and to assess the skin for any edema or areas of excoriation. The patient's leg bag or larger urine collection bag should also be emptied at least every 8 hours, or more frequently as needed.

Protective Pants. For female patients unable to control urination, a device such as an external catheter has not been developed. As an alternative to indwelling catheterization, some female patients as well as some male patients use protective pants. Also known as incontinent briefs, protective pants are typically disposable, waterproof briefs lined with soft, absorbent material. The briefs are open at the sides with tape or Velcro closures to facilitate application for patients who are confined to bed or have difficulty moving, turning, or pulling on clothes. It is important to change the protective pants frequently to avoid odor and to prevent skin irritation from prolonged exposure to moisture. The patient should bathe daily. Each time the protective pants are changed, the perineal area should be cleansed and examined for any areas of irritation.

Urinary Catheterization

Urinary catheterization involves inserting a small tube, called a catheter, through the urethra into the bladder, to allow urine to drain out. The most frequently used method is urethral catheterization, but urine can also be removed through a suprapubic catheter. When catheters remain in place to drain urine over a period of time, they are referred to as **indwelling** (or retention) **catheters.**

PROCEDURE 37–3. Applying a Condom Catheter

■ Purpose
1. Provide a means of collecting urine and controlling incontinence without the risk of infection that an indwelling urinary catheter imposes.

■ Assessment
- Identify patients who require control of incontinence.
- Assess mental status of patient to determine ability to cooperate with procedure.
- Inspect penis for irritation or areas of skin breakdown from previous incontinence.
- Determine patient's activity level and need of leg bag or continuous drainage system for urine collection.

■ Equipment
Soap, warm water, towel.
Commercially packaged condom catheter with adhesive.
Disposable gloves.
Urine collection bag with drainage tubing or leg bag with straps.

■ Procedure
1. Close room door or bedside curtain. Explain procedure to patient.
   Rationale: Provides privacy and encourages cooperation.
2. Wash hands.
3. Assist patient to supine position with only genitalia exposed.
   Rationale: Provides patient comfort and privacy.
4. Put on disposable gloves. Wash genitals with soap and water. Towel dry.
   Rationale: Removes secretions to prevent skin breakdown. Catheter adheres best if skin is thoroughly dry.
5. Trim or shave excess pubic hair from base of penis, if necessary.
   Rationale: Excess hair adheres to the condom adhesive, interferes with a good seal, and is uncomfortable when condom is removed.
6. Apply thin film of skin protector on penis shaft (usually found in commercially packaged condom catheter kits). Allow to dry for 30 seconds.
   Rationale: Protects sensitive penile skin from irritation and provides better adherence to the adhesive liner.
7. Peel paper backing from both sides of adhesive line and wrap spirally around penis shaft.
   Rationale: Spiral wrap prevents a constricting tourniquet effect of the adhesive strip on the penis which could impede circulation.

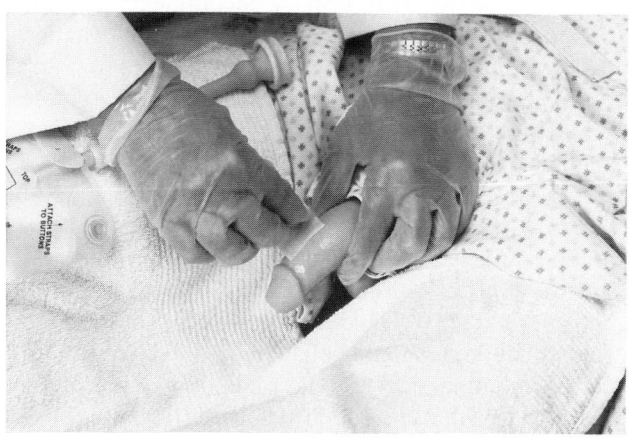

Step 6

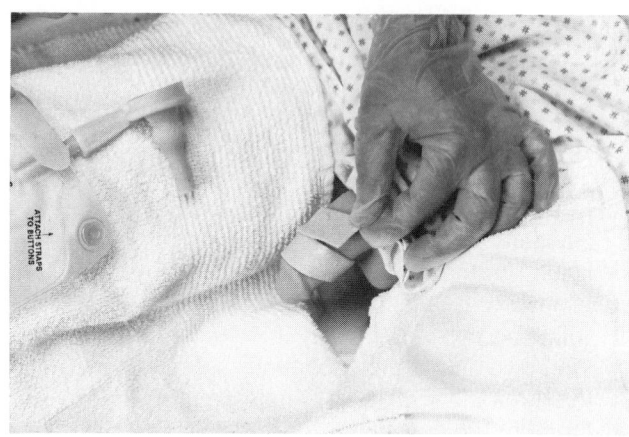

Step 7

8. Place funnel end of pre-rolled condom against glans of penis. Unroll the sheath the length of the penis, over the adhesive liner.

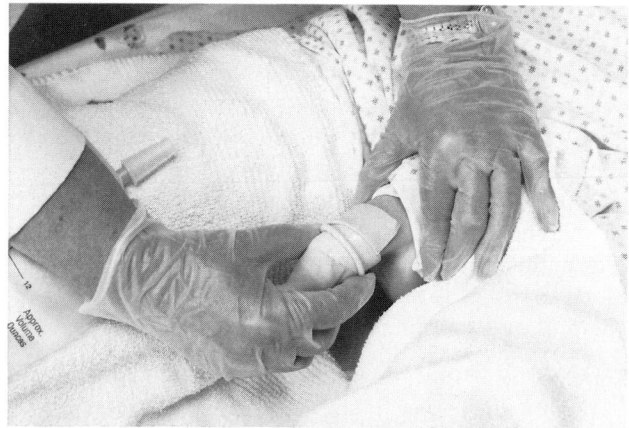

Step 8

(continued)

PROCEDURE 37–3. Applying a Condom Catheter *(continued)*

9. Attach funnel end of condom to collection system. Secure system below level of condom, avoiding kinks or loops in the tubing.
Rationale: Allows free drainage and observation of color and quantity of urine.

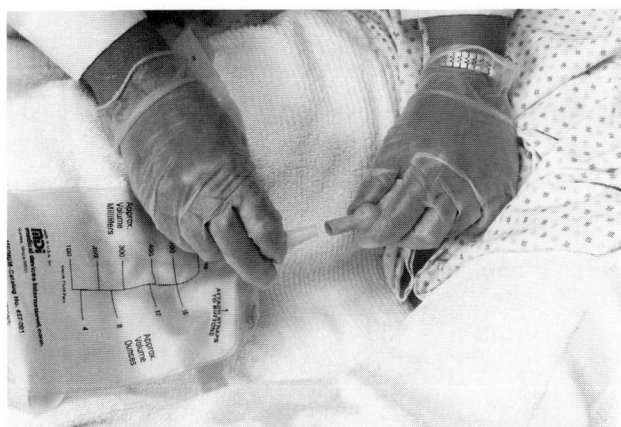

Step 9

10. Discard used supplies and wash hands.
11. Observe penis 15 to 30 minutes after application of condom, for swelling or changes in skin color.
Rationale: Swelling or discoloration of penis indicates condom is too tight and should be removed and reapplied in a larger size.
12. Document procedure and observations.

■ **Lifespan Considerations**
• Condom catheters are not indicated for use in children.

■ **Home Care Modification**
• Patients using condom catheters at home should be taught how to empty and care for their drainage collecting bag. Additionally, the patient should be taught how to attach their condom to a leg bag to allow physical activity without fear of embarrassment from urine incontinence.

When a urethral catheter is inserted temporarily to empty urine from the bladder and then removed, it is referred to as an in-and-out catheterization. If in-and-out catheterization is performed on a routine, scheduled basis for a particular patient, it is known as intermittent catheterization.

Indications for Catheterization. A urethral catheter may be inserted when the patient is experiencing difficulty with urination, such as with incontinence or urinary retention. A catheter may also be inserted when accurate assessment of urinary output is necessary, such as after trauma, burns, or surgery. Surgical patients may have a catheter in place for a few days to permit tissues to heal and edema to subside. For patients having urologic surgery, the catheter provides a means to irrigate the bladder or instill bladder medications. Catheterization may also be necessary to collect a urine specimen or to assess how much urine is left in the bladder after an person has voided.

Types of Catheters. Urinary catheters are usually made of rubber, plastic, or nylon. A straight rubber catheter with only one lumen is used for in-and-out and intermittent catheterization procedures. When an indwelling catheter is required, a double lumen known as a Foley is most commonly used (Fig. 37-7). A Foley catheter contains one lumen to remove the urine, and a second, smaller lumen to inflate a small balloon that keeps

the catheter from falling out of the bladder. The balloon is located near the insertion tip of the catheter and can be inflated and deflated with a syringe. A third type of catheter, a triple-lumen indwelling catheter, is inserted when a patient requires an indwelling catheter, not only to remove urine from the bladder, but also for the administration of medications or irrigating fluid. A triple-lumen catheter is usually used after urologic or prostatic surgery (Fig. 37-8).

Urinary catheters are available in different sizes. The selection of the proper size is important to aid in the prevention of trauma to urethral tissues. A catheter smaller than the external meatus should be used to mini-

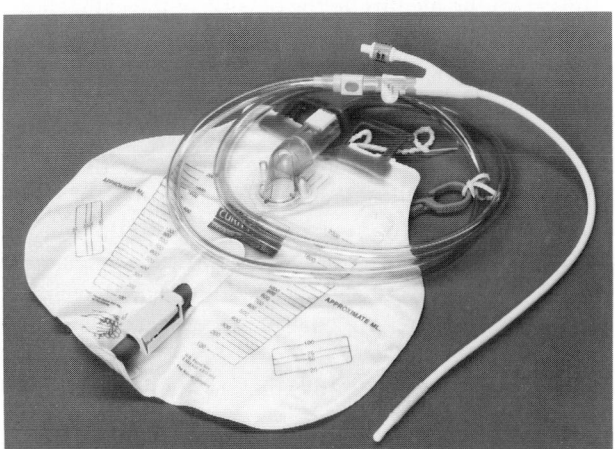

Figure 37–7. Foley catheter.

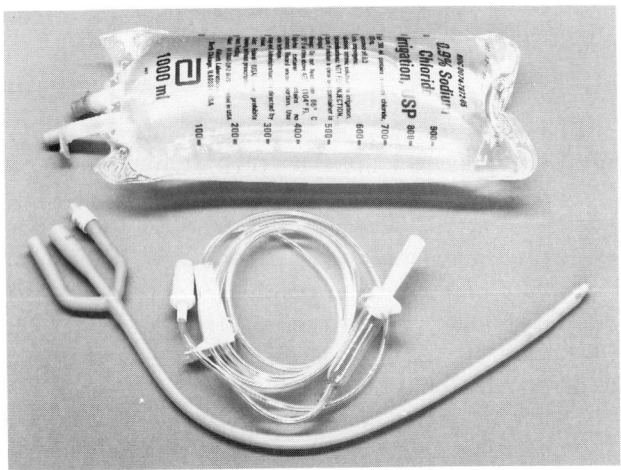

Figure 37–8.   Three-way Foley catheter.

mize trauma. Catheters are sized on the French scale of numbers, according to the diameter of the lumen. On this scale, the larger the lumen size, the larger the French number. Available adult sizes range from #14 to #22, with sizes #18 and #20 commonly used for men, and sizes #16 and #18 commonly used for women.

Catheterization. To avoid introducing microorganisms into the urinary system, which is sterile, strict aseptic technique must be employed whenever a urinary catheter is inserted. Procedure 37-4, "Inserting a Straight or Indwelling Catheter," outlines the correct technique for catheterization.

Risks of Catheterization. Any break in sterile technique during catheter insertion carries with it the risk of infection to the bladder, ureters, and, eventually, kidneys. In addition, with an indwelling catheter, the risk of infection continues and increases as long as the catheter remains in place. The indwelling catheter must be connected to a closed drainage bag to prevent the migration of microorganisms up the inside of the catheter lumen to the bladder. What still can occur, even with the use of a closed drainage system, is the migration of microorganisms from the meatus up the outside of the catheter and drainage tubing toward the bladder.

Another risk of urethral catheterization is trauma to the urethral tissues, which can also contribute to an eventual infection. Men are particularly at risk for tissue trauma because of the length and the curvature of the male urethra. Particular care must be taken to insert the catheter along the normal contour of the urethra to avoid trauma to the tissues. For men in particular, the normal curve of the urethra can be straightened somewhat by elevating the penis to a position perpendicular to the body.

A third risk of urethral catheterization, both in-and-out and indwelling, involves removing a large amount of urine from the bladder at one time. When the urinary bladder is distended with urine beyond 400 to 500 mL,

compression of the blood vessels in the bladder wall occurs. If the bladder is quickly emptied of amounts greater than 700 mL by catheterization, those blood vessels that have been compressed dilate and fill with blood. This can lead to a sudden decrease in the overall circulating blood supply, and can cause the patient to feel faint. As a response to this risk, and as a precautionary measure, if urine is still flowing after 700 mL have been removed from the bladder, the catheter is typically clamped for 30 to 60 minutes to allow the vessels in the bladder wall to accommodate. The tubing is then unclamped to complete the removal of urine. A recent study (Bristoll, 1989) with a small sample (six patients) indicated that rapid bladder decompression may not have clinically significant adverse physiologic effects. More research into this area is needed.

Care of Indwelling Catheters. Because the presence of an indwelling urethral catheter increases a patient's risk for acquiring a urinary tract infection, special care must be taken by nursing personnel to minimize that risk. The catheter, drainage collection tubing, and bag comprise a closed drainage system that preferably should not be disconnected except to change to a new closed system. The retention catheter and collection bag and tubing should be changed as frequently as necessary, as indicated by the presence of increasing sediment in the urine and along the catheter tubing (Roe, 1985). The drainage collection bag should be emptied through the outlet port at the bottom of the bag at least every 8 hours, more frequently if necessary, because pooled urine is an excellent growth medium for microorganisms.

To prevent pulling or kinking of the catheter, it should be taped securely to the body in a fashion which keeps the catheter securely in place, but with enough slack to allow movement by the patient. The catheter should be taped to the inner aspect of the thigh of the female patient or to the lower abdomen of the male patient. It is important to tape the catheter to the abdomen of the male patient rather than the leg to prevent irritation at the penile–scrotal angle. In addition, sometimes a water-soluble lubricant is applied to the meatus to decrease irritation of the urethra.

The drainage collection bag and tubing should be kept below the level of the bladder to maintain proper drainage and prevent pooling or backflow. Most collection bags have a one-way valve at the insertion of the tubing into the collection bag. The collection bag should be attached to the frame of the bed, with the tubing slack coiled and the bag attached to bed frame, not the siderail, and it should not rest on the floor. The tubing should be coiled on the bed and attached to the bed linens in such a way that there are no dependent loops. The collection bag and tubing come equipped with means to attach both the collection bag to the bed frame and the tubing to the bed linens.

(Text continues on page 1077)

PROCEDURE 37–4. Inserting a Straight or Indwelling Urinary Catheter

■ Purpose
1. Monitor urinary function, prevent or relieve bladder distention.
2. Provide continuous bladder drainage.
3. Obtain sterile urine specimens.
4. Measure residual urine.
5. Provide a means for irrigating the bladder with fluids or medication.

■ Assessment
• Reasons for patient requiring catheterization.
• Bladder distention.
• Patient's physical ability to tolerate positioning.

■ Equipment
A light source.
Prepackaged, sterile catheterization kits that generally include: the catheter (the most commonly used adult indwelling catheter is the Foley catheter, size 16 French with a 5-cc balloon), cotton balls, lubricant, disposable forceps, cleansing Betadine solution, specimen cup, gloves and drapes, and drainage bag.
Extra catheter and sterile gloves.

■ Procedure
1. Explain the procedure and rationale to patient.
2. Provide the patient with opportunity to perform personal perineal/penile hygiene. Assist patient as necessary.
   Rationale: Strict asepsis must be maintained to reduce the possibility of introducing a urinary tract infection. Initial cleansing rids body of gross contamination.
3. Wash your hands.
   Rationale: Prevents transfer of microorgamisms.

■ Procedure

Inserting Catheter for a Woman
1. Position in dorsal recumbent position (supine with knees flexed). Externally rotate thighs. Side lying is an alternative position.
2. Drap legs to midthigh with bath blanket.
   Rationale: Provides privacy and prevents chilling which aid in patient relaxation.
3. Set up light source.
   Rationale: Adequate lighting and correct positioning is crucial for clear visualization of the urinary meatus.
4. Open the catheterization tray.
5. Put on sterile gloves.

6. Slide sterile drape under female patient's buttocks. Protect gloved hands with corners of drape or ask patient to lift hips so drape can be slid under.
7. Open sterile lubricant and lubricate catheter tip. Open cleansing solution and pour over half of the sterile balls. Open the sterile specimen container. Inflate balloon with pre-filled syringe to check for defective balloon. Aspirate fluid back into syringe and leave attached.
   Rationale: Attention to preparation of tray decreases chances of contaminating sterile hands or equipment before procedure is completed.
8. Place nondominant hand on labia minora and gently spread to expose urinary meatus. Visualize exact location of meatus. During cleansing and catheter insertion, do not allow labia to close over meatus until after the catheter is inserted. (This hand is now considered contaminated.)
   Rationale: If labia closes over the meatus before catheter insertion, the meatus is considered contaminated and must be recleansed.
9. Using sterile hand, pick up antiseptic solution saturated cotton ball with sterile forceps.

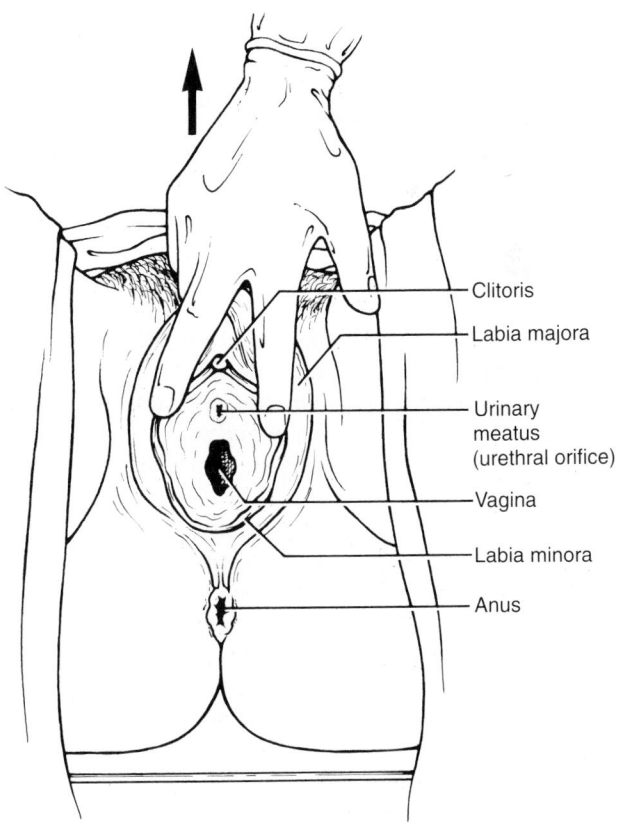

Clitoris
Labia majora
Urinary meatus (urethral orifice)
Vagina
Labia minora
Anus

Step 8

(continued)

PROCEDURE 37–4. Inserting a Straight or Indwelling Urinary Catheter (continued)

10. Cleanse the urinary meatus with one downward stroke. Discard the cotton ball. Repeat this step three to four times.
    Rationale: Cleansing from front to back avoids introducing microorganisms from the rectum to the urinary meatus.

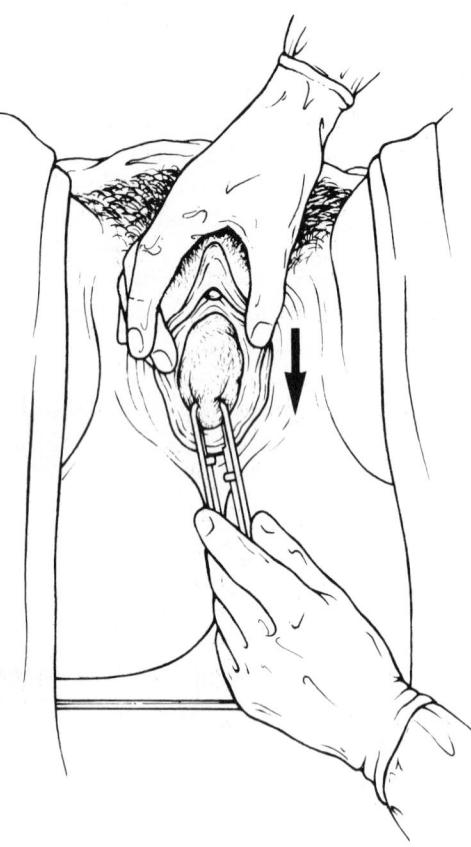

Step 10

11. Use forceps and two dry cotton balls to dry the meatus.
    Rationale: Drying the meatus decreases the slipperiness of the tissues, aids visualization of the meatus, and prevents introducing the cleansing solution into the meatus.
12. With sterile hand, pick up the catheter approximately three inches from the tip and dip into sterile lubricant. Place distal catheter end into sterile basin.
    Rationale: Lubricant facilitates catheter insertion and reduces urethral trauma.
13. Gently insert catheter into urethra (approximately 2 inches) until urine begins to drain.
14. Insert the catheter an additional 1 inch or 2.5 cm. If the catheter enters the vagina by mistake, leave it there as a landmark. Insert a second catheter into the meatus.
15. Obtain urine specimen in sterile container, if ordered.

16. If using a straight catheter: allow bladder to empty, then remove the straight catheter.
17. If using an indwelling catheter: inflate the retention balloon with the prefilled syringe.

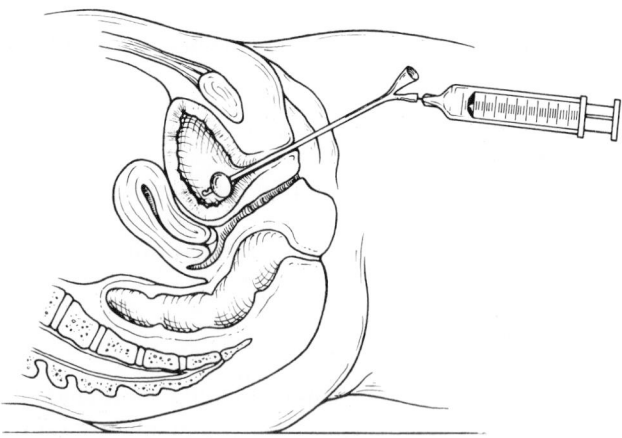

Step 17

18. Check to assure placement by gently pulling on catheter.
19. Connect distal end of catheter to drainage bag.
20. Tape the catheter securely with 1-inch tape to inner thigh with enough give so it will not pull when moving the legs.

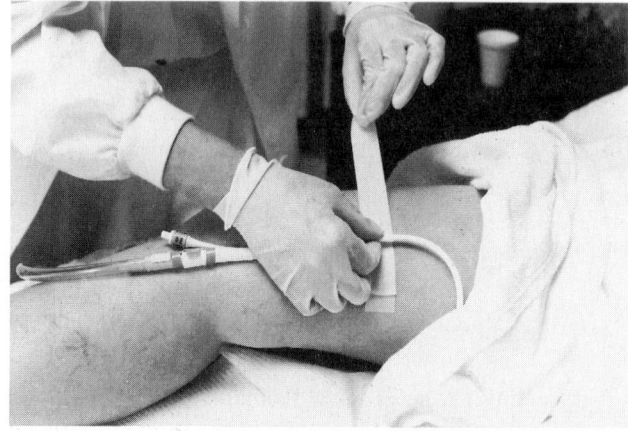

Step 20

21. Attach drainage bag to bed frame, assuring that tubing does not fall into dependent loops or that siderails do not interfere with drainage system.
    Rationale: Dependent loops fill with urine and can prevent free drainage of urine.
22. Remove gloves and wash hands.
23. Record the time procedure was complete, size of catheter inserted, amount and color of urine and any adverse patient responses.

(continued)

PROCEDURE 37–4. Inserting a Straight or Indwelling Urinary Catheter (continued)

■ **Procedure**

Inserting Catheter for a Man

1. Position in supine position.
2. Drape legs to midthigh with bath blanket.
   Rationale: Provides privacy and prevents chilling, which aid in patient relaxation.
3. Open the catheterization tray.
4. Put on sterile gloves. Open sterile lubricant and lubricate catheter liberally. Open cleansing solution and pour over half of the sterile balls. Open the sterile specimen container. Inflate balloon with pre-filled syringe to check for defective balloon. Aspirate fluid back into syringe and leave attached.
   Rationale: Attention to preparation of tray decreases chance of contaminating sterile hands or equipment before procedure is completed.
5. Place the fenestrated drape over the patient's genitalia.
6. With your nondominant hand, hold the penis at a 90-degree angle to his body. If the patient is not circumcised, pull down the foreskin with this hand to visualize the urethral meatus. (This hand is now considered unsterile.)
   Rationale: Holding the penis at a 90-degree angle is important to straighten the urethra and allow for nontraumatic catheter insertion.
7. Using the sterile hand, pick up antiseptic solution-soaked cotton ball with sterile forceps.
8. Cleanse the urinary meatus with one downward stroke or use a circular motion from meatus to base of penis. Discard the cotton ball. Repeat this step at least three to four times.
   Rationale: Same as for female patient.
9. Use forceps to pick up one dry cotton ball to dry the meatus.
10. With sterile hand, pick up the catheter approximately three inches from the tip and dip into sterile lubricant. Place distal catheter end into sterile basin.
    Rationale: Lubricant facilitates catheter insertion and reduces urethral trauma.
11. Gently insert catheter into urethra (approximately 8 inches) until urine begins to drain.
12. Insert catheter an additional 1 inch or 2.5 cm.
    Note: Penile erection may occur during catheterization as a normal physiologic result of handling the penis. This can cause embarrassment to the patient. Continue catheterizing with a fair degree of speed, using a firm but gentle touch. Distraction techniques such as conversation or asking the patient to take a deep breath may be helpful.
13. Obtain urine specimen in sterile container, if ordered.
14. If using a straight catheter: allow bladder to empty, then remove the straight catheter.

15. If using an indwelling catheter: inflate the retention balloon with the prefilled syringe.
    Rationale: To prevent urine collected in catheter from leaking onto bed after removal.

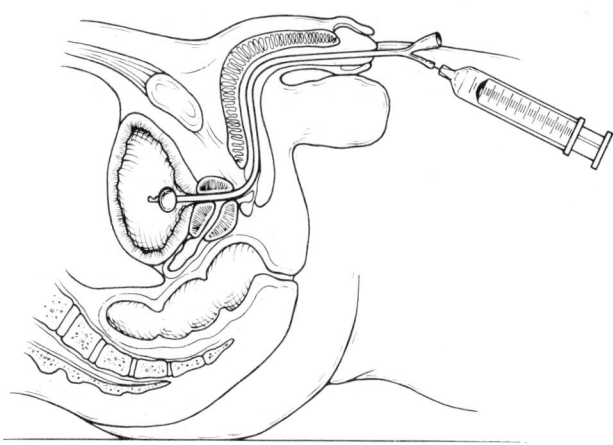

Step 15

16. Check for placement.
17. Connect distal end of catheter to drainage bag.
18. Tape the catheter securely with 1-inch tape to the abdomen to prevent trauma to the penoscrotal angle.

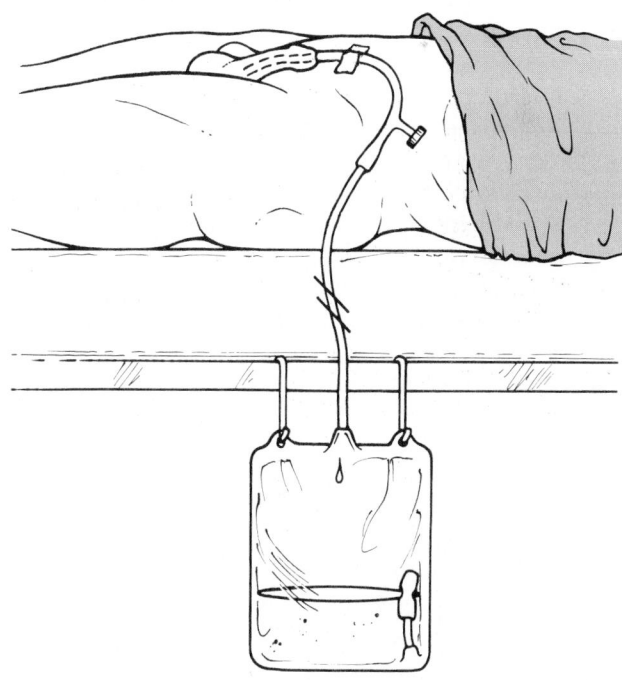

Step 18

(continued)

PROCEDURE 37–4. Inserting a Straight or Indwelling Urinary Catheter *(continued)*

19. In the uncircumcised male, gently replace the foreskin over the glans.
    Rationale: Taping technique prevents trauma to the penile–scrotal angle. If the foreskin is left retracted, it can cause constricting edema and impair circulation to the penis.
20. Attach drainage bag to bed frame, coiling tubing to ensure that tubing does not fall into dependent loops.
21. Wash hands.
22. Record the time procedure was complete, size of catheter, amount and color of urine, and any adverse patient responses.

■ **Procedure**

Removing an Indwelling Catheter

1. Wash your hands.
2. Don clean, disposable gloves.
   Rationale: To prevent transfer of microorganisms from patient's urine to the nurse.
3. Clamp the catheter (optional).
   Rationale: To prevent urine collected in catheter from leaking onto bed after removal.
4. Insert hub of syringe into balloon inflation tube of catheter and draw out all liquid. Size of balloon is indicated on catheter, most commonly less than 10 cc are used. Larger balloons (25 cc) may be used after prostatic or urologic surgery.
   Rationale: The balloon must be completely deflated to prevent trauma to the urethra as catheter is removed.
5. Ask patient to breathe in and out deeply. Gently remove catheter as patient exhales.
   Rationale: Provides distraction and exhalation prevents tightening of abdominal and perineal muscles as catheter is withdrawn.
6. Assist patient to cleanse and dry genitals.
7. Measure and document urine in drainage bag and time of catheter removal.
8. Wash hands.

■ **Safety Alert**

• Strict adherence to sterile technique is necessary to prevent introduction of microorganisms into the urinary tract.
• Trauma and pain are minimized by pre-procedure patient teaching to gain cooperation, adequate lighting for visualization of the urethral meatus, and selection of the proper size catheter. Distraction techniques are useful during insertion to reduce catheter resistance by relaxing the bladder sphincter.
• If catheterizing a distended bladder, clamp the catheter after 700 mL of urine have drained. Wait 30–60

minutes before completing decompression. Removing all of the urine may cause a shift in intra-abdominal pressure and sufficient shift of blood from central circulation to the abdominal vessels that the patient becomes dizzy.

■ **Lifespan Considerations**

Children

• Catheterization can be a frightening painful procedure for a small child. It should be completed in the treatment room so the child's bed remains a "safe" area.
• An assistant may be necessary to help the child remain still during the procedure.
• Locating the urethral meatus on young girls takes extra care since the vaginal opening is more anterior than in grown women.
• A variety of sizes of catheters are available for use in children.

The Older Woman

• The labia of women atrophy after menopause. The skin folds can feel loose and slippery when cleansing prior to insertion.
• Arthritis and other age-related musculoskeletal conditions may make it difficult for the older woman to maintain position for insertion without an assistant.

The Older Man

• The prostate gland often hypertrophies with aging, pressing in at the urethral–bladder junction. Always catheterize gently; if resistance is met, change the angle of the penis and advance catheter again. If resistance continues, stop the procedure and notify the patient's physician.

■ **Home Care Modifications**

• Patients may return home with an indwelling catheter. Home health nurse follow-up is recommended.

Infection

• Instruct patients in signs/symptoms of urinary tract infection, and directions for who to notify. Symptoms include fever, chills, cloudy, foul-smelling urine, and possible burning sensation around the catheter.
• Patients should wash their hands before and after touching any part of their urinary drainage system.
• It is mandatory that thorough cleansing of the urinary meatus and catheter be done with warm water and soap at least twice a day. The uncircumcised male should retract the foreskin and cleanse the entire glans well.

(continued)

PROCEDURE 37–4. Inserting a Straight or Indwelling Urinary Catheter *(continued)*

- To help prevent infection with long-term catheter use, 1 g ascorbic acid per day may be ordered to acidify the urine. Cranberry juice is also recommended to lower urine pH, but six to eight glasses per day are necessary to accomplish this.

Urinary Drainage Bags
- Small bags that attach to the leg are available to increase independence in the ambulating patient.

- Bed-hanging, larger-volume collection bags are used at night.
- Check and follow home agency guidelines for changing the catheter and collecting tubing and drainage bags.

The perineal area and the catheter should be cleansed at least twice daily to remove normal secretions and to help prevent infection. Because specific directions for catheter care vary among agencies, it is important to check agency policy. Most agencies suggest the use of soap and water for cleansing, but some recommend the use of povidone–iodine for cleansing, followed by the application of iodophor ointment to the meatus. In either case, the perineal area is cleansed thoroughly, the meatus washed carefully, and the area rinsed and dried thoroughly. To avoid bringing organisms from the rectum forward toward the meatus, it is important to cleanse the perineal area from front to back in the woman. During catheter care, the patient is assessed for any complaints of perineal irritation or burning, and the area is inspected for redness or excoriation. The color of urine in the tubing and the presence or absence of mucus is noted.

When caring for the patient with an indwelling catheter, it is important for the nurse to monitor intake and output and encourage adequate oral intake. Foods such as meats, eggs, whole grain breads, cranberries, prunes, and plums should be encouraged, since they tend to produce acid urine. An acidic urine environment may inhibit the growth of certain microorganisms and decrease the incidence of infection.

Urinary Catheter Irrigation. The purpose of catheter irrigation is to cleanse the lumen of the catheter tubing to promote patency of the tube. The purposes of irrigation of the urinary bladder include the instillation of solution to help remove mucus, blood clots, or other tissue in the bladder (particularly after genitourinary surgery), and the application of medication to the bladder wall. A physician's order is required before either procedure is performed. In addition, the physician will prescribe the type and amount of solution to be administered and either the closed or open method of irrigation.

The closed method of irrigation is performed without disrupting the closed drainage system using a triple-lumen indwelling urethral catheter (Fig. 37-9). One lumen is used to inflate the balloon of the catheter to keep it securely inside the bladder, one lumen is used for the removal of urine into a closed drainage system, and the third lumen is connected to a container of sterile irrigating solution. The specified type and amount of irrigating solution is administered via a continuous drip at a rate prescribed by the physician or by written protocol. The catheter lumen used for the removal of urine can be clamped until the prescribed solution has been instilled, and then opened to allow drainage, or it can be left open

---

Safety Alert

- Avoid applying a condom catheter too tightly because this can interfere with blood flow to the distal end of the penis. Remove condom catheters daily to inspect penile skin for signs of decreased circulation or skin breakdown.
- Maintain strict asepsis during urethral catheter insertion or irrigation to decrease the incidence of urinary tract infection.
- Attach urinary drainage bags to bed *frames* and never to bedrails to prevent accidental pulling and extreme tension on the tubing when the siderails are raised up and down. This can result in mucosal damage.
- Frequently monitor patients receiving continuous bladder irrigation. Empty the urinary drainage bag when approximatley 1000 cc full; a bulging bag of urine can cause a back pressure, preventing proper outflow of urine, which can cause urinary retention and unrelieved bladder distention.
- Securely tape and take care not to kink tubing under the patient when repositioning in bed. Catheter or drianage bag tubing that is kinked or flattened when the patient lies on it can prevent proper outflow of urine and lead to urinary retention.

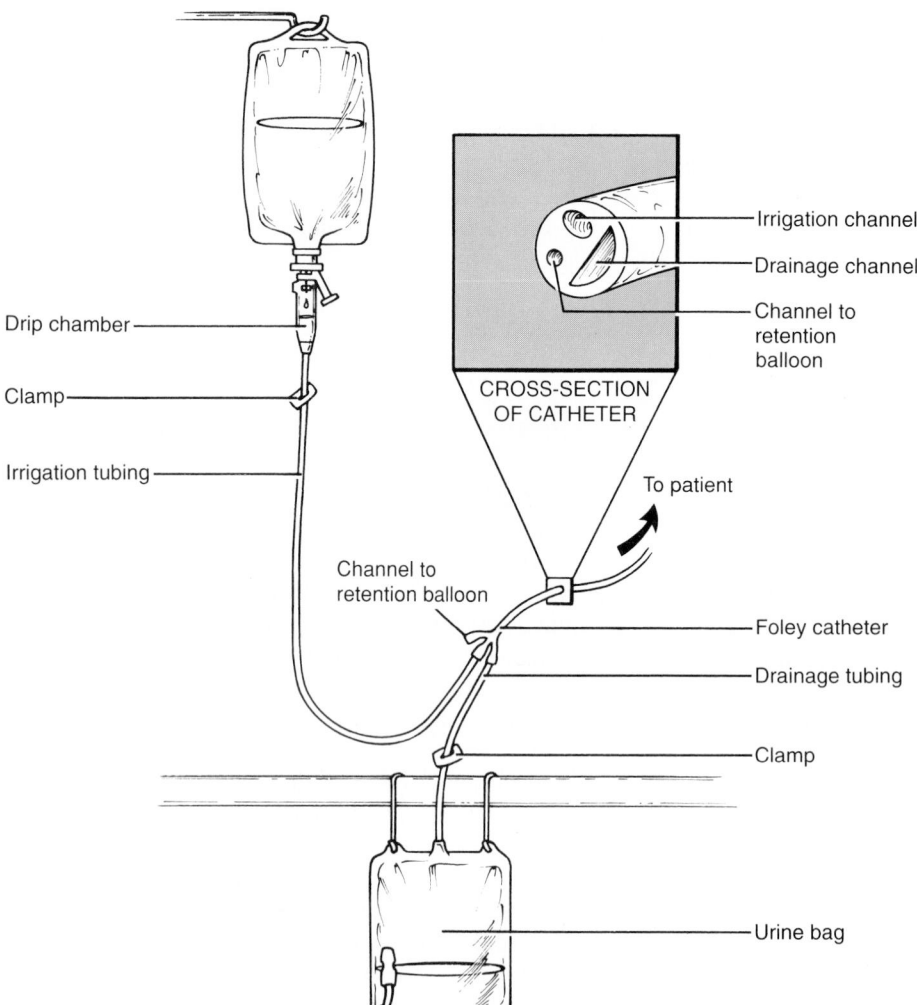

Drip chamber

Clamp

Irrigation tubing

Channel to
retention balloon

CROSS-SECTION
OF CATHETER

Irrigation channel

Drainage channel

Channel to
retention
balloon

To patient

Foley catheter

Drainage tubing

Clamp

Urine bag

Figure 37–9. Closed irrigation system showing the triple-lumen catheter tubing.

to allow outflow of urine throughout the procedure (Fig. 37-10). Throughout the closed method of irrigation, the catheter and drainage tube remain connected to decrease the risk of entry of microorganisms into the system, which could cause an infection. See Procedure 37-5 for a description of continuous bladder irrigation.

The open method of irrigation, which is associated with an increased risk of urinary tract infection, is performed with the double-lumen indwelling urethral catheter. After cleansing the junction between the urethral catheter and the drainage tubing, and using sterile technique, the catheter and the drainage tubing are disconnected. Using a sterile syringe, usually an asepto syringe, the prescribed type and quantity of solution is administered slowly, either by gravity or gentle pressure, into the catheter tubing. The irrigating solution is then allowed to drain by gravity from the catheter. This procedure may be repeated depending on the amount of solution to be instilled and the physician's order. After completion of the irrigation, the catheter and drainage tubing are connected again. Care must be taken throughout the procedure to maintain sterile technique

because of the increased risk of urinary tract infection associated with this procedure.

With both the closed and open methods of catheter and bladder irrigation, it is important to assess the response by the patient to the procedure. Any complaints of pain or discomfort should be noted, as well as the quantity, color, and characteristics of the fluid draining out of the bladder. In addition, note whether the amounts of solution entering the bladder and flowing from it seem to be in appropriate proportions. In most circumstances, the irrigation procedure is painless.

Removal of Indwelling Catheter. The removal of the indwelling urethral catheter is a simple procedure using medically aseptic technique. Care must be taken to avoid trauma to the urethra and discomfort for the patient. In addition, the patient must be informed about what many patients frequently experience after catheter removal. After assembling the necessary equipment (an absorbent pad, disposable gloves, a 10- or 25-mL syringe depending on the size of the catheter balloon, and paper towels and linen for perineal care), explain the pro-

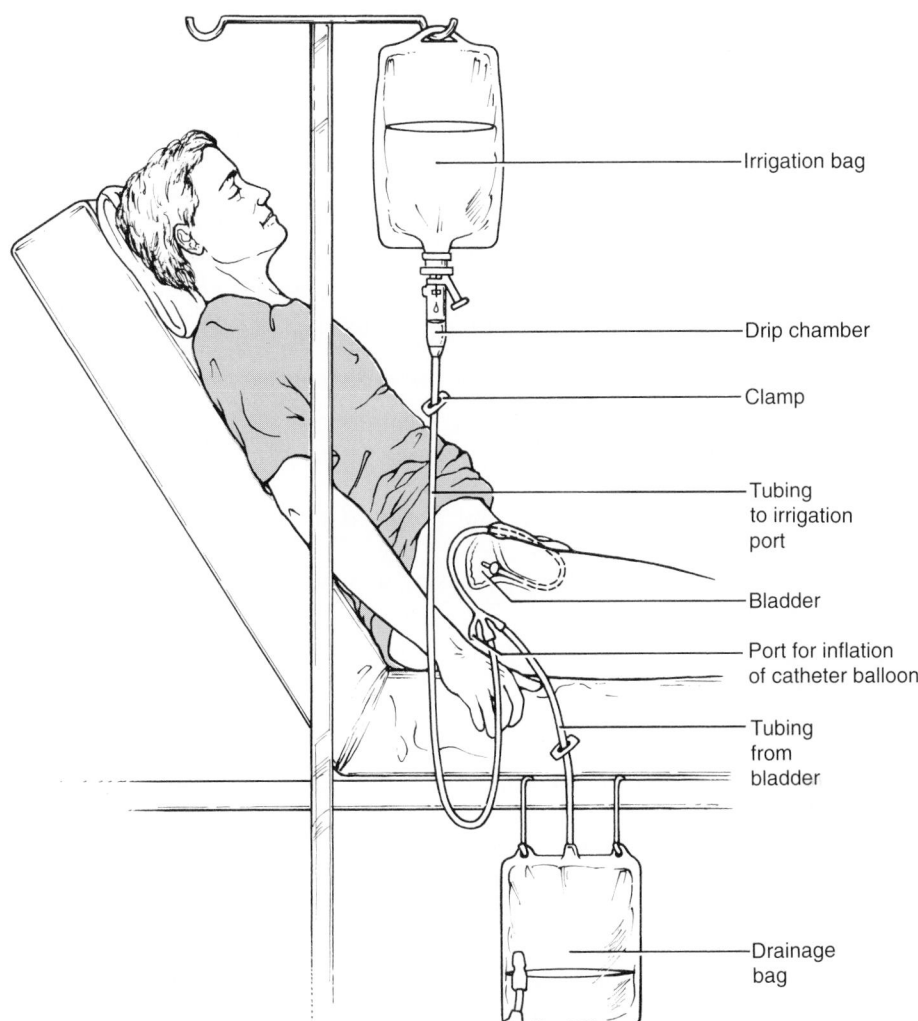

- Irrigation bag
- Drip chamber
- Clamp
- Tubing to irrigation port
- Bladder
- Port for inflation of catheter balloon
- Tubing from bladder
- Drainage bag

Figure 37–10.   Irrigating an indwelling catheter using continuous irrigation.

cedure and position the patient to allow visualization of the perineum. Remove the tape that has secured the catheter tubing to the patient's body. Put on gloves. Insert the syringe into the entry port of the lumen of the catheter that was used to fill the balloon, and then aspirate all fluid from the balloon. Avoid using scissors to cut this portion of the tubing and remove the fluid, as this prevents an accurate assessment of whether or not the balloon is completely empty. If the tubing is obstructed and it has been cut with scissors, aspiration of remaining fluid is difficult, and trauma to the urethra may occur.

After aspirating the fluid from the balloon, instruct the patient to inhale deeply, and then remove the catheter slowly and carefully. As the catheter is removed, pinch the tubing to prevent dribbling of urine onto the patient's bed linens, and then allow the urine to drain into the collection bag. Wrap the catheter in paper towels, then measure and record the amount of urine remaining in the collection bag at the time of catheter removal.

After removing the catheter, assess the perineum and meatus for any signs of redness or irritation, and then

provide perineal care. Inform the patient that it is not uncommon to experience some amount of dribbling of urine after catheter removal, particularly if the catheter has been in place for several days. The patient should be encouraged to drink plenty of liquids to distend the bladder, and should expect to void within the next 6 to 8 hours. The nurse must continue to assess the patient's intake and output, note the time of catheter removal, and also the time 8 hours later when the patient is due to void. If the patient has difficulty reestablishing voluntary control of urination the physician should be notified, because it may become necessary to insert an in-and-out catheter to remove retained or **residual urine.**

Suprapubic Catheter. A suprapubic catheter (Fig. 37-11), designed exclusively for suprapubic catheterization, is a narrow-lumen tube with a curl at the distal end that helps keep the catheter from being expelled by the bladder. It is inserted by the physician into the patient's urinary bladder from an abdominal entry point just above the symphysis pubis. Suprapubic catheterization can be performed with the patient in his or her hospital

---

■ Purpose

1. Maintain patency of the urethral catheter by removing blood clots and cellular debris.
2. Instill medications into the bladder.

■ Assessment

- Review chart for physician's order for type of solution and irrigation rate.
- Determine purpose of irrigation.
- Assess type of catheter already present. Continuous bladder irrigation requires use of a three-way retention catheter.
- Assess urine for amount, color, and presence of mucus, sediment, or blood clots.
- Assess patient for bladder distention, spasms, or pain.

■ Equipment

Sterile irrigating solution.
Infusion tubing.
IV pole.
Three-way retention catheter—present in patient's bladder.
Sterile drainage bag and tubing.
Clean, disposable gloves.

■ Procedure

1. Close room door or pull curtains around bed, and drape patient with bath blanket.
   Rationale: Provides for privacy.
2. Explain procedure to patient.
   Rationale: Reduces anxiety and increases cooperation.
3. Don disposable clean gloves. Empty and record amount of urine in drainage bag. Dispose of soiled gloves.
   Rationale: Provides for accuracy of intake and output records before and during bladder irrigation.
4. Wash your hands.
   Rationale: Reduces transmission of microorganisms.
5. Connect sterile tubing to irrigation solution using aseptic technique. Hang solution container on IV pole.
6. Flush fluid through tubing, maintaining sterility of the distal end. Close the flow clamp.
   Rationale: Expels air from the tubing.
7. Connect input port of the three-way catheter to the irrigating tubing. The other port is connected to the drainage tubing.
8. Open the flow clamp on the irrigation tubing and adjust the drip as ordered.
   Note: If a flow rate is not specified, adjust the rate to keep the urine clear of mucus and blood clots (about 40 to 60 drops/minute).
   Rationale: Maintains patency of the catheter.
9. Tape the catheter securely with 1-inch tape (for woman to inner thigh, for man to the abdomen).
   Rationale: Prevents trauma to urethra.
10. Assist patient to comfortable position.
11. Inspect the drainage for color, clarity, and amount.
12. Wash hands and document procedure and observations.
13. Measure and record intake and output every two hours or per agency protocol.
    Note: The drainage includes both irrigation solution and urine. Actual urine output is calculated by subtracting the amount of irrigation infused from the amount of drainage obtained.

---

bed under local anesthesia, or it can be performed in the operating room with the patient under generalized anesthesia and in conjunction with bladder or vaginal surgery.

In addition to the curl at the distal end of the tubing, which helps to keep the catheter from being expelled, suprapubic catheters are also kept in place by sutures at the abdominal entry point or by a form of body retention seal, which is a part of each catheter. The catheter tubing is then connected to a closed urinary drainage system. When the suprapubic catheter is to be removed, the sutures and/or body retention seal are removed and, as the catheter is guided out of the bladder, the bladder muscles contract over the entry site and seal off the opening made into the bladder. The abdominal entry point is then cleansed and a sterile dressing applied according to agency policy.

Advantages of suprapubic catheterization include association with a lower rate of urinary tract infection than with urethral catheterization, and potential increased comfort for the patient. In addition, when a patient has a suprapubic catheter, it can be easier to evaluate bladder emptying and residual urine. The catheter is first clamped, and the patient voids normally. After voiding, the catheter is then unclamped and the amount of residual urine assessed. This avoids the need for catheterization to assess residual urine volumes after the indwelling catheter is removed.

Complications that can occur with suprapubic catheters include obstruction of urine flow from the bladder due to accumulation of sediment or clots, or the bladder wall closing over the catheter tip. The small lumen size of the suprapubic catheter also increases the incidence of tube kinking and obstruction. The catheter can become

Patient Teaching

Instruct the patient as follows:

- Female patients, wipe the perineum in a front-to-back motion, to prevent the introduction of microorganisms from the anal area into the urinary meatus, which can cause urinary tract infection.
- If you experience incontinence, restrict your intake of coffee, tea, or alcohol, because of the diuretic effect of these liquids, which may result in unpredictable voiding.
- Keep urinary drainage bags below the level of the bladder so gravity can assist the outflow of urine from the bladder. A drainage bag elevated above the bladder risks urine backflow into the bladder, which increases potential urinary tract infection.
- Increase oral fluid intake to promote sufficient urine flow and prevent urinary stasis and infection.
- If you have just had a catheter removed, dribbling small amounts of urine for a short time is not uncommon.
- If urinary dribbling persists beyond 24 hours, increase oral fluid intake and use perineal strengthening exercises.

dislodged or trauma to the bladder wall can occur during catheterization. Nursing assessment of a patient with a suprapubic catheter includes frequent observations of the patient's urine as to its color, clarity, and quantity. In addition, the nurse must assess the patient's fluid intake, temperature status, level of comfort, and condition of the abdominal insertion site.

Bladder Credé

Bladder credé involves manually compressing the walls of the bladder with the hands. This technique is helpful in promoting complete bladder emptying, especially in patients who have neurologic impairment that contributes to urinary retention. Hands are placed on the abdomen below the umbilicus and above the symphysis pubis, with the fingers pointed down toward the bladder. As the hands are pressed into the bladder, the patient tightens the perineal muscles and performs the Valsalva maneuver (holds breath while bearing down).

Urinary Diversion

Although specific nursing care must be individualized according to the specific urinary diversion performed, there are many principles guiding general care of the urinary diversion. Accurate assessment of fluid intake and output, color of the urine, and the presence of sediment or blood clots is important. The stoma should also be carefully inspected for color and skin integrity around the stoma.

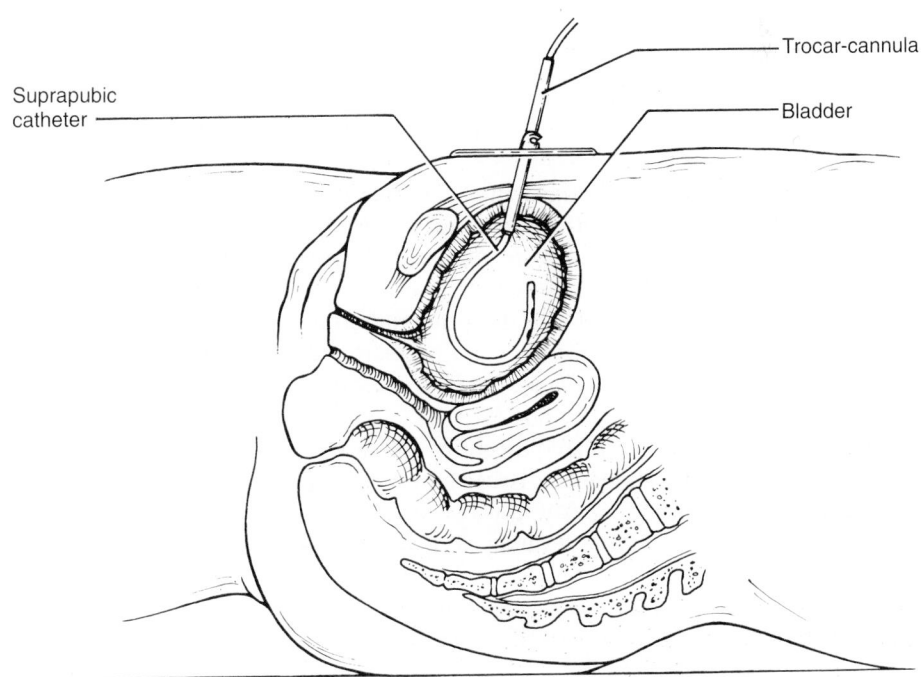

Figure 37–11. Suprapubic catheter.

During the postoperative period after a urinary diversion, special considerations are necessary. Sometimes the physician has placed special splinting catheters, called stents, inside the ureters to keep them patent and maintain urine flow during the initial postoperative period. The stents protrude out of the stoma and urine should flow out of both stents and also from the stoma. The stents are usually removed after 5 to 10 days. The nurse should assess the stents and make sure they are not accidentally dislodged.

Frequently a referral is made to an enterostomal therapist, a nurse who is a specialist in the care of patients with urinary or bowel diversions. Often the enterostomal therapist assesses the patient preoperatively, marking the recommended stoma site on the patient's abdomen. Postoperatively the enterostomal therapist fits the patient's stoma with the appropriate appliance, provides wound care to the stoma site, and begins to teach the patient about stoma care. If the patient has a continent urinary diversion, instruction in self-catheterization are also needed.

The nurse also offers emotional support to both the patient and family members. Often a urinary diversion has been performed because of serious medical problems with which the patient and family may need assistance understanding and accepting. Urinary diversion may alter body image or impair self-esteem. Learning independent management of the stoma takes time and practice. Teaching sessions should be individualized for each patient and include family or significant others when appropriate.

Renal Dialysis

Renal dialysis involves using a semipermeable membrane to remove fluid, electrolytes, and other waste products from the body that are normally removed by healthy kidneys. It is used in instances of renal failure to allow the kidneys time to heal and help prevent further complications of the disease process. In instances of irreversible renal failure, dialysis is necessary to sustain life. Dialysis may be preformed as a temporary or permanent measure, depending on the renal impairment. Hemodialysis and peritoneal dialysis are two types of renal dialysis.

Peritoneal Dialysis. When waste products, electrolytes, and excessive fluid are removed from the body using the peritoneum as diffusing membrane, it is referred to as peritoneal dialysis. A solution called dialy-

---

Nursing Research

Selected Nursing Research Studies

Bristoll, S. L., Fadden, T., Fehring, R. J., Rohde, L., Smith, P. K., & Wohlitz, B. A. (1989). The mythical danger of rapid urinary drainage. *American Journal of Nursing, 89,* 344–345.

Creason, W., et al. (1989). Prompted voiding therapy for urinary incontinence in aged female nursing home residents. *Journal of Advanced Nursing, 14,* 120–126.

Handerson, J. (1989). Intermittent clean self catheterization in clients with neurogenic bladder resulting from multiple sclerosis. *Journal of Neuroscience Nursing, 21,* 160–164.

Newman, E., & Price, M. (1985). External catheters: Hazards and benefits of their use by men with spinal cord lesions. *Archives of Physical Medicine and Rehabilitation, 66,* 310–312.

Ramphal, J. (1987). Urinary incontinence among nursing home patients: Issues in research. *Geriatric Nursing, 8,* 249–254.

Sadowski, A., et al. (1988). A survey of clean indwelling catheters in long term care. *Urologic Nursing, 9*(1), 15–17.

Possible Topics for Nursing Inquiry

- How often should long-term indwelling catheters be changed?
- What are the major predictors for gerontologic incontinence?
- Does complete urinary drainage of amounts in excess of 1000 mL adversely affect blood pressure and heart rate?
- How accurate is noninvasive ultrasonic equipment in measuring residual urine volume?
- For which population group is bladder credé effective to enhance complete bladder emptying?
- How frequently is perineal care performed for patients having indwelling catheters? Does the frequency of perineal care impact the incidence of UTIs for patients with indwelling catheters?
- Does the use of a leg bag drainage system increase the incidence of infection for patients with indwelling catheters?

sate is infused into the peritoneal cavity by means of a catheter. The dialysate contains water, glucose, and normal serum electrolytes. As dialysate is instilled, waste products from the blood diffuse across the semipermeable peritoneal membrane into the dialysate solution. In this way, diffusion filters from the blood high levels of electrolytes, fluid, and waste products. Because the dialysate contains glucose in higher concentration than the blood, excess fluid is drawn from the blood by the process of osmosis. Blood remains free of toxins and excessive fluid for a period of time, until once again dialysis is necessary to return the body to homeostasis.

The nurse observes and records the amount and color of the dialysate that is returned. Typically dialysate drainage is initially bloody, but should quickly clear to become straw-colored. Vital signs are monitored frequently, as well as changes in mentation or level of comfort. Nursing interventions for the patient undergoing peritoneal dialysis include assisting with the placement of the peritoneal catheter, caring for the abdominal wound at the catheter insertion site, and administering and withdrawing the dialysate solution prescribed by the physician. Additional nursing responsibilities include assessment and implementation of any teaching the patient may need regarding the dialysis procedure.

Hemodialysis. Hemodialysis is the removal of fluid, electrolytes, and waste products from the body via access to the circulating blood. During hemodialysis, the patient's blood is pumped from an artery into the dialysis machine. Here, the blood flows through a dialyser, which serves as a semipermeable membrane, and is bathed by dialysate solution. As blood flows through the semipermeable membrane, waste products and electrolytes diffuse into the dialysate. Excess fluid is removed by a process called ultrafiltration, which provides a hydrostatic pressure gradient. After passing through the dialyzer, the blood is returned to the body through venous access.

Special catheters are used for arterial and venous access for hemodialysis and, once inserted, they can be left in place for many dialysis procedures. In between dialysis procedures, heparinized normal saline is injected into the catheter to prevent clotting. The catheter is then capped and covered with a sterile dressing. Care must be taken not to dislodge the catheter, since direct arterial access can result in extensive bleeding. Grafts connecting the venous and arterial circulation can also be performed and serve as an access route for hemodialysis. Blood pressure or any invasive techniques should always be performed on the unaffected arm.

Nursing interventions for the patient undergoing hemodialysis are similar to interventions for the peritoneal dialysis patient. Careful monitoring is essential. The patient undergoing hemodialysis is weighed before the procedure is begun and afterward to assess the quantity of fluid removed. Fluid and electrolyte status is closely monitored by measuring intake and output, serum electrolytes, lung sounds, and weight changes. Patients may report symptoms of dizziness, diaphoresis, and nausea. Adverse reactions include headache, increased blood pressure, decreased pulse rate, and marked neurologic changes.

Discharge Planning and Home Care

Whenever a patient has experienced an alteration in urinary elimination during hospitalization, the nurse needs to develop a discharge plan designed to assist the patient in home management of the problem or prevention of future problems. This plan must be implemented before the patient's discharge. The goals of discharge planning are effective patient education, and the initiation of contacts with community resources for effective follow-up care.

The focus of patient education is twofold: prevention of altered urinary elimination problems, and care of specialized equipment.

Prevention of problems in urinary elimination can be fostered by emphasizing the factors that promote urinary elimination. Specifics about maintaining adequate fluid intake, allowing sufficient time and privacy for voiding, recognizing and responding to body signals, and decreasing external stressors can be useful information. Teach patients to recognize early signs and symptoms of altered urinary elimination, and individualize the information to teach prevention and recognition of problems for which the patient is most at risk. Teach patients how any medication they must take will affect urinary elimination, and advise them of any dietary or activity restrictions.

Care of specialized equipment at home will not be necessary for all discharged patients. However, some patients will be sent home with devices to manage temporarily or permanently an alteration in urinary elimination. Patients and their families may need to be taught the correct methods to care for indwelling urethral or suprapubic catheters, how to manage urinary diversion devices, or how to perform intermittent straight catheterization. The nursing staff at many hospitals has developed standardized teaching plans using prepared audiovisual aids to assist in teaching the care of complex home-care equipment.

It is possible that patients or their families will not be able to master the care of specialized equipment or techniques during hospitalization. Therefore consideration of the need for contacts with resource people in the community for follow-up and home management care is necessary. Nurses can visit patients in their homes on a routine basis to assess progress in the management of their health care needs. These nurses can be associated with the discharging hospital, but are more likely to be associated with a city or county health agency, or with an

Nursing Management Plan
The Patient with Urge Incontinence

Nursing Diagnosis: Urge incontinence related to decreased bladder capacity secondary to urethral sphincter stretching by recent 2.5 week use of indwelling catheter postoperatively TURP as manifested by strong urinary urge with incontinence, frequency, dribbling, and nocturia.
Patient Goal: Patient will reestablish control over voiding.
Patient Outcome Criteria

- Patient remains continent for 2-hour intervals over next 48 hours.
- Patient voids 4 to 5 times a day, remaining continent through hospital stay.
- Patient verbalizes the importance of fluid intake and complies with prescribed intake.

Nursing Intervention	Scientific Rationale
1. Measure and record I&O.	1. To assess for pattern of urinary output, relationship of intake to episodes of incontinence, relative overall fluid balance, success of bladder training.
2. Percuss and palpate lower abdomen after an incontinent episode. Straight catheterize for post void residual volume (PVR), if necessary.	2. To rule out urinary retention and overflow incontinence as the primary urinary alteration.
3. Review patient regimen. Suggest use of alternative medicines if necessary. Increase fluid intake to 1500 to 2000 mL per day.	3. Some medications may adversely affect urinary elimination. Adequate hydration is necessary to cause bladder filling and trigger the normal stretch/contraction response.

4. Regulate fluid intake according to following pattern:
0700 to 1500
  Breakfast: 400 mL
  Lunch: 400 mL
  At will: *360* mL
  Total: 1160 mL
1500 to 2300
  Dinner: 400 mL
  At will: *240* ml
  Total: 640 ml
Note: No fluid intake after 2000
2300 to 0700
  If desired, after 0500 180 mL
Total 180 ml
24-hour total 1980 mL
	4. Concentration of most fluids during daytime hours will decrease nocturia.

5. Begin bladder training routine:	
5a. Assist patient, as necessary, to bathroom to void every 1.5 hours during daytime, every 4 hours at night. Decrease between-voiding intervals to 1 hour if patient is initially unable to consistently remain continent for the longer intervals. Planned voiding schedule: 0730 1300 1930 0900 1500 2100 1030 1630 allow to sleep until 0200 1200 1800 allow to sleep until 0600	5a. To allow bladder to refill between voidings and gradually retrain the normal bladder stretch/contraction response.

(continued)

Nursing Management Plan
The Patient with Urge Incontinence (continued)

Nursing Intervention	Scientific Rationale
5b. Encourage the patient to "hold" his urine if he experiences the urge to void before the next scheduled voiding time.	5b. Suppressing urge to void assists in retraining of voluntary contraction of external urethral muscles.
5c. Increase between voiding intervals by 0.5 hours after patient has successfully remained continent for 24 hours.	5c. Gradual retraining to achieve fewer voids with larger amounts, a more normal pattern.
6. Post voiding schedule in patient's room. Change prn. Include details of current voiding schedule at change of shift report.	6. To increase patient and staff compliance.

Patient Goal: Patient will maintain adequate perineal muscle control.
Patient Outcome Criteria

- Patient performs Kegel exercises five times per day during hospital stay.
- Patient states understanding of purpose of Kegel exercises after teaching session and repeats two days later.

Nursing Intervention	Scientific Rationale
1. Teach patient perineal muscle strengthening exercises and tell them to perform them 10 times every 2 to 3 hours during the day.	1. To strengthen skeletal perineal muscles and increase voluntary contraction of urethral sphincter.
2. Explain rationale for increased fluid intake, voiding schedule, and perineal exercises.	2. To decrease patient knowledge deficit and increase compliance.
3. Explain that patient now knows effective methods to prevent or control future incontinence problems.	3. Knowledge can affect behavior.

independent home health-care agency. The hospital-based nurse should be involved in the decision to make referrals to community agencies.

The home health-care nurse evaluates the patient's progress, assesses for signs and symptoms of any deteriorating condition requiring physician referral or hospitalization, and continues to provide individualized patient teaching and emotional support.

EVALUATION

Specific outcome criteria are the evaluative tools used to measure the attainment of patient goals; nursing interventions are the management tools used to achieve the goals. Examples of outcome criteria are listed below. Some criteria may be appropriate for more than one goal. It is important to identify specific outcome criteria

that will uniquely measure the attainment of the *patient's* goal.

Goal
Patient will maintain strengthened or adequate perineal muscle control.

Possible Outcome Criteria
- Patient performs Kegel exercises five times per day during hospital stay.
- Patient states understanding of purpose of Kegel exercises after teaching session and repeats 2 days later.

Goal
Patient will reestablish control over voiding.

Possible Outcome Criteria
- Patient remains continent for 2-hour intervals over next 48 hours.

- Patient voids four to five times a day, remaining continent through hospital stay.
- By discharge, patient recognizes the urge to void in time to use the toilet or commode.

Goal
Patient will demonstrate understanding of procedures necessary to promote optimal urinary function.

Possible Outcome Criteria
- Patient verbalizes understanding of nurse's instructions after teaching session.
- Patient practices proper self-catheterization technique during teaching sessions and twice in the next 48 hours.
- Patient demonstrates proper application of stoma appliance before discharge.
- Patient identifies proper care of catheter before discharge.

Key Concepts

- Normal kidneys, ureters, bladder, and urethra are important for normal urinary function.
- Filtration, reabsorption, and secretion are processes involved in urine formation.
- The voluntary process of micturition is stimulated by stretch of the detrusor muscle as the bladder fills with urine.
- Two hundred fifty to four hundred milliliters of clear, yellow, aromatic urine per void is considered normal.
- Kidneys mature and voluntary control over urinary elimination is achieved as the child approaches school age; kidney function declines in the elderly due to normal age-related changes.
- Many factors, such as fluid intake, loss of body fluid, dietary intake, body position, and psychologic state, can affect normal urinary elimination.
- Potential alterations in urinary function can be caused by obstruction, infection, hypotension, neurologic injury, decreased muscle tone, pregnancy, surgery, medications, or diversions in structures of the urinary tract.
- Manifestations of altered urinary function include dysuria, polyuria, oliguria, urgency, frequency, nocturia, hematuria, pyuria, urinary retention, urinary incontinence, and enuresis.
- Physical assessment of urinary function includes inspection of urine, and percussion and palpation of the bladder for residual urine.
- Diagnostic tests and procedures that are helpful in identifying urinary dysfunction include urine analysis, urine for culture and sensitivity, specific gravity,

BUN, creatinine, cystoscopy, and urodynamic studies.
- There are six approved NANDA nursing diagnoses that identify problems in urinary function.
- Nursing measures to promote normal urinary function include adequate fluid intake, preventing urinary tract infections, and promoting optimum perineal muscle tone.
- Nursing interventions for urinary retention include bladder credé, in-and-out catheterization, and intermittent catheterization.
- Nursing interventions for urinary incontinence include bladder training, use of external and internal catheters, and the use of protective pants.
- Discharge planning and patient teaching are important when urinary dysfunction is present.

References

Bristoll, S. L. (1989). The mythical danger of rapid urinary drainage. *American Journal of Nursing, 89,* 344–345.

Brunner, L. S., & Suddarth, D. S. (1988). *Textbook of medical–surgical nursing* (6th ed.). Philadelphhia: J. B. Lippincott.

Conti M. T., & Eutropius, L. (1987). Preventing UTI's: What works? *American Journal of Nursing, 87,* 307–309.

Cox, C. (1988). Nosocomial urinary tract infections. *Urology, 32*(3), 210–215.

Fritz, M. (1989). Noninvasive bladder volume measurement. *Urologic Nursing, 9*(1), 8–9.

Guyton, A. C. (1986). *Textbook of medical physiology* (7th ed.). Philadelphia: W. B. Saunders.

NANDA (1990). *Taxonomy I revised 1990, with official nursing diagnoses.* St. Louis, MO: North American Nursing Diagnosis Association.

National Institutes of Health. (1988). Consensus development conference statement: Urinary incontinence in adults. 7(5).

Patrick, M., Woods, S., Craven, R., et al. (1991). *Medical–surgical nursing: Pathophysiological concepts* (2nd ed.). Philadelphia: J. B. Lippincott.

Roe, B. (1985). Catheter care: An overview. *International Journal of Nursing Studies, 22*(1), 45–56.

Turner, S., & Plymat, K. (1988). As women age: Perspectives on urinary incontinence. *Rehabilitation Nursing, 13*(5).

Yu, L. C. (1987). Incontinence stress index: Measuring psychological impact. *Journal of Gerontological Nursing, 13*(7), 18–25.

Bibliography

Alterescu, V. (1986). Theoretical foundations for an approach to urinary incontinence. *Journal of Enterstomal Therapy, 13,* 105–107.

Andreoli, T. E., Carpenter, C. Plum, F. (Eds.). (1986). *Cecil's essentials of medicine.* Philadelphia; W. B. Saunders.

Bates, B. (1990). *A guide to physical examination.* Philadelphia: J. B. Lippincott.

Birdsall, C. (1986). How do you manage peritoneal dialysis? *American Journal of Nursing, 86,* 592–596.

Brogna, L., & Lakaszawski, M. L. (1986). The continent urostomy. *American Journal of Nursing, 86,* 160–163.

Carpenito, L. J. (1989). *Nursing diagnosis: Application to clinical practice.* Philadelphia: J. B. Lippincott.

Corbett, J. V. (1987). Laboratory tests and diagnostic procedures with nursing diagnoses (2nd ed.). Norwalk, CT: Appleton and Lange.

Creason, W. S., et al. (1989). Prompted voiding therapy for urinary incontinence in aged female nursing home residents. *Journal of Advanced Nursing, 14,* 120–126.

Gever, L. N. (1984). Anticholinergics and what to teach your patients about them. *Nursing 84, 14*(9), 64.

Greengold, B. A., & Ouslander, J. G. (1986). Bladder retraining. *Journal of Gerontological Nursing, 12*(6), 31–35.

Hahn, K. (1987). The many signs of renal failure. *Nursing 87, 17*(8), 34–41.

Hellerstein, S. (1987). An end to enuresis. *Emergency Medicine, 87,* 31–43.

Henderson, J. (1989). Intermittent clean self catheterization in clients with neurogenic bladder resulting from multiple sclerosis. *Journal of Neuroscience Nursing, 21*(3), 160–164.

Irrgang, S. J. (1986). Classifications of urinary incontinence. *Journal of Enterstomal Therapy, 13*(2), 62–65.

Jacobs, M., & Geels, W. (1985). *Signs and symptoms in nursing.* Philadelphia: J. B. Lippincott.

Kaschak-Newman, D., & Smith, D. (1989). Incontinence: The problem patients won't talk about. *RN, 52*(3), 42–45.

Kniep-Hardy, M., et al. (1985). Managing indwelling catheters in the home. *Geriatric Nursing, 6*(5), 280–285.

Loughlin, K. R., & Whitemore, W. F. (1987). Managing prostate disorders in middle age and beyond. *Geriatrics, 42*(7), 45–56.

Mattheson, M. K. (1990). *Pharmacotherapeutics: A nursing process approach* (2nd ed.). Philadelphia: F. A. Davis.

Maynard, F., & Glass, J. (1987). Management of the neurogenic bladder by clean intermittent catheterization: 5 year outcomes. *Paraplegia, 25,* 106–110.

Mezzanotte, E. J. (1987). A checklist for better discharge planning. *Nursing 87, 17*(10), 55.

Miller, V. G. (1986). Diabetes: Let's stop testing urine. *American Journal of Nursing, 86,* 54.

Newman, E., & Price, M. (1985). External catheters: Hazards and benefits of their use by men with spinal cord lesions. *Archives of Physical Medicine and Rehabilitation, 66,* 310–312.

Nurse's Drug Alert. (1988). Does cranberry juice help urinary infections? *12*(11), 87.

Peterson, T. (1987). Autonomic dysreflexia. *Nursing 87, 17*(8), 33.

Petrillo, M. H. (1987). The patient with a urinary stoma. *Enterostomal Therapy, 22*(2), 263–279.

Plymat, K. R., et al. (1988). In home management of urinary incontinence. *Home Health Care, 6*(4), 30–34.

Ramphal, J. (1987). Urinary incontinence among nursing home patients: Issues in research. *Geriatric Nursing, 8*(5), 249–254.

Ruge, C. A. (1987). Catheter-related UTI's: What's the best way to prevent them? *Nursing 87, 17*(12), 50–51.

Sadowski, A., et al. (1988). A survey of clean indwelling catheters in long term care. *Urologic Nursing, 9*(1), 15–17.

Shapiro, T., & Stephen, R. (1985). Enuresis: Treatment and overtreatment. *Pediatric Nursing* May/June, 203–206.

Stenwall, M. (1987). Drugs affecting the cardiovascular system—Part 4: Diuretics. *Pharmacy Syllabus, University of Washington,* Spring.

Switters, D. M. (1989). Assessing leakage from around the urethral catheter. *Urologic Nursing, 9*(3), 8–10.

Voith, A. M. (1986). A conceptual framework for nursing diagnoses: Alterations in urinary elimination. *Rehabilitation Nursing, 1*( ), 18–21.

Whippo, C. C. (1989). Bacteriuria and urinary incontinence in aged female nursing home residents. *Journal of Advanced Nursing, 14*(3), 217–225.

Whitman, S., & Kursh, E. D. (1987). Curbing incontinence. *Journal of Gerontological Nursing, 13*(4), 35–40.

Wilde, M. (1986). Living with a Foley. *American Journal of Nursing, 86,* 1121–1123.

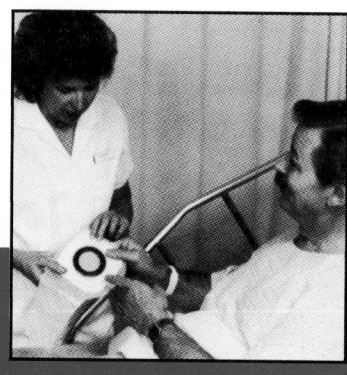

Bowel Elimination

38

Normal Bowel Function
  Anatomy of the Gastrointestinal Tract
  Normal Function of the Intestine
    Motility
    Absorption
    Mucus and Vitamin Production
    Defecation
  Characteristics of Normal Feces
  Normal Functional Bowel Pattern
  Factors Affecting Normal Bowel Elimination
  Lifespan Considerations
Altered Bowel Function
  Potential for Altered Function
    Dietary Factors
    Fluid Intake
    Ignoring the Urge to Defecate
    Fear of Pain
    Lifestyle Changes
    Immobility
    Medications
    Diagnostic Procedures
    Surgery
    Fecal Diversion
  Manifestations of Altered Bowel Function
    Constipation
    Fecal Impaction
    Diarrhea
    Fecal Incontinence
    Flatulence
    Distension
  Impact of Bowel Dysfunction on Activities of Daily
    Living
Assessment
  Subjective Data
    Functional Pattern Identification
    Risk Identification
    Dysfunctional Identification
  Objective Data

Physical Assessment
Diagnostic Tests and Procedures
Nursing Diagnoses and Patient Goals
  Diagnostic Statement: Colonic Constipation
    Definition
    Defining Characteristics
    Related Factors
  Diagnostic Statement: Perceived Constipation
    Definition
    Defining Characteristics
    Related Factors
  Diagnostic Statement: Diarrhea
    Definition
    Defining Characteristics
    Related Factors
  Diagnostic Statement: Bowel Incontinence
    Definition
    Defining Characteristics
    Related Factors
  Related Nursing Diagnoses
  Patient Goals
Implementation
  Nursing Interventions to Promote Health and
    Function
    Patient Teaching
  Nursing Interventions for Altered Bowel Function
    Laxatives
    Antidiarrheal Agents
    Antiflatulent Agents
    Enemas
    Rectal Tubes
    Nasogastric Intubation
    Fecal Impaction Removal
    Bowel Training
    Fecal Collecting Devices
    Stoma Management
  Discharge Planning and Home Care
Evaluation
Key Concepts

The elimination of waste from the bowel is an essential function of the human body. Defecation is the process by which the solid waste products of digestion are eliminated from the bowel. The waste product itself is called feces or stool.

The major nursing responsibilities associated with bowel elimination include assessing bowel function and possible risk factors that could cause bowel dysfunction in the patient; promoting normal bowel health and function; and performing nursing interventions to manage alteration in normal bowel function.

Such responsibilities span many age groups and different health settings. For example, the nurse might need to teach new parents the color and consistency of stool to expect from their newborn, or help a family cope with an elderly parent who has recently developed fecal incontinence. The nurse can work in industry to develop an education program to alert workers to the symptoms of colorectal cancer. In acute care settings the nurse is responsible for working independently and collaboratively to assess and manage bowel function. For example, the nurse may assess the return of bowel motility during the postoperative period for a patient who has had an appendectomy; individualize a bowel management program for a patient who has had a stroke; and teach a patient how to manage and adjust to a new colostomy. The nurse should have an adequate knowledge of normal bowel function, and factors that can alter normal function, to provide optimum care for all patients.

NORMAL BOWEL FUNCTION

Normal bowel function depends on many factors. Normal physiologic function of the lower gastrointestinal tract must be present. Other factors such as diet, fluid intake, lifestyle, body position, and privacy affect normal bowel function.

Anatomy of the Gastrointestinal Tract

The final formation of feces occurs in the lower portion of the gastrointestinal tract, the large intestine; however, the type and amount of food and fluids ingested at the upper end of the gastrointestinal tract have a definite effect on the amount and consistency of the waste produced (Fig. 38-1).

Food and fluids enter the mouth; the food is mixed with salivary enzymes and the process of digestion begins. The bolus of food is propelled to the pharynx, down the esophagus, and into the stomach, where secretions from the stomach further break down and digest the food.

From the stomach the food enters the small intestine, a hollow, tubelike organ comprised of smooth muscle. It is approximately 2.5 cm (1 in) wide and 6 m (20 ft) long, and has three anatomic divisions: the duodenum, the jejunum, and the ileum. It takes approximately 3 to 10 hours for the contents to leave the small intestine and enter the large intestine. The large intestine is comprised

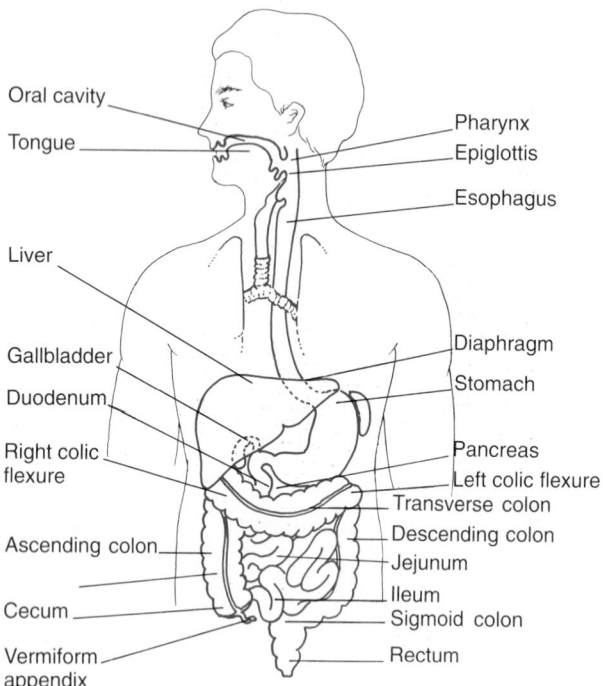

Figure 38–1. Structures of the entire length of the gastrointestinal tract: mouth to anus.

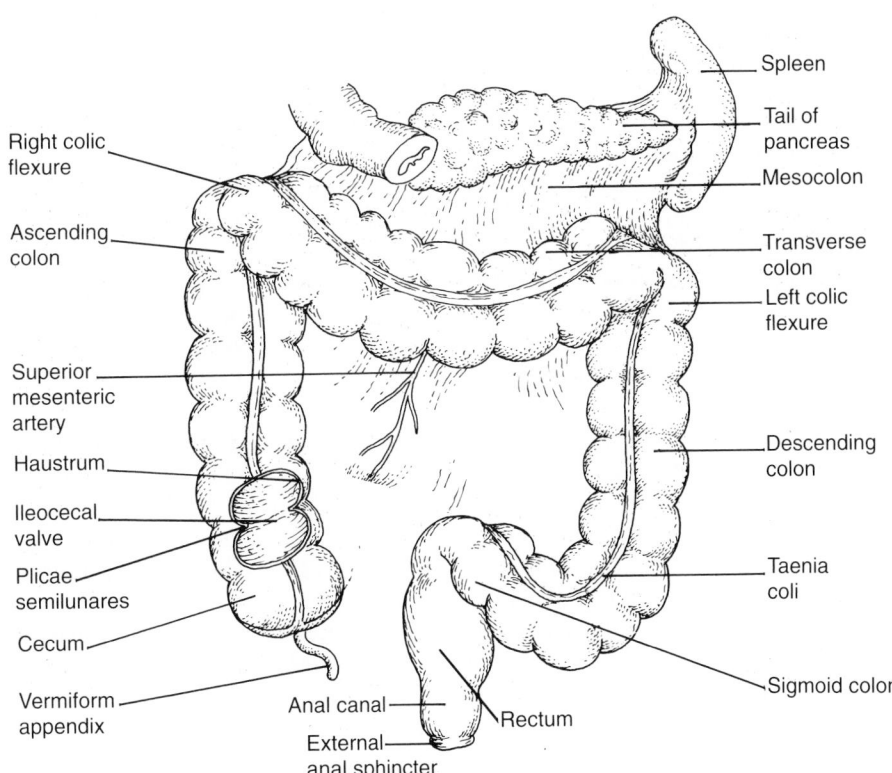

Figure 38–2. Segments of the large intestine: ascending colon, transverse colon, and sigmoid colon.

of smooth muscle and is about 6 cm (2.5 in) wide and 1.5 m (5 ft) long in the average adult. The large intestine consists of the cecum, colon, rectum, and anus. Muscle fibers within the intestine are both circular and longitudinal; this permits circumferential and lengthwise changes in size and shape, and is important in gut motility.

At the junction of the ileum and the cecum is the ileocecal valve, which serves two purposes: to slow down movement of semidigested food into the large intestine, thus allowing more time for the absorption of nutrients

to occur in the small intestine; and to prevent the backflow of fecal contents from the large intestine into the small intestine.

The colon, the major portion of the large intestine, has four parts, the ascending, transverse, descending, and sigmoid (Fig. 38-2). The rectum is the portion of the large intestine that immediately follows the sigmoid colon. The length of the rectum is about 10 to 12 cm (4 in). The rectum is normally empty, but is capable of considerable distention to accommodate stool.

The anus, the last portion of the large intestine (Fig.

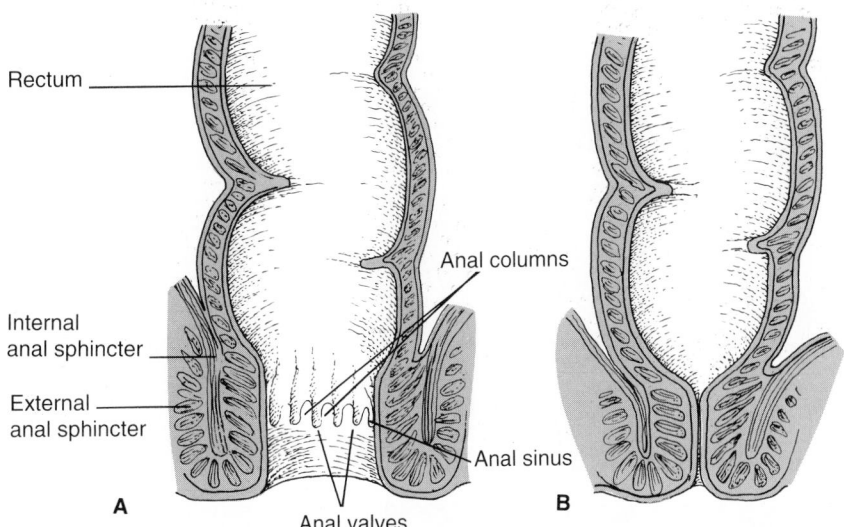

Figure 38–3. Anal sphincter. **A:** Open position. **B:** Closed position.

38-3), serves as an exit passageway for the feces. It is about 5 cm (2 in) long and has two sphincters, the internal sphincter and the external sphincter. The internal anal sphincter is smooth muscle that lies within the anus, and is under involuntary neural control. The external sphincter surrounds and extends beyond the internal sphincter and is comprised of striated muscle; it is under voluntary neural control. Both sphincters are normally in a contracted (closed) position.

Normal Function of the Intestine

The main function of the intestine is to absorb fluid and nutrients so that these can be used by the body. To facilitate the absorption and transport of solid nutrients, the intestine mechanically and chemically breaks down foodstuffs into smaller units. Muscular activity helps to propel the contents through the intestine, as well as aiding in mixing the contents with digestive enzymes. The intestines also produce mucus and certain vitamins important in body functioning. Defecation, the act of expelling waste from the body, is also a function of the intestinal tract.

Motility

Two types of movements, segmentation and peristalsis, occur within the intestine and are responsible for assisting with absorption and transportation of waste products the full length of the intestines (Fig. 38-4). During segmentation, alternating contraction and relaxation of the intestine's smooth muscle occurs. Segmentation mixes the products of digestion in the small intestine, thereby exposing partially digested food to all surface areas of the gut. This type of movement slows the passage of intestinal contents to permit more complete digestion and absorption of nutrients. Segmental contractions in the large intestine are sometimes referred to as haustral

contractions (each segment within the large intestine is a haustrum). Intestinal motility is more sluggish in the large intestine than the small intestine.

The second type of movement, **peristalsis,** assists with the propulsion of intestinal contents along the entire length of the small and large intestines. Peristalsis is reflexively induced by the walls of the intestine. An especially strong stimulus of peristalsis occurs when partially digested food enters the duodenum from the stomach; this strong contraction of colonic smooth muscle serves to propel fecal contents from the transverse colon to the sigmoid colon and the rectum. This duodenocolic reflex is especially strong when food or fluids enter the duodenum after several hours of not eating, especially about 15 minutes after breakfast (Guyton, 1987).

Nervous system input affects the rate of intestinal motility. The intestine is supplied by parasympathetic and sympathetic nerve innervation. Sympathetic stimulation slows down peristalsis and delays passage through the intestine, whereas parasympathetic stimulation increases gut motility and emptying.

Absorption

Partially digested food (also known as chyme) is emptied from the stomach into the small intestine. It is in the small intestine that the digestion process is completed and the absorption of nutrients and fluids begins. Most absorption of nutrients and electrolytes occurs in the duodenum and jejunum, but some vitamins, iron, and fluid are absorbed in the ileum.

Approximately 1500 mL of chyme enters the large intestine each day. Here the final absorption of nutrients, especially the absorption of fluid and electrolytes, occurs. The amount of absorption that occurs depends on the speed at which the intestinal contents move through the colon; the longer that intestinal contents remain in the colon, the greater the absorption of fluid and electrolytes. Reabsorption mainly occurs in the as-

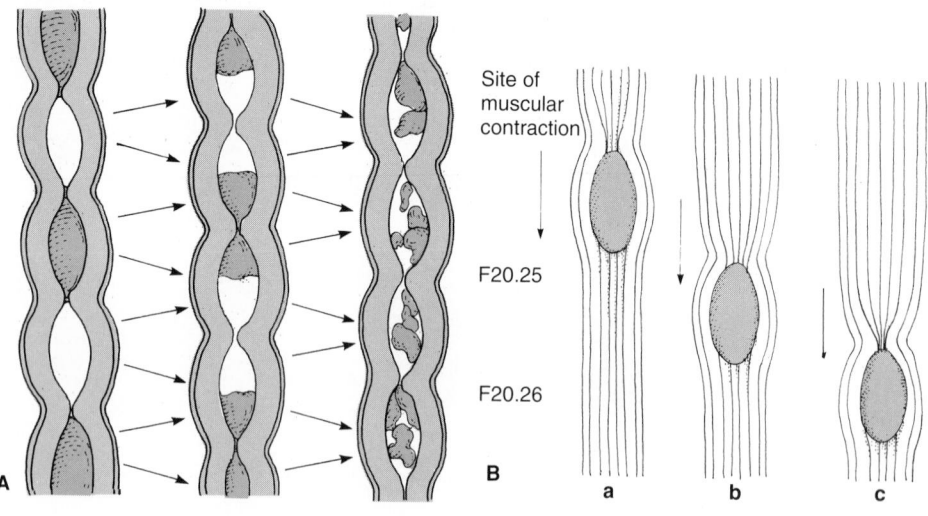

Figure 38-4. Intestinal motility. **A:** Segmentation in small intestine. **B:** Peristalsis in large intestine.

cending and transverse colon. Sodium is actively absorbed; chloride is passively absorbed with the sodium. Therefore, an osmotic gradient exists, causing the absorption of water. The intestinal contents that enter the ascending colon are liquid. When the contents leave the transverse colon, they are of a semi-solid, mushy consistency, and can be called feces. Although the distal colon's principle function is storage of feces, some sodium, chloride, and water will continue to be absorbed during storage. Approximately 80 to 150 mL of fluid from the 1500 mL that entered the large intestine each day will remain unabsorbed, for elimination with other fecal contents (Guyton 1987).

Mucus and Vitamin Production

The large intestine secretes mucus, which protects the walls of the large intestine from digestive acids, and from acids formed by bacteria within the feces. Mucus also serves to lubricate the contents of the colon, thereby decreasing the chance of mechanical trauma to the intestinal wall as the stool moves through the distal end of the colon. Mucus also holds together the fecal mass.

Many bacteria are present in the colon. Bacilli such as *Escherichia coli* and *Enterobacter aerogens* predominate, although some cocci are also normally present (Ganong, 1989). Some of the bacteria serve useful purposes. Bacterial activity is responsible for the formation of vitamins, including vitamins K, B12, thiamine, and riboflavin. Gases are also formed in the colon as a by-product of bacterial activity.

Defecation

The process of defecation begins when peristalsis propels feces into the rectum and causes rectal distention. This rectal distention or stretch begins a series of smooth muscle responses that can trigger bowel evacuation. When stool distends the rectum, parasympathetic afferent nerve fibers in the sacral segment of the spinal cord are stimulated. This stimulation causes contraction of the descending and sigmoid colon, rectum, and anus, and also relaxes the internal anal sphincter. This stimulus–response is a sacral reflex, not under voluntary control; it is called the **defecation reflex.** Defecation will automatically occur unless the external anal sphincter (a striated muscle under voluntary control) is kept contracted. In the presence of the defecation reflex, the external anal sphincter can remain contracted until the person decides that the time and place for defecation is appropriate. At that time, the person can voluntarily relax the external anal sphincter. Defecation is assisted by taking a deep breath against a closed glottis (to move the diaphragm down), contracting the abdominal muscles (to increase intra-abdominal pressure), and contracting the pelvic floor muscles (to push the feces downward). These actions are called the Valsalva maneuver. A strong

defecation reflex can successfully evacuate stool present from the descending colon on down to the anus.

Characteristics of Normal Feces

The feces consist of 75% water and 25% solids. The solids include bacteria, undigested fiber, fat, inorganic matter, and some protein. Table 38-1 lists the percentages of the constituents of the normal feces. The bacteria are mostly bacilli—*E. coli* and *E. aerogens*. Cellulose is the major undigested fiber left in the feces after the process of digestion and absorption have occurred. If dietary intake of fiber is small, less stool per day is produced. The fat in feces is from unabsorbed dietary fatty acids, fat formed by bacteria, and fat in the sloughed epithelial cells.

The normal color of feces is brown. The brown color is caused by the chemical conversion of bilirubin, an orange or dark-yellow bile pigment, into urobilin and stercobilin (brown pigments) by intestinal bacteria enzymes. The characteristic odor of feces comes from solids produced by bacterial decomposition of proteins in the intestine. Hydrogen sulfide, a gas produced by bacterial activity, also contributes to fecal odor. The feces normally have a soft consistency and cylindrical form that approximates the shape of the rectum. About 150 to 300 g of feces are produced each day.

Normal Functional Bowel Pattern

The normal bowel elimination pattern is highly individualized. The frequency of defecations can normally range from one to two per day to once every 2 to 3 days. The normal character of stool is soft, formed, and brown in color. Stool's color can be affected by the ingestion of certain foods; for example, beets may give stool a reddish color. Ingestion of certain medications can also affect the color and consistency of stool. Table 38-2 compares normal and abnormal feces.

TABLE 38–1

Constituents of Normal Feces

Constituents	Percent
Water	75
Solids	25
Bacteria	30
Undigested food fiber and dried constituents of digestive juices	30
Fat	10–20
Inorganic matter	10–20
Protein	3

Adapted from: Guyton, A. C. (1987). *Human Physiology and Mechanisms of Disease* (4th ed.), p. 516. Philadelphia: W. B. Saunders.

TABLE 38–2

Comparison of Normal and Abnormal Characteristics of Feces

	Normal	Abnormal
Frequency	Variable Usual range: 1–2 per day to 1 every 2–3 days	Dependent on usual pattern Guideline: >3 per day; <1 every 3 days
Color	Brown	Black, tarry Reddish-brown, maroon Clay-colored Yellow–green
Consistency	Soft, formed	Hard Loose, liquid High mucus content
Shape	Cylindrical	Narrow, pencil-thin
Amount	100–300 g/day	<100 g/day >300 g/day
Odor	Aromatic; pungent	Foul; objectionable

Factors Affecting Normal Bowel Elimination

Many factors affect normal bowel elimination. Diet and fluid intake, body position, privacy, and lifestyle changes can all change normal bowel patterns.

Nutrition. Diet influences bowel elimination. The 25% of feces that is solid contains a combination of bacteria, inorganic material, some fat and protein, and the undigested residue of food. It is the undigested residue of food that provides the bulk to feces, and this comes chiefly from food with a high cellulose or fiber content. Cellulose or fiber is contained in plant foods. Examples of foods in the high-fiber category are fresh fruits and vegetables with the skins and outer coverings intact, and cereal grains without the outer covering of bran removed. A person who consumes approximately 800 g of any combination of fruits, vegetables, and grains will most likely have sufficient bulk in the stools to allow for easy defecation.

Since 75% of the feces is water content, fluid intake will also have a great deal of influence on stool consistency. While the kidneys have a more direct role in regulating body fluid balance, the intestines also play a role in the absorption of fluid. The ascending colon in particular absorbs water as the fecal contents pass through the large colon. The body cells' need for water is a higher priority than stool consistency. When the body needs to conserve fluid, more water will be absorbed from the large intestine to meet bodily needs. A fluid intake of approximately 1500 to 2000 mL per day is necessary to meet the cells' needs and have enough left over to promote a soft stool consistency. Storage time in the large colon also affects stool consistency. The longer feces remain in the large colon, the more water will be

absorbed; the result is a stool that is harder and drier. Conversely, feces that do not spend sufficient time in the large colon will have a watery consistency and be a source of fluid loss for the person.

Body Position. A sitting or semi-squatting position is the most advantageous position for bowel elimination. This position assists gravity in the elimination of the feces, and also makes it easier to contract the abdominal and pelvic muscles, thus providing external pressure to the large intestine and encouraging evacuation of its contents.

Privacy. Most people require a certain degree of privacy to feel comfortable psychologically during the act of defecation. Deferring defecation until one reaches a toilet is considered essential for everyone past the age of 3 or 4 years. Although part of the defecation reflex is involuntary, the external anal sphincter is under voluntary control, and a person can ignore the urge to defecate until he or she feels the time and place for defecation is appropriate.

Lifestyle and Habits. Many people develop a pattern with respect to the timing of bowel elimination. For many people, the ingestion of food or fluid first thing in the morning will stimulate an urge to defecate. Over time, a pattern of bowel elimination every morning can be established and would be considered a normal pattern of bowel elimination for that person. Some people are ritualistic, using the same method to promote a regular pattern of bowel elimination, while other people have no set pattern except to respond to the defecation urge whenever it occurs.

Lifespan Considerations

Newborn and Infant

The newborn usually evacuates stool within 24 to 48 hours after birth. This stool, which is softly formed and dark-greenish in color, is called meconium. Meconium is the partially dried intestinal secretions that have accumulated in the infant's large intestine before birth.

By about the third day after birth, the characteristics of the infant's stool will begin to reflect the type of milk in the diet. If an infant is fed breast milk, the stools will be bright yellow, of a soft, unformed consistency, and have an unobjectionable odor. If the infant is fed formula, which is usually cow's milk, the color of the stools will be dark yellow or tan, of a slightly more formed consistency than is associated with breast milk, and will have a strong, somewhat objectionable odor. The digestive and absorptive capacities of the infant's gastrointestinal system are not mature at birth, and intestinal contents pass through the system more quickly than in the older child and adult. The infant's stools are loose because of the slower rate of absorption of fluids in the large intestine. Stools become firmer as the infant's gastrointestinal system matures, and with the introduction of more solid foods.

Frequency of bowel elimination will vary individually in infants, as it does in adults. Stool may be passed with every feeding, or just once a day, or even only once every 3 days. As the infant becomes older, he or she may seem to have bowel movements in a more regular or identifiable pattern. The infant cannot control bowel elimination until the central nervous system becomes more mature.

Toddler and Preschooler

It is during toddlerhood, usually between 22 to 36 months, that a child is ready to learn voluntary control of bowel elimination. By this time, the central nervous system has developed to a point where voluntary control of bowel elimination is possible. At some time between 12 and 18 months the myelinization of the sacral spinal cord segments, which control the anus, becomes complete. When this occurs, the toddler can recognize that stool is present in the rectum. A good indicator of the maturation of the spinal cord is when a toddler can walk independently.

The duodenocolic reflex is strong in toddlers and preschoolers. Any ingestion of food may stimulate a bowel movement, and toddlers and preschoolers may normally have more than one bowel movement per day. Water absorption in the large intestine does not occur as quickly in the toddler and preschooler as it does in the older child and adult; therefore, the consistency of the toddler's and preschooler's stool may normally be loose.

Successful bowel training—deferring defecation until reaching an acceptable waste receptacle—usually will not occur before the age of 22 months. Until that age, a toddler's rectum and colon cannot hold large amounts of feces. Training is easier when the number of bowel movements per day has decreased to one or two. Also before the age of 22 months, many toddlers do not have sufficient vocabulary to communicate the need to defecate, and would not remember to do so before actually defecating. A toddler also needs to understand he or she has control over certain bodily functions. It is not until a child can recognize rectal distention, *and* has the ability and willingness to momentarily defer defecation, *and* can also communicate the need to defecate, that he or she is ready for bowel training. In the American culture, most parents believe that children are emotionally, socially, and physically mature enough to begin toilet training for bowel movements somewhere between the age of 24 to 36 months; most children have attained bowel control before age 4 years. Bowel control is usually achieved before bladder control.

The toddler is curious about the products his or her body produces. It is not unusual that at some time during toddlerhood smearing or playing with feces will occur. It is appropriate to let the toddler know that smearing feces is not an acceptable practice; encourage an alternative substance, such as modeling clay or fingerpaints in a matter-of-fact manner that does not destroy the child's self-esteem.

Privacy for bowel movements is a value learned early in our culture. Young toddlers who are not yet toilet trained will sense the urge to defecate and then hurry to another room, or hide behind a couch or other piece of furniture to squat down for a bowel movement. The older preschooler who has mastered the voluntary control of bowel movements usually prefers the privacy of his or her own bathroom at home, rather than public restrooms.

Child and Adolescent

School-age children are bowel trained and are approaching the bowel elimination habits of adults. Stool is brown in color and softly formed. Consistency and frequency depend on intake of sufficient fluids, fiber in the diet, and the amount of daily exercise. School-age children, including adolescents, may choose to defer defecation until they are in the privacy of their own bathroom at home. Continuous practice of this bowel habit puts the child at risk for a decreased responsiveness of the bowel to rectal distention and eventual constipation.

Adult and Older Adult

By the time a person has reached adulthood, a bowel elimination pattern that is normal or typical has developed. Bowel elimination pattern depends on diet, fluid intake, and level of activity. Deviations from typical daily routine can result in short-term alterations in bowel elimination. A return to the status quo or typical daily routine usually ensures a return to the typical bowel elimination pattern.

The motility of the gastrointestinal tract slows with aging; it is therefore not unusual for the frequency of bowel movements to decrease. Intestinal contents remain in the large intestine for a longer period of time, leading to a greater absorption of fluid from the feces. Older adults need to increase the amount of fluids and high-fiber foods in the diet to prevent the formation of a harder stool.

Because of physiologic changes that occur in the gastrointestinal tract with aging, the elderly are at risk for thinking they are constipated when in fact they are experiencing symptoms associated with normal aging. Some people have a strong belief that a daily bowel movement is essential to health. Therefore, when normal age-related bowel changes occur, the elderly person may resort to a laxative to restore the "normal" pattern of daily bowel evacuation. Long-term use of laxatives can lead to a decreased ability of the large intestine to respond to rectal distention; the laxative-dependent bowel will empty only with the chemical stimulation from the laxative. Unfortunately, this type of laxative abuse is common among the elderly. It is far better to educate the elderly to recognize that decreased frequency of bowel elimination is a normal fact of aging for many people, and to encourage a change in dietary habits and an increase in activity level to prevent a change in stool consistency. A decrease in strength of the striated external sphincter muscles occurs with aging. This leads to decreased sphincter control and increases the possibility of fecal incontinence.

ALTERED BOWEL FUNCTION

In addition to understanding normal bowel function, the nurse must become knowledgeable about factors that can contribute to altered bowel status. The nurse, through his or her assessment skills, helps to identify those patients at risk for bowel dysfunction so that preventive measures can be instituted.

Potential for Altered Bowel Function

Many factors have the potential to disrupt normal bowel patterns. Often more than one factor may be present before disrupted bowel function is actually seen. The nurse assesses the potential risk for bowel dysfunction by assessing the presence of the following: inadequate diet, food intolerances, inadequate fluid intake, ignoring the urge to defecate, lifestyle changes, immobility, diagnostic procedures, general surgery, or surgical interventions creating a fecal diversion.

Dietary Factors

A person whose diet is deficient in high-fiber foods will generally have less frequent bowel movements, stools with less bulk, and may experience some difficulty in bowel elimination (Brown, et al., 1990). Ingestion of large amounts of certain foods, such as fresh fruits, may produce loose stools.

Food intolerances may also alter bowel function. Many people have difficulty digesting lactose (the sugar contained in milk products) into its component sugars, glucose and galactose. The digestion of lactose requires the presence of a sufficient quantity of the enzyme lactase in the small intestine. If a person is lactase deficient, alterations of bowel elimination, including the formation of gas, abdominal cramping, and diarrhea, can follow the ingestion of milk products.

Some people are unable to digest gluten, a protein found in wheat, rye, barley, and buckwheat. For these people, ingestion of a gluten-containing food results in the retention of carbohydrates and fats, as they cannot be digested and absorbed through the intestine. The person experiences abdominal **distention** and a bloated feeling, along with a diarrhea of bulky, greasy stools.

For people without a food intolerance, the ingestion of certain specific foods can still alter normal bowel patterns. Over time and with experience a person may recognize that the ingestion of a particular food results in uncomfortable bowel elimination. For example, eating hot, spicy foods predisposes some people to increased peristaltic transit through the gastrointestinal tract. This can result in loose or watery stools, sometimes accompanied by abdominal cramping, and usually with a burning sensation in the anal area as the stool exits.

Fluid Intake

An average fluid intake of 1500 to 2000 mL per day is usually necessary to maintain normal bowel patterns. Usually this means people should drink six to eight glasses of water or other fluids daily. Some fluids are obtained through solid foods, as well as through the metabolism of foodstuffs. When a person loses excessive water from causes such as high fevers, profuse diaphoresis, or other abnormal drainage, usual fluid intake may not be sufficient. When fluid intake is inadequate, stools become harder and more difficult to pass. Ingestion of large amounts of fruit juices may predispose some people to diarrhea.

Ignoring the Urge to Defecate

The defecation reflex and the urge to defecate will subside after a few minutes if the initial urge is ignored. The feces will then remain in the rectum until another mass colonic movement propels more stool into the rectum; this may not occur for several hours or more. While the feces remain in the colon and rectum, water will continue to be absorbed from the feces by the intestinal mucosa. A harder and drier stool that may be more difficult to evacuate will result. Eventually, as a person continually denies the defecation reflex, recognition of the urge to defecate becomes more difficult, and the defecation reflex gets weaker and subsides in time. Rather than relying on inherent body signals to initiate defecation, this person may have to depend on alternative methods. Stimulating a weak defecation reflex by the Valsalva maneuver, the persistent use of laxatives or enemas, or manual disimpaction of stool are examples of alternative methods.

Fear of Pain

People who experience pain during defecation may choose to deny the urge to defecate, which can lead to constipation. People at risk for delaying defecation due to pain include those with rectal or anal pathologies, including hemorrhoids or fissures, post-perineal surgery patients, postpartum women, and those with chronic constipation.

Hemorrhoids are enlarged or varicose veins in the anal canal. Pain and rectal bleeding are sometimes associated with hemorrhoids, and these may lead to frequent denial of the defecation reflex to decrease pain associated with defecation. An anal fissure is an ulcerous crack or splitting of the anal mucosa. Bleeding and pain occur as the stool passes the fissure.

Lifestyle Changes

Alterations in a person's lifestyle or pattern of daily living can have an effect on bowel elimination. Vacations or travel are often a significant enough alteration in the daily routine to cause alterations in bowel elimination.

Lifestyle changes that cause either acute or chronic feelings of anxiety, anger, fear, depression, excitement, or other strong emotions can lead to an altered bowel elimination pattern. Any acute stress or change in a person's lifestyle can increase bowel motility and mucus secretion. The result may be a sudden increase in frequency of bowel movements, with the stool containing large amounts of mucus. Hospitalization, a change in job, a disruption in personal or family relationships, and anticipation of final exams are just a few examples of situations that can stimulate acute stress. Chronic exposure to stress can slow bowel activity, resulting in decreased frequency of bowel movements. Chronic depression is an example of a chronic stressor that slows bowel activity and frequency of bowel movements.

Immobility

Any limitation of normal or usual physical activity can increase the risk of constipation. Decreased physical activity can increase the risk of bowel elimination problems. Decreased physical activity of the large skeletal muscle groups slows overall body activity, including colonic peristalsis. Weakened abdominal and pelvic muscles are not as effective in assisting normal defecation.

Medications

There are a number of medications whose primary purpose is not to affect bowel elimination but can increase the person's risk for bowel elimination problems. Examples of these types of drugs include narcotics and iron preparations (constipation), antibiotics (diarrhea), and antacids (constipation or diarrhea).

Diagnostic Procedures

Some radiologic and endoscopic procedures require cleansing of the large bowel of its fecal contents by laxative medications or enemas before the procedure. The thorough cleansing of the large bowel alters the normal pattern of elimination for 2 or 3 days after the test. When the person's usual diet is resumed, the normal bowel elimination pattern usually reemerges. If barium is used as the radiopaque contrast material, then postprocedure stools will take on a chalky white or tan color until all of the barium has been eliminated from the gastrointestinal tract. Barium hardens if permitted to remain in the colon and causes impaction of stool. Laxatives are frequently ordered after the diagnostic test to facilitate barium removal.

Surgery

Surgical intervention can place the patient at risk for altered patterns of bowel elimination. General anesthetics have a slowing effect on the motility of the gastrointestinal tract. Patients who have undergone a surgical procedure using general anesthesia will usually experience a period of decreased bowel functioning for approximately 24 to 48 hours postoperatively.

Patients who have had abdominal surgery, especially surgery on a portion of the gastrointestinal tract, will require 3 or 4 days for bowel activity to return to normal. Preoperatively, these patients are often given laxatives or enemas to cleanse the large intestine of feces. Also, their diet may have been restricted to low-residue (low-fiber) food for a day or two preoperatively. Intraoperatively, the bowel is exposed to air and manipulation, further leading to decreased bowel motility postoperatively.

Postoperative use of narcotic analgesics, decreased levels of activity, and fear of pain will further inhibit normal bowel motility. Postoperative patients are not allowed food and fluids orally until there is evidence of the return of active bowel motility.

Fecal Diversion

The presence of all or part of the large colon is not necessary to maintain life. It is possible to surgically remove all or part of the colon, rectum, and anus and to bring the proximal portion of the remaining bowel up through the abdominal wall to the abdominal skin surfaces. The portion of the intestine brought through the abdominal wall is known as a **stoma.** When this surgery is performed, it is referred to as a fecal diversion, because the normal route for feces is altered. Fecal diversions can be permanent or temporary.

Which bowel segment is used to form the stoma will depend on the location of the bowel pathology. For example, if the person has rectal cancer, the segment of bowel removed will be the cancerous rectum. The healthy, noncancerous sigmoid colon, which is the segment of the bowel just proximal to the rectum, can be used to form the stoma. This bowel diversion surgery that brings a segment of the large colon out to the abdominal skin is called a **colostomy.** It is also possible that the entire length of the large colon is so diseased that the next healthy proximal segment of intestine is the ileum. When a portion of the ileum is used to make the stoma on the abdomen, the procedure is called an **ileostomy.** Figure 38-5 illustrates fecal diversions.

People with stomas, whether colostomies or ileostomies, have altered bowel elimination. These people no longer evacuate feces through the anus, but rather feces exit the body through the stoma. The consistency of the stool is affected by the length of functioning intestine that remains after the surgery. When an ileostomy is created, the large intestine is no longer available to absorb water from the stool. Thus, stool produced from an ileostomy is liquid and contains large quantities of electrolytes. A descending colostomy, in which only the rectum has been removed, produces stool that is soft in consistency, and elimination may be controlled with daily colostomy irrigations. This often permits a person to return to a pattern of bowel evacuation similar to that experienced before surgery.

Modern methods of surgery have been developed over the last decade that are less disruptive to normal bowel patterns when fecal diversion is necessary. An ileoanal reservoir attaches an ileal pouch to the anal canal, bypassing the large intestine. This permits a person to evacuate feces, usually five to six times a day, through the anus (Watt, 1985; Rolstad, 1986). A Kock pouch or continent ileostomy is another recent development in fecal diversions. A pouch is made from 30 cm of ileum with an outlet valve. Although this procedure requires a stoma, feces can be drained at the convenience of the patient, rather than continually draining into a pouch, as occurs in the traditional ileostomy (Watt, 1985).

Manifestations of Altered Bowel Function

Common manifestations of altered bowel function include constipation, fecal impaction, diarrhea, fecal incontinence, flatulence, and abdominal distention. The nurse works independently and collaboratively with other health-care team members to identify and treat these bowel problems.

Constipation

Constipation is the infrequent, sometimes painful passage of hard, dry stool. This occurs when stool moves through the large intestine too slowly or remains in the large intestine too long. The longer contact time with the intestinal mucosa allows more absorption of water from the feces. The use of the term "constipation" is relative to the person's normal defecation pattern. Constipation involves a change in stool consistency (harder and drier

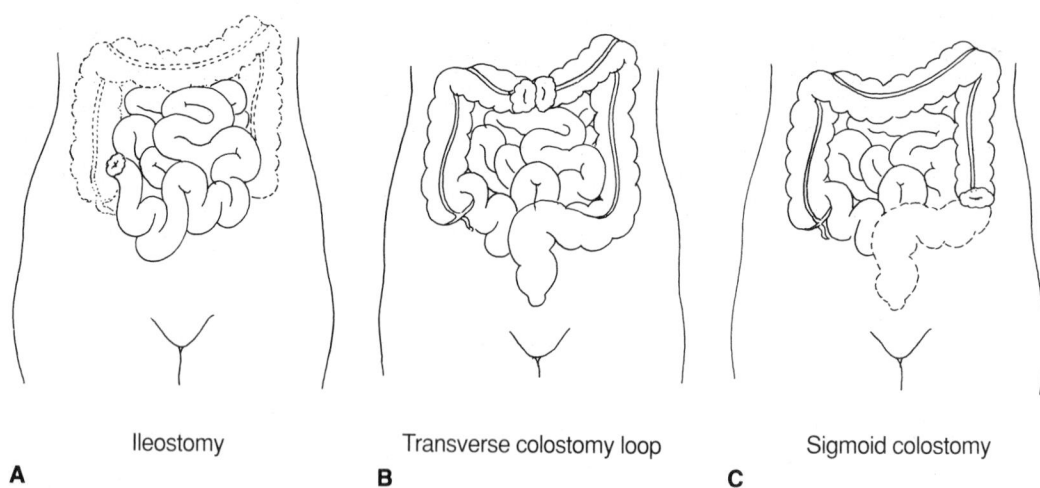

| Ileostomy | Transverse colostomy loop | Sigmoid colostomy |
| A | B | C |

Figure 38–5. Intestinal diversions: ileostomy, transverse colostomy, sigmoid colostomy.

Nursing Research

Selected Nursing Research Studies

Ewing, G. (1989). The nursing preparation of stoma patients for self care. *Journal of Adv Nursings, 14,* 411–420.

Gawron, C. L. (1989). Body image changes in the patient requiring ostomy revision. *Journal of Enterostomal Therapy, 16*(6), 256–263.

Heitkemper, M., & Marotta, S. (1985). Role of diets in modifying gastrointestinal neurotransmitter enzyme activity. *Nursing Research, 34*(1), 19–23.

Heitkemper, M., Shaver, J., & Mitchell, E. S. (1988). Gastrointestinal symptoms and bowel patterns across the menstrual cycle in dysmenorrhea. *Nursing Research, 37*(2), 108–113.

Hu, T. (1990). The cost effectiveness of disposable versus reusable diapers: A controlled experiment in a nursing home. *Journal of Gerontological Nursing, 16*(2), 19–24, 36-7.

Wallston, B. S., et al. (1987). Choice and predictability in the preparation of barium enema: A person-by-situation approach. *Research in Nursing and Health, 10,* 13–22.

Whitehead, W. E., et al. (1989). Constipation in the elderly living at home: Definition, prevalence, and relationship to lifestyle and health status. *Journal of the American Geriatrics Society, 37,* 423–429.

Possible Topics for Nursing Inquiry

- Does biofeedback therapy decrease stress-induced diarrhea?
- Does the use of videotaped instruction, rather than written instruction, increase patient compliance with stomal self-management?
- Do perineal muscle-strengthening exercises help decrease incidence of fecal incontinence in alert geriatric patients?
- Does the ingestion of apple juice in adult populations increase the incidence of diarrhea episodes?
- Comparison of different nasogastric taping methods to prevent nasal skin excoriation.
- Does right side-lying position versus left side-lying position affect the effectiveness of enema administration?
- Incidence of independent initiation of a bowel training program for high-risk patients among nursing staff.

than usual) and a change in frequency (less than usual). The causes of constipation are many; often they are a combination of one or more of the following factors.

Inadequate dietary fiber can be a factor leading to constipation. A diet with a large quantity of refined foods or other low-residue foods is likely to be deficient in bulk-producing fiber. A diet low in natural fiber will result in a less bulky stool, which encourages sluggish colonic movement and distention. In addition, a fluid intake of less than 1000 mL per day will also contribute to drier stool formation and lead to constipation.

People who consistently delay bowel evacuation risk developing constipation. Unreasonable privacy requirements, unavailability of toilet facilities during travel, an unwillingness to interrupt other activities, and embarrassment about using a bedpan, are just a few reasons why people might delay bowel evacuation.

Other factors that contribute to constipation are decreased physical activity, and chronic stress. Continual use of laxatives to trigger bowel evacuation weakens natural bowel responses to fecal distention, resulting in chronic constipation. Medications used for other purposes that have side effects slowing gastrointestinal activity will also contribute to constipation. Finally, one of the physiologic changes that occurs with aging is the slowing of the motility of the gastrointestinal tract. The older adult is physiologically predisposed to developing constipation.

Fecal Impaction

A fecal **impaction** is the accumulation of hardened feces in the rectum (Fig. 38-6). The word impaction implies that the stool is lodged or stuck in the rectum: there is an inability to voluntarily evacuate the stool. A fecal impaction is usually the result of untreated and unrelieved

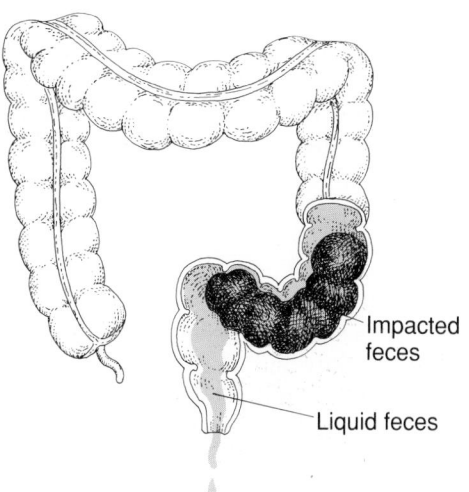

Figure 38–6. Fecal impaction in the sigmoid colon. Liquid stool may pass around hard fecal plug.

constipation. As stool remains in the rectum and sigmoid colon, water is absorbed from the stool, making it drier, harder, and more difficult to pass. More feces continue to be made and accumulate in the colon proximal to the impacted stool. The rectum and large colon are capable of considerable distention to accommodate large amounts of stool.

Fecal impaction is suspected when there is a history of an absence of a regular bowel movement for several days (3 to 5 or more), followed by the passage of liquid or semi-liquid stool. The person is often incontinent of the liquid stool, complaining of an inability to perceive urge. The passage of liquid stool also does not provide subjective relief of rectal and abdominal fullness. The passage of semi-liquid stool is the result of the seepage of unformed fecal contents around the impacted stool in the rectum; the pressure from the large volume of accumulated fecal contents forces liquid feces to the anus. This liquid or semi-liquid stool is not diarrhea, but is sometimes confused with it. Fecal impaction is confirmed by the presence of hardened stool in the rectum upon digital palpation.

Symptoms similar to those experienced with constipation are also present—a subjective feeling of rectal and abdominal fullness or bloating, an urge to defecate but an inability to pass stool, and a generalized feeling of malaise. Loss of appetite, and nausea or vomiting, are typical as well. Abdominal distention is often apparent.

The causes of fecal impaction are usually the same as those for constipation. Frequent denial of the urge to defecate, inadequate dietary fiber or fluids, and laxative abuse causing impaired colonic motility are typical. A nontypical cause of fecal impaction is the hardening of barium, a radiopaque substance used in radiologic examination of the gastrointestinal tract. Patients who have swallowed barium or received a barium enema should be monitored for complete evacuation of barium after the radiologic procedure. Some clinic or hospital protocols require the use of laxatives for 1 or 2 days after the procedure to ensure complete evacuation of the white, chalky barium from the gastrointestinal tract.

People with fecal impactions will need medications or special treatments to remove the impacted stool. Laxatives, enemas, or manual removal of the stool are possible measures.

Diarrhea

Diarrhea is manifested by frequent evacuation of watery stools. Diarrhea is usually associated with increased gastrointestinal motility and, therefore, a rapid passage of fecal contents through the lower gastrointestinal tract. The feces do not remain in the colon long enough for the usual amount of water to be absorbed, resulting in the evacuation of feces with a high water and electrolyte content. It is the consistency of the stool, being less formed and more watery than normal, that is the more

definitive symptom than the increased frequency. An increased frequency usually, but not always, accompanies the change in consistency of stool in diarrhea. Most people feel the urge to defecate when the volume of feces in the rectum approaches 300 mL (Alterescu, 1986). In addition to having a high water content, diarrhea stools may also have increased mucus; both of these factors contribute to increased volume. The extra volume and the rapidity with which it reaches the rectum cause rectal distention, resulting in the intense urge to defecate. Diarrhea stools may vary in color from light brown to yellow to green.

Diarrhea is often accompanied by abdominal cramping and an intense urge to evacuate fecal contents, nausea (with or without vomiting), and a painful burning sensation at the anus. Diarrhea stool is usually acidic, and it is this high acid content that is responsible for the burning sensation at the anus. Frequent passage of these acidic stools can cause inflammation of the skin surrounding the anus, and result in bleeding and breakdown of the perianal skin.

The causes of diarrhea can be many and varied. Any disease process that causes inflammation of the intestinal tract can lead to diarrhea. Specific microorganisms or the toxins they produce can inflame the intestines, resulting in diarrhea. The inflammation irritates the intestinal mucosa to increase its secretions and motility. A large volume of water becomes available to flush out the offending organism or toxin and move it quickly out of the body.

Medications can cause diarrhea. Overuse of laxatives, medications for the relief of constipation, can lead to diarrhea. Antacids taken to decrease stomach acidity, especially those containing magnesium, often lead to diarrhea. Also, some antibiotics are notorious for causing a diarrhea side effect. The medication irritates the bowel mucosa, leading to an increase in bowel motility and secretion. Antibiotics can also promote diarrhea by inhibiting the growth of normal intestinal flora. Normal intestinal flora inhibit the growth of *Clostridium difficile*. When broad-spectrum antibiotics are administered and normal flora altered, *C. difficile* can proliferate and release toxins that cause antibiotic-associated diarrhea (Mathewson, 1991).

Lifestyle changes causing acute stress and anxiety can result in episodes of diarrhea. Acute stress may increase parasympathetic stimulation to the large intestine. The stimulation increases colonic motility, decreasing the transit time of the feces through the intestines. In addition, intense parasympathetic stimulation to the large intestine increases mucus secretion; the diarrhea stools associated with high stress usually have a high mucus content. In severe stress, the volume of mucus is so great that the volume of mucus alone is enough to stimulate a defecation reflex. A stool with little usual fecal material but high in mucus content is possible.

Traveler's diarrhea often follows the ingestion of unfamiliar food or local water while on a trip to a different area or country. Often a water-borne foreign strain of *E. coli* is responsible for intestinal inflammation.

Food intolerances, such as lactase deficiency or gluten intolerance, or specific food allergies, often precipitate a diarrheal response. Apple juice can be a cause of chronic diarrhea for some children (Hyams & Leichter, 1985). Parenteral tube feedings may have a high osmotic load and precipitate a diarrheal response.

Fecal Incontinence

Fecal incontinence is the involuntary elimination of bowel contents. Fecal incontinence is often associated with neurologic, mental, or emotional impairments. Patients with injury to the cerebral cortex may have difficulty perceiving a distended rectum or initiating the motor responses required to complete defecation voluntarily. People who have sustained sacral spinal cord injury or have neurologic diseases that impair the nerve supply to the rectum and anal sphincters (e.g., multiple sclerosis) may also be unable to initiate the natural defecation reflex.

Patients who are disoriented or confused may have lost the social inhibition that prevents immediate fecal evacuation. In the absence of voluntary contraction of the external anal sphincter, the immediate evacuation of the rectum follows rectal distention.

Diarrhea predisposes a person to fecal incontinence. Sometimes the volume of feces is so large and the defecation urge so intense that the person cannot maintain sphincter contraction long enough to access toilet facilities and remove the necessary clothing. People with a fecal impaction may be incontinent of liquid stool seeping around the impaction.

Flatulence

Flatus is the accumulation of gas in the gastrointestinal tract. Gas enters the gastrointestinal tract from three sources: swallowed air, bacterial action in the large intestine, and diffusion from the blood (Guyton, 1987).

Excessive swallowing of air sometimes occurs with anxiety, rapid food or fluid ingestion, improper use of drinking straws, ingestion of large amounts of carbonated beverages, gum chewing, candy sucking, and smoking. Swallowed air is usually eliminated by burping or belching.

Gases produced by bacterial activity in the large intestine are eliminated through the anus. About 7 to 10 L of gases are produced each day, but only 0.6 L is expelled as flatus (Guyton, 1987). When larger than usual quantities of flatus are expelled, it is most often a result of increased colonic motility secondary to intestinal irritation. The colonic activity propels the gases toward the anus before they have time to be absorbed by the intestinal mucosa. Certain foods tend to produce gas more

than others. Cabbage, onions, and legumes (beans) often increase the amount of flatus produced in the intestine. Many other high-fiber foods that are recommended to promote normal bowel elimination can cause excess flatus production when the intake of these high-fiber foods is not introduced into the diet gradually.

Distention

An accumulation of excessive amounts of flatus and liquid or solid intestinal contents causes abdominal distention. Subjectively, the person will complain of abdominal fullness and discomfort and the inability to pass flatus or stool. Visual inspection of the abdomen reveals a distended or a convexly stretched abdomen. Depending on the amount of flatus and fluids in the intestines, the abdomen can appear only slightly distended or taut and stretched. Auscultation of bowel sounds may indicate either hypoactive bowel sounds or a combination of hypoactive and hyperactive bowel sounds. Percussion of the distended abdomen reveals tympanic sounds over areas of the abdomen filled with excessive gas, and a duller sound over areas filled with fluid or solid intestinal contents.

Bowel obstruction causing a blockage of the passage of flatus and intestinal chyme or feces is a primary cause of abdominal distention. Paralytic ileus, abdominal infections, and abdominal tumors are types of bowel obstructions that can produce abdominal distention.

Long periods of bedrest or relative inactivity can slow peristalsis and lead to accumulation of flatus in the large intestine. Peristalsis also slows after surgery with general anesthesia. In particular, bowel surgery where the bowel is manipulated will cause decreased peristalsis for approximately 24 to 72 hours postoperatively, with abdominal distention as a possible consequence. Constipation and fecal impaction also may lead to abdominal distention.

Impact of Bowel Dysfunction on Activities of Daily Living

The excretion of solid bodily waste is an important activity and function of daily living. Independent and acceptable toileting behaviors are important in our culture. People who have difficulty with independent toileting or adequate control of bowel function may experience anxiety or alterations in self-concept.

Alterations in bowel function can potentially alter family and social relationships. The fear of sudden episodes of loose stool necessitates staying close to bathroom facilities. For some, this may mean calling in sick to work or avoiding social obligations outside the home. Frequent hospitalization and decreased work efficiency can cause significant financial strain and family stress.

Alteration in bowel function can affect sexual function. The fear of loose stool or flatus during sexual activity can cause much anxiety and decrease sexual spontaneity. The presence of an ostomy frequently requires an adjustment period for both partners. Decreased energy reserves also negatively affect sexual function.

Nutritional status is affected by alterations in bowel function. Constipation causes bloating, which decreases appetite. Diarrhea often necessitates rest of the gastrointestinal tract by eliminating all oral intake or limiting intake to clear fluids. The person with alterations in bowel function may be unable or unwilling to shop for or prepare food. Blood loss associated with frequent diarrhea can further deplete energy levels. Interference with restful sleep can occur when frequent night wakings are necessary, and pain and discomfort can also contribute to exhaustion.

ASSESSMENT

Asking questions about a person's bowel habits is potentially an embarrassing situation for the patient and the beginning nursing student. Bowel elimination is considered a private function; however, the nurse who intends to give the best possible nursing care must get factual information both from the patient's perspective and through direction observation. The nurse should keep in mind that bowel elimination is a vital part of human functioning; it is therefore essential that the nurse have a sufficient data base to form a plan of care. If the nurse uses a matter-of-fact approach in interaction with the patient, the patient's embarrassment can often be eased.

Subjective Data

A focused functional assessment of bowel elimination includes obtaining subjective data from the patient by asking a series of purposeful questions, and making a mental note of the patient's nonverbal communication, such as facial expression, body language, and tone of voice. On first interaction with a patient, this information is often collected by conducting a nursing history. In later interactions with the patient, the nurse may focus his or her collection of subjective data on important considerations for that specific patient.

Collection of subjective data will assist the nurse in identifying the patient's functional bowel pattern, identifying any factors that place the patient at risk for developing bowel dysfunction, and identifying any actual dysfunctional patterns that are currently present in the patient.

Functional Pattern Identification

To determine the patient's current bowel elimination pattern, the nurse needs to obtain information from

current medical records, the patient, or his or her significant other. The nurse needs answers to the following questions:

What is the patient's usual pattern of bowel elimination?
What is the usual character of the stool?
Does the patient routinely use any aids to defecation?
When was the patient's last bowel movement?
Are there any recent changes in the patient's normal bowel pattern?

Aids to defecation may include ingestion of a hot liquid (coffee or tea) first thing in the morning, prune juice, bran cereal or bran muffins, and medicinal aids such as over-the-counter stool softeners and laxatives. Some people may routinely use small- or large-volume enemas. The specific aid to defecation and its frequency of use should be determined.

Other data that aid the nurse in determining the client's pattern of bowel elimination include the many psychosocial factors that affect bowel elimination, such as information about the patient's emotional mood, and his or her special concerns and fears.

It is important to assess if the patient has a family or other social support system. Because bowel elimination problems can be stressful, patients usually welcome familiar people around for support and reassurance.

The nurse also assesses the patient's intellectual or educational level, which is important in devising a successful teaching plan. The patient's motivation to learn and attention span should be considered.

Risk Identification

The nursing history includes the gathering of information that identifies factors placing the client at risk for developing alterations in normal bowel elimination function. Areas of risk to be assessed include dietary factors, such as adequacy of fiber and water intake; ignoring the urge to defecate; factors or conditions that may alter the patient's mobility pattern; diagnostic procedures, especially those involving the use of radiographic contrast material such as barium; surgical procedures; fear of pain on defecation; and lifestyle changes.

A patient needs good teeth to chew high-fiber foods such as fresh fruits and vegetables. Poor dentition with concomitant difficulty with chewing may lead to an insufficient intake of this food group, and place the patient at risk for constipation. A patient who has difficulty chewing or swallowing may be placed on a liquid diet administered through a feeding tube. Patients receiving tube feedings may be at risk for constipation or diarrhea.

Dysfunctional Identification

To determine if the patient has a bowel elimination dysfunction, it is necessary to assess their beliefs about "normal" bowel function. Some people believe that a normal bowel pattern is a bowel movement every day; they might further believe that a laxative or enema is necessary to correct any deviations from this pattern. A person's psychological concept of whether or not he or she has a bowel elimination dysfunction will depend on the person's beliefs about "normal" bowel elimination and whether his or her current pattern fits these beliefs. While a patient may believe he or she has an altered bowel elimination pattern, the nurse's analysis of the data may differ. Knowing the patient's beliefs about "normal" bowel patterns often directs subsequent nursing intervention.

Dysfunctional patterns can be identified as significant differences from the patient's normal pattern or a pattern that is outside the standards for bowel function. For instance, if a person usually has a bowel movement each day and states the absence of stool for the last 5 days, the nurse may identify a dysfunctional pattern of bowel elimination. Also, a dysfunctional pattern may be identified if a patient states he or she normally has a bowel movement every 3 weeks, since this does not fall within normal bowel status.

Objective Data

Objective data about the patient's bowel elimination pattern is gathered through physical assessment of the patient as well as through diagnostic and laboratory testing. Objective data will also be used to augment subjective data gathered in determining the patient's current pattern of bowel function, risk for bowel dysfunction, and actual bowel function.

Physical Assessment

Visual inspection of the feces and physical assessment of the abdomen and perirectal area provide data on the status of the patient's bowel elimination. The physical examination techniques used are inspection, auscultation, percussion, palpation, and measurement of abdominal girth. A comparison of normal and abnormal findings on physical examination of the abdomen and perirectal area is given in Table 38-3.

Inspection. When examining the patient's abdomen, the nurse begins with inspection. The nurse observes the abdomen for contour and symmetry. The abdomen's contour is normally convex (i.e., slightly rounded). The abdomen may be flat in a muscular or athletic person. An abdomen that appears hollow or scaphoid is not normal and may be associated with malnutrition. An abdomen that appears more than slightly rounded is called protuberant or distended; an abdomen may be protuberant because of excess subcutaneous fat, pregnancy, or accumulation of fluid or gas. The nurse notes any signs of obvious asymmetry, comparing the contour of the right side of the abdomen to the left side of the abdomen, and the upper quadrants to the lower quadrants. The normal abdomen shows no obvious signs of asymmetry.

Auscultation. Auscultation of the abdomen must be performed before percussion or palpation. Percussion or palpation of the abdomen may stimulate intestinal activity and therefore change the quality of frequency of bowel sounds. If the patient has a nasogastric or intestinal tube connected to suction, the suction should tempo-

---

TABLE 38-3
Comparison of Normal and Abnormal Findings on Physical Examination of the Abdomen and Perirectal Area

	Normal	Abnormal
Abdomen		
Inspection		
Contour	Convex or flat	Hollow or scaphoid; distended
Symmetry	Symmetrical	Asymmetrical
Auscultation	Bowel sounds present in all four quadrants every 5-15 seconds	Bowel sounds not present in all four quadrants Hypoactive bowel sounds—every 15-30 seconds Hyperactive bowel sounds—continuous or more than every 5 seconds Absent bowel sounds—no sounds in 1-2 minutes
Percussion	Hollow, tympany in LUQ (stomach)	Dull, tympany in quadrants other than LUQ
Palpation	Soft	Firm distention Presence of mass
Perirectal		
Inspection	Intact, nonreddened skin	Excoriated, reddened skin Hemorrhoids Bleeding
Palpation	No stool or only soft, brown stool present in rectum	Presence of hard stool Bleeding

rarily be shut off so that the sound of suction is not misinterpreted as bowel sounds. Bowel sounds, which are a result of peristalsis throughout the intestine, will be heard through the stethoscope as a bubbling or gurgling noise. Everyone has heard his or her stomach "growl" without the benefit of a stethoscope. This loud type of bowel sound is termed **borborygmi.** Bowel sounds heard through the stethoscope will sound similar, only quieter. The diaphragm of the stethoscope should be placed on the patient's abdomen. If the patient complains of pain in the abdomen, the stethoscope should be placed on that quadrant last. Normally bowel sounds are heard in each of the four quadrants within 5 to 15 seconds of placing the diaphragm on the abdomen; infrequent bowel sounds suggest decreased gastrointestinal peristalsis and motility. Hypoactive bowel sounds in a patient with previously normal bowel sounds indicate a patient at risk for developing a bowel elimination problem, such as constipation or perhaps a bowel obstruction. Hypoactive bowel sounds in a patient with previously absent bowel sounds suggest that intestinal peristalsis is beginning to return to normal.

An absence of bowel sounds means that the nurse has listened in each of the four quadrants for at least 1 to 2 minutes and heard no bowel sounds; it is the rare clinical nurse who has the time to listen to a patient's abdomen for 8 minutes. Clinically, most nurses define absent bowel sounds as no sounds heard within 30 seconds for each quadrant. This method requires the nurse to auscultate bowel sounds for only 2 minutes to document absent bowel sounds. A patient who has undergone abdominal surgery may have hypoactive or absent bowel sounds for a period up to 24 to 72 hours postoperatively. Bowel sounds should gradually return and are an indication that normal peristalsis has begun. A continued absence of bowel sounds beyond 72 hours may signal paralytic ileus, a condition in which the bowel is temporarily paralyzed and distention occurs.

Abnormal bowel sounds also include hyperactive sounds; continuous bowel sounds or sounds heard more frequently than every 5 seconds can be termed hyperactive. Patients with diarrhea usually have hyperactive, high-pitched bowel sounds, which indicate hypermotility in the intestines. A patient who has a bowel obstruction may have a combination of hypoactive and hyperactive bowel sounds, with hypoactive bowel sounds below the level of the obstruction and hyperactive bowel sounds above the level of the obstruction.

A time-efficient method for charting the findings of auscultation during an abdominal examination is the use of a small drawing. The drawing is a simple cross to define four quadrants. Plus or minus signs are placed in each of the four areas of the cross to represent the presence or absence of bowel sounds heard during the auscultation of the abdomen. This method of charting can be written and interpreted quickly and easily. Samples of this type of charting appear in Figure 38-7.

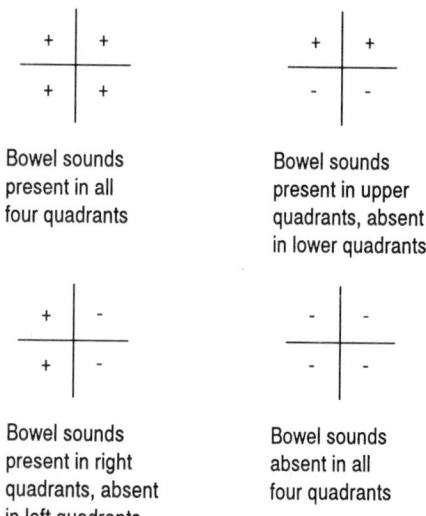

Figure 38–7. Charting findings from auscultation of bowel sounds.

Percussion. Percussion is used to identify air, fluid, or solid masses in the abdomen. Percussion is usually used when an abnormality has been identified during inspection or auscultation. The nurse begins percussion in the quadrant that was first auscultated. It is normal to hear a high-pitched hollow sound, called tympany, over the left upper quadrant (LUQ). The stomach is in the LUQ and contains more air than the small and large intestines. The normal percussion sound heard in the other three quadrants is a hollow sound not quite as high-pitched as tympany, reflecting the fact that there is a mixture of air and fluid in the intestines. When an abdomen is abnormally distended with air (or gas), tympanic percussion notes may be heard throughout the abdomen. When an abdomen contains an excess fluid accumulation, duller, lower-pitched sounds will be heard over the fluid-filled areas. A mass or feces in the large intestine would produce a dull sound.

Palpation. Palpation is the last physical assessment technique used in the examination of the abdomen. Palpation of the abdomen is not reliable in eliciting data about aspects of normal bowel elimination. If the history indicates problems in normal bowel elimination, or if abnormal findings have been observed during inspection, auscultation, or percussion, the nurse may wish to use light palpation. In light palpation the examiner uses the warmed fingertips of one hand to press on the abdomen firmly enough so as not to cause a tickling sensation to the patient but at the same time gently enough so as not to cause discomfort to the patient. The nurse palpates all four quadrants of the abdomen in a systematic manner. Instructing the patient to flex his or her knees during this part of the examination often helps the patient to relax abdominal muscles and results in less discomfort for the patient. From light palpation, the nurse can determine the firmness or softness of the abdominal muscles, the relative degree of abdominal distention, or perhaps the presence of abdominal masses.

A special technique called deep palpation is also part of the abdominal physical examination. During deep palpation, the examiner uses both hands and special techniques to assess deep abdominal masses and specific abdominal organs such as the liver and spleen. It is recommended that beginning nursing students not perform deep palpation independently. If possible, they should take the opportunity to observe the technique performed by a more experienced practitioner.

Measurement of Abdominal Girth. An assessment technique that the nurse can perform independently is the measurement of abdominal girth. A plastic tape measure that is marked in either inches or centimeters is wrapped around the patient's abdomen and the measurement recorded. Comparison of abdominal girth measurements over time is an objective way of determining whether abdominal distention is increasing, decreasing, or remaining unchanged. For the comparison of abdominal girth measurements to be valid, the abdomen must be measured at the same circumference each time. The nurse marks an "X" with a marking pen on the patient's abdomen at the point of greatest distention, ensuring that when the patient's abdomen is remeasured, it will be at the same location.

Perirectal Examination. Examination of the perirectal area completes the physical assessment. The patient needs to be side-lying with one or both knees flexed forward. The nurse needs disposable exam gloves and a packet of water-soluble lubricant.

The nurse inspects the perianal integument. The normal finding is perianal skin intact without any signs of excoriation or redness. There should be no evidence of bleeding, and hemorrhoids will not normally be present.

Abnormal findings during the inspection of the perianal area include the presence of excoriation (red, bleeding, tender skin). Excoriated perianal skin can be caused by the frequent evacuation of diarrhea stools. Another abnormal finding is the presence of hemorrhoids; hemorrhoids can be a result of the evacuation of hard, constipated stools over time. The presence of blood at the perianal skin is also an abnormal finding. If the person has recently evacuated a constipated stool past hemorrhoids, it is possible to see evidence of bleeding.

Palpation of the rectal area is the next part of the physical assessment. To perform a digital examination of the rectum, the nurse needs to separate the patient's buttocks, and insert the lubricated index finger of the gloved hand into the patient's anus and rectum. The finger is aimed in the direction of the patient's umbilicus, while feeling against the sides of the rectal wall and at the tip of the finger for any signs of stool in the rectum. If any stool is felt, the nurse determines if it is hard or soft in

consistency. It often helps the patient to relax the anal sphincter if the nurse slightly distracts the patient by requesting him or her to inhale deeply as the nurse inserts the finger. The patient is asked to slowly exhale as the nurse quickly assesses the rectum.

Sometimes, as the nurse's finger enters the rectum, the patient may exhibit a temporary loss of sphincter control and stool will involuntarily be released from the rectum. This is especially true for the weak elderly and for infants and small children. For these patients, the nurse places a disposable pad under the patient's buttocks before performing the digital examination.

The normal finding during the digital exam is the absence of hard stool in the rectum. A comparison of normal and abnormal findings on physical examination of the abdomen and perirectal area appears in Table 38-3.

Diagnostic Tests and Procedures

There are two laboratory tests commonly performed on stool specimens for diagnostic purposes: the hemo-occult test and the stool culture. Other diagnostic procedures include radiologic examinations and endoscopic examinations. The nurse assists with these procedures and uses information gained to develop a plan of care.

Collecting Stool Specimens. Whether a stool specimen is tested by the nurse or the laboratory, it is often the nurse's responsibility to collect it. First the nurse must explain to the patient the need for a stool sample. If the patient is able to ambulate to the bathroom, a clean bedpan or other container used for obtaining specimens should be placed on the toilet. If the patient is unable to ambulate to the bathroom, the nurse ensures that a bedpan or bedside commode is readily available in the patient's room. When obtaining a specimen for stool culture, the nurse informs the patient that it is best if urine is not mixed with the stool in the bedpan. The male patient can easily use a urinal to prevent this from occurring, but it will be more difficult for the female patient. The nurse may need to have two bedpans ready in the room, one to be used for urine and the second to be used for the stool specimen.

Hemoccult Test. Heme refers to blood, and occult means hidden or not visible on inspection. Testing the stool for hidden blood is called a hemo-occult (hemoccult) or **guaiac** test. The nurse can easily perform this diagnostic test. A small amount of stool is placed on a card or slide made especially for this purpose, and a few drops of a chemical developer are then placed on the slide. The nurse then observes for a color change. Blue is a positive diagnostic finding, indicating the test is positive for the presence of occult blood in the stool sample. The absence of a color change or any color other than blue is a negative diagnostic sign, indicating the absence of occult blood in the stool sample. Guaiac testing is a simple procedure (see Procedure 38-1, "Assessing Stool for Occult Blood"), but the nurse should be sure to read the instructions that accompany the hemo-occult slide and developer and follow them every time for accurate results.

The stool is tested for occult blood to check for pathologic sources of bleeding from the gastrointestinal tract. Gastrointestinal bleeding could be caused by peptic or small intestinal ulcers, or tumors of the gastrointestinal tract. If there is blood on the surface of the stool, it is likely to be secondary to bleeding from hemorrhoids, and is not occult. If blood is mixed in the stool mass itself, its likely source is intestinal. When collecting a stool specimen for occult blood, a stool sample obviously contaminated by hemorrhoidal blood should not be used.

Other false positive results on a hemo-occult test can occur if a patient has recently taken medications known to cause irritation to the gastric mucosa. People who routinely take aspirin or other nonsteroidal anti-inflammatory drugs or steroid medications should avoid taking these medications for 3 days before a stool specimen is collected; the ingestion of rare red meat in large quantities for 3 days before hemo-occult testing can also cause a false positive result. False negative results can occur if the patient has taken more than 2 to 4 g of vitamin C in 24 hours before the test.

Stool Culture. The other laboratory test performed on stool is that for the culture of specific infectious organisms. The stool normally has a high bacteria count as a result of normal intestinal flora. A stool culture is performed to distinguish atypical intestinal organisms present in the stool sample. Examples of atypical infectious organisms that might be cultured from a stool sample would be *Salmonella* or *Shigella* species. When these organisms are present in the intestine, they usually cause diarrhea; specific antibiotics are necessary to kill the offending organism and stop the diarrhea. A special kind of stool culture sometimes necessary is the testing of the stool for ova (eggs) and parasites. A stool specimen should be sent to the laboratory soon after the patient defecates (i.e., while the stool is still warm), where it can be tested for specific parasitic organisms or their eggs, such as *Giardia lamblia* or *Entamoeba histolytica,* that could cause diarrhea.

Radiologic Procedure. There are several diagnostic tests available that aid in identifying specific pathologies associated with alterations in bowel elimination. These tests are either radiologic (x-ray) procedures, using barium as a contrast medium, or are procedures performed by physicians using specialized instruments that provide direct visualization of the lower gastrointestinal tract.

The small and large intestines can be visualized on x-ray if a radiopaque substance, barium, is swallowed or instilled in the rectum. The small bowel x-ray is usually done in conjunction with the x-ray of the upper gastrointestinal tract. The patient must swallow barium, a white liquid with a definite chalky taste. The radiologist can monitor the progress of the barium from esophagus though ileum. Still x-ray pictures can be taken at any time as the barium progresses through the gastrointestinal system. The lower gastrointestinal tract can be radiologically visualized by instilling the barium through the rectum, and thus the term "barium enema" is often used for this procedure. The radiologist can visualize the colon as the barium travels from the rectum back toward the ascending colon.

The purpose of these two radiologic procedures is to visualize the segments of the small and large bowel for signs of abnormalities in shape, motility, and functioning. Examples of abnormal findings are the presence of tumors, diverticuli, obstruction, or filling defects.

For the bowel segments to be maximally visualized, the bowel must be as free as possible from fecal contents. Patients need to take a combination of oral and rectal laxatives the day before and the morning of the procedure; tap-water enemas can sometimes be substituted for the laxative regimen. The patient's oral intake is also restricted, usually beginning at midnight on the day of the test. The patient is NPO and may not have food or fluids until the procedure is finished; oral medications are also withheld until the procedure is completed if withholding the medications will not cause adverse risk for the patient. The nurse is responsible for informing the patient of the necessary preparation regimen and purpose of the procedure, and may also be responsible for administering the laxatives or enemas and for maintaining the patient's NPO status.

When the patient returns from the procedure, he or she may again eat and drink. The nurse must be aware that barium left in the bowel after the procedure can harden and become extremely difficult to eliminate. Therefore, the nurse should encourage the patient to take a laxative such as milk of magnesia, 1 ounce for 1 or 2 days after the x-ray, until no more white-colored barium stool is passed.

Endoscopic Examination. Endoscopic examination, or **endoscopy,** of the large colon is another means of diagnosing colon abnormalities. A flexible fiberoptic instrument called a proctoscope or a sigmoidoscope is inserted through the anus and rectum up to a distance of 65 cm; the procedure is called proctoscopy or sigmoidoscopy. The lower segment of the colon can be directly visualized by the physician. The bowel is examined for the presence of severe inflammation or for tumors. Often, the barium enema does not offer sufficient diagnostic information for the sigmoid and rectum, and the sigmoidoscopy or proctoscopy is necessary. During this procedure, the patient must be in a knee-chest position, which is an uncomfortable and somewhat embarrassing position for most people. Patients also feel the urge to

PROCEDURE 38–1. Assessing Stool for Occult Blood

■ Purpose
1. Screens patients who are at risk for developing gastrointestinal bleeding due to medical history or medication side effects.
2. Screens for early-stage colon cancer.

■ Assessment
- Review patient's medical and drug history for risk factors for gastrointestinal bleeding.
- Assess patient's understanding of need for the procedure and his/her ability to cooperate.
- Note patient's dietary history and need for any modifications before the test. Rare meats can cause false positive test results for occult blood. Some physicians may restrict red meat for 72 hours prior to the test.

■ Equipment
Bedpan, bedside commode, or toilet hat to catch stool.
Disposable exam gloves.
Tongue blade or wooden applicator stick.
Pre-packaged Hemoccult cardboard slide, developing solution or hematest tablets, guaiac filter paper, and several drops of water.

■ Procedure
1. Ask the patient to void before collecting the stool specimen.
   Rationale: Urine mixed with stool sample could dilute stool sample so occult blood is not detected. If urine has red blood cells, the test results might be positive, but the source would be masked.
2. Assist patient onto bedpan, commode, or to bathroom. Provide privacy and leave call bell within reach.
3. Once the patient has passed stool and is clean and comfortable, don disposable gloves and obtain small amount of stool with a tongue blade or wooden applicator.

■ Procedure

Hemoccult Slide Test
1. Open flap of slide and apply a very thin smear of stool onto first window.
   Rationale: The guaiac filter paper is very sensitive to blood content, so only a small sample is needed.
2. Using second applicator, obtain a second sample from a different area of the stool. Smear thinly on second window of slide.
   Rationale: Blood may not be equally distributed throughout stool sample. Testing only from one area may not reveal true test results.

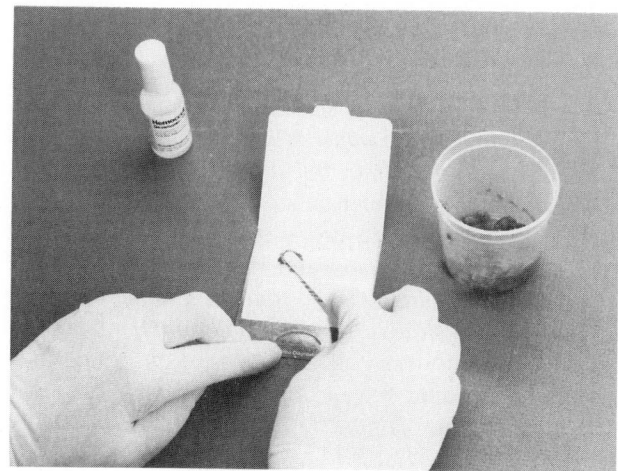

Step 1

Note: Physicians frequently order three different stools to be guaiac-tested.
3. Close slide cover. Open flap on reverse side and apply two drops of hemo-occult developing solution onto each window.
   Rationale: The developing solution penetrates the stool sample to react chemically with the blood.

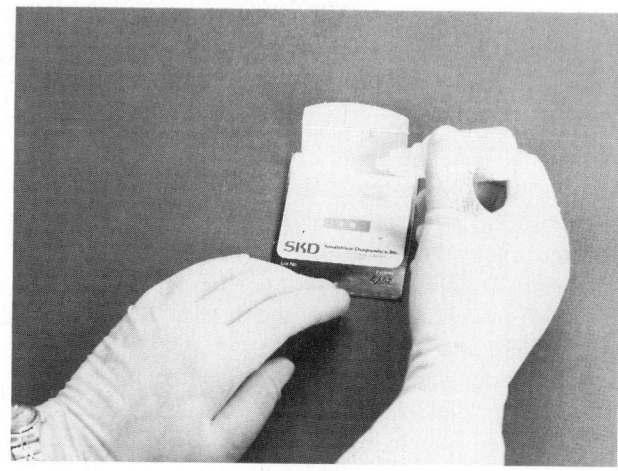

Step 3

4. Wait 30 to 60 seconds. Read test results.
   Rationale: Test is guaiac positive indicating the presence of blood if the filter paper has a bluish discoloration. The test is guaiac negative if there is no color change.

(continued)

■ **Procedure**

Test with Hematest Tablets
1. Apply small smear of stool onto guaiac filter paper. *Rationale: Guaiac paper is highly sensitive to blood content so only a thin smear is needed.*
2. Place hematest tablet on stool sample.
3. Apply two to three drops of water onto hematest tablet. Hold paper so water runs onto guaiac paper. *Rationale: Hematest tablet contains a solid developing solution which dissolves with addition of water.*
4. Read test results within 2 minutes by observing color of guaiac paper. *Rationale: Test is positive if filter paper has a bluish discoloration. Test is not valid after 2 minutes.*
5. Remove gloves, wash hands, and document.

■ **Lifespan Considerations**

Infants and Children
• A child who is not toilet trained cannot cooperate with stool specimen collection. The specimen can be obtained from a diaper if it is not contaminated with urine.
• If the child is having watery diarrhea, place a plastic liner inside the diaper and use a cotton swab to obtain the specimen.

■ **Home Care Modifications**
• If patient is asked to collect stool sample at home, instruct patient to prepare slide with sample, close cardboard flap, write name on slide, and return to the office or clinic for specimen developing.

defecate when the fiberoptic probe is inserted into the rectum, another embarrassing feeling for most people. For patients who are too weak to be examined in the knee-chest position, a side-lying position with the upper leg flexed (Sims position) can be used, although with this position visualization of the sigmoid is not as easy for the examiner.

The nurse's responsibilities include educating the patient before the procedure. The nurse explains the purpose of the examination, the position necessary for the procedure, and sensations likely to be felt during the procedure. Also, the patient must alter his or her diet before the test, and is limited to clear liquids the evening before and the morning of the test. Laxatives, rectal suppository, or small-volume enema may also be required to clean out the lower colon of stool before the procedure. After the procedure, the patient will likely be tired and perhaps hungry and thirsty; the nurse offers rest, food, and fluids.

The upper portion of the large colon can also be directly visualized by a fiberoptic probe. The colonoscope, a flexible fiberoptic instrument, can be advanced up to 180 cm, up to the point of the ileocecal valve. The purpose of this procedure is to directly visualize a greater segment of the large colon, again observing for the presence of severe inflammation or tumors along the entire length of the large colon.

Patient preparation is again an important nursing responsibility. The patient alters his or her diet; clear liquids may be recommended for up to 3 days (72 hours) before the procedure. Laxatives will be necessary for a day or two before the test so that the entire length of the colon will be cleared of feces, and a small-volume enema will be necessary the morning of the procedure. The

colonoscopy will take longer and produce more discomfort than the sigmoidoscopy or the proctoscopy; therefore, the patient is given intravenous medications for pain, to reduce bowel spasm, and to produce light anesthesia. The patient is in the Sims position for the procedure. After the procedure, the patient needs rest, but must be closely monitored by the nurse for signs of rectal bleeding or the onset of continuous, dull abdominal pain, perhaps indicating colonic perforation.

The patient must sign a written consent before an endoscopic procedure. Biopsy (a cutting of a small piece of colon mucosa or tumor) or polypectomy (complete surgical removal of colonic tumor) can be done at the time of endoscopy.

NURSING DIAGNOSES AND PATIENT GOALS

Specific information from the nursing assessment will assist the nurse in identifying potential and actual problems in the area of bowel elimination. NANDA nursing diagnoses concerning bowel elimination include Colonic Constipation, Perceived Constipation, Diarrhea, and Bowel Incontinence. Before 1988, Altered Bowel Elimination was an accepted nursing diagnosis, but was found to be too broad for clinical use (Carpenito, 1989).

Diagnostic Statement: Colonic Constipation

Definition

Colonic constipation is the state in which an individual's pattern of elimination is characterized by hard, dry stool that results from a delay in passage of food residue (NANDA, 1990).

Defining Characteristics

Hard formed stool; defecation frequency less than usual (less than every 3 days); reported feeling of rectal fullness or pressure; straining or pain on defecation; palpable impaction; decreased bowel sounds; abdominal pain, back pain, headache; anorexia (NANDA, 1990).

Related Factors

Constipation can be related to painful defecation, immobility, or changes in lifestyle. Physiologic disruption from neurologic impairment, endocrine disorders, ileus, or hemorrhoids can cause constipation. Constipation can also result from treatment protocols such as surgery, the use of constipating medications (e.g., narcotics, anticholinergics, diuretics, iron preparations, and anesthetics), or the abuse of laxatives. Lifestyle alterations such as lack of regular exercise, immobility, inadequate fluid intake or roughage in the diet, fear of pain with defecation, or lack of privacy can disrupt normal bowel patterns. Maturational factors such decreased gastric motility in the elderly, or anxiety concerning toilet training in the toddler can also lead to constipation (Carpenito, 1989).

Diagnostic Statement: Perceived Constipation

Definition

Perceived constipation is the state in which an individual makes a self-diagnosis of constipation and ensures a daily bowel movement through abuse of laxatives, enemas, and suppositories (NANDA, 1990).

Defining Characteristics

Expectation of a daily bowel movement with the resulting overuse of laxatives, enemas, or suppositories; expected passage of stool at the same time every day (NANDA, 1990).

Related Factors

A sudden change in normal bowel status, together with inadequate knowledge, can motivate a person to overuse medical therapies to ensure a daily evacuation of stool. This is more likely to occur if the person tends to be obsessive–compulsive in behavior or have a long-held belief that deviation from a stool every day is unhealthy (NANDA, 1990).

Diagnostic Statement: Diarrhea

Definition

Diarrhea is the state in which an individual experiences a change in normal bowel habits characterized by the frequent passage of loose, fluid, unformed stools (NANDA, 1990).

Defining Characteristics

Loose, liquid stools; increased frequency of defecation; urgency to evacuate stool; abdominal cramping or pain with evacuation; increase in volume or fluidity of stools (NANDA, 1990).

Related Factors

The related factors typically associated with diarrhea are categorized as untoward side effects. Examples include medications (magnesium antacids, laxatives, antibiotics), physiologic disorders (ulcerative colitis, Crohn's disease, irritable bowel syndrome, lactose intolerance), or an infectious process (*Shigella,* giardiasis). Stress and anxiety can lead to diarrhea, as can an excessive intake of high-fiber foods. Untoward side effects is a nonspecific label for many causative and contributing factors; the nurse should state a specific causative factor whenever possible (Carpenito, 1989).

Diagnostic Statement: Bowel Incontinence

Definition

Bowel incontinence is the state in which an individual experiences a change in normal bowel habits characterized by involuntary passage of stool (NANDA, 1990).

Defining Characteristics

Involuntary passage of stool (NANDA, 1990).

Related Factors

The related factors associated with incontinence are often neurologic impairments or mental or emotional disorders. Examples of neurologic disorders that may lead to bowel incontinence include spinal cord injury, cerebrovascular accident, brain injury, brain tumor, multiple sclerosis, Alzheimer's disease, and comatose conditions. Examples of mental or emotional disorders that may cause fecal incontinence include severe mental depression, acute anxiety, or stress. A severe attack of diarrhea may result in an episode of bowel incontinence. A fecal impaction may be the cause of the involuntary passage of liquid stool (Carpenito, 1990).

Related Nursing Diagnoses

The impact of dysfunctional bowel status can contribute to or cause many potential or actual problems for the patient. Emotionally, altered bowel function can cause Anxiety, Self-Esteem Disturbance, or Ineffective Individual Coping. Knowledge Deficit is often present as a person learns to cope with new treatment modalities. Pain can result from constipation, diarrhea, or abdominal distention. Alteration in bowel status can disrupt physiologic homeostasis by contributing to Fluid Volume Deficits, Altered Nutrition, Decreased Cardiac Output, and Impaired Skin Integrity with increased chance for infection. Interference with sleep patterns and sexual activity can also occur.

Patient Goals

The direction of planning the nursing management for bowel function will depend on the time frame established to achieve the goals. Short-term goals are intended to be achieved within hours or days; a long-term goal is more realistic when the problem will take longer than 2 or 3 days to resolve.

The overall goals for patients with bowel elimination pattern disturbances are:

The patient will demonstrate a normal pattern of bowel elimination without evidence of constipation, diarrhea, fecal incontinence, or distention.
The patient will have an absence of preventable complications or adverse consequences from altered bowel elimination.
The patient will participate in a program to maintain and promote an acceptable pattern of bowel elimination.

The time frame for the patient to achieve the goal of a normal pattern of bowel elimination depends on the particular alteration involved. For example, constipation can usually be relieved in 1 or 2 days, whereas relief of diarrhea or incontinence is not always achievable in this time frame. The etiologic factors associated with the dysfunction also dictate the realistic time frame in which a goal can be accomplished.

The potential complications from bowel elimination dysfunction vary with the specific alteration involved. Some potential complications include the following: an alteration in cardiac output as a result of constipation and straining at stool; an alteration in cardiac output as a result of vagal nerve stimulation during digital rectal examination; fluid volume and electrolyte deficit resulting from diarrhea; impaired skin integrity resulting from diarrhea or incontinence; fear, anxiety, and possible altered coping accompanying unpredictable diarrhea; impaired social interaction or social isolation; self-care deficit; and an alteration in health maintenance when patients are unable to manage their bowel elimination dysfunction.

The promotion of an acceptable bowel elimination pattern is, realistically, a long-term goal. In actual clinical practice, it is often subject to short-term management. Patient teaching is one of the major management tools used to achieve this goal.

IMPLEMENTATION

Once the nurse has identified a nursing diagnosis involving a bowel elimination dysfunction, he or she can work independently to help restore function, or collaboratively with other health-care team members. The nurse also has a significant role in identifying patients at risk for potential alterations in bowel function and initiating appropriate health teaching to promote optimum health.

Nursing Interventions to Promote Health and Function

Patient Teaching

Patient teaching is an important nursing intervention for assisting patients to maintain normal bowel elimination. The nurse teaches the patient to promote a normal ac-

---

Patient Teaching

Instruct the patient as follows:

- Drink eight glasses of water per day, increase fiber in your diet, and increase daily exercise to maintain normal bowel patterns.
- Don't introduce high-fiber foods into the diet too quickly; such an action may cause excessive flatus formation or diarrhea.
- Avoid the use of drinking straws when flatulence or abdominal distention is a problem.
- If you take loperamide hydrochloride (Imodium) or diphenoxylate hydrochloride (Lomotil) for diarrhea, be cautious about driving or other activities which require mental alertness. These drugs may cause drowsiness.
- Empty an ostomy pouch when one-quarter to one-half full; the weight of a full pouch will break the appliance seal.
- Change a colostomy pouch when the bowel is least likely to emit stool—for example, first thing in the morning before eating or drinking.

ceptable bowel pattern through adequate diet and fluid intake, and adequate exercise. The nurse also teaches the patient to avoid common causative factors for bowel elimination problems such as laxative abuse, food intolerances, excessive stress, and lack of response to normal body signals.

Diet. The nurse should encourage the patient to consume a sufficient daily intake of high-fiber foods, as dietary fiber is necessary to provide bulk to stool. The nurse can provide the patient with a list of high-fiber foods, which include fresh or cooked fruit and vegetables with their skins, whole-grain breads and cereals, and fruit and vegetable juices. The patient's food preferences should be discussed. The nurse can assist the patient in selecting foods from a list, identifying those foods that he or she will most likely incorporate into his or her lifestyle. The dietitian can be consulted for a more extensive list of high-fiber foods and recipes using these ingredients. Unprocessed bran flakes can be added to cooked or processed cereals; the patient will need to start with small amounts (1 or 2 teaspoonfuls) to determine if bran causes any intestinal irritation or flatulence. Unprocessed bran is capable of absorbing eight times its weight in water. The amount of bran is gradually added to the diet to achieve an acceptable bowel elimination pattern. The daily intake of approximately 800 g of high-fiber foods (e.g., any combination of five or six servings of fruit or vegetables, and whole-grain bread or cereal) is encouraged. A sandwich with two slices of whole-grain bread, served with a large fresh vegetable salad and two pieces of fruit would provide five servings of high-fiber foods.

Fluids. An intake of approximately 1500 to 2000 mL of fluids per day will promote a pattern of normal bowel elimination. The nurse should discuss with the patient his or her fluid preferences and find a way to encourage the intake of about 8 to 10 glasses of fluid per day.

Some fruit and vegetable juices provide extra bulk because of their high pulp or fiber content. A glass of prune juice is equivalent to more than one serving of the dried fruit, has high magnesium content, and is an excellent source of fluid to promote bowel elimination. Hot fluids, such as coffee, tea, or hot water with lemon juice can sometimes successfully encourage an increase in intestinal motility.

Activity and Exercise. A sufficient amount of daily exercise is necessary to promote general body muscle tone. Exercise also encourages normal smooth muscle functioning, which is important for normal intestinal functioning. If a patient has a relatively sedentary lifestyle, the nurse can explore reasonable alternative ways for him or her to incorporate an increased level of activity in his or her lifestyle. Walking is an excellent exercise in which most people, including hospitalized patients,

can participate. The nurse should encourage isotonic or isometric exercises to increase abdominal muscle tone; an example of these exercises is the alternate contraction and relaxation of the abdominal muscles for about eight to ten repetitions. The many variations of sit-up exercises isometrically tone and strengthen the abdominal muscles. The nurse assists the patient on bedrest to perform range of motion exercises until he or she can perform more independent activities.

Bowel Habits. Many people recognize that their bodies have a regular time for bowel elimination; some people have a bowel movement every day, some twice a day, and some once every 2 days. Often people have a bowel movement at the same time of day or after a certain regular stimulus. The duodenocolic reflex is a strong reflex, especially when food or hot liquid is ingested after of period of fasting, such as after a night's sleep. The ingestion of breakfast or a cup of coffee, tea, or any liquid is stimulus enough for some people to activate the duodenocolic reflex. The nurse teaches patients to listen to their body signals, as ignoring the urge to defecate can lead to constipation.

Nursing Interventions for Altered Bowel Function

Nurses have important responsibilities in the management of altered bowel elimination. Nursing interventions are individualized to reestablish optimal bowel function. Problems in altered bowel elimination include constipation, diarrhea, fecal incontinence, flatulence, abdominal distention, and fecal diversion.

Interventions are individualized for each bowel problem. Constipation is treated with laxatives, suppositories, enemas, and, if chronic in nature, a bowel management program. Management of diarrhea includes treating the underlying cause, bowel rest, and antidiarrheal medications. Fecal incontinence is managed by instituting a bowel training program and using fecal collection devices. Distention is treated with increasing activity, using rectal tubes and return-flow enemas. If distention persists, nasogastric decompression may be necessary. Stoma management consists of fecal collection through stoma appliances and stoma irrigation.

Laxatives

Oral **laxative** medications are usually the first treatment of choice to promote evacuation of hardened stool from the bowel. Table 38-4 contains a list of the common oral laxatives and stool softeners. The nurse is responsible for knowing the purpose, therapeutic dose range, therapeutic effects, side effects, contraindications, and nursing implications of all medications administered. The nurse should

---

Selected Nursing Interventions for Common Bowel Problems

Constipation

- Increase fluid intake
- Increase dietary fiber
- Increase activity and exercise
- Provide laxatives
- Provide suppositories
- Administer enemas
- Initiate bowel management program

Diarrhea

- Treat underlying cause
- Provide bowel rest; limit oral intake
- Administer antidiarrheal medications

Fecal Incontinence

- Initiate bowel management program
- Provide fecal collection devices

Flatulence and Distension

- Administer antiflatulence medication
- Increase activity
- Place rectal tubes
- Administer return-flow enemas
- Provide nasogastric decompression

---

consult a pharmacology or nursing medication text for more extensive details whenever necessary.

Oral laxatives take longer to produce an evacuation of stool than do laxatives given rectally, but are preferred by most patients for their ease of administration and the more gradual effect on intestinal motility.

Laxatives may be given in the form of a rectal suppository. A **suppository** is a medication prepared in a base (e.g., glycerin), which, when inserted into the rectum, melts and can be absorbed for systemic or local effects. Many suppositories are used to promote normal bowel evacuation, but other drugs that do not affect bowel status (such as aspirin) can be administered in suppository form. A suppository is administered when a quick (15 to 60 minutes) effect is desired. When administering a rectal suppository, the nurse needs the medication, a packet of water-soluble lubricant, and a pair of disposable gloves. If the patient cannot ambulate independently to the bathroom, the nurse also places a bedside commode or bedpan in convenient reach before administering the suppository.

Placement of disposable underpads on the bed may be advisable whenever the patient's motor or mental abilities are compromised. The patient should assume a side-lying position. With gloved hands, the nurse removes the outer wrapper from the suppository and covers the suppository with lubricant. While separating the patient's buttocks, the nurse locates the anus and inserts the suppository past the internal sphincter. For the adult, the internal sphincter is at approximately 4 inches, or at the end of the nurse's index finger. The nurse should guide the suppository with his or her index finger aiming in a slightly upward direction toward the umbilicus. The pointed or rounded end of the suppository is inserted first, with the suppository resting on rectal mucosa; some nurses advocate inserting a suppository flat end first. A suppository melts at body temperature and releases its medication as it rests against the rectal mucosa. The nurse should be sure the suppository is not inadvertently deposited into stool that might be present in the rectum, since this will prevent absorption by the rectal mucosa.

Antidiarrheal Agents

Medications that act directly on the intestine to slow bowel motility or to absorb excess fluid in the bowel are called antidiarrheals. Table 38-5 lists the antidiarrheals most commonly administered. Absorbants and bulk-forming agents change the consistency of the stool to relieve diarrhea; they cause few adverse systemic effects and are considered safe for general use. Opiates and antispasmodics act systemically to decrease intestinal motility. They must be used with caution in certain conditions such as bacterial gastroenteritis.

Medications may also be used to relieve the underlying problem. For example, antibiotics are administered when an infectious microorganism is responsible for diarrhea. Steroids may be given to decrease the inflammation in the exacerbation of a chronic inflammatory bowel disease.

Antiflatulent Agents

Antiflatulent agents, such as simethicone, are used to relieve gas. Simethicone coalesces gas bubbles in the intestine; it does not prevent the formation of gas, but does allow the passage of gas present in the gastrointestinal tract by either belching or expelling flatus. Antiflatulent medication is often given in combination with an antacid. Suppositories that increase intestinal motility can also relieve accumulated intestinal flatus.

Enemas

Stool can be removed from the bowel by a procedure called an enema. An **enema** is the cleansing of a portion of the large bowel by insertion of fluid rectally. Enemas can be small-volume, containing a laxative medication (approximately 150 mL), or large-volume, containing only ordi-

TABLE 38–4

Medications Used to Relieve Constipation

Name	Action
Stool Softeners	
Surface-Active Agents	
Dioctyl sodium sulfosuccinate (DOSS)	↓ Surface tension of feces in colon → softer and bulkier stool
Docusate calcium (Surfak)	
Lubricant	
Mineral oil (M.O.)	Lubricates and softens stool in colon → easier evacuation of stool
Laxatives	
Mechanical Stimulation of Colon	
Osmotic Agents	
Magnesium hydroxide (milk of magnesia [MOM])	↑ Bulk in LGI by the osmotic action of the mineral salt to attract water → rectal distention (mechanical stimulation of defecation reflex)
Magnesium citrate	
Magnesium sulfate (epsom salt)	
Other Bulk-Forming Agents	
Metamucil	Nonabsorbable fibers attract water in LGI → rectal distention (mechanical stimulation of defecation reflex)
Effersyllium	
Chemical Stimulation of Colon	
Castor oil	Chemical properties of medication stimulate LGI to ↑ peristalsis → evacuation of colon contents
Phenothalein (Exlax)	
Bisacodyl (Dulcolax)	
Cascara	
Senna	
Aloes	
Suppositories	
Glycerin	Attracts water and softens stool
Bisacodyl (Dulcolax)	Chemically stimulates LGI to ↑ peristalsis
Small-Volume Enemas	
Phosphosoda (Fleets)	Osmotically attracts water to ↑ colonic distention
Oil retention	Lubricates and softens stool in rectum

LGI, lower gastrointestinal tract.

nary tap water or saline (up to 1000 mL for the adult) (Fig. 38-8). (See Procedure 38-2, "Administering an Enema.")

Small-Volume Enemas. Small-volume enemas are commercially prepared and usually administered when an oral laxative has not produced sufficient return of stool or when a rapid evacuation time is preferred. The laxative solution is hypertonic, osmotically drawing water from colonic mucosa to cause water retention in the lower colon, and it also increases peristalsis. The volume of fluid itself also distends the rectum to trigger a defecation reflex.

An oil retention enema is a small-volume enema containing a quantity of mineral oil. The purpose of the mineral oil is to soften any hardened stool that is in the rectum and make the stool easier to pass. An oil retention enema is usually given only when a fecal impaction is suspected.

Small-volume enemas come from the manufacturer in disposable containers with prelubricated tips (see Fig. 38-8A). When administering a small-volume enema, the nurse is sure to use disposable gloves, underpads on the bed as necessary, and has a bedpan, commode, or bathroom accessible. The patient should be side-lying, with bed in low position. The patient usually experiences the urge to defecate within 5 to 10 minutes after administration of the enema.

Large-Volume Enemas. Large-volume enemas cleanse the bowel of stool by distention of the bowel with up to 1000 mL fluid for the adult (15 to 60 mL are recommended for an infant; 240 to 360 mL for a child). Warm tap water or saline is used as the cleansing agent; saline is the only fluid recommended for infants and children

TABLE 38–5

Medications Used to Relieve Diarrhea

Name	Action
Absorbants	
Kaolin	Absorbs excess fluid and bowel irri-
Kaopectate	tants; provides soothing effect to irri-
Attapulgite	tated bowel
Bismuth	
Bulk-Forming Agents	
Metamucil	Attracts water to absorb excess fluid
Effersyllium	
Opiates	
Paregoric	↓ Intestinal motility
Codeine	↑ Intestinal water and electrolyte ab-sorption
Synthetic Opiates	
Lopermide hydrochloride (Imodium)	↓ Intestinal motility
Diphenoxylate hydrochloride (Lomotil)	↓ Intestinal motility
	↑ Intestinal water and electrolyte ab-sorption
Antispasmodics	
Atropine	↓ Intestinal motility
Tincture of belladonna	

Table adapted from Heitkemper, M., & Brubacher L. (1986). Nursing strategies for common gastrointestinal problems. In M. Patrick, et al. (Eds.), *Medical–Surgical Nursing: Pathophysiological Concepts*. Philadelphia: J. B. Lippincott.

(Nurse's Drug Alert, 1987). The large volume of fluid inserted into the bowel causes distention and stimulates the defecation reflex. The large-volume enema can be used as a treatment for constipation or as a method of cleansing the bowel before bowel x-rays or surgery.

The nurse needs to gather the necessary equipment, including an enema bucket or bag connected to plastic tubing, disposable gloves, disposable underpads for the bed, water-soluble lubricant, and the solution (see Fig. 38-8*B*). A bedpan, commode, or access to a toilet should also be available. The patient is positioned as for administration of a suppository or small-volume enema. The nurse flushes or primes the tubing with the solution all the way to the tip of the tubing to prevent air from inadvertently being injected into the rectum; air will cause a degree of discomfort for the patient. The nurse inserts the lubricated tip of the tubing approximately 4 inches, aiming toward the umbilicus, and slowly instills

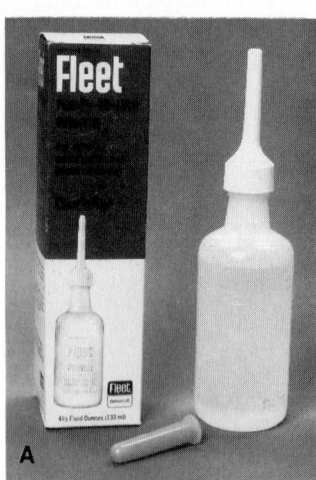
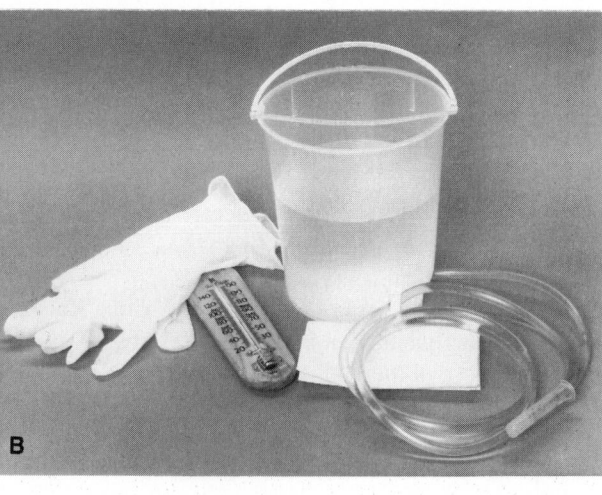

Figure 38–8. Equipment for common enemas.
A: Small-volume enema.
B: Large-volume enema.

PROCEDURE 38-2. Administering an Enema

■ Purpose

1. Relieves constipation or aids removal of fecal impaction.
2. Cleanses the bowel in preparation for diagnostic or surgical procedures.
3. Evacuates feces in patients with hemiplegia, quadriplegia, or paraplegia.
4. Acts as a route for medication administration.

■ Assessment

- Assess patient's past and present elimination history: presence of hemorrhoids, external and internal.
- Review physician's order, and determine the purpose for the enema to guide selection of the solution.
- If constipation or impaction is suspected, palpate abdomen for distention, and perform digital rectal exam.
- Determine patient's understanding of purpose of enema, what to expect during the procedure, and how he or she can help.
- Assess patient's developmental level and if additional assistance is needed to hold the patient while the enema is administered.

■ Equipment

Enema container with appropriately sized tubing (adults—size 22–32 Fr, children—size 14–18 Fr, infants—size 12 Fr, or a bulb syringe).
Possible solutions: Normal saline, tap water, soap solution, medications, commercially prepared bulb enema.
Disposable gloves.
Water-soluble lubricant.
Personal hygiene items: soap, towel, water.
Waterproof bed protector.
Clean bedpan or commode, and toilet paper. Children may use potty chair or diaper.

■ Procedure

1. Provide patient with privacy by closing curtains or door.
   Rationale: Reduces embarrassment for the patient and increases his or her ability to relax during the procedure.
2. Have patient lie on left side (Sim's position) with right knee flexed. Children and adults with poor sphincter control may be placed in dorsal recumbent position on a bedpan.
   Rationale: Sim's position improves retention of enema by allowing solution to flow by gravity along the natural sigmoid colon curve.
3. Place waterproof towel under patient's buttocks.
   Rationale: Prevents soiling of the linen.
4. Cover patient with bath blanket, exposing only the rectum.
   Rationale: Provides privacy, warmth, and increases ability to relax.
5. Put on disposable gloves.

■ Procedure

Large-Volume Enema

1. See steps 1 to 5.
2. Fill enema bag with 750 to 1000 mL lukewarm solution (105 to 110°F, for child—500 mL or less, 100°F). Check temperature of solution with bath thermometer or by pouring small amount over your own inner wrist.
   Rationale: Damage to the intestinal mucosa can occur if temperature of solution is too warm. Cold solutions are difficult to retain and can cause abdominal cramping.
3. Open clamp on tubing and flush solution to remove the air. Reclamp tubing.
   Rationale: If air is instilled into the rectum, the patient may experience cramping and discomfort.
4. Lubricate 2 to 3 inches of the tip of rectal tube with water-soluble lubricant.
   Rationale: Allows smooth insertion of the rectal tube and minimizes trauma to the mucosa.
5. Separate the buttocks to visualize the anus. Observe for external hemorrhoids, ask patient to take a slow, deep breath, and gently insert the rectal tube, directing the tip toward the umbilicus (adult—3 to 4 inches, child—2 to 3 inches, infant—1 to 1.5 inches).
   Rationale: Prevents injury to the intestinal mucosa by directing the tube toward the natural curve of the bowel.
6. Continue holding the tube in the rectum. With other hand open the clamp and allow solution to slowly enter the patient. Raise container 18 inches above the anus, allowing solution to flow in slowly over a period of 5 to 10 minutes. If patient complains of cramping or pain, have patient breathe deeply and lower bag until the sensation stops.
   Rationale: Slow instillation reduces patient discomfort from bowel distention and cramping, thereby allowing a greater volume of solution to be retained.

(continued)

PROCEDURE 38–2. Administering an Enema *(continued)*

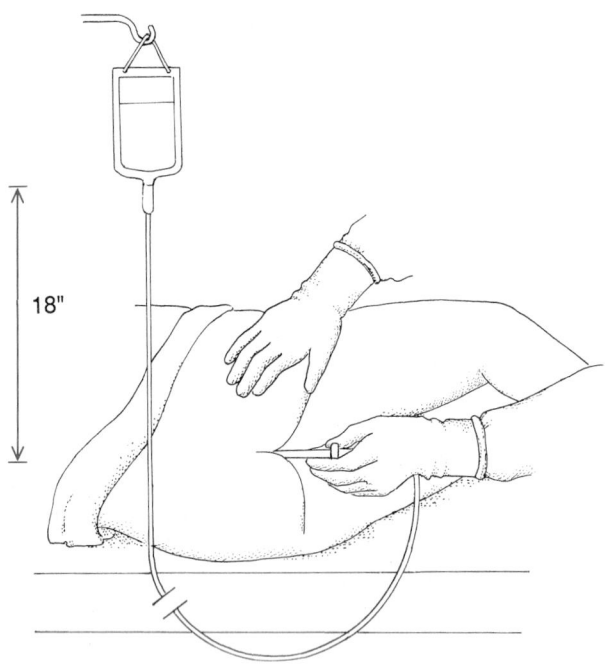

18"

Step 6

7. Reclamp tubing when all solution has infused.
   Rationale: Prevents air from entering the rectum.
8. Remove tube gently and have patient squeeze buttocks together firmly for several minutes until the urge to defecate caused by tube removal has passed.
9. Have patient retain solution as long as possible.
   Rationale: Longer retention of solution enhances more effective stimulation of peristalsis and evacuation of bowel contents.
10. Assist patient to bathroom, commode, or bedpan. Place call bell within reach. Provide privacy until all of the solution has been expelled.
11. Visually inspect character of the feces and solution.
    Rationale: If enemas are ordered "until clear" as preparation for diagnostic testing, it is essential to assess expelled solution for fecal material. Allow patient to rest, then repeat as necessary.
12. Assist patient to position of comfort.
13. Assist with cleansing of patient as needed. Provide materials for patient to wash hands. Open windows or provide air freshener if needed. Clean and dispose of equipment as necessary. Remove gloves and wash hands.
    Rationale: Prevents the spread of microorganisms and increases patient comfort.

■ Procedure

Small-Volume Enema

1. See steps 1 to 5 at beginning of Procedure.
2. Remove protective cap from prelubricated catheter tip. You may add more lubricant if necessary.
   Rationale: Allows smooth insertion of the rectal tip and minimizes trauma to the mucosa.
3. Separate the buttocks to visualize the anus. Observe for hemorrhoids and gently insert rectal tip into rectum. Advance 3 to 4 inches in an adult, directing the tip toward the umbilicus.
   Rationale: Prevents injury to the intestinal mucosa by following the natural curve of the bowel.
4. Squeeze bottle to empty contents into the rectum and colon (approximately 240 mL solution).
   Rationale: Prepackaged solutions are usually hypertonic and require only small volumes to stimulate defecation. Not to be used in children!
5. Maintain pressure on the bottle until you withdraw it from the rectum.
   Rationale: Releasing the pressure while the bottle is still in the rectum will cause the liquid to be drawn back into the bottle.
6. Continue same as with Large-volume enema.

■ Lifespan Considerations

Infants and Children

- Children who are not toilet trained are incontinent. Other children may be unable to control their rectal sphincter sufficiently to retain enema solutions. Administer with the bedpan in place.
- For children under 2 years of age, the physician should order the amount of solution to be administered.
- Children and infants do not usually receive tap water or prepackaged hypertonic enemas because fatal water intoxication or circulatory depletion could occur.

Older Adults

- If adult is incontinent, place clean, dry waterproof linen under his or her buttocks until after enema solution has been expelled and buttocks are cleaned. The skin of older adults macerates easily from prolonged contact with moisture. Check frequently for newly expelled stool and clean as necessary.

■ Home Care Modifications

- Patients should be taught not to rely on enemas to maintain bowel regularity. Enemas *do not* treat the cause of irregularity, and if used frequently can result in dependence on enemas for defecation, as they can disrupt normal elimination reflexes.

the solution into the patient's rectum. The nurse controls the amount and speed of the instillation by opening and closing the tubing clamp and by adjusting the height of the enema bucket. Opening the clamp and raising the bucket will increase the rate of flow of the solution into the rectum. Conversely, closing the clamp or lowering the enema bucket will decrease the rate of flow. If the patient complains of abdominal discomfort and cramping, the nurse momentarily stops the flow of solution. To successfully cleanse the bowel of stool, the average adult will need to tolerate approximately 350 to 500 mL of solution instilled before expelling the enema. When the patient cannot tolerate any more solution per rectum, the nurse stops the enema and assists the patient as necessary to the bedpan, commode, or toilet. A large-volume enema can be repeated up to three times in succession. Guidelines for repetition of a large volume enema include the patient's statement that he or she still feels there is more stool in the bowel that needs to be evacuated; the presence of large pieces of stool in the enema returns; and the water in the enema returns is heavily stool-colored. A step-by-step guide is given in Procedure 38-2.

Return-Flow Enema. The return-flow enema is used to relieve accumulated flatus. The nurse uses the same equipment as for the large-volume enema; however, only 300 to 500 mL of warm tap water is necessary. The nurse proceeds in the same way as for the large volume enema. When the patient indicates he or she feels abdominal discomfort or cramping, the nurse lowers the enema reservoir (the bag or bucket) and allows the water to return through the tubing into the reservoir. Flatus will also return, as evidenced by the bubbling of the water in the bucket. The nurse continues to repeat the procedure until there is no more evidence of flatus being expelled, or the patient states definite relief. This procedure may take 15 to 20 minutes to be effective. The return-flow enema can be repeated as necessary for relief of flatus.

Rectal Tubes

A rectal tube may be used if increased activity or medication does not relieve flatulence.

A rectal tube is a short piece of plastic tubing, similar to the tubing used for large-volume enemas. The lubricated tip of the tube is inserted about 4 inches into the patient's rectum and left in place for about 15 to 20 minutes or until the patient states relief. The gas in the rectum can pass from the rectum through the tube and into a collecting device, such as a bag.

Abdominal pain is the predominant adverse consequence of flatulence. It is wiser to relieve the cause of the pain by the use of rectal tubes or antiflatulence agents than to administer pain medications. Narcotic analgesics in particular will slow intestinal motility and compound the problem.

Nasogastric Intubation

Nasogastric intubation may be ordered by the physician for a variety of bowel problems. The nurse is responsible for inserting the nasogastric tube, assessing the patient during the period of nasogastric intubation, and providing nursing care that ensures proper tube function and patient comfort.

Purposes. A nasogastric tube is a thin, pliable plastic tube that can be inserted into a patient's nose and threaded into the stomach (see Fig. 38-9 for illustration of nasogastric placement). A nasogastric tube may be placed for different reasons, namely, gastric decompression, gastric analysis, gastric lavage, or gastric gavage.

Gastric Decompression. Gastric decompression may be accomplished through nasogastric intubation. Decompression relieves the stomach and intestines of pressure caused by the accumulation of gastrointestinal air and fluid. The nasogastric tube is connected to suction to facilitate decompression of the stomach contents.

Gastric decompression is indicated for a bowel obstruction, paralytic ileus, or when surgery is performed on the stomach or intestine. In each situation, potential or actual accumulation of fluid and gas in the intestine can cause abdominal distention, discomfort for the patient, and serious physiologic alterations. The tube usually remains in place until normal bowel function has returned, which is evidenced by the return of active bowel tones.

Gastric Analysis. Gastric analysis can be accomplished by testing stomach contents aspirated through a nasogastric tube. The nurse inserts a nasogastric tube in a patient who has been NPO for 6 to 8 hours. Gastric contents are aspirated and gastric acidity is determined. A histamine injection is given subcutaneously to stimulate stomach secretions. Stomach contents are then aspirated every 10 to 20 minutes until three posthistamine samples are obtained. The nasogastric tube is then usually removed.

Gastric Lavage. Gastric lavage is the irrigation of the stomach. In cases of accidental poisoning and accidental or intentional drug overdoses, swift removal of stomach contents is necessary. If the patient cannot swallow an emetic medication, gastric lavage will be necessary. In this situation, a nasogastric tube is inserted both to aspirate gastric contents and to instill a rinsing solution (usually normal saline) into the stomach to dilute the toxic substances. Patients with gastric bleeding are sometimes treated with an iced saline lavage. Iced saline is instilled and aspirated through the nasogastric tube to empty the stomach of blood and slow the bleeding at its source.

Gastric Gavage. Gastric gavage delivers liquid food into the stomach through the nasogastric tube for patients unable to obtain nutritional requirement through adequate oral intake. This type of nutrition is called gastric gavage or enteral nutrition. Nasogastric tubes for

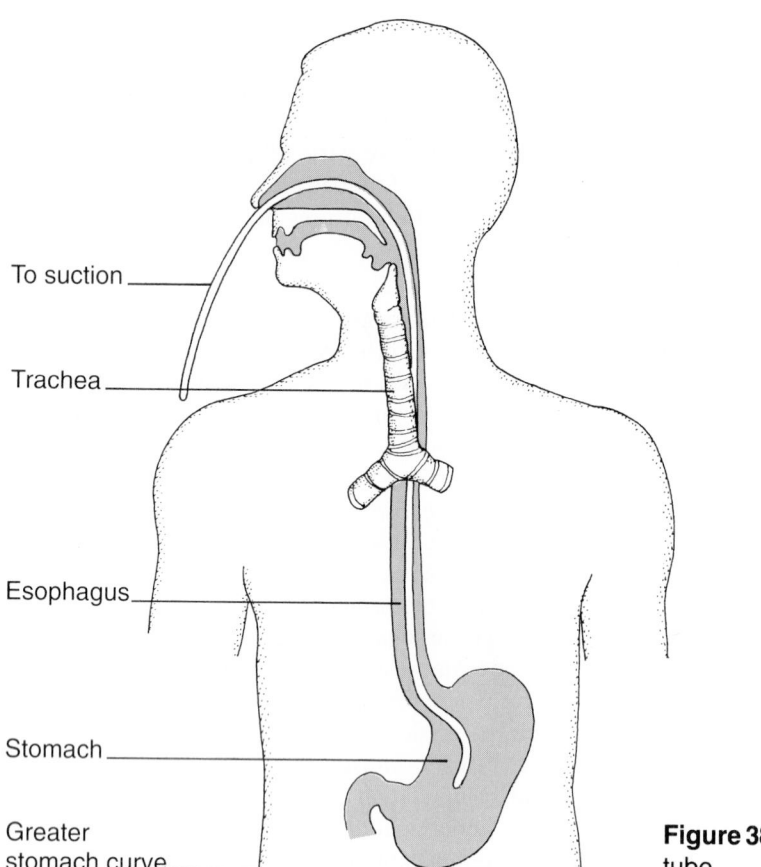

To suction

Trachea

Esophagus

Stomach

Greater stomach curve

Figure 38–9. Proper placement of the nasogastric tube.

feeding are intended to be used for a longer period of time than nasogastric tubes used for decompression or lavage, and therefore are smaller in diameter and made of a more pliable material. Nasogastric feeding tubes and the nursing care associated with enteral nutrition are discussed in Chapter 33.

Medication Administration via Nasogastric Tube. Medication intended for oral consumption can be administered through a nasogastric tube. A liquid form of the medication is preferred, but many tablets can be crushed, mixed with water, and safely administered through the tube. All nasogastric medication administration should be followed with water to clear the tube and ensure the medication has reached the stomach.

Equipment

Nasogastric Tubes. The two most commonly used nasogastric tubes are the single-lumen Levin tube and the double-lumen gastric sump tube (Fig. 38-10).

The Levin tube is a single-lumen tube sized according to the French method; sizes 14 to 18 Fr are typical adult sizes, with a length of 120 cm (48 in). The Levin tube is plastic or rubber and can be used for gastric decompression, analysis, lavage, or gavage. Small openings at the tip end of the tube allow for fluid flow in or out of the tube, and markings at specific points on the tube serve

as measurement guidelines for length of tube to be inserted.

The gastric sump tube is a clear plastic, double-lumen tube also sized according to the French method. Gastric sump tubes are the preferred tube for decompression. The larger lumen is connected to suction and a drainage container to collect the aspirated gastric contents, and the smaller second lumen terminates in a blue vent, often called the tube's "pigtail." The blue vent is always open to the air, providing continuous atmospheric air irrigation. Markings along the length of the tube serve as guides for depth of insertion. Both lumens have openings at the tip end to allow for fluid or air flow in and out of the tube.

Nasointestinal Tubes. When intestinal decompression for mechanical or nonmechanical bowel obstruction is the desired outcome, a longer tube capable of advancing the length of the intestine is used. As with nasogastric tubes, single- or double-lumen tubes are available.

The Harris tube (6 ft) and the Cantor (10 ft) are single-lumen tubes intended for intestinal decompression. Both tubes have mercury-weighted bags attached to the tip of tube. The weight of the mercury assists the tube in passing from the pylorus of the stomach into the duodenum. The weighted tip and the natural peristalsis of the intestine keep the tube advancing through the intestine.

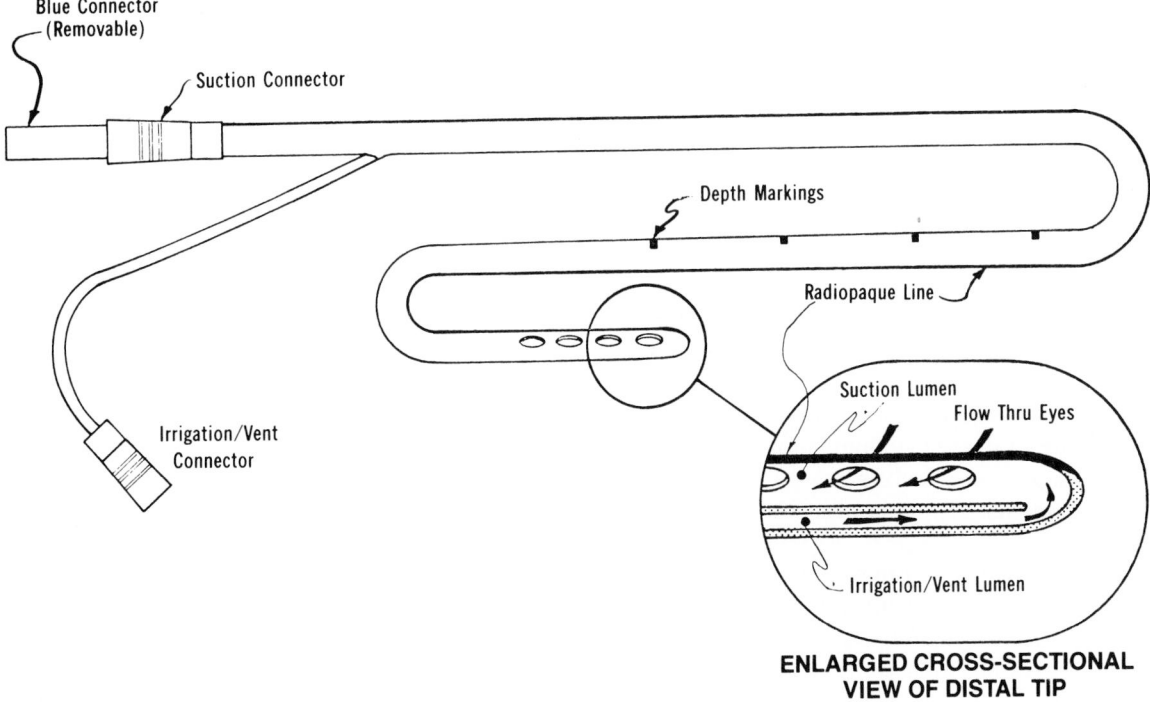

Figure 38–10. Double-lumen gastric sump tube. (Courtesy of National Catheter Co., Argyle, NY.)

The Miller-Abbot is a double-lumen, 10-ft tube. One lumen drains or decompresses the intestine; the second lumen is used to inflate the balloon at the tip of the tube with mercury. Therefore, the double-lumen tube allows for insertion of the mercury after the tip of the tube has passed through the nose and into the stomach.

Nasointestinal tubes are inserted in the same manner as nasogastric tubes. When the tip of the tube has reached the stomach, the tubing is not taped to the patient's nose. The patient can be positioned on the right side, allowing gravity and the mercury bag to enhance passage of the tube into the duodenum. In a few hours, passage of the tube into the small intestine should be verified by x-ray. If the tube has not advanced on its own, the tube can be manually advanced from the stomach into the duodenum under fluoroscopy by the physician or radiologist. Patient activity, position changes in bed, or ambulation encourage increased intestinal peristalsis and self-advancement of tube along the length of the intestine. Markings along the length of the tube help to estimate progress of the tube through the intestine.

Nasointestinal tubes can be attached to a bag positioned below the patient's torso to achieve a drainage of intestinal contents by gravity. Suction, either continuous or intermittent, can also be applied and connected to a collecting device.

Suction. Subatmospheric or negative pressure is applied to nasogastric tubes to pull air or fluid out of the stomach. Most hospitals have wall-outlet suction at the patient's bedside. A suction regulator is inserted into the wall unit. The suction gauge can be set at mm Hg of pressure: 20 to 40 mm Hg = low suction; 80 to 120 mm Hg = high suction. Suction can be regulated as continuous or intermittent on the gauge. Intermittent suction provides for suction at preset time intervals—up to 60 seconds—followed by set intervals of no suction. Connecting tubing is attached between the patient end of the nasogastric tube and a collecting device. The collecting device is connected by tubing to the suction regulator.

In health-care facilities without wall-outlet suction, portable suction units are available. These portable units usually provide only for intermittent suction at a "low" or "high" setting.

Continuous suction greater than 25 mm Hg can lead to irritation of the gastric mucosa if the mucosa are inadvertently "sucked" against one of the openings at the tip of the nasogastric tube. Gastric irritation is most likely to occur when a single-lumen Levin tube is connected to medium or high suction. The blue air vent of a double-lumen sump tube is designed to minimize gastric irritation associated with suction pressure; the blue air vent is left open to the air, allowing air under atmospheric pressure to continually flow into the stomach. As long as the air vent is patent, air will continuously irrigate the distal tip of the tube, keeping the gastric mucosa from tightly adhering to the larger outlets of the suction lumen. To be effective as an air vent, the pigtail must be kept at a level above the patient's stomach; otherwise, gravity will allow gastric contents to flow out of the stomach. Whenever gastric contents or the irrigation fluid enters the air vent, it must be cleared with 5 to 10 mL of air to re-establish air irrigation. Some gastric sump tubes come with an anti-reflex valve (ARV). When the ARV is firmly in place in the blue air vent of the double-lumen sump tube, spillage of gastric contents from the blue pigtail is prevented regardless of pigtail position.

Low continuous suction (30 to 40 mm Hg) is recommended for double-lumen tubes, but may be increased as needed to stimulate flow of gastric contents. Low intermittent suction only is recommended for single-lumen tubes. High suction is not recommended for single-lumen tubes because of high risk of gastric irritation.

The double-lumen sump with ARV is becoming the most frequently used nasogastric tube for decompression. Nurses prefer the second lumen for its continuous air irrigation and ARV, and decreased risk of gastric irritation with higher suction levels.

Nursing Care. Nursing responsibilities in the care of the nasogastric and nasointestinal tubes include accurate placement of the tube, monitoring for adequate suction to drain stomach or intestinal contents, maintaining patency of the tube, monitoring and recording the patient's intake and output, and providing adequate skin (nares) and oral care.

Accurate Placement. Accurate placement of the tube is important to ensure patient safety. Inserting a nasogastric tube is a nursing procedure. The nurse explains the purpose of the tube to the patient before inserting it, and lets the patient know that discomfort may be felt as the tube passes the gag reflex. Patients usually experience a transient nausea, and indeed some patients vomit at this point. Once the tip of the tube passes the gag reflex, the patient can assist in advancing the tube down the esophagus by swallowing. The nurse gently guides the tube with each patient swallow to the predetermined mark on the tube. Refer to Procedure 38-3, "Inserting a Nasogastric Tube," for a detailed description of the technique. Accurate placement is verified by aspiration of gastric contents, listening over the LUQ with a stethoscope for the "burp" as 5 to 10 mL of air is instilled by syringe into the tube, or by x-ray visualization.

Maintaining Suction. Maintaining suction is important when nasogastric tubes are used for gastric decompression. The nurse uses the lowest suction that will achieve successful drainage, checks the suction gauges every 4 hours for proper setting, and looks at the drainage tubing every hour to assess if gastrointestinal contents are flowing in the direction of the collection container. To test suction, the nurse may temporarily disconnect the tubing at the junction between the nasogastric and drainage tubing to hear the "whoosh" of suction and feel the suction at his or her fingertip. The nurse replaces any nonfunctioning suction units.

Tube Patency. Tube patency is important to ensure proper functioning of the inserted tube. Occasionally thick or solid particles of gastrointestinal contents plug the holes of a nasogastric or nasointestinal tube; the tube then ceases to drain gastrointestinal contents, even with properly functioning suction. When a tube is clogged, there will be minimal drainage in the tubing or collecting receptacle. The patient may begin to complain of nausea, which does not occur with a properly functioning system. The abdomen may appear distended. The nurse can irrigate the tube with isotonic normal saline to dislodge particles or viscous gastrointestinal contents from the tip of the tube. A physician order is required for irrigation when surgery on the stomach has occurred. When irrigating a double-lumen nasogastric tube, the nurse can instill irrigating solution in either lumen. If using the blue air vent, the nurse need not disconnect suction during irrigation, but must remember to clear the air vent with 10 mL of air after the procedure. Air will clear the blue lumen of fluid and restore continuous air irrigation. The nurse ensures that the anti-reflex valve in the blue air vent is replaced after irrigation.

If a tube does not appear to be draining well even after irrigation, its placement may need to be checked. To do this, the nurse slightly advances or alternately pulls back on the tube and assesses for any increase in drainage. Changing the position of the patient also sometimes improves nasogastric drainage.

Monitoring Intake and Output. Monitoring intake and output, including the amount, color, and type of gastrointestinal drainage, is measured and recorded every 8 hours. Gastrointestinal contents contain essential body fluids and electrolytes, including water, H^+, K^+, Na^+, Cl^-, HCO_3^- and Mg^{++}. The loss of fluids and electrolytes can lead to fluid volume deficit and metabolic acid–base imbalances. In addition, a patient with a nasogastric or nasointestinal tube for decompression will be NPO. Any fluids swallowed would be immediately returned via the tube; any food swallowed would eventually clog the tube. Patients with nasogastric or nasointestinal tubes will be on IV therapy to supply needed fluids and electrolytes. It is the responsibility of the nurse to record all intake and output and monitor fluid and electrolyte status.

Nares and Oral Care. Nares and oral care is an important nursing concern for the patient with gastrointestinal intubation. Skin irritation and breakdown at the nares can be prevented by appropriate taping of the tube and frequent skin care. The application of water-soluble lubricant to the nares provides moisturizing relief to dry skin. An oil-based lubricant (e.g., petroleum jelly) can inadvertently cause aspiration of oil particles into the lungs, and can lead to lipid pneumonia.

The nurse pins the tubing to the patient's gown to prevent constant tension and pulling on the tube, allowing enough slack so the patient can turn his or her head side-to-side without pulling on the tubing.

Frequent oral hygiene can prevent the consequence of dry mouth associated with nasogastric intubation. Patients often become mouth-breathers when a tube is in

PROCEDURE 38–3. Inserting a Nasogastric Tube

■ **Purpose**

1. Decompresses the stomach to relieve pressure and prevent vomiting.
2. Provides a means for irrigating the stomach (lavage).
3. Provides access to gastric specimens for laboratory analysis.
4. Provides a route for delivering liquid enteral feedings (gavage) in patients who can't swallow.

■ **Assessment**

- Identify patient's need for nasogastric intubation.
- Assess patient's mental status and ability to understand and cooperate with procedure.
- Review medical history for nosebleeds, deviated septum, nasal surgery.
- Assess nostrils for size, lesions, obstructions, or deformities.
  Note: Have patient breathe through one nostril while occluding the other. The tube should be inserted through the most patent nostril.

■ **Equipment**

Nasogastric tube of appropriate size (Adult: 14–18 Fr, Infant/children: 5–10 Fr).
Water-soluble lubricant.
20 to 50 mL syringe with catheter tip or adapter.
Glass of tap water with straw.
Towel.
Stethoscope.
Basin of ice to stiffen catheter if it is rubber.
Hypoallergenic tape.

■ **Procedure**

1. Identify patient, explain procedure.
   Note: Insertion is not painful, but it is uncomfortable because the gag reflex is usually stimulated.
   Rationale: Patient is more cooperative when the procedure is understood.
2. Provide privacy by closing curtains or room door.
3. Raise bed to high-Fowler's position, cover chest with towel, and place emesis basin near.
   Rationale: Elevated head protects against aspiration.
4. Wash hands.
5. Determine length of tubing to be inserted by measuring nasogstric tube from tip of ear lobe to tip of nose, then to tip of xyphoid process. Mark tubing with adhesive tape or note striped markings already on the tube.
   Rationale: This measure determines approximate length of esophagus from nares to stomach, which varies between patients.
6. Lubricate tip of tube with water soluble lubricant.
   Rationale: A water-based lubricant will be reabsorbed if tube inadvertently enters the lung. Never use an oil-based lubricant because respiratory complications may ensue.
7. Gently insert tube into nostril. Advance toward posterior pharynx by aiming back and toward ear.
   Rationale: Following natural contour prevents trauma to nasal mucosa.
8. Have patient tilt head forward and encourage patient to drink water slowly. Advance tube without

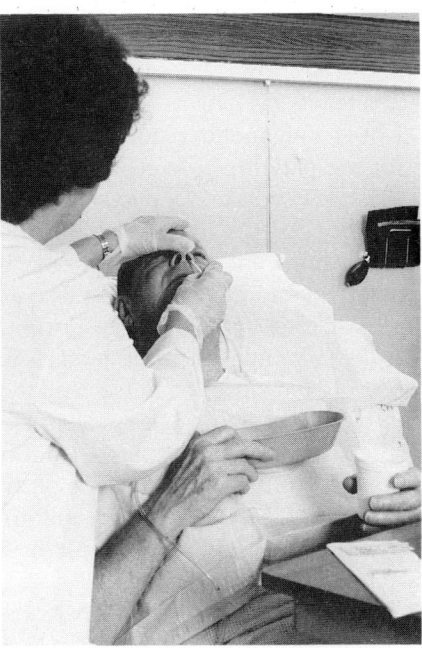

Step 7

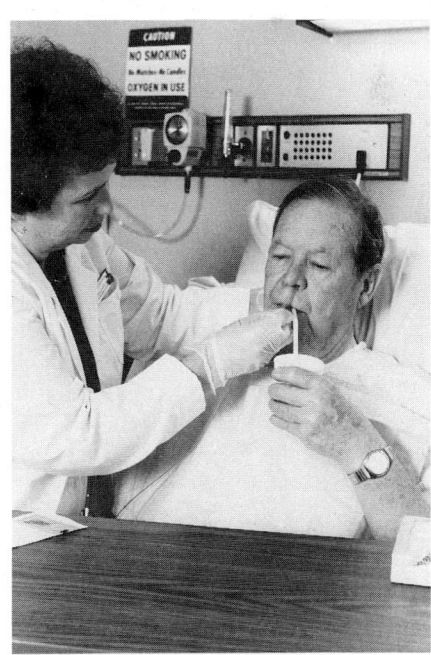

Step 8

(continued)

PROCEDURE 38–3. Inserting a Nasogastric Tube *(continued)*

---

using force as patient swallows. Advance tube until desired insertion length is reached.
Rationale: Forward tilt of head facilitates passage of tube into esophagus and not the larynx. Swallowing moves epiglottis over the larynx and facilitates tube passage.

9. Assess placement of tube:
   a. Aspirate gastric content with 20 to 50 mL syringe.
   Rationale: Gastric content is yellow to green in color and usually present in amounts greater than 10 mL.
   b. Auscultate over epigastrium while injecting 10 to 20 mL air into nasogastric tube.
   Rationale: Bubbling is heard if tube is in stomach.

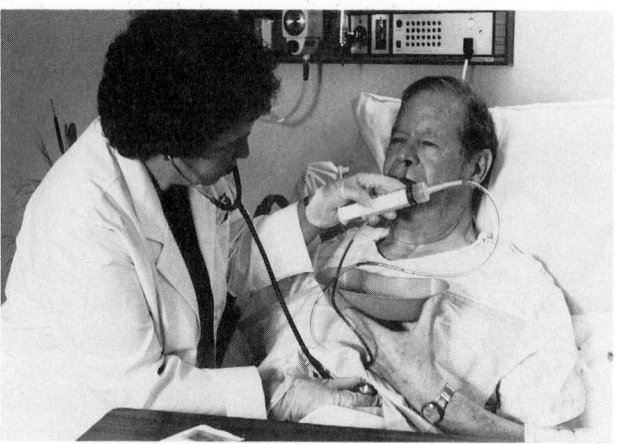

Step 9B

10. If placement in stomach is not verified, advance tube 5 cm and repeat assessment in step 9.
11. Secure tube by taping to bridge of patient's nose. Anchor tubing to patient's gown.
   Rationale: Correct taping prevents the tube from dislodging or pulling and traumatizing the nostril.
12. Clamp end of tubing or attach to suction, as ordered by physician.
13. Wash hands, provide for patient's comfort, and remove equipment.
14. Establish and document a nursing plan for daily care of the nasogastric tube:
   a. Inspecting nostril for irrigation.
   b. Cleansing nare around tube.
   c. Changing adhesive as required to prevent skin irritation or pressure sores on nare from the tube.
   d. Increase frequency of oral care since patients with nasogastric tubes often mouth breathe and may be NPO.

■ **Lifespan Considerations**

Infants
• Measurement of tube length in children under one year of age is from the tip of the nose to the ear lobe, then to point halfway between xyphoid process and umbilicus.

---

the nose. Sucking on ice chips or hard candies, if approved by the physician, can also provide some relief.

The nurse encourages patients who are able to brush their teeth frequently. An oral swab soaked in a solution of one-half water and one-half mouthwash is refreshing to many patients. Use of lemon glycerin oral swabs or swabs soaked in full-strength mouthwash should be avoided. The immediate relief provided by the swab is sometimes followed by rebound dryness. The nurse offers lubricant for the lips to prevent drying and cracking.

Fecal Impaction Removal

Removal of fecal impactions is a nursing responsibility. Manual removal of an impaction can be a cause of embarrassment for the patient. The nurse explains the purpose and necessity of the procedure, telling the patient before beginning what will be done. The nurse proceeds

in a matter-of-fact manner to reduce anxiety and embarrassment for the patient.

The equipment necessary for manual removal of fecal impaction includes plenty of disposable gloves, packets of water-soluble lubricant, several disposable underpads to protect the bed and floor, two bedpans, and a commode if the patient is capable of transferring to it. It is possible for the large intestine to distend to hold a large amount of stool, and since the nurse cannot accurately predict the volume before beginning the procedure, it is best to be prepared to remove a large quantity of stool. The nurse may want to wear some type of washable or disposable covering over his or her uniform because some stool is likely to spill or splash onto the nurse's clothes at some time during the procedure. The odor of the stool can be strong, and an open window or other form of ventilation should be provided.

The nurse begins the procedure with the patient in the

side-lying position. The double-gloved, lubricated index finger is inserted into the rectum. With a gentle hooking motion of the index finger, the nurse removes some of the stool from the rectum. The removal of stool begins slowly, but as the hardened stool that is blocking the lumen of the rectum is removed the remaining stool is often quite loosely formed and will pass quickly. The bedpan should be ready to place under the patient so that he or she can evacuate stool into it if possible; the stool may come so quickly that the patient is unable to control its evacuation. The nurse continues to remove stool manually until he or she can no longer feel stool at the fingertip, and the patient is not voluntarily evacuating any more stool. The nurse removes and disposes of collected stool and soiled linens, and provides hygiene care for the patient. Removal of a fecal impaction is a tiring procedure for the patient, so the nurse provides uninterrupted time and a restful environment after the procedure.

Nursing interventions to prevent complications in the management of fecal impaction include effective yet gentle insertion of the gloved index finger into the patient's rectum when performing digital examination and manual removal of stool. Excess vagal stimulation during digital examination and removal of stool can precipitate cardiac arrhythmias in weak patients or those with cardiovascular disease. Forceful pressure against the rectal mucosa can cause damage to the bowel tissue.

Bowel Training

A long-term approach to the control of bowel elimination may be necessary. Patients who are in the rehabilitation phase of a neurologic impairment (e.g., paralysis, stroke, head injury) are at high risk for constipation and/or fecal incontinence. These patients are usually on a bowel-training program, the intent of which is to maintain a soft stool consistency and develop over time a routine method of stool evacuation. The routine is repeated at the same time of day with the same techniques to train and control the bowel's evacuation time. An example of a classical bowel-training program for neurologically impaired patients is shown in Figure 38-11.

Bowel training may require weeks to months of persistence before success is attained. Reassurance and verbal expressions of confidence in the patient contribute to success of the program. Patient teaching about normal bowel function and factors to promote a soft stool consistency are helpful.

For patients whose anal sphincter control is weak, but not lost, a variation of the classical bowel-training program is used. Stool softeners and an increase in dietary fiber are used to maintain a soft stool consistency, but instead of the routine use of suppositories and digital stimulation, more emphasis is placed on capitalizing on the patient's own defecation signals. Careful assessment and documentation of the timing of incontinent episodes

Safety Alert

- Never leave a patient on a toileting device without a mechanism for summoning assistance; straining with defecation can lead to cardiac arrhythmias or vertigo and thus potential falls and injury.
- Do not administer a laxative to patients with undiagnosed abdominal pain; the resultant increase in peristalsis can rupture an inflamed bowel and cause peritonitis.
- Never administer more than three large-volume tap-water enemas in succession; excess absorption of the hypotonic solution by colonic mucosa leads to fluid and electrolyte imbalance.
- Use warm water (100 to 105°F, 37.7 to 40.5°C) for enemas. Cold water may lead to a decrease in temperature; hot water can cause burns to intestinal mucosa.
- Use the hooking motion of the index finger during manual disimpaction of stool carefully to avoid perforation of the rectum.
- Teach patients to exhale slowly during defecation, to avoid the Valsalva maneuver. This will avoid venous return and increase intracranial pressure, which can be dangerous for selected patients.
- Use low-level suction with nasogastric tubes; high suction can damage gastric mucosa by drawing it into the openings at the tip of the tube.

is done for several days. From then on, the patient is assisted to the toilet at a time that has been identified as "routine" for the individual patient; it often coincides with a duodenocolic mass movement after eating. The intent is to establish a regular defecation time using the patient's natural physiologic function.

Fecal Collecting Devices

In cases where bowel training is not successful or when the fecal incontinence is considered intractable, a drainable fecal collector may be used. The drainable fecal collector is similar to an ostomy appliance. It consists of a collecting pouch and a skin-protective barrier designed to adhere firmly to the perineum, anal cleft, and inner surfaces of the buttocks (Mowlam, North, & Myers, 1986). The pouch has a drainage outlet that can be connected to an additional collecting device for collecting large amounts of liquid stool. If a formed stool collects in the pouch, the drainage outlet can be cut off with

Date	Time	Related Meal or Fluid	Type of Suppository and Time	Comments: How, Where, Level of Independence
8/10	0800	Breakfast containing fiber	0830 Suppository with digital stimulation	Can transfer independently to bedside commode

1. Time bowel program to occur 20 to 30 minutes after eating a meal or at least drinking some warm fluid.
2. Begin program by inserting a well lubricated suppository past the external and internal anal sphincters.
3. 0 to 20 minutes after inserting suppository, transfer patient to commode or toilet (unless the program is to be done in bed).
4. At 15-minute intervals starting approximately 30 minutes after suppository insertion, perform rectal massage or digital stimulation. This is done by gently inserting a well-lubricated gloved finger into the anal canal. Then using a gentle cicular motion the rectal wall is stretched to help stimulate the defecation reflex. The rectal stretching must be done gently and slowly to prevent trauma and to allow enough stimuliu for the reflex emptying to occur.

Figure 38–11. Classic bowel training program.

scissors, the stool emptied, and the end of the pouch resealed with a plastic clamp.

Diapers are considered appropriate management for the nontoilet-trained infant or child. Protective pants, called incontinent briefs, are sometimes used to contain intractable fecal incontinence in the adult.

Stoma Management

Stoma management is a group of nursing interventions that may be necessary after fecal diversion. Nursing responsibilities for patients with stomas include stoma assessment, and management of feces collection via an ostomy appliance or through stoma irrigation. Many hospitals have enterostomal therapists, nurses with specialized training, to assist patients and support other nurses in the care of patients' fecal diversions.

Stoma Assessment. After surgery, the stoma and abdominal incision may be covered with a sterile dressing. When the dressing is removed or when changing appliances over the stoma, the nurse should assess the stoma for color and position. The stoma should exhibit a healthy pink color; a dusky pink color or cyanosis can indicate an absence of adequate circulation to the stoma. The stoma must remain pink and healthy to function properly. The stomal mucosa must remain on the abdominal surface. If the stoma retracts, there is potential for feces entering the abdominal cavity and causing peritonitis. The stoma should also be inspected for bleeding and drainage.

Management of Feces Collection. Patients with ileostomies and colostomies that continuously drain liquid stool will need an ostomy appliance over the stoma at all times. A large selection of ostomy appliances is available (Fig. 38-12). Usually when the enterostomal therapist visits a new ostomy patient, he or she inspects the condition of the stoma and discusses the alternatives for feces collection. The diameter of the stoma must be measured accurately for an appliance with the correctly sized opening to obtain proper fit. An opening that is too small may constrict the stoma and be a source of inadequate circulation, whereas an opening that is too large will allow stool to leak onto the abdominal skin. The enzymatic juices contained in the liquid stool will cause maceration and eventual skin breakdown.

The back surface of the ostomy appliance contains a

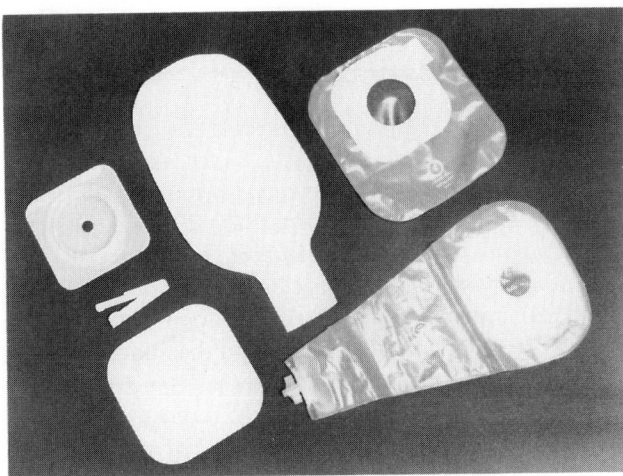

Figure 38–12.   Ostomy appliances.

sticky substance that will adhere to the abdominal skin. The appliance is usually also taped for extra security.

The ostomy bag should be emptied of fecal contents when it is about one-fourth to one-third full. If the bag is permitted to become too full, the weight of fecal contents will disrupt the seal of the ostomy appliance, causing leakage of stool. The odor of the stool may be strong and offensive, especially to a new ostomate. The nurse can spray a deodorant in the room before emptying the pouch. Alternatively, the nurse can spray a fragrance on gauze 4 × 4 pads and let the patient sniff the gauze at his or her discretion (Alterescu, 1985). The bag has an opening secured by a clip or rubber band. The clip or band is removed and the bag is opened over the toilet. The appliance can also be emptied into a bedpan or other collecting device laid on the bed if the patient is unable to get out of bed. As with all procedures in which the nurse will handle feces, disposable gloves must be worn. The emptying of an ostomy appliance is a clean, not a sterile procedure. The bag should be rinsed with clean, warm tap water after emptying. A large (60 mL) syringe works well for this purpose. Air is eliminated by compression of the bag and the clip or rubber band is reapplied to close the bag. The bag is checked for leaks from the stomal area and the condition of the stoma is assessed. If the ostomy appliance leaks fecal contents where it is attached to the skin, the entire bag will need to be removed and replaced. The nurse cleanses the abdominal skin surrounding the stoma, inspects the stoma's appearance, dries the abdominal skin, and applies a new ostomy appliance (see Procedure 38-4, "Applying a Fecal Ostomy Pouch").

If the ostomy is continuously draining fecal material, changing the bag will need to be quick and well-planned. A sterile or clean gauze 4 × 4 pad may need to be placed temporarily over the stoma to collect a small amount of fecal contents as the skin is dried and the new bag is

placed. The 4 × 4 must be removed before the bottom of the bag is clipped shut.

Stomal Irrigation. Bowel training to achieve a predictable evacuation of stool from a sigmoid colostomy can be assisted by stomal irrigation, as the bowel can be trained to evacuate feces only at times of irrigation. Stomal irrigation is similar to giving a large-volume enema through the stomal opening instead of through the anus. More specialized equipment is necessary, but the principle of instilling fluid into the colon to cause distention and a resultant elimination of feces is the same. See Procedure 38-5, "Irrigating a Colostomy," for specific guidelines. The evacuation of the colon at predictable times allows the ostomate a sense of control over his or her body and environment. Patients with sigmoidostomies who have achieved reliable bowel training may be able to eliminate the continuous use of a fecal collection pouch. They can wear a specialized covering over the stoma between bowel evacuations to protect it from clothing irritation.

Because a stomal irrigation is essentially an enema, it can be administered to relieve constipation or as a method of bowel cleansing before diagnostic procedures or tests.

Discharge Planning and Home Care

A patient is assessed on admission for any contributing factors that place him or her at high risk for alterations in bowel elimination. During the course of hospitalization, nursing measures to prevent potential bowel problems are instituted. Teaching that helps the patient to prevent bowel alterations during and after hospitalization is begun as soon as the patient's condition permits. Whenever a patient is admitted for problems in bowel elimination or has experienced an alteration in bowel elimination during hospitalization, planning for home management and prevention of future problems is even more important. The goals of discharge planning are effective patient teaching and the initiation of contacts with community resources when appropriate.

To develop a teaching plan that will meet the patient's unique needs, the nurse needs to consider factors in the patient's home environment that could hinder compliance. Does the patient have adequate access to toilet facilities? If the patient has to use a walker or wheelchair for mobility, will these devices fit through the bathroom doorway? Are there any steps that need to be negotiated to get to the bathroom? Is there someone available to assist the person to the bathroom or with special interventions such as enema administration? Sometimes the use of a bedside commode at home can be helpful in preventing fecal incontinence for a person with mobility or access problems.

(Text continues on page 1129)

PROCEDURE 38–4. Applying a Fecal Ostomy Pouch

■ Purpose
1. Contains drainage and odors for the comfort of the patient and allows accurate assessment of output during hospitalization.
2. Protects the peristomal skin from excoriation.
3. Provides visualization of the stoma and sutures during the postoperative period.

■ Assessment
- Observe color and amount of drainage from stoma.
- Assess existing bag for leakage and note appearance of stoma and incision to determine need to change pouch. Pouches do not have to be changed if not leaking and if the skin barrier is intact.
- Inspect condition of peristomal skin for erythema, excoriation, ulceration, or fistulas before selecting type of skin barrier to apply.
- Note presence of skin folds, creases, scars, and abdominal softness or firmness before selection of pouch.
- Enterostomal therapy specialists are available for consultation at many hospitals to assist in the assessment and planning of ostomy care.

■ Equipment
A clean, drainable pouch and clamp.
Skin barrier.
Warm water, wash cloth and towel, skin cleanser or mild soap.
Plastic bag in which to dispose old pouch.
Hypoallergenic paper tape.
Disposable gloves.

■ Procedure
1. Close curtains around bed or close door to patient room.
   Rationale: Provides privacy.
2. Explain procedure to the patient.
3. Don disposable gloves. Gently remove old appliance. If disposable, discard. If reusable, set aside for washing.
4. Wash skin thoroughly around stoma with skin cleanser or soap and water.
   Rationale: Bacteria in the fecal secretions can cause infection in the incisional area, as well as irritate the skin.
5. Rinse skin thoroughly and blot dry.
   Rationale: Soap residue or dampness can interfere with pouch adhesion, resulting in leakage. Blotting the area dry minimizes trauma to the stoma.
6. Observe condition of peristomal skin, the stoma, and the sutures. Teach the patient to make these observations daily.

Rationale: Allows for monitoring for complications. The stoma is at risk for necrosis during the first postoperative week, as evidenced by dark, dry color and lack of bleeding. The peristomal skin is at risk for breakdown from irritating fecal secretions and infection is more easily corrected if detected early.

7. Prepare clean pouch: Measure stoma and trace circle 1/8-inch larger than stoma on the adhesive paper backing. Cut the stoma pattern.
   Rationale: Pattern cut slightly larger than barrier avoids risk of paper cuts to stoma and ensures a tight seal with the barrier.
8. Prepare skin barrier: Measure stoma and cut hole in barrier the same size as the stoma. Be sure edges are rounded.
   Rationale: Close fit of barrier around stoma prevents fecal secretions from contacting and irritating the skin.
9. If stoma is located in an abdominal crease or the skin is irregular, use a paste barrier to fill the irregularity.
   Rationale: Minimizes leakage by providing a smooth surface for applying the skin barrier.
10. Remove paper backing from the pouch adhesive faceplate. Center and apply the nonadhesive side of the barrier over skin.
    Rationale: Provides a tighter, leakproof seal by reducing the wrinkling that can occur if the pouch is applied alone.
11. Remove paper backing from the barrier. Center the barrier/pouch unit over the stoma and apply, smoothing out from the center.
12. "Picture frame" the faceplate with hypoallergenic tape.
    Rationale: Provides extra reinforcement against leakage.
13. Fold over bottom edge of pouch and clamp.
14. Dispose of old appliance. Clean and store any reusable supplies.
15. Wash hands.
16. Document noted observations.

■ Lifespan Considerations
- The very young and the elderly often are not able to perform their own ostomy care. Any patient who is not able to change his or her pouch independently should have a family member instructed in this procedure.
- Postoperative necrosis of the stoma occurs more commonly in obese patients. The physician should be notified immediately if this is seen.

(continued)

PROCEDURE 38–4. Applying a Fecal Ostomy Pouch *(continued)*

- New ostomy patients often experience the stages of grief as they try to adjust to their new body image. Good nurse–patient communication is essential to help the patient develop a positive attitude about living with an ostomy.
- Young children and infants adjust more readily to lifestyle changes from ostomies than do adolescents and adults.

■ Home Care Modifications
- Patients should have the name and phone number of an enterostomal therapist, community support groups, or other resource people to call if they have questions or problems after discharge.

PROCEDURE 38–5. Irrigating a Colostomy

■ Purpose
1. Regulates the time of evacuation of stool from the colon if the colostomy is in the sigmoid or descending position.
2. Cleanses the colon before a procedure or surgery.

■ Assessment
- Assess permanence of colostomy and location along the large intestine.
- Complete abdominal assessment. Palpate abdomen for distention. Auscultate for bowel sounds.
- Assess current frequency and character of stool. Assess bowel habits prior to surgery.
- Assess stoma for complications (i.e., prolapsed stoma, peristomal hernia).
- Assess patients' mental status, their understanding of the procedure, and their ability to learn to perform the procedure.
- Assess patients' manual dexterity and physical ability to tolerate sitting upright for long periods of time.

■ Equipment
Irrigating catheter with cone.
Water container, warm water.
Irrigating sleeve with belt.
Water-soluble lubricant.
Personal care items.
New appliance and skin barrier.
Clean, disposable gloves.

■ Procedure
1. Prepare patient by explaining procedure.
2. Plan appropriate time for procedure. (Approximately 1 hour after a meal, when patient will be uninterrupted for 45 minutes.)
   Rationale: Coordinate irrigation with normal time of duodenocolic reflex after meals.
3. Assist position to comfortable position. If ambulatory, have patient sit on toilet. If on bedrest, have patient lie on side.
4. Close bathroom door or bed curtains.
   Rationale: Provides privacy and encourages patient relaxation and cooperation.
5. Don gloves.
   Rationale: Gloves prevent exposure from body substances.
6. Remove and dispose of used pouch. Clean stoma and surrounding skin with warm water and soft cloth.
7. Apply irrigating sleeve. Place sleeve into toilet. If procedure is done in bed, place sleeve in bedpan.
8. Fill container with 500 to 1000 mL warm water (105 to 110° F).
   Rationale: 500 to 1000 mL water is needed to distend the colon sufficiently to trigger peristalsis. Cold water may cause cramping; hot water could damage the mucosa.
9. Connect cone to irrigating tube and run water through entire legnth of tubing.
   Rationale: Flushes air from the tubing.
10. Apply water-soluble lubricant to cone tip.
    Rationale: Prevents trauma to the stoma.

(continued)

PROCEDURE 38–5. Irrigating a Colostomy *(continued)*

11. Insert cone firmly into stoma toward direction of bowel lumen. Stoma may have to be digitally inspected with a gloved, lubricated finger before irrigation to determine direction of bowel lumen. *Rationale: The stoma is easily traumatized. Inserting cone toward bowel facilitates introduction of the irrigating solution.*

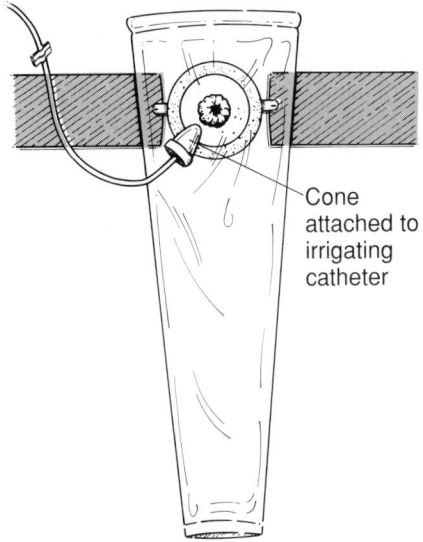

Cone attached to irrigating catheter

Step 11

12. Slowly begin flow of water into stoma, readjust position of cone gently with increasing firmness until there is no leakage around cone. *Rationale: A tight seal is necessary to sufficiently distend the bowel with water to stimulate peristalsis and bowel evacuation.*

13. Adjust height of water container to deliver 1000 mL water in 10 to 15 minutes. The bottom of the container should be even with the patient's shoulder if he or she is in sitting position. If patient complains of cramps, slow or temporarily stop infusion without removing cone. *Rationale: Too rapid instillation can result in cramping, weakness, vertigo, or syncope.*

14. Clamp tubing and remove cone, closing top of sleeve. Small gush of fluid should return into sleeve followed by intermittent spurts. If return is slow, pour warm water over stoma, massage abdomen, or have patient drink a warm liquid. *Rationale: Once bowel is sufficiently distended to stimulate defecation, contraction of muscles with peristalsis should result in intermittent spurts of fluid and feces.*

15. When majority of feces and water have been evacuated, dry and seal bottom of sleeve. Small amounts of fecal return may continue for another 20 to 45 minutes.

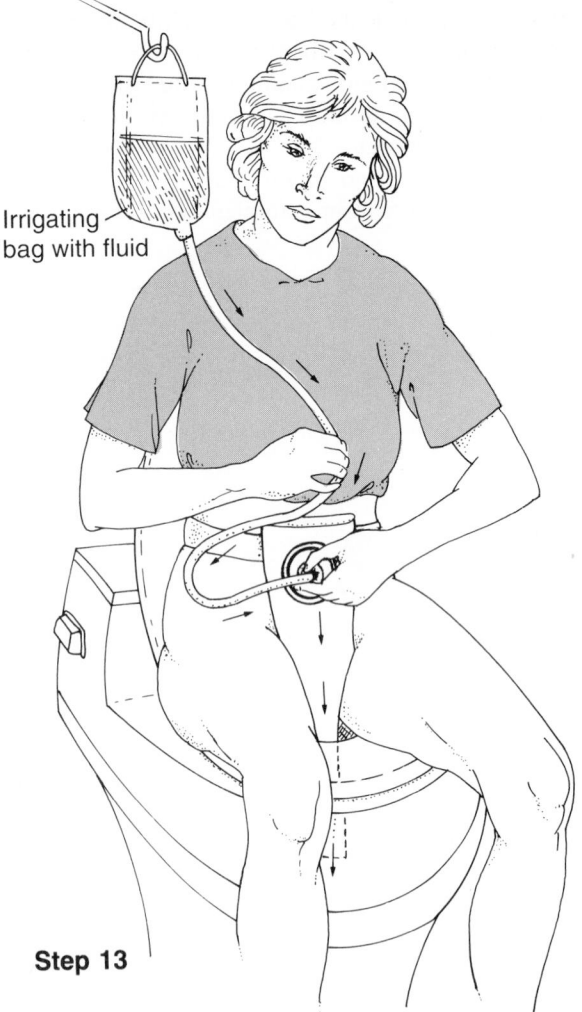

Irrigating bag with fluid

Step 13

Rationale: Wearing closed sleeve allows patient to ambulate while preventing leakage.

16. Remove and dispose of gloves, but reglove before beginning following steps.

17. When bowel evacuation has ceased, remove sleeve and set aside for cleansing.

18. Clean stoma and skin with warm water.

19. Apply skin barrier and new pouch.

20. Rinse sleeve with soap and water. Air dry. *Rationale: Some sleeves are disposable, but most are intended for reuse.*

21. Remove and dispose of gloves.

■ Lifespan Considerations

- Infants and children must have physician orders to determine when to irrigate and amount of irrigant.

■ Home Care Modifications

- Bowel training can take weeks to months. It is easy for the patient and family to grow discouraged with the process. Long-term support from a home health nursing service may be required.

The nurse should assess hindrances to the acquisition or preparation of foods necessary to prevent constipation. Will someone be able to help in food preparation? Does the person have questions about the types of foods to be encouraged or avoided to prevent constipation? Writing a list to guide food choices at home or consulting the hospital dietitian may be necessary.

Are there any financial constraints? Does the patient have health insurance and does it cover the necessary medications or special equipment? If the assessment notes potential problems with financial or social support resources, consultation with the hospital social worker should occur as soon as possible after the patient's admission. The social worker is knowledgeable about the many community agencies available for assistance, and can begin making contacts with the community agencies that will best meet the patient's unique needs after discharge.

Patients or their families may need assistance and advice in the management of specialized equipment and techniques. New ostomates and patients at high risk for fecal incontinence will especially need assistance in the home management of their bowel alterations. Enterostomal therapists are often responsible for the majority of patient teaching of new ostomates; however, the nurse must reinforce the concepts of stoma management and be available to answer questions.

The patient can be referred to ostomy organizations within the community. A member of an ostomy organization, who also has an ostomy and has satisfactorily adjusted to the necessary lifestyle changes, will visit the new ostomy patient. The first visit can be arranged before hospital discharge or can occur when the patient is at home. The "old" ostomate can be a source of support and advice for the "new" ostomate.

Home health nurses visit patients in their homes on a routine basis to assess progress in the management of their health-care problems. These nurses can be associated with the discharging hospital, but more likely are associated with a city or county health agency, or with an independent home health-care agency. The hospital-based nurse should be involved in the decision to make referrals to community agencies and in the communication of nursing care needs to the home-care agency.

The home health-care nurse evaluates the patient's progress, assesses for signs and symptoms of any deteriorating condition requiring physician referral or hospitalization, and continues to provide individualized client teaching and emotional support.

EVALUATION

Specific outcome criteria are the evaluative tools used to measure the attainment of patient goals. Nursing interventions are the management tools used to achieve the goals. Examples of outcome criteria are listed below.

Note that some criteria are appropriate for more than one goal; it is important to identify specific outcome criteria that will most uniquely measure the attainment of the individual patient's goal.

Goal
The patient will demonstrate a normal pattern of bowel elimination without evidence of constipation, diarrhea, fecal incontinence, or abdominal distention.

Possible Outcome Criteria
- Patient has a bowel movement within 24 hours and then every other day.
- Patient has a decrease in loose stools from four to five per day to one to two per day within 2 days.
- Patient demonstrates a stool consistency changing from liquid to semi-soft within 24 hours.
- Patient has a bowel movement every morning after suppository and digital stimulation.
- Patient expels flatus rectally when gas pains are present.
- The abdomen appears flat and nondistended.
- The patient has an absence of hardened stool in rectum on digital examination within 2 days.

Goal
The patient will have an absence of preventable complications or adverse consequences from altered bowel elimination.

Possible Outcome Criteria
- The perianal skin remains intact throughout hospital stay.
- The patient verbalizes that he or she is exhaling properly during defecation after instruction.
- The patient washes hands after bowel movements during hospitalization.
- The patient expresses satisfaction with success of bowel training program within 1 week.
- The patient demonstrates normal bowel sounds present in all four quadrants within 2 days.

Goal
The patient will participate in a program to maintain and promote an acceptable pattern of bowel elimination.

Possible Outcome Criteria
- The patient demonstrates softly formed, brown stool approximately every 1 to 2 days.
- The patient verbalizes that he or she eats bran muffin or bran cereal every day at next appointment.
- The patient performs effective relaxation technique at next appointment.
- The patient requests assistance to toilet at scheduled time during the day.
- The patient drinks 1500 mL of fluid per day, as evidenced on chart each day.

Nursing Diagnosis: Constipation related to immobility manifested by straining and inability to pass stool for 3 days.

Patient Goal: Patient will demonstrate a normal pattern of bowel elimination.

Patient Outcome Criteria

- Patient has a formed brown stool within 24 hours and every 1 to 2 days during hospitalization.

Nursing Intervention	Scientific Rationale
1. Notify dietary to increase high fiber foods in patient's meals.	1. High fiber foods increase the amount of bulk in the lower gastrointestinal tract and results in softer, easier to eliminate stools.
2. Increase fluid intake to 2000 mL/day.	2. A fluid intake of 2000 mL in 24 hours is necessary to promote the formation of soft stools.
3. Assist patient to ambulate (within medically prescribed guidelines) at least or three times daily.	3. Increased physical activity promotes increased gastrointestinal motility.
4. Assist patient to bedside commode or toilet. Fit commode or toilet with raised seat if needed.	4. The sitting position promotes a more physiological position for bowel elimination. A raised seat may be necessary to assist the patient with sitting.
5. Provide privacy but do not compromise patient safety.	5. Many people require a degree of privacy during bowel elimination.
6. Inspect patient's abdomen and auscultate for bowel sounds every shift.	6. To provide essential data for assessment of bowel elimination status.
7. Administer stool softeners and laxatives as necessary per bowel management program.	7. Daily administration of stool softeners can prevent constipation for patients in high risk groups. Laxatives can stimulate the evacuation of bowel contents on an as needed basis.
8. Record patient's bowel movements in the patient's record.	8. To provide essential data about patient's current bowel elimination pattern.

Patient Goal: Patient will participate in a program to maintain and promote an acceptable pattern of bowel elimination.

Patient Outcome Criteria

- Within 24 hours, patient states at least three methods to be used to promote a normal bowel elimination pattern.

Nursing Intervention	Scientific Rationale
1. Plan bowel management program.	1. Patient's current problem of constipation and her restricted mobility place her at high risk for further constipation.
2. Teach patient about methods to promote normal bowel elimination: high fiber diet; increased fluid intake; increased physical activity; avoiding denial of defecation reflex; use of stool softeners; sitting position for bowel movements.	2. Increased knowledge leads to increased compliance and more successful outcomes.
3. Plan with patient for daily routine after discharge with respect to bowel elimination. Discuss patient's likes/dislikes/intolerances of high fiber foods and types of fluids. Discuss plans for physical activity within medically prescribed restrictions.	3. Individualized plan promotes compliance and successful outcomes.

- The patient demonstrates correct stoma pouch application by discharge.

Evaluation includes assessing the patient and comparing the patient's current condition to the established outcome criteria as a measure of goal attainment. Continuation, modification, or termination of the nursing plan of care is implemented based on the systematic evaluation of patient progress.

Key Concepts

- The formation of feces, the solid waste product of digestion, occurs in the large intestine.
- Defecation, the process of eliminating feces from the body, is initiated by reflexes in response to intestinal distention.
- Defecation is under voluntary neural control.
- Many lifestyle habits influence the stool consistency and the pattern of bowel elimination.
- Physiologic alterations of the intestines can adversely affect bowel elimination.
- The manifestations of altered bowel elimination are constipation, impaction, diarrhea, incontinence, flatulence, and abdominal distention.
- The characteristics of feces and bowel elimination patterns change during the lifespan.
- A focused nursing assessment of bowel elimination includes patient history, inspection of stool characteristics, and physical examination of the abdomen and perirectal area.
- The nurse has collaborative responsibilities in laboratory examination of the feces and other diagnostic procedures.
- The nurse can diagnose and collaboratively treat altered bowel elimination.
- Nursing care of patients with identified alterations in bowel elimination is designed to:
  - Relieve alterations in bowel elimination.
  - Prevent complications that can be caused by alterations in bowel elimination.
  - Promote an acceptable pattern of bowel elimination.
- Nursing actions in the care of persons with altered bowel elimination are independent and collaborative.
- Altered bowel elimination can be a source of physiologic, psychological, and social distress.
- Discharge planning considers the home environment and the unique learning needs of the patient and family.
- Continuation, modification, or termination of nursing strategies is based on systematic evaluation of patient response to therapy.

References

Alterescu, V. (1986). Theoretical foundations for an approach to fecal incontinence. *Journal of Enterostomal Therapy, 13,* 44–48.
Brown, M. K., et al. (1990). Gentler bowel fitness with fiber. *Geriatric Nurse, 11*(1), 26–27.
Carpenito, L. J. (1989). *Nursing Diagnosis: Application to Clinical Practice* (3rd ed.). Philadelphia: J. B. Lippincott.
Ganong, W. F. (1989). *Review of Medical Physiology* (14th ed.). Los Altos, CA: Lange Medical Publications.
Guyton, A. C. (1987). *Human Physiology and Mechanisms of Disease* (4th ed.). Philadelphia: W. B. Saunders.
Heitkemper, M., & Brubacher, L. (1986). Nursing strategies for common gastrointestinal problems. In M. Patrick, M. L., Woods, S. L., Craven, R. C., et al. (Eds.), *Medical–Surgical Nursing: Pathophysiological Concepts.* Philadelphia: J. B. Lippincott.
Hyams, J., & Leichter, A. (1985). Apple juice: An unappreciated cause of chronic diarrhea. *American Journal of Diseases of Children, 139,* 503–505.
Mathewson, M. (1991). *Pharmacotherapeutics: A Nursing Process Approach* (2nd ed.). Philadelphia: F. A. Davis.
Mowlan, V., North, K., Myer, C. (1986). Managing fecal incontinence. *Nursing Times, 82*(48), 55–59.
NANDA (1990). *Taxonomy I revised 1990, with official nursing diagnoses.* St. Louis, MO: North American Nursing Diagnosis Association.
Nurse's Drug Alert. (1987). *The Nurses' Handbook of Drug Alerts and Clinical Implications.* New York: M. J. Powers.
Rolstad, B. S. (1986). Ileoanal reservoir: An overview for patients. *Ostomy Quarterly, 23,* 81–83.
Watt, R. C. (1985). Why is it created? *American Journal of Nursing, 85,* 1241–1245.

Bibliography

Alterescu, K. B. (1985). What about special procedures? *American Journal of Nursing, 85,* 1363–1367.
Alterescu, V. (1985). What do you teach the patient? *American Journal of Nursing, 85,* 1250–1253.
Anderson, B. J. (1986). Tube feeding: Is diarrhea inevitable? *American Journal of Nursing, 86,* 704–706.
Avoiding enema-related colonic necrosis. (1990). *Nurse's Drug Alert, 14*(4), 25.
Bayless, T. M., et al. (1988). Help your IBD patient help himself . . . effects of inflammatory bowel disease. *Patient Care, 22*(16), 139–141, 144, 146–148.
Becker, K. L., & Stevens, S. A. (1988). Performing in-depth abdominal assessment. *Nursing 88, 18*(6), 59–63.
Beller, L. C., & Neunaber, K. L. (1986). The "simple" valsalva maneuver. *American Journal of Nursing, 86*(4), 398.
Byrne, C. J., Saxton, D. F., Pelikan, P. K., et al. (1986). *Laboratory Tests: Implications for Nurses and Allied Health Professionals* (2nd ed.). Menlo Park: Addison-Wesley.
Calandrino, C. (1989). Barium enema procedure for the pediatric patient. *Radiologic Technology, 60*(3), 209–214.
Church, J. M. (1986). The current status of the Kock Continent Ileostomy. *Ostomy/Wound Management, 4,* 32–35.
Clarke B. (1989). Making sense of . . . bowel preparation for diagnostic procedures. *Nursing Times, 85*(5), 46–47.
DeSantis, L. (1988). Cultural factors affecting newborn and infant diarrhea. *Journal of Pediatric Nursing, 3*(6), 391–398.
Doering, K. J., & LaMountain, P. (1984). Flowchart to facilitate caring for ostomy patients. Part 1: Preop assessment. *Nursing 84, 14,* 54.
Edes, T. E., et al. (1990). Diarrhea in tube-fed patients: Feeding formula not necessarily the cause. *American Journal of Medicine, 88*(2), 91–93.
Ellickson, E. B. (1988). Bowel management plan for the homebound elderly. *Journal of Gerontological Nursing, 14,* 16–19.
Englert, D. M., & Guillory, J. A. (1986). For want of lactase. *American Journal of Nursing, 86*(8), 902–906.
Ewing, G. (1989). The nursing preparation of stoma patients for self-care. *Journal of Advanced Nursing, 14,* 411–420.

Fischbach, F. (1988). *A Manual of Laboratory Diagnostic Tests* (3rd ed.). Philadelphia: J. B. Lippincott.

Gastrointestinal disorders exam. (1989). *Journal of Practical Nursing, 39*(3), 39–47.

Gawron, C. L. (1989). Body image changes in the patient requiring ostomy revision. *Journal of Enterostomal Therapy, 16*(6), 256–263.

Gilligan, P. H. (1986). Diarrheal disease in the hospitalized patient. *Infection Control, 7,* 607–609.

Hu, T., et al. (1990). The cost effectiveness of disposable versus reusable diapers: A controlled experiment in a nursing home. *Journal of Gerontological Nursing, 16*(2), 19–24, 36–37.

Hoshiko, B. R. (1990). Valsalva maneuver as a possible risk factor for pulmonary embolism. *Orthopedic Nursing, 9*(1), 56–62.

Johns, C. (1985). Encopresis. *American Journal of Nursing, 85,* 153–156.

Kaltreider, D. L., et al. (1990). Can reminders curb incontinence? *Geriatric Nurse, 11*(1), 17–19.

Lewis, B. (1985). Streamlining the process of elimination. *American Journal of Nursing, 85,* 774.

Luz, et al. (1990). Ethnic differences in physiological responses associated with the Valsalva maneuver. *Research in Nursing and Health, 13*(1), 9–15.

McConnell, E. A. (1987). Meeting the challenge of intestinal obstruction. *Nursing 87, 17,* 34–41.

McConnell, E. A. (1990). Assessing abdominal pain in postoperative patient. *Nursing 90, 20*(3), 86–88.

McLane, A. M., et al. (1986). Empirical validation of defining characteristics of constipation: A study of bowel elimination practices of healthy adults. *Classification of Nursing Diagnosis, Proceedings of Sixth Conference,* 448–455.

Mezzanotte, E. J. (1987). A checklist for better discharge planning. *Nursing 87, 17,* 55.

Miller, J. (1985). Helping the aged manage bowel function. *Journal of Gerontological Nursing, 11,* 37–41.

Nornhold, P. (1986). Decreased cardiac output from valsalva maneuver. *Nursing 86, 16,* 33.

Quinless, F. W. (1988). Nurse's guide to successful bowel training. *Nursing 88, 18*(11), 32.

Resnick, B. (1985). Constipation: Common but preventable. *Geriatric Nurse, 6,* 213–215.

Rice, P. S., et al. (1989). Understanding idiopathic chronic constipation: An understated problem. *Gastroenterological Nursing, 12*(2), 90–97.

Rowland, M. A. (1989). When drug therapy causes diarrhea. *RN, 52*(12), 32–35.

Schroy, P. C., et al. (1988). Video endoscopy by nurse practitioners: A model for colorectal cancer screening. *Gastrointestinal Endoscopy, 34,* 390–394.

Shea, M., & McCreary, M. (1984). Early postop feeding. *American Journal of Nursing, 84,* 1230–1231.

Smith, C. E. (1988). Assessing bowel sounds: More than just listening. *Nursing 88, 18,* 42–43.

Smith, D. E. (1985). Detecting acute abdominal distention. *Nursing 85, 15*(9), 34–39.

Smith, M. J., Goodman, J. A., & Lockwood-Ramsey, N. L. (1987). *Child and Family: Concepts of Practice* (2nd ed.). New York: McGraw-Hill.

Stephany, T. (1988). Home care hospice bowel regimen. *Home Health Nurse, 6*(4), 40–41.

Thomas, D. W. (1989). Bloody diarrhea in children. *Gastroenterological Nursing, 12*(2), 100–103.

Whitehead, W. E., et al. (1989). Constipation in the elderly living at home: Definition, prevalence, and relationship to lifestyle and health status. *Journal of the American Geriatrics Society, 37,* 423–429.

Williams, S. G., et al. (1990). Constipation in the long-term facility. *Gastroenterological Nursing, 12*(3), 179–182.

VanderLaan, R., et al. (1989). The use of a programmatic approach by clinical nurse specialists to promote a change in clinical practice . . . in the area of bowel management. *Perspectives, 13*(4), 6–11.

UNIT X
Sleep and Rest

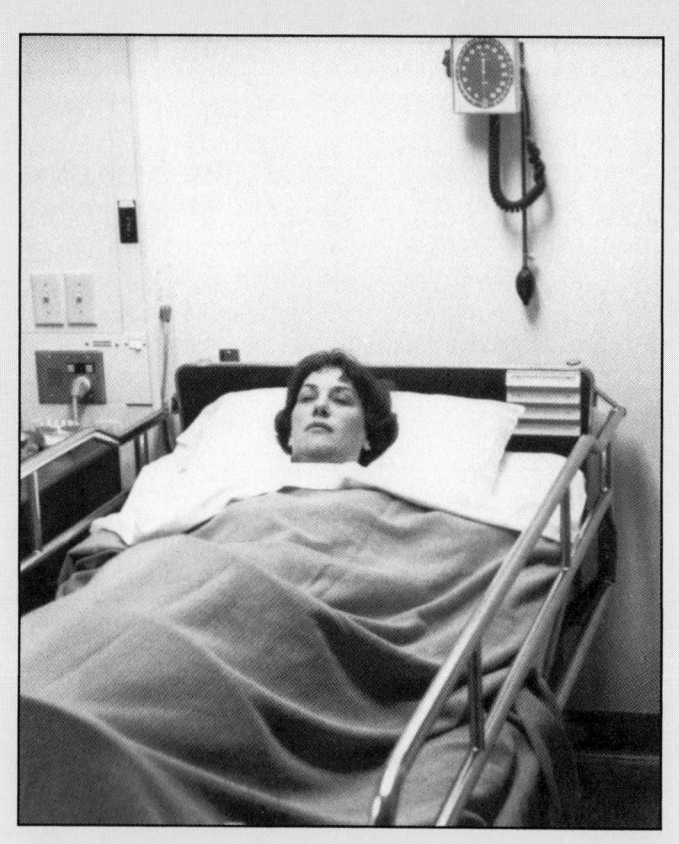

CHAPTERS

39 Sleep and Rest

U nit X examines the sleep and rest area of human function. It
is one that, for the most part, is taken for granted unless it
becomes problematic. Yet adequate rest, sleep, and relaxation are
essential for maintaining healthy function and critical for restoring
and supporting health. Additionally, it is an area of function that
presents patient needs for which nurses intervene on a daily basis.

The single chapter in this unit considers the principles and concepts surrounding sleep and rest. Normal sleep and rest function
varies greatly from patient to patient. Additionally, many patients
experience sleep pattern disturbances while in a health-care facility.
To help the patient adequately meet his or her sleep and rest needs,
it is essential for the nurse to carefully assess normal sleep patterns as
well as nighttime routines. In addition, nurses need to assist patients in
maintaining normal patterns of function whenever possible.

Using a nursing process format, this chapter explores nursing
interventions to promote health and function as well as the many
independent nursing interventions for sleep pattern disturbances.
Meeting patient's sleep and rest needs is essential for normal,
healthy function in all areas.

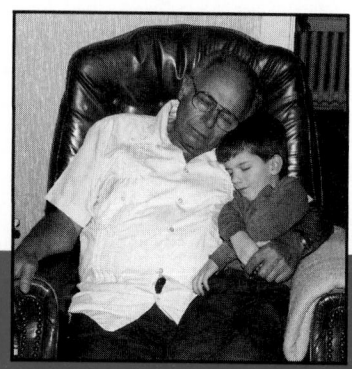

Sleep and Rest

LEARNING OBJECTIVES

Upon completion of this chapter, the student will be able to do the following:

- Describe the five stages of sleep.
- Identify factors that affect sleep and rest.
- Describe normal patterns of sleep and rest throughout the lifespan.
- Conduct an assessment interview regarding usual sleep patterns, risk for disturbance, and problems.
- Develop a daily schedule with a patient incorporating his or her unique needs and patterns for sleep and rest.
- Discuss interventions to promote rest and sleep.
- Develop a nursing care plan for a person with sleep pattern disturbance.

KEY TERMS

Circadian rhythms
Fatigue
Hormonal dysynchrony
Hypnotic
Insomnia
Narcolepsy

Nightmare
Night terrors
NREM sleep
Parasomnias
Rest
REM sleep
Sleep

Sleep apnea
Sleep deprivation
Sleep latency
Sleep–wake cycle
Sleepiness
Somnambulism

39

Normal Sleep/Rest Function
    Normal Physiologic Function
        Electrophysiologic Approach
        Neurotransmitter Balance
        Hormonal Approach
    Characteristics of Normal Sleep/Rest Function
        Awareness of Need
        Restoration and Protection
        Psychological Function
        Circadian Rhythm
    Normal Functional Sleep/Rest Pattern
    Factors Affecting Sleep and Rest
        External Stimuli
        Internal Stimuli
    Lifespan Considerations
Altered Sleep/Rest Function
    Potential for Altered Sleep Function
        Distractions
        Illness
        Drugs
        Mood States
    Manifestations of Altered Sleep Function
        Insomnia
        Narcolepsy
        Sleep Apnea
        Sleep-Related (Nocturnal) Myoclonus
        Altered Sleep–Wake Patterns
        Parasomnias
    Impact of Sleep Dysfunction on Activities of Daily
        Living

Assessment
    Subjective Data
        Functional Pattern Identification
        Risk Identification
        Dysfunctional Identification
    Objective Data
        Physical Assessment
        Diagnostic Tests
Nursing Diagnosis and Patient Goals
    Diagnostic Statement: Sleep Pattern Disturbance
        Definition
        Defining Characteristics
        Related Factors
    Related Nursing Diagnoses
    Patient Goals
Implementation
    Nursing Interventions to Promote Health and
        Sleep/Rest Function
        Minimal Stimuli
        Environment Modification
        Intimacy and Security
        Sleep Rituals
        Beliefs About Sleep
    Nursing Interventions for Altered Function
        Rest
        Judicious Use of Hypnotics
    Discharge Planning and Home Care
Evaluation
Key Concepts

One-third of human life is spent sleeping. Periods of rest may account for another major portion of the lifespan. However, the significance and mechanisms of this function remain largely a mystery. Sleep has long been assumed to have a restorative function, and until recently was thought to be a passive state of decreased stimulation. It is now known that active physiologic processes are involved. Sleep and rest are important in health and illness, although the relationships are not clearly understood.

NORMAL SLEEP/REST FUNCTION

Sleep is a naturally occurring altered state of consciousness characterized by decreased awareness and responsiveness to stimuli. It is distinguished from abnormal states of consciousness by being readily reversible. With **rest,** awareness of the environment is maintained but motor or cognitive response is decreased. Whereas sleep is a total body system phenomenon, the state of rest may involve the total system or only a part. Thus, the person

TABLE 39–1.

Characteristics of the Sleep Stages

Stage	Physiological Correlates	Biochemical Correlates	EEG	Dreaming	Sleep Disorders	Subjective Awareness	Rebound
1 Light	Muscle relaxation Rolling eye movements Respiration even ↓ pulse		Gradual loss of alpha waves			Floating Idle images If awakened, may say was not asleep	No
2 Transition to REM	Eyes may appear to roll		Bursts of sleep spindles Sharp slow waves			Awakens easily May report was thinking or daydreaming	No
3 Deep— slow-wave	Muscles very relaxed but tone maintained Respirations even	Growth hormone Serotonin	Delta (slow-wave) May show responses to outside stimuli but person not aware Spindles present	Less dramatic, more realistic May lack plot	Somnambulism Night terrors Enuresis	Requires stronger stimuli to waken	No
4 Deep— slow-wave	BP↓, T↓, P↓ ↓ urine secretion ↓O$_2$ consumption of muscle Snoring may occur						Yes, priority
REM	Lowest muscle tone Fasciculations ↑BP, ↑P, fluctuating respiration ↑vaginal secretion ↑cerebral blood flow ↑O$_2$ consumption	Episodic cortisol and ACTH Catecholamine	Desynchronized Extremely active Similar to wakefulness	Content vivid Full-color Auditory Implausible settings Frequently involve paralytic component	Nightmares	Difficult to awaken except with significant stimuli	Yes

sun-bathing on a beach during summer vacation may be experiencing a generalized state of rest associated with decreased mental and physical activity, whereas a person with an injured arm in a sling is resting that body part but otherwise may be relatively active mentally and physically.

Normal Physiologic Function

The physiology of sleep can be discussed in relation to three basic research approaches, each of which has provided building blocks for developing concepts relating to mechanisms and functions of sleep.

Electrophysiologic Approach

Polygraph recordings of electrophysiologic changes in brain waves (electroencephalogram), eye movements (electro-oculogram), and muscles (electromyogram) show five sleep stages. The first four stages are classified as **non-rapid eye movement (NREM) sleep,** in contrast to the other stage, REM or paradoxical sleep, in which rapid eye movement is characteristic (Table 39-1).

Stage 1. Stage 1 is the transitional stage between drowsiness and sleep, indicated by a shift from alpha waves to low-voltage, fast theta waves on the electroencephalogram (EEG). Muscles relax, respirations become even, and pulse decreases. This stage usually lasts only a few minutes, and, if awakened, the person may say he or she was not asleep.

Stage 2. Stage 2 is still a relatively light sleep from which the person is easily wakened. Bursts of sleep spindles appear on the EEG (Fig. 39-1). Rolling eye movements continue and snoring may occur.

Stages 3 and 4. Stages 3 and 4 constitute "deep" sleep, sometimes termed slow-wave sleep or delta sleep after characteristic waves seen on EEG (see Fig. 39-1). These two stages are differentiated primarily by the amount of delta waves, and are usually discussed together (Hauri, 1982). During slow-wave sleep the muscles are relaxed but tone is maintained, respirations are even, and blood pressure, pulse, and temperature decrease, as do formation of urine and oxygen consumption of muscle. These are the stages during which snor-

ing, sleepwalking (somnambulism), and bedwetting (enuresis) are most likely to occur. Stronger stimuli are required to awaken people during these stages. Dream content tends to be realistic and may be without plot; these are the dreams in which one drives to work or phones a friend, and, when awakened, wonders if it was really done!

REM Sleep. REM sleep closely resembles wakefulness except for very low muscle tone, indicated by a reduction in amplitude of the EMG (Fig. 39-2). The rapid eye movements from which it receives its name are documented through EOG recording, but may also be noted by careful observation of tiny eye movements detectable through the closed lids. The brain waves as recorded on EEG are similar to those of the awake state (see Fig. 39-1). Blood pressure and pulse rate show wide variations, and may fluctuate rapidly. Respirations are

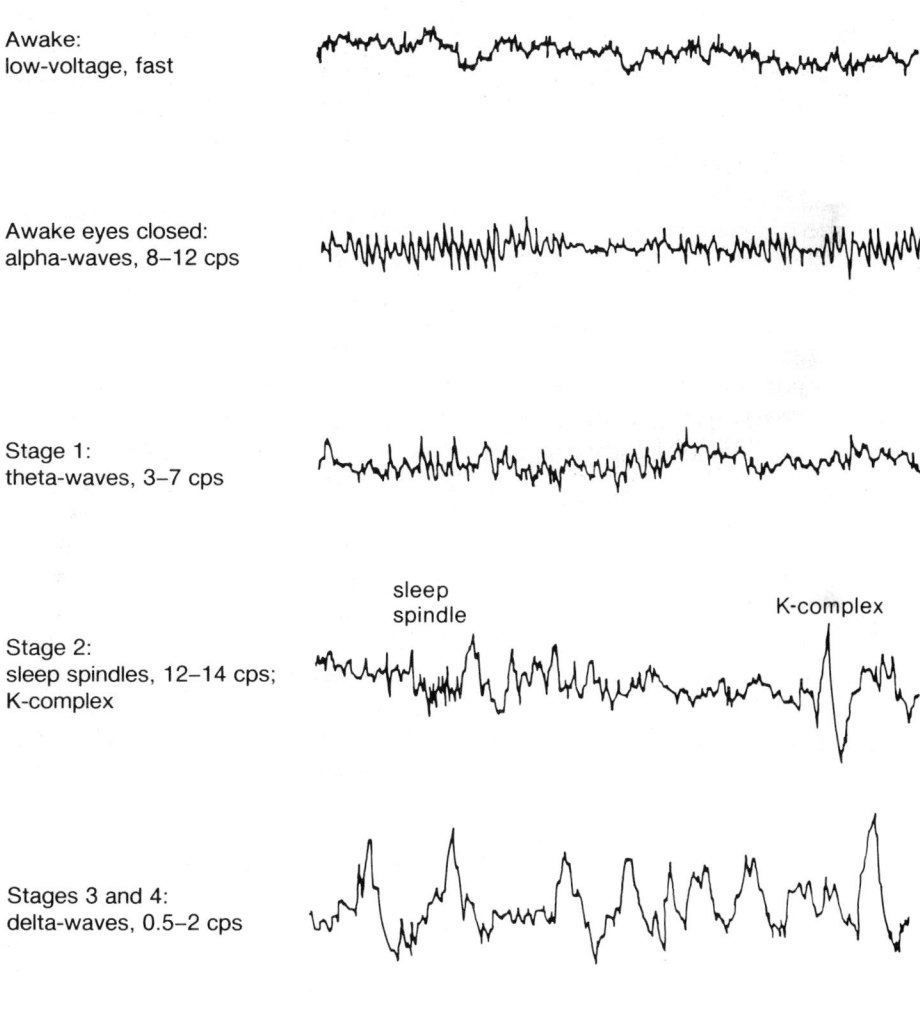

Awake: low-voltage, fast

Awake eyes closed: alpha-waves, 8–12 cps

Stage 1: theta-waves, 3–7 cps

Stage 2: sleep spindles, 12–14 cps; K-complex

Stages 3 and 4: delta-waves, 0.5–2 cps

REM: low-voltage mixed frequency sawtoothed waves

Figure 39–1. Characteristic electroencephalogram wave forms by sleep stage. (Courtesy University of Washington School of Nursing, Sleep Laboratory)

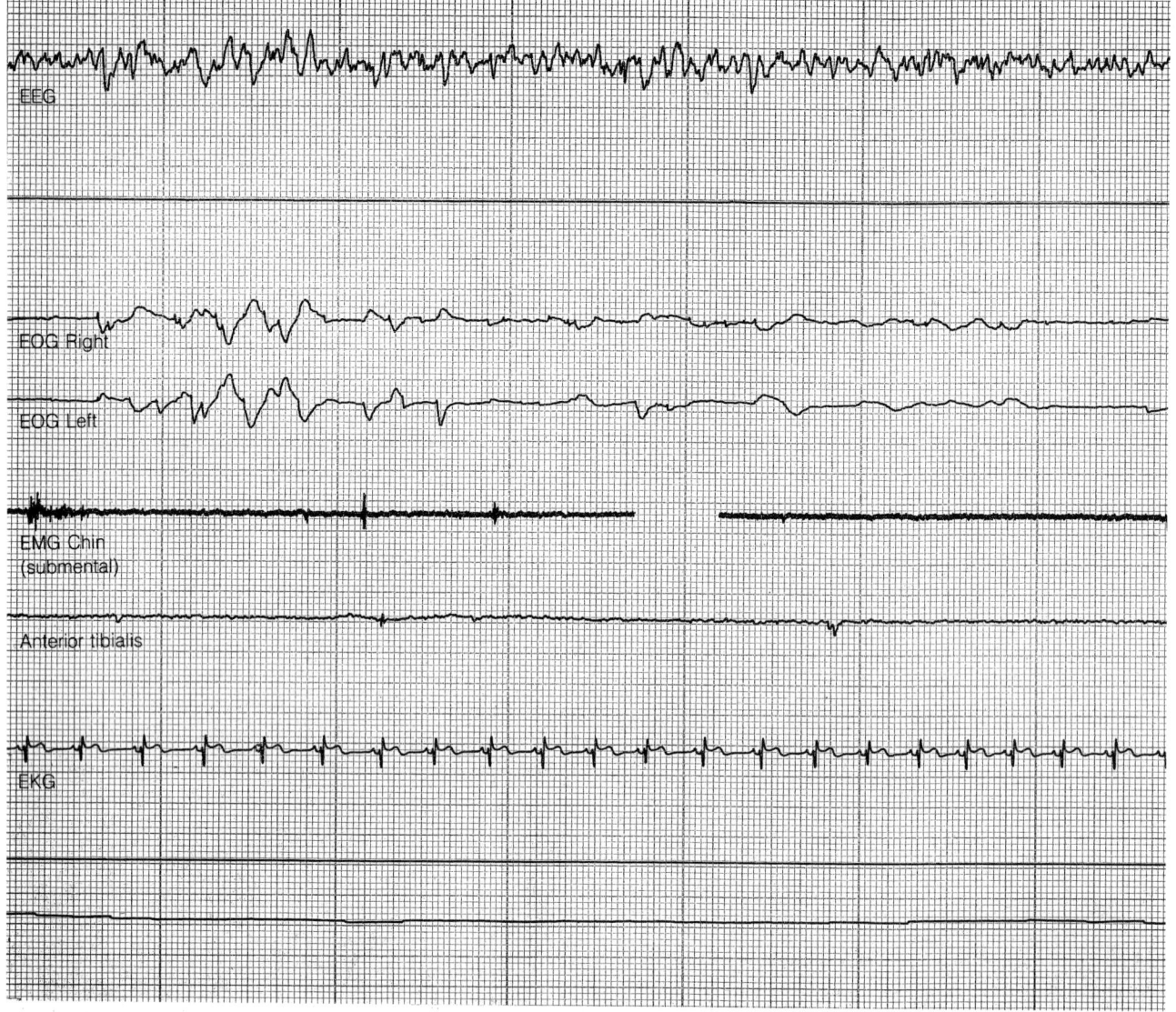

Figure 39–2.   REM sleep on polygraph recording. Note the rapid, low-amplitude waves on the EEG, eye movements on EOG, and minimal muscle activity on EMG. (Courtesy of Alberta Lung Association Sleep Centre, Calgary, Alberta, Canada.)

irregular and oxygen consumption increases. Thermoregulation is lost. Vaginal secretions increase in women and erections may occur in men. Dreams occurring during REM sleep tend to be vivid and implausible, often including a sense of being unable to move.

Sleep Rhythm. Electrophysiologic recordings of nocturnal sleep show a rhythmic pattern of approximately 90-minute cycles during which people progress in sequence through the sleep stages. The usual pattern is fairly rapid progression through stages 1 to 4 and then back through stages 3 and 2, from which REM is then entered (Fig. 39-3). During the early part of the night, periods of slow-wave sleep (stages 3 and 4) are longer. In contrast, the time spent in REM during the first cycle may be only 3 to 4 minutes, whereas toward morning it may be as much as 45 minutes, balanced with shorter periods of slow-wave sleep in which stage 4 may not be present. If awakening occurs, the cycle begins again with stage 1. If the awakening was brief, the tendency is to reenter the type of cycle from which the person was aroused. Thus, an early morning awakening may be followed by return to one or more cycles in which a high percentage of REM is present. In situations where REM deficiency is suspected it is therefore more helpful for the nurse to encourage persons to return to sleep immediately after an early awakening than to plan on napping in the afternoon.

Neurotransmitter Balance

Sleep is an active process involving the reticular activating system (RAS) and a dynamic interaction of neurotransmitters. The RAS consists of a network of interconnecting neurons in the medulla, pons, and midbrain, with projections to the spinal cord, hypothalamus, cerebellum, and cerebral cortex (Gilman & Newman, 1987). It literally fills in the spaces in the brain stem among the major tracts, bringing in sensory messages and relaying motor ones. Thus, it is in a strategic location for stimulation from a wide variety of inputs. The RAS includes the ascending facilitatory area, which is intrinsically active, and a less well understood bulbar inhibitory area, which appears to be particularly involved in decreasing muscle tone during REM sleep (Porth, 1990; Riley, 1985).

As with other parts of the nervous system, communication between neurons primarily involves the release of specific neurotransmitters from axon terminals and their attachment to specific receptors on other cells. Serotonin is a major neurotransmitter associated with sleep. Produced in the Raphe nuclei in the brain stem, this neurotransmitter is derived from its precursor, tryptophan, a naturally occurring amino acid. Serotonin is thought to decrease the activity of the RAS, thereby inducing and sustaining sleep. Another neurotransmitter, the catecholamine norepinephrine from the locus ceruleus (also in the brain stem), appears to be required for REM sleep. The role of acetylcholine and other neurotransmitters is less well understood (Robinson, 1986).

Hormonal Approach

Sleep–wake patterns appear to be affected by and to affect certain hormone levels. Melatonin from the pineal gland is secreted in enormous quantities during sleep. Its apparent rhythm-setting function seems to be closely related to darkness and light. It takes 2 weeks of altered sleep time before secretion of melatonin again matches with the sleep period. Adrenocorticotropic hormone (ACTH) secretion from the pituitary is high during the early part of the sleep period, and levels of cortisol, its target hormone from the adrenal cortex, rise toward the end of the nocturnal sleep period. This pattern also remains stable in relation to clock time in spite of variations in sleep time (e.g., shift work), unless these changes are sustained for up to 2 weeks.

Growth hormone and prolactin levels are closely tied to actual sleep time, changing immediately in relation to variations in the sleep period. Secretion of both hormones increases early in the sleep period.

The significance of this **hormonal dysynchrony,** in which hormonal levels adjust at different rates to alter-

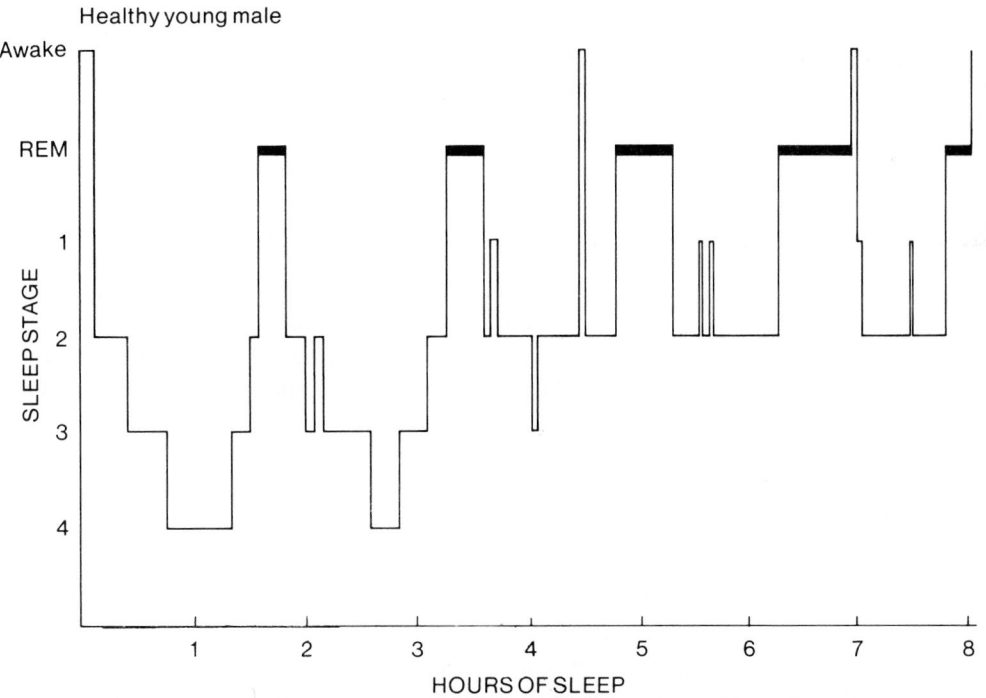

Figure 39–3.   Typical sequence of sleep stages in a young, healthy adult man. Progression occurs through a sequence of 1-2-3-4-3-2 and into REM. Note increased amount of REM sleep and absence of stage 4 towards end of sleep period. (Courtesy University of Washington School of Nursing, Sleep Laboratory)

ations in the timing of the sleep period, is not clearly understood, but is an important research area particularly in relation to shift work and jet travel.

Characteristics of Normal Sleep/Rest Function

Awareness of Need

Awareness of the need for sleep and rest is most commonly associated with the states of **sleepiness** and **fatigue.** These states often overlap. Sleepiness refers to an urge of varying intensity to go to sleep. It may occur in response to too little or too much sleep, or lack of adequate sensory stimulation. Fatigue is a subjective state of weariness in which physical activity is accompanied by intense or rapid tiring. It is a common human response to illness, suggesting the need to conserve energy through rest and sleep.

Restoration and Protection

Sleep and rest are believed to have restorative and protective functions. Adam and Oswald (1984), the leading proponents of the restorative theory, have provided research evidence that shifts in the hormonal balance facilitate physical restoration through the processes of anabolism (synthesis of cell constituents) during sleep. Horne (1980), on the other hand, suggests that the main purpose of sleep may be energy conservation for parts of the body other than the brain. Periods of physical and mental rest are known to reduce metabolic rate and the sense of fatigue.

Psychological Function

Psychological functions of sleep, as described by Gaarder and Chase (1971), are thought to include:

- Sorting and discarding of neurophysiologic data. Much of short-term memory is filled with inconsequential detail that is sifted through and discarded. A person can usually remember what was eaten for breakfast that day or how long the bus took to come, but a month later those data will probably be beyond recall (unless something special happened that day).
- Character reinforcement and adaptation. The REM stage of sleep in particular appears to be important for mental and emotional stability. Through REM dreaming a reprocessing of knowledge and memories is thought to occur. An increased need for REM sleep has been found in people experiencing stress, worry, or new learning situations.

Circadian Rhythm

Biologic rhythms that follow a cycle of about 24 hours are termed **circadian rhythms** from the Latin words *circa* (about) and *dies* (day) (Porth 1990). The **sleep–wake cycle** is an example, and is closely linked with other circadian rhythms such as body temperature. While a person sleeps, core body temperature drops, often reaching the 24-hour low around 4:00 AM. When the sleep period shifts, for instance when the person moves to another time zone, temperature fluctuations also shift to match the new sleeping patterns after a week or so. The superchiasmatic nucleus, located above the optic chiasm in the anterior hypothalamus, has been found to provide the "clock" for most circadian rhythms, including the sleep–wake cycle (Riley, 1985). It receives direct input from the retina regarding environmental cues as to darkness and light.

In situations where environmental cues to time are largely removed, circadian rhythms are maintained, but duration may extend to 25 or more hours and may become less synchronized. Experimental conditions typically involve controlled artificial light and removal of all indicators of time. Nurses are sometimes involved with people who have established life patterns in which environmental cues to time are decreased to the point at which erratic sleep and temperature cycles develop. People living alone without regular occupational or social contact are at risk. Although rare, some people have natural circadian rhythms extending to 50 hours or more (Wirz-Justice & Pringle, 1987).

Normal Functional Sleep/Rest Pattern

The well rested person is mentally alert, energetic, and spontaneous. Daytime activity, even of a monotonous nature, is maintained with a minimum of drowsiness.

The range of "normal" sleep duration is great. In a study using data from health questionnaires completed by over one million adult Americans, the most commonly reported usual sleep duration was 8.0 to 8.9 hours for both men and women of all ages (45%) (Kripke, et al., 1979). The next most common range was 7.0 to 7.9 hours (32%). An average of less than 6 hours per night was reported by 2% of the men and 3% of the women. Some 8.6% of men and 8.2% of women reported more than 9 hours.

Short sleepers, that is, those who sleep for less than 6 hours in 24, tend to be efficient, hardworking people. Winston Churchill required little nighttime sleep, relying instead on his ability to take brief but renewing naps. Long sleepers, that is, those who sleep for more than 9 hours in 24, have a higher percentage of REM sleep, and there is some suggestion that as a group they are more creative. Albert Einstein was a long sleeper.

The range of normality with respect to sleep patterns is also broad. Generally, most people require 10 to 30 minutes to fall asleep; this period of time required to fall asleep is called **sleep latency.** A regular sleep latency of less than 5 minutes suggests excessive sleepiness. Sleep latency of longer than 30 minutes may be accompanied by some sense of frustration with the time taken to get to sleep.

Changes of position during sleep typically occur 20 to 40 times during the night (DeKoninck, Gagnon, & Lallier, 1983). For people with impaired physical mobility, the normally unconscious act of changing positions during sleep may require awakening, conscious planning and effort, or the assistance of the bed partner or care provider. The institutional norm of turning patients every 2 hours scarcely meets the physiologic norm of natural position changes during sleep. Such simple interventions as the use of satin sheets have been found to help persons with impaired physical mobility turn more easily.

One to two awakenings per night are common for young adults; the frequency and duration of awakenings tends to increase with age. The final awakening is often spontaneous, even in North American society, where alarm clocks symbolize the precision of occupational and educational schedules. The well rested person generally awakens with a sense of refreshment and energy for the day.

Daytime naps and rest periods are infrequent among North American adults and older children, except as associated with illness, pregnancy, or "catching up" on a day off. In warmer climates, however, the midday rest period is a cultural expectation. Rest breaks in the more industrialized nations have tended to be associated with the use of stimulants such as the caffeine in coffee or the nicotine in cigarettes. The value of mini-rests in the form of stretching exercises, focusing thoughts or vision on a pleasant scene away from the work station, or going for a walk have been recognized more recently.

Factors Affecting Sleep and Rest

Need. The need for sleep and rest fluctuates according to developmental, individual, and situational variables. Developmental variables are discussed in the section on Lifespan Considerations. Individual variations occur in relation to total sleep need and in relation to preferred schedule. Numerous situational variables are superimposed on developmental considerations, need, and individual variables affecting sleep and rest patterns (Shaver & Giblin, 1989).

It has been hypothesized that humans may require less sleep than they have habitually (Horne, 1980). This concept of lower sleep need is supported by studies that have shown that students in the latter part of the 20th century

average 1.5 hours less sleep per day than their counterparts in 1910 (Hauri, 1982). The unresolved question is whether this represents less need for sleep or a chronic state of **sleep deprivation,** or lack of sleep.

It is important that people attune themselves to their own specific patterns rather than aiming for the mythical standard of 8 hours a night. As a general rule, the person who falls asleep fairly quickly on going to bed, awakens feeling refreshed, and functions with minimal daytime sleepiness can be assumed to be getting adequate sleep.

Individual variations also occur as to the preferred portion of the 24-hour period used for sleeping. Morning people are those who awaken early and easily, feel at their best in the early part of the day, and who prefer to retire early in the evening. Evening people find they function best later in the day, and are often wide awake and looking for activity late in the evening. Adjustments to variations in the timing of the sleep period, as occur with shift work, seem to be more readily tolerated by evening people (Floyd, 1984).

External Stimuli

Stimuli for Comfortable Sleep. Reduction of environmental stimuli, particularly light and noise, facilitates sleep. People vary in their sensitivity to different stimuli, and appear to vary in the intensity and degree of fluctuation of sensory input required. Some people seem to require a slight elevation of sensory input, sleeping better when surrounded by low-level noise such as a radio playing, after drinking coffee, or after exercising.

Bed Partner. Awakening or a lightening of sleep pattern often occurs when the bed partner changes position or snores. Presence of the habitual partner may provide a sense of security; absence of the habitual partner may be disturbing. As discussed in the next section, the nature, quality, and present state of the relationship may be factors that contribute to the effect of the presence or absence of the partner. For those who habitually sleep alone, the presence of another person may be disturbing.

Internal Stimuli

Nutritional Factors. Hunger disturbs the sleep of some people, whereas others have difficulty sleeping after a large meal. Ingestion of L-tryptophan, a precursor of serotonin found in protein foods such as milk, beef, eggs, wheat flour, and corn, has been found to decrease sleep latency and increase stage 4 sleep (Hartman, 1979). Sleep patterns tend to be disturbed during periods of either rapid weight loss or gain.

Elimination. The need to void is one of the most frequent internal stimuli to disturb sleep among the general population. Children can be assisted in establishing the habit of voiding as part of bedtime preparations. Limiting fluid intake after supper may decrease this nocturnal stimuli.

Exercise and Core Body Temperature. Current research suggests that habitual exercise contributes to deeper and longer sleep (Hauri, 1982, Montgomery, et al., 1982). In physically fit people, light-intensity exercise seems to decrease sleep latency and intensive exercise increases the proportion of slow-wave sleep (Horne & Staff, 1983). The basis for increased slow-wave sleep after vigorous exercise may be related to an increase in core body temperature. A daytime period of passive heating, as in a sauna or tub of warm water, has been shown to produce effects similar to those of vigorous exercise on the amount of slow-wave sleep (Horne & Staff, 1983). These findings suggest a promising area for nursing research regarding the value of a warm bath for enhancing the quality of sleep. The relationships between exercise and sleep are more complex than they may first appear, however. Contrary to what might be expected from the previous discussion, bedrest also increases slow-wave sleep by mechanisms not understood (Hauri, 1982).

Vigilance. Another factor affecting sleep is the perceived need to maintain vigilance. Parents and others in protective roles seem able to establish a variable noise threshold in which they may respond to the faintest sound of a toddler changing position in the next room, and yet sleep through a thunderstorm. Hospital patients, such as those recently disconnected from cardiac monitoring equipment, may deliberately prevent themselves from entering the deeper stages of sleep for fear of succumbing to a complication that might go unnoticed by nursing staff.

Lifestyle and Habits. Certain bedtime rituals become such a habitual part of preparation for sleep that to interfere with them is to interfere with sleep itself. Some rituals, such as a warm bath or a snack, may have a physiologic basis. The effectiveness of bedtime habits is also linked with decreasing arousal. Participation in a repetitive routine such as putting out the dog, winding the clock, and changing into night attire become associated with the expectation of sleep. These routines are disrupted during travel or hospitalization.

Lifestyle patterns influencing the sleep–wake schedule, such as time of rising, are closely linked with societal and occupational expectations. A regular time of rising is one of the most effective means of improving sleep quality and synchronizing circadian rhythms with clock time (Hauri, 1982). Toddlers who are having difficulty settling into a bedtime routine can be helped by maintaining an early and consistent rising time and being allowed to stay up in the evening until they are sleepy enough to

settle with quieting activities. Adults who have difficulty getting to sleep should also be encouraged to maintain a consistent rising time, going to bed later if necessary, rather than laying awake for long periods.

Lifespan Considerations

Developmental variations in sleep patterns are evident. Circadian rhythms develop in the first few months of life, are well established through childhood and adulthood, but gradually decrease with advancing age. The polyphasic two-to-one ratio of sleep to wakefulness characteristic of infants gradually shifts to the biphasic one-to-two ratio of adulthood.

Newborn and Infant

Two major sleep states can be observed in newborns. Quiet sleep is characterized by closed eyes, regular respirations, and absence of eye and body movements. Active sleep is manifested by eye movements observable through the closed lids, other body movements, and irregular respirations. Of the three waking states, quiet awake, active awake, and crying, quiet awake would seem to correspond to a state of rest in adults. Newborns sleep an average of 16 to 17 hours per day, divided into about seven sleep periods distributed fairly evenly day and night (Riley & Ferber, 1985).

Infants' sleep patterns differ from those of adults in that the sleep cycle is shorter (50 to 60 minutes), the proportion of active or REM sleep is higher (approximately 50%), and the initial stage is active rather than NREM (Keefe, 1987). Between 1 and 2 months of age, NREM sleep becomes differentiated into stages 1 to 4 (Riley & Ferber, 1985).

One of the infant's major adaptive tasks is to establish sleep–wake patterns compatible with the environment. Most infants are sleeping through the night by 3 months, but nocturnal awakenings continue to be frequent during the latter half of the first year.

The number of sleep periods continue to drop from four to five per 24-hour day at 3 months of age to one nighttime period and two naps at 6 months (Riley & Ferber, 1985). Total sleep time averages 14 to 15 hours, but there is wide variability among infants (Edgil, Wood, & Smith, 1985).

Toddler and Preschooler

By 1 year of age napping has usually been reduced to once or twice a day. Some sleep disturbance is observed in almost all children between 1 and 2.5 years of age; it is thought to be related to the rapidly developing mental abilities of the child. Getting the child to fall asleep is the most frequently reported problem, but frequent awakenings and occasional night terrors may also occur (Gates, et al., 1989). Total sleep time drops from an average of 13 to 14 hours at age 2 to 12 hours by the end of the fifth year, mainly because of the elimination of the afternoon nap. REM sleep drops to about 30%, which is still higher than for adults. The percentage of slow-wave sleep is also higher through childhood, whereas the amount of stage 1 sleep is less.

Child and Adolescent

Sleep and rest needs fluctuate somewhat for school-age children and adolescents in relation to growth spurts and activity patterns. REM content gradually drops to about 20% at puberty. Adolescents actually require slightly more rest than they did before puberty. The cardiovascular and respiratory systems mature less rapidly than other systems, contributing to fatigue from inadequate oxygenation (Murray & Zentner, 1989).

Adult and Older Adult

Adults vary widely in the number of hours of sleep that they require and in their preferred portion of the 24-hour period for sleeping. By middle age, the frequency of nocturnal awakenings tends to increase, and the satisfaction with the quality of sleep tends to decrease. Situational variables, such as job-related stress, parenting responsibilities, and illness probably account for much of the variation seen among people in early to middle adulthood (Verran, et al., 1988).

As people age, the amount of stage 4 sleep decreases significantly (Fig. 39-4). The intranight distribution of REM sleep becomes more even and the percentage decreases. Older men tend to have decreased stage 3 sleep as well, and have more difficulty maintaining sleep toward the end of the sleep period (Robinson, 1986). Circadian rhythms become less prominent with increasing age. Sleeping patterns may become polyphasic, with a shorter nocturnal period plus daytime naps. Core body temperature may no longer show the usual circadian changes. If external cues to time also decrease, as with institutionalization, the cognitively impaired elderly may develop sundowner's syndrome, characterized by nocturnal wakefulness and agitation. It is thought that this may be related to a drop in stimulation level to the point at which the cognitively compromised patient can no longer maintain contact with reality.

Time spent napping and time in bed increase with advancing age (Hayter, 1985). Daytime napping does not appear to interfere with nighttime sleep for these older adults. Total time in bed gradually increases because of napping, longer sleep latency, increases in the number and length of awakenings, and general fatigue. Even healthy people over the age of 85 show a significant increase in total sleep time, and usually change to an earlier bedtime.

Older adults frequently express concern about taking longer to fall asleep, awakening more frequently, daytime sleepiness, and needing longer to adjust to changes in schedule. The nurse can help them to recognize that these changes are a natural part of aging, and to establish or maintain a schedule of rest and activity that meets their individual needs and preferences (Kearnes, 1989; Dinner, et al., 1989)

ALTERED SLEEP/REST FUNCTION

Potential for Altered Sleep Function

Distractions

Noise. People chronically exposed to high noise levels have less slow-wave and REM sleep with more stage 1 and awakenings than their counterparts who live in quieter neighborhoods (Hauri, 1982). Women and older people are more likely to be awakened by noise (Hansell, 1984). As might be expected, the awakening threshold varies with the stage of sleep, with stage 1 being the most vulnerable.

Noise levels recorded in a critical care unit between 10:15 PM and 3:00 AM ranged from 72 to 75 decibels, the equivalent of a noisy office (Snyder-Halpern, 1985). In subsequent testing with volunteer subjects, critical care unit noise from mechanical sources (e.g., suction machines, alarms) was even more disturbing than sounds from staff and patients. Nurses can modify the noise level in hospital environments by keeping equipment noise to a minimum, avoiding unnecessary conversation, and closing doors when possible.

Light. Control of light is usually adequate in home environments. This is not true for shift workers and young children during summer evenings in the northern latitudes. In acute care environments, control of light becomes a nursing responsibility often overlooked in the complexity of meeting other patient needs.

Temperature. The benefits of cool versus moderate sleeping room temperatures are matters of personal preference; however, it has been shown that excessive warmth (above 24°C or 75°F) increases restlessness (Hauri, 1982). During REM sleep thermoregulation is impaired and shivering does not occur.

Environment. Generally, in a new environment sleep latency is increased; total sleep time and proportion of REM are decreased. Those who have chronic difficulties sleeping may associate certain objects in the environment, such as their bed, with poor sleep. These people report sleeping better away from home. In the hospital environment, certain objects in the room may be associated with pain. If a sleeping room doubles as a work

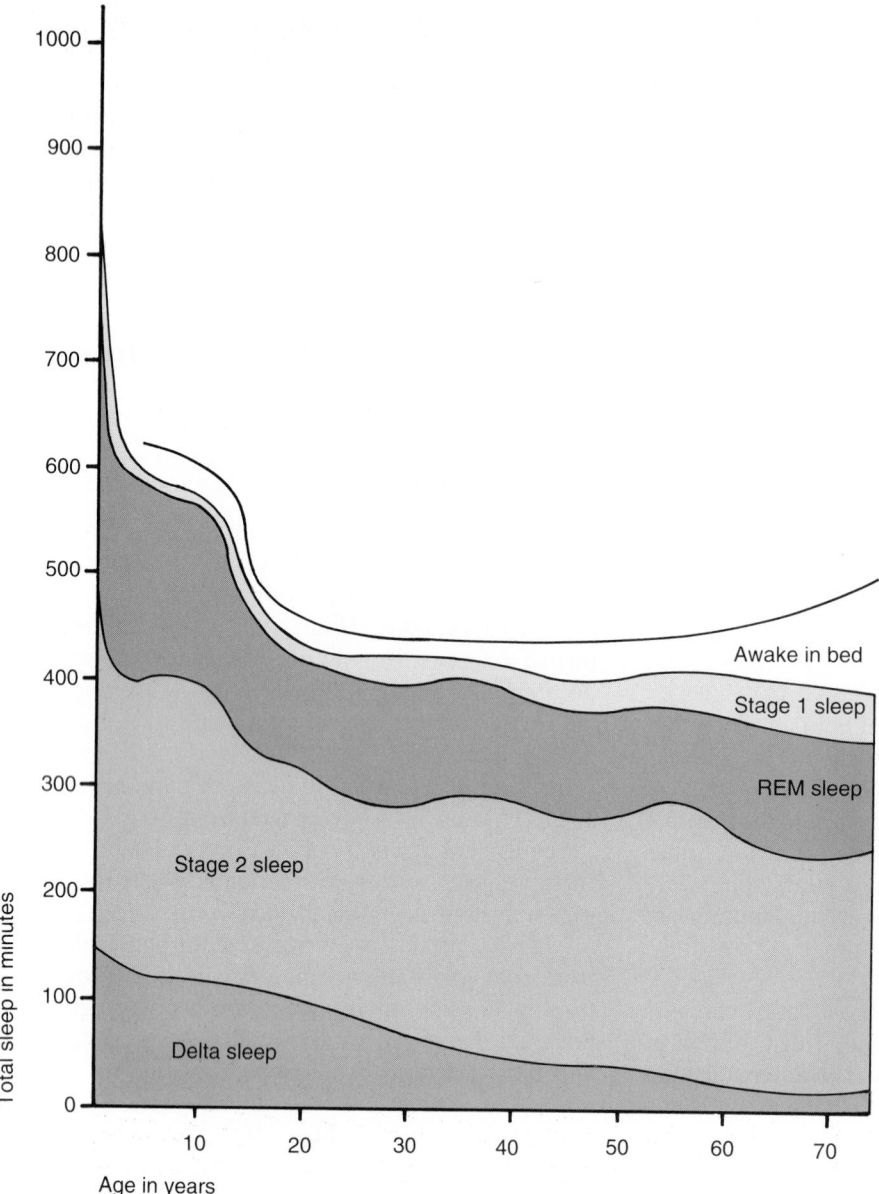

Figure 39–4. Schematic representation of the changes in sleep stages by age. Note that the elderly spend more time in bed than other adults but have less deep sleep. (Adapted with permission from Williams, R. L., Karacen, I., & Hursch, C. J. (1974). *Electroencephalography (EEG) of human sleep: Clinical applications.* New York: Wiley)

area, the room may become associated with work rather than sleep. Objects of play in the child's room may disturb the child's sleep and rest.

Caregiving. The frequent awakenings associated with parenting may contribute to chronic sleep pattern disturbance. It is not unusual to hear mothers speak of never getting more than an hour's sleep at a time over a period of 1 or more weeks when caring for a sick child or a colicky baby. The associated REM deprivation may make coping even more difficult.

Caregivers are among the most frequent disturbers of sleep in institutional settings. In critical care environments patients are awakened frequently for various assessments and treatments. Where possible, these activ-

ities should be clustered to provide periods of 1.5 to 2 hours of undisturbed sleep time. The nurse may have to assume a patient advocacy role in coordinating interruptions from the many disciplines involved in patient care.

Disruptions in Relationships. Disruptions to primary relationships are commonly associated with sleep pattern disturbance. Bereaved people often report the night period as their most difficult. Children who are away from home are frequently homesick at bedtime. Marital discord may contribute to sleep disturbance in children as well as in the involved adults. Security needs are heightened at bedtime for persons of all ages.

Shift Work. Frequent changes in the sleep–wake schedule, such as occur with shift work, contribute to shorter and more fragmented sleep and a high incidence of fatigue (Akerstedt, 1984). The dysynchrony of trying to sleep at times when the body's circadian rhythm is set for wakefulness is thought to be the main reason for the disturbed sleep. Fatigue is secondary to the disturbed sleep. Nurses are among the 20% of the population in industrialized countries involved in shift work, as are many of the people for whom they care (Akerstedt, 1984). Research on the effectiveness of various shift schedules has been inconclusive, suggesting the need for further investigation.

Illness

During acute and chronic illness, patients are particularly vulnerable to loss of stage 3 sleep. Conditions involving pain have long been known to disturb sleep. Current research indicates that body system disturbances also have an effect on sleep, and vice versa. Ventilatory responses to hypoxia and hypercapnea decrease during REM sleep. Although diaphragmatic function is essentially unchanged during REM sleep, the intercostals and other accessory muscles lose substantial activity (Johnson & Remmers, 1984). Thus, the pattern of frequent arousals seen in people with chronic obstructive lung disease may be the body's adaptation to maintain adequate oxygenation. Hypnotics should be used cautiously, if at all, with people experiencing ineffective breathing patterns or impaired gas exchange. Often, low doses of oxygen are required by these patients at night.

Variations in blood pressure and heart rate associated with REM sleep and the relative frequency of myocardial infarctions occurring at night may be related (Hauri, 1982). Similarly, the low systemic blood pressure during slow-wave sleep may be a contributing factor to the frequent nighttime occurrence of strokes from cerebral thrombus formation. The pain and discomfort of angina or dyspnea occurring during the night can disturb sleep.

People with a history of seizure activity risk increased occurrence of seizures following sleep deprivation or with variable sleep habits. Sleep may be disturbed by seizure activity; some epileptic patients have seizures only at night. The recording of brain waves during sleep is an important method for diagnosing the site of abnormal electrical activity.

Hormonal changes contribute to a variety of sleep pattern disturbances. Hyperthyroidism causes fragmented short sleep with an excess of the slow-wave stages, while hypothyroidism seems to cause excessive sleepiness with a lack of slow-wave sleep (Hauri, 1982). The tremendous fatigue often reported after hysterectomy may be related to the loss of estrogen. Administration of estrogen to postmenopausal women has been shown to decrease sleep latency almost as effectively as some hypnotics, and to increase the percentage of REM sleep in contrast to most hypnotics (Schiff, et al., 1979).

Skin conditions such as eczema have been shown to contribute to sleep onset delay, frequent awakenings, and reduction of stages 3, 4, and REM during the first part of the night (Williams, 1988). The itching and discomfort associated with hives, insect bites, and other skin lesions also disturb sleep.

Hospitalization as a result of illness adds a number of additional factors that may disturb sleep. In a survey of 143 adult patients on medical–surgical units, "difficulty finding a comfortable position" and "pain" were identified as the most common stimuli disturbing sleep in hospital. Anxieties arising from the illness and hospitalization, such as those relate to tests and surgery, diagnosis, and impact on family and job, were other frequently identified reasons for disturbed sleep (Fig. 39-5).

Drugs

Sleep patterns are vulnerable to disturbance from medications taken to facilitate sleep, alcohol, medications used to treat other conditions, and other chemicals. **Hypnotics,** or "sleeping pills," the very medications used to decrease sleep latency and improve sleep maintenance, are among those medications most prone to disturb sleep architecture. REM sleep is most vulnerable.

Alcohol is probably the oldest and most commonly used chemical for promoting sleep. A moderate single dose causes early onset of sleep but increases wakefulness in the last half of the night. With acute intoxication, REM sleep is suppressed; slow-wave sleep may initially increase. Abrupt withdrawal in the heavy drinker may trigger massive REM rebound. Recovered alcoholics continue to have decreased slow-wave sleep and gross cycle disturbance even after 1 or 2 years of abstinence (Hauri, 1982).

Other medications also affect sleep patterns. Morphine, for example, increases the time spent awake during the sleep period and shortens total sleep time by decreasing both REM and stages 3 and 4. Antidepressants suppress REM sleep also (Orr, 1985). Dilantin, used in the treatment of epilepsy, often causes insomnia (Rodin, 1983).

The effects of caffeine on the central nervous system (CNS) may last for up to 20 hours, delaying sleep onset and affecting sleep patterns even in those who believe that they are not affected by it (Hauri, 1982). The half-life of caffeine in the elderly is even longer, making them particularly vulnerable to its effects. Nicotine, another mild CNS stimulant, accounts for the poorer sleep observed in heavy smokers compared with nonsmokers.

Mood States

Anxiety frequently delays sleep onset. The tension associated with psychological stress may also contribute to

%	10	20	30	40	50	60	70	80	90	100

Difficulty finding a comfortable position	XXXXXXXXXXXXXXXXXXXXXX
Pain	XXXXXXXXXXXXXXXXXXX
Worry about test/surgery	XXXXXXXXXXX
Worry about family, job, managing at home	XXXXXXXX
Worry about diagnosis/ getting well	XXXXXXXX
Discomfort from dressing, cast, etc.	XXXXXXXX
Being awakened for treatments	XXXXXXXX
Noise from other patients	XXXXXXXX
Too much light	XXXXXXXXX
Fear of dislodging tubing	XXXXXXXX
Lack of exercise	XXXXXXX
Temperature	XXXXX
Noise from TV/radio	XXXXX
Unfamiliar environment	XXXXXXX
Disrupted habits	XXXXX
Noise from nursing station	XXXXXXX
Uncomfortable bed	XXXX
Napping	XXX
Sleeping alone	XXX

Figure 39–5.   Percentage of patients identifying selected stimuli as disturbing to sleep in hospital. (From Reimer, M. A. (1985). *Nursing interventions perceived by patients and their nurses as facilitating nocturnal sleep in hospital.* Unpublished manuscipt)

maintenance or early-awakening insomnia. Depression usually results in disturbed sleep. Both the depression and sleep pattern disturbance may be linked to neurotransmitter imbalance. The depressed person is also more likely to be distressed by poor sleep (Hauri, 1982).

Manifestations of Altered Sleep Function

Signs and symptoms associated with sleep deprivation are fatigue, headache, nausea, increased sensitivity to pain, decreased neuromuscular coordination, general irritability, and inability to concentrate. Eventually, disorientation and hallucinations may occur with the breakthrough of "mini-sleeps," which further interfere with functioning.

Selective disruption of specific stages of sleep results in distinct symptom patterns. Those deprived of REM sleep become agitated and impulsive, whereas deprivation of slow-wave sleep results in withdrawal and vague physical complaints. Tolerance of musculoskeletal pain in particular is significantly decreased after deprivation of slow-wave sleep. When deprived of stage 1, 2, or 3 sleep, the body makes no effort to recover those specific stages, but there seems to be a mechanism that gives priority to recovering stage 4 sleep and REM as soon as the opportunity is given.

Insomnia

Insomnia is a perceived difficulty in sleeping. The persistent insomnia experienced by those who refer to themselves as insomniacs reflects a pattern of perceived difficulty with sleeping over months to years.

Patterns of insomnia can also be classified as onset insomnia (prolonged sleep latency), maintenance insomnia (multiple awakenings), and early-awakening insomnia. When polygraph recordings of insomniacs have been compared to those of self-defined good sleepers, both have been found to be within normal range. Insomniacs consistently underestimated total sleep time, but were accurate in identifying the pattern of insomnia and actually underestimated the number of awakenings. Thus, the problem of insomnia appears to be more of a lack of quality than quantity.

Narcolepsy

Narcolepsy is a disorder of excessive daytime sleepiness characterized by short, almost irresistible daytime sleep attacks, usually of 10 to 15 minutes' duration, and abnormal manifestations of REM sleep (Hauri, 1982). Onset usually occurs in adolescence. Narcolepsy is thought to be a disturbance between REM sleep and wakefulness-triggering systems, in which REM sleep intrudes into wakefulness (Hauri, 1982). Most narcoleptics go almost immediately into REM sleep at the beginning of the sleep period. Episodes of profound weakness during intense emotion, called cataplexy, are reported by 70% of narcoleptics. Other common signs related to disturbed REM mechanisms include episodes of feeling paralyzed when falling asleep or awakening, and vivid hallucinations (Hauri, 1982; Walsleben, et al., 1989).

Sleep Apnea

Sleep apnea refers to recurrent periods of absence of breathing for 10 seconds or longer, occurring at least five times per hour (Weaver & Millman, 1986). Three types of sleep apnea are recognized: obstructure, central, and mixed.

Obstructive Sleep Apnea. Obstructive sleep apnea involves collapse of the upper airway in spite of respiratory effort. With sleep, the muscles of the upper airway relax, occluding an airway that may be already narrowed because of obesity, jaw structure, or enlarged soft tissue structures. With arousal, voluntary control of the upper airway muscles is restored, relieving the obstruction.

The person, often a heavy-set man, may be partially roused up to a couple of hundred times a night. Symptoms are excessive daytime sleepiness, and bed partner reports of apneic periods, heavy snoring, and restless sleep. Common treatments include nasal airway positive pressure applied through a nose mask, or uvulopalatopharyngoplasty, the surgical removal of the uvula, posterior portion of the soft palate, and tonsils (Weaver & Millman, 1986). Weight control and relief of nasal congestion may be effective in milder cases.

At least 1% of the adult male population has obstructive sleep apnea. About 5% of the most severely affected of these patients fit the classical description of Pickwickian syndrome, but obesity is not always present nor are all patients male (Hauri, 1982; Metzler, et al., 1990).

Central Apnea. Central apnea during sleep occurs because of neurogenic failure to trigger respiratory effort. It is most commonly seen with neurologic conditions such as stroke or brain stem involvement. Severely affected patients may require ventilatory support at night.

Mixed Apnea. Mixed apnea, a combination of the two preceding types of sleep apnea, is especially common in the elderly. Manifestations and treatment are similar to those for obstructive sleep apnea.

Use of hypnotics, alcohol, or antihistamines by sleep apnea patients can be dangerous, as the responsiveness to oxygen desaturation is further reduced, therefore further increasing the duration of the apneic spells.

Sleep-Related (Nocturnal) Myoclonus

The periodic leg movements of sleep-related (nocturnal) myoclonus involve repetitive dorsiflexion of the foot and flexion of the knee during sleep at a rate up to once every

15 to 20 seconds. The resultant mini-arousals disrupt sleep, leading to excessive daytime sleepiness, or in some cases insomnia.

Altered Sleep–Wake Patterns

Altered sleep–wake disorders include transient disruptions such as the jet lag syndrome, and persistent disorders such as delayed sleep phase syndrome. Jet lag tends to be worst after east-to-west travel across time zones, and affects poor sleepers and the elderly more than good sleepers (Hauri, 1982). Delayed sleep phase syndrome is a less common but more problematic mismatch of personal circadian rhythm with societal expectations. Some people who function best by going to bed in the early hours of the morning and sleeping into the afternoon find occupations and partners to match. Other people with this disorder find that the continued struggle to rise hours earlier than their internal clock dictates is not made easier by simple treatments such as establishing a consistent rising time. These people can be helped to achieve a phase shift through chronotherapy, in which they progressively delay sleep onset by 2 hours per week until they eventually work around to a more functional schedule (Hauri, 1982).

Parasomnias

Parasomnias are activities that are normal during waking but abnormal during sleep, such as sleepwalking (**somnambulism**), talking, and bedwetting (enuresis). These generally occur during slow-wave sleep and are most frequent in children. There is often a family history of similar behaviors.

Occasional episodes of sleepwalking in children are fairly common, usually beginning before age 10 and stopping by age 15. Behavior during a sleepwalking episode may be semipurposeful, such dressing or going to the bathroom, but lacking in coordination and appropriateness, such as voiding in the closet. Occurrence in adults is frequently associated with stress and anxiety (Hauri, 1982). Parents and family members may need assistance in providing a safe environment to decrease the potential for injury.

Night terrors, another type of parasomnia, are repeated, sudden awakenings accompanied by screaming, acute anxiety, and disorientation (Gates, et al., 1989). They occur mainly among children, and are associated with incomplete arousal from slow-wave sleep early in the night. They are different from **nightmares,** or bad dreams which occur during REM sleep.

Attempts to awaken people from the parasomnias of slow-wave sleep should be discouraged. Help in the event of night terrors or somnambulism should be given only to the extent that it is accepted, and the person should be encouraged to return to sleep as the event subsides (Ferber, 1985).

Enuresis is not limited to slow-wave sleep, although almost two-thirds of all episodes occur in the first third of the night (Ferber, 1985). The incidence in boys decreases from 18% at age 5 to 5% by age 12. Enuresis is less common in girls and tends to disappear earlier.

Impact of Sleep Dysfunction on Activities of Daily Living

Sleep pattern dysfunction affects most activities of daily living to a varying degree. Closely linked to quality of life is the sense of feeling well rested and refreshed, with energy available for activity. Thus, adequacy of sleep and rest directly affects and is affected by the activity exercise pattern.

Role performance and social interactions may become disrupted in the presence of sleep pattern dysfunction. Irritability and impaired concentration accompany sleep deprivation. The excessive sleepiness associated with disorders such as sleep apnea pose serious safety risks for those driving and operating hazardous machinery. Snoring often disturbs the bed partner, who not infrequently seeks the refuge of another bedroom. Lack of sleep impairs coping and cognitive responses.

ASSESSMENT

Sleep pattern disturbances in health and illness are frequent sources of concern to people. It is easy in the hospital situation for nurses to become preoccupied with assessments and treatments associated with the presenting illness. Likewise, in community practice the diabetic's foot care or the new mother's ability to breastfeed may overshadow the concerns those people have regarding unsatisfactory sleep or inadequate rest. However, the professional nurse can play a pivotal role in helping people assess and meet their needs for sleep and rest.

The nurse is frequently involved with situational variations in functional health patterns. The change in environment and anxieties associated with hospitalization frequently result in sleep pattern disturbance.

Subjective Data

The single most important criterion for adequacy of sleep and rest is the patient's statement. The state of feeling rested is a highly subjective one. As discussed earlier, individual requirements for sleep vary widely. Besides the sense of feeling rested, people usually consider the congruency between their expectations and experience in relation to total sleep time, time in bed before sleep onset, number of awakenings, and time of final awakening. The history is the most important component of assessment of sleep and rest.

Functional Pattern Identification

Determine the person's usual sleep and rest patterns through questions such as:

How many hours of sleep do you usually get?
What time do you usually go to bed? Get up?
What helps you get to sleep?
What makes it hard for you to sleep?
How do you feel when you awaken?
How much sleep do you believe you should be getting?
What helps you relax?
How often do you nap? Take rest periods?

Risk Identification

Look for developmental and situational changes (environmental, physical, social) that may increase the need for or interfere with sleep and/or rest. Assess caffeine and alcohol intake, and involvement in shift work.

Dysfunctional Identification

Validate with the person as to whether or not getting adequate sleep and rest is perceived as a problem. If a problem is identified, determine whether it is chronic or situational, what has helped, and what has made it worse. In situations of chronic disturbance it may be useful to interview the sleep partner as well. Questions should be directed toward elaboration of the presenting concern. For example, if the person is concerned about daytime sleepiness, the nurse should inquire regarding a history of snoring, awakenings accompanied by gasping, apneic periods that may have been observed by the partner, restlessness, and impact on activities associated with work, driving, and social interactions.

Having the person keep a sleep diary may be useful as an assessment and as an intervention. By giving the person responsibility for monitoring his or her own health pattern, the nurse may help the person diagnose the problem and related factors or to recognize that the severity is less than originally perceived.

Young and middle-aged adults in the habit of sleeping late on days off sometimes express concern about sleep disturbances at the beginning of their work week, which they may attribute to job stress. Reviewing a sleep diary maintained for a couple of weeks may help them to realize that when they average out total sleep time they are meeting their perceived requirements.

Objective Data

Physical Assessment

Observe for circles under the eyes, yawning, nodding, and slowness of response. Irritability, impaired concentration, and word-finding difficulties may be indicative of sleep pattern disturbance, but may also occur because of other problems.

Adequacy of rest after activity is often measured through return of heart rate and other physiologic parameters to baseline levels (Alteri, 1984). The nurse should monitor vital signs after patient- or caregiver-initiated activity for return to baseline resting levels in the severely compromised patient.

Diagnostic Tests

People with severe sleep problems or excessive daytime sleepiness should be referred to a sleep laboratory for more thorough investigation. Polygraph recordings can be made, including evaluation of other parameters such as oxygen saturation, in suspected sleep apnea.

NURSING DIAGNOSIS AND PATIENT GOALS

To formulate the nursing diagnosis the nurse must cluster the data, sifting out the incidental from the significant. For example, in this author's investigation of presleep rituals, 72% of the respondents reported habitually watching television before going to bed, yet only 26% of them considered this activity important in getting to sleep (Reimer, 1985). Thus, the absence of a television in a patient's hospital environment may be of little significance. The same patient's seemingly casual comment regarding how the children at home are managing "without a disciplinarian around" may be a significant clue to sleep-disturbing anxiety. Diagnostic statements should describe the problem as specifically as possible.

Diagnostic Statement: Sleep Pattern Disturbance

Definition

Sleep pattern disturbance is "disruption of sleep time (that) causes discomfort or interferes with desired lifestyle" (Cox, et al., 1989, p. 331).

Defining Characteristics

Verbal complaints of difficulty falling asleep; awakening earlier or later than desired; interrupted sleep; verbal complaints of not feeling well rested; changes of behavior and performance (increasing irritability, restlessness, disorientation, lethargy, or listlessness); physical signs (mild fleeting nystagmus, slight hand tremor, ptosis of eyelids, expressionless face, dark circles under eyes, frequent yawning, changes in posture); thick speech with mispronunciation and incorrect words (NANDA, 1990).

Related Factors

Sensory alterations: internal (illness, psychological stress); external (environmental, social cues) (NANDA, 1990).

Related Nursing Diagnoses

Fatigue, in the NANDA classification, is defined as "an overwhelming sense of exhaustion and decreased capacity for physical and mental work" (Cox, et al., 1989, p. 269). Some defining characteristics such as irritability and impaired concentration are shared, but Cox and associates suggest that Fatigue is a subjective state that persists in spite of apparently adequate quantity of sleep (Cox, et al., 1989).

Other diagnoses such as inadequate rest are not yet part of the standard list, but may need to be used as part of diagnostic statements.

Patient Goals

Patient goals for sleep pattern disturbance are specifically stated in terms such as minutes before sleep onset, hours of unbroken sleep, or verbal statement of feeling refreshed on wakening. Examples of specific patient goals are:

Patient will report fewer problems with falling asleep.
Patient will report feeling more rested.
Patient will demonstrate physical signs of being rested.

Involving people in setting their own goals for sleep and rest is a useful way of helping them explore what is realistic for their developmental stage, lifestyle, and state of health.

IMPLEMENTATION

Nursing Interventions to Promote Health and Sleep/Rest Function

Minimal Stimuli

Establishing a quiet, darkened environment modified according to the person's preferred level (e.g., low light) may be a source of comfort for children, people in the hospital, or those in another strange environment. People with impaired physical mobility should be assisted with voiding before retiring. Male patients appreciate having a urinal within reach. Children often need to be reminded to go to the bathroom before going to bed. Fluids may need to be restricted in the evening. Simple relaxation exercises can be taught for use at bedtime.

The single most important intervention for chronic sleep pattern disturbance may be to establish a consistent rising time. Getting up is subject to voluntary control, whereas falling asleep usually is not. Slightly decreasing the time in bed solidifies sleep and along with a consistent rising time will finally lead to more regular times of sleep onset (Spielman, Saskin, & Thorpy, 1987).

For the socially and occupationally isolated in the community, counseling may be required regarding the maintenance of routines. For the acutely ill patient, the nurse can enhance cueing by turning lights down at night, keeping window drapes open during the day where possible, and providing verbal cueing regarding time of day.

Environment Modification

The nurse should reserve the sleeping room for sleep whenever possible, and encourage children to play in other areas. Opportunities should be provided for the hospitalized patient to get out of his or her room during the day where feasible, and objects associated with work, conflict, pain, or sleeplessness should be removed.

Intimacy and Security

A bedtime hug for a child, the shared bed of a marriage partner, and an enjoyable evening with a friend are a few ways in which people may enhance sleep quality for one another. If social isolation is suspected as an cause of Sleep Pattern Disturbance, the nurse may need to assist the person in making social contacts.

In the institutional setting, a backrub provides the warmth of human touch as well as physical relaxation (Fakouri & Jones, 1987). Allowing family members to sit at the bedside and having them bring in a favorite blanket or stuffed animal are other ways of enhancing security. Assurance of frequent checks by nursing staff, prompt response to the call bell, and a caring manner can do much to allay the fears of the anxious patient.

For those with faith in God, prayer and reading of scripture often facilitates a sense of peacefulness and subsequent sleep onset. Other persons may find meditation helpful. A sensitive assessment of the person's values and beliefs (see Chapt. 49) helps the nurse maximize strengths.

Sleep Rituals

Rituals play an important role in facilitating sleep in home and hospital environments. Whether it is the bedtime story for the toddler or a cup of tea for the elderly couple, the regular association of certain activities with the end of the waking period is one of the most effective ways of creating the expectation of sleep.

A routine of "settling" patients in institutional settings can provide a similar marking of the end of the day. Assisting with washing of hands and face, a gentle massage, plumping of pillows, and provision of an extra blanket may be incorporated. The nurse can use this time as an opportunity to help patients focus on small goals accomplished during the day, the visit of a loved one, or whatever else is helpful to settle the mind as well as the body.

Beliefs About Sleep

People should be helped to assess their individual sleep needs and to anticipate developmental changes. Middle-aged and older persons can be helped to realize that shorter unbroken sleep periods are normal for their age. Likewise, insomniacs (and potential ones) may benefit from the assurance that they can function on relatively little sleep. Parents may need anticipatory guidance regarding the wide variability in sleep needs of individual children (Edgil, Wood, & Smith, 1985).

Nursing Interventions for Altered Function

In spite of major advances in medical therapeutics, rest remains one of the most common symptomatic treatments for a wide variety of disease conditions. "Rest the affected part" is a standard intervention for almost any condition.

Rest

The person who has suffered myocardial ischemia as a result of a blood clot is placed on a strict regimen of restricted activity. To maintain a resting state for the heart once the initial period of pain has subsided challenges the nurse's creativity. The patient is helped to realize that while he or she may "feel great," the damaged heart needs further rest, with a gradual return to the previous or a decreased activity level. The nurse also has a major role in helping such patients make more lasting lifestyle changes to incorporate more rest and relaxation.

Research on the amount of rest required after various activities provides a basis for nurses to make decisions in implementing care. Alteri studied ten male patients 8 to 20 days after myocardial infarction to determine the length of time required for vital signs to return to the preactivity baseline (Alteri, 1984). Climbing one flight of stairs required 7 minutes to recover, a 10-minute walk on a level surface required 10 minutes to recover, and showering took 30.5 minutes to reach the preactivity baseline. She also found that participants consistently expressed the feeling that they had recovered long before their vital signs returned to normal.

Maintaining traction to "rest" a patient's fractured femur or instilling eye drops to temporarily paralyze and thus rest the eye following surgery are further examples of ways in which nurses help patients meet situationally induced changes in rest requirements.

Judicious Use of Hypnotics

Hypnotics may be useful as a short-term intervention during situationally induced sleep pattern disturbance. For example, hypnotics are usually ordered preoperatively to ensure adequate rest before surgery. When hypnotics are ordered prn (as necessary) in the hospital environment, the nurse has the responsibility of deciding with the patient if and when they should be taken. Many patients expect to be given a sleeping pill in the

---

Nursing Research

Selected Nursing Research Studies

Alley, J., & Rogers, C. (1986). Sleep patterns of breast-fed and non-breast-fed infants. *Pediatric Nursing, 12,* 349–351.

Fontaine, D. K. (1989). Measurement of nocturnal sleep patterns in trauma patients. *Heart and Lung, 18,* 402–410.

Keefe, M. (1987). Comparison of neonatal night-time sleep–wake patterns in nursery versus rooming-in environments. *Nursing Research, 36,* 140–144.

Robers, P. A., et al. (1988). Nurse administration of sleep medication: A comparison of registered nurses and licensed practical nurses. *American Journal of Public Health, 78,* 1581–1583.

White, M. A., et al. (1988). Distress and self-soothing bedtime behaviors in hospitalized children with non-rooming-in parents. *Maternal Child Nursing Journal, 17*(2), 67–77.

Possible Topics for Nursing Inquiry

- What are the long-term effects of chronic sleep deprivation?
- Does a warm tub bath change the quality and quantity of sleep?
- How long does it take a patient's vital signs to return to resting baseline after having an occupied bed made?

Selected Nursing Interventions for Common Sleep Problems

Sleep Pattern Disturbance

- Identify factors affecting the quality of sleep.
- Minimize stimuli by having a darkened, quiet room with low lights.
- Encourage sleep rituals, such as a gentle back-rub, plumping of pillows, and eliminating distracting sound.
- Relieve discomfort through position changes, pain medications, or other measures.
- Reduce factors affecting safety by having call light near at hand, bed in the lowest position, and using a nightlight.
- Encourage contact with family or other significant others who provide the patient with a sense of intimacy and security.

---

hospital, but they may not require it. Other interventions should be tried first.

In making decisions and teaching patients regarding the use of hypnotics, the nurse should consider the following principles:

- All hypnotics require judicious use, as they interfere with normal sleep architecture to some degree. REM sleep is most vulnerable. Therefore, signs of selective stage deficit may be evident, even though total sleep time has increased through hypnotic use. Patients can be taught that a night or two of increased dreaming (REM rebound) after the drug is discontinued is not unusual. Tapering withdrawal in long-term users can prevent REM rebound.
- All hypnotics impair waking function as long as they are pharmacologically active. Perception of daytime drowsiness and impairment of psychomotor skills fades more rapidly than do the actual effects (Dement, Seide, & Carskadon, 1982). Therefore, people in the community environment who are taking hypnotics should be taught about the half-life of the drugs and warned to avoid driving or handling machinery while the drug is in their system. Safety precautions should also be taken in home and hospital when those who have taken a hypnotic want to get up to the bathroom at night.
- The effectiveness of hypnotics decreases over a 4-week period, so long-term users are probably being affected more by expectation of sleep associated with taking a pill than by the active drug (Spielman, Saskin, & Thorpy, 1987). It is therefore important to teach these

people alternative sleep-promoting strategies and prepare them for the possible short-term rebound effects that may follow withdrawal.
- Certain people are at increased risk from the use of hypnotics. The time required for the elderly to metabolize long-acting benzodiazepines is greatly increased. Arousal because of decreased oxygen levels is depressed after the administration of hypnotics. Therefore the nurse must use particular caution in administering ordered hypnotics to the elderly or to those whose pulmonary function is compromised.

Table 39-2 shows how knowledge of the specific properties of each hypnotic can help the nurse determine implications for assessment and teaching. The chart is not intended to be exhaustive, but rather to highlight the need for nurses to be knowledgeable about the hypnotics their patients are taking.

Discharge Planning and Home Care

Hospitalized patients usually associate improved sleep with returning to their home environment, however, they often underestimate their needs for rest when recovering from illness or surgery. The nurse may need to help them plan for periods of rest and for energy conservation. For those patients who will need assistance during the night, the sleep and rest needs of the home caregiver must also be considered in discharge planning.

EVALUATION

The nurse evaluates the degree to which sleep pattern disturbance or inadequate rest has been resolved according to the patient goals initially established. Examples of outcome criteria for the patient goals are listed below.

Goal
Patient will report fewer problems with falling asleep.

Possible Outcome Criteria
- Within 7 days, patient reports decrease in sleep latency to 10 to 15 minutes.
- Within 7 days patient reports less anxiety regarding falling asleep.

Goal
Patient will report feeling more rested.

Possible Outcome Criteria
- Within 10 days patient verbalizes feeling less fatigued.
- As observed by nurse by tenth day, patient demonstrates nonverbally increased restfulness (less dozing, more animation in activity).

TABLE 39-2.
Selected Hypnotics: Their Properties and Nursing Implications

Hypnotic	Properties	Nursing Implications
Benzodiazepines		
Triazolam (Halcion)	Onset rapid Half-life 2.5 hours	Useful for onset insomnia Little hangover effect Rebound insomnia frequent
Flurazepam (Dalmane)	Onset rapid (17 minutes) Half-life 74–160 hours	Good for onset and maintenance insomnia Maximum effectiveness not until third night Less rebound effect because of long half-life but more hangover
Temazepam (Restoril)	Onset 1–2 hours Half-life 9–12 hours	Poor for onset insomnia Most effective for maintenance or early awakening insomnia Hangover effect Safer for elderly
Other		
Chloral hydrate	Rapid onset Half-life 4–12 hours May cause gastric upset	Useful for onset insomnia Safer for children, elderly Give with full glass of water, milk

Goal
Patient will demonstrate physical signs of being rested.

Possible Outcome Criteria
- By seventh day, patient has decrease in circles under the eyes, excessive yawning, or slowness of response.
- Within 10 days, patient reports to nurse that he or she feels rested following activity.

Validation should occur with the patient particularly for this functional health pattern because of the subjectivity and individual variations in what it takes to have adequate rest and satisfying sleep.

Key Concepts

- Sleep is a naturally occurring, altered state of consciousness characterized by awareness and responsiveness to stimuli, and by being readily reversible.
- Rest is a physical and emotional state of decreased muscle and cognitive activity.
- Sleep and rest have restorative, protective, and energy-conserving functions.
- Psychological functions of sleep include reprocessing of memories and character reinforcement.

- The two main types of sleep are NREM (quiet sleep) and REM (rapid eye movement sleep).
- NREM sleep consists of four stages: stage 1, transitional; stage 2, light; stages 3 and 4, and deep, slow-wave sleep.
- REM sleep is similar to wakefulness in terms of brain activity, but muscle tone is low and vital signs fluctuate widely.
- Adults progress through stages 1-2-3-4-3-2-REM in 90-minute cycles.
- Infants have sleep cycles that last about 50 minutes.
- Guidelines for evaluating adequacy of sleep are awakening with a feeling of being refreshed and the absence of daytime sleepiness.
- Factors affecting sleep and rest include environmental stimuli, nutrition, exercise, illness, and hospitalization.
- Common disorders of sleep include disorders of initiating and maintaining sleep (insomnia), excessive daytime sleepiness, disorders of the sleep–wake cycle, and parasomnias.
- Sleep patterns change throughout the lifespan, with the very young and the very old requiring the most sleep.
- Anticipating changes in sleep patterns and needs for rest can contribute to promotion of a healthy balance between rest and activity, and a recognition that sleep pattern changes are developmentally normal.

Nursing Management Plan
The Patient with Sleep Pattern Disturbance

Nursing Diagnosis: Sleep pattern disturbance related to positional discomfort secondary to low back pain and manifested by wakening every 1 to 2 hours to turn, difficulty getting back to sleep, and expressed feelings of inadequate rest.

Patient Goal: Patient will use a sleep pattern that allows him to feel well rested.

Patient Outcome Criteria

- Patient has periods of 3 to 4 hours of undisturbed sleep within 2 days, as observed by the nurse.
- Patient expresses feeling more rested by the end of this week.

Nursing Intervention	**Scientific Rationale**
1. Offer backrub at bedtime and during the night when assisting with turns.	1. Muscle tension increases pain and arousal; backrubs help relaxation.
2. Assess mattress comfort with patient.	2. Adequate support is important in reducing back pain but too firm a surface can cause more wakenings and more stage 1 sleep.
3. Keep radio with earphones within reach during the night.	3. Some people find low-level stimuli help them get to sleep, especially because they mask strange sounds of hospital environment.
4. Alternate supine position with side-lying when assisting with position changes (unless contraindicated or uncomfortable for patient).	4. Poor sleepers have been found to spend more time on their backs with the head straight. This position may be more comfortable for some patients with back pain, however.
5. Increase activity during the day. If patient is on bedrest arrange to take bed to sunroom.	5. Daytime activity and change of environment help in cuing sleep–wake patterns.
6. Cluster assessments and treatments required during the night to coincide with times when the patient is already awake for position change.	6. Sleep cycles average 90 minutes. A sleep latency of 20 to 30 minutes means that patients should be given up to 2 hours of undisturbed time whenever possible.

References

Adam, K., & Oswald, I. (1984). Sleep helps healing. *British Medical Journal, 289,* 1400–1401.

Akerstedt, T. (1984). Work schedules and sleep. *Experientia, 40,* 417–422.

Alteri, C. A. (1984). The patient with myocardial infarction: Rest prescriptions for activities of daily living. *Heart and Lung, 13,* 355–359.

Cox, H., Hinz, M., Lubno, M., et al. (1989). *Clinical applications of nursing diagnosis.* Baltimore: Williams & Wilkins.

De Koninck, J., Gagnon, P., & Lallier, S. (1983). Sleep positions in the young adult and their relationship with the subjective quality of sleep. *Sleep, 6,* 52–59.

Dement, W., Seide, W., & Carskadon, M. (1982). Daytime alertness, insomnia and benzodiazepines. *Sleep, 5*(Suppl.), 28–45.

Dinner, D. S., et al. (1989). Help for geriatric sleep problems, *Patient Care, 23*(8), 74–80, 84–85.

Edgil, A., Wood, K., & Smith, D. (1985). Sleep problems of older infants and preschool children. *Pediatric Nursing, 11,* 87–89.

Fakouri, C., & Jones, P. (1987). Relaxation RX: The slow stroke back rub. *Journal of Gerontological Nursing, 13*(2), 32–35.

Ferber, R. (1985). Sleep disorders in infants and children. In T. Riley (Ed.), *Clinical aspects of sleep and sleep disturbance* (pp. 113–157). Toronto: Butterworth.

Floyd, J. (1984). Interaction between personal sleep–wake rhythms and psychiatric hospital rest-activity schedule. *Nursing Research, 33,* 255–259.

Gaarder, K., & Chase, C. (1971). Control of states of consciousness. *Archives of General Psychiatry, 25,* 429–435.

Gates, D., et al. (1989). Night terrors: Strategies for family coping. *Journal of Pediatric Nursing, 4*(1), 48–53.

Gilman, S., & Newman, S. (1987). *Essentials of clinical neuroanatomy and neurophysiology* (7th ed.). Philadelphia: F. A. Davis.

Hansell, H. N. (1984). The behavioral effects of noise on man: The patient with "intensive care unit psychosis." *Heart and Lung, 13,* 59–65.

Hartman, E. (1979). L-tryptophan and sleep. In P. Passouant & I. Oswald (Eds.), *Pharmacology of states of alertness.* Toronto: Pergamon Press, pp. 75–84.

Hauri, P. (1982). *The sleep disorders: Current concepts* (2nd ed.). Kalmazoo, MI: Upjohn.

Hayter, J. (1985). To nap or not to nap? *Geriatric Nursing, 6,* 104–106.

Horne, J. A. (1980). Sleep and body restitution. *Experientia, 36,* 11–13.

Horne, J. A., & Staff, L. H. (1983). Exercise and sleep: Body-heating effects. *Sleep, 6*(1), 36–46.

Johnson, M. W., & Remmers, J. E. (1984). Accessory muscle activity during sleep in chronic obstructive pulmonary disease. *Journal of Applied Physiology, 57,* 1011–1017.

Kearnes, S. (1989). Insomnia in the elderly. *Nursing Times, 85*(47), 32–33.

Keefe, M. (1987). Comparison of neonatal nighttime sleep–wake patterns in nursery versus rooming-in environments. *Nursing Research, 36,* 140–144.

Kripke, H., Simons, R., Garfinkel, L., et al. (1979). Short and long sleep and sleeping pills: Is increased mortality associated? *Archives of General Psychiatry, 36,* 103–116.

Metzler, D. J., et al. (1990). When to worry if your patients can't sleep . . . Sleep apnea. *RN, 53*(3), 52–57.

Montgomery, I., Trinder, J., & Paxton, S. (1982). Energy expenditure and total sleep time: Effect of physical exercise. *Sleep, 5*(2), 159–168.

Murray, R. B., & Zentner, J. P. (1989). *Nursing assessment and health promotion through the life span* (4th ed.). Englewood Cliffs, NJ: Prentice-Hall.

NANDA (1990). *Taxonomy I revised 1990, with official nursing diagnoses.* St. Louis, MO: North American Nursing Diagnosis Association.

Orr, W. (1985). Sleep pathophysiology in medicine and surgery. In T. Riley (Ed.), *Clinical aspects of sleep and sleep disturbance* (pp. 159–180). Toronto: Butterworth.

Porth, C. (1990). Pathophysiology: *Concepts of altered health states* (3rd ed.). Philadelphia: J. B. Lippincott.

Reimer, M. (1985). *Nursing interventions perceived by patients and their nurses as facilitating nocturnal sleep in hospital.* Unpublished manuscript.

Riley, T. (1985). Biological organization of sleep. In T. Riley (Ed.), *Clinical aspects of sleep and sleep disturbance* (pp. 11–37). Toronto: Butterworth.

Riley, T., & Ferber, R. (1985). Behavioral aspects of sleep. In T. Riley (Ed.), *Clinical aspects of sleep and sleep disturbance* (pp. 39–60). Toronto: Butterworth.

Robinson, C. (1986). Impaired sleep. In V. K. Carrieri, A. M. Lindsey, & C. M. West (Eds.), *Pathophysiological phenomena in nursing.* Philadelphia: W. B. Saunders, pp. 390–417.

Rodin, E. (1983). Carbamazepine (Tegretol). In T. Browne & R. Feldman (Eds.), *Epilepsy: Diagnosis and management* (pp. 203–213). Toronto: Little, Brown & Co.

Schiff, I., Regestein, Q., Tulchinsky, D., et al. (1979). Effects of estrogens on sleep and psychological state of hypogonadal women. *Journal of the American Medical Association, 242,* 2405–2407.

Shaver, J. L. F., & Giblin, E. C. (1989). Sleep. *Annual Review of Nursing Research, 7,* 71–93.

Snyder-Halpern, R. (1985). The effect of critical care unit noise on patient sleep cycles. *Critical Care Quarterly,* 41–51.

Spielman, A. J., Saskin, P., & Thorpy, M. J. (1987). Treatment of chronic insomnia by restriction of time in bed. *Sleep, 10,* 45–56.

Verran, J. A., et al. (1988). Do patients sleep in the hospital? *Applied Nursing Research, 1*(2), 95.

Walsleben, J., et al. (1989). Disorders of excessive daytime sleepiness. *Nurse Practitioner, 14*(3), 11–12, 15–16.

Weaver, T., & Millman, R. (1986). Broken sleep. *American Journal of Nursing, 86,* 146–150.

Williams, R. (1988). Sleep disturbance in various medical and surgical conditions. In R. Williams R & I. Karacan (Eds.), *Sleep disorders: Diagnosis and treatment* (2nd ed.). Toronto: Wiley, pp. 265–291.

Wirz-Justice, A., & Pringle, C. (1987). The non-entrained life of a young gentleman at Oxford. *Sleep, 10,* 57–61.

Bibliography

Coco, P. (1990). Bereavement questions and answers . . . various sleep pattern disturbances related to grief. *Advances in Clinical Care, 5*(2), 44.

Culver, B. H. (1989). Pulmonary responses to sleep. *Respiratory Care, 34,* 510–516.

Davis-Sharts, J. (1989). The elder and critical care: Sleep and mobility issues. *Nursing Clinics of North America, 24,* 755–767.

Emra, K. L., et al. (1989). When your patient tells you he can't sleep. *RN, 52*(9), 79–80, 82, 84.

Fontaine, D. K. (1989). Measurement of nocturnal sleep patterns in trauma patients. *Heart and Lung, 18,* 402–410.

Hanly, P. J., et al. (1989). Respiration and abnormal sleep in patients with congestive heart failure . . . Cheyne-Stokes respiration. *Chest, 96,* 480–488.

Johnson, S. E. (1989). Sleep pattern disturbance: Defining characteristics observable in practice. In *Classifications of Nursing Diagnoses, Proceedings of the Eighth Conference.* 368–370.

Kedas, A., et al. (1989). A critical review of aging and sleep research. *Western Journal of Nursing Research, 1*(2), 95.

Littrell, K., et al. (1989). Promoting sleep for the patient with a myocardial infarction. *Critical Care Nursing, 9*(3), 44, 46–49.

Littrell, K. et al. (1989). Sleep in the C.C.U.: The impossible dream? *Nursing 1989, 19*(11), 32U, 32X 32Z.

Robers, P. A., et al. (1988). Nurse administration of sleep medication: A comparison of registered nurses and licensed practical nurses. *American Journal of Public Health, 78,* 1581–1583.

Roberts, A. (1990). Senior systems . . . older patients and their medication . . . sleep and sleep difficulties in later life: Part 46. *Nursing Times, 86*(11): Systems of Life No. 181:61–64.

Trevelyan, J. (1989). Now I lay me down to sleep . . . mysteries surrounding sleep. *Nursing Times, 85*(47), 34–35.

White, M. A., et al. (1988). Distress and self-soothing bedtime behaviors in hospitalized children with non-rooming-in parents. *Maternal and Child Nursing Journal, 17*(2), 67–77.

Willis, J. (1989). A good night's sleep. *Nursing Times, 85*(47), 28–29.

UNIT XI
Cognition and Perception

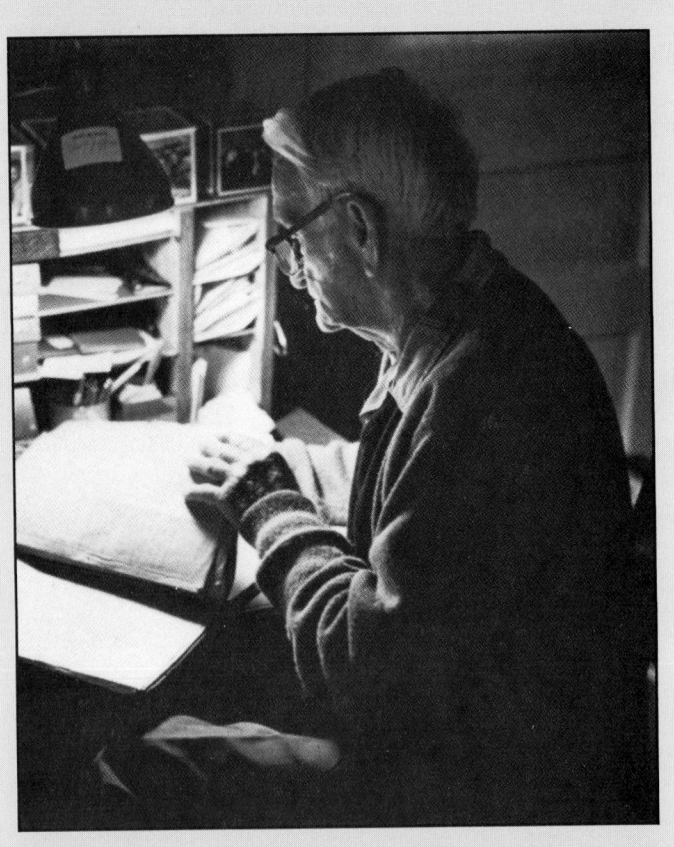

CHAPTERS

40 Pain Perception and Comfort

41 Sensory Perception

42 Cognitive Processes

Cognition and perception affect many other aspects of function; they are of particular concern in the elderly population. Unit XI explores these areas of human function and the nursing responsibilities associated with them.

The first chapter considers all aspects of pain perception and comfort. Pain relief is a primary nursing responsibility that involves both independent nursing actions and nursing interventions resulting from physician's orders. Holistic nursing care is essential to adequately address pain relief. The next chapter discusses sensory perception. Intact and functioning senses are essential for meaningful interaction with the environment. The challenge for the nurse is to avoid both deprivation and overload. Many elderly patients enter the health care system with decreased sensory function, although this may not be the reason they seek health care.

The final chapter in this unit explores cognitive processes. Normal cognitive function is necessary to meaningfully process information. Many patients who enter a health care facility have altered thought processes to some degree. The nurse must be able to meet the needs of patients who cannot always make their needs known. This chapter details the knowledge and skills essential for caring for these patients.

The chapters in this unit discuss issues relating to how well a patient perceives stimuli and interacts with his or her environment. As the population ages, the number of patients with these nursing care needs will increase.

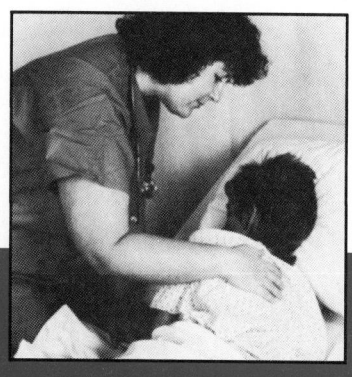

Pain Perception and Comfort

LEARNING OBJECTIVES

Upon completion of this chapter, the student will be able to do the following:

- Discuss how pain sensations are transmitted.
- Describe how the body facilitates or inhibits the transmission of pain.
- Describe the components of a comprehensive nursing database for a patient in pain.
- Describe alternate methods of pain relief based on individual needs.

- Describe the types, actions, and side effects of analgesics.
- List nursing implications for various classes of drugs used for pain management.
- Develop a nursing management plan for surgical patients with problems related to pain.

KEY TERMS

Acute pain
Addiction
Agonist
Antagonist
Chemoreceptors

Chronic pain
Endorphins
Nociceptor
Pain
Pain threshold

Pain tolerance
Proprioceptors
Substantia
  gelatinosa
Thermoreceptors

40

Normal Function of Pain
  Anatomy
    Peripheral Physiology
    Spinal Cord and Central Pathways
  Normal Physiology of Pain
    Pain-Producing Substances
    Endogenous Opiates
    Spinal Reflexes
    Pain Theories
  Characteristics of Pain
    Location
    Intensity
    Quality
    Onset and Duration
    Associated Characteristics
  Normal Function of Pain Perception
  Factors Affecting Normal Pain Function
    Pain Threshold
    Pain Tolerance
    Fear
    Fatigue
    Lack of Knowledge
    Culture, Values, and Beliefs
  Lifespan Considerations
Altered Function Resulting in Pain
  Potential Causes of Pain
    Biologic Factors
    Chemical Factors
    Physical Factors
    Psychogenic Factors
  Manifestations of Pain
    Increased Blood Pressure
    Increased Heart Rate
    Increased Respiratory Rate
    Dilated Pupils

    Perspiration and Pallor
    Increased Blood Glucose
    Verbal and Nonverbal Indications of Pain
    Increased Muscle Tension
  Impact of Pain on Activities of Daily Living
Assessment
  Subjective Data
    Functional Pattern Identification
    Risk Identification
    Dysfunctional Identification
  Objective Data
    Physical Assessment
    Diagnostic Tests and Procedures
Nursing Diagnoses and Patient Goals
  Diagnostic Statement: Pain
    Definition
    Defining Characteristics
    Related Factors
  Diagnostic Statement: Chronic Pain
    Definition
    Defining Characteristics
    Related Factors
  Related Nursing Diagnoses
  Patient Goals
Implementation
  Nursing Interventions to Promote Health and
    Function
  Nursing Interventions for Altered Comfort
    Positioning and Hygiene
    Noninvasive Pain Relief
    Pharmacologic Management
    Invasive Pain Management
  Discharge Planning and Home Care
Evaluation
Key Concepts

Pain, one of the most complex human experiences, is an invisible phenomenon affected by the interaction of physiologic, psychological, social, cultural, and spiritual factors. Because pain is a highly individual experience, the basis for pain management by the nurse is simply the patient's definition of pain. "Pain is whatever

the experiencing person says it is, existing whenever he says it does" (McCaffery, 1968).

Pain is one of the most common and compelling reason that people seek health care. The nurse has daily encounters with patients who anticipate pain or who are in pain, and understanding the phenomenon of pain and contemporary pain theories helps the nurse to intervene effectively.

NORMAL FUNCTION OF PAIN

Anatomy

Pain is the result of a complex pattern of stimuli generated at the pain site and transmitted to the brain. The perception in the subcortical or cortical level of the brain is the result of many different inputs, including psychological and physiologic ones. Sensory receptors of pain, or **nociceptors,** are free nerve endings in the tissue that respond to physiologic stimuli. Receptors that respond to temperature changes (**thermoreceptors**), chemical fluctuations (**chemoreceptors**), or position or movement (**proprioceptors**) may become nociceptors if the stimuli that excite them are sufficiently strong.

Peripheral Physiology

Nociception (the sensory detection and neural transmission of noxious events) develops after an environmental stimulus damages tissues, or when mechanical, thermal, or chemical stimuli activate injury-sensitive receptors deep in body tissues. Nociceptors are found in the skin, blood vessels, subcutaneous tissue muscle, fascia, periosteum, viscera, joints, and other structures. They generate impulses that are transmitted along peripheral fibers to the central nervous system (Fig. 40-1).

Two types of peripheral nerve fibers (axons) are responsible for transmitting pain sensations from the tissues to the nervous system: A-delta fibers and C-fibers. A-delta fibers give rise to bright, sharp, well-localized pain that is immediately associated with the injury. Slow-conducting C-fibers cause pain that is dull, poorly localized, and persistent, although it arises slowly after injury.

The difference between A-delta and C-fiber nociception can best be described as fast versus slow pain. For example, if a sharp object falls on your foot, a fast, sharp pain alerts you to the injury. This is caused by stimulation of the A-delta fibers. After the object is moved from the foot, a low, burning, dull, aching sensation occurs. This sensation, which causes more intense suffering and persists for a longer period, is caused by stimulation of the C-fibers.

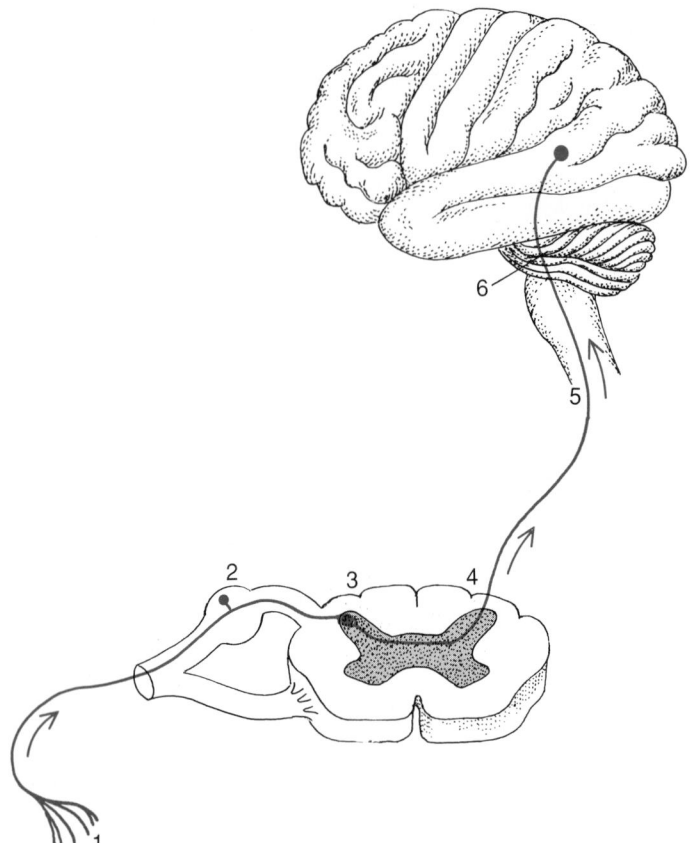

Figure 40–1. Pain stimuli are transmitted from pain receptors (1) via sensory nerves into the dorsal root ganglia (2). The impulse enters the spinal cord and synapses, crosses the cord, and terminates in neurons in cells of substantia gelatinosa (3). Signals then rise to the spinothalamic tract, (4) through the reticular formation (5) and areas of the midbrain (6) to the thalamus (7) and the postcentral gyrus (8), where pain is perceived.

Spinal Cord and Central Pathways

There are numerous pain pathways to the brain. The peripheral nerve fibers enter the dorsal roots of the spinal cord posteriorly, ascend or descend one or two cord segments, and terminate in neurons in the dorsal horns of the spinal cord called the **substantia gelatinosa.** Most signals pass through one or more neurons before reaching long-fibered neurons that cross to the opposite side of the cord. Ascent to the cortex is then completed by way of the dorsal column system and the spinothalamic system.

The major function of the dorsal column system is to transmit information that requires rapid and accurate processing, fine gradations of intensity, and discrete localization. It also transmits fine touch and pressure, vibration, and the kinesthetic or muscle sense.

The spinothalamic tract, also called the pain tract, transmits sensations of pain and temperature, gross information on touch and pressure, sexual sensations, and the sensations of tickle and itch. The spinothalamic tract is divided into three pathways:

The ventral tract transmits general sensations of touch and pressure that require little intensity discrimination and localization on the body surface.

The lateral tract transmits aching, burning, and thermal sensations.

The spinoreticular tract ascends through the reticular formation in the brain stem to areas of the midbrain and eventually ends in the thalamus. The reticular activating system activates most of the nervous system to create a sense of excitement, urgency, or self-defense associated with pain.

Normal Physiology of Pain

The afferent message (message sent) initiated by the nociceptive receptors is subject to modulation (both enhancement and inhibition) at all levels of the nervous system. Pain-producing or pain-enhancing substances, spinal substances, spinal reflexes, and descending inhibitory pathways all affect transmission before the signals reach the higher brain centers. After the signals reach the higher brain centers, psychological factors may influence the pain perception.

Pain-Producing Substances

Nociceptors are usually stimulated by mechanical, chemical, or thermal means. Cellular or tissue injury stimulates nociceptors to release one or more chemical substances that combine with receptors on their surface to cause an impulse. Several agents have been proposed as likely receptor substances, including substance P, cholecystokinin, vasoactive intestinal polypeptide, somatostatin, bradykinin, and histamine. In addition, the inflammatory process leads to the formation of prostaglandins, which in turn enhance the effects of bradykinin on the nociceptors. Thus, the pain of inflammation is generally attributed to the effects of chemical substances on free nerve endings.

Endogenous Opiates

Recent studies have shown that the body has its own natural opiates, or **endorphins.** The effectiveness of several pain-relief measures is related to the release of these endorphins (Holaday, 1985). They are thought to inhibit the release of substances that transmit pain impulses and that alter pain perception. Three groups of endogenous opiates have been identified: enkephalins, endorphins, and dynorphins (Table 40-1).

Spinal Reflexes

Some sensory impulses that enter the spinal cord produce a reflex response via motor fibers to a muscle near the pain site. The muscle then contracts in a protective action (for instance, a pinprick causes immediate withdrawal of the extremity). Nociception may be enhanced by spinal reflexes that affect the environment of the

---

TABLE 40–1
Endogenous Opiates

Type	Location	Function
Enkephalins	Brain stem, limbic system, hypothalamus, adrenal glands, gastrointestinal tract	Inhibit release of substance P, a neurotransmitter that enhances transmission of pain impulses. Half-life, 2 minutes.
Endorphins	Hypothalamus, midbrain, limbic system	Similar to enkephalins but far more potent. Half-life, 4 hours.
Dynorphins	Pituitary, hypothalamus, spinal cord	Analgesic effect 50 times greater than beta-endorphins.

nerve endings in question. For example, trauma may provoke an efferent (motor) reflex that produces muscle spasm in the injured area and causes more nociception.

Pain Theories

No single pain theory explains the complexity of the pain phenomenon. There are four major pain theories that try to explain how pain is transmitted and perceived. Two of these are considered traditional theories (specificity and pattern). The remaining two are considered contemporary theories; they are the gate control theory and the endogenous mechanism of pain inhibition theory.

Traditional Theories. The *specificity theory* proposes that pain results when specific pain receptors are stimulated. Proponents of this theory believe that there is a direct relationship between receptor type, fiber size, and the pain experienced. This theory has been criticized because pain production and perception vary between people and even within the same person at different times (Kim, 1980). This theory does not explain the varying degrees of pain, the effect of emotions, and the inability to locate specific pain receptors.

The *pattern theory* arose because of deficiencies in the specificity theory. This theory proposes that pain results from the transmission of nerve impulses that originate from and are coded at the peripheral stimulation site, rather than from adequate stimulation of specific receptors. A key concept in this theory is that after tissue injury, circuits can be established in the spinal interneurons that enable the pain to be perceived, even though the stimuli that initiated the pain are no longer present. The reverberating circuit might explain the phenomenon of *phantom pain* (pain felt in a body part that is no longer present, such as an amputated foot).

Contemporary Theories. The *gate control theory,* developed by Melzack and Wall (1965), incorporates some aspects of both the specificity and pattern theories. According to this theory, the dorsal horn acts as a gate, closing to prevent impulses from reaching the brain or opening to allow impulses to be transmitted to the brain (Fig. 40-2). In simple terms, when the gate is open, pain impulses flow through and pain is felt. When the gate is closed, pain impulses are stopped. The opening and closing of the gate is influenced by the activity of the large A-delta fibers, the small C-fibers, the reticular formation in the brain stem, and the cerebral cortex (Melzack & Wall, 1965; 1983).

Because small fibers carry pain impulses, it is proposed that when tissue damage occurs, simultaneous activity, such as heat, cold, or touch, in adjacent large fibers could modulate small-fiber transmission. Once pain is transmitted to the cerebral cortex, perception is affected by the patient's mental state, emotions, and past experience.

Therapeutic implications of the gate control theory include the following (McCaffery, 1968):

- Pain can be controlled (the gate can be closed) by selectively influencing the A-delta fibers by techniques such as cutaneous nerve stimulation.
- Pain can be controlled by decreasing C-fiber input.
- Pain can be controlled by counterirritation with electric current, vibration, heat, cold, or tactile stimulation, all of which create toleration for greater noxious stimuli.
- Drugs may affect excitation or inhibition of substantia gelatinosa activity.

There are sensory, emotional, and cognitive dimensions to pain, providing a rationale for many noninvasive nursing actions.

Although this theory is the basis for various pain interventions discussed later in this chapter, it remains controversial and is criticized as having insufficient experimental support.

The *endogenous opiates* theory emphasizes the role of biochemicals in pain modulation. Enkephalins and en-

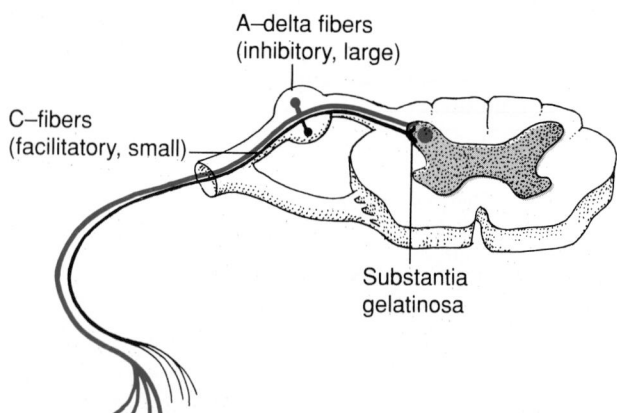

A–delta fibers
(inhibitory, large)

C–fibers
(facilitatory, small)

Substantia
gelatinosa

Figure 40–2. The gate control theory. Small fibers carry pain impulses that may be modulated by other sensations in the large fiber, thus closing or opening the gate to the transmission of pain.

dorphins primarily act at neuron synapses to influence the integration of pain and activation of the brain's analgesic system (Hendler & Fenton, 1979). Researchers studying these biochemicals have not agreed on their mechanisms of action.

Characteristics of Pain

Pain is usually described in relation to location, intensity, onset, and duration. Pain is a highly individualized experience. One person's description of pain may differ from another's, even though the pain stimuli are the same.

Location

Superficial pain that emanates from the skin or from tissues close to the surface is usually localized, and the patient can accurately identify that location. However, when pain originates from deeper structures, accurate identification becomes more difficult. Pain from the abdominal area (also called visceral pain) may originate from the abdominal or pelvic organs, liver, spleen, or kidney. Visceral pain tends to be a dull, aching pain that is diffuse (poorly localized).

Additional terms to help the nurse locate the source of the pain are proximal or distal, medial or lateral, anterior or posterior, right or left, and upper or lower quadrant.

The nurse may need to explain these terms to the patient to get accurate information, just as "abdominal" may need to identified as "tummy" or "belly."

Pain may be described as *referred* when the location where the pain is felt is not necessarily where the pain is originating. For example, pain in the abdomen may be referred to the shoulder and back; thus, the patient may describe back or shoulder pain as the primary sensation.

Intensity

Terms used to describe pain severity include mild, slight, moderate, intermittent, spasmodic, or constant. Pain intensity may also be described on a numerical scale: for example, on a scale of 1 to 10, 1 would be free of pain and 10 would be the worst pain imaginable.

Pain intensity may vary among patients, depending on their previous experience with pain, personal expectations, ability to be distracted or to concentrate on other things, and level of consciousness. Fear of the consequences of reporting pain intensity (hospitalization, tests, diagnoses) may cause patients to minimize their reported pain.

Quality

Many patients find it easier to use an analogy than to find words that describe the pain. For example, a headache may be "pounding like a hammer," or chest pain may be "like an elephant sitting on my chest."

Onset and Duration

The words "acute" and "chronic" are often used to designate the two main types of pain onset and duration. Because the cause, pathophysiology, symptoms, diag-

---

Descriptions of Pain

Location

Localized vs. diffuse	Right vs. left
Proximal vs. distal	Upper vs. lower
Medial vs. lateral	Phantom
Anterior vs. posterior	Referred

Intensity

Mild
Slight
Moderate
Intermittent
Spasmodic
Constant

Quality

Boring	Penetrating
Burning	Piercing
Constant	Pounding
Cramping	Radiating
Crushing	Sharp
Dull	Shooting
Excruciating	Spasms
Hammering	Stabbing
Intermittent	Tearing
Knifelike	Throbbing
Lancinating	Tingling

Onset and Duration

Acute
Chronic
Intractable

Associated Characteristics

Visual disturbance	Muscle spasms
Nausea and vomiting	Anger and aggression
Fatigue and depression	Withdrawal
Anorexia	Regression

nosis, and treatment of these two types of pain are different, it is important to understand the difference between the two.

Acute pain occurs abruptly after an injury or disease and persists until healing occurs. Acute pain may also be associated with anxiety and fear. If acute pain is not effectively managed, it may progress to a chronic state.

Chronic pain lasts for a prolonged period of time. It is associated with prolonged tissue pathology or pain that persists beyond the normal healing period for an acute injury or disease. Depression related to the pain is not uncommon. Many times there is no demonstrable pathology, and the persistence of pain does not necessarily mean that the original organic damage has failed to heal.

Intractable pain is a type of chronic pain that is resistant to cure or relief. Patients with intractable pain often describe it as all-consuming and interfering with their quality of life. Examples of causes of intractable pain are arthritis or incurable cancer.

Associated Characteristics

Other characteristics and symptoms may be related to pain. For example, people who have migraine headaches often experience visual disturbances, nausea, and vomiting. Fatigue, depression, anorexia, and muscle spasms may be other characteristics related to pain. Although pain may produce sadness and depression, it is not uncommon for pain to be related to anger and aggressive behavior, as a way of "fighting back" against the pain. At the other extreme, the person in pain may withdraw from the pain by minimizing interaction with the environment and other people. Regression to earlier stages of development may occur (e.g., a school-age child may revert to toddler-type behaviors).

Normal Function of Pain Perception

Although pain is a great source of human misery, it serves an important biologic purpose: it helps to minimize injury and often serves as a protective mechanism to prevent injury. For instance, pain makes a person pull a hand away from a hot stove, and right lower abdominal pain warns the person of a possible diseased appendix, thus prompting early medical intervention. People who are born without the ability to feel pain do not usually survive past early childhood: death occurs because the lack of warning of disease delays prompt treatment.

Factors Affecting Normal Pain Function

Factors affecting pain can make it more intense, as shown in Figure 40-3.

Pain Threshold

The amount of pain stimulation a person requires before feeling pain is that person's **pain threshold.** A person's pain threshold is remarkably uniform throughout life, although the phenomenon of adaptation may occur. The same stimulus that once caused intense pain can also produce only mild pain; for instance, plunging a hand into hot water causes intense pain, but immersing the hand in cool water, then gradually heating the water,

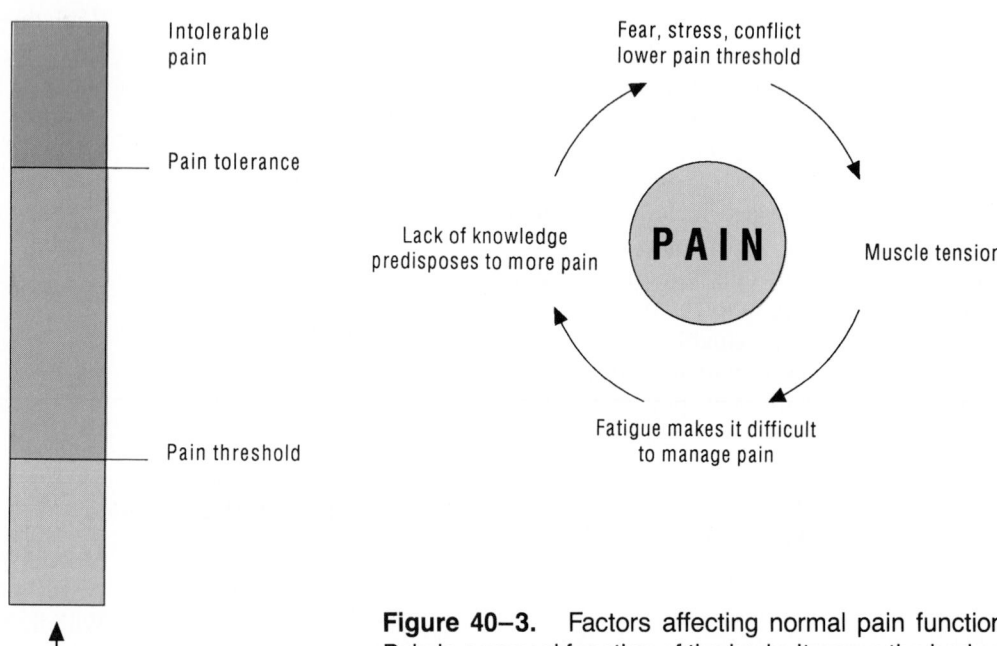

Figure 40–3.   Factors affecting normal pain function. Pain is a normal function of the body. It warns the body of injury and disease. Factors can lower the pain threshold and pain tolerance, and a cycle of pain can follow.

produces mild pain. The pain threshold can also be dramatically changed by the person's state of consciousness (i.e., anesthesia).

Pain Tolerance

Pain tolerance is the highest intensity of pain that the person is willing to tolerate. Some people can tolerate severe pain without intervention, but others can tolerate only minimal discomfort.

Fear

Fear of pain can lower the pain threshold because of the heightened focus on pain. Fear increases muscle tension, which increases pain perception and intensity. For instance, a toddler fearing an injection will cry and tense his or her muscles, thus intensifying the experience.

Fatigue

Pain can be fatiguing, and fatigue can predispose the patient to pain. Exhaustion and lack of sleep contribute to a chronically tired state in which it is difficult to manage pain. What might be tolerable pain to a well-rested person may be intolerable to a fatigued person.

Lack of Knowledge

Fear of the unknown may worsen pain because of the tension and anxiety that the patient brings to the situation. The patient may experience more pain if he or she fears the diagnosis, does not understand the treatments, or does not know enough about the decisions that need to be made.

Culture, Values, and Beliefs

Cultural beliefs about pain can strongly influence a person's response to a painful stimulus. Many cultures see pain tolerance as a virtue; often men are expected to tolerate pain more stoically than women. Health-care providers need to recognize the patient's cultural beliefs and not impose their own judgments.

Lifespan Considerations

Newborn and Infant

A neonate or infant cannot verbally report pain. Although it was formerly believed that infants' neurophysiologic systems were too immature to transport pain impulses, researchers have learned that infants can perceive pain, although measuring it is difficult. Studies have shown that neonates do respond to pain with increased sensitivity even after a few days of age, with full

behavioral response by 3 to 12 months (McCaffery, 1980). More recent studies showed that within 3 seconds of a heel lance, the infant began to cry and cried for an average of 3 minutes, with a heart rate of 50 beats per minute over baseline (Owens, 1986a). As infants develop more motor control, they try to pull or roll away from the pain and show general physical resistance. The behavioral or emotional reactions of the parents or the nurse may influence the infant's response.

Toddler and Preschooler

Toddlers cannot identify the pain they are experiencing or its source. Older toddlers and preschoolers are developing the ability to describe, identify, and locate sources of pain, and can begin to use terms to define the intensity and severity. Associated characteristics are important in this age group: lethargy, fatigue, anorexia, and regression are commonly associated with pain.

During this stage of development, the child is achieving a sense of autonomy. Because pain can be a source of fear and a threat to the child's security, the child responds with crying, anger, physical resistance, or withdrawal. It is difficult to reason with a child of this age about pain and its cause or management; thus, the child may withdraw from attachments for fear of being hurt again. Although parents are the child's greatest source of comfort and support, the child may appear ambivalent toward them, as though blaming them for the pain. The nurse must encourage and support the parents and help them understand the child's response.

Child and Adolescent

School-age children develop a sense of competence and industry. They begin to turn to rationalization as an attempt to explain what happens in their lives. Faced with a painful situation, the child tries to be "brave" and rationalize the pain and is more responsive to explanations about the pain than a younger child. School-age children can identify the general location and quality of pain. If pain persists, the school-age child may temporarily regress to an earlier stage of development in an attempt to handle the situation. For example, the young school-age child may temporarily lose bladder control and may revert to comfort measures such as thumbsucking, nail-biting, and favorite toys.

Because adolescents are developing an identity and personal independence, their physical appearance and abilities are important. When coupled with concern about peer relationships, adolescents demonstrate careful self-control and may be reluctant to acknowledge pain. To recognize or "give in" to pain may seem a sign of weakness. For example, a high-school football player may know that his knee is injured, but he may prefer to deny the pain in an effort to be a "team player" and not let down his team, coach, or school.

Adult and Older Adult

Adult responses to pain vary. For some adults, like adolescents, giving in to pain may be a sign of weakness or failure; hence, they may ignore the normal warning function of pain. Other adults may respond to the warning and take appropriate action, such as making lifestyle changes and getting a medical check-up. Pain may also be an expression of depression or another psychological dysfunction, or may be used for secondary gain (that is, pain may be the route the adult uses to gain attention or some other benefit). Fear of what the pain may indicate prevents some adults from taking action.

The older adult presents unique problems. An elderly person may not report pain due to decreased sensation or perceptions (McGuigan, 1970). Instead, associated characteristics and symptoms may provide the early indications of pain. Anorexia, nausea, and vomiting may appear to be the primary problems, but they may actually be the associated indicators of pain. Associated characteristics such as lethargy, cognitive dysfunction, and loss of appetite may indicate pain even when the older adult cannot verbalize it.

A condition that would produce acute pain in a younger person may remain virtually undetected in an elderly person until complications occur. For example, an elderly person experiencing a myocardial infarction may complain of excess gas, an upset stomach, or extreme fatigue rather than the crushing chest pain identified by younger adults. Thus, the complication of congestive heart failure may be the first indicator of the primary problem.

ALTERED FUNCTION RESULTING IN PAIN

Although pain is a normal function of the body, it also indicates a dysfunction. The four categories of causes of pain—biologic, chemical, physical, and psychogenic—may act alone or together (Watts, 1975).

In the biological, chemical, and physical causes of pain, the two major pathophysiologic processes that contribute to pain are inflammation (a nonspecific defense to any type of injury) and ischemia (the deprivation of oxygen to tissues). Cells react the same way (showing ischemic changes and inflammation) even though the cause of pain may be different (e.g., injury, tumor, burn, infection).

Inflammation brings with it chemical mediators that stimulate nerve endings. These factors include histamine, kinins, serotonin, and prostaglandins. They are released as the result of cell injury and contribute to the accumulation of more fluid and cells, causing increasing distention or edema of the affected tissues. The distended tissues place more pressure on nerve endings, causing additional pain (Porth, 1990).

The process by which ischemia causes pain, although not fully understood, is believed to be similar to that of inflammation. The oxygen-deprived cells exhibit the same response as cells that suffer other injuries. Therefore, the release of chemical mediators and the presence of cellular swelling are the most probable contributors to pain.

Potential Causes of Pain

Biologic Factors

Biologic causes of pain are due to disease, microorganisms, or cell injury. Tissue damage may be actual or impending. Pain of biologic origin may be caused by alterations in essential life processes such as cell growth, oxygenation, nutrition, transport, metabolism, and regularity of response mechanisms. Examples of biologic causes of pain are angina in coronary artery disease, obstruction of organs by tumors, pleural pain in pneumonia, and joint pain in rheumatoid arthritis.

Chemical Factors

Chemical causes of pain include substances released by pathologic processes (i.e., peptic ulcer disease with hydrochloric acid release, inflammation with prostaglandin release) and cytotoxic agents that damage or destroy tissues and cells (i,e., lead, alcohol, drugs, poisons).

Physical Factors

Physical causes of pain include trauma, temperature extremes, electrical burns, and radiation injuries.

Psychogenic Factors

Psychogenic causes are generally described as emotional factors, independent of peripheral stimulation, that cause a person to feel distressed. No anatomic or physiologic cause can be detected to explain the intensity and duration of the pain. The diagnosis of a psychogenic cause is made when a person's apparent discomfort exceeds that usually expected with a given noxious stimulus (Fordyce, 1976).

Pain of psychological origin is as real as any other pain. All types of pain have some psychological overlay and may evoke an emotional response. Anxiety commonly occurs with acute pain, and depression is a common emotional response with chronic pain.

Manifestations of Pain

Common manifestations of pain include physiologic and behavioral responses. Observable physiologic signs of discomfort include increased blood pressure, heart rate, and respiratory rate; dilated pupils; and pallor and perspiration.

An increase in blood glucose may also be measured.

Behavioral responses to pain are subjective and depend on the patient's report or on interpretation of the patient's nonverbal communication. Behavioral responses include report of pain; crying, moaning; rubbing of painful parts; frowns and grimaces; fatigue; and increased muscle tension.

The autonomic nervous system regulates most of the functions involved in the manifestations of pain (Table 40-2). This system is composed of the sympathetic nervous system (the adrenergic system, which maintains homeostasis and provides defense) and the parasympathetic nervous system (the cholinergic system, which conserves and restores basic functions).

The sympathetic nervous system regulates the observable physiologic signs of pain. The neurotransmitters in this system that contribute to these responses are epinephrine and norepinephrine. This system responds to perceived threats, such as pain, with physiologic manifestations in an attempt to maintain homeostasis. It is also the system involved in the fight-or-flight response when the body perceives a threat (see Fig. 47-2).

Increased Blood Pressure

The increase in blood pressure that accompanies acute pain is believed to be due to peripheral vasoconstriction. This is the body's response to the shift of blood away from the periphery (skin, extremities) to the viscera (heart, lungs, kidney) when the body perceives a threat.

Increased Heart Rate

The increased heart rate is the body's attempt to increase the available oxygen and circulating fluid volume to the tissues determined to be in danger as a result of pain. The shunting of blood from the periphery to the vital organs (brain, heart, liver, kidney) is an effort to preserve the body's life-support systems.

Increased Respiratory Rate

An increase in the respiratory rate is an effort to increase the amount of oxygen available to the heart and circulation. Increased respiration also helps eliminate carbon dioxide from the circulation.

Dilated Pupils

Dilatation of the pupils is an effort to increase visual acuity. The improved accommodation for far vision is to help the person to protect himself or herself or to move away from the pain, if possible.

Perspiration and Pallor

Perspiration and pallor reflect the shift of circulating blood from the skin to the vital organs. Increased perspiration also helps regulate body temperature.

Increased Blood Glucose

Increasing the amount of glucose in the blood increases the available energy for responding to the situation. Glucose is released from the liver to the blood to increase available oxygen. Glycogen, stored in skeletal muscle, the skin, and some of the glandular tissues, can be broken down to glucose by the process of glycogenolysis.

Verbal and Nonverbal Indications of Pain

Indicators of pain can be verbal (reporting of pain, moaning, crying) and nonverbal (body positioning, grimaces, frowns, rubbing of painful areas). Nonverbal behaviors indicate the location of pain and perhaps its duration, but verbal reports indicate more clearly its location, intensity, onset, and duration.

TABLE 40–2

Physiologic Response to Stimulation of the Autonomic Nervous System

Response	Sympathetic (low to moderate pain)	Parasympathetic (severe pain)
Skin color	Pallor	Pallor
Blood pressure	Increased	Decreased
Pupils	Dilated	Constricted
Skeletal muscle	Increased	Decreased
Respiratory rate	Increased	No effect
Heart rate	Increased	Decreased
Perspiration	Increased	No effect
Urinary output	Decreased	No effect
GI peristalsis	Decreased	Increased
Mental activity	Increased	No effect
Basal metabolism rate	Increased	No effect

Increased Muscle Tension

The increase in muscle tension shown by body positioning is part of the body's fight-or-flight response as well as a guarding reaction to protect against further pain. Prolonged muscle tension also contributes to fatigue, which affects the person's response to pain.

Impact of Pain on Activities of Daily Living

Pain generally causes decreased energy, which affects all aspects of daily living. The patient in pain often finds it difficult to perform basic daily activities. The ability to be independent and self-sufficient is important in our culture, and people who have difficulty with independent living may experience anxiety or alterations in self-concept.

Pain can make it difficult for the patient to fall asleep or stay asleep, and the resulting lack of sleep then contributes to fatigue, which predisposes the patient to more pain. Pain itself can also be fatiguing. The physiologic and behavioral responses to acute pain cause exhaustion, but in chronic pain, adaptation takes place and a more chronic fatigue is seen.

It is important to remember that sleep does not indicate pain relief. After experiencing pain for an extended time, the patient becomes too tired to talk or cry and falls asleep. Patients in pain may close their eyes and appear to be asleep, but actually may just be conserving energy or focusing on something else to make the pain bearable.

Basic hygiene activities (bathing, dressing, eating, grooming) may be mildly or severely affected depending on the location and degree of pain. Household activities may also be difficult to perform. Pain, particularly chronic pain, can interfere with the person's ability to concentrate on work or school. Pain may be increased with physical activity such as leisure activities, walking, or driving.

Patients with pain may focus on their pain and thus be unable to explore outside interests and relationships. This may alter family and social relationships, and prolonged pain can lead to family deterioration. Decreased energy also hinders sexual functioning.

ASSESSMENT

An accurate diagnosis of the cause of pain is the cornerstone of nursing management. Without an accurate diagnosis, it is impossible to select the best therapy. Ongoing assessment is crucial in formulating an effective, current management plan for the patient in pain.

The nurse must obtain facts from the patient and from direct observation. Because of the person's response and expression of pain, the nurse may find it difficult to remain objective and nonjudgmental. It is important to remember that pain is whatever the patient says it is and occurs whenever the patient says it does.

Subjective Data

A focused functional assessment of pain includes a thorough nursing history. The nurse must review the patient's current functional health status, past relevant life experiences, physical assessment, medical history, and diagnostic test results to establish a baseline and to seek clues to the reason for pain. Although physicians prescribe many pain-management techniques, the nurse is responsible for assessing, administering, monitoring, and evaluating the effectiveness of these techniques and initiating independent nursing measures for pain relief.

An accurate assessment requires the nurse to do the following:

- Listen to the patient's description.
- Observe physiologic signs.
- Observe psychological symptoms.
- Understand the meaning of pain to the patient.
- Identify the patient's coping methods.

Functional Pattern Identification

Collecting subjective data helps the nurse identify the patient's pain pattern and the potential and actual risks present in the patient. To determine the pain pattern, the nurse needs information from the patient (or a significant other) and from current medical records. The nurse will need answers to these questions:

- What is the meaning of pain and suffering for the patient?
- How does the patient describe the pain?
- Can the patient quantify the pain?
- How has the pain hampered the patient's physical activities?
- Does the pain affect self-care, job, or leisure activities?
- Does the pain interfere with personal relationships?
- Does the pain keep the patient from sleeping at night?
- Does it awaken the patient? If so, for how long?
- Does the patient relate pain to alterations in other body functions, such as appetite, elimination, menses, or sex?
- How does the patient usually cope with pain (medications, home remedies, rest, or other therapies)?
- What are the patient's expectations in relation to the pain?

Understanding the meaning of pain to the patient, the patient's expectations, and the effect of pain on the patient's life helps the nurse determine the patient's pattern of pain and pain management.

Other data to help the nurse assess the functional pattern include the presence or absence of the patient's family or other support systems, the patient's educational and intellectual level, and other factors that may be stressful or affect the patient's mood, concerns, and fears. The nurse needs to remember that his or her own attitudes about pain may influence assessment of the patient's pain.

Risk Identification

The nursing history helps identify factors that place the patient at risk for pain. Important information to obtain is how the patient has been socialized to respond to and cope with pain, and the patient's age. Young and elderly patients are at greater risk: the young cannot communicate the location or degree of pain, and the elderly may have decreased sensation or perception of pain. Nurses may inadvertently place the patient at risk by their own personal values and socialization.

Pain Behaviors. The behaviors observed with pain are the result of how the central nervous system processes the original pain sensation. Other factors that affect the patient's perception of and risk for pain include:

- The patient's attitude toward pain
- The value the patient places on withstanding pain
- Social, cultural, and economic factors
- The patient's psychological and physiologic state.

Patients in pain respond in a variety of ways. The response may be different from the nurse's personal or professional customs but may be acceptable and even desirable in the patient's culture. Personal meanings attached to pain arise from individual and cultural experiences; some cultural and family influences that shape a patient's attitude toward pain are listed in the display. These teachings may influence people throughout their lives, regardless of their validity.

Understanding the meaning of pain to a patient may take time. It requires trust and good listening and observation skills. Obtaining this information is useful because it clarifies pain for the patient and helps the nurse and patient set realistic goals.

Coping Skills. Observing a patient's behavior and response to illness gives the nurse clues about how the patient copes. The nurse must assess methods that have been helpful to the patient in the past and those that can be useful in the hospital. This allows staff members to help the patient develop new positive skills. This assessment is important in the patient with acute pain, but it is essential in the patient with chronic pain to help him or her to develop positive coping methods. When assessing coping strategies, the integrity of the patient's nervous system, level of consciousness, age, physical state,

---

> ### Cultural and Familial Role Modeling Related to Pain
>
> #### Children Learn*
>
> - What pains are and are not appropriate to talk about.
> - Appropriate and inappropriate behavior when in pain.
> - What circumstances cause pain and should be avoided.
> - Methods to avoid or relieve pain.
> - Reasons we experience pain (e.g., punishment, testing, bad thoughts).
> - Possible consequences of pain.
>
> #### Cultural Influences on Pain†
>
> - How one person learns to respond to pain may differ from what someone else has learned.
> - Each person considers how he or she learned to respond to pain as natural and correct.
> - Cultural background may influence our attitude and behavioral response to pain more than the intensity of pain itself.
> - Similar responses to pain do not necessarily reflect similar attitudes toward pain.
> - Cultural expectations may include appropriate, acceptable, and effective behavioral response; when, how, and by whom pain should be treated; and the meaning or significance of pain.
>
> * Jaffee, J. H., & Martin, W. R. (1990). Opioid analgesics and antagonists. In A. Gilman, T. W. Rall, A. S. Nis, et al. (Eds.), *Goodman and Gilman's pharmacological basis of therapeutics* (8th ed., pp. 485–521).
> † McCaffery, M. (1979). *Nursing management of the patient with pain.* Philadelphia: J. B. Lippincott.

---

fatigue, and length of suffering must be considered, because they may affect the patient's ability to tolerate pain.

The Nurse's Attitudes. An accurate risk assessment is affected by the nurse's attitudes toward pain and the manner in which they are expressed (Holm, et al., 1989). If the nurse and the patient perceive pain differently, this can result in major conflicts and increased pain risk for the patient. For instance, Jacox (1979a), in a study of more than 100 patients with various types of pain, found that many did not say they were in pain until the pain was severe; some did not verbally communicate at all. The nurse who assumes that a patient will always report pain may be contributing to the patient's discomfort; more active and careful questioning about pain is necessary.

One study on an orthopedic unit (Weiner, 1975) found that many nurses failed to listen to, understand, or provide comfort care to patients in pain. Staff members tended to force patients into legitimizing and enduring their pain by placing a high value on stoicism ("being a good patient").

Obtaining a pain profile on admission to determine the patient's routines and previously effective pain-relief methods is helpful. However, this can be threatening to nurses who are uncomfortable when patients with chronic pain try to advise them about effective or ineffective interventions. If the nurse feels threatened, a negative or antagonistic nurse–patient relationship may be established.

Dysfunctional Identification

Understanding pain from the patient's perspective helps the nurse identify the source and meaning of the pain. To determine the patient's level of pain, it is necessary to assess the patient's beliefs about the normal function of pain. Some people believe that no pain should be present unless something terrible is happening to their body. They may also believe that medication is necessary to correct any deviation from this pattern. Remembering that pain is what the patient says it is helps the nurse to analyze the presenting data. For example, if the patient usually experiences no pain and now reports severe pain, the nurse must accept that subjective data as presented by the patient.

Objective Data

Objective data about the patient's pain are gathered through ongoing physical assessment; diagnostic or screening tests cannot quantify the degree of pain. Objective data are used to augment the subjective data.

Physical Assessment

Physiologic responses to pain are the result of the activation of the autonomic nervous system (ANS). Usual responses of the ANS and parasympathetic nervous system (PNS) are listed in Table 40-2. With acute pain, the general responses observed are tachycardia, elevated blood pressure, increased respiratory rate, diaphoresis, and gastric distress. With chronic pain, these responses may be modified or absent.

Vital Signs. Assessing the patient's vital signs is important for obtaining baseline information, particularly before a potentially painful procedure or situation. The ANS responses to acute pain are evident in the vital signs, with increases in heart rate, respiratory rate, and

blood pressure, and diaphoresis. For patients who have difficulty expressing pain or cannot do so, the vital sign readings and comparisons may prove valuable for evaluation.

Location. The nurse should ask the patient to identify the location of the pain by describing where the pain is, pointing to the site, or showing on a drawing where the pain is.

Angina pain is usually described as beginning in the sternal area of the chest and radiating to the neck, jaw, and left arm. Angina is often preceded by exertion, overeating, or stress. It may begin gradually, build to a peak, then recede. Tachycardia, dizziness, nausea, vomiting, and diaphoresis may accompany it. The nurse must learn the frequency of angina attacks and how the patient obtains relief.

Intermittent claudication is cramping in the leg muscles that occurs with intermittent interruption of circulation brought on by exercise. It is relieved by rest. Occlusive peripheral artery disease and neurologic dysfunctions are two factors that cause narrowing of arteries leading to the legs, resulting in insufficient circulation to the muscles. Assessing how far the patient can walk or how many stairs he or she can climb provides information on the extent of circulation interference.

Phantom pain occurs when the patient perceives pain in an amputated limb. For example, the patient may describe ankle pain, even though he or she knows that the ankle is not present. Although such pain is probably the result of innervation at the amputation site, assessing what the patient thinks induced the pain, how long it lasts, and what if anything relieves it helps the nurse clarify this symptom.

Neuralgia is an intense burning pain that radiates along a peripheral nerve or dermatome plane. For example, a neuralgia may occur along a nerve emanating from the spinal nerve ganglia, causing intense burning, hypersensitivity, or severe shooting pain. Assessing the patient's idea of what may have initiated the pain helps determine the management.

Intensity. Ask the patient to describe the intensity of the pain, using a numerical scale. This number should be recorded for future comparison. A child can be asked to select the number of chips or marbles (out of 10) that reflects his or her pain. When a more definitive assessment of pain is needed, the McGill–Melzack Pain Questionnaire can be used (Wilkie, et al., 1990). As shown in the display, each description is assigned a numerical value, and the sum is the pain rating index. The present pain intensity is based on a scale of 0 to 5.

Quality. Ask the patient to describe the pain quality, and listen for terms such as those listed earlier in the

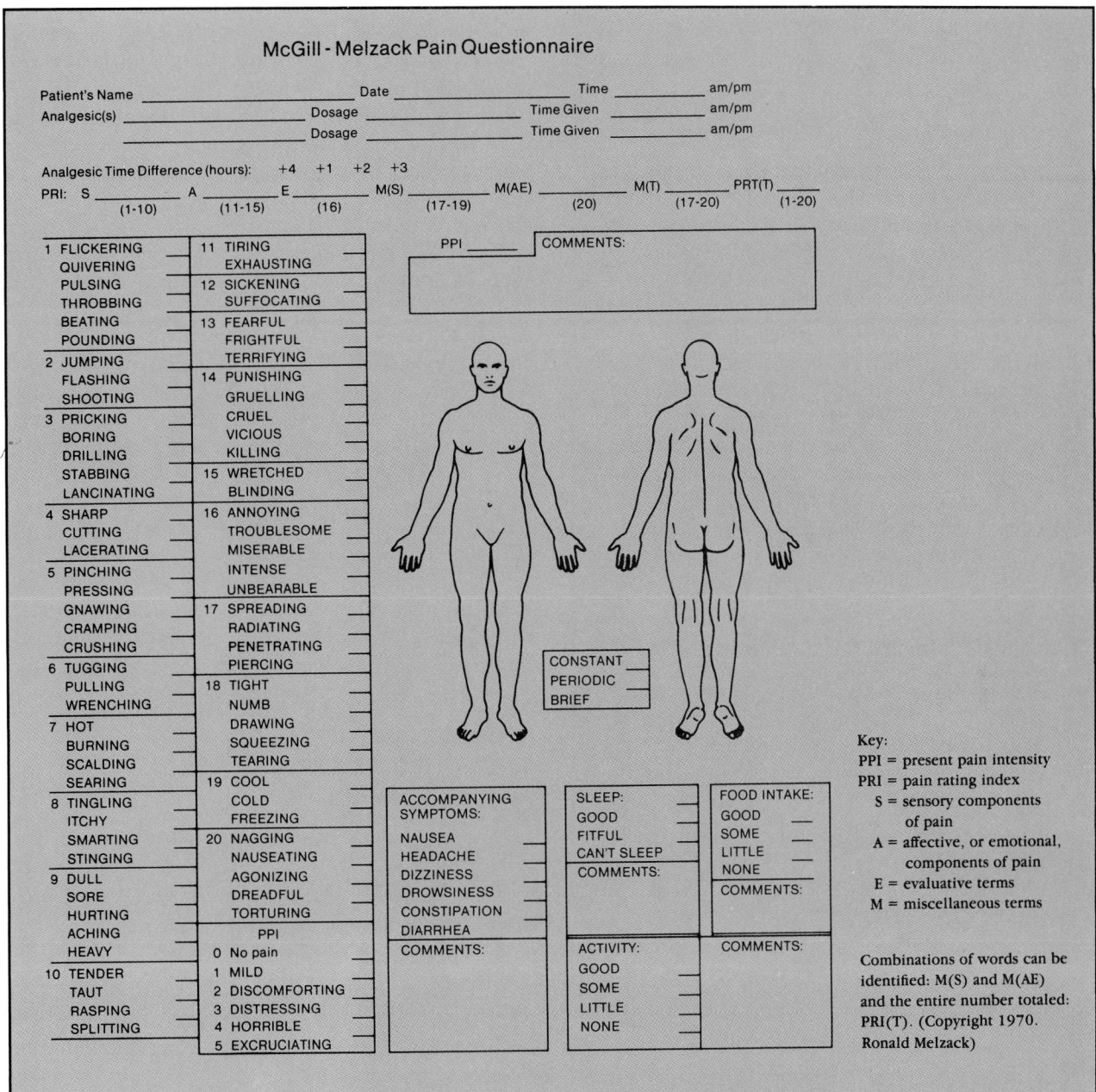

chapter. Asking open-ended questions encourages patients to use their own words and prevents the nurse from inadvertently "leading" the patient. The patient's exact description should be used in documentation.

Onset and Duration. Assessing when the pain began is important in determining whether the patient's pain is acute or chronic. Acute pain has a sudden onset that the patient can pinpoint, but the patient with chronic pain describes the onset in more indefinite terms. The duration of pain is described using terms such as brief, transient, continuous, steady, or constant. Listen carefully for the patient's description of the onset of pain (acute or chronic), its duration (constant, intermittent, spasmodic), and its variations (rhythmicity, intensity).

Associated Characteristics. Be alert to related symptoms that may give additional clues about the pain. Nausea and vomiting, anorexia, fatigue, depression, or withdrawal are not uncommon with pain. The presence of these symptoms should be assessed in relation to the potential for or presence of pain. Relieving the pain may

Nursing Research

Selected Nursing Research Studies

Bever, P. K. (1987). Premature infants' response to touch and pain: Can nursing make a difference? *Neonatal Network, 6*(3), 13–17.

Levin, R. F., et al. (1987). Nursing management of postoperative pain: Use of relaxation techniques with female cholecystectomy patients. *Journal of Advanced Nursing, 12,* 463–472.

Mills, N. M. (1989). Pain behaviors in infants and toddlers. *Journal of Pain Symptom Management, 4,* 184–190.

Radwin, L. E. (1987). Autonomous nursing intervention for treating the patient in acute pain: A standard. *Heart & Lung 16,* 258–266.

Wilkie, D. J., et al. (1990). Use of the McGill Pain Questionnaire to measure pain: A meta-analysis. *Nursing Research, 39*(1), 36–41.

Possible Topics for Nursing Inquiry

- Does preoperative teaching of noninvasive techniques (i.e., relaxation, distraction) lead to decreased use of drugs postoperatively?
- Does the patient experience more or less respiratory depression if usual postoperative narcotics are given on a regularly scheduled versus prn basis?
- Do patients experience less pain if they control analgesia administration?

also relieve these associated characteristics. For example, relieving pain may allow the patient to relax and rest, thus diminishing the fatigue that may be associated with pain.

Physical Expressions of Pain. Observe the patient's facial expressions, body movements, and emotional reactions to pain. Wincing, frowning, and grimacing can indicate pain. Body movements may represent protective actions to decrease the pain, and body movements may increase with pain (rubbing, splinting, or elevating the painful extremity, or frequently changing position). For example, a woman in labor rhythmically rubs her abdomen. As pain increases, total body activity decreases, and eventually the patient lies still and is quiet. This decrease in activity may delay recovery, as when the postoperative patient refuses to ambulate, turn, cough, or deep-breathe.

Pain evokes emotional responses that may be expressed as depression, anger, fear, anxiety, sadness, excitement, denial, or regression. A wide range of verbal responses (moaning, sighing, screaming, crying, and repetition of words or phrases) can be a result of pain. However, such restlessness, moaning, and grimacing can be misleading: the patient may not be in pain, but instead may be disoriented, hypoxic, or febrile or having a medication reaction.

Any of these ways of expressing pain may be absent in stoic patients or those with prolonged chronic pain (Jacox, 1979a). Remember that lack of pain expression does *not* mean lack of pain, as patients adapt physically and psychologically to pain (McCaffery, 1979). Therefore, the nurse must actively solicit information about pain to reach an accurate assessment. Observe accurately and listen; never judge or jump to conclusions.

Diagnostic Tests and Procedures

Although tests cannot quantify the degree of pain, procedures can validate painful events (for instance, an electrocardiogram shows a myocardial infarction after chest pain). Other diagnostic tests may be done that relate to the specific pain source.

NURSING DIAGNOSES AND PATIENT GOALS

There are two NANDA categories of pain: Pain and Chronic Pain.

Diagnostic Statement: Pain

Definition

Pain is a state in which an individual experiences and reports the presence of severe discomfort or an uncomfortable sensation (NANDA, 1990).

Defining Characteristics

Subjective. Communication (verbal or coded) of pain descriptors (NANDA, 1990).

Objective. Guarding behavior, protective; self-focusing; narrowed focus (altered time perception, withdrawal from social contact, impaired thought process); distraction behavior (moaning, crying, pacing, seeking out other people and/or activities, restlessness); facial mask of pain (eyes lack luster, "beaten look," fixed or scattered movement, grimace); alteration in muscle tone (may span from listless to rigid); autonomic responses not seen in chronic stable pain (diaphoresis, blood pressure and pulse change, pupillary dilation, increased or decreased respiratory rate) (NANDA, 1990).

Related Factors

Injury agents (biologic, chemical, physical, psychological) (NANDA, 1990).

Diagnostic Statement: Chronic Pain

Definition

Chronic pain is a state in which the individual experiences pain that continues for more than 6 months in duration (NANDA, 1990).

Defining Characteristics

Major. Verbal report or observed evidence of pain experienced for more than 6 months (NANDA, 1990).

Minor. Fear of reinjury; physical and social withdrawal; altered ability to continue previous activities; anorexia; weight changes; changes in sleep patterns; facial mask; guarded movement (NANDA, 1990).

Related Factors

Chronic physical/psychosocial disability (NANDA, 1990).

Related Nursing Diagnoses

Although Pain and Chronic Pain are the obvious nursing diagnoses for the person in pain, assessment may indicate that the patient has other problems related to the pain. For instance, Anxiety, Ineffective Individual Coping, Ineffective Family Coping, Altered Health Maintenance, Impaired Home Maintenance Management, and Sleep Pattern Disturbance may be related to pain. If the patient suffers from chronic pain, additional nursing diagnoses may be defined, including Self-Care Deficit, Self-Esteem Disturbance, Hopelessness, Impaired Physical Mobility, Sexual Dysfunction, and Spiritual Distress. If the patient is taking medications for pain, other nursing diagnoses may be evident, such as Constipation and Altered Thought Processes.

Patient Goals

Once the causes are identified, goals and nursing interventions can be designed. The overall goal in pain management is for the patient to seek interventions that maximize his or her quality of life. The specific goals for the patient in pain are:

Patient will report a reduction in pain.
Patient will identify factors that precipitate pain.
Patient will identify techniques to decrease pain.

The interventions then can be directed specifically toward eliminating or reducing pain, decreasing suffering, improving coping mechanisms, identifying and reducing precipitating factors, and decreasing dependency on analgesics by using alternative pain-relief measures.

Usually a realistic goal for the patient in acute pain is to reduce pain; complete elimination of pain is expected with recovery and healing. However, total elimination of pain may be unrealistic with chronic pain because over time physical, behavioral, and emotional adaptation has taken place. Therefore, it is important to identify the type and degree of pain relief the patient finds acceptable and possible to achieve. The patient with chronic pain needs to learn that the pain will recur or that no interventions will cancel it entirely. Adapting daily activities to the pain may be a goal for this patient.

Since results are not always predictable, confidence and enthusiasm on the nurse's part increase the chances that a pain-relief measure will be successful. If the patient knows that numerous methods are available, he or she will not be devastated if one fails.

IMPLEMENTATION

Nursing Interventions to Promote Health and Function

Although pain may be unavoidable, patients can be taught ways of anticipating and managing painful procedures or situations to decrease anxiety and fear and to allow them to become active participants in preventing pain and in recovery.

Recognizing pain-inducing situations and factors is the first step in preventing pain. For instance, someone who gets migraine headaches may be aware that certain foods such as chocolate induce a migraine. Increased knowledge about the ways that sports or other recreational activities can aggravate pain allows the person to modify his or her activities to prevent pain and promote function. Adequate warm-up activities to stretch muscles and limber up joints before sports help prevent pain during and after the activity. Using appropriate posture and mechanics at work can help preserve function and prevent pain by avoiding strained muscles and other types of injury.

Patients with chronic pain can be taught lifestyle changes to avoid precipitating pain and dysfunction. For instance, the patient with chronic lower-back pain should be taught proper lifting and bending techniques and exercises to decrease muscle contraction and increase back muscle strength (see Chap. 29). The patient can be taught to decrease dependency on analgesics by using alternate pain-relief measures.

Patient teaching is an important nursing intervention for helping patients prevent and manage pain. For example, if a patient is scheduled for a potentially painful procedure, the nurse can discuss techniques (relaxation

---

Selected Nursing Interventions for Common Pain Problems

Preventing Pain

- Encourage appropriate use of body position and mechanics during work and recreation.
- Assist the patient in identifying factors that precipitate or aggravate pain.
- Provide comfort measures for the patient on bedrest, such as eliminating wrinkles in sheets, avoiding constrictive clothing, and changing positions.
- Provide careful skin hygiene to prevent pain from pressure, excoriation, or irritation.
- Give anticipatory explanation of the amount of pain that can be expected during a procedure or activity.

Acute Pain

- Listen actively to the patient's description of pain.
- Formulate a plan of managing pain with the patient.
- Teach the patient to minimize pain by splinting the area for pain with a pillow before activities, such as moving or coughing.
- Encourage the use of distraction by focusing on pictures, reading, or music.
- Promote the use of cutaneous stimulation, such as massage, heat and cold, acupuncture or acupressure, and contralateral stimulation.

- Explore the use of relaxation techniques, such as meditation, progressive relaxation, or guided imagery with the patient.
- Use pharmacologic methods of pain control judiciously; give adequate medication to relieve pain; use medication when pain begins so analgesics can be most effective; and monitor effectiveness of medication.
- Promote periods of uninterrupted rest after pain relief measures.

Chronic Pain

- Acknowledge the patient's pain.
- Encourage the patient to maintain a log of factors relating to pain, such as activities that precede pain, length and duration of pain, and therapies used to relieve pain.
- Teach the patient to use distraction, cutaneous stimulation, and relaxation techniques alternately and monitor for pain relief effects.
- Promote a schedule of rest and activity during the day to minimize pain.
- Refer to appropriate resources and support services for evaluation.

---

exercises, deep breathing, distraction) that will decrease the pain and improve coping mechanisms.

Nursing Interventions for Altered Comfort

Nursing management of pain includes noninvasive and invasive measures and the administration of analgesics. Being familiar with these techniques helps the nurse decide which ones to use, when to initiate them, and what outcomes to expect.

Positioning and Hygiene

Basic comfort measures take on new importance for the patient on bedrest. For patients who spend many hours in bed, the bed itself and the patient's position may contribute directly to pain. Sheets tend to bunch up under the patient, creating pressure and discomfort. Tightening sheets regularly or changing them, if needed,

can make the patient more comfortable. Repositioning on a regular schedule can also help the patient feel more comfortable. The pressure areas created by lying in one position too long can be painful. If not contraindicated, backrubs can contribute to relaxation and comfort. Giving a backrub also allows the nurse to spend a few minutes with the patient, listening attentively and continuing the ongoing pain assessment.

Anything that can be constrictive contributes to pain, such as gowns that twist or bind, support hose, or wrist restraints used to prevent tubes from being pulled out inadvertently. Restraints and support hose must be removed regularly to assess the pressure on the skin and other problems that may be causing pain. Gowns must be the correct size for the patient and should be checked for comfort whenever the patient's position is changed.

Areas of irritation or excoriation may be sources of pain. Patients who require a bedpan or who are incontinent of urine or stool are at risk for skin impairment if perineal hygiene is not carefully managed. Skin that may

- Thoroughly assess the patient (i.e., past experience with drugs, medical and surgical history, patient expectations) before any interventions for pain are instituted.
- Carefully monitor the patient's level of consciousness, respiratory rate and quality, and vital signs before and after drugs are given.
- Gain knowledge and become skillful at safely administering pharmacologic and nonpharmacologic pain-relief methods.
- Research potential interactions before giving any analgesic.
- Before applying heat or cold therapies, consider the patient's age, level of consciousness, intellectual ability, health problems, and the condition of the affected skin surface.
- Ensure that equipment functions correctly.
- Know the agency's policy about assessment, evaluation, and invasive and noninvasive pain-relief methods.

be exposed to secretions from gastrostomy sites, ileostomies, or colostomies is also at risk for skin impairment.

Anticipatory Guidance. Fear and dread may enhance or precipitate pain. The nurse can help by giving an honest explanation of what the patient can expect. Even if the nurse says that there probably will be pain, the patient can usually manage the pain better knowing what to expect and how to manage it.

The nurse can teach the preoperative patient how to cope with postsurgical pain and how to improve mobility, because early ambulation and pulmonary hygiene are important after surgery. Some techniques include:

Splinting the incision with pillows to decrease muscle tension at the site.

Positioning techniques such as moving side to side, transferring to the side of the bed and to the chair, and proper walking posture.

Premedicating with narcotics before activities. The patient should be taught to request medication when the pain begins so that analgesics can be more effective and can prevent escalating pain.

Noninvasive Pain Relief

The term "noninvasive" often designates external pain-relief measures that do not physically invade the body but have internal effects such as muscle relaxation or

promotion of a more homeostatic autonomic nervous system response. However, acupuncture or menthol lotion, both of which penetrate the skin, are also considered noninvasive techniques. Noninvasive interventions work by altering the opening of the pain control gate, inhibiting the transmission of pain to the cortex. The release of endorphins may also be responsible for the effectiveness of these measures (McCaffery, 1979).

The effectiveness of noninvasive measures also depends on the nurse–patient relationship. The patient's confidence in these methods and willingness to try them may be boosted if he or she trusts the nurse and believes that the nurse cares. A positive approach that the patient believes in and trusts may elicit a placebo effect in about 30% of patients (McCaffery, 1979). General guidelines for noninvasive therapies are shown in the display.

The major noninvasive pain relief measures are distraction, cutaneous stimulation, and relaxation.

Distraction. Distraction is useful when patients are undergoing brief periods of sharp, intense pain, such as

Guidelines for Noninvasive Pain Therapies

- Consider noninvasive therapies when:
  - Anxiety is augmenting pain levels and physiologic response.
  - Patient wants more active participation in pain management.
  - Patient or physician wants to decrease or eliminate use of medications.
  - Pharmacologic or invasive methods are not producing adequate pain relief.
  - Family and friends want to be involved.
  (When in doubt about the safety of a method or legality of independent nursing action, obtain a physician's order.)
- Communicate on the care plan and/or tell all health-team members, family, and friends what technique will be used, its purpose, how it is individualized to the patient's preferences, and needs, and when to use the technique. This will reinforce the technique.
- Anticipate patient needs by starting measures before the pain begins. Practice techniques before they are needed if possible (i.e., preoperatively, before the procedure).
- Recognize the importance of the nurse–patient relationship on the patient's willingness to try and to have confidence in the technique.
- Appreciate that a combination of methods that allows for flexibility often is most efficient.

From McCaffery, M. (1979). *Nursing management of the patient with pain*. Philadelphia: J. B. Lippincott.

dressing changes, wound debridement, or biopsy. The pain relief tends to be temporary, lasting only through the distraction exercise (i.e., the Lamaze method for the woman in labor). Complex stimuli are useful for mild to moderate pain, but as the intensity of pain increases the stimuli must be simplified.

Distraction may be visual (reading, looking at pictures), auditory (playing an instrument, listening to music), or tactile (stroking a pet, rocking). It is more effective if the distraction is something the patient enjoys doing.

Cutaneous Stimulation. Cutaneous stimulation is done to relieve acute or chronic pain. Techniques such as pressure, massage, vibration, heat, cold, and plain or menthol ointments have been proven safe and effective. All these methods have the added benefit of distracting and relaxing the patient; they also help to establish or extend the nurse–patient relationship (see Chap. 11). Usually only massage and contralateral stimulation without counterirritants can be independently initiated by nurses, although other techniques have nursing implications when prescribed by a physician.

The theoretical basis for the effects of stimulation has not been determined, but the analgesic effects are thought to be caused by activation of large A-delta fibers and inhibition of smaller C-fibers, thus closing the gate to pain impulses or stimulating endorphin production (Doehring, 1989).

The effects of cutaneous stimulation are variable and unpredictable, and patience is required while various methods are tried and adjusted. Some patients' pain is relieved until long after stimulation; others find that their pain returns to pretreatment levels immediately after therapy. In still others, stimulation may not relieve pain or may actually cause further pain when the therapy is abandoned. A technique should be tried more than once before deciding that it does not work.

Cutaneous stimulation should be moderate in frequency and duration and its use should be determined by the extent of pain relief. Areas that can be used are the skin over or near the pain site; trigger or acupuncture points; and peripheral nerves.

Massage. *Massage,* or rubbing a painful area, may relax muscles and reduce tension, but it is contraindicated over broken skin, mucous membranes, or rashes. Massage can be performed with counter-irritants such as mustard plasters, poultices, and liniments. Menthol products are the most common over-the-counter irritants, but the smell of menthol may be offensive to some patients. Most menthol products contain methyl salicylate, which is absorbed through the skin to cause the analgesic effect. The immediate sensation is of warmth or sometimes coolness that may last for hours. The sensation may be intensified by increasing the strength of the menthol, prolonging the massage, and ensuring that pores are open. If the ointment relieves the pain, wrapping the painful area in plastic will prolong relief.

Heat and Cold. *Heat and cold* may be used to reduce muscle spasm and decrease pain by elevating the patient's pain threshold. But except for decreasing muscle spasm and increasing the pain threshold, heat and cold have opposite effects on the body. Heat (from a hotwater bottle, heating pad, moist pad, warm bath, or the sun) increases inflammation, blood flow, edema, and bleeding at a site and is especially effective for joint and muscle pain. Cold (from crushed ice in a towel, ice bag, reusable gel pack, frozen paper cup of ice, bag of frozen peas, and Popsicles) decreases the inflammatory response, blood flow, and edema and relieves chronic migraines and back pain. The relief is achieved by decreasing sensory pain impulses to the brain and motor impulses to muscles in the painful area (McCaffery, 1980).

Precautions when using heat or cold stimulation include the following:

- Do not use it over areas of impaired circulation.
- Avoid extremes of temperature, which can cause burns or frostbite.
- Do not use heat over a new injury; it may cause increased bleeding and edema.
- Discontinue use if stimulation increases pain.

Contralateral Stimulation. In *contralateral stimulation,* the opposite area is stimulated with cold, heat, or menthol to relieve pain (for instance, the left hand is stimulated when the right hand is painful). It is effective when the painful area cannot be reached because of a cast or bandages, when the affected skin is too sensitive to touch, or when phantom pain is present. Contralateral massage may be useful for muscle cramps, spasms, or itching. The precautions are the same as for heat and cold and for massage.

Acupuncture. *Acupuncture* involves the insertion of stainless-steel needles into the body, either near the nerves in the painful area or at body points indicated by traditional Chinese acupuncture charts. The needles are placed at specific points but at various depths and angles, and are rotated between the practitioner's thumb and index finger with a slight downward pressure to produce pain relief (Hasset, 1980). A modified acupuncture technique is *acupressure,* in which the acupuncture points are pressed and massaged.

Acupuncture and acupressure are thought to work by stimulating the release of endorphins. This theory is based on evidence that naloxone, a narcotic antagonist, reverses the pain-relieving effects of acupuncture in some patients (Owens, 1986b).

The advantages of acupuncture are its simplicity and its ability to produce analgesia sufficient to perform surgery in some patients. As an anesthetic, acupuncture is superior to anesthesia because it does not affect blood pressure or cause respiratory tract complications. Disadvantages include a high failure rate, the risk of infection due to unsterile needles, and the need for an experienced acupuncturist. Its potential for pain relief is still being investigated in the United States, although it is widely used in China and the Soviet Union. Acupuncture is being used during dental procedures and in patients with tension headaches or migraines, peptic ulcer pain, low back pain, and arthritis.

Transcutaneous Electrical Nerve Stimulation. Transcutaneous electrical nerve stimulation (TENS) is used as an adjunct in the overall management of acute and chronic pain. The TENS unit consists of a palm-sized, lightweight, battery-operated stimulator that generates a mild electrical impulse. Two to four electrodes are taped to the skin near or over a pain zone, and the patient controls the electrode output to produce a sensation that is pleasant and relieves pain. The location of the electrodes and the voltage, frequency, and duration of the stimulus are determined by the patient's response. Tingling, buzzing, or vibrating sensations are initially felt, and some patients find them unpleasant or intolerable. Correct electrode placement and precise output adjustment are essential for this method to be successful.

The advantages of TENS are:

- It appears to produce increased blood flow.
- It may allow the patient to decrease or eliminate pain medications.
- It is nonaddictive.
- It does not interfere with the patient's daily activities.

Skin problems are the major adverse side effect. Skin irritation can be caused by tape irritation or an allergy to the tape or the gel; using hypoallergenic tape, a stockinette-type dressing, or a belt may help. Rashes from the gel may be remedied by changing to another gel, using cortisone cream by itself or mixed with the gel, rotating the electrode sites, and cleaning the electrodes daily with soap and water.

The patient must use TENS only as the physician has prescribed; using TENS for new pain could lead to a delay in diagnosis and treatment. TENS should not be used by patients who have pacemakers because it may interfere with or inhibit the output of some demand-type pacemakers. Electrodes should not be placed over the eyes, over the carotid sinus (could precipitate a vasovagal reaction), and over the anterior neck or mouth areas (could cause spasms and the danger of airway closure). Safety has not been proven for the first trimester of pregnancy, but TENS has been used on the lower back during childbirth (McCaffery, 1979).

Increased pain has been reported in some patients after TENS; this is thought to be due to histamine release. The pain can be abolished by changing the frequency stimulation to 80 Hz or below 106 Hz (Thompson, 1986).

TENS is thought to cause analgesia by stimulating A-delta fibers to block unmyelinated C-fibers, thus blocking noxious stimuli from the periphery, or by stimulating endorphins (Amato, 1983; Hargreaves, et al., 1989).

Relaxation. Relaxation techniques are useful pain-relief measures. Most call for a combination of a quiet environment, a comfortable position, a passive attitude, and a focus of concentration such as a word, sound, or breathing pattern. Except for hypnosis and biofeedback, they are usually initiated independently by a nurse who has additional training in their use.

Relaxation can counteract the effects of the fight-or-flight response and promote mental and physical freedom from tension and stress. Physical and mental tension can aggravate any pain; in fact, they may cause conditions such as headaches and back pain. Relaxation therapies promote a sense of detachment: the patient feels a sense of control over the pain in a particular body part. Other benefits of relaxation are:

- It enables the patient to fight fatigue and sleep restfully, thus increasing his or her energy.
- It complements other pain-relief techniques.
- It allows the patient to cope more effectively with the same intensity of pain.
- It improves the patient's mood and flexibility.
- It produces physiologic changes (decreased muscle tension, increased blood flow, decreased heart and respiratory rate).

Relaxation training is not without problems. Many patients require booster sessions to refamiliarize themselves with procedures they may have forgotten. Some patients with chronic pain may resort to excessive use of relaxation procedures to escape from normal stresses of daily living: the technique itself becomes a debilitating pain behavior (Kiblich & Warfield, 1985).

Meditation. Meditation is a technique in which the person focuses on a single thought or sound; Transcendental Meditation is a popular form. *Yoga* is a combination of meditation and stretching exercises. *Progressive relaxation* is a technique of discriminating between tension and relaxation of specific muscles from head to toe. In *autogenics,* or passive progressive relaxation, the person repeats certain phrases silently to induce relaxation without discriminating between tension and relaxation. Autogenics can be useful with a cardiac patient because tensing the muscles might add work for the heart; visualizing relaxation of muscles could decrease pain.

Guided Imagery. Guided imagery is a technique in which the person focuses on a pleasant, relaxed mental image as a way to decrease the intensity of pain or as a substitute for pain. The image of a healing ball of energy that reduces pain is sometimes used.

Hypnosis. Hypnosis heightens a person's susceptibility to suggestion and alters the subject's state of consciousness. It blocks the awareness of pain through suggestions or by substituting another feeling for pain, altering the meaning of pain, increasing the tolerance for pain, and in extreme cases disassociating perception of the body from the person's awareness (Large & James, 1988). In general, about 20% of hypnotized patients with moderate to severe pain achieve total relief (Amato, 1983). Common myths about hypnosis limit its acceptance. It can be expensive and time-consuming, and practitioners require advanced training.

Biofeedback. In *biofeedback,* the patient learns voluntary control over autonomic functions, such as heart rate, hand temperature, and muscle tension. Electrodes are placed on the patient's body, and auditory or visual feedback (i.e., lights, sounds, digital or graphic readings) provides the patient with information about muscle relaxation, heart rate, blood pressure, and skin temperature. After baseline data are obtained, the patient is taught relaxation and deep-breathing exercises. The relaxation decreases pain by decreasing anxiety and increasing the patient's sense of control over pain. With practice, the patient learns to call on the skills at will. This technique has been found helpful in patients with hypertension, muscle tension, tension headaches, migraines, temporal mandibular joint syndrome, insomnia, chronic pain, and stress-related disorders. Motivation is an important component in its success, because it requires extensive training.

Pharmacologic Management

Analgesic medication is the most common approach to the management of pain.

Types of Analgesics. These drugs may be separated into three groups (Table 40-3):

Nonnarcotic analgesics. Used for mild to moderate pain, they alter pain perception by interfering with the transmission of painful stimuli from peripheral sites.

Narcotic-type analgesics (opiates). Used for moderate to severe pain, they alter perceptive and subjective responses to pain at cerebral levels.

Adjuvant analgesics. These are chemically and pharmacologically diverse drugs that can be considered together because they are used to enhance the analgesic effects of narcotics.

Although analgesics are ordered by the physician, the nurse is responsible for giving the drugs, evaluating their effectiveness, and notifying the physician if the relief obtained is inadequate. The display gives an overview of the nurse's responsibility in the use of analgesics.

Nonnarcotic Analgesics. Nonnarcotics depress pain perception, reduce the patient's response to pain, or relax muscle spasm. These drugs have analgesic or anti-inflammatory actions; they are used principally for mild to moderate pain. Aspirin is generally effective for pain arising from the integumental structures, such as bone, joint, or muscle. Other agents used include combina-

---

Nurses' Responsibility in the Use of Analgesics

- In hospitals, the nurse usually determines if and when an analgesic is given. Because analgesics are usually ordered prn, the nurse must judge how often the analgesic is given.
- Often the nurse must select the appropriate analgesic when more than one is prescribed. With various drugs and various routes of administration, the nurse needs to know about the drugs' potency and absorption.
- The nurse should have sound pain assessment skills to evaluate the effectiveness of the analgesic after each administration.
- The nurse is the health-team member most likely to observe side effects from the analgesic. Close observation minimizes the risk for the patient.
- The nurse must report promptly and accurately to the physician when a change in medication is needed.
- In home care, in office and clinic settings, and after discharge, the nurse is responsible for advising the patient about analgesic use.

From McCaffery, M. (1979). *Nursing management of the patient with pain.* Philadelphia: J. B. Lippincott.

---

tions with phenacetin and caffeine, and propoxyphene. Because aspirin and acetaminophen are so readily available without prescription, their effectiveness is often underestimated.

Corticosteroids are useful for pain related to inflammation and for treating young, otherwise healthy patients with sports-related pain that does not respond to nonsteroidal anti-inflammatory drugs (NSAIDs) (Chapman & Bonica, 1983). Steroids can also be useful for various inflammatory conditions (such as active rheumatoid arthritis, ulcerative colitis, and iritis) and can be injected at the site of inflammation or given by other routes. NSAIDs such as indomethacin and ibuprofen are often prescribed for low back pain, migraine headaches, and dysmenorrhea.

Narcotic Analgesics. The narcotic analgesics are a group of both naturally occurring and synthetic agents that can relieve severe pain in the conscious state. Narcotics are used for postoperative or trauma analgesia and are the mainstay of pain management for cancer. Their action on opiate receptors appears to be responsible not only for pain relief, but also for the development of tolerance, respiratory depression, and dependence (psychological and physical).

Narcotic **agonists** are drugs that bind to specific opiate receptors in certain brain areas to produce analgesia. Morphine is the prototype. Other compounds, known as

TABLE 40–3

Drug Actions and Nursing Implications

Category/Drug	Action	Nursing Implications
Nonnarcotics		
Acetylsalicylic acid (ASA)	Analgesic: Blocks prostaglandin synthesis, thus decreasing sensitivity of peripheral pain receptors to mechanical or chemical activation. Antipyretic: Decreases outflow of vasoconstrictor impulses from hypothalamus, thus promoting vasodilation, sweating, and heat loss. Anti-inflammatory: Decreases capillary permeability and leakage of fluid into surrounding tissues; interferes with release of enzymes. Other actions decrease platelet aggregation.	Because gastric irritation is the major side effect of ASA, it should be given on a full stomach (although this delays absorption and pain relief). Stomach upset can also be avoided by taking enteric-coated ASA, which isn't absorbed until it reaches the intestine. Over several days or after several doses, ASA may cause ringing in the ears (tinnitus). This reflects damage to the auditory nerve and means the dose should be reduced immediately. ASA should never be given with oral anticoagulants, methotrexate, probenecid, or sulfinpyrazone because significant drug interactions will occur.
Acetaminophen	Analgesic and antipyretic. Elevates the pain threshold and reduces sympathetic outflow from hypothalamic temperature-regulating center. Weak antidiuretic action. Exerts no significant anti-inflammatory effect and does not produce gastric erosion, inhibition of platelet aggregation, or prothrombin depression.	Must be used with caution in people with known liver disease because it may cause liver toxicity. Chronic use is associated with analgesic nephropathy.
Corticosteroids (e.g., hydrocortisone, prednisone, dexamethasone)	Anti-inflammatory. Stabilize tissue membranes, and inhibit capillary dilation and permeability.	Give with food or milk and urge patients to advise physician if gastric irritation persists, as drug can cause gastric ulceration. Supplemental antacids may alleviate the distress. Inform patients to notify physician if excessive weight gain, edema, hypertension, muscle weakness, bone pain, sore throat, fever, cold, infection, mood changes, or visual disturbances occur. Observe diabetics closely during steroid therapy, as hyperglycemia or loss of blood sugar control could occur.
Nonsteroidal anti-inflammatory drugs (NSAIDS) (e.g., ibuprofen, naproxen, tolmetin, indomethacin)	Analgesic, anti-inflammatory, and antipyretic effects. Block synthesis and possibly release of prostaglandins. The principal advantage of these drugs is a somewhat lower incidence of the milder forms of GI distress that commonly occur with high-dose salicylate use (excluding indomethacin).	Observe patients with a history of GI problems for signs of gastric intolerance (e.g., dyspepsia, epigastric pain, nausea, cramping). Stop drug if symptoms persist. Reversible and preventable renal insufficiency is associated with most of the NSAIDs. Patients most at risk for this problem are those with congestive heart failure, renal disease, cirrhosis with ascites, and those over 60. Some patients may respond to only one of the several available nonsteroidal agents. Try different derivatives at 2- to 3-week intervals before concluding that this type of drug is ineffective.
Narcotic Agonists/Antagonists		
Agonists: pentazocine, halbuphine, butorphanal Antagonists: naloxone, levallorphan	These drugs act as both narcotics (agonists) and antagonists (drugs that counteract narcotic effects).	May precipitate withdrawal in people who have been receiving narcotics. If given with a narcotic, they may antagonize the analgesic effects of the narcotic and provide poor pain relief.

(continued)

TABLE 40-3

(continued)

Category/Drug	Action	Nursing Implications
Narcotic Agonists/Antagonists		Side effects of agonists include drowsiness, respiratory depression, occasional nausea, and CNS effects such as hallucinations. Naloxone is the drug of choice to counteract respiratory depression induced by narcotics. Large doses will reverse the analgesic effects of narcotics as well as the respiratory depression. If clinical signs of pain (e.g., sweating, increased heart rate) are noted, the antagonist should be stopped.
Narcotic Analgesics Naturally occurring opium alkaloids (morphine, codeine) Semisynthetic derivatives (hydromorphone, oxycodone, oxymorphone) Entirely synthetic derivatives (meperidine, methadone)	Modulate or stimulate opioid receptors within the CNS. Principal effects are calming and anxiety reduction in severe pain. Narcotics alter the perception of pain to a much greater extent than the sensation of pain. This euphoric state is responsible for the desire to repeat the drug, ultimately leading to habituation.	Morphine provides satisfactory pain relief in about 70% of patients with moderate to severe pain. However, if morphine fails to relieve pain or produces side effects (i.e., nausea), better pain relief with fewer side effects may be achieved by changing to another narcotic. Meperidine, while effective in many patients with acute pain, must be used cautiously because of possible CNS toxicity, including irritability, muscle twitching, hallucinations, seizures, and disorientation, especially in patients with renal or hepatic dysfunction. Poor oral absorption and short duration of action preclude its use in chronic pain. Methadone is particularly useful in managing severe chronic pain such as cancer because it is only mildly sedating after the initial few days, has a long duration of action, and is absorbed well from the GI tract.

narcotic **antagonists,** block the narcotic receptors or displace the agonists from these sites. Narcotic antagonists can reverse the depressant effects of opiates, such as respiratory depression, and are used to treat acute narcotic overdoses.

There are three reasons why pain is undertreated with narcotics:

• The fear of causing respiratory depression
• The fear of causing addiction
• The failure to apply basic pharmacologic knowledge (McCaffery, 1979).

Respiratory depression is uncommon and is easily observed and treated with a narcotic antagonist such as naloxone. It occurs most often after acute administration of a narcotic and is associated with other signs of central nervous system depression, such as sedation

and mental clouding. Maximal respiratory depression occurs within 7 minutes of intravenous (IV) administration, within 30 minutes of intramuscular administration, and within 60 minutes of oral administration.

When giving the initial dose, the nurse should closely observe the patient for pain relief and respiratory depression; observation is also needed when the patient is asleep, because sleep causes respiratory depression and effects are additive. The nurse should also monitor patients with a decreased respiratory reserve of effort (for instance, those who have undergone thoracic or upper abdominal surgery). Because breathing causes considerable pain in these patients, they often do not breathe deeply, and this can lead to atelectasis and pneumonia. In these patients, narcotics may actually increase respiratory activity by relieving the pain associated with breathing (Watts, 1975).

Patients in respiratory depression can initially be

treated by encouraging the patient to increase the rate and depth of breathing. If the patient cannot follow instructions or is apneic, artificial ventilation is needed until naloxone, the narcotic antagonist of choice for treating respiratory depression, is given. Naloxone can be given safely without causing withdrawal symptoms or counteracting all the analgesic effect of the narcotic. Naloxone should be given IV at 0.1 to 0.2 mg every 3 to 5 minutes until respiration is reestablished at 16 breaths per minute.

Narcotics can also cause circulatory problems. If circulation to an injection site is inadequate (i.e., due to chilling, paralysis, or edema), drug absorption may be delayed. When normal circulation returns, an excessive amount of the narcotic may be suddenly absorbed, resulting in respiratory depression. Narcotics may seriously lower the blood pressure of patients with cardiovascular depression from hypotension, cardiac disease, or decreased blood volume from hemorrhage (Rusy, 1974). Patients receiving narcotics immediately after major surgery should be closely monitored if their blood pressure is low. However, severe pain can lower the blood pressure as well; thus, close observation and small IV narcotic doses are necessary.

Adjuvant Analgesics. Several medications can be used as adjuvants to narcotic analgesia, including antipsychotic drugs, antidepressants, antianxiety drugs, and stimulants (amphetamines and related compounds) (Atkinson, et al., 1985) The combination of an antipsychotic (particularly a phenothiazine) and a narcotic is widely used to treat postoperative pain because it is believed that antipsychotic medications potentiate (or extend the effect of) analgesia and reduce narcotic-induced emesis. However, studies have shown that these so-called potentiators do not actually prolong opiate effects. Their value may be in reducing extreme anxiety or agitation (McCaffery, 1979).

Antidepressant drugs are best used to treat pain-associated anxiety, because they have no direct analgesic effect. Their use should be restricted to short-term treatment (1 to 4 weeks) of self-limited acute pain syndromes or exacerbations of recurring pain (Kocher, 1976). There is some evidence that mild stimulants such as caffeine may be useful adjuvants to analgesia.

Combining narcotic and nonnarcotic analgesics is logical and effective, because pain is attacked by two different mechanisms at two different levels (the peripheral and the central nervous systems). This approach allows better pain control without increasing the narcotic dose.

Addiction and Tolerance. Narcotics can produce **addiction** (physical and psychological dependence on the drug). Despite recent studies suggesting that medical use of narcotics rarely leads to drug abuse or iatrogenic addiction, fear of addiction is still a major consideration limiting the use of narcotics in hospitalized patients. Most postoperative or traumatic pain can be relieved with adequate doses of narcotics. Addiction is not a

concern if the drugs are given for less than a week, and it is important to guard against undermedication.

Some degree of physical dependence develops in most patients who receive narcotics regularly for more than a few days. A person who is physically dependent on a narcotic-type drug responds to abrupt discontinuation or to administration of a narcotic antagonist with characteristic withdrawal symptoms: anxiety, nervousness, irritability, and alternating chills and hot flashes. A prominent withdrawal sign is "wetness," including salivation, lacrimation, rhinorrhea, profuse perspiration, and gooseflesh. At the peak of withdrawal, patients may experience nausea and vomiting, abdominal cramps, insomnia, and rarely multifocal myoclonus. Abstinence symptoms usually occur within 6 to 12 hours and peak at 24 to 72 hours after cessation of morphine; a delayed onset is seen with drugs with long half-lives, such as methadone.

A narcotic is discontinued by reducing the dose over 1 to 2 days to prevent withdrawal. Clonidine is useful for counteracting the side effects of withdrawal.

Tolerance develops when a given dose of a narcotic becomes less effective on repeated administration; larger doses are needed to produce the original effect. Tolerance is *not* addiction, but involves physiologic changes related to drug metabolism and the nervous system's adaptation to the drug action. Intermittent use of narcotics does not usually lead to significant tolerance. If tolerance develops after prolonged daily use, especially on a preventive basis, the effective dosage may level off (that is, the effective dosage may reach a plateau from time to time).

Once tolerance has developed, the most direct recourse for maintaining pain relief is to increase the narcotic dose. In cancer patients with severe pain, narcotic analgesics should not be used sparingly or "saved to the last." Researchers have been unable to demonstrate any analgesic ceiling for the potent narcotics (Houde, 1974). Often, patients can be switched to another narcotic; cross-tolerance among narcotic-type analgesics appears incomplete (Jaffe & Martin, 1990).

Other Side Effects. Other side effects of narcotics are constipation, nausea and vomiting, and sedation. Constipation is the most common adverse effect. Narcotics act at multiple sites in the gastrointestinal tract and spinal cord to reduce intestinal secretions and decrease peristalsis. Tolerance to constipation does not develop at the same rate as tolerance to the other side effects. Patients taking routine doses of a narcotic should drink at least two liters of fluid daily, get daily exercise, eat a high-fiber diet, and take daily stool softeners.

Nausea and vomiting appear to be caused by stimulation of the medullary chemoreceptor zone and resultant stimulation of the nearby vomiting center, and stimulation of the vestibular part of the ear (McGuigan, 1970). Substituting an equianalgesic dose of another narcotic may reduce or stop nausea and vomiting, or an antiemetic may be given with the narcotic. Many patients become tolerant to this side effect in a few days, if it is not severe. The phenothiazines (prochlorperazine, chlorpromazine, and hydroxyzine), dimenhydrinate, and diphenhydramine control nausea in different ways.

Sedation and drowsiness, which occur in most patients receiving narcotics, is useful in some clinical situations, such as before anesthesia. Excessive sedation may be countered by reducing the dose and increasing the interval between doses. In addition, other central nervous system depressants should be discontinued, such as sedative–hypnotics and antianxiety agents, which potentiate the sedative effects of narcotics. However, fatigue and insomnia may be caused by the pain itself: a narcotic dose may allow the patient to sleep. In the patient taking regular narcotics, drowsiness may occur for the first 2 or 3 days and is usually temporary (Ajeman, 1977).

Guidelines for Pharmacologic Management. Generally, intramuscular or subcutaneous administration of a narcotic is appropriate for only a few days because subcutaneous and muscle tissue can quickly become irritated. Oral narcotics are useful for the patient in prolonged pain, and also for the patient whose acute postoperative pain cannot be controlled on nonnarcotics, if the gastrointestinal tract is healthy enough to ensure absorption and minimal problems with nausea and vomiting (Halpern & Bonica, 1976). See the display for guidelines on the nursing management of acute postoperative pain.

The frequency with which a patient receives a narcotic for pain is left largely to the nurse's discretion. However, this PRN (from the Latin *pro re nata,* as needed) approach should not preclude preventive pain relief. With acute or chronic pain, narcotics are given at fixed intervals before the pain returns (that is, before the analgesia wears off). Thus, the patient's anticipation of pain is eliminated, and the patient's anxiety decreases, controlling the vicious cycle of increasing pain with anxiety (see Fig. 40-3). This method may contribute to decreased pain and a decreased need for analgesia.

Patient-controlled analgesia (PCA), in which patients give themselves doses of narcotic analgesics, is a new approach that allows patients to become more involved in their own care (Gooch, 1989). Clinical studies show that it is safe and effective, and that selected patients tend to take only as much drug as they need for pain control (Sheidler, 1987). The small, frequent IV doses given in PCA systems tend to relieve pain without excessive sedation because they do not produce the wide variations in blood levels of analgesics seen with conventional therapy (Fig. 40-4).

The PCA system has a safety feature to prevent accidental overdoses. Even though the patient may push the button for another dose, the device cannot deliver another full dose until the correct amount of time, as preset by the physician, has elapsed. This lock-out time should not be so long that the patient must wait in pain between doses, however.

In patients with severe acute or prolonged pain that cannot be controlled by any other route, a continuous IV or subcutaneous infusion may be used. This method, used most often in terminal cancer patients, provides a steady blood level of the analgesic (Dolby & Whitestone, 1985). The patient must be observed closely for the first 24 hours for respiratory depression and hypotension. Terminally ill patients may remain alert and pain-free with close supervision.

Older patients are more susceptible to drug effects and may more readily experience confusion, excessive sedation, or respiratory depression from narcotics (McCaffery, 1985). With age, the liver and kidneys become less efficient at clearing drugs from the system, and this can lead to accumulation of the drug in elderly patients.

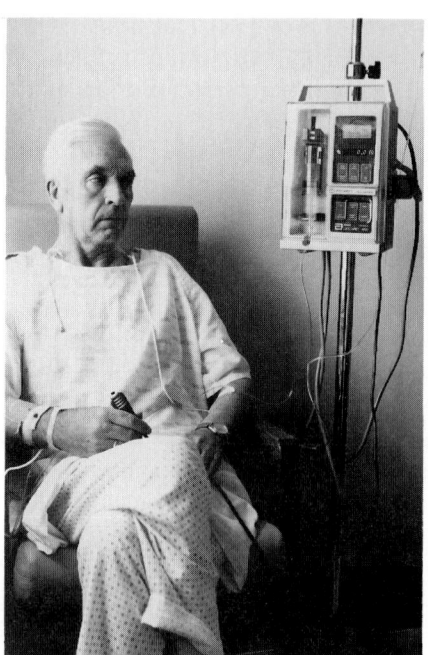

Figure 40–4. Patient-controlled analgesia (PCA) allows the patient to self-administer only as much medication as needed to control pain.

Guidelines for Acute Postoperative Pain

- Assess the patient's physiologic and psychological response to pain, both verbal and nonverbal.
- Give narcotics around the clock, not prn, for the first 36 hours after surgery.
- Give analgesics before or as soon as pain returns.
- Give analgesics before activities such as ambulation or incentive spirometer use.
- Be aware of potentiators.
- Individualize the drug and dosage.
- Monitor and record the patient's response using a pain scale routinely and prn.

Because elderly patients tend to take more drugs, there is an increased risk of drug interactions. Therefore, titration (adjusting the dosage based on the patient's response) is mandatory.

Use of Placebos. Placebos have traditionally been used in selected situations to differentiate functional from organic pain. Pain relieved by a placebo was considered to be psychogenic in origin (McCaffery, 1982). Recent research suggests that a positive placebo response does not prove that a patient's pain is functional: it is now thought that placebos may act directly to change the biochemical processes involved in the sensation of pain. It has been proposed that placebos may relieve pain by causing the body to release endorphins (Fields, 1978).

It is important for the nurse to have a positive attitude about how much pain relief the patient can expect from an analgesic. The nurse who explains the drug's effects optimistically to the patient may find that that the drug works more effectively.

Invasive Pain Management

When intractable pain cannot be controlled by analgesics, as in advanced cancer or excessive pain with tic douloureux (trigeminal neuralgia), surgical intervention to interrupt pain pathways may be necessary. Severe postoperative pain also can be controlled by injecting opiates directly into or by the spinal cord. Table 40-4 summarizes common invasive interventions.

Proper patient and family teaching is essential before any surgical procedure. They must understand the procedure, risks, possible complications, and possible duration of pain.

Discharge Planning and Home Care

Increasingly, pain management is being done at home, and economic trends suggest that even cancer patients with pain will soon be managed without hospitalization. Pain experts agree that a combination of drug and non-

TABLE 40-4
Invasive Pain Management Interventions

Technique	Advantage	Limitations/Precautions	When Used
Nerve roots or pathway interrupted or destroyed: Neurectomy—peripheral sensory nerves Sympathectomy—sympathetic ganglia Rhizotomy—dorsal root ganglia Cordotomy—anterolateral spinothalamic tract	May decrease or eliminate pain	May leave permanent damage (i.e., paralysis, loss of control of the elimination process and sensation)	Intractable pain (i.e., advanced cancer or tic douloureux [trigeminal neuralgia])
Nerve blocks (injected with anesthetic to interrupt nerve pathway)	May decrease or eliminate pain	Pain relief variable	Intractable pain (i.e., celiac block for GI malignancy)
Alcohol injections via transnasal or transphenoid approach of pituitary gland	Nontraumatic, easily performed, inexpensive	Pain relief variable; complications are signs of pituitary inactivation: hypopituitarism, steroid deficiency, decreased libido.	Intractable pain from bony metastases from breast and prostate that are estrogen-sensitive.
Injections of opiates into central nervous system at thoracic or lumbar area via a catheter placed in either the epidural space (space just outside dura mater; analgesic must filter through dura throughout the CSF and spinal cord) or subarachnoid space (contains the CSF)	Catheters can be left in place for months or years. Patient or caregiver can give injections or have intermittent or continuous pump placed to deliver narcotics. This allows independence and allows patient to go home and into community. May decrease or eliminate pain.	Preservative-free narcotic is used to avoid damage to spinal cord or nerve roots. A pump increases the cost of therapy. Preservative-free narcotics are costly. Complications may include nausea/vomiting, urinary retention, pruritus, and respiratory depression, which naloxone can reverse. Close nursing monitoring for somnolence and respiratory depression for the first 24 hours is imperative.	Acute pain (i.e., postoperative thoracic or abdominal surgery, post-cesarean section, phantom pain), chronic intractable pain

---

Patient Teaching

Instruct the patient as follows:

- When visiting the physician, take all your medications so the physician knows what you are taking and how often.
- If you have an unusual reaction, contact the physician.
- When pain occurs, write down any events you think may be related.
- Anticipate painful events and alter your behavior to prevent or minimize pain.
- Ask if you are allowed to drive a car or operate machinery while taking your medication.
- Keep the drugs away from children.
- Tell the physician if you are breastfeeding or think you may be pregnant.

---

drug strategies provide the best home management (Ferrell & Schneider, 1988).

For patients with chronic pain, home pain management is critical in determining their functional ability and quality of life. Chronic pain may immobilize patients, hindering their daily activities, relationships, sleep, and appetite. Family members often provide complex symptom management; outpatient and home-health nurses assess the interventions and test new interventions.

It is the nurse's responsibility to teach home pain management to the patient and family before discharge. The postoperative patient needs information on the healing process and should be encouraged to get adequate rest and nutrition, to avoid fatigue, and to increase mobility. These factors affect patient comfort and enhance recovery. The patient should know how long recovery should take so that medical intervention can be sought if complications occur.

Patients taking analgesics must understand the correct dosage and common side effects and how to avoid or manage them. They should know that analgesics may produce changes in judgment, perception, and coordination; this may preclude driving or operating machinery.

Breastfeeding mothers need to know whether the drug is present in their milk and whether it may affect the infant. At home, analgesics must be kept in a safe, childproof bottle away from children or others.

EVALUATION

An important part of the nurse's role in pain management is accurately evaluating the effectiveness of pain-

relief measures by observing and questioning the patient. The nurse never simply assumes that nursing interventions have been successful. Depending on the results, the measures may be modified or an alternate approach tried.

Specific outcome criteria are used to measure the attainment of patient goals. Although some examples of outcome criteria are presented, it is essential to develop outcome criteria for each patient.

Goal
The patient will report a reduction in pain.

Possible Outcome Criteria
- Patient states within a half-hour of the intervention that there is less pain.
- Within 2 hours of the intervention, patient rates pain as lower than the previous rating on a scale of 1 to 10.
- Within 1 hour of the intervention, patient's facial expressions and body positioning, as observed by the nurse, indicate decreased pain.

Goal
The patient will identify factors that precipitate pain.

Possible Outcome Criteria
- At the next appointment, patient describes factors that precipitate pain.
- At the next appointment, patient describes physical states that aggravate pain.
- On the next shift, patient identifies sources of pain to the nurse.

Goal
The patient will identify techniques that decrease pain.

Possible Outcome Criteria
- At the next appointment, patient identifies the medication regimen that controls pain optimally.
- Within 24 hours, patient defines behavioral interventions that help to control pain.

Key Concepts

- Pain is a subjective experience that is whatever the patient says it is and occurs whenever the patient says it occurs.
- Although pain is a source of human misery, it also minimizes injury and warns of disease.
- All pain-relief measures are based on a thorough ongoing assessment.
- Establishing trust between the nurse and patient enhances the effectiveness of pain-relief measures.
- Sedation does not always indicate pain relief.

Nursing Management Plan
The Patient Experiencing Pain

Nursing Diagnosis: Pain related to surgical incision manifested by nonverbal communication of pain.
Patient Goal: Patient will experience reduced pain.
Patient Outcome Criteria

- Patient identifies cause of pain and appropriate relief measures for pain.
- Patient reports pain immediately at each occurrence.
- Patient states pain is relieved or minimized within half an hour of occurrence.

Nursing Intervention	Scientific Rationale
1. Evaluate preoperative comprehensive pain assessment.	1. The most important component of pain is an ongoing, accurate, thorough pain assessment.
2. Solicit techniques that have previously been found to be helpful.	2. Individual techniques that a patient has used in the past enhance pain relief.
3. Establish a trusting relationship.	3. An effective nurse/patient relationship enhances all pain-relief measures because it conveys "I care—you can trust me."
4. Instruct patient to promptly report pain so relief measures can be instituted before severe pain occurs. Use therapeutic approaches for the prevention of severe pain, not the relief of severe pain.	4. Relief measures are instituted based on patient's verbal report of pain and regular patient assessments. This also informs patient of the expectation to communicate when in pain, since many ethnic and cultural influences often discourage or prohibit expression of pain.
5. Assess level of pain using a self-rating scale of 0 to 10.	5. To obtain data that determines how this person reports pain intensity.
6. Allow rest periods during day and periods of uninterrupted sleep at night when possible. Keep environment quiet.	6. Rest facilitates comfort and sleep, reduces stress, relieves muscle tension, and increases relaxation. Fatigue may enhance pain by lowering pain tolerance.
7. Collaborate with patient to initiate the appropriate noninvasive pain relief measure(s). a. Instruct in distraction technique (specify). Example: engage in conversation or turn radio on to favorite station during abdominal dressing change.	7a. Focus attention away from pain and increased pain tolerance results.
b. Instruct in cutaneous stimulation (specify). Example: give back rub after turning and before bedtime.	b. Stimulates skin to close the gate to pain impulses and stimulating endorphins.
c. Instruct in relaxation techniques (specify). Example: have patient take slow, deep breaths when turning.	c. Slow, deep breaths reduce muscle tension and the intensity of pain and nausea. Change of position increases circulation and decrease muscle tension.
8. Provide optimal pain relief with prescribed analgesics.	8. Optimal pain relief decreases anxiety and fear, both of which increase pain. Goal is to use a preventative approach to avoid severe pain.
a. Individualize medication regimen. After surgery, IM or IV narcotics are usually used for moderate to severe pain for first 48 hours to act on the central nervous system. Then oral route is used after bowel tones are present. Either oral narcotics alone or combined with non-narcotics, which act on the peripheral	

(continued)

Nursing Management Plan
The Patient Experiencing Pain *(continued)*

Nursing Intervention	Scientific Rationale
nervous system, may be used for mild to moderate pain. Collaborate with doctor to five narcotics around the clock instead of prn in the first 24 hours to maintain narcotic blood levels and provide good pain relief.	
b. Assess response to medications.	b. Ongoing assessment of severity of pain before and pain relief after medication is important. Rule of thumb is: IV—check response in 15 minutes; IM—check response in 30 minutes; PO—check response in 60 minutes. This identifies if the drug or dose is sufficient for the patient's pain.
c. Monitor for and minimize common side effects of medications (specify).	c. Respiratory depression, constipation, nausea, vomiting, and dry mouth can be caused by narcotics.

- Because patients may not always report pain, the nurse must assess them regularly.
- Patients of all ages experience pain, but the way they express pain differs with age.
- The nurse should be able to recognize physiologic, psychological, and nonverbal ways of expressing pain.
- Lack of pain expression does not always mean lack of pain.
- Noninvasive pain-relief measures can augment the effectiveness of pharmacologic or invasive methods.
- The nurse's optimistic attitude about expected pain relief helps produce a positive result.
- Educating the patient and family about pain reduces anticipatory fear and anxiety, thereby increasing the patient's tolerance to pain.
- Using a preventive approach for pain relief is more beneficial than waiting until pain becomes severe.
- Intramuscular and intravenous routes should be used for severe pain, intramuscular for moderate to severe pain, and oral for mild to moderate pain.

References

Ajeman, I. (1977). An oral morphine mixture for intractable pain. *Canadian Family Physician, 23*, 1506–1507.

Amato, M. (1983, November). Pain management. TENS: Does it work? *The Coordinator*, 14–23.

Atkinson, J. H., Kremer, E., & Garfin, S. (1985). Psychopharmacological agents in the treatment of pain. *Journal of Bone and Joint Surgery, 76A*(2), 337–342.

Carpenito, L. (1989). *Nursing diagnosis—application to clinical practice* (3rd ed., pp. 112–132). New York: J. B. Lippincott.

Chapman, C. R., & Bonica, J. J. (1983). *Acute pain.* Upjohn Scope.

Chapman, D. R. (1984). New directions in the understanding and management of pain. *Social Science and Medicine, 19*, 1261–1277.

Doehring, K. M. (1989). Relieving pain through touch. *Advances in Clinical Care, 4*(5), 32–33.

Dolby, V. V., & Whitestone, S. T. (1985). Continuous morphine drip for intractable pain control. *National Intravenous Therapy Association, 8*, 415–416.

Ferrell, B., & Schneider, C. (1988). Experience and management of cancer pain at home. *Cancer Nursing, 11*(2), 84–90.

Fields, H. L. (1978). Secrets of the placebo. *Psychology Today, 12*(6), 172.

Fordyce, W. (1976). *Behavioral methods for chronic pain and illness.* St. Louis: C. V. Mosby.

Gooch, J. (1989). Who should manage pain—patient or nurse? *Professional Nurse, 4*, 295–296.

Halpern, L. M., & Bonica, J. J. (1976). Analgesics. In W. Modell (Ed.), *Drugs of choice 1976–1977* (pp. 195–232). St. Louis: C. V. Mosby.

Hargreaves, A., & Lander, J. (1989). Use of transcutaneous electrical nerve stimulation for postoperative pain. *Nursing Research, 38*(3), 159–161.

Hasset, J. (1980). Acupuncture is proving its point. *Psychology Today, 14*(7), 81.

Hendler, N. H., & Fenton, J. S. (1979). *Coping with chronic pain.* New York: Clarkson Potter.

Holaday, J. (1985). *Endogenous opiates and their receptors: Current concepts.* Upjohn.

Holm, K., Cohen, F., & Dudas, S. (1989). Effect of personal pain experience on pain assessment. *Image: Journal of Nursing Scholarship, 21*(2), 72–75.

Houde, R. W. (1974). The use and misuse of narcotics in the treatment of chronic pain. In J. J. Bonica (Ed.), *Advances in neurology* (4th ed., pp. 527–536). New York: Raven.

Jacox, A. K. (1979a). Assessing pain. *American Journal of Nursing, 79*(5), 895–900.

Jacox, A. K. (Ed.). (1979). *Pain: A source book for nurses and other health professionals.* Boston: Little, Brown & Co.

Jaffe, J. H., & Martin, W. R. (1990). Opioid analgesics and antagonists. In A. Gilman, T. W. Rall, A. S. Nis, et al. (Eds.), *Goodman and Gilman's pharmacological basis of therapeutics* (8th ed., pp. 485–521).

Kim, S. (1980). Pain: Theory, research and nursing practice. *ANS, 2*(2), 43–59.

Kocher, R. (1976). Use of psychotropic drugs for the treatment of chronic severe pain. In J. J. Bonica & D. Albe-Fessard (Eds.), *Advances in pain research and therapy* (1st ed., pp. 579–582). New York: Raven.

Kulich, R. J., & Warfield, C. (1985, Dec. 15). Relaxation in the management of pain. *Hospital Practice,* 117–121.

Large, R. G., & James, F. R. (1988). Personalized evaluation of self-hypnosis as a treatment for chronic pain: A repertory grid analysis. *Pain, 35*(2), 155–169.

Malseed, R. T. (1985). *Pharmacology: Drug therapy and nursing considerations* (2nd ed., pp. 137–146). Philadelphia: J. B. Lippincott.

McCaffery, M. (1968). *Cognition, bodily pain and man–environment interactions.* Los Angeles: University of California.

McCaffery, M. (1979). *Nursing management of the patient with pain.* Philadelphia: J. B. Lippincott.

McCaffery, M. (1980). Relieving pain with noninvasive techniques. *Nursing '80, 10*(12), 55–57.

McCaffery, M. (1982). Would you administer placebos for pain? *Nursing '82,* 80–85.

McCaffery, M. (1985). Narcotic analgesia for the elderly patient. *PRN Forum—Pain Research News,* March–April, 1–2.

McGuigan, J. E. (1970). Anorexia, nausea and vomiting. In C. M. MacBryde & R. D. Blacklow (Eds.), *Signs and symptoms: Applied pathologic physiology and clinical interpretation* (5th ed., pp. 369–380). Philadelphia: J. B. Lippincott.

Meinhart, N. T., & McCaffery, M. (1983). *Pain: A nursing approach to assessment and analysis.* New York: Appleton-Century-Crofts.

Melzack, R., & Wall, P. D. (1965). Pain mechanisms: A new theory. *Science, 150,* 971–979. November.

Melzack, R., & Wall, P. D. (1983). *The challenge of pain.* New York: Basic Books.

NANDA (1990). *Taxonomy I revised 1990, with official nursing diagnoses.* St. Louis, MO: North American Nursing Diagnosis Association.

Owens, M. E. (1986a). A crying need. Infants perceive pain. *American Journal of Nursing, 86*(1), 73–94.

Owens, M. E. (1986b). Assessment of infant pain in clinical settings. *Journal of Pain Symptom Management, 1*(1), 29–31.

Pagliaro, L. A., & Pagliaro, A. M. (1983). *Pharmacologic aspects of aging.* St. Louis: C. V. Mosby.

Perry, S. W., & Heidrich, G. (1981). Placebo response: Myth and matter. *American Journal of Nursing, 81,* 721.

Porth, C. M. (1990). *Pathophysiology* (3rd ed.). Philadelphia: J. B. Lippincott.

Raft, D., Smith, R., & Warren, N. (1986). Selection of imagery in the relief of chronic and acute clinical pain. *Journal of Psychosomatic Research, 30,* 481–488.

Rusy, B. F. (1974). Individualization of narcotic analgesic therapy. *Medical Clinics of North America, 58,* 1137–1141.

Sheidler, V. R. (1987). Patient-controlled analgesia. *Current Concepts in Nursing, 1*(1), 13–16.

Thompson, J. M. (1986). *Clinical nursing* (pp. 1971–1975). St. Louis: C. V. Mosby.

Watts, G. T. (1975). Inadequate analgesia. *Lancet* (March 22), 678.

Weiner, C. (1975). Pain assessment on an orthopedic ward. *Nursing Outlook, 23,* 508–516.

Wilkie, D. J., Saverda, M., Holzemer, W., et al. (1990). Use of the McGill pain questionnaire to measure pain: A meta-analysis. *Nursing Research, 39*(1), 36–41.

Bibliography

Balfour, S. E. (1989). Will I be in pain? Patients' and nurses' attitudes to pain after abdominal surgery. *Professional Nurse, 5*(1), 28–30.

Beebe, A., McBride, R., & Gal, P. (1989). Pain: its assessment and treatment. *Journal of Practical Nursing, 39*(2), 17–27.

Chettiar, T. R. (1989). Expanding nursing practice . . . pain and stress management center. *Journal of Urology Nursing, 8,* 557.

Dalton, J. A. (1989). Nurses' perceptions of their pain assessment skills, pain management practices and attitudes toward pain. *Oncology Nursing Forum, 16,* 225–231.

Empting-Koschorke, L. D., Hendler, N., Kolodny, A. L., & Kraus, H. (1990). Non-drug management of chronic pain: what today's pain clinics have to offer. *Patient Care, 24*(1), 165–168.

Fisher, K., Nurse, M., Kennedy, P. (1989). Teaching nurses behavioral methods for pain management: A pilot study. *Behavioral Psychotherapy, 17,* 283–289.

Gyldenvand, T., & Tunick, P. (1989). Validation of the nursing diagnosis Alteration in Comfort: Chronic Pain. In R. M. Carroll-Johnson, ed. *Classification of nursing diagnoses: Proceedings of the eighth conference* (pp. 284–290). Philadelphia: J. B. Lippincott.

Kendrick, E. D. (1989). Pain: A review of physiological and management options. *Home Health Nurse, 7*(6), 9–17.

McCaffery, M., Ferrell, B., O'Neil-Page, E., Lester, M. (1990). Nurses' knowledge of opioid analgesic drugs and psychological dependence. *Cancer Nursing, 13*(1), 21–27.

McGuire, L. (1990). The power of non-narcotic pain relievers. *RN, 53*(4), 28–36.

Mills, N. M. (1989). Pain behaviors in infants and toddlers. *Journal of Pain and Symptom Management, 4*(4), 184–190.

Morgan, M. L. (1988). Where does pain control fit? Evaluation by charge nurses of pain management by staff nurses. *Kansas Nurse, 63,* 4–5.

Nolan, M. F. (1990). Pain: The experience and its expression. *Clinical Management, 10*(1), 22–25.

Pigeon, H. M., McGrath, P. J., Lawrence, J., MacMurray, S. B. (1989). Nurses' perception of pain in the neonatal intensive care unit. *Journal of Pain and Symptom Management, 4*(4), 179–183.

Simon, J. M. (1989). A multidisciplinary approach to chronic pain. *Rehabilitation Nursing, 14*(1), 5.

Thiederman, S. (1989). Stoic or shouter, the pain is real. *RN, 52*(6), 49–51.

Thorpe, D. M. (1989). Pain assessment: Matching the tool to patient needs, Part I. *Dimensions in Oncology Nursing, 3*(2), 19–25.

Van der Does, A. J. (1989). Patients' and nurses' ratings of pain and anxiety during burn wound care. *Pain, 39*(1), 95–101.

Walker, J. M., Campbell, S. M. (1989). Pain assessment, nursing models and the nursing process. *Recent Advances in Nursing, 24,* 47–61.

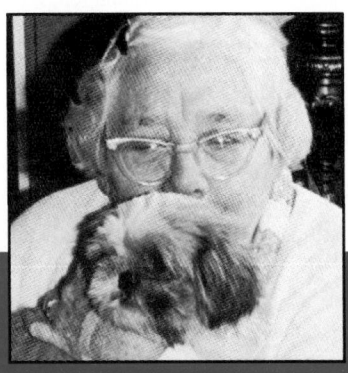

Sensory Perception

41

Normal Sensory Perception Function
  Normal Function of Sensory Perception
    Sensory Awareness
    Input by Senses
  Characteristics of Normal Sensory Perception
  Normal Functional Sensory Pattern
    Sensoristasis
    Adaptation
  Factors Affecting Normal Sensory Perception
  Lifespan Considerations
Altered Sensory Function
  Potential for Altered Sensory Function
    Sensory Overload
    Sensory Deprivation
    Sensory Deficit
  Manifestations of Altered Sensory Function
    Anxiety
    Cognitive Dysfunction
    Hallucinations and Delusions
    Depression and Withdrawal
  Impact of Dysfunction on Activities of Daily Living
Assessment
  Subjective Data
    Functional Pattern Identification
    Risk Identification
    Dysfunctional Identification

  Objective Data
    Physical Assessment
    Diagnostic Tests and Procedures
Nursing Diagnosis and Patient Goals
  Diagnostic Statement: Sensory/Perceptual
    Alterations
    Definition
    Defining Characteristics
    Related Factors
  Related Nursing Diagnoses
  Patient Goals
Implementation
  Nursing Interventions to Promote Sensory Health
    and Function
    Patient Teaching
    Procedure Preparation
    Nurse–Patient Interaction
  Nursing Interventions for Altered Sensory Function
    Stimulation Provision
    Stimulation Reduction
    Sensory Aids
    Safety
  Discharge Planning and Home Care
Evaluation
Key Concepts

Because of today's stepped-up pace, people often feel they do not have time to deal fully with one demand before the next one is nipping at their heels. The average person in American society has daily exposure to 65,000 more stimuli (demands) than ancestors of 100 years ago (Schafer, 1987). Human beings uniquely deal with these demands through senses and higher cognitive processes (the latter is discussed in Chapter 42).

Sensing stimuli is basic to human functioning, growth, and development. Any alteration in sensory function places a person at risk for more serious mental and physical health deficits unless coping take place.

Nurses encounter patients with preexisting sensory alterations, as well as patients experiencing new alterations due to the stress of the health-care environment and present illness. Assessment of sensory function and risk factors for sensory alterations is necessary for all patients, but especially for older adults who frequently have visual and hearing impairment. Nursing interventions for sensory alteration are aimed at teaching patients to make optimal use of their sensory function, preparing patients for procedures in the health-care environment, maintaining effective interaction with the patient, reducing or providing stimulation as appropriate, introducing sensory aids, and ensuring safety.

NORMAL SENSORY PERCEPTION FUNCTION

Normal Function of Sensory Perception

Sensory perception depends on the sensory receptors and the reticular activating system as well as functioning nervous pathways to the brain. Awareness of stimuli is influenced by the reticular activating system. Stimuli are received through the five senses: sight, hearing, touch, smell, and taste. Kinesthetic and visceral senses are stimulated internally.

Sensory Awareness

Awareness of the world at large depends on the **reticular activating system** (RAS), located between the nerve centers of the medulla oblongata in the brain stem. The RAS is responsible for bringing together information from the cerebellum and other parts of the brain and from the sense organs. It is stimulated by sensory, visceral, kinesthetic, and cognitive input (Lee, 1991). Multiple stimuli received by the senses reach the RAS, which selects certain impulses to be conducted to the cerebral cortex of the brain to be perceived.

When the nervous system is oriented to a stimulus and receptive toward it, the neurons of the RAS arouse the brain, facilitating information reception (Vander, Sherman, & Luciano, 1990). The RAS is highly selective; for example, a parent may be awakened in the middle of the night at the slightest murmur of an infant in a bedroom down the hall, but may sleep through the sound of loud traffic noises outside the bedroom window. Destruction of the RAS produces coma and the electroencephalograph (EEG) pattern characteristic of sleep (Vander, Sherman, & Luciano, 1990).

Input by Senses

Sensory function begins with reception of stimuli. The senses receiving stimuli externally are vision, hearing, smell, taste and touch. Receptor organs are the eyes, ears, olfactory receptors in the nose, tastebuds of the tongue, and nerve endings in the skin. The kinesthetic and visceral senses receive stimuli internally. Receptors are nerve endings in the skin and body tissues. The kinesthetic sense influences awareness of the placement and action of body parts, whereas visceral stimuli affect awareness related to the body's large interior organs. Vision, hearing, smell, and taste are termed special senses. Touch, kinesthetic (or proprioceptive) sensation, and visceral sensation are termed somatic senses (Guyton, 1986).

After stimuli are received, they are perceived with the help of the RAS. Sensory **perception** is a conscious process of selecting, organizing, and interpreting sensory stimuli, and depends on intact and functioning sense organs, nervous pathways, and brain (see Chapter 42 for more information on cognitive function).

Characteristics of Normal Sensory Perception

Characteristics of normal sensory perception are the normal measures in quality and quantity of the special and somatic senses. Characteristics of normal vision are visual acuity at or near 20/20, full field of vision, and tricolor vision (red, green, blue). The characteristic of normal hearing is auditory acuity of sounds at an intensity of 0 to 25 decibels, at frequencies of 125 to 8000 cycles per second. The characteristic of normal taste is discrimination of sour, salty, sweet, and bitter; that of normal smell is discrimination of primary odors such as camphoraceous, musky, floral, pepperminty, ethereal, pungent, and putrid. The characteristics of somatic senses include discrimination of touch, pressure, vibration, position, tickling, temperature, and pain (Guyton, 1986).

Normal Functional Sensory Pattern

A normal pattern of sensory perception is common to all human beings in that the person sees, smells, hears, tastes, feels, and responds to stimuli adequately. Normal patterns differ among people as well, however.

Sensoristasis

Each person has his or her own comfort zone or a zone of optimum arousal (Schafer, 1987; Carter, 1981). This comfort zone varies from person to person and is the range at which a person performs at his or her peak. **Sensoristasis** is the term used when a person is in a state of optimum arousal—not too much and not too little. The RAS is viewed by some theorists as a monitor for sensoristatic balance (Carter, 1981).

Adaptation

Beyond the point of sensoristasis, sensory adaptation occurs. Sensory receptors adapt to repeated stimulation by responding less and less and, eventually, the brain will not perceive constant stimulation, as in background traffic noise. Varied and irregular stimuli will still be perceived, however.

There are two necessary time periods crucial in helping a person to deal with new stimuli, lead time and afterburn (Schafer, 1987). Lead time is the period of time each person needs to prepare for an event emotionally and physically. Afterburn is the time needed to think about, evaluate, and come to terms with the activity after it happens. The necessary amount of lead time and afterburn is different for each person. Lead time and afterburn help a person process stimuli so he or she is not overwhelmed and can respond appropriately.

Factors Affecting Normal Sensory Perception

Environment. Sensory stimuli in the environment affect one's sensory perception. For example, a consistently noisy environment such as a school cafeteria may cause a teacher not to notice the noise, but the same teacher may perceive a loud television set very differently in his or her own home, which is usually quiet.

Previous Experience. Previous experience affects sensory perception in that people become more alert to new stimuli or old stimuli that evoked a strong response. For example, one may drive to work by the same route each day, noticing little along the way. Or one may be listening to the radio inattentively until a favorite song is played, then listen to every word. A new experience, such as hospitalization, may cause a patient to perceive a barrage of threatening new stimuli.

Lifestyle and Habits. Lifestyle affects sensory perception. One person may enjoy a lifestyle of abundant stimulation, surrounded by many people, frequent changes, bright lights, and noise, whereas others prefer less contact with crowds, quiet, and a slow-paced routine. People with different lifestyles perceive stimuli differently.

Cigarette smoking causes atrophy of tastebuds, decreasing sensory perception of taste. Chronic alcohol abuse may lead to peripheral neuropathy, a functional disorder of the peripheral nervous system that results in sensory impairment.

Illness. Certain illnesses affect sensory perception. Diabetes and hypertension cause changes in tiny blood vessels and nerves, leading to visual deficits and decreased sensation of touch in the extremities. Cerebrovascular disorders impair blood flow to the brain, possibly blocking sensory perception in the brain. Pain, fatigue, and stress caused by illness also affect perception of stimuli.

Medications. Some antibiotics, including streptomycin and gentamicin, can cause damage to the auditory nerve, impairing hearing. Central nervous system depressants such as narcotic analgesics decrease awareness and impair perception of stimuli.

Lifespan Considerations

Sensory perception is a crucial consideration in the very young and the elderly populations.

Newborn and Infant

Sensory perception is rudimentary at birth, and requires repeated stimulation for the nervous system to mature and discrimination within the senses to develop. Most stimulation is perceived by touch in the newborn and infant, who need to feel objects in the environment and learn to feel comfortable with their own bodies in space. They respond to holding, cuddling, soothing, rocking, and changing position. The newborn sees only gross patterns of light and dark or bright colors, but vision becomes more discriminating as the infant develops.

Toddler and Preschooler

A child's growth, development, and attachment are directly linked with sensory stimulation. Vision is fundamental to the growth of the mind, but full acquaintance with the world includes exploration with all the senses (Gesell & Ilg, 1949). As the child grows, he or she reacts to a world of persons and things (Gesell & Ilg, 1949); lack of meaningful stimulation can lead to developmental and motor delays (Chaze & Ludington-Hoe, 1984). Successful adaptation to change occurs when stimulation is not too much or too little.

The toddler is an explorer, learning through investigation of the environment by seeing, hearing, touching, tasting, smelling. The preschooler seeks in more organized play to perceive and respond to stimuli through the senses, as in singing and story-telling.

Child and Adolescent

Children and adolescents are experiencing rapid changes in their world, and learning is occurring at an accelerated pace. Reading and listening to school lessons dominate a child's day. School-aged children and adolescents are learning to make independent responses based on what is perceived through the senses, such as crossing the street when the light turns green or reporting a fire when smelling smoke.

Adult and Older Adult

Adults' sensory perception function is at its peak; however, as people reach middle age, they begin to notice certain changes in their sensory system. Eyesight diminishes, sounds become more muffled, and deterioration in the other sensory systems occurs. Marked decrements in sensory/perceptual behaviors begin as people approach 60 to 70 years of age (Corso, 1981). This reduction in efficiency means that older people cannot process sensory input as rapidly as they did when they were young (Corso, 1981; Lee, 1991); because of this slowing down, they need more time to deal with stimulating events.

ALTERED SENSORY FUNCTION

Potential for Altered Sensory Function

If a person experiences more sensory stimulation than he or she is used to or can make sense of, distress and sensory overload may occur. On the other hand, if a person experiences less than the usual stimulation, that person is below his or her optimum state of arousal and may be at risk for sensory deprivation.

Reactions to sensory overload or sensory deprivation are special challenges that nurses frequently encounter in themselves and patients. Sensory overload and deprivation can lead to perceptual, cognitive, and decisional problems. It is often difficult to separate where one area begins and another ends. For example, when a person's senses are bombarded with seeing, feeling, and hearing too much information at one time, it may be difficult to perceive accurately, think clearly, or make a good decision.

When the RAS is overwhelmed with input, a person may experience sensory overload, and feel confused, anxious, and unable to take constructive action. When the RAS fails to recognize a stimulus because it is below the threshold level or lacks relevant meaning to the person, sensory deprivation may occur, and the person experiences boredom, depression, restlessness, and vivid sensual imagery, including hallucinations (Lee, 1991; Haber, et al., 1987).

Sensory Overload

Sensory overload occurs when a person is unable to process or manage the intensity or quantity of incoming sensory stimuli. The person feels overwhelmed by the excessive input from the environment and does not feel in control (Haber, et al., 1987; Carter, 1981; Lee, 1991). For example, the woman who goes to her doctor for a routine check-up and is told that she may have a malignant breast tumor, may not process additional stimuli correctly due to the shock of that message. She may not perceive additional information about scheduling a biopsy and the surgical options for dealing with the lump, depending on whether it is nonmalignant or malignant.

Sensory Overload in the Health-Care Setting. Nurses need to understand the common, everyday occurrences in the health setting that can contribute to sensory overload in their patients. Such occurrences fall into three main categories: internal factors, imparting information, and the environment.

Internal Factors. Internal factors, such as thinking about impending surgery or the meaning of a medical diagnosis, can contribute to anxiety and cognitive overload so that the person cannot process additional stimuli (Fig. 41-1). Pain, medication, lack of sleep, worry, and brain injury can also contribute to a person's vulnerability to sensory overload.

Imparting Information. Imparting information to a patient may lead to sensory overload. Some examples include teaching a patient about a procedure, informing a patient about a diagnosis, making requests of a patient, or helping the patient solve a problem.

The Environment. The environment of the health-care setting, being unfamiliar to the patient, provides a higher than usual amount of sensory stimulation (see Fig. 41-1). A patient newly admitted to the hospital, for

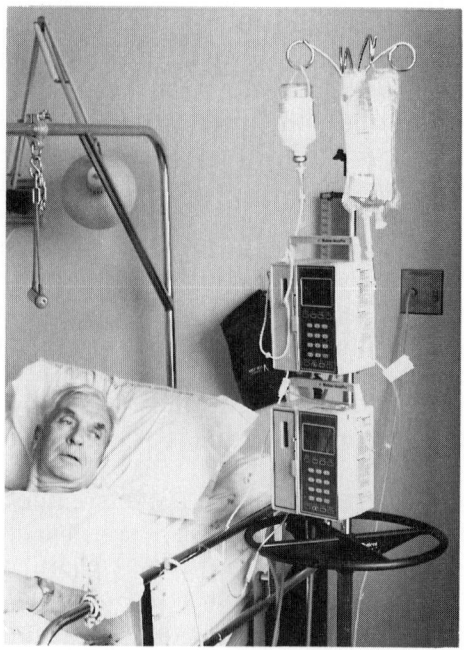

Figure 41–1. Anxiety related to medical diagnosis, prognosis, treatment, and equipment can contribute to sensory overload.

example, may have to cope with adjusting to a new roommate who is a stranger, having the television on more than usual, bright lights, hospital noises and intrusions, meeting many new staff, having the bed move up and down at someone else's bidding, waiting for someone to answer the call light, uncontrolled pain, and having strangers touch and probe very private areas of the body. Patients in intensive care units often exhibit symptoms of sensory overload because of the high degree of light, noise, and activity around the clock (Fig. 41-2).

Sensory Deprivation

Although **sensory deprivation** can be thought of as the opposite of sensory overload, they have many elements in common—think about the paradoxical statement, "The silence was deafening." When we speak about sensory deprivation, we generally mean a lessening or lack of meaningful sensory stimuli, monotonous sensory input, or an interference with the processing of information (Lee, 1991; Lego, 1984; Haber, et al., 1987).

Sensory deprivation (understimulation) can be just as disruptive as sensory overload. Cognitive and emotional deterioration can occur when stimuli are reduced below a person's optimum level of stimulation (Schafer, 1987). One common source of sensory deprivation is a sudden drop-off in stimuli when a person moves from a fast-paced to a slow-paced environment (Schafer, 1987). Each person's tolerance of and reaction to a lessening or lack of meaningful sensory stimuli will be different, of

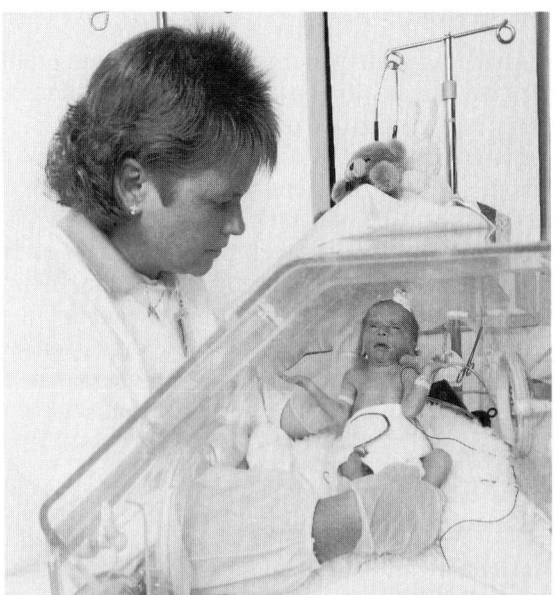

Figure 41–2. Lights and frequent activity may cause sensory overload in a premature infant or in the neonatal intensive care unit. (Photo courtesy of University of Washington School of Nursing.)

course, but in the extreme case, there is a gross misperception of events and personality changes.

Sensory Deprivation in the Health-Care Setting. Any time a patient experiences an interference with or a diminution of sensory input, that person may be at risk for sensory deprivation. In the hospital situation, such occurrences fall into two general categories: altered sensory reception and deprived environments.

Altered Sensory Reception. Altered sensory reception for the patient occurs under such conditions as spinal cord injury, brain damage, changes in receptor organs, sleep deprivation, and chronic illness. The person does not receive adequate sensory input because there is an interference with the nervous system's ability to receive and process stimuli. This inability can also lead to secondary problems, as in the following example:

> *Ralph Wilson suffered a spinal cord injury in an automobile accident, leaving him paraplegic; one day he decided to sneak a cigarette while no one was looking. He accidentally dropped the lighted match on his knitted slipper and burned his foot because he could not feel the heat when his slipper began to smolder.*

The elderly are especially susceptible to sensory deficits, as shown in the following example:

> *Cassie Taylor, 86 years old, stopped attending her assigned groups on the geriatric–psychiatric unit. She spent most of her time sitting in her*

room, and she became more depressed and began to show signs of confusion. As the staff compared notes about Cassie's day, they were able to intervene to assist her to increase her socialization and communication with others.

Deprived Environments. Deprived environments can have a negative effect on a person's sensoristasis. A person who is immobilized for any reason or who is in isolation is being deprived of the usual amount of stimulation, and may show manifestations of sensory deprivation (Fig. 41-3). Consider the following situation:

> *Patrick Matthews, an active and popular college baseball star, was admitted for a retinal detachment after being hit in the head by a baseball. He talked a great deal to the staff about his concerns, and the staff all commented on what a likable person he was. After surgery, he was put on bedrest and both eyes were bandaged. He was given a private room to minimize distractions and overstimulation.*

> *After the first day, Patrick stopped putting on his call light, did not engage in conversation with the nurses, and refused to contact his family and friends.*

> *On the second night after his surgery, Patrick showed signs of having hallucinations that a roommate was talking to him, and delusions that he was being poisoned through his meals.*

> *Patrick's verbal communication with the staff and his family had diminished dramatically since his hospitalization. He could not see; he was unable to check things out visually and was experiencing perceptual distortions. He had misinterpreted sounds outside of his room. He changed from being a likable, open person to being angry and suspicious.*

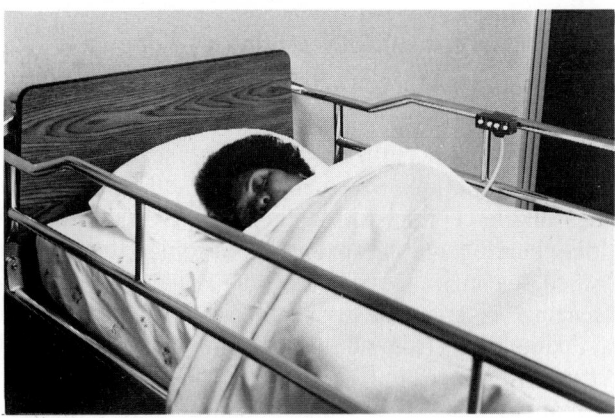

Figure 41–3. Isolation and lack of mobility may contribute to sensory deprivation.

Patrick was showing signs of sensory deprivation. He had been used to a very active, stimulating life and was suddenly put into a very nonstimulating, abnormally quiet environment. To compensate for temporary loss of sight, his senses of hearing and taste became more acute, leading to misinterpretations of sounds and taste of his food. His personality changed drastically.

Sensory Deficit

Sensory deficit is impaired function in sensory reception or perception. The deficit may be blindness due to disease of the eyes such as glaucoma. In this example reception is affected. Spinal cord injuries and strokes cause loss of tactile sensation. This affects perception because of disruption in nerve pathways and/or the brain.

Compensation for the deficit usually occurs when loss of function is gradual. The person often changes behavior to adapt to sensory deficit, such as turning a functioning ear toward a speaker to hear, or measuring temperature of bathwater with a thermometer if there is decreased sensation of the extremities. Physiologic compensation occurs as well, with the remaining senses becoming more acute. For example, a blind person may develop a more acute sense of smell or hearing.

Sensory Deficit in the Health-Care Setting. A sudden loss of sensory perception through a sensory deficit may cause total disorientation. Compensation does not occur immediately. In the health-care setting a sensory deficit may be incurred temporarily or permanently through illness or treatment. Temporary bandaging following eye surgery may render a patient totally unable to care for himself or herself. Nasal packing that temporarily eliminates the sense of smell affects taste and may lead to anorexia. The patient with sudden loss of lower extremity sensation through a spinal cord injury in a motor vehicle accident will be at risk for injury to the lower extremities.

Manifestations of Altered Sensory Function

Anxiety

Altered sensory perception frequently leads to anxiety, just as anxiety can further lead to additional altered sensory perception. An elderly woman living alone, with poor hearing, may be anxious about going to bed at night since she might not hear a smoke alarm, the phone ringing, or someone trying to break into the house. Anxiety stems from not being able to interact fully with the environment due to sensory deficit, fear of embarrassment when trying to communicate with others, or misinterpretation of information perceived through the senses.

Cognitive Dysfunction

Disturbances in remembering, reasoning, and problem solving may occur with sensory overload. Decision-making may be irrational or dysfunctional.

Other common behaviors indicative of cognitive dysfunction include disorientation, verbalizing disconnected thoughts, complaining of too much going on, an inability to think, poor work performance, and complaints of sleeplessness and fatigue (Gordon, 1987).

Sensory deprivation causes a reduction in mental capabilities as well (Toffler, 1970). Mind wandering occurs, along with fantasy activity. The person may have difficulty maintaining concentration and logical thinking.

Hallucinations and Delusions

Hallucinations are sensory impressions that are based on internal stimulations and have no basis in reality. Hearing voices when no one is there is a typical auditory hallucination. **Delusions** are beliefs that are not based in reality and reflect an unconscious need or fear, e.g., believing the hospital food is poisoned. Both hallucinations and delusions have been documented in cases of sensory deprivation, sensory overload, and sensory deficits such as hearing and vision loss (Goldberger, 1982). For example, an elderly woman is suddenly hospitalized. Her glasses are misplaced and the battery is weak in her hearing aid. She may not understand why strange people come into her room at night, and she may have difficulty toileting herself, so she soils her bed. Her sensory deficits cause her to misinterpret stimuli and distort reality. She has delusions that she is in a prison, the nurses are guards, and other prisoners are trying to take advantage of her, and she hallucinates that her dead sister is telling her to join her in heaven.

Depression and Withdrawal

Depression may result from sensory deficits or sensory deprivation. Helplessness and loss of self-esteem lead to depression and withdrawal. The patient who is on isolation precautions may show signs of poor appetite, sleeplessness, and loss of interest in activities or interaction with others as he or she becomes depressed, leading to further sensory deprivation.

Impact of Dysfunction on Activities of Daily Living

Sensory perception dysfunction may have profound effects on activities of daily living (ADL). Visual deficits cause problems with self-care activities as basic as dressing, toiletry, and preparing meals. Moving about outside the home may be impossible without special aids or a helping hand. Hearing deficits restrict people from watching television, listening to the radio, and answering the telephone; safety hazards exist for deaf pedestrians. Many jobs are prohibited for people with sensory deficits, and driving is not allowed. This restricts the environments in which they may move about safely and makes them dependent on others. People with taste and smell deficits may lose interest in eating. Those with sensory deficits of touch are at risk for burns and injuries to the extremities. People with cognitive dysfunction from sensory overload or deprivation may exhibit poor judgment and problem solving during everyday activities.

ASSESSMENT

Nursing assessment should explore the patient's sensory perception through subjective and objective data collection. Assessment for sensory perception focuses on the patient, the environment, and interaction between the patient and others. Subjective data include normal sensory function identification, identification of risk factors, and identification of dysfunctional sensory perception. Family and friends may provide helpful data about changes in the patient's behavior that indicate problems in sensory perception. Objective data are collected through physical examination of the neurologic system and special senses, as well as diagnostic tests. Information gained from nursing assessment leads to formation of nursing diagnoses and interventions to optimize the individual patient's sensory function.

Subjective Data

Functional Pattern Identification

To determine a patient's normal functional pattern of sensory perception, the nurse first asks a general question, such as "How do you spend a typical day?" This question can give the nurse a feel for the level of stimulation the patient usually experiences on a daily basis and the patient's response to that stimulation.

The nurse should next assess how the patient responds to change. Since health-care settings have a lot of change occurring, it is useful to find out how the patient manages these. Asking, "Have there been any recent changes in your life?" can lead to an informative discussion of the degree of complexity of the changes and the responses of the patient.

Next an investigation of the living and social situation of the patient, as well as the modes of transportation the person uses will give the nurse a further idea of the degree of complexity of the patient's life and the level of independence. Questions such as, "With whom do you live?" and "Do you prepare your own (your family's)

meals?", and "When you want to go someplace, how do you get there?" (mode of transportation), give the nurse important information about the daily functioning of the patient.

Finally, questioning can center on the person's lifestyle and habits. What kinds of food are you used to? If the usual diet consists of highly spiced foods, a hospital menu may seem dull and uninteresting, and affect the patient's appetite since it does not meet the usual needs of the patient in the area of gustatory stimulation. How much alcohol does the person drink daily or weekly? How much sleep is the person used to? What is the usual time the patient retires and arises? Knowledge of other factors includes educational level, hobbies and interests, and what jobs the person holds or has held. Table 41-1 gives examples of general and specific questions to elicit information about the patient's interaction with his environment.

Risk Identification

To collect data about risk factors for sensory perception dysfunction, the nurse elicits information about the patient's age, culture and language, level of activity, medical history, and medications. The nurse must also assess the degree of stimulation in the health-care environment in light of the patient's experiences (see the display on risk factors).

Elderly patients are more at risk for sensory deficits due to normal physiologic changes of aging, especially in hearing and vision. Patients with cultural and language barriers may be at risk for sensory deprivation. The nurse should ask about the patient's level of activity; immobilization due to physical disability restricts the usual amount of stimulation the patient may be used to. Medical history includes history of present illness, any chronic illnesses, past hospitalizations, accidents, and surgeries. History of sensory deficits such as visual and hearing impairment place the patient at risk for sensory deprivation. History of illnesses such as diabetes, hypertension, stroke, or spinal cord injury also place the patient at risk for sensory deficits. The patient's past experience with the health-care environment determines the affect of stimulation on the patient. Lack of experience with an intensive care unit or isolation precautions may place the patient at risk for sensory overload or deprivation during hospitalization. Medications the nurse should assess for include central nervous system depressants, such as narcotic analgesics and sedatives, or large doses of antibiotics that may affect hearing.

Dysfunctional Identification

During the nursing assessment the nurse collects data about actual sensory perception problems. Does the patient have difficulty with vision or hearing? How are the patient's senses of smell, taste, and touch? If prob-

TABLE 41–1

General and Specific Questions About the Patient and Environment

General Question	Specific Questions
How do you spend a typical day?	Do you go to school? Do you work outside the home? Do you watch TV, listen to the radio, read the newspaper? How often do you talk to friends and family?
Have there been any recent changes in your life?	Have you experienced any changes such as loss of a loved one, change of a job, a friend moving away, new baby in the house? How are you adjusting to the change?
What are your living arrangements like?	With whom do you live? What is the size of your home? Do you cook and care for family members? Do you live in a neighborhood? How convenient is shopping? Do you have transportation?
What are your interests and habits?	What are your hobbies? Are you involved in sports? Do you smoke, how much? Do you drink alcohol, how much? Do you use any recreational drugs? How much sleep do you need, how much do you get? Do you like to go out? What types of food do you eat?

Risk Factors in the Health-Care Environment for Sensory Perception Dysfunction

Sensory Overload

Room close to nurse's station _____
ICU or intermediate unit _____
Bright lights _____
Use of mechanical ventilator _____
Use of ECG monitor _____
Use of oxygen _____
Use of IVs _____
Other equipment _____
Roommate _____
Frequent treatments _____

Sensory Deprivation

Private room _____
Eyes bandaged _____
Bedrest _____
Sensory aid not available (hearing aid, glasses) _____
Isolation precautions _____
Few visitors _____

---

lems are identified, the nurse should determine when the problem started, its severity, and what the patient has done about it. This information will prove useful in helping the patient adapt to the health-care environment.

The nurse should also question the patient about manifestations the sensory dysfunction may have caused. Is the patient anxious, depressed, withdrawing from social contact? Does the patient have difficulty concentrating, making decisions, remembering? Has the patient ever experienced hallucinations or delusions?

Objective Data

Physical Assessment

The focus of the physical assessment is to determine if there is any impairment in the senses. It is important to include assessment of the following: auditory, visual, taste, smell, touch, somatic senses, and mental status examination. Mental status data can be collected as the nurse takes the patient history. Mental status data should include level of consciousness orientation, attention span, memory, and cognitive skills. See Chapter 18 for more information on assessment.

To collect objective data about the sensory system systematically, the nurse first inspects, then performs simple tests. The nurse inspects the head for any abnormalities of the eyes, ears, nose, or mouth, and inspects the extremities for any burns or injuries. See Table 41-2 for a list of tests to assess sensation.

Diagnostic Tests and Procedures

There are several laboratory findings of which the nurse needs to be aware. Electrolyte imbalances, alterations in blood chemistry, such as elevated ammonia or blood urea nitrogen, and toxic levels of drugs that affect the central nervous system can alter sensoristasis (Kim, McFarland, & McLane, 1987; McFarland and Wasli, 1986). Special visual and auditory acuity tests may also be ordered. Neurologic tests such as nerve conduction studies, computed tomographic scanning of the brain, and cerebral angiography may be performed to determine the cause of sensory deficits.

NURSING DIAGNOSIS AND PATIENT GOALS

The accepted NANDA nursing diagnosis for sensory overload, deprivation, and deficit is Sensory/Perceptual Alterations. These may include visual, auditory, kinesthetic, gustatory, tactile, or olfactory alterations. The nurse uses data from the assessment to determine the presence or risk for any of these disruptions in normal sensory perception function.

Diagnostic Statement: Sensory/Perceptual Alterations

(Specify visual, auditory, kinesthetic, gustatory, tactile, olfactory).

Definition

Sensory/Perceptual Alteration is a state in which an individual experiences a change in the amount or patterning of oncoming stimuli accompanied by a diminished, exaggerated, distorted, or impaired response to such stimuli (NANDA, 1990).

Defining Characteristics

Disoriented in time, in place, or with persons; altered abstraction; altered conceptualization; change in problem-solving abilities; reported or measured change in sensory acuity; change in behavior pattern; anxiety; apathy; change in usual response to stimuli; indication of body-image alteration; restlessness; irritability; altered communication patterns.

Other possible characteristics include complaints of fatigue; alteration in posture; change in muscular tension; inappropriate responses; hallucinations (NANDA, 1990).

TABLE 41–2

Physical Assessment of Sensory Function

Sense	Technique for Assessment
Vision	Use Snellen chart to measure visual acuity (or have patient read newspaper, menu, or whatever is available). Test visual fields.
Hearing	Whisper numbers in each ear, while occluding the other, ask patient to repeat.
	Perform Weber and Rinne tuning fork tests.
	Observe patient's conversation with others.
Smell	With eyes closed, have patient identify three odors such as coffee, tobacco, and cloves, one nostril at a time, while occluding the other nostril.
Taste	With eyes closed have patient identify three tastes such as lemon, salt, and sugar, waiting 1 minute and giving sips of water in between. Have patient close eyes for all tests.
Somatic sensation	Test light touch of extremities with a wisp of cotton.
	Test sharp and dull sensation using the point and blunt end of a pin.
	Test two-point discrimination using two pins held close together.
	Test hot and cold sensation using test tubes filled with warm and cold water.
	Test vibration sense using a tuning fork over joints.
	Test position sense by moving the patient's fingers or toes.
	Test stereognosis by giving the patient a common object (quarter, paperclip) to identify by feel.

Related Factors

Altered environmental stimuli, excessive or insufficient; altered sensory reception, transmission and/or integration; chemical alterations, endogenous (electrolyte), exogenous (drugs, etc.); psychological stress (NANDA, 1990).

Related Nursing Diagnoses

Other nursing diagnoses may be identified for the patient with sensory alterations. The following are possible problems: Body Image Disturbance, Chronic Low Self-Esteem, Diversional Activity Deficit, Fatigue, Altered Growth and Development, High Risk for Injury, High Risk for Poisoning, Self-Care Deficits, and Sleep Pattern Disturbance. If the sensory alterations are the result of spinal injury, additional nursing diagnoses may be the following: Dysreflexia, Impaired Home Maintenance Management, Altered Role Performance, or Impaired Skin Integrity.

Patient Goals

Patient goals are individualized, but focus on achieving optimal sensory function. The patient goals for Sensory/Perceptual Alterations are the following:

The patient will demonstrate an understanding of contributing factors by reducing or eliminating them.

The patient will demonstrate an understanding of interventions and rationale by using this information as foresight in maintaining sensoristasis.

The patient will demonstrate achievement of sensoristasis through a decrease in the symptoms of sensory overload/deprivation.

The patient will demonstrate achievement or maintenance of self-care.

The patient will maintain safety.

IMPLEMENTATION

Nursing Interventions to Promote Sensory Health and Function

Nurses can promote sensory function of patients in the health-care environment by preparing patients for procedures and by providing effective interactions with the patient.

Patient Teaching

Nurses can promote sensory health and function by teaching patients at risk ways to prevent sensory loss as well as by teaching general health measures to health care consumers. Teaching topics include frequent eye examinations and tight control of chronic illness such as diabetes (see the accompanying patient teaching display).

Nurses should teach health-care consumers the importance of sensory function and the roles of sensory receptors and the central nervous system in receiving and perceiving stimuli. Preventing sensory dysfunction will enable the person to interact with the environment at an optimal level. Yearly eye examinations, more often if problems arise, help promote optimal visual function. Other measures to prevent visual dysfunction include avoiding eyestrain and eye infection or injury. Prevention of hearing loss may be achieved through prompt recognition and treatment of ear infections and immunization in childhood against illnesses such as rubella.

The older adult who is at risk for sensory loss due to physiologic changes of aging should be taught to have

---

> ### Patient Teaching
>
> Instruct the patient as follows:
>
> - Obtain routine medical check-ups.
> - Seek early attention for any potential sensory problems to prevent sensory misperceptions.
> - Obtain a yearly eye examination (more frequently if problems arise) to prevent visual sensory deficits.
> - Increase or reduce sensory stimulation as necessary in order to have an optimal balance in sensory perception.
> - If you have diabetes or high blood pressure, maintain tight control of blood sugar and blood pressure through self-monitoring, mediation compliance, diet, and medical follow-up to avoid related sensory disturbances.
> - Seek medical attention for signs of ear infections in your children to avoid hearing problems that interfere with perception.
> - Provide regular immunizations for your children, and maintain a record, to prevent auditory and other sensory losses.

routine check-ups and seek attention for any developing problems. He or she may delay medical attention, fearing that hearing loss is inevitable when simple ear irrigation may dislodge impacted cerumen and restore hearing. Patients with chronic illnesses such as diabetes and hypertension should be taught the importance of tight control of blood sugar and blood pressure, respectively. Control can help prevent tactile and visual dysfunction. Self-monitoring of blood sugar or blood pressure, compliance with medications, diet control, and medical follow-up are essential.

Procedure Preparation

A primary concern of the nurse is to prevent symptoms of sensory overload in the health-care environment. The patient is especially at risk for sensory overload when unfamiliar procedures are taking place. Overstimulation can be prevented by preparing the patient before a procedure, using a technique called **sensation (sensory) information.** The purpose of this intervention is to alleviate distress responses of the patient to threatening stimuli and improve the patient's coping through stimulation of the cognitive processes. The technique involves objectively and specifically describing to a patient, in serial order, what they typically (rare or atypical events are not to be included) will see, hear, smell, taste, or feel (tactile) in a particular situation, from the patient's point of view, not from the observer's viewpoint (Horsley & Crane, 1981; Sime, 1985).

It is important for the nurse to have a good understanding of this technique before using it. In general, sensation information is useful when a patient feels threatened by a procedure. The patient must make that appraisal, not the nurse. Patients who indicate a high level of anxiety before a procedure seem to benefit more than those with low levels of anxiety. Finally, what patient outcomes are desired? Sensation information will not help the patient achieve new coping skills, but it may enhance his or her current coping mechanisms (Sime, 1985).

Other interventions to help prevent sensory overload include educating a patient about why a procedure will be done, who will do it, and how long it will take. Helping a patient gain a sense of control by such interventions as establishing a schedule for routine care, providing a calendar and clock, and allowing choices whenever possible, can also reduce the risk of sensory overload (Lee, 1991).

Nurse–Patient Interaction

Nurse–patient interaction needs to be individualized to promote sensory health function. Those patients at risk for sensory deprivation may need frequent interaction initiated by the nurse, while others may not. In any case, appropriate stimuli provided by the nurse include addressing the patient by name, introducing and reintroducing oneself as necessary, explanation of all activities, and acknowledgment of leaving and when the nurse will return. Length, frequency, and content of interactions should be based on individual needs. Talking to the patient, showing the patient equipment or articles used in care, encouraging the patient to smell and taste food on the meal tray, and touching the patient are appropriate stimuli while interacting with the patient.

Nursing Interventions for Altered Sensory Function

Nursing interventions for patients with altered sensory function may focus on enhancing stimulation or reducing stimulation to minimize sensory deprivation or sensory overload, respectively. Sensory aids can be provided to minimize a patient's sensory deficit. Nurses must also intervene to provide safety for the patient who is at risk for injury due to sensory dysfunction.

Stimulation Provision

Providing Meaningful External Stimuli. Providing meaningful external stimuli can help a patient overcome sensory deprivation or sensory deficit. Playing the televi-

Nursing Research

Selected Nursing Research Studies

Horsley, J. A., & Crane, J. (1981). *Distress Reduction Through Sensory Preparation.* New York: Grune and Stratton.

Rosswurm, M. A. (1989). Assessment of perceptual processing deficits in persons with Alzheimer's disease. *Western Journal of Nursing Research, 11,* 458–468.

Dannenbaum, R. M., et al. (1990). Evaluating sustained touch-pressure in severe sensory deficits: Meeting an unanswered need. *Archives of Physical Medicine and Rehabilitation, 71,* 455–459.

Possible Topics for Nursing Inquiry

- Does location of the room make a difference in sensory overload/deprivation?
- Will assisting the patient to gain a sense of control related to the environment reduce the risk of sensory overload?
- What nursing interventions are most successful in reducing symptoms of sensory deprivation/overload?

sion or the radio occasionally, playing music for brief periods, encouraging the use of a clock and calendar, encouraging use of the patient's clothing, putting up colorful pictures, encouraging visitors, opening the drapes, and placing the bed or chair so the patient can readily see or hear the activities in the hall and when someone enters the room, all provide stimulation.

Frequently Interacting with the Patient. Frequently interacting with the patient may also help. Discussing scheduling of care and placement of equipment, encouraging self-care activities, providing tactile stimulation through back-rubs, combing and brushing the patient's hair (or encouraging the patient to do so), reading to the patient, speaking slowly and clearly, and identifying yourself verbally and with a name tag are meaningful interactions. It may also be necessary to reorient the patient frequently to person, place, and time. Because the patient may be having difficulties in concentrating, he or she may need repeated direction to accomplish even simple tasks. The nurse must add stimulation slowly so the patient is not overwhelmed, and should include a variety of stimuli and keep the amount of sensory input at a moderate level. Orienting the patient to the environment can help the patient avoid experiencing misinterpretations. Visiting the patient often and letting the patient know when the nurse will return helps the patient overcome a feeling of isolation. Providing a calendar and a clock to assist the patient in keeping track of time helps keep the patient in touch with activities of the unit. A roommate for a patient experiencing sensory deprivation can help a great deal. Preparing the patient for any procedure that may add to the sensory deprivation, such as being restricted to bedrest, gives the patient time to think of alternatives to sensory stimulation.

The nurse can encourage the patients to provide self-stimulation. Self-stimulation, such as singing, reading, and talking into a tape recorder and playing it back, can be helpful. Encouraging maximum use of the available senses can help a person adjust. Self-care and activity are also means of self-stimulation.

Encouragement of physical movement can assist the patient to use up his or her restless energy and can prevent symptoms of sensory deprivation. Encouraging the patient to move around in the bed or walk around the room, sit in a chair, do ADLs as independently as possible, and do exercises in the room or in bed if not able to get up, all provide stimulation to the patient's senses.

Stimulation Reduction

Reducing stimulation may be necessary for patients experiencing sensory overload. The nurse can plan care to reduce sensory overload in the areas of imparting information, reducing environmental stimuli, and assisting the patient to deal with internal factors (see the display on nursing interventions to reduce sensory overload). Measures such as reducing extraneous noise, lights, room clutter, interruptions, pain, and stress all reduce stimulation.

Patients in sensory overload may neglect their ADLs to the point that the nurse needs to assist them. Such assistance can be problematic because it can add further to sensory overload. With this in mind, the nurse can

---

Nursing Interventions to Reduce Sensory Overload

Imparting Information

- Introduce new information gradually to allow time for the patient to process the meaning.
- Speak in a slow, unhurried manner.
- Keep hospital/medical jargon to a minimum.
- Use several sensory pathways whenever possible rather than overloading one pathway (i.e., state your name *and* wear a name tag)
- Have the patient repeat back information so you know the patient has a correct understanding.
- Provide for frequent rest periods when the patient is undisturbed.

Reducing Environmental Stimuli

- Dim lights or provide dark glasses.
- Avoid loud noises or provide ear plugs.
- Refrain from bumping the bed, or moving or touching the patient unnecessarily.
- Turn off the TV set.
- Ask staff to hold conversations out of hearing range of the patient.
- Request other personnel not to disturb the patient for unessential tasks (i.e., housekeeping).
- Encourage the patient to use earphones to listen to soothing music or relaxation tapes to block out other noises.

- Plan a routine of care so the patient knows when and what to expect (post the schedule for the patient wherever possible).
- Limit visitors as necessary.
- Reduce noxious odors: empty commode or bedpan immediately after use, keep wounds clean and covered, use room deodorizer when indicated, and provide good ventilation.
- Provide a private room until the patient can tolerate a roommate. Use preventive measures to guard against sensory deprivation.

Internal Factors

- Provide time for the patient to discuss his or her thoughts. Correct misperceptions.
- Orient the patient, when indicated, to person, place, and time.
- Provide for rest and sleep periods to prevent exhaustion.
- Provide for the possibility of increasing the dose and frequency of pain medication until pain management can be achieved through other means (see Chap. 40).
- Help the patient use stress-reduction behaviors to relieve anxiety (see Chap. 47).

best help the patient by assisting only with the immediately essential ADLs (e.g., moving, eating, toileting, and resting), and adding additional tasks as the patient is able to cope.

Sensory Aids

When a patient experiences a sensory deficit, availability of sensory aids help promote optimal function of that and other available senses (e.g., hearing aids in good working order, clean eyeglasses, good oral hygiene). In addition to providing actual physical and situational sensory aids, the nurse should enlist significant others whenever possible to assist the patient in dealing with the deficit (see the display for sensory aids listed by sense). Sensory aids can be used in the health-care environment and taught to patients for use at home. When one sense is lost, sensory aids can be used for other senses to enhance general stimulation. For example, a blind patient should be encouraged to savor the aroma, taste, and texture of food.

Selected Nursing Interventions for Common Sensory Problems

Sensory Overload

- Address the patient by name and introduce yourself.
- Minimize unnecessary noise, light, or distractions.
- Describe any procedures or tests to the patient.
- Encourage uninterrupted periods of sleep and rest.
- Provide orienting cues for the patient, such as clocks, calendars, and windows.
- Support accurate interpretations of perceptions.

Sensory Deprivation

- Encourage the patient's use of sensory aides, such as eyeglasses or hearing aids.
- Identify barriers to communication and sensory perception.
- Address the patient by name and touch the patient during communication.
- Communicate frequently with the patient to maintain meaningful interactions.
- Modify the environment to provide meaningful sensory stimulation.
- Promote uninterrupted periods of sleep and rest.
- Provide a structured routine and activities.

Safety

Implementing safety precautions is another group of nursing interventions for patients with sensory perception dysfunction. Sensory deficits, as well as the cognitive effects of sensory deprivation or sensory overload, place the patient at risk for injury from the environment. The nurse should implement actions such as assisting patients with ambulation, use of bed siderails, night lights, call system, restraints, and frequent or continuous observation as necessary.

The nurse must teach patients with sensory deficits how to ensure safety at home. For example, patients with decreased sensation to temperature in the extremities should have their hot water heater temperature adjusted and must test water temperature with a thermometer before bathing. They should be taught to inspect their legs and feet for any injuries or pressure sores they cannot feel. Patients with decreased sense of smell should be taught the danger of using gas and chemicals. For example, cleaning with ammonia in a confined space such as a bathroom may cause the patient to be overcome by fumes before he or she can smell them. A patient may not smell a gas leak in the home, but if a stove or gas heater is not working properly, it should be reported promptly. Food should be inspected for freshness, since the patient may not smell spoiled meat or dairy products. Patients with hearing and visual deficits need to take additional safety precautions as well. See Chapter 25 for more information on safety.

Discharge Planning and Home Care

In today's world of rising costs and shorter hospital stays, a patient may be discharged while still adjusting to his or her condition. This may be a new or worsening sensory deficit, or an illness or treatment that causes sensory deprivation or sensory overload. Planning should be initiated while the patient is still hospitalized to help him or her adjust to sensory dysfunction. Planning includes patient teaching, enlisting the help and cooperation of family and friends, assembling sensory aids and equipment, contacting home health services, and locating additional support groups as needed.

Assessment of the patient's home environment helps determine what will be needed to help the patient adapt to his or her sensory dysfunction. The nurse can teach the patient and family how to interact with the home environment, using other scenes and sensory aids to adapt and remain safe. The patient may need much help during the adaptation process, but eventually become independent. At first, the patient may need help with basic care and hygiene; however, ongoing nursing assessment will determine the need for further interventions.

It is important to keep in mind that as family roles may suddenly change (e.g., the breadwinner becomes the

(Text continues on page 1206)

Sensory Aids

Vision

- Eyeglasses with the proper prescription, cleaned and in good repair
- Adequate room lighting, drapes open
- Sunglasses or window shades to reduce glare
- Literature with large print
- Uncluttered environment, no furniture rearranging
- Clock with large numbers
- Telephone dial with large numbers
- Magnifying glass
- Bright, contrasting colors in environment
- Color coded dials on appliances, medication bottles, etc.
- Braille, recorded books, seeing-eye dog, etc., as necessary

Hearing

- Hearing aid in good repair with working battery
- Speaking slowly and distinctly in full view of patient, no mouth covering or gum chewing
- Avoidance of background noise
- Amplified phone ringer, doorbell, smoke alarm, etc.
- Head set for telephone communication
- Closed-caption television

Smell

- Fresh food served for meals
- Fresh flowers or fragrance in the room
- Others wearing light perfume or fragrance
- Notice of environmental smells

Taste

- Fresh food, seasoned appropriately, not overcooked or overprocessed to preserve texture
- Foods served at appropriate temperature and time of day
- Note smell as well as taste of food
- Sips of water between foods
- No mixing of foods

Touch

- Therapeutic touch
- Massage (self or nurse)
- Turning and repositioning
- Hairbrushing and grooming (self or nurse)
- Activity around environment
- Amount of pressure individualized to patient's comfort level
- Articles of care and clothing of various textures

Safety Alert

- When assisting a visually impaired patient with ambulation, stand on the patient's hand-dominant side, about 1 foot in front of him or her. Have him or her grasp your arm with the nondominant hand, and use the patient's dominant hand to feel around him or her for barriers or landmarks.
- Maintain an uncluttered environment for a visually impaired patient.
- Organize self-care articles within patient's reach and orient him to their location.
- Make sure the nurse call system is operating and within reach.
- Never rearrange furnishings without orienting the patient.

- Don't rely on a hearing-impaired patient to notify you of an alarm from an IV pump or malfunctioning cardiac monitor. Teach the patient to visually identify kinked IV tubing or a loose ECG lead and check these patients frequently.
- Test the temperature of bath or basin water before a patient with altered tactile sensation bathes.
- Teach a patient with altered taste and smell to avoid ingesting outdated food by checking expiration dates on food packages and visually inspecting the food for color and texture.

Nursing Management Plan
The Patient with Sensory/Perceptual Alterations

Nursing Diagnosis: Visual sensory/perceptual alteration related to temporary decrease in visual sensory input manifested by fear of body-image alteration, irritability, withdrawal, and misinterpretation of sensory stimuli.

Patient Goal: Patient will demonstrate an understanding of the sensory deprivation experience.

Patient Outcome Criteria

- Within 8 hours, patient accurately describes this eye injury and expected medical outcome, i.e., full visual recovery.
- During hospitalization, patient freely discusses problems with the staff, asking appropriate questions
- Before discharge, patient describes his or her behavioral changes and relates them to temporary deficit.
- Before discharge, patient explains his or her behavior changes to family.

Nursing Intervention	Scientific Rationale
1. Introduce self from doorway before entering room and explain reason for being there.	1. To avoid startling the patient and prevent misperceptions.
2. Post schedule for day on wall for all staff, visitors, and family to follow. Review schedule with patient for his input.	2. A schedule assists the patient to know what is going to happen and helps the patient with orientation and anxiety reduction.
3. As rapport and trust build, invite the patient to share his or her concerns about recovery; answer questions and correct misconceptions.	3. By getting the concerns out in the open, the nurse can help the patient separate fears from reality.
4. Encourage patient to identify his or her frustrations and anxieties related to being temporarily "blind," and to ask questions about his or her environment.	4. To provide reassurance, orient patient to his or her environment, and provide a variety of sensory stimulation.
5. Hold a conference with the patient's family to promote mutual discussion of the experience. Encourage patient to teach the family what he or she understands about sensory deprivation.	5. To evaluate the understanding of sensory deprivation and to do additional teaching related to concerns of family about home management.

Patient Goal: Patient will demonstrate achievement of sensoristasis through a decrease in the symptoms of sensory deprivation.

Patient Outcome Criteria

- Before discharge, patient uses various sensory pathways to increase sensory variation.
- Before discharge, patient reports no difficulty related to misperceiving sensory stimuli.
- During hospitalization, patient visits with family/friends for a minimum of 15 minutes per visit.

Nursing Intervention	Scientific Rationale
1. Schedule 5-minute conversations every hour on the hour while awake, for the first 24 hours.	1. To provide cognitive and sensory stimulation gradually and at a time the patient can count on, so the patient is not overwhelmed.
2. Orient to any noises that can be misinterpreted, e.g., the air-conditioner thermostat on the wall, the noises from the pneumatic-tube system (especially loud at night), the chimes indicating a fire drill, the sound of the food cart being wheeled in at meal times.	2. To minimize misperceptions and help the patient stay focused in reality.

(continued)

Nursing Management Plan
The Patient with Sensory/Perceptual Alterations (continued)

3. After the first 24 hours, on day and evening shifts a minimum of two and maximum of four staff per shift, other than assigned caretakers, should talk with the patient for a minimum of 10 minutes. Post a schedule in the front of the patient's chart to sign up for these social visits.

4. Teach the patient about the importance of gradually increasing input from other sensory pathways when vision is temporarily unavailable; include teaching about: self-stimulation such as counting, singing, and using a tape recorder to talk into; isometric exercises; tactile stimulation; auditory variation, gustatory and olfactory stimulation.

3. To build trust, reduce anxiety, provide cognitive stimulation, and sensory variation.

4. To provide information about management of sensory deficit, to increase stimulation gradually, and to prevent further sensory deprivation or overload.

---

care receiver), family members may need as much help and support as the patient, for their own issues and concerns. Social services may be enlisted to help with financial problems related to the patient's sensory dysfunction. Occupational therapy is a referral that can also help the patient adapt to a sensory dysfunction. Nurses are in a unique position to assess the patient's needs before discharge and organize services that can continue the patient's care after discharge.

EVALUATION

Evaluation of the care of a patient with sensory perception dysfunction is based on the goals that were individually designed for that patient. Outcome criteria are looked at to see if goals were achieved. For a patient with sensory/perceptual alteration, was sensoristasis achieved? Were contributing factors to sensory dysfunction reduced or eliminated? Can the patient describe the interventions and rationale so that this information can be used in the future to deal with sensory dysfunction? Was self-care maintained? Was safety maintained? Examples of positive outcome criteria for a patient at risk for sensory overload follow.

Goal
The patient will demonstrate an understanding of contributing factors by reduction or elimination of them.

Possible Outcome Criteria
• Patient uses ear plugs and eyeshades during sleep next three nights.

• Patient limits television and radio use to 1 to 3 hours per 8-hour period for next 48 hours.
• Patient asks appropriate questions about care before and during treatment in next 24 hours.

Goal
The patient will demonstrate an understanding of interventions and rationale by using this information as foresight.

Possible Outcome Criteria
• During next 24 hours, patient describes procedures to nurse before they are done, including what he or she might see, hear, feel, smell, or taste; gives rationale for procedure; and asks questions.

Goal
The patient will demonstrate achievement of sensoristasis through a decrease in the symptoms of sensory overload/deprivation.

Possible Outcome Criteria
• Patient demonstrates ability to concentrate by listening to explanation of medications, asking appropriate questions, and repeating medication schedule every time medication is given in next 24 hours.
• Patient sleeps 5 to 7 hours each night without awakening every night until discharge.
• Patient oriented to person, place, and time during visiting hours for remainder of day as reported by nurse.
• Patient listens to relaxation tape with earphones when housekeeping personnel are cleaning room.

Goal

The patient will maintain safety.

Possible Outcome Criteria

- Patient accurately uses siderails, night light, and call system during next 12 hours.
- Patient reports absence of injuries throughout remainder of hospital stay.

Goal

The patient will demonstrate achievement of maintenance of self-care.

Possible Outcome Criteria

- Patient bathes and performs adequate oral care daily during remainder of hospital stay.
- Patient performs toileting independently and safely during next 24 hours.
- Patient ambulates in hall three times a day for 15 minutes.
- Patient feeds self all the food and liquid on the tray for next three meals.

Key Concepts

- Senses include vision, hearing, taste, smell, and touch. Senses related to touch are the somatic senses of kinesthesia, or position sense, and visceral, or deep sensation.
- The reticular activating system controls arousal and awareness to stimuli.
- The characteristics of normal vision include acuity, field of vision, and color vision.
- Sensoristasis refers to a person's optimum state of arousal through stimulation.
- Adaptation occurs when stimulation becomes constant.
- Sensory perception generally decreases over 60 to 70 years of age.
- Factors that affect normal sensory perception include type of environment one is used to, previous experience, lifestyle, habits such as smoking and drinking, illness such as diabetes and hypertension, and medications such as central nervous system depressants.
- Altered sensory function can occur due to sensory overload, sensory deprivation, or sensory deficits. Sensory overload occurs when a person is unable to process the intensity or quantity of incoming stimuli, as with a patient in an intensive care unit. Sensory deprivation is a lack of meaningful stimuli, often occurring when a patient is on isolation precautions.
- Sensory deficits that occur gradually often bring about behavior changes and sharpening of other senses to help the person adapt.

- Anxiety, cognitive dysfunction, depression, and hallucinations and delusions are manifestations of sensory perception dysfunction.
- Nursing assessment of sensory perception function includes subjective information about the patient and his or her usual environment, as well as physical examination for vision, hearing, taste, smell, and the somatic senses of touch, pressure, position, vibration, pain, and temperature.
- Patient goals for the nursing diagnosis of Sensory/Perceptual Alterations include the achievement of sensoristasis, reduction of contributing factors, description of intervention and rationales, achievement of self-care, and maintenance of safety.
- Patient teaching about eye examinations and treatment of ear infections may help promote sensory function.
- Preparation of patients for procedures should include sensory experiences to prevent sensory overload.
- Nurses must provide appropriate stimulation for patients, while reducing excess stimulation for sensory deprivation/sensory overload, respectively.
- Sensory aids may be physical, such as glasses, hearing aids, large print books, and sound amplifiers; or situational, such as speaking directly in front of a hearing-impaired patient, or encouraging a patient to smell as well as taste food.
- Safety must be maintained while the patient is hospitalized by assisting the patient with ambulation and care, using siderails, night lights, call system, restraints, and frequent observation.

References

Carter, F. M. (1981). *Psychosocial Nursing* (3rd ed.). New York: Macmillan.

Chaze, B. A., & Ludington-Hoe, S. M. (1984). Sensory stimulation in the NICU. *American Journal of Nursing, 84*(1), 68–71.

Corso, J. F. (1981). *Aging Sensory Systems and Perception.* New York: Praeger.

Gesel, A., & Ilg, F. (1949). *Child Development.* New York: Harper Brothers.

Goldberger, L. (1982). Sensory deprivation and overload. In L. Goldberger & S. Breznitz (Eds.), *Handbook of Stress.* New York: The Free Press.

Gordon, M. (1991). *Manual of Nursing Diagnosis 1991–92.* New York: McGraw-Hill.

Guyton, A. C. (1991). *Textbook of Medical Physiology* (8th ed.). Philadelphia: W. B. Saunders.

Haber, J., Leach, A. M., Scheedy, S. M., et al. (1987). *Comprehensive Psychiatric Nursing* (3rd ed.). New York: McGraw-Hill.

Horsley, J. A., & Crane, J. (1981). *Distress Reduction Through Sensory Preparation.* New York: Grune & Stratton.

Kim, M. J., McFarland, G. K., & McLane, A. M. (1987). *Pocket Guide to Nursing Diagnosis* (2nd ed.). St. Louis: C. V. Mosby.

Lee, K. A. (1991). Sensory overload, sensory deprivation, and sleep deprivation. In M. L. Patrick, S. L. Woods, R. F. Craven, et al. (Eds.), *Medical–Surgical Nursing: Pathophysiological Concepts* (2nd ed.). Philadelphia: J. B. Lippincott.

Lego, S. (Ed.). (1984). *The American Handbook of Psychiatric Nursing.* Philadelphia: J. B. Lippincott.

McFarland, G. K., & Wasli, E. L. (1986). *Nursing Diagnoses and Process in Psychiatric Mental Health Nursing.* Philadelphia: J. B. Lippincott.

NANDA (1990). *Taxonomy I revised 1990, with official nursing diagnoses.* St. Louis, MO: North American Nursing Diagnosis Association.

Schafer, W. (1987). *Stress Management for Wellness.* New York: Holt, Rinehart and Winston.

Sime, A. M. (1985). Sensation information. In M. Snyder (Ed.), *Independent Nursing Interventions.* New York: John Wiley.

Toffler, A. (1970). *Future Shock.* New York: Random House.

Vander, A. J., Sherman, J. H., & Luciano, D. S. (1990). *Human Physiology: The Mechanisms of Body Function* (5th ed.). New York: McGraw-Hill.

Bibliography

Barry, P. D. (1990). *Mental Health and Mental Illness* (4th ed.). Philadelphia: J. B. Lippincott.

Baradel, J. G. (1985). Humanistic care of the patient in seclusion. *Journal of Psychosocial Nursing and Mental Health Services, 2,* 9–14.

Beck, C. M., Rawlins, R. P., & Williams, S. R. (1988). *Mental Health–Psychiatric Nursing* (2nd ed.). St. Louis: C. V. Mosby.

Bernardini, L. (1985). Effective communication as an intervention for sensory deprivation in the elderly client. *Topics in Clinical Nursing, 1,* 72–81.

Berry, K. N. (1987). Let's create diagnoses psychiatric nurses can use. *American Journal of Nursing, 87*(5), 707–708.

Birckhead, L. M. (1989). *Psychiatric/Mental Health Nursing.* Philadelphia: J. B. Lippincott.

Campbell, E. G., Williams, M. A., & Mlnarczyk, S. M. (1986). After the fall—confusion. *American Journal of Nursing, 86*(2), 151–154.

Carpenito, L. J. (1985). Altered thoughts or altered perceptions? *American Journal of Nursing, 85*(11), 1283.

Cook, J. S. (1987). *Essentials of Mental Health Nursing.* Reading, MA: Addison-Wesley.

Grazier, S. (1988). The loneliness barrier . . . patients in isolation. *Nursing Times, 84*(41), 44–45.

Hayes, A. W. (Ed.). (1985). *Toxicology of the Eye, Ear, and Other Special Senses.* New York: Raven Press.

Kee, C. C. (1990). Sensory impairment: Factor X in providing nursing care to the older adult. *Journal of Community Health Nursing, 7*(1), 45–52.

Loomis, M. E., O'Toole, A. W., Brown, M. S., et al. (1987). Development of a classification system for psychiatric/mental health nursing: Individual response class. *Archives of Psychiatric Nursing, 1*(1), 16–24.

Rogers J. C., et al. (1987). Maude: A case of sensory deprivation. *American Journal of Occupational Therapy, 41,* 673–676.

Thomas, K. A. (1989). How the NICU environment sounds to a preterm infant. *Maternal–Child Nursing Journal, 14,* 249–251.

Cognitive Processes

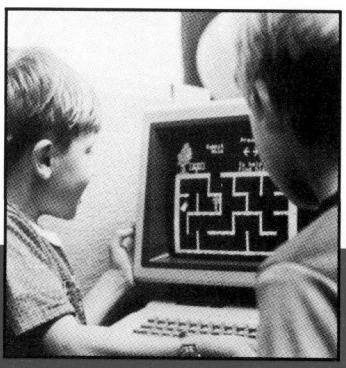

Cognitive Processes

LEARNING OBJECTIVES

Upon completion of this chapter, the student will be able to do the following:

- Identify the components of cognitive and thought processes.
- Describe the characteristics of normal cognition.
- Identify the cognitive factors that are a part of each of the stages of the lifespan.
- Recognize factors that affect normal cognitive function.
- Describe components of potential altered cognition.
- Identify manifestations of altered thought processes.
- Use the nursing process in the care of the person experiencing altered thought processes.
- Appreciate the types of resources available to families of individuals with altered thought processes.

KEY TERMS

Cognition
Comprehension
Confusion
Delirium
Delusions
Dementia
Disorientation

Disorganized
 thinking
Hallucinations
ICU psychosis
Intelligence
Judgment
Learning

Orientation
Perceiving
Reality orientation
Reminiscence
 therapy
Sundown
 syndrome
Thinking

Normal Cognitive Function
  Anatomy
  Normal Physiologic Function
    Perception of Information
    Consciousness
    Thoughts
    Memory
  Characteristics of Normal Cognition
    Intelligence
    Reality Perception
    Communication
    Judgment
    Orientation
    Recall and Recognition
  Normal Cognitive Functional Pattern
    Perceiving
    Thinking
    Learning
    Remembering
  Factors Affecting Normal Cognitive Function
    Adequate Blood Flow
    Nutrition and Metabolism
    Fluid and Electrolyte Balance
    Sleep and Rest
    Organizing Incoming Stimuli
  Lifespan Considerations
Altered Cognitive Function
  Potential for Altered Cognition
    Inadequate Blood Flow
    Altered Nutrition and Metabolism
    Fluid and Electrolyte Imbalance
    Infectious Processes
    Inadequate Sleep and Rest
    Inability to Organize Incoming Stimuli
    Degenerative Processes
  Manifestations of Altered Function
    Disorganized Thinking
    Impaired Thought Processes

    Impact of Dysfunction on Activities of Daily Living
Assessment
  Subjective Data
    Functional Pattern Identification
    Risk Identification
    Dysfunctional Identification
  Objective Data
    Physical Assessment
    Diagnostic Tests and Procedures
Nursing Diagnosis and Patient Goals
  Diagnostic Statement: Altered Thought Processes
    Definition
    Defining Characteristics
    Related Factors
    Related Nursing Diagnoses
    Patient Goals
Implementation
  Nursing Interventions to Promote Cognitive Health
    and Function
    Healthy Lifestyle Promotion
    Memory Improvement
    Maintenance of Learning Skills
  Nursing Interventions for Altered Cognitive
    Function
    Fluid Intake and Nutrition
    Mobility
    Safety
    Therapeutic Communication
    Reality Orientation
    Socialization Therapies
    Family Support
  Discharge Planning and Home Care
    Home Care
    Day and Respite Care
    Long-Term Care
Evaluation
Key Concepts

Nurses in any practice setting may work with people experiencing temporary or irreversible impairment of cognitive function and thought processes. The nurse plays a central role in identification of cognitive impairment and ongoing assessment of the impact on self-care and safety. Nursing interventions are focused on preventing or minimizing contributing factors, compensation for deficits, and promoting optimal function. Planning and evaluating nursing care require an understanding of normal cognition, factors that place a person at risk for impairment, and effective interventions that can be individualized. This chapter concentrates on the components of cognitive function and thought processes, factors that affect normal function, situations of altered function, and the related nursing care.

NORMAL COGNITIVE FUNCTION

Cognition is the systematic way in which a person thinks, reasons, and uses language. Each instant of awareness can be defined as a thought, and awareness itself can be defined as consciousness. Memory is the capability of recalling a thought at least once and usually again. Learning is the capability of the nervous system to store memories. The cerebral cortex coordinates consciousness, thoughts, memory, and learning. All four functions are inseparable (Guyton, 1986).

Anatomy

For information to be processed, the person must be able to perceive the information. Perception of information and environment enters the person's awareness through the special senses and uses the four cognitive processes: consciousness, thoughts, memory, and learning. Intact structure and perceptual functioning of the cerebral cortex are required for a person to be able to take in information through the senses of perception, assimilate and interpret that information in the cerebral cortex, and proceed to an appropriate response cognitively.

The major means of sensory input is through the eyes and ears. The eyeball (Fig. 42-1), a mobile, spherical structure located in the orbit of the skull, is composed of the sclera (the white outer fibrous layer), the uvea (the vascular layer), and the retina (the neural layer). The interior chambers are filled with clear media (the aqueous and vitreous humors) through which light is transmitted to the retina. Visual information is carried to the visual cortex by neuronal axons from the retinal ganglion cells, which form the optic nerve (Porth, 1990).

The ear (Fig. 42-2) consists of the external ear (the auricle and the external acoustic meatus or ear canal), the tympanic membrane, the middle ear (the ossicles and the eustachian tube), and the inner ear (the cochlea, vestibule, and semicircular canals). Sound is transmitted through the auricle and ear canal to the tympanic membrane, which vibrates freely. The vibration is transmitted to the ossicles (malleus, incus, and stapes), which continue the sound transmission to the labyrinth or inner ear. Sound moves through the fluid of the inner ear to the apex of the cochlea and the organ of Corti.

The reticular activating system (RAS), which controls central nervous system activity, is a diffuse formation of cells and fibers that extends from the brain stem and projects upward and throughout the cerebral cortex. Its location is illustrated in Figure 40-1. It is active in sleep and rest (Chap. 39) and pain response (Chap. 40). The nervous system, including cranial nerves (see Chap. 18),

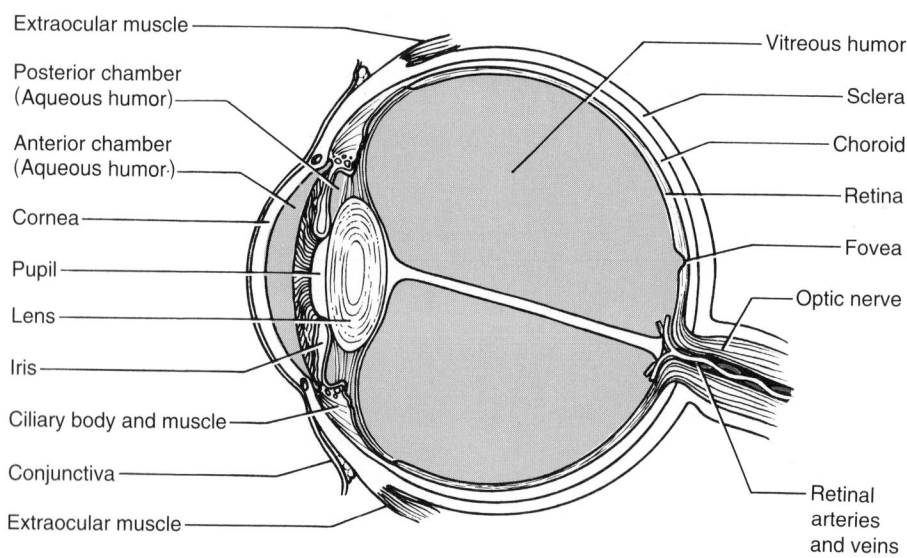

Extraocular muscle

Posterior chamber (Aqueous humor)

Anterior chamber (Aqueous humor·)

Cornea

Pupil

Lens

Iris

Ciliary body and muscle

Conjunctiva

Extraocular muscle

Vitreous humor

Sclera

Choroid

Retina

Fovea

Optic nerve

Retinal arteries and veins

Figure 42–1. Cross-sectional view of structure of the eye.

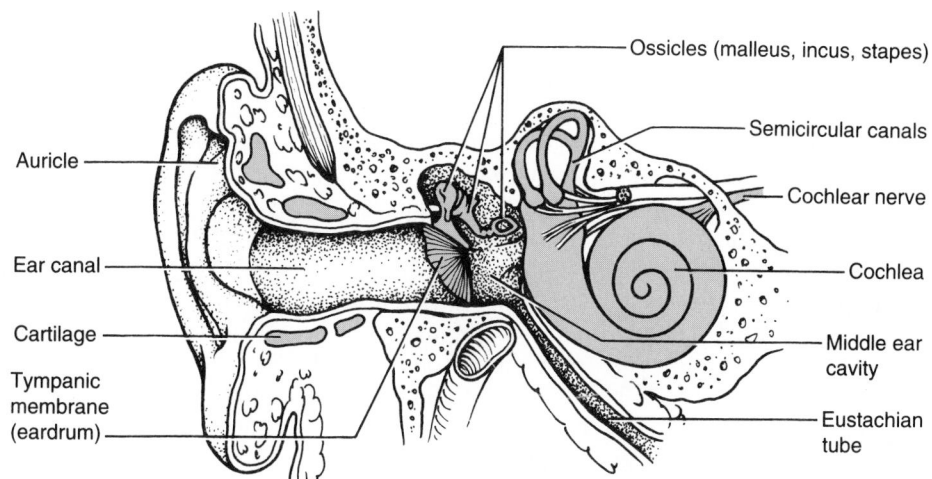

Figure 42–2. Cross-sectional view of structure of the ear.

must be intact for full cognition. Language centers are in the left hemisphere of the brain, and are illustrated in Figure 44-1.

Normal Physiologic Function

Perception of Information

Perception of reality or orientation includes the awareness of time, place, situation, and the self. It is the knowledge of how the self and the environment interact on the continuum of time and transform sensory information into meaning (Schuster & Ashburn, 1986). This phenomenon is complex and depends on functioning sense organs, neurotransmission, and intact central processing.

Sense organs contributing to perception include vision, hearing, touch, taste, and smell. Sensory receptors can be classified into three groups: exteroceptors (distance senses); proprioceptors (near senses); and interoceptors (deep senses) (Schuster & Ashburn, 1986). Neurotransmission occurs when the stimuli to the sense organs are converted to neural impulses and transmitted to the appropriate area for central processing and translation.

Exteroceptors. The exteroceptors include vision and hearing. Vision allows people to perceive and learn about their world from the time of birth throughout life, assuming it remains intact. Vision permits abstract concepts to be linked with concrete objects, thus aiding the learning and memory processes. Hearing, also present from birth, links concepts with frequency, intensity, and duration of sounds. Both eyesight and hearing enable the person to enhance awareness of environment and experiences to amplify cognitive development.

Vision requires the brain-related functions of photo-

reception, visual sensation, and perception for full function. The primary visual cortex, located in the calcarine fissure of the occipital lobe, is the location where visual sensation is first experienced. The nearby associational visual cortex, along with previous learning, adds meaningfulness to the visual perception.

Hearing, involving the vibration of sound waves, is the external stimulus to which the ear responds. The hair cells of the organ of Corti translate the sound waves to nerve impulses, transmitting the impulses on to the primary and associational auditory cortex of the brain's temporal lobe (Porth, 1990). These areas of the brain are necessary for the meaningfulness of sound to occur and for integration of past experience and current auditory information in the hearing process.

Proprioceptors. Proprioceptors include somatic senses (touch, temperature, pain), taste, and smell. Proprioceptive sensations have to do with the physical state of the body, including the relative position of the different parts of the body, the detection of heat and cold, and the sense of pain. While located in the inner ear, the semicircular canals have a proprioceptive function in relation to the equilibrium. See Chapter 29 for a detailed discussion of the function of the semicircular canals.

Somatic senses are activated by touch, pressure, heat, cold, or pain. The resulting nerve impulses enter the spinal cord through the posterior roots. Depending on the sensation, the impulse is transmitted to the brain through either the dorsal column system or the spinothalamic system. The dorsal column transmits sensory information that must be transmitted rapidly, incorporates fine gradations of intensity, and is discretely localized. The spinothalamic system carries information that lacks fine gradations, has less exact localization, or does not need rapid transmission.

Taste is a function of the taste buds of the tongue, and includes sweet, sour, salty, and bitter components. The sensation of taste is transmitted via the fifth cranial nerve to the taste area of the cerebral cortex. Smell is located in the olfactory membrane, and is the least well understood of the special senses. The sensations of smell are transmitted to the olfactory areas of the brain for perception and translation. Taste and smell seem to be closely related, since diminished function in one generally affects the function of the other (Guyton, 1986).

Interoceptors. Interceptors are deep senses arising from the viscera of the body and the deeper tissues such as bone. These sensations are from internal organs, and relate to changes in body position and motions of the musculoskeletal system, as well as to maintaining position in space. The regulation of organic function (e.g., metabolism, fluid balance) contributes to the sense of balance and proprioception. Neural transmissions from the interoceptors travel through the spinal cord to the related central processing structure (Guyton, 1986).

Consciousness

The RAS is divided into facilitatory and inhibitory areas. The facilitatory area is intrinsically active, and produces an increase in muscle tone in the body. The inhibitory area causes a decrease in muscle tone, and permits decreased activity and sleep after prolonged wakefulness. When the facilitatory and inhibitory areas are in balance, the person is neither excited nor inhibited, and is conscious. Consciousness, a state of awareness and full responsiveness to stimuli, relies on an intact RAS in the brain stem. Cognition, the ability to respond to the environment, relies on an intact cerebral cortex (Porth, 1990).

Thoughts

Each thought results from a momentary pattern of stimulation of many parts of the nervous system at the same time. This stimulation involves, most importantly, the cerebral cortex, thalamus, rhinencephalon, and the upper reticular formation of the brain stem. The stimulated areas of the rhinencephalon, thalamus, and reticular formation give thought its crude nature, such as pleasure, displeasure, pain, and comfort. The stimulated area of the cortex determines discrete characteristics of thought (what is seen in the visual field), discrete patterns of sensation (texture of objects), and other specific characteristics (Guyton, 1986).

Memory

Memory is an equally complex process. For the nervous system to provide memory, it must provide or create the same pattern of stimulation that composes current thoughts, but at some time in the future. This means that

current thoughts are placed in storage with enough cueing or coding to allow retrieval at will at some future point in time.

There are basically two types of memory, temporary and lasting. Temporary memory is also referred to as short-term, immediate, or intermediate, and is retained for only brief periods of time. Lasting memory is also known as long-term or prolonged memory. It is believed that there is a difference in the actual neural stimulation and in the synapses of the neurons that contribute to which type of memory occurs.

Short-term memory consists only of local reverberating electrical impulses. Electrical activity is generated by incoming material recorded by the brain. This activity is brief, shallow, and easily dissipated before being imprinted to the long-term memory. Some bits of information excite a great deal of electrical activity, which overflow the boundaries of the short-term memory, leading to actual alteration of synapses.

Long-term memory provides long-term storage of cognitive material, and holds up well with the aging process. As the boundaries of the short-term memory are exceeded, alteration of synapses occurs, creating long-term retention with potential retrieval.

The hippocampi, located within both temporal lobes and part of the limbic system, play a role in pushing information into retention rather than allowing it to be dissipated and forgotten. The hippocampi discriminate between trivia and relevant information to commit to long-term memory, thus performing an important intellectual function. The ability to focus on some things and forget others is essential to intelligent behavior (Guyton, 1986). Assimilating experiences and new information is a process involving memory. The hippocampi play a vital role in retaining new knowledge and preventing dissipation of the information.

Characteristics of Normal Cognition

The characteristics of the normal cognitive function, including intellectual function, perception of reality, communication, and insight or judgment, are revealed in many aspects of daily life. The interrelated and integrated functions of cognition are required to allow people to perform the processes necessary to carry out activities of life.

Intelligence

Intelligence is the measurable product of intellectual functioning. Intellectual function consists of memory, comprehension, and concentration. Memory was discussed previously. Comprehension is a part of learning. Concentration is the ability to screen out extraneous stimuli to focus on a task. People depend on intellectual function to be able to learn in school settings, in vocational surroundings, and in their living environments. Society evaluates and values people in terms of intellectual function abilities.

Reality Perception

Perception of reality, or **reality orientation,** includes the awareness of time, place, situation, and the self. It is the knowledge of how the self and the environment interact on the continuum of time, and transform sensory information into meaning (Schuster & Ashburn, 1986). This phenomenon is complex and depends on functioning sense organs (vision, hearing, touch, taste, and smell), neurotransmission, and intact central processing. People with sensory impairments, such as blindness or hearing deficit, may compensate by increasing the acuity of other senses.

Communication

Communication involves the use of language to store, process, and communicate thought content. Language development depends on a nurturing environment during childhood, when language is developed, and can be affected by sociocultural experiences throughout life. Language uses words, and words vary in use and meaning, depending on a person's age, education, culture, socioeconomic background, and geographic region.

Judgment

Judgment, or insight, the process of reasoning, is the ability to process incoming stimuli and determine the complex meanings that encompass many aspects of a situation. For example, a person driving down the street may see a truck blocking the road ahead. The person determines that the truck is an obstacle and that evasive action is required to prevent a crash. The term "insight" is often used to express perceptions people make about behavior or feelings. For example, recognizing that craving chocolate when studying for exams is an indicator of stress is an insight. The correlation between craving and studying and the recognition of being anxious about doing well in school lead to the insight. This is an example of a complex reasoning process.

Orientation

Orientation is the basic process by which people know their location in the dimensions of time and place. Orientation also includes the ability to know who one is as a person and in relation to other people. People tend to take these abilities for granted until they experience confusion about orientation. On a simple level, one can become confused about one's orientation, or experience **disorientation,** when on vacation and awakening in a new setting, and momentarily forgetting where one is.

Recall and Recognition

Recall and recognition are abilities used to retrieve the information in the long- and short-term memory. Recall involves the ability to retrieve information directly or by relating it to other information (e.g., seeing a person and "recalling" his or her name accurately). Recognition is the ability accurately to relate something currently in the environment with what is in the memory (e.g., seeing a rose and "recognizing" it as a type of flower). People depend on these abilities to perform in school, on the job, and in everyday life. Recall and recognition are skills that can be learned and that need to be practiced to keep them actively useful.

Normal Cognitive Functional Pattern

Cognition is the process of knowing, thinking, and learning, a complex information processing by which sensory input, past experiences, awareness, and emotions are integrated and made meaningful for the person; it enables the person to interact with the environment in a purposeful way. Cognitive function consists of perceiving, thinking, reasoning, and remembering, by which a person comprehends. Thought processes using judgment, insight, planning, and problem-solving abilities involve cognition and cognitive function. Normal cognitive and thought process functions require integration of all of these facets.

Perceiving

Perceiving is the process of recognizing and interpreting sensory stimuli that function as a basis for understanding, knowing, or learning. In perception, a person uses the integrated information obtained through vision, hearing, touching, taste, or smell in concert with past experiences to create understanding or make sense of the environment. An example of perceiving is hearing a phone ring, seeing the phone, touching and holding the receiver, listening to the person speaking, interpreting the meaning in the cerebral cortex, and responding in an appropriate manner. There is integration of the motor activities of handling the phone, sensory activities of seeing and hearing, and central perceptual activities of interpretation resulting in meaningful interaction.

Thinking

Thinking is the process of sorting, organizing, and categorizing information to form mental concepts or perceptions. Thinking is forming ideas or arriving at conclusions. Reasoning is following a logical sequence of thought, starting with what is known and proceeding to a conclusion.

There are different types of thinking of which a person is capable. Concrete thinking involves objects or groups of things that can be perceived by the senses. An example of concrete thinking is the proof of the arithmetical proposition that 1 + 1 = 2 by attaching the numbers to objects, such as apples. Abstract thinking is a higher level thinking that involves a thought or idea apart from any material object. For example, the idea of beauty is a value attributed to a flower, but is not a concrete object in itself. A maxim, such as "People who live in glass houses shouldn't throw stones," is an example requiring abstract thinking for a veiled or abstract truth to be interpreted from the use of concrete objects and terms.

Learning

Learning is the process of acquiring knowledge, and, as such, is a multidimensional process that depends on symbols, language, classifications, concepts, and other concrete operations, along with abstract functions. **Comprehension** is the capacity for understanding and reasoning. (A complete discussion of the concept and process of learning is beyond the scope of this chapter.) For learning to be useful, the person needs to develop strategies for encoding or categorizing the information in the memory so that the information can be recalled as needed.

Remembering

Memory is a complex biochemical storage system that is not yet completely understood. Experiences, ideas, and images are chemically coded and integrated for later retrieval (Freiberg, 1987). The content of long-term (or distant) memory, which is the storehouse of a person's knowledge, depends on the perceived value and significance of the past event. Specific significant life events, such as weddings or the birth of a child, hold greater value and memory potential. Short-term memory (current or "scratch pad"), which is the immediate, working memory, is easily affected by emotional stress (Foreman, Gillies, & Wagner, 1989). The reason some items are moved from short- to long-term memory is not clear, but is probably related to the perceived value of the information and its relation to other memories.

Factors Affecting Normal Cognitive Function

Cognitive processes can be affected by many factors, physiologic, emotional, or environmental. Whether these factors affect normal cognition or thought processes depends on elements such as a supportive and nurturing environment and on the presence of appropriate sensory input.

Adequate Blood Flow. All cells require a continuous oxygen supply and a stable extracellular environment of fluid and electrolytes to function optimally. Oxygenation depends on three factors: respiratory and circulatory function, and hemoglobin production. During respiration, oxygen enters the alveoli, diffuses across capillary membranes to enter the pulmonary venous system, and binds with hemoglobin. Oxygen, bound to hemoglobin in the arterial blood, is transported to brain cells. The brain accounts for 20% of the total oxygen uptake of the body, and requires a constant, ample supply to support brain cell life.

Nutrition and Metabolism. Nutrition affects normal cognitive function because of the brain cells' need for glucose for metabolic energy, iron for hemoglobin, and other nutrients for optimal functioning. The efficiency with which oxygen is delivered to the cells is related to hemoglobin production, which requires an adequate dietary intake of iron. To maintain a stable level of serum glucose, the pancreas monitors glucose levels in the blood, producing or withholding insulin as required for a steady state. The brain, which consumes 25% of the glucose used by the body, requires a steady supply of glucose. Vitamins and minerals are essential for effective neurologic functioning and neurotransmitter activity.

Fluid and Electrolyte Balance. The brain cells require a constant extracellular environment of fluid and electrolytes for optimal function. In the brain, as elsewhere, cellular processes depend on the active and passive movement of water and charged particles across cell membranes (see Chap. 32). The brain is protected by the blood–brain barrier, a shield that prevents or delays the entry of certain substances from the blood into the brain. The blood–brain barrier protects the brain cells from substances other than normal fluid and electrolytes, which could damage sensitive nerve cells. Maintenance of a dynamic state of fluid balance and electrolyte levels provides the ideal internal environment for neurologic function.

Sleep and Rest. Sleep has a restorative function, allowing the person to regain energy for cognitive functions, such as concentrating, organizing, remembering, and reasoning (see Chap. 39). Rapid eye movement (REM) sleep seems to be particularly important for mentally restoring the person for efficient cognitive functioning.

Organizing Incoming Stimuli. The basic cognitive processes of perceiving, thinking, reasoning, and remembering depend on the ability to receive and organize stimuli. The amount of stimuli in the environment, either increased or decreased, can influence normal cognition. For example, one student preparing for exams in an environment of noisy students, television, and loud music may find it very difficult to organize the stimuli and do effective studying. At the same time, another student may find that some background noise assists with concentration, depending on the level of distraction.

Perceptual ability, which contributes to cognitive functioning, declines as a normal part of aging as sense organ functions diminish. For example, the older person needs more light to see an object, has more problem with light glare, and experiences loss of accommodation for near objects (presbyopia). Hearing diminishes, especially in the high-frequency range, and acuity of sense of touch declines. These normal changes affect the ability to organize incoming stimuli.

Lifespan Considerations

Cognitive development is a complex process that is affected by physiologic health and the quality of the social and physical environment. The rate at which a person proceeds through the usual stages of cognitive development can be strongly affected by the environment. People need emotional security, human interaction, and a variety of sensory experiences to develop optimally. Jean Piaget is the most widely recognized theorist in cognitive development, although the work of other theorists, such as Erikson (1963) and Havighurst (1972), contributes to the understanding of cognitive development throughout the lifespan.

Newborn and Infant

The newborn and infant are in the sensorimotor period, in which sensory experience is the major task (Piaget, 1969). The infant interacts with his or her environment in a reflexive or accidental manner, and is beginning to develop very early concrete thinking skills. The child's language skills are not developed, and thoughts or needs are expressed through behavior (Fig. 42-3).

The cognitive developmental work of infancy is carried out through exploration of the environment and through play. The infant learns to connect some behaviors with expected responses. For example, moving a toy in a certain way may cause a pleasing sound to occur. The infant may have learned that through play, but, with repetition and maturity, is able to remember and repeat the action to have it occur at will. In the same manner, an infant begins to assimilate language, linking specific words and sounds with an object of meaning, such as "Mama" or "bottle." Providing stimulation through varied objects, different sounds, and face-to-face communication and interaction enhances cognitive development (Freiberg, 1987).

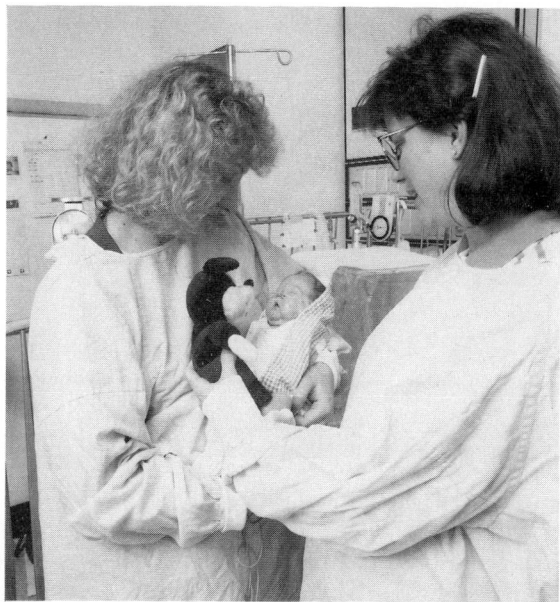

Figure 42–3. The nurse provides anticipatory guidance to new parents for stimulating cognitive and perceptual development. (Photo courtesy of University of Washington School of Nursing.)

Toddler and Preschooler

The young child develops object permanence and begins to label familiar items. The child learns that an object has permanence and constancy, and gives the object a name, using it to represent the object to others (Piaget, 1969). Perceptual ability in vision and hearing is necessary to obtain an understanding of the environment as a basis of thinking. Language and cognition develop side by side. The child is concrete in thinking patterns and demonstrates pronounced egocentrism, or self-concern. The world is viewed from the child's point of view only, and in a concrete manner.

The process of reasoning begins as the child tries to make sense of the world. As a part of cognitive development, the child develops confidence in abilities and gains independence through the encouragement of parents in each new area of learning (Erikson, 1963). Positive, nurturing play environments that encourage imaginative play, interaction, questioning, and use of language and symbols, while at the same time reinforcing earlier knowledge, will foster cognitive development in the preschooler (Fig. 42-4).

Child and Adolescent

The school-age child can carry out complex mental operations such as addition, subtraction, grouping, classifying, and ordering (Piaget, 1969). The multiple dimensions of objects and symbols are understood and represented mentally, and the child can encode stimuli for later retrieval. The child understands conservation,

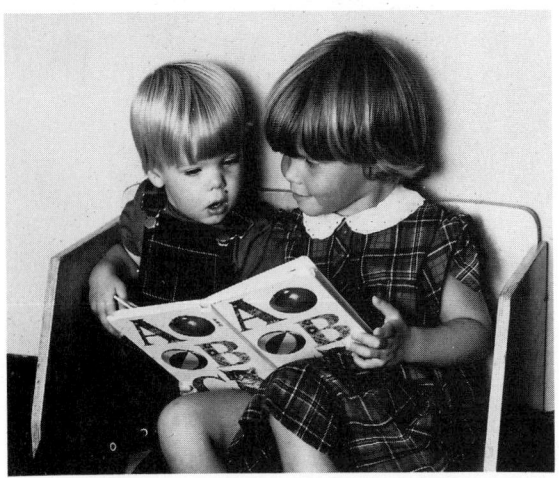

Figure 42–4. Play activities that incorporate language help to develop cognitive abilities in preschoolers. (Photo courtesy of University of Washington School of Nursing.)

or the idea that the properties of an object can stay the same if one or another is altered. For example, if an equal volume of fluid is poured into two differently shaped containers, the young child will perceive that the volume of water has changed, while the older child will see a change in shape but a constant volume. This shift in comprehension indicates the ability to incorporate abstract thinking with concrete processes. At this age, the child receives great pleasure in accomplishments that result from new learning and thinking skills (Erikson, 1963). Learning and play environments that reward the achievements of the child contribute positively to cognitive development.

Adolescence is a particularly difficult time for the development of thinking processes, as it is a time of enormous emotional stress from a variety of sources, including struggling to develop a sense of separateness from parents and a strong need to identify with a peer group (Erikson, 1963). Abstract reasoning and logical judgment are two functions that the adolescent endeavors to develop with increasing maturity.

During adolescence, the person develops the ability to think abstractly and perform complex processes in his or her head. The adolescent is able to hypothesize situations and solutions as well as conceptualize nonconcrete ideas (Piaget, 1969). Classification, serialization, spatial abilities, verbal skills, and abstract relationships are cognitive capacities being developed by the adolescent. Providing opportunities for independent thinking and decision-making encourages increased maturity in cognitive development.

Adult and Older Adult

Throughout young and middle adulthood, the person is steadily gaining in rational thinking abilities, formal and informal educational opportunities, career development, and life experiences. As the adult feels progressively more competent with cognitive management of life, the less rigid and more flexible he or she is able to become. Making decisions and adjusting to changes are managed with less life disruption. Creativity and productivity in work contribute to continual cognitive development and innovative use of integrated abstract and concrete thinking.

Aging is part of the life-long developmental process (Fig. 42-5). In our society, "old" is usually formally defined as being over 65, and the fastest-growing segment of the population consists of those over age 85. Aging is a time when people may feel an attainment of purpose or accomplishment in an area of expertise (Erikson, 1963). Although the older adult still faces developmental tasks such as retirement and change in relationships (Havighurst, 1972), he or she is also a repository of knowledge, wisdom, and cognitive competence. Seeking opportunities to continue to use the accumulated knowledge of a lifetime by volunteering or consulting assists in maintaining cognitive abilities.

As a person ages, cognitive function remains relatively unchanged in the absence of trauma or specific dysfunction, although processing of information may require more time. While problems with thought processes are more common in older adults, they are generally related to a decrease in coping reserves or to a specific problem, and are not a normal part of aging.

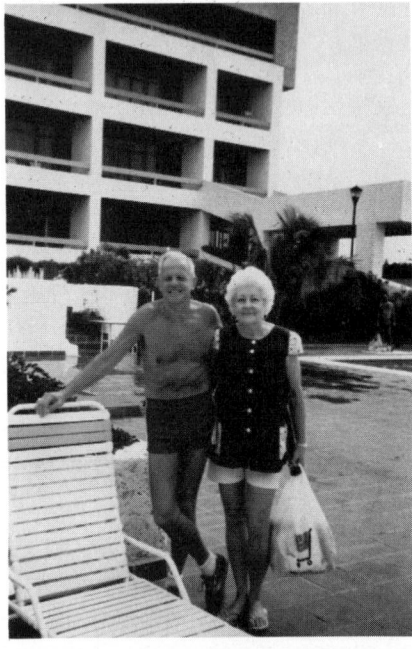

Figure 42–5. With aging, adults can continue to use wisdom and cognitive abilities in all aspects of life. (Photo courtesy of University of Washington School of Nursing.)

ALTERED COGNITIVE FUNCTION

Cognition is a complex process. Multiple, varied stimuli are perceived, organized, and integrated with previous knowledge and experience. The outcome of this process is an appropriate, adaptive behavioral or emotional response. Anything that interrupts this complex process can result in impaired thinking.

Potential for Altered Cognition

Cognitive function is affected by physiologic, psychological, and environmental stress. Any physiologic abnormality that affects the cellular environment can interfere with brain function and produce mild mental clouding, disorientation, or, in extreme cases, profound **delirium** (mental confusion or disorientation) or coma (Porth, 1990).

Inadequate Blood Flow

Any interruption in blood flow to brain cells causes cellular hypoxia and results in changes in function. A chronically inadequate supply to the brain causes cell dysfunction and deterioration of mental processes (Porth, 1990). Any disease process that interferes with alveolar ventilation, pulmonary circulation, cardiac function, or the production of normal hemoglobin can result in hypoxia and decreased cognitive function.

Altered Nutrition and Metabolism

People with inadequate nutritional status often develop low hemoglobin levels and anemia. Abnormal hemoglobin can be produced in people with specific genetic disorders, such as sickle cell anemia. Hypothermia and hypothyroidism, disorders in which metabolic processes are impaired and oxygen cannot be used optimally, can also cause hypoxia (Porth, 1990). Inadequate intake of glucose or impaired use of glucose by the body will limit the quantity of glucose available for the metabolic demands of the brain.

Fluid and Electrolyte Imbalance

Disturbances in the concentration of intracellular and extracellular water and electrolytes can cause cellular dysfunction, which can be manifested by changes in mental status. Such disturbances can have a variety of causes, including abnormal losses of body fluids, dietary deficiencies, acute and chronic disease, and altered effects of medication. Although any disturbance in fluid or electrolyte balance can cause delirium or **confusion** (impairment of cognitive processes), a few are more common (Porth, 1990). They are hyponatremia and hypernatremia (sodium variations in the serum), hyper-

calcemia (elevated serum calcium level), and hypoglycemia and hyperglycemia (abnormal serum glucose levels).

Accumulated metabolic by-products, the end products of metabolism, if not eliminated from the body, can be toxic to central nervous system function. Impaired function of the kidney, liver, or both together can impair the ability to break down and excrete such potential toxins. Ammonia, a by-product of protein metabolism, is usually converted by the liver into urea, which is excreted by the kidney. Liver dysfunction can interfere with this process and cause elevated ammonia levels, producing a delirium known as hepatic encephalopathy. Kidney dysfunction can result in elevated levels of urea, which also causes confusion and lethargy (Porth, 1990).

Infectious Processes

Infectious processes of the central nervous system and the subsequent inflammatory response of nerve cells are obvious causes of cognitive impairment. Infections elsewhere in the body can also cause mental status changes. Any person with a severe infection in the circulation (e.g., bacteremia, septicemia) may experience central nervous system effects, including lethargy and confusion. Common sources for bacteremia or septicemia include the urinary tract, the respiratory system, and any open wounds (Porth, 1990). In the elderly, altered cognitive function may be the earliest indication of an infectious process.

Inadequate Sleep and Rest

Lack of sleep, or sleep deprivation, can cause various disruptions, including irritability, decreased calculation and problem-solving skill, poor concentration, or impaired memory. Everyone has experienced feeling dull and slow after having a sleepless night or staying up too late. Rotating shifts can cause similar problems, particularly if the person has to change shifts frequently without adequate time to adjust to a new sleep pattern. These changes in normal sleep patterns may result in inadequate amounts of REM sleep, which may impair both learning and memory as well as the subjective feeling of being rested.

Inability to Organize Incoming Stimuli

Emotional stress or discomfort can lead to disorganized thinking, memory impairment, and poor judgment. A person learning of an injury to a loved one, finding out about a failed exam, or planning a wedding can have difficulty maintaining the usual level of cognitive performance. Concentration and problem-solving are also difficult when a person is in pain, has a full bladder, or experiences other discomfort. These sometimes minor everyday problems can combine and accumulate, creating enough stress to impair thinking.

Affective disorders, such as depression, interfere with cognitive function and can contribute to altered thought processes. Affective disorders can disrupt physiologic functions by interfering with sleep, rest, and nutrition, as well as cognitive functions, such as perceiving, thinking, reasoning, and remembering. With aging, the older person generally experiences a need for more time to perform mental operations, although this does not interfere with either the ability to learn new things or to carry out activities of daily living. While the brain undergoes some degenerative changes, with the ventricles enlarging slightly and brain weight decreasing, significant cognitive impairment in an older person is never normal, but is an indication of a disorder.

Environmental Stress. The stress of an unfamiliar environment can affect the basic cognitive processes of orientation and level of arousal, which depend on the ability of the cerebral cortex to receive and organize incoming stimuli (Kane, Ouslander, & Abrass, 1989). There are numerous stimuli in any environment, some of which are attended to and some ignored. Through a complex perceptual process, habituation or familiarization occurs to routine background stimuli, such as the feel of clothing and the tick of a clock. As a result, the person is not "overloaded" with meaningless input. The brain can also conjure up input when none is available. People experiencing inadequate sensory input are at risk for cognitive dysfunction, such as visual and auditory hallucinations, as the brain attempts to stimulate itself (see Chap. 41 for a complete discussion of sensory function).

Hospitalization removes people from the surroundings and daily activities that are familiar and provide orienting cues, placing them in an environment of strange noises, sights, feelings, and procedures (Fig. 42-6). All of these unfamiliar stimuli demand attention, as habituation has not had time to develop. This state of sensory overload can overwhelm the person's ability to find meaning, and a state of perceptual dysfunction occurs. There are plenty of stimuli present, but none of them make any sense (Foreman, 1989).

Pharmacologic Agents. Pharmacologic agents, or medications, that primarily act on the central nervous system, such as anticonvulsants, antidepressants, anti-anxiety agents, antipsychotics, and hypnotics, can impair thinking and cause confusion. Discontinuing or decreasing the dosage of these medications will often improve cognitive function within a few days. It is worth noting that medications commonly prescribed to manage agitated or confused behavior, such as haloperidol and benzodiazepines, may cause a paradoxical increase in confusion in some people, especially the elderly.

Drugs that do not have primary pharmacologic effects

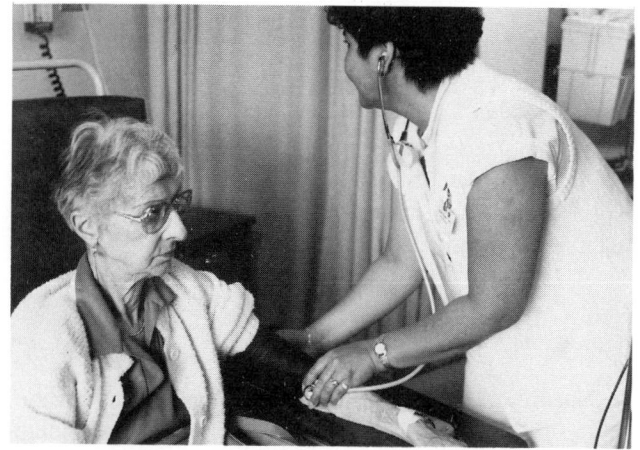

Figure 42–6. Older adults may be at risk for cognitive dysfunction related to unfamiliar environments and procedures.

on the central nervous system can also cause confusion, either alone or in combination with other drugs (Kane, Ouslander, & Abrass, 1989). The mechanism is variable and not always well understood. In some cases, such as with strong diuretics, the drug predisposes the person to another physiologic cause of confusion—hyponatremia. The display lists some drugs that have confusion as a common side effect. In practice it is wise to consider almost any medication as a possible contributing factor to mental status changes.

Toxicity states can occur with overdosage of a medication or alcohol and can lead to confusion. Overdosage of drugs that at normal levels have no central nervous system effects, can potentially cause significant mental status changes. Overuse of drugs affecting the central nervous system alone or in combination with alcohol will also impair thinking.

Degenerative Processes

Any process that contributes to the degeneration of the cells of the brain may ultimately affect cognitive function and thought processes. The causes of degeneration may be related to an organism (viral or bacterial), aging, or unknown sources. The potential end result of the degeneration is impaired thought processes in judgment, insight, planning, and problem-solving, ranging from mild disability to severe dysfunction that may be incompatible with normal cognitive function.

It is important to clarify the terms used to describe degenerative processes related to cognition. Senility, which literally means the process of aging, is a term used in common language to describe cognitive impairments that are mistakenly thought to be a normal part of the aging process. Actually, significant memory and problem-solving impairment is not a part of normal aging, but rather indicates a pathologic process (Kane, Ouslander, & Abrass, 1989). The term "senile dementia" has no

Drug Groups that May Cause Confusion, with Examples of Each Group	
Analgesics	Hypoglycemics
Narcotics	Insulin
Propoxphene	Sulfonylureas
Morphine	Nonsteroidal Anti-inflammatory
Antihistamines	Indomethacin
Diphenhydramine	Anti-Parkinsonism
Antihypertensives	L-dopa
Methyldopa	Carbidopa
Propranolol	Psychotropics
Antimicrobials	Benzodiazepines
Gentamicin	Tricyclic antidepressants
Isoniazid	Haloperidol
Cardiovascular	Hypnotics
Digitalis	Barbiturates
Lidocaine	Chloral hydrate
Diuretics	Others
Thiazides	Cimetidine
Furosemide	Steroids
Anticonvulsants	Ranitidine
Phenytoin	Antiemetics
Carbamazepine	Metoclopramide
Phenobarbital	Promethzine
	Prochlorperazine

place in current nursing practice. Another confusing term that should not be used is "organic brain syndrome," which implies a cognitive impairment caused by a physiologic disorder. The term is often used to include temporary states of confusion as well as permanent dementias, but it is more commonly used to describe dementias that have not been fully evaluated.

Dementia, a specific irreversible dysfunction which has the potential to alter cognitive functioning, is a progressive deterioration of the brain characterized by confusion, disorientation, and severely impaired intellectual function, judgment, insight, memory, planning, and problem-solving. People with a degenerative dementia experience a gradual decline in all cognitive processes, as contrasted to confusional states, which may be reversible dysfunctions (Table 42-1). There are many potential causes for dementia, such as trauma, circulatory interferences, genetic predisposition, alterations in neurotransmitters, and infectious agents. The most common form of dementia is senile dementia of the Alzheimer's type (SDAT), which is a primary neuronal degeneration of unknown cause. It occurs at all ages of adulthood, but increases in incidence with aging, affecting 5% to 10% of people over age 65 and 20% of people over age 75 (Katzman, 1987; Reifler, et al., 1986).

Manifestations of Altered Function

Disorganized Thinking

A person experiencing disturbed thought processes or **disorganized thinking** does not interact appropriately with others or with the environment, and may have an altered perception of reality. Thinking, learning, reasoning, and remembering do not occur in an orderly fashion. Disorganized thinking may be manifested by inappropriate interactions and conversations with others, talking or gesturing to oneself, performing inappropriate activities, or other confused or bizarre behavior. Regression, hallucinations, and delusions are common manifestations of disorganized thinking.

Cognitive impairment frequently interferes with perception of reality, which is based in life experience, personal relationships, and environment. When thought processes become altered, it may be difficult to separate accurately altered perceptions from reality. **Delusions** (fixed false beliefs) and **hallucinations** (perceptions arising from the person's own thoughts) are examples of altered reality. Both of these responses are attempts to cope with or manage stresses or physiologic dysfunctions that impair cognition.

TABLE 42–1

Differences Between Confusion and Dementia

Feature	Confusion	Dementia
Onset	Rapid, often at night	Usually insidious
Duration	Hours to weeks	Months to years
Course	Fluctuates over 24 hours; worse at night; lucid intervals	Relatively stable
Awareness	Always impaired	Usually normal
Alertness	Reduced or increased; tends to fluctuate	Usually normal
Orientation	Always impaired, at least for time; tendency to mistake unfamiliar for familiar place or person	May be intact; little tendency to confabulate
Memory	Recent and immediate; intact if dementia is absent	Recent and remote common knowledge
Thinking	Slow or accelerated; may be dreamlike	Poor in abstraction, impoverished
Perception	Often misperceptions, especially visual	Misperceptions often absent
Sleep–wake cycle	Always disrupted; often drowsiness during the day, insomnia at night	Fragmented sleep
Physical illness or drug toxicity	Usually present	Often absent, especially in primary degenerative dementia

Adapted with permission from Dr. J. Lipowski and the *American Journal of Psychiatry 140*(11):1432. © 1983, American Psychiatric Association.

In disorganized thinking, the content of the person's speech may not make any sense in the context of the conversation, or a sentence may contain multiple unrelated ideas. Interactions with people with disorganized thinking are difficult, as these people are unable to follow a logical sequence or respond in a rational, predictable way. The patient who ignores the meal tray but tries to eat the tissue box with a spoon, or who asks to go to the bathroom but resists assistance to get out of bed, displays impaired reasoning processes. People with chronic disorganized thinking related to mental illness require specialized nursing management, a subject beyond the scope of this chapter.

Impaired Thought Processes

Judgment, insight, planning, and problem-solving can be affected by attention span deficits, memory impairments, and abnormal levels of arousal. Most affected people have aspects of all three elements, and the severity can fluctuate.

Attention Span Deficits. Attention span and concentration are easily impaired by stress and illness. People with a short attention span are highly distractable and cannot screen out competing stimuli. These people will not be able to stay on a conversational topic, or will stop in mid-sentence to look out the window to watch a bird.

This distractibility interferes with the ability to learn new things and to perform activities of daily living.

Memory Impairment. Memory impairment is a concern for old and young alike. Long-term memory, that which has been accumulated over many years, is less affected by situational and emotional stress. Significant impairment of long-term memory usually indicates a central nervous system disorder or a severe confusional state. Short-term memory, that which is of recent events, is much more sensitive to stress. For example, hospitalized patients may have little recall of conversations with health-care professionals, as the stress of illness and coping with hospitalization interfere with the usual functioning of memory.

Level of Arousal Alterations. Arousal is a person's level of reactivity to incoming stimuli. Level of arousal is an integration of neurosensory and cognitive processes. Some situations, particularly hospitalization, interfere with normal integration. There are two well identified confusional states caused by environmental stress and altered levels of arousal—sundown syndrome and ICU (Intensive Care Unit) psychosis (Foreman, 1989; Francis, Martin, & Kapoor, 1990; Ballard, 1981).

Sundown Syndrome. **Sundown (or Sundowner's) syndrome** is a state of disorientation and agitation that occurs at night in institutionalized people who are oriented during the day. It is a temporary state of confusion that cycles with the sun (Beel-Bates & Rogers, 1990). The exact cause is unknown, but it is likely that the person's tenuous hold on reality requires a certain level of arousal, or sensory input (Kane, Ouslander, & Abrass, 1989). At night there is less light, less activity, and fewer caregivers, resulting in less availability of orienting stimuli. The syndrome is often associated with a disturbance in sleep–wakefulness patterns as well (Evans, 1987).

ICU Psychosis. **ICU psychosis** has been defined as a reversible global clouding of consciousness with poor attention span and impaired cognitive processes. It is usually manifested 2 to 5 days after entering the intensive care environment and resolves a few days after leaving, although some patients may develop a longer-term dysfunction (Ballard, 1981). The ICU is a particularly risky sensory environment due to the constant activity level, noises from machines and alarms, frequent intrusive procedures, and lack of difference between day and night because of lights and routines, all of which provide the patient with little meaningful input (Williams, 1989; Chyun, 1989).

Impact of Dysfunction on Activities of Daily Living

Memory, judgment, problem-solving, and the ability to process sensory stimuli appropriately are essential to the performance of any activity. For example, brushing one's teeth requires remembering where the supplies are and how the procedure is done, as well as deciding when to do it. Mild cognitive impairment can be compensated for with written reminders, posted schedules, occasional supervision, and change in occupation or living situation. When cognitive impairment interferes with the ability to perform essential activities safely and appropriately, continued independent living is threatened. This is the critical outcome of altered thought processes—the loss of independence, altered self-concept, and impaired role performance.

Everyone has an individual lifestyle that requires a unique set of skills to maintain. For instance, the daily life of a woman juggling child care and a career in a large city requires skills that are different from those needed by a migrant worker. Social support networks are also individual. The mild memory impairment of an elderly woman living with her husband in a retirement community may have little impact on daily living, while the same degree of memory loss may have major lifestyle implications for a single person employed at a low-income job.

When health-care professionals talk about activities of daily living, they are usually referring to basic skills that are essential to personal safety and hygiene, such as dressing, toileting, feeding, mobility, and bathing. The next level of skills includes complex tasks necessary to meet survival needs and maintain a healthy environ-

ment. Shopping, cooking, arranging transportation, managing money, and following medical regimens are examples of such instrumental or complex skills. Impaired cognition and thought processes interfere with the ability to accomplish and manage consistently these activities needed to carry out daily life. Alterations in thought processes become critical when the impact on daily living is perceived to be a problem by the affected person or significant others.

ASSESSMENT

Functional assessment is an essential aspect of nursing care for cognitively impaired patients to discern their capability to function safely within their environment. Determining how a person functions and the quality of his or her social and physical environment guides the development of outcome criteria and nursing interventions.

Subjective Data

Subjective information about cognitive function is often available from many sources. In addition to the affected person, family members, neighbors, friends, support service providers, and health professionals who know the person well are good resources. Previous medical records may contain anecdotal data and subjective assessments that can give clues to previous function. Gathering subjective data about cognitive ability is a time-consuming process that usually involves multiple brief, planned interactions with a variety of people. It is helpful to keep a general assessment framework in mind (see the display for an example) so that key areas are not forgotten. The situation can be especially complex when the patient is hospitalized and unknown to the staff. Nurses, physicians, and social workers may individually gather information from many sources, which is shared collaboratively. Nurses are in the best position to gather data related to the patient's normal pattern of function, the areas of risk, and the areas of actual dysfunction. It is important that all health-team members document essential subjective data so a consistent assessment can be made and a collaborative approach developed.

Functional Pattern Identification

When assessing thought processes, the nurse gathers information on the functional pattern, the patient's usual cognitive function and its impact on everyday living, or the baseline cognitive function. This information is best obtained by using the framework and resources described previously. The significance lies in the impact of thought processes in relation to function in daily living, not in the impairment itself. For example, an elderly woman may tell the nurse that she does not remember the names, dosages, and purposes of her medications. On the surface, it may seem that she would have a problem with medication management without that information. With further questioning, the nurse learns that she identifies her pills by color, uses a medication management system that has pills grouped in daily dosage units, and that her granddaughter, a registered nurse, oversees her medication management. This woman and her family have developed an effective system to compensate for a mild cognitive deficit.

Detecting mild to moderate memory impairment on interview or during casual conversation can be difficult. People who are aware of and embarrassed by their poor memory can become expert at giving vague answers and steering the conversation into "safe" territory. It is advisable to use a formalized approach to memory testing if an impairment is suspected. A nonjudgmental, warm, and friendly demeanor is important to put the person at ease.

Assessing perception of reality includes determining the individual's orientation to time, place, and person. This is sometimes referred to as "Orientation × 3." To assess these data, the nurse asks the patient questions pertaining to time: the year, the day, the date, or approximate time of day, depending on which question(s) is appropriate for the person. Place is determined by asking the patient questions related to city or location. Person is assessed by asking the patient for his or her name. Orientation generally becomes dysfunctional in that order, with time orientation showing deficit first, and deficits in orientation as to the patient's own identity being the last and most severe form of dysfunction in orientation.

In assessing reality, it is important to clarify what is going on in the environment that may be contributing to the indications of disorganized thinking. An elderly woman may be calling for her son and not understanding why he won't come in to see her when she saw him go by her door. In exploring what may be going on in the

---

Nursing Assessment of Thought Processes

Current Cognitive Function

    Objective Tool—Mini-Mental Status or Pfeiffer

    Subjective Evaluation
Attention
Ability to answer questions
Appropriateness of affect

History and Time Course of Cognitive Impairment

Previous difficulties with thinking or perception
When current symptoms began and how they evolved; include information from family and friends

Presence of Contributing Factors

    Chronic or Acute Illness
Laboratory abnormalities
CNS disorders
Multisystem disease

    Use/Abuse of Medications
Drugs with CNS effects
Drugs with CNS side effects
Drugs with potential for toxicity
Use of recreational drugs or alcohol

Sensory Impairment
Vision
Hearing

    Quality of Physical and Social Environment
Family support
Frequency and number of social contacts
Availability of transportation
Adequacy of financial resources
Nutritional status
Living situation

    Presence of Psychological Stressors
Bereavement
Major life change
Lack of financial resources
Family crisis
Loss of independence
Serious illness

    Family History of Dementia or Mental Illness

Current Functional Status

Ability to perform ADLs
Amount of assistance currently available in the home
Ability to exercise good judgment
Safety of home environment

environment, the nurse may realize that the woman did not have her glasses on and that the man who walked by her door had the same build as and similar clothes to her son's. As a result, she misperceived the information she had. If a nurse is not thorough in assessment, it might lead to the wrong conclusion about the patient, attaching a label of "confused" when there is actually a difficulty with perception. The nurse needs to be careful that personal perceptions of reality do not overshadow ability to monitor another person's perception of reality.

With elderly persons, it may be easy to dismiss changes in mentation as being a "normal part of aging." Patients and families need to understand that cognitive impairments are never "normal," and, if a person is experiencing changes, these changes should be evaluated by a health-care professional. The earlier that families can intervene by reinforcing reality, adjusting diet, or seeking care for diagnosed problems, the less likely it is that the patient will experience a major confusional state or other cognitive problems.

Risk Identification

Risk identification is the process of assessing for physiologic, psychological, and environmental factors that increase the likelihood of experiencing impaired thought processes. Some selected common risk factors for these three categories are shown in the accompanying display. The degree of risk from each category will depend on the individual patient. A nurse working in an acute care setting will focus on physiologic variables, with some attention to environmental concerns. A community health nurse making a home visit to an elderly patient will include a detailed assessment of social and psychological support systems, as well as physiologic assessment.

The presence of multiple risk factors does not always lead to dysfunction. Individual strengths and resources can enable a person to withstand multiple stressors. An important part of a nursing assessment is the identification of existing and potential coping resources. Interventions can then be designed to support and develop these resources. An example is an elderly woman with sensorineural hearing loss who is hospitalized for treatment of a fracture. Risk factors for this patient include altered perceptions related to an unfamiliar environment, altered sleep and rest, and a hearing deficit. These environmental stresses and risk factors usually manifest as a shortened attention span, irritability, impaired sense of time, and, possibly, confusion. During the assessment, the nurse learns that the woman's hearing aid is at home and that she has several family members and supportive friends. Asking a family member to bring in the hearing aid and a few familiar objects from home, and encouraging frequent contact, will decrease the risk of dysfunction.

Medications can be a primary risk factor for altered

Selected Risk Factors for Cognitive Impairment

Physiologic

Fluid imbalance
Electrolyte imbalance
Pain
Decreased oxygen supply to the brain
Renal or hepatic failure
Inadequate blood flow
Neurologic impairment
Systemic infection
Medication toxicity

Psychological

Grief response to losses
Change in socioeconomic situation
Loss of element(s) of support system
Depression/anxiety

Environmental

Unfamiliar environment/routine
Altered sensory input
Mobility restriction

---

thought processes, either alone or in combination with other drugs or substances. Patients and their families need to know the expected actions of medications, potential side effects, potential interactions, and indications of toxicity. Many instances of altered cognitive function can be traced directly to the addition of a new medication, toxic levels of a usual medication, or unexpected interactions with other substances. (See the display of drug groups given earlier.) Patients and families need to be alert to subtle changes in cognition and mental status (e.g., mild confusion or forgetfulness) in relation to their pharmacologic therapies.

Dysfunctional Identification

Information gathered in the functional pattern identification and the risk identification are analyzed to determine if dysfunction is present for a specific patient. As previously mentioned, difficulty in performing activities of daily living can indicate critical dysfunction. When identifying the presence of dysfunction, it is vital to document assessed data in clear terms that are well understood by others. Instead of using vague terms like "slightly confused" or "poor attention span," the nurse should describe the behaviors of the deficits precisely, using anecdotes when appropriate. Phrases like "oriented to self only," "needs verbal cueing to wash face," and "when given toothbrush, combed hair with it" provide clear information for identifying dysfunction.

Objective Data

The physical assessment skills of inspection, palpation, percussion, and auscultation may not seem relevant to cognitive function, but these skills, along with diagnostic tests, are essential in identifying the physiologic causes of delirium.

Physical Assessment

Assessment of physiologic function provides clues as to the source of altered thought processes. Since the earliest clinical signs of changes in the levels of oxygen, electrolytes, and metabolic by-products are lethargy, mild confusion, and impairment of thinking, it is important to assess those components. Cognitive changes are often nonspecific and most obvious to those who know the affected person well. For this reason, it is important to elicit information from family and friends as well as from the patient.

Respiratory Function:

- Assess rate, rhythm, depth of normal respirations.
- Assess lung and breath sounds.

Cardiovascular Function:

- Assess rate, rhythm, and quality of heart beat.
- Evaluate oxygen-carrying capacity of the blood (e.g., presence of adequate hemoglobin).

Nutrition:

- Assess the adequacy of protein, iron, sodium, and calcium intake.
- Assess the adequacy of fluid intake.
- Assess for presence of a previously identified nutritional disorder.

Medication History (whereas this information is usually obtained as subjective data, the nurse may need to seek other objective sources for this information if the patient has altered thought processes):

- Obtain a careful history from the patient or caregiver of *all* medications (including over-the-counter preparations, home remedies, and others) taken by the patient.
- Be alert to new medications added or stopped recently.
- Assess alcohol intake.

Other physiologic functions that are vital to assess are sleep and rest, motor activity, and adequacy of performance of activities of daily living, as disturbances in these functions may affect cognitive function.

Sleep and Rest:

- Determine if the patient has felt rested after a night's sleep.
- Assess changes in life events, patterns, or the current environment that may affect the quality of sleep and rest.

Motor Activity:

- Assess behavior for the presence of agitation or withdrawal from activity.
- Evaluate recent patterns of mobility, whether increased or decreased.

Activities of Daily Living:

- Identify the level of independence in hygiene, grooming, food preparation and intake, and home maintenance.
- Assess problem-solving abilities, such as money management, use of telephone, and interactions with needed services.

Observation. Observation is a useful means for identifying cues to impaired thinking. A disheveled appearance, disorganized speech, and abnormal movements are obvious indicators of dysfunction, especially when they are a change in status from baseline. Difficulty with eye contact, a tendency to tell the same story over and over, disproportionate responses to stress or stimuli, and emotional lability can also indicate difficulty with thought processes. At times, these behavior changes can be subtle, and repeated observation for consistency or inconsistency of behaviors is necessary to identify dysfunction. The assessment of cognitive function in infants and young children is complicated by several factors. Because the child's language skills are not fully developed, and there is difficulty expressing thoughts, observation of behavior becomes the primary data source.

Diagnostic Tests and Procedures

Physiologic Tests. The physiologic causes of confusion can be the result of disorders of multiple systems. Their diagnosis and management require multiple tests and procedures, from simple urinalysis to highly technical scans. In everyday practice in the acute-care setting, readily available tests, such as weight, vital signs, serum electrolytes, complete blood count, cultures, and measures of oxygen saturation are used by nurses to identify potential contributors to impaired cognition. Monitoring these parameters allows the nurse to identify imbalances and plan early interventions to prevent complications.

Arterial Oxygen. Arterial oxygen level is best determined by measuring arterial blood gases. An oxygen partial pressure greater than 60 mm Hg reflects adequate oxygenation. A noninvasive technique for assessing oxygenation is pulse oximetry, either ear or finger, which measures oxygen saturation (the percentage of hemoglobin that is bound to oxygen). A saturation of 90% correlates with a partial pressure of 60 mm Hg, given a normal level of hemoglobin. If a low (less than 90%) value is determined, oxygen therapy and further evaluation may be indicated.

Electrolytes. Electrolytes can be measured to determine their contribution to altered cognition. A serum sodium level less than 135 mEq/L or greater than 145 mEq/L may result in mental status impairment. Mild confusion can progress to agitation or confusion, with hallucinations or delusions, followed by stupor and coma, if the condition is untreated. Because brain cells can adapt to slow changes, severity of symptoms is related to how rapidly the sodium level drops.

An elevated level of serum calcium (greater than 5.8 mEq/L) can cause severe defects in cell conduction activity, with cognitive manifestations of lethargy or decreased level of consciousness.

Serum Glucose. Serum glucose levels below 70 mg/dL typically cause shakiness or nervousness, but can progress to cause altered cognition. While the measurement of serum glucose from venipuncture is the most accurate, the widespread availability of capillary blood glucose monitoring has promoted more reliable self-assessment of serum glucose.

Urea. Urea, converted from ammonia by the liver, is a by-product of protein metabolism, and is excreted by the kidney. Liver disease can interfere with this process and cause elevated ammonia levels (or blood urea nitrogen). A blood urea nitrogen (BUN) level greater than 50 mg/dL can produce a specific confusion known as hepatic encephalopathy, which will progress to coma if untreated. Renal disease can result in elevated levels of urea, which also cause confusion and lethargy.

Toxic Levels of Drugs. Toxic levels of drugs can result from an impaired ability to metabolize or excrete the drug. Serum levels of many drugs can be measured to determine therapeutic and toxic ranges. People with impaired hepatic or renal function are at risk of drug toxicity and require dosage reduction and regular monitoring of drug levels.

Tests of Cognitive Function. Intellectual function consists of short- and long-term memory, comprehension, and concentration. These are straightforward abilities, easily tested and converted to objective measurements with standardized tools. Intelligence or IQ tests attempt to measure intellectual function. These tests rely on verbal ability and vocabulary with a structured questioning format. They are standardized to the vocabulary and cultural experience of white, middle-class Americans, and have questionable validity when administered to other ethnic and socioeconomic groups. It is important to remember that standardized tests of verbal ability are not sensitive to sociocultural differences and so should not be used to assess "normality" for all groups. The primary usefulness of standardized tests is that each person using them assesses the same information, thus providing a common base of information and quantification for comparison.

Because of their limited attention span, it is difficult for children to cooperate with tedious assessment procedures. Assessment tools used with children focus on the observation of behavior, especially behavior elicited by a standard set of stimuli.

Standardized tools are available for the objective assessment of mental status. Two examples are the Pfeiffer Short Portable Mental Status Questionnaire (Pfeiffer, 1975) and the Mini Mental Status Exam (Folstein, Folstein, & McHugh, 1975). A score of 7 or less on the Pfeiffer or 20 or less on the Mini Mental Status Exam indicates significant cognitive impairment. These tools are most useful when given on an outpatient basis to healthy people repeatedly over time, allowing identifica-

Pfeiffer Mental Status Questionnaire

1. What is today's date? _____
2. What day of the week is it? _____
3. What is the name of this place? _____
4. What is your telephone number? _____
   If none, what is your address? _____
5. How old are you? _____
6. When were you born? _____
7. Who is the President of the U.S. now? _____
8. Who was the President before him? _____
9. What is your mother's maiden name? _____
10. Subtract 3 from 20 and keep going down to 0.

Total number of errors _____

From Pfeiffer, E. (1975). A short portable mental status questionnaire for the assessment of organic brain deficit in elderly patients. *Journal of the American Geriatrics Society, 23,* 433–443.

Mini-Mental State Examination

Maximum Score	Score	
		Orientation
5	( )	What is the (year) (season) (date) (day) (month)?
5	( )	Where are we: (state) (county) (town) (hospital) (floor)?
		Registration
3	( )	Name 3 objects: 1 second to say each. Then ask the patient all 3 after you have said them. Give 1 point for each correct answer. Then repeat them until he learns all 3. Count trials and record. (trials _____).
		Attention and Calculation
5	( )	Serial 7's (begin with 100 and count backwards by 7). 1 point for each correct answer. Stop after 5 answers. Alternatively spell "world" backwards.
		Recall
3	( )	Ask for the 3 objects repeated above. Give 1 point for each correct answer.
		Language
9	( )	Name a pencil, and watch (2 points) Repeat the following: "No, ifs, ands, or buts." (1 point)
		Follow a 3-stage command: "Take a paper in your right hand, fold it in half, and put it on the floor." (3 points)
		Read and obey the following: Close your eyes (1 point)
		Write a sentence (1 point)
		Copy design (1 point)
<u>30</u>	__	Total score
		Assess level of consciousness along a continuum:
		Alert Drowsy Stupor Coma

From Folstein, M. F., Folstein, S. E., & McHugh, P. R. (1975). "Mini-Mental state": A practical method of grading the cognitive state of patients for the clinician. *Journal of Psychiatric Research, 12,* 189–198. Copyright 1975, Pergamon Press, Ltd.

tion of changes from baseline. Administering these tools during an acute confusional state can help quantify daily changes, but without a premorbid baseline and in the absence of physiologic imbalance, little can be determined about the patient's change from baseline function. There is a specific battery of tests used to diagnose dementia.

NURSING DIAGNOSIS AND PATIENT GOALS

Diagnostic Statement: Altered Thought Processes

Definition

A state in which an individual experiences a disruption in cognitive operations and activities (NANDA, 1990).

Defining Characteristics

Inaccurate interpretation of environment; cognitive dissonance (disorganized thinking); distractibility; memory deficit/problems; egocentricity (self-centered or existing only as created in the mind); hyper- or hypovigilance (attention dysfunction); inappropriate nonreality-based thinking (NANDA, 1990).

Related Factors

NANDA is developing related factors. Etiologic factors can be physiologic, environmental, and emotional in nature. Physiologic factors include alterations in oxygenation and biochemical components, genetic-related disorders, and dementias. Environmental factors include change in surroundings, routine, significant others; altered sensory input (too much or too little); abuse/misuse of alcohol or drugs; and fear of unknown. Emotional factors include anxiety, depression, loss of family or friends, family conflict, or separation.

Related Nursing Diagnoses

The diagnosis Sensory/Perceptual Alterations is related to factors that may interfere with cognition and thought processes. The range of other factors that can affect cognition encompasses a multitude of nursing diagnoses. Altered Nutrition: Less Than Body Requirements, Hypothermia, Hyperthermia, Altered Tissue Perfusion, Fluid Volume Excess, Fluid Volume Deficit, Decreased Cardiac Output, Impaired Gas Exchange, Fatigue, Sleep Pattern Disturbance, and Pain are nursing diagnoses that can have direct physiologic effects on cognition and thought processes.

Impaired Social Interaction, Social Isolation, Ineffective Individual Coping, Dysfunctional Grieving, Anxiety, and Fear are nursing diagnoses that may make primary or secondary contributions to alterations in cognition and thought processes.

Patient Goals

The goals for the patient with altered thought processes should focus on providing an environment that supports existing impairments, does not predispose to new impairments, and protects the patient from harm. Goals need to be individualized, taking into consideration the patient's history, areas of risk, evidence of dysfunction, and related objective data. Examples of patient goals for the patient with a reversible confusion include:

The patient will express a realistic perception of reality.
The patient will demonstrate return to previous level of cognition.
The patient will have absence of injury related to the confusion.

Examples of patient goals for the patient with irreversible confusion include:

The patient will experience adequate support to compensate for deficits.
The patient will participate in a safe, protected environment.

IMPLEMENTATION

Appropriate nursing interventions will vary with the nature of the cognitive impairment. Preventing dysfunction, along with providing for patient safety and minimizing factors that contribute to dysfunction, are central goals of nursing care (Nagley & Dever, 1988).

Nursing Interventions to Promote Cognitive Health and Function

Instituting preventive measures and recognizing persons at risk for experiencing altered thought processes are relevant activities for nurses in the community and in acute, long-term, and home-care settings. Promoting a healthy lifestyle, improving memory, and maintaining learning skills are particularly useful interventions for healthy cognitive functioning.

Healthy Lifestyle Promotion

To promote healthy cognitive function, maintaining a lifestyle that includes adequate nutrition, rest, regular exercise, stress management, and social activity is essential. A balanced diet with sufficient protein, iron, and other nutrients is required for production of hemoglobin, which carries the oxygen in the blood. In addition to the relationship between nutrition and oxygen availability to the brain cells, a dynamic fluid and electrolyte balance is needed for cells to function optimally. Serum imbalances of water, sodium, calcium, and glucose can be prevented through adequate fluid intake throughout the day, in conjunction with a balanced diet. For people who have known dysfunctions that may place them at risk for some serum imbalances, such as a person with diabetes mellitus, teaching the importance of regulation of the dysfunction, recognizing early indications of imbalances, and initiating preventive dietary or fluid therapy are primary interventions. Chapters 32 and 33 present complete discussions of interventions for promoting fluid and electrolyte balance and balanced nutrition.

Oxygen perfusion to brain cells is enhanced through the practice of regular exercise. Regular exercise provides cardiovascular conditioning, improves circulation throughout the body, and contributes to a sense of well-being and refreshment. (See Chap. 29 for a more complete discussion of the benefits of exercise.) Encouraging people to develop the habit and practice of vigorous exercise contributes positively to cognitive functioning. Depending on the person, the exercise may range from energetic walking to more active sports, such as jogging, tennis, or other activities.

Equally important as getting sufficient exercise is having adequate sleep and rest. Fatigue, from inadequate sleep or interrupted sleep cycles, usually results in loss of REM sleep, manifested by the lack of feeling rested. Encouraging people to maintain regular sleep patterns will assist them in obtaining sufficient sleep and feelings of being rested when they are awake. Counseling the person to provide an environment that is conducive to rest and sleep is an important consideration for enhancing sleep. Chapter 39 presents additional nursing interventions for promoting sleep and rest.

Stress management can contribute to healthy cognition through minimizing distractions, improving rest, and enhancing concentration. Stress is managed by developing effective coping skills that allow the person to channel stress in a way that is productive or that dissipates the resulting tension. Exercise, as previously discussed, is one type of coping skill that the nurse can encourage. Chapter 47 presents a variety of coping skills and mechanisms from which the nurse can draw in assisting the person with stress management.

Many aspects of thought processes and cognitive function are cognitive skills that have been developed throughout life. These skills, like all others, need to be practiced regularly to be maintained. Social interaction is one such skill in which the person needs to participate for a variety of reasons, including enjoying the association of human contact, stimulation of conversation, and confirmation of personhood. Nurses can use social interaction on a one-on-one basis with the patient and can encourage opportunities for social interaction with others in informal group situations. These interactions

can provide feedback to the patient related to reality orientation, self-concept, and sensory perception.

The person with a chronic illness who is functionally able to live in the community can easily become socially isolated and sensory-deprived at home. Any person who depends on others for mobility, is isolated, and has a poor social support system is at risk for developing cognitive dysfunction. Preventive interventions that the nurse can use include referral for home nursing care and providing information about community services. Examples of community services that the nurse can incorporate in preventive interventions include subsidized transportation, senior centers, adult day care, congregate meal programs, community mental health centers, and volunteer opportunities.

For people with sensory impairments, there are a number of assistive devices the nurse can recommend that can help maintain and promote cognitive function. People who have hearing difficulties can often be fitted with hearing aids to allow them to participate in more interactive situations, which help promote cognitive stimulation. Telephone companies can provide equipment to assist with communication, and television now offers "closed caption" programs with printed captions that permit hearing-impaired people access to cognitive stimulation from televised programs. Talking books and other services from public libraries help supplement cognitive input for the visually impaired.

Memory Improvement

The fear of losing one's cognitive abilities is often focused on concerns about the quality of memory. Fatigue, stress, and illness may temporarily affect the efficiency with which a person is able to store information in or retrieve it from the memory. An initial intervention by the nurse can be reassurance that, in most situations, there is no organic basis for simple, occasional forgetfulness, and that reducing stress, relieving fatigue, or recovery from illness may eliminate the temporary memory difficulty.

For people with minimal memory problems, memory training programs or devices may be a beneficial intervention. Memory training programs focus on the personal abilities and compensatory capabilities of the person to stimulate cognitive function. The nurse can encourage the person to participate in memory training or to use principles of memory enhancement. Focusing attention deliberately on the information to be remembered helps to reduce stress and minimize distractions. Using both visual and auditory senses provides two important sources of perceptual input for cognition. Making lists, using mnemonic devices (use of formulas or patterns of letters to aid in remembering), and developing other association techniques can assist the person with remembering tasks or information. The regular practice or rehearsal of retrieving information from the memory helps maintain the skill of retrieval. For example, doing crossword puzzles regularly helps many people rehearse the skill of retrieval of knowledge and information from the long-term memory.

Maintenance of Learning Skills

For the child and young person in formal education, developing the skill for learning is nearly as important as the knowledge actually learned. These learning skills need to be practiced, reinforced, and used throughout life. The nurse can strengthen these skills in situations requiring teaching. People learn better when the relevance of the information is apparent; for example, if a person has experienced side effects of a medication, the learning related to potential effects of other medications has increased relevance because of the desire to prevent problems in the future.

Learning is increased when it is meaningful and linked with previous learning. To illustrate, if the nurse wants to teach a person about the importance of exercise for the body, associating various body parts with analogous parts in an automobile may increase the meaningfulness, due to the link with previous knowledge. As another example, for a person needing to learn about medications, the classifications and generic names of drugs will not be as meaningful as the color, shape, and size of the medication and the frequency with which it is to be taken.

When teaching the elderly, simplicity, clarity, and relevance are important considerations. The nurse should center on a single topic at a time to allow focused attention. Minimizing environmental distractions and sounds assists the person in the learning process. Providing learning materials and approaches that use vision, hearing, and touch will help the older person have perceptual input from several sources. Chapter 21 presents more detailed information related to patient teaching.

Nursing Interventions for Altered Cognitive Function

When the diagnosis of Altered Thought Processes has been identified, the nurse can intervene to help restore or improve cognitive function. The nurse has both an independent and a collaborative role in identifying patients at risk for cognitive dysfunction, and for initiating appropriate teaching for the patient and family. The nurse, as the health-care professional with the most patient contact, is in the best position to monitor changes in cognitive function, to communicate these to the health-care team, and to intervene as appropriate.

Cognitive deficits that are the result of irreversible neurologic deficits are rarely responsive to medical treatment. Nursing interventions designed to improve function include the same measures and activities as for the

patient with reversible cognitive changes. The major focus of nursing care is creating an environment that provides appropriate sensory stimulation, adequate assistance with activities of daily living, and protection from physical injury.

Fluid Intake and Nutrition

Because shifts in nutrients, electrolytes, and fluids contribute to cognitive changes, monitoring the food and fluid intake of patients is an essential nursing intervention. People who are ill often do not feel like eating and may not find food appealing. Patients should be allowed to choose foods that they particularly like, with supportive encouragement and monitoring by the nurse so that the diet is reasonably well balanced.

Similarly, patients may not experience thirst even when increased fluid intake is needed. Keeping fluids within easy reach of the patient, along with reminders to drink, are simple approaches. Fluid intake and output records are useful to observe for a pattern of fluid intake.

Reversible Confusion

- Orient patient to environment.
- Introduce self and others to the patient.
- Provide physical contact (e.g., hand on arm) when communicating with the patient.
- Reduce extraneous noise, light, and other distractions.
- Provide reality orientation with calendars, clocks, and other cues.
- Explain procedures, sounds, and equipment to the patient.

Irreversible Confusion

- Establish a stable, structured environment.
- Employ reality orientation and memory cues consistently.
- Provide for safety within the environment.
- Encourage the patient and family to accept the patient's level of functioning.
- Use the patient's name frequently.
- Establish physical contact with the patient during communication.
- Refer the patient and family to resources and support services.

The most accurate guideline for the adequacy of food and fluid intake is regular measurement of body weight. For patients at risk for fluid imbalances, a regular schedule of weighing will need to be established.

Patients and families will need health teaching regarding the factors that place them at risk for food and fluid imbalances. The diabetic who may have fluctuations in serum glucose needs to understand appropriate diet and medication management. The person who is taking diuretics requires an understanding of the effects and side effects of the medication, and that water should not be withheld unless specifically prescribed by the physician. Patients who have any identified risk factors for the development of cognitive dysfunction should receive health teaching related to the problems, along with warranted supportive nursing care.

Patients with irreversible cognitive impairment need particularly close monitoring of food and fluid intake. With the loss of judgment, some patients do not respond to the normal signals from appetite, thirst, or satiety, so that they may not eat or drink unless reminded, may overeat, may eat inappropriate things, or may forget

how to perform the mechanical process of eating. Sitting with these patients while they eat, reminding them to eat, and assisting them with the mechanics of eating may be useful interventions. Socialization opportunities when eating at a table with others often help to reinforce desired behaviors and activities.

Mobility

Encouraging mobility in patients who have a tendency to be isolated or withdrawn serves several useful purposes. The physical activity of moving stimulates improved ventilation and improved cardiovascular function, with improved oxygenation to the brain as a result. Not only is oxygenation improved, but the person also generally feels better physically and personally. Socialization is often one aspect of increased mobility. As a person moves around more, even on a hospital unit, contact with other people is increased. Contact with other people and varied environments provides more stimulation and reinforcement of reality.

Since it is often difficult to determine what is most meaningful for the patient, providing sensory stimulation for all of the senses is an important consideration, particularly for those patients with irreversible cognitive changes. In addition to hearing and seeing, the nurse should make use of touch through personal contact and varied fabric textures, taste through varieties of food and beverages, and smell through food and flowers.

Safety

A person with altered thought processes is at risk for injury and requires nursing intervention to ensure safety. For example, when a person is hospitalized, the location is unfamiliar, routines are strange, and the person is undoubtedly ill. This patient may temporarily lose orientation and think he or she is at home or somewhere else, and be at risk for falling while trying to get out of bed or while going to the bathroom. Safety measures

Safety Alert

- Supervise patients with confusion during ambulation and other activities because they may have altered judgment as to where they are.
- Be sure that the environment is free from unnecessary obstructions to prevent potential falls.
- Provide structure and predictable routine whenever possible to minimize distractions and potential accidents.
- Provide adequate lighting for safe ambulation within the environment.

such as orienting the patient to the room, the nurse call system, and the lights help to prevent accidents and injuries. Safety is discussed in Chapter 25.

For the patient with progressively impaired judgment, safety becomes a primary concern. In an institutional setting, safety measures for the patient with irreversible cognitive changes involve having the bed at the lowest level; frequent observations to assist the patient in getting out of bed to go to the bathroom or for other reasons; supervision of wandering behavior; and providing secured locks or alerting systems for elevators and doors that allow security for the patients and avoid accidental wandering away.

Restraints, physical or chemical, are generally not useful in maintaining safety. Studies have demonstrated that agitated behaviors tend to increase after the application of restraints (Werner, et al., 1989), the desire for wandering behaviors becomes intensified (Rader, 1987, 1991), and falls are not prevented (Janelli, 1989). Many long-term care facilities are becoming more creative in their management of safety, providing innovations such as an enclosed courtyard with unlimited access for the patients with dementia so that they can wander within a protected confine.

Patients with irreversible cognitive changes, that is dementia, become upset and distressed by changes in routine and environment. For this reason it is beneficial for the care environment to be as predictable as it can be. This includes having meals, baths, treatments, and other activities at regular times with as many familiar staff people as practical. If changes are necessary, remember that the patient with dementia needs additional support and reassurance as an essential element of nursing care.

Therapeutic Communication

Therapeutic communication means that the nurse respects the individuality of patients and uses modes of communication to convey that respect. Therapeutic communication can be used in assessment to obtain accurate information, but it is equally important in ongoing interactions between the nurse and the patient. These communication techniques are presented in detail in Chapter 17, and the student will want to be familiar with, if not skillful in, using them.

Therapeutic communication enables the nurse to reevaluate and to intervene consistently using as accurate patient-based information as possible. Regular use of these communication techniques allows the nurse to detect cognitive changes whenever they occur, so that interventions are as free from personal bias on the part of the nurse as they can be.

Reality Orientation

Reality orientation is a nursing technique to assist the patient in restoring awareness of reality. A hallmark in reinforcing reality for hospitalized patients is to provide those environmental cues on which people depend for orientation to time and place (Rockwood, 1989). Having the change in lighting match the usual day and night cueing is very helpful. Patients who are in specialized units with few windows and lights on throughout the 24 hours have greater difficulty relying on environmental cues.

Clocks and calendars that allow the patient to know the date, day of the week, and time of day are important sources of input for reality orientation. Additional interventions that can promote reality orientation include responding to alarms on monitors promptly, allowing uninterrupted sleep periods when possible, and encouraging visits from family and friends. Contact with familiar objects, such as family photographs, a particular chair, or special books, is also useful in maintaining contact with reality.

Allowing the patient the maximal advantage in relation to sensory–perceptual data is equally important in reinforcing reality. If the patient normally wears glasses or a hearing aid, the nurse needs to be sure that these are available to the patient. If the information that the patient takes in is as accurate as possible, interpreting and responding to reality is easier.

Although patients with irreversible changes such as dementia will not return to previous levels of cognitive functioning, the nurse needs to assist the patient in maintaining current levels of functioning for as long as possible. Reality orientation is an appropriate intervention, using as many possible modalities to accomplish this, such as clocks, calendars, radio, TV, or personal contact.

Teaching Tips for Reality Orientation

- Use cues for reality data, such as clocks, calendars, verbal reminders.
- Address the patient by name often to strengthen personal identification.
- Do not reinforce references to nonreality as in hallucinations or delusions.
- Speak clearly and in short simple statements.
- Maintain a predictable routine or schedule for the patient.
- Promote the addition of familiar objects in the room.
- Encourage visits and meaningful interaction with family and friends.
- Positively reinforce small changes in behavior that indicate increasing orientation to reality.
- Promote continuity of care by having familiar staff with the patient whenever possible.

Socialization Therapies

Socialization therapies can take many forms, such as music, recreation, and reminiscence. The purpose of these therapies is to encourage the patient to expand contact with other people in social settings in an effort increase cognitive stimuli. For some people, the contact within usual social groups, such as Senior Citizen Centers, volunteer groups, church groups, or recreation groups, may provide beneficial stimulation.

For patients who are at risk for being isolated or may require a more protected environment, reality orientation groups or day care centers may provide the same type of human contact and stimulation. Developing an ongoing relationship with the people who staff these groups or centers provides continuity of care and consistent support for cognitive function.

Reminiscence Therapy. In **reminiscence therapy,** the patient uses recall of the past to assist in clarifying meaning in the present or reconciling conflict. It is a particularly useful therapy for the elderly in contributing to successful aging through maintaining self-esteem and reinforcing cognitive function. This therapy requires facilitation by a nurse or other health professional who is skilled in group process and in reminiscence therapy.

Recreation Therapy. Recreation therapy involves using recreation or hobbies to increase contact with meaningful experiences and with other people. It is another way of using familiar objects or abilities from the past to help the person ascribe meaning. While recreation therapy may be prescribed, a nurse may use recreation or hobbies as appropriate to the individual patient in an effort to stimulate cognitive function.

Music Therapy. Music therapy can be a type of recreation therapy in that it is used to make cognitive contact with the person through the familiarity of music. The music may be in the background, used for exercise, or group sings. Both the music itself and the socialization and recreation inherent in group opportunities for music are stimulating for the patient. Some therapists may use music in a specific, prescriptive fashion; however, nurses can use music as a part of nursing care as deemed appropriate.

Family Support

Patients with reversible alteration in thought processes, and their families, are often anxious and fear long-term confusion. The nurse can reassure the patient and family that, in most cases, cognitive function will improve with time. Families can be encouraged to participate actively in the planning and care of the patient, with the goal of preventing or minimizing altered thought processes through collaboration in the interventions previously discussed.

Nurses provide care and support for the families of dementia patients as often as for the patients themselves. Families have a difficult time adjusting to the fact that their loved one is losing or has lost all memory of them and their lives together. The grief process begins before the death of the patient with dementia. In essence, the person that the family once knew and interacted with is no longer present mentally but yet is present physically. The nurse can employ nursing interventions that aid the family in their grief process, as discussed in Chapter 46.

Discharge Planning and Home Care

With shorter hospital stays, patients may be discharged before dysfunctions in cognition and thought processes have returned to normal. As a consequence, careful discharge planning is imperative. If the patient is returning home with family as caregivers, the planning may need to range from informal teaching to arranging for support services to assist the family. Support groups, such as the Alzheimer's Disease and Related Disorders Association (ADRDA), can be very beneficial for caregivers and families by putting them in contact with others who share similar situations.

Home Care

Home-care services, including nursing and homemakers, can be arranged before the patient is discharged. Medicare and some health insurance will assist in the cost of these services. Home care eases the transition from the protected setting of the hospital, with many staff people, to the home, where there are fewer people to call on.

For the mildly cognitively impaired patient, return to home may be useful in reversing the dysfunction, as a result of the familiar environment and customary routines. The person who has a more severe impairment may require more frequent home visits for nursing care and for homemaking help.

If impaired cognitive function interferes with the ability to perform higher-level skills (such as managing medications and home maintenance), support systems can usually be created to promote safety and independence. For people with minor memory problems, there are many ways to support and compensate for memory function, such as making lists of medications to take, things to do, or appliances to turn off. Maintaining organization in the home and in routines provides a predictable environment with fewer distractions, so that memory functions more effectively. For people with moderate impairment, resources like chore service, volunteers, subsidized van service, Meals on Wheels, grocery delivery, and increased family involvement can be arranged.

Day and Respite Care

Day care and respite care are two support services that are very useful for irreversibly cognitively impaired people and their caregivers. Fatigue is a constant companion of caregivers of progressively impaired family members. One means of managing that fatigue is having access to services that allow the caregiver some time away from caregiving, while providing the impaired person with health and rehabilitative services. The caregiver can feel that the impaired family member is benefitting from the alternative care, and, at the same time, the caregiver can have much-needed rest and personal time.

Day Care. Day care is an alternative to residential long-term care, and can provide assistance in caregiving for the caregiver who must work, while furnishing the patient with a structured atmosphere for socialization, rehabilitation services, and health care. People with severe cognitive impairment have poor judgment and inadequate problem-solving skills, are at risk for injuring themselves and others, and are vulnerable to becoming victims of crime. The availability of a safe environment and constant supervision during the day benefits the patient and the caregiver, and delays the need for institutional care.

Respite Care. Respite care provides care for the patient for periods ranging from several days up to 1 or 2 weeks. This allows the caregiver to rest, handle business matters, or take a trip without excessive concern about the family member's care. If the caregiver can have regular periods of respite, it is easier to cope with the stress of continual caregiving.

Long-Term Care

A person with a progressive cognitive impairment or dementia will often need the more consistent support of a long-term care setting, in which there is 24-hour supervision of care, structured environment, and extended health services. Caregivers need the support and reinforcement of nurses and health-care providers as the decision for admission to long-term care is made. This is not a decision that families make easily or casually. Generally, families have given care at home until their health and personal resources simply will not permit them to continue. Families should be supported and assured that they have made the right decision, whatever that decision ultimately is.

For the patient, admission to long-term care can be a very positive move. The patient will have contact with more people, objects, and situations, all of which provide increased stimulation. The full-time care allows the patient's environment to be structured and predictable, which may actually increase the level of cognitive functioning, even if this is temporary. The actual process of relocation can be stressful, but the patient can be helped in coping with it through diligent orientation and unhurried repetition. The caring attitude of the professional caregivers is essential for both the patient and family.

EVALUATION

Specific outcome criteria are the means of measuring the achievement of patient goals. Examples of outcome criteria for cognitive function in the patient with reversible confusion are listed below. Outcome criteria need to be individually personalized to the particular patient so that they will measure the attainment of the specific patient's goals.

Goal
The patient will express a realistic perception of reality.

Possible Outcome Criteria
- By discharge, patient identifies orientation to time, place, and person.
- Within 2 days, patient participates appropriately in self-care activities.

Goal
The patient will demonstrate return to previous level of cognition.

Possible Outcome Criteria
- By discharge, patient performs previous activities of daily living, as acknowledged by spouse.
- By discharge, patient demonstrates ability to carry out intellectual functions of which they were capable at appointments 6 months ago.

Goal
The patient will have absence of injury related to confusion.

Possible Outcome Criteria
- Within 48 hours, patient reports absence of falls related to cognitive dysfunction.
- Within 1 week, patient reports absence of bruises, cuts, abrasions, or other signs of injury or harm.

Goal
The patient will experience adequate support to compensate for deficits.

Possible Outcome Criteria
- Before discharge, patient demonstrates adequate nutrition, safety, and mobility.
- Before discharge, patient receives support services as needed to offset needs presented by cognitive deficits.

Goal
The patient will participate in a safe, protected environment.

Nursing Management Plan
The Patient with Altered Thought Processes

Nursing Diagnosis: Altered thought processes related to biochemical imbalances and sensory deprivation manifested by lack of orientation to place and time and inability to manage ADLs.
Patient Goal: Patient will regain baseline cognitive function.
Patient Outcome Criteria

• Patient will be oriented to self, place, and time during hospital stay.
• Patient's family will state that patient's mental status has returned to pre-illness level by discharge.

Nursing Intervention	Scientific Rationale
1. Assess and record mental status every shift.	1. Regular assessment promotes recognition of changes in condition and allows determination of effectiveness of interventions.
2. Reorient as necessary. Provide orientation cues such as a clock, calendar, and a sign with room number.	2. Frequent reorientation and use of cues compensates for the short-term memory loss that occurs with cognitive impairment.
3. Encourage patient to be out of bed for meals when possible. Establish a consistent bedtime routine.	3. Providing an ADL routine that is similar to that followed at home can help minimize the strangeness of hospital environment.
4. Assign consistent caregivers when possible.	4. Minimizing the number of caregivers allows the patient to recognize staff and feel comfortable with their care.
5. Encourage family and friends to visit; put cards and flowers where patient can see them.	5. The ability to recognize family and friends persists even in state of severe confusion. Presence of loved ones can be reassuring and can minimize the negative effects of the hospital environment.
6. Encourage patient to participate in ADLs as much as possible.	6. To help the patient regain a sense of control and give the nurse an opportunity to assess functional ability.

Possible Outcome Criteria
• During hospitalization, patient demonstrates the absence of injury from environmental hazards.
• During hospitalization, patient demonstrates nonagitated behavior and other indications of comfort with the environment.

Evaluation includes assessing the patient's cognitive function and comparing the patient's progress with the individually established outcome criteria as a measure of the patient's goal attainment. The nursing care plan for the patient with altered thought processes is continued, modified, or concluded based on this systematic evaluation of the individual patient's functioning.

Key Concepts

■ Cognition is the process of knowing, thinking, and learning; it is the complex information processing by

which sensory input, past experiences, awareness, and emotions are integrated and made meaningful for the person and enables him or her to interact with the environment in a purposeful way.
■ To provide comprehensive nursing care, nurses need to be aware of factors affecting normal cognitive function, such as physiologic state, infectious processes, medications, personal and environmental stressors, and affective states.
■ Manifestations of altered cognition include disorganized thinking, attention deficits, memory impairment, and impaired thought processes.
■ For the person with altered thought processes, activities of daily living are disrupted, and the amount of support in the living situation must be assessed.
■ The nurse needs to determine how a person functions, along with assessing the quality of the social and physical environment, to guide the development of the nursing process.
■ Identifying risk factors for impaired thought processes will assist the nurse in defining the actual dys-

function and the appropriate interventions.

■ Thorough assessment of physiologic and psychosocial function is essential in identifying causes of altered thought processes.

■ The nursing diagnosis, Altered Thought Processes, is defined as a state in which a person experiences a disruption in cognitive operations and activities.

■ Nursing goals should focus on providing an environment that supports function, does not cause new impairments, and protects the patient from harm.

■ If the nurse is aware of potential risk for dysfunction, preventive interventions will concentrate on minimizing those factors and supporting the patient and/or caregivers.

■ Among many supportive interventions for the impaired patient is reality orientation, used to reinforce and restore awareness of reality.

■ People with altered thought processes require careful discharge planning and home care, with referral for families to long-term care, day care, or respite care as appropriate.

References

Ballard, K. (1981). Identification of environmental stresses for patients in surgical ICU. *Issues in Mental Health Nursing, 3,* 89–108.

Beel-Bates, C. A., & Rogers, A. E. (1990). An exploratory study of sundown syndrome. *Journal of Neuroscience Nursing, 22*(1), 51–52.

Chyun, D. (1989). Patients' perceptions of stressors in intensive care and coronary care units. *Focus on Critical Care, 16,* 206–211.

Erikson, E. H. (1963). *Childhood and society* (2nd ed.). New York: Norton.

Evans, L. (1987). Sundown syndrome in institutionalized elderly. *Journal of the American Geriatrics Society, 35,* 101–108.

Folstein, M., Folstein, S., & McHugh, P. (1975). Mini-mental status. *Journal of Psychiatric Research, 12,* 189–198.

Foreman, M. (1989). Confusion in the hospitalized elderly: Incidence, onset, and associated factors. *Research in Nursing and Health, 12,* 21–29.

Foreman, M., Gillies, D. A., & Wagner, D. (1989). Impaired cognition in the critically ill elderly patient: Clinical implications. *Critical Care Nursing Quarterly, 12,* 61–73.

Francis, J., Martin, D., & Kapoor, W. (1990). A prospective study of delerium in hospitalized elderly. *Journal of the American Medical Association, 263,* 1097–1101.

Freiberg, K. (1987). *Human development: A life-span approach* (3rd ed.). Boston: Jones and Bartlett.

Guyton, A. C. (1986). *Textbook of medical physiology* (7th ed.). Philadelphia: W. B. Saunders.

Havinghurst, R. J. (1972). *Developmental tasks and education* (3rd ed.). New York: David McKay.

Janelli, L. M. (1989). Physical restraints: How little we know. *Nursing Homes, 38*(10), 10–12.

Kane, R., Ouslander, J., & Abrass, I. (1989). *Essentials of geriatrics.* New York: McGraw-Hill.

Katzman, R. (1987). Alzheimers disease: Advances and opportunities. *Journal of the American Geriatrics Society, 35,* 69–73.

Nagley, S., & Dever, A. (1988). What we know about treating confusion. *Applied Nursing Research, 1,* 80–83.

NANDA (1990). *Taxonomy I revised 1990, with official nursing diagnoses.* St. Louis, MO: North American Nursing Diagnosis Association.

Pfeiffer, E. (1975). A short, portable mental status questionnaire for the assessment of organic brain deficit in elderly patients. *Journal of the American Geriatrics Society, 23,* 433–443.

Piaget, J. (1969). *The psychology of the child.* New York: Basic Books.

Porth, C. (1990). *Pathophysiology: Concepts of altered health states* (3rd ed.). Philadelphia: J. B. Lippincott.

Rader, J. (1987). A comprehensive staff approach to problem wandering. *The Gerontologist, 27,* 756–760.

Rader, J. (1991). Modifying the environment to decrease use of restraints. *Journal of Gerontological Nursing, 17*(2), 9–13.

Reifler, B., Larson, E., Teri, L., et al. (1986). Dementia of the Alzheimers type and dementia. *Journal of the American Geriatrics Society, 34,* 855–859.

Rockwood, K. (1989). Acute confusion in elderly medical patients. *Journal of the American Geriatrics Society, 37,* 150–154.

Schuster, C., Ashburn, S. (1986). *The process of human development* (2nd ed.). Boston: Little, Brown.

Werner, P., Cohen-Mansfield, J., Braun, J., et al. (1989). Physical restraints and agitation in nursing home residents. *Journal of the American Geriatrics Society, 37,* 1122–1126.

Williams, M. A. (1989). Physical environment of the intensive care unit and elderly patients. *Critical Care Nursing Quarterly, 12*(1), 52–60.

Bibliography

Billig, N., et al. (1989). Diagnostic dilemma: Is it dementia? *Patient Care, 23*(7), 192–195, 203–204.

Cattell, R. B. (1963). Theory of fluid and a crystallized intelligence: A critical experiment. *Journal of Educational Psychology, 36,* 1–22.

deSimone, E. M. (1989). The hospitalized elderly: A nursing perspective. *Recent Advances in Nursing, 23,* 36–44.

Downs, F. (1974). Bedrest and sensory disturbances. *American Journal of Nursing, 74,* 434–439.

Eisdorfer, C., & Wilkie, F. (1973). Intellectual changes. In L. Jarvik, C. Eisdorfer, & J. Blum (eds.): *Intellectual functioning in adults.* New York: Springer.

Evans, L. K. (1989). Nursing the hospitalized dementia patient. *Journal of Advanced Medical Surgical Nursing, 1*(2), 18–31.

Horn, J. L. (1982). The aging of human abilities. In B. Wolman (ed.): *Handbook of developmental psychology.* Englewood Cliffs, NJ: Prentice-Hall.

Jackson, C., Ellis, R. (1971). Sensory deprivation as a field of study. *Nursing Research, 20,* 46–58.

Lipowski, Z. (1983). Transient cognitive disorders in the elderly. *American Journal of Psychology, 140,* 1426–1436.

Moore, T. (1989). Sensory deprivation in the ICU. *Nursing, 43,* 269–276.

Noyes, L. E. (1989). Caregiving techniques for dementia patients. *Caring, 8*(8), 18–21.

Schaie, K. W., & Strothers, C. R. (1968). The effects of time and cohort differences on the interpretation of age changes in cognitive behavior. *Multivariate Behavior Research, 3,* 259–294.

Schaie, K. W. & Hertzog, C. (1983). Fourteen-year cohort-sequential analyses of adult intellectual development. *Developmental Psychology, 19,* 531–543.

Talley, J. (1987). Geriatric depression: Avoiding the pitfalls of primary care. *Geriatrics, 42,* 53–66.

Tyumchuk, A. J., Ouslander, J. G., & Rader, N. (1986). Informing the elderly: A comparison of four methods. *Journal of the American Geriatric Society, 34,* 818–822.

Wilkie, F., & Eisdorfer, C. (1974). Terminal changes in intelligence. In E. Palmore (ed.): *Normal aging: Reports from the Duke logitudinal studies, 1970–1973.* Durham, NC: Duke University Press.

Wolanin, M., & Phillips, R. (1981). *Confusion: Prevention and care.* St. Louis: C. V. Mosby.

Wondolowski, C., et al. (1989). Guidelines for nursing management in Alzheimer's care. *Journal of Advanced Medical Surgical Nursing, 1*(2), 76–87.

U N I T XII

Self-Perception and Self-Concept

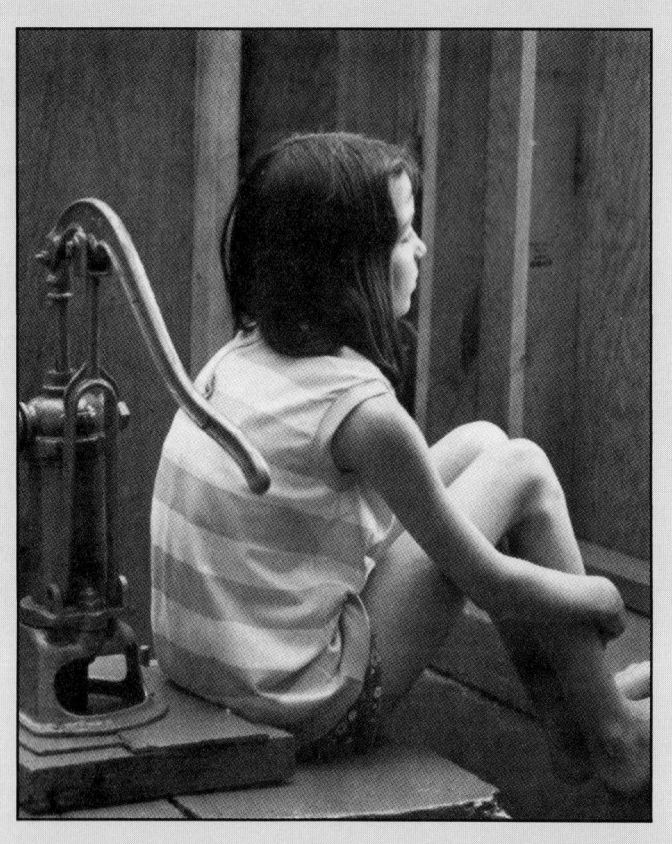

CHAPTERS

43 Self-Concept

U nit XII discusses the self-perception and self-concept areas of human function. Beginning at birth, a person's perception of himself or herself affects actions and pursuits. People tend to act in accordance with their internal self perception. Therefore, a patient's self-concept affects all aspects of patient care.

The content in the single chapter in this unit focuses on the principles and concepts of self-perception with an eye toward helping the nurse understand the effect self-perception has on a patient's sense of worth and, ultimately, the choices he or she makes. A patient's self-concept can be a strength and can positively influence other areas of function. Conversely, a negative self-concept can result in self-esteem disturbances, body image disturbances, altered role performances, or personal identity disturbances. Such patient responses greatly interfere with normal function and affect all activities of daily living.

Using a nursing process format, this chapter presents an introductory discussion of self-concept as a patient need requiring nursing attention. An understanding of how human responses affect self-concept and the impact of self-concept on the patients's responses allows the nurse to incorporate this awareness into all aspects of patient care.

This chapter emphasizes nursing interventions to promote health and function to maximize patient strengths. Additionally, a beginning discussion of altered function and appropriate nursing interventions helps the nurse provide sensitive, holistic care.

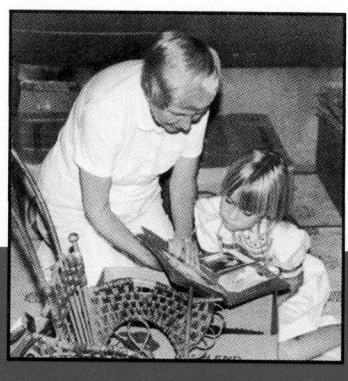

Self-Concept

LEARNING OBJECTIVES

Upon completion of this chapter, the student will be able to do the following:

- Describe the normal function of self and self-concept.
- Define self-concept, self-perception, self-knowledge, self-expectation, social self, and self-evaluation.
- Discuss factors affecting self-concept.
- Identify potential factors for altered self-concept.
- Identify manifestations of altered self-concept.
- Discuss how self-concept develops throughout the lifespan.
- Apply theory to assess for self-concept functioning.
- Plan care for a person with an altered self-concept.

KEY TERMS

Body image
Identity
Role
Self

Self-concept
Self-esteem
Self-evaluation
Self-expectation

Self-knowledge
Self-perception
Social self

43

Normal Function of Self
  Characteristics of Normal Self-Concept
    Self-Concept and Self-Perception
  Normal Functional Self-Concept Patterns
    Positive Body Image
    Self-Esteem
    Strong Personal Identity
    Role Performance
  Factors Affecting Normal Self-Concept
    Biologic Make-Up
    Culture, Values, and Beliefs
    Previous Experience
    Developmental Level
    Illness
    Altered Self-Concept
  Lifespan Considerations
Altered Self-Concept
  Potential for Altered Self-Concept
    Stressful Life Events
    Inadequate Coping Resources
    Incompleted Developmental Tasks
    Role Transition
    Illness, Trauma, and Surgery
  Manifestations of Altered Function
    Self-Care Deficit
    Emotional and Behavioral Changes
    Anxiety and Depression
    Self-Destructive Behavior
  Impact of Dysfunction on Activities of Daily Living
Assessment
  Subjective Data
    Functional Pattern Identification
    Risk Identification
    Dysfunctional Identification

  Objective Data
Nursing Diagnoses and Patient Goals
  Diagnostic Statement: Body Image Disturbance
    Definition
    Defining Characteristics
    Related Factors
  Diagnostic Statement: Self-Esteem Disturbance
    Definition
    Defining Characteristics
  Diagnostic Statement: Personal Identity
    Disturbance
    Definition
    Defining Characteristics
  Diagnostic Statement: Altered Role Performance
    Definition
    Defining Characteristics
    Related Factors
    Related Nursing Diagnoses
    Patient Goals
Implementation
  Nursing Interventions to Promote Health and
    Function
    Identification of Strengths
    Sense of Self
    Development of Self-Concept
  Nursing Interventions for Altered Self-Concept
    Therapeutic Relationship
    Self-Evaluation
    Behavioral Change
  Discharge Planning and Home Care
Evaluation
Key Concepts

A 36-year-old married woman had her first child 3 months ago. The woman experienced no deviations from normal birth. The pregnancy was planned and both she and her husband adjusted to parenthood effectively. During her pregnancy the woman had a weight gain of 40 pounds; after the birth she lost 15 pounds. Before pregnancy, the woman's body image was close to her perceived ideal, and she thought of herself as a thin, attractive young woman. Having fulfilled various roles successfully, including retail clerk, wife, daughter, and friend, she expected to be an adequate-to-good mother. This woman maintained a reality-based identity; she knew who she was and who she was not. The woman respected herself and had moderately high self-esteem. Since giving birth her body image has changed. She describes herself as "slightly fat" and states that her breasts are "too large." The woman feels tired. She has returned to part-time work and has established a warm and satisfying relationship with the baby. Her personal identity has remained intact. This woman feels OK about herself and is coping with her altered body image, new role, and lessened sense of esteem by doing aerobics and attending a mother's support group.

The woman's sense of self has changed. As she continues to adapt to life changes, her body image, self-esteem, personal identity, and role performance will evolve. Self-concept is dynamic and is influenced by experiences and expectations. A sound self-concept is a prerequisite for mental health.

Nursing responsibilities associated with self-concept include self-knowledge, assessment of self-concept, promotion of adequate self-concept functioning, and intervening when self-concept is at risk or altered. If the nurse possesses a healthy self-concept, he or she will be better equipped to deal with patient's unique and varied needs. Conversely, if nurse's self-concept is dysfunctional, he or she will be unable to meet the patients' needs. In fact, the task of coping with such a nurse may actually add to the work of the patient.

NORMAL FUNCTION OF SELF

The concept of self has been examined by many disciplines because of its importance in understanding human behavior. **Self** is elusive, and can be defined variously; it may be defined as a person's unique dimensions, potential, and purposes (Rogers, 1961). **Self-concept** is the mental image one has of oneself; it is the person's meaning when stated as "I" or "me." Self-concept is the frame of reference that influences how one handles life situations and relationships.

Maslow's hierarchy of human needs was discussed in Chapter 12. Esteem and self-actualization are the highest needs in the hierarchy; self-concept is critical to both.

Characteristics of Normal Self-Concept

People with a healthy self-concept exhibit a clear sense of self and others; they have an understanding of who they are in the real world. They can and do distinguish themselves as separate individuals, with strengths and weaknesses. These people acknowledge their emotions and have energy available to bring meaning into life. The person with a healthy self-concept has a realistic view of others and an ability to relate to them in a satisfying manner, including the capacity for intimate and loving relationships. The person with a healthy self-concept is able to deal with the realities and problems of life with appropriate coping behaviors.

Self-Concept and Self-Perception

Whereas self-concept is the mental image of self, **self-perception** is a filtering process (Gary & Kavanagh, 1991) that evaluates events and enters them in the subconsciousness. Such filtering "prevents feelings of guilt, anxiety, and unworthiness from surfacing." (Gary & Kavanagh, 1991).

How one perceives oneself has several dimensions: self-knowledge, self-expectations, social self, and self-evaluation (Fig. 43-1).

Self-Knowledge. **Self-knowledge** or self-awareness involves a basic understanding of oneself, a cognitive perception. It is a consciousness of one's abilities: cognitive, effective, and physical. Self-knowledge involves basic facts (age, weight, sex) and qualities (sincere, athletic, intelligent) related to who one is.

Self-Expectation. **Self-expectation** involves the "ideal" self—the self a person wants to be. It is the setting of goals for present and future. If they are realistic goals, the person may attain them; however, unrealistic goals can be defeating. Self-expectation is based on the limits of the person's awareness. For instance, if the person watches a great deal of television, that person may have as goals to be thin, to be beautiful, to be popular with the other sex, and to be wealthy with a beautiful home. If a person spends time reading, knowledge may be an expectation. Self-expectation is influenced by significant others. If a mother pushes a son to be a physician, the son may have this as an expectation or may set up an expectation of failure because of lack of interest.

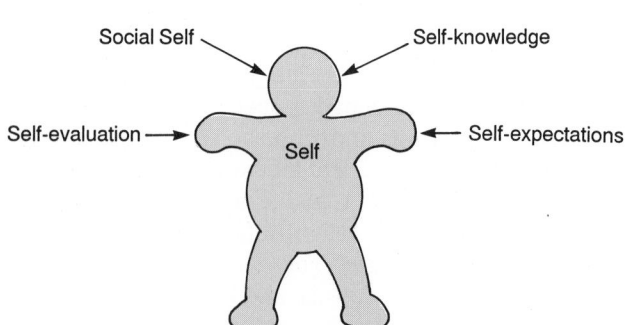

Figure 43–1. Self-perception involves various dimensions.

Social Self. One never fully knows how others see one's self. One can only guess how one is seen, and the guess may be far from reality. Conversely, people tend to wear masks in their social obligations; they tend to hide the true self. The Sunday church self may be different from the partygoer. On an interview a person may hide feelings of aggression, which are later revealed on the job. **Social self** is how one sees oneself in relation to social situations, including behavior and interaction with others.

Self-Evaluation. **Self-evaluation** is the conscious assessment of the self, leading to self-respect or self-worth. "Have I met my expectations? Do I like what I see in the mirror? what I know? how I act?" Self-evaluation involves the aforementioned dimensions. It also involves self-esteem, which will be discussed shortly.

NORMAL FUNCTIONAL SELF-CONCEPT PATTERNS

The mental image of one's self comprises body image, self-esteem, personal identity, and role performance. The whole of self represents more than the total of the four components. The instance of the woman who delivered the baby clarifies these components. Her body image, self-esteem, personal identity, and role performance changed with pregnancy and delivery. Her ideal self changed. But, because her self-concept was healthy, she can evaluate and make necessary changes; she can cope and adapt to the dynamics of self-concept.

Positive Body Image

The human body is the physical manifestation of self in the real world. How one pictures one's body and how one feels about one's body describes **body image.** Body image includes the total conscious and unconscious disposi-

tion toward one's body. It is the unifying concept behind feelings about one's size, sex, and sexuality; the way one looks; the way one's body functions; and whether one's body can help one accomplish goals. Sexual satisfaction is positively correlated with positive body image (Berscheid, et al., 1973).

Body image is influenced by culture and social experience. In American culture, because of media influence, beauty, health, and youth are valued. Each person has a picture of how he or she hopes he or she might look, an idealized body image. Additionally, each person has an awareness of how he or she really looks, a mirrored image. When the real image is close to the ideal image, the person experiences positive regard for self. These positive feelings about body image are part of self-esteem.

Self-Esteem

Self-esteem is the judgment that one makes regarding one's self. It is the result of self-evaluation of worth. Self-esteem is affective in nature, but it is made up of both thoughts and feelings. Stanwyck (1983, p. 11) defined self-esteem as "how I feel about how I see myself." Two sources for esteem are the self and others (Fig. 43-2). Self-esteem develops throughout childhood and adolescence, to become more stable in adulthood.

Early in life, the child accepts the parents' evaluation as his or her own. Then the child incorporates others' appraisals and expectations to form a self-ideal, and then slowly begins self-evaluation. The person emerges into adulthood with a basic or core self-esteem. Coopersmith (1967) identified antecedents of high self-esteem: parental acceptance, clear expectations, limitations, and freedom to express opinions. From these four antecedents, fundamental criteria by which people's self-appraisals are made have been proposed. These include:

- Power, the ability to influence people and events—the sense that my opinion counts and will be listened to
- Meaning, the sense of being valued and worthwhile—my existence matters to others
- Competence, the ability to achieve personal goals—personal success
- Virtue, behaving in a manner consistent with personal values—adherence to a moral or ethical standard

Core self-esteem is the person's consistent, overall appraisal of self. The person acts in ways or perceives events in ways that tend to support his or her level of self-esteem. Although core self-esteem is relatively stable, people do change their perceptions of self based on current experience. Such an example is the woman described at the beginning of this chapter. This changing self-esteem has been called functional self-esteem (Norris & Kunes-Cornell, 1985).

The person with adequate self-esteem has learned to

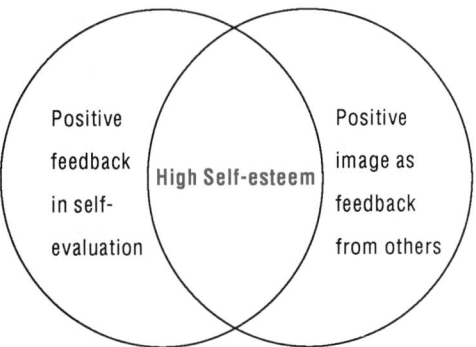

Figure 43–2. High self-esteem develops when there is positive feedback from both self and others.

cope with personal deficiencies and to maximize strengths; this person is self-accepting. The person with high self-esteem accepts others, experiences less anxiety, and functions effectively in social situations.

Strong Personal Identity

Identity is an organizing principle of the self, the awareness that one is a distinct individual separate from others. The person with a strong sense of personal identity has integrated self-esteem, body image, and various roles into an integrated, whole self-concept. This whole or "I" is not associated with any one aspect of the person. Identity provides the person with a sense of continuity through time. "I am not the person I was yesterday, but there are similarities and consistency that provides links for today and the future."

The concept of boundaries is central to identity. Actual body boundaries (this is my hand; that is your hand) and ego boundaries, (this is my thought or feeling, not your thought or feeling) must be intact for a person to have personal identity. The person must be able to differentiate self from others to possess mental health.

Role Performance

A person fills many roles in a lifetime. **Role** is defined as the expected characteristic behavior of a person in a social position. Roles are ascribed or assumed. A role is ascribed when the person has no choice. An example of an ascribed role is daughter; because the person is born female, she becomes a daughter. A role is assumed when the person selects it by choice. Assumed roles include career and family roles; an example is the person who chooses to be a nurse. Roles overlap and the person must combine many roles to achieve a unified pattern for functioning. When the person perceives self as adequate in various roles, self-esteem is enhanced. Roles are discussed in Chapter 45.

Factors Affecting Normal Self-Concept

Many factors affect self-concept, both positively and negatively, including biologic make-up; coping and stress tolerance; culture, values, and beliefs; previous experience; and developmental level.

Biologic Make-Up. One's biologic make-up comprises many characteristics that affect self-concept. Sex, height, weight, skin color, and attractiveness or unattractiveness are set characteristics that are self-perceived and perceived by others to help form self-concept (Fig. 43-3). These factors also affect what a person experiences. For example, men often have more opportunities to play competitive sports, enhancing self-concept, whereas women may be barred from playing certain

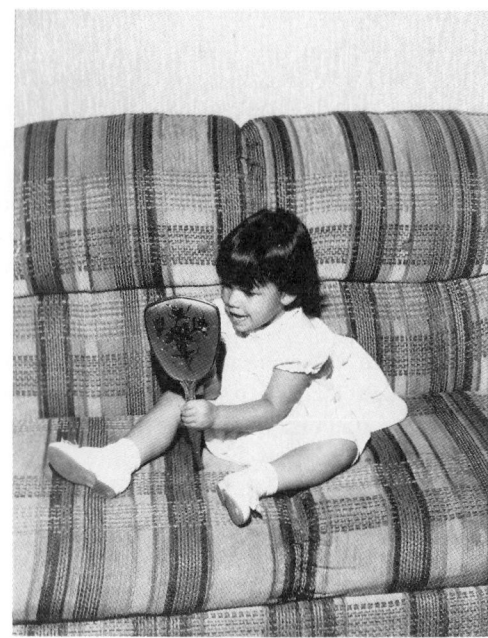

Figure 43–3. One's sex, skin color, hair color, and eye color affect self-perception and percention by others.

sports. The woman who is athletically inclined may perceive her sex and abilities as inferior, thus damaging her self-concept. Likewise, someone who is black in a predominantly white society may have difficulty securing a positive self-concept if others' perceptions are discriminatory. However, a person who is tall, slender, and attractive may easily develop a positive self-concept, since these are favorably perceived qualities.

Culture, Values, and Beliefs. Children grow up internalizing the culture, values, and beliefs to which they are exposed. The degree to which they can subscribe to those norms affects self-concept. The media (television, radio, newspapers, and magazines) provide daily lessons on the norms of American culture. Dietary, childbearing, health, and religious practices are norms that may vary among ethnic groups in the American culture, however. Integration of cultural practices and American beliefs can lead to a healthy self-concept. An adolescent who cultivates an interest in ethnic music and dance but still shares a love of rock music with his peers will have a strong identity and self-esteem.

Coping and Stress Tolerance. Coping and stress tolerance influence self-concept. People who are able to adapt to stress and resolve conflicts through coping tend to develop healthy self-concepts. Internal resources, such as a sense of humor and productivity under pressure, as well as external resources, such as strong support groups, enhance coping. A single mother who has a strong family support group may master the roles of parenthood, financial provider, and activist for women's rights, enhancing self-esteem and likewise strengthening performance in these roles. Poor stress tolerance may lead to crisis, however, damaging self-concept.

Previous Experience. Because self-concept is a complex, ever-changing personal perspective on the person's relationship with the world, self-concept is affected by one's previous experiences with the world.

Experiences will include opportunities for success and failure. If the person meets with success, he or she will begin to feel self-esteem and role satisfaction, and will begin to expect success. The person will also learn what and who he or she can influence. These experiences teach the person expectancies (Rotter, 1966). An expectancy is a belief that one's behavior will lead to a given response. Two expectancies that are incorporated into the self are expectancy for success and locus of control. Expectancy for success means the person has a belief that personal behavior will lead to something desired. Locus of control can be either internal or external. A person with external locus of control perceives that outcomes happen because of luck, chance, or the influence of powerful others; a person with internal locus of control believes that personal behavior influences outcome, and that he or she can achieve desired results. These expectancies develop from life experiences, and influence the self. For instance, if a person believes that luck brought about the outcome, then the person would not feel increased esteem because of the outcome, whereas a person with internal locus of control would. A person with strong internal locus of control may be threatened by illness because it shakes belief in personal control; however, self-concept can be preserved by the person's belief that subsequent health-seeking behavior will bring about wellness.

Experience also allows the person to develop and use coping strategies. As the person experiences stress in life, he or she uses the coping skills that fit with his or her view of self and the world. The person who is able to use health coping mechanisms that worked in the past will reinforce self-esteem with future successful coping.

Developmental Level. Developmental level influences self-concept from infancy through older adulthood. Whereas the newborn has no separate sense of self and the young child is learning that his or her identity is separate from others, the adolescent must deal with body image changes as secondary sex characteristics develop. Each developmental level brings unique experiences that can reinforce or alter self-concept, as discussed more fully in the previous section. Accomplishment of key tasks at each level enhances self-concept.

Illness. Positive self-concept is usually based on a healthy self; self-esteem and body image can be adversely affected by acute and chronic illness, trauma, or surgery. Even physical changes associated with normal aging may alter self-concept. Successful coping during illness, however, may enhance self-esteem. For example, a cancer patient who tolerates chemotherapy, is able to hold down a job, and becomes closer to his or her family, may emerge feeling emotionally stronger, more resourceful, and with a more positive self-concept than before the illness.

Altered Self-Concept. In addition to understanding normal self-concept functioning, the nurse must be aware of factors that place people at risk for dysfunctional self-concept, and manifestations of that dysfunction. Potential for altered self-concept function may arise from stressful life events, inadequate coping, incomplete developmental tasks, role transition, and illness, trauma, or surgery. Manifestations of altered function include self-care deficit, emotional and behavioral changes, anxiety and depression, and self-destructive behavior.

Lifespan Considerations

Each stage of development implies special considerations for the nurse interacting with patients or families. Knowledge of these considerations helps the nurse plan and implement appropriate interventions that will foster the development of positive self-concept.

Theorists in lifespan development were discussed in Chapter 14 and in Table 14-1. Prominent for theories regarding development of self-concept are Freud (1920/1966), Piaget (1969), Erikson (1963), Havighurst (1972), and Kohlberg (1969). Sullivan (1953) discussed an interpersonal theory. Four of these theorists (Freud, Sullivan, Erickson, and Havighurst) and their theories related to development of self-concept are given in Table 43-1.

Newborn and Infant

The newborn has an undifferentiated self; the newborn does not experience a separate existence from others. The mother's self-concept, her sense of competence in the new mothering role, and the amount and intensity of anxiety she feels are transmitted to the newborn (Fig. 43-4). When the mother is reasonably calm, and communicates warmth and acceptance to the baby, the basis for a positive self-concept is established.

The family as well as the newborn experience dramatic changes during the neonatal period. These changes have the potential to affect the self-concept of the infant. The mother shifts from being pregnant and having a pregnant body to not being pregnant. If the mother chooses to breastfeed, she has further body image changes, and concerns about milk production, sexuality, and competence. If she chooses not to breastfeed, she may experience guilt or doubt concerning the mothering role. Dur-

TABLE 43–1

Theories of Self-Concept Development

	Freud: Psychodynamic (1920/1966)	Sullivan: Interpersonal (1953)	Erickson: Ego (1963)	Havighurst: Tasks (1972)
Newborn/ Infant	Oral stage, 0–3 months; child is undifferentiated from mother	Infancy: beginning self-concept formed; security = good me; anxiety = bad me; Overwhelming anxiety or deprivation = not me	Trust vs. mistrust; adequate mothering helps infant establish trust in self and others	Task: establishes physiologic stability
Infant	3 months to 1–½ years; child begins to distinguish his or her body from objects (people and things) in the environment	Infant has no separateness from caretaker		
Toddler	Anal stage; personal identity pronounced "I"; role performance in family learned	Early childhood: beginning differentiation; if relationship adequate, child begins to integrate good me, bad me, and not me into self-concept	Autonomy vs. shame; Personal identity: body image and self-esteem develop as child experiences self-control through exploration in the world	Tasks: learns body image through walking, talking, control of waste
Preschooler	Phallic stage; sex role, body image and personal identity become more clearly differentiated		Initiative vs. guilt; beginning role established through sexual identity development and family relationships	Learns own sex role and identity through above tasks
School-age child	Latency; role performance is primary work of this stage; body image problems may manifest if previous stages not resolved successfully	Juvenile; the process of individuation occurs as peer relationships develop. The individual learns competition, compromise, and collaboration	Industry vs. inferiority; socialization and competence are developing, helping continued growth of self-concept	Tasks: learns physical skills for games; roles, i.e., sex, student and friend; values
Adolescent	Genital stage; body image is altered as the individual establishes self as sexual being; separation from parents leads to enhanced sense of identity; role choices are made	Identity, body image, and role continue to develop or be redefined as individuation progresses	Identity vs. role confusion; search for self	Tasks: acceptance of body and sex role; independence from parents; occupational preparation and other roles learned, i.e., marriage, citizen
Adult	Individual works on conflicts/lacks from previous developmental stages		Intimacy vs. isolation; primary task role related: acquisition of love, sexual fulfillment and closeness	Tasks: marriage, parenting, occupation
			Generativity vs. self-absorption; as person concerns self with next generation(s), new sense of identity develops, increasing self-comfort and integration of varied roles	Tasks: adjusting to physiologic changes; role with aging parents

(continued)

TABLE 43–1

(continued)

	Freud: Psychodynamic (1920/1966)	Sullivan: Interpersonal (1953)	Erickson: Ego (1963)	Havighurst: Tasks (1972)
Older Adult			Integrity vs. despair; individual accepts personal accomplishments or feels decreased worth; body image changes as the person experiences physical alterations associated with old age, i.e., decreased sensory acuity	Tasks: adjusts to decreased physical strength, retirement, possible death of self or spouse, decreased income

ing this same time the mother is shifting in existing roles and developing new roles.

The father also experiences shifts in roles and development of new roles; his new relationships must be integrated into his identity. Relationships with others are altered during this time. Extended family may either help or confuse role transition. Friends may treat the couple differently. Siblings of the newborn experience shifts in role also. Healthy acceptance and working through changes during this period set the stage for positive self-concept development. The infant begins to understand self as a separate body, and that feelings (i.e., hunger) are his or her own. As the infant begins to distinguish self from others, self-concept begins to develop. As the infant interacts with meaningful others, he or she begins to read the wants of others.

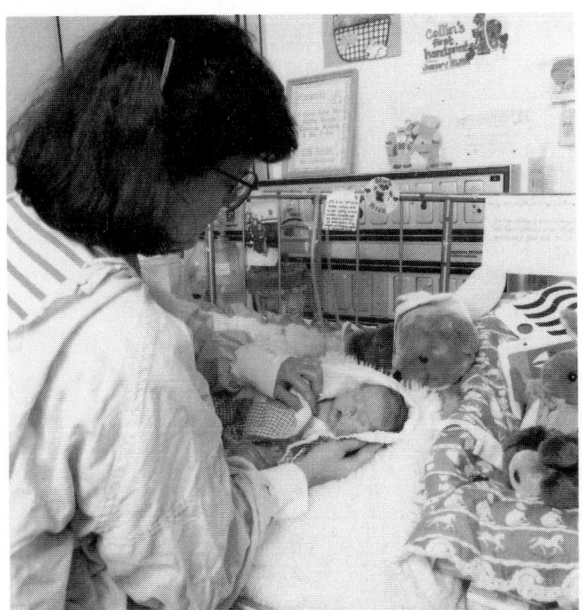

Figure 43–4. The identity of a newborn infant is integrated with the identity of the mother. (Photo courtesy of University of Washington School of Nursing.)

For example, when Mom smiles and plays patty-cake, Mom smiles even more when the infant smiles and makes noises. This is the beginning of learning social role expectations. During this stage the child learns to sit, stand, and possibly walk. This managing of body allows the infant to experience the world in different ways, and teaches the child body boundaries. Bodily control helps to establish a beginning sense of separateness from others. Through play, the infant learns to control aspects of his or her environment. For instance, early during this stage the infant bats at objects, such as colorful items on a mobile. Later, the infant grasps items, and toward the end of this phase may be able to stack two blocks. This play helps the child with very beginning identity, just as social control (i.e., smiles) helps the child with beginning role.

Additionally, the infant begins communication through symbols, that is, a smile means good, a cry means bad, "ma-ma" is associated with the mothering one, and the infant begins to respond to his or her name. The infant accomplishes these developmental tasks through interaction with caregivers and through exploration.

Toddler and Preschooler

The toddler has a rudimentary body image. Although the toddler knows self as separate from others, there is no clear definition of where the body ends. For example, the child may not want to flush the toilet after defecating; the stools are part of the child. The child is not aware of specific influences, only general feelings or thoughts. However, the toddler understands others' responses to behavior; thus, excessive punishment leads to bad feelings and praise leads to good feelings. These feelings gradually become incorporated into the toddler's self-concept.

Self-concept continues to develop actively during preschool years. The preschooler's sense of self becomes more defined as he or she realizes that he or she is separate and unique. During this stage of development, the child exhibits great sexual curiosity; the child is aware that he or she is different from others. In addition to this sense of sexual self, the preschooler's body image is incorporating both spatial relationships and increased coordination of his or her body.

The preschooler's sense of how he or she relates to others is more defined than in previous stages. The child's roles in the family and the world are beginning to take shape. During this stage, the child may share in older siblings' accomplishments or perceive himself or herself as not as good because he or she cannot achieve the same things. If a new baby is added to the family, the preschooler may respond with anger, jealousy, or regression. The family's response to the child's reaction influences his or her role performance and self-esteem.

Because of the preschooler's great amount of curiosity, he or she is learning body parts and names as well as attitudes about his or her body and self. If the preschooler's questions are discounted, met with great anxiety, or if the child is given misinformation, the child may develop a negative self-concept or poor body image.

Child and Adolescent

The school experience can strongly reinforce or alter the child's body image, sense of self, and identity. Teachers and peers become important influences on self-concept. Basically, the child compares self to peers and measures looks, abilities, and social self with them. Because of the rapid change and growth of this stage, the child's self-concept remains quite flexible, and changes are very individual. Figure 43-5 illustrates the flow of a child's self-concept development from age 6 to 12 years.

Through life experiences, children "place values on feelings and on themselves as individuals, and they make decisions about how to behave. When significant others accept an individual's expression of feelings, the self grows and thrives, and the individual feels valued and loved simply for existing. Thus the self and its feelings become part of the developing self-concept . . . " (Gary & Kavanagh, 1991).

The adolescent experiences remarkable changes. The body grows rapidly, and secondary sex characteristics and hormones appear. Both necessitate rapid change in the adolescent's view of self. The adolescent must incorporate these changes to establish a coherent body image. Peers and role models such as sports or media stars strongly influence self-concept. Clothes, hairstyles, and the way the person moves are extensions of body image; these are greatly influenced by peers. Sexual changes and peer group expectations regarding sexual behavior may lead to a sexually active role.

As the adolescent seeks added responsibility, the parents need to learn new methods of parenting. Striving for independence can be felt as a conflict for all family members. The adolescent may act in ways that seem to

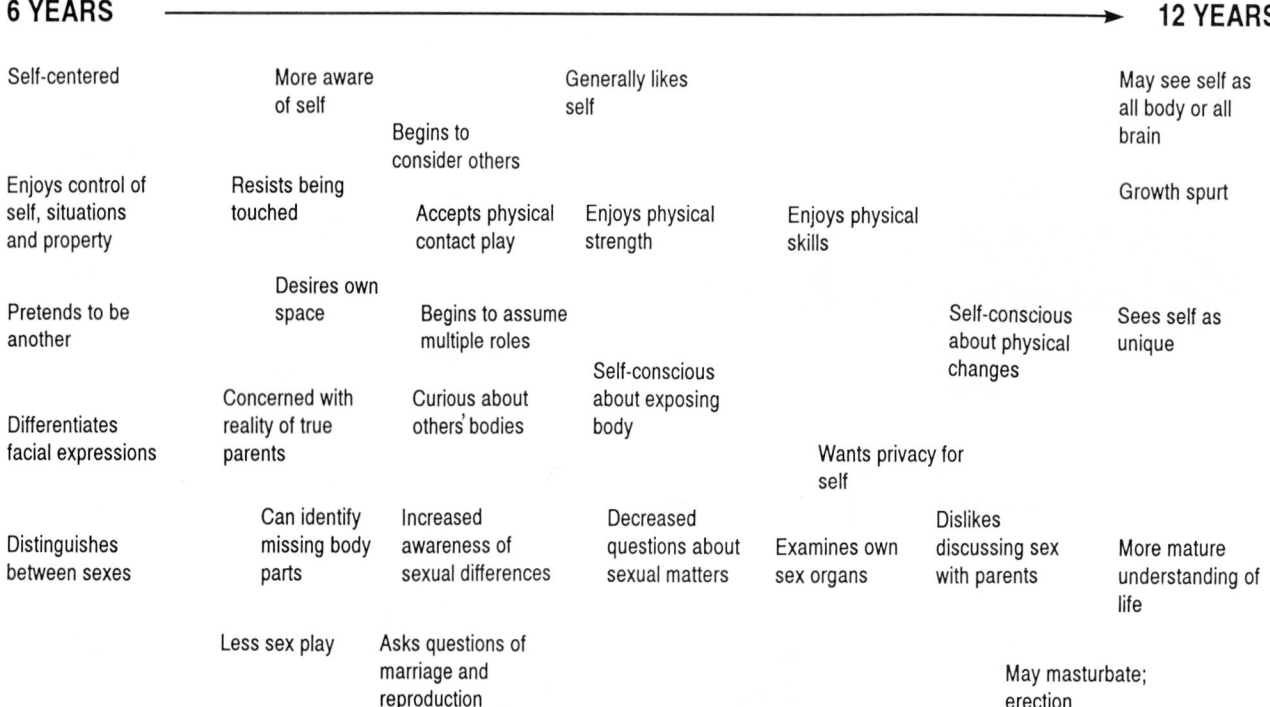

Figure 43–5. Self-concept development on a continuum from age 6 to 12 years. Attributes are approximate on the continuum. Although there is general consistency in development, each child is unique.

be in direct opposition to values and expectations of the family. This behavior occurs because the adolescent's chief developmental task is to develop and define personal identity.

Near the end of adolescence, the person chooses a career or a career path which will influence self-concept for the rest of life. In American society *what* the person does is often seen as *who* the person is. Occupation determines status, economic freedom, and much about lifestyle.

Adult and Older Adult

Adults continue to modify self-concept. The young adult moves away from the conforming peer group with a strong sense of self, a struggled-for personal identity. This is modified through life experiences. Common life experiences for early adulthood include forming intimate relationships, choosing a career, establishing a home base, and starting a family. Much of assumed role formation happens early in the adult stage of life.

During the fourth and into the fifth decade the person may question the fit of the identity chosen and experienced. The person may examine the meaning of self and contemplate the parts of self not previously explored. Roles and options taken and those discarded are examined as the person looks for more meaning in life. This process has been called an "authenticity crisis" by Sheehy (1974). The outcome of this authenticity crisis is renewal or resignation. With renewal, the person emerges from the crisis with an expanded sense of self. If resignation is the outcome of the crisis, the person's self remains defined by the narrow constraints of the roles he or she participates in. The sixth and early seventh decades leave the person living with the outcome of the authenticity crisis.

Retirement requires extraordinary changes in role performance and self-esteem. Since career roles have much to say about who a person is, the retired person is often described by who he or she *was,* implying the person no longer has value. Devaluing the person in this manner greatly affects self-esteem.

Body image is also affected later in life by physical changes such as decreased strength, lost skin turgor, and decreased sensory acuity. Because of America's value of youth, lowered self-esteem is experienced with the changed body image. Sensory changes also affect personal identity. If the environment does not provide feedback, the person may have difficulty determining what is or is not part of self.

When an older person accepts self, the person has found meaning in life. If contributions in the form of perspectives are accepted by others, especially younger members, self-esteem is enhanced. If the older person is treated as if he or she has no more to contribute, self-esteem is damaged.

Potential for Altered Self-Concept

Stressful Life Events

Most people face numerous stressors in daily life, many occurring simultaneously. Common stressors are financial difficulties, problems on the job, change or loss of a job, relationship concerns, sexuality concerns, divorce, moving, making new friends, loss of a loved one, competition, and making an important decision. Stressful events often challenge the person's identity and self-esteem. One stressor may be so intense as to paralyze the person and damage self-concept, but more often, cumulative stress wears away at self-concept (see Chap. 47). For example, a young couple marries and must move to another city where the husband found a job. They have difficulty buying a house due to the high cost of living in the new area, and immediately have financial difficulties. The wife would like to start a family, but must take a job for which she feels overqualified. They have difficulty making new friends and are overwhelmed by the numerous decisions that have to be made while starting their life together. The husband begins to feel that he is not a good provider and cannot afford the lifestyle he would like. The couple experiences stress in their relationship, and both may feel that self-esteem and identity are damaged.

Inadequate Coping

Inadequate coping can lead to self-concept dysfunction. In the above example, the young couple overwhelmed by stressful life events needs strong coping skills to maintain intact self-concepts. However, lack of support systems and an inability to prioritize and problem-solve contribute to further problems. Some people with inadequate coping develop defensive self-esteem. Defensive self-esteem is a protective mechanism in which the person reports high self-esteem in order to deny negative personal information. The person defends the self against hurt, failure, or anxiety through denial, grandiosity, or projection. This person has a high need for social approval.

Incomplete Developmental Tasks

Incomplete developmental tasks can lead to self-concept dysfunction. Adolescence is a particularly difficult time because of the many physical, emotional, and sexual changes occurring during this period. Adolescents must make decisions about the future, are seeking independence from their parents, and are pressured by peer groups. Body image and identity are not secure, but depend on others' perceptions. Self-esteem is fragile.

When a person has disturbed personal identity, he or she has difficulty stating who he or she is. This person may be unable to differentiate personal thoughts and feelings from those of others. This component of self-concept can be affected by changes in role or body image that are occurring during developmental transition. Relationships are affected by decreases in amount or quality of social interaction. If developmental tasks are not completed, self-concept dysfunction occurs, and may lead to incomplete tasks at a later developmental level.

Role Transition

Throughout a lifetime, a person will be required to make multiple role transitions. Two types of role transition are developmental and situational. Developmental role transitions are commonly associated with aging and growth, such as the transition from student to wage earner. Situational transitions are associated with change in relationships, such as the death of a spouse, necessitating the change in status from married to widowed. Either type of role transition can prompt role problems.

Common problems associated with role are role ambiguity, role strain, and role conflicts. Role ambiguity occurs when the person lacks knowledge of role expectations; this fosters anxiety and confusion. An example of role ambiguity is assuming a new job without an orientation to expected performance and responsibilities. Role strain occurs when the person perceives him- or herself as inadequate or unsuited for a role. This can occur in any role, or because of numerous roles. One example is a contemporary woman fulfilling roles of wife, lover, mother, employee, and professional, and feeling that she is not fulfilling any role the way she feels that she should. Role conflict is related to expectations concerning the role. Role conflict can be described as intrapersonal, interpersonal, or inter-role. Intrapersonal role conflict exists when role expectations conflict with the person's personal values, such as a nurse being asked to assist with an abortion when she feels it is an immoral act. Interpersonal role conflict exists when the person's expectations differ from some significant other's; for example, an adolescent might want to play in a rock band, but his or her parents value intellectual pursuits. Inter-role conflict exists when a person is expected to fulfill two or more roles simultaneously. In the case of the death of a spouse, a widow may become sole wage earner for the family, a single parent, and the caretaker of the house. She may be unsure what is expected of her in a new job, her role as wage earner may conflict with parenting responsibilities, and the combination of roles may be overwhelming. Self-concept can be damaged by such role transition.

Illness, Trauma, and Surgery

Illness, trauma, or surgery produce stress, role strain, reduce self-esteem, and alter body image. Altered body image occurs when the person experiences a disruption in the perception of the body image. Obviously, if the person has an actual loss of a body part or function, he or she will have a disrupted body image until the change is incorporated. Feelings associated with disturbed body image include helplessness, hopelessness, powerlessness, fear of others' reactions, and anger.

Amputation, mastectomy, burns, and facial trauma cause significant change in body structure and appearance. Cardiac disease, which limits activities, renal disease requiring dialysis, and a colostomy all change the function of the body. The ability of the self-concept to remain intact in light of illness, trauma, and surgery varies among people. The person's perception of the alteration and the importance he or she places on the body part or function affected influences body image dysfunction. For example, an athlete who places great importance on his or her long, strong legs for running would be devastated by a neurologic illness that produces weakness, placing him or her in a wheelchair. The athlete experiences decreased self-esteem as well as change in body image.

Manifestations of Altered Function

Manifestations of self-concept dysfunction range from subtle emotional and behavioral changes to full-blown, self-destructive behaviors. Manifestations may occur as an immediate reaction to self-concept dysfunction, or may be revealed years after self-concept development has been altered. See Table 43-2 for case studies of manifestations of altered self-concept.

Self-Care Deficit

People with dysfunctional self-concept may exhibit self-care deficit. People with chronic disease may disregard special diet instructions, not take medications, and not keep follow-up appointments. The hospitalized patient may avoid participation in medical and nursing treatment. Self-care deficit may also be characterized by poor personal hygiene, disregard for health maintenance activities, inappropriate exposure or concealment of parts of the body affected by disease, and lack of health-seeking behavior. The person may refuse to acknowledge health concerns or express feelings of not being worth special care or concern. For example, a middle-aged diabetic woman who has had one leg amputated keeps her lower body covered by a blanket, even in the warm weather. She rarely combs her hair or puts on makeup, and she frequently misses doctor's appointments and eats sweets because she feels she's "not worth it."

Emotional and Behavioral Changes

Emotional changes with self-concept dysfunction include feelings of depersonalization, hopelessness, help-

TABLE 43–2

Examples of Manifestations of Altered Self-Concept

Characteristics	Altered Self-Concept Patterns
Case 1: Self-Care Deficit	
A middle-aged diabetic with right below-the-knee amputation sits in a wheelchair all day with lower body covered by blanket. She misses doctor's appointments, disregards hygiene, and does not follow diet. When asked why, she replies, "I'm not worth it anymore."	Body image Self-esteem
Case 2: Emotional and Behavioral Changes	
A 20-year-old woman undergoing cancer chemotherapy has significant hair loss and 20-pound weight loss. She avoids eye contact with staff, refuses help in bathing and dressing, turns away from the mirror in her room, and refuses visitors. When confronted about her feelings and ability to cope, she seems apathetic.	Body image Identity
Case 3: Depression	
An elderly man is hospitalized for dehydration after the death of his wife. His facial expression is sad, he has no appetite, he complains of having no energy, and he often can be found crying. When asked why he has no visitors, he explains that most of his friends and relatives have died and he socializes little since he retired.	Self-esteem Role performance
Case 4: Self-Destructive Behavior (Alcoholism)	
A 40-year-old male banker is treated for injuries sustained in a car accident. He admits that he was drinking, but not heavily. He insists on discharge against medical advice, stating that he was just laid off and does not have medical insurance. When leaving, he comments, "Why do I have such bad luck?"	Self-esteem Role performance

lessness, alienation, fear of rejection, anger, sadness, shame, guilt, inadequacy, worthlessness, and suspicion of others. Emotional responses may be blunted or inappropriately intense.

Behavioral changes that indicate self-concept dysfunction include lack of interest in activities, inability to make decisions, withdrawal from social situations, isolation, refusal to look in the mirror, refusal to look at an affected body part or discuss a limitation, avoiding responsibility, showing hostility toward others, refusal to make eye contact, and negatively verbalizing about self. Behavior may become more dependent on or independent of others, including health-care providers. A woman who has undergone cancer chemotherapy and has lost her hair and undergone significant weight loss may show emotional and behavioral manifestations of self-concept dysfunction. She may refuse to look in the mirror, assume independence in bathing and dressing to prevent others from seeing her body, avoid eye contact with the staff, refuse visitors by saying she is tired, and seem emotionally apathetic.

Anxiety and Depression

Anxiety and depression are two common psychological disturbances that are manifestations of self-concept dysfunction. Whenever there is a change in body image, problems with roles or identity, and low self-esteem, the person is threatened. This threat is often the cause of great anxiety, and is frequently followed by the grieving process. Negative body image has also been related to depression (Noles, Cash, & Winstead, 1985) and to eating disorders (Ciseaux, 1980). Low self-esteem is frequently evident in major psychiatric disorders such as depression. An elderly man who has recently experienced loss of a job, loss of a wife, and loss of good health may show signs of depression.

Self-Destructive Behavior

Substance abuse (drugs, alcohol), sexual promiscuity, gambling, and overeating can be manifestations of self-concept dysfunction. These self-destructive behaviors numb the pain of self-hate and perpetuate the belief that the person with low self-esteem is a loser (Briggs, 1987). They are addictive behaviors, giving immediate gratification only. The person with low self-esteem and negative self-image cannot change self-destructive behaviors because he or she has difficulty seeing him- or herself in a more positive light. A 40-year-old male alcoholic who attributes loss of a job, financial insecurity, and injuries in a car accident to bad luck is an example of a person with self-destructive behavior.

Impact of Dysfunction on Activities of Daily Living

Alteration of self-concept may have an impact on the simplest activities of daily living (ADLs). People with low self-esteem or altered body image may try to avoid social situations and minimize interactions with others. They may not attend to hygiene needs or keep up their appearances. They may show little interest in recreational activities. Those people with altered body image often have difficulty moving in the environment until they incorporate the change psychologically. They may not maneuver well if the body image change involves a disfigured, amputated, or dysfunctional limb, despite physical rehabilitation.

People with identity dysfunction also lose interest in self-care activities, and often cannot make personal decisions. People with role dysfunction often place excessive demands on themselves to perform daily activities, and are self-deprecating when they cannot meet these demands. The quality of ADLs suffers in people with self-concept dysfunction, and there is a concurrent loss of enjoyment and productivity.

ASSESSMENT

The nurse who assesses the patient's self-concept is better equipped to implement the nursing process. This allows the nurse to assist the person in strengthening self-concept. At times, the patient's self-concept will be an identified strength that the nurse uses to enhance interventions for other nursing diagnoses. The nurse will collect subjective data in the areas of functional pattern identification, risk identification, and dysfunction identification. The nurse will also be alert to objective signs of self-concept dysfunction.

Subjective Data

Collection of subjective data will assist the nurse in identifying the patient's self-concept functioning, as well as assist in identifying risk factors or disturbed self-concept. Data are collected by asking purposeful questions during the initial interactions while collecting a nursing history, or as a focused assessment after caring for immediate needs.

Functional Pattern Identification

Gordon (1987) suggests the following questions be asked about self-concept when doing a nursing history:

How would you describe yourself?
Most of the time, how do you feel about yourself?
Are you experiencing changes in your body or the things you can do?
Is this a problem for you?
Have you or are you experiencing changes in the way you feel about yourself or your body?
Do you find things frequently make you feel angry, anxious, frustrated, afraid, sad, or annoyed? If so, what helps?

Further assessment of roles and relationships is discussed in Chapter 45.

Risk Identification

When assessing a person for risk of self-concept dysfunction, the nurse must consider developmental stage, previous experience, intensity of a stressor or threat, and self-expectations. Certain developmental stages are more risky for self-concept dysfunction. If the patient is an infant, what are the self-concepts of the parents like? Is the patient an adolescent who has had a body image change? Does the change affect sexuality? Assessment of previous experience should include past problems with self-concept and history of unsuccessful coping mechanisms, and lack of resources and support. Intensity of a stressor may help identify risk. Is the patient threatened by a role? By an illness or body image change? How important is good health or performance of a role? How serious is an illness or change in body function?

Assessment of the difference between the real self and the ideal self can also identify risk. What are the patient's expectations? How far is he or she from meeting these expectations? Are expectations unrealistic?

Dysfunctional Identification

Dysfunction identification also involves assessment of the patient's thoughts and feelings. People who do not possess a healthy self-concept are less able to cope with life. These people often express feelings of inferiority, self-doubt, and self-dislike. Does the patient verbalize negative feelings, such as "I don't like myself"; "I'm so ugly now"; "I'm worthless"; or "I'm a terrible mother"? Why does the person feel this way? In what area is the person having a problem—self-esteem, role function, personal identity, or body image?

Objective Data

Objective data about the patient's self-concept are gathered through direct observation. These data include behavioral manifestations such as lack of eye contact, and physical observations such as a missing body part or function. The person may try to conceal a body part, for example bandaging an arm scarred by burns after the burns have healed. The person may exhibit anxious behavior such as hand-wringing and shallow breathing, or grief behavior such as weeping.

While some behaviors may be easily observed, assessing the meaning of these behaviors may be more difficult. For instance, if the person hides a body part, does this manifest body image disturbance or extreme need for privacy?

These data are clues and must be judged with the subjective data to determine risk for or actual disturbances in self-concept. Ongoing observation of the patient's behavior helps identify changes in the self-concept.

NURSING DIAGNOSES AND PATIENT GOALS

NANDA-approved nursing diagnoses to be considered in caring for clients with dysfunctional self-concept are Body Image Disturbance, Self-Esteem Disturbance, Personal Identity Disturbance, and Altered Role Performance.

Diagnostic Statement: Body Image Disturbance

Definition

Body image disturbance is disruption in the way one perceives one's body image (NANDA, 1990).

Defining Characteristics

A or B must be present to justify the diagnosis of Body Image Disturbance. A = verbal response to actual or perceived change in structure and/or function; B = nonverbal response to actual or perceived change in structure and/or function. The following clinical manifesta-

tions may be used to validate the presence of A or B (NANDA, 1990).

Objective. Missing body part; actual change in structure and/or function; not looking at body part; not touching body part; hiding or overexposing body part (intentional or unintentional); trauma to nonfunctioning part; change in social involvement; change in ability to estimate spatial relationship of body to environment.

Subjective. Verbalization of: change in lifestyle; fear of rejection or of reaction by others; focus on past strength, function, or appearance; negative feelings about body; and feelings of helplessness, hopelessness, or powerlessness; preoccupation with change or loss; emphasis on remaining strengths, heightened achievement; extension of body boundary to incorporate environmental objects; personalization of part or loss by name; depersonalization of part or loss by impersonal pronouns; refusal to verify actual change.

Related Factors

Biophysical; cognitive/perceptual; psychosocial; cultural or spiritual (NANDA, 1990).

Diagnostic Statement: Self-Esteem Disturbance

Definition

Self-esteem disturbance is negative self-evaluation/feelings about self or self capabilities, which may be directly or indirectly expressed (NANDA, 1990).

Defining Characteristics

Self negating verbalization; expressions of shame/guilt; evaluates self as unable to deal with events; rationalizes away/rejects positive feedback and exaggerates negative feedback about self; hesitant to try new things/situations; denial of problems obvious to others; projection of blame/responsibility for problems; rationalizing personal failures; hypersensitive to slight or criticism; grandiosity (NANDA, 1990).

Diagnostic Statement: Personal Identity Disturbance

Definition

Personal identity disturbance is inability to distinguish between self and nonself (NANDA, 1990).

Defining Characteristics

To be developed by NANDA.

**Diagnostic Statement:
Altered Role Performance**

Definition

Altered role performance is disruption in the way one perceives one's role performance (NANDA, 1990).

Defining Characteristics

Change in self-perception of role; denial of role; change in others' perception of role; conflict in roles; change in physical capacity to resume role; lack of knowledge of role; change in usual patterns of responsibility (NANDA, 1990).

Related Factors

To be developed by NANDA.

Related Nursing Diagnoses

When making a diagnosis related to disturbed self-concept, the nurse must also consider diagnoses with common defining characteristics. Often these are inherent in dysfunctional self-concept. Among these diagnoses are: Anxiety, Ineffective Individual/Family Coping, Fear, Altered Family Process, Anticipatory Grieving, Hopelessness, Powerlessness, Social Isolation, and Altered Thought Processes.

Patient Goals

The following general areas may be included in the formulation of patient goals:

Patient will integrate a realistic body image.
Patient will express positive feelings about self.

Safety Alert

- Supervise patients with body image disturbance during ADLs and other activities, as they may have altered judgment related to the affected body part.
- Maintain an environment that encourages use of physical strengths without creating potential safety problems.
- Provide a structured and predictable setting for children with altered body image that will support the child's self-concept and self-worth.
- Provide an environment in which a child with an altered body image related to physical disability can risk physical activity without injury.

Patient will distinguish between self and nonself.
Patient will perform in accurate and acceptable role.

Patient goals will become more specific and differ according to the defining characteristics that apply to each patient.

IMPLEMENTATION

Implementation of the nursing care plan focuses on either promotion of a healthy self-concept or change of the altered self-concept. Interventions to promote self-concept include identifying strengths, maintaining a sense of self, and assisting development. Interventions used for altered self-concept function include using a therapeutic relationship, self-evaluation, and behavioral change. Nurses can incorporate these interventions into routine nursing care.

Nursing Interventions to Promote Health and Function

Identification of Strengths

Nurses can promote positive self-concept in their patients by assisting them in identifying strengths (Fig. 43-6). The continued use of internal and external resources helps strengthen identity, role performance, self-esteem, and body image. Various personal strengths include good sense of humor, good communication skills, good problem-solving ability, a nice smile, strong health maintenance patterns, strong values, a hobby, strong social support systems, a stable marriage, enjoyment in work, and a good education. When presented with stressors such as illness or loss of a loved one, the

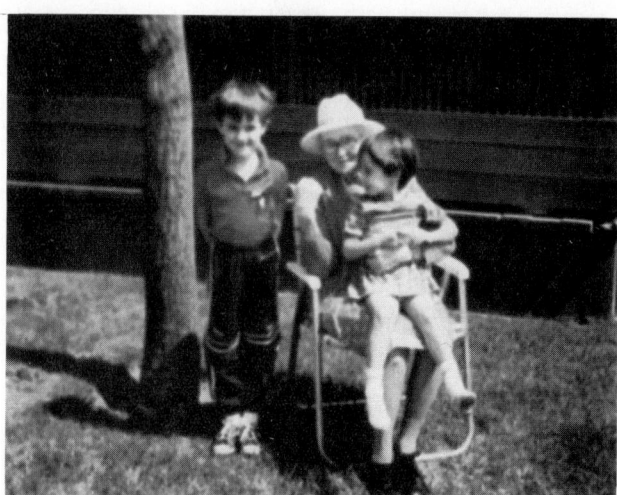

Figure 43–6. Intergenerational relationships in families add stability and strength in the face of changes. (Photo courtesy of University of Washington School of Nursing.)

TABLE 43–3
Developmental Interventions to Promote Self-Concept

Developmental Level	Intervention
Newborn	Assist family in adapting to new roles by establishing therapeutic relationship and educating members.
Infancy	Teach family about infant's need for movement, stimulation, safety.
	Encourage parents to help provide physical care and security to hospitalized infant.
Toddler	Allow toddler to develop skills through exploration.
	Support family and help toddler maintain self-control.
Preschool	Teach preschooler and family health maintenance behaviors.
	Encourage family to stay with the child if hospitalized, and let the child make some decisions about care.
School Age	Allow privacy.
	Teach parents of need for socialization and belonging.
	Allow liberal visitation and age-appropriate activities if hospitalized.
Adolescent	Educate adolescent about sexual health, drug and alcohol use.
	Educate family about identity and body image changes.
	If hospitalized, offer choices in care to maintain autonomy.
Adulthood	Use therapeutic relationship to support the adult and significant other, if hospitalized.
	Support decisions made in relationships and work role.
Older Adult	Treat older adult with respect and allow independence and individuality if hospitalized.
	Help older adult integrate loss of spouse, job, social support network, health, etc.

nurse can point these strengths out to the patient to reinforce self-concept. The patient should be encouraged to cultivate these strengths and use them in the coping process whenever the self is threatened.

Sense of Self

Nurses must treat patients in a respectful, personal manner to help them maintain a sense of self. While hospitalized, patients may experience stress and depersonalization. By respecting the patient's individuality, however, the nurse promotes a positive self-concept. Nurses should pay special attention to their interactions, both verbal and nonverbal, with all patients. Appropriate interventions include introducing oneself to the patient, addressing the patient by name, speaking respectfully, maintaining the patient's privacy, explaining all procedures and nursing activities, and paying attention to the patient's emotional responses.

Development of Self-Concept

The following discussion and Table 43-3 give nursing interventions that assist development and promote self-concept.

Neonatal Period. The nurse's role during this stage is to assist the family in adapting to their new roles and the self-concept related to these roles. Most often, this is accomplished through a therapeutic relationship which allows for exploration of expectations and provides support to deal with anxiety. The nurse educates the family about parental roles, body changes, emotional changes, and family role expectations. When this is done early it provides care that minimizes disturbances in self-concept for all members of the family, including the newborn.

Infancy. The nurse teaches the parents of the infant about the child's need for movement, stimulation, and safety. If a child is hospitalized during this period, an environment that facilitates continued development is crucial. This means having activities that are age-appropriate and health-appropriate, providing safety and security. The parents need to provide as much care as possible for the hospitalized infant. Assisting the parents to decrease their anxiety (to cope with the hospitalization) will assist the infant to feel more secure, foster trust, and promote continued self-concept development.

Toddlerhood. The toddler needs an environment that allows practice of newly developing skills, especially movement-related skills. These skills allow body image and esteem to develop positively. Education for the family includes the knowledge that repetitious positive input and allowing exploration for the toddler support the development of a favorable self-concept. Hospitalization or illness during toddlerhood affects the development of self-concept. The nurse supports the toddler and family by helping the toddler maintain self-control.

Preschool. During the preschool years the nurse educates the family about normal development and supports their establishing an effective environment that facilitates growth. Because the child has increased sexual feelings, the preschooler fears damage to his or her body; therefore the preschooler needs support and education concerning health maintenance behaviors, such as personal hygiene and health-care visits. This can be accomplished through visits to health-care providers with other family members, or through supportive treatment of the child during routine examinations. Hospitalization or serious illness in the preschooler is especially difficult. The preschooler has many fantasies about punishment, abandonment, or physical harm. The nurse combats these fantasies by including the preschooler in decisions as much as possible. Additionally, the family should stay with the child as much as possible. The nurse must remember that the family may respond to the child's hospitalization with guilt, helplessness, and anxiety. The family will need assistance with these feelings in order to aid the child.

School Age. The nurse's role in this stage of development continues to include education and understanding of the child's need for socialization and belonging. Frequently, it is the school nurse who teaches reproduction and health in the school setting. If the child is hospitalized during this period, the nurse must be cognizant of the changing need for privacy in this age group, as well as the child's need to know that he or she still belongs to the family, peer group, etc. Additionally, the school-age child needs information about his or her illness and treatments. Parents again need support and help dealing with their fear and anxiety.

Adolescence. The nurse supports the adolescent and family through the process of assuming roles and establishing independence. The nurse teaches the family about the developmental process and why individual family members may have intense feelings during this period. The adolescent experiments as he or she makes choices to establish identity. Health education for the adolescent includes sexual information concerning birth control, AIDS, and other sexually transmitted diseases. A further concern is drug use and alcohol abuse. The adolescent needs to know the ramifications of choosing drugs or alcohol as a coping style. The adolescent may need assistance to learn and practice alternate coping behaviors.

Often, adolescents are hospitalized on the pediatric unit, which may contradict the person's view of him- or herself as an independent, grown-up person. Offering the adolescent choices regarding care helps the adolescent maintain some autonomy. Feedback about the strengths and weaknesses of the adolescent will help him or her establish a realistic self concept.

Adulthood. The nurse assists the adult with role satisfaction primarily in intimate relationships and occupation. Interventions include use of a therapeutic relationship, structuring the environment to provide for successes, and allowing the person time and support while exploring the meaning of life. A feeling of generativity enhances self-concept. The nurse continues to offer support to significant others.

Older Adult. Older people do not seek care as "old" people but as people with needs. Loss of independence associated with aging often brings loss of self-esteem. The nurse approaches older people as adults and supports appropriate independence and self-care, which enhances self-concept. In working with older people, the nurse's role is to assist in integrating changes, most often loss, into their self-concept. The nurse also enhances self-concept of the older adult by using respect and allowing individuality. Allowing the patient to keep personal belongings, listening to stories told by the patient, respecting privacy, explaining procedures, and allowing the patient extra time to accomplish tasks are some of the interventions aimed at older adults.

Nursing Interventions for Altered Self-Concept

Therapeutic Relationship

Nurses intervene with patients with altered self-concept through a therapeutic relationship. To develop a therapeutic relationship, the nurse must demonstrate great self-awareness and effective communication. The nurse establishes rapport with the patient by conveying a sense of friendship and trust. When the nurse shows empathy, the patient feels that the nurse understands his or her feelings and will care for his or her needs. Once the relationship is established, the nurse uses therapeutic communication techniques, such as active listening, reflection, and reality-based feedback. Through therapeutic communication, the nurse assists the patient with defining self-concept problems and attempting to problem-solve.

Self-Evaluation

Nursing interventions that assist the patient with positive self-evaluation can help change poor self-concept. People with low self-esteem frequently put themselves down and act in ways that perpetuate negative self-evaluation. To break this cycle, the patient needs help in realistically evaluating the self, and developing more positive thoughts and feelings about the self. Emphasis is placed on positive attributes rather than negative behavior. The

---

Selected Nursing Interventions for Common Body-Image Problems

Body Image Disturbances

- Identify the patient's concerns regarding changed body image.
- Provide opportunities to openly discuss feelings related to body image.
- Listen attentively and nonjudgmentally to concerns.
- Demonstrate unconditional acceptance of the patient's altered body image.
- Accept the patient's coping mechanisms for adjusting to the altered body image.
- Promote independent decision-making in as many areas as possible.
- Assist the patient as needed with hygiene and personal grooming.
- Encourage patient to participate in care of affected body part.
- Provide opportunities for success in personal care or in resuming normal activities of daily living.
- Teach family to focus on the patient's abilities, rather than the body image change.
- Refer the patient and family to appropriate support groups.

---

nurse can assist the patient to point out tasks or accomplishments that deserve positive feedback. The nurse offers praise honestly and encourages the patient to do so. The nurse should also be a model for the patient by acting confident, making positive statements, and accepting compliments.

Behavioral Change

Nursing interventions aimed at changing behavior also assist the patient with self-concept problems. General measures that bring about behavioral changes include accepting responsibility for self, defining realistic goals, using resources to enact change, and rewarding positive outcomes. The nurse can help the patient accept responsibility for self by suggesting the patient make "I" statements that reflect his or her thoughts and feelings. For example, for a patient with role performance problems, instead of saying, "nothing ever goes right," a more active statement might be "I can't get the hang of my new job." This is the first step in realizing that the patient may have the power to change behavior.

In helping the patient define realistic goals, the nurse assists the patient in evaluating expectations. If expectations are unrealistic or the discrepancy between the real self and the ideal self is too great, behavior will not change. Goals should be specific, such as "I will ask my boss for a 2-week training period on the new computer system." The nurse helps the patient identify resources to accomplish goals, including, for example, a computer training department at the office, night school courses, or someone to help around the house so the patient can temporarily devote more time to work.

The patient will be more likely to change behavior if he or she feels he or she will be rewarded for more positive behavior. The nurse can point out rewards, such as a feeling of greater competence, less time spent at the office, greater productivity, and praise by others. By assisting the patient with problem-solving, his or her role performance should improve, and self-concept will be strengthened.

Discharge Planning and Home Care

The patient with self-concept disturbance often requires psychosocial assistance beyond basic nursing. The nurse assists the patient with recognizing difficulties and accepting additional therapy. After this, the nurse and patient can initiate plans for additional care, both during and after hospitalization. The goals of discharge planning are effective teaching and referral.

The teaching plan may include where and how to use community resources, such as support groups, or individual teaching concerning stages of loss. Referral may be to a specialized support group such as a group for

---

Patient Teaching

Instruct the patient as follows:

- Encourage family and friends to visit.
- State views and opinions. They have worth and validity.
- Identify strengths and develop them further.
- Learn how to use strengths for successful coping.
- Explore the meaning of life and develop a value system.
- Think positively about one's self.
- Set realistic goals for one's self.
- Learn about community resources and how to use them.
- Develop an interest in people and their personalities.

mastectomy patients, or may be for therapy through a psychiatric nurse specialist, psychologist, or psychiatrist. The physician should be consulted regarding outpatient referrals. If the patient is to receive home health follow-up, communication about the care plan to the home health nurse is essential. For example, home care for the patient after mastectomy should include interventions to help incorporate a change in body image and strengthen self-esteem, if those problem areas were identified while the patient was hospitalized. Whatever interventions initiated in the hospital that work should be described in a home health referral for continuity of care after discharge.

EVALUATION

Specific outcome criteria are the evaluation tools used to measure the attainment of goals in self-concept. If the nurse asks what he or she hopes to see or hear if the interventions he or she chooses are effective, the goals will be behavioral in nature. The nurse then asks under what circumstances the patient will exhibit that behavior, and by when. Such goals are measurable. Since the nurse and patient (in most cases) established goals and outcome criteria, the patient and nurse discuss whether these criteria have been met. Outcome criteria for patient goals discussed earlier in the chapter could be the following:

Goal
Patient will integrate a realistic body image.

Possible Outcome Criteria
- Patient speaks about his or her body within 2 days after surgery.
- Patient views self in mirror within 3 days after surgery.
- Patient assists with dressing changes within 4 days after surgery.

Goal
Patient will express positive feelings about self.

Possible Outcome Criteria
- Patient establishes eye contact with nurse during conversation within 2 days.
- Patient lists negative attitudes and their effect on self by discharge.
- Patient verbalizes feelings of success with self-care activities by discharge.

Goal
Patient will distinguish between self and nonself.

Possible Outcome Criteria
- Patient identifies feelings of depersonalization as related to illness within 2 days.
- Patient states realistic expectations for discharge within 5 days.
- Patient expresses feelings of hope and power over own life within 7 days.

Goal
Patient will perform in accurate and acceptable role.

Possible Outcome Criteria
- Patient expresses interest in caring for newborn within 1 day.
- Patient identifies three coping strategies to help assume new role within 2 days.
- Patient performs basic care of newborn successfully within 3 days.

Nursing Research

Selected Nursing Research Studies

Orr, D. A., Reznikof, M., & Smith, G. M. (1989). Body image, self-esteem, and depression in burn-injured adolescents and young adults. *Journal of Burn Care and Rehabilitation, 9,* 454–461.

Santopinto, M. D. A. (1989). The relentless drive to be ever thinner: A study using the phenomenological method. *Nursing Science Quarterly, 2*(1), 29–36.

Koehler, M. L. (1989). Relationship between self-concept and successful rehabilitation. *Rehabilitation Nursing, 14*(1), 9–12.

Volden, C., Langemo, D., & Adamson, M. (1990). The relationship of age, gender, and exercise practices to measures of health, lifestyle, and self-esteem. *Applied Nursing Research, 3*(1), 77–82.

Possible Topics for Nursing Inquiry

- What nursing interventions permit the greatest reinforcement of positive self-worth and self-concept for the patient with altered body image?
- What nursing interventions place the elderly patient at risk for altered self-concept?
- What is the relationship between a person's coping behavior and successful adaptation to altered body image?

Nursing Management Plan
The Patient with Body Image Disturbance

Nursing Diagnosis: Body image disturbance related to change in physical appearance manifested by patient's refusal to look at body.

Patient Goal: Patient will express improved perception of physical appearance.

Patient Outcome Criteria

- Patient discusses his or her physical changes within 2 days of surgery.
- Patient demonstrates participation in ADLs within 3 days.
- Patient uses coping skills to prepare for changes in physical appearance within 3 days.
- Patient views affected body part within 1 week of surgery.

Nursing Intervention	Scientific Rationale
1. Assess patient's strengths that will positively affect body image, e.g., family relationships.	1. Assessment of factors in the patient that can contribute to improved body image builds on the patient's strengths.
2. Provide opportunities to discuss altered appearance and self-worth.	2. Stating feelings verbally often helps to clarify and provide perspective for the patient.
3. Assist with grooming.	3. When patient is unable physically or emotionally to groom self the nurse's care activities indicate the nurse's concern for the patient's welfare and help to establish rapport.
4. Encourage the patient to participate in self-grooming and to strive for independence.	4. Encouraging participation in self-care provides a sense of control.
5. Encourage identification and use of positive coping strategies.	5. Use of coping strategies that have worked effectively for the patient aids in successful coping with body image.
6. Encourage patient to cultivate positive coping strategies.	6. Use of internal and external resources helps strengthen self-esteem and body image.
7. Provide a mirror for the patient to view self. The patient may want to do so in privacy.	7. Patient must view physical changes before he or she can integrate them into a realistic body image.
8. Provide information and education regarding the altered appearance, support groups, and other resources.	8. Individualized education and information meet the unique needs of the patient.

Key Concepts

- Self-concept is the mental image one has of one's self.
- Characteristics of normal self-concept include the dimensions of self-perception: self-knowledge, self-expectation, social self, and self-evaluation.
- Positive body image, self-esteem, strong personal identity, and role performance are normal functional patterns of self-concept.
- The self-concept of the newborn and infant depends on that of the mother.
- The rapid body growth and sexual development of the adolescent lead to a changing view of self.
- Factors that affect normal self-concept include bio-

logic make-up; culture, values and beliefs; coping and stress tolerance; previous experience; developmental level; and illness.

- Several factors place a person at risk for altered self-concept, including stressful life events, inadequate coping resources, incomplete developmental tasks, role transition, and illness, trauma, or surgery.
- Manifestations of altered self-concept include self-care deficit, emotional and behavioral changes, anxiety and depression, and self-destructive behavior (such as alcoholism, drug abuse, and sexual promiscuity).
- Functional assessment of self-concept involves collection of subjective data through questions such as "How would you describe yourself?" and "How do you feel about yourself?"

■ NANDA-approved nursing diagnoses to be considered in caring for patients with dysfunctional self-concept are Body Image Disturbance, Self-Esteem Disturbance, Personal Identity Disturbance, and Altered Role Performance.

■ Personal strengths the nurse can encourage the patient to cultivate to promote positive self-concept include good sense of humor, good communication skills, strong health maintenance patterns, a hobby, strong social support systems, enjoyment in work, and a good education.

■ Loss of independence associated with aging may bring loss of self-esteem; therefore, the nurse should treat older adults with a sense of respect and individuality.

■ Nurses help patients with low self-esteem by assisting them with realistic self-evaluation and development of more positive thoughts and feelings about themselves.

■ Nurses can also help bring about behavioral change in patients with altered self-concept by assisting them to accept responsibility for themselves, define realistic goals, use resources to enact change, and reward positive outcomes.

References

Berscheid, E., Walster, E., & Bohrnstedt, G. (1973). Body Image. *Psychology Today,* Nov., 119–131.

Briggs, D. C. (1987). Your child's self-esteem: The key to life. In E.Shiff (Ed.), *Experts advise parents.* New York: Delacorte Press.

Ciseaux, A. (1980). Anorexia nervosa: A view from the mirror. *American Journal of Nursing, 80,* 1468–1474.

Coopersmith, S. (1967). *Antecedents of self esteem.* San Francisco: Freeman.

Erikson, E. (1963). *Childhood and Society* (2nd ed.). New York: Norton.

Freud, S. (1920/1966). *Lectures on psychoanalysis* (J. Strachey, ed. and trans.). New York: Norton.

Gary, F., & Kavanagh, C. K. (1991). *Psychiatric mental health nursing.* Philadelphia: J. B. Lippincott.

Gordon, M. (1987). *Manual of nursing diagnosis* (2nd ed.). New York: McGraw-Hill.

Havighurst, R. (1972). *Developmental tasks and education* (3rd ed.). New York: David McKay.

Kohlberg, L. (1969). Stage and sequence: The cognitive developmental approach to socialization. In D. A. Goslin (ed.), *Handbook of socialization: Theory and research.* Chicago: Rand McNally.

NANDA (1990). *Taxonomy I revised 1990, with official nursing diagnoses.* St. Louis, MO: North American Nursing Diagnosis Association.

Noles, S., Cash, T., & Winstead, B. (1985). Body image, physical attractiveness, and depression. *Journal of Consulting Clinical Psychology, 53,* 88–94.

Norris, J., & Kunes-Cornell, M. (1985). Self-esteem disturbance. *Nursing Clinics of North America, 20,* 745–761.

Piaget, J. (1969). The psychology of the child. New York: Basic Books.

Rogers, C. R. (1961). *On becoming a person.* Boston: Houghton Mifflin.

Rotter, J. B. (1966). Generalized expectancies for internal versus external locus of control reinforcement. *Psychology Monographs, 80,* 1–28.

Sheehy, G. (1974). *Passages.* New York: E. P. Dutton.

Stanwyck, D. (1983). Self esteem through the life span. *Family and Community Health, 6*(2), 11–28.

Sullivan, H. (1953). *The interpersonal theory of psychiatry.* New York: W. W. Norton.

Bibliography

Alfano, G. (1988). Oh no, not me. *Geriatric Nursing,* 217.

Antonucci, T., & Jackson, J. (1983). Physical health and self esteem. *Family Community Health, 6,* 1–9.

Branden, N. (1969). *The psychology of self esteem.* Los Angeles: Nash.

Brouse, A. (1988). Easing the transition to the maternal role. *Journal of Advanced Nursing, 13,* 167–172.

Fawcett, J., Bliss-Holtz, V., Haas, M., et al. (1986). Spouse body image changes during and after pregnancy: A replication and extension. *Nursing Research, 35,* 220–223.

Fawcett, J., & Frye, S. (1980). An exploratory study of body image dimensionality. *Nursing Research, 29,* 324–327.

Hardy, M., & Conway, M. (1978). *Role theory: Perspectives for health professionals.* Boston: Appleton-Century-Crofts.

Horgan, P. (1987). Health status perceptions affect health-related behaviors. *Journal of Gerontologic Nursing, 13,* 30–33.

Keteran, S. (1985). Professional and bureaucratic role conceptions and moral behavior among nurses. *Nursing Research, 34,* 248–253.

Kim, M. J., MacFarland, M., & McLane, A. (1984). *Classification of nursing diagnoses: Proceedings of the fifth national conference.* St. Louis: C. V. Mosby.

Kim, M. J., & Moritz, D. A. (1983). *Classification of nursing diagnoses: Proceedings of the third and fourth national conferences.* New York: McGraw-Hill.

Kurtz, R. (1969). Sex differences and variation in body attitudes. *Journal of Consulting and Clinical Psychology, 33,* 625–629.

Lambert, C., & Lambert, V. (1988). A review and synthesis of the research on role conflict and its impact on nurses involved in faculty practice programs. *Journal of Nursing Education, 27,* 54–58.

Lego, S. (1984). *The American handbook of psychiatric nursing.* Philadelphia: J. B. Lippincott.

Long, K., & Hamlin, C. (1988). Use of the Piers–Harris self concept scale with Indian children: Cultural considerations. *Nursing Research, 37,* 43–46.

Mahler, M., Pine, F., & Bergmann, A. (1975). *The psychological birth of the human infant: Symbiosis and individuation.* New York: Basic Books.

McBride, L. (1986). Teaching about body image: A technique for improving body satisfactions. *Journal of School Health, 56,* 76–77.

McGonigle, D. (1988). Making self talk positive. *American Journal of Nursing, 88*(5), 725–726.

McFarland, G., & Wasli, E. (1986). *Nursing diagnosis and process in mental health nursing.* Philadelphia: J. B. Lippincott.

McLane, A. (1987). *Classification of nursing diagnosis: Proceedings of the seventh conference of the North American Nursing Diagnosis Association.* St. Louis: C. V. Mosby.

Meleis, A. J. (1975). Role insufficiency and role supplementation: a conceptual framework. *Nursing Research, 24,* 264–271.

Morris, C. (1985). Self concept as altered by the diagnosis of cancer. *Nursing Clinics of North America, 20,* 611–630.

Murray, R., & Zentner, J. (1975). *Nursing assessment and health promotion through the life span.* Englewood Cliffs, NJ: Prentice Hall.

Quinn-Krach, P., & Hoozer, H. (1988). Sexuality of the aged and the attitudes and knowledge of nursing students. *Journal of Nursing Education, 27,* 359–363.

Reed, G., & Sech, E. (1985). Bulemia: A conceptual model for group treatment. *Journal of Psychosocial Nursing and Mental Health Services, 23,* 16–22.

Rice, M., & Szopa, T. (1988). Group intervention for reinforcing self worth following mastectomy. *Oncology Nurse Forum, 15,* 33–37.

Stuart, G., & Sundeen, S. (1983). *Principles and practice of psychiatric nursing* (2nd ed.). St. Louis: C. V. Mosby.

Sundeen, S., Stuart, G., Rankin, E., et al. (1976). *Nurse–client interaction.* St. Louis: C. V. Mosby.

UNIT XIII
Roles and Relationships

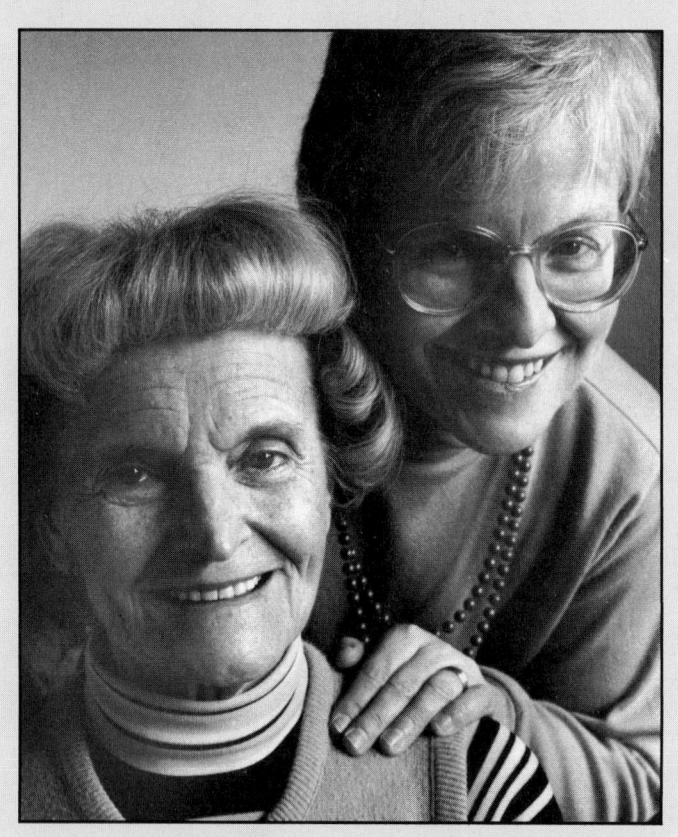

CHAPTERS

44 Communication:
Social Interaction

────────────────────

45 Families and Their
Relationships

────────────────────

46 Loss and Grieving

────────────────────

A person's roles and relationships make up the fabric of his or her life responsibilities. These areas of psychosocial function have a significant impact on health and wellness, and conversely, on other areas of function. Unit XIII explores roles and relationships.

The first chapter discusses the concept of communication as both a human need and a form of social interaction essential in any human relationship. Nurses need to be able to assess a patient's ability to communicate his or her needs to provide holistic nursing care. Most importantly, nurses need to know how to intervene for a patient who has impaired verbal communication and cannot readily make his or her needs known. The chapter emphasizes nursing interventions to promote health and function as well as those for altered function.

The next chapter considers families and their relationships. As health care focuses more on self-responsibility, nurses need to understand and assess family functioning so they can involve families as the primary source of patient support. This chapter provides a beginning discussion of family concepts, featuring holistic nursing interventions to promote family health and function and discussing sources of support for altered family function.

The final chapter discusses loss and grieving. Any loss a patient experiences threatens his or her roles and relationships. Conversely, the loss of a patient produces stress and requires adaptation for the family. Death of a patient or of a patient's loved one requires nursing interventions to promote health and function as well as those to facilitate coping.

This unit focuses on the universal human need for and influence of relationships with others. Both are interwoven with a person's health and well-being.

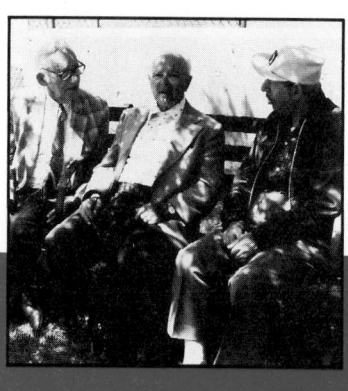

Communication:
Social Interaction

44

LEARNING OBJECTIVES

Upon completion of this chapter, the student will be able to do the following:

- Define communication.
- Identify the areas dominant for language in the left hemisphere of the brain.
- Describe the components of speech and language.
- Describe verbal and nonverbal communication.
- Describe development of language and communication during the lifespan.
- Identify common causes of altered communication.
- Identify the different types of aphasia.

- Discuss the effect of dysfunctional communication.
- Use subjective and objective data in assessing speech and language capabilities.
- Provide interventions facilitating communication.
- Discuss socialization needs of people with altered communication.
- Discuss referral available to people with communication dysfunction.

KEY TERMS

Anomia
Aphasia
Articulation
Coma
Communication

Dysarthria
Language
Laryngectomy
Nonverbal
  communication

Phonation
Resonance
Tracheostomy
Tracheotomy

Normal Communication
   Anatomy of Communication Centers
     Production and Coordination of Communication
   Normal Function of Communication
   Characteristics of Normal Communication
     Verbal Communication: Language
     Nonverbal Communication
   Factors Affecting Normal Communication
   Lifespan Considerations
Altered Communication
   Potential for Altered Communication
     Impaired Speech Apparatus
     Disturbed Articulation
     Cortical Control Interference
   Manifestations of Altered Communication
     Aphasia
     Dysarthria
     Total Loss of Speech
   Impact on Activities of Daily Living
Assessment
   Subjective Data
     Functional Pattern Identification
     Risk Identification
     Dysfunctional Identification

   Objective Data
     Physical Assessment
     Diagnostic Tests and Procedures
Nursing Diagnosis and Patient Goals
   Diagnostic Statement: Impaired Verbal
     Communication
     Definition
     Defining Characteristics
     Related Factors
   Related Nursing Diagnoses
   Patient Goals
Implementation
   Nursing Interventions to Promote Health and
     Function
     Patient Teaching
   Nursing Interventions for Altered Communication
     Function
     Orientation to Surroundings
     Alternative Communication Methods
     Environmental Restrictions
     Coping Measures
   Discharge Planning and Home Care
Evaluation
Key Concepts

Humans are set apart from other organisms by their ability to communicate with one another. The combination of speech and language, along with the senses of vision and hearing, allows humans to receive, interpret, and express ideas, feelings, and needs. Communication brings people together while it sets them apart from one another: it allows individuals to be unique.

The importance of communication in the nurse–patient relationship (therapeutic relationship) was discussed in Chapter 17. Written communication as part of nursing process was discussed in Chapter 10. This chapter discusses the functioning of people through communication in their roles and relationships with others.

NORMAL COMMUNICATION

Communication is the interchange of information between at least two people. There are various types of communication and several elements to the communication process (see Chap. 17). There must be a message delivered from one person (the sender or source) to another (the receiver) (see Fig. 17-2). The message must get the attention of the receiver. Sometimes the sending and receiving of messages occur simultaneously and messages must be separated out. Once a message has been received it must be interpreted. Interpretation is based on language abilities, cultural influences, cognitive function, and past experiences.

Anatomy of Communication Centers

Speech production is a motor activity that requires the coordination of laryngeal and respiratory structures to produce the sound patterns of speech. To understand how motor activity and interpretation are coordinated by the brain, one must look at how the brain functions in relation to speech and language. The brain is divided into two sides, or hemispheres, which are connected and work closely together to monitor and regulate the body's functions. The left hemisphere has been found to be dominant for language function in approximately 90% to 99% of right-handed people (Fig. 44-1). Similarly, in left-handed people, the left hemisphere is dominant for language function 50% to 75% of the time (Pimental, 1986). Additionally, the left hemisphere develops those functions that are closely related to speech and language, including arithmetic ability, verbal ideation and abstraction, and interpretation and understanding of speech.

Production and Coordination of Communication

Speech and vocalization involve the respiratory system, the speech control centers in the cerebral cortex, and the structures of the mouth and nose. Speech is basically composed of the functions of phonation (achieved by the larynx) and articulation (achieved by the mouth).

Phonation. **Phonation** is the process by which humans create vocal sound. Sounds are made when air from the lungs is forced through the oral cavity or nasal passages during exhalation. As forced air moves past the vocal cords (larynx), the vocal folds vibrate.

The vocal pitch, volume, and quality or timbre of phonation are produced at this site. The pitch of the voice can be changed by stretching or relaxing the vocal cords or by changing the mass of the vocal cords' edges by contracting the thyroarytenoid muscles. The volume of the voice is controlled, in part, by the amount of air being forced through the larynx. To force the air through the larynx, the lungs must recoil by means of constriction of the rib cage and contraction of the diaphragm.

Articulation. **Articulation** refers to the enunciation of words and sentences. It is affected by the lips, the tongue, and the soft palate. The movement of the tongue against the palate, the teeth, and the muscles of the mouth and face influences the sound that is made. The lips and the surrounding muscles provide the vault and assist the oral cavity in making rapid changes in shape and size for sound formation and articulation.

The major organs of resonance include the mouth, nose, associated nasal sinuses, pharynx, and the chest. **Resonance** refers to echoing or resounding of sound through various passages. The amount of resonance is reflected in the tone and timbre of the voice. The function of the resonators is demonstrated by the change in voice quality when a person has a severe head cold with congestion.

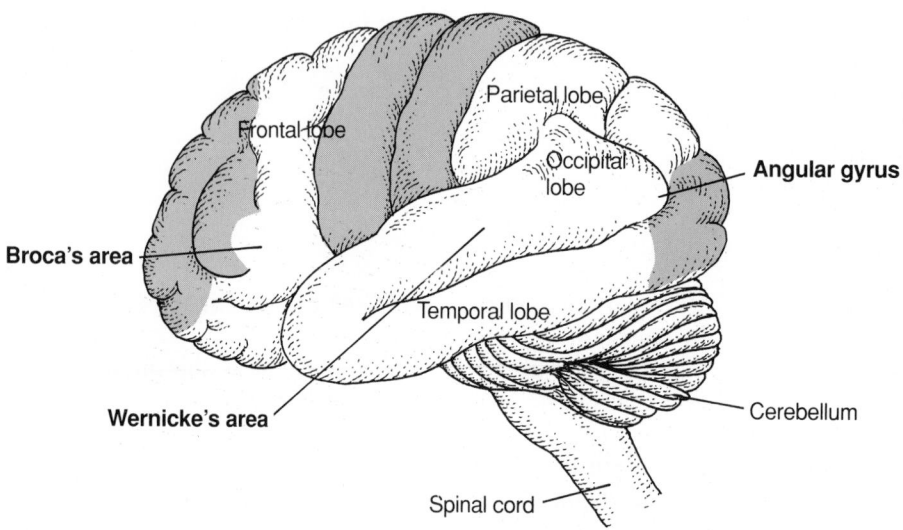

Figure 44–1.   Lateral view of left brain with speech centers. Broca's area allows articulation of words, phrases, and sentences. Wernicke's area allows for comprehension of speech, reading, and writing. Angular gyrus receives incoming sensory stimuli and relates the stimuli to language.

region of the cortex can cause either total or partial inability to speak.

Prerequisites to Adequate Speech Production

Intact Structures for the Physical Production of Sound

- Larynx
- Respiratory structures
- Oral cavity structures
- Nasal cavity structures

Functioning Structures for the Physical Reception of Sound

- Discriminating auditory apparatus
- Receptive speech center

Maturation of the Central Nervous System

- Myelination of major neural pathways
- Growth in functional capacity of the cerebral cortex
- Functioning speech control center in the cerebral cortex

Cognitive Maturation

- Adequate intellectual ability
- Ability to process thoughts

Psychological Stimulation

- Verbal and nonverbal human interaction
- Environmental stimulation

From Broadwell, D., & Saunders, R. (in press). Child health nursing: A comprehensive approach to the care of children and their families. Philadelphia: J. B. Lippincott.

Cortical Control. In addition to vocalization, speech involves the formation in the mind of the thoughts, words, and meanings to be expressed. Thought formation and word choice occur in the sensory areas of the brain. The motor aspect of vocalization is controlled by Broca's area of the dominant hemisphere of the motor cortex. The patterns for control of the larynx, lips, mouth, respiratory system, and other muscles of articulation are controlled by this area of the cortex. The muscular movements that control the actual emission of sound are activated by the facial and laryngeal regions of the motor cortex. Dysfunction or destruction of this

Normal Function of Communication

Communication is essential to social interaction. It enables a person to relate to people in his or her family and community (Fig. 44-2). The communication may revolve around home, work, play, and study. Communication helps a person identify and express roles in those relationships. For instance, a father may discipline a child, an instructor may give instructions for an assignment, or a student may ask questions for clarification of studies.

Communication aids not only in developing the function of social interaction but also supplies a means of expression for other healthy functioning: coping behaviors, self-concept, expression of values and belief (including communication between oneself and a higher being).

Characteristics of Normal Communication

Communication does not occur in a vacuum but is influenced by many factors. It involves both verbal and nonverbal exchanges, which occur simultaneously during a conversation (see Chap. 17).

Verbal Communication: Language

Language is the ability to convey needs, ideas, and feelings through the systematic use of symbols. Humans are unique in being able to use symbolic codes to communicate abstract ideas through a highly refined verbal language (Schuster and Ashburn, 1986).

The interaction and integration of the brain, neural system, and organs of speech biophysically permit humans not only to produce sounds but also to remember what they said in the past and to speak about the future. From early times, humans have sought ways to communicate through verbal symbols of speech, encoding meaning to certain sounds and usages.

The next step was to convert those verbal sounds to a written format that could be deciphered readily by all the members of the group. Pictographs were among the earliest forms of written language, using line drawings or depictions of objects or events to communicate meaning. Hieroglyphics were a sophisticated form of pictographs that combined language and pictures.

Verbal language evolved into special sounds, tones, and inflections peculiar to groups of people. These languages began to take on territoriality, ultimately dividing people into cultures and nations. These languages united the people who used the same language; at the

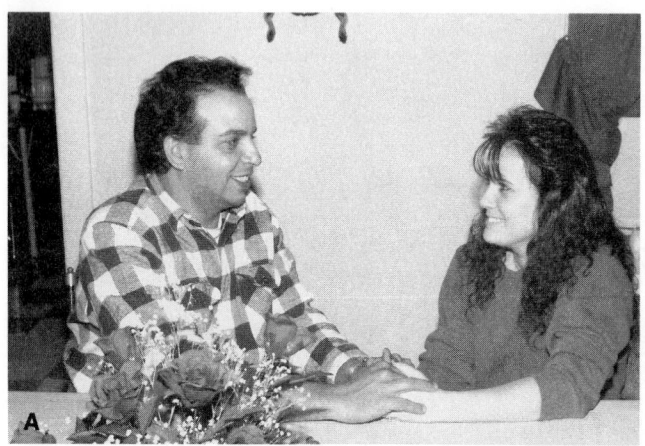

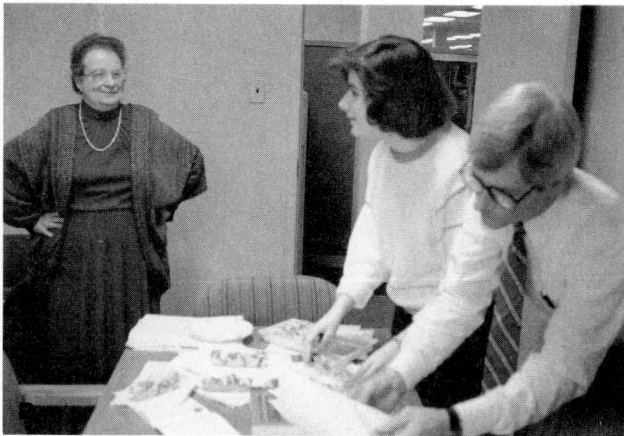

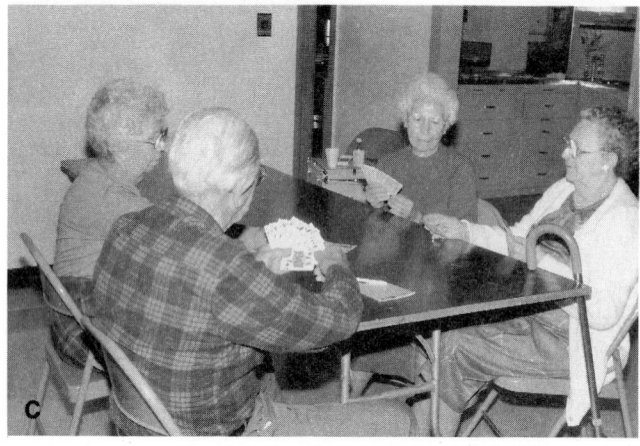

Figure 44–2.   Communication enables development of roles and relationships in social interaction.   **A:** An engaged couple share values and plan for the future.   **B:** A birthday party in the office strengthens working conditions.   **C:** Senior citizens find enjoyment in sharing interests in a senior social group.

same time, it separated people from others who spoke a different language. Speaking, writing, and reading of the language of the group were taught to pass the culture and the language on to future generations.

As civilization evolved, printing by mechanical means further promoted language and allowed people to learn to speak and understand increasing numbers of languages. Books, newspapers, and journals enhanced the spread of information through various languages. Development of the electronic media, beginning with the radio, has promoted the spread of communication throughout the world using satellites, television, telephones, and sophisticated combinations.

Nonverbal Communication

Nonverbal communication is the exchange of messages without using verbal language. Types of nonverbal communication were discussed in Chapter 17 and include such things as eye contact, facial expressions, body posture and movement, gestures, and touch. Nonverbal expression is more likely to be involuntary and less likely to be consciously controlled. Therefore, it is usually a more accurate picture of a person's true communication.

Touch is one of the most effective means of expressing oneself nonverbally. Touch can be used to convey a variety of messages. Touch has many different meanings

and, because of its personal nature, understanding its true meaning may be difficult. Tactile expressions are shaped by familial, regional, class, and cultural influences. Age and sex also play a role in developing meanings that are associated with touch.

Physical closeness between patient and nurse is an essential part of nursing. There is an exceptional amount of touching in the nurse–patient relationship. On the other hand, the use of touch in family relationships is even more personal and conveys a more personal message.

Factors Affecting Normal Communication

Cognition and Perception. Communication is influenced by cognition and by perception of the external world. Cognition, or the act of knowing, occurs through interaction with the world, formal education, and culturalization. Perception refers to the obtaining of knowledge through the senses. The senses of vision and hearing directly affect cognition and the ability to communicate.

Vision allows the person to see the initiation of and response to interaction with another person. The eye transmits electrical impulses from the retina through the optic nerve to the brain where the impulses are translated into images and meanings. This process of visual perception in communication begins in infancy when an infant responds to the caregiver's presence, facial expressions, and other nonverbal behavior. As the person continues through life, communication is affected by the feedback that is visually observed through expressions and body language. The same words or phrases can mean different things with different expressions visually detected by the person who is listening.

Hearing is another primary avenue of perception. The ear carries sound that has been collected in the outer ear through the middle ear to the inner ear. The sound waves are converted to nerve impulses and sent to the brain by way of the auditory nerve. The impulses are translated into meaning, based on the pitch, loudness, and duration of the sound. The expression of meaning and emotion (prosody) is conveyed through pitch, loudness, tonal quality, and inflection. Beginning in infancy, changes in inflection, pitch, and tonal quality clearly convey meaning even without distinguishable words. In turn, the infant understands meaning based on what is heard in spoken tone variation. Throughout life the person listens to the meaning and emotion that is conveyed in speech for a portion of the meaning contained in the words being spoken.

People who have dysfunction of hearing or vision may also have the potential for altered cognition or knowing. If cognition is impaired, communication lacks clarity. The person who is visually impaired loses the information obtained through facial expression and body language, and the person who has a hearing impairment may have little or no input of tone variation to contribute to meaning.

Self-Concept. The perception held of one's self is called self-concept. The way a person feels about himself or herself in relation to the world is conveyed in the person's communication. If a person feels competent and successful and in control of his or her life, the quality of communication reflects that confidence and security.

People who feel disadvantaged or less competent are likely to believe they have little control over their lives. Their self-concept is apt to be correspondingly less confident. If a person sees self as less able to compete in whatever arena (school, work, or play), the person's communication reflects that lack of confidence as well.

The manner in which a person communicates to others is generally mirrored back. If a person communicates confidence and security, that is the response that is received from others. Conversely, if the person communicates insecurity and lack of feelings of control or inadequacy, the responding communication reflects the person's concept of self.

Whether there is any validity in the person's concept of self is a separate question. As a person matures, the person realizes that people vary in personal skills and that one can compensate for other areas. This adapta-

tion and adjustment allow a balanced self-concept and more confident communication.

Culture, Values, and Beliefs. Comprehension and meaning vary among cultures. Communication is often inhibited or blocked as a result. Words and their meanings carry different nuances and significance depending on the culture, values, and beliefs of the individuals.

Although these differences may be particularly noticeable among immigrant groups, they also hold true for groups from different regions within the same country. For example, the same language and some of its meanings may sound different to and be comprehended differently by a person from the southeastern United States than by a person from northeastern states.

Language barriers, whether they are foreign languages or varying dialects of the same language, can result in anxiety, fear, and frustration for people who need to communicate on a daily basis as well as in situations where health care is required. Because communication involves body language along with verbal language, the meaning of body position and expressions can further facilitate or impede communication. Although putting an arm around the shoulder of one person may indicate caring and concern, for a person of another culture that act may be a violation of privacy and an intrusion that blocks communication rather than facilitating it.

A person's values regarding what personal thoughts and feelings are shared with others also affect communication. In this culture, women tend to be more comfortable in communicating feelings than men. This culture values stoicism and emotional reserve in men, so men are less likely to communicate personal thoughts and responses. This reluctance to communicate may actually interfere with effective communication if actual understandings and needs are not shared.

Lifespan Considerations

Each phase of development brings with it unique aspects related to language and communication. Although it is not possible to discuss these complex phenomena completely in this chapter, some interesting points are highlighted here.

Newborn and Infant

The newborn and infant are totally dependent on others for their needs; a lower form of communication is designed to make these needs known to the caregiver. Crying is a form of communication. The newborn's needs must be met promptly, gently, and consistently to lay a foundation of basic trust.

Bonding is essential to the development of basic trust. The primary caregiver is the infant's lifeline. Through this consistent relationship, the infant learns to differentiate self from others, to communicate, and to relate to others. Even young infants respond differently to strangers (Emde, Gaensbauer, & Harmon, 1976; Field, et al., 1984). Around the age of 9 months, infants become more fearful of strangers, especially if strangers are intrusive. The nurse should approach babies in a gentle but secure manner, allowing time for the baby to become accustomed to the nurse. Touch is an important factor in communicating with infants.

Language skills begin with cooing, smiling, and crying and progress to vocalizations that express various emotional states (Hetherington & Parke, 1986). During the babbling period, sounds are produced that form the basis of any language. As the baby matures, he or she begins to understand language and uses words to communicate. Generally a baby's first words are spoken at the end of the first year. The baby also uses gestures such as pointing or tugging at an adult.

Toddler and Preschooler

Children vary in their rate of language acquisition, but there is a uniformity to how all children acquire language. Language is acquired not only in terms of learning principles but also through biologic, environmental, and cognitive factors. A serious change or interruption in any part of these can affect a child's acquisition of language.

By the time an infant becomes a toddler, he has transformed vocalizations and gestures into words to express himself. At the age of 3, a child has about 900 words in his or her vocabulary and can form simple sentences (Hetherington & Parke, 1986).

Another means of expression for children is play. Through play, children learn, explore their environment, develop socially, and learn to cope with stressful situations. Opportunities for play include age-appropriate toys, playmates, and a safe environment.

School Age and Adolescent

Children and adolescents are social beings who seek out and need relationships with peers. As they move into the teen years, they adopt the norms and language uses of their peer group. Communication with peers takes priority over communication with adults. Yet at the same time children and adolescents need adult guidance and protection. In the hospital, peer relationships provide support and companionship.

Adult and Older Adult

Adults depend on communication for dealing instrumentally with the world, managing careers and vocations, maintaining relationships, and carrying out their various roles. Communication conveys thoughts, feel-

ings, and innermost aspects of the human experience.

As a person ages communication becomes increasingly challenged. Diminished vision and hearing are common and can interfere with effective communication. Because these senses generally diminish gradually, older adults develop compensatory mechanisms for adapting to the changes and to the resulting effect on communication.

ALTERED COMMUNICATION

Communication can be impaired by anything that alters brain functioning (such as interrupted circulation, trauma, pressure, or drugs) or impairs articulation and phonation. When there has been an interruption or damage to the speech centers of the brain, communication, both spoken and written, is impaired. The impairment may be either temporary or permanent, depending on the degree of injury.

Temporary dysfunction in communication results from reversible injuries to the speech and cognition centers of the brain or to the organs of speech. Permanent impairment in communication occurs when the speech centers of the brain or the organs of speech have been irreversibly injured.

Interruptions in communication abilities, whether temporary or permanent, affect relationships with others. Clear communication facilitates carrying out of the various roles of a person with family, coworkers, and others. Relationships depend on communication and the interchange of information. When communication is altered, the ability to carry out usual roles becomes less effective.

Potential for Altered Communication

Impaired Speech Apparatus

Impairment of function of the speech apparatus of the larynx, the ability to move air, the use of the tongue and the oral pharynx, and the innervation to each of these structures may alter communication. Cancer of the throat is probably the major risk for impaired phonation. If detected early, cancer of the larynx can be treated with radiation or surgery limited to the exact site; however, extensive malignancies require removal of the whole larynx and the creation of a permanent tracheostoma (external opening to the trachea). Neurologic impairment or muscular dysfunction also have the potential for affecting communication.

Disturbed Articulation

Incoordination or decreased movements of muscles required for articulation can be related to cortical, cerebellar, or cranial nerve dysfunction or from effects of drugs such as alcohol, sedatives, or other medications.

People who have a high cervical (C2, C3 quadriplegia) injury have a permanent tracheostomy and cannot speak because no air will be forced through the vocal cords. They also require ventilatory support. Other neurologic conditions, such as amyotropic lateral sclerosis, multiple sclerosis, and myasthenia gravis, may also lead to inability to speak because of loss of muscle function. These conditions may also necessitate a tracheostomy or ventilatory assistance depending on the severity of the disease. Patients with these diseases have lost the muscle function needed for them to breathe on their own.

Cortical Control Interference

Any substance or event that clouds the sensorium or interferes with usual cortical functioning alters many normal functions, including communication.

Drug Use. Pharmacotherapeutic agents of many types can inhibit or interfere with higher cortical functions. These agents include prescription drugs, alcohol, and illicit drugs. In the early stages or with moderate to heavy dosages, the person may experience impairment in motor control of speech (slowness and slurring) and in comprehension and expression (inability to think of the correct word or response).

Overdosage of drugs potentially can inactivate the speech centers of the brain along with the motor activity required to carry out communication. The degree of damage to these centers determines whether the altered communication is temporary (until the effects of the drug wear off) or permanent. An example of controlled drug use that temporarily interferes with communication is administration of an anesthetic agent, which when appropriately controlled is metabolized by the body in an expected period of time and the patient's communication abilities return.

Stroke. In the United States, 600,000 people per year have a stroke; approximately 200,000 of those die. Average age at onset is 60; it affects all races, both sexes, and all socioeconomic levels (Martin, Holt, & Hicks, 1983). Approximately 20% of all surviving stroke victims need the specialized services of a speech pathologist to help them regain communication skills. The other 80% have only minor or temporary damage to the language centers of the brain (Dreher, 1981). The location of the insult and the extent of damage affect the pattern and severity of the speech impairment.

Head Trauma. About 7 million head injuries are estimated to occur annually in the United States with about 500,000 people admitted to the hospital (Rosenthal, et al., 1990). Most seriously injured patients have major disabilities. Because there are rarely specific injury sites, classification of brain injury and prediction of outcome are difficult. The study of communication disorders secondary to head trauma is in the initial stages. The more severe the head injury, the more likely there is an interruption in communication. Communication problems in head-injured patients are usually compounded by impairments in cognitive function, such as behavior, memory, orientation, and attention.

Coma. The term **coma** or comatose describes people who do not communicate or make meaningful response to stimuli and who do not open their eyes to stimuli. This rapid change in level of consciousness can occur from slow-growing mass lesions (e.g., chronic accumulation of fluid or tumor), metabolic problems (e.g., alterations in serum glucose), or from trauma (e.g., rupture or occlusion of a blood vessel, bleeding, or edema from blows to the head). Altered communication may be either temporary or permanent, depending on the severity of damage from whatever is causing the comatose condition. The person may recover with little or no long-term effects on communication, or may have to learn alternate methods of communication.

Manifestations of Altered Communication

Aphasia

Aphasia is the complete or partial loss of all language modalities, including an understanding of speech (auditory comprehension), reading, speaking, writing, arithmetic, and expression through pantomime. It is an acquired dysfunction of communication that is the result of brain damage, but it does not affect intelligence. Aphasias are produced mostly through damage to the cortical language areas of the dominant left hemisphere (see Fig. 44-1). Rarely, an injury affects one isolated area of speech, but usually all speech and language functions are affected. Anyone who incurs a brain injury or insult could develop aphasia. The most common cause of aphasia is related to an interruption in circulation as a result of a cerebral vascular accident (stroke). Approximately 85,000 new cases of aphasia occur in the United States each year from stroke alone (Albert & Helm-Estabrooks, 1988a).

The manifestation of speech impairment depends on the location and the extent of damage and can range from slight slurring of speech to total loss of communication. Aphasia has been described and categorized based on lesion location and linguistic deficit (Albert, 1988; Albert & Helm-Estabrooks, 1988a and b; Mitchell, et al., 1988). The four most common types of aphasia are expressive (Broca's), receptive (Wernicke's), anomic, and global (Table 44-1).

Expressive Aphasia. Expressive aphasia (also called Broca's, motor, and nonfluent aphasia) is characterized by limited speech that is slow and halting with great effort, reduced grammar, and poor articulation. The

TABLE 44–1

Expression and Comprehension with Major Types of Aphasia

Type of Aphasia	Oral Expression	Written Expression	Comprehension
Expressive (Broca's or motor)	Nonfluent, telegraphic	Limited	Usually good
Receptive (Wernicke's or sensory)	Fluent, speech well articulated, disorganized content	Impaired	Impaired
Anomic	Speech fluent, talks around the subject	Variable, mild to severe impairment	Variable, mild to severe impairment
Global	Speech very poor, meaningless recurrent sounds	Severely impaired	Severely impaired

person knows what he or she wants to say, but cannot find the words needed. Problems with word retrieval are called **anomia.** In expressive aphasia, the person's speech often sounds like a telegraph message, consists of isolated or small groups of words, and lacks tone or inflection.

Because intellect is not necessarily impaired, aphasic patients know what they want to say but are unable to say it correctly. This leads to an extreme sense of frustration and anger. Sometimes the anger shows in physical behaviors, such as pushing objects or people away and shouting. Often the anger is directed at those people who are closest to the patient. This behavior makes it difficult for the spouse or significant others to understand what is happening to the patient.

Writing is also affected and can be as severely, or more severely, impaired than speech.

Receptive Aphasia. Fluent aphasia (also called Wernicke's, sensory, and receptive aphasia) is characterized by speech that is well articulated, has good melody, and has a normal or slightly faster rate. The major manifestations are impaired auditory comprehension and feedback and fluent or hyperfluent, well-articulated, paraphasic speech. Such patients have difficulty understanding spoken and written words. They talk a great deal, but they often do not make sense and their speech lacks specific content. Their ability to read, write, listen, concentrate, or follow instructions is impaired; the level of severity is usually consistent with or worse than the speech impairment.

The patient is unaware of the language impairment and appears euphoric in relation to their language problems. They display little frustration because they are unaware of any problem.

These patients also have a host of symptoms referred to as a right hemisphere syndrome. They often display a neglect of the paralyzed side of their body, even to the point that they do not know that their left arm or leg is really theirs. Behaviorally, these patients are impulsive, lack insight into their deficits, and have poor judgment. Often they are said to have inappropriate behavior,

when actually their behavior is a result of their injury. The combination of these symptoms and behaviors makes language rehabilitation and rehabilitation in general difficult.

Anomic Aphasia. Anomic or amnesic aphasia is characterized predominantly by word-finding problems of a milder nature than expressive aphasia. The speech is fluent and grammatically correct. The communication difficulties arise in using the correct names for particular objects, people, places, or events. If the patient cannot remember the correct name, they talk about the subject until the listener understands what they mean. Auditory comprehension is generally good, although the levels of reading and writing skills are variable and can range from mild to severe. Behaviorally, these patients display anger, frustration, and depression similar to patients with expressive aphasia.

Global Aphasia. Global aphasia results from severe and extensive damage to all language areas (Broca's and Wernicke's) of the brain. These patients have no consistent functional skills in any of the language modalities. They cannot speak or understand speech, nor can they read or write. Some patients' speech consists of meaningless recurrent sounds.

Dysarthria

Dysarthria is a totally separate speech disorder. **Dysarthria** refers to a group of speech disorders that result from a disturbance of motor control, weakness, paralysis, or incoordination of the oral musculature. The disorder is a result of damage to the central or peripheral nervous system. Patients with dysarthria usually have normal auditory comprehension and can select and order words correctly. They do not have a language problem, but rather a motor speech disorder. This disorder causes them to have difficulty saying words and sounds precisely with appropriate stress, loudness, pitch, and control. The result is speech that is described as "slurred," "heavy," or unclear. There are numerous types of dysarthria. The specific type depends on the site of the neurologic lesion.

Total Loss of Speech

Cancer of the larynx is the most common cause of loss of functioning of the larynx. A laryngectomy is the result.

Patients who have had a total **laryngectomy** have had the larynx removed and also the tissues in the area known as the Adam's apple. After the larynx is removed, there is no ability to produce sound and, thus, no ability to speak. The loss of speech is permanent.

Patients who have had a permanent **tracheostomy** (incision through the neck to create a permanent opening in the trachea) have the same difficulty communicating as the patient with a laryngectomy (Fig. 44-3). Some may be able to "mouth" words; others may be able only to blink their eyes in response to yes or no questions. Intellectual functions are not impaired, only the ability to speak.

Loss of function of the larynx can occur temporarily if a tracheotomy is required for emergency care and respiratory ventilation. With a **tracheotomy,** air is diverted through the tracheotomy tube to outside of the body without passing through the larynx. To have laryngeal speech, the person would need to block the tracheotomy tube and allow air to pass through the larynx. After the emergency has subsided and before the temporary tracheotomy tube is removed, this is the action that is used to produce speech. Ultimately, with the removal of the tracheotomy tube, the person can resume usual laryngeal speech.

Impact on Activities of Daily Living

The ability of the person to perform activities of daily living and to participate in usual roles and relationships depends on the degree of impairment to communication. For example, a person whose career depends on speech production and written expression finds that role impaired if he or she has an aphasic dysfunction.

Relationships depend on an interchange of ideas, thoughts, and feelings. The person with altered communication is unable to convey ideas, thoughts, and feelings as clearly, resulting in less intimacy and clarity. When this occurs with friends and acquaintances, they often find it easier to end the relationship or to make it more distant rather than try to bridge the communication problem. Families generally work hard to maintain communication and relationships, although it often becomes a strain on that relationship as well.

People with altered communication may become frustrated with trying to express what they need in relation to hygiene, nutrition, and activities. The affected person may develop problems with continence directly as a result of the difficulty of communicating the need to urinate or defecate.

Some types of aphasia interfere with more than communication. With a specific type of brain damage, the person may also neglect one side of the body. The person needs reminding and assisting in grooming the neglected side of the body and in communicating needs related to that side of the body. Eating may be a problem as well if the person is unable to see or is unaware of half of the food that is presented.

Home maintenance activities such as banking, food shopping, paying bills, and meal preparation are difficult, if not impossible, because these instrumental activities require the communication skills of arithmetic, reading, writing, and spelling. Depending on the degree of dysfunction, the person may be able to do light meal preparation and light housekeeping tasks, but may be unable to do heavy housecleaning and laundry.

Because communication is inseparably integrated with perceptual processes, many people with a communication dysfunction are not able to be independent. These people need support for their ADLs through the provision of a structured environment and around-the-clock assistance.

ASSESSMENT

The ability to communicate is vital to survival. Without communication, a person's physical and psychological health suffers. When encountering a patient with a communication problem, the nurse must rapidly assess the patient's communication difficulties and take steps to intervene. It is particularly important when assessing a patient with communication difficulties to remain attentive and be patient when the person is attempting to communicate. This places the person at ease and encourages the patient to initiate communication.

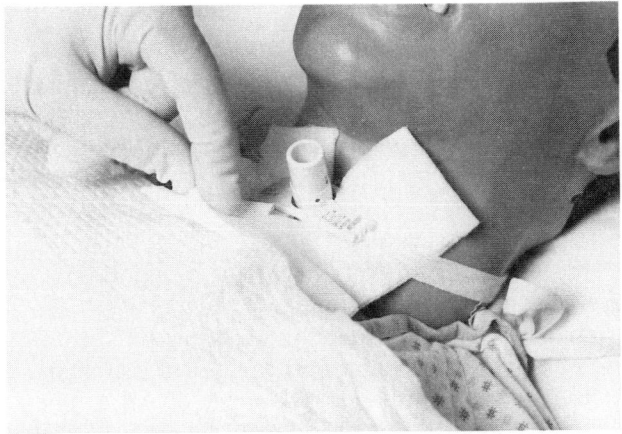

Figure 44–3.   The presence of a tracheostomy tube alters verbal communication.

Subjective Data

The collection of subjective information helps the nurse identify the normal pattern of communication and relationships for the patient, any risk factors that may predispose the patient to alterations in roles and relationships related to communication dysfunction, and any actual dysfunctions in communication, roles, and relationships. If the patient cannot communicate, family or friends may need to provide data regarding communication patterns and abilities.

Functional Pattern Identification

The nurse usually begins the assessment of a person's communication status and ability by obtaining or reviewing their history. In this process, the nurse gains an understanding of the person's normal communication and roles and any factors that may predispose the person to altered communication and relationships.

To determine the patient's current communication pattern, the nurse needs to obtain data from the patient and significant others. An assessment of the patient's ability to communicate should include not only asking questions, but also an assessment of general level of alertness, appropriateness, and emotional state. Assessment of the person's speech patterns and comprehension ability is an important component of the subjective data.

General assessment can begin with an evaluation of how the patient seems to feel about the dysfunction and how the family and significant others view the alteration in communication. Does the patient seem distressed by the inability to communicate, or does the patient appear unconcerned or unaware of a difficulty in communication? Does the communication impairment pose a problem for the spouse or significant other? Is there a disturbance in the person's roles and relationships as a result of the altered communication?

Among the questions that the nurse needs to ask are those listed in the accompanying display. Answers to these questions aid the nurse in determining the patient's previous patterns of communication. To determine the

---

Communication Assessment: Initial Assessment Questions

Is the patient able to speak at all?
If so, if the speech intelligible and appropriate to the situation?
Does the patient use gestures or point in an effort to comunicate?
Is the patient literate?
How much formal education does the patient have?
Is the patient able to speak another language?
Can the patient understand and follow simple one-step commands?
Did the patient have a speech difficulty before this most recent difficulty?
Was the patient previously an active conversationalist or did he or she prefer to listen?

Assessment for Major Types of Aphasia

Verbal Expression
Does the person speak easily, fluently?
Is the content appropriate in context?
Does the person initiate speeh on his or her own?
Is the speech telegraphic (short, choppy)?
Is the speech organized?
Does the verbal output contain recurrent sounds?
Does the person name objects correctly?
Does the person repeat words and phrases easily?

Written Expression
Can the person write own name and address correctly?
Can the person produce a short narrative written paragraph?
Does the written product have appropriate meaning?

Comprehension
Does the person give any indication of hearing impairment?
Does the person answer simple, open-ended questions appropriately?
Does the person answer yes/no questions in appropriate context?
Can the person correctly point to an object that has been named?
Does the person respond appropriately to simple commands?

Nonverbal Expression
Observe for the type of effect (sign of emotion):
  Flat—no sign of emotion
  Labile—wide fluctuation in emotions
Observe gestures for appropriateness to the situation.
Observe for the integrated context of voice tone, emotional expression, body movement.

type of communication disorder that the patient is experiencing, the nurse needs to assess verbal expression, written expression, comprehension, and nonverbal expression. Table 44-1 defines the expected comprehension, verbal and written expression for the four major types of aphasia.

Communication abilities to assess for in the major types of aphasia are also delineated in the display.

Answers to these questions aid the nurse in determining the degree of the patient's communication dysfunction. As the nurse clarifies the alterations in communication, the presence of or potential for disturbances in roles and relationships becomes apparent. This information assists in developing an individual plan of care.

Risk Identification

The patient's history and observed dysfunction may give the nurse information as to whether communication is altered and roles and relationships may be affected. Patients with brain damage from stroke or head injury, impaired speech apparatus as with a laryngectomy or tracheotomy, and other temporary dysfunctions such as drug overdosage and comatose states are at greatest risk for communication impairment. The presence of pathophysiologic factors such as cerebral, neurologic, respiratory, or auditory impairments, and laryngeal infection or edema place the person at high risk for altered communication. Other factors for which the nurse needs to assess are endotracheal intubation, pain medication, oral–facial deformities, and speech problems such as stuttering or lisping, or a language barrier. The inability

to communicate clearly and effectively places the person at risk for interruption of roles and relationships (Fig. 44-4). Lastly, factors such as shyness and lack of privacy and support can be significant barriers to communication and cannot be ignored as causes for impaired communication and altered relationships.

Dysfunctional Identification

The nurse can use the subjective data collected to help identify role and relationship dysfunctions related to communication impairment. Actual communication impairments have aspects of impaired verbal, written, and nonverbal expression and comprehension. The patient or family can provide information regarding the degree of difference from normal patterns of communication. Subjective data need to be validated with objective information gained through the physical assessment and the evaluation of diagnostic results before the actual diagnosis is made.

Objective Data

In addition to gathering subjective data, the nurse also collects objective data concerning the patient's communication abilities through physical assessment of the patient and reviewing related tests.

Physical Assessment

The mouth, tongue, and facial muscles are required to form and articulate words correctly. The patient with altered communication related to impaired motor functioning or brain damage needs to have a thorough assessment of the muscles and organs of speech. Table 18-3 lists assessment methods for cranial nerves.

The tongue receives its motor innervation from the 12th cranial nerve (hypoglossal). Motor control of the tongue can be assessed through instructing the patient to protrude his or her tongue. If there is damage to the hypoglossal nerve, the tongue deviates to the side of the weakness as a result of the strong side pushing the tongue forward unopposed.

The muscles of the face are innervated by the fifth (trigeminal) and seventh (facial) cranial nerves. The motor function of these nerves can be assessed by noting symmetry of facial movement when the patient is asked to show teeth, purse lips, and frown. When the patient's face is at rest, asymmetry of the forehead or cheeks should be noted, along with facial drooping or drooling. A palpable change in the muscle mass of the face may be identified that corresponds with a change in symmetry.

The muscles of swallowing and the gag reflex are supplied by the ninth (glossopharyngeal), tenth (vagus), and eleventh (accessory) cranial nerves. The larynx is supplied by the tenth cranial nerve alone. Motor weak-

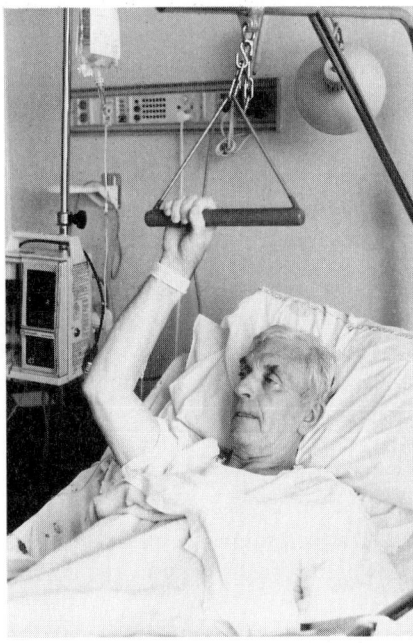

Figure 44–4. An elderly person with impaired verbal communication may be at risk for sensory deprivation.

ness of the soft palate contributes to difficulty in swallowing (dysphagia). Swallowing difficulties may be identified by history as well as by physical assessment. To test for swallowing, the patient should be asked to swallow chips of ice. The ice gives some substance for the patient to manipulate in the mouth, yet if he or she is unable to swallow successfully, it introduces only water into the mouth.

The presence of the gag reflex can be assessed by lightly touching a tongue blade to one side of the palatal arch and then the other. An absence of the gag reflex can be due to nerve damage.

Impairment in the use of the larynx is immediately obvious in the presence of an endotracheal tube or tracheostomy or a ventilator. Because the movement of air bypasses the laryngeal function, the patient is unable to communicate verbally. The nurse needs to assess if the patient is able to use other modes of communication, such as gestures, codes using eye blinks or hands, or written notes.

Indications of motor impairment validate communication alterations observed in the subjective data. Linking the identified objective and subjective data assists in defining the specific problem and appropriate care.

Diagnostic Tests and Procedures

The patient with altered communication is evaluated by a speech pathologist who does a detailed assessment of speech, expression, and comprehension. The results of this assessment contribute to the plan of care for the patient as well as to establishing communication with the patient.

NURSING DIAGNOSIS AND PATIENT GOALS

The accepted NANDA nursing diagnosis for a patient with communication problems is impaired verbal communication. The diagnosis can be further defined into specific categories based on the cause and defining characteristics.

Diagnostic Statement: Impaired Verbal Communication

Definition

Impaired verbal communication is the state in which an individual experiences a decreased or absent ability to use or understand language in human interaction (NANDA, 1990).

Defining Characteristics

Patient is unable to speak dominant language; speaks or verbalizes with difficulty; does not or cannot speak; stutters; slurs words; has difficulty forming words or sentences; has difficulty expressing thought verbally; and exhibits inappropriate verbalization, dyspnea, and disorientation (NANDA, 1990).

Related Factors

Decrease in circulation to brain; brain tumor; physical barrier (tracheostomy, intubation); anatomic defect, cleft palate; psychological barriers (psychosis, lack of stimuli); cultural difference; developmental or age related (NANDA, 1990).

Related Nursing Diagnoses

Because communication alterations may interfere with roles and relationships, related nursing diagnoses include Altered Family Processes, Altered Parenting, Parental Role Conflict, Altered Role Performance, Impaired Social Interactions, Social Isolation, and Grieving. The specific disturbances in roles and relationships determines which, if any, of these related diagnoses are appropriate to consider.

Patient Goals

The formulation of patient goals should include both short-term and long-term goals. Short-term goals are directed at establishing a communication system that allows the patient to have basic needs met. Long-term goals focus on the patient's ability to live with the limitations of impaired communication and accept the changes in lifestyle and self-concept that affect roles and relationships.

The potential complication with any diagnosis of impaired communication is that the patient's basic and immediate needs may go unmet. These needs could be life-threatening or could be fairly routine. Perhaps the most traumatic complication is the social isolation that comes from being unable to express one's thoughts, feelings, or emotions. This inability to express one's self often manifests itself in anger, rage, depression, or withdrawal. These behaviors may also be seen in the spouse, family, or significant others who have also lost the ability to communicate and are experiencing an interruption in relationships.

Examples of short-term goals for the patient with impaired verbal communication include:

The patient will communicate basic needs.
The patient will demonstrate improved ability to express self.
The patient will demonstrate increased ability to understand.
The patient will verbalize experiencing less frustration with communication.

IMPLEMENTATION

A central focus of nursing implementation for the patient with impaired verbal communication is preventing alterations in roles and relationships and supporting effective relationships. Relationships are affected by the ability to communicate effectively thoughts, feelings, needs, and other intimate aspects of life. When one's ability to understand other people's communications and to verbally respond to those communications is disrupted, the usual relationship with those people is also disrupted. Nursing interventions need to reflect cognizance of those relationships and of their importance to the patient as an individual.

Nursing Interventions to Promote Health and Function

Through general health promotion, the nurse provides guidance for optimum health and communication and helps minimize dysfunctional relationships. Patient teaching revolves around the causes of impaired communication. Prevention of cerebrovascular disease and accidents causing trauma to the brain or muscles of the speech organs are high on the agenda.

Patient Teaching

Preventing cardiovascular disease, which can lead to cerebrovascular disorders, has several aspects that each person can personally influence. Prevention initially involves exercise and a low-fat diet (see in Chaps. 29 and 33). A dietitian should be consulted to help the patient plan menus, change recipes, and learn to read labels on food. A regular program of exercise should be developed after consultation with a physician. Serum cholesterol should be monitored regularly to determine the effects of following a low-fat diet and an exercise program. Patients who have high blood pressure should be encouraged to maintain their current medication regimen, to check their blood pressure routinely, and to follow up with their physician.

Smoking increases the chance of heart disease and throat cancer. The nurse needs to educate the patient about the numerous health risks associated with smoking. Patients should be encouraged to quit and often find that support of some type is useful. The early warning signs of throat cancer are nagging cough and chronic hoarseness. Awareness of the warning signals can be helpful with early detection or prevention of throat cancer.

The most frequent causes of communication impairment in young adults are brain injuries and spinal cord injuries. Eighty percent of spinal cord injuries occur before the age of 40 (Porth, 1990). Motor vehicle accidents account for nearly half of all head injuries in the 15- to 24-year-old age group (Kalsbeek, et al., 1980).

Patient Teaching

Instruct the patient as follows:

- Stop smoking to prevent cerebrovascular disease.
- Wear seatbelts to avoid head injury.
- Use helmets for biking and skateboards to prevent head trauma.
- Swim with a buddy in case help is needed and to prevent injury.
- Do not dive into shallow or unknown waters to prevent spinal cord injury.
- Avoid alcohol and drug use to protect cerebral function.
- Eat a low-fat diet to minimize the occurrence of cardiovascular disease.
- Plan a regular regimen of exercise to promote cardiovascular fitness.
- Monitor blood pressure and serum cholesterol regularly to avoid vascular disorders.
- Continue taking prescribed medications unless the physician has been consulted.

The brain-injured adult can experience aphasia or dysarthria; spinal cord-injured patients could require a temporary or permanent tracheostomy depending on the level of their injury.

Drug use contributes to the potential for impairment in communication and relationships. Experimenting with drugs (e.g., alcohol, marijuana, cocaine) may begin during school-age years and adolescence and may impair school roles and family relationships. Programs of drug education are increasing in numbers and in community support. Nurses need to serve as role models by actively supporting these programs.

Because of their age, young adults tend to engage in sports and activities that may place them at greater risk for injury. Yet this group is often resistant to preventive education. A public safety awareness program stressing helmet use with motorcycles, use of seatbelts, use of proper protective sports equipment, and the avoidance of alcohol and drugs may help in reducing injuries. Prevention programs that start in the elementary schools may be the most effective in preventing unsafe behavior.

Nursing Interventions for Altered Communication Function

The plan of care developed by the nurse assists the patient with the ability to express needs and feelings to

---

**Selected Nursing Interventions
for Common Communication Problems**

Impaired Verbal Communication

- Establish a calm, structured environment.
- Maintain a consistent approach with the patient using a normal tone of voice.
- Address the patient by name and speak to person as an adult.
- Ask the patient to repeat words that are unclear.
- Allow the patient adequate time for response and for speech.
- Ask only questions that require short answers.
- Promote use of alternate means to express self, such as gestures, pointing to pictures or a word-board, or writing.
- Teach family to communicate with the patient at appropriate rates of speed and only one person at a time.

Impaired Hearing Ability

- Limit environmental interferences by minimizing noise from equipment, loudspeakers, and visitors.
- Establish contact with the patient to focus the patient's attention before speaking.

- Speak slower and distinctly without excessive loudness.
- Use visual cues along with speech to enhance understanding.
- Assist the patient in referral for or in obtaining assistive listening devices.

Impaired Ability to Understand

- Orient the patient to time, place, and person.
- Establish a calm, structured environment and routine.
- Address the patient by name and introduce yourself when entering room.
- Minimize environmental distractions, both visual and auditory.
- Ask questions or give information in small segments.
- Listen patiently to content and context of responses.
- Encourage socialization activities that are not over-stimulating.

---

the nurse, family, and others. Nursing interventions need to be directed toward maintaining communication and relationships (Keller et al., 1989).

Orientation to Surroundings

The nurse needs to have special consideration for the patient who has difficulty with understanding, such as those with fluent or Wernicke's aphasia (see display). The patient who is experiencing impaired communication may also be experiencing some confusion related to this unfamiliar state. Maintaining a structured environment assists the patient in adapting to this alteration and in reestablishing communication. The presence of a calendar and a clock large enough to be seen by the patient and kept current assists the patient in orientation to time.

A structured routine minimizes the number of factors on which the patient must focus. Sequenced events, a consistent daily schedule, a calendar readily available, and frequent orientation to the schedule contribute to structure for the patient. Predictability in the environment allows the patient to conserve energy for the com-

munication impairment and its related relationship difficulties.

The nurse must orient these patients to person, place, and time. To assist with orientation, ask the patient why he is in the hospital, or where he is, gently correcting a false answer. Encourage the person to look to the affected side by approaching from the affected side and calling the patient's name. Refer to the patient's body parts on the affected side, having the patient rub or touch the affected side. When the patient is eating, encourage the patient to look for food on the tray on the affected side and make sure that food is not pocketed in the affected cheek. Keep the patient oriented to task by constantly cueing him to what he is doing. The patient may be impulsive and have poor judgment; therefore, do not take the patient's word that he can do an activity, watch him do it.

Alternative Communication Methods

The nurse needs to develop a plan of care that provides the patient with Broca's or nonfluent aphasia with an effective, efficient means with which to communicate.

Selected Nursing Interventions for Communicating with Patients with Comprehension Deficits

- Keep distractions at a minimum.
- Remove unnecessary items from the patient's visual field so that he or she can focus on the task at hand.
- Turn off the television or radio.
- Limit the number of visitors at one time.
- Instruct family and visitors to only have one person talk to the patient at one time; do not carry on more than one conversation.
- Redirect the patient frequently to the task at hand. It may be necessary to move into the patient's visual field to get his or her attention.
- Break tasks into small steps.
- Use auditory and visual cues. Repeat the names of objects as they are touched.
- Gently correct errors.
- Monitor the patient for safety. Do not overestimate the patient's abilities.
- Reorient frequently.

The patient who has difficulty speaking may benefit from having others use gestures and facial expressions to give additional clues. Encourage the patient to use any means available to express himself. Other methods of communication that may be helpful include offering the patient pictures at which to point, having the patient use gestures, or letting him show you what he wants. The patient's writing and reading skills may be impaired along with speech; therefore, these skills may not be useful alternatives.

If it is difficult to understand what the patient has said, be honest and let the patient know. Ask the patient to try again and perhaps use gestures to assist with understanding. If the patient tries again and you still do not understand, take a rest, and come back to it in a few minutes. Do not pressure the patient; some symptoms get worse if the patient is fatigued, upset, or anxious. Be alert to the patient's daily schedule, allow for adequate rest at night and naps during the day.

For patients who have lost the ability to produce sound due to a laryngectomy, communication may be restored through the use of sophisticated electronic or computer communication devices or an electronic larynx. In these cases, it is useful for the nurse to learn to use these devices.

As a result of increasing computer technology, communication augmentation systems have become more common (Keith, 1987). These systems are designed to support, enhance, or augment the communication of people who are not independent verbal communicators. Patients who have severe motor difficulties, such as patients with dysarthria, may use these communication augmentation systems.

The Patient with a Laryngectomy. Patients who are to undergo a laryngectomy should address the issue of communication preoperativley. The patients should be given a choice of how they wish to communicate—by wordboard, flashcards, or writing. This method should be delineated explicitly in the care plan. It would be beneficial for the patient to practice lip speaking (forming words with the mouth). By preoperatively addressing how the patient wishes to communicate, the anxiety level is greatly reduced. The nurse also needs to watch the speaker's lips, because articulation should not be affected by surgery. The patient should be referred to a speech therapist for either esophageal speech or an electronic larynx. If the patient already is using esophageal speech, extraneous environmental noise should be eliminated because esophageal speech is quieter and less intelligible than normal speech. The patient who uses esophageal speech has a low-pitched monotone with no melody to phrases. The patient also has no air reservoir so there are short burps of speech. Gestures may enhance speech and communication. Learning to use esophageal speech or an electronic larynx can be frustrating, yet, once the patient has adapted to using a new communication system, there are few restrictions on their ability to perform activities of daily living.

Patients with a laryngectomy need to learn a new breathing system as well as learning how to keep the

Safety Alert

- Remove clutter or unnecessary items from the patient's room or bed table.
- Orient patient to surroundings.
- Place call button within patient's reach.
- Encourage the patient to use any means available to express self and needs.
- Develop a system for signaling emergencies.
- Be sure you understand the patient's method for communication.
- Do not pressure the patient if he or she is tired.
- Do not allow patients to perform activities by themselves unless you have observed them perform the activity and are sure they can perform the activity alone safely.
- Keep the tracheostomy stoma clean and clear.

Nursing Research

Selected Nursing Research Studies

Sarvela, P. D., et al. (1989, October). Knowledge of communication disorders among nursing home employees. *Nursing Homes, 38*(1/2), 21–24.

Scura, K. W. (1988, October). Audiological assessment program. *Journal of Gerontologial Nursing, 14*(10), 19–25.

Smith, A., et al. (1989, January) The relation between perceptual and language deficits in stroke patients. *British Journal of Occupational Therapy, 52*(1), 8–10.

Possible Topics for Nursing Inquiry

What are indicators of role alterations in persons with impaired verbal communication?

What form of communication is most effective in dealing with patients in a coma?

What nursing interventions contribute to effective communication with patients experiencing temporary loss of verbal speech?

stoma open and clean. Patients may shower using a stoma shield, but they cannot swim. If there are no other physical difficulties, the patient should be able to return to work and home management.

The Patient with a Tracheostomy. The patient who has a temporary tracheostomy or is temporarily intubated should be reassured that he or she will be able to talk again once the tube is removed. Often the patient is hoarse for a period of time after tube removal. While the patient is intubated, a temporary communication system should be agreed on by the nurse and patient using whatever means are available.

The patient who has a permanent tracheostomy and is ventilator-dependent may have limited resources to implement a communication system. Often these patients have neuromuscular or neurologic diseases, which limit their ability to use gestures, write, or point. Lip speaking or an eye blink is usually the only means of communication.

The Patient with Dysarthria. The patient who has impaired verbal communication related to dysarthria has slow, slurred speech that is difficult to understand. To facilitate communication with these patients, the nurse should face the patient to read their lips. Communication could be augmented by gestures, written messages, a communication board, or flashcards. The patient should be encouraged to slow speech, to speak louder, and to take a breath between sentences. Ask the patient to repeat words that are unclear. If the patient appears fatigued, ask only questions that require short answers. Some of these patients may have highly specialized computer equipment for communication, but this is an exception more than the norm. Establishing a specific care plan and a routine for delivering care reduces the amount of time the patient would otherwise need to explain his or her care to others.

Environmental Restrictions

The number of visitors with whom the patient has to communicate may add to the level of frustration for the patient with impaired verbal communication. Increased numbers of people and noise in the environment can interfere with cognitive function and understanding. A quiet environment allows the patient to focus on understanding and on speaking or communicating.

The nurse may find that environmental restrictions are advantageous in assisting communication with the patient. Be aware of excessive noise levels caused by equipment, loudspeaker systems, or other patients. Limit the number of visitors present at any given time. Teach visitors how to communicate with the patient, such as only one person speaking at a time and avoiding carrying on another conversation simultaneously in the room.

Coping Measures

The nurse can assist the patient with Broca's or non-fluent aphasia in coping with impaired communication by explaining to the patient what happened, that they had a stroke, that the stroke causes language problems, and that anger and sadness are normal reactions. Patients need to understand and be prepared for wide emotional swings (lability), which are common and decrease with recovery. The nurse should remain calm and not show a negative reaction to the outburst if it occurs, but rather give calm, quiet reassurance and support.

The patient who understands what has occurred but has great difficulty in expressing self may be at risk for depression. A depressed patient may refuse therapy and food and ignore family and friends. Sometimes reassurance is not enough to overcome depressive feelings. The physician needs to be consulted if depression is suspected so that other therapy may be employed.

Discharge Planning and Home Care

Discharge planning for maintaining relationships despite alterations in communication begins the day the nurse first assesses the patient in the hospital or clinic. In planning discharge care for such a patient, the nurse may consider referrals to a speech pathologist for communication deficits and cognitive evaluation and training. Referral should be made to occupational therapy to plan for activities of daily living and to physical therapy for mobility evaluation and training. The nurse's thorough assessment provides the physician with an understanding of the necessity of the referrals. The family must be included in assessment and planning (see display).

Because the hospital stay may be short, evaluation of nursing interventions and teaching may not be accomplished in the hospital. Therefore, it is necessary to ensure follow-up through a public health or visiting nurse referral, or to an appropriate clinic or community program. These programs need to adapt the patient's care plan based on the needs he or she develops when back in the community.

Community self-help groups, such as Stroke Clubs, The Multiple Sclerosis Society, The National Spinal Cord Injury Society, and The International Association of Laryngectomies, can be beneficial to the patient and family in reestablishing and maintaining relationships through communication. These groups offer patients support and provide them with tips to make role adjustment easier and to improve the quality of relationships.

EVALUATION

Outcome criteria are the evaluative tools used to measure goal attainment. Nursing interventions allow patients to attain goals. Nursing interventions must be specific to the patient goal, although some nursing interventions are applicable to more than one goal.

Goal
The patient will communicate basic needs.

Possible Outcome Criteria
- Patient demonstrates improved ability to express needs by practicing using a new method (gestures, writing, blinking, or electronic device) with nurse before discharge.

Goal
The patient will demonstrate improved ability to express self.

Possible Outcome Criteria
- Patient engages in spontaneous social interactions and conversations with hospital personnel and visitors as observed by nurse before discharge.

Goal
The patient will demonstrate increased ability to understand directions.

Possible Outcome Criteria
- Patient demonstrates an understanding of simple one-step commands by following through with the given command at the next teaching session with the nurse.

Goal
The patient will verbalize experiencing less frustration with communication.

Possible Outcome Criteria
- Patient verbalizes to nurse a decrease in frustration with communication problems before discharge.
- Patient expresses a decrease in feelings of isolation and depression before discharge.

The evaluation of the effect of nursing interventions on patient goals includes an assessment of the patient in relation to the outcome criteria. Continuation, modification, or termination of nursing interventions depends on the assessment. This process may be ongoing depending on the cause of the communication impairment.

Family Teaching: Patients with Expression Deficits

Instruct the patient's family as follows:

- Anticipate the patient's needs by asking if he or she needs something so that the patient will be less frustrated with trying to communicate.
- Use one- or two-word phrases and simple word commands to simplify the communication process.
- Use gestures with demonstrations to help clarify meaning.
- Encourage the patient to speak by allowing him enough time to speak so that he may regain confidence in speaking.
- Acknowledge the frustration the patient displays so that his or her feelings are validated and understanding is expressed.
- Give positive feedback to attempts at speech to encourage the patient's efforts.
- Ignore profanity, understanding that it represents an expression of communication disorder.
- Delay conversation with the patient if fatigue is apparent because fatigue interferes with communication and speech.
- Speak to the patient on an adult level because cognition may be unaffected even with impaired communication.

Nursing Management Plan
The Patient with Impaired Verbal Communication

Nursing Diagnosis: Impaired verbal communication related to decreased cerebral circulation manifested by difficulty in speaking and in expressing comprehension/understanding.
Patient Goal: Patient will establish an effective means of communication.
Patient Outcome Criteria

- Patient demonstrates improved ability to express himself or herself before discharge.
- Patient demonstrates improved ability to understand within 1 week.
- Patient experiences decreased frustration with communication by discharge.

Nursing Intervention	Scientific Rationale
1. Assess the patient's ability to comprehend, speak, read and write • Ask simple questions. • Ask the patient to repeat single words and sentences. • Have patient name simple objects. • Ask the patient to write his or her name or copy a sentence. • Have the patient read words or phrases.	1. These exercises help the nurse determine the specific form of aphasia. The specific type of aphasia must be identified before a care plan can be developed.
2. Create an atmosphere that is quiet, relaxed, and supportive. • Remove or decrease any extraneous noise. • Speak to the patient in a normal tone of voice. • Speak on an adult level. • Listen to the patient and wait for him or her to attempt to communicate. • Establish and maintain eye contact. • Assume that the patient can understand. Do not talk about the patient in his or her presence. • Delay conversation when the patient is tired or frustrated.	2. Tension decreases comprehension and inhibits the motor programming for articulation. • Extraneous stimuli decrease attention. • Increasing the loudness of your speech does not increase comprehension. Hearing loss is not part of the aphasia syndrome. • Aphasia does not affect intelligence. • Rushing the patient by interrupting, finishing sentences, or appearing hurried increases his or her frustration and make speech even more difficult. • Allows the patient to make use of both verbal and nonverbal cues to help in comprehension. • Shows your patient basic respect. Intelligence is not affected by aphasia. Talking about the patient in his or her presence is upsetting. • Persons with aphasia become easily fatigued. Attempting conversation when the patient is fatigued makes it more difficult.
3. Use techniques that increase comprehension. Be a role model. • If the patient wears glasses or a hearing aide, encourage their use. • Modify your speech. Speak slowly using adult language. • Do not change the subject rapidly or ask multiple questions in succession. • Match your verbal and nonverbal behavior.	3. These techniques enhance communication and decrease frustration for the patient.

(continued)

Nursing Management Plan
The Patient with Impaired Verbal Communication (continued)

Nursing Intervention	Scientific Rationale
4. Use techniques that enhance communication.	
• Phrase questions so they can be answered with yes or no responses.	• Simple questions can facilitate communication, but an aphasic patient may be confused by verbal symbols and may say yes but nod his or her head no.
• In a group have only one person talk at a time.	• The patient will become more confused if they need to follow a multisided conversation.
• Encourage the use of gestures, pantomime, pictures, writing, or flash cards. Write key words on cards.	• Approaching the patient through whatever sense is stronger helps facilitate communication.
• Rephrase messages to validate the response. If you do not understand the patient, be honest and attempt the message again.	• Pretending you understand when you do not will frustrate the patient even more.
5. Encourage and use techniques to improve speech.	5. Use of these techniques decreases frustration at communication attempts.
• Have the patient slow the rate of speech and say each word clearly.	
• Encourage the use of short phrases.	
• Explain when words are not clear.	
• Avoid topics that are controversial.	
• If the patient makes an error do not correct.	
• Give positive feedback for attempts at communication.	
6. Acknowledge the patient's frustration.	6. Understanding the patient's frustration and communicating this understanding permits the patient to accept the situation and learn to work through the speech difficulties.
• Explain that the stroke caused language difficulty and that feelings of frustration are normal.	
• Maintain a calm, positive attitude.	
• Use reassurance and touch to communicate your understanding.	
• Encourage and use a sense of humor.	
• Allow tears.	
• Ignore profanity, recognize it for what it represents.	
• Allow the patient to make choices about his or her care.	
7. Initiate health teaching and referrals.	7. Early intervention and treatment can reduce the frustration and isolation that accompanies aphasia.
• Consult a speech therapist.	
• Teach family and significant others techniques for improving communication.	

Key Concepts

- Disorders in communication can markedly disrupt the quality of life for the person affected and the person's family.
- Speech problems, when they occur, usually result in long-term difficulties and role disruptions, which may never be completely resolved.
- Establishing an effective communication system and maintaining relationships are priorities.
- In adults. the main cause of impaired communication is brain damage. Other major causes are cancer and neurologic disorders.
- Aphasia is the inability to express oneself.

- Four different types of aphasia are presented: expressive, receptive, anomic, and global.
- Dysarthria is not an aphasia, but is a speech disorder related to difficulty in articulation.
- Communication disorders affect behavior and relationships.
- The plan of care involves collaboration of nursing, speech therapy, and other disciplines, as needed.
- Nursing management of people with impaired communication is directed at:

Developing a reliable means of communication to enable the person to communicate basic need.

Enhancing the person's self-esteem.

Instructing the patient and family in the cause of the deficit and methods to optimize communication and relationships.

Promoting feelings of self-worth for the person.

Discharge planning considering the long-term and ongoing needs of patient and the family.

References

Albert, M. (1988). Aphasia is now treatable. *Hospital Practice, 23*(11A), 31–38.

Albert, M., & Helm-Estabrooks, N. (1988a). Diagnosis and treatment of aphasia: Part I. *Journal of the American Medical Association, 259*(7), 1043–1047.

Albert, M., & Helm-Estabrooks, N. (1988b). Diagnosis and treatment of aphasia: Part II. *Journal of the American Medical Association, 259*(8), 1205–1210.

Dreher, B. (1981). Overcoming speech and language disorders. *Geriatric Nursing, 2*(5), 345–349.

Emde, R. N., Gaensbauer, T. J., & Harmon, R. J. (1976). Emotional expression in infancy: A biobehavioral study. *Psychological Issues 10*(37) New York: International.

Field, T. M., Cohen, D., Garcia, R., & Greenberg, R. (1984). Mother–stranger face discrimination by the newborn. *Infant Behavior and Development, 7,* 19–25.

Hetherington, E. M., & Parke, R. D. (1986). *Child psychology: A contemporary viewpoint.* New York: McGraw-Hill.

Kalsbeek, W. D., McLaurin, R. L., Harris, B. S. H., & Miller, J. D. (1980). The national head and spinal cord injury survey: Major findings. *Journal of Neurosurgery (Suppl.) 53,* S19–S31.

Keith, R. L. (1987). *Speech and language rehabilitation* (3rd ed.). Danville, IL: Interstate Printers & Publishers.

Keller, C., et al. (1989, October). Psychological response in aphasia: Theoretical considerations and nursing implications. *Journal of Neuroscience Nursing, 21*(5), 290–294.

Martin, N., Holt, N. B., & Hicks, D. (1983). *Comprehensive rehabilitation nursing.* New York: McGraw-Hill.

Mitchell, P. H., Hodges, L. C., Muwaswes, M., & Walleck, C. A. (1988). *AANN's neuroscience nursing.* Norwalk, CT: Appleton & Lange.

NANDA (1990). *Taxonomy I revised 1990, with official nursing diagnoses.* St. Louis, MO: North American Nursing Diagnosis Association.

Pimental, P. A. (1986). Alterations in communication. *Nursing Clinics of North America, 21*(2), 321–337.

Porth, C. (1990). *Pathophysiology: Concepts of Altered Health States,* 3rd ed. Philadelphia, J. B. Lippincott.

Rosenthal, M., Griffith, E. R., Bond, M. R., & Miller, J. D. (1990). *Rehabilitation of the head injured adult* (2nd ed.). Philadelphia: F. A. Davis.

Schuster, C. S., & Ashburn, S. S. (1986). *The Process of Human Development.* Boston: Little, Brown & Co.

Weinhouse, I. (1981). Speaking to the needs of your aphasic patient. *Nursing, 11*(3), 34–36.

Bibliography

Buckwalter, K. C., et al. (1989, December). Increasing communication ability in aphasic/dysarthric patients. *Western Journal of Nursing Research, 11*(6), 736–747.

Chovaz, C. (1989, March). Nursing the hearing impaired patient. *Canadian Nurse, 85*(3), 34–36.

Harrison, L. L. (1990, March–April). Minimizing barriers when teaching hearing-impaired clients. *Maternal Child Nursing, 15*(2), 113.

Nelson, G. B. (1988, November). Assessment and intervention for communication problems in home health care. *Journal of Home Health Care Practice, 1*(1), 61–76.

Rambur, B. A. (1989, January). Sudden hearing loss. *Nurse Practitioner, 14*(1):8, 11, 14.

Sarvela, P. D., et al. (1989, October). Knowledge of communication disorders among nursing home employees. *Nursing Homes, 38*(1/2), 21–24.

Schluter, L. A. (1989). Care provider guidelines for adapting hearing aids and instructing the elderly in their use. *Physical and Occupational Therapy in Geriatrics, 7*(4), 71–81.

Scura, K. W. (1988, October). Audiological assessment program. *Journal of Gerontological Nursing, 14*(10), 19–25.

Smith, A., et al. (1989, January). The relation between perceptual and language deficits in stroke patients. *British Journal of Occupational Therapy, 52*(1), 8–10.

Thibodeau, L. (1989, October). Facilitating communication in nursing homes through the use of assistive listening devices. *Nursing Homes, 38*(1/2), 25–28.

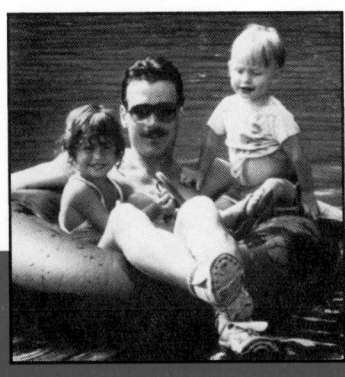

Families and Their Relationships

LEARNING OBJECTIVES

Upon completion of this chapter, the student will be able to do the following:

- Describe variations in normal family and social relationships.
- Identify factors affecting alterations in family and social relationships.
- Differentiate the possible effects of acute and chronic illness on family and social relationships.
- Discuss lifespan considerations for family and social relationships for selected age groups.
- Describe manifestations of dysfunctional families.

- Differentiate subjective and objective data needed to assess alterations in family and social relationships.
- Identify nursing diagnoses and related goals commonly used with altered family and social relationships.
- Describe nursing interventions to promote family and social relationships.
- Describe nursing interventions for the dysfunctional family.
- Explain how evaluation of nursing care would be accomplished.

KEY TERMS

Anticipatory guidance
Blended family
Cohabited family

Communal family
Extended family
Nuclear family

Single-parent family
Social isolation
Role strain

45

Normal Family Function
  Characteristics of a Normal Family
    Family Structure
    Family Function
  Normal Functional Family Pattern
  Factors Affecting Normal Family Function
  Lifespan Considerations
Altered Family Function
  Potential for Altered Function
    Acute Illness
    Chronic Illness
    Traumatic Experiences
    Substance Abuse
  Manifestations of Altered Family Function
    Social Isolation
    Abuse
    Separation and Divorce
    Role Strain
    Emotional Problems in Children
  Impact of Family Dysfunction on Activities of
    Daily Living
Assessment
  Subjective Assessment
    Functional Pattern Identification
    Risk Identification
    Dysfunctional Identification
  Objective Data
Nursing Diagnoses and Patient Goals
  Diagnostic Statement: Altered Family Processes
    Definition

Defining Characteristics
Related Factors
Diagnostic Statement: Ineffective Family Coping:
  Disabling
Definition
Defining Characteristics
Related Factors
Diagnostic Statement: Ineffective Family Coping:
  Compromised
Definition
Defining Characteristics
Related Factors
Diagnostic Statement: Altered Parenting
Definition
Defining Characteristics
Related Factors
Related Nursing Diagnoses
Patient Goals
Implementation
  Nursing Interventions to Promote Family Health
    and Function
    Reinforcement of Family Strengths
    Support
    Anticipatory Guidance
  Nursing Interventions for Altered Family Function
    Problem Solving
    Referral
  Discharge Planning and Home Care
Evaluation
Key Concepts

Family patterns in Western cultures have undergone considerable change in the past two centuries. Two hundred years ago, children were raised in extended families that encompassed several generations of family members living in close proximity. Large families were desired; members were interdependent, and socialization was accomplished as traditions passed from one generation to the next. At the end of the 20th century, family structures are more varied. The small, traditional family unit known as the nuclear family is prominent. There are also blended types of families, extended families, single-parent families, cohabitated families, communal families, and other variations.

Although nurses deal with individual people, those people are integral parts of families. Families influence the health perceptions and practices of their members. Nurses must understand the importance of family functioning to positively affect the health status of the person.

NORMAL FAMILY FUNCTION

A family is a social group whose members share common values, occupy specific positions, and interact with each other over time. Adults bear and rear children, engage in economic and political cooperation, and care for the elders.

Characteristics of a Normal Family

Although there is no one true "normal" family model, families have some common structural and functional characteristics. Family structure is described by who the members are and what their relationships are to one another.

Function is what the family does. Structure and function vary from one family to another, as well as within a family over time.

Family Structure

Although the traditional structure of the family in America today is that of the nuclear family, a variety of family structures exist. Family members do not always live together in one household, but are linked together by relationships.

Nuclear Family. **Nuclear family** members include the adult man and woman, who are married, and their children (Fig. 45-1). Members live under the same roof, usually until the children leave home to work and support themselves or to attend college. In 1990, 26% of the nation's 93.3 million households were composed of a married couple and children under age 18 (U.S. Bureau of the Census, 1990). Variations exist in the nuclear family when couples remain childless due to infertility or personal choice, and when older children move back in with parents after a trial period of independence.

Traditional roles in the nuclear family have been the man as breadwinner outside the home, and the woman as responsible for physical provision of the home and children. The number of traditional families remained stable over the last 20 years, ranging from 24.2 million to 26 million (U.S. Bureau of the Census, 1990).

Extended Family. Members of the **extended family** include the nuclear family as well as grandparents,

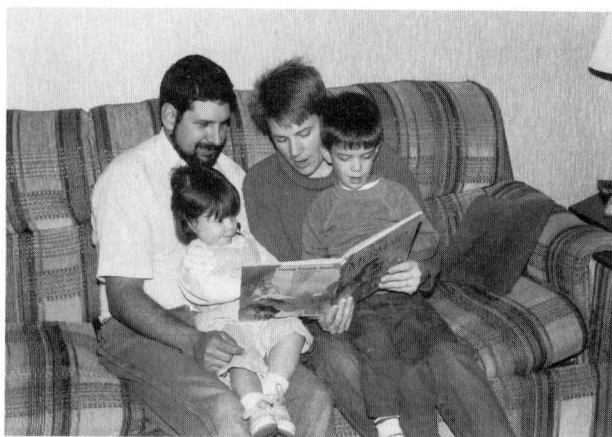

Figure 45–1. The nuclear family consists of the married husband and wife and one or more children, living together in one household.

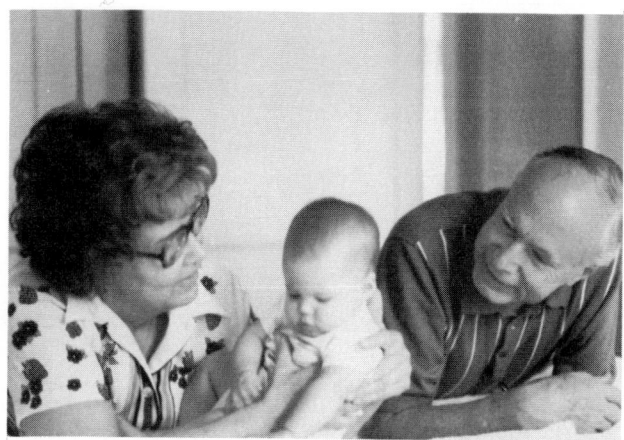

Figure 45–2. As part of the extended family, grandparents contribute to nurturing young children.

aunts, uncles, and cousins (Fig. 45-2). They may or may not live under the same roof, and exert a varying amount of influence on one person. Extended family often consists of three or more generations.

Single-Parent Families. **Single-parent families,** composed of one parent and one or more children, are growing due to high separation and divorce rates (Fig. 45-3). There were 9.7 million single parents in the United States in 1990, 41% more than 10 years earlier. Death of a spouse, desertion, and unwed pregnancy or adoption also result in single-parent families. These families may experience financial strain and an overburdened parent due to lack of support systems. Women head more single-parent families than men, by a margin of 5:1 (U.S. Bureau of the Census, 1990).

Blended Family. Members of a **blended family** (or stepfamily) include children living with one birth parent and one nonbirth parent, as well as the offspring of a nonbirth parent. Each member faces the challenge of forming new relationships with the new members.

Cohabitated Family. **Cohabitated family** structure includes people living together without the formal or legal bond of marriage. Couples include men and women living together as a trial to marriage or as an alternative to marriage, or gay or lesbian couples. Cohabitated families may include children.

Communal Family. A **communal family** includes a number of members who share a common bond such as religious affiliation, ideology, economic needs, or a situation such as attending college. Membership may be short-term, creating instability in the family unit.

Other Families. Still other variations in family structure exist, including commuter marriages, where one member may live away from the rest of the family part of the time to work or go to school; single adults living

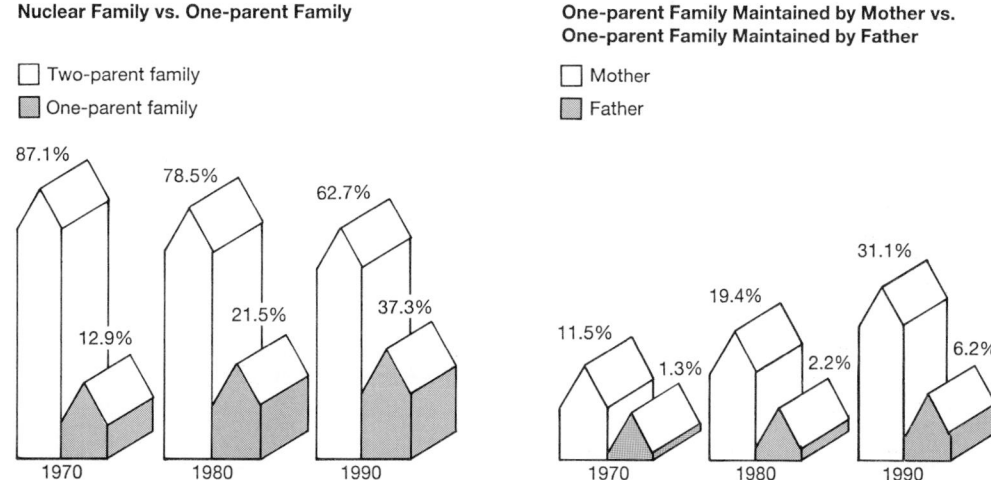

Figure 45–3.   The changing American family.

alone, either as those who have not married, or as the elderly who have launched their families; and two-career families.

Some families have adopted or cared for foster children. Many families have adopted children of a race different from their own, including orphans from southeast Asia, South America, and eastern Europe (Fig. 45-4).

Family Function

Family function is not identical for all families; however, all families exist to meet some common goals. The usual functions of families involve communication, problem solving, goal setting, physical and economic care, sexual intimacy, reproduction, socialization, education, nurturing, and caring. Besides the physical bonds of blood relationships, family members experience emotional bonds. Emotional bonds provide support and security for members, fostering growth and development.

Physical Provision. Physical provision or care is a common need for all members of the family, but greater for children or those members of the family who are more dependent. Physical provision includes food, clothing, shelter, and health care. A normal, functioning family would have some members providing comfort and safety for others. Certain members would cook, clean, shop for food and clothing, and possibly feed and bathe other members. Those being cared for and those doing the caring may change due to situations such as illness, and family maturation.

Economic Provision. One or more family members provides for monetary funds to provide basic necessities such as food and clothing, as well as luxuries and provisions for the future, such as college tuition. Families usually share the funds earned by members. Two-career families are increasingly common due to today's economic climate and standard of living. About 67% of the female population in the United States participates in the work force (U.S. Bureau of the Census, 1990).

Sexual Intimacy. Most couples in families need sexual intimacy. This includes married and cohabiting men and women, and gay and lesbian couples. Sexual intimacy is a basic human need and developmental concern that can be met within a family.

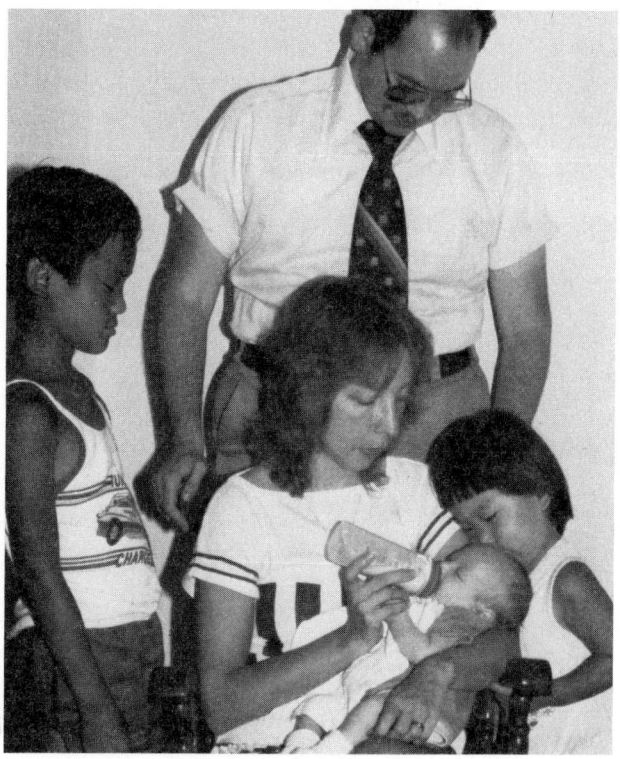

Figure 45–4.   A family of parents, two adopted older children, and the new baby. The adopted children share in the joys of a growing family.

Reproduction. Reproduction is not a function of all families; it is more often a choice rather than a given in family life. Many couples postpone childbearing, eliminate it, or are unable to accomplish it. Alternate methods of having children such as adoption, foster parenthood, use of donor sperm, and surrogate mother programs exist to accomplish this goal.

Education. Education, whether formal or informal, is a function of all families. Parents discipline children, teach them how to begin to care for themselves and get along in the world, and send them to school for formal education. Older members share with younger members information they have learned through living, and younger members in turn teach older members about the changing world. Education not only involves information, but techniques for problem solving and coping, as well as attitudes and values. Education is an ongoing and lifelong function in many families.

Socialization. Socialization is a function in all families, especially in close extended families (Fig. 45-5). Gathering together at the dinner table or converging for holiday celebrations are prime opportunities for socialization in the family. Through socializing, family members learn to get along, learn appropriate behavior in various situations, and express culture, tradition, and religious beliefs.

Nurturing and Support. Families provide nurturing and support to members, from initial bonding at birth to old age and death. Nurturing and support may be provided through the emotional tasks of love, belonging, and affection, as well as through the provision of safety and security for growth. Caplan (1990) describes ten support functions of the family and social groups. These

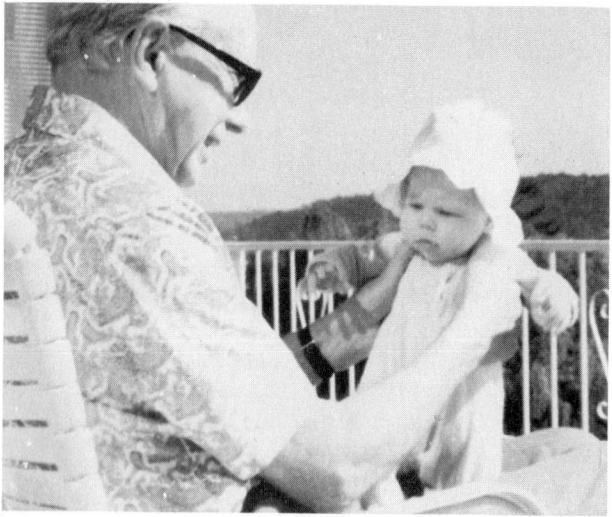

Figure 45–5. Grandparents participate in the socialization of infants.

include providing information, providing feedback, transmitting attitudes, beliefs, and values, guiding problem solving, providing practical services, providing a safe, comfortable environment, providing standards, helping to establish identity, assisting in emotional development, and fostering mutual support by family and community professionals.

Normal Functional Family Pattern

A normal functional family meets the family's developmental tasks and guides family members in accomplishing tasks according to their age bracket. Family development is discussed in Chapter 14, and Table 14-1 presents the developmental cycle of stages and tasks.

Factors Affecting Normal Family Function

Factors that may affect family and social relationships include culture beliefs, economic status, lifestyle, previous life experience, and external stressors such as illness. Age is discussed separately under "Lifespan Considerations."

Culture, Values, and Beliefs. Cultural traditions have an impact on the family as it functions in Western society. Components of a sociocultural dimension include ethnic patterns, language, food customs, patterns of communication, role expectations, health-care beliefs, childrearing practices, availability of extended family support, and religious beliefs and practices. The nurse may encounter much variation in family structure and function among non-Western cultures; each of these variations can have an affect on the person's health status. For example, the extended family is basic to Native American society; children and the elderly are valued, and childrearing is a group endeavor. Extended family is essential as a support system to help families cope when stressors such as illness occur.

The African American or black population has traditionally had families with a matriarchal focus, often involving several generations in childrearing. A strong sense of family is valued. With Mexican Americans, machismo, or the emphasis on proving masculinity through sexual potency, has historically been a predominant cultural value. Women have had lower status than men, but family unity is strongly supported.

Asian American families continue to stress traditional values of loyalty and obedience to parents. The value placed on education has perhaps accounted for the rising middle-class status accorded many Asian families. Elders and men have high status within the family. Traditional submissiveness of women has created a significant role conflict for more recent generations of Asian American women. Strict control of social interactions is valued to avoid "loss of face."

Religious customs also dictate how children grow up in families. The bar mitzvah is considered the "rite of passage" in the Jewish religion. Strict fundamentalist religions rear children with corporal punishment. Mormons emphasize strong family ties.

Families pass down these attitudes about male and female roles and childrearing through the generations; they also pass on beliefs and practices about health, illness, and health care. Even those people born and raised in traditional American society may exhibit behavior arising from a variety of cultural beliefs.

Economic Status. A clear economic influence on family and social relationships can be observed as people with marginal incomes struggle to survive. Economic constraints often create problems in maintaining a family's lifestyle following divorce, change in employment, or with a change from two wage-earners to one. Resentment toward society or toward other members of the family for forcing a below-standard lifestyle may arise. According to Burns (1984), functioning in single-parent families will be difficult when they have limited support, without psychological and economic resources.

Lifestyle. The mobility of families can affect relationships as parents move from job to job and children move from school to school. Support persons and friendships change. Lack of extended family support systems due to geographic distance can increase the strain on parents following relocation. The need to have two incomes has created the "latch-key" practice in childrearing, in which children are responsible for their own care and supervision after school. The family's lifestyle in terms of rest and relaxation, nutrition, smoking, drug and alcohol use, and exercise, influences the health status of all the members and the choices the children will make as they become adults.

Previous Life Experience. Previous life experience greatly affects a family's functioning. Children learn about relationships almost exclusively from their parents and early family life. They will carry ideas to their own future families about how to form relationships, how to make decisions and solve problems, what are accepted roles for men and women, how to raise children, how to use resources, and how to show affection. Some coping strategies, such as taking an alcoholic beverage to numb mental pain and stress, may have been accepted in a person's previous life experience and yet destroy present family relationships.

Coping and Stress Tolerance. Any stress on the entire family or an individual member greatly affects functioning. Acute or chronic illness of a member may alter roles and relationships within the family. For example, in a family with a seriously ill father, the mother may become the economic provider and a child may provide care and

nurturing for the father. Other stresses, such as loss of a family member, involvement in a natural or manmade disaster, or an accident, also alter family functioning. Some families have the ability to grow due to a crisis, others experience dysfunction; some families live with constant stress, others experience little change or stress.

Lifespan Considerations

An understanding of normal growth and development can be a reference point for understanding families.

Newborn and Infant

A process of infant–parent attachment or bonding following birth is critical to family development. Factors that affect the process of attachment may include availability of both parents following birth, flexibility of schedules, feelings about the birth, comfort in parenting roles, emotional responsiveness of infant and parents, financial security, other demands such as care of another child, and presence of supportive others.

By 8 months of age the infant usually becomes attached to the primary caregiver, developing "trust," as described in Erikson's (1963) classic theory of development. The process of socialization can be supported by an interactive family environment. If there are changes in the infant's environment, such as illness of the primary caretaker or of the infant, necessitating hospitalization, inconsistencies can impede the infant's development.

Toddler and Preschooler

Beginning to walk imparts mobility, and increasing cognitive ability adds curiosity. Protection from harm is an important focus for these adventurous years. At the same time, the development of self-control characteristics can strain family interactions as parent–child power struggles, often accompanied by temper tantrums, become the norm. Promoting independence within established limits should be encouraged. Sibling rivalry may escalate as the egocentric toddler resents the dominance of older children and the attention given to younger children in the family. Despite the power struggle, the toddler remains attached to the parent, and from age 18 to 24 months severe separation anxiety may be noted when the mother or primary caregiver leaves the child. Hospitalization involving separation at this time may be especially traumatic, and the toddler may regress into an earlier developmental stage.

Psychosocial development escalates during the preschool years. Identification with the man/woman role is developed as the preschooler interacts differently with the parent(s). The parent of the opposite sex becomes a focus for love, while aggression may be directed toward the parent of the same sex. Consistent involvement with people of both sexes enhances the preschooler's development.

Associative play, with interaction but little organization, evolves into cooperative play as the child nears school age. Cooperative play, along with preschoolers' generally increasing social skills, helps them to develop mutually supportive roles with siblings, even though rivalry continues.

The preschool years are crucial for development of initiative, the ability to begin actions independently. Stable family relationships can enhance the development of creativity. The preschooler can be prepared for changes through playing out feelings and focusing attention on the event one part at a time. The family should reassure the children that changes are not their fault.

Significant others can expand the socialization process as the preschooler develops an ability to separate from home and family. The preschooler still needs both independence and security. Fear of separation remains and may be reinforced by parental anxiety.

Child and Adolescent

The school years are a time of change for both the child and the family. A need for association with peers, usually of the same sex, is enhanced. The role of "best friend" takes on importance. Family atmosphere continues to provide a sense of security as the child moves away from obvious signs of dependence on parents. Sibling rivalry is still present, but continues to resolve unless parents make comparisons among children for differing levels of ability.

Children's perceptions of their own abilities are significant as they seek to accomplish the task of "industry" (Erikson, 1963) and avoid feeling inferior. Fears of illness, injury, punishment, and death of self or significant others are evidenced during this age period. Phobias and ritualistic "good luck" behaviors may be used as adaptive mechanisms by the child. Parental understanding, rather than denial of phobias, is important.

In some cultures, puberty, following completion of identifiable "rites of passage," signals the assumption of adult roles. American culture is not as clear in defining the steps for transition into adulthood. To the extent that independence is desirable, alterations in family and social relationships are normal and inevitable in adolescence.

Psychosocial development is closely related to changes in physical development during adolescence. Peer group identity is strongly desired; the adolescent strives to look and act like the group. Stability in the home environment and supportive relationships with significant others can help an adolescent avoid "role confusion" (Erikson, 1963).

Adult and Older Adult

According to Erikson (1963), the chief developmental tasks of the adult period are "intimacy," involving commitment to others, and "generativity," focusing on productivity. An adult's development is strongly influenced by both social and job-related concerns. Critical life junctures such as marriage, cohabitation, becoming a parent, career advancement, and mobility affect the development of both intimacy and generativity.

A decision to remain single does not exclude development of intimate relationships. Nevertheless, the young adult usually leaves a family of origin, often to form a family of procreation. Social relationships with peers remain important for the young adult's feeling of identity. The need for peer group support may be intertwined with such serious problems as substance abuse, sexually transmitted diseases, unwanted pregnancies, and abortion. The family's acceptance is necessary to help in dealing with these serious health problems.

In the middle years, relationships with children gradually change as children develop independence, and relationships with a significant partner change as each matures. Menopause in the woman and climacteric in the man can precipitate crises in the family, requiring role adjustment. Relationships with aging parents may result in conflict, frustration, or anger as the elderly become more dependent.

Changes in family structure occur as children leave home (and sometimes return), as death occurs, and as new relationships are formed. Changes related to retirement, death of a family member, and decreasing social contacts, alter family and social structure because usual roles must be changed.

ALTERED FAMILY FUNCTION

Potential for Altered Function

Acute and chronic illness, traumatic experiences, and substance abuse all potentially alter family function. Family function may only be mildly altered and affect just some of the members, or the entire family may be thrown into crisis. Family bonds may actually be strengthened by a crisis, however, when members become more committed to common goals of the family. Table 45-1 lists common stressors that contribute to altered family function.

Acute Illness

Acute illness may place sudden demands on the family. The ill member often looks to the family for validation that he or she is sick; with validation from the family, the ill member can seek health care. Roles may be changed as the ill member becomes dependent on other members for physical care, nurturing, and economic security. The

TABLE 45-1

Sources of Family Conflict

Source	Problem Areas
Finances	Lower socioeconomic status; income inadequate to meet needs; disagreement on money management
Occupation	Unemployment; semiskilled status, task-sharing when both adults working
Culture/religion	Mixed religious or cultural background; in-laws; disagreement on childrearing practices
Education	Incongruent levels of education, especially if school dropout
Residence	Mixed rural/urban background; relocation for benefit of only one family member; isolated
Sexual	Dissatisfaction with intimacy level; disagreement on family planning
Substance abuse	Difference in values; physical/psychological changes due to chemical addiction
Social ties	Dissimilar selection of friends; single versus couple focus in friendships
Situational	Fatigue; loss; illness; separation, trauma, disaster
Developmental	Change in family stage (Duvall, 1977); change in individual stage (Erikson, 1963)

ill member's self-esteem may drop as he or she feels he or she is no longer a valuable member of the family.

Other members may temporarily sacrifice their own needs to provide for the needs of the ill member. Needs such as sexual intimacy may go unmet. Problems arise when role adjustments are not made and family or individual needs go unmet. One member in particular may feel overburdened by the situation. For example, when a construction worker is hospitalized for acute back pain, his wife may have to go to work full time to provide for the family economically. The children may be left alone before and after school, and housework may be left undone. The wife tries to fit in around her work schedule visits to her husband, meal preparation, and chauffeuring the children. She is anxious about her husband's condition, as well as how the children are managing on their own. Consequently, her own physical needs for sleep and nutrition, as well as the family's need for nurturing, may go unmet. Depending on the severity of the illness and how suddenly it occurred, the family needs increased nurturing at this time. Stability of the family structure is essential when one or more members is absent, as with the hospitalized husband and working wife. However, some flexibility is needed to share roles and still meet needs such as economic provision and physical care.

Chronic Illness

Because chronic illness is of longer duration, it can influence the family to a greater extent than acute illness. The course of chronic illness may require both individual and family adaptation to changes in lifestyle and roles, and often may result in an increasing degree of dependence on others. Actions by family or significant others can be supportive, but behaviors such as overprotection can be problematic.

Because of the inherent dependency of children, their illness provokes yet other adjustments in the family. The birth of an infant with a congenital defect or the diagnosis of a child with a chronic illness or developmental disability is traumatic, and may result in severe stressors to family relationships. The ability of a family to function will influence the child's ability to develop and cope, and will affect the course of the illness or disability (Masters, Cerreto, & Mendlowitz, 1983). A congenital birth defect that would initially be stressful but is ultimately correctable could have less impact on family and social relationships than would a chronic illness or developmental disability requiring lengthy family involvement with treatment.

Common stressors with regard to childhood illness include vague worry, dealing with pressures from relatives and others, social or travel restrictions on family members, and concern about neglect and resentment of siblings (Satterwhite, 1978). Family roles and social relationships change to meet the needs of the family system as well as the ill child and family members.

Parents with disabled or chronically ill children often express negative feelings about themselves, such as guilt, anxiety, inadequacy, failure, and helplessness (Waisbren, 1980). Denial may be necessary initially as a family struggles with the initial shock of the child's illness or disability, but after the problem is acknowledged, the goal is to return life to "normal."

Traumatic Experiences

Trauma, because of the stress and disruption of normal interactions it entails, can alter family relationships. Traumatic experiences can be physical, such as a gunshot wound, or emotional, such as robbery; can involve one person or many; and can be caused by humans (e.g., surgery) or nature (e.g., flood).

Personal involvement or having a family member or significant other involved in a disaster, such as severe fire, flood, hurricane, or car, train, or plane accident, is associated with loss of control and role change. The role of the survivor is fraught with conflicts. Family members may experience guilt over ideas that they were responsible or that they should have been the victim. One family member may blame another for contributing to the event. The victim may experience difficulty concentrating as the event is relived, or may move from numbness to awareness of the event.

Substance Abuse

The consequences for the family of coping with substance abuse are multiple. For each person afflicted with alcoholism, there are family members who also suffer social and emotional problems associated with the alcoholic's lifestyle disruption. The alcoholic and possibly the family will deny that there is a problem with alcoholism. A spouse or child often becomes an "enabler," one who keeps the family functioning, even on a dysfunctional level. The enabler takes over tasks the alcoholic cannot accomplish, cares for the alcoholic, and makes excuses for them to "cover their tracks." This enables the alcoholic to keep drinking and contributes to the deterioration of the family unit.

Drug abuse also alters family function. Economic destruction may play a greater role in the family of a drug abuser than in that of an alcoholic, due to the higher cost of illegal drugs compared with alcohol. Since drug use is less socially acceptable than alcohol use, the drug abuser and family may be isolated from the community. The threat of drug testing in the workplace may prevent the drug abuser from holding a job, and further disrupts family economic security. Arrest and incarceration may completely disrupt the family unit.

Both alcohol and drug abuse may lead to physical problems from the effects of the substance, as well as injury incurred while intoxicated. Chronic liver disease, poor nutrition, and eventual heart failure are common in alcoholics. Intravenous drug abusers suffer from frequent infections, hepatitis, and possibly AIDS. Family dynamics are further altered by these illnesses.

Manifestations of Altered Family Function

Manifestations of altered family function include social isolation, abuse, separation and divorce, and role strain. Separation and divorce may be solutions, as well.

Social Isolation

Social isolation may result when family members are separated, when there is poor communication within families, or when a family or its members are not accepted by others. Isolation can be physical or psychological. Separation may result from hospitalization, job commitment, or going away to college. Today, many young nuclear families or single adults are separated from their extended families because they have been forced to seek employment elsewhere. They may feel isolated in a new town without the usual family support. Daily demands of job, parenting, home maintenance, college studies, and finances may overburden the person or family members involved. They may not know where to turn for support if they have depended on family in the past. Geographic distance or desire to be independent may make family contact difficult, worsening isolation.

Older adults are facing their final years away from their children and grandchildren, and may be living alone after their spouses are deceased. They may feel isolated by a society that values youth.

Poor communication within a family can isolate individual members. Consider the following example. After the loss of a child, the parents try quickly to get back into a normal routine. They do not involve the sibling in funeral activities and do not cry or talk about their child's death, in an attempt to spare the sibling from pain. The remaining child, who is confused about death, thinks the parents must blame her for the other's death and are punishing her by not involving her. She feels guilty, and imagines that her parents do not love her. She becomes isolated from the family, and from friends as well.

Another form of isolation that families and their members experience occurs when they are not accepted socially or fear such rejection. They may be discriminated against because of race, color, religion, or ethnic origin, or because of stigma associated with illnesses such as AIDS (Fig. 45-6). Fear of isolation by the community, in the workforce, or by others causes further tension within the family.

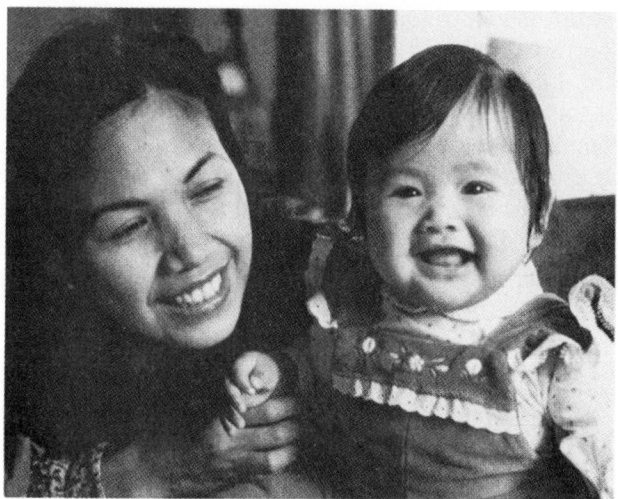

Figure 45–6. The entrance of Mexican–Americans into politics, new perspectives on their culture, and new opportunities have helped Mexican–American families come out of isolation into the "American" culture.

Abuse

Family abuse and violence is a social problem of increasing significance. Abuse may be physical, sexual, emotional, or economic. It may be aimed at the spouse, children, older parents, or grandparents. Factors that contribute to abuse in families include unemployment, substance abuse, chronic illness, inadequate housing, and lack of education and other resources. Family abuse is not limited to lower socioeconomic levels, however, and it is often passed down through the generations in a family; an abused child often grows up to abuse members of his or her own family. The number of child maltreatment cases reported in the United States is about 330 per 1000 population (U.S. Bureau of the Census, 1990).

Abusive family dysfunction is often manifested in parenting behaviors. There may be a lack of attachment (bonding), evidenced by failure to care for the physical or emotional needs of a child or by verbalized resentment or indifference toward the parenting role. Evidence of neglect or physical abuse may be noted, as well as "failure to thrive." Rigidity in role expectations may be present in both parents, inhibiting flexibility in meeting the child's needs.

Sexual abuse of children is another area of concern. Emotional turmoil escalates when the abuse is not reported; or if reported, is ignored to avoid shaming a family member. The child is often confused about the appropriateness of the abuser's behavior and may feel he or she is to blame.

Older adults are also victims of abuse. As they become physically dependent, they may be neglected or verbally and financially abused by their own children. Immobility or sensory disabilities may prevent them from seeking help.

Separation and Divorce

Divorce or separation may be a positive solution to a dysfunctional family situation, or a manifestation of the families' altered function. A major interruption in the developmental process occurs when the family unit is broken by separation or divorce. An ever increasing number of families are being thus affected. The most common form involves the mother and children forming a family unit, while the father moves into a separate environment. A problem that can lead to further dysfunction is role overload for the custodial parent. Shared custody has been attempted to reduce the strain on a single parent, but there is no single solution best for all families.

Remarriage after divorce accounts for one-third of all marriages in the United States (U.S. Bureau of the Census, 1990). Blended families thus formed are also at risk for dysfunction as ties to previous marriages are maintained or broken, and extended family ties are questioned.

Role Strain

Role strain is a manifestation of altered family function when changes in roles are chosen or forced on family members by changing events or development in the family. For example, when a husband becomes chronically ill and unable to work, the wife may become the primary economic provider. She may experience role strain, as she must refocus from being the primary caretaker of the children and house to being a business person. The husband may experience stress as he gives up his role as economic provider and spends more time at home. Children may be reassigned tasks as well, including some physical care for the father.

Giving up familiar roles and taking on new roles may be chosen, as in the case of a two-career family deciding to give up the wife's career for her to stay home and raise children. Family developmental stages call for changing roles periodically; however, role strain develops when family members cannot adapt and needs are not met. Inherent decision-making power influences role strain. Altered roles and resultant role strain can further impede interactions within the family and between the family and society.

Emotional Problems in Children

A variety of emotional and developmental problems can be manifestations of a dysfunctional family. Parenting may suffer whenever family function is altered. Problems with bonding and attachment may arise, and children may have difficulty with emotional development. Depending on the age of the child when family conflict arises, psychosocial development is arrested at that level, according to Erikson's (1963) eight stages of development. For example, if family tension arises while a child is an adolescent and the family does not function adequately, the adolescent may not complete the task of establishing identity. He may be left confused, indecisive, and unable to make plans for the future. He may not satisfactorily complete successive tasks of intimacy and generativity.

The ability of the family to teach, nurture, educate, and socialize offspring is important, according to many developmental models. Emotional problems are often displayed by behavior inappropriate for age or situation. Acting out may occur in the form of temper tantrums, poor school performance, or sexual promiscuity. See Chapter 13 for more information on development.

Impact of Family Dysfunction on Activities of Daily Living

Family dysfunction can have an impact on activities of daily living. To examine changes in family and social relationships related to illness of one family member, consider the following example. A 42-year-old single mother is diagnosed with lung cancer after repeated colds and a bout with pneumonia. In the immediate crisis following the diagnosis, decisions as to how to share the diagnosis with 15- and 11-year-old daughters, whether to ask the grandmother to come and "keep house" during the period of treatment, and what kind of treatment (surgery, radiation, chemotherapy) to choose, all have to be made.

Family relationships will change as usual roles are adjusted. Someone must continue the cooking, cleaning, chauffeuring of children to activities, and so forth. The patient will have to decide whether or not to take a leave of absence from her teaching job or just a few weeks of sick leave. Who in the family will make decisions about discipline, spending money, organizing the home? What will be the financial impact of an extended illness? As the illness moves from an acute to a chronic stage, what options are available for extended care? The grandmother may need to return to her own job. Will friends be available to support the family? Will they feel comfortable continuing to interact with a "cancer patient?" Changes in daily activities are inevitable.

ASSESSMENT

Family assessment can be accomplished in terms of development, wholeness, communication, and support. Subjective and objective data should be recorded. Subjective data are gathered by interviewing the patient and family members, and objective data are gathered by observing family interactions as well as by performing the physical examination. Functional patterns, risks, and family dysfunction are identified through nursing assessment. This serves as a basis for making nursing diagnoses and formulating interventions.

Subjective Assessment

The accompanying questionnaire can be used to assess family function. Usual patterns, risks, and areas of dysfunction may be identified.

Functional Pattern Identification

A systems assessment, in terms of wholeness, communication, and support, can incorporate gathering data on the ability of the family to meet its physical needs, such as food, shelter, health maintenance, etc.; its psychological needs, such as love and belonging, and emotional stability; and its sociocultural needs or interactions within the family and with society (Murray & Zentner, 1989).

Wholeness, communication, and support can also be noted in family interaction patterns in terms of the roles each member assumes. Assessment would include, but

---

Assessment of Family Function, Risk, and Dysfunction Identification

Functional Pattern Identification

Tell me about your family life.

Who are the members of your family?
How are the physical needs of food, shelter, health care, met?
Does each member have assigned tasks?
What is the financial status of the family?
What are the roles of different members?
How does the family communicate?
Who makes decisions in the family?
What does the family do socially or for recreation?
Are members supportive of each other?
What are your family goals? Personal goals?

Risk Identification

What are the potential sources of stress in your family?

How do you feel about your new role?
Are there any financial problems in the family?
Do you have adequate health insurance?
How healthy are other family members?
How did your parents cope with problems in your family when you were growing up?
Is there a history of alcoholism in your family? child abuse?
What other support systems do you have?
Are there communication problems in the family?
Are there relationship problems among members?
Do you feel as though your needs are being met?

Dysfunction Identification

Tell me about the problems in your family.

Are you experiencing role strain?
Describe the abuse you've been experiencing.
How long have you been separated?
Are your children experiencing any emotional problems since you've been ill?
Is your husband denying your child's illness?
What family needs are going unmet?

not be limited to, a study of the relationships between husband and wife, or parent and child; role-relationships of commune members could also be included in an interactional study of family structure and function in meeting individual and group needs. Communication patterns would be considered the key to an interactional approach.

The subjective factors of the actual and perceived roles of family members include work roles and responsibilities in current life situations. Patient identification of satisfaction or disturbances in family, work, or social relationships, and responsibilities related to these roles, should also be assessed. See the display for a list of questions to ask to determine the pattern of family function.

Risk Identification

History-taking to identify areas of risk or potential problems can use both open-ended and focused questioning. Questions related to potential sources of stress in the areas of roles, finances, lifestyle, previous experience, and general health can help identify risk. A general question such as "what are the potential sources of stress in your family?" can be followed by specific questions (see the Display).

Developmental stage of the family should also be taken into account when assessing risk of a family for dysfunction. For example, the birth of a child is a critical point in family development. Perinatal information can be gathered through open-ended questions such as "How did you feel when you realized you were pregnant?" Further information can be obtained with direct questions such as "Who is available to help you after the baby is born?" Reaction to the birth will depend on multiple factors such as whether the pregnancy was planned or desired, whether the child is the first, second, third, etc., whether there is physical space for an additional child, whether the family finances are adequate, whether resource persons are available, and whether the relationship between partners was of short or long duration before the birth.

Subjective Assessment of Family/Social Relationships

Family Structure and Function

- Description of patient's family unit—age, sex, etc.
- Patient's responsibilities in the household?
- Persons responsible for decision within patient's household
- Management of finances?
- Ways in which family responsibilities are distributed?
- Patterns of eating, sleeping, and health practices?

Family/Social Interaction

- Most significant person in patient's life?
- Availability of significant others to patient?
- Any other people that patient can turn to if necessary?
- Number of friends?
- Patient's socialization with friends, neighbors, relatives?
- Description of patient's neighborhood, neighbors.

Indicators of Change

- Any major change in patient's role(s) or responsibilities (explain)?
- Patient's anticipated future changes in the coming years.

- Preparations made for these changes?
- Any family stressors—how they are being handled?

Parental Role Function (If Person Is a Parent)

- Patient's relationship with his or her children?
- Any plans to expand his or her family?
- Comparison of parenting patterns to those of client's parents, e.g., discipline (explain)?

Occupational Role Factors

- Patient's occupation (include work role and responsibilities)?
- Hours worked per week—interference from work with other aspects of patient's lifestyle?
- Ability of patient's income to maintain patient's lifestyle?

Leisure Time Management

- Usual activity pattern? Joint activites?
- Vacations taken and frequency?
- Patient's plans for retirement—if retired, is patient enjoying it?

Cultural Factors

- Ethnic/religious background.
- Similarity of family values.

Adapted from University of Scranton Guide to Care Plan Assessment.

Characteristic risk factors for potential alterations in parenting include unrealistic expectations of self or a child, lack of an appropriate role model, history of a parent having been abused as a child, inability to complete the bonding process, an inadequate support system, the presence of stress, a skill or knowledge deficit, growth and development delay in a child, and unmet psychosocial needs of a child or parent.

Dysfunctional Identification

Dysfunctional family functioning can be identified when there is a significant difference from a normal pattern of functioning. Inability to express or accept emotions, lack of respect or support for other family members, and inability to adapt to change are contributing factors for alterations in family functioning.

When a child is hospitalized, the parental role as caretaker alters. This may be evidenced by verbalization of feelings of inadequacy, guilt, anxiety, failure, helplessness, and powerlessness. Parents may also express concerns about the effect of the child's illness on siblings and the financial burden of illness. Noncompliance with treatment may be manifested in situations involving denial, when parents refuse to acknowledge that there is a problem. Denial may be used as a mechanism to maintain or restore "normality" in family life, but can indicate dysfunction if it deters a family from dealing with the situation (see the display for suggested questions that identify dysfunction).

Objective Data

Objective data for assessing family function include observation of family interactions and individual members' behaviors, as well as the physical examination. Behavioral signs of family dysfunction may include labile emotions, withdrawal, irritability, poor sleeping and eating, inability to concentrate, and dependency. The nurse should observe family communication patterns. How do members relate to each other and how effectively do they communicate? Observation includes who does the talking, who remains silent, are they listening to one another, how disagreements are handled, how decisions are made, and what the nonverbal communication is. Observation of who visits, how often, and how the patient responds can also help the nurse assess the family.

Physical assessment includes inspection, palpation, auscultation, and percussion, performed systematically. While assessing physical health, the nurse looks for family dysfunction clues. The nurse should pay special attention to injuries or bruises, which may indicate physical abuse; enlarged liver and other signs of chronic alcoholism; track marks indicating intravenous drug injection; signs of stress such as weight loss, fatigue, and impaired cognitive function; and multiple acute and chronic physical problems.

NURSING DIAGNOSES AND PATIENT GOALS

Careful assessment of members and the family as a whole may identify actual or potential problems. NANDA has identified the following accepted nursing diagnoses in family problems: Altered Family Processes, Ineffective Family Coping: Disabling; Ineffective Family Coping: Compromised; and Altered Parenting.

Diagnostic Statement: Altered Family Processes

Definition

Altered Family Processes is the state in which a family that normally functions effectively experiences a dysfunction (NANDA, 1990).

Defining Characteristics

Family system unable to meet physical needs of its members; family system unable to meet emotional needs of its members; family system unable to meet spiritual needs of its members; parents do not demonstrate respect for each other's views on childrearing practices; inability to express/accept wide range of feelings; inability to express/accept feelings of members; family unable to meet security needs of its members; inability of the family members to relate to each other for mutual growth and maturation; family uninvolved in community activities; inability to accept/receive help appropriately; rigidity in function and roles; a family not demonstrating respect for individuality and autonomy of its members; family unable to adapt to change/deal with traumatic experience constructively; family failing to accomplish current/past developmental task; unhealthy family decision-making process; failure to send and receive clear messages; inappropriate boundary maintenance; inappropriate/poorly communicated family rules, rituals, symbols; unexamined family myths; inappropriate level and direction of energy (NANDA, 1990).

Related Factors

Situation transition and/or crises; developmental transition and/or crisis (NANDA, 1990).

Diagnostic Statement: Ineffective Family Coping: Disabling

Definition

The state in which the behavior of a significant person (family member or other primary person) disables his or her own capacities and the patient's capacities to effec-

Nursing Research

Selected Nursing Research Studies

Anderson, C. L. (1987). Assessing parenting potential for child abuse risk. *Pediatric Nursing, 13,* 323.

Bartek, J. K., Lindeman, M., Newton, M., et al. (1988). Nurse-identified problems in the management of alcoholic patients. *Journal of Studies on Alcohol, 49,* 62.

Fisk, N. B. (1986). Alcoholism: Ineffective family coping. *American Journal of Nursing, 86,* 586.

Lasky, P., Buckwalter, K. C., Whall, A., et al. (1985). Developing an instrument for the assessment of family dynamics. *Western Journal of Nursing Research, 7,* 40.

Mengel, M. (1987). The use of the family APGAR in screening for family dysfunction in a family practice center. *Journal of Family Practice, 24,* 394.

Possible Topics for Nursing Inquiry

* Is there a relationship between a family's developmental stage and their family APGAR score?
* Do nurses who use the family APGAR screening tool to evaluate family functioning develop more family-related diagnoses?
* Does using the Parenting Profile Assessment Tool versus an open-ended questionnaire increase the reporting of child abuse risk in a Public Health Clinic?
* Is there a relationship between socioeconomic status and nurses' use of referral as an intervention in families dealing with chronic childhood illnesses?

tively address tasks essential to either person's adaptation to the health challenge (NANDA, 1990).

Defining Characteristics

Neglectful care of the patient in regard to basic human needs and/or illness treatment; distortion of reality regarding the patient's health problem, including extreme denial about its existence or severity; intolerance; rejection; abandonment; desertion; carrying on usual routines, disregarding patient's needs; psychosomaticism; taking on illness signs of patient; decisions and actions by family which are detrimental to economic or social

well-being; agitation, depression, aggression, hostility; impaired restructuring of a meaningful life for self, impaired individualization, prolonged over-concern for patient; neglectful relationships with other family members; patient's development of helpless, inactive dependence (NANDA, 1990).

Related Factors

Significant person with chronically unexpressed feelings of guilt, anxiety, hostility, despair, etc.; dissonant discrepancy of coping styles for dealing with adaptive tasks by the significant person and patient or among significant people; highly ambivalent family relationships; arbitrary handling of family's resistance to treatment, which tends to solidify defensiveness as it fails to deal adequately with underlying anxiety (NANDA, 1990).

Diagnostic Statement: Ineffective Family Coping: Compromised

Definition

The state in which a usually supportive primary person (family member or close friend) is providing insufficient, ineffective, or compromised support, comfort, assistance, or encouragement which may be needed by the patient to manage or master adaptive tasks related to his or her health challenge (NANDA, 1990).

Defining Characteristics

Subjective. Patient expresses or confirms a concern or complaint about significant other's response to his or her health problem; significant person describes preoccupation with personal reaction, (e.g., fear, anticipatory grief, guilt, anxiety, to patient's illness, disability, or to other situational or developmental crises); significant person describes or confirms an inadequate understanding or knowledge base which interferes with effective assistive or supportive behaviors (NANDA, 1990).

Objective. Significant person attempts assistive or supportive behaviors with less than satisfactory results; significant person withdraws or enters into limited or temporary personal communication with the patient at the time of need; significant person displays protective behavior disproportionate (too little or too much) to the patient's abilities or need for autonomy (NANDA, 1990).

Related Factors

Inadequate or incorrect information or understanding by a primary person; temporary preoccupation by a significant person who is trying to manage emotional conflicts and personal suffering and is unable to perceive or act effectively in regard to patient's needs; temporary family disorganization and role changes; other situational or developmental crises or situations the significant person may be facing; little support provided by patient, in turn, for primary person; prolonged disease or disability progression that exhausts supportive capacity of significant people (NANDA, 1990).

Diagnostic Statement: Altered Parenting

Definition

The state in which a nurturing figure experiences an inability to create an environment which promotes the optimum growth and development of another human being (NANDA, 1990).

Defining Characteristics

Abandonment, runaway, verbalization, cannot control child, physical and psychological trauma; lack of parental attachment behaviors, inappropriate visual, tactile, auditory stimulation; negative identification of infant/child's characteristics or negative attachment of meanings to infant/child's characteristics; constant verbalization of disappointment in gender or physical characteristics of the infant/child; verbalization of resentment towards the infant/child or to role inadequacy; inattentive to infant/child needs; verbal disgust at body functions of infant/child; noncompliance with health appointments for self and/or infant/child; inappropriate or inconsistent discipline practices; frequent accidents; frequent illness; growth and development lag in the child; history of child abuse or abandonment by primary caretaker; verbalizes desire to have child call him/herself by first name versus traditional cultural tendencies; child receives care from multiple caretakers without consideration for the needs of the infant/child; compulsively seeking role approval from others (NANDA, 1990).

Related Factors

Lack of available role model; ineffective role model; physical and psychosocial abuse of nurturing figure; lack of support between/from significant other(s); unmet social/emotional maturation needs of parenting figures; interruption in bonding process, i.e., maternal, paternal, other; unrealistic expectation for self, infant, partner; perceive threat to own survival, physical and emotional; mental and/or physical illness; presence of stress (financial, legal, recent crisis, cultural move); lack of knowledge; limited cognitive functioning; lack of role identity; lack or inappropriate response of child to relationship; multiple pregnancies (NANDA, 1990).

Related Nursing Diagnoses

When a family is dysfunctional, other problems may arise for members of the family. Related nursing diagnoses include Anxiety, Decisional Conflict; Fear; Grieving: Anticipatory/Dysfunctional; Low Self-Esteem: Chronic/Situational; Parental Role Conflict; Powerlessness; Altered Role Performance; Impaired Social Interaction; Social Isolation; Spiritual Distress; High Risk for Violence.

Patient Goals

Goals are designed to develop alternative desired responses for patients. Patient goals are often derived from identification of the contributing factors and are designed to indicate an improvement in adaptation. General goals can be identified for family functioning and then individualized for each patient situation and the nursing diagnoses that have been identified. Goals should be realistically attainable and measurable.

Patient-centered goals for patients or families experiencing problems with family functioning include:

Patient will identify instances in which intrafamily communication has been achieved.
Patient or family will demonstrate awareness of other members' needs for physical care, economic security, education, and nurturing.
Patient will demonstrate knowledge of effective coping mechanisms.
Patient will demonstrate accomplishment of the developmental stages of the family.

The general goals are individualized for the care plan by adding a time frame, such as "by discharge" or "within 7 days." Nursing interventions or nursing orders are written based on what can be done to achieve the goal, when it can be done, where it can be done, how often, and for how long it should be done.

IMPLEMENTATION

Nurses can intervene with the patient, the family, or both to promote family health and function or to care for the dysfunctional family. To promote family health and function, the nurse teaches and supports. Interventions for the dysfunctional family include referral, counseling, and help with problem solving. The more members of the family the nurse can involve, the greater the potential impact on the family.

Nursing Interventions to Promote Family Health and Function

The family that is at risk for altered function may be helped by identifying strengths, reinforcing positive be-

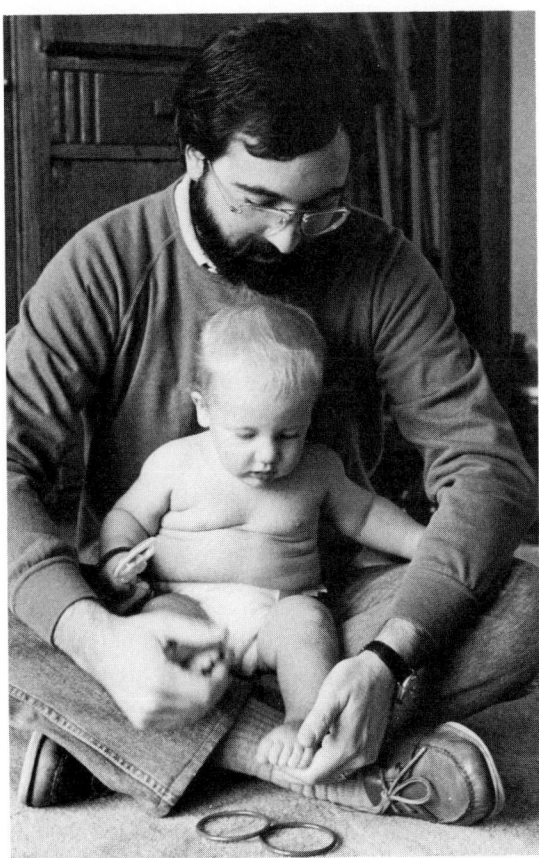

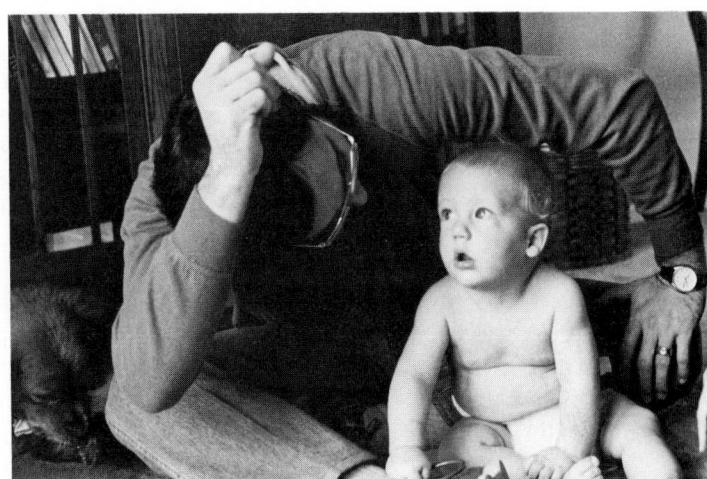

Figure 45–7.   Although the father was traditionally viewed as the authority figure and breadwinner, the father's role now includes attachment to his infant and involves feelings of tenderness and gentleness. These strengths should be supported by the nurse.

haviors and resources, and providing support. The emphasis is on prevention of family dysfunction.

Reinforcement of Family Strengths

The nurse can help the patient or family identify its own areas of strength. These include effective communication, good parenting practices, mutual support of members, flexible roles, general stability, healthy coping mechanisms, and presence of good support systems (Fig. 45-7). Identification of strengths will help the family realize that it has resources to draw from for daily functioning, as well as for when crises develop. Focus is on the strengths rather than weaknesses of the family. The nurse can point out examples of strengths to the patient, such as the ability of a husband to take care of the children while the wife is hospitalized, or spiritual support provided by a priest or minister from the community visiting the patient. The patient and family should also be encouraged to think of examples of strengths themselves, and how these strengths can be drawn on if needed.

Support

The nurse can support the patient and family in actions that promote family functioning. The nurse acts as a support system by listening to and educating the patient

and family. With serious or chronic illnesses, close bonds may be formed between the nurse and patient and family, so they may naturally look to the nurse for emotional support. The nurse also helps them identify other

---

Patient Teaching

Instruct the patient as follows:

- Identify your family's strengths and use them when dealing with family problems.
- Seek outside support when there are problems. Outside support is a strength rather than a weakness.
- Use clear communication, clarify ideas, and listen to one another.
- Use positive (rather than negative) coping mechanisms to deal with family stress.
- Use problem-solving techniques to work through your problems: recognize general problem area; gather information pertaining to it; define specific problem(s); discuss means of solving the problem(s); decide on which means you will use and set goals; periodically evaluate your progress and make further plans.

sources of support in their lives. These may include extended family, religious affiliations, work groups, peers, and community groups. Once identified, contact with support groups can be strengthened to help the family function. The family should be assured that use of support systems is a strength rather than weakness.

Anticipatory Guidance

Anticipatory guidance is a technique that combines teaching and support. Rather than focusing on what has happened in the course of an illness, the nurse prepares the patient and family for what is going to happen and why. A proven example of anticipatory guidance is childbirth preparation. Anticipatory guidance is especially helpful for developmental issues. Family development and child development can be fostered by guiding the family through what is expected to occur and what actions can be helpful. Specific information should be taught, so the family knows what to expect. See Table 13-1 for a list of developmental tasks and parental focuses that can be used to guide the childrearing family.

Birth of a premature infant, or a history of the parents having been abused, may affect parenting roles and normal family functioning. General nursing interventions using anticipatory guidance include:

- Provide a safe and accepting environment for discussion.
- Offer anticipatory information of expectations for child development.
- Identify a positive support system for parents to contact if problems arise.
- Provide opportunities to observe parent–child interactions.
- Discuss parenting strategies and alternatives if problems arise.

The caregivers need to be helped to understand the child's development and express their feelings about their own parenting roles. Opportunities for physical and emotional contact need to be provided. Culturally based child-care practices can also be important. For example, if a grandmother is afforded a primary responsibility in advising the family, it is appropriate to support this cultural tradition unless the advice is injurious. Teaching should be directed towards all people who are involved in the child's care.

Nursing Interventions for Altered Family Function

Once altered family functioning has been identified, interventions focus on adapting behaviors that will return the family to normality. The nurse can help the family with problem solving, offer referrals, and suggest family counseling if necessary.

Problem Solving

Nurses can help dysfunctional families attain goals by assisting them in problem solving.

Interventions aimed toward resolving a family conflict must first identify the willingness of participants to acknowledge a problem, and their ability to communicate. Communication practices, such as allowing each member to speak, listening, and expressing feelings as well as events, should be stressed. Nursing interventions to foster problem solving would then include:

- Clarify the conflict with participants
- Help participants identify contributing factors
- Correct misconceptions
- Provide concrete feedback based on nursing observations
- Assist participants to develop solutions
- Support decision-making among participants.

The nurse should focus on helping the participants develop self-awareness and to identify a working method to solve problems. The family should be led through problem solving while being taught how to conduct the

---

Selected Nursing Interventions for Common Family Problems

Family Coping
- Identify decision-making style in the family.
- Encourage open discussion among family members.
- Identify coping mechanisms within the family.
- Teach communication skills for expressing concerns.
- Support use of counseling for the family to improve communication.
- Identify self-help and support groups appropriate for the family dysfunction.
- Refer to parenting groups or classes if needed.

Problem-Solving Needs
- Clarify the actual conflict among the participants.
- Assist participants in identifying contributing factors.
- Correct and clarify misconceptions.
- Provide concrete feedback based on nursing observations.
- Assist participants in developing solutions.
- Support decision-making among participants.

process themselves. The nurse should guide the family in solving a small problem first, providing reassurance that they can deal with larger problems.

Along with improving communication and problem solving, coping mechanisms should be strengthened (see Chap. 47). The nurse can assist the family in identifying what coping mechanisms worked in the past, as well as what coping mechanisms may be detrimental, such as use of alcohol.

Referral

The nurse may be able to refer the patient and family within the immediate health-care system to find help for areas of dysfunction. Members of the social service department or spiritual ministry may help families with unmet needs. Clinical nurse specialists, nutritionists, and physical and occupational therapists may provide information and training for the patient and family to meet physical care needs.

Examples of self-help and support groups that are often community-based include Alcoholics Anonymous, Al-Anon, Al-Ateen, Narcotics Anonymous, cancer support groups, Compassionate Friends, stroke support groups, and Alzheimer support groups. These groups can help the family work out problems by providing information and emotional support. Parenting groups also are available.

Although people tend to handle their children as they were treated themselves, parenting behaviors can be learned. Professional referrals and peer support groups can be sources of help to people experiencing difficulty in a parenting role. Self-help groups for parents include Parents without Partners, La Leche League International, and Parent Effectiveness Training. Numerous "support groups" listed in the blue pages of phone books are valuable resources for referrals. Rollins (1987) has compiled a comprehensive list of these groups, their activities, and resources.

Other referrals the nurse may have to initiate are those to psychiatric programs, police, drug and alcohol treatment programs, social workers, department of child protective services, and shelters for battered women. When a family is in crisis, the nurse is obligated to ensure the safety of individual members through notification and referral to the appropriate groups. Evidence of suspected child abuse necessitates notification of the police and referral to appropriate agencies.

Ongoing counseling may be necessary for families with chronic stressors such as chronic illness, substance abuse, loss of family member, role strain, or separation or divorce. Family or marital counseling focuses on members interacting with one another rather than on counseling any one person. Roles and relationships are examined, communication and problem solving are fostered, and bonds are strengthened. Nurses can be instrumental in leading patients and families to counseling if

---

Safety Alert

- If you suspect child abuse, notify the police or local child protective services agency. Tell the family that you are acting as an advocate for the child and you are legally responsible to report your suspicion.
- Enlist the help of social services to assist the family.
- Find resources for child care, paying medical bills, and providing other basic needs while a parent is hospitalized.
- Refer an abused spouse to the police or temporary shelter when safety is threatened.
- Point out the deleterious effects of alcohol or drug abuse on the person and family, and refer the person to a substance abuse treatment program.

---

members are unable to overcome dysfunction within the family without outside help.

Discharge Planning and Home Care

Alterations in family and social relationships often must be dealt with in the home environment, placing stress and additional responsibility on family members. When the causative factor is illness, it is necessary before discharge to assess the home environment for supports and barriers to provision of appropriate care and quality of life. Family members can differ in their willingness to assume additional responsibilities. Referrals to social agencies such as Home Health Care may be needed to assure adequate support for a person or family.

Discharge planning should address specific needs, types of assistance and equipment needed, who needs to be taught what, and alternative support availability. Teaching family members techniques of care to meet physical needs can assist in adaptation to the role of caregiver. Teaching should also include signs of risk factors for complications to promote confidence in caring for a patient at home. Providing the family with the name and phone number of someone to contact with questions can ease adaptation to the home setting.

Use of an interdisciplinary approach should include referrals to social workers, counselors, spiritual advisors, community resource centers, and self-help support groups as needed. Community self-help groups such as Al-Anon or an ostomy club can provide support and practical advice and assistance, both before and after discharge.

EVALUATION

Evaluation is an ongoing process of determining progress toward the stated goals that were described in the planning phase. For alterations in family, expected outcome criteria would focus on patient and family communication, family needs, use of coping mechanisms, and family development. The following are examples of possible outcome criteria for general goals.

Goal
Patient will identify instances in which intrafamily communication has been achieved.

Possible Outcome Criteria
- By discharge, each family member engages in conversation while visiting patient, as observed by nurse.
- By discharge, other members listen while family member is talking, as observed by nurse.
- Patient relates that content of conversations includes feelings within 48 hours.
- Patient identifies nonverbal communication as being consistent with verbal messages within 48 hours.
- Patient expresses use of alternatives such as telephone and letter writing when personal visits are not possible during hospital stay.

Goal
Patient or family will demonstrate awareness of other members' physical care, economic security, educational needs, and nurturing.

Possible Outcome Criteria
- Within 48 hours, patient states that children are being cared for, bills are being paid, children are attending school, and family members are attending social functions.
- Within 48 hours, family members display affection toward one another, as observed by nurse.

Goal
Patient will demonstrate knowledge of effective coping mechanisms.

Possible Outcome Criteria
- During first counseling sessions, patient discusses family coping mechanisms that worked in past.
- During first counseling session, patient states coping mechanisms that were detrimental in past.
- By discharge, patient verbalizes coping mechanisms that he or she will use in future.

Goal
Patient will demonstrate accomplishment of developmental stages of the family.

Possible Outcome Criteria
- Patient exhibits appropriate parenting behaviors (holds infant, maintains eye contact, smiles at infant) by discharge.
- Patient maintains family contact by displaying pictures of children in room within 48 hours.
- Patient discusses children with spouse within 48 hours.

Key Concepts

- Although the traditional nuclear family is common, many other family structures exist, including extended families, single-parent families, and blended families.
- Families function in their own unique ways, but usually have common goals. Some needs that families provide for include physical care, economic provision, sexual intimacy, reproduction, education, and socialization.
- Factors that affect family function include culture, economics, lifestyle, previous life experience, and stress and illness.
- Families and their relationships change in reaction to both acute and chronic illness. Roles may be redefined to meet individual and family needs.
- Common manifestations of altered family function include social isolation, separation or divorce, abuse, and emotional problems in children.
- Both objective and subjective data are useful for assessment of family dysfunction. Assessment seeks to identify normal family patterns of function, families at risk for dysfunction, and actual dysfunction.
- Patient goals and nursing interventions focus on the family members and the family unit when caring for dysfunctional families. Goals involve improved communication and coping mechanisms, fulfilled needs of the family, and accomplished development of the family.
- A multidisciplinary approach is useful in intervention of altered family and social relationships. Interventions to promote family functioning include reinforcement of family strengths, support, and anticipatory guidance. Interventions for the dysfunctional family may include referral, problem solving, and counseling.
- Evaluation of nursing care is accomplished by comparing outcomes with criteria established during the planning stage.

References

Burns, C. E. (1984). The hospitalization experience and single parent families. *Nursing Clinics of North America, 19,* 285.

Caplan, G. (1990). Loss, stress, and mental health. *Community Mental Health Journal, 26,* 27.

Nursing Management Plan
The Infant and Family with Altered Parenting

Nursing Diagnosis: Altered parenting related to anxiety, lack of knowledge, money, and paternal support manifested by developmental delay in infant; mother crying easily; verbalized inadequacy of knowledge, finances, and husband.

Family Goal: Child will experience nurturance as caregiver(s) increase parenting skills.

Family Outcome Criteria

- Mother demonstrates decreased anxiety with increased confidence in caretaking behaviors within 1 month.
- Infant demonstrates progress in development within 1 month.
- Family seeks external resources within 2 weeks.

Nursing Intervention	Scientific Rationale
1. Assess mother's knowledge of child-care techniques by questioning and observation. Be nonjudgmental. Encourage expression of feelings.	1. Verbal responses can be validated by objective data. Need to identify without provoking resentment.
2. Reinforce positive caregiving and focus on positive behaviors.	2. Encourages mother and decreases anxiety.
3. Role-model effective stimulation techniques (low cost), such as having mother explore body parts, use colors, talk to and hold infant.	3. Stimulation is important for developmental growth. Sounds, body parts, and color are recognizable by 6 months.
4. Explore with mother ways to involve all family members in meeting infant needs consistently and securely.	4. By decreasing passivity infant can be helped to trust. Likelihood of compliance increased if all members involved.
5. Initiate a plan to develop parenting skills by providing information and alternative opportunities for mother–child interaction with feedback.	5. Information on realistic expectations and solutions can promote effective coping. Practice reinforces.
6. Explore possible sources of support. Offer to make initial contacts. Fear of authorities may inhibit initiating action.	6. Support needs to be ongoing for change to be maintained.
7. Refer for home-visit care.	7. To continue assessment and support.

Duvall, E. (1977). *Family development* (5th ed.). Philadelphia: J. B. Lippincott.

Erikson, E. (1963). *Childhood and society.* New York: Norton.

Masters, J. C., Cerreto, M. C., & Mendlowitz, D. R. (1983). The role of the family in coping with childhood chronic illness. In T. G. Burish & L. A. Bradley (Eds.), *Coping with chronic disease: Research and applications.* New York: Academic Press.

Murray, R. B., & Zentner, J. P. (1989). *Nursing assessment and health promotion strategies through the life span* (4th ed.). Norwalk, CT: Appleton & Lange.

NANDA (1990). *Taxonomy I revised 1990, with official nursing diagnoses.* St. Louis, MO: North American Nursing Diagnosis Association.

Rollins, J. A. (1987). Self-help groups for parents. *Pediatric Nursing, 13,* 403.

Satterwhite, B. B. (1978). Impact of chronic illness on child and family: An overview based on five surveys with implications for management. *International Journal of Rehabilitation Research, 1,* 7.

United States Bureau of the Census. (1990). *Statistical abstract of the United States: 1990.* Author: Washington, DC.

Waisbren, S. E. (1980). Parent's reactions after the birth of a developmentally disabled child. *American Journal of Mental Deficiency, 84,* 345.

Bibliography

Aguilera, D., & Messick, J. (1990). *Crisis intervention theory and methodology* (6th ed.). St. Louis: C. V. Mosby.

Bakke, K., & Pomietto, M. (1986). Family care when a child has late stage cancer: A research review. *Oncology Nursing Forum, 13*(6), 71.

Bloch, B. (1983). Bloch's assessment guide for ethnic/cultural variations. In M. S. Orque, B. Bloch, & L. S. A. Monrroy (Eds.), *Ethnic nursing care: A multicultural approach.* St. Louis: C. V. Mosby.

Burish, T. G., & Bradley, L. A. (Eds.). (1983). *Coping with chronic disease: Research and applications.* New York: Academic Press.

Carpenito, L. J. (1989). *Nursing diagnosis: Application to clinical practice* (3rd ed.). Philadelphia: J. B. Lippincott.

Carter, E. A., & McGoldrick, M. (Eds.). (1980). *The family life cycle: A framework for family therapy.* New York: Gardner Press.

Croog, S. H. (1983). Recovery and rehabilitation of coronary patients: Psychosocial aspects. In D. S. Krantz, A. Baum, & J. E. Singer (Eds.), *Handbook of psychology and health: Cardiovascular disorders and behavior* (Vol. 3). Hillsdale, NJ: Erlbaum.

Davis, F. (1963). *Passage through crisis: Polio victims and their families.* Indianapolis, IN: Bobbs-Merrill.

Ebersole, P., & Hess, P. (1990). *Toward healthy aging: Human needs and nursing response* (3rd ed.). St. Louis: C. V. Mosby.

Fisk, N. B. (1986). Alcoholism: Ineffective family coping. *American Journal of Nursing, 86,* 586.

Foxall, M. J., Ekberg, J. Y., & Griffith, N. (1985). Adjustment patterns of chronically ill middle-aged persons and spouses. *Western Journal of Nursing Research, 7,* 425.

Goetting, A. (1982). The six stages of remarriage: Developmental tasks of remarriage after divorce. *Family Relationships, 31,* 213.

Gordon, M. (1987). *Manual of nursing diagnosis 1986–1987.* New York: McGraw-Hill.

Horowitz, M. J. (1986). *Stress response syndromes* (2nd ed.). New York: Wiley.

Knafl, K. A., & Deatrick, J. A. (1986). How families manage chronic conditions: An analysis of the concept of normalization. *Research in Nursing and Health, 9,* 215.

Suchman, E. A. (1979). Stages of illness and medical care. In E. G. Jaco (Ed.), *Patients, physicians, and illness* (3rd ed.). New York: Free Press.

Waechter, E. H., Phillips, J., & Holaday, B. (1985). Nursing care of children (10th ed.). Philadelphia: J. B. Lippincott.

Wortman, C. B. (1985). Social support and the cancer patient. (Workshop conference on methodology in behavioral and psychosocial cancer research). *Cancer, 53,* 2339.

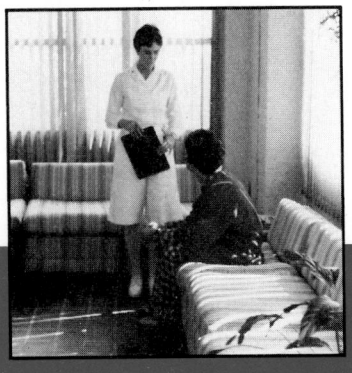

Loss and Grieving

46

Normal Grief Function
  Characteristics of Normal Grief and Loss
    Loss and Grief
    Models of Grief
    Comparison of Grief Reactions to Types of Loss
    Loss: Crisis or Transition
  Normal Functional Grief Pattern
  Factors Affecting Normal Function
  Lifespan Considerations
Altered Grieving Function
  Potential for Altered Grieving Function
  Manifestations of Altered Grieving Function
    Impact of Grieving Dysfunction on Activities of
    Daily Living
Assessment
  Subjective Data
    Functional Pattern Identification
    Risk Identification
    Dysfunctional Identification
  Objective Data
    Physical Assessment
Nursing Diagnoses and Patient Goals
  Diagnostic Statement: Anticipatory Grieving

    Definition
    Defining Characteristics
    Related Factors
  Diagnostic Statement: Dysfunctional Grieving
    Definition
    Defining Characteristics
    Related Factors
  Related Nursing Diagnoses
  Patient Goals
Implementation
  Nursing Interventions to Promote Health and
    Grieving Function
    Patient Teaching
    Working Through Grief Stages
    Support Groups
    Care of the Deceased
  Nursing Interventions for Altered Grieving
    Function
  Discharge Planning and Home Care
    Referral
    Hospice Programs
Evaluation
Key Concepts

Loss and grief are universal experiences; each person experiences various losses from birth until death. These losses vary in importance, from insignificant losses that cause minor and brief distress, to major losses that cause intense and long-lasting distress. Grief is a normal response to loss: it is the price that humans pay for becoming attached to people, objects, or beliefs.

NORMAL GRIEF FUNCTION

Characteristics of Normal Grief and Loss

Loss and Grief

Loss is a normal part of the human experience. Some losses are the result of normal development, whereas other losses are the result of non-normative events. Whether a loss is the result of an expected developmental event or an unexpected, non-normative event, grief is a necessary and normal reaction to loss. The presence of grief indicates attachment to the lost object or person. Through the grief process the person is able to sever attachment to the lost person or object and become attached to other persons or objects.

Loss. Loss is defined as the experience of parting with an object, person, belief, or relationship that is valued; the loss necessitates a reorganization of one or more aspects of the person's life. Losses range from minor ones, such as the loss of a wallet, which necessitates only minor adjustments, to major ones, such as the death of a loved one, which necessitates major adjustments. The intensity and duration of grief depend on numerous factors, including the significance of the loss, the person's personality, and the availability of support.

Losses are part of the normal developmental cycle. At birth the infant loses the warmth and security of the mother's womb. Later, the infant loses the comfort and gratification of the mother's breast. When a sibling is born, the child loses his or her place as the baby or the youngest in the family. Physical losses, such as loss of teeth, follow. Each loss has both negative and positive aspects. For example, by no longer being the youngest in the family, the child gains certain rights and responsibilities, but the child also loses the undivided attention of his or her mother and the special privileges attached to being the youngest in the family.

Many developmental milestones that are ordinarily perceived as desirable events have a component of loss to them. Graduation from high school signifies completion of a major portion of the adolescent's education, and a movement into the world of adults, with its greater freedoms and choices, but it also means the loss of important peer and teacher relationships, and the loss of the routine and security of the high school environment. Marriage is generally perceived as a gain of love, status, and security, but it may also result in a number of losses, such as loss of freedom, loss of individuality, and loss of the single life-style.

Individual patterns of coping with losses are established early in life. Parents often want to protect children from experiencing the pain of loss; however, such protection interferes with the child's development of skills to cope with loss. The person who has learned in childhood that loss is a natural part of life, and that grief is a normal response to loss, will be better prepared to cope with major losses later in life. On the other hand, a major loss, or too many minor losses, early in life often has a harmful effect on the child's personality development, and on the child's ability to cope with losses and develop intimate interpersonal attachments.

Types of Loss. Losses may be categorized in a number of ways: objective vs. subjective; actual vs. perceived; material vs. psychological; or expected vs. unexpected. An objective loss is one that is readily recognized by others as a loss, whereas a subjective loss is one that is not readily apparent to others but is perceived by the person as a loss. A material loss is a loss of some tangible object or possession, whereas a psychological loss is a loss of something that has no physical form but has important symbolic meaning.

Objective or material losses include loss of a body part; loss of body function (paralysis); loss of money; loss of job (retirement); or loss of home (relocation, fire, or disaster). Subjective or psychological losses include loss of a relationship (by death, divorce, or termination of a friendship); loss of hope; loss of a dream; loss of a sense of immortality; or loss of a sense of invulnerability.

Many losses have both material and psychological components. For example, loss of a job results in the material loss of income, but it may also result in numerous psychological losses, such as loss of status, loss of self-esteem, loss of relationships with coworkers, loss of meaning for living, and loss of structure in daily routines. Loss of health may be objectively observable to the person and to others, or it may be unobservable, to self or others. Loss of health often precipitates many other losses, such as loss of ability to work or to perform in one's marital or parental role, or inability to continue in social and recreational activities. Loss of health may be a precursor to loss of life and therefore loss of health may initiate grieving for the person's anticipated death.

Loss of the breast by surgery provides an example of the complex interaction of the various types of loss. Loss of the breast has both objective and subjective components; the removal of the breast results in physical loss of a body part, but it may also result in some loss of function (inability to nurse a child or decreased strength in the arm) or loss of self-image, or perceived loss of potential for dating or for marriage, and thus the loss of the anticipated future. While the objective loss is the same—loss of the breast—the significance of the loss varies greatly from person to person based on the subjective meaning of the loss as perceived by the person. Thus, objective losses are often accompanied by subjective losses. However, subjective losses may occur in the absence of an objective loss. The significance of the loss is determined by the individual's perception of the loss and the meaning he or she ascribes to the loss.

Grief. **Grief** is the characteristic pattern of psychological and physiologic responses a person experiences after the loss of a significant person, object, belief, or relationship. Grief encompasses the entire range of physical, psychological, cognitive, and behavioral responses to a loss, and incorporates the loss into the personality and makes resolution of the loss possible.

Bereavement is a state of desolation that occurs as the result of a loss, particularly the death of a significant other. Bereavement manifestations are the person's total response to a loss and include emotional, physical, social, and cognitive responses.

Mourning encompasses the socially prescribed behaviors after the death of a significant other. Such behaviors vary from culture to culture. Mourning behaviors are socially conventional bereavement behaviors, and do not necessarily indicate the presence or absence of grief. Examples include wearing black clothing, or a black veil or arm-band.

Types of Grief. Two major types of normal grief have been identified: conventional grief, which occurs after a loss, and anticipatory grief, which occurs in anticipation of a loss.

Anticipatory grief is the characteristic pattern of psychological and physiologic responses a person makes to the impending loss (real or imagined) of a significant person, object, belief, or relationship. Although there is little agreement on the exact nature of anticipatory grief (Fulton & Gottesman, 1980; Rando, 1986), there is general agreement that anticipatory grief facilitates coping with loss when the loss actually occurs. Forewarning of a loss should not be confused with anticipatory grief, because it is possible to be forewarned of a loss and not engage in anticipatory grief.

Models of Grief

Normal grief is a multifaceted response to loss. Many researchers and theorists have attempted to describe the characteristics of normal grief and the grief process. Professionals from many disciplines, including nursing, have developed models of grief. Some have proposed stage models of grief, while others have rejected stage models and proposed task models of grief. Still others have proposed models of subconcepts such as bereavement, guilt, and helpfulness in the bereaved. Each of these models provides a framework for understanding the grief process; which model a practitioner chooses to use will influence the nursing process.

Models of grief are useful in guiding nursing care of people experiencing loss. These conceptual models provide understanding of the normal grief process and can be used to provide directions for interventions. They are also useful in helping to identify grief reactions that are outside the normal range.

Some of the problems that arise from use of grief models are due to the inappropriate application of these models, not to limitations in the models themselves. There are no clear-cut stages of grief nor are there any exact time-tables; furthermore, people tend to move back and forth from one stage to another. It is inappropriate and insensitive to expect everyone to conform to a specific model, and to imply that the patient or the staff has failed if the patient does not conform to the model.

Several models of grief have been developed; they are outlined in the display and discussed below. Three popular stage models of grief are those proposed by Engel (1964), Kübler-Ross (1969), and Parkes (1986).

Engel's Model. Engel (1964), one of the first to study

Models of Stages of Grief

Popular Early Models

Engel's Model
1. Shock and disbelief
2. Developing awareness
3. Restitution
4. Resolving the loss
5. Idealization
6. Outcome

Kübler-Ross' Model
1. Denial
2. Anger
3. Bargaining
4. Depression
5. Acceptance

Parkes' Model
1. Numbness
2. Yearning
3. Disorganization
4. Reorganization

Nursing Models

Murphy (1983)
Organized variables that influence bereavement responses

Richter (1984)
Interpersonal support, religious–spiritual belief, and interpersonal coping are resources that, when combined with caring approach of the nurse, can promote health after bereavement

Dimond (1981)
Complexity of grief and the interrelatedness of many intervening factors with bereavement processes and outcomes

Demi (1984)
Incorporates the stage theory of grief, crisis theory, and stress theory

Miles and Demi (1983–1984)
Bereavement guilt

Rigdon, Clayton, and Dimond (1986)
Helpfulness in the aged bereaved

Grief Cycle Model

1. Shock
2. Protest
3. Disorganization
4. Reorganization

grief, proposed six phases of the grief process: (1) shock and disbelief, (2) developing awareness, (3) restitution, (4) resolving the loss, (5) idealization, and (6) outcome. In the shock–disbelief stage, the survivor either refuses to accept the loss, or shows intellectual acceptance of the loss but denies the emotional impact. Developing awareness occurs as the reality and meaning of the loss penetrate the person's consciousness. The numbness of the first phase is replaced with feelings of intense psychological pain, often expressed through crying and anger. The next phase, restitution, consists of the work of mourning and includes the various funeral and religious rituals. The next phase, resolving the loss, occurs intrapsychically as the grieving person focuses energy on thoughts of the deceased. In the phase of idealization, first, all negative feelings toward the deceased are repressed, then, through identification, the survivor incorporates certain characteristics of the deceased into his or her own personality. Gradually, the grieving person's psychological dependence on the deceased diminishes and his or her interest in new relationships returns. According to Engel, the resolution of grief takes 1 year or more.

Kübler-Ross' Model. Kübler-Ross (1969) proposed five stages of grief: (1) denial, (2) anger, (3) bargaining, (4) depression, and (5) acceptance. The denial stage is similar to that proposed by Engel. Anger in the second stage may be directed toward fate, God, family members, health-care providers, or others. Bargaining occurs as the patient seeks to delay the dreaded event; the patient bargains with God for more time, and, in return, promises to do something to repay God for this favor. Depression occurs when the patient acknowledges the reality and inevitability of his or her impending death. In the fifth and final stage, acceptance, the patient comes to terms with the loss, begins to detach from supportive persons, and to lose interest in worldly activities.

Parkes' Model. Parkes (1986) proposed four stages of grief in his model: (1) numbness, (2) yearning, (3) disorganization, and (4) reorganization. In the numbness stage, the bereaved survivor is so overwhelmed by the trauma that denial must be used as a psychological defense. This stage is generally of brief duration. The next stage, yearning, is characterized by intense psychological distress, with thoughts focusing on the deceased. The yearning stage generally lasts several months. The disorganization stage follows, and is characterized by severe depression, social withdrawal, and lack of interest in people and activities. Reorganization generally begins 6 to 9 months after the loss, and is characterized by a gradual renewal of interest in people and activities, and return of a sense of meaning in life. Parkes proposed that this progression through the stages of grief (after the death of a significant other) normally takes 2 or more years.

While Engel and Parkes applied their models primarily to the bereaved, Kübler-Ross applied her model primarily to the dying, which may account for some of the differences between the models. All three saw shock and denial as the first reaction; however, there is little similarity between the models' subsequent stages.

Kübler-Ross' model has gained wide acceptance in nursing and other disciplines, probably because she was a pioneer in developing sensitive, compassionate care for the dying. Her work provided the impetus for increased attention to the needs of the dying and the bereaved, and had an influence on the later development of hospice programs.

Nursing Models. Several nurses have also developed models of grief. Murphy (1983) organized the variables that influence bereavement responses into a model of grief. Richter (1984) proposed relationships between the variables that affect grief and health outcomes; in this model, interpersonal support, religious–spiritual belief, and interpersonal coping are resources that, when combined with the nurse's caring approach, can promote health after bereavement. Dimond's (1981) model indicated the complexity of grief by showing the interrelatedness of many intervening factors with bereavement processes and outcomes. Demi (1984) proposed a model of grief that incorporates the stage theory of grief, crisis theory, and stress theory.

Nurses have also developed models of grief subcon-

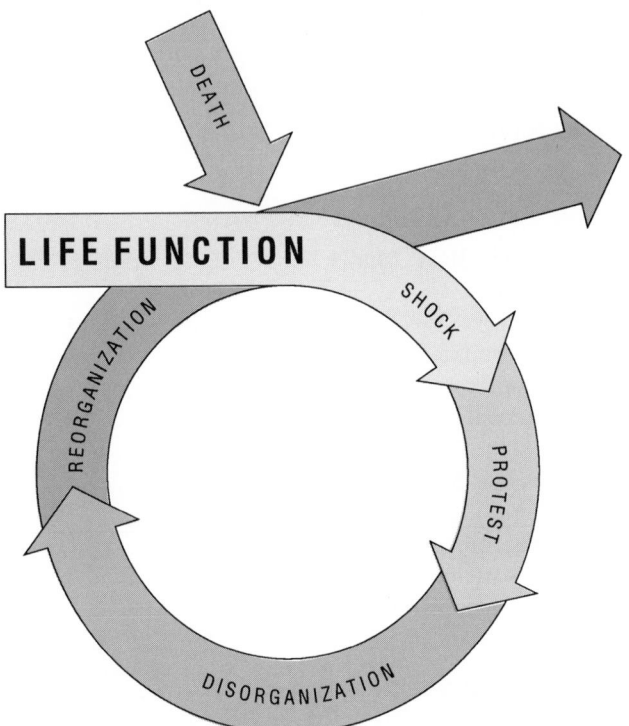

Figure 46–1. Grief cycle. From Demi, A. (1981). *Bereavement support group: Leadership manual.* Littleton, CO: Grief Education Institute.

cepts. Miles and Demi (1983–1984) developed a theory of bereavement guilt, and Rigdon, Clayton, and Dimond (1987) developed a theory of helpfulness in the aged bereaved. Each of these models is useful in guiding practice in specific types of bereavement situations.

Grief Cycle Model.   The grief cycle model (Fig. 46-1), which was derived from Parkes' (1986) theory of grief, provides a model that can be used to guide practice with the bereaved. It can also be used, with minor modifica-

tions, to guide practice with people who have experienced other types of loss. The grief cycle model assumes that, before a major loss, the person is functioning on a relatively unchanging level.

Shock.   When a loss occurs, the first reaction is shock; concurrent with shock is a drop to a lower level of functioning. The shock stage may last several hours to several days. The most common manifestations of the shock stage are listed in Table 46-1. People vary greatly in their responses to loss; some of the manifestations listed are

TABLE 46-1

Major Functional Manifestations During Grief

Category	Shock Stage	Protest Stage	Disorganization Stage	Reorganization Stage
Cognitive	Slowed thinking Disorganized thinking Blocking of thoughts Wish to join deceased Thoughts of suicide	Preoccupation with thoughts of deceased Searching for deceased Dreams (pleasant or unpleasant) Hallucinations Concerns about health and safety of others Continued death wishes	Difficulty making decisions Aimlessness Loss of interest in people Loss of interest in work Loss of interest in usual activities Life perceived as meaningless Focus on memories and reminders of deceased	Realistic memory of deceased Comfortable when remembering deceased Return to previous level of ability
Denial	Denial of the reality of the loss Denial of the significance of the loss			
Emotional	Blunted affect Emotional outbursts May appear unaffected Euphoria Numb emotionally Feeling of unreality	Sadness Anger Guilt Relief Anxiety Yearning for deceased Presence of deceased felt	Depression Loneliness Meaninglessness Decreased self-esteem Apathy	Feels life has meaning Able to experience pleasure

Physical	Numbness
	Hyperactivity
	Underactivity
	Immobility
		Pain in heart
		Sleep problems
		Appetite problems
		Weight loss
		Neglect of appearance
		Fatigue
		Lethargy
			Continued sleep and appetite problems
			Restlessness
			Decreased sexual interest/satisfaction
			Aimless activity
			Decreased resistance to illness
			Accident prone
			Poor health habits
			  Increased alcohol intake
			  Increased drug use
			  Increased tobacco use
				Renewed vigor
				Restoration to previous level of health
				Improved health habits
				Sexual drive renewed

Social	Passive Unaware of others Focus on supporting others	Dependent on others Help and advice of others sought	Withdrawn Contact with other people avoided Initiative severely diminished Interest in social activities absent	New or renewed social relationships New or renewed activities Development of close relationship with at least one other person

polar opposites, such as hyperactivity and underactivity. Thus, not all of these characteristics are exhibited simultaneously by one person.

Protest. The second stage, protest, generally starts in the first week and continues through the third month. The person continues to drop in his or her level of functioning. During this period there is intense physical and psychological distress. The common characteristics of this stage are listed in Table 46-1.

Disorganization. The disorganization stage starts around the third month and continues for 3 to 6 months. The person continues to drop in his or her level of functioning and sinks to the lowest level of functioning during this stage. This stage is characterized by feelings of depression and social withdrawal. The manifestations of this stage are listed in Table 46-1.

Reorganization. The reorganization stage starts at approximately the sixth month and generally continues for at least 1 year, but may continue for a much longer period of time. Many people will continue in this phase for the rest of their lives. The major characteristics of this stage are listed in Table 46-1. During reorganization, the person gradually increases his or her level of functioning. People who have sufficient resources during this period are likely to continue to improve their level of functioning, and often emerge from the grief cycle at a higher level of functioning than before the loss. On the other hand, people who experience many stressors during the grief period, and who have limited resources, are often unable to recover fully from the grief experience, and thus will continue to function at a lower level than before the loss.

Caution must be used to prevent interpreting the grief cycle model too literally. In reality, the stages are not as discrete as the model implies, and there is much individual variation in the grief process. It is helpful to use the model as a general guide, however, while keeping in mind the fact that people may vary greatly in their responses to loss and still fall within the normal response range.

Comparison of Grief Reactions to Types of Loss

Only a few researchers have attempted to compare reactions to types of losses. Parkes (1986) compared grief reactions after the loss of a significant other by death with loss of a limb by amputation, and Fried (1962) compared reactions to death of a spouse with reactions to the loss of a home through relocation. Both of these researchers found a number of similarities in grief reactions after these diverse losses.

Parkes (1986) found a similar pattern of reaction in amputees and in widows. The first reaction was the gradual process of realization, then a stage of alarm, and next an urge to search and recover the lost loved object. The process was less obvious in the amputee than in the widow, but it was nevertheless present. One of the problems for the amputees was that society did not expect them to mourn the loss of a leg, and thus they received little support in their grieving process. The bereaved were preoccupied with thoughts of the deceased, while the amputees were preoccupied with thoughts of their altered body image. Both groups of subjects pined painfully for the world that was no longer theirs. The widowed envied other couples, and the amputees envied intact people. Both groups of people felt anger at physicians and nurses.

Parkes found that, at 1 year after surgery, 26% of the amputees were still depressed and withdrawn, and most were making little use of their prosthesis. Parkes concluded that the psychosocial transition from intact person to amputee is a time-consuming process similar to the transition from married status to widowhood.

Two researchers investigated the effect of loss of one's home by relocation (Fried 1962; Marris, 1975). Fried (1962) studied Boston slum dwellers after their forced geographic relocation, and found that, while their reactions to the loss of their homes varied widely, the general pattern was congruent with a grief reaction. Common manifestations were feelings of loss, continued longing, depressive feelings, displaced anger, and idealization of the lost place. Marris (1975) studied Nigerian slum dwellers and found similar effects after their relocation. Marris proposed that the loss of one's home was as devastating as the death of a family member.

Loss: Crisis or Transition

Some theorists propose that a major loss results in a life crisis, whereas others propose that a major loss results in a life transition. Caplan's (1964) and Lindemann's (1944) early conceptualizations of bereavement as a life crisis were oversimplifications. Crisis theory (Caplan, 1964) is based on the following propositions:

The psychobiologic forces for change during a crisis operate for a relatively short period of time (a few weeks).

The outcome of a crisis is not predetermined but rather is determined by the balance of stressors and resources available during the crisis.

During a crisis, a person has a heightened desire for help.

During a crisis, the person is more susceptible to the influence of others.

In the intervening years, Caplan (1974) realized the inappropriateness of the proposition that a major loss can be resolved in a few weeks. Consequently, he developed a life transition theory, in which he proposed that there are several crisis periods during the course of mourning, which are more appropriately perceived as life transition periods than as a single crisis. He recognized that some people will continue the psychological work of mourning for the rest of their lives and still be within the normal range of grieving.

Normal Functional Grief Pattern

Grief has several important functions:

- To make the outer reality of the loss into an internally accepted reality
- To sever the emotional attachment to the lost person or object
- To make it possible for the bereaved person to become attached to other persons or objects.

Although grief is often very painful, it is both normal and necessary. In contrast, inability to grieve is abnormal.

Factors Affecting Normal Function

Many factors influence people's reactions to loss, the course of the grief process, and the ultimate recovery from grief. These factors include characteristics of the loss itself, personal resources, personal stressors, sociocultural resources, and sociocultural stressors.

According to crisis theory (Caplan, 1964), the outcome of a loss experience is not predetermined, but rather, is determined by the balance of stressors and resources present during the grief period. Thus, a person who has few stressors and many resources is likely to be able to cope well with a loss, whereas a person who has many stressors and few resources is likely to have difficulty coping with a loss.

Characteristics of the Loss. People have a tendency to ascribe their own values and feelings to others, and thus incorrectly assume that a specific loss is or is not traumatic to a specific person without first ascertaining the meaning of the loss to that person. Loss of a finger would have very different meanings to a classical guitarist and to a manual laborer. Divorce may be extremely undesired and cause intense grief in one person, or it may be welcomed and thus cause little or no grief reaction in another.

When it is a loved one that is lost, regardless of the mode of loss (e.g., death, divorce, or separation), numerous aspects of the relationship affect the grief process. These aspects include such factors as the intensity of the relationship, the symbolic meaning of the relationship, the amount of ambivalence in the relationship, and the availability of others to fulfill some of the roles of the lost person.

The circumstances under which the loss occurred also affect the grief process. A loss that occurs under violent or frightening conditions is much more difficult to cope with than a loss that occurs under more peaceful conditions. For example, a death that occurs as a result of homicide or suicide is usually more stressful than a death that occurs due to natural causes. Another stressor is the perception that the grieving person in some way caused or contributed to the loss. For example, when a parent buys a child a bicycle and the child is maimed or killed in a bicycle accident, the parent may blame himself or herself for the accident.

Personal Resources and Stressors. Each person enters a loss situation with a unique combination of personal resources and stressors. What is a resource for one person may be a stressor for another. For example, health status may be either a resource or a stressor: the person who has good nutrition, good health habits, and a generally high level of wellness has a major advantage over the person who has poor nutrition, poor health habits, both chronic and acute diseases, and a history of emotional illness.

Personal resources and stressors that influence response to a loss include coping skills, previous experiences with loss, emotional stability, spiritual beliefs, physical health, individual developmental stage, family developmental stage, and socioeconomic status.

Research indicates that socioeconomic status is one of the major factors related to ability to cope with loss. People with higher levels of education, higher income, and higher job status tend to have better outcomes after a major loss. This may not be a causal relationship, but rather may be due to the fact that people who are healthier mentally and physically are more likely to be in higher socioeconomic classes.

Additional factors that may influence outcomes are the number of other crises that the person experienced in the time periods preceding and after the loss. Other losses may produce a pile-up effect that may overwhelm the person's capacity to cope with these multiple stressors.

Sociocultural Resources and Stressors. The sociocultural resources and stressors that influence grief reactions also vary widely from person to person. Sociocultural resources include the social support that is available from family, friends, coworkers, and formal institutions (Fig. 46-2). Absence of these social supports creates additional stressors for the grieving person. In some instances the presence of these supports can also be stressors, particularly if the resource people are not able to empathize with the grieving person. The overall sociocultural environment influences outcomes. If a community is able to deal with loss, and has reasonable expectations of the survivors, this reduces stress; however, if the community tends to blame the survivors for their plight (as in the case of AIDS), or if the community has unrealistic expectations, the grieving person will have much more difficulty coping with the loss.

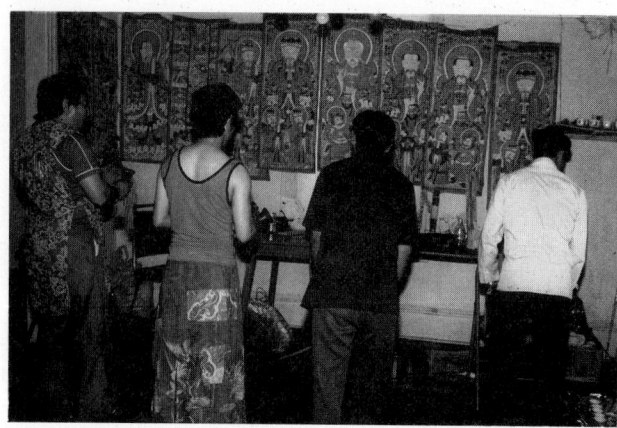

Figure 46–2. A Mien shaman and his assistants present offerings to the gods at a grandmother's home after she died in a hospital. (Photo courtesy of Marjorie A. Muecke, Seattle, WA.)

Community resources such as self-help groups, hospice bereavement programs, pastoral counselors and other clergymen, and health-care professionals are necessary resources to help those who have experienced a loss.

Lifespan Considerations

Reactions to loss vary across the lifespan. The interaction of grief and life cycle stage is complex. Grief may interfere with the achievement of developmental tasks, and developmental tasks may interfere with the grieving process. Thus, the person's developmental stage must be considered when assessing reactions to loss and planning interventions.

The impact of a traumatic event depends heavily on the developmental stage during which the event occurs. Children's reactions to loss differ markedly from adults' reactions, both in their specific characteristics and in their duration. Children tend to grieve in a piecemeal fashion. Losses are so painful to the young that they are able to endure distressing emotions for only brief periods of time; they grieve for intermittent periods of time, but their grief work extends over many years. Since children's distressing emotions are often expressed as anger or behavior problems, these signs are often not recognized as grief manifestations. The overwhelming need for love and security promptly motivates the child to search for and find a replacement for the lost loved person or loved object.

Newborn and Infant

To develop a concept of life and death, of being and nonbeing, one has to have cognitive function and have begun the socialization process. The newborn, thus, has no concept of life and death.

"The ability to sense alterations in existence during the cycles of wakefulness and sleep is likened to a beginning understanding of the physical states of 'being' and 'nonbeing.' The game of 'peek-a-boo,' ironically, an old English game meaning 'alive or dead,' introduces the child to the death-related concepts of absence and presence. The child's delighted reaction represents relief from the terror of being briefly separated from physical reality" (Waechter, Phillips, & Holaday, 1985).

As the infant develops, he or she begins to distinguish the primary caregiver from other people. The infant responds to the mother's or father's voice and face. The infant's concept of death or loss is related to feelings of separation anxiety. This occurs when the mother is out of sight during early infancy, but levels off when the infant learns (as in peek-a-boo) that the mother still exists although she cannot be seen. Nevertheless, this recognition that mother will return initiates another realization that the mother *may not* return. Thus, the developmental task of developing a sense of trust works to nullify the anxiety that the caregiver will not return. Other characteristics of grief and loss in the infant are given in Table 46-2.

Toddler and Preschooler

Cognitive powers are evidenced by 18 to 24 months. Cognitive meaning intensifies the toddler's experience of separation anxiety. The developmental task of developing a sense of autonomy occurs during toddlerhood. This task helps the toddler break the tie with mother. She can now be out of sight for some time without the toddler being unduly concerned. However, since the toddler vacillates between being independent and being clinging, the separation still gives the toddler a fear of maternal loss or abandonment. Other characteristics of grief and loss in the toddler are given in Table 46-2.

Preschoolers develop an increasing awareness of themselves as separate physical and emotional beings. With this deepening awareness of "self" comes the vague realization that one's identity may cease to exist. Although preschoolers sense their own vulnerability and begin to make the distinction between being alive and dead, they still cannot grasp the finite limits imposed by death (Waechter, Phillips, & Holaday, 1985).

Preschoolers develop their concepts from their experiences. If the child watches television, many life concepts may develop from what they see. People die and reappear in another show, and this is how the preschooler sees death. The preschool child has some beginning cognitive understanding of death, but perceives death as reversible, avoidable, and occurring in degrees.

Preschoolers think of death as a long sleep. They cannot differentiate infinite and finite. The death of a pet or a family member plays an important part in developing a concept of death, although their cognitive ability does not allow a clear understanding. At first they

TABLE 46–2

Characteristics of Childen Across the Lifespan Regarding Loss and Death Concept

Developmental Age	Developmental Task	Characteristics and Concepts
Infant	To develop a sense of trust	Dependent on those around him or her to meet his or her basic needs No intellectual capacity to comprehend death Experiments with concepts of absence/presence and being/nonbeing Anxiety separation from primary caregiver
Toddler	To develop a sense of autonomy	Less dependent, learning to separate from primary caregiver Egocentric Fully explores concepts of absence/presence and being/nonbeing May misinterpret illness as punishment for being bad Fears abandonment or separation from family
Preschooler	To develop a sense of initiative	Expanding his or her social environment Egocentric, influenced by magical thinking Death concept involves a temporary departure or sleep Fears family separation
School-aged child	To develop a sense of industry	Less egocentric; views world from external point of view Death concept is equated with old age and violence Death is personified Concept evolves rapidly until aware that death is irreversible, permanent Fascinated with physiologic phenomena and death rituals May believe in spiritual continuation Fears own possible death
Adolescent	To develop a sense of identity	Working toward being independent and self-sufficient Looking toward the future, establishing career, and personal life goals Moving into adulthood Death is viewed as a universal, inevitable process that is permanent

ask straightforward questions, but later begin to develop an aversion to it.

Psychoanalysts believe that children cannot complete the work of mourning until they have a realistic concept of death. Since it is generally agreed that preschool-aged children have a very limited understanding of death, they are unable to complete mourning until they are older. See Table 46-2 for more information on the preschooler.

Child and Adolescent

The school-aged child gradually develops a more realistic concept of death. In the early school years, the child perceives death as unnatural, reversible, and avoidable; the child may also personify death (e.g., perceives death to be a person or an animal). At about 9 years of age, the child's concept of death matures, and the child perceives death realistically as irreversible, universal, inevitable, and natural.

Society reinforces concepts of life and death. By school age, children have usually been touched by death in some way (i.e. a family member, classmate, friend's family, a pet, or a news story). Some children live in

violent neighborhoods where death is common, and some live in abusive families where injury and hospitalization may occur. The modern school curriculum includes discussions about war and death if these are prominent in the news or a traumatic local event occurs. The religious institution teaches about spiritual life and heaven and hell. Christian denominations observe the death, birth, and resurrection of a savior. The school child eventually realizes that death is an event no one escapes. See Table 46-2 for further characteristics of children regarding loss and grief.

As age increases, the child's understanding of death becomes more realistic. A high level of cognitive development allows the adolescent to view life and death with an adult understanding. Adolescents begin to develop a philosophy of life and death. "Nevertheless, the thought of one's own death is extremely overwhelming, and consequently, is suppressed. Adolescents are already in the midst of a developmental crisis during which they experience constant change" (Waechter, Phillips, & Holaday, 1985).

Adolescents generally have the capacity to mourn fully, but they are at greater risk for poor outcomes than adults because of the numerous other stressors and development changes they experience during this stage of the life cycle.

Adult and Older Adult

In contrast to children, adults tend to grieve more intensely and more continuously, but for a relatively shorter period of time. Furthermore, adults generally do not seek an immediate replacement for the lost loved person, but rather move toward this after achieving some resolution of their grief.

Young adults often experience many losses within a short period of time, which makes them particularly at risk for poor outcomes. They may experience the death of a family member for the first time in their lives, or the ending of their schooling and consequent separation from peers, or broken relationships, or failure in their attempt to achieve a satisfying job. The suicide rate for 20- to 24-year-olds is second only to the rate for the aged. Special attention must be given to meet the needs of this at-risk group.

Middle-aged adults who have a relatively stable lifestyle and adequate support systems generally cope well with loss; however, an untimely loss, such as the death of a child or the death of a spouse, may be extremely stressful, because this is perceived as out of the normal sequence of events.

Aged adults are generally at higher risk than other adults for poor outcomes after major losses. The elderly often experience numerous losses, sequentially or simultaneously. At a time when their stressors are the highest, their resources are often the most meager. Deaths of relatives and friends, retirement, impaired health of self or family members, and decreased economic resources are all common stressors for the elderly. As their social network shrinks due to deaths and illnesses of family members and friends, they have fewer support networks available to them. Thus, the elderly may need to rely more on health-care providers to assist them in coping with their losses.

Community resources such as self-help groups, hospice bereavement programs, pastoral counselors and other clergyman, and health-care professionals are necessary resources to help those who have experienced a loss.

ALTERED GRIEVING FUNCTION

Dysfunctional grief is grief that falls outside the normal response range and may be manifested as exaggerated grief, prolonged grief, or absence of grief. In dysfunctional grief, the grieving person often becomes stuck in one stage of the grief process and is unable to progress to the next stage or stages. Furthermore, the grieving person expends so much energy either repressing the grief or dealing ineffectively with the grief that little time or energy is left to invest in normal growth and development.

Potential for Altered Grieving Function

The potential for altered function is affected by the stressors and resources that the person experiences during the loss, by the piling up of stressors that occurred before the loss, and by the accumulation of resources before the loss. If the stressors outweigh resources, then the person is at risk for altered functioning. Particularly at risk are those with several concurrent losses, few support systems, poor coping skills, and previous unresolved losses.

Manifestations of Altered Grieving Function

In a recent study of bereavement experts' perceptions of "grief that falls outside normal parameters," Demi and Miles (1987) found that more than 30 different terms were commonly used to label dysfunctional grief. The most commonly accepted terms were pathologic grief, unresolved grief, dysfunctional grief and prolonged grief.

Many symptoms that have generally been considered abnormal or dysfunctional were identified as components of the normal grief process. At 1 year after bereavement, most experts believed that the grief manifestations listed in the Display were within normal parameters.

Bereavement experts reported that they consider almost all bereavement manifestations to be normal during the early stages of grief, but consider most of the manifestations to be abnormal if they continue beyond 3 years after bereavement. Some of the symptoms considered normal during the early bereavement period but abnormal if present beyond 3 years are listed in the display.

Impact of Dysfunction on Activities of Daily Living

Dysfunctional grief leads to dysfunction in everyday life activities. The person may be too tired or too depressed to concentrate on daily household chores or personal hygiene. Crying, loss of appetite, and sleep disturbance add to the grieving dysfunction and loss of energy. The adult may no longer be able to maintain a job or provide a safe and healthy home atmosphere, and the child may be unable to keep up with schoolwork. Social isolation may add to the family's dysfunction. An added stress may be that, because of involvement of "self" in grieving, the family becomes unable to communicate with each other.

Normal and Abnormal Grief Manifestations

Normal at 1 Year Postbereavement

- Excessive or persistent expression of affect
- Inability to experience joy
- Clinical symptoms of depression
- Inability to form new relationships
- Inability to speak of the deceased without intense emotion
- Hearing or seeing the deceased
- Feelings of emptiness or meaninglessness

Abnormal if Present Beyond 3 Years

- Leaving the deceased's room and belongings intact
- Reporting physical symptoms similar to those the deceased had before death
- Talking about the loss as if it just happened
- Inability to remember or talk about the deceased
- Being preoccupied with thoughts of the deceased
- Talking or acting as if the deceased were still alive
- Experiencing physical illness that seems to be related to the loss

ASSESSMENT

Questions about losses (actual and anticipated) need to be incorporated into the assessment of every patient. Frank physical illness may be the result of a loss, actual or anticipated; often the patient does not connect the presenting symptom with the loss. On the other hand, physical illness or accident may result in loss, both actual and anticipated. Some patients recognize the effect of loss or anticipated loss, while others completely deny the loss and its meaning. The skillful nurse will recognize the relationship of loss to health status and will help the patient recognize and acknowledge this connection also.

Subjective Data

Nurses must be cautious not to interpret a single behavior as dysfunctional grief. Many behaviors previously thought to be dysfunctional are being recognized as normal components of grief.

Observation and assessment of a grieving person at a single point in time is not a good way to assess the normality of the grief response. A much better way to assess the normality of a grief response is to follow the grieving person over time and observe whether grief manifestations are increasing, remaining the same, or diminishing. Furthermore, one must assess the entire constellation of grief manifestations and not overemphasize any specific symptom.

To distinguish between a normal grief reaction and a dysfunctional grief reaction, one must assess the severity of the symptoms and the pattern of change over time. Many of the symptoms previously reported as signs of dysfunctional grief are believed to be normal components of the grief process and therefore are not discussed here. Data to be collected are listed in the display.

Functional Pattern Identification

Historical events that should be assessed include the nature of the relationship with the deceased and the circumstances of the loss. When interviewing a patient, it is helpful to start the interview with some general, nonthreatening questions before moving in to ask questions about the loss. However, a major factor in understanding the loss reaction is assessing the relationship to the lost person/object. The nurse needs to know:

- What was the physical and psychological significance of the lost person/object?
- Was the loss unexpected or expected?
- Did the survivor contribute or perceive that he or she contributed to the loss?

The nurse also needs to assess the patient's personal resources and personal stressors. Personal resources are strengths within the person that contribute to a healthy pattern of grieving. Personal stressors are limitations within the person that may inhibit healthy grieving. Personal stressors and resources include personality characteristics, coping skills, communication skills, physical health status, spirituality, and previous experiences with loss. To assess personal stressors and resources, one needs to know the following:

- Does the patient have a history of emotional illness?
- What coping behaviors does the patient usually use?
- How well does the patient communicate with others?
- What previous losses has the patient experienced?
- How did the patient cope with these previous losses?
- Are any of these previous losses still unresolved?
- Does the patient have any physical health problems?
- What are the patient's spiritual beliefs and how do they influence his or her reactions to loss?

The nurse also needs to assess sociocultural resources and stressors. Sociocultural resources are the assets that

---

Subjective Data Collection

Nature of the loss: _____.

Meaning of the loss to the patient: _____.
_____.

Patient's usual pattern of coping with loss: _____.
_____.

Availability of resources: _____.
_____.

Other stressors (preceding or concurrent with loss):
_____.
_____.
_____.

Physical symptoms:
  Sleep patterns _____.
  Appetite _____.
  Tightness in throat and chest _____.
  Heart palpitations _____.
  Pain in chest _____.
  Frequent sighing _____.
Emotional symptoms:
  Sadness _____.
  Guilt _____.
  Anger _____.
  Relief _____.

Anxiety _____.
Loneliness _____.
Wishing to die _____.
Suicidal ideation _____.
Subtance use:
  Alcohol _____.
  Illegal drugs _____.
  Prescribed drugs _____.
  Caffeine _____.
  Nicotine _____.
Socal behavior:
  Ability to function in roles (family, work, and social roles)
  _____.
  _____.

Cognitive behavior:
  Preoccupation with thoughts of loss _____.
  Seaching for lost person/object _____.
Spiritual:
  Loss of faith _____.
  Anger at God _____.

---

are available to the patient from the interpersonal environment, and include social support, practical support, and cultural traditions and customs. Sociocultural stressors are strains and tensions exerted on the patient by the social and cultural systems. Adequate social support is a key factor in the prevention of dysfunctional grieving. Family members, peers, friends, coworkers, and employers can function as either resources or stressors. Cultural traditions also may be either resources or stressors. For example, if the cultural tradition dictates a long mourning period and the bereaved person is ready to move into the reorganization stage of grief, this may create feelings of conflict. However, it is more likely that sociocultural expectations will be that the bereaved person stop grieving and get "back to normal" long before the bereaved person is capable of doing so. To assess sociocultural stressors and resources, the following questions need to be asked:

- What social supports are available to the grieving person?
- Does the grieving person perceive these supports as helpful?
- What are the traditional rituals for dealing with this type of loss?
- To what extent did the grieving person participate in the sociocultural rituals and how satisfied were they with the rituals?
- Do any of the social and cultural traditions conflict with needs of the grieving person?

Risk Identification

The risk for dysfunctional grief can be identified through analysis of the resources and stressors that the patient is experiencing. Patients with many stressors and few resources are at greatest risk. The severity of the loss and the degree of anticipation of the loss also affect risk; losses that affect many aspects of the person's life, and losses that are unanticipated are more stressful. The nurse must always keep in mind the patient's perception of the loss; what is perceived as a minor loss by one person may be perceived as a major loss by another.

Physical health and psychosocial adjustment are intricately intertwined. The bereaved are known to be at greater risk for mortality and morbidity than are comparable nonbereaved persons. Research reveals that the greatest increase in mortality after bereavement has been due to suicide, accidents, and homicide (Kaprio, Koskenvuo, & Rita, 1987). In addition, men are particularly at risk for dying of cardiovascular disease. This increased risk of mortality is greatest in the first month after bereavement, remains elevated throughout the first year of bereavement, then drops to normal range by the end of the second year of bereavement (Kaprio, Koskenvuo, & Rita, 1987).

Dysfunctional Identification

It is difficult to identify dysfunction based on a single contact with a patient. People with normal grief may display many diverse and intense signs and symptoms. Nurses must avoid inappropriately placing a label of dysfunctional grief on a normal process. Generally, dysfunction can only be identified after several contacts with the patient over an extended period of time. If a person remains in complete denial of the loss, or if the person's grief symptoms continue unabated over a long period of time, the person is likely to be having a dysfunctional grief process.

Objective Data

Grief may manifest itself in many diverse physiologic and psychological signs that are directly observable. Many of these signs are identical to the signs of depression; consequently, it is very difficult to differentiate between normal grieving and depression. Currently, there is no laboratory test to assess the presence of grieving, but there are a few paper-and-pencil tests that are helpful in assessing grief symptomatology, such as the Grief Experience Questionnaire (Sanders & Mauger, 1979), the Bereavement Experience Questionnaire (Demi & Schroeder, 1985), the Impact of Event Scale (Zilberg, Weiss, & Horowitz, 1982), the Texas Inventory of Grief (Fauschingbaur, DeVaul, & Zisook, 1977), and the Beck Depression Inventory (Beck, 1972).

Physical Assessment

Many of the subjective manifestations of grief have concomitant objective manifestations:

- Dejected physical appearance
- Slowed motor function
- Weeping
- Outbursts of anger
- Emotional blunting
- Unkempt appearance
- Sleep disturbance
- Appetite disturbance (excessive weight loss or gain)
- Preoccupation with thoughts of that which was lost.

NURSING DIAGNOSES AND PATIENT GOALS

Anticipatory Grieving and Dysfunctional Grieving are the two approved nursing diagnoses relevant to loss and

grief (McLane, 1987). A number of nurses believe that another diagnostic category should be added, Normal Grieving (Carpenito, 1989). The rationale for adding this diagnosis is that normal grieving results in numerous physical, emotional, and social consequences that can be ameliorated through nursing interventions.

Diagnostic Statement: Anticipatory Grieving

Definition

Anticipatory Grieving is defined as the state in which an individual or group experiences feelings in response to an expected significant loss (Carpenito, 1989).

Defining Characteristics

Potential loss of significant object; expression of distress at potential loss; denial of potential loss; guilt; anger; sorrow; choked feelings; changes in eating habits; alterations in sleep patterns; alterations in activity level; altered libido; altered communication patterns (NANDA, 1990).

Related Factors

Related factors have yet to be developed for this diagnosis.

Diagnostic Statement: Dysfunctional Grieving

Definition

Dysfunctional Grieving is defined as the state in which an individual or group experiences prolonged unresolved grief and engages in detrimental activities (Carpenito, 1989).

Defining Characteristics*

Verbal expression of distress at loss; denial of loss; expression of guilt; expression of unresolved issues; anger; sadness; crying; difficulty in expressing loss; alterations in: eating habits, sleep patterns, dream patterns, activity level, libido; idealization of lost object; reliving of past experiences; interference with life functioning; developmental regression; labile affect; alterations in concentration and/or pursuits of tasks (NANDA, 1990).

Related Factors

Actual or perceived object loss (object loss is used in the broadest sense); objects may include: people, posses-

* Caution must be exercised in using these characteristics to diagnose Dysfunctional Grief since many of the characteristics are components of the normal grief process (Demi & Miles, 1987).

sions, a job, status, home, ideals, parts and processes of the body (NANDA, 1990).

Related Nursing Diagnoses

In addition to the diagnoses of Anticipatory Grieving and Dysfunctional Grieving, patients who have experienced a major loss may also be found to have the nursing diagnoses based on functional health given in Table 46-3.

Patient Goals

Development of patient goals centers around the stage of grief the patient is in and whether the grief is normal, anticipatory, or dysfunctional. The patient should have input in deciding what personal needs are for the moment. Short-term and long-term goals are needed. The following patient goals are samples of what may need to be addressed with this patient.

The patient will move toward resolution of diverse emotions.
The patient will accept the reality of the loss.
The patient will reinvest emotional and physical energy in meaningful persons and activities.

TABLE 46–3

Nursing Diagnoses Related to Grief and Based on Functional Health

Functional Health Area	Nursing Diagnoses
Health perception/ health management	Altered health maintenance High risk for injury
Nutrition/metabolism	Altered nutrition: Less than body requirements
Activity/exercise	Activity intolerance Diversional activity deficit Impaired home maintenance management
Sleep/rest	Sleep pattern disturbance
Cognition/perception	Knowledge deficit Decisional conflict
Self-perception/ self-concept	Anxiety Fear Hopelessness Self-esteem disturbance
Sexuality/reproduction	Sexual dysfunction
Coping/stress tolerance	Ineffective individual coping Impaired adjustment Ineffective family coping: Compromised
Values/beliefs	Spiritual distress

Nursing Research

Selected Nursing Research Studies

Field, D. (1989). Nurse's accounts of nursing terminally ill on a coronary care unit. *Intensive Care Nursing, 5*(3), 114–122.

Fraser, S. et al. (1990). Survivors recollections of helpful and unhelpful emergency nurse activities surrounding sudden death of a loved one. *Journal of Emergency Nursing, 16*(1), 13–16.

Gilbert, K. R. (1989). Interactive grief and coping in the marital dyad. *Death Studies, 13*(6), 605–626.

Lattanzi-Licht, M. E. (1989). Bereavement services: Practice and problems. *Hospice Journal, 5*(1), 1–28.

Lockard, B. E. (1989). Immediate, residual, and long term effects of a death education instructional unit on the death anxiety level of nursing students. *Death Studies, 13*(2), 137–159.

Possible Topics for Nursing Inquiry

- What are the long-term effects of specific nursing therapies with grieving children?
- Do specific nursing activities provide definable support for families of terminally ill patients?
- What coping mechanisms do critical care nurses employ when caring for critically ill patients?

IMPLEMENTATION

Nurses are frequently in close contact with many patients who are experiencing a major loss; therefore, nurses have many opportunities to provide care for grieving persons. Since grief is frequently both devastating and long-lasting, there are generally many opportunities for nursing interventions throughout the grief process. Normal grieving will be discussed, as managing dysfunctional grieving is beyond the scope of the beginning student.

Nursing Interventions to Promote Health and Grieving Function

Nursing interventions to promote normal grieving should occur before a loss occurs or is anticipated to occur.

Patient Teaching

Nurses should teach parents to begin loss education during early childhood. Preschoolers should be taught about the normality of loss and grief through exposure to naturally occurring events. A visit to a nursing home, the death of a distant relative, the death of a goldfish, the loss of a favorite toy, or the loss of a friend all provide opportunities to discuss the natural life cycle and loss in nonthreatening ways. The parent or other relative who can talk about loss honestly and openly, in terms that the child can understand, will help the child establish a healthy attitude toward loss and will serve as a role model for the child.

Loss education should continue throughout childhood and adolescence. Nurses should continue their role in educating parents about ways to help children deal with grief and loss (see the display). Parents should be encouraged to include children in mourning rituals; however, children should never be forced to participate in such rituals. Parents should also be encouraged to allow children to express their diverse feelings about various losses. Gradual exposure to loss and death situations concurrent with appropriate preparation and support will prepare the child to cope with losses later in life.

Nurses should also be directly involved in education of children about grief and loss. Nurses should incorporate grief education naturally into their contacts with children in various health-care settings, such as schools, hospitals, physician's offices, and clinics.

Working Through Grief Stages

Nursing interventions for grieving should be based on the stage of grief that the patient is experiencing. The following discussion and the display list these interventions. Further interventions are found in the Nursing Management Plan at the end of the chapter.

During the shock phase, nursing interventions should focus on protecting the patient from physical harm and on getting the patient to accept the reality of the loss. During this phase the nurse should help the patient to mobilize normal support systems; for example, the nurse should help the patient to contact family members and to tell them about the loss. Patients may act out impulsively, or may have decreased reaction times, and therefore effort must be taken to prevent the patient from self-harm (suicide attempts) and from accidents. It is generally helpful to have a family member present when the patient is notified of a loss, or an anticipated loss, and to have this person drive the patient home; this is particularly important when the loss is unanticipated. Patients should be encouraged to use coping behaviors that have been helpful to them in the past, such as participation in religious activities, or talking with a friend or relative. If the loss was a death, patients should be encouraged to participate in funeral and mourning rituals.

Patient Teaching

Instruct the parent as follows:

DOs
- Know your own feelings and beliefs.
- Be honest.
- Begin at the level the child is on.
- Include child in family rituals related to death and mourning.
- Encourage expression of feelings.
- Provide security and stability.
- Encourage remembrance of deceased.
- Recognize that child grieve differently than adults.
- Expect the child to alternate between grieving and normal functioning.
- Talk openly about death and feelings it generates.
- Introduce death concepts into conversation naturally.

DON'Ts
- Praise stoicism.
- Encourage forgetting of the deceased.
- Force the child to participate in grief and mourning rituals.
- Emphasize the likeness of the child to the deceased.
- Compare the child to the deceased.
- Use euphemisms.
- Protect child from exposure to experiences with death.

During the protest phase, nursing interventions should focus on getting the patient to express thoughts and feeling about the loss, and maintaining the patient's normal health status. Interventions include those listed in the display on the next page.

During the disorganization phase, emphasis should be placed on getting the patient to accept the reality of the loss and to begin reorganization of his or her life. Interventions instituted during the shock phase should be continued. Additional interventions are included in the display on the next page.

During the reorganization phase, emphasis should be placed on helping the patient to continue reorganizing his or her life, and to find new or renewed meaning in life. Some losses, such as the death of a spouse, or a spinal cord injury or blindness, require a major reorganization of many life activities, while other losses, such as reproductive sterility or amputation of a finger, may require reorganization in only a few areas. Patients who

---

Selected Nursing Interventions to Help the Patient Move Through Grief Stages

Interventions During Shock Phase

- Help patient mobilize a support system.
- Protect patient from physical harm.
- Have a family member present when notifying patient of a loss.
- Have someone drive patient home.
- Help patient establish coping behaviors used in past.
- Encourage patient to participate in mourning rituals.

Interventions During Protest Phase

- Encourage expression of diverse feelings (sadness, loneliness, anger, guilt, resentment, relief).
- Encourage remembering and talking about that which was lost.
- Provide anticipatory guidance regarding the normal grief process.
- Provide role models who have successfully coped with similar loss.
- Encourage patient to use existing support systems.

- Identify new support systems.
- Discourage use of alcohol, drugs, and caffeine.
- Promote appropriate sleep habits.
- Promote good nutrition.
- Refer for complete physical examination.
- Encourage participation in religious rituals.
- Encourage use of previous healthy coping behaviors.
- Introduce new coping behaviors.

Interventions During Disorganization Phase

- Continue interventions begun in shock phase.
- Refer patient to self-help groups.
- Refer patient for individual or group counseling.

Interventions During Reorganization Phase

- Refer patient for career counseling.
- Refer patient to educational programs.
- Refer patient to social activity programs.

---

experience a greater degree of life reorganization may need additional interventions (see the display above).

Support Groups

Common problems for those experiencing loss are intense emotional distress, lack of social support, and prolonged grief. To prevent these problems from occurring, patients should be encouraged (early in the grief process) to participate in befriender programs or self-help support groups. Befriender programs, such as the Widow-to-Widow program (Silverman, MacKenzie, & Pattipas, 1974) and the Reach-to-Recovery program for mastectomy patients, provide one-to-one support by nonprofessionals who have experienced a similar loss and have made a satisfactory recovery from the loss. These befriender programs provide role modeling, education, and emotional support. Self-help support groups serve the same functions as befrienders; however, the help is less individualized and is primarily provided in a group setting. Furthermore, the support group is composed of people in various stages of recovery from their grief.

Care of the Deceased

Nursing care continues after the death of the patient. Concern for dignity in the care of the body as well as sensitivity to the needs of the deceased patient's family are within nursing's responsibility. Immediately after the patient's death has been certified, family members may wish to spend some time alone with the patient's body. In an effort to limit exposure to the disturbing sight of equipment and medical supplies, the nurse should remove unneeded items, and clean, position, and cover the patient. Allowing the family time alone with the patient may be an important step for them in the grief process. Some families may appreciate the presence of a nurse, spiritual leader, other family members, or friends. Other families may feel comforted by spending this time alone. Religious and ethnic beliefs and customs should be observed as far as possible.

The physical care of the body includes bathing as needed to remove drainage and secretions. The patient's eyelids should be gently closed. Dentures (if any) can be inserted in the mouth, and a rolled towel or washcloth placed under the chin to help keep the mouth closed. The body needs to be aligned as normally as possible before rigor mortis develops (about 4 to 6 hours after death). Jewelry and other valuables need to be removed and given to the family along with other personal belongings, and their disposition should be noted in the medical record.

When the patient's body has been prepared and the family leaves, the nurse should place appropriate identification tags on the wrist and ankle of the patient's body. The body is then taken to the hospital's morgue, or is removed from the room by the mortician.

If there have been special instructions from the patient's family regarding donor use of the patient's organs, the nurse will need to take immediate measures to preserve the donor organs, either by notification of the appropriate medical teams or by placement of ice packs. When an autopsy is desired, the physician will request written permission from the family. While the general aspects of care after death remain the same in all facilities, there may be specific guidelines and policies for each individual facility of which the nurse needs to be aware.

Nursing Interventions for Altered Grieving Function

Patients experiencing dysfunctional grief need professional help to resolve problems. This help generally takes one of two forms: individual therapy, or professionally led support groups. This type of help may be prescribed, in addition to self-help. Professional support is particularly important if the patient has inadequate support systems. Many nurse–therapists specialize in grief therapy.

Discharge Planning and Home Care

When a patient has experienced a major loss, or is anticipating such a loss, adequate discharge planning and home care are essential. Since the grief process extends over a long period of time, the severity of the patient's grief may not be obvious during hospitalization. Nurses may misperceive the patient's shock and denial, and conclude that the patient is "unaffected by the loss." Actually, the patient who appears unaffected by a loss is particularly in need of follow-up care, since he or she may have a delayed grief reaction.

Referral

Discharge planning should include referral to befriender programs, self-help groups, professionally led support groups, public-health nurses, or hospice programs, depending on the patients' specific needs and the community resources. Patients should also be encouraged to continue their contact with their primary health-care provider (physician or nurse), since the grief process often decreases resistance to disease and exacerbates existing illnesses.

Hospice Programs

Hospice programs are particularly important resources for the terminally ill and their families. **Hospice** refers to both a place where people can go to receive care when they are terminally ill, and to a philosophy of care for the terminally ill. The goal of the hospice program is to promote the highest possible quality of life for the patient and family throughout the terminal illness and at the time of death.

There are two major types of hospice programs, inpatient programs and home-care programs. All hospice programs are based on the principles listed in the display.

One of the unique aspects of hospice care is the attention given to the grief of the dying patient and to the grief of the family members. Hospice caregivers assist the patient in coping with numerous losses and in facing impending death. They also facilitate anticipatory grieving of family members, and provide bereavement care after the patient has died. Thus, hospice programs are important community resources that contribute to continuity of care for grieving patients.

EVALUATION

Below are listed some general goals and outcome criteria for a grieving patient that can be used as a guide for

(Text continues on page 1330)

Principles of the Hospice Program

- The quality of life is more important than the quantity of life.
- The family is the unit of care.
- Many of the needs of the dying patient can be met at home.
- Hospice services must be available 24 hours per day.
- Since the patients needs cannot always be met in the home, appropriate inpatient services must be available.
- Because of the complex needs of dying patients and their families, services are provided by an interdisciplinary team.
- Interventions focus on the management of physical and psychosocial needs of patients and family members.

Nursing Management Plan
The Patient Who Is Grieving

Nursing Diagnosis: Grieving (normal) related to actual loss of significant person manifested by expression of unresolved issues.

(During the shock stage)

Patient Goal: Patient will move toward resolution of diverse emotions.

Patient Outcome Criteria

- Patient cognitively accepts the reality of death within 1 week.
- Patient participates in funeral and mourning rituals within 1 week.
- Patient expresses emotional affect in discussion, facial expressions, and reactions within 72 hours.
- Patient uses family and friends for social support in resolving emotional responses within 1 week.

Nursing Intervention	Scientific Rationale
1. Encourage mourner to see deceased and allow mourner to touch or hold the deceased, if desired.	1. Cognitive recognition of the reality of death is necessary before beginning to work on acceptance of the emotional significance of the death.
2a. Provide anticipatory guidance regarding physical appearance of the deceased. b. Encourage mourner to participate in grief and mourning activities that are congruent with their sociocultural and spiritual/religious beliefs.	2. Cognitive acceptance of the death is facilitated by participating in funeral and mourning rituals.
3. Notify the family members of the death in person in a private setting whenever possible.	3. Trauma of notification of the death can be eased by sensitive attention to family members' needs.
4. Encourage mourner to express diverse feelings, e.g., guilt, sadness, relief, numbness, anger.	4. Open expression of feelings facilitates gradual resolution of these feelings; some feelings are perceived as socially unacceptable.
5. Encourage mourner to talk about the deceased and to ask questions about the death.	5. Preoccupation with thoughts of the deceased is a normal part of the grief process; talking about the deceased's life and death begins breaking emotional bonds with the deceased.
6. Provide anticipatory guidance on the grief process, including common thoughts, feelings, and behaviors; emphasize that there is no one right way to grieve.	6. Most people have little knowledge about the normal grief process, and it is reassuring for them to know that what they are experiencing is normal.
7. Assist mourner with making decisions regarding urgent postdeath responsibilities; help mourner contact family members and other support persons.	7. Bereaved person is often in crisis and needs the emotional and practical support from family and other support persons.
8. Protect the mourner from deliberate or unintentional harm, e.g., inquire about suicidal thoughts; encourage mourner not to drive own car immediately after learning of the death.	8. Bereaved are at greater risk of mortality and morbidity, particularly from accidents and suicide.

(continued)

Nursing Management Plan
The Patient Who Is Grieving (continued)

(During the protest stage)
Patient Goal: Patient will begin acceptable transition to life without deceased.
Patient Outcome Criteria

- Patient recognizes and accepts emotional feelings as acceptable within 2 months.
- Patient begins transition to new roles within 2 months.
- Patient experiences minimal deterioration of physical health during first 3 months after death of loved one.

Nursing Intervention	Scientific Rationale

1. Encourage mourner to remember and talk about both the negative and positive memories of the deceased.
    Use counseling skills of empathy, warmth, and positive regard.
    Facilitate reality testing.
    Assess need for individual or family counseling.
	1. The process of breaking bonds with the deceased continues over an extended period of time.
	    Counseling skills can be used to elicit unrecognized thoughts and feelings.
	
	    Bereaved people who have numerous stressors and few resources benefit from professional therapy.

2. Teach support persons about the emotional needs of the bereaved.	2. Adequately prepared support persons can augment professional services or may be the only intervention needed.
3. Provide appropriate reading materials on the grief process.	3. Identification with other bereaved persons can be therapeutic.
4. Reinforce use of healthy coping skills.	4. During a crisis, a person may be too overwhelmed to use his or her usual coping skills; therefore the nurse must help them remember these skills.
5. Assess for suicidal ideation.	5. Transition to new roles is a major stressor for the bereaved; role models and education on the new roles facilitates ease in role transition.

6. Encourage patient to assume some new roles, to relinquish other roles, and to allow support persons to fill some of the deceased roles.
    Provide role models for new roles (e.g., widow-to-widow befriender)
    Recommend participation in self-help or mutual help support groups.
	6. The death of a significant other precipitates role changes.
	
	    Patients often do not know how to function in new roles; role models can show them how to function.

7. Teach problem-solving skills related to new roles.	7. New roles require diverse problem-solving skills.
8. Provide appropriate reading materials on practical aspects of role transition (e.g., financial management, automobile maintenance, child care, home maintenance).	8. Seeing things in written form helps to reinforce ideas and knowledge; books become references.
9. Encourage complete physical assessment.	9. The risk of increased mortality and morbidity is highest during the early bereavement period but continues throughout the first year of bereavement.
10. Promote good health habits (e.g., nutrition, rest, avoidance of alcohol and tobacco).	10. Good health habits and early identification of health problems may prevent serious illness.

(continued)

Nursing Management Plan
The Patient Who Is Grieving *(continued)*

(During the disorganization stage)
Patient Goal: Patient will reinvest emotional and physical energy in meaningful persons and activities.
Patient Outcome Criteria

- Patient emotionally accepts the loss within 9 months, as disclosed by patient.
- Patient experiences improved functioning in new roles within 9 months.
- Patient discusses with nurse a search for new meaning in life within 9 months.
- Patient/family verbalizes experiencing increased family cohesiveness within 9 months.

Nursing Intervention	Scientific Rationale
1. Assist patient in decision-making regarding disposal of deceased's belongings.	1. During the disorganization stage the patient recognizes the emotional significance of the loss and begins to accept the meaning of the loss.
2. Support patient's expression of grief (e.g., cemetery visits, memorial services, visiting places of special meaning to deceased).	2. Activities focusing on the unresolved grief can facilitate resolution of the loss.
3. Normalize thoughts and feelings.	3. Same as above.
4. Use role-play to work through unresolved issues.	4. Same as above.
5. Encourage patient to express thoughts and feelings through writing.	5. Same as above.
6. Enhance previous coping skills.	6. New roles continue to cause stress; effort must be directed toward strengthening bereaved's intrapersonal and interpersonal competence.
7. Introduce additional coping techniques.	7. Same as above.
8. Support independent problem-solving skills.	8. Same as above.
9. Keep support systems mobilized.	9. Same as above.
10. Encourage to delay major decisions until out of acute grief.	10. Same as above.
11. Support patient's reevaluation of the meaning of his or her life.	11. The death of a loved one leads the bereaved to question the meaning of life.
12. Encourage participation in spiritual/religious activities.	12. Same as above.
13. Encourage patient to participate in social and recreational activities.	13. Same as above.
14. Teach family members that each person expresses grief differently and resolves his or her grief at a different speed.	14. The family functions as a system; death of a family member affects all parts of the system.
15. Encourage open family communication about the loss and the feelings engendered.	15. Each subsystem affects other subsystems and the system as a whole.
16. Identify and reinforce the strengths of each family member.	16. Strengthening any part of the system has a positive effect on other subsystems and on the system as a whole.
17. Encourage family members to provide support to each other.	17. Same as above.
18. Mobilize extra family support systems.	18. Friends, coworkers, and others can supplement support received from family members.

(continued)

Nursing Management Plan
The Patient Who Is Grieving (continued)

(During the reorganization stage)
Patient Goal: Patient will increase level of physical, emotional, social, and spiritual level of functioning (previous level or higher level of functioning)
Patient Outcome Criteria

- Patient resolves emotional reactions to the loss within 2 years.
- Patient reports satisfaction with new roles within 2 years.
- Patient reports finding new meaning in life within 2 years.
- Patient reports achievement of personal growth within 2 years.
- Patient reports improved coping skills within 2 years.

Nursing Intervention	Scientific Rationale
1. Avoid unrealistic expectations for mourner to recover quickly.	1. Resolution of grief after the death of significant other often takes 2 to 5 years. By the end of the first year, the bereaved should have resolved the major portion of his or her grief but will continue to reexperience grief on anniversaries.
2. Remind patient that it is normal for grief feelings to be rekindled by trigger events such as holidays and anniversaries.	2. Same as above.
3. Support renewal of old friendships/interests and development of new friendships/interests.	3. Meeting with friends and finding new activities eases the emotional loss and give new meaning to life.
4. Use gentle confrontation to deal with unresolved feelings towards deceased.	4. It is important to deal with all feelings before the grief period can end.
5. Facilitate recognition of own strengths and limitations.	5. Knowing yourself aids in acceptable functioning.
6. Encourage continued participation in support group.	6. Support is still needed from people with similar problems.
7. Support continued involvement in religious, social and recreational activities.	7. By end of second year, bereaved should have found a satisfactory level of health and functioning.
8. Praise patient for satisfactory achievement of roles.	8. By end of second year, bereaved should be functioning satisfactorily in roles.
9. Encourage reevaluation of diverse meanings in life.	9. The search for meaning continues for a long period of time after resolution of other aspects of grief.
10. Support changes in patient's behavior and life style.	10. The crisis of bereavement often produces profound personal growth.
11. Reinforce use of a variety of coping skills.	11. Bereaved persons often report greatly increased coping skills after resolution of grief and also report a sense of confidence that since they managed to handle their grief satisfactorily, they will be able to handle any other stressor satisfactorily.

evaluation. However, the nurse must constantly keep in mind the fact that evaluation must be individualized based on the patient's specific needs and goals. Thus, these goals and outcome criteria are presented as suggestions, to be amended based on knowledge about the specific patient.

Goal
The patient will recognize and express diverse emotions.

Possible Outcome Criteria
- Within 7 days, patient expresses diverse emotions, such as sadness, anger, guilt, loneliness, or relief.
- Within 14 days, patient states that experienced emotions are normal components of the grief process.

Goal
The patient will move toward resolution of diverse emotions.

Possible Outcome Criteria
- Within 6 months, patient states decreased frequency and intensity of painful emotions.
- Within 9 months, patient expresses decreased frequency of preoccupation with thoughts of the lost loved one/object.

Goal
The patient will recognize reality of the loss.

Possible Outcome Criteria
- Within 4 weeks, patient discusses the loss and its meaning.
- Within 4 weeks, patient discusses potential life changes necessary because of the loss.
- Within 6 months, patient disposes of articles no longer needed (e.g., paraplegic gives away skis, widow gives away deceased spouse's clothing).
- Within 12 months, patient plans for major life changes to accommodate the loss (e.g., selling home, taking new job).

Goal
The patient will recognize need for help and seek help appropriately.

Possible Outcome Criteria
- Within 24 hours, patient reaches out to family and friends for emotional and practical help.
- Within 2 months, patient uses family and friends for social support.
- Within 6 months, patient uses community resources for support.
- Within 12 months, patient assumes major responsibility for self.

Goal
The patient will retain or regain physical health status.

Possible Outcome Criteria
- Patient does not use sleeping pills, alcohol, caffeine, tobacco, or tranquilizers as crutches to ease the pain.
- Within 3 months, patient follows prescribed medical regimen and adheres to healthful behaviors.
- Within 12 months, patient states that he or she has returned to normal eating, sleeping, and exercise habits.

Goal
The patient will reinvest emotional and physical energy in meaningful persons and activities.

Possible Outcome Criteria
- Within 9 months, patient participates in new activities.
- Within 12 months, patient reports making necessary changes in social, recreational, and occupational spheres.
- WIthin 12 months, patient identifies renewal of old friendships and development of new friendships.
- Within 24 months, patient expresses sense of satisfaction with life and a sense of meaning in life.

Evaluation is an ongoing process that includes assessing the patient and comparing the patient's status to the outcome criteria. During this process the nurse must keep in mind the long-term nature of grief, and that progress toward these outcomes may be very slow, but nevertheless, within the normal range. The nurse must use astute clinical judgment to determine if the patient is making satisfactory progress toward the goals; if the patient is not making satisfactory progress, then the nursing care plan must be revised.

Key Concepts

- Loss is a universal experience, and grieving is a normal response to loss.
- Models of the grief process provide direction for nursing assessment.
- The grief process is similar regardless of the type of loss experienced.
- A major loss results in a long-term life transition.
- The characteristics of the loss, personal resources and stressors, and sociocultural resources and stressors affect the normal grief process.
- The outcome of a loss experience is not predetermined, but rather, is determined by the balance of stressors and resources present during the grief period.

■ Risk of dysfunctional grieving can be identified through analysis of the stressors and resources that the patient is experiencing.

■ Response to loss is influenced by the person's stage of development.

■ Physical health and psychosocial adjustment during the grief process are intricately intertwined.

■ Nursing interventions should be based on knowledge of the long-term nature of the grief process.

■ Many grief manifestations, identified in the literature as dysfunctional, are considered to be components of the normal grief process.

■ Caution should be used in labeling a client as having dysfunctional grieving.

■ Discharge planning must consider the long-term nature of the grief process.

■ Hospice programs are important community resources that provide family-focused support for clients who are experiencing grieving.

References

Beck, A. (1972). *Depression: Causes and treatment.* Philadelphia: University of Pennsylvania Press.

Caplan, G. (1964). *Principles of preventive psychiatry.* New York: Basic Books.

Caplan, G. (1974). Foreward. In I. Glick, R. Weiss, & C. M. Parkes (Eds.), *The first year of bereavement* (pp. vii–xi). New York: Wiley.

Carpenito, L. (1989). *Nursing diagnosis: Application to clinical practice* (3rd ed.). Philadelphia: J. B. Lippincott.

Demi, A. (1984). Hospice bereavement programs: trends and issues. In S. Schraff, ed. *Hospice: the nursing perspective* (pp. 131–151). New York: National League for Nursing.

Demi, A., & Miles, M. (1987). Parameters of normal grief: A Delphi study. *Death Studies, 11,* 397–412.

Demi, A., & Schroeder, M. (1985). *Bereavement experience questionnaire.* Paper presented at Measurement of Clinical and Educational Nursing Outcomes Conference, New Orleans, LA.

Dimond, M. (1981). Bereavement and the elderly: A critical review with implications for nursing practice and research. *Journal of Advanced Nursing, 6,* 461–470.

Engel, G. (1964). Grief and grieving. *American Journal of Nursing, 64*(9), 88–100.

Faschingbauer, T., DeVaul, R., & Zisook, S. (1977). Development of the Texas Inventory of Grief. *American Journal of Psychiatry, 134,* 696–698.

Fried, M. (1962). Grieving for a lost home. In L. J. Duhl (Ed.), *The environment of the metropolis.* New York: Basic Books.

Fulton, R., & Gottesman, A. (1980). Anticipatory grief: a psychosocial concept considered. *British Journal of Psychiatry, 137,* (45–54).

Kaprio, J., Kaskenvuo, M., & Rita, H. (1987). Mortality after bereavement. *American Journal of Public Health, 77,* 283–287.

Kubler-Ross, E. (1969). *On death and dying.* New York: Macmillan.

Lindemann, E. (1944). Symptomatology and management of acute grief. *American Journal of Psychiatry, 101,* 141–148.

Marris, P. (1975). *Loss and change.* Garden City, NY: Doubleday.

McLane, A. (1987). *Classification of nursing diagnoses.* St. Louis: C. V. Mosby.

Miles, M. S., & Demi, A. S. (1983–1984). Sources of guilt in bereaved parents: Toward the development of a theory bereavement guilt. *Omega, 14,* 299–314.

Murphy, S.A. (1983). Theoretical perspectives on bereavement. In P. L. Chinn (Ed.), *Advances in nursing theory development* (pp. 191–206). Rockville, MD: Aspen.

NANDA (1990). *Taxonomy I revised 1990, with official nursing diagnoses.* St. Louis, MO: North American Nursing Diagnosis Association.

Parkes, C. M. (1986). *Bereavement: Studies of grief in adult life* (2nd ed.). New York: International Universities Press.

Rando, T. (1986). *Loss and anticipatory grief.* Lexington, MA: Lexington.

Richter, J. M. (1984). Crisis of mate loss in the elderly. *Advances in Nursing Science, 6*(4), 45–53.

Rigdon, I., Clayton, B., & Dimond, M. (1987). Toward a theory of helpfulness for the elderly bereaved: An invitation to a new life. *Advances in Nursing Science, 9*(2), 32–43.

Sanders, C., & Mauger, P. (1979). *A manual for the Grief Experience Inventory.* Tampa, FL: University of Florida.

Silverman, P., MacKenzie, D., Pattipas, M., et al. (1974). *Helping each other in widowhood.* New York: Health Sciences.

Waechter, E. H., Phillips, J., & Holaday, B. (1985). *Nursing care of children* (10th ed.). Philadelphia: J. B. Lippincott.

Zilberg, N., Weiss, D., & Horowitz, M. (1982). Impact of event scale: A cross validational study and some empirical evidence supporting a conceptual model of stress response syndromes. *Journal of Consulting and Clinical Psychology, 50*(3), 407–414.

Bibliography

Attig, T. (1989). Coping with mortality: An essay on self-mourning. *Death Studies, 13,* 361–370.

Beaton, J. L., et al. (1990). Life and death decisions: The impact on nurses. *Canadian Nurse, 86*(3), 18–19, 21–22.

Blunt, K. L. (1989). Grief observations. *Journal of Urologic Nursing, 8*(4), 752–753.

Carter, S. L. (1989). Themes of grief. *Nursing Research, 38,* 354–358.

Cecchini, J. A. L. (1990). Reach out and touch . . . dealing with dying patients and their families. *Imprint, 37*(1), 73.

Coco, P. (1989). Bereavement questions and answers: When a patient dies I feel so inept. Please tell me what I can do to help the grieving family. *Advances in Clinical Care, 4*(6), 11.

Davis, C. B. (1989). The use of art therapy and group process with grieving children. *Issues in Comprehensive Pediatric Nursing, 12*(4), 269–280.

Field, D. (1989). Nurse's accounts of nursing terminally ill on a coronary care unit. *Intensive Care Nursing, 5*(3), 114–122.

Fraser, S., et al. (1990). Survivors recollections of helpful and unhelpful emergency nurse activities surrounding sudden death of a loved one. *Journal of Emergency Nursing, 16*(1), 13–16.

Gifford, B. J., et al. (1990). Supporting the bereaved. *American Journal of Nursing, 90*(2), 48–55.

Gilbert, K. R. (1989). Interactive grief and coping in the marital dyad. *Death Studies, 13,* 605–626.

Lattanzi-Licht, M. E. (1989). Bereavement services: Practice and problems. *Hospice Journal, 5*(1), 1–28.

Lockard, B. E. (1989). Immediate, residual, and long term effects of a death education instructional unit on the death anxiety level of nursing students. *Death Studies, 13,* 137–159.

Lyons, G. J. (1988). Bereavement and death education: A survey of nurses' views. *Nursing Education Today, 8*(3), 168–172.

Robinson, P. J., et al. (1989). Differentiating grief and depression. *Hospice Journal, 5*(2), 39–53.

Rognlie, C. (1989). Perceived short and long term effects of bereavement support group participation at the Hospice of Petaluma. *Hospice Journal, 5*(2), 39–53.

Rosen, S. L. (1990). Stillbirth: What the nurse should and should not do. *Imprint, 37*(1), 65–67.

Youll, J. W. (1989). The bridge beyond: Strengthening nursing practice in attitudes towards death, dying, and the terminally ill, and helping the spouses of critically ill patients. *Intensive Care Nursing, 5*(2), 88–94.

UNIT XIV

Coping and Stress Management

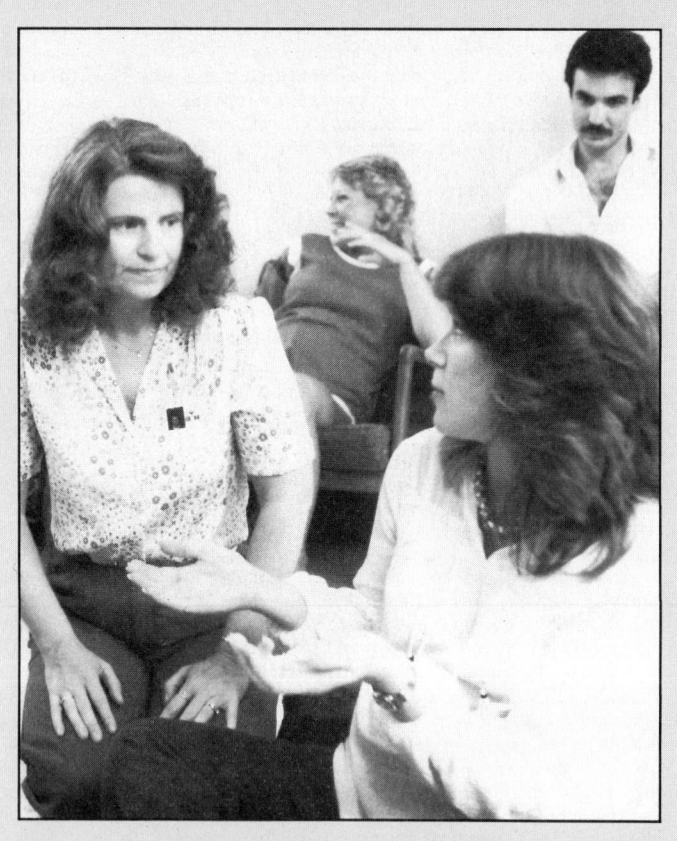

47 Stress, Coping, and Adaptation

Stress, coping, and adaptation are daily facts of life for patients and nurses. Stress affects how patients perceive and meet needs and has an impact on every other area of function. Unit XIV discusses the coping and stress tolerance area of function.

The single chapter in this unit explores the theories and concepts about stress and the many factors that affect coping and stress tolerance. Using the nursing process as a framework, the chapter emphasizes assessment for stressors and previous coping patterns and interventions to maximize effective stress management. Nursing interventions are particularly important in this area of human function since the degree to which the patient manages stress tolerance and coping can be either health promoting or illness producing. The chapter focuses on holistic nursing interventions to promote health and function and also details the many independent nursing interventions that can be used for a patient who has ineffective coping.

The content covered in this unit provides the knowledge base and skills needed to assist or support patients in reducing or managing stress through effective coping and also assists the nurse as he or she manages the stress of daily life.

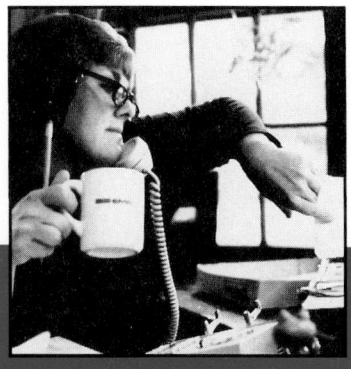

Stress, Coping, and Adaptation

LEARNING OBJECTIVES

Upon completion of this chapter, the student will be able to do the following:

- Describe the three stages of the general adaptation syndrome.
- Identify physiologic signs and symptoms of stress.
- Identify psychological responses to stress.
- List examples of biophysical and psychosocial stressors.
- Give examples of mediating variables that influence the person's ability to cope with stress.
- Identify stress management techniques that the nurse can use to assist the person to adapt to stress.

KEY TERMS

Adaptation
Burnout
Coping
Coping mechanism
Fight-or-flight
    response
General adaptation
    syndrome
Homeostasis
Local adaptation
    syndrome
Mental health
Stress
Stressor

47

Normal Coping and Adaptation to Stress
  Normal Function of Stress and Coping
    Homeostasis
  Characteristics of Normal Coping and Adaptation
    Stress as a Stimulus
    Stress as a Response
  Normal Pattern of Coping and Adaptation
  Factors Affecting Normal Stress and Coping
  Lifespan Considerations
Altered Coping and Adaptation to Stress
  Potential for Altered Coping
    Involuntary Relocation
    Dysfunctional Families
    Dysfunctional Lifestyles
    Dysfunctional Defense Mechanisms
    Sensory Deficits
  Manifestations of Altered Coping
    Addictive Behaviors
    Physical Illness
    Anxiety and Depression
    Violent Behavior
  Impact of Coping Dysfunction on Activities of
    Daily Living
Assessment
  Subjective Data
    Functional Pattern Identification
    Risk Identification
    Dysfunctional Identification
  Objective Data

    Physical Assessment
    Diagnostic Tests and Procedures
Nursing Diagnosis and Patient Goals
  Diagnostic Statement: Ineffective Individual
    Coping
    Definition
    Defining Characteristics
    Related Factors
  Related Nursing Diagnoses
  Patient Goals
Implementation
  Nursing Interventions to Promote Health and
    Function
    Stress Management for Nurses
    Stressor Reduction
    Addressing Perfection
    Supportive Internal Messages
    Assertiveness
    Lifestyle Changes
    Exercise
    Relaxation Techniques
  Nursing Interventions for Altered Function
    Relaxation Training
    Environment Modifications
    Crisis Intervention
  Discharge Planning and Home Care
Evaluation
Key Concepts

S tress is an inherent part of life. It is unavoidable, essential, and problematic. Stress can be the stimulus for constructive change and positive growth, or it can result in illness, disease, and, possibly, death. **Coping** is a problem-solving process that the person uses to manage the stresses or events with which he or she is presented. Coping with stress in a successful manner requires **adaptation** (the process by which the human system modifies itself to conform to the environment). Therefore, the ability to cope with and adapt to stress is a crucial determinate of human well-being.

The major nursing responsibilities associated with coping and adaptation to stress include: assessing the patient's ability to cope with the stressors present in the environment; identifying risk factors that could lead to ineffective coping; promoting effective coping and stress management; and performing nursing interventions to manage ineffective coping when it occurs. Additionally, nurses must recognize and cope effectively with stress in their own lives.

NORMAL COPING AND ADAPTATION TO STRESS

Throughout history humans have experienced stressful lives. Like all organisms, they have faced demands from their environment that necessitated changes in them to ensure survival. For many years this process was assumed to occur as a series of starts and stops, in which constancy and stability were assumed to prevail until some danger or threat occurred, at which time the organism changed in some way, then entered another period of stability where it remained until again faced with a demand for change. In fact, both the organism and the environment are involved in a process of continual change.

Normal Function of Stress and Coping

Today more than ever people live in a world full of change, one that requires many adjustments. Some of these adjustments are made with little effort, and some are made subconsciously. Others require major efforts to accomplish. These demands, changes, adjustments, and efforts are what is referred to when we talk about coping and adaptation to stress.

Homeostasis

Walter B. Cannon (1935), an American physiologist, created the term **homeostasis** to refer to the coordinated physiologic processes that maintain most of the steady states in the organism. He applied the term homeostasis

mainly to the self-regulation of physiologic processes within the body, such as heart rate, blood pressure, body temperature, and fluid and electrolyte balance. Today, the concept of homeostasis has been expanded to include external as well as internal environments, and to include psychosocial as well as physiologic balance.

Physiologic Homeostasis. Physiologic homeostasis is that condition in which the internal environment of the body is relatively constant. This relative constancy, essential for the survival and proper functioning of cells, is maintained through continual changes in such internal physiologic processes as heart rate, blood pressure, body temperature, fluid and electrolyte balance, blood glucose concentration, and blood oxygen level.

Although homeostasis is simple in principle, in actuality it is wonderfully complex. Numerous interrelated control mechanisms involving virtually all tissues and organs of the body interact to maintain the delicate homeostatic balance. Neuroendocrine integration functions in a central role. The neuroendocrine response includes the activities of the autonomic nervous system and the endocrine system, mediated by the hypothalamic–pituitary–adrenal axis.

In general, the nervous system regulates the rapid muscular and excretory activities of the body, whereas the endocrine system regulates mainly the slower-react-

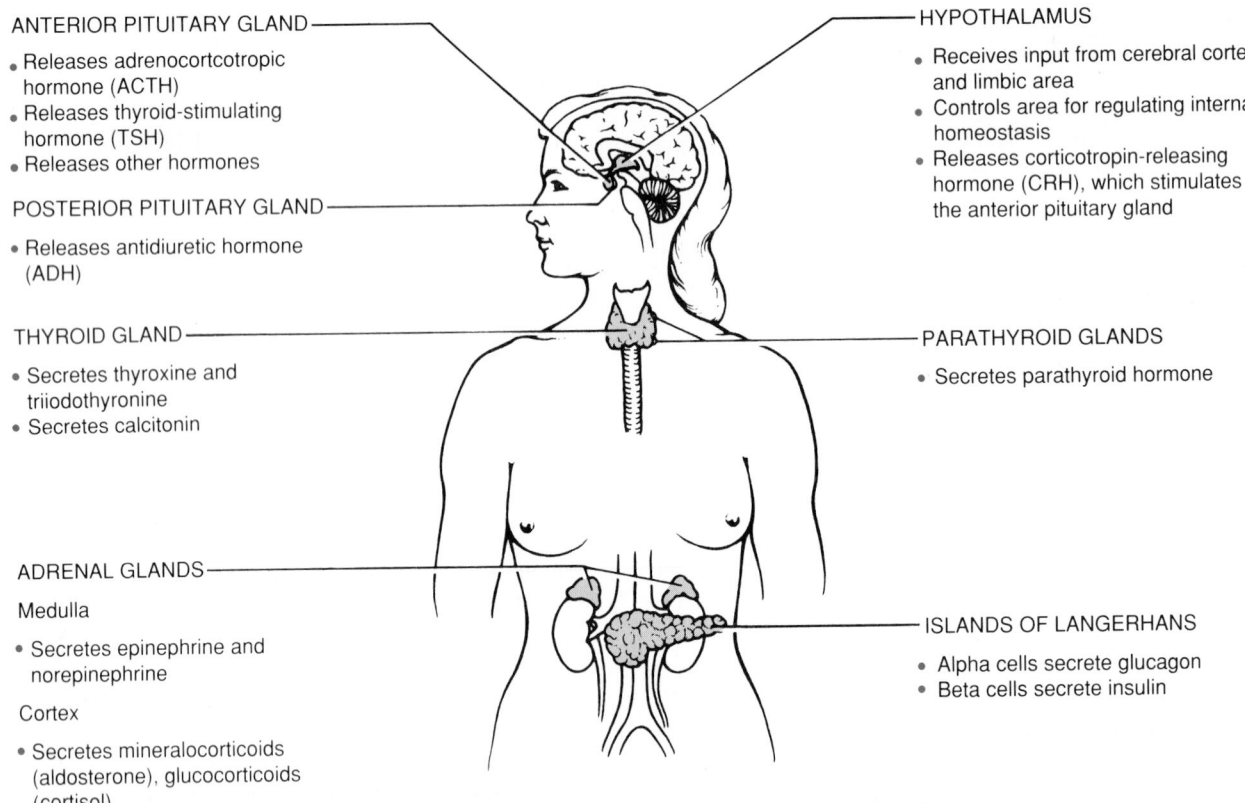

Figure 47–1. Location of specific endocrine glands that affect the body's adaptation to stress.

ing metabolic functions. Other important regulatory mechanisms include the renal, cardiovascular, respiratory, gastrointestinal, and musculoskeletal systems.

Autonomic Nervous System. The autonomic nervous system (ANS) plays a major role in homeostatic control. The ANS regulates the visceral functions of the body, such as smooth muscles of the blood vessels and digestive tract, cardiac muscle, and glands such as the digestive organs, liver, pancreas, and adrenal medulla. The two divisions of the ANS are the parasympathetic and sympathetic systems. The parasympathetic system is generally responsive to an internal need for restoration and conservation, and promotes digestion and elimination. The sympathetic system functions as an emergency system, responding to sudden demands or threats. The resulting physiologic changes prepare the body for increased energy expenditure. Some of the sympathetic responses include increases in heart rate, blood glucose, blood flow to skeletal muscles, and mental arousal.

Endocrine System. The endocrine system is another important homeostatic regulatory mechanism. The functions of five major endocrine glands will be reviewed: pituitary, adrenal, thyroid, parathyroid, and pancreas. The endocrine glands secrete chemical substances called hormones, which are specific mediators that alter cell activity some distance from their source. Figure 47-1 shows location and function of specific endocrine glands that affect the body's adaptation to stress.

Psychosociologic Homeostasis. Psychosociologic homeostasis refers to a state of mental or emotional well-being. **Mental health** is often defined in terms of mastery in areas of interpersonal relationships, as well as role fulfillment and achievement in the realms of work, family, and community. In addition, the person must have a positive sense of self-esteem and self-worth.

Human beings are open systems, constantly interacting with the environment. Several approaches address helping the person maintain a state of dynamic equilibrium, or psychological homeostasis. For instance, Maslow's human needs (see Chap. 12) should be met to maintain equilibrium.

Levine and Scotch (1970) report that various broad sociocultural phenomena, derived from sociologic, anthropologic, and epidemiologic data, can serve as sources of stress. These sources include:

- Differences between the structure of the person's family and those families that predominate in the social environment
- Varying aspects of the life cycle of families
- Role conflict
- Work-related stressors
- Social isolation
- Socioeconomic class and race.

Lazarus (1981) developed the Everyday Hassles Scale (EHS) to help identify and rank everyday stressful events (see the display). The EHS contains both "hassles" that create stress and "uplifts" that promote a sense of well-being. People may have different awarenesses of hassles and uplifts.

Knowing the nature of potential psychosociologic stressors provides the means of anticipating possible problems and the related psychological reactions.

Characteristics of Normal Coping and Adaptation

Stress is normal. People talk about the stress in their lives on a daily basis. Work, relationships, family, school, and

---

Lazarus's Everyday Hassles Scale

The following scale rank orders "hassles," which contribute to stress and "uplifts," which contribute positively to stress management, as evaluated by several middle-aged patient groups. The nurse may determine the patient's hassles and uplifts for purposes of providing anticipatory guidance. Individual patients may perceive hassles and uplifts differently from the groups studied by Lazarus.

Hassles (Rank Ordered)

1. Feeling concerned about weight.
2. Worrying about health of a family member.
3. Worrying about rising cost of living.
4. Dealing with home maintenance.
5. Having too many things to do.
6. Misplacing or losing things.
7. Doing yard work or outside home maintenance.
8. Worrying about property, investment, or taxes.
9. Worrying about crime.
10. Feeling concern about physical appearance.

Uplifts (Rank Ordered)

1. Relating well to spouse or lover.
2. Relating well with friends.
3. Completing a task.
4. Feeling healthy.
5. Getting enough sleep.
6. Eating out.
7. Meeting responsibilities.
8. Visiting, telephoning, or writing someone.
9. Spending time with family.
10. Home pleasing to you.

Adapted from Lazarus, R. S. (1981). Little hazards can be hazardous to your health. *Psychology Today, 15*(7), 58–62.

illness are all possible sources of stress. Even though stress is a term in common usage, it is a word that is difficult to define. The term **stress** is used in varying ways; stress may be considered a stimulus, or it may be considered a response to a particular stimulus. A broader concept of stress encompasses many interacting factors, such as stimulus, response, appraisal of the threat, and coping styles (Mason, 1975).

Stress as a Stimulus

When viewed as a stimulus, stress is defined as an event or set of events causing a disrupted response (Lyon & Werner, 1987). In 1953, Wolff described disease states caused by life stress resulting from disruption in lifestyles and relationships, deprivation of human needs, and failure to act in ways to eliminate the cause of the distress.

Holmes and Rahe (1967) studied the relationship between specific life changes, such as divorce or death of a spouse, and the subsequent onset of illness. These life change events were rated according to their perceived stressfulness and the degree of adaptation required. Holmes and Rahe (1967) developed tools called the Social Readjustment Rating Scale (SRRS) and the Schedule of Recent Experiences (SRE) to measure the number and magnitude of life change events, both positive and negative, experienced by the subject within a certain time frame. They found that the higher the person's cumulative score, the greater was the likelihood of that person developing a serious illness within 1 to 2 years. The SRRS is shown in Table 18-9.

Although the SRE has been used extensively, current researchers advise caution in its use, as there are significant differences in a person's perception and subsequent rating of stressful life events. Variables, such as age, gender, marital status, and ethnic origin can influence this tool's results. Thus, a critical factor in evaluating the impact of stressful life events is the person's perception of that event.

Stress as a Response

Hans Selye, who has written several books on the stress response, defined stress as "the nonspecific response of the body to any demand upon it" (Selye, 1974, p. 27). He used the theoretical framework that stress is a response to a certain stimulus.

Selye used the term "stressor" to differentiate between the stress-producing agent and the response to stress. A **stressor** is the stimulus or agent that evokes a stress response in the person. A stressor is anything that places a demand on the person for change or adaptation. Stressors may be biophysical, psychological, or social–cultural.

Stressors can be viewed by the person as positive or negative. Selye (1974) referred to pleasant events as eustress from the Greek prefix *eu*, meaning good or positive. One example might be going to college, which the person views as positive and desirable, but is also stressful, because it involves changes in one's routine and requires adaptation to those changes. Negative or undesirable events are referred to as distress. Examples might include being fired from a job, having an argument with a close friend, or being hospitalized. Pleasurable events seem to evoke the same physiologic reactions as negative stressors.

Selye (1974) termed this undifferentiated physiologic reaction "nonspecific response," meaning that the body goes through a number of biochemical changes and readjustments without regard to the nature of the stress-producing agent. Because the physiologic response to the stressful agent seemed to be universal in all organisms, he referred to this pattern of defense as the general adaptation syndrome. The following section discusses these changes and readjustments; they are outlined in Figure 47-2.

General Adaptation Syndrome. The nonspecific response to stress is termed the **general adaptation syndrome** (GAS). The GAS is a generalized adaptive response to states of stress, and consists of three stages: alarm, resistance, and exhaustion (Selye, 1974, p. 38).

Alarm Reaction. The alarm reaction, also called the **fight-or-flight response,** is the body's initial response to stress, in which its defenses are alerted and the person is prepared for "fight or flight." This preparation includes the secretion of hormones and the response of target organs.

The hormones epinephrine and norepinephrine, secreted by the adrenal glands, trigger an increase in blood pressure and in the heart and respiratory rates, which increases oxygen availability and blood flow to muscles to prepare for defense by either fight or flight. Increased mental alertness and pupillary dilation to improve visual acuity are additional effects of the hormonal influence. Epinephrine increases the blood sugar level, and cortisol, also secreted by the adrenals, stimulates the process of gluconeogenesis (the conversion of proteins and fats into glucose by the liver), making additional energy available to the skeletal muscles of the body. The conversion of proteins and fats to simpler substances (glucose) is referred to as a catabolic process (Vander, 1990).

In the alarm reaction, the body is preparing to act in response to the stressor with which it has been presented. This stage may last only a few minutes or may continue for several hours. A stress situation that is longer-lasting or in which a more serious threat is perceived causes the body to move to the next stage, the stage of resistance.

Stage of Resistance. In the stage of resistance, the body attempts to adapt to the stressor and mobilizes coping mechanisms. Stabilization occurs in the body's heart and respiratory rates, blood pressure, and hormone levels. The body begins coping with the new state of adaptation, trying to return to normal function.

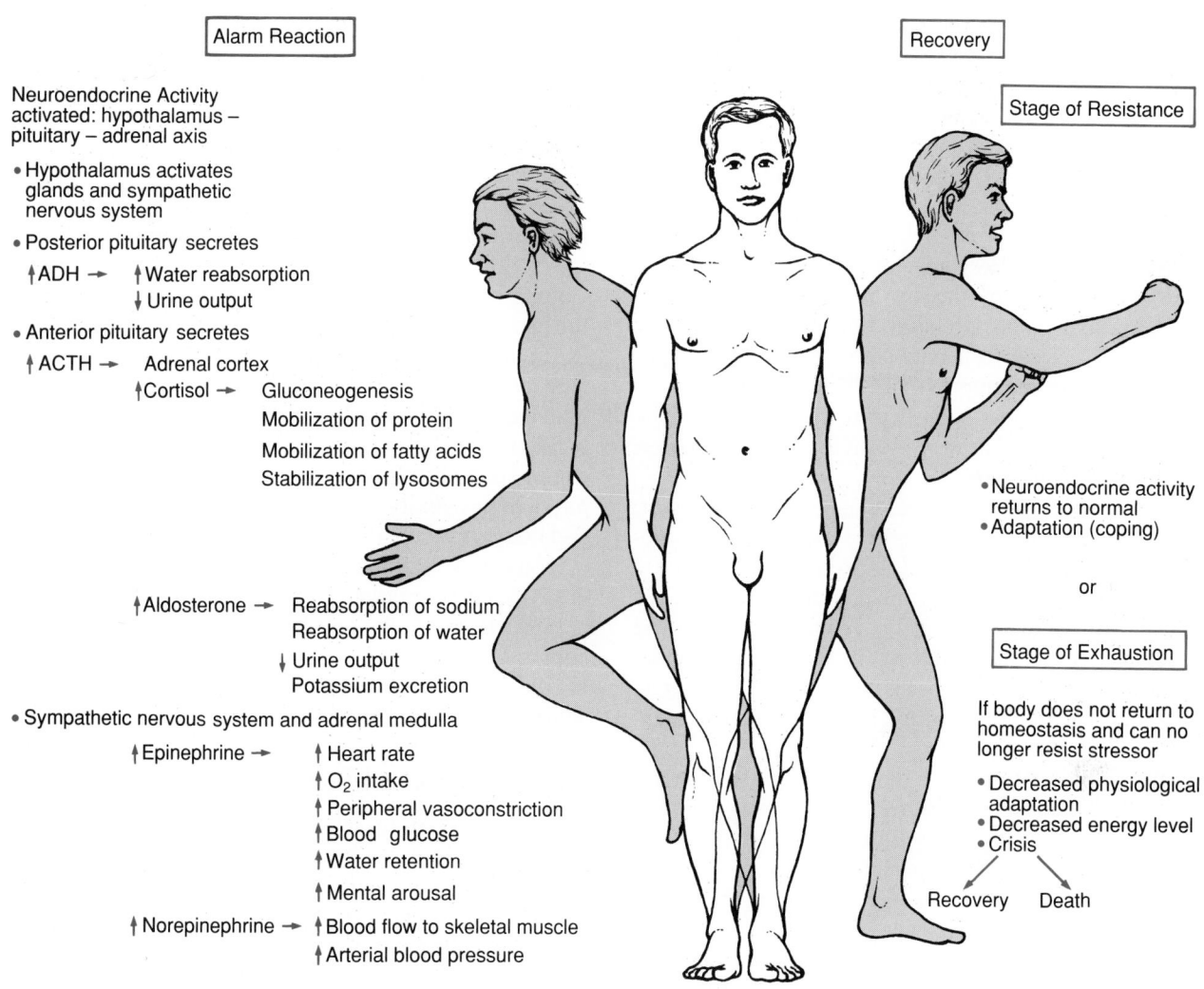

Figure 47–2.   General adaptation syndrome.

If the stressor has not been removed or if the effects of the stressor lead to continued inability to adapt, then the body's attempt to return to normal will be incomplete, and the physiologic adaptation will not return the body to its previous homeostatic state.

Stage of Exhaustion. When the body can no longer resist the stressor or cannot maintain its adaptation, it moves to the stage of exhaustion. In this stage the body's ability to respond to the continuing stress is diminished or depleted. If the body has sufficient energy resources for continued adaptation, then rest, recovery, and return to normal may be the end result. If the adaptation is not adequate or if the body is unable to mobilize further defense, then exhaustion ensues, and death may be the outcome.

Finite Adaptability. According to Selye (1974), the general adaptation syndrome demonstrates that the body's adaptability, or adaptation energy, is finite.

He compared the three stages of the GAS to the human lifespan. In childhood, there is lowered resistance and excessive response to any kind of stimulus. During adulthood, the body has adapted to most commonly encountered agents, and there is increased resistance. With aging, there is a loss of adaptability and eventual exhaustion, ending with death.

Local Adaptation Syndrome. The localized response to stress is referred to as the **local adaptation syndrome** (LAS). In the LAS, a localized area of the body, such as a body tissue, organ, or part, can respond to the stress of pain, inflammation, or trauma. The LAS is differentiated from the GAS by being localized, not systemic; short-term; adaptive; and restorative to localized homeostasis. The LAS has three stages as well, but they occur locally, rather than generally, as in the GAS. During the LAS, the following changes occur:

Blood vessels dilate in the inflamed area.

Fibrous connective tissue proliferates to prevent spread of potential pathogens into the blood stream.

Cells proliferate to repair or replace damaged tissue.

Chemical substances are secreted from the blood and connective tissue to neutralize toxins and destroy any bacteria present (Selye, 1974).

Psychosociologic Response. A person's response to stress is influenced by the use of coping strategies, or coping skills. When stressful events are successfully managed by effective coping, the person experiences personal growth and improved problem-solving abilities. People who are most successful in coping tend to be flexible and to use a variety of strategies to adapt to new situations and stressors.

Cognitively, a person perceives an event or stressor, appraises it as a threat or nonthreat, and calls on automatic coping responses. Reappraisals of the threat are made to determine if a discrepancy exists between the degree of threat and the person's coping capacity. The person may respond by reducing the emotional response through an appropriate discharge of emotions, direct actions, or through defenses (Lazarus and Folkman, 1980).

One way of attempting to cope with stress is to use defense mechanisms simply to withdraw from the stress. Defense mechanisms are self-protective, unconscious processes that enable the person to deny or distort a stressful encounter, and thus decrease feelings of anxiety (Wilson & Kneisl, 1983). There are a number of ways that people try to do this, including denial, increased time spent sleeping, daydreaming, and fantasizing. Table 47-1 lists and defines the common coping mechanisms. If the stress is more than the person can or wants to deal with, one method of coping is to withdraw to some activity that is viewed as comforting and nonstress-ful. For example, while one is sleeping, stress can be avoided or responding to it can be delayed, assuming that the stress does not keep one awake. Daydreams and fantasies allow the person to withdraw mentally to a more pleasant, less stressful scene.

Normal Pattern of Coping and Adaptation

Coping successfully with stress requires **adaptation,** or the process of the person's effort to manage internal and external demands. **Coping** is often described as a problem-solving process or strategy that the person uses to manage the out-of-the-ordinary events or situations with which he or she is presented. Coping may be entirely cognitive in nature, but it is more likely to be a psycho-physiologic activity involving an integration of the mind and body. As such, it is a major process in the successful response to stress and crucial to the person's continued growth and adaptation.

Lazarus and Folkman (1980) described two types of coping processes: problem-oriented—the manipulation of the person–environment relationship that is the source of stress; and emotion-focused—the regulation of stressful emotions.

Examples of problem-oriented coping include:

- Making out a time schedule for studying, and sticking to it
- Applying for job at another company because your current position is too demanding
- Trying to find out more about an illness, such as diabetes, so it can be managed better.

Examples of emotion-focused coping include:

- Accepting sympathy and understanding from a friend in the loss of a family member

TABLE 47–1

Common Defense Mechanisms

Compensation	The attempt to achieve respect or recognition in one activity as a substitute for inability to achieve in another endeavor.
Denial	Refusing to believe or accept something as it is but rather as one wishes it to be.
Displacement	Transfering emotion away from the person or situation that incited the emotion to an inappropriate person or object.
Introjection	Taking into one's personality the characteristics of another.
Projection	Attributing one's own thoughts, emotions, characteristics, or motives to another.
Rationalization	Concealing the motive for behavior by giving some socially acceptable reason for the action.
Regression	Return to behaviors more appropriate to an earlier stage of development.
Repression	Immersing something in the subconscious or unconscious level of thought.
Sublimation	Release of libido in socially acceptable behavior rather than using it to obtain sexual gratification.
Suppression	Consciously dismissing something from the mind and thoughts.

- Releasing tension after a hard day at work by meditating, crying, or taking a walk
- Blaming someone else, such as a spouse or teacher, for the situation you are in.

Bell (1977) divided **coping mechanisms** (activities or measures for managing stress) into two groups: long-term and short-term. Long-term coping mechanisms are positive, constructive ways of dealing with stress and can be effective over long periods of time. Short-term coping methods are temporary measures that reduce stress and tension; however, if used over long periods of time, they may have a detrimental effect on the person, and lead to maladaptive behavior.

Examples of long-term coping mechanisms include:

- Working out the stress through physical exercise
- Talking with others about a problem (friend, counselor)
- Relying on belief in a higher power
- Seeking additional information about a situation
- Drawing on past experience
- Developing alternative plans for handling the situation.

Examples of short-term coping mechanisms include:

- Smoking
- Alcohol use
- Overeating
- "Pill-popping"
- Excessive coffee intake.

Factors Affecting Normal Coping and Adaptation

In the course of life, there are many events and situations that occur as a normal part of living. While these events are within the realm of normal living, they still may produce stress, requiring a person to be able to cope and adapt to them. Among these events are transitions or changes (such as attending school, moving, marriage, and childbearing), and lifestyle factors (such as nutrition, exercise, and fitness).

Roles and Relationships. For a child who has felt secure and has experienced only minimal stress, attending school for the first time can be filled with real or perceived stress, with which the child must cope. On a larger scale, the student who moves to new schools and levels of education (middle school, high school, college) learns to cope and adapt to the stresses connected with each new advancement and with increasing maturity.

In our mobile society, many families find that frequent moving and relocation for career purposes is a way of life. Each move has its own unique stresses related to

closure of family life in one community and beginning of family life in a new community. Not only is there the physical relocation, but there is also separation from the family's emotional ties and support systems within the community. Most families can develop these relationships in time in their new community, but it is generally a stressful time, even when everything goes well.

As people mature and move into the developmental tasks of adult life, the transitions related to those events require adequate coping and adaptation. The selection of a mate, marriage, and childbearing are examples of those transitional events. Generally, the marriages of young adults are happy occasions, but even so, families are faced with the stresses of decisions relating to the actual event, to the new alliance, and to separation from the previous parent–child relationship. The newlyweds face the stresses of changing their previous relationships with their families, developing the new marriage relationship, and making decisions relating to day-to-day life. When a child is born, new stresses accompany the expansion of the family, even when the baby is anticipated with great delight. There are now new demands on both marriage partners in terms of emotions, dependencies, time, and money. Childbearing demands a new set of coping strategies to adapt successfully.

Nutrition and Metabolism. Today, more and more people are concerned about the quality of their dietary intake. Not only are the total calories of concern, but so is the nutrient content of the food. When the body has adequate nutrients and does not experience the malnutrition of being either undernourished or overfed, the nutritional resources give the body more reserve with which to respond to stress. Imbalances in the intake of essential nutrients can enhance the stress response, making the effects more exaggerated than usual. A person who is poorly nourished as a result of either overeating or undereating may be less well prepared to face a stressful situation.

Activity and Exercise. When an adequate nutritional state is further combined with a regular program of exercise, the resulting fitness benefits the person physiologically and psychologically. The benefits of exercise include improved cardiovascular conditioning, weight control, muscle tone, and sense of well-being. Since many chronic illnesses have some relation to one or more of these factors, exercise programs can be effective in decreasing these outcomes of stress. Regular patterns of exercise provide people with a ready outlet for stress before it becomes prolonged or chronic.

A person who is fit generally has developed lifestyle habits that allow an outlet for stress on a regular basis. The exercise routine permits the person to cope with the normal, day-to-day stresses so that adaptation occurs in smaller increments. This modulated approach to the daily stresses of life prevents the accumulation of many little things to a point where the person can no longer cope.

Sleep and Rest. To be rested and relaxed, a person needs a pattern of adequate sleep. When a person is anticipating stress or experiencing stress, it is particularly important to be rested and relaxed. Given the busy schedules of many persons, sleep and rest are often insufficient, therefore compromising their ability to manage stress.

Safety and Security. The amount of threat perceived as compared to the degree of security a person feels affects response to stress. For example, if a student is failing a class in school and feels very insecure about how his or her parents will react, the student will experience greater stress than if he or she felt secure about the support and understanding of his or her parents. The effect of stress-producing situations, such as giving birth, acute illness, or role changes, depends on the person's perception of the event, adequate support, and effective coping mechanisms.

Previous Experience. Past experience with stressors can influence the response and adaptation to present stressful encounters. Responses to stressors may be learned, often from other family members. For instance, a child may develop a fear of heights because the father also had this phobia.

Previous exposure to a stressful situation may also help the person to cope with similar situations. For example, as mentioned above, a person who has been hospitalized before may find the experience much less stressful than the patient who has never been hospitalized.

Lifespan Considerations

Newborn and Infant

The newborn and infant depend largely on reflex responses for coping with their environment and the stresses that are presented. For example, if a newborn is hungry, he or she will cry and be physically active as a means of reflexively coping with the situation and attempting to do something about it. The parent learns to respond to the infant's communication and participates in a mutual coping adaptation by giving the infant food. As the infant continues to develop, new coping strategies are gradually learned to fit various situations, though these are generally limited to reflex and sensory functions, and responses to stress may be excessive.

At this stage of development, the infant depends totally on the parent for physiologic needs, safety, and loving attachment. These needs, if met, ameliorate the effect of stress and provide the basis for coping.

Toddler and Preschooler

During the toddler and preschool stages of development, the child's physical development becomes more stable. The child learns to develop coping strategies for relatively simple events, such as coping with not getting something that he or she wants at the exact time that he or she wants it. While learning to handle a slight delay in getting wants and needs met may seem like a small accomplishment, it sets a pattern from which the child can expand to other situations later in life.

Parents are still an important part of the child's frame of reference in terms of handling stress and adapting to situations. Because the child is developing coping strategies, the child may still experience excessive response to stressful situations. He or she depends on parents for safety and limit-setting to define the boundaries within which stress can be handled.

Child and Adolescent

The schoolaged child is expanding his or her world, moving out of the totally protected realm of home into the experience of school and interactions with others. There are new stresses presented in classroom situations, structured play, and interactions with other children and adults. The child must learn to adapt to these stresses and to cope with new experiences and rules. At this age, the child can identify stressors and begin to reason with parents and others about how to cope with them, drawing from past development and developing new approaches.

During the period of adolescence, the person moves toward achieving emotional independence from the parents, develops a sexual identity, acquires values, and achieves socially responsible behavior. Achieving these tasks is stress-producing in itself, requiring the adolescent to use the coping strategies developed thus far and to develop new ones continually. Physiologically, the adolescent has adequate reserves for responding to stress. Psychological maturation is a primary task of adolescence, requiring adaptation of behavior and development of new coping mechanisms. While separation from parents is in progress the adolescent still needs the security and boundaries provided by parents and family.

Adult and Older Adult

Adults are relatively stable physiologically and able to handle stress efficiently in most cases. However, the various demands of adulthood (occupation, lifestyle, relationships, family, etc.) create more stress on a daily basis. The coping skills developed throughout life are drawn on, and new ones are developed. Previous exposure to a stressful situation may help the person to cope with similar situations in a more adaptive manner. For example, a person who has been hospitalized before may find the experience much less stressful than the patient who has never been hospitalized. For parents, bringing a new baby into the home may present stress, and having that same child grow up and leave home may present stress on another level. These stresses may stimulate positive change and growth.

As a person ages, stress does not decrease. Among the stresses of aging are retirement, decline in physical energy, decrease in financial potential, loss of family and friends, and, possibly, relocation. Older adults must adapt to these stresses and changes at a time when individual reserves and strength are less than when younger. When the general adaptation syndrome is initiated in the elderly, there is much more concern that the stage of exhaustion may end in death, rather than rest and recovery.

Nursing Research

Selected Nursing Research Studies

Kleehammer, K., Hart, A. L., Keck, J. F. (1990). Nursing students' perceptions of anxiety-producing situations in the clinical setting. *Journal of Nursing Education, 29*(4), 183–187.

Wallace, A. (1989). An active role for patients in stress management. *Professional Nurse, 5*(2), 65–66, 68–59,72.

Diekmann, J. M. (1988). An evaluation of selected "I Can Cope" programs by registered participants. *Cancer Nursing, 11*(5), 274–282.

Cochran, J., et al. (1989). A comparison of nurses' and patients' perceptions of intensive care unit stressors. *Journal of Advanced Nursing, 14*(12), 1038–1043.

Della Sega, C. (1990). Coping with caregiving: Stress management for caregivers of the elderly. *Journal of Psychosocial Nursing and Mental Health Services, 28*(1), 15–16, 19–22, 40–41.

Possible Topics for Nursing Inquiry

- What are early indicators of ineffective coping in adolescents of single-parent families?
- What are effective coping strategies in patients who have experienced disfigurement due to surgery?
- What nursing interventions can be used to minimize ineffective coping in patients who require frequent procedures and treatment?

ALTERED COPING AND ADAPTATION TO STRESS

In addition to being knowledgeable about the function of stress and the factors that affect stress and coping, the nurse needs to differentiate normal coping with stress from altered coping situations, and identify their resulting manifestations and impact on people.

Potential for Altered Coping

The same factors that create stress in day-to-day living, and can be considered normal, can also have other facets that become potential factors for altered coping and adaptation. These include transition factors (such as involuntary relocation, hospitalization, divorce, loss, or domestic abuse) and lifestyle factors (such as fatigue, illness, or death).

Involuntary Relocation

Even under the best of circumstances, relocation can be stressful, but when the move is involuntary, the potential for stress is greatly increased. For example, while moving may be necessary for career reasons, there are many families that may be fragile in some way (e.g., a disabled child, health problems, disturbed adolescents), and have developed needed and useful support systems in their present community. A move may be viewed as very stressful and disrupting, interfering with coping strategies and preventing adaptation.

In another example, an elderly person may be faced with the realization that living independently is no longer an option, but is denying it. Family or other support systems may have to help the elderly person make the decision to move to an environment where there is improved safety and more support for daily living activities. This involuntary relocation can produce overwhelming stress and altered coping for the elderly person.

Another form of involuntary relocation is hospitalization. A person is not admitted to a hospital without a specific health reason, either physiologic or psychological. Depending on the problem, there may be a mild amount of stress or a great amount, both of which require the use of coping skills and patterns to manage the problem. The health problem may overwhelm the person's previous patterns of coping, leading to or adding to a dysfunctional state of stress.

Dysfunctional Families

Although families can be a great source of support, they can also be the source of distress and altered coping. Many marriages end in separation and divorce, which can be either amicable or bitter. Divorce, particularly when there are dependent children, can lead to altered coping as a result of the stressful situation, and can require new adaptation strategies. Children in particular feel the stress of the loss of a secure environment, and can respond with altered coping and adaptation, either behaviorally or physically. Adolescents are particularly vulnerable to instability, which can lead to serious consequences from the resulting altered coping.

Stresses from other sources often have their outlet in the family. When individual coping strategies are not adequate, that outlet may take the form of physical abuse. The abuse of one spouse by another (usually the wife by the husband) or the abuse of a child by a parent are often the outcome. The awareness of domestic abuse has increased in recent years, and more service agencies and support services are becoming available.

Dysfunctional Lifestyles

The absence of adequate nutrition, rest, exercise, and fitness can predispose the person to fatigue, illness, and perhaps death. A person who has a lifestyle pattern of poor nutrition, insufficient rest, and an irregular exercise routine is prone to experience altered coping and adaptation as a result of inadequate physiologic reserves. In these circumstances, the person may overreact psychologically to stress-producing situations, as in the domestic abuse described above, and the neuroendocrine response may be compromised, as well.

Dysfunctional Defense Mechanisms

Coping mechanisms may keep the person from dealing with stress realistically. Daydreams, increased sleeping, denial, or fantasies can be dysfunctional when the person resorts to them rather than confronting the stress and actively problem-solving. While defense mecha-nisms help to avoid pain, modify strong emotions, or relieve anxiety, overuse can be self-defeating and interfere with coping and adapting abilities.

Sensory Deficits

Deficits or impairments in the senses can alter the person's ability to cope with and respond effectively to stress. Sensory deficits in vision and hearing interfere with the ability to interact with the environment and with other people. It becomes increasingly difficult to make judgments when under stress, to know what coping options exist, or to adapt to changes that challenge sensory–perceptual abilities. Inability to see what is occurring in the environment or to hear sounds accurately can lead to misperception and the potential for altered coping.

Manifestations of Altered Coping

Altered coping may be manifested in a variety of ways, including use of alcohol and drugs, excessive smoking, increased sleeping, overeating, avoidance and withdrawal, daydreaming and fantasizing, and illness. Table 47-2 gives examples of expressions of stress in patients.

Addictive Behaviors

Alcohol has long been used as a means of trying to alter reality and awareness. The phrase "crawling into a bottle" illustrates the attempt to withdraw from stress and problems with the intake of alcohol. In recent years, excessive use of drugs, both prescription and "street" drugs, has joined alcohol use as an attempt to escape stress. The results of excessive use of both alcohol and drugs are addiction, dependency, psychological prob-

TABLE 47–2

Possible Expressions of Stress in Patients

Psychosocial Expressions		Physiological Expressions
Behaviors	*Emotions*	
Crying	Anger, anxiety	Back, neck, or shoulder pain
Decreased motivation	Nervousness	Breathing irregularities
Decreased self-esteem	Moodiness, depression	Elevated blood pressure
Decreased intellectual processes	Emotional instability	Change in appetite
Forgetfulness	Irritability	Stuttering, trembling
Impulsive behavior	Fears, phobias	Jaw tension
Inability to make decisions	Feeling out of control	Sexual dysfunction
Learning disabilities	Frustration	Constipation or diarrhea
Poor concentration	Feelings of worthlessness	Irregular heartbeat
		Muscle cramps, spasms
		Stomach, digestive disorders
		Sweating, skin problems
		Tension headaches
		Insomnia or fatigue

lems, and physiologic sequelae, and, probably, more stress and less effective coping. Adolescents are at particular risk for substance abuse as a result of their vulnerable stage of development.

Smoking is also an addictive behavior, with nicotine being the addictive substance. People, frequently adolescents, often begin smoking in an effort to portray a certain image (older, macho, or more sophisticated), and end up being addicted and finding it difficult to stop. When stressed, people often increase the amount of smoking, both to handle the stress via the nicotine and to provide a physical outlet by having something to do with their hands when they are upset. Smoking is an ineffective coping strategy for stress. Physiologic alterations, such as lung problems and cardiovascular disorders, are the end result of chronic smoking.

The use of food can be an addictive behavior in much the same way as smoking, in that the person seeks the immediate pleasure of food to avoid the discomfort caused by the stress. The problem of overeating has no simple cause or explanation. As with sleeping and daydreams, food offers many people a pleasurable escape from stressful situations. The behavior may work in the short term; however, in the long term, overeating leads to obesity, which has significant health consequences. People with a substance abuse or overeating manifestation of stress and altered coping require a comprehensive treatment program to address their coping and adaptation problems.

Physical Illness

Prolonged stress and exposure to the effects of the neuroendocrine hormones can lead to physiologic dysfunction. Selye (1974) found that, as a result of prolonged stress, the adrenal glands become enlarged, lymphatic structures (thymus, spleen, and lymph nodes) atrophy, and the stomach develops deep ulcerations. These indications seem to illustrate an overstimulation of the adrenals, a decline in immune system function, and an increased risk for cell and tissue damage. While there is controversy over the exact relation of stress to illness, there is evidence that a person can mediate his or her heart rate and blood pressure through effective application of coping strategies. Increased blood pressure and heart rate are manifestations of the effect of the adrenal hormones.

Anxiety and Depression

Stress can cause anxiety, a subjective reaction to a real or imagined threat. The sense of uneasiness or dread may range from mild to severe, and may be manifested by lack of sleep, poor nutrition, excessive caffeine intake or smoking, or physical illness.

The extreme response to prolonged stress may be depression and suicide. People with poor coping mecha-

nisms or inadequate support may see suicide as a desirable way to end stress and depression. Because of the inherent instability of the adolescent years, adolescents who are experiencing various kinds of stress have a higher rate of suicide than the general population.

Violent Behavior

People with poor impulse control or with inadequate coping mechanisms may respond to stress through acting out in violent or abusive ways. For example, a man who has a stressful situation at work may come home and behave violently with his wife or children as an outlet for the stress. Wife battering and child abuse are common forms of violent behavior related to altered coping.

Impact of Coping Dysfunction on Activities of Daily Living

The manifestations of altered coping can interfere with the person's activities of daily living (ADLs). The use of addictive substances, such as alcohol, drugs, and nicotine, to handle stress ultimately leads to more problems, not only with stress management, but with the simple activities that are a part of daily living. The outcomes of alcohol and drug use contribute to cognitive impairments, which make personal hygiene, home maintenance, and school and work performance difficult. Smoking and other substance use diverts income to support those activities instead of the needs of the person or household.

As stress becomes prolonged or overwhelming, it can dominate the awareness of the person, or the person may try to withdraw from it. In either event, the activities of studying, cooking, cleaning, personal hygiene, and care of clothing may become less important. If that occurs, stress may actually increase as a result both of the changes in ADLs and of the further compromise of the person's reserves.

Stress may interfere with the person's employment if it prevents him or her from performing optimally in his or her current education or position, or from obtaining a new position. While the presence of some stress may serve to heighten performance, a large amount of stress may severely impair performance.

ASSESSMENT

Many patients with health problems are faced with many stressors, and have varying ways of coping with them. It is important that the nurse have an understanding of the methods or strategies used by the patient, so that nursing care can be appropriately individualized.

Subjective Data

The focused functional assessment of coping and adaptation includes obtaining subjective data from the patient through a series of purposeful questions and interviews, and through observation and mental notation of the patient's nonverbal communication, such as body position, facial expressions, gestures, and voice and speech. The nursing history is one of the earliest sources of these data, and in continued interactions, the nurse becomes increasingly focused in the specific considerations for that particular patient.

Subjective data assist the nurse in identifying the patient's functional coping and adaptation patterns and strategies, identifying any factors that place the patient at additional risk for ineffective coping, and identifying any actual dysfunction that may be present.

Functional Pattern Identification

To assess the patient's coping and adaptation pattern, the nurse needs to obtain information from the patient, family or significant other, and health-care providers. Because there are many sources for stress with which the patient may be required to cope or adapt, it is helpful to determine the source of stress: physiologic, psychological, environmental, or sociocultural (Fuller & Schaller-Ayers, 1990).

Physiologic Stress. Physiologic stress produces a physiologic response. Consequently, it is important to inquire about physiologic responses, such as the patient's feelings of fatigue, adequacy of sleep, appetite, bowel elimination patterns, and level of physical activity. Assessment of physical responses to stress is discussed more fully under "Objective Data." Changes in normal patterns of these or other physiologic activities may be an expression of ineffective coping.

Psychological Stress. Psychological stress is generated from the person's thoughts and feelings about specific events or perceptions of events. For a person facing a health problem or hospitalization, there may be stresses related to loss of personal control or a sense of powerlessness over the situation. The patient may exhibit behavioral responses such as denial, ambivalence, suspicion, hostility, regression, depression, or withdrawal. Asking the patient to tell the nurse what factors the patient is feeling concerned about, what problems the patient is able to identify, and what feelings the patient is experiencing about specific problems, is a beginning approach to obtaining information for both the patient and the nurse. If the nurse can help the patient bring some clarity to stressful feelings and problems, there is a better basis for both of them to plan purposeful nursing interventions.

Environmental Stress. Environmental stress may be related to relocation or unfamiliarity with the setting. The change in surroundings, with new sounds, smells, and sights may produce stress for a patient. In a hospital or long-term care facility, there is also a loss of privacy, change in daily activities, and change in the level of sensory stimulation (either more or less). The nurse should ask questions that determine the patient's response to the environment, define sources of stress for the patient, and reveal areas that both the nurse and the patient think may be amenable to mutual planning.

Sociocultural Stress. Sociocultural stress may be related to family, financial, career, and spiritual concerns. The nurse needs to elicit information about specific concerns the patient may have about the care of the family during hospitalization, whether his or her job or career will be affected, what kind of financial support is available from job, insurance, or spouse, and how the current situation fits in with spiritual beliefs and values. This information alerts the nurse to the type of planning and collaboration that may be necessary for this patient.

Risk Identification

The nursing history includes the collection of information that identifies factors that place the patient at risk for ineffective coping and adaptation. Areas of risk to be assessed include transition factors, such as moving and relocation, situations involving separation (e.g., divorce, child custody, prison), and hospitalization; and lifestyle factors, such as fatigue, malnutrition, and illness.

Many of the factors that place a patient at risk for ineffective coping may actually be positive factors in relation to long-term outcomes, but that does not eliminate the possibility that ineffective coping may occur in the short term. For example, a woman leaving an abusive marriage may have very positive outcomes as an end result, but she may be at risk for ineffective coping during the transitional period, in which she is adapting to her new situation and reestablishing herself, and perhaps her children, in a new life.

Some risk factors have a direct relationship to the reason that a particular patient may be encountering a health problem, however. If a patient has a history of an eating disorder, such as anorexia or bulimia, the resulting malnutrition may predispose the patient to related health problems. The nurse will find it very useful in caring for the patient if specific risk situations that may be present for the patient can be identified.

Dysfunctional Identification

To determine if the patient has a coping dysfunction, it is necessary to assess the patient's beliefs about normal levels of stress and usual coping behaviors or strategies.

Some people have a high tolerance for stress and are so accustomed to living with an elevated level of stress that what may be identified as extremely stressful by another person is considered as rather ordinary. There are also correspondingly wide ranges of variation in coping behaviors and strategies employed by different people. To gain the most accurate understanding, it is important that the nurse not insert his or her bias and personal coping expectations into the assessment, but stay open to learning how the patient identifies the situation.

Dysfunctional patterns can be identified as significant differences from the patient's normal behavior for coping with stress, and as coping and adaptation patterns that are outside the range of normal for a particular patient. For example, if a person usually handles stress at the job by doing hard physical activity in a gym, but now finds that his or her response to on-the-job stress has become fatigue and excessive sleep, then a dysfunctional pattern has been identified.

Objective Data

Physical Assessment

As a result of the activation of the autonomic nervous system and the endocrine system, physiologic responses may occur and be observed in the physical assessment. Because there may be many other reasons for some of the responses, the nurse must be careful not to assume that the cause of some physical findings is stress alone, when there may be other contributory causes.

Cardiovascular System. The cardiovascular system is the target system for the effects of epinephrine and norepinephrine, which include increased heart rate, vasoconstriction of peripheral organs, and increased oxygen consumption by the heart. The manifestations of prolonged stimulation by these hormones may include:

- An increase in the heart rate at rest related to direct stimulation of the myocardium, which may be described as "pounding in the chest" or palpitations
- An increase in systolic blood pressure related to peripheral vasoconstriction
- Arrhythmias related to ischemia (tissue oxygen lack and increased energy demand), noted in an irregular heartbeat or in rhythm changes
- Angina, or chest pain, and changes in the electrocardiogram related to ischemia
- Migraine headaches related to vasoconstriction.

Respiratory System. The respiratory system is affected by norepinephrine, leading to increased rate of breathing and to bronchiolar dilation. Hyperventilation accompanied by a feeling of "air hunger," dizziness, and tingling in the hands and feet are generally the most common physical manifestations.

Gastrointestinal System. The gastrointestinal system is a common target system in stressful situations. Whereas the nervous system activity usually slows motility, people experiencing stress often report loss of appetite, nausea, vomiting, and increased peristaltic activity. Increased peristalsis is manifested by increased bowel sounds, increased secretion of hydrochloric acid (HCl) in the stomach, and increased number of bowel movements. The increase in HCl may also contribute to the nausea and vomiting and, in combination with cortisol, to gastrointestinal ulcer formation.

Musculoskeletal System. The musculoskeletal system responds to stress by exhibiting increased tenseness in the larger muscles, and shakiness and tremor in smaller muscles. The muscle tenseness is related to the "fight-or-flight" preparation of the general adaptation syndrome to ready the body to protect itself. Prolonged tenseness can lead to muscle spasm, particularly in the back.

Integumentary System. The skin, or integumentary system, manifests the peripheral effects of norepinephrine and epinephrine by being diaphoretic (moist) and cool, and by exhibiting smooth muscle tenseness ("making the hairs stand on end").

Diagnostic Tests and Procedures

There are no simple laboratory tests to determine the amount of stress. The presence of stress-related hormones (epinephrine, norepinephrine, and cortisol) can be determined through laboratory tests, and from their existence the presence of stress can be inferred. Objective data about the patient's coping and adaptation are gathered by means of structured interviews and coping and stress assessment tools. These types of laboratory tests are evaluated in conjunction with other data related to measuring stress. These tools attempt to identify and quantify stressors and coping patterns, as described under "Subjective Data." Formal assessment tools include instruments such as the Social Readjustment Rating Scale (Holmes & Rahe, 1967), Everyday Hassles Scale (Lazarus, 1981), and the Coping and Stress Tolerance Pattern: Interview Guidelines (Fuller & Schaller-Ayers, 1990). The former two appear earlier in the chapter; the latter appears here. These instruments help identify behaviors and feelings that may relate to the amount of stress and the corresponding vulnerability to illness and dysfunction. The scales, which turn subjective factors into objective numbers, may be used by the nurse in some situations, or they may be used by a psychosocial clinical nurse specialist, a consultant, or a psychologist. The interview guide can be employed usefully by all nurses.

The Coping and Stress Tolerance Pattern: Interview Guidelines

A structured interview guide may be used to facilitate data collection. The headings provided on this screening interview form correlate with major interview areas discussed in the text and may be deleted when creating forms to record data in practice settings.

Nature of Stressors

Major changes/losses in the past year _____

Situations that cause stress: At the present time _____

In the past _____

Perception of Stressors/Stress

What does this problem/stressor/loss mean to you? _____

Have stressful situations been good or bad for you? _____

How have stressful situations affected you? (physically and emotionally) _____

Coping Strategies

How do you relieve tension and deal with stress?

Talk to others _____   Try to solve the problem _____   Blame someone else for the
Try to forget _____   Try to relieve tension with   problem _____
Do something to get mind off   alcohol _____ drugs _____   Seek help _____
  problems _____   overeating _____   Other (describe) _____
Pray _____   Go to sleep _____   _____
Do nothing _____   Accept the situation _____   _____

Is there someone you rely on to help you solve problems? _____

Is there something the nurse can do to make hospitalization (clinic visits, home visits, etc.) less stressful?

Resolution of Stress

Do you usually solve your problems? _____

Do the methods you just described for relieving tension usually help? _____

From Fuller, J., & Schaller-Ayers, J. (1990). *Health assessment: A nursing approach.* Philadelphia: J. B. Lippincott.

NURSING DIAGNOSIS AND PATIENT GOALS

There are seven categories of diagnoses related to coping and adaptation currently approved as nursing diagnoses. These diagnoses include: Impaired Adjustment, Defensive Coping, Ineffective Denial, Ineffective Family Coping: Disabling, Ineffective Family Coping: Compromised, Family Coping: Potential for Growth, Post-Trauma Response, and High Risk for Violence. One diagnosis will be presented in this text: Ineffective Individual Coping.

Diagnostic Statement: Ineffective Individual Coping

Definition

Ineffective Individual Coping is defined as impairment of adaptive behaviors and problem-solving abilities of a person in meeting life's demands and roles (NANDA, 1990).

Defining Characteristics

Verbalization of inability to cope or inability to ask for

help*; inability to meet role expectations; inability to meet basic needs; inability to problem-solve*; alteration in societal participation; destructive behavior toward self or others; inappropriate use of defense mechanisms; change in usual communication patterns; verbal manipulation; high illness rate; high rate of accidents (NANDA, 1990).

Related Factors

Situational crises; maturational crises; personal vulnerability (NANDA, 1990).

Related Nursing Diagnoses

In addition to the previously mentioned nursing diagnoses related to ineffective coping, dysfunctional grieving and post-trauma syndrome may also be related to ineffective coping. When a person moves beyond normal grieving (see Chap. 46), continued inability to cope with a loss leads to dysfunctional grieving in connection with ineffective coping. A trauma victim has been exposed to extraordinary stress or to repeated stresses, usually with threats to personal safety; in the period after the trauma, the person may reexperience the traumatic event, resulting in manifestations of ineffective coping.

Patient Goals

The goals for the patient with ineffective individual coping need to be individualized, taking into consideration the patient's history, areas of risk, evidence of dysfunction, and related objective data. Examples of patient goals include:

The patient will identify sources of stress in his or her life.
The patient will identify usual personal coping strategies for stressful situations.
The patient will define the effect of stress and coping strategies on activities of daily living.

For the patient who has related nursing diagnoses and more complex problems with stress, coping, and adaptation, the patient goals will need to be adjusted accordingly, along with the time frame in which they can be realized.

IMPLEMENTATION

Once the nursing diagnosis of Ineffective Individual Coping has been identified, the nurse can intervene independently to help restore function, or collab-

*Critical

Safety Alert

- When you are experiencing an unusual amount of stress, take extra precaution while operating motor vehicles, as you may be easily distracted.
- Be aware of alcohol intake and the amount of smoking, as it may be easy to overdo as a result of stress.
- If eating is a coping mechanism, keep a journal of food intake so that when your are experiencing stress, any extra food consumption will be easily recognized.
- If specialized types of stress reduction and coping strategies are to be used, be sure that you learn them from expert clinicians.

---

oratively with other health-team members. The nurse can assist the patient in recognizing signs and symptoms of stress, identifying the sources of distress, and choosing an appropriate course of action. The patient may not be able to recognize that muscle tension, or feelings such as depression and anxiety, are related to stress. Because the stress response is highly complex and individual, the management of that response must also be individualized. Stress management techniques that are effective for one person may not be helpful for another. The nurse can assist the patient in finding the techniques that are most effective. The nurse also has a significant role in identifying people at risk for ineffective coping and initiating appropriate teaching to promote optimum health.

Nursing Interventions to Promote Health and Function

Helping the patient recognize and manage stress is an important aspect of health maintenance and disease prevention. Learning to adapt to stress requires self-appraisal and recognition of one's own manifestations of stress; this is true for nurses as well as patients.

Stress Management for Nurses

Nurses must be aware of their own stress levels. Nursing practice often involves working in a stressful environment. In addition to dealing with people who are dependent and needy, the nurse has to adjust to working odd hours, weekends, and holidays. Inpatient units are often crowded, noisy, and understaffed. Nursing literature describes two conditions that frequently occur in nurses: burnout and tedium.

Burnout is the result of working with people who are demanding and needy, which often creates conflict within the nurse and leads to depletion of energy and low morale. Tedium is the result of environmental factors that create conflicts or place demands on the nurse. Burnout and tedium are often characterized by physical and emotional depletion, negative self-concept, negative attitudes, and feelings of helplessness and hopelessness (Pines, Aronson, & Kafry, 1981).

To manage personal stress, the nurse must first recognize the existence of stress, along with personal manifestations of stress. Learning to admit that increased fatigue, anger, disorganization, or other behavior changes may be related to an increased level of stress is one step. Noting changes in lifestyle factors, such as smoking, alcohol or other substance use, or changes in eating behavior may provide further acknowledgment of the presence of stress.

Once the nurse is able to recognize the ways in which he or she responds to stress, the nurse can then attend to the times when stress is most pronounced, and to the situations that stimulate a stress response. When the nurse is familiar with sources and manifestations of stress, then he or she can take positive action to prevent, manage, and alleviate stress so that effective coping strategies can be instituted. The accompanying display lists ways to deal with daily pressures and stresses, and to promote effective coping for nurses.

Stressor Reduction

The nurse needs to be sensitive to responses from the patient that assist in recognizing the presence of stress, its source, and its meaning to the patient. By clarifying

---

Stress Management Suggestions for Nurses

- Get out of bed 15 minutes earlier to have more time to prepare for the day.
- Establish a regular program of exercise and activity to focus energy expenditure.
- Eliminate or restrict the amount of alcohol, caffeine, and other mood-altering substances as a means of managing stress.
- Learn to accept failure, your own and others, and turn it into a constructive experience.
- Develop techniques for assertiveness to have more feelings of personal control.
- Develop support systems among colleagues and friends to bolster personal resources.
- Have an optimistic view of the world, believing that most people are doing the best that they can.

---

these parameters, the nurse and the patient are formulating an approach either to reducing the stressor or removing it entirely. Through health teaching and learning what is causing the stress, the patient can then develop strategies for coping and adapting.

For example, the working mother who is tired from putting in overtime and does not have enough time to spend with her family may find herself feeling angry, excessively fatigued, and short-tempered with her children. She may be helped to realize that the mood changes she is experiencing are stress-induced, and that examples of coping strategies may be changing jobs to better accommodate her family's needs as well as her own, asking her spouse for help, or hiring part-time help.

Addressing Perfection

Faulty perceptions in one's belief system can contribute to the stress response. Often, perfectionistic "shoulds, oughts, and musts" only enhance the person's response to stress. An example is the person who tells himself or herself: "I must never make a mistake" or "I should always clean the house before going to work." Helping the patient realize that a desire for perfection or unrealistic self-expectations are stress-inducing is an important nursing intervention. Being realistic about self-expectations and remembering that relationships are more important than things or tasks can help reduce stress.

Supportive Internal Messages

The internal dialogue whereby a person describes and interprets the world is referred to as self-talk, or internal messages. Internal messages have a definite impact on one's daily functioning and self-concept. A constant stream of negative self-messages can lead to generalized feelings of inferiority and self-doubt. Instead of being defeated by negative internal messages, one can learn to control them by using supportive messages to help cope with difficult situations. Changing internal messages involves these three steps:

- Identifying what one says when the situation occurs (self-talk).
- Evaluating how rational/irrational these messages are.
- Replacing the negative messages with supportive coping statements, and integrating them into daily life. (Nakagawa-Kogan, et al., 1979)

For example, a person interviews for a job but is not hired. Instead of saying, "I blew it, I'm a failure; I'll never get the job I want," these statements can be restructured into supportive self-statements such as, "I feel disappointed that I didn't get this job. I know I presented myself well. I have the ability to get the job

Patient Teaching

Instruct the patient as follows:

- Exercise to release tension in muscles.
- Get adequate sleep and rest to re-energize the body.
- Eat a balanced diet to give energy for body and mind.
- Manage time appropriately to increase sense of control and organization.
- Be assertive to increase self-esteem and personal control.
- Learn relaxation techniques (breathing, progressive relaxation, or visualization) to release tension and quiet the mind.
- Do something for others to get your mind off yourself and boost your self-esteem.
- Laugh to release tension and relax mind and body.

I want." The nurse can encourage the patient to examine internal messages and practice rephrasing those that are negative or irrational.

Another behavioral strategy useful for gaining control over self-defeating thoughts is called "thought stopping." Thought stopping can be accomplished by using the following technique:

- Say "stop," inwardly or out loud, when a negative or self-defeating thought crosses the mind (e.g., "I'll never be able to find a job").
- Substitute a positive, assertive statement for the negative thought (e.g., "I have the skills needed to get the job I want").
- If using the word "stop" is ineffective, place a rubber band around the wrist and snap it whenever negative, unwanted thoughts occur.

Assertiveness

Another technique useful in changing one's behavior in response to a stressful encounter is assertiveness. Assertive behavior enables the person to act in his or her own best interests, to stand up for him- or herself, to express his or her feelings openly and honestly, and to exercise his or her rights without infringing on the rights of others. Assertiveness is a learned behavioral skill that requires practice. A nurse who recognizes a person who has difficulty expressing feelings or getting his or her needs met might suggest that this person enroll in a class or workshop in assertiveness training.

Lifestyle Changes

Adequate rest and nutrition are important components of a person's personal resources in managing stress and effective coping. One is more capable of handling the stressful events of everyday life if the body is not fatigued or malnourished. Encouraging the patient to get adequate sleep and nutrition, to limit or eliminate smoking, to cut down on coffee consumption, and avoid depending on "pill-popping" (such as aspirin or tranquilizers) will promote healthier management of stress.

Exercise

A technique that helps counter the effects of the stress response is physical activity or exercise. Vigorous physical exertion helps to release tension from the muscles, and is a natural outlet when the body is in a fight-or-flight state of arousal. There are two broad categories of exercise, aerobic exercise and low-intensity exercise (Davis, Eshelman, & McKay, 1982). Aerobic exercise involves sustained activity of the large muscle groups and places an increased demand on the cardiopulmonary system. Examples of aerobic exercise include running, bicycling, swimming, cross-country skiing, brisk walking, and rowing.

Low-intensity exercise is not vigorous and provides little benefit to the cardiovascular system. However, it can be used to increase muscle strength and flexibility and to prepare the sedentary person for more vigorous aerobic exercise. Examples include calisthenics, slow walking, gardening, and housecleaning.

A regular program of exercise is an important component of health. For the patient, exercise may take the form of active or passive range of motion, either encouraged or performed by the nurse. Additional possible benefits of exercise are shown in the display.

Health Benefits of Exercise

- Improves muscular strength, endurance, and flexibility.
- Improves cardiovascular efficiency.
- Lowers resting heart rate.
- Reduces blood cholesterol levels.
- Reduces general anxiety and depression.
- Reduces chronic fatigue and insomnia.
- Lowers body weight by burning calories and suppressing appetite.
- Increases absorption and use of food.
- Improves appearance and self-image.

Relaxation Techniques

Another method of decreasing physiologic arousal is through relaxation techniques. The physiologic reactions of the GAS, described earlier in this chapter, cause activation of all body systems. During this state, muscle tension and a heightened sense of awareness begin to compete with a state of relaxation. The body has the ability to elicit the "relaxation response," which is in direct opposition to the responses of the GAS. The relaxation response was first described by the Harvard researcher, Dr. Herbert Benson (1976). He discovered that meditation brought about an integrated set of physiologic changes, in opposition to the fight-or-flight response, including lowered oxygen consumption, heart rate, respirations, and blood lactate. Several techniques have been shown to elicit the relaxation response, including deep breathing, progressive relaxation, autogenics, visualization, meditation, yoga, and biofeedback. Some selected advanced stress management techniques are presented in Table 47-3.

Deep Breathing. Breathing is an important element of the relaxation response. As stress and tension mount during the day, breathing becomes shallow and irregular, and the heart rate accelerates. Poorly oxygenated blood contributes to lethargy, tension, and depression. When one is relaxed, breathing slows and deepens, and the heart rate returns to normal. Because breathing is the easiest physiologic system to control, one can use slow, deep breathing to trigger the relaxation response. In fact, many relaxation techniques begin by having the person slowly inhale and exhale for a few minutes.

As an incentive to practice deep breathing, one might associate it with something commonly done during the day, such as answering the phone or looking at the clock. Frequently, the act of taking a few deep breaths before a stressful situation can decrease fear and anxiety, allowing for a more relaxed frame of mind.

Progressive Relaxation. Progressive relaxation consists of systematically tensing and relaxing various mus-

TABLE 47–3

Selected Advanced Stress Management Techniques

Autogenic Training	A systematic technique teaching the body and mind to respond to verbal commands, allowing the person to achieve a deep state of relaxation through self-suggestion (or self-hypnosis).
Visualization and Imagery	An attempt to affect an unconscious process by using a conscious suggestion, or a mental picture of the desired change (Mason, 1980).
Affirmations	Strong, positive, feeling-rich statements about a desired change to reinforce and increase the effectiveness of visualization; can be done silently, spoken aloud, written down, or chanted. For example, a person who has a strong sense of time urgency might use this affirmation: "I am relaxed and centered. I have plenty of time for everything."
Meditation	An age-old technique from Eastern religious traditions to achieve a deep state of mental and physical relaxation. Four elements include: a quiet place; a comfortable position; an object to dwell on, such as a word or symbol; and a passive attitude.
Biofeedback	A specialized form of relaxation technique in which the person learns to monitor physiologic processes, feed back a measure of that function, and exert control over autonomic functions. Information, such as heart rate, muscle tension, and finger temperature, is translated into an auditory or visual signal that the person senses, and through these signals the person learns to discriminate between tension and relaxation.
Therapeutic Touch	The use of touch as a means of anxiety and stress reduction, relief of pain, and comfort.
Massage	The manipulation of soft tissue, generally using the hands, to provide stimulation and relaxation and to reduce stress and anxiety.
Yoga	A form of exercise (often combined with meditation) to foster relaxation, mental alacrity, and good health.

cle groups in the body, moving from head to toe. Many people do not realize that their muscles are in a state of chronic tension. Progressive relaxation provides a method of identifying particular muscle groups and distinguishing between sensations of tension and relaxation. The steps involved in doing progressive muscle relaxation are shown in the display.

There are other specialized forms of relaxation techniques that require training, expertise, and supervised practice for the nurse to be skillful in using them with patients.

Nursing Interventions for Altered Coping Function

Many of the techniques that promote healthy coping function can also be used for situations of altered function. An advantage of using techniques for controlling stress and promoting effective coping when one is well is that the person has the skill to employ these techniques when altered function exists.

Relaxation Training

The nurse may encounter many stressful situations, in both inpatient and outpatient settings, where it is appropriate to teach, or to remind the patient to use, relaxation techniques. Patient situations where relaxation training might be used include:

- Before and after diagnostic tests
- During childbirth
- After surgery to help manage postoperative pain
- During recovery from a myocardial infarction
- Calming an anxious or agitated person on the psychiatric unit
- Before a painful procedure, such as an intramuscular injection or inserting an intravenous line.

It is becoming a common practice for many inpatient and outpatient settings to have relaxation tapes available for patients' use. Relaxation tapes may be purchased, or the patient may want to make his or her own personal recording. Taking a few deep breaths before a procedure can decrease the patient's anxiety. For example, before a

---

Progressive Muscle Relaxation Technique

Progressive relaxation is a self-taught or instructed exercise that involves learning to constrict and relax muscle groups in a systematic way, beginning with the face and finishing with the feet. This exercise may be combined with breathing exercises that focus on inner body processes. It usually takes 15 to 30 minues and may be accompanied by a taped instruction that directs the person concerning the sequence of muscles to be relaxed.
1. Wear loose clothing; remove glasses and shoes.
2. Sit or recline in a comfortable position with neck and knees supported; avoid lying completely flat.
3. Begin with slow, rhythmic breathing.
   a. Close your eyes or stare at a spot and take in a slow deep breath.
   b. Exhale the breath slowly.
4. Continue rhythmic breathing at a slow steady pace and feel the tension leaving your body with each breath.
5. Begin progressive relaxation of muscle groups.
   a. Breathe in and tense (tighten) your muscles, and then relax the muscles as you breathe out.
   b. Suggested order for tension–relaxation cycle (with tension technique in parentheses).
      Face, jaw, mouth (squint eyes, wrinkle brow)
      Neck (pull chin to neck)
      Right hand (make a fist)
      Right arm (bend elbow in tightly)
      Left hand (make a fist)
      Left arm (bend elbow in tightly)
      Back, shoulders, chest (shrug shoulders up tightly)
      Abdomen (pull stomach in and bear down on chair)
      Right upper leg (push leg down)
      Right lower leg and foot (point toes toward body)
      Left upper leg (push leg down)
      Left lower leg and foot (point toes toward body)
6. Practice technique slowly.
7. End relaxation session when you are ready by counting to three, inhale deeply, and saying, "I am relaxed."

From Carpenito, L. J. (1980). *Nursing diagnosis: Applications to clinical practice.* Philadelphia: J. B. Lippincott.

painful procedure or intramuscular injection, ask the patient to take two or three slow, deep breaths. Usually patients will experience less discomfort if they are in a relaxed, calm state of mind.

Environment Modifications

The nurse needs to be aware of stressors in the environment, making changes and adjustments whenever possible to reduce the sensory overload and assist the patient with coping and adaptation. For the hospitalized patient, the environment, which affords little privacy and is unfamiliar, may be the source of the stress. Increased noise levels, constant lights, and unfamiliar procedures all contribute to stress.

The nurse may be instrumental in making modifications in the environment that assist the patient in managing the stress of the situation and in coping with the environment. Organizing nursing care to decrease disturbance to the patient, having as few extra lights on as possible, and keeping down the level of conversational tone in the hallways are a few examples.

Crisis Intervention

An acute health problem, illness, loss, or trauma may precipitate a crisis in a person's life. A crisis suggests a situation in which usual coping strategies are ineffective, and the person is disorganized or unable to problem-solve appropriately. For resolution of a crisis to occur, the patient needs assistance in realistic perception of the problem or stress; adequate support during the crisis and its resolution, from family, friends, clergy, and health-care providers, including nurses; and support while relearning or reinstituting coping strategies. Nursing assists in meeting these needs as a part of nursing management.

Discharge Planning and Home Care

When a person is convalescing from a stress-producing situation, there is increased vulnerability to other stresses and to ineffective coping. It is at this time that continued support for coping and adaptation are particularly important. Support groups can be effective at this time; these can be informal, such as the family, friends, and spiritual sources, or the groups can be formal in nature. For example, the Alzheimer's Disease and Related Disorders Association (ADRDA) is composed of people who have had members of their family diagnosed with Alzheimer's disease, a progressive senile dementia. A group such as this can be particularly helpful for someone experiencing the stress associated with caring for a person with that diagnosis, and can offer many useful ideas for coping strategies and effective adaptation.

There are many support groups that offer that type of assistance for many specialized problems and needs. It is useful for the nurse to be aware of these groups and to develop networks with other health professionals to link patients to them appropriately.

EVALUATION

Specific outcome criteria are the evaluative tools for measuring the attainment of patient goals. Nursing interventions are the means for achieving the goals. Examples of the outcome criteria are listed below. Outcome criteria need to be specifically tailored to the individual patient so that the criteria will uniquely measure the attainment of patient's goals.

Goal
The patient will identify sources of stress in his or her life.

Possible Outcome Criteria
- The patient defines events that create personal stress by listing them before next meeting with the nurse.

Nursing Management Plan
The Patient With Ineffective Individual Coping

Nursing Diagnosis: Ineffective individual coping related to situational crises manifested by inability to manage stressors.

Patient Goal: Patient will identify cause of current problems and usual personal coping strategies for stressful situations.

Patient Outcome Criteria

- Patient verbalizes feelings related to present emotional state within 24 to 48 hours.
- Patient identifies recent stressful life events or sources of stress during first week.
- Patient identifies signs and symptoms of current stress.
- Within a week, patient identifies current coping patterns and consequences of such behavior.

Nursing Intervention	Scientific Rationale
1. Assess causative and contributive factors by discussing with client (i.e., loss, grieving, inadequate support, recent life changes).	1. Assessment of causative factors provides the nurse with information on which to develop a treatment plan.
2. Assess the person's present coping status: Determine onset of symptoms and correlation with recent life changes Assess for risk of self-harm.	2. Identification of current coping skills helps the nurse to assess adequacy/inadequacy of coping.
3. Encourage the patient to evaluate the effectiveness of current coping skills.	3. Personal understanding of coping skills and outcomes reinforces use of acceptable coping or encourages the patient to look for alternatives in coping.

Patient Goal: Patient will demonstrate appropriate coping strategies.

Patient Outcome Criteria

- Patient makes environmental changes to reduce stress within 1 to 3 months.
- Patient practices several new coping skills, i.e., relaxation techniques, assertiveness, exercise, talking about feelings, thought stopping, affirmations.
- Patient assesses effectiveness of social support network and, if inadequate, take steps to correct lack of support within 1 to 3 months.

Nursing Intervention	Scientific Rationale
1. Assist patient to problem solve in a constructive manner.	1. Development of healthy coping strategies helps to eliminate or reduce stress and decrease possibility of chronic illness.
2. Help patient identify problems in environment that are stressful. Discuss how to change them, if this is possible.	2. Patient may need help in knowing how to make necessary changes.
3. When there are problems the patient cannot control directly, help him or her identify stress-reducing techniques that can be used.	3. In addition to identifying techniques, the patient needs to understand them and learn proper skills for their usefulness.
4. Assist patient in identifying social support network. Encourage patient to develop this support if it is helpful Assist patient in finding support groups to meet his or her needs.	4. People need external as well as internal resources for coping.

- The patient demonstrates anticipation of stressful situations by discussing them with the nurse before they occur.
- The patient identifies the difference between positive and negative sources of stress in next discussion with the nurse.

Goal

The patient will identify usual personal coping strategies for stressful situations.

Possible Outcome Criteria

- The patient names at least ten personal coping patterns to the nurse during the hospital stay.
- The patient describes techniques used to reinforce previous responses or to establish new responses in the next teaching session with the nurse.
- The patient consciously initiates effective stress management techniques during a stressful period, as observed by the nurse.

Goal

The patient will define the effect of stress and coping strategies on ADLs.

Possible Outcome Criteria

- The patient identifies specific ADLs affected by the presence of stress by describing them to the nurse within 24 hours.
- The patient describes how specific coping strategies interfere with or promote ADLs after the next teaching session with the nurse.
- The patient demonstrates new coping skills effective in managing stress and assisting ADLs to the visiting nurse at the first home visit.

Evaluation includes assessing the patient and comparing the patient's current progress with the individually established outcome criteria as a measure of the patient's goal attainment. The nursing care plan is continued, modified, or concluded based on this systematic evaluation of the individual patient.

Key Concepts

- Stress is an inherent part of life that may have positive or negative effects.
- Coping with stress successfully requires adaptation, or a change in response to stress.
- Homeostasis is the coordinated physiologic processes that maintain most of the steady states in the person.
- Integration of the autonomic nervous system and the endocrine system plays a major role in homeostatic control.

- Stress may be considered as an event or set of events that can be either a stimulus or a response.
- When stress is a stimulus, it may cause a disrupted response.
- The multisystem response to stress is referred to as the general adaptation syndrome (GAS).
- The three stages of the GAS are the alarm reaction, stage of resistance, and stage of exhaustion.
- The local adaptation syndrome (LAS) is a localized expression of the three stages of the GAS.
- The physiologic response to stress is mediated by the hypothalamic–pituitary–adrenal axis.
- Coping is a problem-solving process that the person uses to manage the stresses or events with which he or she is presented.
- People of all ages and levels of development encounter stress, and need to cope and adapt.
- Coping and adaptation are affected by transition and lifestyle events.
- Transition factors can include relocation, marriage, childbirth, and school.
- Lifestyle factors can include nutrition, rest, exercise, and previous learning.
- Altered coping may be manifested by use of alcohol and drugs, excessive smoking, increased sleeping, withdrawal, and illness.
- Manifestations of altered coping can interfere with the person's effective management of activities of daily living.
- A focused nursing assessment of coping and adaptation includes the history of the patient's previous coping methods, areas of risk for ineffective coping, and identification of a coping and adaptation dysfunction.
- Nursing interventions include assisting the patient to develop effective coping strategies to promote healthy adaptation to stress, and supporting the patient in using those strategies in unusually stressful situations.
- Discharge planning and home care needs to include the use of support persons or groups to maintain effective coping strategies.

References

Bell, J. M. (1977). Stressful life events and coping methods in mental-illness and wellness behaviors. *Nursing Research, 26*(2), 136–141.

Benson, H. (1976). *The relaxation response.* New York: Avon Books.

Cannon, W. B. (1935). Stressors and strains of homeostasis. *American Journal of Medical Sciences, 189,* 1.

Davis, M., Eshelman, E. R., & McKay, M. (1982). *The relaxation and stress reduction workbook.* Oakland, CA: New Harbinger.

Fuller, J., & Schaller-Ayers, J. (1990). *Health assessment: A nursing approach.* Philadelphia: J. B. Lippincott.

Holmes, T. H., & Rahe, R. H. (1967). The social readjustment and rating scale. *Journal of Psychosomatic Research, 11,* 213–218.

Lazarus, R., & Folkman, S. (1980). An analysis of coping in a middle-aged community sample. *Journal of Health and Social Behavior, 21,* 219–239.

Lazarus, R. S. (1981). Little hazards can be hazardous to your health. *Psychology Today, 15*(7), 58–62.

Levine, S., Scotch, N. (1970). Social stress. Chicago: Aldine Publishing Co.

Lyon, B., & Werner, J. (1987). Stress: ten years of practice-relevant research. In H. Werley & J. Fitzpatrick, eds. *Annual review of nursing research.*

Mason, J. W. (1975a). A historical view of the stress field, Part 1. *Journal of Human Stress, 1*, 6–12.

Mason, J. W. (1975b). A historical view of the stress field, Part 2. *Journal of Human Stress, 1*(2), 22–36.

Nakagawa-Kogan, H. et al. (1979). *Training manual for the management of stress response program.* Seattle, University of Washington, School of Nursing, Psychosocial Nursing Department.

NANDA (1990). *Taxonomy I revised 1990, with official nursing diagnoses.* St. Louis, MO: North American Nursing Diagnosis Association.

Pines, A., Aronson, E., & Kafry, D. (1981). *Burnout from tedium to personal growth.* New York: Free Press.

Selye, H. (1974). *Stress without disease.* Philadelphia: J. B. Lippincott.

Vander, A. J. (1990). *Human physiology: The mechanisms of body function* (5th ed.). New York: McGraw-Hill.

Wilson, H. S., & Kneisl, C. R. (1983). *Psychiatric nursing.* Menlo Park, CA: Addison-Wesley.

Wolff, H. G. (1953). *Stress and disease.* Springfield, IL: Thomas.

Bibliography

Aldana, S. G., et al. (1989). The relationships of physical activity and perceived stress. *Health Values, 13*(5), 34–37.

Barnfather, J. S., et al. (1989). Evaluation of two assessment techniques for adaptation to stress. *Nursing Science Quarterly, 2*(4), 172–182.

Biley, F. C. (1989). Stress in high dependency units. *Intensive Care Nursing, 5*(3), 134–141.

Caty, S., et al. (1989). Helping hospitalized preschoolers manage stressful situations: The mother's role. *Child Health Care, 18*(4), 202–209.

Cohen, L. H. (1988). *Life events and psychological functioning.* Newbury Park: Sage Publications.

Conway, F. J., et al. (1989). Cultural complexity: The hidden stressors. *Journal of Advanced Medical Surgical Nursing, 1*(4), 65–72.

Doswell, W. M. (1989). Physiological responses to stress. *Annual Review of Nursing Research, 7*, 51–69.

Eccles, A. M. (1990). Using humor to relieve stress. *Point of View, 27*(1), 8–9.

Engels, G. L. (1975). A unified concept of health and disease. In T. Million (Ed.), *Medical behavior science.* Philadelphia: W. B. Saunders.

Everly, G. S. (1989). *A clinical guide to the treatment of the human stress response.* New York: Plenum Press.

Friedman, M., & Rosenman, R. H. (1974). *Type A behavior and your heart.* New York: Alfred A. Knopf.

Ganter, R. K. (1990). Positive stress for health care providers. *Caring, 9*(1), 18–20, 22.

Guzzetta, C. E. (1989). Effects of relaxation and music therapy on patients in a coronary care unit with presumptive acute myocardial infarction. *Heart and Lung, 18*, 609–616.

Holmes, T. H. (1984). *Life change events research, 1966–1978.* New York: Praeger.

Holroyd, K. A., & Lazarus, R. S. (1982). Stress, coping, and somatic adaptation. In L. Goldberger & S. Breznitz (Eds.), *Handbook of stress.* New York: Free Press.

Jacobs, D. (1989a). Assessing stress: Step toward relief, part 1. *OR Manager, 5*(2), 3.

Jacobs, D. (1989b). Stress reaction: Positive or negative, part 2. *OR Manager, 5*(3), 10.

Leidy, N. K. (1989). A physiologic analysis of stress and chronic illness. *Journal of Advanced Nursing, 14*, 868–876.

Lieberman, M. A. (1982). The effects of social supports on responses to stress. In L. Goldberger & S. Breznitz (Eds.), *Handbook of stress.* New York: Free Press.

Maslow, A. (1954). *Motivation and personality.* New York: Harper Brothers.

Mason, L. J. (1980). *Guide to stress reduction.* Los Angeles: Peace Press.

Nyamathi, A., et al. (1989). Maladaptive coping in the critically ill population with acquired immunodeficiency syndrome: Nursing assessment and treatment. *Heart and Lung, 18*, 113–120.

Pelletier, K. (1977). *Mind as healer, mind as slayer.* New York: Dell.

Ramsey, J. M. (1982). *Basic pathophysiology.* Menlo Park, CA: Addison-Wesley.

Roberts, S. L. (1987–1988). A framework for coping with stress and its application in patient care. *Nursing Forum, 23*(3), 101–107.

Sedgwick, R. (1975). Psychological responses to stress. *Journal of Psychiatric Nursing and Mental Health, 13*(5), 20.

Selye, H. (1978). On the real benefits of eustress. *Psychology Today, 10*, 69.

Selye, H. (1982). History and present status of the stress concept. In L. Goldberger & S. Breznitz (Eds., *Handbook of stress.* New York: Free Press.

Smith, J. G. (1990). *Cognitive–behavioral relaxation training.* New York: Springer.

Smith, M., & Selye, H. (1979). Reducing the negative effects of stress. *American Journal of Nursing, 79*, 1953.

Sutterly, D. C. (1979). Stress and health: A survey of self-regulation modalities. *Topics in Clinical Nursing 1*(1), 8.

Wolfer, J. A., et al. (1989). *Using nursing research: Pediatric surgical patients' and parents' stress responses and adjustment as a function of psychologic prearation and stress-point nursing care.* NLN Publication #15-2232, 155–172. New York: National League for Nursing.

UNIT XV
Sexuality and Reproduction

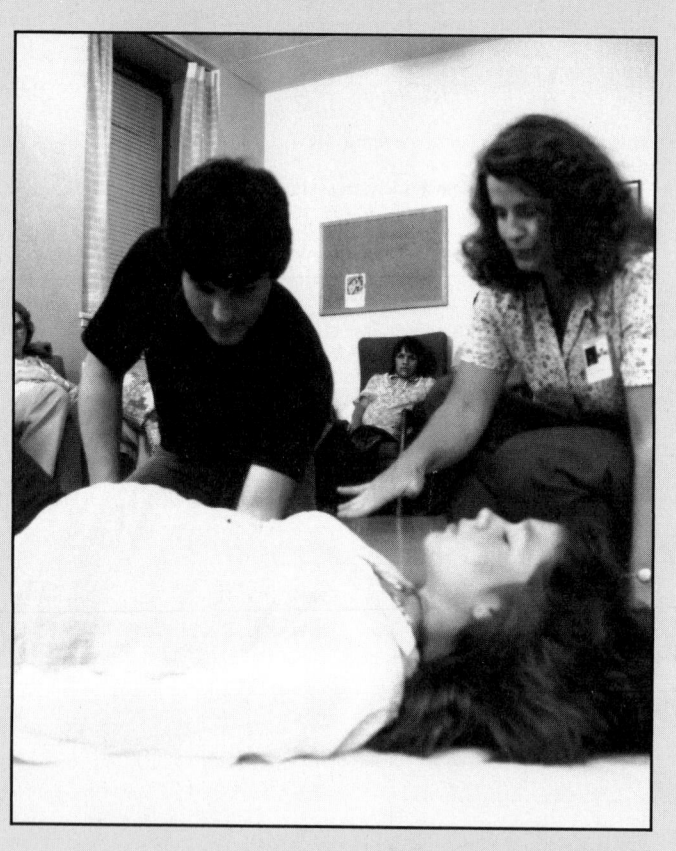

48 Human Sexuality

The single chapter in this unit discusses the sexuality and reproduction area of human function. Sexuality is a basic human need and one that concerns many patients when illness threatens their normal function. It is also a subject that creates discomfort for many nurses.

This chapter explores the physiologic and psychosocial components of sexuality. The discussion encourages nurses to explore their own feelings about sexuality. This is particularly important because normal function varies. Additionally, nurses may find themselves in situations where they must generate the conversation. The content in this chapter helps the nurse learn to avoid being judgmental when assessing and interviewing in this area of function.

Holistic nursing interventions and empathetic caring are essential for effective care for patients with sexuality needs. This chapter offers nursing interventions that promote health and function as well as a beginning discussion of holistic nursing interventions for patients with altered function.

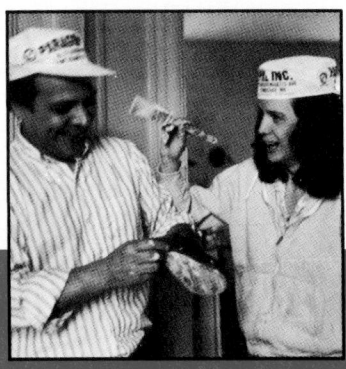

Human Sexuality

LEARNING OBJECTIVES

Upon completion of this chapter, the student will be able to do the following:

- Describe the anatomy of the male and female reproductive systems.
- Discuss sexual expression; sexual orientation; gender identity and roles; menstruation, and conception, pregnancy, and birth.
- Describe the male and female sexual response cycles.
- Discuss sexuality at all stages of the life cycle.

- Discuss factors that affect normal sexual functioning.
- Describe common risks and alterations in sexuality.
- Understand the nursing process as it relates to people with altered sexual functioning.
- Perform breast self-examination or testicular self-examination.

KEY TERMS

Bisexual
Climacteric
Clitoris
Dyspareunia
Foreskin
Heterosexual
Homosexual

Human sexual
    response
Impotence
Masturbation
Menarche
Menopause
Orgasm

Prepuce
Premature
    ejaculation
Sexuality
Transsexual
Vaginismus

48

Normal Human Sexuality
  Anatomy
    Male Reproductive System
    Female Reproductive System
  Normal Function of Male and Female Reproductive
    Systems
    Sexual Expression
    Menstruation and Ovulation
    Conception, Pregnancy, and Birth
    Milk Production
  Characteristics of Normal Sexuality
    Sexual Orientation
    Gender Identity and Roles
    Sexual Response
  Normal Sexual Functional Pattern
  Factors Affecting Sexuality
    Health Management
    Roles and Relationships
    Cognition and Perception
    Culture, Values, and Beliefs
    Self-Concept
    Coping and Stress Tolerance
    Previous Experience
  Lifespan Considerations
Altered Sexual Function
  Potential for Altered Sexuality
  Manifestations of Altered Sexuality
    Sexual Abuse
    Inhibited Sexual Desire
    Impotence
    Ejaculatory Dysfunction
    Orgasmic Dysfunction
    Dyspareunia
    Vaginismus

  Impact of Sexual Dysfunction on Activities of
    Daily Living
Assessment
  Subjective Data
    Functional Pattern Identification
    Risk Identification
    Dysfunctional Identification
  Objective Data
    Physical Assessment
    Diagnostic Tests and Procedures
Nursing Diagnoses and Patient Goals
  Diagnostic Statement: Sexual Dysfunction
    Definition
    Defining Characteristics
    Related Factors
  Diagnostic Statement: Altered Sexuality Patterns
    Definition
    Defining Characteristics
    Related Factors
  Related Nursing Diagnoses
  Patient Goals
Implementation
  Nursing Interventions to Promote Health and
    Function
    Patient Teaching
    Contraceptive Use
  Nursing Interventions for Altered Function
    Levels of Activities of Daily Living
    Counseling
    Referral
  Discharge Planning and Home Care
Evaluation
Key Concepts

Currently there is increased openness regarding sexual matters, although reservations still exist on the part of some to discuss sexuality. The nurse's challenge is complex in today's social context of more open sexual expression combined with more fears of sexually transmitted diseases, particularly AIDS.

Nurses see patients in many settings, some not directly involved with sexuality, but may be confronted in any setting with patients' concerns regarding their sexuality. Thus, sexual issues should be part of the patient history. Some common problems can be dealt with in the health-care facility; more advanced problems, however, require specially trained personnel. Each nurse must be aware of personal expertise and limitations. In addition, he or she must be aware of his or her personal attitude, and make sure that this does not interfere with the care rendered.

NORMAL HUMAN SEXUALITY

Sexuality includes function of the sexual organs, as well as a person's perceptions of his or her own functioning and sexual expression and preference. Human sexual response is highly variable and greatly influenced by many factors. These may include psychological, emotional, and cultural factors; and values and moral views, as well as comfort with one's body and quality of one's relationship with the other person, assuming one is involved in a relationship. People not involved in sexual relationships still regard themselves as sexual beings.

Anatomy

Although sexuality is not synonymous with reproduction, the reproductive organs are involved in human sexual response. For purposes of clarity, the male and female reproductive systems are discussed separately.

Male Reproductive System

The male reproductive system, as illustrated in Figure 48-1A, is composed of both external and internal organs. The external organs include the penis and scrotum. The penis is a cylindrical, pendulous, erectile organ. It is composed of the shaft and glans. The shaft contains the urethra, the outlet for urine from the urinary bladder. The glans is the cone-shaped head of the penis; it is covered with loose skin called the **prepuce** or **foreskin.** In the uncircumcised man, the glans can be retracted for intercourse and cleaning. In the circumcised man, the glans is exposed because the foreskin has been removed surgically.

The scrotum is the loose, pouchlike sac that contains the testes. The testes are the male gonads, reproductive glands that produce male cells, or spermatozoa, and testosterone, the male hormone.

The internal organs include the prostate gland and seminal vesicles. These are glands that produce and store most of the seminal fluid. The combination of seminal fluid and spermatozoa form semen, the secretion discharged from the urethra during orgasm.

Female Reproductive System

The female reproductive system includes external and internal organs, as illustrated in Figure 48-1B and C. External genitalia include the mons pubis, labia majora, labia minora, clitoris, urethral meatus, Skene's and Bartholin's glands, and the vaginal orifice. Collectively, these external anatomic parts are referred to as the vulva.

The mons pubis is a pad of fatty tissue that lies over the bony prominence called the symphysis pubis. The labia are the fleshy borders of the external genitalia. The labia majora lie on either side of the vaginal opening, forming the lateral borders. The labia minora are thinner folds that lie just inside the labia majora.

The **clitoris** is a small erectile body lying just above the urinary meatus and partially covered by the meeting of the labia minora. The clitoris corresponds to the male penis in its physiologic function of orgasm. Skene's glands lie inside of and on the posterior of the urethra, and Bartholin's glands are small mucous glands on the lateral wall of the vestibule of the vagina.

The internal genitalia include the ovaries, fallopian tubes, uterus, and vagina (Fig. 48-1C). The ovaries are two almond-shaped bodies lying on either side of the pelvic cavity, which contain ova and female hormones, specifically estrogen and progesterone. Fallopian tubes are narrow ducts of about 4.5 inches (11.4 cm) in length. They extend laterally on either side of the uterus, and terminate in finger-like projections near but not touching the ovaries.

The uterus is a muscular, pear-shaped organ that lies between the sacrum and the symphysis pubis. It consists of three areas: the fundus or upper portion; the cavity, which is hollow; and the lower end, the cervix, which connects the uterus to the vagina. The uterus is an expandable organ.

The vagina is a musculomembranous tube that forms a passageway from the uterus to the vulva. It is located between the urinary bladder and the rectum. The vagina represents a potential space—that is, the walls of the vagina, which are normally in contact, will stretch for sexual intercourse or the birth of a baby.

Breasts. The female breasts are considered organs of reproduction because they are directly influenced by the reproductive hormones, estrogen and progesterone, and because they are organs of lactation. Also called the mammary gland, each breast is composed of fatty and glandular tissue and consists of 15 to 20 lobes (Fig. 48-2). Each lobe drains through a lactiferous duct that opens on the tip of the nipple. The nipple is surrounded by a circular, pigmented area called the areola; the color of the areola is a pale to deep pink. Breast size varies from woman to woman and through the lifespan, after development in adolescence.

Normal Function of Male and Female Reproductive Systems

The male reproductive system is responsible for the generation, maturation, and ejaculation of spermatozoa. The female reproductive system is responsible for cyclic maturation and release of an ovum, and preparation of the uterus for implantation of a fertilized ovum, should fertilization occur.

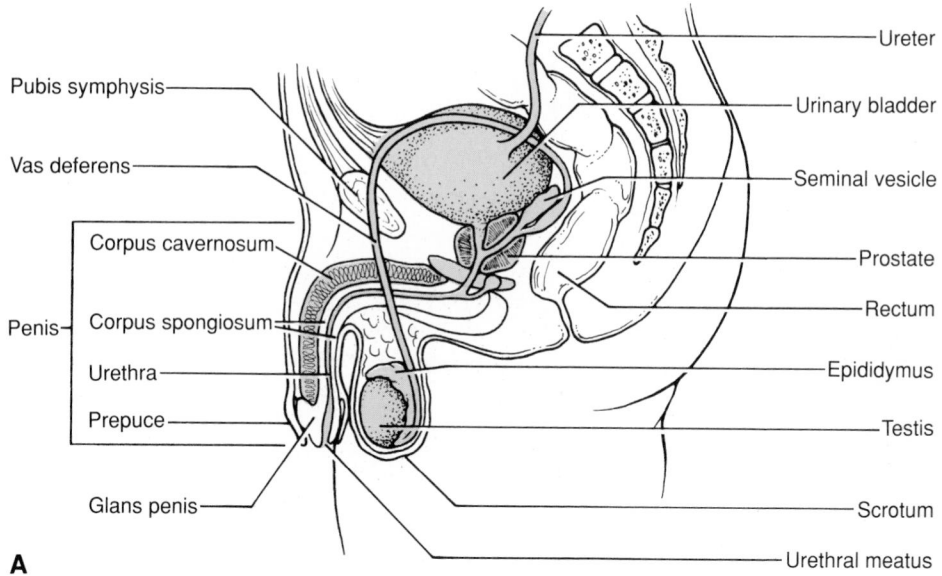

Ureter
Urinary bladder
Seminal vesicle
Prostate
Rectum
Epididymus
Testis
Scrotum
Urethral meatus

Pubis symphysis
Vas deferens
Corpus cavernosum
Penis
Corpus spongiosum
Urethra
Prepuce
Glans penis

A

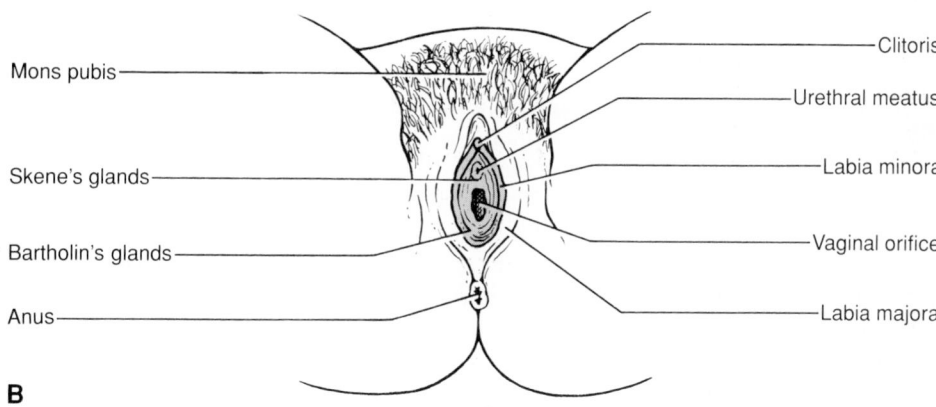

Mons pubis
Skene's glands
Bartholin's glands
Anus

Clitoris
Urethral meatus
Labia minora
Vaginal orifice
Labia majora

B

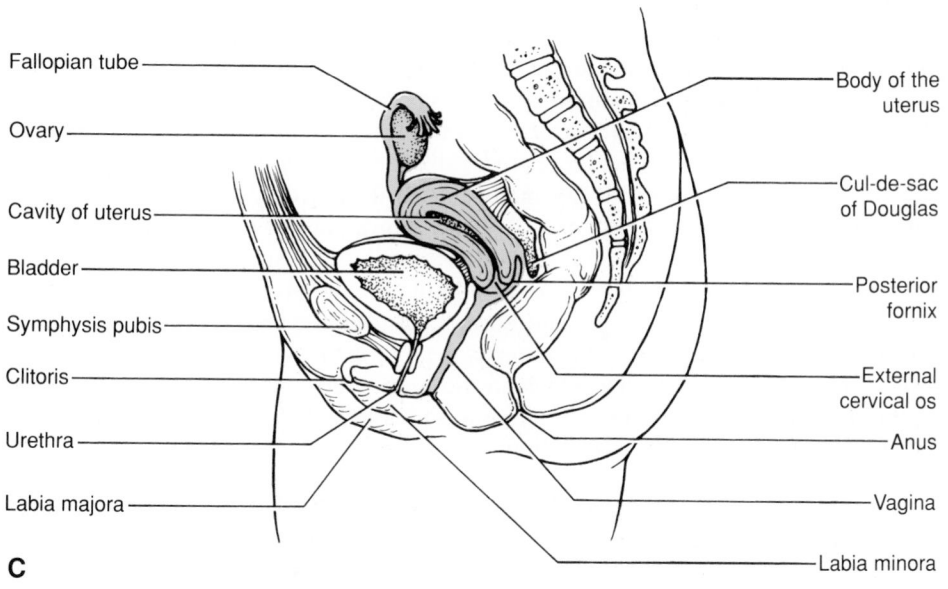

Fallopian tube
Ovary
Cavity of uterus
Bladder
Symphysis pubis
Clitoris
Urethra
Labia majora

Body of the uterus
Cul-de-sac of Douglas
Posterior fornix
External cervical os
Anus
Vagina
Labia minora

C

Figure 48–1. Anatomic cross-section of external and internal genitalia. **A:** Male genitalia; **B:** external female genitalia; **C:** internal female genitalia.

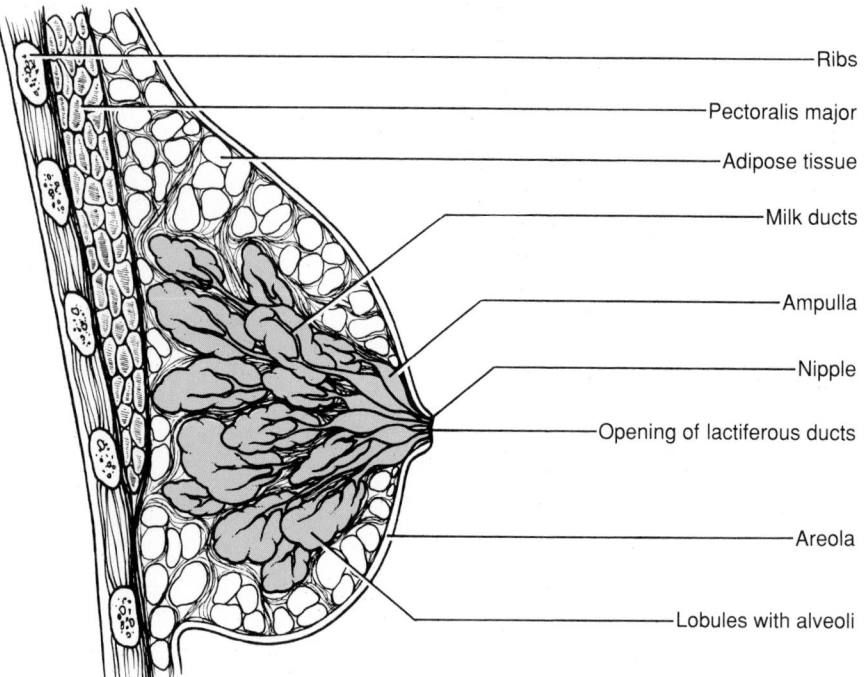

Ribs

Pectoralis major

Adipose tissue

Milk ducts

Ampulla

Nipple

Opening of lactiferous ducts

Areola

Lobules with alveoli

Figure 48–2. Breast structure and organs of lactation.

Reproduction is only one part of sexuality. Human beings can be sexual—can engage in sexual relationships—without the occurrence of reproduction.

Sexual Expression

Sexual expression varies among people. Various positions for coitus and stimulation may be used, without any particular one being considered "normal." The frequency of sexual expression also varies, with no determined "normal" frequency. In addition, the amount and kind of foreplay (activity before sexual intercourse) may vary greatly. Some people engage in **masturbation** (self-stimulation), whether it is mutual masturbation with a partner or masturbation without a partner. Others choose celibacy, although they still may consider themselves to be sexual, perhaps in a more spiritual form.

Menstruation and Ovulation

Menstruation is a physiologic process that occurs in women and is essential to their reproductive function. Sexual expression can occur in the absence of menstruation (e.g., a woman with Turner's syndrome or a woman who has gone through menopause). Because of its direct connection with reproduction, however, it is appropriate to discuss menstruation in this chapter. Menstruation is a cyclic, periodic discharge of a bloody fluid from the uterus through the vagina during the reproductive years of a woman's lifetime. The length of a cycle may vary from woman to woman, and even within one woman. The cycle repeats itself approximately every 28 days,

although much variation can occur and still be considered normal.

Menstruation depends on the interplay of various hormones. The hypothalamus secretes gonadotropin-releasing hormone (GnRh), which stimulates the pituitary gland to secrete follicle-stimulating hormone (FSH) and luteinizing hormone (LH) (Fig. 48-3A). These hormones stimulate the ovaries to produce estrogen and progesterone, which are necessary for stimulation of the target organs (vagina, breast, uterus) in preparing the body for a possible pregnancy. If pregnancy does not occur, the levels of estrogen and progesterone fall, menses ensues, and the feedback mechanism begins again with a new menstrual cycle.

The menstrual cycle is discussed in terms of the ovarian cycle and the endometrial or uterine cycle. The ovarian cycle consists of the follicular phase, the ovulatory phase, and the luteal phase (Fig. 48-3B). The follicular phase is estrogen-dominant; during this phase the follicles mature, with usually only one follicle reaching full maturity. This follicle, or oocyte, ruptures from the ovary at the time of ovulation. At this point the estrogen level loses its dominance and progesterone becomes the dominant hormone during the second half of the cycle, or the luteal phase. During this phase, the progesterone levels become elevated, preparing the uterus for possible implantation and maintenance of a fertilized ovum.

The endometrial or uterine cycle is divided into the proliferative and secretory phases (Fig. 48-3C). The proliferative phase refers to the proliferation of the endometrium, or uterine lining, as the dominant hormone, estrogen, influences such growth. During the secretory

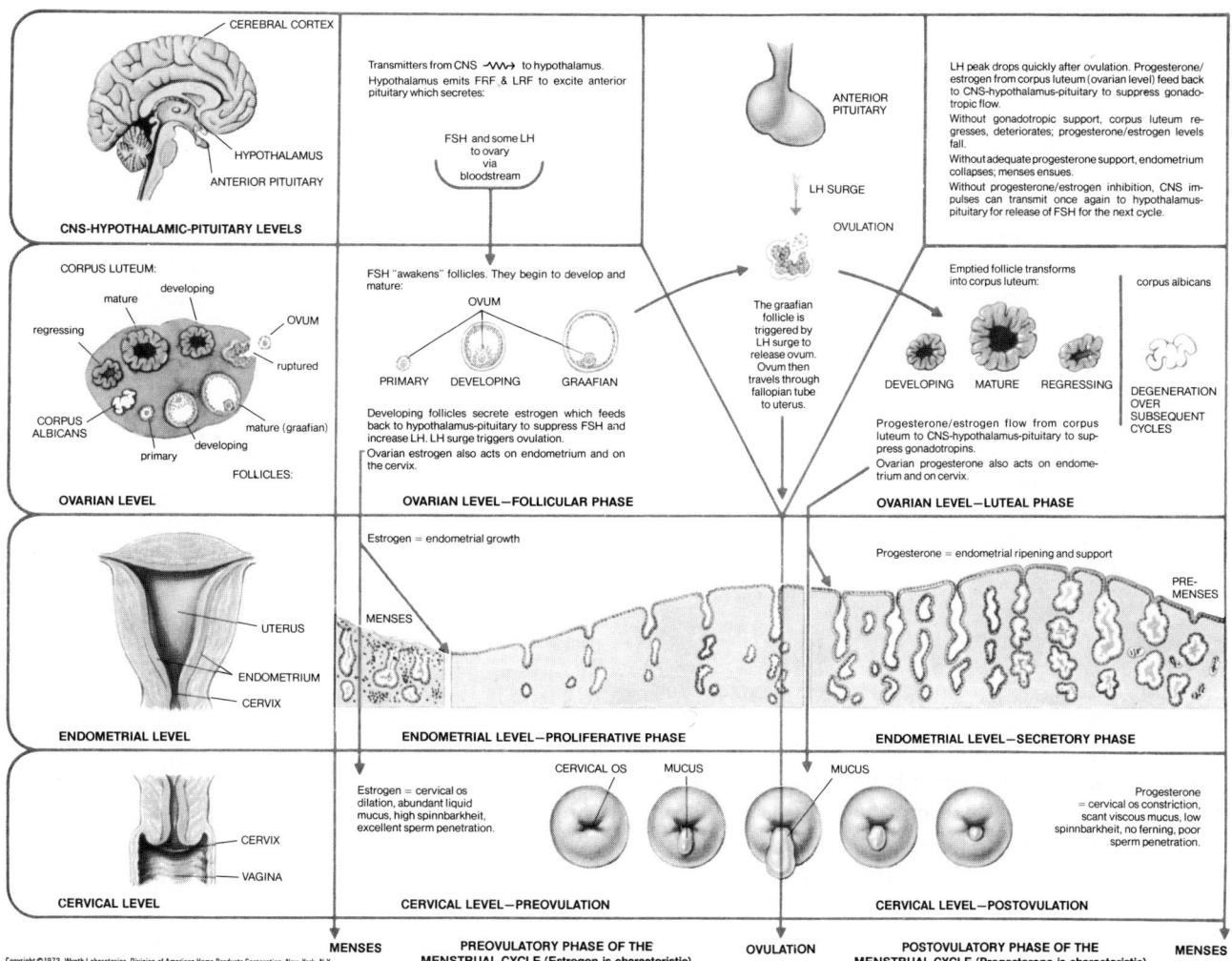

Figure 48–3. The normal menstrual cycle. The hypothalamus activates the pituitary to release hormones, which stimulate the ovaries to produce estrogen and progesterone (**A**). These hormones set in action the menstrual cycle, which is subdivided into the ovarian cycle (**B**) and the endometrial or uterine cycle (**C**). The cervix prepares for sperm penetration and fertilization (**D**). (Courtesy of Wyeth Laboratories, Philadelphia, PA.)

phase, which is progesterone-dominant, the endometrial glands continue to grow, becoming edematous and dense, in preparation for implantation and maintenance of a fertilized ovum.

Hormones also affect the uterus at the cervical level (Fig. 48-3D). Under the influence of estrogen, the cervical mucus becomes more watery, alkaline, and stretchy, resembling the quality of egg whites. This quality is conducive to sperm survival, thus preparing for the possibility of conception.

Conception, Pregnancy, and Birth

For conception and reproduction to occur, several complicated factors must be in full operation. First, the man must produce fully matured spermatozoa in enough numbers and with enough motility to penetrate the cer-

vix and ascend the uterus and fallopian tubes. This transportation occurs by way of cervical mucus, which becomes alkaline and thus receptive to the sperm. When the spermatozoa reach the fallopian tubes, they undergo capacitation, a process in which the surface characteristics of the sperm change, releasing enzymes that enhance their ability to penetrate the ovum.

The occurrence of ovulation must correspond to the process described above, because there is a time period of only a few days in which the woman can be impregnated. In ovulation, a mature follicle is released from the ovary into one of the fallopian tubes (see Fig. 48-3). The fimbriae or finger-like projections at the end of each fallopian tube assist in extracting the ovum from the ovary and bringing it into the fallopian tube.

Fertilization of one ova with one spermatozoon normally occurs in the outer third of the fallopian tube.

After fertilization occurs, the fertilized ovum undergoes several cell divisions and moves down toward the uterus, where it implants in the uterine wall.

The first 2 weeks after fertilization are critical; many pregnancies do not continue beyond this point because of a defective ova or spermatozoon or because of hormone imbalances. If a pregnancy continues following these complex factors and potential risks, the embryo develops rapidly. The average length of pregnancy, counted from the time of conception, is approximately 267 days or 38 weeks, but may vary by about 2 weeks in either direction.

Birth is a normal process that occurs in three stages of labor. Although the initiation of labor and birth is not entirely understood, labor involves stimulation by hormones that cause the uterus to contract, thus pushing the fetus through the birth canal after a number of hours of labor.

Milk Production

With pregnancy, the breasts undergo physiologic and anatomic changes. They enlarge and become more sensitive. The nipples enlarge, becoming darker, and the sebaceous glands in the areola hypertrophy. Later in pregnancy (during the second half), colostrum may begin to be secreted by the alveolar cells. Colostrum is a yellowish fluid, considered a precursor to actual milk, containing important nutrients for the newborn.

Milk production occurs under the influence of prolactin, glucocorticoids, insulin, and parathyroid hormone. Estrogen and progesterone actually inhibit milk production, and thus, at birth, with the delivery of the placenta, the levels of estrogen and progesterone fall dramatically.

Characteristics of Normal Sexuality

Sexual Orientation

It is essential that, when working with patients, nurses understand and appreciate that various forms of sexual orientation exist. As mentioned earlier under the section on "Sexual Expression," there is not one "normal" way of being in relation to sexuality and sexual orientation. Some people are **heterosexual,** relating sexually to members of the opposite gender. Others are **bisexual,** relating to both men and women in a sexual way. Others are **homosexual,** relating sexually to members of the same gender. Still others may abstain totally from sexual relations, either permanently or temporarily.

Gender Identity and Roles

One's gender identity and corresponding roles that one takes on influence sexuality. It is important for the nurse to understand the person's perception of his or her gender, and what that gender means to the person in terms of identity and roles.

Sometimes actual biologic gender does not coincide with gender identity; this is so in the case of people who are **transsexuals.** A man who is a transsexual views himself as a woman trapped in a man's body, and the reverse is true for a female transsexual. Social roles are often very confusing for transsexuals. Some may marry and have families, but others may never do so. Some seek medical intervention in the form of hormones and surgery to change their physical gender.

Sexual Response

The **human sexual response** was first studied scientifically by Masters and Johnson (1966). They found that humans undergo four distinct phases of sexual response, as outlined in Table 48-1. These phases are referred to as excitement, plateau, orgasm, and resolution. The excitement phase begins as a result of various stimuli, both physiologic and psychological. If there are no distracting stimuli, this phase will continue and will intensify as the person begins the plateau phase, in which there is increased sexual tension. If this sexual tension continues, still without distracting stimuli, **orgasm,** or the involuntary climax of this tension, occurs. During orgasm the person experiences involuntary contractions and release of the vasocongestion that occurs in the phases leading to orgasm. The resolution phase refers to the period after orgasm, in which physiologic changes occur that allow the body to return to its preexcitement state. These phases will be discussed more specifically as they are experienced by both men and women.

Male Sexual Response. Masters and Johnson (1966) found one pattern of sexual response in men, although according to Woods (1984), it is unlikely that male sexual response occurs without variation. This predominant pattern, as described by Masters and Johnson, and Woods, includes a rapid excitement phase, a short plateau phase with orgasm occurring immediately, and a resolution phase, which includes an obligatory refractory period.

Excitement. The excitement phase is characterized by rapid erection of the penis, with tensing and thickening of the scrotal skin and elevation of the scrotal sac. Additionally, there is shortening of the spermatic cords, resulting in partial elevation of both testes toward the perineum. The vasocongestion that occurs during this phase is responsible for the erection of the penis, as well as the thickening of the scrotal skin and the elevation of the scrotal sac. The testes increase in size as they are partially elevated. The man may experience nipple erection during the excitement phase. During the excitement phase it is not unusual for the man to partially lose his penile erection and regain it. He is also subject to distractions that may interfere with this phase.

Plateau. The plateau phase involves a thickening of the circumference of the penis at the coronal ridge, and an

TABLE 48–1

Phases of the Human Sexual Response Cycle

Phase	Changes in Man	Changes in Woman
Excitement	Rapid penile erection Partial elevation of testes Increased size of testes Nipple erection	Enlargement of clitoris Vaginal lubrication Expansion of vagina Enlargement of breasts Nipple erection Sex flush
Plateau	Thickening of circumference of penis Continued increase in size of testes Fluid from Cowper's glands Sex flush Muscle contraction Hyperventilation Increased heart rate Increased blood pressure	Retraction of clitoris Increased size of labia minora Elevation of uterus Muscle contraction Hyperventilation Increased heart rate Increased blood pressure
Orgasm	Expulsive contractions of urethra Ejaculation	Contractions of orgasmic platform Possible gushing of fluid
Resolution	Rapid loss of vasocongestion Decreased size of penis Decreased size of testes Descent of testes into scrotum Refractory period	Return of clitoris to normal size and position Decreased size of orgasmic platform Relaxation of vagina No refractory period

Adapted from Masters, W. H., & Johnson, V. E. (1966). *Human sexual response.* Boston: Little Brown.

increase in size of the testes by about 50% more than their nonstimulated size (Woods, 1984). A couple of drops of fluid appear at the urethral meatus. This fluid is produced from the Cowper's glands, and contributes to lubrication. In addition to mucoid-producing lubrication, this fluid may contain some active spermatozoa. The man may experience nipple erection, and a sex flush, characterized by a maculo-papular rash over the epigastric area, may appear during the latter part of the plateau phase. The plateau phase also consists of an increase in voluntary and involuntary muscle contraction, hyperventilation, increased heart rate, and elevated blood pressure.

Orgasm. Orgasm is the climax of the plateau phase, and consists of expulsive contractions of the entire length of the urethra. The initial three or four contractions are the strongest, and they subsequently decrease. Concurrently, the force of ejaculation is greatest with the first several contractions and decreases thereafter. Ejaculation can be viewed as composed of two stages (Woods, 1984). The first stage consists of expulsion of seminal fluid substrate from the seminal vesicles into the prostatic urethra. The second stage consists of expulsion of the seminal fluid from the prostatic urethra to the urethral meatus.

Resolution. The fourth and final phase, resolution, occurs immediately after orgasm and consists of an initial rapid loss of vasocongestion with an accompanying decrease in the size of the penis. The scrotum becomes less congested, and the testes descend back into the scrotum

and decrease to their preexcitement size. Disappearance of the sex flush and of nipple erection, if they occurred, is apparent.

Men experience an obligatory refractory period, during which they are unable to be restimulated to erection. The length of this period varies individually.

Female Sexual Response. Although they found only one response pattern in men, Masters and Johnson (1966) found some variability in the patterns of sexual response among women. Some women experience a plateau phase with several peaks, without actually experiencing orgasm. Others experience a definite orgasm, and still others experience multiple orgasms. Masters and Johnson believe that many other patterns in addition to these three exist in women's sexual response.

Excitement. The excitement phase in women consists of enlargement of the clitoris and vaginal lubrication occurring in response to vasocongestion. The vaginal space expands in the inner one-third portion, and the uterus may become elevated. The vaginal orifice opens as the labia majora and minora either separate or move away slightly. The woman may also experience nipple erection and enlarging of the breasts. She may experience a sex flush, similar to that described earlier for men.

Plateau. The plateau phase involves retraction of the clitoris under the clitoral hood. The labia minora increase in size as a result of vasocongestion, and the vagina itself expands in width and depth. Full elevation of the uterus with concurrent rising of the cervix occurs. Nipple erection may continue, and the sex flush, if it has occurred, may spread. There is an increase in both voluntary and involuntary muscle contraction, and hyperventilation, increased heart rate, and increased blood pressure occur.

Orgasm. The orgasmic platform, or the outer third of the vagina and the labia minora, is the location of primary response during the orgasmic phase. Contractions occur very quickly and strongly in this area during orgasm. After the initial three to six contractions, the intensity and frequency of the contractions decrease. The woman experiences an increased respiratory rate, increased heart rate, and increased blood pressure. Controversy exists as to whether women experience an expulsion of fluid during orgasm. Some research reports that women have described feeling that there was a gushing of fluid along with orgasm (Belzer, 1981).

Resolution. The resolution phase includes a return of the clitoris to normal size and position. Vasocongestion dissipates, with resulting decrease in size of the orgasmic platform and relaxing of the vagina.

The woman does not have an obligatory refractory period and may experience multiple orgasms in a short period of time.

Normal Sexual Functional Pattern

People have a need to be loved (see Fig. 12-1). Sexuality involves much more; it also affects self-esteem, roles and relationships, values and beliefs, and coping. The World Health Organization (1975) has defined sexual well-being as the following three elements:

- A capacity to enjoy and control sexual behavior in accordance with a social and personal ethic
- Freedom from fear, shame, guilt, false beliefs, and other psychological factors inhibiting sexual response and impairing sexual relationships
- Freedom from organic disorder, disease, and deficiencies that interfere with sexual and reproductive functions.

Factors Affecting Sexuality

Human sexual response is highly variable and greatly influenced by many factors. These may include health management, roles and relationships, cognition and perception, culture, values and beliefs, self-concept, coping and stress tolerance, and previous experience. As described previously, not all people are involved in sexual relationships, but they still regard themselves as sexual beings.

Health Management. Managing one's health influences one's sexuality. Sleep, rest, adequate nutrition, and posi-

tive mental outlook all contribute to pleasure in one's sexual life.

Roles and Relationships. The quality of a person's relationship with a sexual partner has a strong influence on the quality of the sexual relationship. Love and trust may be key factors in facilitating one's comfort with sexuality and sexual relations with the person with whom one shares mutual love and trust. The experience of a sexual relationship is often greatly influenced by the relationship one has with the person with whom one engages in sex.

Cognition and Perception. Psychological factors include such aspects as certain mental images being triggered in the mind, leading to sexual arousal. One's emotional state may have a great influence on one's sexual response. For example, someone who is depressed may be less sexually arousable or less concerned with sex overall than someone who is not depressed.

In addition, one's knowledge or lack of knowledge regarding sexuality will influence sexual functioning; misper-

---

Nursing Research

Selected Nursing Research Studies

De Santis, L. (1987). Parental attitudes toward adolescent sexuality: transcultural perspectives. *Nurse Practitioner, 12*(8), 43–48.

Taylor, M. E. (1985). Qualitative and quantitative strategies for exploring the progress of sex education for the handicapped. *Health Education, 16*(3), 16–19.

Webb, C. (1988). A study of nurses' knowledge and attitudes about sexuality in health care. *International Journal of Nursing Studies, 25*(3), 235–244.

Yarber, W. L. (1986). The relationship between the sexual attitude of parents and their college daughters' or sons' sexual attitudes and sexual behavior. *Journal of School Health, 56*(2), 68–72.

Possible Topics for Nursing Inquiry

- What are cultural indicators of sexual activity among adolescents?
- How does the sexual health concept of a specific ethnic group affect compliance with treatment programs?
- What factors have a relationship with access to sexual health information and education?

ceptions about sexuality often adversely affect one's sexual functioning.

Culture, Values, and Beliefs. Cultural factors include society's predominant views of sexuality, with those views comprising the social context within which persons experience sexuality. Values and morals also have a great impact on one's sexuality. Subscribing to particular values related to sexuality, such as whether or not one condones sex outside of marriage, will have direct relationship to one's own sexuality. Religious beliefs may affect a person's views of contraception, abortion, and sex education.

Self-Concept. One's view of self has a direct impact on one's sexuality. A person who feels decreased self-esteem and lacks confidence in himself or herself may experience a negative effect on his or her sexual functioning. The person may have a decreased sexual drive or, conversely, may attempt to compensate for this negative self-concept by overemphasizing involvement in sexual relations.

Coping and Stress Tolerance. A person's level of tolerance for stressful situations and ways of coping with these situations influence self-concept, and, in turn, influence sexual functioning. As noted in the paragraph above, one's sexual functioning is affected by one's self-concept.

Previous Experience. Previous experience with sexuality or ideas about sexuality influences one's current sexual functioning. For example, a woman who has been sexually abused in the past will, most likely, have repercussions from that experience that negatively affect her current sexual functioning. A more subtle example is that of a man or woman who has grown up with many cultural taboos related to sexuality, and finds it difficult later on to engage in a healthy sexual relationship.

Lifespan Considerations

Mims and Swenson (1980) have outlined the stages of the life cycle with reference to sexuality, and Woods and Stamer (1984) have recently adapted their work. This section is based largely on the work of Mims and Swenson, and Woods and Stamer. It examines sexuality at each developmental stage of life, emphasizing physiologic, emotional, and social aspects of sexuality.

Prenatal

At fertilization, when the ovum and spermatozoon unite, the chromosomal formation is determined. The sperm carries either an X or a Y chromosome to combine with the X chromosome supplied by the ovum. An XX combination becomes a female and an XY combination becomes a male, at about the fifth or sixth week of prenatal life. Hormonal influences play an important part in determin-

ing gonadal sex. In addition to the presence of an XY zygote, androgens must be present and cells must be sensitive to androgens in order for male genitalia to form. Lack of sensitivity to androgens, even in the presence of an XY genotype, will lead to development of female genitalia.

If genetic errors occur leading to ambiguous genitalia, parents will have difficulty assigning gender to their newborn. Under normal circumstances, parents automatically interact with their child according to the child's gender. Problems such as ambiguous genitalia, or lack of particular sex hormones may create serious problems for parents in relating to their child as male or female, and may create serious problems for the child as he or she grows up.

Newborn and Infant

It is particularly important for parents to touch and cuddle their newborn and infant. This is considered crucial for normal psychosexual development. The development of trust should occur in this period, paving the way for future healthy interpersonal relationships. Parents normally relate to their infants as either male or female, which has consequences for later development. Because infants are very sensitive to touch, it is common for them to explore their own bodies, often their own genitalia, and it is important for parents to recognize this as a normal developmental process.

Toddler and Preschooler

As a child becomes a toddler, learning to walk and gaining independence from parents, he or she begins to explore his or her body even more. The toddler begins to develop a concept of his or her own body, and sexual identity is part of this body image. The toddler may engage in masturbation, and parents need to be reassured that this is normal behavior, and, in fact, healthy for normal development.

As a child becomes preschool-age, he or she begins to engage in further exploration of the body. Playing with friends as well as exploring one's own body is normal. A child at this age will be curious about body parts, and may often ask questions related to such things as where babies come from, breast feeding, and physical differences between grown men and women and young boys and girls.

Child and Adolescent

During elementary school age, children continue to learn certain sex role behaviors and usually maintain friendships with same-sex friends. Children continue to learn about anatomy of their bodies, particularly their genitals, and continue to engage in masturbation, a normal and healthy activity. Mims and Swenson (1980) state that all children experiment with heterosexual and homosexual roles.

Adolescence is a turbulent time, after the relative calmness of the school-age stage of psychosexual development. The adolescent not only copes with development of identity and independence from parents, but concurrently experiences a surge of hormonal changes, leading to the physiologic changes of puberty. Tanner Stages, as shown in the display, clarify sexual development and help in assessment of adolescents.

A key point in the development of the adolescent girl is the beginning of menstruation. The first menstrual period is termed **menarche.** The accompanying development of breasts and of an adult female shape and proportions coincide with puberty. Adolescent girls become concerned with these physical changes, often equating them with acceptance, confidence, and popularity as well as with sexual identity.

Adolescent boys begin to experience such things as nocturnal emissions. The adolescent boy assumes a masculine sexual identity and behaviors based on role models and on personal expectations. At this age, boys are often competitive in all areas of life, and, particularly, in sexual activity.

The adolescent's engagement in sexual experimentation is not without consequences. Teenage pregnancy is an increasing problem. Sexually transmitted diseases and interpersonal relationship conflicts, as well as pregnancy, are common occurrences during adolescence.

Adult and Older Adult

The period of adulthood, between the tumultuous changes of adolescence and the later years during the climacteric, spans about 35 years. Many changes occur during this time, such as becoming involved in an adult intimate relationship, raising children, letting children go, and beginning to experience aging. Adults have the responsibility of educating their children about sexuality, and they have

---

Stages of Sexual Development (Tanner)

Male

Stage I
- Prepubertal state; no changes noted

Stage II
- Long, downy hair at base of penis
- Testes increase in size
- Circumference of penis increases
- Scrotal reddening and textural changes of skin
- No changes in tone or pitch of voice
- No axillary or facial hair present

Stage III
- Increased lengthening of penis
- Enlargement of testes
- Enlargement of scrotum
- Sparsely distributed pubic hair; darker, coarser, and curly
- Voice begins to change
- Axillary hair begins to appear
- Downy facial hair on upper lip

Stage IV
- Circumference of penis increases
- Facial hair on upper lip and chin becomes coarser
- Presence of perianal hair
- Presence of axillary hair
- Voice begins to deepen

Stage V
- Adult sex characteristics present

Female

Stage I
- Prepubertal; slight elevation of papillae of breasts

Stage II
- Sparse, downy long hair on labia
- Labia majora thicken
- Thickening of vaginal epithelium tissue
- Lowering of vaginal pH
- Breast tissue enlarges slightly; elevation around papillae, areolar diameter enlarges

Stage III
- Enlargement of uterus
- Vaginal pH drops
- Onset of menses
- Continued enlargement of breast and areola
- Appearance of coarse, curly pubic hair
- Labia enlarge
- Axillary hair begins to appear

Stage IV
- Uterus enlarges
- Ovulation occurs
- Axillary hair present
- Projection of papillae and areolae
- Pubic hair has adult appearance
- Vaginal discharge

Stage V
- Adult characteristics present

much influence in shaping their children's attitudes toward sexuality. Adults will often continue to grapple with their own struggles around sexuality and sexual behavior if they have not developed a high enough comfort level with their own sexuality. Many myths persist surrounding sexuality and sexual behavior; many stereotypes abound as people fear certain aspects of sexuality, such as homosexuality. Adults, therefore, often also need guidance from health-care professionals, as they struggle with their own conflicts regarding values and beliefs about sexuality.

During adulthood, many women and their mates experience pregnancy. Although this can also occur during adolescence, it is more predominant during adulthood. Pregnancy poses many developmental issues related to sexuality. In addition, it may pose sexual difficulties between partners, due to fear of sexual intercourse during pregnancy or contraindication of sexual intercourse due to high-risk conditions during pregnancy. For couples who wish to become pregnant but are unable to because of infertility problems, sexual issues may arise as well, caused by the need for them to have sexual intercourse according to a rigid schedule.

The **climacteric** refers to the period of time in which changes occur in the transition from middle age to old age. Although the term climacteric is usually used in relation to women as they experience menopause, Mims and Swenson (1980) use this term as a generic term to refer to the 15- to 20-year interval between middle age and old age. During this period both men and women experience changes that are significant in their lives and their sexuality. **Menopause** is the permanent cessation of menstrual activity. It normally occurs between the approximate ages of 40 and 55, but may be surgically induced.

Certain physiologic changes occur as a result of decreasing amounts of estrogen in women during the climacteric. Some women require estrogen replacement, which is controversial. Physiologic changes occur in men also. Specific effects can be noted in relation to the sexual response cycle as described by Masters, Johnson, and Kolodny (1988). During the excitement phase, women experience slower and decreased amounts of lubrication, while men experience slower erection and decrease in the firmness of erection. Women undergo a certain amount of atrophy, and thus the clitoris becomes smaller, and men may need more direct genital stimulation during the excitement phase. During the plateau phase, the vaginal canal does not increase in size as much as it did earlier, and the uterus does not become as elevated as it did previously. Men experience a decrease in the amount of Cowper's gland secretion, are able to maintain an erection longer before ejaculation, and have decreased testicular elevation. The orgasmic phase may become shortened for women and may not occur for men, as their need to ejaculate is decreased. Men also experience a decreased force and volume of the ejaculate. Men experience a longer refractory period, and both men and women experience more rapid return to nonengorgement of the genitals.

ALTERED SEXUAL FUNCTION

Certain conditions directly related to sexuality have a direct influence on a person's ability to engage in mutually satisfying sexual relations. Conditions other than those mentioned in this section also may have a direct impact on sexuality.

Potential for Altered Sexuality

Many factors can predispose a person to disruption of normal patterns of sexuality. Such factors are pregnancy, infertility, and abortion; alterations in gender identification; environment; illness; and surgery.

Pregnancy, Infertility, and Abortion. Pregnancy clearly alters sexual functioning. Although sexual intercourse is not contraindicated during a normal, low-risk pregnancy, sexual drive is often affected. It is common for women to have a decreased sexual drive during the first trimester, when they are fatigued and may feel nauseated. In addition, they may worry about miscarriage during the first trimester, and thus fear having sexual intercourse. During the second trimester, many women experience a surge of energy and a corresponding increase in sexual drive. The third trimester may again be a time of decreased sexual drive as the woman's abdomen grows, making it difficult to have sexual intercourse comfortably. It must be noted, however, that there is much variation in this pattern, and not all women respond in the same way. Men may also vary in their sexual desires. Some men find their pregnant wives sexually attractive, whereas others are apprehensive about having sexual relations with their pregnant wives for fear of harming their wives or the fetuses.

Infertility is often a stressor on a couple's sexual relationship. Infertile couples must have sex on a rigid schedule, according to when the woman is ovulating. Sex becomes programmed and loses its spontaneity. In addition, couples feel that they are having sex for a specific purpose rather than for enjoyment and mutual satisfaction. They often feel that they are being judged for how well they have sex, in that pregnancy will symbolize "successful" sex and lack of pregnancy will symbolize "failure." Many couples report that normal sexual relations resume after time has elapsed or infertility treatments are discontinued.

Women who have experienced unwanted pregnancies and subsequent abortions may feel apprehensive about having sexual intercourse. They may be fearful of having another unwanted pregnancy, they may not trust their contraceptive method, or they may continue to misuse or not use contraception while having sexual intercourse.

Alterations in Gender Identification. Alterations in gender identification may have either a small or a significant effect on one's sexual functioning. As mentioned earlier, some transsexuals marry and have children, and thus function in their socially prescribed sexual roles, while feeling trapped in those roles and experiencing much unhappiness. Other transsexuals do not function in socially prescribed roles.

Environment. Environment can have a large impact on one's sexual functioning. A hospitalized patient, particularly one undergoing long-term hospitalization, may find it inhibiting to have sexual relations with a partner or to masturbate within the confines of a hospital room. Lack of privacy becomes a major issue. The same is true for people in nursing homes.

Environment is a factor for people who are not hospitalized. Living in crowded conditions may preclude privacy. Fears about environmental pollutants affecting fertility may influence sexuality.

Illness. Illness poses a threat to normal sexual functioning. A person with cardiac problems may fear overexertion from engaging in sexual relations. Although this fear may not be based on physiologic principles, it can still be inhibiting to both sexual partners. A person with a sexually transmitted disease may fear transmitting the disease to a partner, or, conversely, a person may fear contracting a sexually transmitted disease from a partner. Although safer sex guidelines may be followed, this fear can often inhibit sexual relations.

Pain and disorders of the joints may make normal sexual intercourse uncomfortable. Disability caused by motor accidents has created a sizable population with spinal cord injuries (paraplegia and quadriplegia). People with any of these problems must find alternate methods of sexual functioning.

Medication. Some medications affect the ability to perform sexually. Ball (1985) discusses these medications according to the categories of approved social drugs (e.g., alcohol) and nonapproved social drugs (e.g., opiates, marijuana, sedative–hypnotics, cocaine and amphetamines, amyl nitrite, LSD, cantharides, and yohimbine). He also notes that many conventional therapeutic drugs may adversely affect sexual functioning. Such drugs are antihypertensives, antipsychotic tranquilizers, antidepressants, neurotransmitters, and hormones.

Surgery. Examples of surgical procedures that have an effect on sexuality are cesarean births, hysterectomy, and mastectomy. Women who have cesarean births may experience a longer recovery period than women who have vaginal births, and may feel less desire to resume sexual relations. A woman who has had a cesarean birth may also feel that she was a "failure" during the labor and birth process, even though this is an irrational thought. Such thoughts may affect her sexual functioning.

A woman who has had a hysterectomy may feel that her femininity has been adversely affected. Again, this is irrational in the sense that women with hysterectomies are certainly able to engage in sexual intercourse and have

orgasms, but the meaning of the hysterectomy to the woman may be so negative that it adversely affects her sexual functioning.

A woman who has had a mastectomy may also feel that her femininity has been adversely affected, particularly in a society in which the breasts are highly emphasized as sexual objects. A woman's view of herself may be negatively affected by having had a mastectomy, and this, in turn, will often negatively affect her sexual functioning.

Manifestations of Altered Sexuality

Alterations in normal patterns of sexuality can be seen in the following manifestations: sexual abuse, inhibited sexual desire, impotence, premature ejaculation, inability to ejaculate, organic dysfunction, dyspareunia, and vaginismus. The nurse can play a key role by assessing alterations in sexuality and assisting in prevention of problems as well as coping with problems that exist.

Sexual Abuse

Some people manifest altered sexual functioning by being sexually abusive to others, whether it be children, spouses, acquaintances, or unknown people. Seventy-five percent of sexual abusers of children are men. Sexual abuse results in sexual problems for the abused person as well.

Inhibited Sexual Desire

A lack of or inhibited sexual desire can be subjective. Since there is no "normal" for frequency of sexual relations, it is difficult to determine what frequency reflects a decreased or inhibited sexual desire. A key feature is that the person's partner is not satisfied with the frequency of sexual relations. Thus, the importance of role relationships is evident in discussing sexual dysfunctions. Often, inhibited sexual desire in one partner goes hand in hand with inhibited desire in the other partner, although it is more common for the desires of each partner to be incongruent, and hence it is viewed as a problem. Many factors contribute to inhibited sexual desire, among them physical factors such as taking certain medications, neurologic problems, hormonal imbalances, as well as psychological factors such as depression, and interpersonal difficulties. Sometimes it is quite difficult to determine whether depression is a result of inhibited sexual desire or if it is, in fact, a cause of inhibited sexual desire and consequent marital problems. In addition, a history of sexual abuse or incest, pain with intercourse, or vaginismus may be factors leading to inhibited sexual desire.

Impotence

Impotence, the inability to attain or maintain an erection long enough to have satisfactory sexual intercourse, is often troubling to a man. Most cultures highly value a man's "virility," and erectile dysfunction is a manifestation of his "failure to perform" as a man. Impotence can be primary or secondary. Primary impotence refers to a man who has never been able to achieve an erection necessary for intercourse; secondary impotence refers to a man who in the past has been successful in attaining and maintaining erection, but who has subsequently developed difficulty in this area.

Causes of impotence, whether primary or secondary, can be physiologic, psychological, or a combination. Certain manifestations may indicate the probability that the problem is secondary to a physiologic factor or a psychological factor. For example, if a man is able to attain erection in certain sexual situations but not others, or if he has erections during sleep or has experienced periods in which he had no erection difficulties, the problem is probably due to psychological factors. If erection is not possible in any of these situations, however, the problem is probably due to physical factors.

Ejaculatory Dysfunction

Premature Ejaculation. **Premature ejaculation** is a relatively recent phenomenon, according to Hogan (1985). This is not because the condition itself has only occurred recently, but because in the Victorian era, women predominantly viewed sex as something to endure; the sooner the sex act was over, the better. Today, however, with women desiring sexual satisfaction as well, it is often unacceptable if a man ejaculates early and does not allow for the woman to reach orgasm. Premature ejaculation is a relative definition, depending on the subjective responses of both partners, that is, whether or not both partners are satisfied. It is a condition in which the man is unable to maintain an erection long enough for satisfactory intercourse to occur. It is believed that premature ejaculation is caused by anxiety on the part of the man and fear of failure in the sex act.

Inability to Ejaculate. Inability to ejaculate actually refers to inability to ejaculate in the vagina. This condition is not as common as premature ejaculation. The cause of ejaculatory incompetence may be primary or secondary. Primary causes include psychological disturbances; secondary causes may be related to interpersonal problems with one's sexual partner, or organic causes such as lumbar sympathectomy or antiadrenergic drugs, such as guanethidine or methyldopa (Hogan, 1985).

Orgasmic Dysfunction

Difficulty achieving orgasm is common in women. Historically, orgasm was differentiated according to vaginal or clitoral orgasm, with vaginal orgasm considered to be the more mature, according to psychoanalytic thought. Masters and Johnson (1966) have found that this dichotomy is misleading, however, since orgasm occurs through vaginal or clitoral stimulation. In addition, it has been found that the Grafenberg spot, in the anterior portion of the vagina halfway between the vaginal opening and the cervix, is another area capable of stimulation to orgasm. Difficulty with attaining orgasm may be caused by lack of information, lack of adequate stimulation, or problems in an intimate relationship. Sometimes women feel pressure to have an orgasm to please their partners, and some partners feel pressure to "bring" their female partner to orgasm so that they will know they have been "successful" in the sex act. This kind of pressure may inhibit the woman's ability to attain an orgasm.

Dyspareunia

Dyspareunia, or painful intercourse, is thought to occur regularly in 1% to 2% of adult women (Masters, Johnson, & Kolodny, 1988). These researchers approximate that 15% of adult women occasionally experience pain with intercourse. Dyspareunia is commonly caused by organic problems including lack of adequate lubrication at the opening to the vagina or within the vaginal walls, usually due to inadequate sexual arousal, drugs (antihistamines, certain tranquilizers, marijuana, alcohol), or estrogen deficiency. In addition, vaginal infections may lead to painful penetration on intercourse. Barrier methods of contraception may be irritating to the vagina, causing painful intercourse. Pelvic diseases may also cause pain.

Vaginismus

Vaginismus is involuntary contraction of the muscles surrounding the vaginal orifice, such that penetration may be impossible and very painful. This is an uncommon condition, occurring in about 2% to 3% of women (Masters, Johnson, & Kolodny, 1988). There usually is no concurrent anatomic abnormality, and rarely is there a physiologic abnormality, although these must be ruled out. Generally, vaginismus is the result of psychological problems, namely fear of penetration due to a negative association with it, such as rape and sexual abuse, or fear of men or of sexual intercourse. The woman develops a conditioned reflex in certain situations (e.g., attempted sexual intercourse or during a pelvic examination) in which her vaginal muscles involuntarily contract, precluding penetration.

Impact of Sexual Dysfunction on Activities of Daily Living

Because sexuality is integral to one's life, any sexual dysfunction can have a major impact on activities of daily living. Emotionally, one may suffer from a decrease in self-esteem and in self-confidence, and interpersonal relationships may be affected. The consequences are that a person may have less emotional energy to concentrate on important aspects of daily living, or may be slow and careless in accomplishing daily, routine tasks. Physically, although a person may function normally, one's view of the physical self may be adversely affected.

ASSESSMENT

Functional assessment involves the nurse collecting subjective and objective data regarding normal sexual function, risk factors for sexual dysfunction, and any present sexual dysfunction(s). Such an assessment is made by asking direct questions, observing nonverbal behavior, and evaluating information obtained through physical assessment and diagnostic and laboratory tests.

The content of the history is also important, although the technique and approach influence the content obtained. Hogan (1985) includes a thorough outline of important content to elicit in a sexual history. This outline is reproduced as an example of necessary information (Table 48-2); however, it is essential to point out that not all patients need to be questioned on all areas in this outline. The nurse must assess which areas are appropriate for the individual patient with whom he or she is working.

Subjective Data

Subjective data are gathered through a careful nursing history. Although the data elicited in a sexual history are important, the approach used in eliciting the data is often equally, if not more, important. The process of interacting with a patient around his or her sexual concerns provides an excellent opportunity for the nurse to put the patient at ease, encourage the patient to ventilate any pent-up feelings, and listen actively to any concerns the patient may have. If a sexual history is approached in a humanistic, open manner, it can have therapeutic value as well as being a source for essential information. Nonverbal cues can be noticed as well.

The nurse should know the slang terms for sexual functions and organs (Hogan, 1980; Poorman, 1988). Some professionals believe that it is beneficial to use the patient's terminology to communicate better; however, others believe that professionals should use formal terminology so patients know that the professional is, indeed, a professional. What is clear is that professionals should be sure they understand what their patients are saying, patients need to understand what the professionals are saying, and professionals should clarify terminology with the patients if they are not sure they are communicating correctly.

A technique in interacting with patients is to ask less sensitive questions initially, gradually progressing to more sensitive areas. For example, initial questions such as "When did you begin menstruating?" are much less threatening than such questions as "What is your sexual orientation?" or "How satisfied are you with your sex life?"

Functional Pattern Identification

Specific questions regarding the patient's normal functional status will yield information about functional patterns. The nurse must approach the patient in an open manner, asking open-ended, nonjudgmental questions. Some examples are: "How often do you masturbate?" instead of saying, "Do you ever masturbate?" The first question allows the person permission to state that he or she masturbates, whereas the second question may suggest a more judgmental attitude to a "yes" answer.

Assessment of the patient's psychosocial status is part of the sexual history, but it is discussed separately to reinforce the importance of doing such an assessment. Often, assessing a problem with sexuality is highly subjective since it depends on the patient's perspective on the problem or potential problem. For example, an assessment of inadequate frequency of sexual relations is meaningless unless placed within the context of the patient's perceptions of what adequate frequency means to him or her. Psychosocial assessment includes the patient's perception(s) of his or her sexuality. In addition, it includes an assessment on the part of the health-care provider, based on data elicited, of the patient's psychosocial functioning. Outlook on life, social support, role relationships, and family functioning are all aspects of a psychosocial assessment.

Risk Identification

A careful history should reveal clues to the nurse about those patients at risk for altered sexual function.

Pregnancy, Infertility, and Abortion. Although pregnancy is generally a time of anticipation, that is not always the case. Unwanted pregnancies occur and can create many problems for the people involved. Although unwanted pregnancies are more common among adolescents, they can occur in adult years as well. In assessing the pregnant woman, the nurse needs to be careful not to let personal assumptions influence the assessment. The nurse should phrase questions to determine what the pregnancy means to this woman, how she feels about it, how her partner feels (if she has a partner), and what her plans are.

When a pregnancy is lost, either by miscarriage or voluntary termination, the nurse needs to assess the effect of the loss on the individual woman. In both voluntary and involuntary abortion, a sense of loss is generally present. Sensitive assessment will assist the patient and nurse in planning the type of support from which the patient can receive the greatest benefit.

The nurse should be particularly sensitive to the stress placed on infertile couples. Assessing the feelings of both spouses is essential; there may be guilt, self-blame, or other feelings that are present and affecting the situation. Inquiring about past illnesses, infections of the reproductive system, and previous non-term pregnancies may provide useful assessment and counseling information.

Alterations in Gender Identification. For patients experiencing alterations in gender identification, the nurse needs to be tactful and discerning in assessment. While the beginning nurse will not have many opportunities to work

TABLE 48–2

Data to Be Collected by Nursing History for All Patients/Clients

Data	Significance of Data	Nursing History Question
Age	Identifies period in life cycle.	In what year were you born; month, day?
Sex	Each sex may react differently to life events. Highlight gender identity problems.	[Usually is evident by dress, otherwise:] What sex do you consider yourself to be?
Education, occupation	Sexual practices may be related to education—socioeconomic class; change in occupation may contribute to role disturbances.	How far did you go in school? What do you do for a living? What change has there been in your ability to do your job?
Significant others	Other sources of support, stable or otherwise.	What persons do you consider most helpful right now? In what way? Are they available?
Quality of relationship with significant others	Relationship may be supportive, negative, or punitive, and these affect ability to cope with sexual problems.	Are there any differences in the way you get along with these people since you have been ill or hospitalized (or recently)?
Interests, hobbies	Indicates other support systems and avocational interests that contribute to self-esteem.	What do you do with your free time? What leisure and work activities are important to you? How are these being affected now?
Spiritual/religious/philosophical beliefs	Sexual practices may be related to beliefs. Guilt may occur if religious beliefs are compromised. Conflict and anxiety may be experienced by patient if different practices are suggested by nurse.	With what religious denomination are you affiliated? Can you describe any spiritual or other beliefs that are helpful to you now? Do you have or want the support of a clergyman (minister, priest, rabbi)?
Health problems, medical conditions, surgical procedures in past and anticipated in the future; medication therapy	Some medical problems, surgical treatment, or medications result in sexual dysfunction (physiologic changes). Anxiety over outcome or change in body image may lead to functional problems.	What illness and/or surgery have you had in the past? Did they affect your usual way of living or work? Did they affect sexual function? Do you expect this illness/hospitalization will have effects on your usual way of living or work? In what ways? What medications do you take?
Changes in role relationships and ability to carry out the usual sexual role	Change in ability to carry out what is perceived as the usual sexual role may cause anxiety, depression, and/or sexual dysfunction.	What difference has there been in your functioning in the family? Describe. Can you do your usual tasks or jobs? Describe. Have there been any changes in your relationship (with the way you get along) with others (male, female, significant others)?
Potential changes in ability to carry out usual sexual role	Expectations of problems may cause problems (self-fulfilling prophecy).	What changes do you expect after you get home (or in the future)?
Change in perception of self as male or female due to illness or life events	Anxiety and sexual dysfunction may result from threat to gender identity.	How do you expect this illness (or life event) to affect how you see yourself as a man/woman?
Existing or potential sexual dysfunction	Elicits problems (sexual dysfunction).	Has there been or do you expect to have any changes in sexual functioning (sex life) because of (illness, life events)? Describe.

Note: Wording of the questions is changed depending on educational level of the patient/client.
From Hogan, R. (1985). *Human sexuality: A nursing perspective* (2nd ed.) (pp. 162–163). New York: Appleton-Century-Crofts.

with these patients, it is useful to be aware of the assessment needs, including the patient's feelings about self, how others regard the patient, the treatments and medications, and other feelings that may be present in this situation.

Environment. Lack of privacy, especially that which occurs in acute and long-term care, is a concern. Sensitive assessment of the patient's response to the environment is essential. Since acute-care settings involve relatively short stays, long-term care settings are where the nurse will particularly encounter and need to assess the effect of the environment on sexuality. Assessing the need for privacy for the patient is a necessary part of nursing assessment in nursing homes and other long-term care settings.

Illness. Assessment of present illness, past illnesses, chronic conditions, and medications is an integral part of assessing sexuality. Illness may have created some constraints on sexual relations or on sexual performance. Attentive assessment by the nurse may reveal areas of previously unspoken concern that can be dealt with (Schover, 1988). Careful assessment may reveal misconceptions about the advisability of having sexual relations, as with patients with cardiac problems. Obtaining this information may assist the nurse and the patient in planning further assessment or counseling.

If the illness the patient is concerned about is a sexually transmitted disease, the nurse needs to do a diligent assessment of the person's feelings regarding the diagnosis, fears related to the consequences, and anxiety about future sexual relations. A nonjudgmental approach to assessment will support the patient in clarifying and focusing the aspects of greatest concern.

Surgery. Surgical procedures that relate to the reproductive organs often create sexual concern. Procedures such as prostate resection, mastectomy, and hysterectomy may initiate apprehension regarding sexuality, desire, disfigurement, and future sexual relations. Thoughtful questioning and listening as part of the assessment may alert the nurse to areas of anxiety as well as to misunderstandings.

Dysfunctional Identification

Dysfunctional patterns can be identified as those significantly different from the patient's or couple's normal patterns, such as difference in desires for frequency of sexual intercourse, lack of interest, or anger, which may indicate an underlying problem. If a problem is detected, an approach to discovering important data regarding that problem is suggested by Annon (1974), and includes eliciting information in several areas. These areas include a description of the current problem, the onset and course of the problem, the patient's perception of what has caused the problem and what prevents the problem from being alleviated, any past treatment and the outcome of that treatment, whether it was medical or professional or self-treat-

ment, and the patient's current expectations and goals of treatment.

Objective Data

Objective data consist of information elicited from physical examination and from diagnostic tests and procedures. This combination yields data important in the nurse's overall functional assessment.

Physical Assessment

A thorough physical examination is important. It should include a complete, systematic, head-to-toe examination, with specific focus on the genital organs or any infectious process that might be a result of sexual activity or might impair sexual activity. Privacy should be provided and careful draping used. Instruments should be warm. Gloves must be worn during physical examination of the genitals.

Physical examination includes inspection and palpation, as described in Chapter 18. The role of the nurse in examination of the genitals varies with nursing preparation and the type of health-care facility. The nurse may perform the assessment or assist another clinician.

Examination of Male Genitalia. The nurse helps the male patient into a position for examination of the penis, scrotum, and testicles. A side-lying position with the knees bent exposes the genitals for examination. Genitals are inspected and palpated. Distribution of hair in the area is observed.

Careful attention to any skin masses, lesions on the skin, discharge from the penis, or anal/rectal abnormalities is essential. Attention to absence or atrophy of the testicles and the presence of the foreskin or of circumcision is also important. The location of the urethra will indicate whether or not hypospadia exists; hypospadia is an abnormal congenital opening of the urethra on the undersurface of the penis rather than the center of the glans penis.

Male breasts are observed for deviations from normal. Although rare, breast cancer can occur in men.

Examination of Female Genitalia. The female patient is helped into the lithotomy position (see Fig. 20-2). The nurse ensures that the patient is comfortable. External genitalia are inspected for normal and abnormal characteristics, including hair distribution and development of the genitals.

A complete pelvic examination is necessary, and includes checking for pelvic masses, pelvic tenderness, vaginal discharge, other signs of infection, and vaginal or vulvar lesions. The pelvic examination is conducted in two parts: a speculum examination and bimanual palpation. The speculum examination views the vagina and cervix. The speculum is a two-bladed instrument that, after its insertion in the vagina, is expanded for viewing. It is helpful if the patient relaxes to minimize discomfort. The speculum should be warmed before insertion. Samples and smears for culture are taken while the speculum is in place. As the speculum is withdrawn, the clinician views the vaginal walls.

In bimanual palpation, the clinician places the index and middle fingers of one hand into the vagina, while placing the other hand on the lower abdomen. The cervix, ovaries, and uterus are palpated by this method.

A breast examination is included with the assessment of the reproductive organs. The breast examination is discussed in Chapter 18 and illustrated in Figure 18-18. The clinician checks for size, symmetry, contour, color, lesions, and nipple discharge. This is also a good time to teach the woman how to do a breast self-examination, which is discussed under "Interventions" in this chapter.

Diagnostic Tests and Procedures

In conjunction with the physical examination, certain diagnostic tests are often performed. Blood work to detect anemia or infection may routinely be ordered. Cultures to detect sexually transmitted diseases such as gonorrhea or chlamydia may be indicated. For women, a Pap smear would probably be done if one had not been done within the past 6 months to 1 year. Depending on the nature of the problem or potential problem, certain other tests may be performed at the discretion of the health-care provider. A summary of various diagnostic tests and procedures is given in Table 48-3.

NURSING DIAGNOSES AND PATIENT GOALS

The NANDA-approved nursing diagnoses in the area of sexuality are Sexual Dysfunction and Altered Sexuality Patterns. Also included in this pattern is Rape-Trauma Syndrome, although this diagnosis will not be discussed in this chapter because it is beyond the scope of the information presented here. The nurse uses data from the assessment of sexual function to determine the presence of or risk for any of these alterations in normal sexual functioning.

Diagnostic Statement: Sexual Dysfunction

Definition

Sexual Dysfunction is the state in which an individual experiences a change in sexual function that is viewed as unsatisfying, unrewarding, inadequate (NANDA, 1990).

Defining Characteristics

Verbalization of problem; alterations in achieving perceived sex role; actual or perceived limitation imposed by disease and/or therapy; conflicts involving values; alteration in achieving sexual satisfaction; inability to achieve desired satisfaction; seeking confirmation of desirability; alteration in relationship with significant other; change of interest in self and others (NANDA, 1990).

TABLE 48–3
Diagnostic Tests and Procedures of the Reproductive Systems

Test/Procedure	Description
VDRL (Venereal Disease Research Laboratories)	Blood test to detect syphilis ♀ ♂
Chlamydia culture	Cervical culture to detect chlamydia ♀ ♂
Gonorrhea culture	Cervical culture to detect gonorrhea ♀ ♂
Wet preparation (KOH—potassium hydroxide) (NS—normal saline)	Slide preparation from vaginal secretions to detect *Candida*, (*Monilia*), *Gardnerella*, *Trichomonas* ♀
Pap smear	Slide preparation from endocervical secretions to detect cellular changes in cervix, cervical cancer ♀

Related Factors

Biopsychosocial alteration of sexuality; ineffectual or absent role models; physical abuse; psychosocial abuse, e.g., harmful relationships; vulnerability; values conflict; lack of privacy; lack of significant other; altered body structure or function (pregnancy, recent childbirth, drugs, surgery, anomalies, disease process, trauma, radiation); misinformation or lack of knowledge (NANDA, 1990).

Diagnostic Statement: Altered Sexuality Patterns

Definition

Altered Sexuality Patterns is the state in which an individual expresses concern regarding his or her sexuality (NANDA, 1990).

Defining Characteristics

Major. Reported difficulties, limitations, or changes in sexual behaviors or activities (NANDA, 1990).

Related Factors

Knowledge/skill deficit about alternative responses to health-related transitions, altered body function or structure, illness or medical; lack of privacy; lack of significant other; ineffective or absent role models; conflicts with sexual orientation or variant preferences; fear of pregnancy or of acquiring a sexually transmitted disease; impaired relationship with a significant other (NANDA, 1990).

Related Nursing Diagnoses

Other diagnoses may be relevant to patients with sexual difficulties. Such diagnoses are Altered Family Processes, Rape-Trauma Syndrome, Altered Role Performance, Ineffective Individual or Family Coping, and Spiritual Distress.

Patient Goals

Goals for the patient or couple with sexual dysfunction should be individualized, depending on patient assessment. General goals for most patients include:

The patient/couple will recognize symptoms of sexual dysfunction.
The patient/couple will decrease symptoms of altered sexual functioning.
The patient/couple will express satisfaction with level of sexual functioning.

IMPLEMENTATION

The nurse plays a key role in assisting patients with any of the diagnoses listed above. The nurse functions independently, particularly in the areas of teaching and anticipatory guidance. At times, however, the nurse may need to refer patients to other health-care providers, for example if a major sexual dysfunction is noted.

Nursing Interventions to Promote Health and Function

Concerns about sexual issues may or may not be obvious to the nurse. Patients may enter the health-care system for a primary problem unrelated to sexuality. Nurses must put patients at ease, develop rapport, and allow patients to discuss any issues of concern. The nurse must be nonjudgmental, allowing patients to ventilate their feelings, concerns, and fears. Often, nurses can clear up misconceptions and dispel myths that may be interfering with an adult's sexual relationship or acceptance of his or her own sexuality.

Patient Teaching

Anticipatory guidance is a major role of the nurse. Nurses assist patients in anticipating outcomes and consequences, as well as helping them to devise plans to cope with or manage such outcomes and consequences (Fig. 48-4).

Self-Awareness. Nurses can assist people in becoming more aware of their bodies and how their bodies function. Exploring and understanding the body are essential in assisting both men and women to achieve healthy sexual

---

Selected Nursing Interventions for Common Sexuality Problems

Concerns about Sexuality

- Explore feelings and fears related to sexuality.
- Discuss the patient's expectations in regard to sexuality.
- Assist the patient in becoming more aware of own body.
- Teach self-examination techniques.
- Encourage sex education and responsible sex.
- Promote open communication between the patient and partner.
- Support appropriate counseling for the patient or partner.

relationships. Women need assistance in understanding their anatomy. The use of a mirror during a pelvic exam is one way of beginning this process; a second way is encouraging women to examine themselves with a mirror. Understanding the anatomy of their genitals may help women understand how their bodies respond to sexual stimulation and what helps them to achieve orgasm. Women need to understand what happens to their bodies during menstruation, pregnancy, and menopause.

Men also need assistance in becoming more aware of their bodies. Understanding their anatomy, and particularly what kind of stimulation causes them to have an

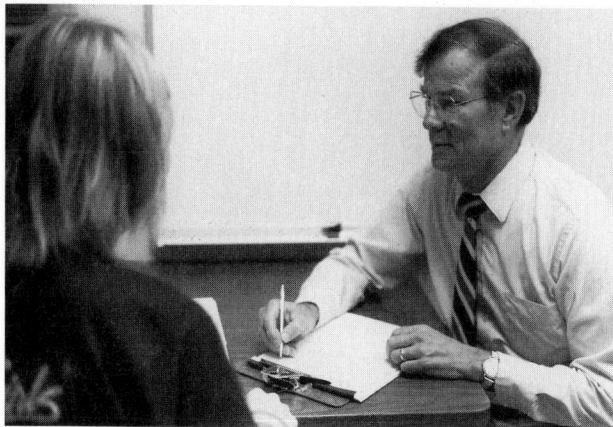

Figure 48–4.   School or clinic nurses help young people understand the consequences of their sexual activities. (Courtesy of Overlake Hospital Medical Center, Bellevue, WA.)

erection, will assist them in developing healthy sexual relationships.

Self-Examination. As part of developing awareness of their own bodies, men and women need assistance in learning techniques of self-examination. Men should be taught to perform testicular self-examination and women

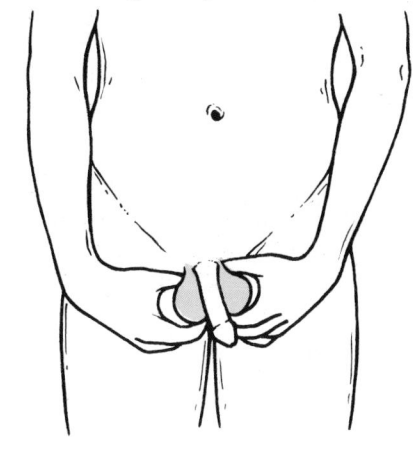
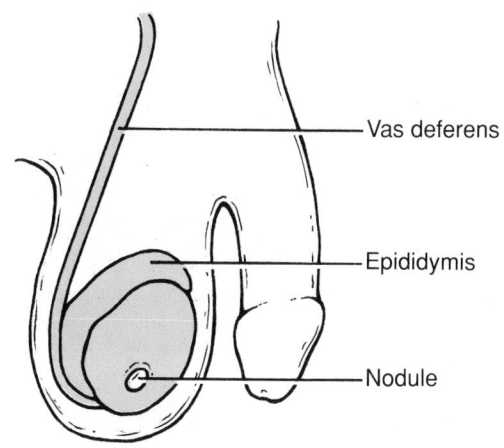

Why Do the Breast Self-Exam?

There are many good reasons for doing the breast self-exam (BSE) each month. One reason is that breast cancer is most easily treated and cured when it is found early. Another is that if you do BSE every month, it will increase your skill and confidence when doing the exam. When you get to know how your breasts normally feel, you will quickly be able to feel any change. Another reason is that it is easy to do.

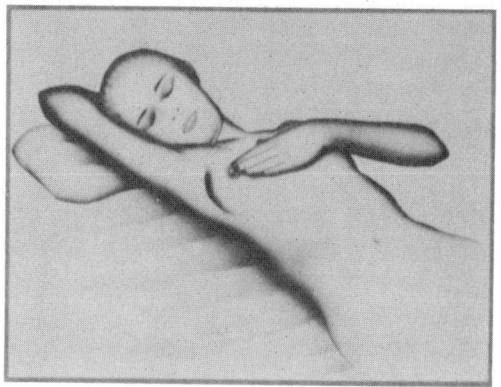

When To Do BSE

The best time to do BSE is about a week about your period, when breasts are not tender or swollen. If you do not have regular peiods or sometimes skip a month, do BSE on the same day every month.

Now, How To Do BSE

1. Lie down and put a pillow under your right shoulder. Place your right arm behind your head.
2. Use the finger pads of your three middle fingers on your left hand to feel for lumps or thickening. Your finger pads are the top third of each finger.
3. Press firmly enough to know how your breast feels. If you're not sure how hard to press, ask your health care provider, or try to copy the way your health care provider uses the finger pads during a breast exam. Learn what your breast feels like most of the time. A firm ridge in the lower cure of each breast is normal.
4. Move around the breast in a set way. You can choose either the circle (A), the up and down line (B), or the wedge (C). Do it the same way every time. It will help you to make sure that you've gone over the entire breast area, and to remember how your breast feels each month.
5. Now examine your left breast using right hand finger pads.
6. If you find any changes, see your doctor right away.

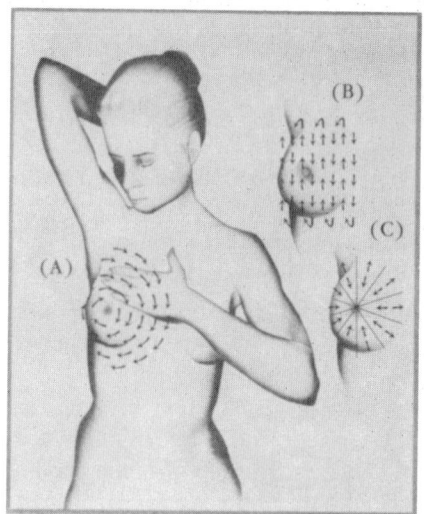

For Added Safety

You might want to check your breasts while standing in front of a mirror right after you do your BSE each month. See if there are any changes in the way your breasts look: dimpling of the skin, or changes in the nipple, redness or swelling. You might also want to do an extra BSE while you're in the shower. Your soapy hands will glide over the wet skin, making it easy to check how your breasts feel.

Remember: BSE could save your breast—and save your life. Most breast lumps are found by women themselves, but, in fact, most lumps in the breast are not cancer. Be safe, be sure.

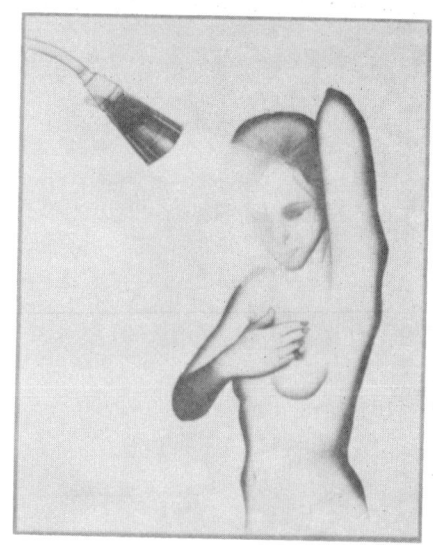

Reprinted by permission of the American Cancer Society, Inc.

to perform breast self-examination, as illustrated in the accompanying displays.

Kegel Exercises. Self-awareness for the woman also involves control of the muscle of the pelvic floor. The nurse can teach the simple steps necessary during assessment or in a teaching situation. The exercises involve contraction and release of the pubococcygeus muscle, which is contracted when one prevents urine flow or a bowel movement. Muscles always work better when they are in good shape. Muscle tone can be restored in about 6 weeks of regular practice of the Kegel exercises. Benefits of Kegel exercises are increased vaginal lubrication during sexual arousal, enhanced sexual excitement, stronger gripping of the base of the penis, more rapid postpartum recovery of the pelvic floor muscles, increased flexibility of episiotomy scars, and relief of constipation (May & Mahlmeister, 1990). Kegel exercises are also used in bladder training. Steps of the Kegel exercises are listed in the accompanying display.

Sex Education. Sex education needs to be encouraged by nurses. Although nurses work with patients on a one-to-one basis, it is also appropriate that they become involved at the community level. By supporting and encouraging sex education in the schools, nursing is taking a stance in support of educating people about their own bodies and sexuality.

Parents of preschool children need guidance in becoming comfortable answering questions, as well as in volunteering information that may not have been directly asked for by their child(ren). During adolescence, both the adolescent and the parents need guidance. Adolescents need reassurance that their confusing and conflicting feelings are often normal, and they need to be treated with patience as they vacillate between wanting to be taken care of and wanting to assert their independence. Parents need assistance in dealing with the mood swings and unpredictability of their adolescents. They need reassurance and support regarding their approach to their adolescent children. In addition, parents need help in maintaining their own intimate relationship with one another during a turbulent time, one that often points out their own aging as their children are growing older.

Responsible Sex. Teaching men and women to participate in responsible sex is important. Specifically, advising limiting the number of sexual partners and advising the use of condoms in a nonmonogamous relationship are very important.

If the nurse can present, in a nonjudgmental manner, the importance of limiting sexual contacts, he or she should do so. If such a discussion is going to defeat the purpose of the counseling or teaching session, however, the importance of hygiene and condom use must be stressed. Condoms should always be used in nonmonogamous relationships and male homosexual relationships, and in other relationships that have the potential for AIDS transmission. Much has been said in the media about "safe sex," and the nurse should build on this groundwork. Potential sexual partners need to be encouraged to talk openly with one another about how to have safer sex, and to be honest with one another about any history of sexually transmitted diseases.

As part of responsible sex teaching, the nurse teaches patients about the prevention of sexually transmitted diseases (STDs). Some STDs are easily treatable, whereas others are not (e.g., herpes, HIV/AIDS). At this time AIDS is considered incurable and ultimately fatal. Thus, the importance of teaching about prevention of STDs cannot be overemphasized.

Contraceptive Use

Decisions regarding family size and spacing are possible largely because of the variety of birth control methods available. Child spacing, limit of family size, and timing of the first birth are recognized as preventive health measures (May & Mahlmeister, 1990). Health measures must be addressed especially in the adolescent, because of the rise in adolescent pregnancy and births.

Men and women need to become aware of various contraceptive methods available to them. Patients may approach the nurse for information and counseling regarding family planning; therefore, the nurse needs a working knowledge of family planning and contraceptives. Some nurses may work in family planning clinics, where their

---

Kegel Exercises

1. Locate the muscles surrounding the vagina by sitting on the toilet and starting and stopping the flow of urine.
2. Test the baseline strength of the muscles by inserting a finger in the opening of the vagina and contracting the muscles.
3. Exercise A—Squeeze the muscles together and hold the squeeze for 3 seconds. Relax the muscles. Repeat.
4. Exercise B—Contract and relax the muscles as rapidly as possible 10 to 25 times. Repeat.
5. Exercise C—Imaging sitting in a pan of water and sucking water into the vagina. Hold for 3 seconds.
6. Exercise D—Push out as during a bowel movement, only with the vagina. Hold for 3 seconds.
7. Repeat exercises A, C, and D ten times each, and exercise B once. Repeat the entire series three times a day.

From May, K. L., Mahlmeister, L. R. (1990). *Comprehensive maternity nursing: Nursing process and the childbearing family* (2nd ed.) (p. 471). Philadelphia: J. B. Lippincott.

Contraceptive Methods

- Abstinence
- Coitus interruptus (withdrawal)
- Natural family planning
- Hormonal methods
- Intrauterine devices (IUDs)
- Mechanical barriers: diaphragm, cervical cap, vaginal sponge, condom
- Chemical barriers: foam, cream, jelly, suppositories
- Elective abortion
- Surgical sterilization

---

major responsibility is assistance in family planning and contraceptive methods. The adolescent may approach the school nurse for counseling.

It is the nurse's responsibility to be familiar with the various contraceptive methods: their advantages and disadvantages, contraindications, effectiveness, safety, and cost. The best method is the one the couple decides is most comfortable for them to use and will use consistently and correctly.

No perfect contraceptive method exists, but there are several good methods, each with advantages and disadvantages. It is beyond the scope of this text to discuss them in detail, but they are summarized in the following sections.

Natural Family Planning. Fertility awareness is used in natural family planning. Currently there are four methods available, all using some period of abstinence (periodic abstinence). The *calendar rhythm* method uses calculations of menstrual cycles and fertile and infertile periods. The *temperature* method uses the rise in basal body temperature (BBT) to determine ovulation. The *cervical mucus* method involves training the woman by a professional in the differentiation of dryness, moistness, and wetness at the vaginal introitus, and differentiation of types of mucus. The *sympto-thermal* method combines the other techniques. These methods are acceptable to couples who follow the tenets of certain religions. Disadvantages are that the methods require motivation, time, keeping consistent daily records, and abstinence for long periods of time. Miscalculations can occur in any of the methods, and they do not allow for spontaneous sex.

Hormonal Methods. Hormonal methods provide the most effective birth control (after surgery), and they are easy to use. They use estrogen and progestin in various combinations, and are introduced by various means into the female body. Oral contraceptives ("the pill") are the most commonly used, despite years of controversy about them. Mini-pills and postcoital pills are also used. Oral contraceptives and mini-pills are taken daily. Postcoital pills are used "the day after" coitus. After being used in Europe for years, a progestin implant was accepted and introduced to the United States in 1991. Capsules are inserted under the skin of the forearm, and are effective for 5 years. Hormonal methods allow for spontaneous sex and less stress and anxiety. There are side effects for these methods, and they can become expensive if used for a lengthy period of time. For those women taking daily pills, the need to remember to take each pill is critical to the success of the method.

Intrauterine Devices. Intrauterine devices (IUDs) are also controversial. Some IUDs were taken off the market in the 1970s and 1980s. Two remain: Progestasert and ParaGard (Copper T). In this contraceptive method, a small device is inserted in the uterine cavity, where it remains until removed by a health-care worker. The exact mechanics for contraception are not clearly understood. Women who use the IUD must be carefully screened, because there are a number of contraindications. Women who use the IUD must learn danger signals to report to their health-care worker. Infection and ectopic pregnancy are the major considerations.

Barrier Method. Chemical and mechanical barriers are popular with women who cannot or prefer not to use the pill or IUD. Barrier methods are readily available, and some can be bought over-the-counter. Mechanical barriers include diaphragms, cervical caps, vaginal sponges, and condoms. Diaphragms and cervical caps are prescribed and fitted by a professional; both fit over the cervix. The diaphragm must be used with spermicide. In both cases, the woman has to learn correct insertion methods and must plan ahead for sexual encounters, because the devices must be inserted before intercourse. Both seem to be highly effective. Their use may result in discomfort to one or both partners. Infection, including toxic shock syndrome, is among the side effects.

Vaginal sponges that incorporate spermicides may be purchased over the counter. The pillow-shaped sponge fits over the cervix and provides 24-hour protection. Risks seem to be small, although allergies and other side effects can result. The effectiveness is probably a little lower than the diaphragm's. The major form of male birth control is the condom, which ranks in popularity second only to the pill as a contraceptive method. Its importance in prevention of sexually transmitted diseases is an advantage of this method.

Foams, creams, jellies, and suppositories are chemical barriers. These vaginal spermicides act in two ways, blocking and killing sperm. Chemical barriers are bought without prescription and have few, if any side effects; that is their advantage. However, there is some question regarding possible harm to an already implanted embryo.

Elective Abortion. Elective abortion (therapeutic abortion) is considered by some to be a contraceptive method, although this remains controversial. There are several methods for performing an abortion. The rate of complications, such as infection, bleeding, and uterine or cervical trauma may be extremely high in illegal abortions.

Coitus Interruptus. Coitus interruptus, withdrawal of the penis just before ejaculation, has been used for centuries. Although no expense is involved in its use and there are no medical side effects, the effectiveness is not high because of difficulty in using the method.

Surgical Sterilization. Surgical sterilization may be done for both men and women. Female sterilization includes tubal ligation (cutting and tying of the fallopian tubes so ova cannot pass through) and tubal canterization (canterizing or burning the tubes so that ova cannot pass through). Vasectomy is the male form of surgical sterilization. Vasectomy involves cutting the vas deferens, preventing sperm from being ejaculated in the semen. Although both male and female sterilization are considered permanent, there is a slight chance of reversing each.

Nursing Interventions for Altered Function

A holistic approach addresses both physical and psychological issues related to sexual dysfunction. Each patient must be aided in living as full a life as possible, even in the presence of dysfunctions. This is accomplished through counseling and educating regarding a specific problem area, treating a specific problem if appropriate, promoting activities of daily living, referral to appropriate resources, and home management.

Levels of Activities of Daily Living

One of the nurse's responsibilities is to assist patients in achieving and maintaining a level of daily living that reaches their potential. Nurses can be instrumental in suggesting ways of improving patients' levels of activities of daily living despite their sexual dysfunction. For example, nurses play a key role in counseling older adults regarding sexuality and the fact that it is possible for older adults to maintain an active sex life. The nurse gives guidance on modifications, such as using lubricants to counteract the effect of decreased lubrication in women, and to engage in more foreplay to allow more stimulation of the man so that he can more easily have an erection. Also, older adults can be helped to discover alternative forms of sexual expression such as physical closeness and caressing, in addition to sexual intercourse (Fig. 48-5).

Counseling

When treating a person with a nursing diagnosis of Sexual Dysfunction, the nurse should direct his or her intervention toward educating and counseling the patient and his or her partner regarding various patterns of human sexual response. By talking with the patient and allowing the patient to describe and ventilate his or her feelings, the nurse will have a clearer sense of the patient's perspective on the sexual dysfunction. In this way, the nurse will discover what the dysfunction means to the patient

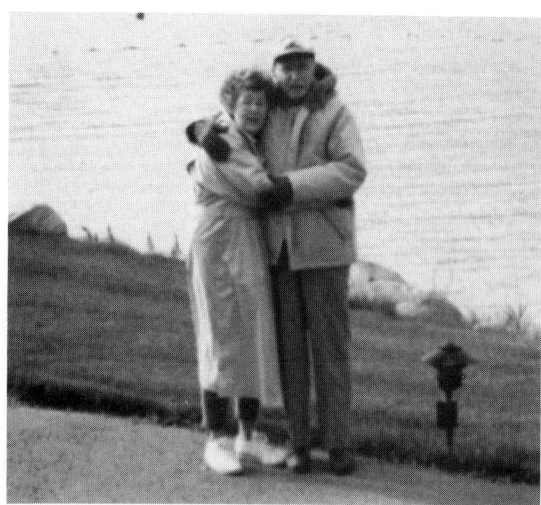

Figure 48–5.   Warmth, intimacy, and companionship are expressions of sexuality. (Photo courtesy of University of Washington School of Medicine.)

and how the patient is responding to it, enabling the nurse to develop interventions that are individualized for that patient.

The PLISSIT Model. One specific technique that nurses can use in working with patients with altered sexual functioning is the PLISSIT Model. The PLISSIT Model was developed by Annon (1974), and is based on learning principles. The acronym stands for the following: P = permission giving, LI = limited information, SS = specific suggestions, and IT = intensive therapy.

Using this approach, nurses begin with nonthreatening actions: permission giving and limited information. If the patient continues to need further therapy or has more serious problems, specific suggestions will be recommended, and, possibly, intensive therapy will be warranted. The belief is, according to this model, that many sexual problems are a result of lack of education, and, therefore, applying learning principles may help alleviate many sexual problems. Table 48-4 gives the principles of the PLISSIT model with examples of how it may be used.

Referral

Nurses may refer patients for further counseling if they deem that to be appropriate. In addition, nurses may refer patients to organizations that educate and provide support to people regarding sexuality.

Discharge Planning and Home Care

Much of the nurse's work with patients suffering from sexual dysfunction involves outpatient settings or, if patients are hospitalized, involves assisting patients in pre-

TABLE 48–4

Principles of the PLISSIT Model with Examples

Acronym	Definition	Example
P =	Permission giving (allowing patient to say what is on her/his mind without value judgments communicated by nurse.)	The patient says, "I need to practice birth control. Too many pregnancies are tiring me out physically and emotionally. But I'm not sure if birth control is right." The nurse may reply, "Some people practice birth control, while others choose not to. It is an individual choice."
LI =	Limited Information (giving/providing the patient with information, but not too much information that would be overwhelming.)	After further questions, the nurse says, "A variety of contraceptives exist, each having advantages and disadvantages. People choose contraceptives that are best for their personal situation."
SS =	Specific Suggestions (giving specific advice to the patient in an attempt to solve the patient's problems or alleviate concerns/worries.)	The nurse gives specific information regarding a variety of contraceptives: advantages, disadvantages, contraindications, side effects, effectiveness, cost, and procedures for each.
IT =	Intensive Therapy (providing more in-depth, perhaps long-term treatment, if problems are not solved with specific suggestions.)	If the patient has had several (planned or unplanned) abortions, she may need intensive, professional help related to using a specific contraceptive; dealing with grief, guilt, self-blame, or other emotional results; fitting for a specific method.

*The PLISSIT Model provides an organized approach to the patient, based on teaching-learning principles.

paring for discharge. Questions regarding sexual functioning are common as patients prepare to return home. Such questions may be common after birth, cesarean section, hysterectomy, or other surgery. The nurse should be prepared to give guidance in such sexual matters. Patients may be referred for group therapy in instances that seem appropriate.

Home visits by nurses may be appropriate to assess how well the patient is doing. Nurses can reinforce specific treatment protocols that may have been prescribed for patients. In addition, nurses can assess how well patients are after the treatment protocols, and can answer any questions that patients may have regarding the treatment. Most important, the nurse serves as a supportive person with whom the patient can develop a trusting relationship. When patients are being followed for sexual problems, many personal issues often are raised as well, and the supportive presence of the nurse is important for the patient's well-being.

EVALUATION

Specific outcome criteria are used to evaluate attainment of patient goals related to sexuality. Criteria may be different from criteria related to ordinary physiologic problems, in that the nurse can observe results in many physiologic problems, but in most instances relies on the patient/couple's verbal report of goal achievement in sexuality. Examples of possible outcome criteria for sexuality are listed here. Criteria may be similar because there is some overlap in goals.

Goal
The patient/couple will recognize symptoms of sexual dysfunction.

Possible Outcome Criteria
• Patient describes male and female reproductive anatomy following next teaching session with the nurse.

**Nursing Management Plan
The Patient with Sexual Dysfunction**

Nursing Diagnosis: Sexual dysfunction related to inability to conceive as manifested by altered sexual satisfaction.
Patient Goal: The patient/couple will restore normal sexual functioning.
Patient Outcome Criteria

- Patient/couple verbalizes increased satisfaction in sexual relationship within 3 months of treatment, as measured by their self-evaluation.
- Patient/couple verbalizes to health care provider that they are more relaxed and feeling better within 6 months.

Nursing Intervention	Scientific Rationale
1. Encourage patient and partner to discuss their current patterns of sexual behaviors, with acknowledgment by the nurse that the patient's complaints are understandable.	1. If the partners are able to discuss their current patterns of sexual behavior and these patterns are acknowledged by the nurse as normal, the couple may feel more relaxed and less concerned about their new sexual patterns.
2. Suggest possible ways for the couple to attain and maintain a close physical relationship even without sexual intercourse if they are uncomfortable with it.	2. If permission is given to have close physical contact without sexual intercourse, the couple may feel more relaxed and less pressured to have unspontaneous sexual intercourse.
3. Give couple permission to "take a vacation" from infertility at times in an effort to restore their previous sexual relationship.	3. Permission to take a vacation from infertility may help restore some spontaneity into their sexual relationship.

- Within 6 months, patient/couple describes normal sexual functioning to nurse, as learned in teaching session.
- Patient identifies specific symptom experiences, including etiology and treatment, as patient talks with nurse in next 6 months.

Goal
The patient will decrease symptoms of altered sexual functioning.

Possible Outcome Criteria
- Within 6 months, patient verbalizes to nurse that symptoms are decreasing.
* Within 1 year, patient and partner report satisfaction with sexual relationship.

Goal
The patient/couple will express satisfaction with level of sexual functioning.

Possible Outcome Criteria
- Within 6 months, patient states success in using alternate method for sexual functioning.
* Within 6 months, patient reports satisfaction with level of sexual functioning.
* Within 1 year, patient's partner reports satisfaction with level of sexual relationship.

Key Concepts

- Nurses require a valid understanding of the reproductive system, sexuality, and sexual orientation, because sexual health is a holistic approach to human health.
- Sexuality includes function of the sexual organs, individual perceptions of functioning, sexual expression, and preferences.
- Sexual activity is highly individual, with wide variation in expression.
- Reproduction depends on the establishment of the menstrual cycle in women and spermatozoa production and motility in men.
- Sexual orientation may be heterosexual, homosexual, or bisexual.
- Human sexuality appears in a variety of forms across the lifespan.
- Factors affecting normal sexual function include health maintenance; roles and relationships; cognition and perception; culture, values, and beliefs; self-concept; coping and stress tolerance; and previous experience.
- Sexual function may be altered by pregnancy, infertility, and abortion; altered gender identification; environment; illness; surgery; or medications.

■ Altered sexuality may be manifested by sexual abuse; inhibited sexual desire; impotence; ejaculatory dysfunction; orgasmic dysfunction; dyspareunia; or vaginismus.

■ Functional assessment by the nurse includes subjective and objective data regarding normal sexual function, risk factors, and sexual dysfunction.

■ The nurse functions independently in areas of teaching and anticipatory guidance, and refers patients with major sexual dysfunction to specialists.

■ Teaching includes self-awareness, self-examination, Kegel exercises, sex education in general, responsible (safe) sex, and contraceptive use.

■ Nursing interventions for altered function include guidance in increasing levels of activities of daily living, assuring privacy, counseling, and referral as necessary.

■ Discharge planning and home care include appropriate assessment and referral.

References

Annon, J. S. (1974). *The behavioral treatment of sexual problems, vol. 1: Brief therapy.* Honolulu: Enabling Systems, Inc.

Ball, W. D. (1985). Drugs that affect sexuality. In R. M. Hogan (Ed.), *Human sexuality: A nursing perspective* (2nd ed.). New York: Appleton-Century-Crofts.

Belzer, E. (1981). Orgasmic expulsions of women: A review and heuristic inquiry. *Journal of Sex Research, 17*(91), 1–12.

Hogan, R. (Ed.). (1985). *Human sexuality: A nursing perspective* (2nd ed.). New York: Appleton-Century-Crofts.

Masters, W., & Johnson, V. (1966). *Human sexual response.* Boston: Little, Brown & Company.

Masters, W., Johnson, V., & Kolodny, R. (1988). *Human sexuality* (3rd ed.). Boston: Little, Brown & Company.

May, K. A., & Mahlmeister, L. R. (1990). *Comprehensive maternity nursing* (2nd ed.). Philadelphia: J. B. Lippincott.

Mims, F. H., & Swenson, M. (1980). *Sexuality: A nursing perspective.* New York: McGraw-Hill.

NANDA (1990). *Taxonomy I revised 1990, with official nursing diagnoses.* St. Louis, MO: North American Nursing Diagnosis Association.

Poorman, S. C. (1988). *Human sexuality and the nursing process.* Norwalk, CT: Appleton and Lange.

Reeder, S. J., & Martin, L. L. (1987). *Maternity nursing: Family, newborn, and women's health care.* Philadelphia: J. B. Lippincott.

Schover, L. R. (1988). *Sexuality and chronic illness.* New York: Guilford Press.

Woods, N. F. (1984). Human sexuality: A holistic perspective. In N. F. Woods (Ed.), *Human sexuality in health and illness* (3rd ed.). St. Louis: C. V. Mosby.

Woods, N. F. (1987). Toward a holistic perspective of human sexuality: Alterations in sexual health and nursing diagnoses. *Holistic Nursing Practice, 1*(4), 1–11.

Woods, N. F., & Stamer, A. F. (1984). Sexuality throughout the life cycle: Prenatal life through adolescence. In N. F. Woods (Ed.), *Human sexuality in health and illness* (3rd ed.). St. Louis: C. V. Mosby.

World Health Organization (WHO). (1975). *Education and treatment in human sexuality: The training of health professionals.* Technical Report Series No. 572. Geneva: Author.

Bibliography

Benson, R. C. (1987). *Current obstetric and gynecologic diagnosis and treatment* (6th ed.). Los Altos, CA: Appleton-Lange.

Dirubbo, N. E. (1987). The condom barrier. *American Journal of Nursing, 87*(10), 52.

Speroff, L. (1987). Which birth control pill should be prescribed today? *Contemp OB/GYN, 29*(3), 102.

Yoos, L. (1987). Adolescent cognitive and contraceptive behaviors. *Pediatric Nursing, 13*(4), 247.

UNIT XVI
Values and Beliefs

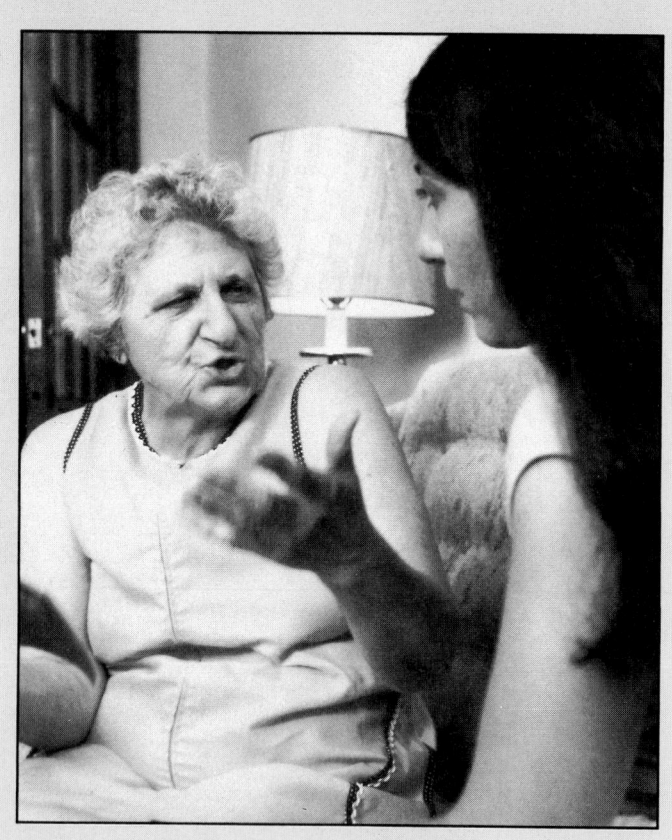

49 Spiritual Health

The values and beliefs area of human function includes those aspects of a person that guide his or her actions and choices. It is this function that governs what a person perceives as important in life.

Chapter 16, Values, discusses the principles and concepts related to values and values clarification. Chapter 49, Spiritual Health, builds on that foundation, exploring the concept of spiritual health. Spirituality encompasses more than just religious beliefs and practices, and meeting a patient's spiritual needs is the essence of providing holistic nursing care.

Using a nursing process format, this chapter provides a beginning discussion of assessment factors about a patient's spirituality. In this way, the nurse can adequately begin to understand and evaluate a patient's spirituality needs. Likewise, the chapter presents an introductory discussion of nursing interventions to promote health and function as well as those for the pateint with spiritual distress.

The content in this chapter focuses on spirituality from the perspective of meeting a pateint's needs for this area of function. By providing this emphasis, the nurse is truly able to incorporate holistic care into every facet of his or her patient encounters.

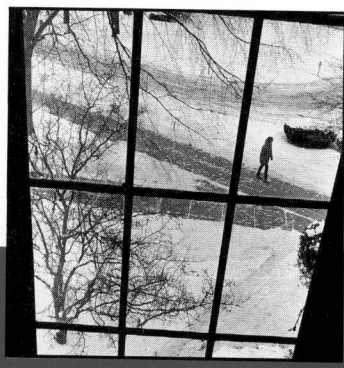

Spiritual Health

49

Normal Spiritual Function
  Characteristics of Normal Spirituality
    Holism
    Spiritual Need
    Spiritual Quest
    Spiritual Well-Being
  Normal Spiritual Functional Pattern
  Factors Affecting Normal Spiritual Expression
    Culture
    Gender
    Previous Experience
    Crisis
  Lifespan Considerations
Altered Spiritual Function
  Potential for Altered Spiritual Function
    Crisis and Change
    Separation from Spiritual Ties
    Moral Issues Regarding Therapy
    Inadequate or Inappropriate Care
  Manifestations of Altered Spiritual Function
    Verbalization of Distress
    Altered Behavior
  Impact of Spiritual Dysfunction on Activities of
    Daily Living
Assessment
  Subjective Data

    Functional Pattern Identification
    Dysfunctional Identification
  Objective Data
Nursing Diagnoses and Patient Goals
  Diagnostic Statement: Spiritual Distress (Distress
    of the Human Spirit)
    Definition
    Defining Characteristics
    Related Factors
  Related Nursing Diagnoses
  Patient Goals
Implementation
  Nursing Interventions to Promote Spiritual Health
    and Function
    Use of Self
    Spiritual Support
    Support of Spiritual Practices
  Nursing Interventions for Altered Spiritual
    Function
    Listening and Supporting
    Referral
    Age-Specific Interventions
  Discharge Planning and Home Care
Evaluation
Key Concepts

There are several kinds of healing. One of these involves the spiritual dimension. The nurse, working with any patient, has the opportunity to participate in that person's spiritual health by promoting spiritual well-being and providing the climate for spiritual healing. All people have a spiritual component that can be developed; however, the ways in which a person's spirituality is expressed depend on the person's family background, society, culture, and particular religion.

As the nurse begins to think about spiritual care, his or her own family background, culture, and religion become integral parts of the nurse–patient interaction. For this reason, the nurse must step back and examine his or her own spirituality, values, and beliefs. Often, this examination leads to reflection on some deeper philosophic questions such as: Who am I? Why am I here? What am I doing? Why am I doing it? How can I justify these things? Reflecting on these questions aids in developing one's personal philosophic base from which to think more clearly about nursing and health. For example, what one believes about the spiritual dimension, is reflected in the way one relates to people.

NORMAL SPIRITUAL FUNCTION

"The **spiritual dimension** is a quality that goes beyond religious affiliation, that strives for inspiration, reverence, awe, meaning and purpose, even for those who do not believe in any god. The spiritual dimension tries to be in harmony with the universe, strives for answers about the infinite, and comes into focus when the person faces emotional stress, physical illness, or death" (Murray & Zentner, 1985, pp. 474–475).

Although all people have this dimension within their being, not all have the same depth or intensity of it in their lives. The spirit or **spirituality** refers to the quality or essence that pervades, integrates, and transcends one's biopsychosocial nature.

Fromm (1968) commented on what it means to be human: "If man were satisfied to spend his life making a living, there would be no problem . . . [however] there is a sphere characteristic of man which one can call the trans-survival or trans-utilitarian sphere . . . He [man] is the only case of life being aware of itself (p. 68)."

Both Assagioli (1971), a psychotherapist, and Tillich (1969), a theologian, describe the human need for synthesis with the Supreme Being or Supreme Other. It appears that all humans have a spiritual dimension, the potential to strive toward unity and a higher consciousness in order to locate meaning and purpose in life.

Characteristics of Normal Spirituality

The major characteristics of normal spirituality include a sense of wholeness and harmony within one's self, with others, and with God, or one's Higher Power as one defines it. The person, according to his or her developmental level, experiences and projects personal security, a strong identity, and a sense of hope. However, this does not mean that the person is totally satisfied with life or has all the answers, for as one's life normally unfolds, there are many situations in which one may experience anxiety, helplessness, or confusion. During these times it is important that the nurse recognize that these experiences of difficult situations often generate spiritual questions, and that assisting a patient with the ensuing spiritual

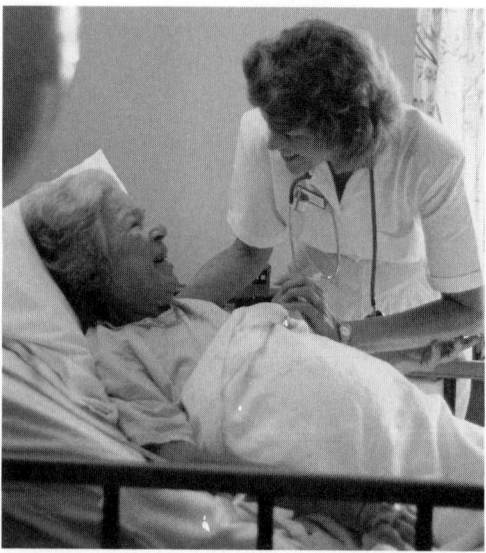

Figure 49–1. In spiritual care, the nurse addresses both the physical and spiritual needs of the patient. (Courtesy of Overlake Hospital Medical Center, Bellevue, WA.)

struggle is a valid and important aspect of maintaining health and giving health care.

Holism

Holism, as discussed in Chapter 11, was defined as the position of reviewing the universe as a system of harmonious interconnectedness rather than a sum of isolated parts. Holism not only integrates mind–body, but also emphasizes spirit. Brallier (1978) states that, "Holistic practitioners take the spiritual aspects seriously. They believe that man is more than a clump of well organized cells, that man has a spirit and that this spark of life energizes the body (p. 645)."

A holistic approach is grounded in the recognition that the spiritual struggle is a valid and important aspect of health and health care (Fig. 49-1). It is the integrating factor of "previously compartmentalized constructs of physical body, rational mind, emotional psyche, and intuitive spirit" (Ruffing-Rahal, 1984, p. 12).

Spiritual Need

Definitions of spiritual need vary depending on the belief system of the author. For example, a general definition is, "The fundamental spiritual need of any sick person is the need to find meaning in the apparently meaningless experience he is going through" (Penrose & Barrett, 1982, p. 38). In contrast, another definition states, "A spiritual need is the lack of any factor or factors necessary to establish and/or maintain a dynamic, personal relationship with God" (Fish & Shelly, 1982, p. 39). In summarizing the various definitions of spiritual need, it appears that a spiritual need represents a normal expression of a person's inner being that seeks meaning in all experience and a dynamic relationship with self, others, and to the supreme other as defined by the person.

Spiritual needs are derived through affective experiences of faith, hope, love, and positive experiences that serve as catalysts of synthesis and meaning. A composite list of spiritual needs so far identified in the literature includes trust, forgiveness, love and relatedness, faith, creativity and hope, meaning and purpose, and grace.

Spiritual Quest

Life may be looked on as a spiritual quest, not only to answer the philosophic questions given at the beginning of this chapter, but also to seek a higher level of consciousness or a deeper awareness of spiritual life. For example, the Twelve Step program of Alcoholics Anonymous identifies recovery as a spiritual journey; members of this group practice a spiritual discipline to live in a more meaningful way, day by day. Recovery begins "through a 'leap of faith' which says that there is no meaning to be found other than that which is beyond one's self; that which transcends man's ability to know—that which is God (Kreidler, 1984, p. 175). Chapman (1986) also includes the idea of search in defining optimal spiritual health. Spiritual health includes " . . . our ability to discover and articulate our own basic purpose in life, learn how to experience love, joy, peace and fulfillment . . . (p. 41)."

Spiritual Well-Being

Spiritual well-being is a condition marked by an affirmation of life, peace, harmony, and a sense of interconnectedness with God, self, community, and environment that nurtures and celebrates wholeness (Moberg, 1979). In the hierarchy of human needs, spiritual well-being appears to connote fulfillment of needs beyond the self-actualization level. For example, Hunglemann and co-workers' (1985) study of older adults also found that harmony and interconnectedness were the two major determinants of spiritual well-being with healthy, as well as with terminally ill patients. The subjects all expressed a belief in a Supreme Being, had some means of communication with that entity such as individual or group prayer and worship, and all also had an extensive social support system of ongoing, meaningful personal relationships.

Normal Spiritual Functional Pattern

Part of a person's spiritual functional pattern relates to his or her values, beliefs, and faith. Beliefs may range from atheism—the denial of the existence of God—to agnosticism—the belief that the reality of God is unknown and unknowable—or to theism—the belief that the reality of God is personal, without a body, perfect in all things, and creator and sustainer of the universe. For example, Christians, Jews, and Muslims are all theists, though each group further delineates distinctive beliefs about God's nature and activity (Richardson & Bowden, 1983). **Faith,** however, is more than belief; it is the way that beliefs are acted out in one's life. It involves "one's dynamic way of making meaning" (Fowler, 1981). It is the personal expression of living out one's spiritual dimension (Fig. 49-2). Thus, beliefs, faith, and values are interconnected, because what one sets one's heart on, believes in, or lives out is also what one values. Faith is central to the way the person makes meaning.

The expression of spirituality, often through a specific religious group, usually follows an established order of practices. These practices may range from simple meditation and relaxation to more formal worship, such as church services or rituals at shrines. Many observances take place within the home, in privacy or with the family. Some traditions involve special foods or ceremonies as part of the celebration of special holy days. These celebrations hold symbolic meaning and a sense of deep mystery or miracle to those who follow the religion.

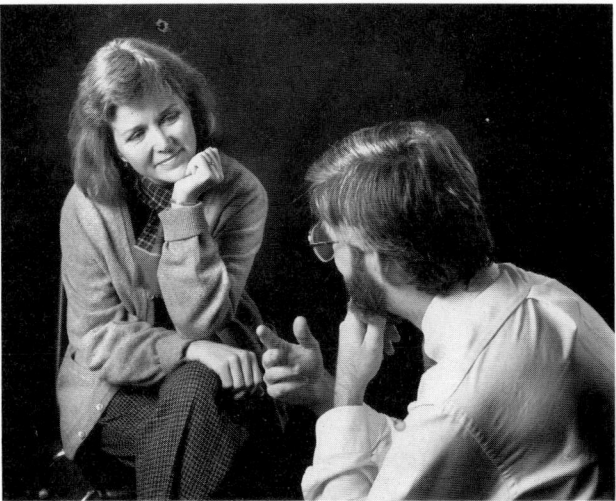

Figure 49–2.   One's spiritual dimension is lived out in one's belief, faith, and values. (Courtesy of Seattle Pacific University, Seattle, WA. Photo by Jon Warren.)

Some people may practice their form of spirituality daily, whereas others may formally observe only one or two holy days; still others may answer a "call" to full-time service in a specific religious group. Whatever the spiritual or religious beliefs the person holds and practices, these beliefs fulfill the following needs:

- Give meaning to life, illness, other crises, and death
- Contribute a sense of security for present and future
- Guide daily living habits
- Drive acceptance or rejection of other people
- Furnish psychosocial support within a group of like-minded people
- Provide strength in meeting life's crises
- Give healing strength and support

All the major religions of the world are found in the United States and Canada. The major groups include Christianity, Judaism, Hinduism, Buddhism, and Islam. These groups have many branches, which represent the occurrence of historical events. For example, when the ancient Roman Empire fell, the church was divided, becoming the Eastern Orthodox Church and the Roman Catholic Church. Still later, the Roman Catholic Church was split again, forming the Anglican Church or the Church of England, when King Henry VIII of England decided to rule the church himself in place of the Pope. During the Protestant Reformation, begun by a monk named Martin Luther, more Christian groups were formed, including such denominations as Lutheran, Presbyterian, and Methodist. Today, a fourth Protestant group, the Baptists, is the largest denomination in the United States. Judaism has three main branches: Reformed, Conservative, and Orthodox. Islam also has several branches in the United States. The newest form of Islam, the American Muslim Mission, sometimes called the Black Muslims, developed out of the West African slave trade.

Most religious groups have a spiritual leader. That person may range from a pastor, priest, or rabbi, educated in spiritual direction or pastoral counseling, to a shaman or spiritual healer, trained in ancient cultural traditions, as in such groups as Native Americans and many Southeast Asian groups. This leader is often the center of the spiritual or religious community, encouraging the group by leading in worship, teaching, and healing.

Factors Affecting Normal Spiritual Expression

There are a number of factors that affect the person's expression of spiritual needs. These include such things as culture, gender, and previous experience. Individual reactions vary, depending on personality style and past coping styles. Other contributing factors to spiritual health include: appropriate religious education, a firm spiritual identity, a dynamic and adaptable belief system, maintenance of belief systems in times of adversity or under questioning by others, recognition of spiritual assistance when needed, empathy for others' beliefs and values, and a sense of spiritual fulfillment (Houldin, Saltstein, & Ganley, 1987).

Culture. Attitudes, beliefs, and values arise out of one's sociocultural background. Usually, but not always, people follow the spiritual and religious traditions of the family. The child learns the importance of religious practices, including moral values, from the family's relationships and participation in religious forms. In an interfaith marriage, the child may follow the practices of one parent over the other. Some parents try to instill the strengths of both religions in their offspring.

Often, a person's religious preference is tied to the family's ethnic background. For example, many Italians are Roman Catholics, many Scandinavians are Lutherans, and many East Indians are Hindus. Whatever the religious tradition or belief system the person follows, however, the inner spiritual experience is uniquely personal.

Gender. One's spiritual expression also depends on the society's and religious group's beliefs and teachings about gender or expected behaviors in male and female roles. If one's religion has dietary laws, it probably is the woman's responsibility to see that the family follows the laws. A person's organized religion may also determine how each sex dresses, and whether one wears a head covering. In some cases, the spiritual leader is always male. Some mainline religions are now encouraging women to assume pastoral positions, however; this change rises from political processes, particularly the equal rights movement.

Previous Experience. Fowler (1981) and others observe that many people direct their lives based on values that have been appropriated more or less uncritically. If something disruptive occurs, the person's "meaning-in-life assumptions" are called into question. This is sometimes called a "test of faith." Thus, it would appear that if one's faith and values are confronted, then the deeper spiritual needs will arise. During a crisis period, past coping styles or learned ways of handling situations are likely to be in evidence. These coping patterns can be healthy and adaptive, or they can be maladaptive. Additionally, the life experiences in general are an influence. Such experiences may be related to age, but not necessarily.

Crisis. A crisis may strengthen a person's spirituality. This often happens when people face death, for example, as a soldier on a battlefield or a terminally ill patient. One study (Reed, 1986) has shown that terminally ill patients or those who have life-threatening medical diagnoses demonstrate that spirituality is potentially a very significant variable. When these patients confronted their own mortality, reliance on spiritual assets such as faith and prayer increased compared with nonterminally ill hospitalized patients or healthy, nonhospitalized people. The disorienting experience of being near death enabled members of this group to reorient their lives spiritually, and in one sense there was healing.

Lifespan Considerations

The expression of the spiritual dimension is also influenced by the person's level of growth and development. Fowler (1981), building on the theories of Erikson and Piaget, has formulated a theory of faith development as the person's integrating center of valuing. Fowler's theory does not address the content of a person's faith, such as a specific religious belief system, but looks at faith as another way of knowing the world, a spiritual knowing based on the particular phase of psychological and cognitive development. The stages of faith knowing have parallels with the stages of cognitive development of Piaget and psychosocial development of Erikson. Table 49-1 is adapted from *Stages of Faith* (Fowler, 1981). The following discussion integrates faith stage concepts with growth and development, and identifies spiritual needs arising from these stages.

Newborn and Infant

Trust in the caregiver is the basis not only for development of a sense of safety, security of self in the world, and interpersonal relationships, but is also the basis for faith development. Human beings' initial knowing of the world is through relationships; if basic trust needs are met by parents who themselves are secure and have a sense of meaning and commitment, infants will sense

TABLE 49–1

Stages of Human Development: Optimal Parallels

Eras (years)	Erikson	Piaget	Fowler
Infancy (0–1.5)	Trust (hope) Autonomy (will)	Sensorimotor	Undifferentiated Primal
Early childhood (2–6)	Initiative (purpose)	Intuitive/Preoperational	Intuitive Projective
Childhood (7–12)	Industry (competence)	Concrete Operational	Mythic-Literal Faith
Adolescence (13–21)	Identity (fidelity)	Formal Operational	Synthetic-Conventional
Young Adulthood (21–35)	Intimacy (love)		Individuative-Reflective Faith
Adulthood (35–60)	Generativity (care)		Conjunctive Faith
Maturity (60–)	Integrity (wisdom)		Universalizing Faith

Adapted from Fowler, J. (1981). *Stages of faith* (p. 52). New York: Harper and Row.

this kinesthetically and incorporate this feeling into their "innermost being." This sense of trust will later broaden and deepen into trust in the world, the universe, and a "higher power."

Toddler and Preschooler

The first stage of faith development is Intuitive–Projective, which is characterized by a continuing differentiation of self from others and an awakening of consciousness and memory. The introduction of language and gestures facilitates the ability to participate in some rituals of faith in the parents' religious belief systems. Children will respond to the routine of grace before meals, bedtime stories and prayers, special celebrations, and holy days if these are offered as a consistent, natural part of family life. The child also responds positively to those who treat their questions about the world, life, and death seriously. Although children do not know about such matters in a rational way, they intuitively sense the deeper spiritual questions of existence.

Child and Adolescent

In childhood, children notice the difference between themselves as individuals and others in like or in different groups. Belonging and acceptance in one's own group is very important for children, although they are still primarily oriented to the parents' authority. They continue to be sensitive to good–bad issues, often trying to "make-up" for wrongdoing in a concrete, literal way (Fowler, 1981).

Children at these ages can now think in a historical perspective, and see themselves as a part of their family tree. The use of "story" is a major strategy for bringing meaning to experience. It is a period when the lore, legends, language, and symbols of a particular religious group are best presented. Wishes, needs, facts, and fantasy may appear somewhat confused, but again, the child is attempting to make sense out of the world. This period is the Mythic–Literal period.

The major change in adolescence is the beginning of or the potential for the ability to think abstractly, conceptualize, and synthesize. Adolescents can ask more sophisticated, philosophic questions, testing the truth, evaluating others' behavior, and noting the incongruities. It is a time during which they develop their own personal style, based on their beliefs, attitudes, and values. Although the adolescent is individually involved in this personal synthesis of identity, it is carried out mainly in the peer group, where mutuality and interpersonal relationships have a major impact. This process is therefore both individualistic and conventional, insofar as it conforms to the peer group. Authority has moved away from the parents to the peer group. Thus, the name for this stage is Synthetic–Conventional.

Adult and Older Adult

In this stage, the Individuative–Reflective, the young adult is moving away from the conforming peer group and clarifying boundaries of selfhood and commitment. This shift away from the group is often precipitated by an encounter with people or groups other than those that supported the person in the previous stage. One's values, beliefs, and attitudes change as a result of interacting in a more pluralistic setting. Some of the situations precipitating this upheaval include experiences such as a new job, international travel, advanced study or education, or a new religious affiliation. In addition, this is intertwined with achievement of intimate relationships, choosing a career, and perhaps starting a family. The faith challenge during this stage is to establish one's own sense of faith and commitment based on personal experience and reflection on personal meaning in life (Fowler, 1981).

The middle years are fulfilled through productive activity—in Erikson's term, generativity. However, it is still a time of growth and renewed questioning, in some ways very similar to adolescence. This time the adult is not dealing with group conformity as much as with a broader world view. The older adult notices the polarities or extremes in life; these include such things as young and old, rich and poor, masculine and feminine, war and peace, constructive and destructive, and self-awareness and self-denial. These tensions, enhanced or precipitated by personal and environmental situations, demand integration and resolution; this is referred to as Conjunctive Faith (Fowler, 1981).

The final stage of faith, Universalizing, is seldom achieved by most people; usually only great leaders, such as Gandhi, Martin Luther King, and Mother Theresa appear to have reached this world view. One's social perspective expands to include everyone as God's children, and there is a more radical living out of one's vision of the earth community. Terms such as justice, love, and compassion describe the goals of this person.

ALTERED SPIRITUAL FUNCTION

Many factors can effect a change in a person's spiritual health and well-being; however, those life situations to which the person is personally connected are subjective. For example, one person's sense of meaning may be challenged by a job change, while another's may be influenced by a broken relationship.

Potential for Altered Spiritual Function

Crisis and Change. Just as crisis may strengthen one's faith, it may also deal it a blow. Many people do not consciously reflect on their personal philosophy of life. They live life as if it were going to continue forever. "Often it is not until the crisis, illness, aging, loss, limitation or suffering occurs that the illusion [or security] is shattered . . . Therefore, illness, suffering, aging, loss, and ultimately death, by their very nature, become spiritual experiences as well as physical and emotional experiences" (Grandstrom, 1985, p. 12).

Crisis may be related to pathophysiologic changes, the treatment required, or situations affecting the person. The diagnosis of an illness that may be debilitating, disfiguring, or terminal can lead to the person's questioning his or her personal belief system. Sudden trauma, miscarriage, or stillbirth may cause the person to doubt the presence of a Higher Being. The various treatments required for trauma and illness can lead to a sense of isolation or uncertainty. Many treatments generate additional problems, such as amputation, surgery, medication effects, dietary restrictions, and other procedures.

Personal changes resulting from death or illness of a loved one, opposition to personal religious beliefs by significant others, or change in personal status can become other sources of spiritual distress. Being hospitalized can interrupt the person's usual religious practices at a time when they are needed the most, thus adding to the patient's spiritual distress.

Separation from Spiritual Ties. The experience of being a patient in the hospital or a resident in a retirement or nursing home can be shattering initially. One is isolated, to some extent, from personal freedom, personal privileges, and social support systems. The person may be isolated in a private room without familiar surroundings, and may feel insecure. Daily living habits may be changed. The person may not be able to attend formal services, have the accoutrements of the faith, or receive the support of the familiar group. This separation from spiritual ties places the person at risk for altered spiritual function.

Moral Issues Regarding Therapy. For most of the major religions, the healer and the healing process are seen as parts of God's way of working in the world. However, certain religious groups object to some modern medical interventions. For example, Jehovah's Witnesses do not accept blood transfusions because of their belief in Old Testament teachings. Some Christians do not condone abortion because of their belief that the soul enters the body at conception. The Amish may refuse expensive treatment because the cost would impose a severe financial hardship on the community. There are many other medical procedures that may be affected by religious teachings, such as right-to-die decisions, organ transplants, circumcision, birth control, sterilization, autopsies, and handling of the deceased. Some groups, such as the Christian Scientists and the Amish, have been legally exempted from immunizations; however, many medical decisions are reviewed on a case-by-case basis, depending on the patient's age and the imminence of death. The choice to treat may be difficult to make if the religious beliefs say "no" and the health-care system says "yes." Many hospitals now have an ethics committee that can clarify and review such situations, so that more adequate and informed decisions can be made.

Inadequate or Inappropriate Care. Peterson (1985) states, "There are some pitfalls . . . to be avoided in providing spiritual care . . . The first is doing nothing . . . [and the second] is to jump in too quickly (p. 26)." Generally, when people become patients they depend on the nurse and the health-care team. Nurses attempt to overcome this inherent dependency by being a patient advocate, and by involving the patient as much as possible in mutual goal-setting and care-planning. However, the patient is a captive audience. Thus, either of the aforementioned positions may result in inadequate or inappropriate care.

There are several reasons why nurses may avoid spiritual care. These include insecurity in their own spiritual lives, assigning less value and importance to spiritual care, having little or no educational preparation in spiritual care, or believing that it is the clergy's territory. Grandstrom (1985) elaborates on these reasons when she identifies five fairly complex values issues between nurses and patients:

- Pluralism: nurses and clients embrace a wide spectrum of beliefs and creeds
- Fear: fear relating to not being able to handle situations, intruding on client's privacy, or becoming confused in one's own belief and value system
- Awareness of Own Spiritual Quest: what gives meaning, purpose, hope, and sense of love in one's own life
- Confusion: confusion over differences between religious and spiritual concepts
- Basic Attitudes: attitudes relative to illness, aging, and suffering

Mathai (1980) studied spirituality in relation to nurses' own coping strategies when dealing with suffering patients. She concluded that nurses who function in a spiritual vacuum feel frustrated, helpless, and anxious when caring for suffering patients. Since relief of suffering is a critical and essential goal in nursing, there is a clear need to help nurses face and work effectively with this situation. Kreidler (1984) states that, "nurses need reassurance that groping for meaning in suffering . . . [is] . . . a sign of strength . . . Our spiritual distress when facing suffering must be explored and understood if we are to be able to minister to our patients' needs (p. 174)." And again, Kreidler (1984) states, "Spiritual distress is met through the encouragement and preservation of life coupled with the belief that every human life does have meaning; that no one ever lives, suffers or dies in vain (p. 175)."

Thus, nurses need opportunities to reflect on their own philosophy and belief systems. Useful questions (Richardson & Noland, 1984) for this kind of reflection include:

What do I believe?
What gives meaning to my life?
How is my belief system working for me?
Is my behavior compatible with my belief system?
How does my belief system relate to my future?
Is there a relationship between my belief system and my health-care behavior?

Manifestations of Altered Spiritual Function

A variety of behaviors and expressions should alert the nurse that patients may be experiencing spiritual concerns. Table 49-2 is a compilation of several authors' categorizations regarding adaptive and maladaptive expressions of spiritual needs (Houldin, Saltstein, & Ganley, 1987; Highfield & Cason, 1983; Sundborg, 1985; Williams, 1971). The seven areas of spiritual need identi-

fied earlier are included. Although this list is seminal in its development, it may aid the nurse in examining potential spiritual distress. The distress may be manifested in the patient or may appear in the support person or family.

Verbalization of Distress

The person suffering spiritual dysfunction may verbalize that distress or express a need for help. The manifestation may be precise: "I feel guilty because I should have realized earlier he was having a heart attack." A person may state that he or she misses Sunday church services and the beautiful music of the choir, or may say, "I've never missed a service in 20 years." The manifestation may be more subjective, as in the case of the patient's rambling speech about life, death, and worth. A patient may ask the nurse to pray for him or her or to notify a spiritual leader of his or her illness.

Altered Behavior

A change in behavior may be a manifestation of spiritual dysfunction. A patient who is nervous about the outcome of a diagnostic test or who shows anger after hearing the results may be suffering from spiritual distress. Some people will become more introspective; they may reason out the situation and search for facts in available literature. Some will react emotionally and seek out information and support from friends and family. Still others may appear not to "hear," and show no outward signs of recognition of the problem, but it may surface in sleeplessness or lack of concentration. Guilt, fear, depression, and anxiety may indicate altered spiritual function. Table 49-2 gives other specifics.

Impact of Spiritual Dysfunction on Activities of Daily Living

In one sense, the activities of daily living may not appear to vary from patient to patient. All patients need some orientation and understanding of the structure of their day; however, the attitude and mood of patients toward their day influence their acceptance and expectation of care. Patients may go through the motions of daily living, but their involvement in living is changed. Their "spirit" level has changed. For example, if the patient is experiencing spiritual distress related to love and relatedness, he or she may refuse to cooperate with the health regimen or not ask for help. If the patient questions the pain or the meaning of illness, or expresses no reason to live, he or she may be expressing spiritual distress related to loss of meaning and hope. Thus, it is the process of daily living, rather than the actual tasks, that is influenced by spiritual distress.

TABLE 49–2

Adaptive and Maladaptive Expressions of Spiritual Needs

Needs	Signs of Maladaptive Behavior or Patterns	Signs of Adaptive Behavior or Patterns
Trust	Uncomfortableness with self-awareness Gullibility Inability to be open to others Feels that only certain people and certain places are safe Expects people to be unkind and undependable Wants needs met promptly, cannot trust to wait Lack of openness to God Fears God's intentions	Trust in self and own endurance Accepts that others will be able to meet needs Trust in life even if evidence is against it Acceptance of outcome of life Openness to God
Forgiveness	Feels illness is a punishment Feels God is judgmental Feels that forgiveness is qualified by behavior Is unable to accept self Either self-blaming or projecting of blame onto others Feels others are judging him Self-destructive behavior	Accepts self and others as fallible Nonjudgmental Views illness realistically Experiences self-forgiveness Offers to forgive others Accepts God's forgiveness Realistic perspective on the past
Love and Relatedness	Fears dependence Does not call on others for help Refuses to cooperate with health regimen Worries about separation from the rest of the family Self-rejecting or false pride and selfishness Inability to believe that self is lovable by God, lacks love relationship with God Dependent, magical relationship with God Feelings of distance and separation from God Expresses ambivalent feelings about God	Expresses feelings of being loved by other/ God Able to accept help Self-accepting Seeks the good of others
Faith	Lack of faith in a transcendent power/God Fear of death/life after death Senses isolation from faith community Bitterness, frustration, and anger with God Unclear values, beliefs and goals Values conflicts Lack of commitment	Dependency on divine wisdom/God Motivated for growth Expresses satisfaction with explanation of life after death Expresses need to enter into and/or understand larger drama of human history/ existence Expresses need for the symbolic, ritual Expresses need for sense of a shared faith/ community
Creativity and Hope	Expresses fear of loss of control Expresses boredom Lacks vision of possible alternatives Fearful of therapy Despairing Cannot help self or accept help Cannot enjoy anything Has put life/major decisions on hold	Asks for information about condition Talks about condition realistically Uses time during hospitalization/illness constructively Seeks ways for self-expression Finds comfort in inner self being rather than physical self or worldly criteria Expresses hope in the future Open to the possibility of peace
Meaning and Purpose	Expresses no reason to live Cannot find any meaning in suffering Questions the meaning of suffering Questions the purpose of illness Cannot form goals or has unattainable goals Abuses drugs/alcohol Jokes about life after death	Expresses contentment with life Expresses that life is lived in accordance with value system Accepts or uses suffering for self understanding Expresses meaning in life/death Expresses commitment and goal orientation Clearer sense of what is important
Grace	Anxious about the past/future	Alive in the moment/presencing

(continued)

TABLE 49–2
(continued)

Needs	Signs of Maladaptive Behavior or Patterns	Signs of Adaptive Behavior or Patterns
	Oriented towards achievement/production Focused on regrets/remorse Talks about doing better/trying harder Perfectionistic	Sense of blessing/abundance Sense of mercy given beyond self from God Sense of harmony/wholeness

Adapted from Highfield, M. F., & Cason, C. (1983). Spiritual needs of patients: Are they recognized? *Cancer Nursing, 3*(7), 188–189; Houldin, A., Salstein, S., & Gandy, K. (1987). *Nurisng diagnosis for wellness. Philadelphia: J. B. Lippincott Co.,* pp. 141–143; Sundborg, S. (1985, October 16). *From perfection to grace: Spirituality—being stuck . . . getting free* (talk). Seattle University, Seattle, WA.

ASSESSMENT

Stoll (1979) cautions that the timing of the spiritual assessment is important, and that it should come after the psychosocial assessment. Then, if the patient has some questions about this portion of the interview, the nurse can explain that one's spiritual beliefs are also an important part of maintaining health.

Subjective Data

Functional Pattern Identification

Several nurses have developed spiritual assessment tools. Stoll's (1979) "Guidelines for Spiritual Assessment" is probably the most widely recognized tool. Four areas are identified, and questions for each are suggested: (1) concept of God or Deity, (2) source of hope and strength, (3) religious practices and rituals, and (4) relationship between spiritual beliefs and state of health. Some of the questions include:

- Is religion or God significant to you?
- To whom do you turn when you need help?
- Do you feel your faith (religion) is helpful to you? If yes, tell me how.
- Has being sick (or what has happened to you) made any difference in your feeling about God or the practice of your faith?

Fish and Shelly (1978) also developed an assessment tool; the questions are similar to Stoll's, but the following represent some differences in focus:

- Why are you in the hospital?
- Has being ill affected your outlook in any way?
- Has your illness affected your relationship to the most significant person(s) in your life?
- Has being ill affected the way in which you view yourself?
- What is your greatest need at this time?

Tools have also been modified for various popula-

tions. For example, Still (1984) uses different questions to assess children's spiritual needs. Some of the questions include:

- How do you feel when you are in trouble?
- To whom do you turn when you are scared (in addition to your parents)?
- What are the favorite things you like to do when you are happy? When you are sad?
- Do you know who God is? What is He like?

An example for spiritual assessment accompanies this text.

In addition to the collection of data using assessment tools, other cues can be drawn from sensitive observation and listening. Other cues regarding children's spiritual needs might include the refusal to attend activities, preoccupation with another's situation or illness, reference to Sunday School, statements made in passing by the parents about God's will, and symbolic drawings (Shelly, 1982b).

In one sense, all patients who are suffering from ill health are at risk for spiritual distress. They may be physically separated from sources of spiritual help, such as a faith community where relationships are maintained and rituals of worship are performed. They may be emotionally separated as well, especially if they have not led a self-examined life. Even for those who have spiritual strengths, however, the time of illness and attendant crises bring on increased anxiety. Certainly those patients with critical or terminal illnesses, who are facing death or other profound physical changes, face ultimate, meaning-in-life questions. Westberg (1956) identifies nine situations indicative of a patient at spiritual risk:

- One who is lonely and has few, if any visitors
- One who expresses some apprehensions and fears
- One whose illness may have some connection with his or her emotions or religious attitudes
- One who is facing surgery
- One whose surgery or illness forces him or her to change his or her way of living

Spiritual Assessment

Patient Name _____ Date _____

Days in Treatment _____ Religious Preference _____

Marital Status _____   Children _____   Age _____

Part I. Spiritual Assessment Guide: In the beginning, share with the patient that people have several personal aspects, such as physiologic, emotional, and spiritual, and that this is an interview dealing with the spiritual needs. If the patient appears to be very uncomfortable, clarify his or her concern and listen.

1. Spiritual Ecology of Childhood
   A. Developmental History: Examples of some questions might be: Describe some early memories of how your family "kept" Sunday (or Saturday) or other Holy Days. How did you feel about yourself? your family? God? Eternity? Who taught you about spiritual things? Can you remember any religious symbols, hymns, stories that had an impact on you? How did these experiences change as you got older?
   B. Current religious practice: Do you participate in a religious organization? Do you pray or meditate, or participate in some spiritual exercise?
2. Awareness of the Spiritual: Patient's awareness of some universal power greater than him- or herself and his or her experience of that power. What do you think or feel about God? Is there an image or a song that expresses how you feel?
3. Meaning and Purpose: Patient's concept of the direction his or her life has taken, the present direction, and who is responsible for its direction. What meaning does your life have for you right now? When you're feeling down or discouraged, what gives life meaning?
4. Faith and Trust: Patient's ability to accept life's uncertainties and his or her willingness to trust and be trustworthy. How do you view the changes in your life? If you were to get a box labeled "Your Next Major Change," what would you do with it?
5. Forgiveness and Grace: Patients acceptance of others and self that allows him or her to confess and admit mistakes. What does the word "sin" mean to you?

6. Hope and Creativity: Patient's desire to make changes in life/lifestyle. When you think of the future, how does it make you feel?
7. Love and Relatedness: Patient's quality of relationships with family, friends, work associates, community, self, and God. How would you describe your relationship with people?
8. Crises and Peak Experiences: Patient's coping abilities and strengths. Have you ever had a time of crisis or suffering when you felt life had no meaning? What happened to you during these times? Did you feel the same or different after these experiences? Did you try to get help from any idea or person? Was there a spiritual thought or expression that was helpful to you during this time? Have you ever had moments of great joy or breakthrough? How has this affected you? Is there any spiritual image, music, or art that expresses your experience?

Part II. Closing: Since this interview will stimulate a lot of thoughts and feelings, be sure to offer some clarification and summary time. Is there anything we haven't discussed that you would like to add? Do you have any questions?

Adapted from Davis, M C. (1981). Another look at spiritual assessment: A behavior adaptation model currently in use in a chemical association. *45*, 19–26; and Leean, C. (1985). *Faith development in the adult life cycle*. Module 2 (Rev.). Prepared for the Religious Education Association of the United States and Canada.

- One who seems to be doing more than the average amount of thinking about the relationship of his or her religion to his or her health
- One whose pastor is unable to call on him or her, or who has no church affiliation and so would receive no pastoral care
- One whose illness has obvious social implications
- One whose illness is terminal

Dysfunctional Identification

The discovery of actual spiritual distress depends on the nurse's observation of the patient's responses, both verbal and nonverbal, to the nursing history interview. Patients need to be assisted in understanding that the nursing history is a review of their whole being, and that the questions will be wide-ranging, including not only physical and emotional health, but spiritual health as well. Patients who appear angry, anxious, depressed, or defensive when the spiritual questions are asked may need to hear something like, "I can see from your response that you might not have expected these questions; however, they do let you know that we are interested in how you are experiencing your current situation. Do you have a question or concern in this area?" Some patients may appear relieved to know that the spiritual aspect of their being is worthy of the nurse's concern. Still other patients may indicate that they have a spiritual concern, but that they will deal with it in their own time and way.

Identifying which spiritual need is lacking is related to the nurse's ability to "listen with a third ear." This means that the content or facts of the interview, in combination with the nonverbal behavior, evolve into a theme or a feeling tone such as distrust, judgment, isolation, or bitterness. These themes can then be linked with spiritual needs such as trust, forgiveness, love and relatedness, and faith.

Objective Data

There are objective data that can be helpful in assessing spiritual health; however, because of the qualities of the spiritual dimension, the nurse must verify the objective assessment with subjective information. Sometimes, in a patient reluctant to verbalize, the objective data are the only clues of a difficulty.

The nurse can glean much information about the patient from general appearance, facial expression, eye contact, body posture and movement, sleeplessness, anxiety, crying, and inappropriate humor or anger. Materials such as religious articles, books, cards, and pictures also indicate the spiritual dimension, as do visitors from the church or clergy.

NURSING DIAGNOSES AND PATIENT GOALS

Spiritual Distress is the nursing diagnosis used for acknowledging and identifying the spiritual dimension and needs of patients.

Diagnostic Statement: Spiritual Distress (Distress of the Human Spirit)

Definition

Spiritual Distress is disruption in the life principle that pervades a person's entire being and integrates and transcends one's biologic and psychosocial nature (NANDA, 1990).

Defining Characteristics

Expresses concern with meaning of life/death and/or belief systems;* anger toward God; questions meaning of suffering; verbalizes inner conflict about beliefs; verbalizes concern about relationship with deity; questions meaning of own existence; unable to participate in usual religious practices; seeks spiritual assistance; questions moral/ethical implications of therapeutic regimen; gal-

* Critical

Nursing Research

Selected Nursing Research Studies

Carson, V., et al. (1986). The effects of didactic teaching on spiritual attitudes. *Image, 18*(4), 161–164.

Dennis, P. M. (1991). Components of spiritual nursing care from the nurse's perspective. *Journal of Holistic Nursing, 9*(1), 27–41.

Sodestom, K. E., & Martinson, I. M. (1987). Patient's spiritual coping strategies: A study of nurse and patient perspectives. *Oncology Nursing Forum, 14*(2), 41–46.

Possible Topics for Nursing Inquiry

- What are spiritual needs?
- Do there need to be additional spiritual care nursing diagnoses?
- What are modalities for teaching spiritual caregiving?

lows humor; displacement of anger toward religious representatives; description of nightmares/sleep disturbances; alteration in behavior/mood evidenced by anger, crying, withdrawal, preoccupation, anxiety, hostility, apathy, and so forth (NANDA, 1990).

Related Factors

Separation from religious/cultural ties; challenged belief and value system, e.g., due to moral/ethical implications of therapy, due to intense suffering (NANDA, 1990).

Related Nursing Diagnoses

Because of the variety of causes, manifestations, and results of spiritual distress, other nursing diagnoses may be evident. Possible diagnoses include the following: Anxiety; Decisional Conflict; Ineffective Denial; Dysfunctional Grieving; Altered Family Processes; Fatigue; Fear; Hopelessness; Noncompliance; Parental Role Conflict; Personal Identity Disturbance; Powerlessness; Altered Role Performance; Self-Esteem Disturbance; Sleep Pattern Disturbance; and Social Isolation.

Patient Goals

The goals for the patient with spiritual distress should focus on providing an environment that supports the person's usual religious practices and beliefs. Goals need to be individualized, taking into consideration the patient's history, areas of risk, evidence of dysfunction, and related objective data. Examples of goals for the patient with spiritual distress include:

The patient will express acceptance of current life situation.
The patient will participate in spiritual practices that are personally supportive.

IMPLEMENTATION

Some of the qualities essential in implementing spiritual care are commitment to the nurse–patient relationship, good communication skills, trust, empathy, self-awareness, and an acceptance of a broad definition of spirituality. This is the qualitative aspect of providing spiritual care, and it largely depends on the individual nurse for assessing and meeting spiritual needs.

Although the qualitative aspects play a large part in performing nursing interventions, implementation also includes continuing data collection, maintaining current documentation, and collaborating with the health-care team. These steps are important because they ensure

---

Safety Alert

- Be aware of your patients' spiritual or religious beliefs.
- Be aware of any religious beliefs or practices that may be violated by various treatments and therapies.
- Be mindful of religious beliefs regarding diet or dietary restrictions. Such knowledge may prevent nutritional problems or spiritual distress.
- Be attentive to the patient's religious practices or preferences regarding death, especially if death is imminent.
- Be aware of significance of clothing, jewelry, and other apparel. Some clothing may have religious significance for the patient.
- Care needs to be taken in regard to removal or disposal of clothing.

---

consistency and continuity in patient care. Spiritual care is not one individual nurse's project.

The process should affirm the individual (Piepgras, 1984). If the nurse has been an effective communicator, then either facilitating the patient's use of his or her own spiritual resources or finding someone else to help the patient will more naturally evolve. The timing will not be forced, but will demonstrate sensitivity and empathy.

Nursing Interventions to Promote Spiritual Health and Function

Spiritual care can be defined as a mutual process that is a potentially healing or integrating experience in which the patient's spiritual needs are met. The word "potential" is inserted here, because Penrose and Barret (1982) state: "Ultimately, it is God (or the Supreme Being as one understands it) who fulfills spiritual needs; people are merely His channels to this end (p. 39)."

Use of Self

Spiritual care occurs in the context of the nurse–patient relationship. This relationship does not only consist of talking with patients; it is the purposeful use of self to help another person grow in his or her ability to face reality and discover potential solutions to problems. Spiritual care is a relationship that the nurse perceives as a valuable part of therapy and to which a commitment exists (Valliot, 1970).

Qualities such as trust and empathy are partially built on good communication skills and an understanding of the processes and phases of the nurse–patient relationship. For example, making oneself and one's time available to the patient is necessary to build trust in the initial phase of the relationship. Through active listening, the nurse can gain an understanding of the patient's perspective, and thus be more sensitive to a variety of needs, including spiritual needs. Without the establishment of trust and empathy in the first phase of the relationship, the nurse will not be able to discern the deeper concerns, such as meaning and purpose.

In discussing spiritual care of the elderly, Peterson (1985) states that "being" with the patient is a much more important aspect of spiritual care than "doing" (Fig. 49-3). "Sharing in people's lives is still one of the greatest privileges and responsibilities of nursing (p. 27)." This supports the idea of Burkhardt and Nagai-Jacobson (1985), who state "That the very definition of spiritual issues implies not answers, but the need to struggle with the questions . . . (p.193)" Thus, involvement in the meeting of spiritual needs is a very personal one for both the nurse and the patient.

Spiritual Support

Nurses also need to have a broad definition of spirituality so that they can be discerning with a variety of patients. Nurses cannot rely on their own spiritual traditions; they must also be knowledgeable about other spiritual expressions and other religious traditions that express these needs (Ozmon & Craver, 1981).

The expression of spiritual needs and the level or depth of spiritual care will vary with the patient. Therefore, the nurse needs to be sensitive to this variability and offer appropriate care.

Peck (1981) describes situations in which spiritual faith and belief are beyond the scope of scientific explanation, yet appear to be helpful. She states that the nurse should "do nothing to destroy a constructive faith already present . . . " The nurse should support and build on the patient's faith. If faith is removed the patient will lose hope, and without the will to live, one is frequently

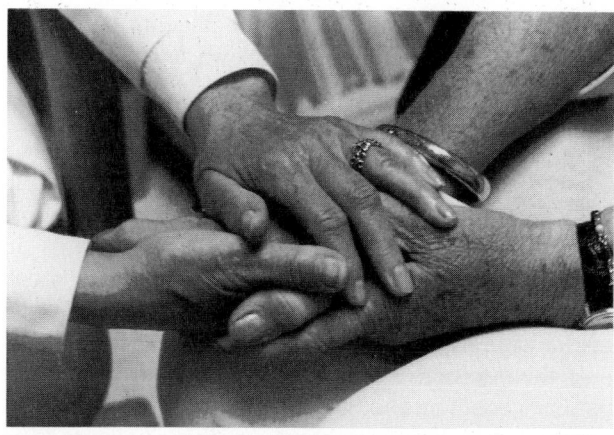

Figure 49–3.   Being with the patient when the patient needs someone is an important aspect of spiritual care. (Courtesy of Overlake Hospital Medical Center, Bellevue, WA.)

beyond the help of the most potent medical powers. Shelton (1981) offers a moderating statement by saying,

> . . . encouraging patients to elaborate on the emotional and spiritual aspects of their faith enhances their growth and personality integration. It is important, however, that these conversations not be judgmental or controversial. If patients feel accepted and affirmed in their religious beliefs, the possibility of their opening up other, perhaps more intimate, areas of concern is increased . . . (p. 58).

Piepgras (1984) gives the major principle in dealing with the ethical issue of personal witness in the nurse–patient relationship.

> Discussion should be confined to the patient's ideas, the patient's needs, and to whatever level of religious terminology and frame of reference the patient wishes to use. Personal witness by the nurse should be used, if at all, only after a common ground and easy dialogue have been established between the patient and the nurse (p. 2613).

Support of Spiritual Practices

During the assessment, the nurse should have obtained information regarding the patient's spiritual needs and religious preference. To facilitate the meeting of spiritual needs through specific religious practices, the nurse should also become familiar with the various religious groups within the community. Special religious considerations include beliefs about birth, death, sacraments, diet, holy days, and holy objects; a full description of these cannot be covered in this text. For example, dietary practices reflect dietary laws, such as no pork or beef, as well as celebration of holy days by fasting or feasting. If the food required is so specialized that the dietary de-

---

Patient Teaching

Instruct the patient as follows:

- Alert the nurse to preferences related to spiritual beliefs and customs, so that religious practices will not be interrupted.
- Ask the nurse to notify your religious leader or pastor, if you have one, so you can have all the spiritual support you need.
- Keep near you religious articles that may have significance or are a source of comfort.

partment cannot accommodate the patient's needs, the family may ask to bring in their own food. Table 49-3 gives a brief overview of the major religious groups' practices related to health.

Generally, it is the patient's right to be able to practice personal spiritual expressions in private, such as reading holy scriptures, praying, or meditating while in the hospital. The wearing of special amulets or garments on areas exposed to tests, treatments, or surgery may call for a special consultation with the family and spiritual leader rather than automatically removing them.

If the spiritual leader or healer plans to visit, the patient's room and religious articles should be readied appropriately. If the sacraments or other rituals are to be performed, the bedside stand or table may need to be cleared.

Nursing Interventions for Altered Spiritual Function

In considering the implementation of spiritual care, the nurse must prioritize emergent patient needs. For example, basic survival needs, such as maintaining an airway, take priority over growth needs that have to do with self-actualization. However, if the patient has found no meaning in suffering, is experiencing hopelessness, or is unable to take part in his or her faith community, the spiritual dimension can become a central need. The patient may have regained physical strength, but the spirit remains unfulfilled.

Listening and Supporting

The simplest definition of spiritual care is care (support, comfort, help) given that meets spiritual needs. Shelly (1982) summarizes spiritual care as follows:

Spiritual care is an integrating factor in health care. Respecting and encouraging a person's spiritual and religious interest and concerns enhances the healing process. Spiritual support includes communicating love, forgiveness, meaning, purpose, and hope in a time of discouragement and anxiety (p. 15).

Thus, active listening with empathy and sensitivity becomes one of the most valuable interventions for the nurse. Through purposeful listening, the nurse allows the patient to define personal spiritual questions and to direct the type of support that would be most useful at that point in time (Fig. 49-4).

The following situation, adapted from Frye and Long (1985), illustrates the intervention of listening and support as an integral part of spiritual caregiving.

Robert was a junior medical student. He is the son of a practicing physician and the eldest of four children. He is a handsome, popular, young man with a keen, satirical sense of humor.

On January 10, 1984, Robert was scheduled to be at his first family practice clinic. He never made it. Traffic was heavy on the freeway. He found himself in between a truck and a semi-trailer, with cars on either side. He swerved into an adjacent freeway lane, rear-ending a large truck. The impact propelled him off and under his motorcycle, resulting in instant unconsciousness. When he arrived at the emergency room, both pupils were fixed and the outlook was grim.

The next 5 months were a battle. Fluctuating intracranial pressures with complications, pervading depression, and thoughts of suicide haunted him.

Having deeply religious parents and a strong background in religious education, Robert

---

Selected Nursing Interventions for Common Spirituality Problems

Spiritual Distress

- Listen empathetically and sensitively.
- Encourage verbalization about faith and hope.
- Identity the patient's personal coping mechanisms.
- Arrange for opportunities for privacy to express spiritual beliefs.
- Assist with requested spiritual practices.
- Refer to appropriate resources for spiritual support.

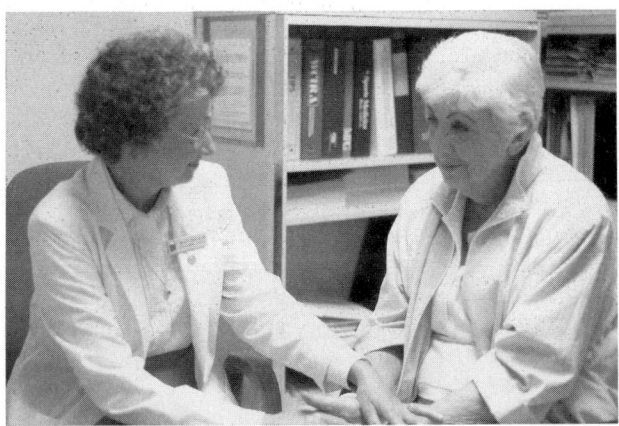

Figure 49–4. Listening and supporting is an important nursing intervention. (Courtesy of Overlake Hospital Medical Center, Bellevue, WA.)

TABLE 49–3

Practices of Major Religious Groups Related to Health

Religious Faiths	Dietary Rules	Birth Control and Abortion	Organ Transplants	Death and Dying
Observant Jews	Orthodox Jews observe Kosher dietary laws; Reform Jews usually do not observe dietary restrictions.	Orthodox Jews do not encourage birth control; abortion may be performed only to save mother's life.	Organ transplants generally not permitted by Orthodox or Reform Jews without rabbinical consent.	Advocate use of life support without heroic measures. Believe that family or friends should be with the dying patient. There are special procedures for care of the body after death.
Roman Catholics	Observe fasting and abstinence from meat on certain Holy Days. Hospitalized patients are excused from dietary obligations.	Birth control prohibited except for abstinence and natural family planning. Abortion is prohibited.	Organ donation and transplantation are acceptable.	Each Roman Catholic should have the anointing of the sick as well as the Eucharist and penance by a priest before death.
Mainline Protestants (e.g., Baptist, Nazarene, Lutheran, Methodist, Presbyterian, Episcopal)	Use of alcohol and tobacco is forbidden by many denominations. Episcopalians may observe fasting and abstinence from meat on some days.	Birth control is generally left as a matter of personal choice. Abortion is generally discouraged, but there may be some exceptions.	Organ donation and transplantation are acceptable.	Notification of clergy, Scripture reading, and prayer are appropriate.
Islam (Muslims)	Pork and alcohol are forbidden.	Contraception is permitted by Islamic law. Abortion is forbidden.	Donation of body parts or organs is generally not allowed. Vigilant attitude is required to avoid misuse.	Believe family should be with the dying patient so they can read the Koran and pray. There are special procedures for care of body after death. Men wash male bodies and women wash female bodies and perform a variety of other rituals.
Other Western Faiths				
Christian Science	Alcohol and tobacco are prohibited.	Personal choice.	Donations of organs unlikely.	A Christian Science practitioner may be called.
	Special Concerns: Normally do not seek medical care.			
Jehovah's Witnesses	Use of alcohol and tobacco discouraged.	Birth control is personal choice. Abortion is opposed.	Organ transplant is a personal decision but must be cleansed with a nonblood product.	No special practices.
	Special Concerns: Blood transfusions are not allowed.			
Church of Jesus Christ of Latter Day Saints (Mormons)	Abstinence from tobacco, alcohol, and caffeine-containing			Church elder should be notified.

(continued)

TABLE 49–3

(continued)

Religious Faiths	Dietary Rules	Birth Control and Abortion	Organ Transplants	Death and Dying
	beverages such as coffee, tea, cola.			

Special Concerns: A sacred undergarment must be worn at all times.

Religious Faiths	Dietary Rules	Birth Control and Abortion	Organ Transplants	Death and Dying
Seventh Day Adventists	Alcohol, tobacco, coffee and tea prohibited. Most members are vegetarians.	Personal choice.	Personal choice.	No special practices. Clergy may be notified.

Other Eastern Faiths

Religious Faiths	Dietary Rules	Birth Control and Abortion	Organ Transplants	Death and Dying
Hinduism represents a 5000-year tradition. It has many different beliefs and practices depending upon the culture and tribal unit. One of the medical traditions is the Ayurveda system. Illness and wellness are viewed as a state of balance. In this world view the human being is continuous with the environment.	Ranges from complete vegetarian to restrictions on certain foods, such as poultry and milk products. Traditional foods include many legumes, yogurt, and spices. There is also a belief system of "hot" and "cold" food, depending on how the body responds. Balancing tastes is also important, e.g., sour, bitter. In some places, to refuse food means that one is angry or hurt.	All of life is sacred, so generally not practiced; however, there is preference for male children and female infant sacrifices have been known. There may be some concern that amniocentesis could be used to preference males. Since India has a population problem, both birth control and abortion are permitted but not generally practiced. Abortion has been legal since 1972.	In the Hindu tradition, often ancient myths are reinterpreted to fit current circumstances. At present, there is no information available as to how this procedure is viewed; however, the wealthy may go to other countries for medical care.	There is a belief in reincarnation, so that life never ends. Untimely death is regarded with fear and sorrow. The family participates in mourning rituals both before and after mortal death. At death, some place the body on the floor or the earth, to facilitate the soul's journey. Cremation is the common practice; fire purifies the body, the family gives the ashes to the holy waters.

(continued)

seemed to have the spiritual strengths to deal with this crisis . . . until one day when the depth of his loneliness and doubt surfaced . . .

His nurse approached him, suspecting that he needed permission and acceptance of doubt of the validity of previous convictions. (There was) an outpouring of questions. Where was God when he needed Him? Why had God let him down?

Many conversations followed with Robert's mother, the nurses, doctor, therapists, and chaplain . . . Family, friends, and staff supported him in his questions . . . Robert identified with the story of Job and began to talk of his hope, too . . .

As part of this denial of his former convictions, Robert frequently requested pain medication during the day to help him sleep. He stated, "I just don't want to be awake." The nurse con-

fronted him, asking him if he was truly in pain or trying to escape from the realities of his situation . . . She recommended that they work together on a different approach.

Referral

The nurse should be comfortable in listening to the patient's spiritual needs and in hearing religious requests. If the patient or family members ask for prayer or scripture reading, and the nurse is comfortable in doing that, the nurse should identify the special focus or topic before he or she begins. When the patient and family appear to have no religious tradition, the nurse may ask to assist the patient or family in a quiet, reflective moment. The nurse may also respond to a request to see the hospital chaplain, or initiate a referral to see one. For an effective referral, it is helpful if the nurse has a working knowledge of the chaplaincy program and knows the

TABLE 49–3

(continued)

Religious Faiths	Dietary Rules	Birth Control and Abortion	Organ Transplants	Death and Dying
Buddhism began in the 6th Century B.C. in northeast India and expanded along trade routes to the South, Southeast Asia, China, and Japan and in the latter 19th century to the West. The medical system that was used is the Ayurveda system. The path of health is right living and thinking. There are many different Buddhist groups who follow different leaders.	Diet is an issue of balance, similar to Hindu beliefs. Alcohol and other drugs are forbidden because they can lead to moral carelessness. The laity may consume fairly heavily, however, and recent attempts at reform have not been taken seriously.	There is ambiguity about when life begins so there is no clear-cut view on abortion. They are against killing or injuring humans and animals. Both birth control and abortion have been known and practiced. The practice may not reflect the faith as much as current social and political policies.	At present there is no stated view about organ transplants. The principles guiding such decisions would include: "all is interdependent (family, donor, health care persons, society) and suffering." Personal communication from Ronald Nakasone, Ph.D., Institute of Buddhist Studies, Berkeley, CA)	Life is a temporary state as a combination of body/mental elements, thus death is temporary also; it is necessary for rebirth. Family needs to be present, certain prayers need to be said by the priest. The color white means death, so the use of white by health-care persons may cause increased anxiety for some patients/families. Priest visits family home every day for prayers until burial. Prayers are said at certain times and up to 1 year after death, and then every year.

Special Concerns: Most Buddhists have no hesitation about seeking medical advice from non-Buddhist physicians. Thus, some see medical interventions, such as organ transplants, as a technologic issue only.

Derived from Anles, P. (1989). Medicine and Living Tradition of Islam. In L. E. Sullivan (Ed.), *Healing and restoring, health and medicine in the world's religious traditions* (p. 189). New York: Macmillan; Carson, J. B. (1989). *Spiritual dimensions of nursing practice* (pp. 76–112). Philadelphia, W. B. Saunders; Desai, P. N. (1989). *Health and medicine in the Hindu tradition*. New York, Crossroad Publishing Company; Kitagawa, J. M. (1989). Buddhist Medical History. In L. E. Sullivan (Ed.), *Healing and restoring, health and medicine in the world's religious traditions* (pp. 9–32). New York: Macmillan.

chaplain(s) personally. The chaplain is also a resource for finding representatives for other religious groups as well.

Age-Specific Interventions

Nursing interventions need to be tailored to the stage of faith development of the individual patient.

Newborn and Infant. Hospitalization and illness potentially disrupt the infant's basic trust in parents. At this stage, it is the nurse's role to support the spiritual needs of the parents, which in turn will meet the needs of the infant. This can best be done by listening, offering support, and promoting stability in the family support system. To accomplish this, the parents must be encouraged to be present with the infant as much as possible and involved in the caring process (Betz, 1981; Shelly, 1982b).

Toddler and Preschooler. Carrying out established routines and responding to concrete questions are important considerations with the toddler and preschooler. The role of the nurse is to support the family in carrying out the rituals of faith. If the family is not available to do this, then it is helpful if the nurse can carry them out. For example, bedtime, often a difficult transition for children at this age, but especially so in the hospital, is a crucial time of the day to offer support (Betz, 1981, Shelly, 1982b).

Children in early childhood are also very sensitive to good–bad issues. They should not be told that painful or scary treatments are in any way a punishment, even though they might feel that. It should be affirmed that they are still loved by their parents, the nurse, and God or Jesus, or whatever is appropriate given the source of the family's faith (Shelly, 1982b).

Child and Adolescent. The nurse continues to be of

major support to the family unit, carrying out the familiar religious rituals in the health-care setting. It is also important that the nurse clarify fact and fantasy when it comes to all of the medical interventions and procedures (Betz, 1981; Shelly, 1982b). Often, a "story" about a similar situation will aid in this reality-orienting process. Generally, local libraries have a variety of books in which children experience going to the health clinic or the hospital. Again, it is imperative that the child not associate illness and hospitalization with wrongdoing and punishment, becoming in the process more anxious about themselves and fearful of their surroundings. Acceptance and clarification of the experiences are the effective modes in offering meaning to the child.

Development of a personal style and interaction with peers remain priorities even when the adolescent is ill. The nurse can be available to the adolescent's peers, involving them by encouraging them to remain available, either through visits, letters, or telephone. If a long-term illness, accident, or some other severe condition is involved, other networks of support might also be useful, such as the school or the church. For example, the youth group might make a commitment to be a communication link for the adolescent while he or she is in the hospital. It is also possible that the peers might need an opportunity to explore their own responses to illness and accidents in order to work through their feelings about life. The youth leaders or the hospital chaplain are resources for this kind of experience.

Adolescents are capable of conceptualizing a personal relationship with God (Betz 1981; Shelly 1982b). In a time of illness, they may question the meaning of the experience, trying to integrate it into their lives, much as many adults would do under similar circumstances. These issues can often be discerned during a nursing history and assessment. The nurse can either follow-up on the data or involve the hospital chaplain or the adolescent's spiritual counselor.

Adult and Older Adult. The young adult is clarifying personal beliefs and commitments based on experience and mentoring relationships. The faith challenge is to establish and reflect on personal faith and the meaning of life. Perhaps it is too much to expect that a nurse can perform a mentoring relationship with many patients. However, in some long-term relationships, being available to listen, support, and validate feelings and experiences would facilitate exploration of meaning-in-life or meaning-in-death experiences. At the very least, it is important for the nurse to understand that young adults have this need, and to be open to explore with the patient possibilities as to who might fulfill this role. In addition, it is also important to continue to be supportive to the patient's family–social network, because these relationships also give meaning to the patient's life (Shelly, 1982b).

During the middle years, the adult becomes more concerned with a broader world-view and more concerned about polarities. The resolution of these polarities is to be able to see the paradoxes and live with them, not threatened by diversity, but open to it. They might be described as "wise-hearted," and in some ways have much to offer others. For example, a young adult nurse might gain personally by spending time with an adult who was working through a paradox of health and illness. By being available to listen, support, and reflect with the patient, the nurse could gain understanding of the patient's struggle. By accepting the possibility of mutuality in the relationship, the nurse has the opportunity to give new meaning and hope to the patient. Risking mutuality demonstrates true respect and care, which in turn enhances the selves of both patient and nurse (Fowler, 1981).

The gerontologic nursing literature has some guidelines for meeting faith or spiritual needs of the older patient (Jourard, 1964; Peterson, 1985; Ruffing-Rahal, 1984). As in other age groups, listening and support are an essential part of the nurse's role as the patient deals with the health–illness situation. An additional aspect could be the use of a life review strategy, in which the patient is given the opportunity to recollect past experiences and come to an understanding of them. As infirmity increases, the older adult may not be able to participate in his or her faith community as much as previously. At this point, the nurse needs to facilitate connections with people or groups in this community who can either visit regularly or assist with transportation. Connections such as this provide meaning and hope for the older person, for some rituals of faith can be satisfactorily performed only in a group setting.

Often, other family members and friends have died in the last few years, and the older adult not only needs to be able to form new relationships with the younger generations, but also may want to come to terms with his or her own mortality. Again, the nurse does not need to have the "answer," but the nurse does need to provide an opportunity for the patient to discuss death and make his or her own choices about how arrangements should be handled (Shelton, 1981).

Discharge Planning and Home Care

The nurse and patient can plan for the patient's needs after discharge. Devotional materials may be provided from the chaplain, a spiritual healer, or from a religious supply store. The patient may want the nurse to make arrangements for a visit by a pastor, priest, or members of the religious community after the person arrives home. In some areas of the United States, churches have developed a parish nurse program. These nurses can assist patients and families, not only in dealing with

---

Nursing Management Plan
The Patient with Spiritual Distress*

Nursing Diagnosis: Spiritual distress related to crisis of illness as evidenced by loss of meaning in life, suicidal thoughts, and overuse of pain medication.

Patient Goal: Patient will express increased understanding and acceptance of current life situation.

Patient Outcome Criteria

- Patient verbalizes feelings of despair, anger, and fear after 3 weeks.
- Patient identifies support provided by staff, family, and friends during periods of questioning and despair after 5 weeks.
- Patient identifies some alternative coping mechanisms other than requesting pain medications after 10 weeks.

Nursing Intervention	Scientific Rationale
1. Offer patient opportunity for one-on-one nurse–patient relationship. Actively listen to the patient. Allow expression of negative feelings.	1. Initiating a one-on-one relationship establishes a climate of acceptance and builds trust and safety.
2. Plan and coordinate a multidisciplinary team conference, including the chaplain. Facilitate a care-planning conference involving the social support network, including family and friends.	2. Initiating a multidisciplinary social network of conferences facilitates a sense of acceptance, love, and belonging.
3. Explore past coping mechanisms, including use of music, scripture, prayer, and relaxation techniques. Help patient identify times when he or she can use a variety of these alternative strategies.	3. Building on past positive coping mechanisms enhances a sense of self-control and self-esteem.
4. Use the "life review" technique focusing on faith/spiritual development. Help patient explore ways to use this experience in a unique way, such as sharing in a group or with medical students or other health-care professional students.	4. By focusing on personal faith/spirit the patient can gain new insights into his or her relationship with God, sensing hope and the potential for creativity or self-actualization.

*Refers to the patient situation of "Robert."

---

appropriate community health care, but in meeting spiritual needs as well. Patients do not need to be members of the church to have a parish nurse visit; they can be referred by geographic area.

If the patient has not met the goals addressing spiritual distress while in the hospital, the nurse and patient should discuss how to restate and reach goals in the home. If the patient has no interest in spirituality or in any religious organization, the nurse may explore other means that address spiritual needs, such as meditation or an appropriate support group. The patient cannot be forced to deal with spiritual issues or assume religious beliefs.

EVALUATION

Specific outcome criteria are the evaluative tools for measuring the attainment of goals for the patient with spiritual distress. Examples of outcome criteria are listed below and use "Robert" (see Listening and Supporting) as the patient example. Outcome criteria need to be specifically tailored to the patient so that the criteria will uniquely measure the attainment of that patient's goals.

Goal
The patient will express acceptance of current life situation.

Possible Outcome Criteria

- Patient verbalizes feelings of despair, anger, and fear after 3 days.
- Patient identifies support provided by staff, family, and friends during periods of questioning and despair after 3 weeks.

Goal

The patient will participate in spiritual practices that are personally supportive.

Possible Outcome Criteria

- Within first week, patient asks to speak to his or her spiritual advisor.
- Patient demonstrates spiritual practices, such as prayer, scripture reading, and the sacraments within 1 week.
- Patient expresses satisfaction with being able to maintain relationships with his or her faith community within 2 weeks.

Key Concepts

- The role of philosophy is not to answer questions but to help people to question and develop a view of life. Spirituality does the same thing, in part.
- The spiritual dimension is the essence of a person. It is expressed in the need to seek meaning in experiences and to make a spiritual journey through life.
- Spiritual well-being is the condition in which a person is at peace with God, self, community, and environment.
- Fowler's stages of faith have parallels to Piaget's stages of cognitive development and Erikson's stages of psychosocial development.
- Nurses may provide inadequate or inappropriate care if they have not fully addressed their own spirituality and spiritual well-being, and if they hesitate to encourage the patient to speak of personal spirituality.
- Altered spiritual function may be expressed in various verbalizations of distress and a variety of altered behaviors.
- Every patient has the right to practice his or her spirituality according to personal preference. The nurse should not be judgmental, but assist the patient in fulfilling those needs.
- Nursing interventions include use of self, spiritual support, support of religious practices, listening and supporting, and referral.

References

Assagioli, R. (1971). *Psychosynthesis.* New York: Penguin Books.

Betz, C. L. (1981). Faith development in children. *Pediatric Nursing, 7,* 22–25.

Brallier, L. W. (1978). The nurse as holistic health practitioner. *Nursing Clinics of North America, 13,* 643–655.

Burkhardt, M., & Nagai-Jacobson, M. G. (1985). Dealing with spiritual concerns of clients in the community. *Journal of Community Health, 2,* 191–198.

Carson, V. B. (1989). *Spiritual dimensions of nursing practice* (pp. 76–112). Philadelphia: W. B. Saunders.

Chapman, L. S. (1986). Spiritual health: A component missing from health promotion. *American Journal of Health Promotion, 1*(1), 38–41.

Fish, S., & Shelly, J. A. (1978). *Spiritual care: The nurse's role.* Downer's Grove, IL: InterVarsity Press.

Fowler, J. W. (1981). *Stages of faith.* San Francisco: Harper & Row.

Fromm, E. (1968). *The revolution of hope.* New York: Harper & Row.

Frye, B., & Long, L. (1985). Spiritual counseling approaches following brain-injury. *Rehabilitation Nursing, 10,* 14–16.

Grandstrom, S. L. (1985). Spiritual care of oncology patients. *Topics in Clinical Nursing, 7*(1), 39–45.

Highfield, M. F., & Cason, C. (1983). Spiritual needs of patients: Are they recognized? *Cancer Nursing, 3,* 187–192.

Houldin, A., Saltstein, W. A., & Ganley, K. M. (1987). *Nursing diagnoses for wellness.* Philadelphia: J. B. Lippincott.

Hunglemann, J., Kenke-Rossi, E., Klassen, L., et al. (1985). Spiritual well-being in older adults: Harmonious inter-connectedness. *Journal of Religion and Health, 24,* 147–153.

Jourard, S. M. (1964). *Transparent self.* New York: Van Nostrand Reinhold.

Kreidler, M. (1984). Meaning in suffering . . . philosophy for nurses. *International Nursing Review, 31,* 174–176.

Mathai, M. K. (1980). *Spirituality in relation to nurses' perception of their own coping strategies when patients are perceived to be suffering.* Ann Arbor, MI: University of Michigan.

Moberg, D. O. (Ed.). (1979). *Spiritual well-being: Sociological perspectives.* Washington, D. C.: University Press of America.

Murray, R. B., & Zentner, J. P. (1985). *Nursing concepts for health promotion* (3rd ed.). Englewood Cliffs, NJ: Prentice-Hall.

NANDA (1990). *Taxonomy I revised 1990, with official nursing diagnoses.* St. Louis, MO: North American Nursing Diagnosis Association.

Ozmon, H. A., & Craver, S. M. (1981). *Philosophical foundations of education* (3rd ed.). Columbus, OH: Charles E. Merrill.

Peck, M. L. (1981). The therapeutic effect of faith. *Nursing Forum, 20,* 153–166.

Penrose, V., & Barret, S. (1982). Spiritual needs: "In sickness I lack myself." *Nursing Mirror, 10,* 38–39.

Peterson, E. A. (1985). The physical . . . the spiritual . . . can you meet all of your patient's needs? *Journal of Gerontological Nursing, 11,* 23–27.

Piepgras, R. (1984). The other dimension: Spiritual help. *American Journal of Nursing, 68,* 2610–2613.

Reed, P. (1986). Spirituality and well-being in terminally ill hospitalized adults. *Research in Nursing and Health, 10,* 335–344.

Richardson, A., & Bowden, J. (1983). *The Westminster dictionary of Christian theology* (p. 562). Philadelphia: Westminster Press.

Richardson, G. R., & Noland, W. P. (1984). Treating the spiritual dimension through educational imagery: Health education. *Health Values, 8,* 25–30.

Ruffing-Rahal, M. A. (1984). The spiritual dimension of well-being: Implications for the elderly. *Home Health Nurse, 2,* 12–16.

Shelly, J. A. (1982a). Spiritual care . . . planting seeds of hope. *Critical Care Update, 9,* 7–15.

Shelly, J. A. (1982b). *The spiritual needs of children: A guide for nurses, parents and teachers.* Downer's Grove, IL: InterVarsity Press.

Shelton, R. L. (1981). The patient's need of faith at death. *Topics in Clinical Nursing, 3,* 55–59.

Still, J. V. H. (1984). How to assess spiritual needs of children. *Journal of Christian Nursing, 1,* 4–6.

Stoll, R. I. (1979). Guidelines for spiritual assessment. *American Journal of Nursing, 79,* 1574–1577.

Sundborg, S. (1985, October 16). *From perfection to grace: Spirituality—being stuck . . . getting free* (talk). Seattle University, Seattle, WA.

Tillich, P. (1969). *What is religion?* New York: Harper and Row.

Valliot, M. C. (1970). The spiritual factors in nursing. *Journal of Practical Nursing, 20,* 30–31.

Westberg, G. (1956). *Nurse, pastor and patient: A hospital chaplain talks with nurses.* Rock Island, IL: Augustina Press.

Bibliography

Conrad, N. L. (1985). Spiritual support for the dying. *Nursing Clinics of North America, 20,* 415–426.

Forshee, T., Wiebe, S., Siegel, M. A., et al. (1984). How we teach spiritual care. *Journal of Christian Nursing, 1,* 20–23.

McCormick, R. A. (1987). *Health and medicine in the Catholic tradition: Tradition in transition.* New York: Crossroad.

Meeks, L. B. (1977). The role of spiritual health in achieving high level wellness. *Health Values, 1,* 222–224.

Parks, S. (1986). *The critical years: The young adult search for a faith to live by.* San Francisco: Harper and Row.

Rahman, F. (1989). *Health and medicine in the Islamic tradition: Change and identity.* New York: Crossroad.

Soeken, K. L., & Carson, V. J. (1986). Study measures nurses' attitudes about providing spiritual care. *Health Progress, 4,* 52–55.

Veninga, R. L. (1985). *A gift of hope.* New York: Ballantine Books.

Appendices

A   Equivalents

B   Laboratory Values

C   Medical Terminology: Prefixes, Roots, and Suffixes

D   Recommended Dietary Allowances, USA

E   Nutrition Recommendations for Canadians

APPENDIX A

Equivalents

Outline of the Metric System

Prefix	Meaning	Example(s)	
Kilo	1000	1 kilogram	1000 grams (g)
Hecto	100	1 hectogram	100 grams (g)
Deca	10	1 decaliter	10 liters (L)
	1	1 gram	
		1 liter	
		1 meter	
Deci	0.1	1 deciliter	0.1 liter (L)
Centi	0.01	1 centimeter	0.01 meter (m)
Milli	0.001	1 milligram	0.001 gram (g)
Micro	0.000001 (10^6)	1 microgram	0.000001 gram (g)
		1 micrometer	0.000001 meter (m)
Nano	0.000000001 (10^9)	1 nanogram	0.000000001 gram (g)
Pico	0.000000000001 (10^{12})	1 picogram	0.000000000001 gram (g)

Spencer, R. T., et al. (1990). *Clinical pharmacology and nursing management* (3rd ed.). Philadelphia: J.B. Lippincott

Approximate Weight Equivalents

Metric	Apothecaries	Metric	Apothecaries
0.0001 gram —0.1 mg—$\frac{1}{640}$ grain ($\frac{1}{600}$ grain)		0.02 gram —20 mg—$\frac{1}{3}$ grain	
0.0002 gram —0.2 mg—$\frac{1}{320}$ grain ($\frac{1}{300}$ grain)		0.025 gram —25 mg—$\frac{3}{8}$ grain	
0.0003 gram —0.3 mg—$\frac{1}{210}$ grain ($\frac{1}{200}$ grain)		0.03 gram —30 mg—$\frac{2}{5}$ grain ($\frac{1}{2}$ grain)	
0.0004 gram —0.4 mg—$\frac{1}{150}$ grain		0.04 gram —40 mg—$\frac{3}{5}$ grain ($\frac{2}{3}$ grain)	
0.0005 gram —0.5 mg—$\frac{1}{120}$ grain		0.05 gram —50 mg—$\frac{3}{4}$ grain	
0.0006 gram —0.6 mg—$\frac{1}{100}$ grain		0.06 gram —60 mg—$\frac{9}{10}$ grain (1 grain)	
0.0007 gram —0.7 mg—$\frac{1}{90}$ grain		0.7 gram —70 mg—$1\frac{1}{20}$ grains	
0.0008 gram —0.8 mg—$\frac{1}{80}$ grain		0.08 gram —80 mg—$1\frac{1}{5}$ grains	
0.0009 gram —0.9 mg—$\frac{1}{75}$ grain		0.09 gram —90 mg—$1\frac{1}{3}$ grains	
0.001 gram —1 mg—$\frac{1}{64}$ grain ($\frac{1}{60}$ grain)		0.2 gram —200 mg—3 grains	
0.0011 gram —1.1 mg—$\frac{1}{60}$ grain		0.3 gram —300 mg—$4\frac{1}{2}$ grains	
0.0016 gram —1.6 mg—$\frac{1}{40}$ grain (1.5 mg)		0.4 gram —400 mg—6 grains	
0.0020 gram —2 mg—$\frac{1}{32}$ grain ($\frac{1}{30}$ grain)		0.5 gram —500 mg—$7\frac{1}{2}$ grains	
0.0022 gram —2.2 mg—$\frac{1}{30}$ grain		0.6 gram —600 mg—9 grains	
0.003 gram —3 mg—$\frac{1}{20}$ grain		0.80 gram —800 mg—12 grains (0.75 gram)	
0.004 gram —4 mg—$\frac{1}{16}$ grain ($\frac{1}{15}$ grain)		1.0 gram —1000 mg—15 grains	
0.005 gram —5 mg—$\frac{1}{12}$ grain		1.50 grams—1500 mg—22 grains	
0.006 gram —6 mg—$\frac{1}{10}$ grain		2 grams—2000 mg—30 grains ($\frac{1}{2}$ dram)	
0.008 gram —8 mg—$\frac{1}{8}$ grain		4 grams —1 dram (60 grains)	
0.01 gram —10 mg—$\frac{1}{6}$ grain		5 grams —75 grains	
0.016 gram —16 mg—$\frac{1}{4}$ grain (15 mg)		30 grams —1 ounce	

Approximate Volume Equivalents: Liquid Measures

Metric	Apothecaries	Metric	Apothecaries
0.06 cubic centimeter	—1 minim	15 cubic centimeters	—4 fluid drams
0.25 cubic centimeter	—4 minims	20 cubic centimeters	—5½ fluid drams
0.3 cubic centimeter	—5 minims	25 cubic centimeters	—⅚ fluid ounce
0.5 cubic centimeter	—8 minims	30 cubic centimeters	—1 fluid ounce
0.6 cubic centimeter	—10 minims	60 cubic centimeters	—2 fluid ounces
0.75 cubic centimeter	—12 minims	100 cubic centimeters	—3½ fluid ounces
1 cubic centimeter	—15 minims	120 cubic centimeters	—4 fluid ounces
2 cubic centimeters	—30 minims	200 cubic centimeters	—7 fluid ounces
3 cubic centimeters	—45 minims	250 cubic centimeters	—8 fluid ounces
4 cubic centimeters	—1 fluid dram	500 cubic centimeters	—1 pint
8 cubic centimeters	—2 fluid drams	1000 cubic centimeters	—1 quart
10 cubic centimeters	—2½ fluid drams		

Note: A cubic centimeter (cc) and a milliliter (mL) are approximate equivalents. The terms are used interchangeably.

APPENDIX B

Laboratory Values*

Laboratory values may vary according to the techniques used in different laboratories.

ABBREVIATIONS

Conventional Units
- kg = kilogram
- gm = gram
- mg = milligram
- μg = microgram
- μμg = micromicrogram
- ng = nanogram
- pg = picogram
- dL = 100 milliliters
- mL = milliliter
- cu mm = cubic millimeter
- fL = femtoliter
- mM = millimole
- nM = nanomole
- mOsm = milliosmole
- mm = millimeter
- μ = micron or micrometer

- mm Hg = millimeters of mercury
- U = unit
- mU = milliunit
- μU = microunit
- mEq = milliequivalent
- IU = International Unit
- mIU = milliInternational Unit

SI Units
- g = gram
- L = liter
- d = day
- h = hour
- mol = mole
- mmol = millimole
- μmol = micromole
- nmol = nanomole
- pmol = picomole

Reference Ranges—Hematology

| Determination | Reference Range | | Clinical Significance |
	Conventional units	SI units	
A₂ hemoglobin	1.5%–3.5% of total hemoglobin	Mass fraction: 0.015–0.035 of total hemoglobin	Increased in certain types of thalassemia
Bleeding time	2–8 min	2–8 min	Prolonged in thrombocytopenia, defective platelet function, and aspirin therapy
Factor V assay (proaccelerin factor)	60%–140%		
Factor VII assay (antihemophiliac factor)	50%–200%		Deficient in classical hemophilia
Factor IX assay (plasma thromboplastin component)	75%–125%		Deficient in Christmas disease (pseudohemophilia)
Factor X (Stuart factor)	60%–140%		Deficient in Stuart clotting defect
Fibrinogen	200–400 mg/dl	2–4 g/dl	Increased in pregnancy, infections accompanied by leukocytosis, nephrosis. Decreased in severe liver disease, abruptio placentae
Fibrin split products	Less than 10 mg/L	Less than 10 mg/L	Increased in disseminated intravascular coagulation

(continued)

Reference Ranges—Hematology
(continued)

Determination	Reference Range		Clinical Significance
	Conventional units	*SI units*	
Fibrinolysins (whole blood clot lysis time)	No lysis in 24 h		Increased activity associated with massive hemorrhage, extensive surgery, transfusion reactions
Partial thromboplastin time (activated)	20–45 sec		Prolonged in deficiency of fibrinogen, factors II, V, VIII, IX, X, XI, and XII, and in heparin therapy
Prothrombin consumption	Over 20 sec		Impaired in deficiency of factors VIII, IX, and X
Prothrombin time	9.5–12 sec		Prolonged by deficiency of factors, I, II, V, VII, and X, fat malabsorption, severe liver disease, coumarin-anticoagulant therapy
Erythrocyte count	Males: 4,600,000–6,200,000/ cu mm	$4.6–6.2 \times 10^{12}$/L	Increased in severe diarrhea and dehydration, polycythemia, acute poisoning, pulmonary fibrosis
	Females: 4,200,000–5,400,000/ cu mm	$4.2–5.4 \times 10^{12}$/L	Decreased in all anemias, in leukemia, and after hemorrhage, when blood volume has been restored
Erythrocyte indices			
Mean corpuscular volume (MCV)	80–94 (cu μ)	80–94 fL	Increased in macrocytic anemias; decreased in microcytic anemia
Mean corpuscular hemoglobin (MCH)	27–32 μμg/cell	27–32 pg	Increased in macrocytic anemias; decreased in microcytic anemia
Mean corpuscular hemoglobin concentration (MCHC)	33%–38%	Concentration fraction: 0.33–0.38	Decreased in severe hypochromic anemia
Reticulocytes	0.5%–1.5% of red cells	Number fraction: 0.005–0.015	Increased with any condition stimulating increase in bone marrow activity (i.e., infection, blood loss [acute and chronic]); after iron therapy in iron deficiency anemia, polycythemia rubra vera
			Decreased with any condition depressing bone marrow activity, acute leukemia, late stage of severe anemias
Erythrocyte sedimentation rate (ESR)—Westergren method	Males under 50 yr: <15 mm/h	<15 mm/h	Increased in tissue destruction, whether inflammatory or degenerative; during menstruation and pregnancy; and in acute febrile diseases
	Males over 50 yr: <20 mm/h	<20 mm/h	
	Females under 50 yr: <20 mm/h	<20 mm/h	
	Females over 50 yr: <30 mm/h	<30 mm/h	
Erythrocyte sedimentation ratio–Zeta centrifuge	41%–54% in both sexes	Fraction: 0.41–0.54	Significance similar to ESR
Hematocrit	Males: 42%–50%	Volume fraction: 0.42–0.5	Decreased in severe anemias, anemia of pregnancy, acute massive blood loss
	Females: 40%–48%	Volume fraction: 0.4–0.48	Increased in erythrocytosis of any cause, and in dehydration

(continued)

Reference Ranges—Hematology
(continued)

Determination	Reference Range		Clinical Significance
	Conventional units	*SI units*	
Hemoglobin	Males: 13–18 gm/dL Females: 12–16 gm/dL	2.02–2.79 mmol/L 1.86–2.48 mmol/L	or hemoconcentration associated with shock Decreased in various anemias, pregnancy, severe or prolonged hemorrhage, and with excessive fluid intake Increased in polycythemia, chronic obstructive pulmonary diseases, failure of oxygenation because of congestive heart failure, and normally in people living at high altitudes
Hemoglobin F	Less than 2% of total hemoglobin	Mass fraction: <0.02	Increased in infants and children, and in thalassemia and many anemias
Leukocyte alkaline phosphatase	Score of 40–100		Increased in polycythemia vera, myelofibrosis, and infections Decreased in chronic granulocytic leukemia, paroxysmal nocturnal hemoglobinuria, hypoplastic marrow, and viral infections, particularly infectious mononucleosis
Leukocyte count	Total: 5000–10,000/ cu mm	$5–10 \times 10^9$/L	Elevated in acute infectious diseases, predominantly in the neutrophilic fraction with bacterial diseases, and in the lymphocytic and monocytic fractions in viral diseases
Neutrophils	60%–70%	Number fraction: 0.6–0.7	
Eosinophils	1%–4%	Number fraction: 0.01–0.04	
Basophils	0%–0.5%	Number fraction: 0.00–0.05	
Lymphocytes	20%–30%	Number fraction: 0.2–0.3	
Monocytes	2%–6%	Number fraction: 0.02–0.06	Elevated in acute leukemia, after menstruation, and after surgery or trauma Depressed in aplastic anemia, agranulocytosis, and by toxic agents such as chemotherapeutic agents used in treating malignancy Eosinophils elevated in collagen disease, allergy, intestinal parasitosis
Osmotic fragility of red cells	Increased in hemolysis occurs in over 0.5% NaCl Decreased if hemolysis is incomplete in 0.3% NaCl		Increased in congenital spherocytosis, idiopathic acquired hemolytic anemia, isoimmune hemolytic disease, ABO hemolytic disease of newborn Decreased in sickle cell anemia, thalassemia
Platelet count	100,000–400,000/ cu mm	$0.1–0.4 \times 10^{12}$/L	Increased in malignancy, myeloproliferative disease, rheumatoid arthritis, and postoperatively, about 50% of patients with unexpected increase of platelet count will be found to have a malignancy Decreased in thrombocytopenic purpura, acute leukemia, aplastic anemia, and during cancer chemotherapy, infections, and drug reactions

Reference Ranges—Serum, Plasma, and Whole Blood Chemistries

Determination	Normal Adult Reference Range		Clinical Significance	
	Conventional Units	**SI Units**	**Increased**	**Decreased**
Acetoacetate	0.2–1.0 mg/dL	19.6–98 μmol/L	Diabetic acidosis Fasting	
Acetone	0.3–2.0 mg/dL	51.6–344.0 μmol/L	Toxemia of pregnancy Carbohydrate-free diet High-fat diet	
Adrenocorticotropic hormone (ACTH) (plasma)—RIA*	Less than 50 pg/mL	Less than 50 mg/L	Pituitary-dependent Cushing's syndrome Ectopic ACTH syndrome Primary adrenal atrophy	Adrenocortical tumor Adrenal insufficiency secondary to hypopituitarism
Aldolase	3–8 Sibley-Lehninger U/dL at 37°C	22–59 mU/L at 37°C	Hepatic necrosis Granulocytic leukemia Myocardial infarction Skeletal muscle disease	
Aldosterone (plasma)—RIA	Supine: 3–10 ng/dL Upright: 5–30 ng/dL Adrenal vein: 200–800 ng/dL	0.80–0.30 nmol/L 0.14–0.90 nmol/L 5.54–22.16 nmol/L	Primary aldosteronism (Conn's syndrome) Secondary aldosteronism	Addison's disease
Alpha-1-antitrypsin	200–400 mg/dL	2–4 g/L		Certain forms of chronic lung and liver disease in young adults
Alpha-1-fetoprotein	None detected		Hepatocarcinoma Metastatic carcinoma of liver Germinal cell carcinoma of the testis or ovary Fetal neural tube defects— elevation in maternal serum	
Alpha-hydroxy-butyric dehydrogenase	Up to 140 U/mL	Up to 140 U/L	Myocardial infarction Granulocytic leukemia Hemolytic anemias Muscular dystrophy	
Ammonia (plasma)	40–80 μg/dL (enzymatic method); varies considerably with method	22.2–44.3 μmol/L	Severe liver disease Hepatic decompensation	
Amylase	60–160 Somogyi U/dL	111–296 U/L	Acute pancreatitis Mumps Duodenal ulcer Carcinoma of head of pancreas Prolonged elevation with pseudocyst of pancreas Increased by drugs that constrict pancreatic duct sphincters: morphine, codeine, cholinergics	Chronic pancreatitis Pancreatic fibrosis and atrophy Cirrhosis of liver Pregnancy (2nd and 3rd trimesters)
Arsenic	6–20 μg/dL; if 50 μg/dL, suspect toxicity	0.78–2.6 μmol/L	Accidental or intentional poisoning Excessive occupational exposure	
Ascorbic acid (vitamin C)	0.4–1.5 mg/dL	23–85 μmol/L	Large doses of ascorbic acid as a prophylactic against the common cold	
Bilirubin	Total: 0.1–1.2 mg/dL Direct: 0.1–0.2 mg/dL	1.7–20.5 μmol/L 1.7–3.4 μmol/L	Hemolytic anemia (indirect) Biliary obstruction and disease	

(continued)

Reference Ranges—Serum, Plasma, and Whole Blood Chemistries
(continued)

| Determination | Normal Adult Reference Range | | Clinical Significance | |
	Conventional Units	SI Units	Increased	Decreased
	Indirect: 0.1–1 mg/dL	1.7–17.1 μmol/L	Hepatocellular damage (hepatitis) Pernicious anemia Hemolytic disease of newborn	
Blood gases Oxygen, arterial (whole blood): Partial pressure (PaO$_2$)	95–100 mm Hg	12.64–13.30 kPa	Polycythemia	Anemia
Saturation (SaO$_2$)	94%–100%	Volume fraction: 0.94–1	Anhydremia	Cardiac decompensation Chronic obstructive pulmonary disease
Carbon dioxide, arterial (whole blood): partial pressure (PaCO$_2$)	35–45 mm Hg	4.66–5.99 kPa	Respiratory acidosis Metabolic alkalosis	Respiratory alkalosis Metabolic acidosis
pH (whole blood, arterial)	7.35–7.45	7.35–7.45	Vomiting Hyperpnea Fever Intestinal obstruction	Uremia Diabetic acidosis Hemorrhage Nephritis
Calcitonin	Basal: nondetectable 400 pg/mL	400 ng/L	Medullary carcinoma of the thyroid Some nonthyroid tumors Zollinger-Ellison syndrome	
Calcium	8.5–10.5 mg/dL	2.125–2.625 mmol/L	Tumor or hyperplasia of parathyroid Hypervitaminosis D Multiple myeloma Nephritis with uremia Malignant tumors Sarcoidosis Hyperthyroidism Skeletal immobilization Excess calcium intake: milk-alkali syndrome	Hypoparathyroidism Diarrhea Celiac disease Vitamin D deficiency Acute pancreatitis Nephrosis After parathyroidectomy
CO$_2$, venous	Adults: 24–32 mEq/L Infants: 18–24 mEq/L	24–32 mmol/L 18–24 mmol/L	Tetany Respiratory disease Intestinal obstruction Vomiting	Acidosis Nephritis Eclampsia Diarrhea Anesthesia
Carcinoembryonic antigen (CEA)—RIA	0–2.5 ng/mL	0–2.5 μg/L	The repeatedly high incidence of this antigen in cancers of the colon, rectum, pancreas, and stomach suggests that CEA levels may be useful in the therapeutic monitoring of these conditions.	
Catecholamines (plasma)—RIA	Epinephrine random: up to pg/mL Norepinephrine, random 100–550 pg/mL Dopamine, random up to 130 pg/mL	Up to 490 pmol/L 590–3240 pmol/L Up to 850 pmol/L	Pheochromocytoma	

(continued)

Reference Ranges—Serum, Plasma, and Whole Blood Chemistries (continued)

| Determination | Normal Adult Reference Range | | Clinical Significance | |
	Conventional Units	*SI Units*	*Increased*	*Decreased*
Ceruloplasmin	30–80 mg/dL	300–800 mg/L		Wilson's disease (hepatolenticular degeneration)
Chloride	95–105 mEq/L	95–105 mmol/L	Nephrosis Nephritis Urinary obstruction Cardiac decompensation Anemia	Diabetes Diarrhea Vomiting Pneumonia Heavy metal poisoning Cushing's syndrome Burns Intestinal obstruction Febrile conditions
Cholesterol	150–200 mg/dL	3.9–5.2 mmol/L	Lipemia Obstructive jaundice Diabetes Hypothyroidism	Pernicious anemia Hemolytic anemia Hyperthyroidism Severe infection Terminal states of debilitating disease
Cholesterol esters	60%–70% of total	Fraction of total cholesterol 0.6–0.7		The esterified fraction decreases in liver diseases
Cholinesterase	Serum: 0.6–1.6 delta pH Red cells: 0.6–1 delta pH	0.6–1.6 U 0.6–1 U	Nephrosis Exercise	Nerve gas intoxication (greater effect on red cell activity) Insecticides, organic phosphates (greater effect on plasma activity)
Chorionic gonadotropin, beta subunit—RIA	0–5 IU/L	0–5 IU/L	Pregnancy Hydatidiform mole Choriocarcinoma	
Complement, human C₃	Males: 88–252 mg/dL Females: 88–206 mg/dL	880–2520 mg/L	Some inflammatory diseases	Acute glomerulonephritis Disseminated lupus erythematosus with renal involvement
Complement C₄	14–51 mg/dL	140–510 mg/L	Some inflammatory diseases	Often decreased in immunologic disease, especially with active systemic lupus erythematosus Hereditary angioneurotic edema
Complement, total (hemolytic)	90%–94% complement		Some inflammatory diseases	Acute glomerulonephritis Epidemic meningitis Subacute bacterial endocarditis
Copper	70–165 μg/dL	11–25.9 μmol/L	Cirrhosis of liver Pregnancy	Wilson's disease

(continued)

Reference Ranges—Serum, Plasma, and Whole Blood Chemistries
(continued)

Determination	Normal Adult Reference Range		Clinical Significance	
	Conventional Units	*SI Units*	*Increased*	*Decreased*

Cortisol—RIA	8 A.M. 7–25 μg/dL
	4 P.M. 2–9 μg/dL
		193–690 nmol/L
		55–248 nmol/L
			Stress: infectious disease,
			  surgery, burns, etc.
			Pregnancy
			Cushing's syndrome
			Pancreatitis
			Eclampsia
				Addison's disease
				Anterior pituitary
				  hypofunction

C-peptide reactivity	1.5–10 ng/mL	1.5–10 μg/L	Insulinoma	Diabetes
Creatine	0.2–0.8 mg/mL	15.3–61 μmol/L	Pregnancy Skeletal muscle necrosis or atrophy Starvation Hyperthyroidism	

Creatine
  phosphokinase
  (CPK)
	Males: 50–325 mU/
	  mL
	Females: 50–250
	  mU/mL
		50–325 U/L
		
		50–250 U/L
			Myocardial infarction
			Skeletal muscle diseases
			Intramuscular injections
			Crush syndrome
			Hypothyroidism
			Alcohol withdrawal delirium
			Alcoholic myopathy
			Cerebrovascular disease	

Creatine
  phosphokinase
  isoenzymes
	MM band present
	  (skeletal muscle);
	  MB band absent
	  (heart muscle)
			MB band increase in
			  myocardial infarction,
			  ischemia	

Creatinine	0.7–1.4 mg/dL	62–124 μmol/L	Nephritis Chronic renal disease	Kidney diseases

Creatinine clearance	100–150 mL of blood
	  cleared for crea-
	  tinine per min
		1.67–2.5 mL/s		

Cryoglobulins,
  qualitative
	Negative		Multiple myeloma
			Chronic lymphocytic
			  leukemia
			Lymphosarcoma
			Systemic lupus
			  erythematosus
			Rheumatoid arthritis
			Infective subacute
			  endocarditis
			Some malignancies
			Scleroderma	

11-Deoxycortisol	1 μg/dL	<0.029 μmol/L	Hypertensive form of
			  virilizing adrenal
			  hyperplasia due to an
			  11-β-hydroxylase defect	

Dibucaine number	Normal: 70%–85%
	  inhibition
	Heterozygote:
	  50%–65%
	  inhibition
	Homozygote:
	  16%–25%
	  inhibition
				Important in de-
				  tecting carriers
				  of abnormal
				  cholinesterase
				  activity who are
				  susceptible to
				  succinyldicholine
				  anesthetic shock

Dihydrotestosterone	Males: 50–210 ng/dL
	Females: none
	  detectable
		1.72–7.22 nmol/L		Testicular femini-
				  zation syndrome

Estradiol—RIA	Females:
	  Follicular:
	    10–90 pg/mL
	  Midcycle:
	    100–500 pg/mL
		
		37–370 pmol/L
		
		367–1835 pmol/L
			Pregnancy	Depressed or fail-
				  ure to peak—
				  ovarian failure

(continued)

Reference Ranges—Serum, Plasma, and Whole Blood Chemistries (continued)

Determination	Normal Adult Reference Range		Clinical Significance	
	Conventional Units	**SI Units**	**Increased**	**Decreased**
Estriol—RIA	Luteal: 50–240 pg/mL	184–881 pmol/L	Pregnancy	Depressed or failure to peak—ovarian failure
	Follicular phase: 2–20 ng/dL			
	Midcycle: 12–40 ng/dL			
	Luteal phase: 10–30 ng/dL			
	Postmenopausal: 1–5 ng/dL			
	Males: 0.5–5 ng/dL			
	Nonpregnant females: <0.5 ng/mL	<1.75 nmol/L		
	Pregnant females: 1st trimester: up to 1 ng/mL	Up to 3.5 nmol/L		
	2nd trimester: 0.8–7 ng/mL	2.8–24.3 nmol/L		
	3rd trimester: 5–25 ng/mL	17.4–86.8 nmol/L		
Estrogens, total–RIA	Females: cycle days: Day 1–10: 61–394 pg/mL	61–394 ng/L	Pregnancy Measured on a daily basis, can be used to evaluate response of hypogonadotropic, hypoestrogenic women to human menopausal or pituitary gonadotropin	Fetal distress Ovarian failure
	Day 11–20: 122–437 pg/mL	122–437 ng/L		
	Day 21–30: 156–350 pg/mL	156–350 ng/L		
	Males: 40–115 pg/mL	40–115 ng/L		
Estrone–RIA	Females: Day 1–10: 4.3–18 ng/dL	15.9–66.6 pmol/L	Pregnancy	Depressed or failure to peak—ovarian failure
	Day 11–20: 7.5–19.6 ng/dL	27.8–72.5 pmol/L		
	Day 21–30: 13–20 ng/dL	48.1–74 pmol/L		
	Males: 2.5–7.5 ng/dL	9.3–27.8 pmol/L		
Ferritin–RIA	Males: 10–270 ng/mL	10–270 µg/L	Nephritis Hemochromatosis Certain neoplastic diseases Acute myelogenous leukemia Multiple myeloma	Iron deficiency
	Females: 5–100 ng/mL	5–100 µg/L		
Folic acid–RIA	4–16 ng/mL	9.1–36.3 nmol/L		Megaloblastic anemias of infancy and pregnancy Inadequate diet Liver disease Malabsorption syndrome Severe hemolytic anemia
Follicle stimulating hormone (FSH)—RIA	Females: Follicular phase: 5–20 mIU/mL	5–20 IU/L	Menopause and primary ovarian failure	Pituitary failure
	Peak of middle cycle: 12–30 mIU/mL	12–30 IU/L		
	Luteinic phase: 5–15 mIU/mL	5–15 IU/L		

(continued)

Reference Ranges—Serum, Plasma, and Whole Blood Chemistries
(continued)

Determination	Normal Adult Reference Range		Clinical Significance	
	Conventional Units	SI Units	Increased	Decreased
Galactose	Menopausal females: 40–200 mIU/mL <5 mg/dL	40–200 IU/L <0.28 mmol/L		Galactosemia
Gamma glutamyl transpeptidase	Males: <45 IU/L Females: <30 IU/L	45 U/L 30 U/L	Hepatobiliary disease Anicteric alcoholics Drug therapy damage Myocardial infarction Renal infarction	
Gastrin–RIA	Fasting 50–155 pg/mL Postprandial: 80–170 pg/mL Zollinger-Ellison syndrome: 200–over 2000 pg/ mL Pernicious anemia: 130–2260 pg/mL (mean 912)	50–155 ng/L 80–170 ng/L 200–over 2000 ng/L 130–2260 ng/L (mean 912)	Zollinger-Ellison syndrome Peptic ulceration of the duodenum Pernicious anemia	
Glucose	Fasting: 60–110 mg/ dL Postprandial (2 h): 65–140 mg/dL	3.3–6.05 mmol/L 3.58–7.7 mmol/L	Diabetes Nephritis Hyperthyroidism Early hyperpituitarism Cerebral lesions Infections Pregnancy Uremia	Hyperinsulinism Hypothyroidism Late hyperpituitarism Pernicious vomiting Addison's disease Extensive hepatic damage
Glucose tolerance (oral)	Features of a normal response: 1. Normal fasting between 60–110 mg/dL 2. No sugar in urine 3. Upper limits of normal: Fasting = 125 1 hour = 190 2 hours = 140 3 hours = 125	3.3–6.05 mmol/L 6.88 mmol/L 10.45 mmol/L 7.70 mmol/L 6.88 mmol/L	(Flat or inverted curve) Hyperinsulinism Adrenal cortical insufficiency (Addison's disease) Anterior pituitary hypofunction Hypothyroidism Sprue and celiac diseases	(High or prolonged curve) Diabetes Hyperthyroidism Primary adrenal cortical tumor or hyperplasia Severe anemia Certain central nervous system disorders
Glucose-6-phosphate dehydrogenase (red cells)	Screening: Decolorization in 20–100 min Quantitative: 1.86–2.5 IU/mL RBC	1860–2500 U/L		Drug-induced hemolytic anemia Hemolytic disease of newborn
Glycoprotein (alpha-1-acid)	40–110 mg/dL	400–1100 mg/L	Neoplasm Tuberculosis Diabetes complicated by degenerative vascular disease Pregnancy Rheumatoid arthritis Rheumatic fever Infectious liver disease Lupus erythematosus	
Growth hormone— RIA	<10 ng/mL	<10 mg/L	Acromegaly	Failure to stimulate with arginine or insulin—hypopituitarism

(continued)

APPENDIX B   LABORATORY VALUES

Reference Ranges—Serum, Plasma, and Whole Blood Chemistries
(continued)

Determination	Normal Adult Reference Range		Clinical Significance	
	Conventional Units	SI Units	Increased	Decreased
Haptoglobin	50–250 mg/dL	0.5–2.5 g/L	Pregnancy Estrogen therapy Chronic infections Various inflammatory conditions	Hemolytic anemia Hemolytic blood transfusion reaction
Hemoglobin (plasma)	0.5–5 mg/dL	5–50 mg/L	Transfusion reactions Paroxysmal nocturnal hemoglobinuria Intravascular hemolysis	
Hemoglobin A1 (Glycohemoglobin)	Nondiabetics & diabetics whose control of glucose is: Good: 4.4%–8.2% Fair: 8.3%–9.2% Poor: >9.2%			
Hexosaminidase, total	Controls: 333–375 mM/mL/h Heterozygotes: 288–644 nM/mL/h Tay-Sachs disease: 284–1232 nM/mL/h Diabetics: 567–3560 nM/mL/h	333–375 µmol/L/h 288–644 µmol/L/h 284–1232 µmol/L/h 567–3560 µmol/L/h	Diabetes Tay-Sachs disease	
Hexosaminidase A	Controls 49%–68% of total Heterozygotes: 26%–45% of total Tay-Sachs disease: 0%–4% of total Diabetics: 39%–59% of total	Fraction of total: 0.49–0.68 0.26–0.45 0–0.4 0.39–0.59		Tay-Sachs disease and heterozygotes
High-density lipoprotein cholesterol (HDL cholesterol)				HDL cholesterol is lower in patients with increased risk for coronary heart disease

Age (yr)	Males (mg/dL)	Females (mg/dL)	Males (mmol/L)	Females (mmol/L)
0–19	30–65	30–70	0.78–1.68	0.78–1.81
20–29	35–70	35–75	0.91–1.81	0.91–1.94
30–39	30–65	35–80	0.78–1.68	0.91–2.07
40–49	30–65	40–85	0.78–1.68	1.04–2.2
50–59	30–65	35–85	0.78–1.68	0.91–2.2
60–69	30–65	35–85	0.78–1.68	0.91–2.2

Determination	Conventional Units	SI Units	Increased	Decreased
17-Hydroxyprogesterone—RIA	Males: 0.4–4 ng/mL Females: 0.1–3.3 ng/mL Children: 0.1–0.5 ng/mL	1.2–12 nmol/L 0.3–10 nmol/L 0.3–1.5 nmol/L	Congenital adrenal hyperplasia Pregnancy Some cases of adrenal or ovarian adenomas	
Immunoglobulin A	Adults: 50–300 mg/dL (in children the normals are lower and vary with age)	0.5–3 g/L	Gamma A myeloma Wiskott-Aldrich syndrome Autoimmune disease Hepatic cirrhosis	Ataxia telangiectasis Agammaglobulinemia Hypogammaglobulinemia, transient Dysgammaglobulinemia Protein-losing enteropathies

Reference Ranges—Serum, Plasma, and Whole Blood Chemistries
(continued)

Determination	Normal Adult Reference Range		Clinical Significance	
	Conventional Units	*SI Units*	*Increased*	*Decreased*
Immunoglobulin D	0–30 mg/dL	0–300 mg/L	IgD multiple myeloma Some patients with chronic infectious diseases	
Immunoglobulin E	20–740 ng/mL	20–740 µg/L	Allergic patients and those with parasitic infestations	
Immunoglobulin G	Adults: 635–1400 mg/dL	6.35–14 g/L	IgG myeloma After hyperimmunization Autoimmune disease states Chronic infections	Congenital and acquired hypogammaglobulinemia IgA myelomas, Waldenstrom's (IgM) macroglobulinemia Some malabsorption syndromes Extensive protein loss
Immunoglobulin M	Adults: 40–280 mg/dL	0.4–2.8 g/L	Waldenstrom's macroglobulinemia Parasitic infections Hepatitis	Agammaglobulinemias Some IgG and IgA myelomas Chronic lymphatic leukemia
Insulin—RIA	5–25 µU/mL	0.2–1 µg/L	Insulinoma Acromegaly	Diabetes mellitus
Iron	65–170 µg/dL	11.6–30.4 µmol/L	Pernicious anemia Aplastic anemia Hemolytic anemia Hepatitis Hemochromatosis	Iron deficiency anemia
Iron-binding capacity	IBC: 150–235 µg/dL TIBC: 250–420 µg/dL % Saturation: 20–50	26.9–42.1 µmol/L 44.8–75.2 µmol/L Fraction of total iron-binding capacity: 0.2–0.5	Iron deficiency anemia Acute and chronic blood loss Hepatitis	Chronic infectious diseases Cirrhosis
Isocitric dehydrogenase	50–180 U	0.83–3 U/L	Hepatitis: cirrhosis Obstructive jaundice Metastatic carcinoma of the liver Megaloblastic anemia	
Lactic acid (whole blood)	Venous: 5–20 mg/dL Arterial: 3–7 mg/dL	0.6–2.2 mmol/L 0.3–0.8 mmol/L	Increased muscular activity Congestive heart failure Hemorrhage Shock Some varieties of metabolic acidosis Some febrile infections May be increased in severe liver disease	
Lactic dehydrogenase (LDH)	100–225 mU/mL	100–225 U/L	Untreated pernicious anemia Myocardial infarction Pulmonary infarction Liver disease	
Lactic dehydrogenase isoenzymes				
Total lactic dehydrogenase	100–225 mU/mL	100–225 U/L Fraction of total LDH:	LDH-1 and LDH-2 are increased in myocardial infarction, megaloblastic anemia, and hemolytic anemia	
LDH-1	20%–35%	0.2–0.35		
LDH-2	25%–40%	0.25–0.4		
LDH-3	20%–30%	0.2–0.3	LDH-4 and LDH-5 are increased in pulmonary in-	
LDH-4	0–20%	0–0.2		

(continued)

Reference Ranges—Serum, Plasma, and Whole Blood Chemistries (continued)

Determination	Normal Adult Reference Range		Clinical Significance	
	Conventional Units	*SI Units*	*Increased*	*Decreased*
LDH-5	0–25%	0–0.25	farction, congestive heart failure, and liver disease	
Lead (whole blood)	Up to 40 μg/dL	Up to 2 μmol/L	Lead poisoning	
Leucine amino-peptidase	80–200 U/mL	19.2–48 U/L	Liver or biliary tract diseases Pancreatic disease Metastatic carcinoma of liver and pancreas Biliary obstruction	
Lipase	0.2–1.5 U/mL	55–417 U/L	Acute and chronic pancreatitis Biliary obstruction Cirrhosis Hepatitis Peptic ulcer	
Lipids, total	400–1000 mg/dL	4–10 g/L	Hypothyroidism Diabetes Nephrosis Glomerulonephritis Hyperlipoproteinemias	Hyperthyroidism

Lipoprotein Phenotype: Summary of Findings in the Primary Hyperlipoproteinemias

Type	Frequency	Appearance	Triglyceride	Cholesterol	Lipoprotein Staining				Secondary Causes
					Beta	*Pre-Beta*	*Alpha*	*Chylomicrons*	
Normal		Clear	Normal	Normal	Moderate	Zero to moderate	Moderate	Weak	
I	Very rare	Creamy	Markedly increase	Normal to moderately increased	Weak	Weak	Weak	Markedly increased	Dysglobulinemia
II	Common	Clear	Normal to slightly increased	Slightly to markedly increased	Strong	Zero to strong	Moderate	Weak	Hypothyroidism, myeloma, hepatic syndrome, macroglobulinemia, and high dietary cholesterol
III	Uncommon	Clear, cloudy, or milky	Increased	Increased	Broad intense band	Extends into beta	Moderate	Weak	
IV	Very common	Clear, cloudy, or milky	Slightly to markedly increased	Normal to slightly increased	Weak to moderate	Moderate to strong	Weak to moderate	Weak	Hypothyroidism, diabetes mellitus, pancreatitis, glycogen storage diseases, nephrotic syndrome, myeloma, pregnancy, and oral contraceptives
V	Rate	Cloudy to creamy	Markedly increased	Increased	Weak	Moderate	Weak	Strong	Diabetes mellitus, pancreatitis, and alcoholism

Types I and II are fat induced; types III and IV are carbohydrate induced; type V is fat and carbohydrate induced.

Lithium	Usual maintenance level; 0.5–1 mEq/L		0.5–1 mmol/L		
Low-density lipoprotein cholesterol (LDL cholesterol)	Age (yr)	mg/dL	mmol/L	LDL cholesterol is higher in patients with increased risk for coronary heart disease	
	0–19	50–170	1.30–4.40		
	20–29	60–170	1.55–4.40		
	30–39	70–190	1.80–4.92		
	40–49	80–190	2.07–4.92		
	50–59	80–210	2.07–5.44		

(continued)

Reference Ranges—Serum, Plasma, and Whole Blood Chemistries
(continued)

| Determination | Normal Adult Reference Range | | Clinical Significance | |
	Conventional Units	*SI Units*	*Increased*	*Decreased*

Luteinizing hormone—RIA	Males: 6–30 mIU/mL
	Females:
	  Follicular phase:
	    2–3 mIU/mL
	  Ovulatory peak:
	    40–200 mIU/mL
	  Luteal phase:
	    0–20 mIU/mL
	  Postmenopausal:
	    35–120 mIU/mL
		1.4–6.9 mg/L
		
		0.5–6.9 mg/L
		
		9.2–46 mg/L
		
		0–5 mg/L
		
		8–27.5 mg/L
			Pituitary tumor
			Ovarian failure
				Depressed or failure to peak—pituitary failure

Lysozyme (muramidase)	2.8–8 μg/mL	2.8–8 mg	Certain types of leukemia (acute monocytic leukemia) Inflammatory states and infections	Acute lymphocytic leukemia
Magnesium	1.3–2.4 mEq/L	0.7–1.2 mmol/L	Excess ingestion of magnesium-containing antacids	Chronic alcoholism Severe renal disease Diarrhea Defective growth
Manganese	0.04–1.4 μg/dL	72.9–255 nmol/L		
Mercury	Up to 10 μg/dL	Up to 0.5 μmol/L	Mercury poisoning	
Myoglobin—RIA	Up to 85 ng/mL	Up to 85 μg/mL	Myocardial infarction Muscle necrosis	
5' Nucleotidase	3.2–11.6 IU/L	3.2–11.6 U/L	Hepatobiliary disease	
Osmolality	280–300 mOsm/kg	280–300 mmol/L	Useful in the study of electrolyte and water balance	Inappropriate secretion of antidiuretic hormone
Parathyroid hormone	160–350 pg/mL	160–350 ng/L	Hyperparathyroidism	
Phenylalanine	1.2–3.5 mg/dL 1st week 0.7–3.5 mg/dL thereafter	0.07–0.21 mmol/L 0.04–0.21 mmol/L	Phenylketonuria	
Phosphatase, acid, total	0–11 U/L	0–11 U/L	Carcinoma of prostate Advanced Paget's disease Hyperparathyroidism Gaucher's disease	
Phosphatase, acid, prostatic—RIA	0–10 ng/mL Borderline: 2.5–3.3 IU/L	0–10 μg/L	Carcinoma of prostate	
Phosphatase, alkaline	Adults: 30–115 mU/mL	30–115 μ/L	Conditions reflecting increased osteoblastic activity of bone Rickets Hyperparathyroidism Liver disease	
Phosphatase, alkaline, thermostable fraction	Thermostable fraction >35%: hepatic disease and combined disease with predominant hepatic component Thermostable fraction between 25% and 35%: combined hepatic and skeletal disease		Hepatic disease	

(continued)

Reference Ranges—Serum, Plasma, and Whole Blood Chemistries
(continued)

Determination	Normal Adult Reference Range		Clinical Significance	
	Conventional Units	SI Units	Increased	Decreased
	Thermostable fraction <25%: skeletal disease with increased osteoblastic activity			
Phosphohexose isomerase	20–90 IU/L	20–90 U/L	Malignancy Disease of heart, liver, and skeletal muscles	
Phospholipids	125–300 mg/dL	1.25–3 g/L	Diabetes Nephritis	
Phosphorus, inorganic	2.5–4.5 mg/dL	0.8–1.45 mmol/L	Chronic nephritis Hypoparathyroidism	Hyperparathyroidism Vitamin D deficiency
Potassium	3.8–5 mEq/L	3.8–5 mmol/L	Addison's disease Oliguria Anuria Tissue breakdown or hemolysis	Diabetic acidosis Diarrhea Vomiting
Progesterone—RIA	Follicular phase: up to 0.8 ng/mL Luteal phase: 10–20 ng/mL End of cycle: <1 ng/L Pregnant: up to 50 ng/mL in 20th week	2.5 nmol/L 31.8–63.6 nmol/L <3 nmol/L Up to 160 nmol/L	Useful in evaluation of menstrual disorders and infertility and in the evaluation of placental function during pregnancies complicated by toxemia, diabetes mellitus, or threatened miscarriage	
Prolactin—RIA	6–24 ng/mL	6–24 μg/L	Pregnancy Functional or structural disorders of the hypothalamus Pituitary stalk section Pituitary tumors	
Protein, total Albumin Globulin	6–8 gm/dL 3.5– gm/dL 1.5–3 gm/dL	60–80 g/L 35–50 g/L 15–30 g/L	Hemoconcentration Shock Multiple myeloma (globulin fraction) Chronic infections (globulin fraction) Liver disease (globulin)	Malnutrition Hemorrhage Loss of plasma from burns Proteinuria
Electrophoresis (cellulose acetate) Albumin Alpha-1 globulin Alpha-2 globulin Beta globulin Gamma globulin	3.5–5 gm/dL 0.2–0.4 gm/dL 0.6–1 gm/dL 0.6–1.2 gm/dL 0.7–1.5 gm/dL	35–50 g/L 2–4 g/L 6–10 g/L 6–12 g/L 7–15 g/L		
Protoporphyrin erythrocyte (whole blood)	15–100 μg/dL	0.27–1.80 μmol/L	Lead toxicity Erythropoietic porphyria	
Pyridoxine	3.6–18 ng/mL			A wide spectrum of clinical conditions such as mental depression, peripheral neuropathy, anemia, neonatal seizures, and reactions to certain drug therapies

(continued)

Reference Ranges—Serum, Plasma, and Whole Blood Chemistries
(continued)

| Determination | Normal Adult Reference Range | | Clinical Significance | |
	Conventional Units	SI Units	Increased	Decreased
Pyruvic acid (whole blood)	0.3–0.7 mg/dL	34–80 μmol/L	Diabetes Severe thiamine deficiency Acute phase of some infections, possibly secondary to increased glycogenolysis and glycolysis	
Renin (plasma)—RIA	Normal diet: Supine: 0.3–1.9 ng/mL/h Upright: 0.6–3.6 ng/mL/h Low salt diet: Supine: 0.9–4.5 ng/mL/h Upright: 4.1–9.1 ng/mL/h	 0.08–0.52 ng/L/sec 0.16–1.00 μg/L/sec 0.25–1.25 μg/L/sec 1.13–2.53 μg/L/sec	Renovascular hypertension Malignant hypertension Untreated Addison's disease Primary salt-losing nephropathy Low-salt diet Diuretic therapy Hemorrhage	Frank primary aldosteronism Increased salt intake Salt-retaining steroid therapy Antidiuretic hormone therapy Blood transfusion
Sodium	135–145 mEq/L	135–145 mmol/L	Hemoconcentration Nephritis Pyloric obstruction	Alkali deficit Addison's disease Myxedema
Sulfate (inorganic)	0.5–1.5 mg/dL	0.05–0.15 mmol/L	Nephritis Nitrogen rentention	
Testosterone—RIA	Females: 25–100 ng/dL Males: 300–800 ng/dL	0.9–3.5 nmol/L 10.5–28 nmol/L	Females: Polycystic ovary Virilizing tumors	Males: Orchidectomy for neoplastic disease of the prostate or breast Estrogen therapy Klinefelter's syndrome Hypopituitarism Hypogonadism Hepatic cirrhosis
T_3 (triiodothyronine) uptake	25%–35%	Relative uptake fraction: 0.25–0.35	Hyperthyroidism TBG deficiency Androgens and anabolic steroids	Hypothyroidism Pregnancy TBG excess Estrogens and antiovulatory drugs
T_3, total circulating—RIA	75–200 ng/dL	1.15–3.1 nmol/L	Pregnancy Hyperthyroidism	Hypothyroidism
T_4 (thyroxine)—RIA	4.5–11.5 μg/dL	58.5–150 nmol/L	Hyperthyroidism Thyroiditis Elevated thyroxine-binding proteins caused by oral contraceptives Pregnancy	Primary and pituitary hypothyroidism Idiopathic involvement Cases of diminished thyroxine-binding proteins caused by androgenic and anabolic steroids Hypoproteinemia Nephrotic syndrome
T_4, free	1–2.2 ng/dL	13–30 pmol/L	Euthyroid patients with normal free thyroxine levels may have abnormal T_3 and T_4 levels caused by drug preparations	

(continued)

Reference Ranges—Serum, Plasma, and Whole Blood Chemistries (continued)

	Normal Adult Reference Range		Clinical Significance	
Determination	*Conventional Units*	*SI Units*	*Increased*	*Decreased*
Thyroid-stimulating hormone (TSH)—RIA		0.3–5 m/IU/L	Hypothyroidism	Hyperthyroidism
Thyroid-binding globulin	10–26 µg/dL	100–260 µg/L	Hypothyroidism Pregnancy Estrogen therapy Oral contraceptives Genetic and idiopathic	Androgens and anabolic steroids Nephrotic syndrome Marked hypoproteinemia Hepatic disease
Transaminase, serum glutamic-oxalo-acetate (SGOT, aspartate amino-transferase)	7–40 U/mL	4–20 U/L	Myocardial infarction Skeletal muscle disease Liver disease	
Transaminase, serum glutamic-oxaloacetate (SGPT, alanine aminotransferase)	10–40 U/mL	5–20 U/L	Same conditions as SGOT, but increase is more marked in liver disease than SGOT	
Transferrin	230–320 mg/dL	2.3–3.2 g/L	Pregnancy Iron-deficiency anemia due to hemorrhaging Acute hepatitis Polycythemia Oral contraceptives	Pernicious anemia in relapse Thalassemic and sickle cell anemia Chromatosis Neoplastic and hepatic diseases
Triglycerides	10–150 mg/dL	0.10–1.65 mmol/L	See *Lipoprotein Phenotype*	
Tryptophan	1.4–3 mg/dL	68.6–147 nmol/L		Tryptophan-specific malabsorption syndrome
Tyrosine	0.5–4 mg/dL	27.6–220.8 mmol/L	Tyrosinosis	
Urea nitrogen (BUN)	10–20 mg/dL	3.6–7.2 mmol/L	Acute glomerulonephritis Obstructive uropathy Mercury poisoning Nephrotic syndrome	Severe hepatic failure Pregnancy
Uric acid	2.5–8 mg/dL	0.15–0.5 mmol/L	Gouty arthritis Acute leukemia Lymphomas treated by chemotherapy Toxemia of pregnancy	Xanthinuria Defective tubular reabsorption
Viscosity	1.4–1.8 relative to water at 37°C (98.6°F)		Patients with marked increases of the gamma globulins	
Vitamin A	50–220 µg/dL	1.75–7.7 µmol/L	Hypervitaminosis A	Vitamin A deficieny Celiac disease Obstructive jaundice Giardiasis Parenchymal hepatic disease
Vitamin B₁ (thiamine)	1.6–4 µg/dL	47.4–135.7 nmol/L		Anorexia Beriberi Polyneuropathy Cardiomyopathies
Vitamin B₆ (pyridoxal phosphate)	3.6–18 ng/mL	14.6–72.8 nmol/L		Chronic alcoholism Malnutrition

(continued)

Reference Ranges—Serum, Plasma, and Whole Blood Chemistries
(continued)

Determination	Normal Adult Reference Range		Clinical Significance	
	Conventional Units	*SI Units*	*Increased*	*Decreased*
Vitamin B₁₂—RIA	130–785 pg/mL	100–580 pmol/L	Hepatic cell damage and in association with the myeloproliferative disorders (the highest levels are encountered in myeloid leukemia)	Uremia Neonatal seizures Malabsorption, such as celiac syndrome Strict vegetarianism Alcoholism Pernicious anemia Total or partial gastrectomy Ileal resection Sprue and celiac disease Fish tapeworm infestation
Vitamin E	0.5–2 mg/dL	11.6–46.4 μmol/L		Vitamin E deficiency
Xylose absorption test	2 hr, 30–50 mg/dL	2–3.35 mmol/L		Malabsorption syndrome
Zinc	55–150 μg/dL	7.65–22.95 μmol/L	Zinc is essential for the growth and propagation of cell cultures and the functioning of several enzymes	

* By radioimmunoassay.

Reference Ranges—Urine Chemistry

Determination	Normal Adult Reference Range		Clinical Significance	
	Conventional Units	*SI Units*	*Increased*	*Decreased*
Acetone and acetoacetate	Zero		Uncontrolled diabetes Starvation	
Acid mucopolysaccharides	Negative		Hurler's syndrome Marfan's syndrome Morquio-Ulrich disease	

Aldosterone	Normal salt:
	  Normal:
	    4–20 μg/24 h
	  Renovascular:
	    10–40 μg/24 h
	  Tumor:
	    20–100 μg/24 h
		
		11.1–55.5 nmol/24 h
		
		27.7–111 nmol/24 h
		
		55.4–277 nmol/24 h
			Primary aldosteronism (adrenocortical tumor)
			Secondary aldosteronism
			Salt depletion
			Potassium loading
			ACTH in large doses
			Cardiac failure
			Cirrhosis with ascites formation
			Nephrosis
			Pregnancy	

Alpha amino nitrogen	50–200 mg/24 h	3.6–14.3 mmol/24 h	Leukemia Diabetes Phenylketonuria Other metabolic diseases	
Amylase	35–260 units excreted per h	6.5–48.1 U/h	Acute pancreatitis	
Arylsulfatase A	>2.4 U/mL			Metachromatic leukodystrophy

(continued)

Reference Ranges—Urine Chemistry
(continued)

Determination	Normal Adult Reference Range		Clinical Significance	
	Conventional Units	**SI Units**	**Increased**	**Decreased**
Bence-Jones protein	None detected		Myeloma	
Calcium	<150 mg/24 h	<3.75 mmol/24 h	Hyperparathyroidism	Hypopara-thyroidism
			Vitamin D intoxication	Vitamin D defi-ciency
			Fanconi syndrome	
Catecholamines	Total: 0–275 μg/24 h	0–275 μg/24 h	Pheochromocytoma	
	Epinephrine:	Fraction total:	Neuroblastoma	
	10%–40%	0.10–8.4		
	Norepinephrine:	Fraction total:		
	60%–90%	0.60–0.90		
Chorionic gonadotropin, qualitative (pregnancy test)	Negative		Pregnancy	
			Chorionepithelioma	
			Hydatidiform mole	
Copper	20–70 μg/24 h	0.32–1.12 μmol/24 h	Wilson's disease	
			Cirrhosis	
			Nephrosis	
Coproporphyrin	50–300 μg/24 h	0.075–0.45 μmol/24 h	Poliomyelitis	
			Lead poisoning	
			Porphyria hepatica	
			Porphyria erythropoietica	
			Porphyria cutanea tarda	
Cortisol, free	20–90 μg/24 h	55.2–248.4 nmol/d	Cushing's syndrome	
Creatine	0–200 mg/24 h	0–1.52 mmol/24 h	Muscular dystrophy	
			Fever	
			Carcinoma of liver	
			Pregnancy	
			Hyperthyroidism	
			Myositis	
Creatinine	0.8–2 gm/24 h	7–17.6 mmol/24 h	Typhoid fever	Muscular atrophy
			Salmonella infections	Anemia
			Tetanus	Advanced de-generation of kidneys
				Leukemia
Creatinine clearance	100–150 mL of blood cleared of creatinine per min	1.67–2.5 mL/s		Measures glomerular filtration rate
				Renal diseases
Cystine and cysteine	10–100 mg/24 h	0.08–0.83 mmol/24 h	Cystinuria	
Delta aminolevulinic acid	0–0.54 mg/dL	0–40 μmol/L	Lead poisoning	
			Porphyria hepatica	
			Hepatitis	
			Hepatic carcinoma	
11-Desoxycortisol	20–100 μg/24 h	0.6–2.9 μmol/d	Hypertensive form of virilizing adrenal hyperplasia due to an 11-beta hydroxylase defect	
Estriol (placental)				Decreased values occur with fetal distress of many conditions, including preeclampsia, placental insufficiency, and poorly controlled diabetes mellitus

Weeks of pregnancy	**μm/24 h**	**nmol/24 h**
12	<1	<3.5
16	2–7	7–24.5
20	4–9	14–32
24	6–13	21–45.5
28	8–22	28–77
32	12–43	42–150
36	14–45	49–158
40	19–46	66.5–160

(continued)

Reference Ranges—Urine Chemistry
(continued)

Determination	Normal Adult Reference Range		Clinical Significance	
	Conventional Units	**SI Units**	**Increased**	**Decreased**
Estrogens, total (fluorometric)	Females: Onset of menstruation: 4–25 µg/24 h Ovulation peak: 28 µg/24 h Luteal peak: 22–105 µg/24 h Menopausal: 1.4–19.6 µg/24 h Males: 5–18 µg/24 h	4–25 µg/24 h 28 µg/24 h 22–105 µg/24 h 1.4–19.6 µg/24 h 5–18 µg/24 h	Hyperestrogenism due to gonadal or adrenal neoplasm	Primary or secondary amenorrhea
Etiocholanolone	Males: 1.9–6 mg/24 h Females: 0.5–4 mg/24 h	6.5–20.6 µmol/24 h 1.7–13.8 µmol/24 h	Adrenogenital syndrome Idiopathic hirsutism	
Follicle-stimulating hormone—RIA	Females: Follicular: 5–20 IU/24 h Luteal: 5–15 IU/24 h Midcycle: 15–60 IU/24 h Menopausal: 50–100 IU/24 h Males: 5–25 IU/24 h	5–20 IU/d 5–15 IU/d 15–60 IU/d 50–100 IU/d 5–25 IU/d	Menopause and primary ovarian failure	Pituitary failure
Glucose	Negative		Diabetes mellitus Pituitary disorders Intracranial pressure Lesion in floor of 4th ventricle	
Hemoglobin and myoglobin	Negative		Extensive burns Transfusion of incompatible blood Myoglobin increased in severe crushing injuries to muscles	
Homogentisic acid, qualitative	Negative		Alkaptonuria Ochronosis	
Homovanillic acid	Up to 15 mg/24 h	Up to 82 µmol/d	Neuroblastoma	
17-hydroxycorti-costeroids	2–10 mg/24 h	5.5–27.5 µmol/d	Cushing's disease	Addison's disease Anterior pituitary hypofunction
5-Hydroxy-indoleacetic acid, qualitative	Negative		Malignant carcinoid tumors	
Hydroxyproline	15–43 mg/24 h	0.11–0.33 µmol/d	Paget's disease Fibrous dysplasia Osteomalacia Neoplastic bone disease Hyperparathyroidism	
17-ketosteroids, total	Males: 10–22 mg/24 h Females: 6–16 mg/24 h	35–76 µmol/d 21–55 µmol/d	Interstitial cell tumor of testes Simple hirsutism, occasionally Adrenal hyperplasia Cushing's syndrome Adrenal cancer, virilism	Thyrotoxicosis Female hypogo-nadism Diabetes mellitus Hypertension Debilitating dis-ease of mild to

(continued)

Reference Ranges—Urine Chemistry
(continued)

Determination	Normal Adult Reference Range		Clinical Significance	
	Conventional Units	**SI Units**	**Increased**	**Decreased**
			Arrhenoblastoma	moderate severity Eunuchoidism Addison's disease Panhypopitu-itarism Myxedema Nephrosis
Lead	Up to 150 μg/24 h	Up to 60 μmol/24 h	Lead poisoning	
Luteinizing hormone	Males: 5–18 IU/24 h Females: Follicular phase: 2–25 IU/24 h Ovulatory peak: 30–95 IU/24 h Luteal phase: 2–20 IU/24 h Postmenopausal: 40–110 IU/24 h	2–25 IU/d 30–95 IU/d 2–20 IU/d 40–110 IU/d	Pituitary tumor Ovarian failure	Depressed or fail-ure to peak—pituitary failure
Metanephrines, total	Less than 1.3 mg/24 h	Less than 6.5 μmol/d	Pheochromocytoma; a few patients with pheochromocytoma may have elevated urinary metanephrines but normal catecholamines and VMA	
Osmolality	Males: 390–1090 mM/kg Females: 300–1090 mM/kg	390–1090 mmol/kg 300–1090 mmol/kg	Useful in the study of elec-trolyte and water balance	
Oxalate	Up to 40 mg/24 h	Up to 456 μmol/d	Primary hyperoxaluria	
Phenylpyruvic acid qualitative	Negative		Phenylketonuria	
Phosphorus, inor-ganic	0.8–1.3 gm/24 h	26–42 mmol/24 h	Hyperparathyroidism Vitamin D intoxication Paget's disease Metastatic neoplasm to bone	Hypoparathy-roidism Vitamin D deficieny
Porphobilinogen, qualitative	Negative		Chronic lead poisoning Acute porphyria Liver disease	
Porphobilinogen, quantitative	0–1 mg/24 h	0–4.4 μmol/24 h	Acute porphyria Liver disease	
Porphyrins, qualita-tive	Negative		See porphyrins, quantitative	
Porphyrins, quanti-tative (copropor-phyrin and uroporphyrin)	Coproporphyrin: 50–160 μg/24 h Uroporphyrin: up to 50 μg/24 h	0.075–0.24 μmol/24 h Up to 0.06 μmol/24 h	Porphyria hepatica Porphyria erythropoietica Porphyria cutanea tarda Lead poisoning (only copro-porphyrin increased)	
Potassium	40–65 mEq/24 h	40–65 mmol/24 h	Hemolysis	
Pregnanediol	Females: Proliferative phase: 0.5–1.5 mg/24 h Luteal phase: 2–7 mg/24 h Menopause: 0.2–1 mg/24 h	1.6–4.8 μmol/24 h 6–22 μmol/24 h 0.6–3.1 μmol/24 h	Corpus luteum cysts When placental tissue re-mains in the uterus after parturition Some cases of adreno-cortical tumors	Placental dysfunc-tion Threatened abor-tion Intrauterine death

(continued)

Reference Ranges—Urine Chemistry
(continued)

Determination	Normal Adult Reference Range		Clinical Significance	
	Conventional Units	SI Units	Increased	Decreased
	Pregnancy: **Weeks of gestation** mg/24 h	μmol/24 h		
	10–12 5–15	15.6–47		
	12–18 5–25	15.6–78.0		
	18–24 15–33	47.0–103.0		
	24–28 20–42	62.4–131.0		
	28–32 27–47	84.2–146.6		
	Males: 0.1–2 mg/24 h	0.3–6.2 μmol/24 h		
Pregnanetriol	0.4–2.4 mg/24 h	1.2–7.1 μmol/24 h	Congenital adrenal androgenic hyperplasia	
Protein	Up to 100 mg/24 h	Up to 100 mg/24 h	Nephritis Cardiac failure Mercury poisoning Bence-Jones protein in multiple myeloma Febrile states Hematuria	
Sodium	130–200 mEq/24 h	130–200 mmol/24 h	Useful in detecting gross changes in water and salt balance	
Titratable acidity	20–40 mEq/24 h	20–40 mmol/24 h	Metabolic acidosis	Metabolic alkalosis
Urea nitrogen	9–16 gm/24 h	0.32–0.57 mol/L	Excessive protein catabolism	Impaired kidney function
Uric acid	250–750 mg/24 h	1.48–4.43 mmol/24 h	Gout	Nephritis
Urobilinogen	Random urine: <0.25 mg/dL 24-hour urine: up to 4 mg/24 h	<0.42 mol/24 h Up to 6.76 μmol/24 h	Liver and biliary tract disease Hemolytic anemias	Complete or nearly complete biliary obstruction Diarrhea Renal insufficiency
Uroporphyrins	Up to 50 μg/24 h	Up to 0.06 μmol/24 h	Porphyria	
Vanillylmandelic acid (VMA)	0.7–6.8 mg/24 h	3.5–34.3 μmol/24 h	Pheochromocytoma Neuroblastoma Coffee, tea, aspirin, bananas, and several different drugs	
Xylose absorption test (5 hour)	16%–33% of ingested xylose	Fraction absorbed: 0.16–0.33		Malabsorption syndromes
Zinc	0.15–1.2 mg/24 h	2.3–18.4 мmol/24 h	Zinc is an essential nutritional element	

Reference Ranges—Cerebrospinal Fluid (CSF)

Determination	Normal Adult Reference Range		Clinical Significance	
	Conventional Units	SI Units	Increased	Decreased
Albumin	15–30 mg/dL	150–300 mg/L	Certain neurologic disorders Lesion in the choroid plexus or blockage of the flow of CSF Damage to the blood–CNS barrier	

(continued)

Reference Ranges—Cerebrospinal Fluid (CSF)
(continued)

| Determination | Normal Adult Reference Range | | Clinical Significance | |
	Conventional Units	SI Units	Increased	Decreased
Cell count	0–5 mononuclear cells per cu mm	$0–5 \times 10^6$/L	Bacterial meningitis Neurosyphilis Anterior poliomyelitis Encephalitis lethargica	
Chloride	100–130 mEq/L	100–300 mmol/L	Uremia	Acute generalized meningitis Tuberculous meningitis
Glucose	50–75 mg/dL	2.75–4.13 mmol/L	Diabetes mellitus Diabetic coma Epidemic encephalitis Uremia	Acute meningitides Tuberculous meningitis Insulin shock
Glutamine	6–15 mg/dL	0.41–1 mmol/L	Hepatic encephalopathies, including Reye's syndrome Hepatic coma Cirrhosis	
IgG	0–6.6 mg/dL	0–66 mg/L	Damage to the blood–CNS barrier Multiple sclerosis Neurosyphilis Subacute sclerosing panencephalitis Chronic phases of CNS infections	
Lactic acid	<24 mg/dL	<2.7 mmol/L	Bacterial meningitis Hypocapnia Hydrocephalus Brain abscesses Cerebral ischemia	
Lactic dehydrogenase	1/10 that of serum	Activity fraction: 0.1 of serum	CNS disease	
Protein			Acute meningitides	
Lumbar	15–45 mg/dL	150–450 mg/L	Tubercular meningitis	
Cisternal	15–25 mg/dL	150–250 mg/L	Neurosyphilis	
Ventricular	5–15 mg/dL	50–150 mg/L	Poliomyelitis Guillain-Barré syndrome	
Protein electrophoresis (cellulose acetate)	% of total:	Fraction:	An increase in the level of albumin alone can be the result of a lesion in the choroid plexus or a blockage of the flow of CSF. An elevated gamma globulin value with a normal albumin level has been reported in multiple sclerosis, neurosyphilis, subacute sclerosing panencephalitis, and the chronic phase of CNS infections. If the blood–CNS barrier has been damaged severely during the course of these diseases, the CSF albumin level may also be elevated.	
Prealbumin	3–7	0.03–0.07		
Albumin	56–74	0.56–0.74		
Alpha$_1$ globulin	2–6.5	0.02–0.065		
Alpha$_2$ globulin	3–12	0.03–0.12		
Beta globulin	8–18.5	0.08–0.185		
Gamma globulin	4–14	0.04–0.14		

Gastric Analysis

Determination	Normal Adult Reference Range		Clinical Significance	
	Conventional Units	*SI Units*	*Increased*	*Decreased*
pH	2	2		Pernicious anemia
Basal acid output	0–6 mEq/h	0–6 mmol/h	Peptic ulcer	Gastric carcinoma
Maximum acid	5–40 mEq/h	5–40 mmol/h	Zollinger-Ellison syndrome	Chronic atrophic gastritis
				Decreased normally with age

Miscellaneous Value

Determination	Normal Value	Clinical Significance	
		Conventional Units	*SI Units*
Acetaminophen	Zero	Therapeutic level 10–20 Mg/mL	10–20 mg/L
Aminophylline (theophylline)	Zero	Therapeutic level 10–20 Mg/mL	10–20 mg/L
Bromide	Zero	Therapeutic level 5–50 mg/dL	50–500 mg/L
Carbon monoxide	0%–2%	Symptoms with 20% saturation	
Chlordiazepoxide	Zero	Therapeutic level 1–3 Mg/mL	1–3 mg/L
Diazepam	Zero	Therapeutic level 0.5–2.5 Mg/dL	5–25 Mg/L
Digitoxin	Zero	Therapeutic level 5–30 ng/mL	5–30 Mg/L
Digoxin	Zero	Therapeutic level 0.5–2 ng/mL	0.5–2 Mg/L

Ethanol	0%–0.01%	Legal intoxication level 0.10% or above
		    0.3%–0.4% marked intoxication
		    0.4%–0.5% alcoholic stupor	

Gentamicin	Zero	Therapeutic level 4–10 Mg/mL	4–10 mg/L
Methanol	Zero	May be fatal in concentration as low as 10 mg/dL	100 mg/L
Phenobarbital	Zero	Therapeutic level 15–40 Mg/mL	10–20 mg/L
Phenytoin	Zero	Therapeutic level 10–20 Mg/mL	10–20 mg/L
Primidone	Zone	Therapeutic level 5–12 Mg/mL	5–12 mg/L
Quinidine	Zero	Therapeutic level 0.2–0.5 mg/dL	2–5 mg/L
Salicylate	Zero	Therapeutic level 2–25 mg/dL	20–250 mg/L
		Toxic level 30 mg/dL	300 mg/L

Sulfonamide	Zero	Therapeutic levels:
		    Sulfadiazine 8–15 mg/dL
		    Sulfaguanidine 3–5 mg/dL
		    Sulfamerazine 10–15 mg/dL
		    Sulfanilamide 10–15 mg/dL
			
			80–150 mg/L
			30–50 mg/L
			100–150 mg/L
			100–150 mg/L

* Reprinted with permission from Suddarth, D.S. (1991). *The Lippincott manual of nursing practice* (5th ed.). Philadelphia: J.B. Lippincott. Prepared by Goodman, D.B.P., MD, PhD, Professor and Department Chief, Department of Pathology and Laboratory Medicine, Hospital of the University of Pennsylvania, Philadelphia, PA.

Medical Terminology: Prefixes, Roots, and Suffixes

Medical terms are made up of components that are derived mostly from Latin or Greek. The root is the main part of the word. Prefixes precede the root and suffixes follow the root to modify its meaning. The roots are presented here with combining vowels that are used to ease pronunciation when a suffix is added.

Prefixes

Prefix	Meaning	Example	Definition of Example
a-, an-	without, not	aseptic	Sterile; free of infection
		anoxia	Lack of oxygen
ab-	away from	abduct	To move away from the midline
acro-	extremity	acromegaly	Disease marked by enlargement of the extremities
ad-	to, toward	adduct	To move toward the midline
ambi-	both	ambidextrous	Able to use either hand
ante-	before	antenatal	Occurring before birth; prenatal
anti-	against	antidote	Substance that neutralizes a poison
auto-	self	autoimmunity	An immune response to one's own body tissues
bi-	two, double	binocular	Pertaining to both eyes
brady-	slow	bradycardia	Slow heart rate
circum-	around	circumduction	Circular movement of a limb at a ball-and-socket joint
co-	together	coherent	Sticking together; logical
contra-	against	contraindication	A condition that makes it inadvisable to use a certain form of treatment
de-	without, removal	dehydration	Removal of water
di-	two, twice	diatomic	Having two atoms
dia-	through	dialysis	Separation of substances by passage through a semipermeable membrane
diplo-	double, two	diplopia	Double vision
dis-	removal, separation	disinfect	Remove infectious organisms from
dys-	abnormal, difficult, painful	dysmenorrhea	Painful menstruation
ecto-	outside	ectopic	Outside the normal position
endo-	within	endoscope	Instrument for viewing the inside of a body space
epi-	above	epigastric	Above the stomach
eryth/r/o-	red	erythema	Redness of the skin
		erythrocyte	Red blood cell
eu-	normal, good, true	eupnea	Normal breathing
ex/o-	out, out of	excise	To remove surgically
extra-	outside, in addition to	extracellular	Outside the cell
hemi-	half	hemiplegia	Paralysis of one half of the body
hetero-	other, different	heterosexual	Pertaining to the opposite sex
homo-, homeo-	same	homograft	Transplant of tissue from same species
		homeostasis	State of internal constancy
hyper-	high, excessive	hypertension	High blood pressure
hypo-	under, decreased	hypoglycemia	Low blood sugar

(continued)

Prefixes
(continued)

Prefix	Meaning	Example	Definition of Example
in, im-	in, within	inhale	To breathe in
		impacted	Held firmly
in-, im-	not	indigestion	Incomplete digestion
		impermeable	Unable to be penetrated
infra-	below	infrared	Pertaining to heat waves beyond the red spectrum
inter-	between	interstitial	Between cells
intra-	within	intracranial	Within the skull
iso-	equal, same	isotonic	Having the same concentration as cellular fluids
juxta-	near	juxtaglomerular	Near the glomerulus of the kidney
leuk/o-	white, colorless	leukemia	Malignant overgrowth of white blood cells (leukocytes)
macro-	large	macromolecule	Large molecule composed of subunits
mal-	bad, poor	malnutrition	Poor nutrition
melan/o-	black, dark	melanin	Dark pigment found in skin, hair, the brain, and the eye
mega/lo-mes-	large, enlarged	megalocyte	Large red blood cell
mes/o-	middle	mesoderm	Middle germ layer of the embryo
meta-	beyond, over, change	metamorphosis	Change in form or structure; passage from one stage to another
micr/o-	small, one millionth	microscope	Instrument for viewing extremely small objects
mon/o-	one	monocyte	White blood cell with a single large nucleus
multi-	many	multipara	Woman who has borne more than one viable fetus
neo-	new	neoplasm	A new, abnormal growth of tissue; a growth or tumor
noct/i-	night	nocturnal	Occurring at night
non-	not	nontoxic	Not poisonous
olig/o-	little, deficiency	oliguria	Decreased amount of urine formation
ortho-	straight, correct	orthopedics	Medical specialty that deals with prevention and correction of deformities
pan-	all	pandemic	Presence of a disease in most of a large population
para-	beside, near	paramedic	Trained medical assistant
per-	by, through	percutaneous	Through the skin
peri-	around	perioral	Around the mouth
poly-	many	polydactyly	Having more than the normal number of fingers or toes
post-	after, behind	postpartum	Occurring after birth
pre-	before	pre-existing	Present or occurring before a given time
prim/i-	first	primigravida	Woman during her first pregnancy
pro-	before	prognosis	Prediction of the outcome of a disease
pseud/o-	false	pseudostratified	Appearing to be in layers
quad/r/i-	four	quadriplegia	Paralysis of all four limbs
re-	back, again	reflux	Backward flow
retro-	backward, behind	retroperitoneal	Behind the peritoneum
scler/o-	hard, hardening	scleroderma	Disease characterized by hardening of the skin
semi-	half	semilunar	Shaped like a half moon
sub-	below, under	subcutaneous	Under the skin
super-	above, excessive	superinfection	Second infection after an initial infection and caused by a different organism
supra-	above	suprapubic	Above the pubis

(continued)

Prefixes
(continued)

Prefix	Meaning	Example	Definition of Example
syn-, sym-	together	synthesis	Union of elements or molecules; a joining of parts
		symmetry	Correspondence in position of parts
tachy-	fast	tachypnea	Rapid respiration rate
trans-	through, across	transfusion	Injection of a substance into the bloodstream
tri-	three	tricuspid	Having three points or cusps
ultra-	beyond	ultrasound	Sound waves beyond the audible range
un-	not	unconscious	Lacking in awareness; insensible
uni-	one	unicellular	Having one cell

Roots

Root	Meaning	Example	Definition of Example
aden/o	gland	adenoma	A neoplasm of glandular epithelium
angi/o	vessel	angioplasty	Surgical repair of a blood vessel
arteri/o	artery	endarteritis	Inflammation of the lining of an artery
arthr/o	joint	arthroscope	Instrument for examining the interior of a joint
audio/o	hearing	audiologist	Specialist in the study and treatment of hearing disorders
bio	life	biopsy	Removal and examination of living tissue
blast/o	immature form, growing form	osteoblast	A growing cell that produces bone tissue
brachi/o	arm	antebrachium	Forearm
bronch/o, bronchi/o	bronchus	bronchogenic	Originating in a bronchus
		bronchiectasis	Chronic dilation of the bronchi
carcin/o	cancer	carcinogen	Agent that causes cancer
cardi/o	heart	cardiomyopathy	Any disease affecting the heart muscle
cerebr/o	brain	cerebrospinal	Pertaining to the brain and spinal cord
cephal/o	head	hydrocephalus	Accumulation of excess cerebrospinal fluid in the brain
cervic/o	neck, cervix	cervical	Pertaining to the neck or cervix
chol/e	bile	cholelithiasis	Presence or formation of gallstones
cholecyst/o	gallbladder	cholecystectomy	Surgical removal of the gallbladder
chondr/o	cartilage	endochondral	Located or occurring within cartilage
cleid/o	clavicle	cleidomastoid	Pertaining to the clavicle and mastoid process
col/o	colon	colostomy	Surgical formation of an opening between the colon and the surface of the body
colp/o	vagina	colpocele	Hernia into the vagina
cost/o	rib	intercostal	Between the ribs
crani/o	skull	craniotomy	Surgery on the cranium
cyst/o	sac, bladder	cystitis	Inflammation of the urinary bladder
cyt/o	cell	cytology	Study of cells
derm, dermat/o	skin	hypodermic	Beneath the skin
		dermatosis	Any skin disease
encephal/o	brain	encephalitis	Inflammation of the brain

(continued)

Roots
(continued)

Root	Meaning	Example	Definition of Example
enter/o	intestine	enterotoxin	Toxin that acts on the cells lining the intestine
gastr/o	stomach	epigastric	Above the stomach
genesis	origin	spermatogenesis	Formation of sperm cells
glomerul/o	glomerulus	glomerulonephritis	Inflammation of the glomeruli of the kidney
gloss/o	tongue	hypoglossal	Under the tongue
hem/o, hemat/o	blood	hemoglobin	The pigment that carries oxygen in red blood cells
		hematoma	Localized collection of clotted blood
hepat/o	liver	hepatomegaly	Enlargement of the liver
hist/o	tissue	histologist	One who studies tissue
hydr/o	water, fluid	hydrophilic	Readily absorbing water
hyster/o	uterus	hysterectomy	Surgical removal of the uterus
ile/o	ileum	ileocecal	Pertaining to the ileum and cecum
ili/o	ilium	iliac	Pertaining to the ilium
kerat/o	cornea, horny layer of the skin	keratoplasty	Plastic surgery of the cornea; corneal grafting
		keratosis	Any horny growth, such as a wart or callus
labi/o	lip, labium	labiodental	Pertaining to the lips and teeth
lact/o	milk	lactogenic	Promoting formation of milk
laryng/o	larynx	laryngospasm	Spasmodic closing of the larynx
lith/o	stone	sialolith	Stone in a salivary gland or duct
lymph/o	lymph	lymphadenopathy	Any disease of a lymph node
mast/o	breast	mastectomy	Surgical removal of a breast
medull/o	central part, medulla oblongata	medullary	Pertaining to the central region of a structure or to the medulla oblongata
men/o	menses	menarche	Beginning of menstrual cycles
mening/o	meninges	meningocele	Hernia of the meninges
metr/o	uterus	endometrium	Lining of the uterus
my/o	muscle	myofiber	Muscle cell
myc/o	fungus	dermatomycosis	Any fungal infection of the skin
myel/o	marrow, spinal cord	myelogenous	Originating in bone marrow
		myelodysplasia	Defective formation of the spinal cord
myring/o	tympanic membrane	myringotomy	Incision of the tympanic membrane
nas/o	nose	paranasal	Near the nose
necr/o	death	necrosis	Death of tissue
nephr/o	kidney	hydronephrosis	Accumulation of fluid in the renal pelvis due to obstruction
neur/o	nerve	neuralgia	Pain along the path of a nerve
ocul/o	eye	oculomotor	Pertaining to eye movements
odont/o	tooth	orthodontics	Branch of dentistry that deals with prevention and correction of irregularities in the teeth
onc/o	tumor, swelling	oncolytic	Destructive of tumor cells
onych/o	nail	paronychia	Infection of the area around a nail
oo	egg, ovum	oocyte	Developing ovum
oophor/o	ovary	oophorectomy	Removal of an ovary
ophthalm/o	eye	exophthalmia	Protrusion of the eyeball
orchi/o, orchid/o	testis	orchiopexy	Surgical fixation of an undescended testis in the scrotum
		orchidoptosis	Dropping of the testis
os, oste/o	bone	ossification	Formation of bone
		periosteum	Membrane that covers bone
ot/o	ear	otosclerosis	Formation of bone tissue in the inner ear leading to hearing loss
ovari/o	ovary	ovariorrhexis	Rupture of an ovary

(continued)

Roots
(continued)

Root	Meaning	Example	Definition of Example
path/o	disease	pathophysiology	Study of the physiology of disease
ped/o	child, foot	pediatrics	Branch of medicine that deals with care of children
		pedometer	Instrument for recording numbers of steps
phag/o	eating	phagocyte	Cell that takes in and destroys waste or foreign particles
phak/o, phac/o	lens of the eye	phacolysis	Destruction of the lens
phleb/o	vein	phlebotomist	One who draws blood from a vein
pneum/o, pneumon/o	lung, air, breathing	pneumothorax	Accumulation of air in the pleural space
		pneumonia	Inflammation of the lung
proct/o	rectum	proctoscopy	Endoscopic examination of the rectum
psych/o	mind	psychogenic	Of mental or emotional origin
ptosis	dropping	blepharoptosis	Drooping of the eyelid
py/o	pus	empyema	Accumulation of pus in a body cavity
pyel/o	pelvis, renal pelvis	pyelography	X-ray study of the renal pelvix and ureter
pylor/o	pylorus	pylorospasm	Spasm of the pylorus
rachi/o	spine	rachiocentesis	Lumbar tap
ren/o	kidney	suprarenal	Above the kidney
rhin/o	nose	rhinorrhea	Discharge of thin mucus from the nose
salping/o	tube, oviduct	salpingectomy	Surgical removal of the oviduct
scler/o	hardening	arteriosclerosis	Hardening of the arteries
splen/o	spleen	splenectomy	Removal of the spleen
thorac/o	chest, thorax	thoracotomy	Surgical incision of the chest wall
thromb/o	blood clot	thrombosis	Formation or presence of a blood clot, usually causing obstruction of a vessel
tox/o, toxic/o	poison	toxoid	Modified bacterial toxin used to produce immunity
		toxicology	The study of poisons
trache/o	trachea	tracheostomy	Surgical creation of an opening into the trachea
trich/o	hair	trichology	Study of hair
ureter/o	ureter	ureterectasis	Dilation of the ureter
urethr/o	urethra	urethrostenosis	Narrowing of the urethra
ur/o	urine	anuria	Lack of urine formation
vas/o	vessel, duct	vasomotor	Pertaining to changes in the diameter of a vessel
vesic/o	urinary bladder	vesical	Pertaining to the urinary bladder

Suffixes

Suffix	Meaning	Example	Definition of Example
-algia	pain	gastralgia	Pain in the stomach
-cele	tumor, hernia, swelling	cystocele	Hernia of the bladder
-centesis	puncture, tap	paracentesis	Surgical puncture of a cavity for removal of fluid
-cide	killing	bactericide	Agent that kills bacteria
-ectasis	dilation, stretching	atelectasis	Incomplete expansion of the lungs
-ectomy	excision	tonsillectomy	Surgical removal of the tonsils
-emia	blood	ischemia	Insufficient blood supply to an area
-esthesia	pertaining to sensation	anesthesia	Loss of sensation
-form	shaped like	cruciform	Shaped like a cross

(continued)

Suffixes
(continued)

Suffix	Meaning	Example	Definition of Example
-gen, -genic	formation, origin, producing	fibrinogen	Substance in the blood that is converted to fibrin during blood clotting
		cardiogenic	Originating in the heart
-gram	record	echocardiogram	Record produced by echocardiography
-graph	recording instrument	pneumograph	Instrument for recording the rate and depth of respiration
-graphy	recording of data	radiography	The taking of x-ray pictures
-iasis	condition	helminthiasis	Infestation with worms
-ism	condition	embolism	Blockage of a blood vessel, usually by a blood clot
-itis	inflammation	pericarditis	Inflammation of the pericardium
-logy	study	etiology	Study of the origin of disease
-lysis	separation, disintegration	hemolysis	Rupture of red blood cells
-malacia	softening	osteomalacia	Softening of the bones
-megaly	enlargement	splenomegaly	Enlargement of the spleen
-meter	measuring instrument	calorimeter	Instruction for measuring heat production
-metry	measurement	pelvimetry	Measurement of the pelvis
-odynia	pain	cephalodynia	Pain in the head; headache
-oid	like, resembling	rheumatoid	Similar to rheumatism
-oma	tumor	sarcoma	Tumor of connective tissue
-osis	condition	narcosis	Unconsciousness due to narcotics
-pathy	disease	myopathy	Any disease of muscle
-penia	lack of	leukopenia	Abnormal decrease in the number of white blood cells
-pexy	surgical fixation	hysteropexy	Surgical fixation of the uterus
-phagia	eating	dysphagia	Difficulty in swallowing
-phil, -philic	attracting	basophil	White blood cell that stains with basic stain
-plasia	formation, molding	hyperplasia	Excessive growth of cells
-plasty	plastic repair	rhinoplasty	Plastic surgery of the nose
-plegia	paralysis	paraplegia	Paralysis of both legs and the lower part of the body
-pnea	breathing	apnea	Absence of breathing
-poiesis	formation, production	erythropoiesis	Formation of red blood cells
-ptosis	dropping	nephroptosis	Dropping of the kidney
-rhage, -rhagia	bursting forth	hemorrhage	Bursting forth of blood
		menorrhagia	Excessive menstrual bleeding
-rhaphy	surgical repair	herniorrhaphy	Surgical repair of a hernia
-rhea	discharge	pyorrhea	Discharge of pus
-rhexis	rupture	amniorrhexis	Rupture of the amnion
-scope	instrument for examining	cystoscope	Instrument for examining the bladder
-scopy	visual examination	bronchoscopy	Examination of the bronchi
-stasis	stoppage of flow	hemostasis	Prevention of blood loss
-stomy	surgical formation of an opening	colostomy	Surgical formation of an opening in the colon
-tomy	incision into	tracheotomy	Incision into the trachea
-trophy	nourishing	atrophy	Wasting or decrease in size of an organ or tissue
-tropic	acting on	gonadotropic	Acting on the gonads
-tripsy	crushing	lithotripsy	Crushing of a stone
-uresis	urination	diuresis	Elimination of large amounts of urine
-uria	urine	hematuria	Presence of blood in the urine

WORD ROOTS ACCORDING TO BODY SYSTEM

Circulatory System
angi/o
arteri/o
cardi/o
hem/o, hemat/o
lymph/o
myel/o
phleb/o
thromb/o
vas/o

Digestive System
chol/e
cholecyst/o
col/o
enter/o
gastr/o
gloss/o
hepat/o
ile/o
lith/o
odont/o
proct/o

Integumentary System
derm, dermat/o
onych/o
trich/o

Musculoskeletal System
arthr/o
brachi/o
cervic/o
chondr/o
cleid/o
cost/o
crani/o
ili/o
my/o
myel/o
os, oste/o
ped/o
rachi/o
sarc/o

Nervous System
audi/o
cerebr/o
encephal/o
kerat/o
medull/o
mening/o
myring/o
neur/o
ocul/o
ophthalm/o
ot/o
phac/o, phak/o
psych/o

Reproductive System
cervic/o
colp/o
hyster/o
labi/o
lact/o
mast/o
men/o
metr/o
oo
oophor/o
orchi/o, orchid/o
ovari/o
salping/o

Respiratory System
bronch/o
laryng/o
nas/o
pneum/o, pneumon/o
rhin/o
thora, thorac/o
trache/o

Urinary System
cyst/o
glomerul/o
nephr/o
pyel/o
ren/o
ureter/o
urethr/o
ur/o
vesic/o

Recommended Dietary Allowances, USA

Summary Table: Estimated Safe and Adequate Daily Dietary Intakes
of Selected Vitamins and Minerals*

		Vitamins	
Category	Age (yr)	Biotin (μg)	Pantothenic Acid (mg)
Infants	0–0.5	10	2
	0.5–1	15	3
Children and adolescents	1–3	20	3
	4–6	25	3–4
	7–10	30	4–5
	11+	30–100	4–7
Adults		30–100	4–7

		Trace Elements†				
Category	Age (yr)	Copper (mg)	Manganese (mg)	Fluoride (mg)	Chromium (μg)	Molybdenum (μg)
Infants	0–0.5	0.4–0.6	0.3–0.6	0.1–0.5	10–40	15–30
	0.5–1	0.6–0.7	0.6–1.0	0.2–1.0	20–60	20–40
Children and	1–3	0.7–1.0	1.0–1.5	0.5–1.5	20–80	25–50
adolescents	4–6	1.0–1.5	1.5–2.0	1.0–2.5	30–120	30–75
	7–10	1.0–2.0	2.0–3.0	1.5–2.5	50–200	50–150
	11+	1.5–2.5	2.0–5.0	1.5–2.5	50–200	75–250
Adults		1.5–3.0	2.0–5.0	1.5–4.0	50–200	75–250

* Because there is less information on which to base allowances, these figures are not given in the main table
of RDA and are provided here in the form of ranges of recommended intakes.
† Since the toxic levels for many trace elements may be only several times usual intakes, the upper levels for
the trace elements given in this table should not be habitually exceeded.

Food and Nutrition Board, National Academy of Sciences—National Research Council Recommended Dietary Allowances, Revised 1989*

Designed for the maintenance of good nutrition of practically all healthy people in the United States

| | | Weight† | | Height† | | Protein | Fat-Soluble Vitamins | | | |
| | Age (yr) | | | | | | Vita-min A | Vita-min D | Vita-min E | Vita-min K |
Category	or Condition	(kg)	(lb)	(cm)	(in)	(g)	(μg RE)‡	(μg)§	(mg α-TE)‖	(μg)
Infants	0.0–0.5	6	13	60	24	13	375	7.5	3	5
	0.5–1.0	9	20	71	28	14	375	10	4	10
Children	1–3	13	29	90	35	16	400	10	6	15
	4–6	20	44	112	44	24	500	10	7	20
	7–10	28	62	132	52	28	700	10	7	30
Male	11–14	45	99	157	62	45	1000	10	10	45
	15–18	66	145	176	69	59	1000	10	10	65
	19–24	72	160	177	70	58	1000	10	10	70
	25–50	79	174	176	70	63	1000	5	10	80
	51+	77	170	173	68	63	1000	5	10	80
Females	11–14	46	101	157	62	46	800	10	8	45
	15–18	55	120	163	64	44	800	10	8	55
	19–24	58	128	164	65	46	800	10	8	60
	25–50	63	138	163	64	50	800	5	8	65
	51+	65	143	160	63	50	800	5	8	65
Pregnant						60	800	10	10	65
Lactating	1st 6 months					65	1300	10	12	65
	2nd 6 months					62	1200	10	11	65

* The allowances, expressed as average daily intakes over time, are intended to provide for individual variations among most normal persons as they live in the United States under usual environmental stresses. Diets should be based on a variety of common foods to provide other nutrients for which human requirements have been less well defined. See test for detailed discussion of allowances and of nutrients not tabulated.

† Weights and heights of Reference Adults are actual medians for the U.S. population of the designated age, as reported by NHANES II. The median weights and heights of those under 19 years of age were taken from Hamill et al. (1979) (see pages 16–17). The use of these figures does not imply that the height-to-weight ratios are ideal.

‡ Retinol equivalents. 1 retinol equivalent = 1 μg retinol or 6 μg β-carotene. See text for calculation of vitamin A activity of diets as retinol equivalents.

§ As cholecalciferol. 10 μg cholecalciferol = 400 IU of vitamin D.

‖ α-Tocopherol equivalents. 1 mg d-α tocopherol = 1 α-TE. See text for variation in allowances and calculation of vitamin E activity of the diet as α-tocopherol equivalents.

¶ 1 NE (niacin equivalent) is equal to 1 mg of niacin or 60 mg of dietary tryptophan.

Reprinted with permission from Recommended Dietary Allowances, 10th edition, © 1989 by the National Academy of Sciences. Published by National Academy Press, Washington, DC.

	Water-Soluble Vitamins						Minerals						
Vitamin C (mg)	Thiamin (mg)	Riboflavin (mg)	Niacin (mg NE)¶	Vitamin B_6 (mg)	Folate (μg)	Vitamin B_{12} (μg)	Calcium (mg)	Phosphorus (mg)	Magnesium (mg)	Iron (mg)	Zinc (mg)	Iodine (μg)	Selenium (μg)
30	0.3	0.4	5	0.3	25	0.3	400	300	40	6	5	40	10
35	0.4	0.5	6	0.6	35	0.5	600	500	60	10	5	50	15
40	0.7	0.8	9	1.0	50	0.7	800	800	80	10	10	70	20
45	0.9	1.1	12	1.1	75	1.0	800	800	120	10	10	90	20
45	1.0	1.2	13	1.4	100	1.4	800	800	170	10	10	120	30
50	1.3	1.5	17	1.7	150	2.0	1200	1200	270	12	15	150	40
60	1.5	1.8	20	2.0	200	2.0	1200	1200	400	12	15	150	50
60	1.5	1.7	19	2.0	200	2.0	1200	1200	350	10	15	150	70
60	1.5	1.7	19	2.0	200	2.0	800	800	350	10	15	150	70
60	1.2	1.4	15	2.0	200	2.0	800	800	350	10	15	150	70
50	1.1	1.3	15	1.4	150	2.0	1200	1200	280	15	12	150	45
60	1.1	1.3	15	1.5	180	2.0	1200	1200	300	15	12	150	50
60	1.1	1.3	15	1.6	180	2.0	1200	1200	280	15	12	150	55
60	1.1	1.3	15	1.6	180	2.0	800	800	280	15	12	150	55
60	1.0	1.2	13	1.6	180	2.0	800	800	280	10	12	150	55
70	1.5	1.6	17	2.2	400	2.2	1200	1200	300	30	15	175	65
95	1.6	1.8	20	2.1	280	2.6	1200	1200	355	15	19	200	75
90	1.6	1.7	20	2.1	260	2.6	1200	1200	340	15	16	200	75

Nutrition Recommendations for Canadians

Recommended Nutrient Intake Based on Age and Body Weight Expressed as Daily Rates

Age	Sex	Weight (kg)	Protein (g)	Vit. A (RE*)	Vit. D (µg)	Vit. E (mg)	Vit. C (mg)	Folate (µg)	Vit. B₁₂ (µg)	Calcium (mg)	Phosphorus (mg)	Magnesium (mg)	Iron (mg)	Iodine (µg)	Zinc (mg)
Months															
0–4	Both	6.0	12†	400	10	3	20	25	0.3	250‡	150	20	0.3§	30	2§
5–12	Both	9.0	12	400	10	3	20	40	0.4	400	200	32	7	40	3
Years															
1	Both	11	13	400	10	3	20	40	0.5	500	300	40	6	55	4
2–3	Both	14	16	400	5	4	20	50	0.6	550	350	50	6	65	4
4–6	Both	18	19	500	5	5	25	70	0.8	600	400	65	8	85	5
7–9	M	25	26	700	2.5	7	25	90	1.0	700	500	100	8	110	7
	F	25	26	700	2.5	6	25	90	1.0	700	500	100	8	95	7
10–12	M	34	34	800	2.5	8	25	120	1.0	900	700	130	8	125	9
	F	36	36	800	2.5	7	25	130	1.0	1100	800	135	8	110	9
13–15	M	50	49	900	2.5	9	30‖	175	1.0	1100	900	185	10	160	12
	F	48	46	800	2.5	7	30‖	170	1.0	1000	850	180	13	160	9
16–18	M	62	58	1000	2.5	10	40‖	220	1.0	900	1000	230	10	160	12
	F	53	47	800	2.5	7	30‖	190	1.0	700	850	200	12	160	9
19–24	M	71	61	1000	2.5	10	40‖	220	1.0	800	1000	240	9	160	12
	F	58	50	800	2.5	7	30‖	180	1.0	700	850	200	13	160	9
25–49	M	74	64	1000	2.5	9	40‖	230	1.0	800	1000	250	9	160	12
	F	59	51	800	2.5	6	30‖	185	1.0	700	850	200	13	160	9
50–74	M	73	63	1000	5	7	40‖	230	1.0	800	1000	250	9	160	12
	F	63	54	800	5	6	30‖	195	1.0	800	850	210	8	160	9
75+	M	69	59	1000	5	6	40‖	215	1.0	800	1000	230	9	160	12
	F	64	55	800	5	5	30‖	200	1.0	800	850	210	8	160	9
Pregnancy (additional)															
1st Trimester			5	0	2.5	2	0	200	0.2	500	200	15	0	25	6
2nd Trimester			15	0	2.5	2	10	200	0.2	500	200	45	5	25	6
3rd Trimester			24	0	2.5	2	10	200	0.2	500	200	45	10	25	6
Lactation (additional)			20	400	2.5	3	25	100	0.2	500	200	65	0	50	6

* Retinol equivalents.
† Protein is assumed to be from breast milk and must be adjusted for infant formula.
‡ Infant formula with high phosphorus should contain 375 mg calcium.
§ Breast milk is assumed to be the source of the mineral.
‖ Smokers should increase vitamin C by 50%.
Nutrition Recommendations: The Report of the Scientific Review Committee 1990, p. 204. Published by the authority of the Minister of National Health and Welfare.

Glossary of Terms

Abduction Movement of a body part away from the midline of the body.

Abrasion Wound in which skin or mucous membranes are rubbed or scraped away.

Abscess Collection of debris from local tissues, dead and dying white blood cells, and bacteria without a blood supply to the center.

Absorption Process by which a medication enters the body.

Abstract thinking Level of thought that involves an idea apart from any material object.

Acid Any substance capable of releasing hydrogen ions in solution.

Acidosis Excessive acidity of body fluids; pH below 7.38.

Acne vulgaris Inflammatory disorder of the sebaceous glands; usually occurs in adolescence.

Action The performance of a specific function, step, or procedure.

Active range of motion Exercise or movement of joints done independently.

Active transport Movement of substances across a cell membrane against an electrochemical gradient.

Activities of daily living (ADLs) Activities frequently performed on a daily basis, such as bathing, grooming, eating, and toileting.

Activity tolerance Physical ability to withstand activity.

Actual nursing diagnosis An existing human response to a health problem identified by the nurse that is amenable to nursing intervention.

Acute Having a short and relatively severe course.

Acute pain Pain that lasts less than 6 months; usually associated with physical findings.

Adaptation Process by which a person changes to conform to the environment.

Addiction A psychological dependence with behavioral pattern of compulsive drug use or physical dependence to maintain self without signs and symptoms of withdrawal.

Adduction Movement of a body part toward the midline of the body.

Adenosine triphosphate (ATP) Nucleotide involved in energy metabolism, required for DNA synthesis, and used to store energy.

Administration Top-level management of an organization.

Adult day care An interdisciplinary service provided in congregate settings during specific daytime hours to disabled or impaired adults who need stimulation, supervision, socialization, or recreational therapy.

Adventitious breath sounds Abnormal lung sounds heard on auscultation.

Adverse effect Secondary effect of a drug (e.g., sensitivity, allergy, or idiosyncratic reactions).

Advocacy Communicating and acting on behalf of the welfare of another, especially a patient in the health-care system; keeping the patient informed about treatment and nursing care.

Aerobic Exercise requiring inspired oxygen for energy; involves elevation of heart rate for an extended period.

Aerosol Fine mist or spray of water, saline, or medication inhaled for therapeutic effects.

Affective Refers to emotional reactions (feeling as opposed to knowing).

Agent First link in the chain of infection; may be a bacteria, virus, fungus, or parasite.

Agonist Drug that has affinity for a receptor and is capable of eliciting a pharmacologic response.

Air embolus Air bubble in the vascular space that may obstruct circulation.

Airway resistance Increased work of breathing caused by narrowing of airway diameter.

Albuminuria Presence of albumin, a protein, in urine.

Aldosterone Adrenal cortex hormone that regulates sodium reabsorption.

Alkalosis Excessive alkalinity of body fluids; pH above 7.42.

Alveoli Spherical, saclike epithelial structures in the lungs through which gas exchange occurs.

Ambulatory care Health-care services (community, personal or combined) provided to a person who is not an in-patient in a health-care institution.

American Nurses Association Professional nursing organization concerned with all aspects of professional nursing; provides standards and leadership for the profession. ANA is comprised of individual state nursing associations and also has nursing specialty bodies representing all nursing practice areas.

Amino acids Building blocks from which proteins are constructed; end-products of protein digestion.

Ampule Small, sealed glass container.

Anabolism Building phase of metabolism in which the body converts simple substances into more complex substances (e.g., tissue repair, growth).

Anaerobic exercise Exercise in which muscles cannot extract enough oxygen, and anaerobic pathways are used to provide additional energy for a short time; useful in endurance training.

Analgesia Blockage of pain.

Analgesic Something that relieves pain.

Anaphylaxis Exaggerated allergic reaction to a foreign substance (drug or food); requires immediate medical intervention.

Anemia Insufficient number of red cells in the blood.

Anergy Inability to mount an immune response; seen in severe nutritional deficits.

Anesthesia Loss of sensation due to injury, disease, or a drug.

Anesthesiologist Physician who specializes in anesthesia administration.

Aneurysm Dilation or weakness of a blood vessel; occasionally seen as a localized ballooning.

Angina Pain and discomfort about the heart, characteristic of myocardial ischemia; severe pain felt in the anterior chest, shoulder, left arm, neck, and jaw.

Angiogram X-ray of blood vessels injected with radiopaque dye.

Anion Negatively charged ion.

Anonymity Protection of a research participant in such a way that the participant cannot be linked to the information provided.

Anorexia Loss of appetite.

Anorexia nervosa Eating disorder in which a person refuses to eat because of a fear of becoming overweight, even in the presence of normal or less than ideal body weight.

Antagonist Agent that blocks drugs from being used at the receptors (e.g., naloxone).

Anthropometric measurements Comparative body measurements (e.g., height and weight, skinfold measurements, limb circumference measurements).

Antibiotic Medication that can prevent the growth of or destroy bacterial organisms.

Antibody Protective substance produced by the body to protect it from an antigen.

Anticipatory grief Pattern of psychological and physiologic responses a person makes to the impending loss (real or imagined) of a significant person, object, belief, or relationship.

Anticoagulation Prevention of clot formation.

Antidiuretic hormone (ADH) Hypothalamic hormone stored in the posterior pituitary that promotes reabsorption of water by the kidney; also called vasopressin.

Antiemetic Drug given to prevent or relieve vomiting.

Antigen Substance that provokes irritation or damage to the body tissues and induces the formation of antibodies.

Antipyretic Medication used to reduce body temperature.

Antiseptic Agent that stops or slows the growth of microorganisms on living tissue.

Anuria Formation and excretion of less than 100 cc of urine in 24 hours.

Aorta Largest artery in the body; carries blood from the left ventricle to the body.

Aphasia Communication disorder that may affect speech, reading, and writing.

Apnea Absence of respiration.

Apneustic respirations Pattern of breathing characterized by a long inspiratory period that is gasping in nature and a short expiratory period.

Aquathermia pad Heating pad through which water circulates; used to apply local heat.

Arrhythmia Abnormal heart rate, rhythm, or pattern.

Arterial blood gases Set of blood tests used to assess acid–base balance and/or respiratory status.

Arteriosclerosis Disease characterized by thickening of arterioles with loss of elasticity and contractility due to fatty deposits and lesions.

Arthroscopy Direct visualization of a joint by insertion of a scope.

Articulation Enunciation of words and sentences.

Ascites Abnormal accumulation of fluid in the abdominal cavity.

Asepsis Absence of disease-producing microorganisms.

Asphyxiation Lack of oxygen, leading to cell death.

Aspiration Act of inhaling fluid or particulate matter into the bronchi.

Assault Threat of touching a person without his or her consent.

Assessment First phase of the nursing process. Data are gathered to identify actual or potential health problems.

Assisted range of motion Exercises that the patient can perform with help from another person.

Ataxia Abnormal lack of muscle coordination.

Atelectasis Collapse of alveoli.

Atrophy Wasting away of an organ, muscle, or body tissue.

Attention span deficit Inability to concentrate; patient is highly distractible and cannot screen out competing stimuli.

Audit Review of records.

Auricle Portion of the ear outside the head; the flap of the ear.

Auscultation Technique of listening to body sounds with a stethoscope.

Auscultatory gap Absence of audible sounds during blood pressure measurement that may cause inaccurate readings.

Autism State in which the patient is withdrawn and preoccupied with inner thoughts, daydreams, fantasies, delusions, and hallucinations.

Autonomy Degree of discretion and independence a practitioner has.

Axillae Armpits.

Bacteremia Presence of bacteria in the blood.

Bacteriocidal Able to kill bacteria.

Bacteriostatic Able to inhibit the growth of bacteria.

Bacteriuria Presence of bacteria in the urine that can cause infection of the urianry tract.

Bandage Piece of gauze or other material used to cover an injured body part.

Barium Contrast medium used in x-rays of the gastrointestinal system.

Barrel chest Increased diameter of the chest caused by air trapping; common in COPD.

Basal body temperature Temperature of the body taken early in the morning before getting out of bed. This temperature rises during ovulation.

Basal metabolic rate Amount of energy used by the body during absolute rest in an awake state.

Base Any substance that can combine with and decrease hydrogen ions in solution; alkali.

Battery Unlawful touching of a person's body without his or her consent.

Bedrest Restriction of activity to resting in bed.

Behaviors Observable actions.

Beliefs Ideas that a person accepts as true.

Belongingness and love needs Developing relationships with others and seeking friendship, love, and intimacy.

Bereavement Response to the death of a significant other.

Binder Large bandage used to support a body part or hold a dressing in place.

Biopsy Specimen of tissue or cells, or the procedure used to obtain the sample.

Biot's respirations Cyclic pattern of breathing characterized by periods of shallow breathing alternating with periods of apnea.

Biotransformation Chemical deactivation of a drug.

Blended family Two parents with unrelated children who are being raised together.

Blood gases Studies performed on arterial blood to evaluate the patient's oxygenation, ventilation, and metabolic (acid–base) status.

Blood pressure Force exerted by the blood against the walls of the blood vessels.

Blood transfusion Administration of blood or blood components into the circulatory system.

Body image Feelings about one's body.

Body mechanics Positioning or movement of the body to prevent or correct problems related to activity or immobilization.

Body substance isolation Protocol that recommends wearing gloves for contact with moist body membranes, nonintact skin, and moist body substances from all patients at all times. Gowns, masks, and goggles should be worn when splashing or soiling of the caregiver's face or clothing with the patient's body fluids is likely.

Bolus Concentrated form of medication given intravenously in a controlled fashion (IV push).

Borborygmus Rumbling sound produced by the normal movement of gas through the intestines (plural: borborygmi).

Bradycardia Abnormally slow heart rate (usually less than 60 beats per minute).

Bradypnea Abnormally slow respiratory rate (usually less than 10 breaths per minute).

Bronchioles Narrow airways that conduct air into alveolar ducts and alveoli.

Bronchospasm Narrowing of the bronchioles caused by tightening of smooth muscles in the airways.

Bronchovesicular breath sounds Muffled, blowing sounds of medium pitch normally heard over the mainstem bronchi.

Bruit Abnormal swishing or blowing sound heard on auscultation of veins or arteries; caused by increased turbulence of blood.

Buccal Pertaining to the inside cheek.

Buffer Compound that helps stabilize the pH of a solution by neutralizing added acid or base.

Bulla Serous skin elevation greater than 1 cm in size or diameter.

Burn Injury caused by exposure to thermal, chemical, electrical, or radioactive energy.

Burnout Depletion of energy and low morale.

Butterfly bandage Butterfly-shaped adhesive strip used to hold wound edges together.

Calorie (kilocalorie) Unit of heat; commonly used to describe the energy value of food.

Capillary Peripheral blood vessel.

Carbohydrates Food group containing simple sugars and complex sugars composed of carbon, hydrogen, and oxygen.

Cardiopulmonary response Pulse, blood pressure, and respiratory rate.

Care plan conference Meeting held to discuss care plan revisions and coordination of care.

Caregiver Person, usually a family member, responsible for providing day-to-day care, especially hygiene, nutrition, supervision and nurturance, for someone who has a functional or instrumental ADL impairment.

Carrier Person from whom a microorganism can be cultured but who shows no sign of disease.

Case finding Activities undertaken to identify people who need health or social services.

Case management Professional approach to providing care in which a patient's services are coordinated by one provider.

Catabolism Breaking-down process of metabolism in which energy is released by converting complex substances to simpler substances.

Catheter Tube placed into a body cavity or vessel for evacuating or injecting fluid.

Cation Positively charged ion.

Cellulitis Reddened area resulting from the inflammatory response with small vessel dilation, leakage of fluid from the endothelium, and WBC infiltration; usually a sign of infection.

Cerebrospinal fluid Fluid that circulates in the subarachnoid space and protects the brain and spinal cord from injury.

Certification Achievement of competence in a specialty area evidenced by successful completion of a variety of testing measures specified by the organization granting certification.

Change-of-shift report Information passed between nurses at change of shift about patient status and care plans.

Charge nurse Nurse responsible for the functioning of a nursing unit for a particular work shift.

Chemical drug name Name that gives a drug's molecular structure.

Chemoreceptors Nerve receptors that respond to chemical changes.

Chemotaxis Chemical attraction of the neutrophil toward the bacterial cell to be phagocytized.

Chemotherapeutic agents Chemicals used for therapeutic purposes in the body, such as antiviral medications and antibiotics; also used to refer to drugs used in cancer therapy.

Chest physiotherapy Treatment designed to facilitate removal of mucus from lungs; usually involves postural drainage.

Cheyne–Stokes respiration Respiratory pattern characterized by periods of respirations of increased rate and depth alternating with periods of apnea.

Chief complaint Patient's specific reason for seeking medical attention.

Cholesterol Type of animal fat;

needed for specific body functions, but an excess is harmful to the arteries.

Chronic Persisting over a long period of time.

Chronic bronchitis Disease characterized by cough, greatly increased mucus production, and chronic inflammation and infection of larger airways.

Chronic obstructive pulmonary disease (COPD) Usually a combination of chronic bronchitis and emphysema.

Chronic pain Pain that lasts more than 6 months.

Chyme Partially digested food and digestive secretions of the stomach and small intestine.

Circadian rhythm Regular occurrence of certain phenomena in cycles of about 24 hours.

Circadian thermal rhythm Fluctuations in normal body temperature occurring over a 24-hour period.

Circle of confidentiality Professionals with whom patient information can be shared.

Circumcision Surgical removal of the foreskin from the head of the penis.

Clean-catch urine sample Small amount of voided urine that has been obtained after the urinary meatus has been cleansed with soap or disinfectant.

Cleaning Physical removal of visible dirt and debris.

Climacteric Menopause.

Clinical judgment Process of evaluating patient cues to make an accurate nursing diagnosis.

Clinical nurse specialist Registered nurse who holds a master's degree in a nursing specialty and has advanced clinical experience.

Clitoris Small erectile organ located just above the urinary meatus in females; plays a key role in female orgasm.

Clustering Combining patient data into meaningful patterns.

Coagulation Blood clotting.

Cognition Thinking and awareness; system by which sensory input, past experiences, and emotions are integrated and made meaningful.

Cognitive Refers to rational thought (knowing as opposed to feeling).

Cognitive function Ability to think, understand, and communicate with the environment.

Cognitive level Degree of ability to know, think, and remember.

Coitus interruptus Withdrawal of the penis from the vagina just before ejaculation; an ineffective means of contraception.

Collaboration Actions taken in coordination with other professionals.

Collaborative health problem Problems based on medical diagnoses, medically ordered treatments, or other related problems that require interdependent standards and activity to be addressed.

Colonization State in which a microorganism is present but no immune reaction or tissue destruction occurs.

Colostomy Opening of a part of the colon onto the abdominal skin surface.

Coma Abnormally deep stupor occurring in illness or as a result of injury. The patient cannot be aroused by external stimuli.

Communal family Related and unrelated people with common goals and beliefs sharing a household.

Communicable disease Disease transmissible between hosts.

Communication Interchange of information.

Communication channel Medium through which a message is sent (e.g., television, writing, speaking).

Community Social group whose members may or may not share common geographic boundaries but interact because of common interests or shared values to meet their needs within a larger society.

Community-acquired infections Infections that are present and symptomatic on admission to the hospital or within 24 hours after admission.

Complete protein Protein that contains sufficient amounts of essential amino acids to maintain body tissues and to promote body growth.

Compliance 1. Adherence to recommended plan. 2. Measure of the "stretchiness" of the lung.

Comprehension Capacity for understanding and reasoning.

Conceptual framework Formal explanation that links concepts and emphasizes relationships among them.

Concrete thinking Objects or groups of things that can be perceived by the senses; objective reality.

Condom catheter (external, Texas) Noninvasive urinary collection device for incontinent male patients; consists of a thin flexible sheath placed over the penis and attached to tubing and a collection bag.

Confidentiality Practice of keeping patient information private.

Confusion Impaired cognition; ranges from mild memory or orientation deficits to profoundly disorganized thinking.

Consultation Conferring with another professional to obtain his or her assessment of a situation or patient.

Consumer Person who engages the services of another while retaining rights and responsibilities related to the service provided.

Consumerism Public's expectation that they will have a voice in determining the type, quality, and cost of care being provided.

Contact Person who has been near an infected person and may have been exposed to an infectious disease.

Contamination State in which microorganisms are present on an inanimate object or on the body surface without tissue invasion.

Continuing education Education beyond basic preparation; purpose is to remain current in knowledge and practice.

Continuity of care Provision of uninterrupted service as a patient moves between settings.

Contraception Any method of preventing pregnancy.

Contract Negotiated agreement between nurse and patient in which roles and responsibilities of each are delineated.

Contractility Force of contraction.

Contracture Shortening or distortion of muscle tissue so that the joint cannot be extended.

Contrast medium Material that appears solid in x-rays; used to outline cavities and blood vessels to show abnormalities.

Controlling Management function that involves checking that plans are being carried out effectively and evaluating the outcomes of the actions.

Coordination Act of assembling and directing activities of others so that services are provided harmoniously.

Coping Problem-solving process a

person uses to manage stresses or events.

Coping mechanism Effort used to manage stress.

Core temperature Internal temperature of the body.

Crackles Abnormal breath sounds; rales.

Credentialing Method of ensuring quality health-care services (e.g., licensure, certification, degrees).

Crepitus Crunching or grating sounds that occur when bones rub against one another during movement.

Critical pathway Standard care plan used to establish and monitor the extent and timing of care; includes key elements such as diagnostic tests, consultations, treatments, activities, procedures, and discharge planning and teaching.

Cue Piece of data, subjective or objective, about a patient.

Cultural relativity Principle that meaning is created by one's culture and truth is culture specific; the same experience may carry different meanings to people of different cultures.

Cultural sensitivity Acceptance of a culture other than one's own.

Culture 1. Behavior and institutions of a given society. 2. Growth of microorganisms in a specialized medium under precise conditions.

Culture shock Failure to comprehend the culture in which one is living.

Data Pieces of information.

Debridement Removal of foreign material or dying tissue from a wound.

Decision-making process Method of analyzing a problem, determining alternatives, and selecting the appropriate action.

Decoding Process of understanding a message.

Decompression Removal of pressure caused by an accumulation of gas and fluids.

Decontamination Removal of potential pathogens.

Decubitus ulcer Breakdown of the surface of body tissue; caused by prolonged pressure on a body part.

Deductive theory Process by which specific predictions are developed from general principles.

Defecation Elimination of solid waste from the bowels.

Defecation reflex Involuntary response of intestinal contraction and anal sphincter relaxation to rectal distention.

Defendant Person being sued or accused.

Deglutition Swallowing.

Dehiscence Accidental separation of wound edges, especially a surgical wound.

Dehydration Condition resulting from excessive loss of body water.

Delirium Reversible disorder of cognition; confusion.

Delusion Belief that is not based in reality and that reflects an unconscious need or fear.

Demands of daily living (DDLs) Responsibilities generated by job, house, car, pets, environment, and so on.

Dementia Cognitive impairment as the result of irreversible organic changes in brain cell function.

Deontology Theory of philosophy that examines our duty to moral law or moral principles.

Dependent variable Variable (or item of interest that varies) that is the outcome; hypothesized to depend on or be caused by another variable.

Depressive pseudodementia Dementialike syndrome due to depression rather than cerebral degeneration.

Dermatitis Various skin conditions involving inflammation.

Dermis Layer of skin beneath the epidermis; composed of dense connective fibers, blood vessels, nerves, hair follicles, and glands.

Detrusor Smooth muscle of the urinary bladder.

Development Process of ongoing change throughout a person's life.

Developmental stages Points in life when old responsibilities are discarded and new ones are taken on.

Developmental tasks Psychomotor, psychosocial, or cognitive skills attained at certain stages of life that are prerequisites for successive skill development.

Diagnosis-related groups (DRGs) Categories or classifications of illnesses, disorders, procedures, or other conditions necessitating hospitalization from which cost of care is predetermined.

Diagnostic process Skills used to make nursing diagnoses.

Diaphragmatic breathing Breathing exercise using the diaphragm to obtain a deep breath.

Diastole Period of rest in the cardiac cycle, when the ventricles are not contracting and the coronary arteries are filling with blood.

Diastolic blood pressure Pressure in the blood vessels during cardiac ventricular relaxation.

Diffusion Movement of molecules from an area of higher concentration to one of lower concentration.

Digestion Mechanical and chemical processes necessary to convert food to an absorbable state.

Direct care Care that requires the professional to interact directly with the patient.

Directing Management function of supervision and ongoing decision-making to get people to carry out plans.

Directive leadership Leadership style in which the leader makes all the decisions and tells subordinates what to do.

Disability Degree of physical or mental impairment.

Discharge planner Health professional who coordinates services for patients making the transition from one health-care setting to another setting.

Discharge planning Process of coordinating, planning, and arranging for the transition from one health-care setting to another setting.

Disinfectant Chemical used to kill microorganisms on lifeless objects.

Disinfection Reduction in the number of microorganisms by physical or chemical means.

Disorganized thinking Disorder manifested by inappropriate interactions and conversations with others, talking or gesturing to oneself, performing inappropriate activities, or other confused or bizarre behavior.

Disorientation Lack of awareness of identity or environment (person, place, time).

Distention Condition of being stretched or inflated.

Distress Too much or too little arousal of a person's mind and body, resulting in harm to the mind or body.

Distressor Demand on the mind or body leading to distress.

Distribution Process by which a drug

passes from the circulation of blood and lymphatic systems across cell membranes to a specified tissue.

Disuse osteoporosis Decrease in bone density due to lack of activity or stress on bones.

Diuresis Formation and excretion of large amounts of urine.

Diuretics Drugs that cause the kidney to form and excrete more urine.

Doppler Hand-held transducer that directs high-frequency sound waves to the organ or vessel being scanned during ultrasonography.

Dorsiflexion Bending at the ankle joint so as to point toes upward.

Drain Device used to remove excess fluid from a wound or body area.

Drug Substance that alters physiologic function with the potential for affecting health.

Dualism Theory that divides concepts into two mutually irreducible elements.

Duodenocolic reflex Involuntary response of intestinal contraction and motility to duodenal distention.

Dysarthria Disorders affecting either single or combined motor control of the muscles of speech.

Dysfunction Action that does not meet expected norms.

Dysfunctional grief Grief that falls outside normal parameters; may be manifested as absence of grief, delayed grief, exaggerated grief, or prolonged grief.

Dyspareunia Painful sexual intercourse.

Dyspnea Breathing that requires marked effort.

Dysuria Painful voiding.

Eczema Inflammatory skin condition characterized by erythema, papules, vesicles, scales, and crusts.

Edema Accumulation of fluid in the interstitial tissues.

Effective communication Transfer of meaning between two or more people.

Elective surgery Surgical procedure performed at the desire of the patient but not needed to preserve life or function.

Electrocardiogram (EKG, ECG) Record of heart action showing specific patterns of electrical activity in the heart muscle.

Electroencephalogram (EEG) Record of electrical activity in the brain.

Electrolyte Chemical compound that dissociates into ions when in solution; usually refers to extracellular sodium, potassium, and chloride.

Embolus Foreign substance, usually a blood clot, circulating in the blood and lodging in small arterial vessels.

Embryo Stage of development from the second week after conception to about 8 weeks, during which time major structures and organs are formed.

Emergent surgery Situation in which surgery must be performed immediately to preserve the function of a body part or the life of the patient.

Empathy Ability to understand how another person sees a situation, while maintaining objectivity.

Emphysema Disease characterized by loss of bronchiolar smooth muscle tone, destruction of alveoli, and air trapping.

Encoding Process of translating the purpose of a communication into a message that can be sent.

Endemic Infectious disease restricted to a particular nation, region, or group; found in a community all the time but does not spread.

Endocardium Innermost layer of the heart muscle; covers all internal surfaces of the heart and is lined by endothelium continuous with that of the blood vessels.

Endogenous (autogenous) From a source inside the patient.

Endorphins Endogenous opiates that alter pain perception.

Endoscopy Procedure allowing visual inspection of hollow body organs using a fiberoptic instrument.

Endothelium Single layer of cells lining the blood vessels and the heart.

Endurance Ability to withstand physical or other stressors over time.

Enema Insertion of fluid into the rectum and colon.

Enteral nutrition Delivery of nutrition into the gastrointestinal system, usually in the form of tube feedings.

Enuresis Bedwetting; involuntary voiding by a child who has otherwise attained control over urinary elimination.

Environment Context in which a person lives; includes social and inanimate characteristics.

Epicardium Serous, external layer of the heart.

Epidemic Disease that breaks out in a large proportion of the population.

Epidemiology Study of the causative agents of disease, occurrence of disease, and distribution of health and disease in populations; also concerned with defining risks for contracting diseases.

Epidermis Thin, avascular, outermost layer of skin.

Erythema Redness of the skin.

Eschar Black, leathery crust of dead tissue covering a wound.

Esophagus Muscular tube connecting the pharynx and the stomach.

Esteem needs Two types: esteem derived from others and self-esteem (feelings of self-worth marked by the perception of confidence, competence, achievement, and productivity).

Ethics Professional standards of behavior related to right and wrong.

Ethnicity or ethnic identity Shared cultural characteristics that symbolize a common group origin.

Ethnocentrism Use of one's own culture to judge the beliefs, behaviors, attitudes, and values of people of another culture.

Etiology Cause or origin.

Evaluation Judgment of the effectiveness of nursing care in achieving patient goals.

Eversion Turning the feet outward so toes are pointed away from the midline.

Evisceration Protrusion of internal organs through an open wound.

Exanthem Skin rash or eruption occurring in certain infectious diseases.

Excitement phase First phase in the human sexual response cycle, according to Masters and Johnson, in which there is initial response to physiologic or psychological stimuli.

Excoriation Loss of superficial skin layers.

Excretion Process by which a drug or waste product is eliminated from the body.

Exogenous From a source other than the patient.

Extension Straightening a joint.

External rotation Lateral rotation of the anterior surface of a limb.

Extracellular fluid compartment (EFC) Body fluid outside the cells; mainly interstitial fluid and plasma.

Exudate Fluid that has penetrated from blood vessels into surrounding tissues as the result of inflammation.

Faith Belief held; a relational phenomenon.

Family Basic human social unit; membership is based on mutual commitment, heredity, or legal arrangements.

Family development tasks Activities that usually occur at pre-expansion, expansion, dispersion, and replacement stages of family life. The failure to accomplish these tasks may identify families at risk for dysfunction.

Fasting Doing without food for a period of time.

Fatigue A subjective state of weariness, lack of energy.

Fats Lipid organic substances composed of carbon, hydrogen, and oxygen.

Febrile With an elevated temperature.

Fecal impaction Hard stool lodged in the rectum.

Feces Solid waste products of digestion; stool.

Feedback loop Output is rerouted back to the system as input.

Fetus Stage of development from 8 weeks after conception to birth.

Fever State in which the body's core temperature rises above the normal level for that person during rest.

Fiber Component of food that adds bulk to the diet and is not broken down by digestion.

Fight-or-flight response Sympathetic physiologic response that prepares a person to fight or to flee from a stressor.

Filtration Passage of a solution through a semipermeable membrane from a region of higher pressure to a region of lower pressure.

Filtration pressure Hydrostatic pressure minus osmotic pressure; determines the direction of flow across a membrane or vessel wall.

Fistula Abnormal tubelike passage between organs or between an organ and the body surface, often as the result of poor wound healing.

Flaccid Without muscle tone or resistance.

Flatus Gas in the gastrointestinal tract.

Flexibility Ability to bend without excessive resistance.

Flexion Bending or being bent so as to decrease the angle between two bones at a joint.

Flora Microorganisms.

Flowsheet Form for charting routine nursing procedures.

Fluid overload Condition of excessive extracellular fluid that can be due to the overadministration of IV fluids.

Fluid volume deficit Abnormal reduction in isotonic extracellular fluid; also called hypovolemia, saline deficit, or isotonic dehydration.

Fluid volume excess Abnormal increase in isotonic extracellular fluid.

Fluoroscopy X-ray visualization of organs or movement within organs.

Foot drop Temporary or permanent plantar flexion due to weakness or paralysis.

Foreskin Loose skin at the head of the penis, removed during circumcision; prepuce.

Fowler's position Semisitting position in bed.

Frequency 1. Measurement of vibrations. 2. Voiding more often than usual.

Functional health patterns A framework for collecting and organizing nursing assessment data to ascertain the strengths of the patient as well as any dysfunctional or potentially dysfunctional patterns that exist.

Gait Character of one's walk.

General adaptation syndrome Response to stress composed of three stages: alarm reaction, stage of resistance, and stage of exhaustion.

General anesthetic Agent used to induce complete loss of sensation and consciousness.

Generic drug name Product or medication not protected by trademark; nonproprietary name assigned to a drug.

Genetics Characteristics determined by the DNA code inherited from biologic mother and father.

Germicide Agent that destroys microorganisms, particularly pathogens; used on both living tissue and inanimate objects.

Glomerular filtrate Plasma fluid that is filtered out by the glomerular capillaries of the nephron and passes in the nephron tubule.

Glucosuria Presence of an abnormal amount of sugar, specifically glucose, in urine.

Glycogenesis Anabolic process of glycogen storage; formation of glycogen from glucose.

Glycogenolysis Catabolic process that converts stored glycogen into glucose so it can be used as an energy source.

Glyconeogenesis Catabolic process occurring in the liver that forms glycogen from noncarbohydrate sources such as amino acids or fatty acids.

Goal 1. Aim or expected end to work toward. 2. Desired outcome of nursing care.

Gram stain Process to identify microorganisms in which a slide of a specimen is stained with identifying chemicals.

Granulation tissue Soft, pink, highly vascularized connective tissue formed during wound repair.

Granulocytes Polymorphonuclear white blood cells: neutrophils, eosinophils, and basophils.

Grief Psychological and physiologic response after the loss of a significant person, object, belief, or relationship.

Ground To connect electricity between an electrical conductor and the ground or earth.

Growth Progressive increase in physical size or psychosocial development.

Guaiac Test to reveal the presence of blood in urine or feces.

Half-life Time required for a drug or substance to lose 50% of its activity through metabolism or elimination.

Hallucination False sensory perception; seeing, hearing, smelling, feeling, or tasting objects that are not there.

Head nurse Department head or manager responsible for all operations of a patient-care unit; provides a vital communication link between the patient, the direct-care providers, and the administration.

Health 1. State of well-being and optimal functioning. 2. Interactive process between the person and the internal and external environment. The person responds to changes in the environment to maintain integrity and harmony.

Health-care delivery system People, institutions, and associated businesses responsible for providing health care to the public.

Health insurance Protection against the cost of medical care and hospitalization.

Health maintenance Positive health behaviors to preserve a current state of health.

Health maintenance organization (HMO) Organization that provides comprehensive health services to members for a set monthly fee.

Health promotion Health behaviors that enhance a person's level of health.

Health status Level of health.

Hematocrit Percent of red blood cells in a given volume of whole blood.

Hematology Study of blood components.

Hematoma Localized accumulation of blood in a body tissue, organ, or space as the result of broken blood vessels.

Hematuria Presence of blood in urine.

Hemoglobin Oxygen-carrying component of the red blood cell.

Heterosexual Person who relates sexually to a member of the opposite sex.

High-level wellness Way of living in which a person strives toward the highest potential in physical, mental, emotional, and spiritual health.

High-risk nursing diagnosis State of being at risk for the development of a health problem amenable to nursing intervention; formerly called a potential nursing diagnosis.

Holism Seeing the universe—and the patient—as a system of connected parts rather than a sum of isolated parts.

Home health aide Person hired to provide basic hygiene for homebound patients.

Home health care Health-care services provided at home.

Home management Ability to maintain oneself in a safe, nurturing home.

Homebound Unable to leave home because of poor health.

Homeless Lacking a permanent residence or having no shelter.

Homeostasis State of balance in the body, including the balance of body fluids and their chemical constituents.

Homosexual Person who relates sexually to a member of the same sex.

Hormonal dyssynchrony Situation in which the circadian rhythms of different hormones adjust to changes in sleeping time at different rates.

Hospice Family-focused health service that provides care for terminally ill patients.

Hospital Information System (HIS) Computer system developed for the needs of hospitals.

Host Person or animal who harbors and nourishes a microorganism.

Human need Physiologic or psychological factor necessary for a healthy existence.

Human sexual response cycle Pattern of physiologic responses to sexual stimulation proceeding from arousal to orgasm.

Humidification Addition of water vapor to inspired air to prevent drying of the respiratory mucosa.

Hydrostatic pressure Pressure exerted by a fluid against the walls of its container (e.g., against vessel walls).

Hypercalcemia High concentration of calcium in the blood.

Hyperextension Extension of a joint beyond its normal (or intended) range of motion.

Hyperkalemia High concentration of potassium in the blood.

Hyperlipoproteinemia Excessive fat-protein molecules in the blood; includes fat-protein combinations such as high-density lipoproteins (HDL), low-density lipoproteins (LDL), and triglycerides.

Hypermagnesemia High concentration of magnesium in the blood.

Hypernatremia High concentration of sodium in the blood; also called water deficit.

Hyperpyrexia Fever that becomes life-threatening.

Hyperresonant Increased propagation of sound on percussion.

Hypertension Abnormally high blood pressure.

Hyperthermia Above-normal core temperature.

Hypertonic Of greater concentration than in body fluids.

Hyperventilation Breathing in excess of metabolic demands, resulting in removal of too much carbon dioxide from the blood; indicated by decreased $PaCO_2$.

Hypnotic Medication that induces or maintains sleep.

Hypocalcemia Low concentration of calcium in the blood.

Hypokalemia Low concentration of potassium in the blood.

Hypomagnesemia Low concentration of magnesium in the blood.

Hyponatremia Low concentration of sodium in the blood; also called water excess.

Hypotension Abnormally low blood pressure.

Hypothermia Below-normal core temperature.

Hypothesis Statement that predicts the relationships between the variables under study.

Hypotonic Of lower concentration than in body fluids.

Hypoventilation Breathing insufficient to meet metabolic demands and adequately remove carbon dioxide from the blood; indicated by elevated $PaCO_2$.

Hypovolemia Abnormally decreased volume of circulating plasma.

Hypoxemia Below-normal amount of oxygen in the blood.

Hypoxia Decreased amount of oxygen available to the tissues.

Hypoxic drive Stimulus to breathe based on decreased PaO_2; found in some COPD patients.

Iatrogenic infection Infection caused as the result of receiving health-care treatment.

ICU psychosis State of delirium and agitation that can occur after several days in an ICU; caused by obtrusive stimuli, sleep deprivation, and acute illness. Usually reverses a few days after leaving the ICU.

Ideal body weight Body weight optimal for functioning and health.

Identity Awareness of self, as separate and distinct from others.

Ileostomy Opening of the ileum onto the abdominal skin surface.

Illness Subjective symptoms of disease such as malaise, nausea, and vomiting.

Illness prevention Positive behaviors to prevent illness or disease; also known as health promotion.

Imagery Focusing the mind on a series of images for self-awareness, relaxation, and healing.

Immobility State in which the patient cannot or does not move.

Immunity Resistance to a specific infection; may be naturally or artificially acquired.

Immunosuppression Unresponsiveness of the body's immune system to the presence of a foreign substance.

Impetigo Highly contagious skin infection characterized by bullae and pustules.

Implementation Action phase of the nursing process, in which nursing care is provided.

Impotence Inability to attain or maintain an erection long enough to have satisfactory sexual intercourse.

Incentive spirometer Breathing exercise device that uses sustained maximal inspiration to prevent or reverse atelectasis.

Incidence Rate or range of occurrence of a disease.

Incident Unusual happening to a patient or visitor at a health-care facility.

Incision Cut or wound made by a sharp instrument, usually during a surgical procedure.

Incomplete protein Protein that does not contain enough amino acid to independently maintain life, build tissue, or promote growth.

Incontinence Inability to control excretion from the bowel or bladder.

Independence Ability to carry out activities of daily living autonomously.

Independent variable Variable that causes or affects the dependent variable.

Indirect care Care provided in which the professional does not interact with the patient; rather, the care is given by people under the professional's direction.

Inductive theory Process by which specific observations lead to more general rules.

Indwelling catheter Tube placed through the urethra into the bladder to drain urine.

Infarction Dead tissue resulting from ischemia due to lack of circulation.

Infection Organ or tissue dysfunction caused by microorganisms.

Infectious disease Process resulting from infection that produces manifestations such as fever, leukocytosis, inflammation, or tissue damage.

Infectivity Ability to invade and multiply within the host.

Infiltration Abnormal or accidental seepage or deposition of a substance into the tissues; accidental administration of IV fluids into subcutaneous tissues that occurs when the needle or catheter becomes dislodged from the vein.

Influence Power to bring about a change in others.

Information processing theory Method of organizing information so that cues can be used to make accurate diagnoses.

Informed consent Legal document giving permission for surgical or diagnostic procedure signed by patient or legal guardian; before signing the physician has explained all aspects of the surgery, including the risks.

Inpatient Patient who occupies a hospital bed.

Insensible evaporation Body water that is continuously being lost through evaporation from the skin and lungs.

In-service education Education provided at a health-care facility to orient and update employees.

Insomnia Difficulty sleeping; may be characterized by trouble falling asleep or staying asleep, or waking too early.

Inspection Systematic visual examination of the patient.

Integument Skin.

Intellectual function Memory, comprehension, and concentration.

Intelligence Measurable product of intellectual functioning.

Intensity Loudness of sound.

Interaction Response or action between a drug and the body cells.

Interdisciplinary Involving members of different fields or specialties, who interact to maximize the effectiveness of health care.

Interferon Protein that retards viral replication. It is produced by body cells on exposure to viruses and it triggers a reaction that neutralizes the virus.

Intermittent positive pressure breathing (IPPB) Treatment that provides deep breaths under pressure

to improve air distribution in the lungs.

Internal rotation Rotation toward the midline of the anterior surface of a limb.

International Council of Nurses Nursing organization concerned with health and nursing care throughout the world.

Intervention Activity carried out by the nurse.

Interview Goal-directed conversation in which the nurse questions the patient.

Intra-arterial Involving administration of a medication within an artery.

Intracellular fluid compartment (IFC) Portion of body fluid contained within the cells.

Intradermal Involving administration of a medication into the dermis.

Intramuscular Involving administration of a medication within muscle tissue.

Intraoperative period Time that starts when the patient is transferred to the operating room and ends with transfer to the recovery area.

Intraspinal Involving administration of a medication within the substance of the spinal column; also called intrathecal.

Intravenous (IV) Involving administration of medication within a vein.

Intravenous therapy Infusion of a fluid into a vein to treat or prevent fluid and electrolyte or nutritional imbalances; may be used to deliver medications or blood products.

Intuition Use of insight, instincts, and clinical experience to make judgments.

Invasiveness Ability of microorganisms to enter tissues.

Inversion Turning the feet inward so toes are pointing toward the midline.

Ion Charged particle formed by the dissociation of electrolytes in solution.

Irrigation 1. The cleansing of a wound or body cavity by flushing with fluid. 2. The cleansing of a tube with solution to clear a blockage.

Ischemia Insufficient blood supply in a body part due to obstruction of circulation.

Isometric exercise Exercise involving muscle contraction without a change in muscle length (often occurs against resistance).

Isotonic Osmotic concentration equal to that of body fluids.

Isotonic exercise Dynamic form of exercise in which there is constant muscle muscle tension, muscle contraction, and active movement.

IV time strip Strip of tape placed on an IV solution container marked to indicate the amount of fluid expected to infuse each hour.

Judgment Process of reasoning; ability to process incoming stimuli and determine meanings that encompass many aspects of a situation.

Kardex Trade name of a care plan documentation system.

Kegel exercises Exercises to strengthen the muscles of the pelvic floor.

Key informant Person who knows and will discuss certain aspects of his or her culture with someone outside that culture.

Kinship Relationship between people based on common blood ties.

Korotkoff sounds Sounds heard during auscultation that indicate the systolic and diastolic blood pressure.

Kussmaul respirations Pattern of breathing characterized by respirations of increased rate and depth.

Kyphosis Exaggerated curvature of the thoracic spine; hunchback.

Labia Fleshy border of the female external genitalia; divided into labia majora and labia minora.

Laceration Wound caused by tearing of body tissue.

Language A prescribed way of using words; a means of expressing thoughts and feelings.

Lacrimal fluid Tears.

Laryngectomy Excision of the larynx.

Laws Standards of human conduct established and enforced by the authority of an organized society through its government.

Laxative Medication that causes bowel elimination.

Leadership Ability to influence others to strive for a goal or to change.

Leadership style Manner in which

the leader interacts with subordinates.

Learning Process of acquiring knowledge; a multidimensional process that depends on symbols, language, classifications, concepts, and other concrete operations along with abstract functions.

Learning nursing care plan Educational tool to help students learn the nursing process.

Lesbian Female homosexual.

Lesion Injured or diseased area of the skin or other body tissue.

Leukocytosis Increase in production of white blood cells.

Leukopenia Insufficiency of white blood cells in the blood.

Liability Responsibility for one's actions; an obligation one is bound to perform.

Licensed practical nurse Person licensed by a state after completing a state-approved nursing program to provide technical nursing care under the direct supervision of a registered nurse.

Licensure Process for ensuring safe practice in nursing. States grant permission via licensure for qualified professionals to practice professional nursing. Qualification is determined by successful completion of the licensure examination developed by each state's board of nursing.

Literature review Process of selecting published materials about the concepts to be examined in a research project.

Local adaptation syndrome Localized expression of the three stages of the general adaptation syndrome.

Long-term care Health-care services provided over a period of time to patients who need ongoing care; generally provided in institutions such as nursing homes.

Lordosis Exaggerated curvature of the lumbar spine; swayback.

Lumbar puncture Puncture, usually between the third and fourth lumbar vertebrae, to obtain cerebrospinal fluid.

Maceration Softening of tissue due to excessive moisture.

Macrodrip IV tubing that delivers 10, 15, or 20 drops per milliliter.

Macula Spotted, nonelevated discoloration of the skin.

Malignant hyperthermia Severe body temperature elevation after administration of certain anesthetics.

Malpractice Professional misconduct; causing harm or injury to a person from lack of experience, skill, knowledge, or judgment.

Mammogram Radiograph of the breast; used to detect breast tumors or cysts.

Managed care Model of nursing care delivery in which the primary nurse uses a predetermined critical pathway to establish and monitor care within an anticipated length of hospital stay.

Management Getting the job done or accomplishing a goal through the functions of planning, organizing, directing, and controlling.

Mastication Chewing.

Masturbation Autostimulation of the genitals.

Maturation Process of development.

Meconium First feces of a newborn.

Medicaid Government-funded health insurance plan that provides financial assistance to the disabled or financially needy.

Medical diagnosis Identified disease or pathologic process; treatment focuses on correcting or preventing specific pathology of specific organs or body systems.

Medicare Federally funded program that provides medical and hospital insurance to people age 65 or older or those who are disabled.

Medication Drug given for its therapeutic effects. All medications are drugs.

Meditation Purposeful quieting of the mind to experience inner peace.

Melanin Pigment found normally in the skin that gives it a brown color and protects it from ultraviolet light.

Menarche First menstrual period.

Menopause Permanent cessation of menstruation.

Mental health Mental or emotional well-being in terms of interpersonal relationships, role fulfillment, and achievement in work, family, and community.

Metabolism 1. Chemical reactions in the cells that produce heat as a byproduct. 2. Breakdown of a drug (usually in the liver) to an inactive form.

Metacommunication Meanings beyond the literal level of communication, such as the roles of the communicators and the context in which the communication is taking place.

Method Procedure a researcher follows to gather and analyze data.

Microdrip IV tubing that delivers 60 drops per milliliter.

Micturition Urination.

Milliequivalent (mEq) Unit used to give the concentration of an electrolyte in solution; commonly expressed as mEq/L.

Minority Smaller segment of a society.

Mode of transmission Way in which a microorganism moves from the source to the host.

Monosaccharides Simple sugars.

Montgomery straps (or ties) Adhesive strips with ties used to hold dressings in place; they allow frequent changes without the need for tape removal.

Moral Involving correct behavior.

Motivation Something that provides drive or incentive.

Mourning Behavior after the death of a significant other. Mourning behaviors vary from culture to culture.

Mucociliary escalator Mucus blanket that lies on top of ciliated cells in airways. It traps bacteria and dust and moves them upward toward the mouth for expectoration.

Mucosa Mucous membrane lining many tubular body structures; capable of secreting mucus.

Multidisciplinary Involving people of different specialties who work together.

Multi-infarct dementia Dementia that results from multiple small infarcts in cerebral vessels.

Myelogram Radiographic procedure to evaluate the subarachnoid space around the spinal cord.

Myocardium Layer of cardiac muscle that forms the walls of the heart.

Myoclonus Uncontrolled muscle movements.

Narcolepsy Sleep disorder characterized by sudden uncontrollable episodes of sleep.

National League for Nursing Organization that serves as the accrediting body for nursing education programs.

Nebulizer Device that breaks liquids into tiny droplets for aerosol therapy.

Necrosis Localized areas of dead tissue, dying leukocytes, bacteria, and cellular debris.

Negative nitrogen balance State in which nitrogen excretion is greater than intake; can occur due to impaired protein synthesis or excessive breakdown (e.g., with intense physical stress).

Negligence Not doing something that a reasonably prudent person would do, or doing something that a reasonably prudent person would not do.

Neonate Infant from birth to about 1 month.

Nephron Functional unit of the kidney; contains the glomerulus and the tubule.

Neutropenia Decrease in the neutrophils in the blood, the white blood cells responsible for quick response to invasion by infectious organisms.

Nightmare Frightening dream occurring during REM sleep.

Night terrors Repeated episodes of sudden wakening accompanied by screaming and acute anxiety, occurring during slow wave sleep.

Nitrogen balance State of equilibrium in which the amount of nitrogen taken in is equal to the amount of nitrogen excreted.

Nits Eggs of lice.

Nociceptors Free nerve endings that sense and respond to potentially noxious thermal, electrical, mechanical, or chemical stimuli.

Nocturnal Occurring at night.

Noncompliance Failure to adhere to a recommended plan.

Noninvasive Not entering a body cavity or breaking the skin.

Nonproprietary name Not protected by trademark; synonymous with generic name.

Non-REM sleep Non-rapid-eye-movement sleep, the four stages of quiet sleep in which brain waves slow but muscle tone is maintained.

Nonverbal communication Messages sent without words (e.g., via gestures, facial expressions, body posture, silence).

Normal flora Microorganisms commonly found in a body location that ordinarily cause no harm to the person.

Nosocomial infection Infection acquired during receipt of health care.

NPO Nothing by mouth; oral food or liquids are forbidden.

Nuclear scan Radiographic procedure in which organs are visualized through the use of radioactive dye.

Nurse administrator Nurse who supervises the organization of nursing care to ensure overall safety and quality; requires at least a baccalaureate degree in nursing.

Nurse anesthetist (CRNA) Nurse who specializes and is certified in the administration of anesthesia.

Nurse educator Nurse responsible for nursing and health-care education in a variety of settings; requires a master's or doctoral degree.

Nurse executive Top administrative nursing position in an organization.

Nurse midwife Nurse with advanced education and certification in the care of women during pregnancy and childbirth.

Nurse practice acts State guidelines that govern the practice of professional nursing.

Nurse practitioner Nurse with advanced education and certification in health assessment. May practice independently in a variety of health-care areas.

Nurse researcher Nurse responsible for continued development of nursing knowledge and improvement of practice through research; usually requires a doctoral degree.

Nursing Profession that involves diagnosis and treatment of human responses to actual or potential health problems.

Nursing centers Free-standing centers that provide nursing services on an independent basis.

Nursing diagnosis Actual, potential, or possible health problem identified by the nurse that is amenable to nursing intervention.

Nursing history Process in which the nurse interviews the patient to elicit a description of his or her current and past health status.

Nursing monitor Review by a nurse of a patient's care or records to determine the extent to which the care or records meet established standards.

Nursing orders Prescribed interventions in the nursing care plan.

Nursing process Systematic approach to providing nursing care using assessment, planning, intervention, and evaluation.

Nursing research Research that focuses on establishing a scientific base for the practice of nursing.

Nursing theory Explanation or description of nursing issues that defines and predicts nursing practice.

Nutrients Foods containing elements for normal body functioning.

Obesity Weight more than 20% over ideal body weight.

Objective data Observable, measurable information that can be validated or verified.

Observation Art of noticing patient cues.

Obstructive disease Lung disorder characterized by narrowed airways, such as asthma, emphysema, or bronchitis.

Occult Hidden; not visible to the naked eye.

Official drug name Name of medication as listed in official publications.

Oliguria Formation and excretion of less than 500 mL of urine in 24 hours.

One-day surgery center Medical facility where admission, surgery, and discharge occur on the same day; also known as a surgicenter.

Open family People who recognize a commitment to each other but are not necessarily related by blood.

Ophthalmoscope Instrument for examining the interior of the eye.

Opportunistic organisms Organisms that invade the tissues when body defenses are suppressed.

Opsonization Preparation of the bacterial cell wall to facilitate engulfment by phagocytes.

Oral administration Given by mouth.

Organizing Arranging the work to be done in small units so it can be accomplished.

Orgasm Climax phase of the human sexual response cycle; the man experiences expulsive contractions of the entire length of the urethra, and the woman experiences contractions in the outer third of the vagina and labia minora, as well as uterine contractions.

Orientation Awareness to time, place, situation, and self.

Orthopnea Ability to breathe easily only when in an upright position.

Orthostatic hypotension Fall in blood pressure associated with a change in position (from lying to sitting to standing).

Osmolality Concentration of solutes in a solution; expressed as milliosmols per kilogram.

Osmolarity Concentration of solutes in a solution; expressed as milliosmols per liter.

Osmosis Movement of a solvent through a semipermeable membrane from a region of lower to higher solute concentration.

Osmotic pressure Pressure exerted by nondiffusible particles in a solution across a semipermeable membrane; tends to hold fluid within its container and is opposed by hydrostatic pressure.

Osteoporosis Reduction in bone mass due to loss of calcium.

Otoscope Instrument for examining the ear.

Outcome criteria Specific, measurable, realistic statement of goal attainment.

Outpatient Patient who is having diagnostic or laboratory tests, receiving therapy, or attending a clinic, but does not occupy a bed.

Ovaries Almond-shaped bodies that contain the female gonads; they lie on either side of the pelvic cavity.

Over-the-counter (OTC) medication Medication that can be bought without a prescription.

Oxygenation Provision of oxygen to the blood or tissues.

PaCO$_2$ Partial pressure of carbon dioxide in arterial blood.

PaO$_2$ Partial pressure of oxygen in arterial blood.

Pain threshold Lowest intensity at which a certain person perceives a stimulus to be painful.

Pain tolerance Highest intensity of pain that the person is willing to tolerate.

Palpation Use of the sense of touch to ascertain the size, shape, and configuration of underlying body structures.

Pandemic Worldwide epidemic.

Papule Small, solid skin elevation.

Paracentesis Puncture of a body cavity (usually the abdomen) to remove fluid.

Paradoxical blood pressure Signifi-

cant decrease in systolic blood pressure with inspiration.

Paraplegia Paralysis of both legs and the lower part of the body.

Parasomnias Group of disorders, such as somnambulism (sleepwalking) and enuresis (bedwetting), involving autonomic and motor activity associated with partial arousal from sleep.

Parenteral administration Medication given by injection, usually intravenously or intramuscularly.

Parenteral nutrition Nutritional elements supplied through an intravenous route, usually into a central vein.

Parenting Process of nurturing children to enhance development.

Participative leadership Style of a leader who involves subordinates in setting goals, solving problems, and making decisions.

Passive range of motion Exercises in which body parts are moved by another person.

Pathogen Microorganism that can harm humans.

Pathogenicity Ability to induce a disease.

Patient Person requiring the services of a health-care provider.

Pediculosis Infestation with lice.

Peer review Evaluation and judgment of performance by other nurses.

Penis Male organ of copulation; urine and semen flow from the body through it.

Perceiving Process of recognizing and interpreting sensory stimuli; basis for understanding, knowing, or learning.

Perceptions How we view ourselves and the world; influenced by culture, religion, family, past experiences, expectations, and knowledge.

Percussion Examination by tapping the body surface with the fingertips and evaluating the sounds obtained.

Perfusion Passing of blood through an area.

Perineal care Cleansing of the perineum.

Perineum Area of the body containing the external pelvic structures: in a girl or woman, the area between the vulva and the anus; in a boy or man, the area between the penis and anus.

Perioperative period Period that begins with the decision to have surgery and ends with recovery.

Peripheral parenteral nutrition Infusion of isotonic lipids into the peripheral vessels to meet nutritive requirements.

Peristalsis Motility and movement of the intestines.

Peritonitis Inflammation of the membranous lining of the abdominal cavity.

pH Measure of the degree of acidity or alkalinity of a solution; as the pH increases, the acidity decreases.

Phagocytosis Process of engulfing microorganisms and other antigens.

Pharmacokinetics Study of how a medication changes as it passes through the body and undergoes absorption, distribution, metabolism, and excretion.

Phlebitis Inflammation or infection of a vein, manifested by redness, swelling, and tenderness along the course of the vein.

Phonation Process by which humans create vocal sounds.

Physical examination Use of one's senses through the techniques of inspection, palpation, percussion, and auscultation to obtain information about the structure and function of body parts.

Physical fitness State of health in which a person can perform normal and strenuous daily activities.

Physiologic needs Needs for air, food, water, elimination, sleep and rest, temperature maintenance, and sex.

Piggyback Diluted intravenous medication given over an intermediate length of time (i.e., 30 minutes).

Placebo Inactive substance given to patient for its psychological benefit.

Plaintiff Person who sues another.

Plan Written nursing diagnoses, outcome criteria, and interventions necessary to provide nursing care.

Planning Management function of deciding what to do, when, where, how, by whom, and with what resources.

Plantar flexion Bending at the ankle so as to point toes downward.

Plateau phase Phase of the human sexual response cycle that follows the excitement phase and precedes the orgasmic phase.

Pleximeter In percussion, the finger placed between the area to be percussed and the finger creating the vibrations.

Plexor Finger creating the vibrations during percussion.

Pneumonia Inflammation of the tissues in the lungs caused by bacteria, viruses, chemicals, fluids, or other irritants.

Pneumothorax Collection of air in the pleural space, usually as a result of perforation of the chest wall or the pleura covering the lung.

Poison Substance or gas that can injure or kill.

Pollution Substances in air, water, or land that are potentially harmful to health.

Polygraph recordings Graphic recordings of electrophysiologic changes in brain waves, eye movements, and muscles.

Polymicrobial infections Infections caused by a variety of organisms growing synergistically, often of mixed anaerobic and aerobic species.

Polysaccharides Complex sugars.

Polyuria Formation and excretion of large amounts of urine in the absence of a concurrent increase in fluid intake.

Portal of entrance Site of deposition of a microorganism.

Portal of exit Means of escape of a microorganism, such as body fluids.

Positive nitrogen balance State in which intake of nitrogen is greater than the amount excreted; occurs in growth, athletic training, or pregnancy.

Positive regard Warmth, caring, interest, and respect for another person; a nonjudgmental attitude toward others.

Possible nursing diagnosis Health problem amenable to nursing intervention that requires additional data collection and validation before it can be confirmed or deleted as a nursing diagnosis.

Postoperative period Phase that begins with transfer to the surgical recovery area and ends with recovery.

Precordium Part of the chest that overlies the heart and lower thorax.

Premature ejaculation Condition in which the man cannot delay ejaculation long enough for the woman to reach orgasm, or for satisfactory sexual intercourse to occur.

Preoperative checklist Form summarizing a patient's preoperative prep-

aration; ensures that all necessary information is in the chart.

Preoperative period Phase that begins with the decision to have surgery and ends with transfer to the operating room.

Prepuce Loose skin at the head of the penis; foreskin.

Prescription Directive written by a physician.

Pressure sore Sore or ulcer caused by prolonged pressure and decreased blood flow to skin and underlying tissue; also known as decubitus ulcer or bedsore.

Prevalence Extent to which a condition exists within a population.

Preventable infection Infection that could have been prevented if some event related to the infection had been altered.

Primary intention Healing process that occurs in wounds with little tissue loss and well-approximated edges; results in minimal granulation tissue and scar formation.

Primary nursing Model of nursing care in which a professional nurse develops a 24-hour nursing care plan and integrates that plan with the therapy plan of other healthcare professionals.

Priority Nursing problem that takes on a position of prominence.

Problem-oriented medical record Charting system in which everyone caring for the patient uses the patient problem list as a guide.

Problem-solving Systematic process that involves identifying and analyzing the problem, determining and weighing possible solutions, choosing and implementing a solution, and evaluating the results.

Pronation 1. Rotation of the forearm, turning the palm to face downward. 2. Assuming a face-down position.

Prone Lying face down.

Proprietary name Name protected by trademark; synonymous with brand or trade name.

Proprioceptors Nerve receptors that respond to position or movement.

Proprioception Awareness of the position and movements of body parts in space, sensed by sensory nerve terminals in muscles, tendons, and the labyrinth of the ear.

Prospective payment Method of reimbursing a fixed dollar amount for patient care based on diagnosis-related groups (DRGs).

Protein Organic compound composed of polymers of amino acids connected by peptide bonds.

Protein-sparing action Body's use of carbohydrates rather than protein as an energy source.

Proteinuria Presence of protein in urine.

Pruritus Severe itching.

Psoriasis Skin disease involving overproduction of epidermal cells.

Psychomotor Relating to muscle movements resulting from a mental process.

Psychosomatic Involving the integration of mind and body.

Puberty Period of life in which the sex organs mature, secondary sex characteristics appear, and reproduction becomes possible.

Pulmonary system System designed for ventilation and gas exchange; includes the lungs, their vasculature, and the structures required for their proper function.

Pulse deficit Mathematical difference between apical and radial pulse.

Pulse pressure Mathematical difference between systolic and diastolic blood pressure.

Purpose statement Clear, concise statement that defines the limits of a study.

Pursed-lip breathing Exhalation of air against resistance that patients with obstructive diseases use to reduce trapping of air; done by forming a small "O" with lips.

Purulent Producing or containing pus.

Pus Thick liquid product of inflammation that contains dead white blood cells, dead liquified tissue, and living or dead bacteria.

Pustule Small pus-filled skin elevation.

Pyuria Presence of pus in urine.

Quadriplegia Paralysis of arms and legs.

Quality assurance Systematic evaluation of health care designed to ensure excellence.

Quality assurance monitors Mechanisms that ensure that acceptable patient care is provided and standards are upheld.

Race Group defined by biologic characteristics (e.g., Asian, black, or caucasian).

Racism Oppression and exploitation of people of a different skin color or ethnic origin.

Radioisotope Radioactive chemical used in diagnostic tests.

Radiopaque Impenetrable to x-ray.

Rales Crackling breath sounds heard on inhalation that indicate fluid in alveoli or alveoli that are partially collapsed between breaths.

Range of motion Extent to which joints and muscles can be moved.

Range-of-motion exercises Systematic movement of joints to maintain flexibility and prevent muscle contractures.

Rationale Reason for a nursing intervention, supported by clinical research.

Reality orientation Nursing technique to help restore the patient's awareness of reality.

Rebound phenomenon In relation to sleep, the tendency for stage 4 and REM sleep to be recovered at the expense of the other stages.

Recall and recognition Abilities used to retrieve information in long- and short-term memory.

Recommended Dietary Allowances (RDAs) Nutritive requirements for kilocalories, proteins, and selected vitamins and minerals determined by research to support health.

Record Permanent document of patient information and care.

Referral Request of another professional to provide a service outside the scope of the professional making the referral.

Regional anesthetic Agent used to induce loss of sensation in a selected body area.

Registered nurse Person licensed by a state to practice professional nursing. Steps toward licensure include completing a state-approved nursing program and passing the state licensure examination.

Rehabilitation Actions taken to restore, to the extent possible, a person to a former state of functioning.

Reliability Degree to which an instrument or test consistently or dependably measures the attribute it is intended to measure.

REM sleep Sleep characterized by rapid eye movements and very low muscle activity.

Reminiscence therapy Use of recall of the patient's past to help clarify meaning in the present or reconcile conflict.

Reporting Sharing of patient information by two or more health-care professionals.

Research design Overall plan for collecting and analyzing data.

Reservoir Place where microorganisms collect, reproduce, and grow.

Residential care Health and social services provided to patients who live in a group-housing setting.

Residual urine Amount of urine remaining in the bladder after voiding.

Resistance In microbiology, lack of response by a microorganism to a drug that is intended to slow its growth or destroy it.

Resolution phase Final phase of the human sexual response cycle; immediately follows orgasm and is marked by rapid loss of vasocongestion.

Resonance Echoing of sound through passages.

Respiration Exchange of carbon dioxide for oxygen in the lungs and in the tissues.

Respiratory failure Inability of the pulmonary system to meet the metabolic demands of carbon dioxide elimination and tissue oxygenation.

Respite care Health-care services provided to a patient to give the regular caregiver a temporary relief from responsibility.

Respondeat superior "Let the master answer"; doctrine in which a hospital is held liable for an employee's negligence.

Rest Physical and emotional state of decreased muscle and cognitive activity.

Restraint Device that prevents a patient from moving or from gaining normal access to a body part.

Restrictive disease Lung disorder characterized by decreased ability to stretch the lungs, such as pneumonia or fibrosis.

Reticular activating system (RAS) Part of the brain responsible for bringing together information from the cerebellum and other parts of the brain and from the sense organs.

Rh factor Group of antigens on the erythrocytes of most people; a person is designated Rh + or Rh − based on the absence or presence of this factor.

Rhonchi   Rumbling breath sounds caused by air passing through secretions in the airways.

Roentgenogram   X-ray.

Role   Expected function and behavior of a person.

Role play   Therapeutic enactment of a problematic situation.

Rotation   Movement of a bone or body part about an axis.

Safety needs   Freedom from fear, anxiety, and danger.

Sanguineous   Pertaining to or containing blood.

Sanitizing   Cleaning an item, generally by use of chemical agents.

Satiety   Satisfaction; often used to describe gratification of hunger or thirst.

Scabies   Highly contagious, inflammatory skin disease caused by mites.

Scoliosis   Abnormal lateral curvature of the spine.

Scrotum   Loose, pouchlike sac in the male external genitalia that contains the testes.

Sebaceous glands   Oil-secreting glands of the dermis.

Secondary intention   Wound healing by filling in with granulation tissue.

Self-actualization   Process of developing one's maximum potential and managing one's life confidently.

Self-awareness   Knowing and caring for oneself; recognizing one's strengths and limitations.

Self-concept   Mental image of oneself.

Self-esteem   Evaluation and judgment of one's worth.

Self-evaluation   Conscious assessment of the self.

Self-expectation   The self a person wants to be.

Self-knowledge   Basic understanding of oneself.

Self-perception   A person's awareness or identification of self; the filtering process of evaluating events and entering them into the subconscious.

Semipermeable membrane   Membrane that permits passage of some molecules in a solution while excluding others.

Sensation information   Telling a patient what he or she will see, hear, smell, taste, or feel in a particular situation.

Sensitivity   Identification of the antibiotic that will destroy specific cultured microorganisms.

Sensoristasis   State of optimal sensory input; differs for each person.

Sensory deprivation   Lack of meaningful sensory stimuli, monotonous input, or interference with the processing of information; leads to behavioral changes ranging from boredom to psychosis.

Sensory overload   State of arousal in which a person cannot manage the intensity or quantity of incoming sensory stimuli.

Sepsis   Poisoning of body tissues; usually refers to bloodborne organisms or their toxic products.

Septicemia   Bacterial infection in the bloodstream, leading to fever, chills, malaise, and collapse; may proceed to septic shock.

Serosanguineous   Containing serum and blood.

Serous   Thin, watery, serumlike.

Sexuality   Person's characteristics and perceptions concerning sexual expression.

Shearing force   Force applied when tissues move against each other, causing stretching of vasculature in the subcutaneous tissues. Occurs when a patient slides up or down in bed.

Shock   Severe circulatory insufficiency.

Shock (electrical)   Interruption of body functions due to electrical current.

Sims' position   Side-lying with the upper leg flexed.

Single-parent family   Family consisting of a parent and child or children.

Skilled nursing facility   Inpatient facility that provides long-term nursing care.

Sleep   Readily reversible state of altered consciousness in which awareness and responsiveness to the environment is decreased.

Sleep apnea   Condition in which, at least five times an hour, the patient stops breathing for 10 seconds or more during sleep.

Sleep deprivation   State of having less sleep than needed.

Sleep latency   Time it takes to go to sleep after going to bed.

Sleep pattern disturbance   Disruption in quantity or quality of sleep, causing discomfort or interfering with life.

Sleep–wake cycle   Alternating periods of sleep and wakefulness in a 24-hour period.

SOAP note   Method of organizing charting entries so that subjective, objective, assessment, and planning information is included in each entry.

Social isolation   State in which a person's desire for interpersonal relationships is perceived as unattainable; negative feelings of being alone.

Social self   One's behavior and interaction with others in social situations.

Social worker   Professional trained to assess and assist people regarding public assistance, social or family crisis, and access to social service programs.

Socialization   Process in which a person is familiarized with the ways of a specific culture or group.

Somnambulism   Sleepwalking.

Somnolence   Sleepiness.

Source   Place from which the infectious agent passes to the host.

Source recording   Type of medical record system in which each healthcare specialty records in a separate area on the chart.

Spasticity   Sudden involuntary increase in muscle tone or contractions due to central nervous system lesions.

Specific gravity   Measure of the weight of a substance in comparison to an equal volume of water; indicates relative concentration of a fluid.

Sphincter   Circular muscle that surrounds and constricts an opening.

Spiritual distress   Condition in which a person's value system, from which he or she draws strength and hope, is disturbed.

Spiritual well-being   Condition marked by an affirmation of life and a sense of unity with God, self, community, and environment.

Spirituality   Personal striving toward unity and God in an attempt to find meaning in life.

Sputum   Expectorated respiratory secretions, including mucus and saliva.

Standards   Statements of the required quality of nursing care that serve as the model for others to follow.

Standing order   Order to be implemented until canceled by a physician or by agency policy.

Stasis Stagnation or slowing of body fluid.

Stat order Directive to be carried out immediately.

Stenosis Narrowing of an opening.

Stereotype Preconceived belief about a person or people.

Sterilization 1. Destruction of all bacteria, spores, fungi, and viruses on an item; accomplished by heat, chemicals, or gas. 2. Rendered unable to reproduce biologically.

Steristrip Small adhesive strip used to hold wound edges in approximation.

Stethoscope Instrument used to amplify sounds produced in the body.

Stimulus Something that rouses the mind or spirit.

Stoma Artificially created opening of bowel on the abdominal skin surface.

Stool Solid waste products of digestion; feces.

Straight catheter Tube placed through the urethra into the bladder to drain urine temporarily.

Strategic planning Planning major long-range goals, objectives, and directions for an organization.

Stress State of arousal of mind and body in response to demands made on the person.

Stressor Stimulus or event that requires coping and adaptation.

Stria Thin streak or line; often associated with stretch marks from pregnancy or obesity (plural: striae).

Stridor Harsh crowing sound heard on inspiration, caused by upper airway obstruction; common in croup.

Stroke Cerebrovascular accident (CVA); involves a sudden onset of hemorrhage, blood clots, or other vascular lesions in the brain.

Stroke volume Amount of blood ejected from each cardiac ventricle with each contraction of the heart.

Subclinical infection Infection that produces an immune response without overt disease.

Subculture Beliefs held by a portion of the larger population (e.g., an occupational or ethnic group).

Subcutaneous Pertaining to the layer of tissue under the dermis.

Sublingual Under the tongue.

Substantia gelatinosa Area in the dorsal horn of the spinal cord that is thought to be the "gate" for pain transmission.

Substrate Substance on which an enzyme works to produce changes.

Suffocation Oxygen deprivation.

Sundown syndrome Nocturnal delirium; state of disorientation and agitation that occurs at night in institutionalized patients who are oriented during the day.

Supination Rotation of the forearm, turning the palm upward.

Suppository Medication inserted into the rectum or vagina.

Suppuration Production or discharge of pus.

Suprainfection State in which susceptible microbes are suppressed by an antibiotic, allowing overgrowth of strains that are resistant to the antibiotic.

Surgery Treatment of disease and injury by invasive manual and operative techniques.

Surgical holding area Area outside the operating room where final preparations are made before surgery.

Suture Material used to stitch together the edges of traumatic or surgical wounds.

Symbiotic Living in harmony, with no harm to host or organism.

Symmetry Correspondence of size, shape, movement, and other qualities on opposite sides of the body.

System Set of interacting parts that make up a whole.

Systems theory Way of viewing the world or an organization in which the parts are seen in relation to the whole.

Systole Period of contraction of the ventricles.

Systolic blood pressure Pressure in the blood vessels during cardiac ventricular contraction.

Tachycardia Abnormally rapid heart rate, usually above 100 beats per minute.

Tachypnea Abnormally rapid respiratory rate, usually more than 20 breaths per minute.

Tangential lighting Light shining from the side to create shadows over the area being examined; accentuates subtle differences in contour and movement.

Taxonomy Classification system to organize information.

Teaching To communicate and impart knowledge by instruction, lesson, or demonstration.

Team conference Gathering of health-care providers to discuss a specific patient.

Team nursing Model of nursing care in which a team of nurses, licensed practical nurses, and nursing assistants are assigned specific functions or procedures to do for a group of patients.

Teleology Theory of philosophy in which the consequences of actions are considered in judging right and wrong.

Terminal ends Values regarded as good in themselves; they transcend immediate needs and shape long-term goals.

Testes Male gonads.

Testosterone Male hormone.

Theory Explanation of the relationships among phenomena.

Therapeutic communication Interactions that help a person express feelings and work out problems.

Therapeutic relationship Human connection that results in healing for at least one of the people.

Thermoreceptors Nerve receptors that respond to temperature changes.

Third spacing Loss of intravascular fluid into an area of the body (a "third space") where it cannot be reabsorbed (e.g., into the abdominal cavity).

Thoracentesis Puncture of the thoracic cavity to remove fluid.

Thought processes Cognitive functions under cerebral cortical control, including short- and long-term memory, use of language, attention span, judgment, and the ability to solve problems

Thrombocytopenia Deficiency of platelets in the blood.

Thrombocytosis Excessive number of platelets in the blood.

Thrombosis Presence of a blood clot that completely or partially obstructs a blood vessel.

Thrombus Blood clot obstructing a blood vessel.

Tidal volume Amount of air moving in and out of the lungs with each breath.

Tissue turgor Ability of the skin to return to normal position after being pinched; reflects skin elasticity and/or hydration status.

Tolerance Decreased physiologic response to repeated administration of a drug; an increase in dosage is needed to maintain a given therapeutic effect.

Topical administration   Application directly to a body site.

Tort   Wrong committed against a person or property; is subject to action in a civil court.

Total parenteral nutrition (TPN)   Administration of hypertonic solutions containing dextrose, proteins, vitamins, and minerals to provide for nutritional deficits; also known as hyperalimentation.

Toxicity   Harmful effect of a drug.

Tracheostomy   Permanent opening into the trachea through the neck.

Tracheotomy   Incision through the neck to create a temporary opening in the trachea; usually performed in an emergency.

Trade name   Synonymous with brand name; name designated by the drug manufacturer.

Transcribe   To write orders and treatments on the nursing Kardex, medication administration records, or treatment records.

Transdermal medication   Topical medication that is released through the epidermis and dermis to the blood.

Transient ischemic attack (TIA)   Temporary cerebral ischemia due to transient interruption in blood supply.

Transient flora   Microorganisms not normally found on the surface of the tissue that have not become attached to the tissue and are not growing or replicating.

Transsexual   Person who psychologically sees himself or herself as a member of the opposite sex.

Tremor   Involuntary trembling or convulsive movement due to alternating contractions of opposing muscle groups.

Tympany   Hollow, drumlike sound heard on percussion over an organ containing air or fluid.

Ultrasonography   Diagnostic technique in which the reflection of sound waves is used to view organs and blood flow.

Unit dose   Individual dose that is packaged and labeled in its own container.

Universal precautions   Practice in which blood and certain body fluids, particularly those containing visible blood, of all patients are considered potentially infectious for bloodborne pathogens.

Urgency   Inability to voluntarily delay voiding.

Urgent care centers   Newer form of health care offered in shopping areas and malls and operating during regular business hours.

Urgent surgery   Surgery performed for a health problem that is not immediately life-threatening.

Urticaria   Hypersensitivity to food, drugs, or emotional factors manifested by pruritus and elevated patches (wheals); hives.

Uterus   Muscular pear-shaped organ in which the fetus develops; womb.

Vagina   Tube extending from the uterus to the vulva; its walls stretch to accommodate the penis in sexual intercourse and the baby at birth.

Vaginismus   Involuntary contraction of the muscles around the vaginal orifice; makes sexual intercourse painful or impossible.

Validation   Re-examining information to check its accuracy.

Validity   Degree to which something measures what it is intended to measure (e.g., Glasgow coma scale).

Valsalva maneuver   Forceful exhalation against a closed glottis, nose, and mouth, as during defecation.

Values   Personal standards for decision-making.

Values conflict   Different views on a decision or course of action.

Values system   Enduring set of personal principles and rules.

Valve   Structure that temporarily closes an opening; flaps or cusps that allow fluid to move in only one direction.

Vasoconstriction   Decrease in diameter of a vessel due to the contraction of smooth muscle cells.

Vasodilation   Increase in diameter of a vessel due to the relaxation of smooth muscle cells.

Venipuncture   Insertion of a needle or catheter into a vein.

Ventilation   Movement of air in and out of the lungs; breathing.

Ventilator   Breathing machine used in patients with respiratory failure.

Verbal ability   Use of language to store, process, and communicate thought content.

Vesicle   Serous skin elevation less than 1 cm in diameter.

Vial   Small plastic or glass bottle for medication.

Virulence   Ability of a microorganism to cause disease; depends on the quality of the environment and the vigor of the organism.

Vitamins   Organic compounds that do not supply energy but are necessary to the body in small amounts for growth, development, maintenance, and reproduction.

Vulva   Collective term for the external female genitalia.

Wheeze   Musical breath sound indicating narrowed airways; commonly heard in asthma and COPD.

Working nursing care plan   Concise, practical working tool for the practicing nurse that focuses on patient needs.

Wound   Break in tissue continuity secondary to trauma or injury.

Wound approximation   Bringing wound edges into close proximity.

Wound healing   Process of restoring tissue to normal structure and function.

Index

Page numbers followed by *f* indicate figures; those followed by *t* indicate tabular material. Nursing diagnoses terminology is capitalized.

A

AACN. *See* American Association of Colleges of Nursing

Abbreviations
in documentation, 151t–152t
in drug orders, 505t
in health-care delivery system, 28
in laboratory values, 1415

Abdellah, Faye Glenn, 14t–15t
perception of human needs, 190

Abdomen, assessment of, 322, 324–327
landmarks for, 322, 326

Abdominal binder, 966, 967f

Abdominal distention, 1101, 1112

Abdominal girth, bowel function assessment and, 1105

Abduction, 701, 703t, 704t

Abduction pillow, 726t

ABO blood groups, 881

Abortion, 1371, 1374
elective, 1382

Abrasion, 940, 940t

Absorbents, 1114t

Absorption
by digestive system, 900
of drugs, 511
intestinal, 1092–1093

Abuse, family function and, 1295

Access devices, for intravenous therapy, 870, 871f

Accidents. *See also* Falls; Injuries; Trauma
altered health maintenance function and, 600

Accommodation, in cognitive development theory, 201

Accreditation. *See also* Joint Commission on Accreditation of Healthcare Organizations
quality assurance and, 36

Accuracy, of charting, 153, 153f

Acetaminophen, 1181t

Acetylsalicylic acid (ASA), 1181t

Achilles reflex, assessment of, 338t

Acid(s), 853
in blood, 854

Acid-base balance, 853–855
acids, bases and pH and, 853–854
acids and bases in blood and, 854
altered, 857–861
activities of daily living and, 861
manifestations of, 860–861
potential for, 858–859

assessment of, 861–866
objective data and, 862–866
subjective data and, 861–862
evaluation and, 886–887
factors affecting, 854–855
interventions and, 867–886
altered acid-base balance and, 868–884
discharge planning and home care and, 884, 886
to promote health and function, 867–868
nursing diagnoses and patient goals and, 866–867

Acidosis, 858

ACLS (advanced cardiac life support), 836

Acquired immune deficiency syndrome (AIDS), 990t
health-care workers with, work restriction and, 437–438
waste disposal and, 438

Active euthanasia, 52

Active immunity, 985

Active listening, 284–285, 285f

Active range of motion, 722

Active transport, fluid and electrolyte movement and, 849

Activities of daily living (ADLs)
body temperature and, 1028
bowel function and, 1101–1102
cardiopulmonary function and, 817
cognitive function and, 1223
coping and adaptation and, 1345
family function and, 1295–1296
fluid and electrolyte and acid-base imbalances and, 861
grieving and, 1318
health maintenance function and, 601
home maintenance management and, 614–615
infections and, 1000
mobility and, 714
pain and, 1170
respiratory function and, 758
safety dysfunction and, 575–576
self-concept and, 1252
sensory perception and, 1196–1197
sexual function and, 1373, 1383, 1383f
sleep and, 1150
spiritual dysfunction and, 1397
urinary elimination and, 1054
values and, 269–270
wound healing and, 950–951

Activity. *See also* Activity–exercise health pattern;
       Exercise(s)
  assessment of, 332
  bowel function and, 1111
  cardiovascular function and, 807
  coping and adaptation and, 1341–1342
  immobility and, 708–711
  respiratory function and, 752
  safety and, 565
Activity–exercise health pattern, 90, 107
  assessing human needs and, 192
  assessment of, 308–320
    cardiovascular, 316–320
    mobility and self-care and, 308–310
    respiratory, 310–316
  in community, 232
  disruption by diagnostic procedures, 394t
  drugs promoting normal function and, 501t
  exercise and immobility and, 708t
  in family, 228
  health maintenance and, 597t
  health problems and anticipatory guidance and,
    212–213
  surgery and, 469
  values and, 263
Activity Intolerance, 717
  altered cardiopulmonary function and, 823
  nursing management plan for, 838
Activity tolerance
  assessment of, 717
  mobility and, 707
Actual nursing diagnoses, 118, 121
Acupressure, 1178
Acupuncture, 1178–1179
Adaptation. *See also* Coping; Coping–stress tolerance
    health pattern; Stress
  assessment and, 1345–1347
    objective data and, 1347
    subjective data and, 1346–1347
  characteristics of, 1337–1340
  in cognitive development theory, 201
  factors affecting, 1341–1342
  functional health patterns and, 1346
  general adaptation syndrome and, 1338–1339
  lifespan considerations and, 1342–1343
  normal pattern of, 1340–1341
  nursing diagnoses and patient goals and, 1348–1349
  sensory, 1192
Addiction
  coping and adaptation and, 1344–1345
  to narcotic analgesics, 1183
Adduction, 701, 703t, 704t
ADH. *See* Antidiuretic hormone
ADLs. *See* Activities of daily living
Admission entries, 161
Adolescent
  bathing and, 661
  body temperature and, 1023
  bowel function and, 1095
  cardiovascular function and, 809
  cognitive function and, 1218
  communication and, 289, 1270
  coping and adaptation and, 1342

  development of, 203t, 207
  diagnostic and laboratory testing and, 404
  family and, 1292
  feeding, 919
  fluid and electrolyte balance and, 853
  functional health assessment of, 345
    auscultation of bowel sounds in, 326
    auscultation of breath sounds in, 316
    auscultation of heart sounds in, 319–320
  functional health patterns and, health problems and
    anticipatory guidance and, 210–219
  grieving and, 1317t, 1317–1318
  health maintenance and, 598–599, 603t
  home maintenance management and, 617–618
  infection control and, 460
  medications and, 556
  mobility and, 705
  needs of, 189
  nutrition and, 908
  pain and, 1167
  patient teaching and, 422, 422f
  resistance to infection and, 987
  respiratory function and, 753
  safety and, 568
  self-care and, 646
  self-concept and, 1246t, 1248–1249, 1256
  sensory perception and, 1193
  sexuality and, 1369–1370
  shampooing hair of, 669
  skin and, 939
  sleep and, 1145
  spiritual function and, 1395, 1408
  surgery and, 473
  urinary elimination and, 1047–1048
  values and, 267
  vital signs in, 375–376
Adult. *See also* Middle adult; Older adult; Young adult
  body temperature and, 1023–1024
  bowel function and, 1095–1096
  cardiovascular function and, 809
  cognitive function and, 1218
  communication and, 289–290, 1270
  coping and adaptation and, 1342–1343
  diagnostic and laboratory testing and, 404
  family and, 1292
  fluid and electrolyte balance and, 853
  functional health assessment of, 345–346
  grieving and, 1318
  health maintenance and, 599
  home maintenance management and, 618
  infection control and, 460
  medications and, 556
  mobility and, 705
  needs of, 189
  nutrition and, 908
  obese, subcutaneous injections and, 540–541
  pain and, 1167
  patient teaching and, 422–423
  resistance to infection and, 987
  respiratory function and, 753
  safety and, 568–569
  self-care and, 646
  self-concept and, 1246t, 1249, 1256

sensory perception and, 1193
sexuality and, 1370–1371
skin and, 939
sleep and, 1145, 1146f
spiritual function and, 1395–1396, 1408
surgery and, 473–474
transferring, 737
urinary elimination and, 1048
values and, 267
vital signs in, 376
Advanced cardiac life support (ACLS), 836
Adverse effects. *See* Side effects
Advice giving, 288
Advocacy, 18
    nurse-patient relationship and, 278–279, 279t
Aerobic exercise, 701
Aerosol therapy, altered respiratory function and,
        770–772
Affective disorders, mobility and, 706
Affective domain of knowledge, 411
Affective teaching methods, 419
Age. *See also specific age groups*
    bathing and, 660–662
    blood pressure and, 365
    body temperature and, 350
    cardiovascular function and, 807
    drug action and, 514
    health maintenance and, 596
    pulse and, 354, 356
    respiratory function and, 361–362, 752
    safety and, 565
    wound healing and, 948–949
Aged. *See* Older adult
Agent, 174
Age spots, 939
Agranulocytes, 983
AIDS. *See* Acquired immune deficiency syndrome
Air, need for, 186
Airborne transmission, 430, 430t
Air embolism
    intravenous therapy and, 879
    total parenteral nutrition and, 929
Air-filled surfaces, 956
Air lock injection technique, 545
Air pollution. *See* Pollution
Airway
    emergency measures for, 788
    obstruction of, 754, 754f
        Heimlich maneuver and, 788, 793–794
        prevention of, 794
Airways
    nasal, 781, 787f
    oral, 781, 787f
AJN (American Journal of Nursing), 9, 503
Alarm reaction, 1338
Albumin, 881
Alcohol
    abuse of, altered nutrition and, 911
    in diet, 902, 904
    respiratory function and, 755
    sleep and, 1147
Aldosterone-angiotensin system, fluid and electrolyte
        balance and, 852

Alignment, of body, 695f, 695–696
    assessment of, 716
Alkali, 853
Alkalosis, 858
Allergens, respiratory function and, 755
Allergic reactions
    to blood transfusion, 882
    medication assessment and, 515–516
    to medications, 513–514
    skin and, 939
Allopathic physicians, 35
Altered Family Processes, 1298
Altered Health Maintenance, 604
Altered Nutrition: Less than Body Requirements, 915
    nursing management plan for, 931
Altered Nutrition: More than Body Requirements, 915
Altered Nutrition: Potential for More than Body
        Requirements, 915
Altered Parenting, 1300
    nursing management plan for, 1305
Altered Role Performance, 1254
Altered Sexuality Patterns, 1378
Altered Thought Processes, 1229
    nursing management plan for, 1236
Altered Tissue Perfusion (Renal, Cerebral, Cardiopulmon-
        ary, Gastrointestinal, Peripheral), 823
    defining characteristics for, 824t
Alternating air surfaces, 956
Alternatives, looking at, 284t, 286, 296f
Altitude, respirations and, 362
Alveoli, 748
Ambulation, 726–732. *See also* Gait
    assisting patient with, 727, 730–731
    infections and, 1010
    mechanical aids and, 727, 729, 731–732, 732f, 733–735
    muscle strengthening for, 732
    respiratory function and, 766–767
    transfer belts and, 727, 732f
Ambulation belts, 727, 732f, 739t
Ambulatory care centers, 32
Ambulatory care settings, infection hazards in, 433
American Association of Colleges of Nursing (AACN),
        statement of values of, 257, 257t
American Hospital Association, Patient's Bill of Rights of,
        48, 53
American Hospital Formulary Service, The, 501–502
American Journal of Nursing (AJN), 9, 503
American Medical Association Drug Evaluations, The, 501
American Nurses Association (ANA), 9, 20, 22
    Code for Nurses of, 42, 43, 46
    Code of Ethics of, 257, 257t
    Commission on Nursing Education, 77
    Commission on Nursing Research, 72–73
    nursing service defined by, 59
    as quality assurance monitor, 145
    research sponsored by, 72
    standards of care set by, 48
    Standards of Nursing Practice of, 21, 84, 112
Amnesic aphasia, 1272, 1272t
Ampules, for parenteral medications, 531, 532f
ANA. *See* American Nurses Association
Anaerobes, 992
Anaerobic exercise, 701

Analgesics, 1180–1185
  addiction and tolerance and, 1183
  adjuvant, 1183
  side effects of, 1183–1184
  types of, 1180, 1181t–1182t, 1182–1185, 1184f
Analytic skills, ethical dilemmas and, 45
Anemia, iron-deficiency, 899
Anesthesia
  general, 487, 488t
    stages of, 487, 488t
  monitoring, 487–488
  regional, 487–488, 488t
  urinary elimination and, 1050
Anesthesiologist, 487
Aneurysms, 810
Angina, 815
  pain and, 1172
Angiography, 398–399
  coronary, 399, 822
  respiratory assessment and, 764
Anions, 846
Anomia, 1272
Anomic aphasia, 1272, 1272t
Anonymity, research and, 77
Anorexia
  altered nutrition and, 909
  immobility and, 711
ANS. See Autonomic nervous system
Anterior chest
  anatomic landmarks of wall of, 310f–311f, 310–311
  auscultation of, 315
Anterior-posterior (AP) diameter, 312
Anthropometric measurements, nutrition and, 913f, 913–914
Anticipatory grief, 1310–1311
Anticipatory Grieving, 1321
Anticipatory guidance
  family function and, 1302
  pain and, 1177
Antidepressants, pain relief and, 1183
Antidiarrheal agents, 1112, 1114t
Antidiuretic hormone (ADH)
  fluid and electrolyte balance and, 851–852
  urinary elimination and, 1046
Antiembolic stockings, prevention of venous return and, 826–827, 828–829
Antiflatulent agents, 1112
Antimicrobials, infections and, 1010–1011
Antipyretics, 1033
Antiseptics, 443, 444t
Antispasmodics, 1114t
Anuria, 1052
Anxiety
  altered sensory function and, 1196
  coping and adaptation and, 1345
  self-concept and, 1251–1251
AP (anterior-posterior diameter), 312
Aphasia, 1271–1272, 1272t
Apical pulse, cardiopulmonary function and, 820
Apnea, 363, 1149
Apneustic respirations, 363
Apocrine glands, 937
Apothecaries' system, 506t, 506–507

Appetite. See Anorexia
Approximation, wound healing and, 945
Aquathermia pads, 974, 975–976
Arm circumference, nutrition and, 914
Arousal, alterations in level of, 1222–1223
Arrhythmia, 809–810
Arterial blood gases, 392
  acid-base balance and, 866
  cognitive function and, 1227
  respiratory assessment and, 763
Arterial puncture, 387
Arteries, 802
  altered cardiopulmonary function and, 816
  dysfunction of, 810, 811f
Arteriosclerosis, 810
Arthropods, 993
Arthroscopy, mobility and, 717
Articles of the Nuremberg Tribunal, 76
Articulation, 1266–1267
  disturbed, 1270–1271
Artificial airways, 781, 785, 787–788
Artificial eyes, care of, 676
ASA (acetylsalicylic acid), 1181t
Ascorbic acid (vitamin C), normal physiologic function of, 895t, 897
Asepsis, 426–461. See also Infection(s)
  barriers and, 445–448
  cleaning, disinfection, and sterilization and, 443–445
  handwashing and, 440–443
  isolation systems and, 448, 450–453
  lifespan considerations and, 457, 460–461
  medical, 439
  surgical. See Surgical asepsis
  universal precautions and, 448–450
Asian Americans, health/illness considerations and, 244
Asphyxiation, 573
Aspiration, enteral tube feedings and, 923
Aspiration diagnostic procedures, 399–402
Aspirin, fever and, 1033
Assault, 49, 52
Assertiveness, stress management and, 1351
Assessment. See Functional health assessment; Nursing assessment; Physical assessment; Physical examination
Assessment parameters, 106
  documentation of, 106
Assessment record
  computerized, 103
  written, 103
Assimilation, in cognitive development theory, 201
Assistant head nurse, 66–67
Associate degree nursing programs, 16
Associate nurse, 13
Ataxia, 707
Ataxic gait, 707
Atelectasis, 753–754
  immobility and, 710
Atherosclerosis, 810, 811f
Athetosis, 707
Athlete's foot, 665t
Atrophy
  of muscle, immobility and, 708–709
  of skin, 947t

Attention span deficits, 1222
Attitudes, 256
    of nurse, toward pain, 1171–1172
    spiritual care and, 1397
Audiovisual aids, patient teaching and, 417, 417f
Auditing, as purpose of patient record, 150
Auditory assessment, 335, 335f, 336f
Auscultation, 101, 306f, 306–307, 307t
    blood pressure measurement and, 370–371, 371f, 371t
    of bowel sounds, 324–326
        bowel function and, 1103–1104, 1104f
        infections and, 1002
    of breath sounds
        infections and, 1002
        respiratory assessment and, 313–316, 314t, 762
    of heart sounds
        cardiopulmonary assessment and, 820
        cardiovascular assessment and, 318–320
    pulse measurement and, 358
Auscultatory gap, 370–371
Automatic ROM equipment, 722
Autonomic nervous system (ANS)
    blood pressure and, 365
    homeostatic control and, 1337
    pain and, 1169, 1169t, 1172
    pulse and, 356
Autonomy, ethics and, 42–43
Autopsy, 54

B

Baccalaureate degree nursing programs, 16
Backrubs, 663, 664
Bacteremia, 994, 996
Bacteria, 428, 992, 993
Bactericidal chemicals, 443
Bacteriostatic chemicals, 443
Balance, 696, 696f, 697f
    assessment of, 309, 716
Bandages, 959, 963–965, 965f
Barium, 395
    bowel function studies and, 1106
Barrier(s), infection control and, 445–448
Barrier family planning method, 1382
Barton, Clara, 9
Basal body temperature, 1021
Basal metabolic rate (BMR), 905, 1019
Base(s), 853
    in blood, 854
Basic discharge plan, 629
Basic four food groups, 902, 903f, 904
Basophils, 983t
Bathing, 642, 655–662, 656t
    age-related considerations and, 660–662
    assisting with bath or shower and, 661
    in bed, 657–660
    methods of, 655–661
Battery, 49, 52
Bed(s)
    bathing patient in, 657–660
    care of, 681–682
    making, 682, 683–688
        occupied bed and, 686–688
        unoccupied bed and, 683–685

for patients unable to turn themselves, 682
    positioning patient in, 723–725
    positions for, 681
    shampooing hair in, 668–669
Bed cradle, 725t
Bedpans, 678, 679–680, 1067–1068, 1068f
Bedside commode, 678, 1067
Bedsores. *See* Pressure sores
Bedwetting, 1053–1054, 1150
Behavior(s), 256
    body temperature and, 1023
    changes in, self-concept and, 1250–1251, 1251t, 1257
    spiritual dysfunction and, 1397
Behavioral goals, 128
Beliefs, 256. *See also* Values–beliefs health pattern
    about sleep, 1153
    communication and, 1269
    culture and, 241
    family function and, 1290–1291
    health maintenance and, 598
    pain perception and, 1167
    self-care and, 645
    self-concept and, 1244
    sexuality and, 1369
Beneficence, 42, 630
Benzodiazepines, 1155t
Bereavement, 1310. *See also* Grieving; Loss
Biceps reflex, assessment of, 338t
Binders, 959, 965–966, 966f, 967f
Biocultural variation, 246–247
Bioethics, decision making and, 38
Biofeedback, pain relief and, 1180
Biologic factors
    causing pain, 1168
    self-concept and, 1244, 1244f
Biopsy, 399–400
    of bone marrow, 400
    of liver, 399
    renal, 399–400
Biotin, normal physiologic function of, 896t
Biotransformation, of drugs, 511
Biot's respirations, 363, 363t
Birth, 1366
Bisexual, 1366
Blacks
    health/illness considerations and, 244
    key informants for, 248
Bladder, urinary. *See* Urinary bladder
Bladder training, 1069
Bland diet, 920
Blended family, 1288
Blood. *See also* Plasma; Plasma chemistries; *headings beginning with term* Serum
    acids and bases in, 854
    altered composition of, 811–812
    viscosity of, altered, 812
    volume of, altered, 812
Blood-body fluid precautions, 451
Blood chemistry studies, 390–391
Blood coagulation studies, 390–391
Blood components, 880–881
Blood cultures, 393
    infections and, 1004

Blood flow
  altered, 810–811
  blood pressure and, 364
  cardiopulmonary function and, 822
  cognitive function and, 1216, 1219
  distribution of, 805, 806f
  through heart, 804–805
Blood glucose, 390–391
  arterial, 1227
  measurement by skin puncture, 389–390
  pain and, 1169
Blood lipids, 391
  cardiopulmonary function and, 821
Blood pressure, 364–373, 807
  abnormalities of, 371–373
  assessment of, 366–373
    equipment for, 366–369, 369f
    methods for, 369t, 369–371, 370f, 371f, 371t
    sites for, 366
  cardiopulmonary function and, 820
  cardiovascular function and, 814
  central venous, fluid and electrolyte imbalance and, 865
  diastolic, 364
  factors affecting, 365–366
  fluid and electrolyte imbalance and, 860
  normal fluctuations in, 366
  pain and, 1169
  paradoxical, 370
  physiologic factors determining, 364
  postural, assessment of, 716
  pulmonary artery, fluid and electrolyte imbalance and, 865
  pulse, 364
  systolic, 364
Blood specimens, collection of, 385–388
Blood tests, urinary elimination and, 1062–1063
Blood transfusions, 880–884
  blood compatibility and, 881
  blood components and, 880–881
  complications of, 882, 884
  donors and, 881–882
  technique for, 882, 883–884
Blood urea nitrogen (BUN), 1062
Blood vessels, 802–803. *See also* Arteries; Capillaries;
      Cardiovascular function; Veins
  normal function of, 805–806
Blue Cross program, 33
B-lymphocytes, 983t
BMR (basal metabolic rate), 905, 1019
Body fluids
  culture of, infections and, 1004
  stasis of, infections and, 998
Body image, 1243
  disturbance in, 1253, 1257, 1259
Body Image Disturbance, 1253
  nursing management plan for, 1259
Body mechanics, 697f, 697–701
  components of, 697, 699
  principles of, 699–701
  proper, using, 698–699
Body odor. *See* Odor(s)
Body position. *See also* Patient positioning
  aids for, 725t–726t

bowel function and, 1094
cardiopulmonary function and, 829–830
cardiovascular function and, 808
infections and, 1010
mobility and, 719–720, 721t–722t, 723–725, 725t–726t
pain and, 1176
respiratory function and, 362, 752, 766–767
urinary elimination and, 1046
Body-substance isolation, 451–452, 453f, 454t
Body systems, assessing before medication administration,
      517–518
Body systems model, organizing data and, 105, 106t
Body temperature, 349–354. *See also* Fever;
      Thermoregulation
  cardiovascular function and, 808
  factors affecting, 350–351, 1022–1023
  measurement of, 351–354, 354, 355–356, 1029
    axillary, 352, 355
    equipment for, 352–353
    factors affecting, 351
    oral, 351–352, 355
    rectal, 352, 356
  normal pattern of, 1021, 1021t
  respirations and, 362
Bone(s), 694. *See also* Musculoskeletal system
  infections of, 996
Bone marrow biopsy, 400
Borborygmi, 1104
Bowel assessment, fluid and electrolyte imbalance and, 865
Bowel elimination, 1088–1131. *See also* Elimination health
      pattern; Feces
  altered, 1096–1102
    activities of daily living and, 1101–1102
    altered nutrition and, 912
    incontinence and, 1101, 1109, 1112
    manifestations of, 1098–1101
    potential for, 1096–1098
  assessment and, 328, 1102–1108
    nursing diagnoses and patient goals and, 1108–1110
    objective data and, 1103–1108
    subjective data and, 1102–1103
  evaluation and, 1129, 1131
  factors affecting, 1094
  gastrointestinal tract anatomy and, 1090f, 1090–1092,
      1091f
  interventions and, 1110–1129
    altered bowel function and, 1111–1125
    discharge planning and home care and, 1125, 1129
    to promote health and function, 1110–1111
  lifespan considerations and, 1095–1096
  normal bowel function and, 1092–1093
  normal functional pattern and, 1093, 1094t
Bowel habits, 1111
Bowel Incontinence, 1109
Bowel incontinence, 1101, 1109, 1112
Bowel preparation, surgery and, 480
Bowel sounds. *See* Auscultation, of bowel sounds
Bowel training, 1123, 1124f
Bradycardia, 358
Bradypnea, 363, 363t
Brain, altered cardiopulmonary function and, 816
Breach of duty, 50–51
Bread, 902

Breasts, 1362, 1364f
Breast self-examination, 1379–1381
Breathing. *See also* Lungs; Respirations; Respiratory
 function
 deep, 767, 768, 769
  stress management and, 1352
 pursed-lip, 767
 work of, increased, 753–754
Breathing pattern
 altered, management of, 780
 normal, 751, 752t
Breath sounds, 313–316, 314t
 abnormal, altered respiratory function and, 758
 adventitious, 313
 auscultation of. *See* Auscultation, of breath sounds
 bronchial, 313, 314t
 bronchiovesicular, 313, 314t
 normal, 313, 314t
 respiratory assessment and, 762
 vesicular, 313, 314t
Brewster, Mary, 9
British Pharmacopeia, 502
Broca's aphasia, 1271–1272, 1272t
Bronchioles, 748
Bronchoscopy, respiratory assessment and, 763–764
Bronchospasm, 754
Brown, Esther Lucille, 9
Bruits, 320
Brushing, of hair, 663f, 663–664
Buccal medication administration, 528, 528f
Buddhism, religious practices of, 1407t
Buffers, acid-base balance and, 854–855
Bulk-forming agents, 1114t
Bulla, 944, 946t
BUN (blood urea nitrogen), 1062
Bunions, 665t
Burnout, 1350
Burns, 572, 943
 minor, first aid for, 958
 prevention of, 584–585
Butterflies, 960

C
Caffeine, sleep and, 1147
Calciferol. *See* Vitamin D
Calcium, 848
 dietary sources of, 869t
 imbalance of, 856–857
 normal physiologic function of, 897–899, 898t
Calendar rhythm method, 1382
Calf pumping exercises, 826
Calluses, 665t
Calorie count, nutrition and, 914
Canada, health-care delivery in, 34
Canadian Nurses Association (CNA), 9, 20, 22
 Code of Ethics for Nursing of, 43, 46
 standards of practice of, 21
Cancer
 altered nutrition and, 911
 infections and, 998
 patient teaching about, 606–607
Candidal infections, of skin, 940
Canes, 727, 732f

Capillaries, 802–803
 dysfunction of, 810
Capillary puncture, 388, 388f, 389–390
Capillary refill time, 819, 820f
Car accidents, 575
Carbohydrates
 digestion of, 900
 metabolism of, 900–901
 normal physiologic function of, 893
Cardiac catheterization, 399, 822
Cardiac enzymes, cardiopulmonary function and, 820–821
Cardiac failure, fluid and electrolyte and acid-base
 imbalances and, 859
Cardiac output, 805
Cardiac workload, immobility and, 709
Cardiopulmonary resuscitation (CPR), 587, 832, 833–837
Cardiovascular function, 800–839, 803, 803f. *See also*
 Arteries; Blood vessels; Capillaries; Circulation;
 Veins
 altered, 809–817
  activities of daily living and, 817
  manifestations of, 813–817
  potential for, 809–813
 assessment and, 316–320, 817–822
  landmarks for, 317, 317f
  objective data and, 819–822
  subjective data and, 817–819
 cardiovascular system anatomy and, 802–803
 evaluation and, 837–839
 factors affecting, 807–808
 interventions and, 824–837
  for altered cardiovascular function, 825–837
  to promote health and function, 825
 lifespan considerations and, 808–809
 normal, 803–806
 normal functional pattern and, 806–807
 nursing diagnoses and patient goals and, 822–824
 stress and, 1347
Career development, 19–20
Caregivers, 628
 needs of, 633
 nurse as, 18, 18f
Caregiving, sleep and, 1146
Care plan conferences, 168
Care planning. *See also* Nursing care plans
 as purpose of patient record, 150
Caries, 643
Case management, home care and, home maintenance
 management and, 631
Case Western Reserve University, 16
Catastrophic health insurance, 33
Categorically needy, 34
Category-specific isolation, 450–451, 454t
Catheter(s)
 infusion rate and, 876
 oxygen, 448f, 449f, 774–775
 urinary
  collection of urine specimen from, 1057, 1060
  external, 1069
  indwelling, 1069, 1072–1077, 1078–1079
  irrigation of, 1077–1078, 1078f, 1079f, 1080
  suprapubic, 1079–1081, 1081f
  types of, 678, 1071f, 1071–1072, 1072f

Cations, 846
CBC. *See* Complete blood count
CDC (Centers for Disease Control), infection control and, 434, 436, 438, 450
Cell migration, wound healing and, 945
Cellular immunity, 984
Center of gravity, 696
Centers for Disease Control (CDC), infection control and, 434, 436, 438, 450
Central apnea, 1149
Central pathways, pain and, 1163
Central venous catheter, 388
Central venous pressure, fluid and electrolyte imbalance and, 865
Cereals, 902
Cerebrospinal fluid (CSF), reference ranges for, 1435–1436
Cerebrovascular accident (CVA; stroke), 816
    communication and, 1271
Certification, quality assurance and, 37
Cerumen, 643
Cervical mucus method, 1382
Change
    cultural, 239f, 239–240
    development and, 198
    spiritual function and, 1396
Change management, as management skill, 63, 64f
Change-of-shift reports, 165, 167
Changing the subject, 288
Chaplains, 36
Charge nurse, 61
    role of, 66
Charitable care, 35
Charting, 150, 152–154. *See also* Documentation; Patient record
    accuracy of, 153, 153f
    completeness of, 153
    conciseness of, 152–153
    confidentiality and, 154
    legibility of, 153
    organization of, 153
    timeliness of, 153–154
CHD. *See* Coronary heart disease
Chemical burns, 943
Chemical factors, causing pain, 1168
Chemical name, of drugs, 500
Chemical safety, intraoperative, 486–487
Chemoreceptors, 1162
Chest, anatomic landmarks of, 310f–311f, 310–312
Chest pain, altered respiratory function and, 757
Chest physiotherapy, 780–781
Cheyne-Stokes respirations, 363, 363t
Chickenpox, 988t
Child. *See also* Adolescent; Infant; Newborn; Preschooler; School-age child
    antiembolic stockings and, 828
    aquathermia pads and, 975
    bathing, 661
    bedpan and, 680
    blood glucose measurement in, 390
    blood pressure assessment in, 368
    blood transfusions and, 884
    body temperature of, 1023
        assessing, 356

bowel function and, 1095
cardiopulmonary resuscitation and, 835–836
cognitive function and, 1217–1218
cold packs and, 973
colostomy irrigation and, 1128
communicating with, 289
condom catheters and, 1071
coping and adaptation and, 1342
coughing and deep breathing exercises and, 769
diagnostic and laboratory testing and, 404
    preparing for, 381
dressing changes and, 963
emotional problems in, family function and, 1295
enemas and, 1116
family and, 1292, 1295
fluid and electrolyte balance and, 853
foot and nail care and, 667
grieving and, 1317, 1317t
health maintenance function and, 598–599, 600–601
Heimlich maneuver and, 794
home maintenance management and, 617
indwelling urinary catheter and, 1076
intravenous infusions and
    infusion rate and, 879
    medication administration and, 552
    monitoring, 873
medications and, 555–556
    dosage calculation for, 521
    intravenous, 552
    oral, 526
needs of, 189
nutrition and, 908
oral care and, 671
ostomy care and, 1126
oxygen delivery systems for, 774t, 777–778
pain and, 1167
patient teaching and, 421–422
preparing for diagnostic and laboratory tests, 381
pulse assessment in, 360
    pulse deficit and, 362
resistance to infection and, 987
respiratory function and, 753
    assessment of, 365
safety and, 568, 583–584, 584f
self-care and, 646
self-concept and, 1246t, 1248, 1248f
sensory perception and, 1193
sexuality and, 1369
shampooing hair of, 669
skin and, 939
sleep and, 1145
spiritual function and, 1395, 1407–1408
strict isolation and, 452
subcutaneous injections and, 540–541
suctioning and, 785, 787
surgery and, 473
total parenteral nutrition and, 925, 928
tracheostomy care and, 791
transferring, 737
urinary elimination and, 1047–1048
urine specimen collection from, 1058–1059, 1060
vital signs in, 375–376
Chlamydia, 990t

Chlamydia culture, 1377t

Chloral hydrate, 1155t

Choosing pattern, nursing diagnosis and, 114

Chorea, 707

Christian Science, religious practices of, 1405t

Chronic Pain, 1175

Church of Jesus Christ of Latter Day Saints, religious practices of, 1405t–1406t

Cicatrix, 946t

Cigarette smoking. *See* Smoking

Circadian rhythms, 1142

Circle of confidentiality, nurse-patient relationship and, 279

Circoelectric bed, 682

Circular turns, 964, 965f

Circulation. *See also* Arteries; Blood vessels; Capillaries; Cardiovascular function; Veins
  body temperature and, 1022, 1025
  coronary, 802
  mobility and, 702
  pulmonary, 803
  skin and, 938
  systemic, 803
  wound healing and, 948

Circulatory maintenance, postoperative, 494

Circulatory overload, blood transfusion and, 882

Circumduction, 701

Civil law, 47

Civil Rights Act, Title VI of, 249

Civil War, nursing during, 9

Clarification, seeking, 284t, 285

Clarity, of communication, 276, 276t

Claudication. *See* Intermittent claudication

Clean-catch urine specimen, collection of, 1057–1058, 1059

Cleaning, asepsis and, 443

Cleansing baths, 655

Clear liquid diet, 920

Client, as alternative term for patient, 180

Climacteric, 1371

Clinic(s), 32
  surgery performed in, 466

Clinical model, of health, 174

Clinical nurse specialists, 19, 19f
  role of, 65, 66

Clinical nursing care plans, 131, 134

Clinitron bed, 682

Clips, wound closure and, 490

Clitoris, 1362

Closed drainage systems, 967, 967f, 968

Clubbing, of digits, 312, 312f
  altered respiratory function and, 758

Clusters, 118–120, 119f

CNA. *See* Canadian Nurses Association

Coagulation studies, 390–391

Cobalamin (vitamin B$_{12}$), normal physiologic function of, 896t, 897

Codes, 52
  resuscitation and, 836

Codes of ethics, 42–43, 46–47

Code team, 837

Cognition. *See also* Cognition–perception health pattern; Cognitive development; Cognitive function
  body temperature and, 1025
  cardiovascular function and, 807

communication and, 1268–1269

health maintenance and, 596

home maintenance management and, 615, 619

immobility and, 713

ischemia and, 816

resistance to infection and, 985

safety and, 565

self-care and, 644–645, 647

sexuality and, 1368–1369

Cognition–perception health pattern, 90, 107
  assessing human needs and, 192
  assessment of, 328–337
    cognitive function and, 329–333
    pain and, 336–337
    sensory function and, 333–336
  in community, 232
  disruption by diagnostic procedures, 394t
  drugs promoting normal function and, 501t
  exercise and immobility and, 708t
  in family, 228
  health maintenance and, 597t
  health problems and anticipatory guidance and, 213f, 213–214
  surgery and, 471
  values and, 263–264, 264t

Cognitive development
  of adolescent, 207
  of infant, 205
  intrauterine, 204
  of middle adult, 208
  of neonate, 204
  of older adult, 209
  of preschooler, 206
  of school-age child, 206
  of toddler, 205–206
  of young adult, 207

Cognitive development theory, 199, 200t, 201

Cognitive domain of knowledge, 410–411

Cognitive function, 1210–1237. *See also* Cognition; Cognition–perception health pattern; Cognitive development
  altered, 1219–1223
    activities of daily living and, 1223
    manifestations of, 1221–1223
    potential for, 1219–1221
  altered sensory function and, 1196
  anatomy and, 1212f, 1212–1213, 1213f
  assessment and, 1223–1229
    objective data and, 1226–1229
    subjective data and, 1223–1226
  assessment of, 329–332
  characteristics of, 1214–1215
  evaluation and, 1235–1236
  factors affecting, 1216–1217
  functional health patterns and, 1215–1216
  interventions and, 1229–1235
    for altered function, 1231–1234
    discharge planning and home care and, 1234–1235
    to promote health and function, 1229–1231
  lifespan considerations and, 1217–1218
  normal, 1212–1218
  nursing diagnoses and patient goals and, 1229
  tests of, 1227, 1229

Cognitive teaching methods, 419
Cohabitated family, 1288
Coitus interruptus, 1383
Cold, common, 988t
Cold applications, 969, 971t
  pain relief and, 1178
  safety with, 971–972, 972t
Cold compresses, 972
Cold packs, 972, 973
Collaborative health problem, nursing diagnosis and, 116t, 117, 117f
Colonic Constipation, 1108–1109
Colonization, bacterial, 993
Color
  of skin, 937
  wound classification by, 957t
Colostomy, 1098, 1098f
Comatose patient, Heimlich maneuver and, 794
Comatose patients
  aquathermia pads and, 976
  communication and, 1271
  eye care in, 676
  oral care and, 672
Comfort. *See also* Pain
  infections and, 1010
  postoperative, 494
Commode, bedside, 678, 1067
Common cold, 988t
Common law, 47
Communal family, 1288
Communicable diseases, 431
Communicable period, 431–432
Communicating pattern, nursing diagnosis and, 113
Communication, 1215, 1264–1284
  altered, 1270–1273
    activities of daily living and, 1273
    manifestations of, 1271–1273
    potential for, 1270–1271
  alternative methods for, 1278–1280
  anatomy of communication centers and, 1266f, 1266–1267
  assessment and, 1273–1276
  characteristics of, 1267–1268
  congruent, 275
  evaluation and, 1281
  facilitating, 283
  factors affecting, 1268–1269
  incongruent, 275
  interventions, 1277–1281
  lifespan considerations and, 1269–1270
  as management skill, 62–63
  metacommunication and, 274
  nonverbal, 62, 274, 1268
  normal function of, 1267, 1268f
  nursing diagnoses and patient goals and, 1276
  of pain, 1169
  patient teaching and, 417–418
  production and coordination of, 1266–1267
  as purpose of patient record, 150
  of spiritual distress, 1397
  therapeutic. *See* Therapeutic communication
  verbal, 274, 1267–1268. *See also* Report(s)
    altered home maintenance management and, 619

altered self-care and, 648
  written. *See* Documentation; Patient record; Reporting
Communication channel, 275
Communication process, 274f, 274–276
  elements of, 275
  language and experience and, 275–276, 276t
  types of communication and, 274–275
Communication skills, developing, 286, 287t
Communicator, nurse as, 18–19
Community, 229–233, 230f
  advanced concepts of, 233
  assessment of, 231t, 233
  definition of, 229–233
  eliciting information related to functional health in, 232
  as nursing practice setting, 17
  responsibility for functional health, 233
  safety in, 567
  as source of values, 259, 259f
  types of, 230, 230t, 233
Community acquired infections, 993
Community-based agencies, 32f, 32–33
Community nutrition programs, 916
Community resources
  assessment of, home maintenance management and, 622–623
  home maintenance management and, 616–617, 619–620, 632t, 633
Complete blood count (CBC), 388–390
  cardiopulmonary function and, 820
Completeness, of charting, 153
Compliance
  assessing before medication administration, 518
  assessment of, 415
Comprehension, 1216
Comprehensive Drug Abuse Prevention and Control Act of 1970, 52, 508
Computed tomography (CT), 396
  infections and, 1005
Computer documentation, 155, 158f
Computerized care plans, 131
Conception, 1365–1366
Conceptual models, 12
  for family, 225–228
  knowledge of, as evaluation skill, 141
  organizing data and, 105t, 105–107
  research and, 73
Conciseness, of charting, 152–153
Condom catheter, 678, 1069, 1070–1071
Conduction
  cardiac, problems of, 809–810
  heat loss and, 1020–1021
Confidentiality
  circle of, nurse-patient relationship and, 279
  ethics and, 43
  of patient record, 154, 168–169
  research and, 77
Conflicts
  among roles, 45
  among values, 267–269
Confusion, 1232
  spiritual care and, 1397
  surgery and, 471
Congenital problems, altered mobility and, 705

Consciousness level, 1214. *See also* Comatose patients
   assessment of, 329, 329t, 333
Consent. *See* Informed consent
Constipation, 1098–1099, 1112
   immobility and, 712
Constipation (nursing diagnosis), nursing management plan
      for, 1130
Constriction, avoiding, prevention of venous return and,
      827, 829
Consumerism, 29
Contact isolation, 451
Contact lenses, care of, 673, 674f–675f, 676
Contact transmission, 429, 430t
Contagious diseases, 431
Contamination, 443
Continuity, of communication, 276, 276t
Continuity of care, discharge planning and, 626
Continuous infusion technique, 552–553
Continuous positive airway pressure, 775, 777
Contraceptives, 1381–1383
Contract(s)
   home maintenance management and, 628
   nurse-patient relationship and, 277–278
Contractility, cardiac, 805
Contractures, 707
   immobility and, 709
Contralateral stimulation, pain relief and, 1178
Contrast media, 395, 395t
Controlled substances, 52, 508t, 508–509, 509t
Controlled Substances Act (CSA), 508t, 508–509, 509t
Controlling, as management function, 61f, 61–62
Contusion, 940t
Convalescent period, 431
Convection, heat loss and, 1021
Conventional judgment, 44–45
Cool-water bath, 656t
Coordinating nursing interventions, 137–138
Coordination (physical), 696–697
   assessment of, 716
   mobility and, 706–707
Coordination (process), discharge planning and, 626
Coordinator, nurse as, 18
Coping. *See also* Adaptation; Coping–stress tolerance
      health pattern; Stress
   altered, 1343–1345
      activities of daily living and, 1345
      manifestations of, 1344t, 1344–1345
      potential for, 1343–1344
   assessment and, 1345–1347
      objective data and, 1347
      subjective data and, 1346–1347
   cardiovascular function and, 808
   characteristics of, 1337–1340
   communication and, 1280
   factors affecting, 1341–1342
   family function and, 1291
   functional health patterns and, 1346
   health maintenance and, 598
   home maintenance management and, 616
   interventions and, 1349–1354
      altered coping and, 1353–1354
      discharge planning and home care and, 1354
      to promote health and function, 1349–1353
   lifespan considerations and, 1342–1343
   mobility and, 704, 713
   normal function of, 1336–1337
   normal pattern of, 1340–1341
   nursing diagnoses and patient goals and, 1348–1349
   pain and, 1171
   safety and, 566
   self-concept and, 1244–1245, 1249
   sexuality and, 1369
Coping mechanisms, 1341
Coping–stress tolerance health pattern, 90, 107
   assessing human needs and, 193
   assessment of, 340
   in community, 232
   disruption by diagnostic procedures, 394t
   drugs promoting normal function and, 501t
   exercise and immobility and, 708t
   in family, 228
   health maintenance and, 597t
   health problems and anticipatory guidance and, 217–218
   surgery and, 472
   values and, 265
Core temperature, 350, 1018
   sleep and, 1144
Corns, 665t
Coronary angiography, 399
Coronary heart disease (CHD), 809
   risk factors for, 812
Cortical control, communication and, 1267, 1271
Corticosteroids, 1181t
Coughing
   altered respiratory function and, 756, 768–770
   controlled, 768–769
Counseling, sexual function and, 1383
CPR (cardiopulmonary resuscitation), 587, 832, 833–837
Crackles, 762
Cranial nerves
   assessment of, 335–336, 337t
   communication and, 1275–1276
Creams, 528–529
Creatinine excretion, nutrition and, 914
Creativity, need for, spiritual dysfunction and, 1398t
Cretinism, 899
Crimes, 51–52
   torts versus, 50t
Crisis, spiritual function and, 1396
Crisis intervention, stress management and, 1354
Crust, skin and, 947t
Crutches, 729, 731–732, 733–735
   gaits for, 731–732, 733–735
Cryoprecipitate, 881
CSA (Controlled Substances Act), 508t, 508–509, 509t
CSF (cerebrospinal fluid), reference ranges for, 1435–1436
CT. *See* Computed tomography
Cue(s), 118–120
   validation of data and, 103–105, 105f
Cue clustering, 118–120, 119f
   cluster interpretation and, 120
   problems in, 119–120
Cultural value orientations, 263–264
Culture, 237–250
   biocultural variation and, 246–247
   characteristics of, 238–241

Culture (*continued*)
   communication and, 1269
   culturally sensitive nursing care and, 243, 245
   definition of, 237
   ethnicity and ethnic identity and, 241–242
   family function and, 1290–1291
   grounding nursing assessments in patient's perspective
      and, 247–248
   health/illness concepts and, 244–245
   health maintenance and, 598
   health variations and, 241
   infections and, 1003
   material, 241
   minority and, 242
   nutrition and, 906
   pain perception and, 1167, 1171
   patient education and, 250, 250f
   patients who do not speak nurse's language and, 248–249
   patient teaching and, 414
   peer, as source of values, 259
   race and, 242
   racism and, 242
   self-care and, 645
   self-concept and, 1244
   sexuality and, 1369
   spiritual function and, 1394
   stereotype and, 243
   subculture and, 242–243, 243f
   values and beliefs and, 241
Culture shock, 239
Culture testing, 392–393
Cutaneous stimulation, pain relief and, 1178–1179
CVA. *See* Cerebrovascular accident
Cyanosis
   altered respiratory function and, 758
   ischemia and, 815
Cystoscopy, 1063–1064

D

Dalmane (flurazepam), 1155t
Damages, 51
Dandruff, 665
DAT (diet as tolerated), 920
Data
   objective, 102, 102t
   organizing, 105t, 105–107
      body systems model for, 105, 106t
   subjective, 102, 102t
   validation of, 103–105, 105f
Data collection, 102–103
   evaluation and, 142–143
   for functional health assessment, 297, 303–307
      interview and, 297, 303
      physical examination and, 303–307
   recording data and, 103
   sources of data and, 102–103
   types of data and, 102, 102t
Day care, cognitive function and, 1235
Day-care centers, 32
DDLs (demands of daily living), home maintenance
      management and, 614–615
Death and dying. *See also* Grief; Grieving; Loss
   care of deceased and, 52, 54, 1324–1325

legal issues and, 52, 54
Death certificate, 52
Debridement, of wounds, 967–968
Decision-maker, nurse as, 18, 18f
Decision-making
   information needed in, 48
   process of, 88
   as source of values, 260
Decoding, in communication process, 275
Decontamination, 443
Decreased Cardiac Output, 823
Decubitus ulcers. *See* Pressure sores
Deep breathing, 767, 768, 769
   stress management and, 1352
Deep cough, 770
Deep tendon reflexes, assessment of, 336, 338t
Deep vein thrombosis, immobility and, 710
Defamation of character, 49
Defecation, 1093
   ignoring urge to defecate and, 1096–1097
Defecation reflex, 1093
Defendant, 50
Defense mechanisms, dysfunctional, coping and adaptation
      and, 1344
Defensive phase, of wound healing, 945
Defining characteristics, in nursing diagnosis, 118
Definition, in nursing diagnosis, 118
Degenerative processes, cognitive function and, 1220–1221,
      1222t
Deglutition, 900
Dehiscence, wound healing and, 950, 950f
Deltoid site, for intramuscular injections, 542, 542f
Delusions, 1196, 1221
Demands of daily living (DDLs), home maintenance
      management and, 614–615
Dementia, 1221, 1222t
Demonstrations, patient teaching and, 419, 420f
Denture care, 672f, 672–673
Deontology, ethics and, 44
Department of Health and Human Services (DHHS), 33
Dependent nursing functions, 17–18
Dependent variable, 75
Depression
   coping and adaptation and, 1345
   self-care and, 648
   self-concept and, 1251t, 1251–1251
   sensory perception and, 1196
Dermatitis, 939
Dermis, 936, 936f
Detrusor muscle, 1043
Development, 196–219
   of adolescent, 203t, 207
   biocultural variation in, 246
   definition of, 197
   functional health and, health problems and anticipatory
      guidance and. *See* Functional health patterns,
      health problems and anticipatory guidance and
   genetics and environment and, 198–199
   health maintenance and, 598
   of infant, 202t, 204–205
   intrauterine, 201, 202t, 204
   of middle adult, 203t, 208
   of neonate, 202t, 204, 205f

of older adult, 203t, 208–209
of preschooler, 202t–203t, 206
principles of, 199
of school-age child, 203t, 206–207
of self-concept, 1245, 1249–1250, 1255t, 1255–1256
   theories of, 1246t, 1247t
theories of, 199–201, 200t
   cognitive development, 199, 200t, 201
   developmental task, 199, 200t, 201
   human needs, 199, 200t, 201
   moral development, 199, 200t, 201
   psychodynamic, 199, 200, 200t
of toddler, 202t, 205–206
of values, 269
of young adult, 203t, 207–208
Developmental framework, for family, 225–226, 226r
Developmental problems, altered health maintenance
   function and, 600–601
Developmental stages, of family, 225–226, 226r
Developmental task theory, 199, 200t, 201
Diabetes mellitus, altered nutrition and, 910
Diagnosis, 30. *See also* Nursing diagnoses
Diagnosis-related groups (DRGs), 29, 35
Diagnostic and Statistical Manual of Mental Disorders
   (DSM-III-R), 113
Diagnostic label, 118
Diagnostic reasoning process, 89
Diagnostic statement, formulation of, 121–122
   actual nursing diagnoses and, 121
   high risk nursing diagnoses and, 122
   possible nursing diagnoses and, 122
Diagnostic tests and procedures, 378–385, 393–403, 394t.
      See also Laboratory tests
   aspiration procedures and, 399–402
   bowel function and, 1097, 1105–1108
   cardiopulmonary function and, 820–822, 821t,
      822f
   cognitive function and, 1226–1229
   communication and, 1276
   coping and adaptation and, 1347
   data collection from, 103
   evaluating electrical conduction, 402–403
   fluid and electrolyte imbalance and, 865–866
   health maintenance and, 604
   individualizing care using data from, 385, 386t
   infections and, 1002–1005
   invasive viewing techniques and, 397–399
   lifespan considerations and, 403–404
   mobility and, 717
   noninvasive viewing techniques and, 393–397
   nursing responsibilities during, 383–384
   nursing responsibilities following, 384–385
   nutrition and, 914
   pain and, 1174
   patient preparation for, 380–383
   potential alteration in normal function due to, 394t
   respiratory function and, 762–764
   sensory perception and, 1199
   sexual function and, 1377, 1377t
   skin and, 953
   sleep and rest and, 1151
   urinary elimination and, 1056–1064
Diarrhea, 1100–1101, 1109, 1112

enteral tube feedings and, 923
infections and, 1000
Diastole, 803
Diastolic blood pressure, 364
Diet. *See also* Food; Nutrient(s); Nutrition–metabolism
      health pattern
   bowel function and, 1096, 1111
   patient teaching about
      fluid and electrolyte balance and, 869, 869t
      to reduce edema, 829
   special, 920–921
Diet as tolerated (DAT), 920
Diet orders, checking before medication administration, 516
Diffusion
   fluid and electrolyte movement and, 848–849
   of gas, 749–750, 750f
Digestion, 900
Digestive system, anatomy of, 892–893
Digits, clubbing of, 312, 312f
   altered respiratory function and, 758
Diploma nursing program, 13
Dipsticks, urine testing and, 1060
Direct contact, transmission by, 429
Directing, as management function, 61, 61f
Directive leadership, 60, 60f
Discharge planner, 625
Discharge planning
   bowel function and, 1125, 1129
   cognitive function and, 1234–1235
   communication and, 1280–1281
   coping and adaptation and, 1354
   family function and, 1303
   fluid and electrolyte and acid-base balance and, 884, 886
   grieving and, 1325
   health maintenance and, 608
   home maintenance management and, 625–626, 629–630
   infections and, 1012–1014
   levels of, 629, 629t
   medications and, 553–554
   mobility and, 735, 740, 742
   nutrition and, 929–930
   pain and, 1185–1186
   postoperative, 495
   respiratory function and, 788, 792, 795
   safety and, 587–588, 588f
   self-care deficits and, 682, 685, 688–689
   self-concept and, 1257–1258
   sensory perception and, 1203, 1206
   sexual function and, 1383–1384
   skin conditions and, 976
   sleep and, 1154
   spiritual function and, 1408–1409
   thermoregulation and, 1034–1035
   urinary elimination and, 1083, 1085
   values and, 270
Discharge preparation, 629–630
Discharge summary, 161, 164f, 165
Diseases. *See also* Illness; *specific diseases*
   communicable, 431
   contagious, 431
   holistic health care and, 177–178
   infectious. *See* Infection(s); Infectious diseases
   risk of, 570–571

Disease-specific isolation, 451, 454t
Disinfectants, 443, 444t
Disinfection, 443, 444t
  effectiveness of, 445
  levels of, 444–445
Disorganization, grief and, 1314
Distraction, pain relief and, 1177–1178
Distribution, of drugs, 511
Disuse osteoporosis, 711
Divorce, family function and, 1295
Dix, Dorothea, 9
DNR (do not resuscitate; no code; no heroics), 52
Doctoral degree programs, 16
Documentation. *See also* Patient record
  abbreviations used in, 151t–152t
  of assessment parameters, 106
  avoiding lawsuits and, 54, 56f
  computer, 155, 158f
  computerized assessment record and, 103
  of diagnostic and laboratory tests, 385
  of functional health assessment, 297, 298f–302f
  legal, as purpose of patient record, 150
  of medication administration, 523, 523f
  of patient teaching, 420–421
  process recording and, 286, 287t
  of vital signs, 375f, 376
  written assessment record and, 103
Donors, of blood, 881–882
Doppler techniques
  blood pressure assessment and, 368
  pulse measurement and, 358, 361f
Dorsal recumbent position, 721t
Dorsogluteal site, for intramuscular injections, 546f,
      546–547, 547f
Dosage
  calculating, 519–521
    for children, 521
    conversions from one system to another and, 520–521
    conversions within a system and, 520
    for intravenous medications, 521
  in drug orders, 504
Drainage, 966–967
  advancing and removing drains and, 967, 969f
  closed drainage systems and, 967, 967f, 968
  of wounds, 953
Drainage-secretions precautions, 451
Draping, intraoperative, 487
Dressing (clothing), 644, 678, 680–681
Dressings, 958–960
  changing, 959–960, 961–964
  methods of securing, 958–595, 959f
  types of, 958, 959t
  wet-to-dry, 964
DRGs. *See* Diagnosis-related groups
Droplet contact, transmission by, 429
Drug(s). *See also* Medication(s); *headings beginning with
      term* Medication
  abuse of, 511
    altered nutrition and, 911
  arterial, 1227
  cardiovascular function and, 813
  communication and, 1271
  controlled substances, 52, 508t, 508–509, 509t
  factors affecting action of, 514–515
  medications versus, 500
  names of, 500
    in drug orders, 504
  pharmacodynamics and, 512–514
  pharmacokinetics and, 511–512
  reference ranges for, 1437
  respiratory function and, 755
  scheduled, 508–509, 509t
  side effects of. *See* Side effects
  sleep and, 1147
  therapeutic effects of, 512, 513f
  types and forms of, 500, 501t, 502t
  wound healing and, 949
Drug enforcement agencies, 508–509, 509t
Drug levels, serum, 392
Drug orders, 504–505, 505t
  abbreviations used in, 505t
  interpretation of, 519
  types of, 504–505
DSM-III-R (Diagnostic and Statistical Manual of Mental
      Disorders), 113
Dullness, percussion and, 305, 305t
Duration, auscultation and, 306
Durkham-Humphrey Amendment of 1952, 507, 508t
Duty, 50
  breach of, 50–51
Dysarthria, 1272–1273, 1280
Dysfunction, holistic health care and, 178–179
Dysfunctional grief, 1318, 1321–1322
Dysfunctional Grieving, 1321–1322
Dyspareunia, 1373
Dyspnea, 364
  altered respiratory function and, 757
  management of, 780
Dystonia, 707
Dysuria, 1051

E
Ear care, 643, 676–677
Eccrine glands, 937
ECG. *See* Electrocardiogram
Echocardiography, cardiopulmonary function and, 822
Economic provision, as family function, 1289
Economics. *See also* Poverty
  health maintenance and, 598
  home maintenance management and, 616
  limited medical and financial resources and, 37
  nutrition and, 906–907
Economic status, family function and, 1291
Eczema, 944
Edema, 327
  altered cardiovascular function and, 816
  cardiopulmonary function and, 819, 820f
  reduction of, 829
Education. *See also* Nursing education; Patient teaching
  as family function, 1290
  as purpose of patient record, 150
  on sexuality, 1381
Educative nursing interventions, 136
Educator, nurse as, 19
EEG (electroencephalogram), 402–403
Ego, 200

EHS (Everyday Hassles Scale), 1337
Ejaculatory dysfunction, 1373
Elaboration, encouraging, 284t, 285
Elbow protectors, 726t
Elderly. *See* Older adult
Elective surgery, 466
Electrical burns, 943
Electrical safety, 580
  intraoperative, 486
Electrical shock, 573–574
Electrocardiogram (ECG), 402, 402f
  cardiopulmonary function and, 821, 822f
Electroencephalogram (EEG), 402–403
Electrolyte replacement, 869
Electrolytes, 390–391, 846–848, 848t. *See also* Fluid and
    electrolyte balance
  cardiopulmonary function and, 821
Electronic blood pressure measurement, 368–369
Electronic thermometers, 353, 353f
Elimination. *See also* Bowel elimination; Elimination health
    pattern; Feces; Urinary elimination; Urine;
    headings beginning with term Stool
  home maintenance management and, 616
  immobility and, 712–713
  need for, 186–187
  postoperative, 494
  sleep and, 1143–1144
Elimination health pattern, 90, 107
  assessing human needs and, 192
  assessment of, 327–328
    bowel elimination and, 328
    urinary elimination and, 327–328
  in community, 232
  disruption by diagnostic procedures, 394t
  drugs promoting normal function and, 501t
  exercise and immobility and, 708t
  in family, 228
  health maintenance and, 597t
  health problems and anticipatory guidance and, 212
  laboratory and diagnostic tests related to, 386t
  surgery and, 470
  values and, 263
Embolism
  immobility and, 710
  pulmonary, 816
Embolus, 710
Embryo, 201, 204
Emergency assessment, 96t, 97
Emergent surgery, 466
Emotional changes, self-concept and, 1250–1251, 1251t
Emotional damages, 51
Emotional problems
  in children, family function and, 1295
  self-care and, 648
Emotional support. *See* Support, emotional
Empathy, 280, 280f, 280t
Emphysema, 754
Encephalitis, 989t
Encoding, in communication process, 275
Endocrine system, homeostatic control and, 1337
Endogenous opiates, 1163
Endogenous opiates theory of pain, 1164–1165
Endogenous pyrogens, body temperature and, 1025

Endoscopy, 398, 398t
  bowel function and, 1106, 1108
Endotracheal tubes, 781
Endurance, muscle atrophy and, 709
Enemas, 1112–1117, 1114f
  large-volume, 1113–1117
  return-flow, 1117
  small-volume, 1113, 1113t, 1116
Energy
  decreased, altered nutrition and, 912
  mobility and, 702
  self-care and, 644, 647
Energy balance, nutrition and, 905, 906
Energy conservation
  altered cardiopulmonary function and, 830–831
  respiratory function and, 792, 795
Enteral tube feedings, 921–923, 922f
  continuous versus intermittent, 923, 924–296
  enteral formulas and, 922
  hazards and complications of, 923
  indications for, 922, 922f
  types of tubes for, 922
Enteric precautions, 451
Enuresis, 1053–1054, 1150
Environment
  body temperature and, 350, 1024
  communication and, 1280
  concept of, 12
  development and, 198
  for functional health assessment, 296–297
  health maintenance function and, 599
  home maintenance management and, 614, 620
  host-agent-environment model and, 174
  nosocomial infections and, 432
  for nursing assessment, 97
  orientation to, communication and, 1278
  patient teaching and, 417
  resistance to infection and, 986
  respiratory function and, 752, 755
  safety and, 566, 567f
  self-care and, 645, 648
  sensory perception and, 1192–1193, 1194, 1195f,
    1195–1196
  sexual function and, 1376
  sexuality and, 1372
  sleep and, 1145–1146, 1152
  stress management and, 1354
Environmental stress, 1346
Enzymes
  cardiac, cardiopulmonary function and, 820–821
  serum, 391–392
Eosinophils, 983t
Epidermis, 936, 936f
  condition of, 938
Equipment
  handling of, infection control and, 448
  safety and, intraoperative, 486
Equivalents, measurement, 1413–1414
Erikson, Erik, psychodynamic theory of, 199, 200, 200t,
    1246t, 1247t
Erosion, of skin, 946t
Erythrocyte sedimentation rate (ESR), 390–391
  infections and, 1003

Eschar, 941
Esteem needs, 188, 224
Ethical issues, 41–45, 49
  analysis of, 45
  decision making and, 38
  ethical philosophy and, 43–44
  home care and, home maintenance management and, 630–631
  moral development and, 44–45
  in nursing research, 76–77
  professional codes of ethics and, 42–43
  role conflict and, 45
  technologic advances and, 29
Ethical principles, 42
Ethics
  definition of, 42
  values and, 258–259
Ethnicity, 241–242
  health/illness considerations related to, 244–245
Ethnocentricity, 240
Ethnographic interview, grounding assessments in patient's perspective and, 247–248
ETT. *See* Exercise tolerance testing
Euthanasia, active, 52
Evaluation, 86, 139–146, 140f
  bowel function and, 1129, 1131
  cardiopulmonary function and, 837–839
  cognitive function and, 1235–1236
  communication and, 1281
  coping and adaptation and, 1354, 1356
  data collection and, 142–143
  family function and, 1304
  fluid and electrolyte and acid-base balance and, 886–887
  grieving and, 1325, 1330
  home maintenance management and, 633, 634t, 635
  in instructional nursing care plans, 133
  intraoperative, 490
  of learning, 420
  measuring goal attainment and, 143f, 143–144
  medications and, 554
  mobility and, 742–743
  nutrition and, 930–932
  outcome, 142
  pain and, 1186
  postoperative, 495
  preoperative, 483–484
  process, 141–142
  quality assurance monitors and, 144–146
  recording judgment or measurement of goal attainment and, 144
  resistance to infection and, 1014
  respiratory function and, 795–797
  reviewing patient goals and outcome criteria and, 142
  revising and modifying nursing management plan and, 144, 144f, 145f
  safety and, 589–590
  of self, 1243, 1256–1257
  self-care deficit and, 689–690
  self-concept and, 1258
  sensory perception and, 1206–1207
  sexual function and, 1384–1385
  skills for, 140–141
  skin and, 976, 978
  sleep and, 1154–1155
  spiritual function and, 1409–1410
  structure, 141
  thermoregulation and, 1035–1036
  urinary elimination and, 1085–1086
  using functional health approach, 146
Evaporation, heat loss and, 1021
Eversion, 701, 703t
Everyday Hassles Scale (EHS), 1337
Evisceration, wound healing and, 950
Exchanging pattern, nursing diagnosis and, 113
Excitement phase, of sexual response, 1366, 1367, 1367t
Excretion. *See also* Bowel elimination; Elimination; Elimination health pattern; Feces; Urinary elimination; Urine; *headings beginning with term* Stool
  digestive system and, 901
  of drugs, 512
Exercise(s), 701. *See also* Activity; Activity–exercise health pattern
  benefits of, 701
  body temperature and, 350, 1025
  bowel function and, 1111
  cardiovascular function and, 807, 813
  coping and adaptation and, 1341–1342, 1351
  deep breathing, 767, 768, 769
    stress management and, 1352
  heat production and, 1019
  immobility and, 708–711
  Kegel, sexual function and, 1381
  for legs, prevention of venous return and, 826, 827f
  range-of-motion, 722, 728–729
  respiratory function and, 362, 752
  safety and, 565
  sleep and, 1144
  types of, 701
Exercise tolerance testing (ETT), 402
  cardiopulmonary function and, 821–822
Exhaustion, general adaptation syndrome and, 1339
Experience
  communication process and, 275–276, 276t
  coping and adaptation and, 1342
  family function and, 1291
  health maintenance and, 598
  safety and, 565–566
  self-concept and, 1245
  sensory perception and, 1193
  sexuality and, 1369
  as source of values, 260
  spiritual function and, 1394
  traumatic, family function and, 1293–1294
Exploring, 285–286
Expressive aphasia, 1271–1272, 1272t
Extended care facilities, infection hazards in, 433–434
Extended family, 1288, 1288f
Extension, 701, 703t, 704t
Exteroceptors, 1213
Eye(s), artificial, care of, 676
Eye care, 643, 673–676
  in comatose patient, 676
Eyeglasses, care of, 673

F

Facilitation, discharge planning and, 626
Faith, 1393. *See also* Spiritual function
Fallopian tubes, 1362

Falls, 572
  mobility and, 707
  prevention of, 581–583, 582f, 583f
  risk for, assessment of, 716
False imprisonment, 49–50
False reassurance, 288
Family, 224–229, 1286–1304
  altered function of, 1292–1296
    activities of daily living and, 1295–1296
    manifestations of, 1294–1295
    potential for, 1292–1294, 1293t
  assessment and, 227t, 228–229, 1296–1298
    objective data and, 1298
    subjective data and, 1296–1298
  characteristics of, 1288–1290
  definition of, 224
  developmental framework for, 225–226, 226t
  discharge preparation and, 630
  dysfunctional, coping and adaptation and, 1343–1344
  eliciting information related to functional health patterns
    in, 228
  evaluation and, 1304
  factors affecting, 1290–1291
  functional health pattern of, 1290
  home maintenance management and, 616, 619–620, 621
  interventions, 1300–1303
  involvement in patient teaching, 416
  lifespan considerations and, 1291–1292
  needs of, 633
  nursing diagnoses and patient goals and, 1298–1300
  pain and, 1171
  as resource, 628
  responsibility for functional health, 229
  stress in, altered home maintenance management and,
    620
  structure of, 1288–1289
  systems framework for, 226, 227f, 228
  value conflicts in, 267–268
Family history, cardiovascular function and, 813
Family members
  as barriers to patient goal attainment, 143
  data collection from, 103
Family planning, 1381–1383
Family support, cognitive function and, 1234
Fat
  in diet, 902, 904
    altered nutrition and, 910
  digestion of, 900
  metabolism of, 901
  normal physiologic function of, 894
Fatigue, 1142
  pain perception and, 1167
  safety and, 566
FDA (Food and Drug Administration), 507–508
Fear
  pain perception and, 1167
  safety dysfunction and, 575
  spiritual care and, 1397
Febrile patient, 1020. *See also* Fever
Febrile reaction, to blood transfusion, 882
Fecal collecting devices, 1123–1124
Fecal diversion, 1098, 1098f
Fecal impaction, 1099f, 1099–1100
  removal of, 1122–1123

Fecal incontinence, 1101, 1109, 1112
Feces. *See also headings beginning with term* Stool
  characteristics of, 1093, 1093t
Federal Food, Drug, and Cosmetic Act of 1938, 507, 508t
Federal Trade Commission (FTC), 508
Feedback
  in communication process, 275
  in systems theory, 87, 87f
Feeding, 643, 677–678
  assisting with, 918–919
Feeding tubes, clogging of, 923
Feeling pattern, nursing diagnosis and, 116
Festinating gait, 707
Fetus, 204
Fever, 1026–1027
  infections and, 999, 999f
  management of, 1032–1034
  phases of febrile episode and, 1026–1027
  resistance to infection and, 984
  respirations and, 362
  types of, 1026, 1027t
Fidelity
  ethics and, 43
  home care and, home maintenance management and,
    630
Fight-or-flight response, 1338
Figure-eight turns, 965, 965f
Filtration
  fluid and electrolyte movement and, 849
  urine formation and, 1045
Filtration pressure, fluid and electrolyte movement and,
    850, 851f
Fingers. *See* Digits
Fire(s), 572
  evacuation and, 586
Fire extinguishers, classes of fires and, 580, 580t
Fire safety, 580, 580t
Fissure, of skin, 947t
Fistula, wound healing and, 950
'Five Ds,' 83
Flaccidity, 706
Flatness, percussion and, 305, 305t
Flatulence, 1101, 1112
Flexion, 701, 703t, 704t
Flora, normal, 982
Flossing, 669–671
Flotation surfaces, 956
Flow rate, of intravenous infusions, calculating, 872, 874
Flowsheets, 161, 162f, 163f
Fluid and electrolyte balance, 846–853
  altered, 857–861
    activities of daily living and, 861
    manifestations of, 860–861
    potential for, 858–859
  arterial, 1227
  assessment of, 861–866
    objective data and, 862–866
    subjective data and, 861–862
  cognitive function and, 1216, 1219
  distribution of, 848–850
  electrolytes and, 846–848, 848t
  evaluation and, 886–887
  factors affecting, 850–852, 852t
  fluid compartments and, 846, 847f

Fluid and electrolyte balance (*continued*)
 interventions and, 867–886
  altered fluid and electrolyte balance and, 868–884
  discharge planning and home care and, 884, 886
  to promote health and function, 867–868
 lifespan considerations and, 852–853
 nursing diagnoses and patient goals and, 866–867
 skin and, 937
 total body water and, 846, 847t
Fluid compartments, 846, 847f
Fluid intake
 bowel function and, 1096, 1111
 cognitive function and, 1231–1232
 fluid and electrolyte balance and, 850–852, 852t
 increasing, fluid and electrolyte balance and, 868
 monitoring, fluid and electrolyte and acid-base balance
  and, 862–864, 864f
 output and, fluid and electrolyte imbalance and, 860
 promotion of, 1066
 restricting, fluid and electrolyte balance and, 868–869
 urinary elimination and, 1046
Fluid loss
 excessive, fluid and electrolyte imbalance and, 858–859
 urinary elimination and, 1046
Fluid orders, checking before medication administration,
  516
Fluid restriction, to reduce edema, 829
Fluid Volume Deficit, 866
 nursing management plan for, 885–886
Fluid volume deficit (FVD), 855, 866, 885–886
Fluid Volume Excess, 866–867
Fluid volume excess (FVE), 855, 866–867
 intravenous therapy and, 879–880
 total parenteral nutrition and, 929
Fluorine, normal physiologic function of, 898t, 899–900
Fluoroscopy, 395
Flurazepam (Dalmane), 1155t
Foam surfaces, 956, 956f
Focus assessment, 96t, 96–97
Focused care providers, 35
Focusing, 284t, 285
Focus on Care, 78
Folic acid (folacin), normal physiologic function of, 895t
Food. *See also* Diet; Feeding; Nutrient(s); Nutrition–
  metabolism health pattern
  basic four food groups and, 902, 903f, 904
  inability to acquire and prepare, 909, 909f
  withholding, 919–920
Food and Drug Administration (FDA), 507–508
Food intake
 fluid and electrolyte balance and, 851
 optimal intake promotion and, 917, 918–919
Footboard, 725t
Foot care, 642, 663, 665t, 666–667
Foreign languages
 communication and, 290
 patient teaching and, 414
Foreskin, 1362
Forgiveness, need for, spiritual dysfunction and, 1398t
For profit hospitals, 30
Four-point gait, 731, 733–734
Fowler's position, 721t
Fractures, of hip, positioning and, 720

Fraud, 49
Frequency
 auscultation and, 306
 urinary elimination and, 1052
Freud, Sigmund, psychodynamic theory of, 199, 200, 200t,
  1246t, 1247t
Friction, decubitus ulcers and, 943
Friends, involvement in patient teaching, 416
Frostbite, 1028
Fruits, 902
FTC (Federal Trade Commission), 508
Full liquid diet, 920
Functional health
 community responsibility for, 233
 family responsibility for, 229
Functional health approach
 evaluation using, 146
 implementation using. *See also* Patient record
 to nursing process, 90, 91f
 planning organized by, 134
Functional health assessment. *See also specific functional
  health patterns*
 components of, 106
 concluding, 343–344
 data collection for, 297, 303–307
  interview and, 297, 303
  physical examination and, 303–307
 individual aspects of functional health and, 307
 lifespan considerations and, 344–346
 organization and documentation of, 297, 298f–302f
 preparation of patient and environment for, 296–297
 purpose of, 296
Functional health patterns, 90. *See also specific functional
  health patterns*
 assessing human needs and, 192–193, 193f
 bowel function and, 1102
 cardiopulmonary function and, 817–818
 cardiovascular, 806–807
 cognitive function and, 1223–1225
 communication and, 1274–1275
 in community, 232
 description of, 106–107
 in family, 228
 family function and, 1296–1297
 fluid and electrolyte and acid-base balance and, 861
 functional health assessment and, 106
 grieving and, 1319–1320
 health maintenance and, 601
 health problems and anticipatory guidance and, 209–219
  activity and exercise and, 212–213
  cognition and perception and, 213f, 213–214
  coping and stress tolerance and, 217–218
  elimination and, 212
  health perception and health management and,
   209–211, 210f, 211f
  nutrition and metabolism and, 211–212
  roles and relationships and, 215–216, 216f
  self-perception and self-concept and, 215
  sexuality and reproduction and, 216–217
  sleep and rest and, 214–215
  values and beliefs and, 218–219
 home maintenance management and, 620
 infections and, 1001

integumentary, 938
laboratory and diagnostic tests related to, 386t
mobility and, 715
nursing diagnoses organized by, 123–125
nutritional, 902–905
    basic four food groups and, 902, 903f, 904–905
nutrition and, 912
organizing data and, 106–107
pain and, 1170–1171
respiratory function and, 759
safety assessment and, 576
self-care and, 649, 649t
self-concept and, 1252
sensory perception and, 1197, 1198t
sexual function and, 1374
sexuality and, 1368
skin and, 951
sleep and rest and, 1150
spiritual function and, 1399, 1401
surgery and, 468–472
thermoregulation and, 1028–1029
urinary elimination and, 1054
values and, 261–265
Functional Incontinence, 1065
Functional incontinence, 1053, 1065
Funding, 33–35
charitable, 35
government involvement in, 33–35
private health insurance and, 33
Fungi, 428, 993
FVD. *See* Fluid volume deficit
FVE. *See* Fluid volume excess

G
Gait
altered, 707
assessment of, 309, 716
crutches and, 731–732, 733–735
normal, 702
GAS (general adaptation syndrome), 1338–1339
Gas diffusion, 749–750, 750f
Gas sterilization, 444
Gas transport, 750
Gastric analysis
nasogastric intubation and, 1117
reference ranges for, 1437
Gastric decompression, nasogastric intubation and, 1117
Gastric gavage, nasogastric intubation and, 1117–1118
Gastric lavage, nasogastric intubation and, 1117
Gastric tubes, oral administration through, 527–528
Gastroenteritis, manifestations of, 1002
Gastrointestinal motility, assessing before medication
        administration, 517
Gastrointestinal tract
infections and, 1000
inflammation of, altered nutrition and, 910
normal anatomy of, 1090f, 1090–1092, 1091f
normal function of, 1092–1093
obstruction of, altered nutrition and, 910
stress and, 1347
Gastrostomy, 921–922, 922f
Gastrostomy/jejunostomy tube, 922
Gate control theory of pain, 1164f, 1164–1165

Gender. *See* Sex; Sexual function; Sexuality–reproductive
        health pattern
Gender identity, 1366
alterations in, 1371–1372, 1374, 1376
Gender roles, 1366
General adaptation syndrome (GAS), 1338–1339
General anesthesia, 487, 488t
stages of, 487, 488t
General damages, 51
Generative activities, in holistic health care, 179–180
Generic care plans, 131
Generic name, of drugs, 500
Genetics, 198
drug action and, 514
Genital herpes, 989t
German measles, 988t
Gerontologic patients. *See* Older adult
Gilligan, Carol, 45
Gingiva, 643
Glasgow Coma Scale, 329, 329t, 333
Glass mercury thermometers, 352, 352f, 353f
Global aphasia, 1272
Gloves
infection control and, 437, 445
sterile, 457, 458–460
Glucose, blood. *See* Blood glucose
Glycogenesis, 900
Goals. *See also* Patient goals
behavioral, 128
long- and short-term, 128
Goldmark Report, 9
Gonorrhea, 989t
Gonorrhea culture, 1377t
Good Samaritan Law, 56
Government
health-care funding and, 33–35
hospitals owned by, 30
Gowns, infection control and, 445–448
Graduate degree programs, 16
Gram-positive bacteria, 992
Gram stain, 392
Granulation tissue, 945
Granulocytes, 880, 983
Grenade drain, 953
Grief, 1310–1311. *See also* Grieving; Loss
models of, 1311–1314
    nursing models and, 1312–1313
    normal functional pattern of, 1315
    stages of, working through, 1323–1324
    types of loss and, 1314
Grief cycle model, 1312f, 1313t, 1313–1314
Grieving, 1308–1331
activities of daily living and, 1318
altered, 1318–1319
    manifestations of, 1318
    potential for, 1318
assessment and, 1319–1321
    subjective data and, 1319–1321
characteristics of, 1310–1311
evaluation and, 1325, 1330
factors affecting, 1315–1316
interventions and, 1322–1325
    for altered function, 1325

Grieving, interventions and (*continued*)
  discharge planning and home care and, 1325
  to promote health and function, 1322–1325
  lifespan considerations and, 1316–1318, 1317t
  nursing diagnoses and patient goals and, 1321–1322
Grieving (nursing diagnosis), nursing management plan for, 1326–1329
Grooming, 644
  altered self-care and, 648
Gross national product, 28
Ground, electrical, 574
Growth. *See also* Development
  abnormal, of skin, 940
  biocultural variation in, 246, 246f
  home maintenance management and, 615
  principles of, 199
Guided imagery, pain relief and, 1179

H
Habit(s)
  bowel function and, 1094
  cardiovascular function and, 808
  health maintenance and, 598
  health maintenance function and, 600
  home maintenance management and, 616
  mobility and, 704
  nutrition and, 905–906
  safety and, 565
  sensory perception and, 1193
  skin and, 938
  sleep and, 1144
Habit retraining, 1069
Hair, 937
  altered, altered nutrition and, 912
Hair care, 642, 663–665, 668–669
Haitian Americans, key informants for, 248
Halcion (triazolam), 1155t
Hall, Lydia E., 14t–15t, 83
  perception of human needs, 190–191
Hallucinations, 1196, 1221
Hallux valgus, 665t
Hand roll, 726t
Hand veins, fluid and electrolyte imbalance and, 865
Handwashing, 440–443
  infection control and, 1011, 1011f
  surgical, 456–457
Hand-wrist splint, 726t
Havighurst, Robert, developmental task theory of, 199, 200t, 201, 1246t, 1247t
Hazards, safety and, 569–570
HCFA. *See* Health Care Financing Administration
Head nurse, 66
Head-to-toe approach. *See* Body systems model
Head trauma, communication and, 1271
Healing. *See also* Wound healing
  by first intention, 945
  by second intention, 945
  by third intention, 945, 947
Health, 173–176. *See also* Diseases; Illness; *specific disorders*
  clinical model of, 174
  concept of, 12

cultural variations in, 241
  definition of, 173
  of employees, infection control and, 435–438
  health belief model of, 174–175, 175f
  high-level wellness model and, 175, 176f
  holistic health model and, 175–176, 176f
  host-agent-environment model of, 174, 174f
Health belief model, 174–175, 175f
Health care
  access to, 37–38
  fragmentation of services and, 37, 37f
  holistic. *See* Holistic health care
  home maintenance management and, 626–628, 627f
  individualizing, 385
  levels of care and, 626–628, 627f
  as right, 28
  routine, 607, 607f
Health-care costs, limited medical and financial resources and, 37
Health-care delivery system, 26–38
  abbreviations used in, 28
  in Canada, 34
  challenges to, 36–38, 37f
  colleagues in, 35–36
  definition of, 27–28
  factors affecting, 28–29, 29f
  funding of services and, 33–35
  infection prevention within, 1008–1009
  settings in, 29–33, 30f–32f
  value conflicts between patient and, 268–269
    resolving, 268–269
Health Care Financing Administration (HCFA), 33–3434
Health-care setting. *See also* Settings
  sensory deficit in, 1196
  sensory deprivation in, 1195f, 1195–1196
  sensory overload in, 1194, 1194f, 1195f
Health-care workers. *See also* Nurse(s); Physicians
  infection control and, 435–438
    monitoring and counseling personnel and, 435t, 435–436
    significant exposure and, 436–437
    transmissible diseases and, 436, 436t
    work restriction and, 437–438, 439t
Health education. *See also* Patient education
  preventive, 412, 412f
Health insurance. *See also* Medicaid; Medicare
  catastrophic, 33
  patient record audits for, 150
  private, 33
  supplemental, 33, 34
Health maintenance, 592–610, 593–594. *See also* Health perception–health management health pattern
  altered, 599–601
    activities of daily living and, 601
    manifestations of, 600–601
    potential for, 599–600
  assessment of, 601–604
    objective data and, 602–604
    subjective data and, 601–602
  characteristics of, 594f, 594–595
  evaluation and, 608–609
  factors affecting, 596–598
  functional, 595–596

interventions and, 605–608, 606f
  for altered function, 607–608
  discharge planning and home care and, 608
  to promote health and function, 605–607
  lifespan considerations and, 598–599
  nursing diagnoses and patient goals and, 604–605
Health maintenance organizations (HMOs), 31
Health management. *See also* Health perception–health
       management health pattern
  immobility and, 707–708
  sexuality and, 1368
Health perception. *See also* Health perception–health
       management health pattern
  immobility and, 707–708
Health perception–health management health pattern, 90,
       106
  assessing human needs and, 192
  assessment of, 307–308
    objective data in, 308
    subjective data in, 307–308
  in community, 232
  exercise and immobility and, 708t
  in family, 228
  health maintenance and, 597t
  health problems and anticipatory guidance and, 209–211,
       210f, 211f
  laboratory and diagnostic tests related to, 386t
  surgery and, 469
  values and, 261
Health promotion, 30, 179–180, 595, 596, 597t
  generative activities and, 179–180
  home maintenance management and, 615, 619
  nurturative activities and, 179
Health promotion centers, as nursing practice settings, 17
Health records. *See also* Patient record
  data collection from, 103
Health-Seeking Behaviors, 604
  nursing management plan for, 609
Health-team members, as barriers to patient goal
       attainment, 144
Health-team reports, data collection from, 103
Hearing
  assessment of, 335, 335f, 336f
  observation and, 98
Hearing aids
  care of, 676f, 676–677
  types of, 676
Heart, 802. *See also* Cardiovascular function
  altered cardiopulmonary function and, 816
  decreased pumping ability of, 809–810
  normal function of, 803–805
Heart attack, 810
Heart disease. *See also* Coronary heart disease
  functional and therapeutic classification of patients with,
       832
  patient teaching about, 605–606
Heart failure, fluid and electrolyte and acid-base
       imbalances and, 859
Heart rate, 806–807
  pain and, 1169
Heart sounds, 318, 318f
  auscultation of. *See* Auscultation, of heart sounds
  extra and abnormal, 318, 320, 320f

Heat applications, 969, 971, 971t
  pain relief and, 1178
  safety with, 971–972, 972t
Heat cradles, 974
Heat cramps, 1027
Heat exhaustion, 1027
Heating pads, 974
Heat lamps, 974
Heat stroke, 1027
Heel protectors, 726t
Height
  drug action and, 514
  measurement of, 321t, 322
  nutrition and, 913–914
Heimlich maneuver, 788, 793–794
Helminths, 993
Helpers, 180
Hematest tablets, 1108
Hematocrit, 390
  specific gravity of, 866
Hematologic tests, 388–392
  mobility and, 717
Hematology, reference ranges for, 1415–1417
Hematomas, wound healing and, 949–950
Hematuria, 1052
Hemiplegic gait, 707
Hemoccult test, 1105–1106, 1107
Hemodialysis, 1083
Hemoglobin, 388, 390
  nutrition and, 914
Hemolytic reactions, to blood transfusion, 882
Hemorrhage, wound healing and, 949
Hemostasis, wound healing and, 945
Hemovac, 953, 968
Henderson, Virginia, 14t–15t
  perception of human needs, 189
Henry Street Settlement, 9
Heparin administration, 540, 541
Heparin lock, 552
Hepatitis A, 990t
Hepatitis B, 990t
Herpesvirus infection
  genital, 989t
  of skin, 940
Heterosexual, 1366
Hierarchy of skills, 265
High-level wellness model, 175, 176f
High Risk for Altered Body Temperature, 1030
High Risk for Disuse Syndrome, 718
High Risk for Infection, 1005
  nursing management plan for, 1013
High Risk for Injury
  alterations in safety and, 578
  nursing management plan for, 589
High risk nursing diagnoses, 118, 122
Hill-Burton Act of 1946, 29
Hinduism, religious practices of, 1406t
Hip fractures, positioning and, 720
Hispanics
  health/illness considerations and, 245
  key informants for, 248
HMM. *See* Home maintenance management
HMOs. *See* Health maintenance organizations

Holism, 29
 definition of, 176
 nursing research and, 73
 spiritual function and, 1392, 1392f
Holistic health care, 176–179
 disease and, 178
 dysfunction and, 178–179
 illness and, 178
 imagery in, 181
 lifestyle modification in, 180
 meditation in, 181
 nursing as therapeutic partnership and, 180, 180f, 181t
 nursing diagnoses for wellness and, 180
 practice of, 177f, 177–178
  informed choices and, 177
  self-responsibility and, 177
  self-worth and, 177–178
 promoting health and preventing illness and, 179–180
  generative activities and, 179–180
  nurturative activities and, 179
  preventive activities and, 179
 stress and, 179
 therapeutic touch in, 181–182
Holistic health model, 175–176, 176f
Holmes and Rahe's Social Readjustment Scale, 340, 341t, 1338
Homan's sign, 820
Home, safety in, 566, 567f
Home assessment, home maintenance management and, 622
Homebound patients, 627
Home care
 bowel function and, 1125, 1129
 cognitive function and, 1234–1235
 communication and, 1280–1281
 coping and adaptation and, 1354
 family function and, 1303
 fluid and electrolyte and acid-base balance and, 884, 886
 grieving and, 1325
 health maintenance and, 608
 home maintenance management and, 630–633
 infection hazards in, 433
 infections and, 1012–1014
 medications and, 553–554
 mobility and, 735, 740, 742
 nutrition and, 929–930
 pain and, 1185–1186
 postoperative, 495
 respiratory function and, 788, 792, 795
 safety and, 587–588, 588f
 self-care deficits and, 682, 685, 688–689
 self-concept and, 1257–1258
 sensory perception and, 1203, 1206
 sexual function and, 1383–1384
 skin conditions and, 976
 sleep and, 1154
 spiritual function and, 1408–1409
 thermoregulation and, 1034–1035
 urinary elimination and, 1083, 1085
Home-care modifications
 ambulation and, 731
 antiembolic stockings and, 829
 aquathermia pads and, 976

 assessing body temperature of, 356
 assessing stool for occult blood and, 1108
 assisting with bathing or shower and, 661
 blood glucose measurement and, 390
 blood pressure assessment and, 368
 body mechanics and, 699
 cardiopulmonary resuscitation and, 836
 cold packs and, 973
 colostomy irrigation and, 1128
 condom catheters and, 1071
 crutches and, 735
 dressing changes and, 963
 enemas and, 1116
 feeding and, 919
 handwashing and, 442
 indwelling urinary catheter and, 1076–1077
 intravenous infusions and, monitoring, 874
 oral medications and, 526
 ostomy care and, 1127
 positioning patient in bed and, 725
 pulse assessment and, 360
 subcutaneous injections and, 540–541
 suctioning and, 785, 787
 total parenteral nutrition and, 925, 928
 tracheostomy care and, 791
 weight measurement and, 324
Home-health agencies, 32–33
Homelessness, 620
Home maintenance management (HMM), 612–635
 altered, 618f, 618–620
  manifestations of, 619–620
  potential for, 618–619
 assessment of, 620–623
  objective data and, 621–623
  subjective data and, 620–621
 characteristics of, 614–615
 evaluation and, 633, 634t, 635
 factors affecting, 615–617
 functional pattern of, 615
 interventions and, 625–633
  for altered home maintenance management, 626–633
  to promote health and function, 625–626
 lifespan considerations and, 617–618
 nursing diagnoses and patient goals and, 623–625
Homeostasis, 178
 stress and, 1336–1337
  physiologic homeostasis and, 1336f, 1336–1337
  psychosociologic homeostasis and, 1337
Homosexual, 1366
Hope, need for, spiritual dysfunction and, 1398t
Hormonal dysynchrony, 1141–1142
Hormones
 body temperature and, 351
 family planning methods and, 1382
 fluid and electrolyte balance and, 851–852
 homeostatic control and, 1337
 menstrual cycle and, 1364–1365, 1365f
 sleep and, 1141–1142
 urinary elimination and, 1046
Hospices, 33
 grieving and, 1325
Hospital(s)
 acute-care, 30

as nursing practice setting, 16–17, 17f
surgery performed in, 466
Hospitalization
 infections and, 994f, 994–996
 values and, 269
Host, 174
 compromised, 996–998
 susceptibility to pathogens, 430
Host-agent-environment model, of health, 174
Host defenses, enhancement of, 1009–1010
Hot packs, 974
Hot-water bath, 656t
Household system, 507, 507t
Huff cough, 770
Human needs. *See* Need(s)
Human response patterns, nursing diagnosis and, 113–116
Human sexual response. *See* Sexual response
Humoral immunity, 984–985
Hydration. *See also* Fluid intake; Fluid volume deficit;
      Fluid volume excess
 abnormal, fluid and electrolyte imbalance and, 860–861
 infections and, 1010
 postoperative, 494
 respiratory function and, 766
Hydraulic lifts, 735, 739t, 740f
Hydrostatic pressure, fluid and electrolyte movement and,
      850
Hygiene, 642
 altered self-care and, 648
 pain and, 1176–1177
 resistance to infection and, 986
Hyperalimentation. *See* Total parenteral nutrition
Hypercalcemia, 857
Hyperextension, 701, 703t, 704t
Hyperglycemia, 893
 enteral tube feedings and, 923
 total parenteral nutrition and, 929
Hyperinflation, respiratory function and, 767–769
Hyperkalemia, 856
Hypermagnesemia, 857
Hypernatremia, 855–856
Hyperpyrexia, 1026–1027
Hyperresonance, 305, 305t
Hypersensitivity reactions. *See* Allergic reactions
Hypertension, 371
 altered cardiovascular function and, 814
 patient teaching about, 605–606
Hyperthermia, 1024
 malignant, 469, 1024–1025
 management of, 1030, 1034
Hyperthermia (nursing diagnosis), 1030
Hypertonic solutions, 850, 850f, 870
Hyperventilation, 763
 management of, 780
Hypnosis, pain relief and, 1179–1180
Hypnotics, 1147, 1153–1154, 1155t
Hypocalcemia, 857
Hypoglycemia, 893
Hypokalemia, 856
Hypomagnesemia, 857
Hyponatremia, 856
Hypotension
 orthostatic. *See* Orthostatic hypotension

urinary elimination and, 1049
Hypothalamus, body temperature and, 1022
Hypothermia, 1027–1028, 1030
 accidental, 1028
 induced, 1027–1028
 management of, 1034
Hypothermia (nursing diagnosis), 1030
Hypothermia blankets, fever and, 1033–1034
Hypothesis, 71
Hypotonic solutions, 850, 850f, 870
Hypoventilation, 763
 management of, 780
Hypoxemia, 773
 levels of, 763
Hypoxia, 763

I
Iatrogenic illness, 177
IBW (ideal body weight), 901
ICD-9-CM (International Classification of Diseases-9-CM),
      113
Ice bags, 972
ICN. *See* International Council of Nurses
ICU (intensive care unit), communicating with patient in,
      290
ICU psychosis, 1223
Id, 200
Ideal body weight (IBW), 901
Identity. *See also* Gender identity
 personal, 1244
Ileal conduit, 1050, 1051f
Ileostomy, 1098, 1098f
Illness. *See also* Diseases; Infection(s); *specific illnesses*
 acute, 430–431
  self-care and, 647
 chronic
  altered health maintenance function and, 600
  fluid and electrolyte and acid-base imbalances
        and, 859
  mobility and, 706
 coping and adaptation and, 1345
 family function and, 1292–1293
 holistic health care and, 177–178
 iatrogenic, 177
 infections and, 998
 self-concept and, 1245, 1250
 sensory perception and, 1193
 sexual function and, 1376
 sexuality and, 1372
 sleep and, 1147, 1148f
 stress-related, 575
 values and, 269
Illness prevention, 30, 179–180, 595, 596t, 597t
Imagery, in holistic health care, 181
Imaginal skills, values and, 265
Immobility
 bowel function and, 1097
 functional health and, 707–714, 708t
Immune system
 infections and, 998
 resistance to infection and, 984–985, 985f
 wound healing and, 948
Immunity, impaired, immobility and, 711

Immunization
infection prevention and, 1008, 1008t
resistance to infection and, 986
Immunocompetence testing, nutrition and, 914
Impaired Gas Exchange, 764–765
Impaired Home Maintenance Management, 623–624
nursing management plan for, 634
Impaired Physical Mobility, 717
nursing management plan for, 741–742
Impaired Skin Integrity, 954
nursing management plan for, 977–978
Impaired Swallowing, 915–916
Impaired Tissue Integrity, 954
Impaired Verbal Communication, 1276
nursing management plan for, 1282–1283
Implementation, 86, 134–139, 135f
definition of, 134
nursing interventions and, 136–139. *See also* Nursing interventions
reassessment and, 135
recording actions and, 139
setting priorities and, 135–136, 136f
skills for, 135
using functional health approach, 139
Impotence, 1372–1373
Impulse conduction, cardiac, 804, 804f
Incentive spirometry, 767, 769, 770f, 771
Incidence, of infection, 992
Incident reports, 165, 587
Incontinence
bowel, 1101, 1109, 1112
urinary, 1053, 1064
Incubation period, 430
Incubator, oxygen therapy and, 774t, 777–778
Independent nursing functions, 18
Independent variable, 75
Index of Activities of Daily Living, 650, 650t
Indirect contact, transmission by, 429
Individual, 223–224, 224f
needs of, 224
Individual care plans, 131
Ineffective Airway Clearance, 764
nursing management plan for, 796
Ineffective Breathing Pattern, 764
Ineffective Family Coping: Compromised, 1299–1300
Ineffective Family Coping: Disabling, 1298–1299
Ineffective Individual Coping, 1348–1349
nursing management plan for, 1355
Ineffective Thermoregulation, 1030
nursing management plan for, 1035
Infant. *See also* Newborn
aquathermia pads and, 975
assessing body temperature of, 356
assessing stool for occult blood and, 1108
bathing, 661
blood glucose measurement in, 390
blood pressure assessment in, 368
blood transfusions and, 884
body temperature and, 1023
bowel function and, 1095
cardiopulmonary resuscitation and, 835–836
cardiovascular function and, 808
cognitive function and, 1217, 1217f

cold packs and, 973
colostomy irrigation and, 1128
communication and, 1270
coping and adaptation and, 1342
coughing and deep breathing exercises and, 769
development of, 202t, 204–205
diagnostic and laboratory testing and, 403–404
preparing for, 381
enemas and, 1116
family and, 1291
feeding, 919
fluid and electrolyte balance and, 852–853
foot and nail care and, 667
functional health assessment of, 344
auscultating heart sounds in, 319
auscultation of bowel sounds in, 326
auscultation of breath sounds in, 316
neurologic assessment in, 333
weight measurement in, 324
functional health patterns and, health problems and anticipatory guidance and, 209–218, 210f, 213f
grieving and, 1316, 1317t
health maintenance and, 598, 603t
Heimlich maneuver and, 794
home maintenance management and, 617
infection control and, 457
intravenous infusions and
infusion rate and, 879
medication administration and, 552
monitoring, 873
medications and, 555
intravenous infusions and, 552
mobility and, 705
nasogastric intubation and, 1122
needs of, 188
nutrition and, 907
oral care and, 671
oral medications and, 526
pain and, 1167
patient teaching and, 421
preparing for diagnostic and laboratory tests, 381
pulse assessment in, 360
pulse deficit assessment in, 362
resistance to infection and, 986
respiration function and, assessment of, 365
respiratory function and, 752–753
safety and, 566f, 567
self-care and, 645
self-concept and, 1246t, 1247, 1255
sensory perception and, 1193
sexuality and, 1369
shampooing hair of, 669
skin and, 938–939
sleep and, 1144
spiritual function and, 1394–1395, 1407
strict isolation and, 452
subcutaneous injections and, 540
suctioning and, 785, 787
surgery and, 473
total parenteral nutrition and, 925, 928
tracheostomy care and, 791
transferring, 737

urinary elimination and, 1047
values and, 266
vital signs in, 375
Infection(s), 574–575
    active versus chronic, 994
    agents causing, 428
    chain of, 428–430, 429f
    cognitive function and, 1219
    hospitalization and, 994f, 994–996
    infectious agents and, 992–993, 998t–991t
    inspection for, 953
    intravenous therapy and, 879
    latent, 431–432
    local versus systemic, 994
    manifestations of, 998–1000, 1002
    microorganisms and, 428–434
    nonspecific symptoms of, 998–999
    nosocomial, 432–433, 987, 993–994
    progress of, 430–432, 431f
    resistance to, 980–1015, 992–1000
        activities of daily living and, 1000
        assessment and, 1000–1005
        characteristics of, 982t, 982–985
        evaluation and, 1014
        factors affecting, 985–986
        interventions and, 1006–1014
        lifespan considerations and, 986–992
        manifestations of infection and, 998–1000
        nonspecific natural defenses and, 982t, 982–984
        nursing diagnoses and patient goals and, 1005–1006
        potential for infection and, 992–998
        specific acquired defenses and, 982t, 984–985
    of skin, 940
    total parenteral nutrition and, 929
    types of, 993–994
    of urinary tract, immobility and, 712
    wound healing and, 949, 950
Infection control, 434–438, 581, 1011–1012
    employee health and, 435–438
    handwashing and, 1011, 1011f
    isolation and, 1011–1012
    recognition of factors and, 434
    regulatory agencies and, 434–435
    respiratory function and, 788
    secretion disposal and, 1012
    sterile technique and, 1011
    universal precautions and, 570
    waste disposal and, 438, 440t
Infection control committees, 434–435, 1009
Infection hazards, in nonacute care setting, 433–434
Infectious diseases, 428, 988t–991t. *See also* Infection(s)
    infection control and. *See* Infection control
    reporting, 435
    significant exposure and, 436–437
Inferences, validation of data and, 103–105, 105f
Infertility, 1371, 1374
Infiltration, intravenous therapy and, 876
Inflammation
    gastrointestinal, altered nutrition and, 910
    infections and, 999
Inflammatory response
    resistance to infection and, 983–984
    wound healing and, 945

Influenza, 988t
Information, giving, 284t, 285–286
Information-processing theory, 88–89, 89f
Informed choice, holistic health care and, 177
Informed consent, 48
    for diagnostic and laboratory tests, 382
    surgery and, 478, 479f, 480
Infusion rate, factors affecting, 875–876
Ingrown nails, 665t
Inhaled medications, 530
Inhalers, metered-dose, 772, 773f
Initial assessment, 96, 96t
Injections
    intradermal, 534, 534f
    intramuscular, 541f, 541–547
        complications associated with, 548t–549t
    subcutaneous, 534, 537, 537f, 538–541
Injuries. *See also* Accidents; Falls; Trauma
    altered health maintenance function and, 600
    neurologic, urinary elimination and, 1049
    prevention of, 719
Inpatient services. *See also* Hospital(s)
    agencies providing, 30–32, 31f
    specialized, 31–32
Input, in systems theory, 87, 87f
Insensible evaporation, 1021
In-service education, 16
Insomnia, 1148
Inspection
    abdominal assessment and, 326
    body temperature and, 1029–1030
    bowel function and, 328, 1103
    cardiopulmonary assessment and, 819
    cardiovascular assessment and, 317–318
    infections and, 1002
    in physical examination, 100–101, 303–304
    respiratory assessment and, 312, 312f, 761
    sexuality-reproduction assessment and, 342
    of skin, 952–953
    urinary elimination and, 327, 1056
    of wound, 952–953
Institutional review boards, research and, 76
Instructional nursing care plans, 130–134
Instrumental skills, values and, 265
Insulin administration, 537, 541
Insurance. *See* Health insurance; Medicaid; Medicare
Intake. *See* Diet; Fluid intake; Food intake; Nutrition
Integration, development and, 198–199
Integumentary system, 937. *See also* Hair; Nails; Skin
    assessment of, fluid and electrolyte imbalance and, 864, 865f
    safety assessment and, 577
    stress and, 1347
Intellectual skills, for implementation, 135
Intelligence, 1214–1215
Intensity, auscultation and, 306
Intensive care unit (ICU), communicating with patient in, 290
Interaction
    altered sensory function and, 1201–1202
    as source of values, 260, 260f
Interdependent nursing functions, 18
Intermittent claudication, 815, 830
    pain and, 1172

Intermittent fever, 1026, 1027t
Intermittent infusion technique, 550–552
Intermittent positive pressure breathing (IPPB), 769
Internal messages, stress management and, 1350–1351
International Classification of Diseases-9-CM (ICD-9-CM), 113
International Council of Nurses (ICN), 9, 20, 22–23
   Code for Nurses of, 46–47
Interoceptors, 1214
Interpersonal skills
   for implementation, 135
   values and, 265
Interpreter. *See* Foreign languages
Intertrigo, 939
Interview, 99t, 99–100
   concluding phase of, 100
   ethnographic, grounding assessments in patient's
      perspective and, 247–248
   introductory phase of, 100
   maintenance phase of, 100
   open-ended, grounding assessments in patient's
      perspective and, 247
   preparatory phase of, 99–100
Intimacy
   as family function, 1289
   sleep and, 1152
Intractable pain, 1166
Intradermal injections, 534, 534f
Intramuscular injections, 541f, 541–547
   air lock injection technique for, 545
   complications associated with, 548t–549t
   deltoid site for, 542, 542f
   dorsogluteal site for, 546f, 546–547, 547f
   rectus femoris and vastus lateralis sites for, 542, 542f,
      545, 546f
   venterogluteal site for, 545, 546f
   Z-track method for, 545, 547, 547f
Intraoperative nursing, 467–468, 484f, 484–490
   assessment and, 484
   evaluation and, 490
   interventions and, 485t, 485–490
   nursing diagnoses and patient goals and, 484–485, 485t
Intrauterine development, 201, 202t, 204
   functional health patterns during, health problems and
      anticipatory guidance and, 209
Intrauterine devices (IUDs), 1382
Intravenous access, surgery and, 480
Intravenous medication administration, 547, 549t, 550–553
   calculating dosages for, 521
   continuous infusion technique for, 552–553
   intermittent infusion technique for, 550–552
   IV push technique for, 547, 550
   patient-controlled analgesia and, 553
Intravenous pyelogram (IVP), 1063, 1063t
Intravenous therapy, fluid and electrolyte imbalance and,
     869–880
   changing bottles and tubing and, 876, 877–879
   complications of, 876, 879–880
   discontinuing, 880
   equipment for, 870f–872f, 870–871, 874f
   infusion rate and, 875–876
   intravenous site care and, 876, 880f
   monitoring, 872, 873–875, 875f, 876f
   purpose of, 869–870
   types of solutions for, 870
Intravenous tubing, 871, 872f
Intuition, 101
   in assessment, 101
Invasion of privacy, 49
Invasive devices, infections and, 997–998
Invasiveness, of pathogens, 429, 992
Invasive pain management, 1185, 1185t
Invasive trauma, risk of, 570
Inversion, 701, 703t
Ions, 846
IPPB (intermittent positive pressure breathing), 769
Iron, normal physiologic function of, 898t, 899
Irrigation
   of colostomy, 1125, 1127–1128
   of wounds, 968, 970–971
Irrigation solutions, 528
Ischemia
   altered cardiovascular function and, 815–816
   pain and, 830
Islam, religious practices of, 1405t
Isolation, 448–453
   blood-body fluid precautions and, 451
   body-substance, 451–452, 453f, 454t
   category-specific, 450–451, 454t
   contact, 451
   disease-specific, 451, 454t
   drainage-secretions precautions and, 451
   enteric precautions and, 451
   infection control and, 1011–1012
   nursing considerations and, 453
   protective, 452
   respiratory, 451
   safety dysfunction and, 575
   strict, 451, 452
   tuberculosis, 451
   universal precautions and, 448–450
Isometric exercise, 701
Isotonic exercise, 701
Isotonic solutions, 850, 850f, 870
Itching, 939, 944
IUDs (intrauterine devices), 1382
IV containers, 870–871
   changing, 876, 877–878
IV controller, 874–875, 876f
IVP (intravenous pyelogram), 1063, 1063t
IV pump, 874–875, 876f
IV push technique, 547, 550
IV solutions, changing, 878–879
IV tubing, changing, 876, 878–879

J
Jackson-Pratt drain, 953
JCAHO. *See* Joint Commission on Accreditation of
    Healthcare Organizations
Jehovah's Witnesses, religious practices of, 1405t
Jejunostomy, 922
Jews, religious practices of, 1405t
Johnson, Dorothy E., 14t–15t
Joint(s), 695. *See also* Musculoskeletal system
   assessment of, 716
   decreased flexibility of, mobility and, 707

infections of, 996
maintaining mobility of, 722, 728–729
movement of, 703t–704t
   terms describing, 701
pain in, immobility and, 709
Joint Commission on Accreditation of Healthcare
      Organizations (JCAHO), 36
   infection control and, 434, 438
   infection prevention and, 1009
   nursing assessment and, 96
   nursing care plans and, 130
   nursing diagnosis and, 112
   nursing process and, 86
   patient record audits conducted by, 150
   planning and, 128
   as quality assurance monitor, 145
   standards of care set by, 48
Joint mobility, assessment of, 310
Journals. *See* Nursing journals
Judgment, 1215
Justice
   ethics and, 43
   home care and, home maintenance management and,
      630

K

Kant, Immanuel, 44
Kardex, 158, 159f
Kefauver-Harris Act of 1962, 507, 508, 508t
Kegel exercises, sexual function and, 1381
Keloids, 947t
Keratoses, 939
Key informant technique, grounding assessments in
      patient's perspective and, 248
Kidney(s). *See also headings beginning with term* Renal
   altered cardiopulmonary function and, 816
   anatomy of, 1042, 1043f
   biopsy of, 399–400
Kidney function studies, cardiopulmonary function and, 821
King, Imogene M., 14t–15t
   perception of human needs, 190
Knowing pattern, nursing diagnosis and, 114, 116
Knowledge
   assessing before medication administration, 518
   baseline, patient teaching and, 414
   domains of, 410–411
   inadequate, altered nutrition and, 909
   pain perception and, 1167
   of self, 1242
   skin and, 938
Knowledge Deficit, medication administration and, 518–519
Kock pouch diversion, 1050, 1051f
Kohlberg, Lawrence, 44–45
   moral development theory of, 199, 200t, 201
Korotkoff sounds, 370, 371f, 371t
Kussmaul respirations, 363, 363t

L

Laboratory tests, 378–393, 385–393. *See also* Diagnostic
      tests and procedures
   blood specimen collection for, 385–388
   cardiopulmonary function and, 820–821
   checking before medication administration, 517

culture and sensitivity testing and, 392–393
   data collection from, 103
   fluid and electrolyte imbalance and, 865–866
   hematologic, 388, 390–392
   individualizing care using data from, 385, 386t
   lifespan considerations and, 403–404
   nursing responsibilities during, 383–384
   nursing responsibilities following, 384–385
   patient preparation for, 380–383
   reference ranges for. *See* Reference ranges
   urine, 392
Laceration, 940, 940t
Lactation, 1366
   medication assessment and, 516
   nutrition and, 907
Language, 1267–1268
   communication process and, 275–276, 276t
   patients who do not speak nurse's language and, 248–249
      communicating with, 290
Lanugo, 938
Large intestine, anatomy of, 892
Laryngectomy, 1273, 1279–1280
LAS (local adaptation syndrome), 1339–1340
Latent infections, 431–432
Lateral chest wall, anatomic landmarks of, 310f–311f, 311
Laws. *See* Legal issues; Legislation
Laxatives, 1111–1112, 1113t
Leadership, 59–60
   in clinical practice roles, 63–66
   nursing management roles and, 66–67
   styles of, 59–60, 60f
   teaching roles and, 67–68
Learning, 410–412, 1216. *See also* Education; Nursing
      education; Patient teaching
   assessing readiness for, 414–415
   of culture, 238–239
   domains of knowledge and, 410–411
   maintenance of learning skills and, 1231
   sequence of events in, 410, 410f
   styles of, 411f, 411–412
Learning needs, assessment of, 413–414, 414t
Lectures, patient teaching and, 419
Legal dilemmas, 41–42
Legal documentation, as purpose of patient record, 150
Legal issues, 45, 47–56. *See also* Legislation
   controlled substances and, 52
   death and dying and, 52, 54, 54f
   Legal issues, avoiding lawsuits and, 54, 56, 56f
   licensure and, 47–48
   medication administration and. *See* Medication
      administration, legal aspects of
   in nursing research, 76–77
   sources of laws and, 47
   standards of care and, 48
   torts and crimes and, 48–52, 50t
Legal principles, 42
Legibility, of charting, 153
Legislation, 29. *See also* Legal issues
   drugs and medications and, 507–508, 508t
   Good Samaritan Law and, 56
   sources of laws and, 47
Lesions, of skin, 944–945, 946t–947t
Leukocytosis, 390, 1003

Leukopenia, 390
Levine, Myra Estrin, 14t–15t
Liability, 51
Libel, 49
Lice, 664–665
Licensed practical nurse (LPN), 13
Licensed vocational nurse (LVN), 13
Licensing, 47–48
  quality assurance and, 36
Lichenification, 947t
Lifestyle
  altered health maintenance function and, 600
  bowel function and, 1094, 1097
  cardiovascular function and, 808
  cognitive function and, promotion of healthy lifestyle
    and, 1229–1230
  dysfunctional, coping and adaptation and, 1344
  family function and, 1291
  health maintenance and, 598
  home maintenance management and, 616
  mobility and, 704
  modification of, in holistic health care, 180
  nutrition and, 905–906
  respiratory function and, 754–755
  safety and, 565
  sensory perception and, 1193
  skin and, 938
  sleep and, 1144
  stress management and, 1351
Lifts, 735, 739t, 740f
Light, sleep and, 1145
Lighting, tangential, 304
Limbs, elevation of, to reduce edema, 829
Liquids. *See also* Intravenous therapy; *headings beginning*
  with term Fluid
  body temperature measurement and, 351
Listening
  active, 284–285, 285f
  communication and, 63
  required for effective use of nursing process, 89–90
  spiritual function and, 1404, 1404f, 1406
Literacy. *See* Reading ability
Literature review, 74
Liver
  anatomy of, 893
  biopsy of, 399
Liver spots, 939
Living wills, 52, 55
Local adaptation syndrome (LAS), 1339–1340
Lockjaw, 991t
Locus of Control Scales, 339
Logrolling, 720, 725
Longevity, increasing, 28, 29f
Long-term care, cognitive function and, 1235
Long-term care facilities, 30–31, 31f
  as nursing practice settings, 17
Long-term goals, 128
Loss. *See also* Death and dying; Grief; Grieving
  characteristics of, 1309–1311
    grieving and, 1315
  crisis vs. transition and, 1314–1315
  types of, grief and, 1314
Lotions, 528–529
Love needs, 188, 224

spiritual dysfunction and, 1398t
Low-flow cough, 770
LPN. *See* Licensed practical nurse
Lumbar puncture, 400, 400f
Lungs. *See also* Breathing; Respirations; Respiratory
  function; Respiratory system
  anatomic landmarks of, 310f–311f, 310–312
  auscultation of, 313–316, 314t
  circulation of, 803
  distribution of air in, 749
  immobility and, 710–711
  restricted movement of, 753–754
Lung scan, 764
LVN. *See* Licensed vocational nurse
Lymph nodes
  infections and, 1000
  palpation of, infections and, 1002
Lysaught Report, 9

M
Maceration, 942
Macrophages, 983t
Macule, 946t
Magnesium, 848
  dietary sources of, 869t
  imbalance of, 857
  normal physiologic function of, 898t
Magnetic resonance imaging (MRI), 397, 397f
  infections and, 1005
Maintenance nursing interventions, 139
Malignant hyperthermia, 469, 1024–1025
Malpractice, 50, 51
Mammography, 395–396
Managed care, 64–66
Management, 60–63
  in clinical practice roles, 63–66
  functions of managers and, 60–62, 61f
  nursing management roles and, 66–67
  skills for, 62–63
  teaching roles and, 67–68
Managers
  beginning, 66
  nurse as, 18
  unit, 66–67
Many-tailed binder, 966, 966f
Masks, infection control and, 445–448
Maslow, Abraham, human needs theory of, 185–188, 186f,
  199, 200t, 201, 224
Massage
  of back, 663, 664
  pain relief and, 1178
Master's degree nursing programs, 16
Mastication, 900
Material culture, 241
Maternalistic approach, 278, 279t
Maturation phase, of wound healing, 945
Meaning, need for, spiritual dysfunction and, 1398t–1399t
Measles (rubeola), 988t
Measles, German (rubella), 988t
Meats, 902
Medicaid, 29, 33–3434
  discrimination prohibition and, 249
  medication administration and, 508
Medical asepsis, 439

Medical diagnosis, nursing diagnosis and, 116t, 116–117
Medical history
  cardiovascular function and, 813
  medication assessment and, 516
Medical Letter, 503
Medically needy, 34
Medical model. *See* Body systems model
Medical records. *See* Patient record
Medical terminology, 1438–1444
  prefixes and, 1438–1440
  roots and, 1440–1442
    according to body system, 1444
  suffixes and, 1442–1443
Medicare, 29, 33–34, 35
  discrimination prohibition and, 249
  medication administration and, 508
  Part A, 33–34
  Part B, 33, 34
Medication(s), 498–557. *See also* Drug(s)
  administration of. *See* Medication administration
  antipyretic, 1033
  blood pressure and, 366
  bowel function and, 1097, 1100
  cardiovascular function and, 813
  cognitive function and, 1220
  distribution systems for, 503
  dosage of. *See* Dosage
  drug orders and. *See* Drug orders
  drugs versus, 500
  evaluation and, 554
  infections and, 998
  interaction of, 514, 514f
  lifespan considerations and, 554–556
  measurement systems for, 505–507
    conversions between, 520–521
    conversions within, 520
  nasogastric intubation for administration of, 1118
  nonprescription, 504
  pain relief and, 1180–1185
  preoperative, 480–481
  prescription, 504
  to promote normal function, 501t
  pulse and, 357
  reference ranges for, 1437
  respirations and, 362
  for respiratory conditions, 772t
  respiratory function and, 788, 792
  self-administered, 503
  sensory perception and, 1193
  sexuality and, 1372
  sleep and, 1147
  sources of information about, 500–502
  therapeutic drug monitoring and, infections and, 1005
  urinary elimination and, 1050
Medication administration, 519f, 519–554
  assessment before, 516–518
  discharge planning and home care and, 553–554
  documentation of, 523, 523f
  'five rights' and, 521–523
  inhaled medications and, 530
  legal aspects of, 507–511
    drug enforcement agencies and, 508–509, 509t
    institutional medication policies and, 510
    laws and, 507–508, 508t
    nurse practice acts and, 509–510
    patient's rights and, 510–511
    substance abuse and, 511
  oral, 523–528, 527f
    advantages of, 526
    buccal, 528, 528f
    contraindications for, 526
    forms of oral medications and, 526–527
    sublingual, 528, 528f
    through tubes, 527–528
  parenteral, 530–533
    advantages and disadvantages of, 531
    drawing up medications and, 533–534, 535–537
    equipment disposal and, 534
    equipment for, 531–533
    heparin administration and, 540, 541
    insulin administration and, 537, 541
    intradermal injections and, 534, 534f
    intramuscular injections and, 541f, 541–547
    intravenous, 547–553, 549t
    mixing medications and, 534, 535–537
    reconstituting medications and, 534
    subcutaneous injections and, 534, 537, 537f, 538–541
  route of, in drug order, 504
  safety and, 519–523
  topical, 528–530
    applied to skin, 528–529
    nasal, 529
    ophthalmic, 529, 529f
    otic, 529, 530f
    rectal, 529–530, 530f
    transdermal, 529, 529f
    vaginal, 530, 531f
Medication assessment, 515–518
  before administration, 516–518
  information collected on admission and, 515–516
  knowledge and compliance and, 518
Medication errors, 523
Medication history, 515
Medication policies, 510
Medication record, 165, 166f
  checking before medication administration, 516
Medication standards, 502–503, 503t
Meditation
  in holistic health care, 181
  pain relief and, 1179
Melanin, 936
Memory, 1214, 1216
  assessment, 333
  cognitive function and, memory improvement and, 1230–1231
  impairment of, 1222
  of older adult, patient teaching and, 423
Menadione (vitamin K), normal physiologic function of, 895t, 896–897
Menarche, 1370
Meningitis, 989t
Menopause, 1371
Menstruation, 1364–1365, 1365f
  cessation of, 1371
  onset of, 1370
Mental health, 1337
Mental health centers, 32

Mental impairments, preparing patient for diagnostic and laboratory tests and, 381
Mental status
  decubitus ulcers and, 942
  fluid and electrolyte imbalance and, 860
Mercury thermometers, 352, 352f, 353f
Message, in communication process, 275
Metabolic acidosis, 858
Metabolic alkalosis, 858
Metabolism. *See also* Nutrition–metabolism health pattern
  cognitive function and, 1216, 1219
  coping and adaptation and, 1341
  by digestive system, 900–901
  of drugs, 511
  heat production and, 1018–1019
  immobility and, 711–712
  increased metabolic demand and, 910–911
  safety and, 565
  skin and, 938
Metacommunication, 274
Methods, of research, 74
Metric system, 506, 506t, 1413
Mexican Americans. *See* Hispanics
Microorganisms, 429. *See also specific microorganisms*
  host susceptibility and, 430
  infection and, 428–434
  mode of transmission of, 429–430, 430t
  portal of entry and, 430
  portal of exit of, 429
  source of, 429
  transient, decrease of, 1009
Micturition, 1045
Micturition reflex, 1045
Middle adult. *See also* Adult
  development of, 203t, 208
  functional health patterns and, health problems and anticipatory guidance and, 210–219
  health maintenance and, 603t
Milia, 938
Milk, 902
  production of. *See* Lactation
Minerals
  normal physiologic function of, 897–900, 898t
  recommended dietary allowances for, 1447
Mini Mental Status Exam, 1227, 1228
Minority, 242
Mixed apnea, 1149
Mobility, 692–743. *See also* Activity; Activity–exercise health pattern; Ambulation; Exercise; Movement
  altered, 705–714
    activities of daily living and, 714
    functional health and, 707–714, 708t
    manifestations of, 706–707
    potential for, 705–706
  assessment of, 308–310, 332, 714–717
    objective data and, 715–717
    subjective data and, 715
  characteristics of normal movement and, 701–702, 703t–704t
  cognitive function and, 1232
  evaluation and, 742–743
  factors affecting, 702, 704
  home maintenance management and, 616, 616f, 619

interventions and, 718–742
  for altered mobility, 719–735
    discharge planning and home care and, 735, 740, 742
    to promote health and function, 718–719
  lifespan considerations and, 704–705
  musculoskeletal system anatomy and, 694–695
  normal physiologic function and, 695–701
  nursing diagnoses and patient goals and, 717–718
  postoperative, 493
  safety assessment and, 577–578
Moisture
  decubitus ulcers and, 942
  in skin, 937
Mongolian spots, 246
Mononuclear cells, 983
Monosaccharides, 893
Mons pubis, 1362
Montgomery straps, 959, 959f
Mood, sleep and, 1147–1148
Moral(s), 42
Moral development, 44–45
Moral development theory, 199, 200t, 201
Moral issues, regarding therapy, spirituality and, 1396
Moralistic responses, 288
Moral values, 45, 256
Mormons, religious practices of, 1405t–1406t
Moro reflex, 333
Motility, intestinal, 1092, 1092f
Motivation
  health maintenance and, 594–595
  for learning, assessment of, 414–415
  patient teaching and, 423
  self-care and, 645
Motor aphasia, 1271–1272, 1272t
Motor vehicle accidents, 575
Motor vehicle safety, 585–586, 586f
Mourning, 1310
Mouth. *See also* Oral care
  assessment of, 322, 322f
  nutrition and, 914
Movement. *See also* Activity; Activity–exercise health pattern; Ambulation; Exercise; Mobility
  coordinated, 696–697
    mobility and, 706–707
  pattern of, nursing diagnosis and, 114
MRI. *See* Magnetic resonance imaging
Mucous membranes
  altered, altered nutrition and, 912
  breaks in, infection and, 996
  intact, infections and, 1009
  resistance to infection and, 985–986
Mucus production, intestinal, 1093
Mumps, 988t
Murmurs, 820
Muscle(s), 694–695. *See also* Musculoskeletal system; Neuromuscular function
  assessment of, 716
  atrophy of, immobility and, 708–709
  cardiac, damage to, 810
Muscle activity, heat production and, 1019
Muscle mass, assessing before medication administration, 517
Muscle strength
  altered mobility and, 706

for ambulation, increasing, 732
   assessment of, 309–310, 716
   immobility and, 708–709
Muscle tension, pain and, 1170
Muscle tone
   abnormal, fluid and electrolyte and acid-base imbalances and, 861
   altered mobility and, 706
   assessment of, 716
   promotion of, urinary elimination and, 1066
   urinary elimination and, 1049
Musculoskeletal system. *See also* Muscle(s); *headings beginning with term* Muscle
   anatomy of, 694–695
   mobility and, 702, 706
   stress and, 1347
Music therapy, 1234
Muslims, religious practices of, 1405t
Myelogram, 400
Myocardial infarction, 810
Myocardium, 802
Myoclonus, sleep-related, 1149

N

Nails, 937
   care of, 642, 663, 665t, 666–667
   clubbing of, 312, 312f
   ingrown, 665t
NANDA. *See* North American Nursing Diagnosis Association
Narcolepsy, 1148–1149
Narcotic(s), control of, 508–509, 509t
Narcotic agonists/antagonists, 1180, 1181t–1182t, 1182–1183
Nares, nasogastric intubation and, 1120, 1122
Narrative nursing progress notes, 158
Nasal airways, 781, 787f
Nasal cannula, 774, 774t, 776–777
Nasal medications, 529
Nasal prongs, 774, 774t, 776–777
Nasogastric decompression, surgery and, 480
Nasogastric intubation, 1117–1122
   equipment for, 1118–1120, 1119f
   medication administration via, 1118
   nursing care with, 1120, 1121–1122
   purposes of, 1117–1118, 1118f
Nasogastric tubes, 1118, 1119f
   oral administration through, 527–528
Nasointestinal tubes, 1118–1120
Nasopharyngeal secretions, suctioning, 782–785
Nasotracheal secretions, suctioning, 786–787
National Center for Nursing Research, 73
National Formulary (NF), 502
National Institutes of Health, 73
National League for Nursing (NLN), 9, 20, 22, 36
National Research Act of 1974, 76
National Student Nurses' Association (NSNA), 20, 22
Native Americans
   health/illness considerations and, 244–245
   key informants for, 248
Natural Death Acts, 52
Natural family planning, 1382
Nausea
   altered nutrition and, 909

enteral tube feedings and, 923
   narcotic analgesics and, 1183–1184
Nebulizers
   hand-held, 771t, 771–772
   pneumatic, 775
Neck veins
   engorged, altered respiratory function and, 758
   fluid and electrolyte imbalance and, 864–865
Need(s), 184–193
   assessing, functional health patterns and, 192–193, 193f
   esteem, 188, 224
   learning, assessment of, 413–414, 414t
   lifespan considerations and, 188–189
   love, 188, 224
   Maslow's theory of, 185–188, 199, 200t, 201, 224
   nursing theory and, 189–192
   physiologic, 185–187, 224
   safety, 187–188, 224
   self-actualization, 188, 224
   for sleep, 1143
      awareness of, 1142
   spiritual, 1392
   spiritual dysfunction and, 1398t–1399t
Needlesticks, 437, 437f, 438f
Negative nitrogen balance, 894
Negligence, 50–51
Negotiation, discharge planning and, 626
Neoplasms, of skin, 940
Nervous system. *See also* Brain; Neurologic assessment; Neurologic injury; Spinal cord
   autonomic. *See* Autonomic nervous system
   body temperature and, 1022, 1024
   mobility and, 702, 705–706
   parasympathetic, pain and, 1172
   sympathetic. *See* Sympathetic nervous system
Neuman, Betty, 14t–15t
Neuralgia, 1172
Neurologic assessment, 330–333
   safety assessment and, 577
Neurologic injury, urinary elimination and, 1049
Neuromuscular function, 705–706
   self-care and, 644, 647
Neurotransmitters, sleep and, 1141
Neutrophils, 983t
   infections and, 1003
Newborn
   bathing, 661
   body temperature and, 1023
   bowel function and, 1095
   cardiovascular function and, 808
   cognitive function and, 1217
   communication and, 1269–1270
   coping and adaptation and, 1342
   diagnostic and laboratory testing and, 403
   family and, 1291
   fluid and electrolyte balance and, 852
   functional health assessment of, 344
      auscultating heart sounds in, 319
      auscultation of bowel sounds in, 325
      auscultation of breath sounds in, 316
      neurologic assessment in, 333
   functional health patterns and, health problems and anticipatory guidance and, 209–218, 210f

Newborn (*continued*)
  grieving and, 1316
  health maintenance and, 598
  home maintenance management and, 617
  infection control and, 457
  medications and, 555
  mobility and, 704–705
  needs of, 188
  nutrition and, 907
  pain and, 1167
  patient teaching and, 421
  resistance to infection and, 986
  respiratory function and, 752
  safety and, 567
  self-care and, 645
  self-concept and, 1245, 1246t, 1247, 1247f, 1255
  sensory perception and, 1193
  sexuality and, 1369
  skin and, 938
  sleep and, 1144
  spiritual function and, 1394, 1407
  surgery and, 473
  urinary elimination and, 1047
  vital signs in, 373, 375
NF (*National Formulary*), 502
Niacin (vitamin B₃), normal physiologic function of, 895t, 897
Nicotine. *See also* Smoking
  sleep and, 1147
Nightingale, Florence, 9, 14t–15t
  perception of human needs, 189
Nightingale Pledge, 256
Nightmares, 1149–1150
Night terrors, 1149–1150
Nitrogen balance
  immobility and, 711
  positive and negative, 894
NLN. *See* National League for Nursing
Nociceptors, 1162
No code (DNR; do not resuscitate; no heroics), 52
Nocturia, 1052
Nodule, 946t
No heroics (DNR; do not resuscitate; no code), 52
Noise, sleep and, 1145
Noncompliance, 518, 605
  assessment of, 415
Noncompliance (nursing diagnosis)
  altered health maintenance and, 605
  medication administration and, 518
Nonfluent aphasia, 1271–1272, 1272t
Nonmaleficence, 42
Nonprofessional involvement, 288–289
Non-rapid eye movement (NREM) sleep, 1138
Nonspecific natural defenses, 982t, 982–984
Nonsteroidal anti-inflammatory drugs (NSAIDS), 1181t
Nontherapeutic responses, 287–289
Nonverbal communication, 62, 274, 1268
Normal flora, 982
North American Nursing Diagnosis Association (NANDA), 112
  nursing diagnosis defined by, 111
Nose care, 643
Nosocomial infections, 432–433, 987, 993–994
  risk factors for, 432f, 432–433

Not-for-profit hospitals, 30
NPO (nothing by mouth), 480, 919–920
NREM (non-rapid eye movement) sleep, 1138
NSAIDS (nonsteroidal anti-inflammatory drugs), 1181t
NSNA (National Student Nurses' Association), 20, 22
Nuclear family, 1288, 1288f
Nuclear scan, 396
Nurse(s)
  attitudes toward pain, 1171–1172
  as barrier to patient goal attainment, 143–144
  death assisted by, 52
  licensing of. *See* Licensing
  stress management for, 1349–1350
  values of, manifestations of, 265–266
Nurse administrators, 20
Nurse anesthetists, 19
  role of, 66
Nurse doctorate programs, 16
Nurse educators, 20, 20f
Nurse executives, 61, 67, 67f
Nurse midwives, 19
  role of, 66
Nurse-patient relationship, 277t, 277–279
  advocacy and, 278–279, 279t
  circle of confidentiality and, 279
  contract-setting and, 277–278
  phases of, 277
  self-care deficits and, 654
  sensory perception and, 1201
Nurse practice acts, 20
  medication administration and, 509–510
Nurse practitioners, 19
  role of, 65, 66
Nurse researchers, 19–20
Nurses' Drug Alert, 503
Nursing
  concept of, 12
  definition of, 11
  as subculture, 242
  team, 63–64, 65, 66
Nursing assessment, 84–85, 94–107, 96f
  assessment skills and, 97t, 97–101
    for interviewing, 99t, 99–100
    intuition as, 101
    for observation, 98–99
    for physical examination, 100–101
  bowel function and, 1102–1108
    objective data and, 1103–1108
    subjective data and, 1102–1103
  cardiopulmonary function and, 817–822
    objective data and, 819–822
    subjective data and, 817–819
  in clinical care plan, 134
  cognitive function and, 1223–1229
    objective data and, 1226–1229
    subjective data and, 1223–1226
  communication and, 281–283, 1273–1276
    objective data and, 1275–1276
    subjective data and, 1274–1275
  of community, 231t, 233
  coping and adaptation and, 1345–1347
    objective data and, 1347
    subjective data and, 1346–1347

data collection for, 102t, 102–103
definition of, 95
during diagnostic and laboratory tests, 383
emergency, 96t, 97
for eye problems, 673
family function and, 227t, 228–229, 1296–1298
    objective data and, 1298
    subjective data and, 1296–1298
fluid and electrolyte and acid-base balance and, 861–866
    objective data and, 862–866
    subjective data and, 861–862
focus, 96t, 96–97
following diagnostic and laboratory tests, 384–385
grieving and, 1319–1321
    subjective data and, 1319–1321
grounding in patient's perspective, 247–248
health maintenance and, 601–604
home maintenance management and, 620–623
    objective data and, 621–623
    subjective data and, 620–621
infections and, 1000–1005
    objective data and, 1001–1005
    subjective data and, 1001
initial, 96, 96t
intraoperative nursing and, 484
for learning, 413–415
for medication administration. See Medication assessment
mobility and, 714–717
    objective data and, 715–717
    subjective data and, 715
nutrition and, 912–914
    objective data and, 913–914
    subjective data and, 912–913
organizing data for, 105t, 105–107, 106t
pain and, 1170–1174
    objective data and, 1172–1174
    subjective data and, 1170–1172
postoperative, 490–491, 492t
    in recovery facility, 490–491, 491t
preoperative, 474, 475t, 476f, 477t
as purpose of patient record, 150
respiratory function and, 759–764
    objective data and, 761–764
    subjective data and, 759–761
of safety, 576–578
    objective data and, 577–578
    subjective data and, 576–577
self-care and, 648–651
    objective data and, 650–651, 651t
    subjective data and, 648–650
self-concept and, 1252–1253
    objective data and, 1253
    subjective data and, 1252–1253
sensory perception and, 1197–1199
    objective data and, 1198–1199
    subjective data and, 1197–1198
setting and environment for, 97
sexual function and, 1374–1377, 1375t
    objective data and, 1376–1377
    subjective data and, 1374–1376
skin and, 951–953
    objective data and, 952–953
    subjective data and, 951–952

sleep and, 1150–1151
    objective data and, 1151
    subjective data and, 1150
thermoregulation and, 1028–1030
    objective data and, 1029–1030
    subjective data and, 1028–1029
time-lapsed, 96t, 97
urinary elimination and, 1054–1064
    objective data and, 1055–1064
    subjective data and, 1054–1055
validation of data for, 103–105, 105f
of values, 269–270
Nursing care, culturally sensitive, 243, 245
Nursing care plans, 155
    behavioral verbs used in, 129
    formulating, as purpose of patient record, 150
    for infant and family with altered parenting, 1305
    instructional, 130–134
        clinical, 134
    for patient at risk for infection, 1013
    for patient at risk for injury, 589
    for patient experiencing pain, 1187–1188
    for patient who is grieving, 1326–1329
    for patient with activity intolerance, 838
    for patient with altered nutrition, 931
    for patient with altered thought processes, 1236
    for patient with body image disturbance, 1259
    for patient with constipation, 1130
    for patient with fluid volume deficit, 885–886
    for patient with health-seeking behavior, 609
    for patient with impaired home maintenance
        management and, 634
    for patient with impaired physical mobility, 741–742
    for patient with impaired skin integrity, 977–978
    for patient with impaired verbal communication,
        1282–1283
    for patient with ineffective airway clearance, 796
    for patient with ineffective individual coping, 1355
    for patient with ineffective thermoregulation, 1035
    for patient with self-care deficit, 690
    for patient with sensory/perceptual alterations,
        1205–1206
    for patient with sexual dysfunction, 1385
    for patient with sleep pattern disturbance, 1156
    for patient with spiritual distress, 1409
    for patient with urge incontinence, 1084–1085
    revising and modifying, 144, 144f, 145f
    types of, 130–131
    writing, 130f, 130–134
Nursing centers, as nursing practice settings, 17, 17f
Nursing diagnoses, 85–86, 110–125
    actual, 118, 121
    for alterations in safety, 578
    altered health maintenance and, 604–605
    bowel function and, 1108–1110
    cardiopulmonary function and, 822–823
    in clinical care plan, 134
    cognitive function and, 1229
    communication and, 1276
    components of, 117–118
    conferences on, 114t
    coping and adaptation and, 1348–1349
    definition of, 111

Nursing dianoses (*continued*)
  development of, 111–112
  family function and, 1298–1300
  fluid and electrolyte and acid-base balance and, 866–867
  formulating diagnostic statement and, 121–122
  grieving and, 1321–1322
  high risk, 118, 122
  home maintenance management and, 623–624
  human response patterns and, 113–116
  identifying patterns and, 118–120, 119f
  intraoperative nursing and, 484–485, 485t
  medications and, 518–519
  mobility and, 717–718
  nutrition and, 915–916
  organized by functional health patterns, 123–125
  other health-care problems and, 116t, 116–117, 117f
  pain and, 1174–1175
  for patient teaching, 415
  possible, 122
  postoperative, 491, 493t
  preoperative, 474
  relationship to entire nursing process, 112f
  resistance to infection and, 1005–1006
  respiratory function and, 764–765
  self-care and, 651–653
  self-concept and, 1253–1254
  sensory perception and, 1199–1200
  sexual function and, 1377–1378
  significance of, 122, 124
  skin and, 954
  sleep and, 1151
  spiritual function and, 1401–1402
  taxonomy of, 112–116
    definition of, 112–113
    development of, 113–116, 114t
  thermoregulation and, 1030–1031
  urinary elimination and, 1064–1065
  validation of, 120–121, 121f
  for wellness, 180
Nursing discharge summary, 161, 164f, 165
Nursing education, 13, 16
  associated degree nursing programs and, 16
  baccalaureate degree nursing programs and, 16
  diploma nursing programs and, 13, 16
  doctoral degree programs and, 16
  graduate degree programs and, 16
  in-service education and, 16
  instructional nursing care plans and, 130–134
  master's degree nursing programs and, 16
  during 19th century, 9
  nurse doctorate programs and, 16
  practical nursing programs and, 13
  professional values and, 257
Nursing interventions
  bowel function and, 1110–1129
    altered bowel function and, 1111–1125
    discharge planning and home care and, 1125, 1129
    interventions to promote health and function and, 1110–1111
  cardiopulmonary function and, 824–837
    altered, 825–837
    interventions to promote health and function and, 825
  in clinical care plan, 134
  cognitive function and, 1229–1235

    altered cognitive function and, 1231–1234
    interventions to promote health and function and, 1229–1231
    discharge planning and home care and, 1234–1235
  for collaborative problems, 136
  communication and, 1277–1281. *See* Therapeutic communication, intervention and
    discharge planning and home care and, 1280–1281
    interventions for altered function and, 1277–1280
    interventions to promote health and function and, 1277
  coping and adaptation and, 1349–1354
    discharge planning and home care and, 1354
    interventions for altered function and, 1353–1354
    interventions to promote health and function and, 1349–1353
  definition of, 129
  evaluation of, 133
  family function and, 1300–1303
    discharge planning and home care and, 1303
    interventions for altered family function and, 1302–1303
    interventions to promote health and function and, 1300–1302
  fluid and electrolyte and acid-base balance and, 867–886
    altered, 868–884
    discharge planning and home care and, 884, 886
    interventions to promote health and function and, 867–868
  grieving and, 1322–1325
    discharge planning and home care and, 1325
    interventions for altered function and, 1325
    interventions to promote health and function and, 1322–1325
  health maintenance and, 605–608, 606f
    discharge planning and home care and, 608
    interventions for altered function and, 607–608
    interventions to promote health and function and, 605–607
  home maintenance management and, 625–633
    altered, 626–633
    interventions to promote health and function and, 625–626
  implementation and, 136–139
  in instructional nursing care plans, 133, 133t
  intraoperative nursing and, 485t, 485–490
  mobility and, 718–742
    altered, 719–735
    discharge planning and home care and, 735, 740, 742
    interventions to promote health and function and, 718–719
  monitoring effectiveness of, as evaluation skill, 141
  nutrition and, 916–930
    discharge planning and home care and, 929–930
    interventions for altered function and, 917, 919–929
    interventions to promote health and function and, 916–917
  pain and, 1175–1186
    discharge planning and home care and, 1185–1186
    interventions for altered comfort and, 1176–1185
    interventions to promote health and function and, 1175–1176
  planning, 129–130
  postoperative, 491–495
  preoperative, 474–483

resistance to infection and, 1006–1014
  discharge planning and home care and, 1012–1014
  interventions for altered function and, 1009–1012
  interventions to promote health and function and, 1006–1009
respiratory function and, 765–795
  altered, 772–788
  discharge planning and home care and, 788–795
  interventions to promote health and respiratory function and, 765–772
safety and
  altered safety function and, 586–587
  discharge planning and home care and, 587–588, 588f
  to promote health and safety function, 579–586
scientific rationale for, 133
self-care and, 653–689
  altered self-care and, 653–682
  discharge planning and home care and, 682, 685, 688–689
  interventions to promote health and self-care and, 653
self-concept and, 1254–1258
  discharge planning and home care and, 1257–1258
  interventions for altered self-concept and, 1256–1257
  interventions to promote health and function and, 1254–1256
sensory perception and, 1200–1206
  discharge planning and home care and, 1203, 1206
  interventions for altered sensory function and, 1201–1203
  interventions to promote health and function and, 1200–1201
sexual function and, 1378–1384
  discharge planning and home care and, 1383–1384
  interventions for altered function and, 1383
  interventions to promote health and function and, 1378–1383
skin and, 954–976
  discharge planning and home care and, 976
  interventions for altered function and, 957t, 957–596
  interventions to promote health and function, 955–956
sleep and, 1151–1154
  altered function and, 1153–1154
  discharge planning and home care and, 1154
  interventions to promote health and function and, 1151–1153
spiritual function and, 1402–1409
  discharge planning and home care and, 1408–1409
  interventions for altered function and, 1404–1408
  interventions to promote health and function and, 1402–1404
thermoregulation and, 1031–1035
  altered thermoregulation and, 1032–1034
  discharge planning and home care and, 1034–1035
  interventions to promote health and, 1031–1032
type of community and, 231t
types of, 136–139, 137t
urinary elimination and, 1066–1085
  altered function and, 1068–1083
  discharge planning and home care and, 1083, 1085
  interventions to promote health and urinary function and, 1066–1068
Nursing journals, 9, 72, 78
  about medications, 503
Nursing management plans. *See* Nursing care plans

Nursing monitors, 145
Nursing practice, 20–23
  nurse practice acts and, 20
  professional organizations and, 20, 22–23
  research and, 77–78
    applications of, 77–78
  standards of practice and, 20, 21
  trends in, 23
Nursing practice settings, 16–17, 17f
Nursing process
  definition of, 83, 84, 85, 85f
  development of, 83–84, 84t
  functional health approach to, 90, 91f
  future trends in, 90–92
  phases of, 84–86. *See also* Evaluation; Implementation; Nursing assessment; Nursing diagnoses; Planning
  professional relevance of, 90
  relationship of nursing diagnosis to, 112f
  requirements for effective use of, 89–90
  theoretical foundations of, 87–89
    decision-making process and, 88
    diagnostic reasoning process and, 89
    information-processing theory and, 88–89, 89f
    problem-solving process and, 87–88, 88t
    systems theory and, 87, 87f
Nursing profession, 5–11, 6f, 7t–8t
  career development and, 19–20
  definitions of, 11, 11t
  evolution of, 6–10
    during early Christian era, 6
    during 18th century, 8
    Greeks and, 8
    during Middle Ages, 8
    during 19th century, 8–9
    during pre-Christian era, 6
    during Reformation, 8
    during Renaissance, 8
    during 20th century, 9–10
  socialization to, 10, 10t
Nursing progress notes, 158–161, 160f
  narrative, 158
  SOAP, 160f, 161
Nursing Research, 72
Nursing research, 70–79, 72f
  applying to practice, 77–78
  characteristics of, 73
  clinical, 77
  definition of, 71
  developing ideas for, 74
  dissemination of results of, 76
  evolution of, 72–73
  knowledge of, as evaluation skill, 141
  legal and ethical issues in, 76–77
  literature review and, 74
  nurses' roles in, 77
  in practice, 75–76
  problem statement and, 75
  research design and, 73–74, 74f
  scientific process and, 73, 73t
  theoretical framework for, 74–75
Nursing roles, 17–19, 18f
  clinical practice, leadership and management in, 63–66
  expanded, 19–20
  management, 66–67

Nursing roles (*continued*)
  medication administration and, 509–510
  in research, 77
  teaching, leadership and management in, 67–68
Nursing rounds, 167
Nursing theory, 12–13, 14t–15t
  practice related to, 13
  single versus multiple, 12
Nurturing
  as family function, 1290
  in holistic health care, 179
Nutrient(s), 892. *See also* Nutrition
  excess intake of, 909–910
  inability to use, 910
  inadequate intake of, 909, 909f
  malabsorption of, altered nutrition and, 910
Nutrient density, 904
Nutrition, 890–932. *See also* Diet; Feeding; Food;
       Nutrient(s); Nutrition–metabolism health
       pattern; Total parenteral nutrition
  altered nutritional function and, 909–912
    manifestations of, 911–912
    potential for, 909–911
  anatomy of digestive system and, 892–893
  assessment and, 912–914
    objective data and, 913–914
    subjective data and, 912–913
  body temperature and, 1025
  bowel function and, 1094
  Canadian recommendations for, 1448
  cardiovascular function and, 812
  characteristics of, 901
    ideal body weight and, 901
    normal laboratory values and, 901
    physical status and, 901
  cognitive function and, 1216, 1219
  coping and adaptation and, 1341
  decubitus ulcers and, 943
  evaluation and, 930–932
  factors affecting, 905–907
  home maintenance management and, 616, 619
  immobility and, 711
  inadequate, infections and, 998
  infections and, 1009–1010
  interventions and, 916–930
    for altered function, 917, 919–929
    discharge planning and home care and, 929–930
    to promote health and function, 916–917
  lifespan considerations and, 907–909
  need for, 186
  normal nutritional functional pattern and, 902–905
    basic four food groups and, 902, 903f, 904–905
  normal physiologic function of digestive system and,
       900–901
    absorption and, 900
    digestion and, 900
    excretion and, 901
    metabolism and, 900–901
  normal physiologic function of nutrients and, 893–900
    carbohydrates and, 893
    fat and, 894
    minerals and, 897–900, 898t
    protein and, 893–894

  vitamins and, 894, 895t–896t, 896–897
  water and, 900
  nursing diagnoses and patient goals and, 915–916
  postoperative, 494
  resistance to infection and, 986
  respiratory function and, 755
  safety and, 565
  safety dysfunction and, 575
  skin and, 938
  sleep and, 1143
  urinary elimination and, 1046
  wound healing and, 947–948
Nutritional supplements, 921
Nutritional tolerance, biocultural variation in, 246
Nutrition–metabolism health pattern, 90, 106
  assessing human needs and, 192
  assessment of, 320–327
    objective data in, 321–327
    subjective data in, 320–321
  in community, 232
  disruption by diagnostic procedures, 394t
  drugs promoting normal function and, 501t
  exercise and immobility and, 708t
  in family, 228
  health maintenance and, 597t
  health problems and anticipatory guidance and, 211–212
  surgery and, 469
  values and, 261, 263

O

Obesity
  altered nutrition and, 912
  antiembolic stockings and, 829
  Heimlich maneuver and, 794
  subcutaneous injections and, 540–541
  wound healing and, 949
Objective data, 102, 102t
Observation
  cognitive function and, 1226
  hearing and, 98
  smell and, 98
  touch and, 98–99
  vision and, 98
Obstructive sleep apnea, 1149
Occlusive dressings, 958, 959t
Occult blood, assessing stool for, 1105–1108
Odor(s)
  of body, biocultural variation in, 246
  of feet, 665t
  in physical examination, 307
  of skin, 938
  of urine, 1046
Official name, of drugs, 500
Older adult
  aquathermia pads and, 976
  assessing body temperature of, 356
  bathing and, 661
  bedpan and, 680
  blood pressure assessment in, 368
  blood transfusions and, 884
  body temperature and, 1024
  bowel function and, 1096
  cardiovascular function and, 809

cognitive function and, 1218, 1218f
cold packs and, 973
communicating with, 289–290
communication and, 1270
coping and adaptation and, 1343
crutches and, 735
development of, 203t, 208–209
diagnostic and laboratory testing and, 404
dressing changes and, 963
enemas and, 1116
family and, 1292
feeding, 919
fluid and electrolyte balance and, 853
foot and nail care and, 667
functional health assessment of, 346
  auscultating heart sounds in, 320
  auscultation of bowel sounds in, 326
  auscultation of breath sounds in, 316
  neurologic assessment in, 333
functional health patterns and, health problems and
  anticipatory guidance and, 211–219, 211f, 216f
grieving and, 1318
health maintenance and, 599, 603t
home maintenance management and, 618
indwelling urinary catheter and, 1076
infection control and, 460–461
medications and, 556
mobility and, 705
needs of, 189
nutrition and, 908–909
oral care and, 671
oral medications and, 526
ostomy care and, 1126
pain and, 1167
patient teaching and, 423
pulse assessment in, 360, 362
resistance to infection and, 987, 992
respiratory function and, 753
safety and, 569
self-care and, 646
self-concept and, 1247t, 1249, 1256
sensory perception and, 1193
sexuality and, 1371
shampooing hair of, 669
skin and, 939
sleep and, 1145
spiritual function and, 1396
surgery and, 474
urinary elimination and, 1048
values and, 267
vital signs in, 376
Oliguria, 1052
One-day surgical centers, 466
One-time order, 505
Open-ended interview, grounding assessments in patient's
  perspective and, 247
Open-ended questions, 284, 284t
Opening remarks, 284, 284t
Operative values, 256
Ophthalmic medications, 529, 529f
Ophthalmologists, 35
Opiates, 1114t
  endogenous, 1163

Opposition (joint movement), 701
Optometrists, 35
Oral airways, 781, 787f
Oral care, 643, 643f, 667, 669–673
  in comatose or unconscious patient, 672
  nasogastric intubation and, 1120, 1122
Oral intake, inadequate, fluid and electrolyte and, 858
Oral medications. *See* Medication administration, oral
Orem, Dorothea E., 14t–15t
  perception of human needs, 190
Organ donation, 54, 54f
Organization
  of charting, 153
  in cognitive development theory, 201
Organizing, as management function, 61, 61f
Organ system dysfunction, altered cardiopulmonary
    function and, 816
Organ system function, drug action and, 515
Orgasm, 1366, 1367, 1367t, 1368
Orgasmic dysfunction, 1373
Orientation, 1215
  communication and, 1278
  to patient unit, safety and, 580
Orientation phase, of nurse-patient relationship, 277
Orlando, Ida Jean, 14t–15t
  perception of human needs, 190
Oropharyngeal secretions, suctioning, 782–785
Orthostatic hypotension, 371–374
  assessment for, 373–374
  immobility and, 709–710
Osmosis, fluid and electrolyte movement and, 849, 849f
Osmotic pressure, fluid and electrolyte movement and,
  849–850, 850f
Osteomalacia, 898–899
Osteopathic physicians, 35
Osteoporosis, 899
  disuse, 711
  patient teaching about, 607
Ostomies, 941
OTC (over-the-counter) medications, 504
Otic medications, 529, 530f
Outcome criteria
  bowel function and, 1129, 1131
  cardiopulmonary function and, 837–839
  cognitive function and, 1235–1236
  communication and, 1281
  coping and adaptation and, 1354, 1356
  family function and, 1304
  fluid and electrolyte and acid-base balance and, 886–887
  grieving and, 1325, 1330
  health maintenance and, 608–609
  home maintenance management and, 633, 634t, 635
  in instructional nursing care plans, 132–133
  intraoperative nursing and, 490
  mobility and, 742–743
  nutrition and, 930–932
  pain and, 1186
  in planning, 128–129, 129f
  preoperative nursing and, 483–484
  postoperative nursing and, 495
  resistance to infection and, 1014
  respiratory function and, 795–797
  reviewing, evaluation and, 142

Outcome criteria (*continued*)
    safety and, 590
    self-care deficit and, 689–690
    self-concept and, 1258
    sensory perception and, 1206–1207
    sexual function and, 1384–1385
    skin and, 976, 978
    sleep and, 1154–1155
    spiritual function and, 1409–1410
    thermoregulation and, 1035–1036
    urinary elimination and, 1085–1086
Outcome evaluation, 142
Outpatient services, agencies providing, 32
Output, in systems theory, 87, 87f
Ovaries, 1362
Over-the-counter (OTC) medications, 504
Overweight. *See also* Obesity
    altered nutrition and, 911
Ovulation, 1364
Oxygen, arterial, cognitive function and, 1227
Oxygenation. *See also* Cardiovascular function; Respiratory
        function
    mobility and, 702
    wound healing and, 948
Oxygen catheters, 448f, 449f, 774–775
Oxygen tents, 778
Oxygen therapy, 772–780
    body temperature measurement and, 351
    in home, 792, 792f
    oxygen administration and, 773, 773f
    oxygen delivery systems and, 773–778, 774t, 775f
        pediatric, 777–778
    safety considerations with, 778–780
Oxyhood, 774t

P

PA. *See* Physician's assistant
Packing, of wounds, 969, 970–971
P_ACO_2, 749
Pain, 1160–1188
    acute and chronic, 1166
    altered function resulting in, 1168–1170
        activities of daily living and, 1170
        manifestations of pain and, 1168–1170, 1169t
        potential causes of pain and, 1168
    assessment and, 336–337, 1170–1174
        objective data and, 1172–1174
        subjective data and, 1170–1172
    cardiovascular function and, 807
    causes of, 1168
    characteristics of, 1165–1166
    in chest
        altered cardiopulmonary function and, 830
        altered respiratory function and, 757
    evaluation and, 1186
    fear of, bowel function and, 1097
    immobility and, 709
    infections and, 999–1000
    interventions and, 1175–1186
        for altered comfort, 1176–1185
        discharge planning and home care and, 1185–1186
        to promote health and function, 1175–1176
    ischemia and, 815

    management of, altered cardiopulmonary function and, 830
    mobility and, 707
    normal function of, 1162–1168
    nursing diagnoses and patient goals and, 1174–1175
    perception of, 1166t, 1166–1167
    relief of, noninvasive, 1177–1180
    self-care and, 647
    substances producing, 1163
    surgery and, 471
    theories of, 1164–1165
    tolerance of, 1167
Pain (nursing diagnosis), 1174–1175
    nursing management plan for, 1187–1188
Pain behaviors, 1171
Pain threshold, 1166–1167
Pallor
    ischemia and, 815
    pain and, 1169
Palpation, 101
    blood pressure measurement and, 371
    bowel function assessment and, 328, 1104–1105
    cardiopulmonary assessment and, 819–820, 820f
    cardiovascular assessment and, 318
    deep, 304, 305f
    light, 304, 304f
        abdominal assessment and, 326–327
        urinary elimination assessment and, 327–328
    of lymph nodes, infections and, 1002
    in physical examination, 304f, 304–305, 305f
    pulse measurement and, 358, 359
    respiratory assessment and, 312–313, 313f, 761
    sexuality-reproduction assessment and, 342–343, 343f
    of skin, 953
    urinary elimination and, 1056, 1056t
Pantothenic acid, normal physiologic function of, 896t
P_AO_2, 749, 750f
PAP (pulmonary artery pressure), fluid and electrolyte imbalance and, 865
Paper thermometers, disposable, 353, 354f
Pap smear, 1377t
Papule, 946t
Paracentesis, 401f, 401–402
Paradoxical blood pressure, 370
Paraffin baths, 974
Paralyzed patients, aquathermia pads and, 976
Parasites, 428, 993
Parasomnias, 1149–1150
Parasympathetic nervous system (PNS), pain and, 1172
Parathyroid hormone (PTH), fluid and electrolyte balance and, 852
Parenteral medications. *See* Medication administration, parenteral
Participative leadership, 60, 60f
Passive immunity, 985, 985f
Passive range of motion, 722
Patch (skin lesion), 946t
Patellar reflex, assessment of, 338t
Paternalistic approach, 278, 279t
Pathogen(s), 428, 982
Pathogenicity, 429, 992
Patient. *See also* Nurse-patient relationship
    connotation of term, 180

Patient advocate, nurse as, 18, 278–279, 279t
Patient-controlled analgesia (PCA), 553, 1184, 1184f
Patient education, culturally sensitive, 250, 250f
Patient goals
    for alterations in safety, 578–579
    altered health maintenance and, 605
    attainment of
        barriers to, 143–144
        facilitators of, 143
        measuring, 143f, 143–144
        recording judgment or measurement of, 144
    bowel function and, 1110, 1129, 1131
    cardiopulmonary function and, 823–824, 837–839
    in clinical care plan, 134
    cognitive function and, 1229, 1235–1236
    communication and, 1276, 1281
    coping and adaptation and, 1354, 1356
    family function and, 1300, 1304
    fluid and electrolyte and acid-base balance and, 867, 886–887
    grieving and, 1322, 1325, 1330
    health maintenance and, 608–609
    home maintenance management and, 624–625, 633, 634t, 635
    in instructional nursing care plans, 132
    intraoperative nursing and, 484–485, 485t, 490
    mobility and, 718, 742–743
    nutrition and, 916, 930–932
    pain and, 1175, 1186
    patient teaching and, 415–416
    in planning, 128
    postoperative, 491, 493t
    postoperative nursing and, 495
    preoperative nursing and, 474, 483–484
    resistance to infection and, 1006, 1014
    respiratory function and, 765, 795–797
    reviewing, evaluation and, 142
    safety and, 590
    self-care and, 653
    self-care deficit and, 689–690
    self-concept and, 1254, 1258
    sensory perception and, 1200, 1206–1207
    sexual function and, 1378, 1384–1385
    skin and, 954, 976, 978
    sleep and, 1151, 1154–1155
    spiritual function and, 1402, 1409–1410
    thermoregulation and, 1031, 1035–1036
    urinary elimination and, 1065, 1085–1086
Patient positioning. See also Body position
    for diagnostic and laboratory tests, 383–384, 384f
    intraoperative, 487
Patient preparation
    for diagnostic and laboratory tests, 380–383
    for functional health assessment, 296, 297
    sensory perception and, 1200–1201
    for surgery, 480–481
Patient record, 149–165
    computer documentation and, 155, 158f
    confidentiality and, 168–169
    nursing entries on, 155–165
        admission entries and, 161
        incident reports and, 165
        Kardex and, 158, 159f

        medication records and, 165, 166f
        nursing care plan and, 155
        nursing discharge summary and, 161, 164f, 165
        nursing progress notes and, 158–161, 160f
    principles charting and, 150, 151t–152t, 152–154, 153f
    problem-oriented, 155, 156f, 157f
    purpose of, 150
    recording nursing interventions in, 139
    source-oriented, 154t, 154–155
Patient responses, knowledge of, as evaluation skill, 141
Patient rooms. See Patient unit
Patient safety, intraoperative, 486–487
Patient's Bill of Rights, 48, 53
    medication administration and, 510–511
Patient scheduling, for diagnostic and laboratory tests, 380
Patient support, during diagnostic and laboratory tests, 383
Patient teaching, 56, 408–423
    about common illnesses, 605–607
    about diet
        fluid and electrolyte balance and, 869, 869t
        to reduce edema, 829
    for acute problems, 412t, 412–413
    altered cardiopulmonary function and, 825–826
    assessment for, 413–415
    audiovisual aids and, 417, 417f
    bowel function and, 1110–1111
    for chronic problems, 413
    communication and, 417–418, 1277
    for diagnostic and laboratory tests, 380, 382, 382f
    documentation of, 420–421
    environment control and, 417
    evaluation of learning and, 420
    grieving and, 1323
    home maintenance management and, 625, 625f
    lifespan considerations and, 421–423
    nursing diagnoses and patient goals and, 415–416
    nutrition and, 916, 917f
    planning for, 415–416
    preoperative, 475, 477–478
    to promote health and function, 412–413
    repetition and, 418
    sensitivity and, 416–417
    sensory perception and, 1200
    sexual function and, 1378–1381, 1379f
    structured teaching sessions and, 417
    teaching-learning process and, 410–412
    teaching methods and, 418–419
    teaching strategies and, 419–420, 420f
Patient transfers, reports and, 167
Patient transport, to recovery facility, 490
Patient unit
    care of, 681–682
    infection control and, 445, 448
    orientation to, safety and, 580
Pattern label, 106
Pattern theory of pain, 1164
PCA (patient-controlled analgesia), 553, 1184, 1184f
Pediculosis, 664–665
Peer culture, as source of values, 259
Peer review, 145–146
    individual, 145–146
    nursing monitors and, 145
PEG (percutaneous endoscopic gastrostomy), 922, 922f

Penis, 1362
Penrose drain, 953
Peplau, Hildegard E., 14t–15t
Perceived Constipation, 1109
Perceiving pattern, nursing diagnosis and, 114
Perception, 198, 1215. *See also* Cognition–perception health pattern; Health perception–health management health pattern; Sensory perception
   communication and, 1268–1269
   health maintenance and, 594, 596
   home maintenance management and, 615
   immobility and, 713
   of information, 1213–1214
   of pain, 1166t, 1166–1167
   of reality, 1215
   resistance to infection and, 985
   safety and, 564, 565
   of self. *See* Self-perception–self-concept health pattern
   self-care and, 644–645
   sexuality and, 1368–1369
Percussion, 101
   bowel function assessment and, 1104
   chest physiotherapy and, 781
   direct and indirect, 305–306, 306f
   in physical examination, 305t, 305–306, 306f
   respiratory assessment and, 313, 761–762
   urinary elimination and, 327, 1056
Percutaneous endoscopic gastrostomy (PEG), 922, 922f
Perfection, stress management and, 1350
Perfusion, of tissues, 805–806
Perineal care, 662f, 662–663
Perioperative nursing, 464–496. *See also* Intraoperative nursing; Postoperative nursing; Preoperative nursing; Surgery
   phases of, 466–468
Peripheral nerves, pain and, 1162, 1162f
Peripheral parenteral nutrition (PPN), 923
Perirectal examination, bowel function assessment and, 1105
Peristalsis, 900
Peritoneal dialysis, 1082–1083
Permeable dressings, 958, 959t
Person, concept of, 12
Personal hygiene. *See* Hygiene
Personal Identity Disturbance, 1253
Personal resources, grieving and, 1315
Personal values. *See* Values
Perspiration, pain and, 1169
Pertussis, 989t
Pfeiffer Mental Status Questionnaire, 1227
Phagocytes, 983, 983t
Phantom pain, 1164, 1172
Pharmacists, 36
Pharmacodynamics, 511, 512–514
Pharmacokinetics, 511–512
Pharynx, anatomy of, 892
Phlebitis, intravenous therapy and, 876, 879
Phonation, 1266
Phosphorus, normal physiologic function of, 898t
Physical assessment. *See also* Physical examination
   bowel function and, 1103t, 1103–1105
   cardiopulmonary function and, 819–820
   cognitive function and, 1226

communication and, 1275–1276
   coping and adaptation and, 1347
   fluid and electrolyte and acid-base balance and, 862–865
   grieving and, 1321
   health maintenance and, 203t, 204, 204f, 602, 602f
   infections and, 1001–1002
   before medication administration, 517–518
   mobility and, 715–717
   nutrition and, 913–914
   pain and, 1172–1174
   respiratory function and, 761–762
   sensory perception and, 1198–1199, 1199t
   sexual function and, 1376–1377
   sleep and rest and, 1151
   urinary elimination and, 1056
Physical development
   of adolescent, 203t, 207
   of infant, 202t, 204–205
   intrauterine, 201, 202t, 204
   of middle adult, 203t, 208
   of neonate, 202t, 204
   of older adult, 203t, 208–209
   of preschooler, 202t–203t, 206
   of school-age child, 203t, 206
   of toddler, 202t, 205
   of young adult, 203t, 207
Physical examination, 100–101. *See also* Physical assessment
   auscultation in, 101, 306f, 306–307, 307t. *See also* Auscultation
   definition of, 100
   for functional health assessment, 303–307
   inspection in, 100–101, 303–304. *See also* Inspection
   palpation in, 101, 304f, 304–305, 305f. *See also* Palpation
   percussion in, 101, 305t, 305–306, 306f. *See also* Percussion
   skin and, 952–953
Physical factors
   causing pain, 1168
   in discharge preparation, 629
   nutrition and, 905
Physical fitness, promotion of, 718f, 718–719
Physical needs, home care and, home maintenance management and, 631, 632t, 633
Physical provision, as family function, 1289
Physical state, patient teaching and, 415
Physicians, 35
   allopathic, 35
   death assisted by, 52
   osteopathic, 35
   reports to, 167–168, 168f
Physician's assistant (PA), 36
Physicians' Desk Reference, The, 501
Physicians' offices, 32
   surgery performed in, 466
Physiologic changes, in older adult, patient teaching and, 423
Physiologic factors, safety and, 565
Physiologic needs, 185–187, 224
Physiologic stress, 1346
Piaget, Jean, cognitive development theory of, 199, 200t, 201
Piers-Harris Self-Concept Scale, 339

Pillow, positioning and, 725t
Placebos, pain relief and, 1185
Plaintiff, 50
Planning, 86, 127–134, 128f. *See also* Discharge planning;
        Nursing care plan
    definition of, 127
    establishing patient goals and outcome criteria and,
        128–129, 129f
    establishing priorities and, 128
    as management function, 61, 61f
    of nursing interventions, 129–130
    organized by functional health, 134
    for patient teaching, 415–416
    writing nursing care plan and, 130f, 130–134
Plantar warts, 665t
Plaque
    atherosclerotic, 810, 811f
    dental, 643
    on skin, 946t
Plasma, altered composition of, 812
Plasma chemistries, reference ranges for, 1418–1431
Plateau phase, of sexual response, 1366–1368, 1367t
Platelet(s), 880
Platelet count, 390
Pleximeter, 305Plexor305–306, 306f
PLISSIT method, 1383, 1384t
Pluralism, spiritual care and, 1397
Pneumothorax, total parenteral nutrition and, 929
PNS (parasympathetic nervous system), pain and, 1172
Poisoning, 572–573, 573f, 574
    emergency care in, 586–587
    prevention of, 585
    toxins and, 992
        in home, 574
Polio, 989t
Pollens, respiratory function and, 755
Pollution
    respiratory function and, 755
    safety and, 567, 571f, 571–572
Polymorphonuclear cells, 880, 983
Polysaccharides, 893
Polyuria, 1051–1052
POMR. *See* Problem-oriented medical record
Positive nitrogen balance, 894
Positive regard, 280–281
Possible nursing diagnoses, 122
Posterior chest
    anatomic landmarks of wall of, 310f–311f, 311–312
    auscultation of, 315–316
Postion. *See* Body position; Patient positioning
Postoperative nursing, 468, 490–495
    assessment and, 490–491, 492t
        in recovery facility, 490–491, 491t
    evaluation and, 495
    interventions and, 491–495
    nursing diagnoses and patient goals and, 491, 493t
    patient teaching and, 413, 477–478, 478t
Postural drainage, chest physiotherapy and, 781
Posture, 695f, 695–696
Potassium, 847–848
    dietary sources of, 869t
    imbalance of, 856
    normal physiologic function of, 898t, 899

Poverty. *See also* Economics
    altered health maintenance function and, 599–600
PPN (peripheral parenteral nutrition), 923
Practical nursing program, 13
Preconventional judgment, 44
Preferred provider organizations, 31
Pregnancy, 1365–1366, 1371, 1374
    fluid and electrolyte and acid-base imbalances and,
        859
    Heimlich maneuver and, 794
    intrauterine development during, 201, 202t, 204
    medication assessment and, 516
    nutrition and, 907
    respiratory function and, 752
    urinary elimination and, 1049–1050
Premature ejaculation, 1373
Prenatal development, sexuality and, 1369
Preoperative checklist, 481, 482f, 483, 483t
Preoperative nursing, 467, 474–484
    assessment and, 474, 475t, 476f, 477t
    evaluation and, 483–484
    informed consent and, 478, 479f, 480
    nursing diagnoses and patient goals and, 474
    patient preparation and, 480–481
    patient teaching and, 412–413, 475, 477–478
    preoperative checklist and, 481, 482f, 483, 483t
Prepuce, 1362
Preschooler
    body temperature and, 1023
    bowel function and, 1095
    cardiovascular function and, 809
    cognitive function and, 1217, 1218f
    communication and, 1270
    coping and adaptation and, 1342
    development of, 202t–203t, 206
    diagnostic and laboratory testing and, 404
    family and, 1291–1292
    feeding, 919
    fluid and electrolyte balance and, 853
    functional health assessment of, 345, 345f
        auscultating heart sounds in, 319
        auscultation of bowel sounds in, 326
        auscultation of breath sounds in, 316
        neurologic assessment in, 333
    functional health patterns and, health problems and
        anticipatory guidance and, 210–218
    grieving and, 1316–1317, 1317t
    health maintenance and, 598, 603t
    home maintenance management and, 617, 617f
    infection control and, 457
    medications and, 555
    mobility and, 705
    needs of, 189
    nutrition and, 907–908
    pain and, 1167
    patient teaching and, 421, 421f
    resistance to infection and, 986–987
    respiratory function and, 753
    safety and, 567–568
    self-care and, 645–646
    self-concept and, 1246t, 1247–1248, 1256
    sensory perception and, 1193
    sexuality and, 1369

Preschooler (*continued*)
  skin and, 939
  sleep and, 1144–1145
  spiritual function and, 1395, 1407
  surgery and, 473
  urinary elimination and, 1047
  values and, 266
  vital signs in, 375
Pressure sores, 941–943
  immobility and, 711–712
  locations of, 943, 944f
  prevention of, 956, 956f
  risk factors for, 941–943, 942f, 943f
  staging, 941, 941f
Preventive activities, in holistic health care, 179
Preventive health education, 412, 412f
Primary nursing, 64, 65
Primary prevention, 596t
Primary sources, 102
Priorities
  implementation and, 135–136, 136f
  patient teaching and, 413
  in planning, 128
Privacy
  bowel function and, 1094
  invasion of, 49
Private-duty nursing, 17
Private rooms, infection control and, 445, 448
P.R.N. orders, 504–505
Problem-oriented medical record (POMR), 155, 156f, 157f
Problem-solving
  family function and, 1302–1303
  as management skill, 62
  process of, 87–88, 88t
Problem statement, 75
Process evaluation, 141–142
Process recording, 286, 287t
Prodromal period, 430
Professionalism
  definition of, 11
  relevance of nursing process for, 90
  values of, 256–257, 257t
    classroom study and, 257
    clinical study and, 257
    socialization and, 257
Professional nurse, 13
Professional organizations, 9, 20, 22–23. *See also specific organizations*
  specialty, 22
Progressive relaxation, stress management and, 1352–1353
Progress notes. *See* Nursing progress notes
Prompted voiding, 1069
Pronation, 701, 704t
Prone position, 721t
Proprietary hospitals, 30
Proprioceptors, 1162, 1213–1214
Prospective payment system, 29, 34–35
Prostate gland, 1362
Protective isolation, 452
Protective pants, 1069
Protein(s)
  complete, 893
  digestion of, 900
  incomplete, 893–894
  metabolism of, 901
  normal physiologic function of, 893–894
  partially complete, 893
Protest, grief and, 1314
Protestants, religious practices of, 1405t
Protozoal infections, 993
Proximate causes, 51
Pruritus, 939, 944
  relief of, 957
Psoriasis, 940
Psychocognitive considerations, in discharge preparation, 630
Psychodynamic theories of development, 199, 200, 200t
Psychogenic factors, causing pain, 1168
Psychological factors, urinary elimination and, 1046–1047
Psychological function, of sleep, 1142
Psychological state
  altered nutrition and, 911
  drug action and, 515
Psychological stress, 1346
Psychomotor domain of knowledge, 410
Psychomotor nursing interventions, 139
Psychomotor teaching methods, 419
Psychosis, ICU, 1223
Psychosocial development
  of adolescent, 203t, 207
  of infant, 202t, 205
  intrauterine, 202t, 204
  of middle adult, 203t, 208
  of neonate, 202t, 204, 205f
  of older adult, 203t, 209
  of preschooler, 202t–203t, 206
  of school-age child, 203t, 206–207
  of toddler, 202t, 206
  of young adult, 203t, 207–208
Psychosocial nursing interventions, 138–139
Psychosocial problems, altered health maintenance function and, 601
Psychosociologic response, to stress, 1340, 1340t
PTH (parathyroid hormone), fluid and electrolyte balance and, 852
Puerto Ricans. *See* Hispanics
Pulmonary artery pressure (PAP), fluid and electrolyte imbalance and, 865
Pulmonary embolism, 816
Pulmonary function tests, 762
Pulmonary toilet, infections and, 1010
Pulse, 354, 357–361
  actors affecting, 354, 356–357
  altered cardiovascular function and, 814
  apical, 357, 359–360
  assessment of, 357–361
  brachial, 357
  cardiopulmonary function and, 820
  carotid, 357
  characteristics of, 354
  femoral, 357
  fluid and electrolyte imbalance and, 860
  infections and, 999
  pedal, 357
  popliteal, 357
  posterior tibial, 358

quality of, 360, 361t
  radial, 357, 359
  rate of, 358
  rhythm of, 358, 360
  temporal, 357
Pulse deficits, 360–361
  assessment of, 362
Pulse pressure, 364
Pulse rate, altered cardiovascular function and, 814–815
Puncture wound, 940, 940t
Punitive damages, 51
Pupillary dilation, pain and, 1169
Pure Food and Drug Act of 1906, 507, 508t
Purpose, need for, spiritual dysfunction and, 1398t–1399t
Purulent drainage, 953
  infections and, 1000
Pustule, 944, 946t
Pyrexia. *See* Fever
Pyrogens, body temperature and, 1025
Pyuria, 1052

Q

Quad cough, 770
Qualifiers, in nursing diagnosis, 118
Quality, auscultation and, 306
Quality assurance, 36–37
Quality assurance monitors, 144–146
Question-and-answer session, patient teaching and, 419
Questionnaires, evaluation of learning with, 420

R

Race, 242
Racism, 242
Radiation, heat loss and, 1020
Radiation injury, 574
  burns and, 943
Radiation safety, 580–581, 581f
  intraoperative, 487
Radiography, 393–396. *See also* Computed tomography;
      Magnetic resonance imaging
  bowel function and, 1106
  cardiopulmonary function and, 822
  contrast media and, 395, 395t
  fluoroscopy and, 395
  infections and, 1005
  mammography and, 395–396
  mobility and, 717
  radioisotope scanning and, 396
  respiratory assessment and, 762
  urinary elimination and, 1063
Radioisotope scanning, 396
Radiopaque media, 395, 395t
Rales, 762
Random urine specimen, collection of, 1056, 1059
Range of motion (ROM)
  active, 702
  full, 701–702, 703t–704t
  maintaining, 722, 728–729
Rapid eye movement (REM) sleep, 1138t, 1139f,
      1139–1140, 1140f
RAS. *See* Reticular activating system
Rash, 944
  infections and, 1000

RDAs (recommended daily allowances), 904
Reabsorption, urine formation and, 1045
Reading ability
  assessment of, 333
  patient teaching and, 415
Reagent strips, urine testing and, 1060
Realism, patient teaching and, 413–414
Reality orientation, cognitive function and, 1233
Reality perception, 1215
Reassessment, implementation and, 135
Reassurance, false, 288
Recall, 1215
Receiver, in communication process, 275
Receptive aphasia, 1272, 1272t
Recharging, closed drainage systems and, 967
Recognition, 1215
Recommended daily allowances (RDAs), 904
Recommended dietary allowances, 904, 1445–1447
Reconstructive phase, of wound healing, 945
Recording. *See* Documentation; Patient record; Reporting
Recovery facility
  assessment in, 490–491, 491t
  interventions in, 492–493
  transport to, 490
Recreation therapy, 1234
Rectal medications, 529–530, 530f
Rectal tubes, 1117
Rectus femoris site, for intramuscular injections, 542, 542f, 545
Recurrent bandaging, 965, 965f
Red blood cell(s), altered, 811
Red blood cell count, 388
Reference ranges, 385, 1415–1437
  abbreviations used in, 1415
  for cerebrospinal fluid, 1435–1436
  for drugs, 1437
  for gastric analysis, 1437
  for hematology, 1415–1417
  laboratory tests and, 385
  for serum, plasma, and whole blood chemistries,
      1418–1431
  for urine chemistry, 1431–1435
Referral, 629
  complex, 629
  family function and, 1303
  grieving and, 1325
  sexual function and, 1383
  simple, 629
  spiritual function and, 1406–1407
Referred pain, 1165
Reflection, 284t, 285
Reflex(es)
  deep tendon, 336, 338t
  defecation, 1093
  micturition, 1045
  Moro, sucking, 333
  rooting, 333
  spinal, pain and, 1163–1164
  sucking, 333
  tonic neck, 333
Reflex Incontinence, 1064–1065
Reflex incontinence, 1053, 1064–1065
Refuse. *See also* Waste disposal
  handling of, infection control and, 448

Regeneration, of skin, 937

Regional anesthesia, 487–488, 488t

Registered nurse, 13

Regression, 646

Regulatory agencies, infection control and, 434–435

Rehabilitation, 30
  altered cardiopulmonary function and, 831–832, 832t

Rehabilitation centers, as nursing practice settings, 17

Rehabilitation goals, home maintenance management and, 624

Relapsing fever, 1026, 1027t

Related factors, in nursing diagnosis, 118

Relatedness, need for, spiritual dysfunction and, 1398t

Relating pattern, nursing diagnosis and, 113

Relationships. *See also* Nurse-patient relationship;
    Roles–relationships health pattern; Therapeutic
    relationship
  coping and adaptation and, 1341
  health maintenance and, 598
  home maintenance management and, 616
  immobility and, 713
  sexuality and, 1368
  sleep and, 1146

Relative immunity, 985

Relaxation
  infections and, 1009
  pain relief and, 1179–1180
  stress management and, 1352t, 1352–1353

Relaxation training, 1353–1354

Religion. *See also* Spiritual function
  nutrition and, 906
  religious group practices and, 1405t–1407t

Relocation, involuntary, coping and adaptation and, 1343

Reminiscence therapy, 1234

Remittant fever, 1026, 1027t

REM (rapid eye movement) sleep, 1138t, 1139f, 1139–
    1140, 1140f

REM rebound, 1154

Renal biopsy, 399–400

Renal buffering, acid-base balance and, 854–855, 856t

Renal calculi, immobility and, 712–713

Renal dialysis, 1082–1083

Renal failure, fluid and electrolyte and acid-base
    imbalances and, 859

Reorganization
  development and, 198–199
  grief and, 1314

Repetition, patient teaching and, 418

Report(s), 165, 167–169
  care plan conferences and, 168
  change-of-shift, 165, 167
  nursing rounds and, 167
  from other departments, 168
  patient transfers and, 167
  to physicians, 167–168, 168f
  telephone, 167

Reporting, definition of, 149

Reproduction. *See also* Sexual function; Sexuality–
    reproductive health pattern
  as family function, 1290

Reproductive system
  female, 1362, 1363f
  male, 1362, 1363f

Rescue feelings, 288

Rescuing, 180, 180f, 181t

Research. *See also* Nursing research
  definition of, 71
  as purpose of patient record, 150

Research design, 73–74, 74f

Reservoir mask, 774t, 775

Residual urine, 1079

Res ipsa loquitur doctrine, 51

Resistance
  general adaptation syndrome and, 1338–1339
  to infection, nosocomial infections and, 432–433
  vascular, blood pressure and, 364

Resolution phase, of sexual response, 1367, 1367t, 1368

Resonance, 305, 305t, 1266–1267

Resources. *See also* Community resources; Support
  home maintenance management and, 615, 628

Respect, home maintenance management and, 630

Respirations, 361–364, 363t, 751. *See also* Breathing;
    Lungs; Respiratory function
  altered cardiovascular function and, 815
  apneustic, 363
  assessment of, 362–364, 365
  Biot's, 363, 363t
  Cheyne-Stokes, 363, 363t
  depth of, fluid and electrolyte imbalance and, 860
  factors affecting, 361–362
  quality of, 363–364
  rate of, 363
    measurement of, 364, 365
  rhythm and depth of, 363, 363t

Respiratory acidosis, 858

Respiratory alkalosis, 858

Respiratory buffering, acid-base balance and, 854

Respiratory cycle, blood pressure and, 370

Respiratory disease, manifestations of, 1002

Respiratory failure, fluid and electrolyte and acid-base
    imbalances and, 859

Respiratory function, 746–797. *See also* Lungs; Respiratory
    system
  altered, 753–759
    activities of daily living and, 758–759
    manifestations of, 755–758
    potential for, 753–755
  assessment of, 310–314, 759–764
    anatomic landmarks of chest and lungs and, 310f–311f,
      310–312
    objective data and, 761–764
    subjective data and, 759–761
  evaluation and, 795–797
  factors affecting, 751–752
  interventions and, 765–795
    for altered respiratory function, 772–788
    discharge planning and home care and, 788–795
    to promote health and respiratory function, 765–772
  lifespan considerations and, 752–753
  normal breathing pattern and, 751, 752t
  normal respiratory system function and, 749–751
  nursing diagnoses and patient goals and, 764–765
  respiratory system anatomy and, 748f, 748–749

Respiratory isolation, 451

Respiratory maintenance, postoperative, 494

Respiratory rate

fluid and electrolyte imbalance and, 860
infections and, 999
pain and, 1169
Respiratory system. *See also* Breathing; Lungs; Respirations; *headings beginning with term* Respiratory
defenses of, 751
infections of, 995–996, 997
stress and, 1347
Respite care, 633
cognitive function and, 1235
Respondeat superior doctrine, 51, 54
Responsible sex, 1381
Rest, 1137, 1153. *See also* Sleep–rest health pattern
cognitive function and, 1216, 1219
coping and adaptation and, 1342
immobility and, 713
infections and, 1009
need for, 187
postoperative, 495
rest, safety dysfunction and, 575
Restatement, 284t, 285
Restoril (temazepam), 1155t
Restraints, fall prevention and, 283f, 582–583
Restrictive diets, 921, 921t
Restrictive lung diseases, 754
Reticular activating system (RAS)
cognitive function and, 1214
sensory perception and, 1192, 1194
sleep and, 1141
Retinol (vitamin A), normal physiologic function of, 894, 895t, 896
Retirement communities, 31
Return demonstration, 410
evaluation of learning with, 420
Reverse isolation, 452
Review of systems. *See* Body systems model
Rh factor, 881
Rhonchi, 762
Riboflavin (vitamin B$_2$), normal physiologic function of, 895t, 897
Richards, Linda, 9
Rickets, 898
Rights
medication administration and, 521–523
of patient, medication administration and, 510–511
Patient's Bill of Rights and, 48, 53
of subjects, research and, 76–77
Ringworm, 665t, 940
Risk(s)
bowel function and, 1102
cardiopulmonary function and, 818
cardiovascular function and, 812–813
cognitive function and, 1225
communication and, 1275, 1275f
coping and adaptation and, 1346
for falls, assessment of, 716
family function and, 1297–1298
fluid and electrolyte and acid–base balance and, 861–862
grieving and, 1320–1321
health maintenance and, 601–602
home maintenance management and, 620–621
identification of, safety assessment and, 576–577

infections and, 1001
mobility and, 715
nutrition and, 912–913
pain and, 1171–1172
respiratory function and, 759–760
self-care and, 649
self-concept and, 1252
sensory perception and, 1197
sexual function and, 1374–1376
skin and, 951–952
sleep and rest and, 1150
of suctioning, 781, 786–787
thermoregulation and, 1029
of tracheostomy, 785
urinary elimination and, 1054–1055
Risk factors
for nosocomial infections, 432f, 432–433
in nursing diagnosis, 118
Roentgenogram. *See* Radiography
Rogers, Martha E., 14t–15t
perception of human needs, 190
Role(s). *See also* Roles–relationships health pattern
coping and adaptation and, 1341
gender, 1366
health maintenance and, 598
home maintenance management and, 616
immobility and, 713
performance of, 1244
sexuality and, 1368
Role conflict, ethical dilemmas and, 45
Role models, as source of values, 259–260
Role-playing, patient teaching and, 419
Roles–relationships health pattern, 90, 107
assessing human needs and, 193
assessment of, 339–340
objective data in, 340
subjective data in, 339–340
in community, 232
disruption by diagnostic procedures, 394t
exercise and immobility and, 708t
health maintenance and, 597t
health problems and anticipatory guidance and, 215–216, 216f
surgery and, 471–472
values and, 264, 265f
Role strain, family function and, 1295
Role transition, self-concept and, 1250
Roller board, 739t
ROM. *See* Range of motion
Roman Catholics, religious practices of, 1405t
Rooting reflex, 333
Rosenberg's Self-Esteem Scale, 339
Rotation
external, 701, 704t
internal, 701, 704t
Rotorest bed, 682
Roy, Sister Callista, 14t–15t
perception of human needs, 190
Rubella, 988t
Rubeola, 988t
Rubor, ischemia and, 815
Rumbles, 762
Rural health centers, 32, 32f

S

Safety, 562–590
  altered safety function and, 569–576
    activities of daily living and, 575–576
    identification of dysfunction and, 577
    interventions for, 586–587
    manifestations of, 572–575
    potential for, 569–572
  altered sensory function and, 1203, 1204
  assessment of, 576–578
    objective data and, 577–578
    subjective data and, 576–577
  characteristics of, 564, 564f
  cognitive function and, 1232–1233
  coping and adaptation and, 1342
  disregard for, 572
  evaluation and, 589–590
  factors affecting, 565–567
  heat and cold applications and, 971–972, 972t
  home maintenance management and, 615, 619
  interventions and, 579–588
    for altered safety function, 586–587
    discharge planning and home care and, 587–588,
      588f
    to promote health and safety function, 579–586
  intraoperative, 486–487
  lifespan considerations and, 567–569
  medication administration and, 519–523
  normal functional pattern and, 564–565
  nursing diagnoses and patient goals and, 578–579
  oxygen therapy and, 778–780
Safety belts, for ambulation, 727, 732f, 739t
Safety needs, 187–188, 224
Salmonella, 991t
SAM (self-administered medications), 503
Sanguineous drainage, 953
Sanitation, safety in, 567
Scales, skin and, 947t
Scar, 946t
Scarlet fever, 988t
Scheduled care, self-care deficits and, 654, 655
Scheduled drugs, 508–509, 509t
Schedule of Recent Experiences, 1338
School(s), infection hazards in, 433
School-age child. *See also* Child
  cardiovascular function and, 809
  communication and, 1270
  development of, 203t, 206–207
  functional health assessment of, 345
    auscultating heart sounds in, 319–320
    auscultation of bowel sounds in, 326
    auscultation of breath sounds in, 316
  functional health patterns and, health problems and
      anticipatory guidance and, 210–218
  health maintenance and, 603t
  infection control and, 457, 460
  mobility and, 705
  self-concept and, 1256
  values and, 266–267
Scientific knowledge, required for effective use of nursing
      process, 89
Scientific process, nursing research and, 73, 73t
Scientific rationale, for interventions, 133

Scrotum, 1362
Scultetus binder, 966, 966f
Scurvy, 897
Sebaceous glands, 937
Secondary prevention, 596t
Secondary sources, 102–103
Secretion (process), urine formation and, 1045
Secretions
  disposal of, infection control and, 1012
  of lung, immobility and, 710–711
  nasopharyngeal, suctioning, 782–785
  nasotracheal, suctioning, 786–787
  oropharyngeal, suctioning, 782–785
Security
  coping and adaptation and, 1342
  sleep and, 1152
Selenium, normal physiologic function of, 898t
Self, 1242
  comfortable sense of, 281
  sense of, 1255
  social, 1243
  use of, spiritual function and, 1402–1403, 1403f
Self-actualization needs, 188, 224
Self-administered medications (SAM), 503
Self-awareness
  holistic health care and, 177
  sexual function and, 1378–1379
Self-care, 640–691
  altered, 646–648
    manifestations of, 648
    potential for, 647–648
  assessment of, 308–310, 648–651
    objective data and, 650–651, 651t
    subjective data and, 648–650
  characteristics of, 642–644
  discharge planning and home care and, 682, 685,
      688–689
  evaluation and, 689–690
  factors affecting, 644–645
  functional patterns and, 644
  interventions and, 653–689
    for altered self-care, 653–682
    to promote health and self-care, 653
  levels of, 649t
  lifespan considerations and, 645–646
  nursing diagnoses and patient goals and, 651–653
  postoperative, 493–494
Self-care deficit, self-concept and, 1250, 1251t
Self-Care Deficit, Bathing/Hygiene, 651–652
  interventions for, 654
  nursing management plan for, 690
Self-Care Deficit, Dressing/Grooming, 652
  interventions for, 654
Self-Care Deficit, Feeding, 653
  interventions for, 654
Self-Care Deficit, Toileting, 652–653
  interventions for, 654
Self-concept, 1240–1260. *See also* Self-perception–
      self-concept health pattern
  activities of daily living and, 1252
  altered, 1245
    manifestations of, 1250–1252, 1251t
    potential for, 1249–1250

assessment and, 1252–1253
characteristics of, 1242–1243
communication and, 1269
development of, 1255t, 1255–1256
evaluation and, 1258
factors affecting, 1244–1245
immobility and, 713
interventions and, 1254–1258
   for altered self-concept, 1256–1257
   discharge planning and home care and, 1257–1258
   to promote health and function, 1254–1256
lifespan considerations and, 1245–1249, 1246t–1249t
mobility and, 704
normal functional patterns of, 1243–1252
nursing diagnoses and patient goals and, 1253–1254
safety dysfunction and, 575–576
sexuality and, 1369
Self-destructive behavior, self-concept and, 1251t, 1252
Self-esteem, 1243f, 1243–1244
   respiratory function and, 795
Self-Esteem Disturbance, 1253
Self-evaluation, 1243, 1256–1257
Self-examination
   sexual function and, 1379–1381
   techniques for, 607
Self-expectation, 1242
Self-knowledge, 1242
Self-perception. *See also* Self-perception–self-concept
      health pattern
   immobility and, 713
Self-perception–self-concept health pattern, 90, 107
   assessing human needs and, 193
   assessment of, 337, 339
      objective data in, 339
      subjective data in, 339
   in community, 232
   disruption by diagnostic procedures, 394t
   exercise and immobility and, 708t
   in family, 228
   health maintenance and, 597t
   health problems and anticipatory guidance and, 215
   laboratory and diagnostic tests related to, 386t
   surgery and, 471
   values and, 264
Self-responsibility, holistic health care and, 177
Self-worth, holistic health care and, 177–178
Semi-Fowler's position, 721t
Seminal vesicles, 1362
Semipermeable dressings, 958, 959t
Semiprone position, 722
Senile lentigines, 939
Sensation information, sensory perception and, 1200–1201
Sensitivity, patient teaching and, 416–417
Sensitivity testing, 392–393
   infections and, 1003–1004
   urine, 1062
Sensoristasis, 1192
Sensorium. *See* Cognition; Cognitive function
Sensory abilities. *See also* Sensory deficits; Sensory perception
   patient teaching and, 415
   safety and, 565
Sensory aids, 334, 1203, 1204
Sensory aphasia, 1272, 1272t

Sensory assessment, 330–332, 333–336
Sensory deficits, 1196
   coping and adaptation and, 1344
   home maintenance management and, 619
   preparing patient for diagnostic and laboratory tests and, 381
   surgery and, 471
Sensory deprivation, 1194–1196
Sensory overload, 1194, 1194f, 1195f
Sensory perception, 1190–1207
   abnormal, fluid and electrolyte and acid-base imbalances and, 861
   altered, 1193–1197
      activities of daily living and, 1196–1197
      manifestations of, 1196
      potential for, 1193–1196
   assessment and, 1197–1199
      objective data and, 1198–1199
      subjective data and, 1197–1198
   characteristics of, 1192
   evaluation and, 1206–1207
   factors affecting, 1192–1193
   interventions and, 1200–1206
      for altered sensory function, 1201–1203
      discharge planning and home care and, 1203, 1206
      to promote health and function, 1200–1201
   lifespan considerations and, 1193
   normal function of, 1191–1193
   nursing diagnoses and patient goals and, 1199–1200
   self-care and, 645, 647
Sensory/Perceptual Alterations, 1199
Separation
   family function and, 1295
   spiritual function and, 1396
Sepsis, 428
Septicemia, 428, 994
Septic reactions, to blood transfusion, 884
Serology tests, infections and, 1004–1005
Serosanguineous drainage, 953
Serous drainage, 953
Serum albumin, nutrition and, 914
Serum chemistries, reference ranges for, 1418–1431
Serum creatinine, 1062–1063
Serum drug levels, 392
Serum electrolytes
   cardiopulmonary function and, 821
   fluid and electrolyte imbalance and, 866
Serum enzymes, 391–392
Serum osmolality, fluid and electrolyte imbalance and, 866
Serum transferrin, nutrition and, 914
Settings. *See also* Health-care setting
   in health-care delivery system, 29–33, 30f–32f
   for nursing assessment, 97
   for nursing practice, 16–17, 17f
   for surgical intervention, 466
Seventh Day Adventists, religious practices of, 1406t
Sex. *See also* Sexuality–reproductive health pattern
   cardiovascular function and, 808
   drug action and, 514
   need for, 187
   nutrition and, 907
   respirations and, 362
   spiritual function and, 1394

Sex education, 1381
Sexual abuse, 1372
Sexual desire, inhibited, 1372
Sexual Dysfunction, 1377–1378
  nursing management plan for, 1385
Sexual expression, 1364
Sexual function, 1360–1386. *See also* Sexuality–
    reproductive health pattern
  altered, 1371–1373
    activities of daily living and, 1373
    manifestations of, 1372–1373
    potential for, 1371–1372
  anatomy and, 1362
    female, 1362, 1363f
    male, 1362, 1363f
  assessment and, 1374–1377, 1375t
    objective data and, 1376–1377
    subjective data and, 1374–1376
  characteristics of, 1366–1368
  evaluation and, 1384–1385
  factors affecting, 1368–1369
  interventions, 1378–1384
    for altered function, 1383
    discharge planning and home care and, 1383–1384
    to promote health and function, 1378–1383
  lifespan considerations and, 1369–1371
  normal, 1362, 1364–1366
  normal functional health pattern and, 1368
  nursing diagnoses and patient goals and, 1377–1378
Sexual intimacy, as family function, 1289
Sexuality, 1362. *See also* Sexual function; Sexuality–
    reproductive health pattern
  immobility and, 713–714
Sexuality–reproductive health pattern, 90, 107
  assessing human needs and, 193
  assessment of, 341–343
    objective data in, 342–343
    subjective data in, 341–342
  in community, 232
  disruption by diagnostic procedures, 394t
  drugs promoting normal function and, 501t
  exercise and immobility and, 708t
  in family, 228
  health maintenance and, 597t
  health problems and anticipatory guidance and, 216
  laboratory and diagnostic tests related to, 386t
  surgery and, 472, 472t
  values and, 265
Sexually transmitted diseases (STDs), 989t–990t, 1381
Sexual orientation, 1366
Sexual response, 1366–1368, 1367t
  female, 1367–1368
  male, 1366–1367
Shampooing, 663, 668–669
Shaving, 665, 665f, 667
Shearing force, decubitus ulcers and, 943, 943f
Shift work, sleep and, 1147
Shigella, 991t
Shivering, body temperature and, 1022–1023
Shock, grief and, 1313t, 1313–1314
Shoe coverings, infection control and, 445
Shortness of breath, altered respiratory function and, 757
Short-term goals, 128

Shower, assisting with, 661
Side effects, 512–514
  allergic reactions and, 513–514
  cumulative, 513
  hypersensitivity reactions and, 513
  idiosyncratic, 513
  interactions and, 514, 514f
  secondary reactions and, 513
  tolerance and, 513
  toxicity and, 513
Side-lying position, 721t
  positioning patient in, 724–725
Siderail, 726t
Sighs, 364
Sign(s). *See* Objective data
Signature, on drug order, 504
Silence, communication and, 284t, 286
Simple oxygen mask, 774, 774t, 776–777
Sims' position, 722
Simulation, patient teaching and, 419–420
Single-parent families, 1288, 1289f
Sitz baths, 656t, 974
Skills
  communication, developing, 286, 287t
  hierarchy of, 265
Skin, 934–979
  altered, altered nutrition and, 912
  altered function of, 939–951
    activities of daily living and, 950–951
    manifestations of, 944–945
    potential for, 939–943
    wound healing and, 945–950
  anatomy of, 936–937
  assessment and, 951–953
    objective data and, 952–953
    subjective data and, 951–952
  assessment of, 327
  body temperature and, 1022, 1025
  breaks in, infection and, 996
  characteristics of, 937–938
  color, temperature, and character of
    biocultural variation in, 246–247
    ischemia and, 815
  edema and, 327
  evaluation and, 976, 978
  factors affecting, 938
  intact, infections and, 1009
  interventions and, 954–976
    for altered function, 957t, 957–976
    discharge planning and home care and, 976
    to promote health and integumentary function, 955–956
  lesions of, 327
  lifespan considerations and, 938–939
  medications applied to, 528–529
  normal functional pattern of, 938
  normal physiologic function of, 937
  nursing diagnoses and patient goals and, 954
  preventing dryness of, 660
  resistance to infection and, 985–986
  temperature and color of, cardiovascular function and, 807
  turgor of, 327

Skin care, 662–664
Skinfold measurements, nutrition and, 914
Skin preparation, for surgery, 480, 481f
    surgical asepsis and, 454, 456
Skin puncture, blood glucose measurement by, 389–390
Skin tags, 939
Skin tests, respiratory assessment and, 764
Slander, 49
Sleep, 1136–1155. *See also* Sleep–rest health pattern
    altered, 1145–1150
        activities of daily living and, 1150
        manifestations of, 1148–1150
        potential for, 1145–1148
    assessment and, 1150–1151
        objective data and, 1151
        subjective data and, 1150
    characteristics of, 1142
    cognitive function and, 1216, 1219
    coping and adaptation and, 1342
    electrophysiological approach to, 1138t, 1138–1140
    evaluation and, 1154–1155
    factors affecting, 1143–1144
    immobility and, 713
    interventions and, 1151–1154
        altered function and, 1153–1154
        discharge planning and home care and, 1154
        to promote health and function, 1151–1153
    lifespan considerations and, 1144–1145
    need for, 187
    normal functional pattern of, 1142–1143
    normal sleep/rest function and, 1137–1145
    nursing diagnoses and patient goals and, 1151
    rhythm of, 1140, 1141f
    safety dysfunction and, 575
Sleep apnea, 1149
Sleep deprivation, 1143
Sleepiness, 1142
Sleep latency, 1143
Sleep Pattern Disturbance, 1151
    nursing management plan and, 1156
Sleep–rest health pattern, 90, 107
    assessing human needs and, 192–193
    assessment of, 328
    in community, 232
    disruption by diagnostic procedures, 394t
    drugs promoting normal function and, 501t
    exercise and immobility and, 708t
    in family, 228
    health maintenance and, 597t
    health problems and anticipatory guidance and,
        maintenance and, 597t
    health problems and anticipatory guidance and, 214–215
    laboratory and diagnostic tests related to, 386t
    surgery and, 470
    values and, 263
Sleep rituals, 1152–1153
Sleep-wake cycle, 1142
    altered, 1149
Sleepwalking, 1149
Sling, 966
Small intestine, anatomy of, 892
Smell sense, observation and, 98
SMI. *See* Supplemental medical insurance

Smoking
    body temperature measurement and, 351
    cardiovascular function and, 812
    respiratory function and, 754–755
    sleep and, 1147
    wound healing and, 949
Soaks, 656t
SOAP note, 160f, 161
Social isolation, family function and, 1294, 1294f
Socialization
    as family function, 1290, 1290f
    to professional nursing, 10, 10t
        professional values and, 257
Socialization therapies, cognitive function and, 1234
Social Readjustment Scale, 340, 341t, 1338
Social Security Act
    amendments to (1965), 29
    amendments to (1983), 34–35
Social self, 1243
Social support. *See* Support, social
Social workers, 36
Sociocultural resources, grieving and, 1315–1316, 1316f
Sociocultural stress, 1346
Sodium, 847
    dietary sources of, 869t
    imbalance of, 855–856
    normal physiologic function of, 898t, 899
Soft diet, 920
Somnambulism, 1149
Source, in communication process, 275
Source-oriented record, 154t, 154–155
Spastic gait, 707
Special damages, 51
Specialized inpatient services, 31–32
Specific gravity, of urine, 1060, 1061
    fluid and electrolyte imbalance and, 866
Specificity, of infectious agents, 429
Specificity theory of pain, 1164
Specimen collection, following diagnostic and laboratory
        tests, 385
Speech, loss of, 1273, 1273f
Speech apparatus, impaired, 1270
Sphygmomanometer, 366, 369f
Spinal cord, pain and, 1163
Spinal reflexes, pain and, 1163–1164
Spiral reverse turns, 965, 965f
Spiral turns, 964, 965f
Spiritual care, inadequate or inappropriate,
        1396–1397
Spiritual dimension, 1391. *See also* Spiritual function
Spiritual Distress, 1401–1402
    nursing management plan for, 1409
Spiritual function, 1390–1410
    altered, 1396–1397
        activities of daily living and, 1397
        manifestations of, 1397, 1398t–1399t
        potential for, 1396–1397
    assessment and, 1399–1401
        objective data and, 1401
        subjective data and, 1399–1401
    characteristics of, 1392–1393
    evaluation and, 1409–1410
    factors affecting, 1394

Spiritual function (*continued*)
  interventions, 1402–1409
    for altered function, 1404–1408
      discharge planning and home care and, 1408–1409
      to promote health and function, 1402–1409
  lifespan considerations and, 1394–1396, 1395t
  normal functional pattern of, 1393f, 1393–1394
  nursing diagnoses and patient goals and, 1401–1402
Spirituality, 1392. *See also* Spiritual function
Spiritual need, 1392
Spiritual practices, support of, 1403–1404, 1405t–1407
Spiritual quest, 1392–1393
  spiritual care and, 1397
Spiritual well-being, 1393
Spirometry, incentive, 767, 769, 770f, 771
Sputum
  assessment of, 762
  production of, altered respiratory function and, 757
Sputum cultures, 393
  infections and, 1004
  respiratory assessment and, 763
Stacked cough, 770
Staff nurse, role of, 63–66
Stairs
  climbing, 735
  descending, 735
Standardized care plans, 131
Standards of care, 48
  informed consent and, 48
  knowledge of, as evaluation skill, 140
  Patient's Bill of Rights and, 48
Standards of practice, 20, 21
Standing order, 504
Staples, 960, 960f
  wound closure and, 489
Stasis dermatitis, 941
Stat order, 505
STDs (sexually transmitted diseases), 989t–990t, 1381
Steam sterilization, 443–444
Stenosis, valvular, 810
Stereotypes, 243
Sterile technique, infection control and, 1011
Sterilization (of equipment), 443–444
  effectiveness of, 445
  levels of, 444–445
Sterilization, surgical, 1383
Steristrips, 960
Stethoscope, 306f, 306–307, 307t
  blood pressure assessment and, 366
  pulse measurement and, 358
Stimulation
  providing, altered sensory function and, 1201–1202
  reducing, altered sensory function and, 1202–1203
Stimuli
  organization of, cognitive function and, 1216–1217, 1219–1220
  sleep and, 1143–1144, 1151–1152
Stockings, antiembolic, prevention of venous return and, 826–827, 828–829
Stock supply, of medications, 503
Stoma, 1098, 1124–1125
  assessment of, 1124
  irrigation of, 1125, 1127–1128
  postoperative necrosis of, 1126

Stomach, anatomy of, 892
Stool cultures, 1106
  infections and, 1004
Stool softeners, 1113t
Stool specimens
  collecting, 1105
  collection from stoma, 1124–1125, 1125f, 1126–1127
Strengths
  of family, reinforcing, 1301, 1301f
  identification of, self-concept and, 1254f, 1254–1255
Stress, 1334–1356. *See also* Coping; Adaptation; Coping–stress tolerance health pattern
  body temperature and, 350–351, 1025
  bowel function and, 1100
  cardiovascular function and, 808, 813
  cognitive function and, 1220, 1220f
  environmental, 1346
  evaluation and, 1354, 1356
  in family, altered home maintenance management and, 620
  family function and, 1291
  fluid and electrolyte imbalance and, 859
  grieving and, 1315–1316, 1316f
  health maintenance and, 598
  holistic health care and, 179
  home maintenance management and, 616
  illnesses related to, 575
  immobility and, 713
  infections and, 998
  normal function of, 1336–1337
  physiologic, 1346
  psychological, 1346
  respirations and, 362
  respiratory function and, 755
  as response, 1338–1340, 1339f
  safety and, 566
  self-concept and, 1249
  sexuality and, 1369
  sociocultural, 1346
  as stimulus, 1338
  urinary elimination and, 1047
  wound healing and, 949
Stress assessment tools, 340, 341t
Stress Incontinence, 1064
Stress incontinence, 1053, 1064
Stress management, for nurses, 1349–1350
Stressors, 1338
  reduction of, 1350
Stress tolerance, self-concept and, 1244–1245
Stretcher, transferring patient to, 736–737
Strict isolation, 451, 452
Stridor, 364
Stroke. *See* Cerebrovascular accident
Structured teaching sessions, 417
Structure evaluation, 141
Stryker frame, 682
Stump bandaging, 965, 965f
Subculture, 242–243, 243f
Subcutaneous injections, 534, 537, 537f, 538–541
Subcutaneous layer, 936, 936f
Subjective data, 102, 102t
  interview and, 297, 303
Subject rights, research and, 76–77
Sublingual medication administration, 528, 528f

Substance abuse, 511
  family function and, 1294
Substantia gelatinosa, 1163
Sucking reflex, 333
Suctioning, 781, 782–787
  of nasotracheal secretions, 786–787
  of oropharyngeal and nasopharyngeal areas, 782–785
Suffocation, 573
Sugar, in diet, 902, 904
Sullivan, Harry Stack, self-concept development theory of, 1246t, 1247t
Summarizing, communication and, 284t, 286
Sundown syndrome, 1222–1223
Superego, 200
Supervisory nursing interventions, 137
Supination, 701, 704t
Supine position, 721t
Supplemental medical insurance (SMI), 33, 34
Supplies, for diagnostic and laboratory tests, 382–383
Support. *See also* Community resources
  emotional
      intraoperative, 486
    skin conditions and, 974–975
  family, cognitive function and, 1234
  family and, 1290, 1301–1302
  home maintenance management and, 615
  social, home maintenance management and, 616, 619–620, 621
  spiritual, 1403, 1404, 1404f, 1406
  of spiritual practices, 1403–1404, 1405t–1407
Support groups, grieving and, 1324
Supportive nursing interventions, 138
Suppositories, 1112, 1113t
Suppuration, 971
Surface temperature, 1018
Surgery, 466–474. *See also* Anesthesia; Intraoperative nursing; Perioperative nursing; Postoperative nursing; Preoperative nursing
  altered nutrition and, 911
  bowel function and, 1097
  classification of, 466, 467t
  elective, 466
  emergent, 466
  fluid and electrolyte imbalance, 859
  functional health and, 468–472
  lifespan considerations and, 473–474
  self-care and, 647
  self-concept and, 1250
  sexual function and, 1376
  sexuality and, 1372
  surgical facilities and, 466
  urgent, 466
  urinary elimination and, 1050
Surgical asepsis, 439, 453–457, 489, 489f
  handwashing and, 456–457
  principles of, 454, 455t
  skin preparation and, 454, 456
  sterile gloves and, 457, 458–460
Surgical recovery unit, interventions in, 493–495
Surveillance nursing interventions, 139
Sustained fever, 1026, 1027t
Sutures, 489, 960, 960f
Swab culture, 393
Swallowing, 900
  impairment of, altered nutrition and, 909
  nutrition and, 914
Swallowing ability, assessing before medication administration, 517
Sweat glands, 937
  body temperature and, 1023
Swinging-to gait, 735
Swing-through gait, 731–732, 735
Symbiotic relationship, 982
Sympathetic nervous system
  heat production and, 1019
  stimulation of, stress and, 340
Symptoms. *See also* Subjective data
Sympto-thermal method, 1382
Syphilis, 989t
Syringes, for parenteral medications, 531–533, 532f, 533f
Systems theory, 87, 87f
  family and, 226, 227f, 228
Systole, 803
Systolic blood pressure, 364

T
Tachycardia, 358
Tachypnea, 363, 363t
Tangential lighting, 304
Tape, to secure dressings, 958–959
Tartar, 643
Tax Equity and Fiscal Responsibility Act of 1982 (TEFRA), 34
Taxonomy, 112–113
  nursing diagnosis, 113–116, 114t
T-binder, 966
Teaching. *See also* Patient teaching
  methods of, 418–419
  strategies for, 419–420, 420f
Teaching roles, 67–68
Team leader, 64, 66
Team nursing, 63–64, 65, 66
Technical skills, for implementation, 135
Technicians, 35
Technologic advances, 28–29
Technologists, 35
Teeth, care of, 643, 643f
TEFRA. *See* Tax Equity and Fiscal Responsibility Act of 1982
Teleology, 43
Telephone drug orders, 505
Telephone reports, 167
Telfa dressings, 958
Temazepam (Restoril), 1155t
Temperature
  body. *See* Body temperature
  of skin, 937
  sleep and, 1145
Temperature family planning method, 1382
Temperature-sensitive strips, 353
TENS (transcutaneous electrical nerve stimulation), 1179
Tepid baths, fever and, 1033
Terminal values, 256
Termination, of nurse-patient relationship, 277
Terminology. *See* Medical terminology
Tertiary prevention, 596t
Testability, of research, 75
Testing, patient teaching and, 419, 420

Tetanus, 991t
Texas catheter, 678, 1069, 1070–1071
Theory, 12–13, 14t–15t
  of cognitive development, 102, 199, 200t
  evelopmental task, 102, 199, 200t
  of human needs, of Maslow, 185–188, 186f, 199, 200t,
      201, 224
  information-processing, 88–89, 89f
  of moral development, 199, 200t, 201
  nursing. *See* Nursing theory
  of pain
    endogenous opiates, 1164–1165
    gate control, 1164f, 1164–1165
    pattern, 1164
    specificity, 1164
  practice related to, 13
  psychodynamic
    of Erikson, 100t, 199, 200, 1246t, 1247t
    of Freud, 100t, 199, 200, 1246t, 1247t
  research and, 74–75
  single versus multiple, 12
  systems, 87, 87f
    family and, 226, 227f, 228
  of value development, 267
Therapeutic baths, 655, 656t
Therapeutic communication, 272–291, 274f
  assessment and, 281–283
  cognitive function and, 1233
  comfortable sense of self and, 281
  communication process and, 274f, 274–276
  empathy and, 280, 280f, 280t
  intervention and, 283–290, 284t
    active listening and, 284–285, 285f
    developing communication skills and, 286, 287t
    exploring and, 285–286
    helping patient get started and, 283–284, 284t
    nontherapeutic responses and, 287–289
    special situations and, 289–290
  nurse-patient relationship and, 277t, 277–279
  nursing process and, 281–291
  positive regard and, 280–281
Therapeutic drug monitoring, infections and, 1005
Therapeutic modalities, mobility and, 706
Therapeutic regimen, nosocomial infections and, 432–433
Therapeutic relationship
  nursing as, 180, 180f, 181t
  self-concept and, 1256
Therapeutic touch, in holistic health care, 181–182
Therapists, 35
Thermal burns, 943
Thermometers, 352–353
  electronic, 353, 353f
  glass mercury, 352, 352f, 353f
  paper, disposable, 353, 354f
  scales of, 353, 354f
Thermoreceptors, 1162
Thermoregulation, 1016–1036. *See also* Body temperature;
      Fever
  altered, 1024–1028
    activities of daily living and, 1028
    manifestations of, 1026–1028
    potential for, 1024–1025
  assessment and, 1028–1030

  objective data and, 1029–1030
    subjective data and, 1028–1029
  evaluation and, 1035–1036
  heat loss and, 1020f, 1020–1021
  heat production and, 1018–1019
  interventions and, 1031–1035
    for altered thermoregulation, 1032–1034
    discharge planning and home care and, 1034–1035
    to promote health, 1031–1032
  lifespan considerations and, 1023–1024
  need for, 187
  nursing diagnoses and patient goals and, 1020–1031
  safety in, 567
  skin and, 937
  surgery and, 469
Thiamine (vitamin B₁), normal physiologic function of,
      895t, 897
Third-party reimbursement, 33
Thoracentesis, 401, 401f
Thought, 1214, 1215–1216. *See also* Cognition; Cognitive
      function
  assessment of, 1224
  disorganized, 1221–1222
  impaired thought processes and, 1222–1223
Three-point gait, 731, 734
Thrills, cardiovascular assessment and, 318
Throat cultures, infections and, 1004
Thrombocytopenia, 390
Thrombocytosis, 390
Thrombus formation
  altered cardiovascular function and, 816
  immobility and, 710
Throughput, in systems theory, 87, 87f
Thyroid hormones, heat production and, 1019
TIA (transient ischemic attack), 816
Tidal volume, 361
Timed voiding, 1069
Time-lapsed assessment, 96t, 97
Timeliness, of charting, 153–154
Time of administration, drug action and, 514–515
Time of day, body temperature and, 350
Time strip, intravenous infusions and, 874, 875f
Tinea pedis, 665t
Tissue perfusion, 805–806
T-lymphocytes, 983t
Tocopherol (vitamin E), normal physiologic function of,
      895t, 896
Toddler
  body temperature and, 1023
  bowel function and, 1095
  cardiovascular function and, 809
  cognitive function and, 1217, 1218f
  cold packs and, 973
  communication and, 1270
  coping and adaptation and, 1342
  development of, 202t, 205–206
  diagnostic and laboratory testing and, 404
  family and, 1291
  feeding, 919
  fluid and electrolyte balance and, 853
  functional health assessment of, 345, 345f
    auscultating heart sounds in, 319
    auscultation of bowel sounds in, 326

auscultation of breath sounds in, 316
neurologic assessment in, 333
functional health patterns and, health problems and
anticipatory guidance and, 210–218
grieving and, 1316, 1317t
health maintenance and, 598
home maintenance management and, 617, 617f
infection control and, 457
medications and, 555
mobility and, 705
needs of, 189
nutrition and, 907–908
pain and, 1167
patient teaching and, 421, 421f
resistance to infection and, 986–987
respiratory function and, 753
safety and, 567–568
self-care and, 645–646
self-concept and, 1246t, 1247, 1255–1256
sensory perception and, 1193
sexuality and, 1369
skin and, 939
sleep and, 1144–1145
spiritual function and, 1395, 1407
surgery and, 473
urinary elimination and, 1047
values and, 266
vital signs in, 375
Toes. *See* Digits
Toilet, 1067
Toileting, 643
assisting with, 678, 679–680
Tolerance
to medications, 513
to narcotic analgesics, 1183
Tonic neck reflex, 333
Toothbrushing, 669f, 669–672
Topical medications. *See* Medication administration,
topical
Torts, 48–51
crimes versus, 50t
intentional, 49–50
unintentional, 50–51
Total body water, 846, 847t
Total Incontinence, 1065
Total incontinence, 1053, 1065
Total parenteral nutrition (TPN), 923–939
bolus or intermittent, 925
changing tubing and dressing and, 927
complications of, 929
continuous, 925
cycling infusions and versus, 929
indications for, 923
intralipids and, 927–928
solutions for, 923, 929, 929f
venous access for, 923, 928f
Touch
observation and, 98–99
therapeutic, 181–182
Toxicity, of medications, 513
Toxins. *See* Poisoning
Toxoids, 986
TPN. *See* Total parenteral nutrition

Trachea, 313, 313f
Tracheostomy, 781, 785, 787–788
care of, 787–788, 789–792
communication and, 1273, 1273f, 1280
Tracheotomy, 1273
Trade name, of drugs, 500
Transcutaneous electrical nerve stimulation (TENS), 1179
Transdermal medications, 529, 529f
Transfer(s), 732, 735, 736–739, 739t
equipment to assist, 739t
to stretcher, 736–737
to wheelchair, 737–739
Transfer belt, 739t
Transfer belts, 727, 732f
Transfer board, 739t
Transfer sled, 739t
Transient ischemic attack (TIA), 816
Transitions, discharge planning and, 625–626
Transsexual, 1366
Trapeze bar, 726t
Trauma. *See also* Accidents; Injuries
family function and, 1293–1294
to head, communication and, 1271
invasive, risk of, 570
mobility and, 706
self-concept and, 1250
Traveler's diarrhea, 1000, 1100–1101
Treatment, 30
Tremor, 707
Triazolam (Halcion), 1155t
Triceps reflex, assessment of, 338t
Trochanter roll, 725t
Trust, need for, spiritual dysfunction and, 1398t
Tuberculosis isolation, 451
Tumor, of skin, 946t
Turgor, 327
Turning schedules, altered mobility and, 719–720, 720f
Turn sheet, 726t
24-hour urine specimens, 392, 1062
collection of, 1059–1060
Two-point gait, 731, 734
Tympany, percussion and, 305, 305t
Typhoid fever, 991t

U
UA. *See* Urinalysis
Ulcers
decubitus. *See* Pressure sores
of skin, 947t
Ultrasonography, 396–397, 397f
Unconscious patient. *See* Comatose patient
Underweight, altered nutrition and, 912
Unit dose, 503
United States Pharmacopeia (USP), 503
Unit managers, 66–67
Universal precautions, 448–450, 570
Urea, arterial, 1227
Ureterostomy, 1050–1051, 1051f
Ureters, 1042–1043
Urethra, 1043
Urge Incontinence, 1064
nursing management plan for, 1084–1085
Urge incontinence, 1053, 1064, 1084–1085

Urgency, urinary elimination and, 1052
Urgent care centers, 32
Urgent surgery, 466
Urinal, 678, 1067, 1067f
Urinalysis (UA), 0162t, 392, 1060, 1062
  infections and, 1003
Urinary bladder, 1043, 1044f
  bladder training and, 1069
  credé of, 1081
Urinary catheterization, 1069, 1071–1081
  indications for, 1071
  risks of, 1072
Urinary diversion, 1050–1051, 1051f, 1081–1082
Urinary drainage bags, 1077
Urinary elimination, 1040–1086. *See also* Elimination
      health pattern; Urine
  altered, 1048–1054
    activities of daily living and, 1054
    manifestations of, 1051–1054
    potential for, 1048–1051
  assessment and, 1054–1064
    objective data and, 1055–1064
    subjective data and, 1054–1055
  assessment of, 327–328
  evaluation and, 1085–1086
  factors affecting, 1046–1047
  interventions and, 1066–1085
    altered function and, 1068–1083
    discharge planning and home care and, 1083, 1085
    to promote health and urinary function, 1066–1068
  lifespan considerations and, 1047–1048
  normal pattern of, 1046
  normal urinary system function and, 1043, 1045
  nursing diagnoses and patient goals and, 1064–1065
  urinary tract anatomy and, 1042f, 1042–1043
Urinary incontinence, 1053, 1064
Urinary Retention, 1065
Urinary retention, 1052–1053, 1065
  assessment of, 1055–1056
Urinary stasis, immobility and, 712
Urinary tract infection (UTI), 994, 995, 1049
  immobility and, 712
  manifestations of, 1002
  prevention of, 1066
Urination, 1045
Urine
  assessment of, 1055
  characteristics of, 1045–1046
  formation of, 1045
  normal output of, 1047t
  obstruction of flow of, 1048
  output of, cardiovascular function and, 807
  residual, 1079
  specific gravity of, 1060, 1061
    fluid and electrolyte imbalance and, 866
Urine chemistry, reference ranges for, 1431–1435
Urine culture, 393, 1062
Urine osmolality, fluid and electrolyte imbalance and, 866
Urine output
  fluid and electrolyte balance and, 851
  fluid intake and, fluid and electrolyte imbalance and, 860
  monitoring, fluid and electrolyte imbalance and,
      862–864, 864f

Urine specimens, collection of, 392, 1056–1060
  devices for, 1066–1068
Urine testing, 392, 1060–1062
Urine volume monitoring, 1064
Urodynamic studies, 1064, 1064t
Urticaria, 944
USP (*United States Pharmacopeia*), 503
Uterus, 1362
UTI. *See* Urinary tract infection
Utilitariansim, ethics and, 43–44

V
Vaccines, 986
Vagina, 1362
Vaginal medications, 530, 531f
Vaginismus, 1373
Validation, of nursing diagnosis, 120–121, 121f
  problems in, 121
Valsalva maneuver, 709
Value(s), 42, 254–270. *See also* Values–beliefs health
      pattern
  action, 260, 261f
  applied ethics and, 258–259
  assessment of, 269–270
  choice, 260, 261f
  communication and, 1269
  culture and, 241
  definition of, 256
  family function and, 1290–1291
  health maintenance and, 598
  hierarchy of skills and, 262–263, 265
  lifespan considerations and, 266t, 266–267
  major categories of, 256
  manifestations of
    functional health and, 261–265
    nurses' values and, 265–266
  moral, 45, 256
  operative, 256
  pain perception and, 1167
  professional, in nursing, 256–257, 257t
  self-care and, 645
  self-concept and, 1244
  sexuality and, 1369
  sources of, 259–260
  terminal, 256
  value and belief patterns and, 256–259
  vision, 260–261, 261f
Value conflicts, 267–269
  resolving, 268–269
Value development theory, 267
Values–beliefs health pattern, 90
  assessing human needs and, 193
  assessment of, 343
  in community, 232
  disruption by diagnostic procedures, 394t
  in family, 228
  health maintenance and, 597t
  health problems and anticipatory guidance and, 218–219
  laboratory and diagnostic tests related to, 386t
  surgery and, 472
  values and, 265
Values clarification, 257–258, 258f
  patient teaching and, 419

Values inquiry, 258, 259f
Value system, 256
Valuing pattern, nursing diagnosis and, 114
Valves, cardiac, 802
    dysfunction of, 810
Variables, dependent and independent, 75
Vastus lateralis site, for intramuscular injections, 542, 545, 546f
VDRL (Venereal Disease Research Laboratories) test, 1377t
Vectorborne transmission, 430, 430t
Vegetables, 902
Vehicle transmission, 429, 430t
Veins, 803
    of neck and hands, fluid and electrolyte imbalance and, 864–865
Venereal Disease Research Laboratories (VDRL) test, 1377t
Venipuncture, 385, 387, 387f, 871–872
Venous congestion, blood pressure and, 370
Venous pooling, 810–811
Venous return, prevention of, 826–829
Ventilation, 749. See also Breathing; Lungs; Respirations; Respiratory function; Respiratory system
    control of, 750–751
Ventilators, 778
Ventrogluteal site, for intramuscular injections, 545, 546f
Venturi mask, 774, 774t, 776–777
Veracity, ethics and, 43
Verbal drug orders, 505
Vesicle, 944, 946t
Vesicostomy, 1051, 1051f
Vials, for parenteral medications, 531, 532f
Vibration, chest physiotherapy and, 781
Vigilance, sleep and, 1144
Violent behavior, coping and adaptation and, 1345
Virulence, 429, 992
Viruses, 428, 992–993
Vision, observation and, 98
Visual assessment, 334, 334f
Visual Sensory/Perceptual Alteration, nursing management plan for, 1205–1206
Vital organs, perfusion of, 806
Vital signs, 348–377, 350t. See also Blood pressure; Body temperature; Pulse; Respirations
    altered cardiovascular function and, 813–815
    assessing before medication administration, 517
    documenting, 375f, 376
    fluid and electrolyte imbalance and, 860, 864
    infections and, 1002
    lifespan considerations and, 373, 375–376
    normal values for, 349, 350t
    pain and, 1172
Vitamin(s)
    fat-soluble, recommended dietary allowances for, 1446
    intestinal production of, 1093
    normal physiologic function of, 894, 895t–896t, 896–897
        fat-soluble vitamins and, 894, 895t, 896–897
        water-soluble vitamins, 895t–896t, 897
    water-soluble, recommended dietary allowances for, 1447
Vitamin A (retinol), normal physiologic function of, 894, 895t, 896
Vitamin B$_1$ (thiamine), normal physiologic function of, 895t, 897

Vitamin B$_2$ (riboflavin), normal physiologic function of, 895t, 897
Vitamin B$_3$ (niacin), normal physiologic function of, 895t, 897
Vitamin B$_{12}$ (cobalamin), normal physiologic function of, 896t, 897
Vitamin C (ascorbic acid), normal physiologic function of, 895t, 897
Vitamin D (calciferol)
    normal physiologic function of, 895t, 896
    synthesis of, skin and, 937
Vitamin E (tocopherol), normal physiologic function of, 895t, 896
Vitamin K (menadione), normal physiologic function of, 895t, 896–897
Volume equivalents, 1414
Voluntary hospitals, 30
Vomiting
    altered nutrition and, 909
    enteral tube feedings and, 923
    narcotic analgesics and, 1183–1184

W
Waddling gait, 707
Wald, Lillian, 9
Walkers, 727, 729, 731
Walking. See Ambulation; Gait
Walking rounds. See Nursing rounds
Walsh, Mary, 83–84
    perception of human needs, 190, 191t
Warm compresses, 972, 974
Warm soaks, 974
Warm-water bath, 656t
Warts, plantar, 665t
Waste disposal, infection control and, 438, 440t
Water
    need for, 186
    normal physiologic function of, 900
Watson, Jean, 14t–15t
    perception of human needs, 191–192
WBC differential, 390
Weight. See also Obesity; Overweight
    altered nutrition and, 911–912
    cardiovascular function and, 813
    drug action and, 514
    fluid and electrolyte imbalance and, 864
    ideal body weight, 901
    measurement of, 321t, 321–324
    nutrition and, 913–914
    respiratory function and, 752
Weight equivalents, 1413
Wellness
    definition of, 174
    high-level wellness model and, 175, 176f
    holistic health care and, 176–179
        disease and, 178
        dysfunction and, 178–179
        holistic practice and, 177f, 177–178
        illness and, 178
        nursing in, 179–182
        promoting health and preventing illness and, 179–180
        stress and, 179
    nursing diagnoses for, 180

Wernicke's aphasia, 1272, 1272t
Wet preparation, 1377t
Wheal, 944, 946t
Wheelchair, transferring patient to, 737–739
Wheeler-Lea Act of 1938, 508
Wheezing, 364, 762
White blood cell(s), 880
  resistance to infection and, 982t, 983, 983t
White blood cell count, 390
  infections and, 1003
White blood cell differential, 390
Whites, health/illness considerations and, 245
WHO (World Health Organization), infection control and, 434
Whole blood, 880
Whole blood chemistries, reference ranges for, 1418–1431
Whole plasma, 880
Whooping cough (pertussis), 989t
Wills, 54
  living, 52, 55
Withdrawal, sensory perception and, 1196
Working phase, of nurse-patient relationship, 277
Workplace
  infection hazards in, 433
  safety in, 566–567
World Health Organization (WHO), infection control and, 434
Wound(s), 937, 940t, 940–941
  accidental, 940, 940t
  agents used to clean, 959
  color classification of, 957t
  debridement of, 967–968
  dressings and, 958–960

  infections of, 994–995, 996f, 996t
    manifestations of, 1002
  irrigation of, 968, 970–971
  minor, first aid for, 957–958
  packing, 969, 970–971
  support for, 960–966
  surgical, 940t, 940–941
Wound care, postoperative, 494
Wound closure, 489–490
Wound cultures, infections and, 1004
Wound healing, 937, 945–950
  complications of, 949–950
  factors affecting, 947–949
  phases of, 945
  types of, 945–947, 948f
Writing skills, required for effective use of nursing process, 89

X

X-rays. *See* Radiography

Y

Young adult. *See also* Adult
  development of, 202t, 207–208
  functional health patterns and, health problems and anticipatory guidance and, 210–219
  health maintenance and, 603t
Yura, Helen, 83–84
  perception of human needs, 190, 191t

Z

Zinc, normal physiologic function of, 898t
Z-track injections, 545, 547, 547f

ISBN 0-397-54669-6

9 780397 546695

90000